Principles and Practice of

Genitourinary Oncology

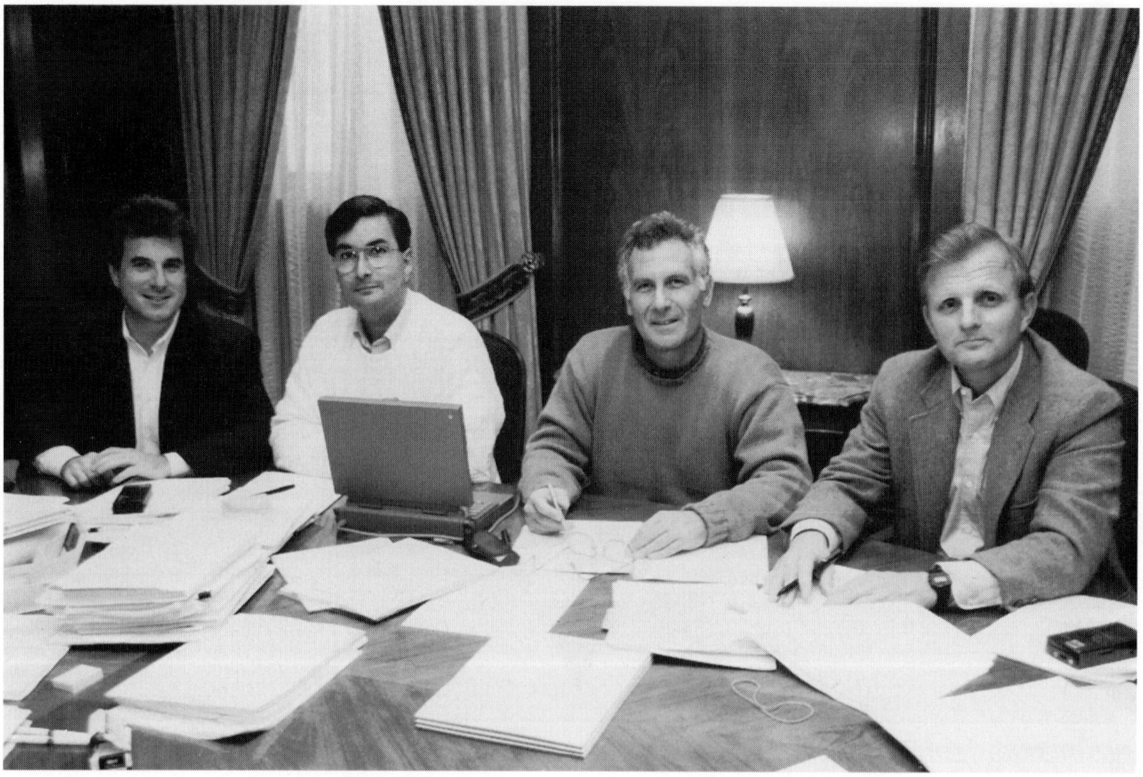

Howard Sher, Derek Raghavan, Steven Leibel, and Paul Lange

Principles and Practice of Genitourinary Oncology

Derek Raghavan, MBBS, PhD, FRACP, FACP
Chief, Departments of Solid Tumor Oncology
and Investigational Therapeutics
Roswell Park Cancer Institute and
Professor of Medicine and Urology
State University of New York at Buffalo
Buffalo, New York

Howard I. Scher, MD
Chief, Genitourinary Oncology Service
Associate Attending Physician
Division of Solid Tumor Oncology
Department of Medicine
Memorial Sloan-Kettering Cancer Center
New York, New York

Steven A. Leibel, MD
Vice Chairman and Clinical Director
Attending Radiation Oncologist
Department of Radiation Oncology
Memorial Sloan-Kettering Cancer Center
New York, New York

Paul Lange, MD, FACS
Professor and Chair
Department of Urology
University of Washington
Seattle, Washington

With 226 Additional Contributors

Lippincott - Raven
PUBLISHERS
Philadelphia • New York

Developmental Editor: Eileen Wolfberg Jackson
Project Editor: Ellen M. Campbell
Production Manager: Caren Erlichman
Production Coordinator: MaryClare Malady
Design Coordinator: Doug Smock
Indexer: Steve Sorenson
Compositor: Maryland Composition Company, Inc.
Printer: Courier Book Company/Westford

Library of Congress Cataloging-in-Publication Data

Principles and practice of genitourinary oncology / Derek Raghavan . . .
[et al.] ; with 226 additional contributors.
p. cm.
Includes bibliographical references and index.
ISBN 0–397–51458–1 (alk. paper)
1. Genitourinary organs—Cancer. I. Raghavan, Derek.
[DNLM: 1. Urogenital Neoplasms. WJ 160 P9573 1996]
RC280.U74P746 1996
616.99′26—dc20
DNLM/DLC
for Library of Congress 96-8893
CIP

Care has been taken to confirm the accuracy of the information presented and to describe generally accepted practices. However, the authors, editors, and publisher are not responsible for errors or omissions or for any consequences from application of the information in this book and make no warranty, express or implied, with respect to the contents of the publication.

The authors, editors, and publisher have exerted every effort to ensure that drug selection and dosage set forth in this text are in accordance with current recommendations and practice at the time of publication. However, in view of ongoing research, changes in government regulations, and the constant flow of information relating to drug therapy and drug reactions, the reader is urged to check the package insert for each drug for any change in indications and dosage and for added warnings and precautions. This is particularly important when the recommended agent is a new or infrequently employed drug.

Some drugs and medical devices presented in this publication have Food and Drug Administration (FDA) clearance for limited use in restricted research settings. It is the responsibility of the health care provider to ascertain the FDA status of each drug or device planned for use in their clinical practice.

9 8 7 6 5 4 3 2 1

In Memoriam

During the development of this book, our field lost several leading clinical scientists, each of whom made vast contributions to our understanding of the biology of genitourinary cancer and to the comfort and survival of our patients. In each instance, the loss of these great men was untimely, and we grieve for them. They taught us by example and inspired us to greater achievements. We will miss them and remember them as our friends, colleagues, teachers, and leaders. We salute them and all others in our field whom we have lost:

Geoffrey Chisholm
William Cooner
Bruce Pearson
Willett Whitmore, Jr.
Alan Yagoda

Contributors

Jan Adolfsson, MD
Department of Urology
Karolinska Hospital
Stockholm, Sweden

Richard J. Andrassy, MD
Professor of Surgery and Pediatrics
The University of Texas Medical School at Houston
Chief, Pediatric Surgery
M. D. Anderson Cancer Center
Houston, Texas

Gerald L. Andriole, Jr., MD
Associate Professor
Division of Urologic Surgery
Washington University School of Medicine
St. Louis, Missouri

Ploutarchos Anezinis, MD
Assistant Professor
University of Crete Medical School
Department of Urology
University General Hospital
Crete, Greece

Mark Austenfeld, MD
University of Kansas Medical School
Kansas City, Kansas

Alberto G. Ayala, MD
Professor and Deputy Chairman
Department of Pathology
The University of Texas
M. D. Anderson Cancer Center
Houston, Texas

Dean Bajorin, MD
Assistant Attending Physician
Department of Medicine
Memorial Sloan-Kettering Cancer Center
New York, New York

J. Bruce Beckwith, MD
Department of Pathology
Loma Linda University
Loma Linda, California

Arie S. Belldegrun, MD
Professor, Department of Surgery
Division of Urology
Center for the Health Sciences
University of California, Los Angeles
Director, Cancer Immunotherapy Program
Jonsson Comprehensive Cancer Center
Los Angeles, California

June L. Biedler, PhD
Member Emeritus
Memorial Sloan-Kettering Cancer Center
New York, New York

Richard Bihrle, MD
Associate Professor
Department of Urology
Indiana University Hospital
Indianapolis, Indiana

Brent Blumenstein, PhD
Senior Statistician
Southwest Oncology Group
Fred Hutchinson Cancer Research Center
Seattle, Washington

Michael J. Boyer, MBBS, PhD, FRACP
Staff Oncologist
Royal Prince Alfred Hospital
Camperdown, New South Wales, Australia

Michael K. Brawer, MD
Department of Urology
University of Washington
Seattle, Washington

Norman E. Breslow, PhD
Department of Biostatistics
University of Washington
Seattle, Washington

James D. Brooks, MD
The James Buchanan Brady Urological Institute
The Johns Hopkins Medical Institutions
Baltimore, Maryland

John S. J. Brooks, MD, MRCPath
Professor of Pathology
Chairman, Department of Pathology
Roswell Park Cancer Institute
Professor and Vice-Chairman
Department of Pathology
State University of New York at Buffalo
Buffalo, New York

Nicholas Bruchovsky, MD, PhD, FRCPC
Professor of Medicine
Head, Department of Cancer Endocrinology
British Columbia Cancer Agency
Vancouver, British Columbia, Canada

Chandra M. Burman, PhD
Department of Medical Physics
Memorial Sloan-Kettering Cancer Center
New York, New York

Paul Cairns, PhD
Division of Head and Neck Cancer Research
Department of Otolaryngology—Head and Neck Surgery
The Johns Hopkins University School of Medicine
Baltimore, Maryland

Peter R. Carroll, MD
Department of Urology
Program in Urologic Oncology
UCSF/Mt. Zion Cancer Center
University of California School of Medicine
San Francisco, California

Robert P. Castleberry, Jr., MD
Professor of Pediatrics
Director, Pediatric Hematology/Oncology
The Children's Hospital of Alabama at Birmingham
Birmingham, Alabama

William J. Catalona, MD
Professor and Chief
Division of Urologic Surgery
Washington University
School of Medicine
St. Louis, Missouri

Michael L. Cher, MD
Wayne State University
Department of Urology
Detroit, Michigan

Nathan I. Cherny, MBBS, FRACP
Pain and Palliative Medicine Physician
Department of Internal Medicine
Shaare Zedek Medical Center
Jerusalem, Israel

Nai-Kong V. Cheung, MD, PhD
Department of Pediatrics
Memorial Sloan-Kettering Cancer Center
New York, New York

Peter L. Choyke, MD
Department of Radiology
Warren G. Magnuson Clinical Center
Bethesda, Maryland

Chen-Shou Chui, PhD
Department of Medical Physics
Memorial Sloan-Kettering Cancer Center
New York, New York

Leland W. K. Chung, PhD
University of Virginia
Department of Urology
Charlottesville, Virginia

Samuel M. Cohen, MD, PhD
Professor and Chair
Department of Pathology and Microbiology
University of Nebraska
Omaha, Nebraska

Michael S. Cookson, MD
Assistant Professor
Division of Urology
University of Kentucky Medical Center
Lexington, Kentucky

William H. Cooner, MD†
Professor of Surgery
Section of Urology
Emory University School of Medicine
Atlanta, Georgia

Carlos Cordon-Cardo, MD, PhD
Director, Division of Molecular Pathology
Department of Pathology
Memorial Sloan-Kettering Cancer Center
New York, New York

Benjamin W. Corn, MD
Clinical Director
Department of Radiation Oncology
Medical College of Pennsylvania
Philadelphia, Pennsylvania

Anthony J. Costello, FRACS
Head, Department of Urology
St. Vincent's Hospital
Melbourne, Australia
Department of Surgery
Melbourne University
Victoria, Australia

† Deceased

E. David Crawford, MD
Professor and Chairman
Division of Urology
University of Colorado Health Sciences Center
Denver, Colorado

Patrick J. Creaven, MBBS, PhD
Attending Physician
Department of Investigational Therapeutics
Roswell Park Cancer Institute
Research Professor
Department of Medicine
State University of New York at Buffalo
Buffalo, New York

Ivan Damjanov, MD
Department of Pathology and Laboratory Medicine
The University of Kansas School of Medicine
Kansas City, Kansas

Giulio J. D'Angio, MD
Department of Radiation Oncology
Hospital of the University of Pennsylvania
Philadelphia, Pennsylvania

Bauke de Jong
Department of Medical Genetics
University of Groningen
Groningen, The Netherlands

Jean B. deKernion, MD
Professor and Chief
Division of Urology
Department of Surgery
Center for the Health Sciences
University of California, Los Angeles
Los Angeles, California

Pieter H. M. De Mulder, MD
St. Radboud University Hospital
Nijmegen, The Netherlands

Louis Denis, MD
Professor and Chairman
Department of Urology
University of Antwerp
A. Z. Middleheim Hospital
Antwerp, Belgium

Robert Devoll, DDS, PhD
Department of Biochemistry
Dental Branch
The University of Texas Medical School at Houston
Houston, Texas

Ethan Dmitrovsky, MD
Assistant Attending
Department of Medicine
Memorial Sloan-Kettering Cancer Center
New York, New York

Colin P. N. Dinney, MD
Departments of Cell Biology and Urology
The University of Texas
M. D. Anderson Cancer Center
Houston, Texas

John P. Donohue, MD
Distinguished Professor and Chair
Department of Urology
Indiana University School of Medicine
Indianapolis, Indiana

Robert Dreicer, MD, FACP
Associate Professor of Medicine and Urology
Associate Director for Clinical Research
University of Iowa Cancer Center
University of Iowa College of Medicine
Iowa City, Iowa

Michael J. Droller, MD
Professor and Chairman
Milton & Carroll Petrie Department of Urology
The Mount Sinai Medical Center
New York, New York

Jean-Pierre Droz, MD
Department of Medical Oncology
Centre Leon Barard
Lyon, France

William J. Ellis, MD
Department of Urology
University of Washington
Section of Urology
Seattle VA Medical Center
Seattle, Washington

Anas M. El-Mahdi, MD, ScD
Professor and Chairman
Department of Radiation Oncology and Biophysics
Eastern Virginia Medical School
Norfolk, Virginia

Jonathan I. Epstein, MD
Professor of Pathology, Urology and Oncology
The Johns Hopkins Medical Institutions
Associate Director of Surgical Pathology
The Johns Hopkins Hospital
Baltimore, Maryland

Christopher Evans, MD
Chief Resident
Department of Urology
University of California
San Francisco, California

William R. Fair, MD
Professor and Chair
Urology Service
Memorial Sloan-Kettering Cancer Center
New York, New York

Cindy Farach-Carson, PhD
Department of Biochemistry
The University of Texas Medical School at Houston
Houston, Texas

Isaiah J. Fidler, DVM, PhD
Departments of Cell Biology and Urology
The University of Texas
M. D. Anderson Cancer Center
Houston, Texas

Robert A. Figlin, MD
Professor, Department of Medicine
Division of Hematology/Oncology
Center for the Health Sciences
University of California
Los Angeles, California

Robert C. Flanigan, MD
Professor and Chair
Department of Urology
Loyola University Medical School
Maywood, Illinois

Kathleen M. Foley, MD
Chief, Pain Service
Department of Neurology
Memorial Sloan-Kettering Cancer Center
New York, New York

Howard P. Forman, MD
Robert Wood Johnson Clinical Scholar, 1994–1996
Department of Radiology
Hospital of the University of Pennsylvania
Philadelphia, Pennsylvania

Richard S. Foster, MD
Associate Professor
Department of Urology
Indiana University Hospital
Indianapolis, Indiana

Yves Fradet, MD
Professor of Urology
Laval University Cancer Research Center
Quebec, Canada

D. Frappaz, MD
Centre Regional Leon Berard
Cedex, France

Mark Frydenberg, MBBS, FRACS (Urol)
Attending Urologist
Department of Urology
Royal Melbourne Hospital
Victoria, Australia

Zvi Fuks, MD
Department of Radiation Oncology
Memorial Sloan-Kettering Cancer Center
New York, New York

Aleksander Giwercman, MD
University Department of Growth and Reproduction
Rigshospitalet
Copenhagen, Denmark

Dorothy Glaves, PhD
Cancer Research Scientist
Department of Medicine
Roswell Park Cancer Institute
Buffalo, New York

Martin E. Gleave, MD, FRCSC
Assistant Professor of Surgery
University of British Columbia
Vancouver, British Columbia, Canada

Gladys M. Glenn, MD
Diagnosis Branch
Division of Cancer Biology, Diagnosis and Centers
National Cancer Institute
Bethesda, Maryland

James R. Gnarra, MD
Urologic Oncology Section
Surgery Branch
Clinical Oncology Program
Division of Cancer Therapy
National Cancer Institute
Bethesda, Maryland

S. Larry Goldenberg, MD, FRCSC
Clinical Professor of Surgery
Division of Urology
University of British Columbia
Vancouver, British Columbia, Canada

Mary K. Gospodarowicz, MD
Professor
Department of Radiation Oncology
Princess Margaret Hospital
Toronto, Ontario, Canada

H. Barton Grossman, MD
Department of Urology
The University of Texas
M. D. Anderson Cancer Center
Houston, Texas

Daniel M. Green, MD
Chairman, National Wilms Tumor Study Group
Department of Pediatrics
Roswell Park Cancer Institute
Buffalo, New York

David Grignon, MD
Department of Pathology
Wayne State University School of Medicine
Detroit, Michigan

Paul E. Grundy, MD
Departments of Pediatrics and Oncology
Cross Cancer Institute and
The University of Alberta
Edmonton, Alberta, Canada

Gabriel P. Haas, MD
Professor and Chair
Department of Urology
State University of New York
Syracuse, New York

Reginald R. Hall, FRCS
Head, Department of Urology
Freeman Hospital
Newcastle-upon-Tyne
United Kingdom

Thomas C. Hamilton, PhD
Fox Chase Cancer Center
Philadelphia, Pennsylvania

Gerald E. Hanks, MD
Professor and Chair
Department of Radiation Oncology
Fox Chase Cancer Center
Philadelphia, Pennsylvania

Ala B. Hamoudi, MD
Clinical Professor of Pathology
Ohio State University
Department of Laboratory Medicine
Children's Hospital
Columbus, Ohio

Harry W. Herr, MD
Attending Physician
Department of Urology
Memorial Sloan-Kettering Cancer Center
New York, New York

Susan Hilton, MD
Department of Radiology
Memorial Sloan-Kettering Cancer Center
New York, New York

Alan Horwich, MD, PhD, FRCR
Professor and Chair
Department of Radiation Oncology
Royal Marsden Hospital
Sutton, Surrey
United Kingdom

Scott F. Howe, MD
Section of Urologic Surgery
University of Nebraska Medical Center
Omaha, Nebraska

Jer-Tsong Hsieh
Assistant Professor of Biochemistry
The University of Texas
M. D. Anderson Cancer Center
Houston, Texas

Robert B. Huben, MD
Chief
Department of Urology
Roswell Park Cancer Institute
Buffalo, New York

Janet E. Husband, MD
Consultant Radiologist
The Royal Marsden NHS Trust
Department of Diagnostic Radiology
Sutton, Surrey
United Kingdom

Maha H. Hussain, MD
Assistant Professor
Division of Hematology/Oncology
Wayne State University
Detroit, Michigan

Sharon Hyland, RN, MSN, NP
Department of Solid Tumor Oncology
Roswell Park Cancer Institute
Buffalo, New York

Julianne Imperato-McGinley, MD
Professor of Medicine
Chief, Division of Endocrinology
Director General Clinical Research Center
Cornell University Medical College
New York, New York

John T. Isaacs, PhD
Professor of Oncology and Urology
The Johns Hopkins University School of Medicine
The Johns Hopkins Oncology Center
Baltimore, Maryland

William B. Isaacs, PhD
The James Buchanan Brady Urological Institute
The Johns Hopkins Hospital
Baltimore, Maryland

Michael A. S. Jewett, MD
Professor and Chair
Division of Urology
University of Toronto
Toronto, Ontario, Canada

Sonny L. Johansson, MD, PhD
Professor and Director of Anatomic Pathology
Department of Pathology and Microbiology
University of Nebraska Medical Center
Omaha, Nebraska

Douglas E. Johnson, MD
Department of Urology
St. Joseph Hospital
Houston, Texas

Steven W. Johnson, MD
Fox Chase Cancer Center
Philadelphia, Pennsylvania

Vijay V. Joshi, MD, PhD, FRCPath
Professor and Director of Pediatric Pathology
Department of Pathology and Laboratory Medicine
East Carolina University School of Medicine
Greenville, North Carolina

Philip W. Kantoff, MD
Assistant Physician
Dana Farber Cancer Institute
Assistant Professor of Medicine
Harvard Medical School
Boston, Massachusetts

Melissa D. Katz, MD
Division of Endocrinology
The New York Hospital
Cornell University Medical College
New York, New York

Susan Kim, MD
Assistant Professor
Division of Radiation Medicine
Roswell Park Cancer Institute and
State University of New York at Buffalo
Buffalo, New York

Michael O. Koch, MD
Associate Professor of Urology
Department of Urology
Vanderbilt University Medical Center
Nashville, Tennessee

James M. Kozlowski, MD, FACS
Associate Professor of Urology
Surgery and Tumor Cell Biology
Director, Genitourinary Oncology Program
Vice Chairman, Department of Urology
Northwestern University Medical School
Chicago, Illinois

Deborah A. Kuban, MD
Associate Professor
Department of Radiation Oncology and Biophysics
Eastern Virginia Medical School
Norfolk, Virginia

M. Vijay Kumar, PhD
Department of Urology Research
Mayo Clinic
Rochester, Minnesota

Brian H. Kushner, MD
Department of Pediatrics
Memorial Sloan-Kettering Cancer Center
New York, New York

Gerald J. Kutcher, PhD
Department of Medical Physics
Memorial Sloan-Kettering Cancer Center
New York, New York

Donald L. Lamm, MD
Professor and Chair
Department of Urology
University of West Virginia Medical Center
Morgantown, West Virginia

Paul H. Lange, MD, FACS
Professor and Chair
Department of Urology
University of Washington
Seattle, Washington

Michael P. LaQuaglia, MD
Department of Pediatrics
Memorial Sloan-Kettering Cancer Center
New York, New York

Edmund C. Lattime, PhD
Associate Professor
Department of Medicine
Division of Neoplastic Diseases
Thomas Jefferson University
Philadelphia, Pennsylvania

Steven A. Leibel, MD
Vice Chairman and Clinical Director
Attending Radiation Oncologist
Department of Radiation Oncology
Memorial Sloan-Kettering Cancer Center
New York, New York

John Levi, MD
Department of Clinical Oncology
Royal North Shore Hospital
St. Leonards, Australia

Ellis G. Levine, MD
Associate Professor of Medicine
Division of Medicine
Roswell Park Cancer Institute
Buffalo, New York

David A. Levy, MD
Fellow, Department of Urology
The University of Texas
M. D. Anderson Cancer Center
Houston, Texas

Robert M. Lifeso, MD
Clinical Professor of Orthopaedic Surgery
State University of New York at Buffalo
Buffalo, New York

Karen Lindsley, MD
Department of Radiation Oncology
University of Washington Medical Center
Seattle, Washington

W. Marston Linehan, MD
Urologic Oncology Section
Surgery Branch
Clinical Oncology Program
Division of Cancer Therapy
National Cancer Institute
Bethesda, Maryland

C. Clifton Ling, PhD
Department of Medical Physics
Memorial Sloan-Kettering Cancer Center
New York, New York

Mark S. Litwin, MD, MPh
Assistant Professor of Surgery, Urology and Public Health
Division of Urology
UCLA Medical School
Los Angeles, California

Brian C.-S. Liu, PhD
Senior Research Scientist
Department of Urology
Mt. Sinai Medical Center
New York, New York

Patrick J. Loehrer, Sr., MD
Professor of Medicine
Indiana University Medical Center
Indianapolis, Indiana

Christopher J. Logothetis, MD
Department of Genitourinary Medical Oncology
The University of Texas
M. D. Anderson Cancer Center
Houston, Texas

Leendert H. J. Looijenga
Laboratory of Molecular Medicine
Genitourinary Oncology Service
Department of Medicine
Molecular Pharmacology and Therapeutics Program
Memorial Sloan-Kettering Cancer Center
New York, New York

Gikas S. Mageras, PhD
Department of Medical Physics
Memorial Sloan-Kettering Cancer Center
New York, New York

Christopher Lee Marsh, MD
Assistant Professor
Department of Urology
Division of Transplantation
University of Washington
Seattle, Washington

Fray F. Marshall, MD
The James Buchanan Brady Urological Institute
The Johns Hopkins Medical Institutions
Baltimore, Maryland

Bruce L. McClennan, MD
Professor of Radiology
Mallinckrodt Institute of Radiology
Washington University School of Medicine
St. Louis, Missouri

W. Scott McDougall, MD
Professor of Surgery
Chief of Urology
Department of Urology
Massachusetts General Hospital
Boston, Massachusetts

Brian E. McGrath, MD
Associate Professor of Orthopaedic Surgery
State University of New York at Buffalo
Department of Orthopaedic Oncology
Buffalo, New York

Roger L. Miesfeld, PhD
Department of Biochemistry
University of Arizona
Arizona Cancer Center
Tucson, Arizona

Gary J. Miller, MD, PhD
Professor
Department of Pathology and Division of Urology
University of Colorado Medical Center
Denver, Colorado

Radhe Mohan, PhD
Department of Medical Physics
Memorial Sloan-Kettering Cancer Center
New York, New York

James E. Montie, MD
Professor, Urologic Oncology
Division of Urology
University of Michigan
Ann Arbor, Michigan

Malcolm Moore, MD
Department of Medicine
Ontario Cancer Institute
Princess Margaret Hospital
Toronto, Ontario, Canada

Robert J. Motzer, MD
Associate Attending Physician
Department of Medicine
Memorial Sloan-Kettering Cancer Center
New York, New York

Robert P. Myers, MD
Department of Urology
Mayo Clinic
Rochester, Minnesota

David M. Nanus, MD
Assistant Professor
Genitourinary Oncology Section
Division of Solid Tumor Oncology
Department of Medicine
Memorial Sloan-Kettering Cancer Center
New York, New York

Perinchery Narayan, MD
Chief, Division of Urology
University of Florida
Gainesville, Florida

William A. Newton, Jr., MD
Department of Laboratory Medicine
Children's Hospital
Columbus, Ohio

Nicola Nicolai, MD
Division of Urology
Istituto Nazionali Tumori
Milan, Italy

Craig R. Nichols, MD
Associate Professor of Medicine
Department of Medicine
Indiana University Medical Center
Indianapolis, Indiana

Andrew C. Novick, MD
Professor and Chair
Department of Urology
Cleveland Clinic Foundation
Cleveland, Ohio

Peter B. Odland, MD
Associate Professor of Dermatology
University of Washington Medical School
Seattle, Washington

Joseph E. Oesterling, MD
Professor and Chairman
Division of Urology
University of Michigan
Ann Arbor, Michigan

J. Wolter Oosterhuis, MD, PhD
Department of Pathology
Dr. Daniel den Hoed Cancer Center
Rotterdam, The Netherlands

Alan W. Partin, MD, PhD
Department of Urology
The Johns Hopkins University School of Medicine
The James Buchanan Brady Urological Institute
The Johns Hopkins Hospital
Baltimore, Maryland

David F. Paulson, MD
Professor and Chief
Division of Urologic Surgery
Duke University Medical Center
Durham, North Carolina

Raymond P. Perez, MD
Assistant Professor
Departments of Solid Tumor Oncology and Investigational Therapeutics
Roswell Park Cancer Institute
Buffalo, New York

Thierry Philip, MD
Directeur
Centre Regional Leon Berard
Cedex, France

Kenneth J. Pienta, MD
Associate Professor
Department of Medicine
University of Michigan
Ann Arbor, Michigan

Luigi Piva, MD
Division of Urology
Istituto Nazionali Tumori
Milan, Italy

Giorgio Pizzocaro, MD
Chief, Division of Urology
Istituto Nazionale Tumori
Milan, Italy

J. Edson Pontes, MD
Professor and Chairman
Department of Urology
Wayne State University School of Medicine
Detroit, Michigan

Russell K. Portenoy, MD
Director, Analgesic Studies
Pain Service, Department of Neurology
Memorial Sloan-Kettering Cancer Center
New York, New York

Derek Raghavan, MBBS, PhD, FRACP, FACP
Chief, Departments of Solid Tumor Oncology and Investigational Therapeutics
Roswell Park Cancer Institute and
Professor of Medicine and Urology
State University of New York at Buffalo
Buffalo, New York

R. Beverly Raney, MD
Professor of Pediatrics
Department of Pediatrics
Chief, Non-Neural Solid Tumor Section
The University of Texas
M. D. Anderson Cancer Center
Houston, Texas

Timothy L. Ratliff, PhD
Director of Genitourinary Research
Department of Urology
Washington University School of Medicine
St. Louis, Missouri

John F. Redman, MD
Professor and Chair
Department of Urology
University of Arkansas College of Medicine
Little Rock, Arkansas

Michael J. Rentzepis, MD
Department of Urology
University of California, Davis
Sacramento, California

Martin I. Resnick, MD
Professor and Chairman
Department of Urology
Case Western Reserve University
School of Medicine
Cleveland, Ohio

Jerome P. Richie, MD
Professor and Chair
Department of Urology
Brigham and Women's Hospital
Harvard Medical School
Boston, Massachusetts

Michael L. Ritchey, MD
Division of Pediatric Surgery
The University of Texas
Houston, Texas

Mark A. Ritter, MD
Associate Professor
Department of Human Oncology
Section of Radiation Oncology
University of Wisconsin
School of Medicine
Madison, Wisconsin

Jae Y. Ro, MD
Professor
Department of Pathology
The University of Texas
M. D. Anderson Cancer Center
Houston, Texas

Robert A. Ross, PhD
Department of Biological Sciences
Fordham University
Bronx, New York

Bruce J. Roth, MD
Associate Professor of Medicine
Division of Hematology/Oncology
Indiana University Medical Center
Indianapolis, Indiana

Randall G. Rowland, MD
Professor
Department of Urology
Indiana University Hospital
Indianapolis, Indiana

Pamela J. Russell, PhD
Associate Professor and Director
Genitourinary Cancer Research Laboratory
Prince of Wales Hospital
New South Wales, Australia

Robert H. Sagerman, MD, FACR
Professor and Director
Radiation Oncology Division
State University of New York Health Science Center at Syracuse
Syracuse, New York

W. Holt Sanders, MD
Section of Urology
The Emory Clinic
Atlanta, Georgia

Richard A. Santucci, MD
Department of Urology
Seattle, Washington

Michael F. Sarosdy, MD
Professor and Chair
Department of Urology
The University of Texas Health Science Center at San Antonio
San Antonio, Texas

Paul F. Schellhammer, MD
Professor and Chairman, Department of Urology
Virginia Prostate Center of Eastern Virginia Medical School and Sentara Cancer Institute
Norfolk, Virginia

Howard I. Scher, MD
Chief, Genitourinary Oncology Service
Associate Attending Physician
Division of Solid Tumor Oncology
Department of Medicine
Memorial Sloan-Kettering Cancer Center
New York, New York

Hans-Joachim Schmoll, MD
Professor
Division of Hematology
Department of Internal Medicine
Hannover University Medical School
Hannover, Germany

Lawrence H. Schwartz, MD
Department of Radiology
Memorial Sloan-Kettering Cancer Center
New York, New York

T. Vincent Shankey, PhD
Associate Professor
Department of Urology
Loyola University Medical School
Maywood, Illinois

Hiroyuki Shimada, MD, PhD
Director, Electron Microscopy
Department of Pathology and Laboratory Medicine
Children's Hospital of Los Angeles
Los Angeles, California

Ramesh A. Shivdasani, MD, PhD
Instructor
Dana Farber Cancer Institute
Instructor in Medicine
Harvard Medical School
Boston, Massachusetts

William U. Shipley, MD
Deputy Director
Massachusetts General Hospital Cancer Center
Needham, Massachusetts

David Sidransky, MD
Director
Head and Neck Cancer Research
Departments of Medicine and Otolaryngology
The Johns Hopkins Oncology Center
Baltimore, Maryland

Stuart E. Siegel, MD
Department of Pediatrics
University of Southern California School of Medicine
Children's Hospital, Los Angeles
Los Angeles, California

Jonathan W. Simons, MD
The James Buchanan Brady Urological Institute
The Johns Hopkins Oncology Center
The Longrifle Center for Molecular Medicine
Baltimore, Maryland

Niels E. Skakkebæk, MD
University Department of Growth and Reproduction
Rigshospitalet
Copenhagen, Denmark

Eila C. Skinner, MD
Assistant Professor
Department of Urology
University of Southern California
Norris Cancer Center
Los Angeles, California

Donald G. Skinner, MD
Professor and Chair
Department of Urology
University of Southern California
Norris Cancer Center
Los Angeles, California

Joseph A. Smith, Jr. MD
William L. Bray Professor and Chairman
Department of Urology
Vanderbilt University Medical Center
Nashville, Tennessee

Mitchell H. Sokoloff, MD
Department of Surgery
Division of Urology
Center for the Health Sciences
University of California
Los Angeles, California

James Spellman, MD
Assistant Professor
Department of Sarcoma-Melanoma Surgery
Division of Surgery
Roswell Park Cancer Institute
Buffalo, New York

Barbara A. Spengler, M.A.
Department of Biological Sciences
Fordham University
Bronx, New York

Gunnar Steineck, MD, PhD
Associate Professor in Oncology
Genitourinary Oncology Service
Division of Solid Tumor Oncology
Department of Medicine
Memorial Sloan-Kettering Cancer Center
New York, New York

Cora N. Sternberg, MD
Chief of Medical Oncology
Department of Medical Oncology
San Raffaele Scientific Institute
Rome, Italy

Martin Stockler, FRACP, MBBS
Department of Medicine
Ontario Cancer Institute
Princess Margaret Hospital
Toronto, Ontario, Canada

Gerrit Stoter, MD
Professor and Chair
Department of Medical Oncology
Dr. Daniel den Hoed Klinick
University of Rotterdam
Rotterdam, The Netherlands

David A. Swanson, MD
Professor of Urology
Department of Urology
The University of Texas
M. D. Anderson Cancer Center
Houston, Texas

William H. Sweatt, MD
The James Buchanan Brady Urological Institute
The Johns Hopkins Oncology Center
The Longrifle Center for Molecular Medicine
Baltimore, Maryland

Anthony J. Swerdlow, MD
Epidemiological Monitoring Unit
London School of Hygiene and Tropical Health
London, United Kingdom

Rodney J. Taylor, MD
Professor of Surgery
Chairman, Urologic Surgery
University of Nebraska Medical Center
Omaha, Nebraska

Patricia J. Terry, MD
The University of Texas Health Science Center at San Antonio
San Antonio, Texas

George Thalmann, MD
Assistant Professor
Urologische Universitaatsklinik
Anna-Seiler-Haus
Inselspital
Bern, Switzerland

Carol J. Thiele, PhD
Cell and Molecular Biology Section
Pediatric Branch
National Cancer Institute
Bethesda, Maryland

Patrick R. M. Thomas, MB, BS
Chairman, Department of Radiation Oncology
Temple University School of Medicine
Philadelphia, Pennsylvania

Ian Thompson, MD
Chief, Urology Service
Brooke Army Medical Center
San Antonio, Texas

Donald J. Tindall, PhD
Department of Urology Research
Department of Biochemistry/Molecular Biology
Mayo Clinic
Rochester, Minnesota

Jeffery Triest, MD
Department of Urology
Wayne State University School of Medicine
Detroit, Michigan

Lawrence D. True, MD
Assistant Professor
Department of Pathology
University of Washington
Seattle, Washington

Donald L. Trump, MD
Professor of Medicine and Surgery
Deputy Director
Pittsburgh Cancer Institute
University of Pittsburgh
Pittsburgh, Pennsylvania

Satish Velagapudi, MD
Associate Chief
Department of Urologic Oncology
Roswell Park Cancer Institute
Buffalo, New York

Judith G. Villablanca, MD
Department of Pediatrics
University of Southern California School of Medicine
Children's Hospital, Los Angeles
Los Angeles, California

Nicholas J. Vogelzang, MD
Professor
Section of Hematology/Oncology
Department of Medicine
University of Chicago
Pritzker School of Medicine
Chicago, Illinois

Cheryl L. Walker, PhD
Associate Professor
Department of Carcinogenesis
The University of Texas
M. D. Anderson Cancer Center
Science Park Division
Smithville, Texas

Kent Wallner, MD
Assistant Attending Radiation Oncologist
Department of Radiation Oncology
Memorial Sloan-Kettering Cancer Center
New York, New York

Patrick C. Walsh, MD
Department of Urology
The James Buchanan Brady Urological Institute
The Johns Hopkins Hospital
Baltimore, Maryland

McClellan M. Walther, MD
Urologic Oncology Section
Surgery Branch
Clinical Oncology Program
Division of Cancer Therapy
National Cancer Institute
Bethesda, Maryland

Philip J. Walther, MD, PhD, FACS
Professor of Urologic Surgery
Assistant Professor of Experimental Pathology
Staff Physician
Duke University Comprehensive Cancer Center
Durham, North Carolina

Yu Wang, MD
Department of Urology
Memorial Sloan-Kettering Cancer Center
New York, New York

Padraig R. Warde, MB, MRCPI, FRCPC
Assistant Professor
University of Toronto
Princess Margaret Hospital
Toronto, Ontario, Canada

Moody D. Wharam, Jr., MD
Professor of Oncology, Radiological Sciences, Neurosurgery and Pediatrics
Director, Division of Radiation Oncology
The Johns Hopkins Oncology Center
Baltimore, Maryland

Gary L. Whipple, MD
Radiation Oncology Division
State University of New York Health Science Center at Syracuse
Syracuse, New York

Ralph deVere White, MD
Professor & Chair
Department of Urology
University of California, Davis
School of Medicine
Sacramento, California

Donna Wilkinson, NP, MS
Department of Urologic Oncology
Roswell Park Cancer Institute
Buffalo, New York

Richard D. Williams, MD
Professor and Chair
Department of Urology
The University of Iowa Hospitals and Clinics
Iowa City, Iowa

Howard N. Winfield, MD
Associate Professor
Department of Urology
Iowa University Hospitals
Iowa City, Iowa

David P. Wood, Jr., MD
Chief of Urologic Oncology
Department of Surgery
University of Kentucky Medical Center
Lexington, Kentucky

Berton Zbar, MD
Laboratory of Immunobiology
National Cancer Institute
Bethesda, Maryland

Michael J. Zelefsky, MD
Department of Radiation Oncology
Memorial Sloan-Kettering Cancer Center
New York, New York

Marcelo Zerati, MD
Instituto de Urologia e Nefrologia
Rio Preto, Brazil

Zuo-Feng Zhang, MD
Department of Epidemiology
Memorial Sloan-Kettering Cancer Center
New York, New York

Preface

For many years, the genitourinary cancers were the Cinderellas of oncology, with an emphasis only on strategies of local control, and with involved clinicians deriving little support or interest from other clinical disciplines, the basic sciences, or funding agencies. In the past two decades, however, the management of genitourinary malignancy has become one of the paradigms of successful care for patients with cancer, blending a much greater focus of basic research with translational and applied components of clinical treatment to produce well-designed trials that have changed treatment standards.

More importantly, this field has become truly multidisciplinary. In the past, clinical or research meetings in the basic sciences, diagnostic specialties, radiation, and medical oncology included small sessions on genitourinary cancer which were regularly attended by a committed but very small cadre of investigators. Educational and research activities in the urologic disciplines provided an important focus on cancer, but with scant input from other basic and clinical sciences. Now, however, academic programs devoted to genitourinary cancer have joined lung cancer and breast cancer in attracting huge audiences at international, national, and regional meetings, with very active support and contributions from the oncology community, both practicing and academic. Cooperative clinical trial groups have focused considerable attention and time on the development of research programs in this domain, and an increasing proportion of national cancer research is being designated for basic and clinical research into cancer of the prostate, the bladder, the kidney, and related sites.

Against this background, we believe that the time is right for a definitive text on the biology and management of the genitourinary cancers, predicated on multidisciplinary research and treatment. We have sought contributions from the international leadership in our field, drawing input from all of the clinical and research disciplines. Where possible, we have combined the expertise and knowledge of multidisciplinary working groups, in an effort to provide both the practicing clinician and the academic researcher with definitive statements of current knowledge and practice, as well as an outline of future endeavors. In particular, we have attempted to address the major controversies, discussing the various points of view and emphasizing balance. We have attempted to be global in our approach, including detailed coverage of advances in the basic sciences, an integrated approach to the diagnosis and treatment of each type of urologic malignancy, detailed discussion of the pediatric genitourinary cancers, and a specific emphasis on the interplay with psychological and support services.

This textbook will stand as a tribute to the many investigators who have labored to increase our understanding of these cancers. It is devoted to the concept that cure will be achieved by multidisciplinary, structured, collaborative research, and it stands as an anthology of the best work in our field.

Derek Raghavan
Howard I. Scher
Steven A. Leibel
Paul H. Lange

Acknowledgments

We gratefully acknowledge the love, support, and forbearance of our families, and the patience and assistance of our secretaries.

Contents

Section I Principles of Oncology

Section II Bladder Cancer

Section III Prostate Cancer

Section IV Testis Cancer

Section V Renal Cancer

Section VI Cancer of the Penis

Section VII Adrenal Cancer

Section VIII Genitourinary Sarcomas

Section IX Pediatric Rhabdomyosarcomas and Soft Tissue Sarcomas

Section X Neuroblastoma

Section XI Wilms' Tumor/Nephroblastoma

Principles and Practice of

Genitourinary Oncology

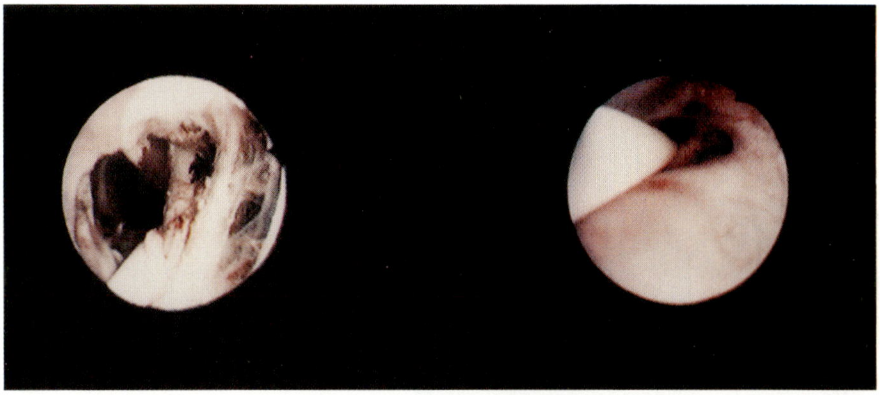

COLOR FIG. 6-1. Apearance of ureterointestinal stricture before incision and dilation *(left)*. Subsequent intraoperative appearance of stricture after electroincision and dilation *(right)*.

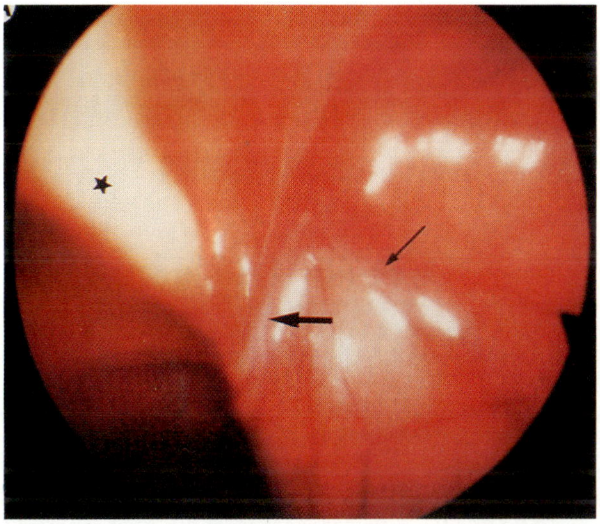

COLOR FIG. 6-4. Appearance of the obturator-iliac region before the initiation of dissection. The right obliterated umbilical artery *(star),* right testicular vessels *(narrow arrow)*, and right vas deferens *(bold arrow)* are shown.

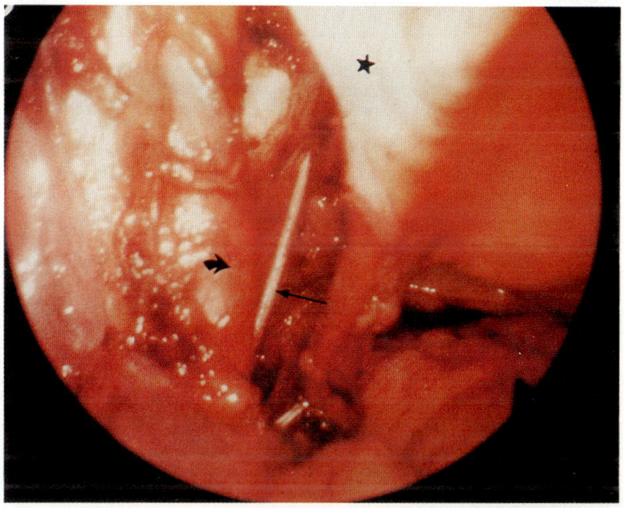

COLOR FIG. 6-5. Completed obturator lymph node dissection on left side. The left obliterated umbilical artery *(star)*, left external iliac vessels *(curved arrow)*, and left obturator nerve *(straight arrow)* are shown.

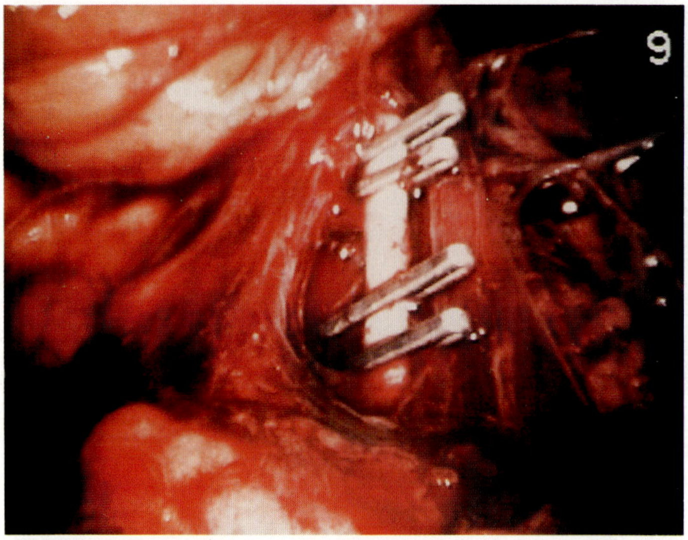

COLOR FIG. 6-8. Double-clipped and transected renal artery.

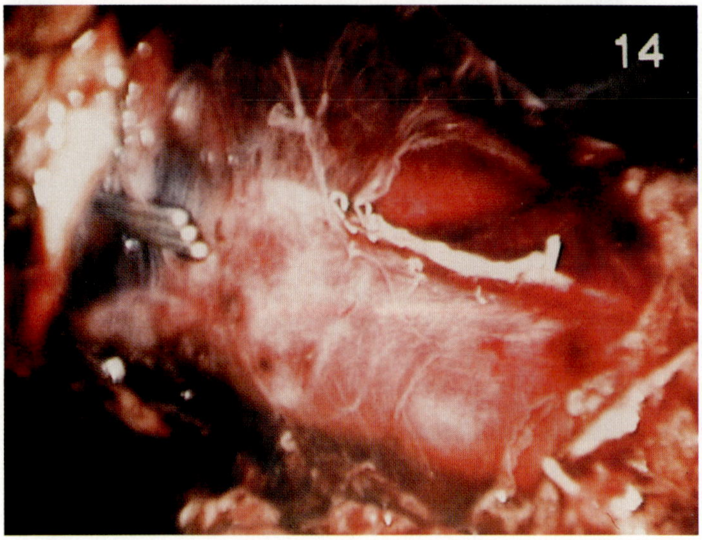

COLOR FIG. 6-9. Transection of the right renal vein with a vascular endo-GIA stapling device leaves three rows of staples at the junction with the inferior vena cava.

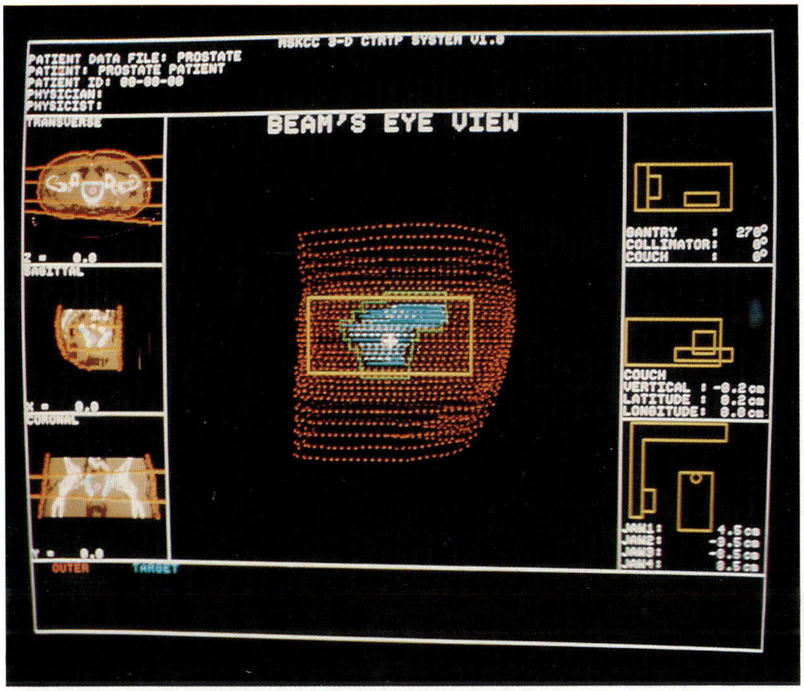

COLOR FIG. 7-3. Beam's-eye view of the prostate, seminal vesicles, and body surface contour shown as wire-frame projections. Reconstruction of the prostate and seminal vesicles *(blue)* and the body surface *(red)* are displayed in relation to the beam path of a lateral irradiation field *(yellow rectangle)*. In this field, a beam aperture *(green line)* representing the leaves of a multileaf collimator is drawn around the target volume. Midplane axial, sagittal, and coronal computed tomographic images with the intersections of the displayed beam in each image are shown on the left, and treatment machine orientation parameters for this field are displayed on the right.

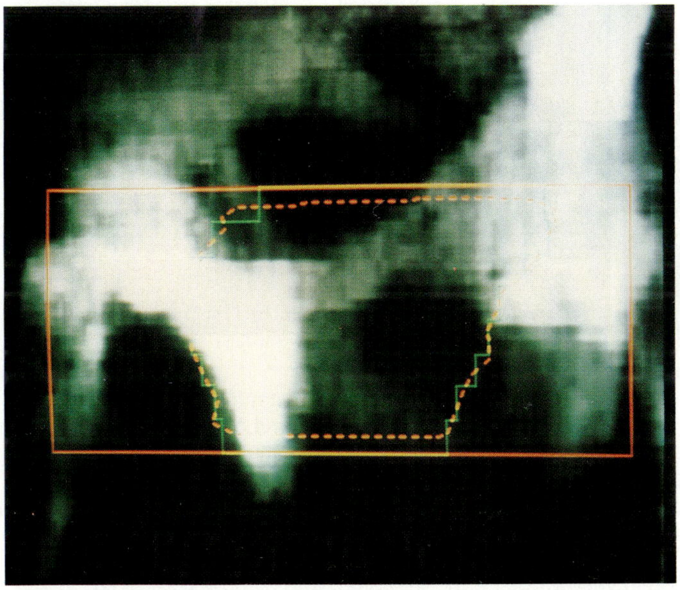

COLOR FIG. 7-4. Digitally reconstructed radiograph (DRR) produced from the planning computed tomography image set. The DRR is superimposed with a treatment field *(solid red line)* with beam aperture shapes for a conventional low melting alloy block *(broken red line)* and for a multileaf collimator field *(green line)*. Radiographic simulator films are obtained for each of the treatment fields, and the beam aperture block outline for each treatment field on the DRR is transferred onto the simulator films, which are used for comparison with treatment portal and verification films.

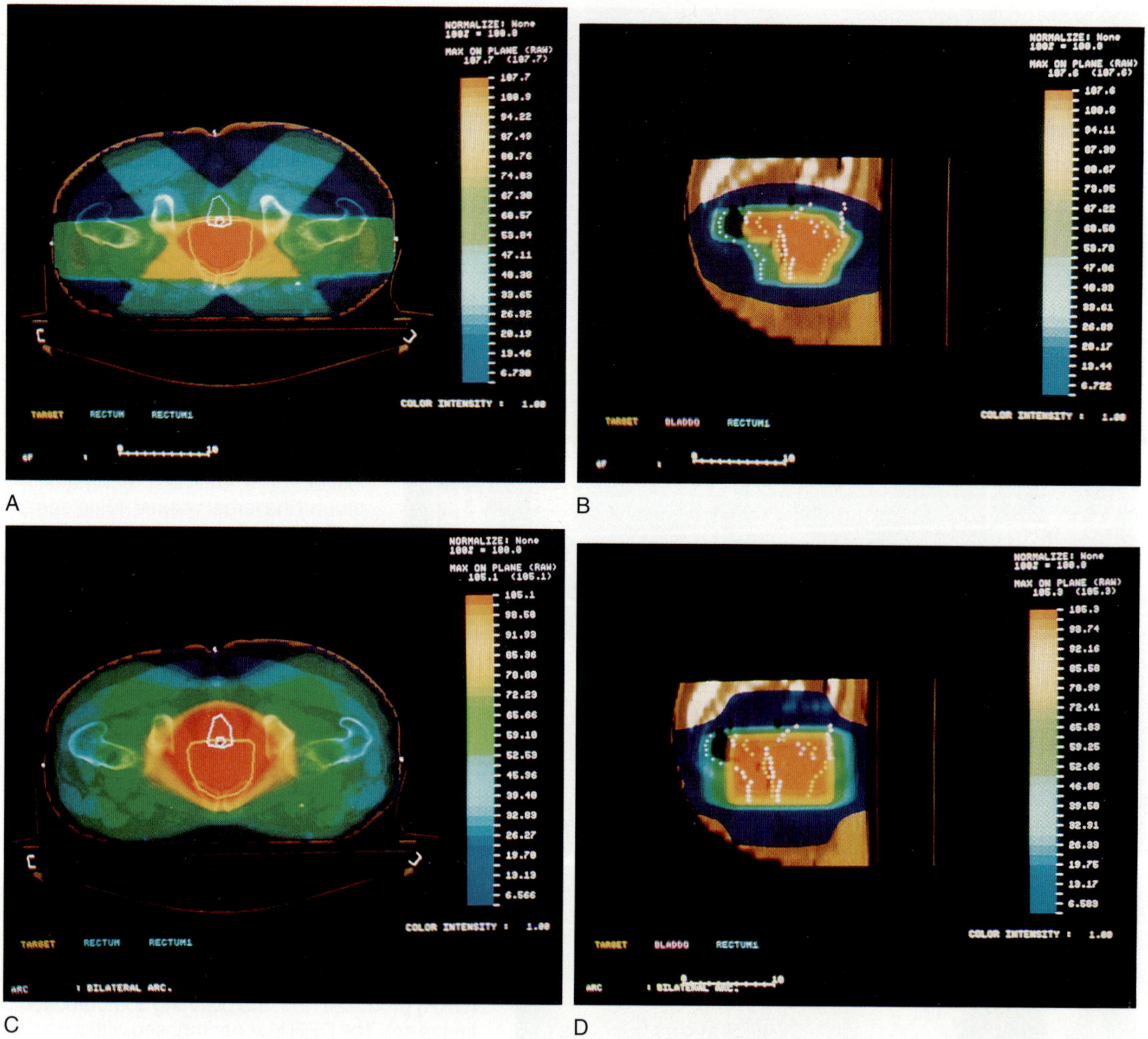

COLOR FIG. 7-5. Comparison of dose distributions for a three-dimensional (3D) conformal six-field plan and a traditional 120-degree bilateral arc rotation plan for a patient with carcinoma of the prostate. Midplane **(A)** axial and **(B)** sagittal color-wash dose-distribution displays of the six-field coplanar 3D prostate treatment plan for 15-mV x-rays, consisting of one pair of lateral and two pairs of oblique fields. In this display, a band of the color spectrum *(right)* corresponds to a range of doses. The prescription dose is normalized to 100%. The red region corresponds to the prescription isodose distribution (100% to 107%), yellow represents approximately 75% to 95%, green represents 50% to 74%, and blue represents 49% or less. The target contour is outlined in yellow dots, and the rectum and bladder **(B and D)** are represented by blue and magenta dots, respectively. Midplane **(C)** axial and **(D)** sagittal color-wash dose-distribution displays for a conventional 120-degree bilateral arc rotational approach. Because this technique does not allow the use of shaped blocks to shield normal tissues, a greater volume of the rectum and bladder receive high radiation doses than with the conformal approach.

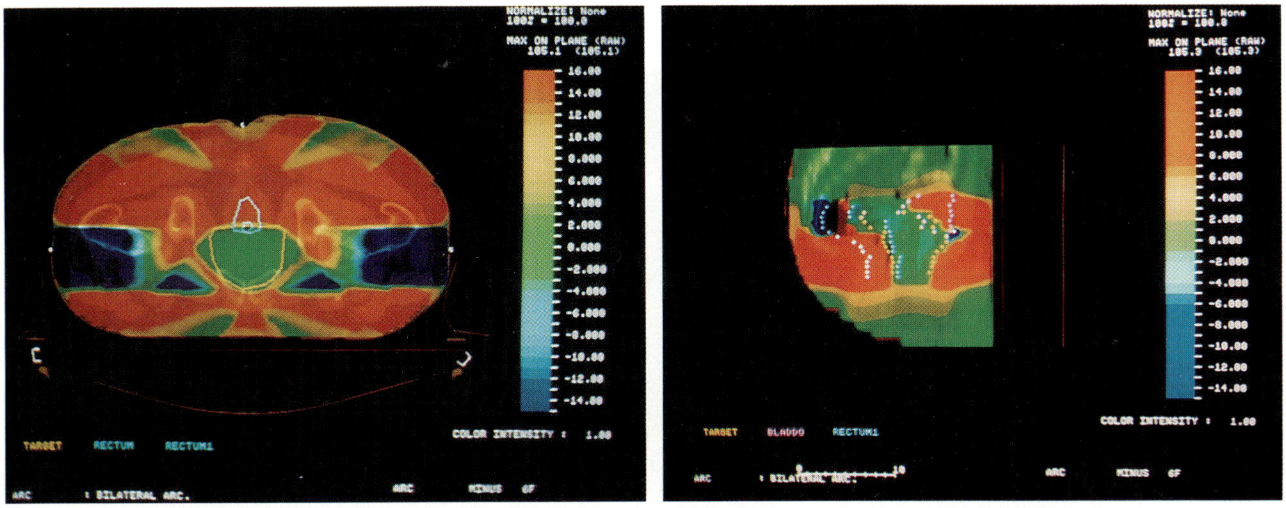

A B

COLOR FIG. 7-6. Midplane **(A)** axial and **(B)** sagittal color-wash displays of the difference in dose distribution between the two treatment plans shown in Figure 7-5. The region that receives a higher radiation dose with the traditional rotational plan than with the conformal plan is shown in red, the region in which the dose is similar is shown in green, and the area in which the dose is lower in the rotational plan than in the conformal plan is shown in blue.

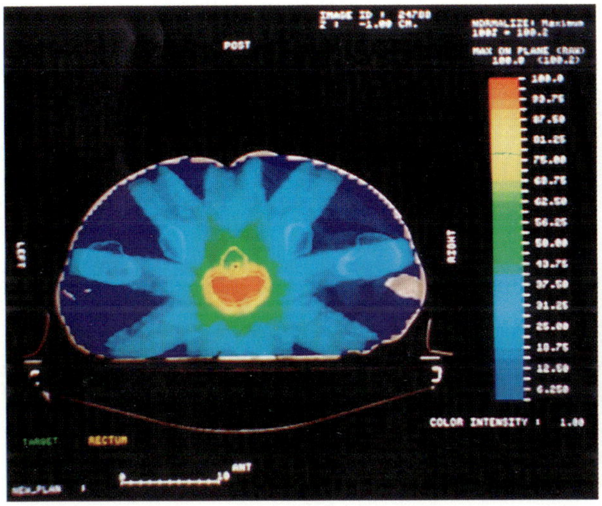

COLOR FIG. 7-8. Axial color-wash dose-distribution display of an inverse treatment plan consisting of nine equiangular intensity-modulated fields for a patient with carcinoma of the prostate. There is marked improvement in the conformality of the dose distribution to the shape of the target volume *(white dots)* compared with the six-field conformal plan shown in Figure 7-5*A*. The objective of this plan was to deliver a dose of 81 Gy to the target volume while limiting the upper dose to the rectum *(yellow dots)* to 60% of the target dose.

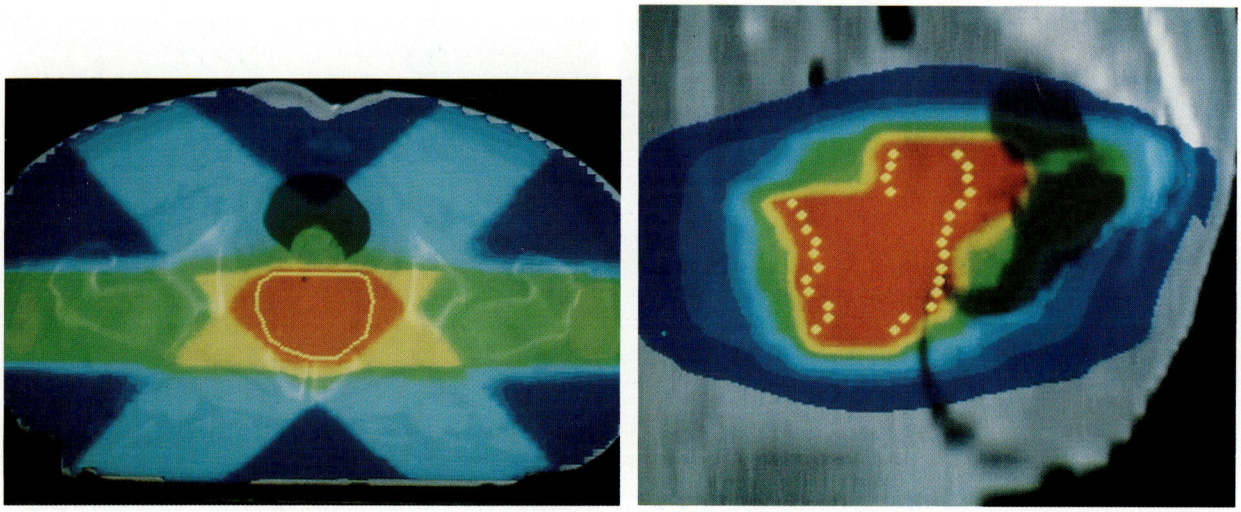

A B

COLOR FIG. 51.1-2. Midplane **(A)** axial and **(B)** sagittal dose-distribution displays of a six-field coplanar prostate treatment plan with 15-mV x-rays, consisting of one pair of lateral and two pairs of oblique fields. In this color-wash display, each band of the color spectrum corresponds to a dose range. The prescription dose is normalized to 100%. The red region represents the prescription isodose distribution (100–101%), while yellow corresponds to approximately 70–80%, green to 45–75%, and blue to 45% or less of the prescription dose. The planning target volume contour is outlined in yellow.

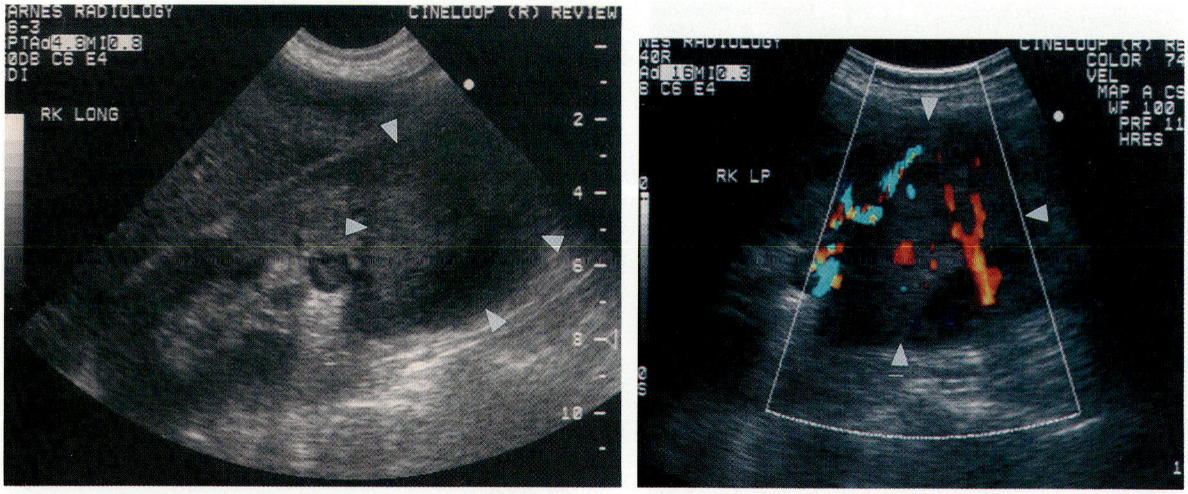

A B

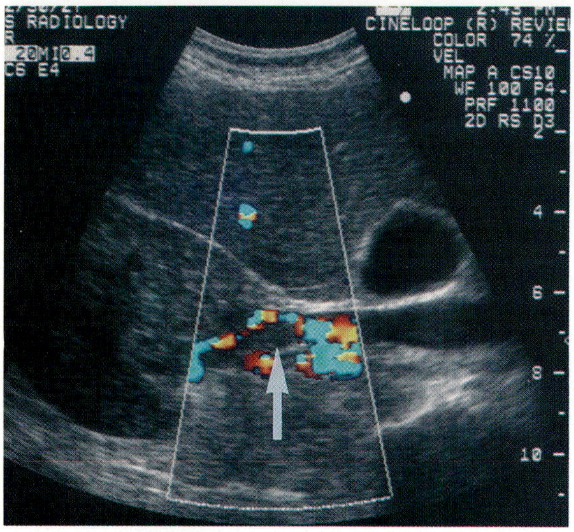

C

COLOR FIG. 80-3. **(A)** Large right lower pole solid mass *(arrowheads)* on a longitudinal sonogram. A computed tomographic scan also showed the mass, but not the right renal vein. **(B)** Longitudinal view of right kidney with color Doppler ultrasound shows flow within the mass *(arrowheads)* confirming the diagnosis of renal cell carcinoma. **(C)** Transverse view through the right kidney and tumor at the level of the right renal vein. Flow around thrombus *(arrow)* in the renal vein is indicated by colored areas (red and blue) within the vein.

SECTION I

Principles of Oncology

Principles and Practice of Genitourinary Oncology, edited by Derek Raghavan, Howard I. Scher, Steven A. Leibel, and Paul H. Lange. Lippincott-Raven Publishers, Philadelphia, © 1997.

CHAPTER 1

Principles of Molecular Biology Techniques

M. Vijay Kumar and Donald J. Tindall

Application of molecular biology techniques has brought about a revolution in the understanding of cell growth and division, mechanisms of development and differentiation, and physiology and pathology of organ systems. Such techniques have been used in every field of modern biology, including disease diagnosis and treatment. In this chapter we describe the use of molecular biology techniques in understanding critical steps involved in cellular functions from transcription to protein synthesis. Furthermore, we delineate some of the techniques that are being used to understand the regulation of genes whose disruption could lead to disease. We provide examples from our own studies of the androgen receptor (*AR*) and prostate-specific antigen (*PSA*) genes to enumerate the principles behind molecular pathways. The purpose of this chapter is not to describe all of the known techniques in molecular biology, but to delineate some of the techniques that will help a novice reader to understand the principles underlying biology of the cell.

REGULATION OF GENE EXPRESSION

Knowledge of how genes are regulated in humans and higher eukaryotes is essential for the understanding of normal development and disease. The unit of inheritance is the gene, which consists of nucleotide sequence encoding genetic information essential for the synthesis of a protein. When a gene is activated, its genetic sequence is translated into a protein. A gene is ''turned on'' when an inducer protein binds the promoter region located at the 5′ end of the gene or when a suppressor protein is released. The first step in protein production is the production of RNA using the DNA sequence as a template, a process termed transcription (Fig. 1-1). The RNA is a single-stranded molecule that is a copy of the anticoding (i.e., antisense or complementary) strand of the double-stranded DNA. The genomic DNA consists of exons and introns, whereas the messenger RNA (mRNA) contains only the exons (see Fig. 1-1). By definition, exons are the regions of DNA that are represented in mRNA and are therefore responsible for encoding a protein. The newly synthesized RNA undergoes a process of maturation (splicing) which results in the formation of mRNA. In this process, the intervening sequences (i.e., introns), are excised and the two ends of the neighboring exon RNA are joined together in the same order as they are in the DNA.[1,2] This process is intramolecular and thus limited to splicing and joining of RNA from the same molecule. The mRNA binds to polyribosomes in the cytoplasm and serves as a template for the synthesis of a protein wherein sequences of three nucleotides in the mRNA (i.e., codons) encode amino acids. The transfer RNAs (tRNAs) carry the amino acids to the translation machinery and attach them sequentially to form a polypeptide molecule. This process is called translation. After their formation, most proteins undergo posttranslational modifications. These modifications include cleavage of a signal peptide sequence to form a mature protein; glycosylation, in which sugar groups are added to the protein; and the formation of secondary and tertiary structures.

In the following sections we discuss in greater detail the three main steps involved in the regulation of gene expression and describe molecular techniques used to understand these mechanisms.

TRANSCRIPTION OF GENES

The functional unit of a gene is divided into the 5′-flanking region, the coding region, including the exons and introns, and the 3′-flanking region.

5′-Flanking Region

Gene transcription is regulated by the binding of proteins to specific DNA sequences.[3–5] Depending on their function, the DNA sequences are termed enhancers, suppressors, or response elements (Fig. 1-2). Although these elements are not capable of initiating transcription, they influence the initiation of transcription by promoters.[6,7] A promoter is defined as a DNA sequence required for accurate and efficient initiation of transcription. In the majority of genes, this region consists of several components:

The capsite element is located near the site of initiation of transcription and is usually denoted as the +1 nucleotide. The nucleotides located upstream of the transcription start site are given negative numbers (−) and those located downstream are given positive numbers (+).

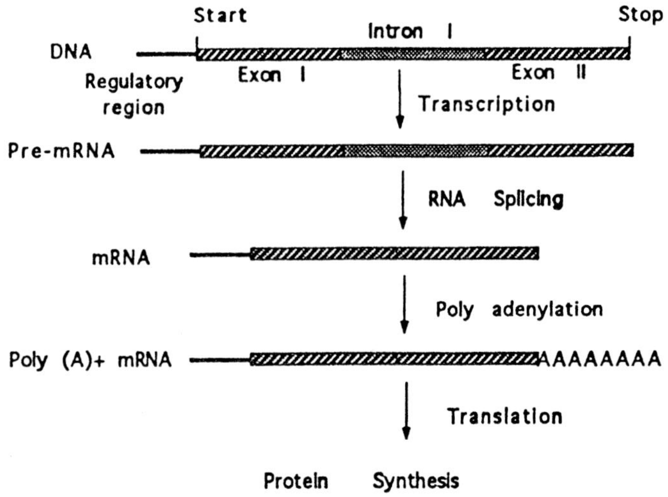

FIG. 1-1. Events involved in the transcription of RNA and translation of protein. The exons are indicated as hatched bars, and the intron is indicated as a stippled bar. The solid line indicates the 5′-regulatory region.

Upstream of the transcription start site, at about −30 nucleotides, is an AT-rich region known as the TATA box.
The CCAAT box is located about −40 to −110 nucleotides upstream of the transcription start site.
A TATA box consists of a consensus sequence, 5′-TATAA/TAA/T-3′, which is a key element in the initiation of transcription.[8–10] An example of this system is the promoter region of the *PSA* gene, which contains a TATA box[11] to which a complex of proteins, including the TATA-binding factors, bind to initiate transcription.[6,12,13]

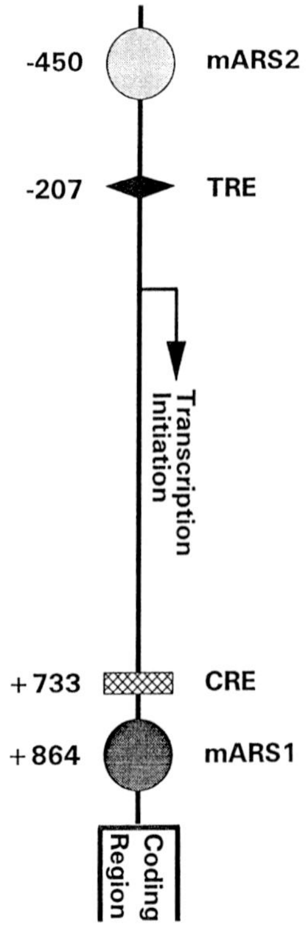

FIG. 1-2. Some of the response elements and suppressors characterized in the 5′-flanking region of the androgen receptor gene. The arrow indicates the primary site of transcription. CRE, cyclic AMP response element; mARS1 and mARS2, the two suppressors on either side of the transcription start site; TRE, TPA response element.

In recent years, several genes have been identified whose promoters do not contain a TATA box.[14–16] A relevant example of this group is the *AR* gene.[17–20] The promoter region of the TATA-less genes is usually rich in GC nucleotides, which initiate transcription at multiple sites. The *AR* gene contains several copies of the sequence GGGGA upstream of the transcription start site and possesses multiple transcription sites.[19,21] Furthermore, in genes with TATA-less promoters, transcription factors bind to the region upstream of the transcription start site to initiate transcription.[14,15] In the *AR* gene, two promoters have been characterized. The 5′-most promoter initiates transcription at two sites that differ by 13 nucleotides.[19,21] A second promoter downstream of the first transcribes a smaller RNA.[22]

Transcription of the *AR* gene is influenced by several regulatory elements present in the 5′-flanking region, including a functional cyclic AMP (cAMP) response element[23,24]; two suppressors, one on either side of the transcription start site[20,21]; and a binding site for the protooncogenes *JUN* and *FOS*.[25]

Coding Region

The coding region of a gene is situated immediately following the 5′-flanking region. Although the DNA is a double-stranded helical structure, only one strand codes for a given protein. The genetic code is read in non-overlapping triplets known as the open reading frame. There are three possible ways of reading the triplets from mRNA and translating these into an amino acid sequence. The translation process is initiated at the ATG codon (for methionine) and comes to a halt when a stop codon or nonsense codon is present in the reading frame (e.g., UAA, UAG, UGA). The 5′ end of the coding region of the gene encodes the N-terminus region of the protein, whereas the 3′ end of the gene encodes the C terminus of the protein. There are 64 possible codons of three bases coding for 20 amino acids; therefore, more than one triplet may code for an amino acid, making it a "degenerate" codon. Thus, a mutation in a nucleotide may or may not affect the protein product. Insertion or deletion of a nucleotide results in a shift of the reading frame and is termed a frame-shift mutation. Examples of these mutations are found in the *AR* gene that result in testicular feminization in mice[26] and androgen-insensitivity syndrome (AIS) in men.[27]

3′-Flanking Region

Similar to the 5′ end, a 3′-flanking region is present downstream of the stop codon. Most eukaryotic mRNAs have a series of adenines (As) at the 3′ end known as the polyadenylic acid or poly (A) tail. The poly (A) sequence in the RNA is not encoded in the DNA but is added as a posttranscriptional modification by the enzyme poly (A) polymerase. The sequence AAUAAA in the mRNA, situated about 11 to 30 nucleotides upstream of the poly (A) tail, is suggested to be the polyadenylation signal. The polyadenylation signal is a highly conserved sequence, and mutations in this sequence results in a lack of the poly (A) tail in the RNA. The presence of the poly (A) tail in the 3′ end of messenger RNA has been effectively exploited in the separation of mRNA from the total RNA population (discussed later).

Analysis of Transcription

There are two aspects of the study of transcription: analysis of RNA and analysis of the DNA in the regulatory region.

RNA Analysis

A typical mammalian cell contains about 10 to 15 μg of RNA, of which about 80% to 85% is ribosomal RNA (rRNA), 15% to 20% is transfer RNA (tRNA), and 1% to 5% is messenger RNA (mRNA). mRNA is analyzed to study its expression or to map the transcription start site. The principle behind some of these techniques is described below.

RNA Extraction

The primary step in the analysis of RNA is to extract total RNA (including rRNA, tRNA, and mRNA) using any of the standard techniques available in the literature. The main impediment in studies involving RNA is that RNA is highly susceptible to degradation by ribonuclease (RNAse). Ribonuclease is a very stable enzyme that does not lose its activity even when boiled in water; therefore, extreme care must be taken to maintain an RNAse-free environment. It is customary to add RNAse inhibitors to the extraction mixture.

To purify mRNA from total RNA, the RNA is separated on a column that contains a short sequence of thymidines (Ts) linked to cellulose, which is capable of binding the poly (A) tail of the mRNA.

Northern Blot Analysis

Northern blot analysis is used to determine the size and amount of mRNA expressed. Either total RNA or mRNA is extracted and electrophoresed on a denaturing agarose gel (Table 1-1). After electrophoresis, the RNA is transferred to nitrocellulose or nylon membrane and noncovalently linked to the membrane by ultraviolet illumination. To locate the RNA of interest, a radiolabeled DNA or RNA probe is hybridized to the Northern blot. The DNA probe is of known sequence and will hybridize to any complementary RNA sequence on the membrane.

S-1 Nuclease Mapping

S-1 nuclease mapping can be used to locate the 5′ or 3′ ends of mRNA and to quantify the amount of mRNA in RNA extractions. This method was developed by Berk and Sharp[28] and was modified for the use of end-labeled probes[29] to facilitate determination of the DNA strand that is being transcribed. The main feature of this method is the use of the enzyme S-1 nuclease, which is a single-strand–specific endonuclease capable of digesting both single-stranded RNA and DNA. The principle of the technique is to hybridize the cDNA probe to mRNA and treat with S-1 nuclease, which will digest all single-stranded regions, including the 5′ or 3′ overhangs and introns. The RNA:cDNA hybrid is then electrophoretically separated on an polyacrylamide gel to determine the size and amount of RNA in the hybrid (Fig. 1-3).

Ribonuclease Protection Assay

In ribonuclease protection assay, radiolabeled RNA, instead of single-stranded cDNA, is used as a probe to detect and quantify specific RNAs.[30,31] The differences between the ribonuclease protection assay and S-1 nuclease mapping are in the preparation of the probes and the use of RNAse instead of S-1 nuclease for digestion of RNA that has not formed an RNA:RNA hybrid (see Fig. 1-3).

The gene of interest or a gene fragment is cloned into a vector containing a phage promoter (e.g., T3 or T7 phage promoter) which enables synthesis of a ^{32}P-labeled RNA in the presence of T3 or T7 RNA polymerase. The sequence to be analyzed is cloned in such a way that the RNA produced by RNA polymer-

Table 1-1. *Blotting techniques used to analyze DNA, RNA, and protein*

Blot	Electrophoresis	Type of gel	Probe
Southern	DNA	Agarose	DNA
Northern	RNA	Agarose	RNA or cDNA
Western	Protein	Polyacrylamide	Protein
Southwestern	Protein	Polyacrylamide	DNA

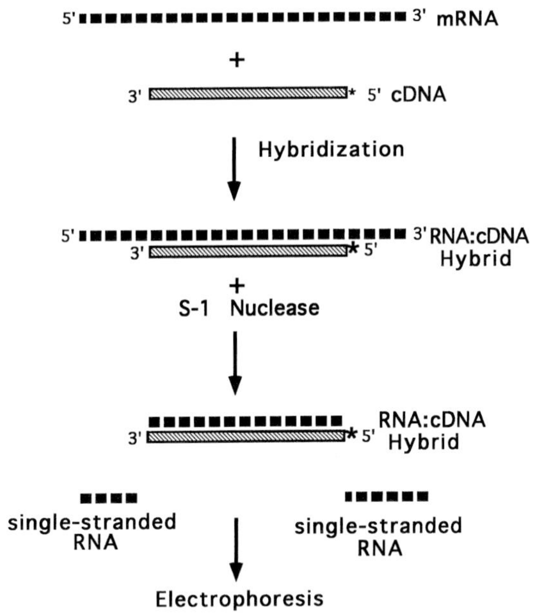

FIG. 1-3. A simplistic protocol for the S-1 nuclease mapping technique. The mRNA is indicated as dashed bars, and the cDNA is indicated as hatched bars. The cDNA is radiolabeled at the 5′ end using γ-^{32}P-ATP (indicated by a star) in the presence of T4 polynucleotide kinase.

ase is complementary to the RNA being analyzed (antisense). The probe RNA is incubated with total or mRNA and allowed to hybridize to form an RNA:RNA hybrid. The unhybridized RNA is digested by the addition of RNAse, and the radiolabeled RNA:RNA hybrid is then detected and quantified by separation on a polyacrylamide gel under denaturing conditions. This method is very sensitive and is capable of detecting picogram quantities of mRNA. Ribonuclease protection assay kits are available from several companies.

In Situ Hybridization

The previously described analyses indicate the levels of RNA in a given tissue. However, if the objective is to determine the differential expression of the same gene in two different cell types, the technique of choice is in situ hybridization. An excellent example is the analysis of expression of a gene in paired prostate tumor and benign cells. For a Northern blot analysis, paired tumor and benign tissue is collected during surgery, quickly frozen, and processed as described previously. However, it should be recognized that the tumor tissue sample is probably not 100% tumor but rather a mixture of benign and tumor cells; therefore, it is rather difficult to evaluate the data. Under these conditions, in situ hybridization is used to localize the mRNA of interest to individual cell types (e.g., benign or tumor). The technique involves collecting the tissue of interest, fixing the sample in 4% paraformaldehyde, and embedding the sample in paraffin after dehydration in graded alcohol solutions. Serial sections are deparaffinized and hybridized using ^{32}P-labeled RNA or a cDNA probe. The positive cells are those containing black grains of radioactive signal.

Polymerase Chain Reaction

Since the first report of specific DNA amplification using the polymerase chain reaction (PCR)[32,33] the technique has transformed DNA analysis both in research and clinical laboratories. Although this technique was originally used to amplify DNA, PCR has found applications in most problems in molecular biology. PCR has been used to identify and sequence unknown DNA that flanks a known segment,[34] to delineate genome walking,[35] to identify point mutations,[36] to identify genomic footprinting,[37] and to reveal mutagenesis to analyze the function of genes and their regulatory elements.[38–40]

In PCR, the DNA sequence of interest is amplified by using two primers flanking the sequence (Fig. 1-4). The first primer is an oligonucleotide complementary to the bottom strand (primer 1; see Fig. 1-4), whereas the second primer is complementary to the top strand (primer 2; see Fig. 1-4). The reaction mixture in a typical PCR consists of the two primers: a template DNA that incorporates the sequence to be amplified (a mixture of dATP, dGTP, dCTP, dTTP) and a DNA polymerase enzyme capable of synthesizing DNA. The first step in PCR is to denature the double-stranded DNA into single strands by heating the DNA to 94°C and then cooling it to about 50°C, a process called annealing (see Fig. 1-4). During the cooling process, the two primers find their complementary sequences and anneal to them. At this stage, the temperature is again raised to about 72°C to enable the DNA polymerase to use the annealed primer as an anchor to synthesize a new strand of DNA that is complementary to the template. These three steps—denaturation, annealing, and extension—constitute a cycle. At the end of one cycle, the two strands of DNA have been amplified once to yield four strands. These four strands serve as templates for the second cycle of amplification, the products of which will be used as templates for further amplification. By the end of a given number of cycles (n), a theoretical maximum of 2^n DNA molecules is produced. Theoretically, one DNA molecule can yield 1×10^{12} product molecules after 40 cycles. Thus, depending on the research requirements of the product, DNA is amplified through 30 to 40 cycles of PCR.

Differential Display Polymerase Chain Reaction

Before the description of differential display PCR (DD-PCR),[41,42] the standard method used for identifying mRNAs that are differentially expressed was the use of subtractive libraries. However, preparation and screening of subtractive libraries was very time consuming and labor intensive and required a known probe. In contrast, the advantages of DD-PCR are many-fold:

It is possible to screen for any differentially expressed gene using random primers instead of known sequences.

The technique is fast and uses microgram quantities of template, enabling work with small samples.

In this technique (Fig. 1-5), total RNA is extracted and mRNA is isolated as described previously. The 3′-end primer for PCR consists of copies of T with additional bases at the 3′ end to yield specificity in binding (e.g., 5′-TTTTTTTTTTTCA). The 5′-end primers are a battery of oligo-

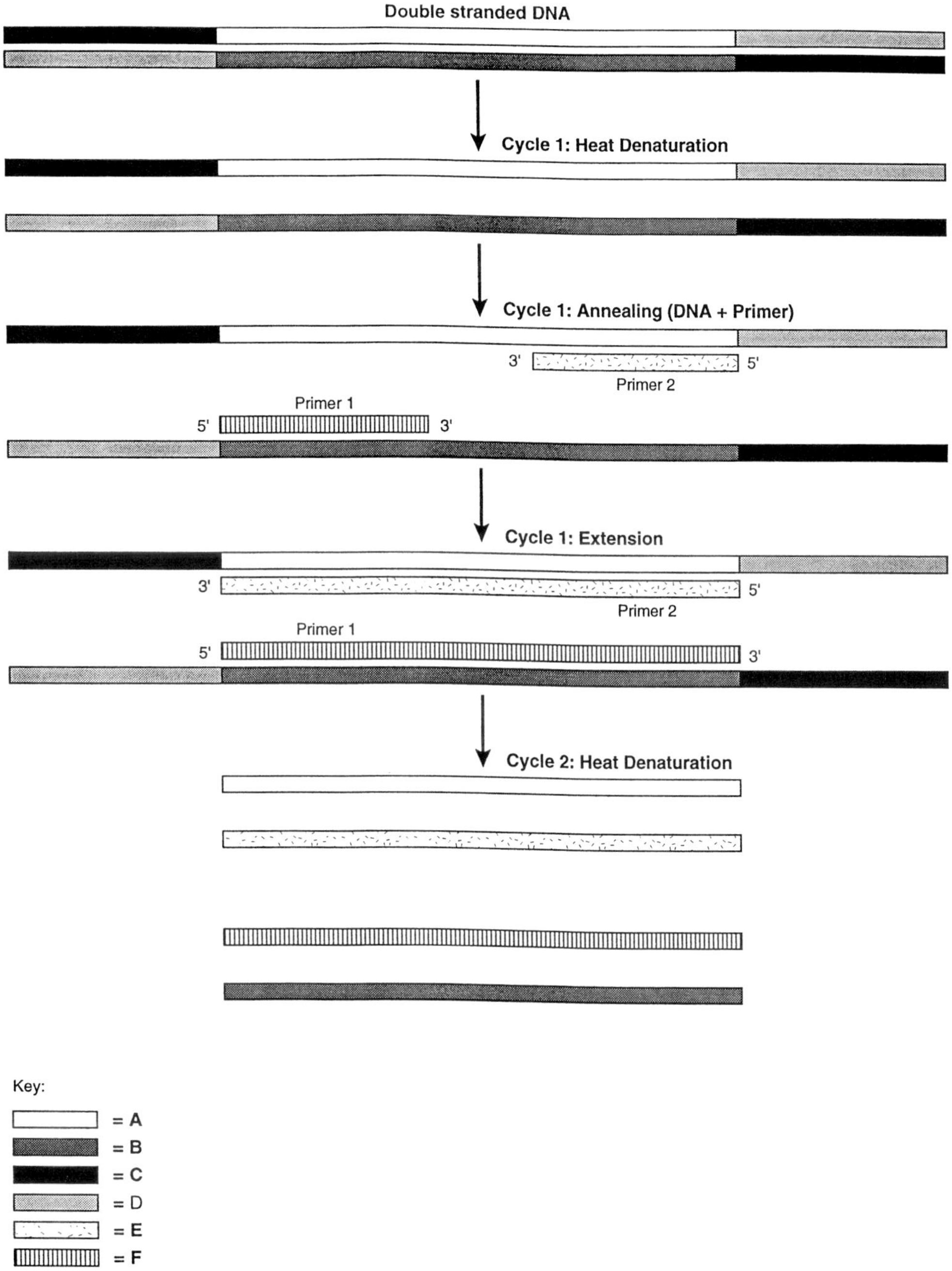

FIG. 1-4. The two strands of template DNA (A, B), the 5′-flanking DNA (C), and the 3′-flanking region (D) are shown. The first step in cycle 1 is heat denaturation (at 94°C) of double-stranded DNA into individual strands. In the second step of annealing, the temperature is lowered to about 42°C, resulting in the binding of primer 1 to the bottom strand; primer 2 will anneal to the top (1) strand because it is complementary to that strand. In the third step, extension, which takes place at about 72°C, the Taq polymerase synthesizes a new strand of DNA using the primers as anchors, resulting in the production of two new strands (E, F). During the second cycle, these steps are repeated, and the two pairs of double-stranded DNA are heat denatured into four single-stranded templates for further amplification.

nucleotides with random nucleotide sequences. Using one of the 3′-end primers and a poly (A)+ RNA as the template, cDNA is synthesized using reverse transcriptase enzyme. The synthesized cDNA is then used as a template for amplification by PCR using the same 3′-end primer that was used to synthesize the cDNA and one of the random 5′-end primers. The amplification reaction is carried out as described previously in the presence of ^{32}P-ATP. The ^{32}P-labeled PCR product is electrophoresed on a polyacrylamide gel in the presence of urea used as a denaturing agent. This gel is similar to the sequencing gel

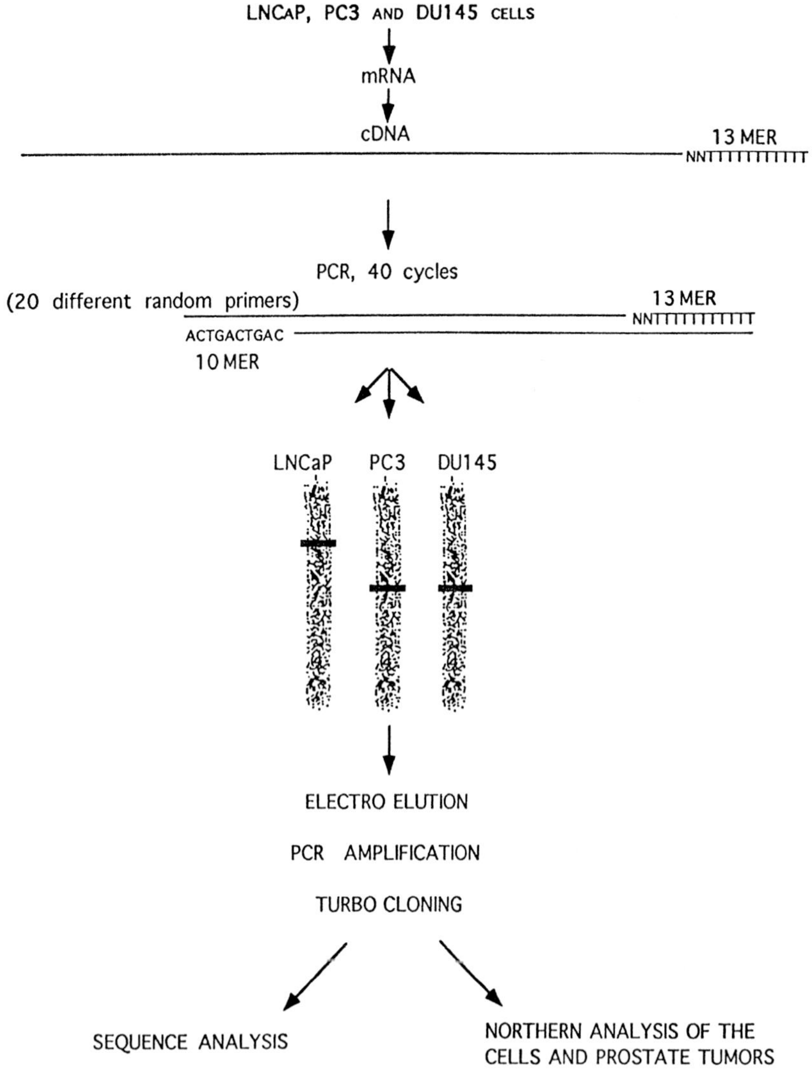

FIG. 1-5. The steps involved in differential display polymerase chain reaction (PCR). In this example, the objective is to identify genes that are differentially expressed in the prostate cancer cell lines LNCaP, PC3 and DU145. Total RNA is extracted, and the mRNA is isolated using an oligo d(T)-cellulose column. The first strand of cDNA is synthesized using a 13-mer poly T primer, which anneals to copies of A added to the 3′ end of the mRNA as a posttranscriptional activity (see Fig. 1-1). The cDNA is synthesized by PCR in the presence of the enzyme reverse transcriptase, which synthesizes cDNA using RNA as a template; this process is called reverse transcriptase–PCR. Using the same 13-mer as the 3′-end primer and one of the 20 random 10-mers as the 5′-end primer, the second strand of cDNA is synthesized by PCR. In this reaction, α-^{32}P-dATP is included to enable radiolabeling of the amplified product, which is electrophoresed on a sequencing gel. In this example, a band is present in the androgen-responsive LNCaP cells that is absent in the androgen-independent PC3 and DU145 cells. Similarly, a common band is present in the PC3 and DU145 cells that is absent in LNCaP. The DNA on the gel corresponding to these bands are collected, electroeluted from the filter paper, PCR amplified, and cloned into a turbocloning vector pCRII (In Vitrogen). This clone is used as a probe to analyze Northern blot analyses of RNA from LNCaP, PC3, and DU145 cell lines to confirm their differential expression.

and therefore is capable of resolving populations of DNA that differ from each other by one nucleotide.

We have used the DD-PCR technique to isolate differentially expressed genes in androgen-dependent and androgen-independent cell lines.[43] In the example provided in Figure 1-5, RNA was isolated from LNCaP, PC3, and DU145 cell lines; the cDNA was synthesized using PCR. A double-stranded cDNA was synthesized, and the product was electrophoresed on a sequencing gel. Bands of interest were isolated, and the DNA was eluted and subcloned for further characterization. This technique is also being used to isolate genes that are turned on or off in prostate cancer cells compared with paired benign samples.

DNA Analysis

The 5′-flanking region of a gene contains most of the key regulatory elements. A gene is usually regulated by the interaction of nuclear proteins, called transcription factors, with the 5′-flanking regions in the promoter of the gene by way of enhancers, suppressor elements, or both. The following paragraphs describe some of the methods used to analyze the 5′-flanking DNA sequence with particular reference to the *AR* gene.

The DNA sequence upstream of ATG but downstream of the transcription start site is known as the 5′ untranslated region, and the sequences upstream of the transcription start site constitute the 5′-flanking region. To analyze the regulation of the *AR* gene, the 1.5-kb 5′-flanking region was isolated and sequenced. Several key regulatory elements were identified by the sequence homology to known regulatory elements and characterized by creating deletion and point mutations and by transient transfection analysis.[20–23,25]

DNA Extraction

The primary step in the analysis of genomic DNA is its extraction from cells. Several protocols, which vary depending on the requirement, are available in the literature. To obtain good quality DNA, it is necessary to limit defragmentation of DNA during extraction. Furthermore, a common contaminant in DNA preparation is RNA, which can be efficiently denatured by incubation with DNAse-free RNAse. Another contaminant

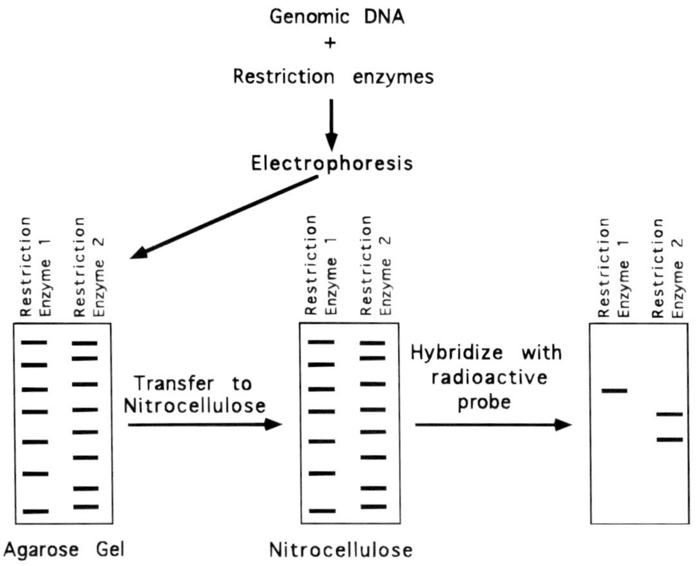

FIG. 1-6. Steps involved in Southern blot analysis of genomic DNA. In this example, genomic DNA was digested with two restriction enzymes in separate tubes and subjected to electrophoresis. The bands generated by restriction enzymes 1 and 2 are different because they generate DNA fragments of different sizes. The DNA fragments are transferred to nitrocellulose and hybridized with a radioactive probe. The restriction enzyme 2 is shown to hybridize to two bands, indicating that a restriction site for this enzyme is present in the region hybridized by the probe. Only one band is seen when the DNA is digested with restriction enzyme 1, which suggests the absence of a recognition site in the region hybridized by the probe and also indicates that the gene of interest is a single-copy gene.

in these preparation is the protein. A common method of deproteinizing DNA preparation is by extraction with phenol and chloroform, which denature protein and dissolve the denatured protein.

Southern Blot Analysis

A list of blotting techniques used to analyze DNA, RNA, and protein is shown in Table 1-1. In 1975, Southern, working at the University of Edinburg, Scotland, described a method for transferring fragments of DNA from agarose gels to nitrocellulose filters which could then be hybridized to radioactive probes.[25] This came to be known as Southern blotting. Subsequently, methods were described to transfer RNA rather than DNA, which was called Northern blotting, and transfer of protein to filters was called Western blotting. A Western blot probed with DNA probe was called Southwestern analysis (see Table 1-1).

Southern blot analysis involves extraction of genomic DNA and fragmentation of this DNA by treating it with restriction enzymes (Fig. 1-6). The restriction digest is subject to electrophoresis in an agarose gel. The DNA from the gel is transferred to a nitrocellulose filter by passive capillary action and is then hybridized using a probe (see Fig. 1-6).

Deletion of 5′-Flanking DNA

Early approaches to the construction of deletion mutants used restriction endonucleases to cleave the DNA, and the cleaved DNA was cloned into a suitable vector, making it important that a convenient restriction site was available at the point of mutation. Subsequently, other enzymes were used to cleave the DNA progressively from the ends (e.g., exonuclease III, Bal 31, DNAse I); however, these techniques are time consuming and labor intensive.

The advantages of using PCR for the generation of deletion mutations[44] include the following:

Deletions at a selected site can be created.
If necessary, both 5′- and 3′-end deletions can be created.
It is easy to generate constructs with nested deletions wherein one end of the mutant is fixed and the other end is progressively deleted (Fig. 1-7).
All the deletion mutants can be cloned at the same site in a vector by incorporating similar restriction sites in the primers.

For the *AR* 5′-deletion mutations, the 5′-end primer complementary to the bottom strand and the 3′-end primer complementary to the top strand were synthesized. Using these two primers and the full-length 5′-flanking sequence as a template, the deletion mutant was amplified and cloned into vectors. By using the same 3′-end primer (primer 4; see Fig. 1-7) and synthesizing several 5′-end primers (primers 1, 2, and 3; see Fig. 1-7) 5′-nested deletions were generated by PCR amplification. A similar strategy can be used to generate 3′-end nested deletions by using a common 5′-end primer (primer P; see Fig. 1-7) and several 3′-end primers (primers X, Y, and Z; see Fig. 1-7).[44]

Transient Transfection of DNA Into Cells

Transient transfection is used as a functional assay to characterize promoters, enhancers, suppressors, or other response elements. To identify and characterize a promoter, the 5′-flanking DNA containing that promoter is cloned into a site upstream of a chloramphenicol acetyl transferase (CAT) cDNA into vectors that contain no promoter. If the objective is to characterize an enhancer, or response-element sequence, the DNA fragment is cloned into vectors that contain a promoter sequence upstream of the CAT cDNA.

For example, to characterize enhancer elements on the *AR* gene, the full-length and deletion constructs were cloned into the pBLCAT3 vector, which does not contain a promoter.[20–23] For analysis of the cAMP response element,[23] TPA-response element,[27] and the suppressor sequences[20,21] of the *AR* gene, the DNA was cloned into the pBLCAT2 vector, which contains a thymidine kinase promoter upstream of a *CAT* gene. The

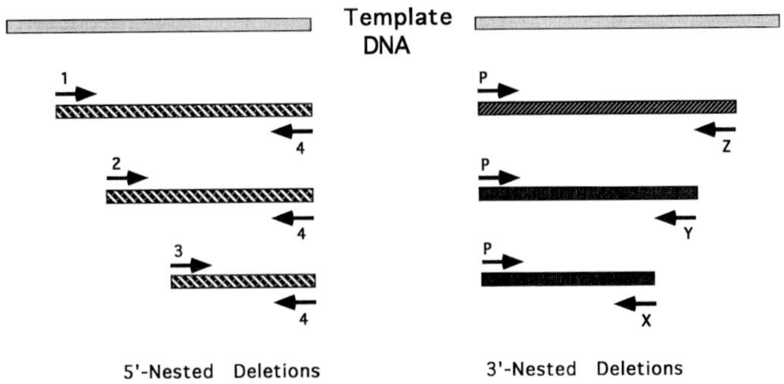

FIG. 1-7. Steps involved in the generation of 5′- and 3′-nested deletions using polymerase chain reaction (PCR). To generate 5′-nested deletions, a common primer (4) is used in all PCR amplifications. The first deletion is generated by using primer 1, which is homologous to the bottom strand. Primer 2 is internal to primer 1, whereas primer 3 is internal to primer 2. Using these primers and the template DNA (*stippled bar*), PCR technique is used to generate 5′-nested deletions. Similarly, using primer P as a common 5′-end primer and nested primers X, Y, and Z, a series of 3′-nested deletions can be generated.

reporter constructs were transfected into cells by either the calcium phosphate technique or electroporation. Generation of calcium phosphate in the culture medium produces a chemical environment that results in DNA attaching to the cell surface, which is then internalized by endocytosis. Electroporation uses an electric field to open pores in the cells through which DNA diffuses. After transfection, the cells were incubated for 24 to 48 hours and harvested, and the proteins were extracted. The protein was assayed for CAT, which is representative of the activity of the promoter or the DNA fragment of interest.

Typically, to account for the amount of DNA internalized during transfection, a vector containing the cDNA for β-galactosidase enzyme was also transfected. After harvesting the cells, β-galactosidase enzyme in the extract was assayed, and all values for CAT activity were normalized to the β-galactosidase activity.

TRANSLATION OF mRNA: OVEREXPRESSION OF FOREIGN PROTEINS

mRNA is translated into protein in the cytoplasm. Amino acids are assembled into proteins on the ribosomes which moves along the mRNA to decipher the codons. A carrier RNA called the transfer RNA (tRNA) is involved in the transfer of an amino acid to the site of production of the protein. The one end of the tRNA matches the codon of the RNA and the other end is attached to a single amino acid. Thus, tRNA is specific to each codon and amino acid. The process of translation involves three major steps: initiation, elongation, and termination. For the initiation of translation, the ribosome must bind to mRNA, forming an initiation complex along with several translation factors. The sequence of steps preceding the formation of a peptide bond between the first and second amino acid is termed initiation. Elongation includes all subsequent steps from the formation of the first peptide bond until the stop of translation in response to the presence of the stop codon. In this process, the amino acids are carried by tRNA to the initiation complex and are attached like beads on a string. When the stop codon is reached, the mRNA is released from the ribosome, and the completed polypeptide chain is released into the cytoplasm. This is known as termination. Upon release from the ribosomes, the peptide assumes the secondary and tertiary structures of the mature protein. Some proteins undergo additional posttranslational modifications such as cleavage of signal sequences in the N-terminus and addition of sugar groups. At this point, the newly synthesized protein is capable of executing its effect on target genes by binding to the DNA of the target gene. For example, the *AR* regulates PSA production by binding to an androgen-response element (ARE) in the 5′-flanking region of the *PSA* gene. The DNA binding sites are specific to a protein in terms of the sequence of the DNA and the number of nucleotides involved in binding. For example, an ARE is a sequence of 12 partially palindromic nucleotides separated by three nonspecific nucleotides. Two molecules of AR bind as a dimer to the ARE, thus turning on the *PSA* gene.[12]

Upon isolation of a full-length cDNA coding for an entire protein, the protein can be produced in large quantities in vitro with cell lysates, in procaryotes, or in eucaryotes.

Cell-Free Translation Systems

In addition to the use of procaryotic and eucaryotic cell systems for overexpression of proteins, cell-free systems have been successfully used for small-scale expression of proteins. The popular systems used are the rabbit reticulocyte lysate and the wheat germ extract. Both of these systems provide the necessary factors to initiate translation and produce full-sized peptide products. The reticulocyte lysate is prepared from New Zealand white rabbits. The reticulocyte is purified to remove contaminating cells, which would alter the translational process, and are treated with nuclease to remove endogenous rabbit mRNA. Thus, the reticulocyte contains tRNA, rRNA, amino acids, and translation initiation, elongation, and termination factors. In our laboratory, we have used the combined transcription translation system (Promega Corporation, Madison, WI) to synthesize mRNA from cloned *AR* cDNA and to produce AR protein.[45]

Procaryotic System

A significant feature of recombinant DNA technology is the ability to overexpress eucaryotic genes in *Escherichia coli*.[46] Several vectors and hosts have been developed. Depending on the requirements, the foreign protein can be expressed in the cytoplasm or secreted through the cell membrane, which is controlled by the sequences present in the vector. Furthermore, the proteins can be expressed as native products or as fusion proteins (i.e., a combination of the procaryotic and eucaryotic proteins).

Eucaryotic Systems

The advantage of an eucaryotic system is that any expressed foreign proteins will undergo posttranslational modifications which are not possible in procaryotic hosts, such as signal sequence cleavage and glycosylation. The two types of systems available for overexpression of foreign protein are insect cells and yeast. We have used the insect cell[47] and yeast[48] systems to overexpress AR proteins.

In the insect cell system, the cDNA of interest is cloned into a plasmid carrying a portion of the baculoviral DNA so that the cDNA is under the control of a strong viral structural protein gene (polyhedron) promoter. The recombinant plasmid is then cotransfected with wild-type baculovirus DNA into an insect cell line derived from *Spodoptera frugiperda*. A natural cell-mediated recombination between homologous regions of the viral and plasmid DNA occurs, which results in replacement of the wild-type viral structure (polyhedron) gene with the plasmid sequences containing the cDNA to be expressed. This technique takes advantage of the fact that the polyhedron is nonessential for viral replication in cell culture. Using the absence of polyhedron as a marker, colonies containing the recombinant plasmid are collected and used for overexpression. To express AR in insect cells, we cloned the *AR* cDNA into pVL1393 transfer vector and overexpressed the protein in *S frugiperda* (SF9) cells.

Another technique used for overexpression of a foreign protein is the use of yeast. Baker's yeast, or *Saccharomyces cerevisiae*, has been used as an excellent expression system to study transcriptional activation of mammalian steroid hormone receptors. We have used this system to overexpress wild-type and mutant AR proteins.[48] This system combines the advantages of eucaryotic expression with the ease of *E coli* system in terms of growth, screening, and analysis. *S cerevisiae* is also known to yield higher expression levels than do insect cells and bacteria, and the secretion of the protein can be targeted.

Western Blot Analysis of Proteins

In Western blot analysis, the protein of interest is mixed with sample buffer containing sodium dodecyl sulfate and β-mercaptoethanol. The sample is electrophoresed on a polyacrylamide gel, and, aided by electric current, the separated proteins are transferred to a nitrocellulose filter by an active transfer process in the presence of buffer and methanol. The filters are then probed with a primary antibody specific to the protein of interest. A secondary antibody, which is conjugated to an enzyme such as alkaline phosphatase or horseradish peroxidase, is used to enable localization of the protein of interest.

POSTTRANSLATIONAL EVENTS

After translation of a regulatory protein in a cell, the protein binds to the target gene to initiate its effect. Several powerful techniques have been developed to understand the nature of protein-DNA interactions, including gel retardation assay and DNAse I protection assay.

Gel Retardation Assay

Gel retardation assay, also called gel shift assay and band shift assay, exploits the property of a protein to bind to a specific DNA sequence. Using this simple technique, it is possible to determine the binding of protein to a particular DNA sequence, to identify specific nucleotides responsible for the interaction, and to verify the specificity of binding of protein to DNA.

In our laboratory, we have used this technique to characterize the TPA-response element (TRE),[25] cAMP response element,[23] and suppressors[20,21] present in the 5′-flanking region of the *AR* gene. As an example, we describe the use of gel retardation assay to analyze TRE. Complementary oligonucleotides containing TRE were synthesized and annealed. The double-stranded oligonucleotide was end-labeled using ^{32}P-ATP. An aliquot of the end-labeled TRE was mixed with nuclear extract in the presence of suitable buffers to enable the protein to bind to DNA. The protein-DNA complex was subject to electrophoresis on a polyacrylamide gel, and the gel was dried and exposed to x-ray film. A positive result in a gel shift assay is the presence of a slower running band compared to the lane in which only the labeled probe is present (i.e., no protein). The specificity of the signal is determined by the addition of varying concentrations of unlabeled oligonucleotides to compete with labeled probe for protein binding. Using this technique, it is also possible to determine the importance of any of the nucleotides in the sequence by synthesizing complementary sequences that incorporate a mutation in the nucleotide of interest. The absence of a shifted band when mutants were used in the gel retardation assay indicate that the site of the mutated nucleotide is critical for interaction of the DNA with the protein.

DNAse I Protection Assay

DNAse I protection assay, or footprinting, is a technique for determining specific sites of the DNA bound by the protein. DNAse I is an enzyme that is capable of hydrolyzing the phosphodiester bond of DNA unless the sequence is protected by the binding of a protein.

In this method, the DNA to be characterized is amplified using PCR, wherein one of the primers used for amplification was end-labeled using ^{32}P-ATP (Fig. 1-8). The ^{32}P-labeled amplified DNA is mixed with varying concentrations of nuclear extract in the presence of suitable buffer. DNAse I is added to this complex, and the reaction product is separated on a sequencing gel that is capable of resolving single-nucleotide differences. The nucleotides bound by the protein are seen as blank spaces on an autoradiogram (see Fig. 1-8, lane 2) compared with the lane in which no protein was added (see Fig. 1-8, lane 1). The blank region is the protected fragment, which can be precisely identified by running a sequencing reaction in the neighboring lanes.

APPLICATIONS OF MOLECULAR BIOLOGY TECHNIQUES

Molecular biology techniques are increasingly being used in diagnosis and treatment of diseases. These techniques have several advantages over earlier techniques. Most molecular biology techniques require only small samples, are less time consuming, and are very sensitive and accurate. A good example of the improvement of molecular biology techniques over preexisting techniques is the diagnosis of infectious diseases. Classic techniques include culture on a Petri dish or biochemical

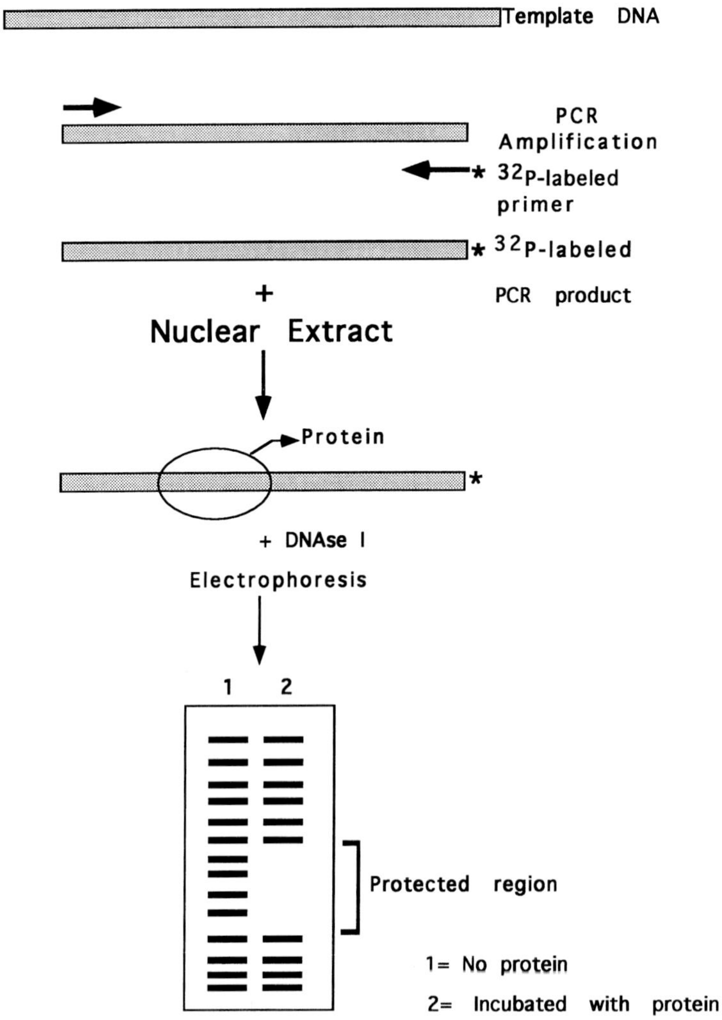

FIG. 1-8. The steps involved in DNAse I protection assay, also known as DNAse I footprinting. The region of interest is amplified using a primer that is end-labeled using γ-^{32}P-ATP, which yields ^{32}P-labeled PCR products. Incubation of PCR product with nuclear extract results in sequence-specific binding of the protein to DNA. Digestion of this product using the enzyme DNAse I and electrophoresis results in generation of a protected region at the site of binding of the protein to the DNA.

tests that indicate the presence of a microorganism. These classic techniques are time consuming, and the information yielded is limited. Using molecular biology techniques, it is comparatively easier to detect procaryotic nucleic acid in the human body using a DNA/RNA probe or PCR. Because PCR is an extremely sensitive technique, it is possible to detect foreign DNA even from a single bacterial colony. Several bacterial and viral diseases are routinely diagnosed using molecular techniques. Furthermore, the biology and life cycle of the infectant can be understood in greater detail by the use of these techniques.

Detection of Genetic Disorders

Perhaps the most dramatic influence of molecular biology is in the diagnosis of genetic disorders. The initiation and success of the human genome project is an indication of the importance of molecular techniques in analyzing human genes. The availability of Southern blotting and in situ hybridization techniques has greatly facilitated the prenatal diagnosis of genetic disorders. Prenatal genetic diagnosis has been further aided by the availability of chromosome-specific probes that enable accurate and sensitive identification of chromosomal aberrations.[49] Another simple technique that has been successfully used in identification of chromosomal disorders is restriction fragment length polymorphism (RFLP).

The greatest impetus to the advancement of molecular biology as a distinct branch of biology was the discovery of restriction enzymes. Restriction enzymes are endonucleases that bind in a sequence-specific manner to double-stranded DNA, which is then cleaved. In RFLP, the DNA is digested using a restriction enzyme, which results in the production of restriction fragments of different lengths. This permits identification of DNA fragments from two chromosomes individually (Fig. 1-9). RFLP has been used to identify polymorphisms and as markers in linkage analysis.[50] Another popular molecular biology technique is DNA fingerprinting, which takes advantage of the fact that the human genome is slightly different for every individual. These differences can be identified by restricting the DNA of interest and then separating it electrophoretically.

Andrology

Molecular techniques are increasingly being used to understand the physiology and pathology of the male reproductive

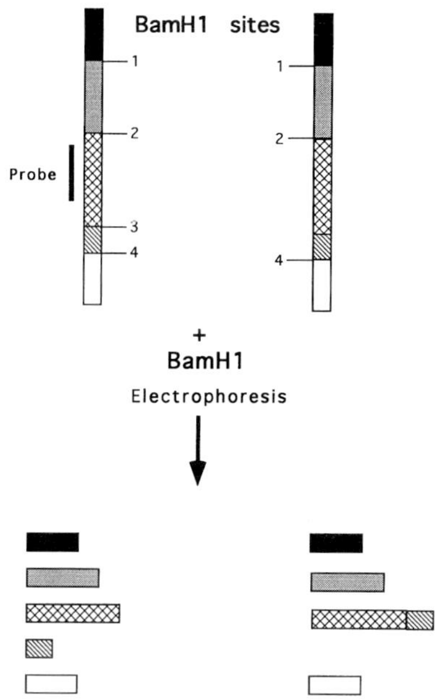

FIG. 1-9. Two chromosomes are shown to possess several recognition sites for the enzyme BamH1. The chromosome on the left has four BamH1 sites, whereas a mutation at site 3 results in only three BamH1 sites in the chromosome on the right. Digestion of these two chromosomes by BamH1 produces the fragments shown at the bottom. The left chromosome produces five fragments, and the right chromosome produces four fragments. The fragments are separated by electrophoresis and transferred to nitrocellulose by Southern blot analysis. Hybridization of the Southern blot with a probe corresponding to the fragment generated by sites 2 and 3 (Probe) displays the differences in restriction fragment length generated by digestion of the two chromosomes with the same restriction enzyme.

system. The *AR* gene is one of the most important genes in the field of andrology. As a mediator of the action of androgens, *AR* is centrally involved in the function of the male reproductive system. Prior to the isolation and sequencing of the *AR* cDNA,[51–53] histochemical and biochemical techniques were used to characterize *AR* in normal and disease conditions. In the following paragraphs we describe some of the advances in the physiology of *AR* and its role in androgen-insensitivity syndrome (AIS) and prostate cancer.

Because of the labile nature of AR protein, progress in understanding the physiology and pathology of *AR* was hampered for several years, during which even the correct size of AR protein could not be ascertained accurately.[54] Knowledge of the molecular structure of the *AR* gene has led to a better understanding of its regulation in normal and disease conditions.

The application of molecular biology techniques have enabled elucidation of the role of *AR* in several disease conditions, including prostate cancer. Mutations in the *AR* gene have been associated with spinal and bulbar muscular atrophy (Kennedy's disease), myotonic dystrophy, and Reifenstein's syndrome.[55–59] The N-terminal domain of the *AR* gene contains three polymeric regions of glutamine, proline, and glycine. The function of these polymeric regions is unclear; however, they have been implicated in transactivation.[60] Using PCR and subsequent sequencing, several point mutations, deletions, and translocations that result in AIS have been discovered in the *AR* gene.[27] AIS is caused by mutations that alter one of the critical functions of the *AR* gene such as steroid binding or DNA binding resulting in feminization. Mutations within the steroid-binding domain prevent *AR* detection by ligand binding assays and are referred to as *AR*-negative. Conversely, several *AR*-positive patients exhibited AIS that was unexplainable until the *AR* mRNA was isolated and sequenced, demonstrating the presence of mutations in the DNA-binding domain. Furthermore, it is known that in testicular feminization syndrome (TFM), the equivalent of AIS in animals, the AR protein was smaller than normal, although the mechanism causing this reduction in size was unknown.[61] With the application of molecular techniques, it was noted that TFM is caused by a single-nucleotide deletion in the transactivation domain of the *AR* gene which caused a shift in the reading frame resulting in the creation of a stop codon upstream of the DNA binding domain.[26] Translation was terminated at the stop codon, resulting in a smaller AR protein. These findings were confirmed using mutation analysis and transient transfections.[45] Similar single-nucleotide deletion mutations in the *AR* gene have been described in patients with AIS.[27]

Prostate Cancer

The use of molecular techniques as diagnostic markers and in identification of mutations in prostate and bladder cancer is described in Chapters 20 and 39. This chapter highlights the impact of molecular techniques in determining the role of the *AR* gene in prostate cancer.

The application of molecular techniques has greatly influenced research in prostate cancer.[62–65] Using PCR to amplify *AR* cDNA from prostate tissue or even from cells collected by microdissection of paraffin sections, mutations in the *AR* gene have been identified.[65–68] Gaddipati and colleagues[68] have discovered in advanced prostate cancers a single-nucleotide change in codon 877 that resulted in change of threonine to alanine. This mutation is similar to the one described in the LNCaP prostatic carcinoma cell line.[69] This mutation causes a loss of specificity of binding of steroids to AR, so that glucocorticoid or progesterone could bind to the steroid-binding domain and thus activate the *AR* gene. Furthermore, somatic mutations have also been found in the ligand-binding domain,[65,66] which indicates that a single change of an amino acid in the ligand-binding domain enhances the transactivation response of mutant *AR*. This could explain progression of prostatic carcinoma even in the absence of testicular androgens.[66]

Future Directions

The available literature clearly indicates that molecular biology will become critical for ascertaining the diagnosis and prognosis of many diseases. Instead of depending on biochemical and histochemical assays alone, in situ hybridization, Northern blotting, and PCR will be used extensively. However, with advances in isolation and characterization of genes in disease conditions, gene transfer and gene therapy will be the molecular biology techniques of the future. Indeed, transgenic mice models are already being extensively used for gene transfer.

Based on the basic knowledge of the structure and function of genes and their mutations in disease conditions (e.g., cystic fibrosis), gene therapy is becoming an option in the treatment of diseases. However, for gene therapy to be successful, the disease must result from defects altering one gene. Introduction of an exogenous gene might correct a genetic defect by random insertion into the genome or by targeting the gene site using tissue-specific sequences. Gene therapy potentially will yield lifesaving treatments for patients with genetic defects.

REFERENCES

1. Cech TR. RNA editing: world's smallest introns? Cell 1991;64:667.
2. Agabian N. Trans splicing of nuclear pre-mRNAs. Cell 1990;61:1157.
3. Herendeen DR, Williams KP, Kassavetis GA, Geiduschek EP. An RNA polymerase-binding protein that is required for communication between an enhancer and a promoter. Science 1990;248:573.
4. Lewin B. Commitment and activation at Pol II promoters: a tail of protein-protein interactions. Cell 1990;61:1161.
5. Buratowski S. The basics of basal transcription by RNA polymerase II. Cell 1994;77:1.
6. Latchman DS. Eukaryotic transcription factors. Biochem J 1990;270: 281.
7. Ptashne M, Gann AAF. Activators and targets. Nature 1990;346:329.
8. Young CYF, Montgomery BT, Andrews PE, Qiu S, Bilhartz DL, Tindall DJ. Hormonal regulation of prostate-specific antigen mRNA in a human prostatic adenocarcinoma cell line, LNCaP. Cancer Res 1991; 51:3748.
9. Xu L, Thali M, Schaffner W. Upstream box/TATA box order is the major determinant of the direction of transcription. Nucleic Acids Res 1991;19:6699.
10. Young CYF, Andrews PE, Montgomery BT, Tindall DJ. Tissue-specific and hormonal regulation of human prostate-specific glandular kallikrein. Biochemistry 1992;31:818.
11. Klobeck H-G, Combriato G, Schulz P, Arbusow V, Fittler F. Genomic sequence of human prostate specific antigen (PSA). Nucleic Acids Res 1989;17:3981.
12. Murtha P, Tindall DJ, Young CYF. Androgen induction of a human prostate-specific kallikrein, hKLK2: characterization of an androgen response element in the 5′ promoter region of the gene. Biochemistry 1993;32:6459.
13. Wingender E. Transcription regulating proteins and their recognition sequences. Crit Rev Eukaryot Gene Expr 1990;1:11.
14. Azizkhan JC, Jensen DE, Pierce AJ, Wade M. Transcription from TATA-less promoters: dihydrofolate reductase as a model. Crit Rev Eukaryot Gene Expr 1993;3:229.
15. Wiley SR, Kraus RJ, Mertz JE. Functional binding of the "TATA" box binding component of transcription factor TFIID to the −30 region of TATA-less promoters. Proc Natl Acad Sci U S A 1992;89:5814.
16. White RJ, Jackson SP. Mechanism of TATA-binding protein recruitment to a TATA-less class III promoter. Cell 1992;71:1041.
17. Baarends WM, Themmen APN, Blok LJ, et al. The rat androgen receptor promoter. Mol Cell Endocrinol 1990;74:75.
18. Tilley WD, Marcelli M, McPhaul MJ. Expression of the human androgen receptor gene utilizes a common promoter in diverse human tissues and cell lines. J Biol Chem 1990;265:13776.
19. Faber PW, King A, van Rooij HCJ, Brinkamann AO, de Both MJ, Trapman J. The mouse androgen receptor: functional analysis of the protein and characterization of the gene. Biochem J 1991;278:269.
20. Kumar MV, Jones EA, Grossmann ME, Blexrud MD, Tindall DJ. Identification and characterization of a suppressor element in the 5′-flanking region of the mouse androgen receptor gene. Nucleic Acids Res 1994; 22:18.
21. Grossmann ME, Lindzey J, Kumar MV, Tindall DJ. The mouse androgen receptor is suppressed by the 5′-untranslated region of the gene. Mol Endocrinol 1994;8:448.
22. Grossmann ME, Lindzey J, Blok LJ, Perry JE, Kumar MV, Tindall DJ. The mouse androgen receptor gene contains a second functional promoter which is regulated by dihydrotestosterone. Biochemistry 1994;33:14594.
23. Lindzey J, Grossmann ME, Kumar MV, Tindall DJ. Regulation of the 5′-flanking region of the mouse androgen receptor gene by cAMP and androgen. Mol Endocrinol 1993;7:1530.
24. Mizokami A, Yeh S-Y, Chang C. Identification of 3′5′-cyclic adenosine monophosphate response element and other cis-acting elements in the human androgen gene promoter. Mol Endocrinol 1994;8:77.
25. Southern EM. Detection of specific sequences among DNA fragments separated by gel electrophoresis. J Mol Biol 1975;98:503.
26. He WW, Kumar MV, Tindall DJ. A frame-shift mutation in the androgen receptor gene causes complete androgen insensitivity in the testicular-feminized mouse. Nucleic Acids Res 1991;19:2372.
27. Lindzey J, Kumar MV, Grossman M, Young C, Tindall DJ. Molecular mechanisms of androgen action. In: Litwack G, ed. Vitamins and hormones, vol 49. New York: Academic Press, 1994:383.
28. Berk AJ, Sharp PA. Sizing and mapping of early adenovirus mRNA's by gel electrophoresis of S1 endonuclease-digested hybrids. Cell 1977; 12:721.
29. Weaver RF, Weissman C. Mapping of RNA by a modification of the Berk-Sharp procedure: the 5′-termini of 15S β-globin mRNA precursor and mature 10S β-globin mRNA have identical map coordinates. Nucleic Acids Res 1979;7:1175.
30. Zinn K, DiMaio D, Maniatis T. Identification of two distinct regulatory regions adjacent to the human β-interferon gene. Cell 1983;34:865.
31. Melton DA, Krieg PA, Rebagliati MR, Maniatis T, Zinn K, Green MR. Efficient in vitro synthesis of biologically active RNA and RNA hybridization probes from plasmids containing a bacteriophage SP6 promoter. Nucleic Acids Res 1984;12:7035.
32. Saiki RK, Scharf S, Faloona F, et al. Enzymatic amplification of beta-globin genomic sequences and restriction site analysis for diagnosis of sickle cell anemia. Science 1985;230:1350.
33. Saiki RK, Gelfand DH, Stoffel S, et al. Primer-directed enzymatic amplification of DNA with a thermostable DNA polymerase. Science 1988;239:487.
34. Jones DH, Winistorfer SC. Sequence specific generation of a DNA panhandle permits PCR amplification of unknown flanking DNA. Nucleic Acids Res 1992;20:595.
35. Jones DH, Winistorfer SC. Genome walking with 2- to 4-kb steps using panhandle PCR. PCR Methods Appl 1993;2:197.
36. Ugozzoli L, Wallace RB. Allele-specific polymerase chain reaction. Methods: Companion Methods Enzymol 1991;2:42.
37. Mueller PR, Wold B. Ligation-mediated PCR: applications to genomic footprinting. Methods: Companion Methods Enzymol 1991;2:20.
38. Bowman S, Tischfield JA, Stambrook PJ. An efficient and simplified method for producing site-directed mutations by PCR. Technique 1990; 2:254.
39. Sarkar G, Sommer SS. The "megaprimer" method of site-directed mutagenesis. Biotechniques 1990;8:404.
40. Jones DH, Winistorfer SC. Site-specific metagenesis and DNA recombination by using PCR to generate recombinant circles in vitro or by recombination of linear PCR products in vivo. Methods: Companion Methods Enzymol 1991;2:2.
41. Liang P, Pardee AB. Differential display of eukaryotic messenger RNA by means of the polymerase chain reaction. Science 1992;257:967.
42. Liang P, Averboukh L, Keyomarsi K, Sager R, Pardee AB. Differential display and cloning of messenger RNAs from human breast cancer versus mammary epithelial cells. Cancer Res 1992;52:6966.
43. Blok LJ, Kumar MV, Tindall DJ. Isolation of cDNAs that are differentially expressed between androgen-dependent and androgen-independent prostate carcinoma cells using differential display PCR. Prostate 1995;26:213.
44. Kumar MV, Tindall DJ. Use of PCR in the analysis of the 5′-flanking region of the androgen receptor gene. In: Sarkar G, ed. PCR in neuroscience, vol 26. New York: Academic Press 1994:324.
45. He WW, Lindzey JK, Prescott JL, Kumar MV, Tindall DJ. The androgen receptor in the testicular feminized (Tfm) mouse may be a product of internal translation initiation. Receptor 1994;4:121.
46. Young CYF, Qui S, Prescott JL, Tindall DJ. Overexpression of a partial human androgen receptor in E. coli: characterization of steroid binding, DNA binding and immunological properties. Mol Endocrinol 1990;4: 1841.
47. Kumar MV, Lindzey J, Lam J, Tindall DJ. Expression of full length mouse androgen receptor in insect cells using baculovirus expression system. 73rd Endocrine Society meeting, June 19–22, 1991.

48. Mak P, Young CYF, Tindall DJ. A novel yeast expression system to study androgen action. Recent Progr Hormone Res 1994;49:347.
49. Dawson DB, Cummins LA, Schaid DJ, et al. Carrier identification of cystic fibrosis by recombinant DNA techniques. Mayo Clin Proc 1989; 64:325.
50. Tefferi A, Thibodeau SN, Solberg LA Jr. Clonal studies in myelodysplastic syndrome using X-linked restriction fragment length polymorphisms. Blood 1990;75:1770.
51. Chang C, Kokontis J, Liao S. Structural analysis of complementary DNA and amino acid sequences of human and rat androgen receptors. Proc Natl Acad Sci U S A 1988;85:7211.
52. Lubahn DB, Joseph DR, Sar M, et al. The human androgen receptor: complementary deoxyribonucleic acid cloning, sequence analysis, and gene expression in prostate. Mol Endocrinol 1988;2:1265.
53. He WW, Fisher LM, Sun S, et al. Molecular cloning of androgen receptors from divergent species with a polymerase chain reaction technique: complete cDNA sequence of the mouse androgen receptor and isolation of androgen receptor cDNA probes from dog, guinea pig, and clawed frog. Biochem Biophys Res Commun 1990;171:697.
54. Johnson MP, Young CYF, Rowley DR, Tindall DJ. A common molecular weight of the androgen receptor monomer in different target tissues. Endocrinology 1987;26:3174.
55. la Spada AR, Wilson EM, Lubahn DB, Harding AE, Fischbeck KH. Androgen receptor gene mutations in X-linked spinal and bulbar muscular atrophy. Nature 1991;352:77.
56. Igarashi S, Tanno Y, Onodera O, et al. Strong correlation between the number of CAG repeats in androgen receptor genes and the clinical onset of features of spinal and bulbar muscular atrophy. Neurology 1992;42:2300.
57. Amato AA, Prior TW, Barohn RJ, Snyder P, Papp A, Mendell JR. Kennedy's disease: a clinicopathologic correlation with mutations in the androgen receptor gene. Neurology 1993;43:791.
58. Nakao R, Yanase T, Sakai Y, Haji M, Nawata H. A single amino acid substitution (Gly743-Val) in the steroid-binding domain of the human androgen receptor leads to Reifenstein syndrome. J Clin Endocrinol Metabol 1993;77:103.
59. Choi WT, MacLean HE, Chu S, Warne GL, Zajac JD. Kennedy's disease: genetic diagnosis of an inherited form of motor neuron disease. Aust N Z J Med 1993;23:187.
60. Gerber H-P, Seipel K, Georgiev O, et al. Transcriptional activation modulated by homopolymeric glutamine and proline stretches. Science 1994;263:808.
61. Young CYF, Jonhson MP, Prescott JP, Tindall DJ. The androgen receptor of the testicular-feminized (Tfm) mutant mouse is smaller than the wild-type receptor. Endocrinology 1989;124:771.
62. Van der Kwast TH, Schalken J, Ruizeveld de Winter JA, et al. Androgen receptors in endocrine-therapy-resistant human prostate cancer. Int J Cancer 1991;48:189.
63. Rinker-Schaeffer CW, Isaacs WB, Isaacs JT. Molecular and cellular markers for metastatic prostate cancer. Cancer Metastasis Rev 1993; 12:3.
64. Foster, CS, McLoughlin J, Bashir I, Abel PD. Markers of the metastatic phenotype in prostate cancer. Hum Pathol 1992;23:381.
65. Newmark JR, Hardy DO, Tonb DC, et al. Androgen receptor gene mutations in human prostate cancer. Proc Natl Acad Sci U S A 1992; 89:6319.
66. Culig Z, Hobisch A, Cronauer MV, et al. Mutant androgen receptor detected in an advanced-stage prostatic carcinoma is activated by adrenal androgens and progesterone. Mol Endocrinol 1993;7:1541.
67. Suzuki H, Sato N, Watabe Y, Masai M, Seino S, Shimazaki J. Androgen receptor gene mutations in human prostate cancer. J Steroid Biochem Mol Biol 1993;46:759.
68. Gaddipati JP, McLeod DG, Heidenberg HB, et al. Frequent detection of codon 877 mutation in the androgen receptor gene in advanced prostate cancers. Cancer Res 1994;54:2861.
69. Veldscholte J, Berrevoets CA, Ris-Stalpers C, et al. The androgen receptor in LNCaP cells contains a mutation in the ligand binding domain which affects steroid binding characteristics and response to antiandrogens. J Steroid Biochem Mol Biol 1992;41:665.

Principles and Practice of Genitourinary Oncology, edited by Derek Raghavan, Howard I. Scher, Steven A. Leibel, and Paul H. Lange. Lippincott-Raven Publishers, Philadelphia, © 1997.

CHAPTER 2

Biology of Metastasis: Studies in Renal Cancer

Colin P. N. Dinney and Isaiah J. Fidler

For many patients with cancer, metastasis has occurred by the time of diagnosis. The major barrier to the effective treatment of their metastases is the biologic heterogeneity of neoplastic cells. This heterogeneity is exhibited in numerous genetic, biochemical, immunologic, and biologic characteristics, such as cell-surface receptors, enzymes, karyotype, cell morphology, growth properties, sensitivities to various therapeutic agents, and ability to invade and produce metastasis.[1–7]

Understanding the mechanisms responsible for the development of the biologic heterogeneity of cancer and the process by which tumor cells invade local tissues and spread to distant organs is a primary goal of cancer research. This review describes the way in which the development of relevant preclinical models for human renal cell carcinoma has facilitated the study of the biology of metastasis.

PATHOGENESIS OF A METASTASIS

The process of cancer metastasis consists of a series of sequential steps, each of which can be rate limiting.[6] After cellular transformation, either unicellular or multicellular, growth of neoplastic cells is progressive, but extensive vascularization must occur if a tumor mass is to exceed 2 mm in diameter.[8] Local invasion of the host stroma by some tumor cells, the next step, can occur by several mechanisms that are not mutually exclusive.[9] For example, thin-walled venules and lymphatic channels, which offer little resistance to penetration by tumor cells, provide the most common pathways for tumor cell entry into the circulation. Detachment of small tumor cell aggregates and embolization occur next. The tumor cells that survive the circulation must lodge in the capillary beds of organs. Extravasation follows, probably by the same mechanisms that influence initial invasion. Proliferation within the organ parenchyma completes the metastatic process (Fig. 2-1). To produce detectable lesions, the metastases must develop a vascular network, evade the host immune system,[2] and respond to organ-specific factors that influence their growth.[10,11] Once they do so, metastatic cells can invade host stroma, penetrate blood vessels, and enter the circulation to produce further metastases, the so-called "metastasis of metastases."[4,5]

Only a few cells in a primary tumor can give rise to clinical metastasis, partly because of the elimination of disseminating tumor cells that fail to complete any step in metastasis.[12] Using radiolabeled B16 melanoma cells, researchers observed that, by 24 hours after entry of the cells into the circulation, <1% of the cells were still viable, and <0.01% of tumor cells placed into the circulation survived to produce metastases.[12] These observations brought into question whether the development of metastases represents the chance survival and growth of neoplastic cells or the selective growth of unique subpopulations of malignant cells endowed with special properties. In other words, can any cell growing in a primary neoplasm produce metastases, or do only specific and unique cells possess the appropriate properties that enable them to metastasize? Most recent data conclude that neoplasms are biologically heteregenous and the process of metastasis is indeed selective.

ROLE OF THE ORGAN ENVIRONMENT

Clinical observations of cancer patients and preclinical studies with experimental rodent tumors have demonstrated that certain tumors produce metastasis to specific organs independent of vascular anatomy, rate of blood flow, or the number of tumor cells delivered to each organ. For instance, the distribution and fate of hematogenously disseminated, radiolabeled melanoma cells in experimental rodent systems amply demonstrate that tumor cells reach the microvasculature of many organs.[12–15] Extravasation into the organ parenchyma and proliferation of tumor cells occur only in certain organs, however. Therefore, the mere presence of viable tumor cells in a particular organ does not always predict that the cells will proliferate to produce metastases.[10,13–16]

The search for the mechanisms that regulate the pattern of metastasis began more than a century ago when, in 1889,[17] Paget questioned whether the distribution of metastases was due to chance. Paget therefore analyzed 735 autopsy records of women with breast cancer, and the nonrandom pattern of visceral metastases suggested to him that the process was not due to chance, but rather, certain tumor cells (the "seed") had a specific affinity for the milieu of certain organs (the "soil"). Metastases resulted only when the appropriate seed and soil were matched.[17]

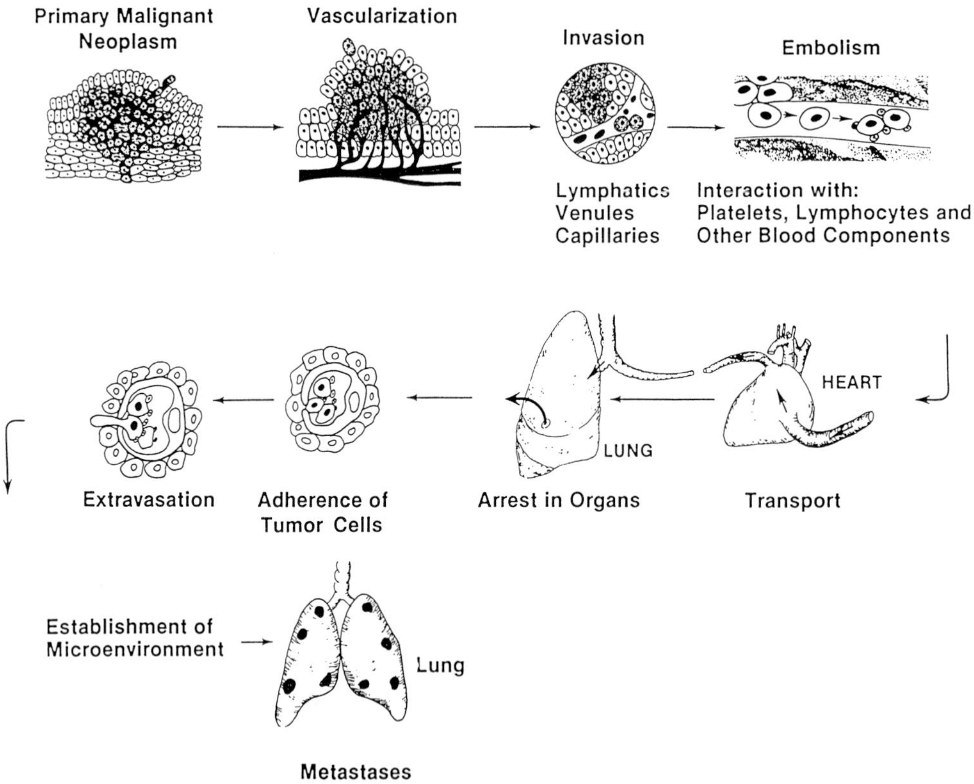

FIG. 2-1. The pathogenesis of cancer metastasis. To produce clinically relevant metastases, tumor cells in a primary neoplasm must complete a series of sequential, selective, and rate-limiting steps.

Experimental data supporting the "seed and soil" hypothesis came from studies on the preferential invasion and growth of B16 melanoma metastases in specific organs.[18] When the B16 melanoma cells were injected into the circulation of syngeneic mice, tumors developed in the lungs and in fragments of lung or ovarian tissue implanted intramuscularly. In contrast, metastatic lesions did not develop in renal tissue implanted as a control organ or at the site of surgical trauma.[18] This study confirmed that the production of metastasis was determined not only by the characteristics of the neoplastic cells, but also by the microenvironment of the host tissue. In vitro experiments demonstrating organ-selective adhesion, invasion, and growth also support Paget's hypothesis.[17] Using the B16 melanoma system, cells with increased capacity for organ adhesion, invasion, and growth have been isolated.[10,19–24] Moreover, experiments with organ tissue-derived soluble growth factors indicate that soil factors can have profound effects on certain tumor cell subpopulations.[10]

Although clinical observations have suggested that carcinomas frequently metastasize through the lymphatic system, and malignant tumors of mesenchymal origin more often spread by the hematogenous route, the presence of numerous venolymphatic anastomoses invalidates this belief.[25] The circulatory anatomy influences the dissemination of many malignant cells; however, it cannot, as Ewing proposed,[26] fully explain the patterns of distribution of numerous tumors. Ethical considerations rule out the experimental analysis of cancer metastasis, as studied in laboratory animals, in patients. The introduction of peritoneovenous shunts for palliation of malignant ascites has, however, provided an opportunity to study some factors affecting metastatic spread in humans.[27,28] Good palliation with minimal complications was reported for 29 patients with various neoplasms. The autopsy findings in 15 patients substantiated the clinical observations that the shunts do not significantly increase the risk of visceral organ metastasis. In fact, despite continuous entry of hundreds of millions of tumor cells into the circulation, metastases in the lung (the first capillary bed encountered) were unusual.[27,28] These results provide compelling verification of the seed and soil hypothesis.

METASTATIC HETEROGENEITY

Populations of cells that differ in metastatic potential have been isolated from the parent neoplasm, a finding that supports the hypothesis that not all the cells in a primary tumor can successfully disseminate. Two general approaches have been used. In the first, metastatic cells are selected in vivo: tumor cells are implanted into mice, and metastatic lesions are harvested. The cells recovered can be expanded in culture or used immediately to repeat the process. The cycle is repeated several times, and the behavior of the cycled cells is compared with that of the cells of the parent tumor. This procedure was originally used to isolate the B16-F10 line from the wild-type B16 melanoma,[20] and it has since also been successful in producing tumor cell lines with increased metastatic capacity from many other experimental tumors.[6] In the second approach, cells are selected for the enhanced expression of a phenotype believed to be important in one or another step of the metastatic sequence, and then they are tested in the appropriate host to determine whether concomitant metastatic potential has been increased or decreased.

The first experimental proof of metastatic heterogeneity in neoplasms was provided by Fidler and Kripke in 1977, in studies with mouse B16 melanoma.[27] Using the modified fluctuation assay of Luria and Delbruck,[28] Fidler and Kripke showed that distinct tumor cell clones, each derived from individual cells isolated from the parent tumor, varied dramatically in their potential to form pulmonary nodules after intravenous inoculation into syngeneic mice. Control subcloning procedures demonstrated that the observed diversity was not a consequence of the cloning procedure.[27]

To exclude the possibility that the metastatic heterogeneity found in the B16 melanoma cells may have been introduced as a result of lengthy cultivation, Kripke studied the biologic and metastatic heterogeneity of a mouse melanoma induced in C_3H mice by long-term exposure to ultraviolet B radiation and painting with croton oil.[29] One mouse thus treated developed a melanoma designated K-1735. The original K-1735 melanoma was established in culture and immediately cloned.[30,31] The clones differed from each other and from the parent tumor in their ability to produce lung metastases. Moreover, the metastases demonstrated significant variability in their size and pigmentation. Metastases to the lymph nodes, brain, heart, liver, and skin were found in addition to lung metastases; those growing in the brain were uniformly melanotic, whereas those growing in other organs generally were not.[30,31]

MODELS FOR HUMAN RENAL CANCER METASTASIS

The concept that neoplasms are heterogeneous and contain subpopulations of cells with different patterns of biologic behavior, including metastatic ability, is no longer controversial. Studies in most rodent tumor systems have also demonstrated that metastasis is a selective process,[20,32,33] metastases can have a clonal origin,[34–38] metastases can develop from the expansion of a single cell,[38] and the host organ microenvironment can profoundly influence the growth of metastatic tumor cells.[6] Although most data on the metastatic heterogeneity of neoplasms and on host-tumor cell interactions during the metastatic process have been derived from studies in nonhuman systems, evidence is now accumulating about the biology of metastasis by cells isolated from surgical specimens of human cancers. In large measure, this accumulation of evidence has been due to recent improvements in the use of in vivo models for the isolation of metastatic subpopulations of human cancer cells and for testing of their metastatic potential. With the discovery of the athymic T cell-deficient nude mouse, its use as a recipient for human xenografts, and its adaptation for the study of human cancer growth and metastasis,[39] many aspects of the biology of human cancer can now be studied. Reports on the metastatic ability of human tumors subsequent to implantation into nude mice have recently increased,[39,40] and several reports have concluded that the metastatic capacity of human tumor cells in nude mice is influenced by variations in experimental techniques.[41,42] Fidler has shown that the capacity to produce metastasis from human tumor cell lines of long duration[43,44] or of recent origin[45–48] depends both on the injection site and on the intrinsic properties of the cells.[39]

An appropriate model for studies of human cancer metastasis must meet two rigid demands: it must use metastatic cells (seed), and it must grow in the relevant organ environment (soil). To study the properties of metastatic subpopulations from surgical specimens of human cancers, methods for their isolation, propagation, and testing must be developed.

The study of the biology of human renal cell carcinoma (HRCC) has been facilitated by the development of relevant in vivo models. Orthotopic implantation of HRCC cells allows for the isolation of tumor cells capable of producing metastasis to the lymph nodes, lung, and other organs. Furthermore, this system allows for analysis of the properties that identify metastatic HRCC under in vivo conditions.

ESTABLISHMENT OF RENAL CANCER CELL LINES

We have used two HRCC cell lines, the SN12 and KG-2, to study the metastatic potential of HRCC. Naito and associates established the SN12 renal cell carcinoma line from a radical nephrectomy specimen of a renal cell carcinoma in a 43-year-old man.[49] A cell suspension with high viability was divided into three aliquots. One was used to produce a tissue culture line designated SN12C. The second was injected subcutaneously in the lateral aspect of the anterior thoracic wall of several nude mice. Two months later, a subcutaneous tumor was excised and dissociated enzymatically. The cells were established in culture, and the line was designated SN12S1. The third aliquot was injected into the kidneys of nude mice. Several weeks later, a large tumor was harvested. In one mouse, a grossly visible tumor nodule was found in the liver, and the peritoneum contained ascitic fluid. Tumor cells isolated from the kidney tumor and the liver nodule were established as individual cell lines in culture and designated lines SN12K1 and SN12L1, respectively. The cell line established from the ascitic cells was designated SN12A1.

The cells of the HRCC lines grew on plastic as monolayer cultures with similar morphologic features. The human origin of all five cell lines was ascertained by detailed karyotypic analysis and isoenzyme determinations. No contamination with mouse cells was found in any of the lines.

Similarly, the KG-2 cell line was isolated from a surgical specimen subsequent to radical nephrectomy in a 58-year-old man. Cells were injected into the subcutis, kidney, cecal wall, and spleen of nude mice. Tumor grew in the subcutis and kidney, and only kidney tumors produced distant metastases.

BIOLOGIC BEHAVIOR OF THE DIFFERENT HRCC LINES

Subsequent experiments showed that the five HRCC SN12 cell lines consisted of cells with different biologic properties, including growth in vivo at ectopic and orthotopic sites and production of experimental and spontaneous metastasis (Table 2-1).[49]

The in vitro tumor cell doubling time did not differ significantly among the cell lines. All lines were tumorigenic at subcutaneous sites, but SN12L1 cells (developed from a metastasis) grew at the fastest rate, whereas SN12A1 cells (ascites) were the

Table 2-1. *Biologic properties of HRCC lines*

HRCC	Growth: In vitro	Growth: Subcutaneous tissue	Growth: Kidney	Metastasis: From in vitro	Metastasis: From subcutaneous	Metastasis: From kidney
SN12–culture	Best	+ +	+ + +	–	+	+ +
SN12–skin	+ +	Best	+ + +	–	Highest	+ +
SN12–kidney	+ +	+ +	+ + +	–	+	+ + +
SN12–kidney–liver	+ +	Best	+ + +	+	+	Highest
SN12–kidney–ascites	+ +	+ +	+ +	–	–	–
KG-2	+ +	+ +	+ + +	+	–	–

slowest. A large part of the subcutaneous tumor was necrotic, irrespective of the tumor cell line and its growth rate.

Injection of the SN12 HRCC cells into ectopic organs, such as the subcutis, peritoneum, or the spleen, produced a high rate of tumorigenicity but not distant metastases. This finding was remarkable because intrasplenic injection has been shown to be optimal for the study of metastatic behavior of human colon carcinoma cells.[45–48] The injection of HRCC cells into the kidney environment produced the highest incidence of tumorigenicity regardless of the cell line, a finding suggesting that the kidney is the best environment for expression of tumorigenicity of HRCC cells. The growth rate of the HRCC cells in the kidney differed among the lines, with SN12L1 cells producing the fastest-growing tumors. The slowest-growing tumors were produced by cells of the SN12C (tissue culture) or SN12A1 (ascites derived) lines. The production of lung metastasis from kidney tumors varied among the lines. A high incidence of lung metastasis was observed with cells of line SN12L1 (derived from a liver metastasis), whereas cells of the SN12A1 line (derived from ascites) produced few lung metastases. Cells from the SN12L1 line were also highly invasive and produced metastases in the omental and mesenteric lymph nodes, pancreas, diaphragm, and seminal vesicles.

These data suggest a correlation between the method for isolation of the HRCC lines and their biologic behavior. The SN12C line was isolated by culture, and these cells exhibited the fastest in vitro growth rate. The SN12S1 cells were isolated from a subcutaneous tumor; they grew well in the subcutis to produce a high incidence of spontaneous lung metastasis. The SN12K1 and SN12L1 cells were isolated from kidney and liver tumors, respectively, and grew readily in the kidney; these cells produced a high incidence of spontaneous lung metastasis. The SN12A1 cells isolated from ascitic fluid were the least malignant of the five lines.

ORTHOTOPIC VERSUS ECTOPIC IMPLANTATION FOR STUDIES OF SPONTANEOUS METASTASIS

The implantation of HRCC cells into the subcutis of nude mice has resulted in tumors that failed to metastasize.[50–57] Therefore, even if HRCC cells growing subcutaneously in nude mice maintain their original morphologic and biochemical characteristics, whether the subcutaneous environment of the nude mouse is appropriate for studies of metastasis is questionable. The ideal in vivo model for studying this disease should allow the interaction of the tumor cells with their relevant organ environment, the kidney. Naito and associates specifically examined this issue by injecting SN12L1 cells (isolated in culture from a liver metastasis produced in a nude mouse by cells from the surgical specimen growing in the kidney) into the subcutis and the kidney.[58] Tumor growth was studied histologically, and the production of metastasis was recorded.

Two weeks after injection of tumor cells, palpable nodules were found at the subcutaneous injection site. These tumors were surrounded by a fibrous capsule. Although the tumors were well vascularized, small areas of necrosis were also found. At this time, the HRCC cells implanted in the kidney were within the renal subcapsular space. Prominent areas of invasive growth into the renal parenchyma were also noted, however. These tumors were free of necrosis and were not encapsulated.

By 4 or 6 weeks after injection, the tumors growing subcutaneously were encapsulated by a fibrous connective tissue. Although the periphery of the tumor mass was well vascularized, central areas of necrosis were prominent. The tumor growing in the kidney was highly invasive, with a moderate degree of vascularization. The tumors were neither necrotic nor encapsulated.

Six weeks after tumor cells were injected into the kidney, most of the renal parenchyma was destroyed by the growing tumor. Grossly apparent pulmonary metastases were found, and the diaphragm, mesenteric and omental lymph nodes, and pancreas contained growing tumors.

Experiments using the KG-2 cell line also found differences between tumors arising from orthotopic implantation and those arising from ectopic implantation. For instance, the morphologic pattern of HRCC growing in the subcutis was different from that of HRCC growing in the kidney.[50] The KG-2 HRCC cell line was highly vascularized (in the patient) and consisted of a clear cell carcinoma with a 20% sarcomatoid component. This histologic pattern was maintained in KG-2 tumors growing in the kidney of nude mice. Metastases also developed in the lung and lymph nodes, so the KG-2 behavior in nude mice recapitulated the clinical behavior. Within the kidney, the tumor retained a predominant clear cell histologic pattern, with only 10% of the tumor composed of a sarcomatoid component. The tumor was well vascularized and grew rapidly, with no evidence of central necrosis or fibrous encapsulation. In contrast, the KG-2 tumor in the subcutis consisted primarily of granular cells (70%), with a minor component of clear (20%) and sarcomatoid (10%) cells. These tumors were not vascularized and had central necrosis and a surrounding fibrous pseudocapsule. Metastasis occurred only in nude mice after orthotopic implantation of cells.[58]

GROWTH IN DIFFERENT ORGAN ENVIRONMENTS SELECTING FOR DIFFERENT SUBPOPULATIONS OF HRCC CELLS

The data discussed in the preceding paragraphs demonstrate that cell lines derived from HRCC by growth in the subcutis or kidney differ in their biologic behavior. Moreover, the biologic behavior of HRCC cells isolated directly in culture differed from that of HRCC cells first grown in nude mice and then established in culture.

To determine whether the different methods of isolation yielded different subpopulations of HRCC cells, the five SN12 lines were subjected to detailed cytogenetic analysis. Cells harvested from semiconfluent cultures were prepared for G- and Q-bandings by well-established techniques.[59] Samples were also stained with Giemsa to determine modal chromosome number and the presence of double-minute chromosomes. Complete karyotypes were prepared from at least 50 metaphase spreads of each cell line, and clonality of a marker (altered) chromosome was further examined when it was present in more than one cell. This detailed cytogenetic analysis indicated that the SN12 lines each consist of unique subpopulations of cells derived from the original HRCC tumor.

Today, with the development of molecular techniques, we have much more sophisticated methods for establishing clonality and clonal dominance within a tumor. Viral and plasmid vectors can be used to insert selectable genetic markers into tumor cells, and clones with unique insertion sites can be tracked as the tumor grows and metastasizes. This technique has been used to determine whether the tumor clones that dominate an SN12C tumor and its metastasis are the same and whether clonal dominance is influenced by the microenvironment.[60] Transduction of the SN12C human renal cell carcinoma line with the *NEO*^{R} gene produced a genetically "tagged" cell population within which individual clones can be identified if they dominate the tumor during its growth in vivo. These experiments showed that clonal dominance is influenced by the organ environment in which the primary tumor grows, that is, distinct clones dominated in the kidney, colon, and subcutaneous sites. In addition, tumors grown in the orthotopic site (kidney) were all populated by the same dominant clones, and each distant visceral metastasis retained the same clonality. SN12C *NEO*^{R} cells grown in an epithelial, ectopic site (colon) produced tumors with unique dominant clones, and their visceral metastases retained the dominant pattern expressed by the parent tumor from which they were derived. In contrast, SN12C tumors growing subcutaneously showed a random pattern of clonal dominance in both their primary and metastatic sites.

Some progress has been made in understanding the molecular mechanisms of the heterogeneity of human neoplasms in vivo. These experiments have reinforced the concept that metastasis depends on the interaction of tumor cells with the appropriate microenvironment. For instance, the inability of the KG-2 cells to produce metastasis from a subcutaneous tumor may have been due to multiple additive factors, among which is vascularization. The growth of tumors and production of metastasis are known to depend on angiogenesis.[61] In many rodent and human cancers, the probability of metastasis increases after vascularization.[61] Of several diffusible cytokines that are mitogenic to vascular endothelium, one produced by many HRCC, basic fibroblast growth factor (bFGF), has been shown to stimulate the proliferation and migration of capillary endothelial cells.[50] Gohji and associates found that, under in vitro conditions, KG-2 cells stained positive for bFGF. The highly metastatic KG-2 LM6 cell lines were most positive. Angiogenesis, however, depended on the organ environment. Regardless of which of the KG-2 lines were injected, subcutaneous tumors were not well vascularized, whereas kidney tumors were. Whether this characteristic was due to differences in levels of bFGF (or other factors) is uncertain.

Singh and associates[62] found that, after the orthotopic and ectopic implantation of both SN12C and the highly metastatic SN12PM6, renal tumors were highly vascularized, as revealed by immunohistochemistry using antibodies to factor VIII, whereas subcutaneous tumors were not. The expression of bFGF in renal tumors was 10- to 20-fold that in subcutaneous tumors. Similar data were obtained at the protein level by using fluorescence-activated cell sorting (FACS), immunohistochemistry, and enzyme-linked immunosorbent assay. bFGF was detected in the urine of mice with HRCC tumors growing in the kidney but not the subcutis. The serum level of bFGF was two- to threefold greater in mice with HRCC tumors in the kidneys. These data strengthen the argument that the organ microenvironment influences the expression level of bFGF in HRCC.

Gohji and associates also showed that highly metastatic renal cell carcinoma cells expressed higher levels of both 72-kd collagenase type IV and urokinase, and these researchers observed a direct correlation between the production of these enzymes and metastatic potential.[63] They examined the effect of the microenvironment on the expression of collagenase type IV and found that the 72-kd collagenase type IV level in the culture supernatants of KG-2 cells was increased by their cultivation with mouse kidney or lung fibroblasts. In contrast, cocultivation of KG-2 cells with mouse skin fibroblasts significantly reduced collagenase type IV activity. Similar results were obtained by culturing KG-2 cells in the medium conditioned by different mouse fibroblasts. Gohji and colleagues investigated the effects on KG-2 cells of cytokines and growth factors known to be produced by fibroblasts of various origins. Cytokines and growth factors tested, bFGF, hepatocyte growth factor, and transforming growth factor-beta, (TGF-β_1) often stimulated collagenase type IV expression by the cultured KG-2 cells. Parallel immunohistochemical analyses revealed that mouse kidney and lung fibroblasts produced higher levels of TGF-β_1 than did skin fibroblasts. These results indicated that collagenase type IV production by KG-2 renal cell carcinoma cells is influenced by the organ microenvironment. Specifically, organ-specific fibroblasts regulate the production of degradative enzymes by KG-2 cells and, hence, profoundly influence their invasive and metastatic capacity. Subsequently, these same investigators found that the incubation of KG-2 with either interferon alpha (IFN-α) or interferon gamma (IFN-γ) suppressed transcription of the 72-kd gelatinase gene and gelatinase activity.[64] These inhibitory effects were independent of their antiproliferative effects and were accompanied by decreased invasion through Matrigel by the metastatic renal cell carcinoma cells.

MODULATION OF TUMOR CELL RESPONSE TO CHEMOTHERAPY BY THE ORGAN ENVIRONMENT

The organ microenvironment can also influence the response of metastases to chemotherapy. Cancer metastases may regress in one organ and may continue to grow in other sites after systemic chemotherapy. Fidler and associates[65] demonstrated this effect in a series of experiments using a murine fibrosarcoma, a murine colon carcinoma, and a human colon carcinoma. The tumor cells were implanted subcutaneously or into different visceral organs. Subcutaneous tumors were sensitive to doxorubicin (DXR), whereas lung or liver metastases were not. In contrast, sensitivity to 5-fluorouracil (5-FU) did not differ between these sites of growth. The differences in response to DXR between subcutaneous tumors (sensitive) and lung or liver tumors (resistant) were not due to variations in DXR potency or DXR distribution. The expression of the multidrug resistance-associated P-glycoprotein, as determined by flow cytometric analysis of tumor cells harvested from lesions in different organs, correlated inversely with their sensitivity to DXR: increased P-glycoprotein was associated with overexpression of *PGY1* (*mdr1*) messenger ribonucleic acid (mRNA). The organ-specific mechanism for upregulating *PGY1* and P-glycoprotein has yet to be elucidated, however. The clinical implications of these observations are obvious and may explain many of the discrepancies between in vivo and in vitro studies designed to evaluate the response of tumor cells to therapy.

SELECTION OF HRCC CELLS WITH HIGH METASTATIC POTENTIAL

The nude mouse can be used to select metastatic subpopulations from heterogeneous, unselected mouse[66] and human[43,47] neoplasms. Naito and associates[67] examined whether the orthotopic implantation (into the kidney) of SN12 cells would provide a more stringent and efficient selection procedure for HRCC. The SN12C cells grew in the kidney and produced spontaneous lung metastases, which were harvested under aseptic conditions. Separate lungs containing multiple metastases were processed to allow establishment of 11 different cell lines, each originating from several metastases.[67] The metastatic potential of the SN12C cells and the 11 lines was then compared by intravenous injection (experimental metastasis) and by implantation into the kidney (spontaneous metastasis). The intravenous injection of SN12C cells did not produce lung tumor colonies. In contrast, the injection of cells derived from spontaneous lung metastases produced a significant number of tumor lung colonies. In the second set of studies, cells were injected into the renal subcapsule. In this experiment, 4 of 11 lines produced a significantly higher number of spontaneous lung metastases than the SN12C cells, and 7 of 11 did not differ from the SN12C line. Naito was thus able to isolate some variant lines with increased metastatic potential from the heterogeneous SN12C HRCC.

EVIDENCE FOR METASTATIC HETEROGENEITY OF HRCC

Naito and associates[68] designed experiments to determine whether metastatic heterogeneity could also be found in HRCC of recent origin. We used the SN12C derived from a surgical specimen of HRCC. Cells from an early in vitro passage were used to produce 11 clonal lines by a double-dilution technique. The metastatic potential of these cells was determined in nude mice after inoculation of cells into the venous circulation or the kidneys.[68] Metastatic heterogeneity was not demonstrable after intravenous injection of tumor cells because the incidence and number of metastatic tumor colonies in the lung were minimal in all the mice injected. These data are in contrast to Fidler's work with the mouse UV-2237 fibrosarcoma, in which the production of experimental metastasis by cells injected intravenously closely agreed with the ability of the cells to produce spontaneous metastasis from a subcutaneous tumor.[69] After injection into the renal subcapsule, 6 of the 11 SN12C clones produced numbers of pulmonary tumor nodules that differed significantly from the SN12C line. Furthermore, the incidence of tumor growth in peritoneal organs varied among the SN12C and the cloned lines and paralleled the ability to produce lung metastasis. Thus, this HRCC line demonstrated metastatic heterogeneity subsequent to injection into the renal subcapsule. As with other human tumors,[39] the demonstration of metastatic heterogeneity in nude mice is influenced both by the intrinsic properties of the tumor cells and by host factors that include organ environment.

HOMEOSTASIS AND CANCER METASTASIS

Factors that control the processes of organ repair and regeneration are known to be organ-specific. For example, subsequent to partial hepatectomy, the liver, but not the kidney, undergoes rapid cell division termed "regeneration." Similarly, subsequent to unilateral nephrectomy, the mouse kidney, but not the liver, compensates by hypertrophy and hyperplasia.

Giavazzi and associates[46] carried out transplantation experiments on human colon carcinoma (HCC) and on HCC cells in nude mice that had been subjected to either nephrectomy, hepatectomy, or abdominal surgery (as a trauma control). The results were intriguing. HCC cells implanted subcutaneously demonstrated accelerated growth in mice that had undergone partial hepatectomy, but not mice that had undergone nephrectomy. Von Eschenbach and colleagues reported that HRCC cells established as micrometastases in the lungs of nude mice underwent a significant growth acceleration subsequent to unilateral nephrectomy but not hepatectomy.[70] In other words, liver regeneration in nude mice stimulated growth of HCC cells, whereas hypertrophy and hyperplasia of the kidney stimulated the growth of HRCC cells.

These results indicate that metastatic cells can respond to physiologic signals produced when homeostasis is disturbed, as in the processes of repair and regeneration. Damage to the organs is followed first by inflammation. Subsequent repair then stimulates the growth of normal cells. Tumor cells that either originate from or have an affinity for growth in this particular organ can also respond to these signals.

CONCLUSIONS

Human renal cancers are heterogeneous for various biologic properties, including invasion and metastasis. The presence of a small subpopulation of cells with a highly metastatic phenotype has important clinical implications for the diagnosis and therapy of cancer. For this reason, researchers must develop animal models for the selection and isolation of metastatic variants from human neoplasms and for testing the metastatic potential of human tumor cells.

Both Naito and Gohji and their colleagues[49,50] implanted HRCC cells (obtained from a surgical specimen) into different organs of nude mice and then recovered the tumors and established each in culture. Their established cell lines differed in their biologic and metastatic properties and had unique karyotypes, indicating that growth in different organs selects for different subpopulations of HRCC. Moreover, the HRCC cells did not metastasize unless they were implanted orthotopically. These findings indicate that the appropriate nude mouse model for studying the biology and therapy of HRCC must be based on the orthotopic implantation of tumor cells.

The data presented here show that metastasis is a highly selective process regulated by several mechanisms. This belief is contrary to the once widely accepted notion that metastasis represents the ultimate expression of cellular anarchy. The view that cancer metastasis is a selective and, hence, regulated process implies that understanding these regulatory mechanisms will lead to better therapeutic interventions.

ACKNOWLEDGMENT

Supported in part by Cancer Center Support Core grant CA 16672 and grant R35-CA 42107 (I.J.F.) from the National Cancer Institute, National Institutes of Health, Bethesda, MD.

REFERENCES

1. Willis RA. The spread of tumors in the human body. London: Butterworth, 1972.
2. Poste G, Fidler IJ. The pathogenesis of cancer metastasis. Nature 1979; 283:139.
3. Fidler IJ, Balch CM. The biology of cancer metastasis and implications for therapy. Curr Probl Surg 1987;24:137.
4. Sugarbaker EV. Cancer metastasis: a product of tumor-host interactions. Curr Probl Cancer 1979;3:1.
5. Weiss L. Principles of metastasis. Orlando, FL: Academic Press, 1985.
6. Fidler IJ. Critical factors in the biology of human cancer metastasis: twenty-eighth G.H.A. Clowes Memorial Award Lecture. Cancer Res 1990;50:6130.
7. Fidler IJ, Poste G. The cellular heterogeneity of malignant neoplasms: implications for adjuvant chemotherapy. Semin Oncol 1985;12:207.
8. Folkman J, Klagsburn M. Angiogenic factors. Science 1987;235:444.
9. Liotta LA. Tumor invasion and metastasis: role of the extracellular matrix. Rhoads Memorial Award Lecture. Cancer Res 1986;46:1.
10. Fisher B, Fisher ER. The interrelationship of hematogenous and lymphatic tumor cell dissemination. Surg Gynecol Obstet 1966;122:791.
11. Nicolson GL. Cancer metastasis: tumor cell and host organ properties important in metastasis to specific secondary sites. Biochim Biophys Acta 1988;948:175.
12. Price JE, Tarin D, Fidler IJ. The influence of organ microenvironment on pigmentation of a metastatic murine melanoma. Cancer Res 1988; 48:2258.
13. Fidler IJ. Metastasis: quantitative analysis of distribution and fate of tumor cell emboli labeled with ^{125}I-5-iododeoxyuridine. J Natl Cancer Inst 1970;45:773.
14. Price JE, Aukerman SL, Fidler IJ. Evidence that the process of murine melanoma metastasis is sequential and selective and contains stochastic elements. Cancer Res 1986;46:5172.
15. Fidler IJ, Gersten DM, Riggs CW. Relationship of host immune status to tumor cell arrest, distribution, and survival in experimental animals. Cancer 1977;40:46.
16. Hart IR, Talmadge JE, Fidler IJ. Metastatic behavior of a murine reticulum cell sarcoma exhibiting organ-specific growth. Cancer Res 1981; 41:1281.
17. Fidler IJ, Talmadge JE. Evidence that intravenously derived murine pulmonary metastases can originate from the expansion of a single tumor cell. Cancer Res 1986;46:5167.
18. Paget S. The distribution of secondary growths in cancer of the breast. Lancet 1889;1:571.
19. Hart IR, Fidler IJ. Role of organ selectivity in the determination of metastatic patterns of B16 melanoma. Cancer Res 1981;41:1281.
20. Fidler IJ. Selection of successive tumor lines for metastasis. Nature (New Biol) 1973;242:148.
21. Nicolson GL, Dulski KM. Organ specificity of metastatic tumor colonization is related to organ-selective growth properties of malignant cells. Int J Cancer 1986;38:289.
22. Raz A, Hanna N, Fidler IJ. In vivo isolation of a metastatic tumor cell variant involving selective and nonadaptive processes. J Natl Cancer Inst 1981;66:183.
23. Talmadge JE, Fidler IJ. Cancer metastasis is selective or random depending on the parent tumor population. Nature 1978;27:593.
24. Talmadge JE, Fidler IJ. Enhanced metastatic potential of tumor cells harvested from spontaneous metastases of heterogeneous murine tumors. J Natl Cancer Inst 1982;69:975.
25. Raz A, Hart I. Murine melanoma: a model for intracranial metastasis. Br J Cancer 1980;42:331.
26. Ewing J. Neoplastic diseases, 6th ed. Philadelphia: WB Saunders, 1928.
27. Fidler IJ, Kripke ML. Metastasis results from pre-existing variant cells within a malignant tumor. Science 1977;197:893.
28. Luria SE, Delbruck M. Mutations of bacteria from virus sensitive to virus resistant. Genetics 1943;28:491.
29. Kripke ML. Speculation on the role of ultraviolet radiation in the development of malignant melanoma. J Natl Cancer Inst 1979;63:541.
30. Fidler IJ, Kripke ML. Metastatic heterogeneity of cells from the K-1735 melanoma. In: Grundmann E, ed. Metastatic tumor growth. Stuttgart: Gustav Fischer, 1980:71.
31. Fidler IJ, Gruys E, Cifone MA, et al. Demonstration of multiple phenotype diversity in a murine melanoma of recent origin. J Natl Cancer Inst 1981;67:947.
32. Talmadge JE, Fidler IJ. Cancer metastasis is selective or random depending on the parent tumor population. Nature 1982;27:593.
33. Price JE, Aukerman SL, Fidler IJ. Evidence that the process of murine melanoma metastasis is sequential and selective and contains stochastic elements. Cancer Res 1986;46:5172.
34. Talmadge JE, Wolman SR, Fidler IJ. Evidence for the clonal origin of spontaneous metastasis. Science 1982;217:361.
35. Ootsuyama A, Tanaka K, Tanooka H. Evidence by cellular mosaicism for monoclonal metastasis of spontaneous mouse mammary tumors. J Natl Cancer Inst 1987;78:1223.
36. Hu F, Wang RY, Hsu TC. Clonal origin of metastasis in B16 murine melanoma: a cytogenetic study. J Natl Cancer Inst 1987;78:155.
37. Talmadge JE, Zbar B. Clonality of pulmonary metastases from the bladder 6 subline of the B16 melanoma studied by Southern hybridization. J Natl Cancer Inst 1987;78:315.
38. Fidler IJ, Talmadge JE. Evidence that intravenously derived murine pulmonary metastases can originate from the expansion of a single tumor cell. Cancer Res 1986;46:5167.
39. Fidler IJ. Rationale and methods for the use of nude mice to study the biology and therapy of human cancer metastasis. Cancer Metastasis Rev 1986;5:29.
40. Sharkey FE, Fogh J. Considerations in the use of nude mice for cancer research. Cancer Metastasis Rev 1987;4:29.
41. Kyriazis APL, DiPersio GJ, Michael GJ, et al. Growth patterns and metastatic behavior of human tumors growing in athymic nude mice. Cancer Res 1978;38:3186.
42. Kyriazis AA, Kyriazis AP. Preferential site of growth of human tumors in nude mice following subcutaneous transplantation. Cancer Res 1980; 40:4509.
43. Kozlowski JM, Hart IR, Fidler IJ, et al. A human melanoma line heterogeneous with respect to metastatic capacity in athymic nude mice. J Natl Cancer Inst 1984;72:913.
44. Kozlowski JM, Fidler IJ, Campbell D, et al. Metastatic behavior of human tumor cell lines grown in the nude mouse. Cancer Res 1984; 44:3522.
45. Giavazzi R, Jessup JM, Campbell DE, et al. Experimental nude mouse model of human colorectal cancer liver metastases. J Natl Cancer Inst 1986;77:1303.
46. Giavazzi R, Campbell DE, Jessup JM, et al. Metastatic behavior of

tumor cells isolated from primary and metastatic human colorectal carcinomas implanted into different sites in nude mice. Cancer Res 1986; 46:1928.
47. Morikawa K, Walker SM, Jessup JM, et al. In vivo selection of highly metastatic cells from surgical specimens of different primary human colon carcinomas implanted into nude mice. Cancer Res 1988;48:1943.
48. Morikawa K, Walker SM, Nakajima M, et al. Influence of organ environment on the growth, selection, and metastasis of human colon carcinoma cells in nude mice. Cancer Res 1988;48:6863.
49. Naito S, von Eschenbach AC, Giavazzi R, et al. Growth and metastasis of tumor cells isolated from a human renal cell carcinoma implanted into different organs of nude mice. Cancer Res 1986;46:4109.
50. Gohji K, Nakajima M, Dinney CPN, et al. The importance of orthotopic implantation to the isolation and biological characterization of a metastatic human clear cell renal carcinoma in nude mice. Int J Cancer 1993;2:23.
51. Katsuoka Y, Baba S, Hata M. Transplantation of human renal cell carcinoma to the nude mouse: As an intermediate of in vivo and in vitro studies. J Urol 1976;115:373.
52. Hoehn WA, Schroeder FH. Renal cell carcinoma: two new cell lines and a serially transplantable nude mouse tumor (NC 65). Invest Urol 1978;16:106.
53. Otto U, Kollermann MW, Kloppel G. Transplantation von menschlichem Nierenadenokarzinomgewebe auf die nackte Maus. Urol Int 1981;36:110.
54. Naito S, Kanamori T, Hisano S. Human renal cell carcinoma: establishment and characterization of two new cell lines. J Uról 1982;128:1117.
55. Otto U, Kloppel G, Baisch H, et al. Transplantation of human renal cell carcinoma into NMRI nu/nu mice. I. Reliability of an experimental tumor model. J Urol 1984;131:130.
56. Otto U, Huland H, Baisch H, et al. Transplantation of human renal cell carcinoma into NMRI nu/nu mice. II. Evaluation of response to vinblastine sulfate monotherapy. J Urol 1984;131:134.
57. Clayman RV, Figenshau RS, Bear A. Transplantation of human renal carcinomas into athymic mice. Cancer Res 1985;45:2650.
58. Naito S, von Eschenbach AC, Fidler IJ. Different growth pattern and biologic behavior of human and renal cell carcinoma implanted into different organs of nude mice. J Natl Cancer Inst 1987;78:377.
59. Pathak S. Chromosome banding techniques. J Reprod Med 1976;17: 25.
60. Staroselsky AN, Radinsky R, Fidler IJ, et al. The use of molecular genetic markers to demonstrate the effect of organ environment on clonal dominance in a human renal cell carcinoma grown in nude mice. Int J Cancer 1992;51:130.
61. Folkman J, Shing Y. Angiogenesis. J Biol Chem 1992;267:10931.
62. Singh RK, Bucana CD, Gutman M, et al. Organ site dependent expression of basic fibroblast growth factor in human renal cell carcinoma cells. Am J Pathol (in press).
63. Gohji K, Fidler IJ, Fabra A, et al. Regulation of gelatinase production in metastatic renal cell carcinoma by organ-specific fibroblasts. Jpn J Cancer Res 1994;85:152.
64. Gohji K, Fidler IJ, Tsan R, et al. Human recombinant interferons beta and gamma decrease gelatinase production and invasion by human KG-2 renal carcinoma cells. Int J Cancer (in press).
65. Fidler IJ, Wilmanns C, Staroselsky AN, et al. Modulation of tumor cell response to chemotherapy by the organ environment. Cancer Metastasis Rev (in press).
66. Pollack VA, Fidler IJ. The use of young nude mice for selection of subpopulations of cells with increased metastatic potential from nonsyngeneic neoplasms. J Natl Cancer Inst 1982;69:137.
67. Naito S, Walker SM, Fidler IJ. In vivo selection of human renal cell carcinoma cells with high metastatic potential in nude mice. Clin Exp Metastasis 1989;7:381.
68. Naito S, Walker SM, von Eschenbach AC, et al. Evidence for metastatic heterogeneity of human renal cell carcinoma. Anticancer Res 1988;8: 1163.
69. Fidler IJ. The Ernst W. Bertner Memorial Award Lecture: the evolution of biological heterogeneity in metastatic neoplasms. In: Nicolson GL, Milas L, eds. Cancer invasion and metastasis: biologic and therapeutic aspects. New York: Raven Press, 1984:5.
70. von Eschenbach AC, Avallone A, Price JE, et al. The biology of renal cancer: the influence of nephrectomy. Eur Urol 1990;18:40.

Principles and Practice of Genitourinary Oncology, edited by Derek Raghavan, Howard I. Scher, Steven A. Leibel, and Paul H. Lange. Lippincott-Raven Publishers, Philadelphia, © 1997.

CHAPTER 3

Clinical Decision Making in Genitourinary Oncology

Martin Stockler and Malcolm Moore

Decision making is fundamental to the practice of medicine. Medical decisions are frequent, complicated, and have important consequences, yet the process of medical decision making is implicit and rarely scrutinized. If, when faced with a problem, everyone made the same decision, the path taken would be of limited interest (assuming a correct decision). Genitourinary (GU) oncologists hold diametric opinions regarding the management of common GU cancers.[1] This disagreement occurs despite the general availability of the evidence on which these mutually exclusive conclusions are based. Diametrically opposed views were revealed in a study in which GU oncologists were used as patient surrogates and were asked what treatments they would select for themselves if faced with various, common GU problems. When North American oncologists were asked to imagine that they had localized prostate cancer, 70% of urologists chose surgery, and 90% of radiation oncologists chose radiotherapy, whereas medical oncologists were almost evenly divided between these two modalities. When asked to imagine that they had symptomatic metastatic bladder cancer, cytotoxic chemotherapy was chosen by 37% of British urologists, by 62% of Canadian urologists, and by 96% of urologists in the United States. Although these specialists were generally aware that controversy existed, they were not prepared to support clinical trials comparing their preferred option with that of others. This unwillingness was due to a conviction that evidence was adequate to indicate the superiority of their chosen treatment.[2] Under these circumstances, the decision-making process is of greater interest.

Divergence of opinion is typical of clinical medicine and is not restricted to GU oncology.[3] Certain developments in GU oncology have resulted in changes in practice that warrant special attention, however. Methods for the early detection of prostate cancer have identified a large population of men with early disease for whom the appropriate management strategy is undefined. The optimal choice of treatment for muscle-invasive bladder cancer is complicated by treatments that are partially effective, have significant adverse effects, may be combined in different ways, and for which reliable comparative data are lacking.

Ideally, clinical decisions should reflect the logical application of accurate, generic information about disease and treatment to the salient details of individual cases. The remainder of this textbook is devoted to the body of generic medical knowledge about GU cancer. This chapter explores the nature of this generic knowledge, the individual factors, and the way in which these elements are combined in making a decision.

CLINICAL DECISIONS

Decision making is the process of choosing among alternatives. Clinical decisions can be considered either diagnostic or therapeutic. To reach a diagnosis, hundreds of pieces of information must be considered: the patient's current and past history, the findings on physical examination, and the results of various tests, as well as the body of generic medical information about health and disease.[4] Diagnostic decisions extend beyond the choice of a provisional diagnosis and a list of differential diagnoses to include the selection of additional tests and information on which subsequent therapeutic decisions will be based. Such information may include the extent of disease (which staging tests?), the nature of the primary tumor (which features: differentiation, nuclear grade, mitotic activity, surface markers, ploidy, oncogene expression, for example?), the values of other prognostic factors (age, serum tumor marker levels) and the presence or severity of comorbid conditions (Is the atypical chest pain important? Is the patient fit to have a cystectomy? To have doxorubicin?).

To make a therapeutic decision, information about the natural course of disease and about both the effectiveness and the adverse effects of possible treatments must be applied to the specifics of the individual case. The extent, severity, virulence, and tempo of disease, the presence of coexisting medical conditions, attitudes about health states (preferences), and psychosocial issues all bear on the decision in an individual patient. Therapeutic decisions may be seen as a choice between intervention and observation, although each obviously implies further choices among specific interventions and modes of observation.

Thus, every clinical interaction includes a multitude of decisions, each intimately dependent on those preceding it. The presenting complaint and the superficial characteristics of a patient influence the line of questioning. The initial history influences the physical examination. The resulting clinical picture affects the choice of investigations. This conglomerate then influences what the physician chooses to tell the patient. The final choice of management strategy then emerges from a complicated and variable interaction between the accumulated information and the preconceptions of the involved parties (physician, patient, and "significant others").

How should we chose among alternatives? Every alternative has a set of possible consequences or outcomes. Possible outcomes of treating localized prostate cancer with radical prostatectomy include the following: cure, locoregional relapse, distant relapse, postoperative pain, impotence, incontinence, deep venous thrombosis, and perioperative death. Alternatives differ in the probabilities with which these outcomes occur. For example, treating localized prostate cancer with radiotherapy has a lower risk of perioperative death or postoperative pain (zero), but a higher risk of radiation proctitis and cystitis (both obviously zero for surgery alone). Outcomes also differ in their desirability. In a patient with localized prostate cancer, cure is highly desirable, perioperative death is highly undesirable, and locoregional relapse and distant relapse are presumably intermediate concerns, as are impotence, incontinence, deep venous thrombosis, radiation cystitis, and proctitis. Thus, the attractiveness of a particular alternative depends on the desirability of its possible outcomes and the probabilities of these outcomes. To chose the best alternative, it seems we must consider (1) all the important outcomes of each alternative, (2) the likelihood of each outcome under each alternative (probabilities), and (3) the desirability of each of the outcomes (utilities). This information must be combined in a fashion that results in a single choice because decisions cannot be avoided (choosing to wait is no less a decision than is choosing to treat).

This simple linear description of decision making as an orderly sequence of single steps is clearly an oversimplification. The process is both iterative, in that individual steps may be repeated many times, and dynamic, in that options change with new information. Each step in the process adds an additional layer of complexity. The first layer of complexity results from the number of aspects to be considered at each step. The second layer of complexity results from the number of steps and their interdependence. The third layer of complexity results from uncertainty that permeates all levels of clinical practice. Uncertainty stems both from our inability to predict the future and from the nature of the information on which decisions are based.

MEDICAL KNOWLEDGE

Biologic processes are inherently unpredictable; forecasts (prognoses) must be couched in terms of probabilities. In a given individual, we cannot know beforehand whether a tumor is destined to relapse without treatment or whether adjuvant treatment will prevent relapse. Individuals live for different lengths of time, suffer different illnesses, react differently to the same illnesses, and respond differently to the same treatments. We know that individuals vary widely even if the clinical picture is precisely defined. The median survival of a group of otherwise well 70-year-old men with bone-dominant metastatic prostate cancer and no visceral metastases who are treated by orchidectomy may be 2 years, but the survival curve includes some men who live for only a few months and others who live for many years. Even if we have a good idea of the *average* effect of a disease, prognostic factor, or treatment, this average is made up of variable and idiosyncratic individual responses. We must be satisfied with statements such as the following: "the probability of relapse following treatment A is X%, and this can be reduced to Y% by the addition of treatment B." The accuracy and precision of our probability estimates are also uncertain because of the effects of bias and random error.

Furthermore, probabilities can only be estimated but not *known* in any absolute sense. Whether one takes the traditional frequentist view of probability as the rate of occurrence in the whole (and therefore infinite) population or the Bayesian view that probability represents the strength of belief in a particular proposition, probabilities are unknowable *parameters* that can only be estimated from finite samples.[5] We cannot *know* the probability of prostate cancer in an asymptomatic man with a given level of prostate-specific antigen (PSA) unless we *know* everybody's PSA level and whether they have prostate cancer. We can *estimate* the probability from a sample (less than everybody). The accuracy of this estimate depends on both the size of the sample and on how closely the sample resembles the population of interest. The bigger the sample, the smaller the effect of chance fluctuations. The influence of chance fluctuations can be illustrated with confidence intervals.[6] Table 3-1 shows the effect of sample size on the confidence intervals of proportions. Even substantial samples produce estimates with wide ranges of plausible values. The play of chance is important but relatively innocent because we can always reduce its effect by taking a bigger sample.

Bias is much more sinister. It occurs when a systematic difference between the study sample and the population of interest affects that which we are trying to estimate. For example, we estimate the incidence of prostate cancer in the whole population from a sample. If the sample has a different age distribution (systematic difference) from that of the population as a whole (population of interest), we will be concerned that a simple estimate (incidence in the sample) differs from the truth (incidence in the whole population). Our estimate of the incidence of prostate cancer from the study sample is confounded by the effect of age. Factors that affect outcome are commonly referred to as prognostic or risk factors.

Imbalances of *known* prognostic factors are a common cause

Table 3-1. *95% Confidence intervals for proportions from different size samples**

Sample Proportion	Sample Size 10	20	40	100	500
0%	0–31	0–17	0–9	0–4	0–1
1	—	—	—	0–6	0–2
5	—	0–25	0–17	2–11	3–7
10	0–45	1–32	3–24	5–18	8–13
20	3–56	6–44	9–36	13–29	17–24
50	19–81	27–73	34–66	40–60	46–54

* Calculated by Fisher's exact method.

of bias. Comparisons of radiotherapy and surgery are typically confounded by selection bias: fitter, younger patients tend to have surgery, whereas older patients with coexisting medical problems tend to have radiotherapy. Comparisons of new treatments with historical controls are fraught with potential bias.[7] Stage migration,[8] improvements in supportive care, improvements in patient selection,[9] and shorter follow-up time all make new treatments look better than their predecessors. Trials of new or intensive interventions frequently have restrictive entry criteria, including age limits, requirements for normal cardiac, renal, hepatic, respiratory, hematologic, and nervous system function, and access to a tertiary or quaternary referral center. The requirement for measurable disease may also select patients destined to do better, regardless of therapy. Those who pass these stringent barriers are a highly selected and atypical subset of patients with the disease (the population of interest). For example, the selection criteria for a recent study of interleukin 2 and lymphocyte-activated killer cells in metastatic renal cancer included a normal cardiac stress test, no symptoms or history of ischemic heart disease, a forced expiratory volume greater than 75% of predicted, and no single metastatic lesion bigger than 100 cm^2, as well as conventional requirements for normal renal, hepatic and hematologic function.[10] Trials of more conservative therapy may also restrict entry to patients with more favorable disease. For example, we can predict that patients able to have a partial nephrectomy for renal cell carcinoma will have less extensive tumors than those requiring radical nephrectomy. Applying the results derived from these highly selected patients to routine clinical practice ignores the importance of these major, systematic differences.

If we already know that a prognostic factor is important, then we can adjust our estimates to take imbalances in this factor into account. These adjustments depend on subgroup estimates, however, which are always less reliable than the overall estimate. In fact, we cannot be sure that an adjusted estimate is closer to the truth than an unadjusted estimate.[11]

To decide whether to adjust for known prognostic factors is difficult. To adjust for unknown factors is impossible. For example, interest is growing in the prognostic potential of various molecular characteristics, such as the presence of cell-surface growth factor receptors, oncogenes, and drug-resistance phenotypes. If some of these characteristics prove to be important and independent prognostic factors, then differences in their distributions will result in bias. Until we know that a factor is important, however, we cannot assess it or adjust for any imbalances. Prognostic factors generally cannot be studied by experimental methods and must be identified by observational studies. A single observational study is inconclusive, and although several confirmatory studies are reassuring, they are still no guarantee against bias. Although we cannot be sure that important prognostic factors remain to be discovered, we strongly suspect their existence as part of the explanation of individual variability.

The only way of dealing with unknown prognostic factors is randomization. Although we cannot assess whether randomization has succeeded in balancing unknown factors, inferential statistics allow us to estimate our confidence in the reliability of the results generated by random allocation. Randomization, when combined with blinded outcome assessment, also provides protection against the preconceptions (subconscious or otherwise) of investigators and patients.[12]

Meta-analysis of all conducted RCTs

Meta-analysis of all published RCTs

2 or more confirmatory RCTs

1 randomized controlled trial (RCT)

Case-control study

Cohort study

Case series

Case report

FIG. 3-1. The hierarchy of clinical evidence.

Levels of evidence in clinical medicine can be regarded as a hierarchy, the pinnacle of which is rarely reached (Fig. 3-1). Unfortunately, much of GU oncology practice is based on the lowest levels of this hierarchy. The GU oncology literature is replete with uncontrolled clinical trials (case reports, case series, phase 1 and 2 trials), with relatively few randomized trials.[13] A common mistake is to regard the results of phase 1 and 2 studies as the basis for clinical decision making. Phase 1 and 2 trials are preliminary tests of tolerability and activity. If the results of these early phase trials are encouraging, the next step should be a randomized controlled trial against standard therapy. Phase 1 and 2 trials are designed to make decisions about the directions for further research, not about individual patient management. To make reliable choices, we require data from reliable comparative studies.

Clinical trials also differ in their focus. The distinction between explanatory and pragmatic trials was first pointed out by Schwartz and Lellouch.[14] Explanatory trials are characterized by narrow inclusion criteria and surrogate outcome measures (such as tumor response rates, time to local failure, or time to recurrence). Pragmatic trials are characterized by broad inclusion criteria and more direct outcome measures, such as overall survival. Explanatory trials are better suited to exploring biology and mechanisms, whereas pragmatic trials are better suited to answering questions about the likely effect of treatment in routine clinical practice.

The criteria by which medical interventions are compared are critically important. From the standpoint of clinical decision making, medical interventions should be judged on two criteria: (1) effects on quantity of life; and (2) effects on quality of life. Surrogate outcomes, as described earlier, may be suitable for defining differences in biologic activity; however, biologic activity is not synonymous with benefit to the patient. Demonstration that tumors shrink with chemotherapy may establish antitumor activity, but does not prove that chemotherapy either prolongs survival or improves quality of life. Local control of tumor and postponement of recurrence may be reasonable goals, but these goals alone do not guarantee benefit to the patient. Overall survival is generally accepted as a definitive outcome. Quality of life is a fundamental concern in clinical oncology: both disease and treatment can have profound effects on quality of life. Physicians are coming to acknowledge the importance of quality of life as a criterion for judging medical interventions, although few trials include quality of life as an end point. Quality of life assessment is particularly relevant when the effects of treatment on overall survival are modest and when treatments can have both major positive and major negative effects on quality of life.[15,16] These characteristics are typical of many radical cancer treatments (for example radical cystectomy, prostatectomy, radical pelvic radiotherapy, adjuvant chemotherapy) and of most palliative treatments.

The body of medical knowledge, as manifest by published medical literature, is growing at an exponential rate, with an estimated doubling time of 19 years.[17] Each month, over 30,000 articles are added to the Medline database. In the first 6 months of 1994, these additions to Medline included over 3500 articles indexed under "urogenital neoplasms," about 700 on "prostatic neoplasms," and 450 on "bladder neoplasms" (these are all limited to clinical studies). Furthermore, Medline only indexes about one-sixth of the world's biomedical journals.[17] In comprehensive efforts to identify *all* the relevant information on specific topics, investigators have consulted computerized databases, references to published works, and the memories of experts.[18,19] Any one of these methods, including a computerized literature search carried out by an information specialist, is unlikely to reveal more than 50% of the available information.[20] For most questions, a concerted search reveals a morass of published information of varying quality and conclusions.

Once identified, evidence must be appraised and synthesized according to scientific merit, rather than according to preconceptions and prejudice. Cognitive psychology has demonstrated that human judgment is vulnerable to systematic errors. Tversky and Kahneman have described and explored cognitive tricks or "rules of thumb" that help us to make quick, but systematically flawed, judgments.[21] Although these studies primarily addressed probabilistic judgments, subsequent work has confirmed that these and other biases also influence judgments of the quality of evidence. Scientists (including physicians) are more likely to overlook methodologic flaws in research if the research appears to address an important question.[22] Favorable judgments are more likely to be given to research supporting earlier beliefs.[23] Our estimates are influenced by the order in which we receive information and by the way in which it is subdivided.[24] In a survey of primary care physicians in the United States and their opinion leaders, fewer than 50% said that they examined the methods section of an article to assess its scientific merit (27% of the whole group, 59% of opinion leaders). About 90% said that they evaluated scientific worth by comparing an article's findings with their own experience. Practical guidelines for coping with medical literature and for critical appraisal are available.[25,26] Expert literature reviews, as published in journals and textbooks, are a popular source of medical information. That literature reviews are prone to the shortcomings of both retrospective research and human judgment constitutes a strong argument for a systematic approach. Comparisons of traditional narrative reviews with more systematic methods reveal wide discrepancies between available evidence and published opinion.[3] As Haynes points out, "Readers looking for a shortcut to understanding evidence about health problems and patient care should at least look for reviews by those who have not taken shortcuts."[27] Critical appraisal is the best protection against shortcuts that prove to be wrong turns.[28]

Many, perhaps most, clinical decisions must be made in the absence of data from randomized controlled trials addressing the relevant clinical issues. Decisions cannot be avoided on the basis of inadequate information, but we must recognize and acknowledge decisions based on weak evidence and accept them as tentative.[29]

INDIVIDUAL PREFERENCES

The need to consider the desirability of outcomes is self-evident; however, the appropriate way to measure and incorporate preferences in decision making is much less obvious. To choose among alternatives, we need to know which one we would like best. The desirability of an outcome depends on how long it lasts (duration), how it feels (quality), and when it occurs (timing). If these three characteristics move together, then decision making is simple. Everything else being equal, we prefer longer life span and better quality of life, with gains brought forward, and losses delayed. Medical outcomes are complicated, however, with trade-offs among length, quality, and timing. The longest life span may be associated with the immediate and persistent discomfort of additional treatment. The discomfort of treatment may be short and severe or long and mild. The treatment with the higher chance of promoting long-term survival may be associated with a lower chance of short-term survival. The desirability of an outcome is an abstract and purely subjective concept. As such, we expect that preferences vary among individuals.

When making a clinical decision, the preferences used must be consistent with those of the patient. The most obvious solution is to ascertain the patient's own preferences directly. Other possible sources include relatives, medical attendants, and survivors of the disease or treatment. Empiric research confirms that the preferences of these groups are systematically different, and therefore, using the preferences of one group to represent those of another introduces bias.[30,31] The appropriate source of preferences for a decision depends on the perspective from which the decision is being made. If the decision is regarding the allocation of resources, the preferences of the whole community (predominantly well people who may not have to face the particular decision, but who will face the economic consequences) may well be most appropriate.

For individual clinical decisions, the appropriate preferences are those of the patient. This question is distinct from the thornier one of who should actually make the decision. Individuals vary in their preferences for information and involvement in decision making.[32,33] Physicians also have differing opinions about their roles in the physician-patient interaction.[34] Some patients are unambiguous in their request that the physician make any medical decision, whereas others make it plain that the physician is simply a source of information that may be taken into account. Furthermore, physicians do not seem to be good judges of their patients' information preferences; physicians underestimate patients' desires for information, but they overestimate patients' desires to make decisions.[35] The physician and the patient both hold unique information critical to reaching a decision. We argue that neither individual should make the decision, but rather that the decision should emerge from an interaction in which both parties are equal participants. Formal approaches to decision making emphasize and reinforce the cooperative nature of the process. This approach also removes the mantle of decision maker from either individual and acknowledges that both sides should be influential. The final arbiter must always be the patient who will suffer (or enjoy) the consequences of the decision.

Patients facing a decision will not have experienced the relevant outcomes when they make their choices. To judge the desirability of an outcome, the subject must be given an accurate picture of what it is like to experience that outcome. This preparation includes thorough disclosure of the inconveniences and toxicities of treatment, as well as the consequences of failed treatment. These descriptions must allow the patient to see beyond the symbolic significance of an outcome (the response to finding out) to appreciate its real significance or actuality (what it is like to experience the outcome). For example, to judge the desirability of life without a urinary bladder, the patient must go beyond the initial response to being told "Your bladder will be surgically removed" (symbolic significance) to consider the details of what life is really like after a cystectomy (actuality). Similarly, to judge the desirability of life with recurrent cancer, the patient needs to imagine what life with recurrent cancer is actually like, rather than what the initial response is to being told "your cancer has come back." The descriptions should cover specific physical, psychosocial, emotional, and functional problems, their likely progress, and what can be done for them. Perhaps the most important and difficult aspects to disclose are a time frame for the outcome, which must be unambiguous and realistic, and the element of uncertainty, which characterizes all medical decisions.

Unfortunately, few data describing the effects of cancer or treatment on quality of life are available. Little direct evidence exists regarding quality of life in GU cancer. Preliminary work has been published in the setting of advanced prostate cancer,[36,37] and some randomized trials include quality-of-life outcomes. Most of the available data refer to side effects of treatment; however, the validity of many of these data is compromised by selection bias, treatment bias, and variable definitions.[18] Some studies including rigorously collected outcome data have highlighted further the problems of traditional case series.[38,39] Such studies are useful, although reliable comparative data depend on unbiased assessment in randomized trials. In the absence of unbiased data regarding quality and quantity of life, we are forced to rely upon biased comparisons of unproved surrogate outcome measures, such as reductions in serum tumor marker levels.

To choose among alternatives, preferences for disparate outcomes must be expressed quantitatively. Methods used to assess individuals' preferences for health states have ranged from a simple request that the individual rate desirability directly (categorical rating) to more complex and indirect techniques such as the time trade-off and standard gamble methods.[40] Different techniques elicit different preference values, a result that is not surprising because each technique asks the subject to answer a slightly different question. The question of which technique is "best" is therefore unresolved despite considerable debate. Investigators generally acknowledge that preference values are sensitive to the way in which they are elicited, and they must therefore be interpreted circumspectly.[41]

Evaluation of formal methods for eliciting preference has also shed light on several aspects of physician-patient communication. Many studies have demonstrated important differences in preferences according to the way in which the information is presented.[42–44] For example, the common practice of describing outcomes in a positive frame (probability of surviving), rather than a negative frame (probability of dying), appears to yield more accurate estimates of preference.[42] Patients' treatment preferences are influenced by false preconceptions about the nature of those treatments.[43] Extensions of this type of research have also demonstrated important differences in physicians' preferences for treatments according to the way in which the results are presented to them.[45,46] These studies emphasize the need for careful consideration of what we say and how we say it, as well as what we ask and how we ask it.

The importance of expressing preferences in a uniform format with particular characteristics stems from the need to compare disparate outcomes. The desirability of a particular outcome depends on both how long it lasts (quantity) and what it feels like (quality). Clinical decisions often involve trade-offs between these characteristics. The decision to take aspirin for a headache involves a comparison of the likelihood of relief and the impact of relief on quality of life with the likelihood of side effects and the impact of side effects on quality of life. The potential for benefit must be weighed against the potential for harm. Typical clinical problems are obviously much more complicated and involve trade-offs between widely divergent outcomes, for example, the short- and long-term effects of surgery compared with those of radiotherapy, or the short- and long-term effects of adjuvant chemotherapy compared with those of reserving further treatment for symptomatic progression.

The desirability of an outcome also depends on its timing—we prefer to bring forward gains and to delay losses. Everything else being equal, immediate relief is preferred to delayed relief, and delayed discomfort is preferred to immediate discomfort. Discounting is probably part of the reason why smokers are reluctant to suffer the immediate discomfort of quitting, despite the obviously substantial risk of much worse discomfort in the future. In deciding whether to undergo adjuvant chemotherapy, the prospect of immediate discomfort must be weighed against the possibility of an increment in survival, a delayed benefit. The same applies to screening and treatment for early-stage prostate cancer. Monetary costs and benefits are discounted over time: we accept that a dollar is worth more to us today than it is in 10 years' time. The need to discount health benefits and risks is widely accepted.[47] Exactly how this should be done is contentious.[48,49]

In the context of clinical decision making, the simplest and most explicit approach is to specify the timing of outcomes. For example, immediate androgen blockade for advanced prostate cancer produces immediate side effects that last as long as the treatment is continued. The effects on preexisting cancer-related symptoms are also likely to be immediate; however, they are transient, lasting about 2 years on average. Androgen blockade may also postpone the development of new symptoms and may prolong survival by a few months; both these benefits are delayed.

The need to choose among outcomes with good and bad aspects across distinct dimensions (quantity and quality) has important ramifications. To *compare* outcomes, quantity and quality can be considered separately. To *choose* among outcomes, quantity and quality must be considered simultaneously; they must be combined into a single dimension or score, so the preferred option, the one with the highest "score," can be identified and selected.

A MODEL

Decision making is vulnerable to bias and error at every level. A good decision requires consideration of all important outcomes, estimation of each outcome's probability, and assignment of a measure of preference to each outcome according to its desirability. This information must be synthesized in such a way that a single option can be chosen. For example, an individual treated with radical cystectomy for muscle-invasive transitional cell carcinoma of the bladder is found to have microscopic metastases in the resected lymph nodes. The possible outcomes without further treatment include cure (if no residual disease is present) or, more likely, symptomatic relapse and subsequent death from recurrent bladder cancer. Adjuvant chemotherapy may reduce the risk of relapse and death from bladder cancer, but it entails the risk of both acute and chronic subjective toxicity (vomiting and peripheral neuropathy, respectively) and a small but real risk of serious morbidity or death (neutropenic sepsis or vascular toxicity).

At the time the decision must be made, all the outcomes are uncertain: we do not know whether residual disease is present, and if it is, we do not know whether adjuvant chemotherapy will be effective, nor do we know how much toxicity the individual will suffer. Individual patient factors alter the probabilities: for example, the presence of symptomatic atherosclerotic disease increases the risk of vascular toxicity, and previous alcohol abuse reduces the probability of severe nausea and vomiting. The values assigned to the outcomes also differ across individuals: a risk-averse 70-year-old patient who wants to attend a grandchild's wedding with a full head of hair in 12 weeks may value 3 months of chemotherapy differently from a bald 45-year-old patient who wants to reach 60.

To chose between adjuvant treatment and observation, the disparate outcomes of length and quality of survival must be combined. Adjuvant chemotherapy causes short-term toxicity, but it may postpone or even prevent relapse. Observation avoids the acute toxicity of chemotherapy, but at the risk of shortened overall survival if adjuvant therapy is efficacious. If the patient goes on to develop advanced disease, palliative chemotherapy may improve cancer-related symptoms, but it causes subjective toxicity; it may delay death from cancer, or it may hasten it from neutropenic sepsis. The behavior of recurrent disease and its response to palliative chemotherapy may be influenced by the previous administration of adjuvant chemotherapy. Immediate effects on quality of life are being weighed against future effects on quantity and quality of life. Such trade-offs are typical of clinical decisions.

Simultaneous consideration of all these issues may seem unrealistically ambitious. If we agree that they are all important, however, then to justify any exclusions is difficult. Most clinical decisions must be made "on the fly" and represent an intuitive response to the overall clinical picture, rather than a conscious consideration of the separate elements of the clinical picture. The informal, clinical-Gestalt decision of an experienced, knowledgeable clinician is likely to reflect the same data and considerations as a formal analytic approach, but because the process remains hidden and implicit, it is not amenable to scrutiny or modification. Any decision is supported by whatever data the individual decision maker found influential. This process conforms with mainstream scientific discourse, which follows a legal-adversarial model in which evidence is selectively amassed to support a preconceived opinion, rather than examined dispassionately to form an opinion.[50] The physician-surrogate data[1] confirm that traditional, informal medical decision making, despite the best intentions, is prey to such prejudices. The complexity of medical decision making and our demonstrated fallibility argue for a more systematic approach.

Several prescriptive models of decision making have been proposed, of which the best known is expected value decision making.[51] A related but simpler model aims to minimize the displeasure associated with bad outcomes.[52] The basis of expected value decision making is that the preferred alternative is the one that yields the highest expected value. Each alternative is described in terms of its possible outcomes; for a given alternative, each outcome has a probability and a utility. The expected value of an alternative is the result of multiplying each outcome's utility with its probability of occurring, and then summing these products. The expected value therefore represents the average outcome of an alternative. If the list of outcomes is exhaustive, the probabilities are accurate, and the utilities are pertinent, then the alternative with the highest expected value is the preferred choice.

That individuals faced with uncertainty make choices that are at odds with expected value decision making should come as no surprise. Prescriptive models, suggesting how decisions *should* be made, must be distinguished from descriptive models, which aim to describe how decisions *are* made. Both these pragmatic models refer to the ordinary conditions of routine practice. Normative models refer to how decisions should be made under *ideal* conditions.[53] These perspectives are useful, distinct, and may yield different conclusions.

Formal methods of decision analysis have two main advantages over informal methods. First, the process is explicit and therefore amenable to scrutiny. The outcomes, probabilities, assumptions, and preferences are all open to inspection and criticism. Second, the process lends itself to validation (or refutation) and modification. To assess the effect of changes in the way the model is defined is simple. What if the probability of relapse without adjuvant treatment is higher? What if adjuvant treatment is more effective? What if the side effects of treatment are more severe? This process of testing the underlying assumptions is known as sensitivity analysis—testing the sensitivity of the decision to changes in the way the model is defined.

SCREENING AND TREATMENT FOR EARLY PROSTATE CANCER

The work done by the Prostate Patient Outcomes Research Team deserves special attention. To assess the value of alternative strategies for early-stage prostate cancer, these investigators first performed a structured review of Medline-referenced English-language literature from 1966 to 1991.[18] This yielded 144 articles that fulfilled predetermined criteria out of an initial pool of 1600 titles. Synthesis of the data revealed some information about complications, but the authors concluded that data were inadequate to draw inferences about the effectiveness of the surgery or radiotherapy. In the absence of randomized data, these investigators performed a formal decision analysis comparing radical prostatectomy, external-beam radiotherapy, and watchful waiting.[54] They modeled for the effects of age, tumor stage, and tumor grade (Gleason score) on the rates of development of distant metastases, of progression from hormone-responsive to hormone-refractory metastatic cancer, and of excess mortality from metastatic cancer, as well as the effect of local treatment (surgery or radiotherapy) on progression to metastatic disease, local control, and GU and bowel symptoms. Effects on quality of life included impotence, incontinence, bowel injury, bladder outlet obstruction, and the effects of both hormone-responsive and hormone-resistant metastatic disease. The effects of different discount rates were also analyzed. These investigators concluded that, although radiotherapy or prostatectomy may be of benefit in younger patients with high-grade tumors, in most cases, the potential benefits are small and sensitive to individual preferences, and for many men, watchful waiting is a reasonable option.

Two independent groups have also looked rigorously at this question. Mold and associates[55] looked at whether to perform a biopsy of an asymptomatic nodule found during a digital rectal examination (DRE) done by a primary care physician in a 65-year-old man. They found that further evaluation and treatment resulted, on average, in a 1.1-month gain in survival but a 3.5-month loss in quality-adjusted survival, and they concluded that DRE should not be performed by primary care physicians as a screening test for prostate cancer. Krahn and associates assessed the clinical and economic effects of screening with PSA, DRE, and transrectal ultrasonography (TRUS).[56] They found that screening with PSA or TRUS prolonged unadjusted survival but shortened quality-adjusted survival, that screening with DRE alone did not improve survival in any group, and that results were sensitive only to estimates of the efficacy of treatment. These investigators concluded that screening asymptomatic men with PSA, DRE, or TRUS was not supported by the evidence, and ''screening may result in poorer health outcomes and will increase costs dramatically.''

CONCLUSIONS

Good clinical decisions require an understanding of the generic data regarding disease and treatment, the specifics of the particular problem, the individual patient's preferences, the nature of trade-offs, and uncertainty. The outcome of every medical decision is uncertain. No matter how carefully we stage a patient's illness, no matter how much we know about a particular management option, we cannot accurately predict the outcome in an individual case. Instead, we must be satisfied with choosing the alternative that produces the *best* outcome on average. The definition of *best* is a question of perspective rather than of absolute truth, and different perspectives are expected to result in different conclusions. The choice of the best decision does not guarantee a good outcome, nor does a bad outcome necessarily imply the wrong decision. Formal methods of decision analysis are complicated and time consuming and may therefore seem impractical. We can argue (particularly on behalf of the subject of the decision), however, that if a decision is worth making, it is worth making well. In any case, a systematic approach is often revealing and is invaluable for directing further research.

REFERENCES

1. Moore MJ, O'Sullivan B, Tannock IF. How expert physicians would wish to be treated if they had genitourinary cancer. J Clin Oncol 1988; 6:1736.
2. Moore MJ, O'Sullivan M, Tannock IF. Are treatment strategies of urologic oncologists influenced by the opinion of their colleagues? Br J Cancer 1990;62:988.
3. Antman EM, Lau J, Kupelnick B, Mosteller F, Chalmers TC. A comparison of results of meta-analyses of randomized controlled trials and recommendations of clinical experts: treatments for myocardial infarction. JAMA 1992;268:240.
4. Eddy DM, Clanton CH. The art of diagnosis: solving the clinicopathologic exercise. N Engl J Med 1982;306:1263.
5. Armitage P, Berry G. Statistical methods in medical research. Oxford: ? Blackwell Scientific Publications, 1987:42.
6. Gardner MJ, Altman DG. Confidence intervals rather than P values: estimation rather than hypothesis testing. Br Med J 1986;292:746.
7. Stockler M. Better right than quick? Med Decis Making 1992;12:76.
8. Feinstein A. The Will Rogers phenomenon: stage migration and new diagnostic techniques as a source of misleading statistics in cancer. N Engl J Med 1985;312:1604.
9. Sacks H, Chalmers TC, Smith H. Randomized versus historical controls for clinical trials. Am J Med 1982;72:233.
10. Weiss GR, Margolin KA, Aronson FR, et al. A randomized phase II trial of continuous infusion interleukin-2 or bolus injection interleukin-2 plus lymphokine-activated killer cells for advanced renal cell carcinoma. J Clin Oncol 1992;10:275.
11. Hemenway D. The second best in statistics. J Clin Epidemiol 1991; 44:957.
12. Senn S. Fisher's game with the devil. Stat Med 1994;13:217.
13. Raghavan D, Tannock IF. Clinical trials in genitourinary oncology: what have they achieved? In: Smith PH, ed. Combination therapy in urological malignancy. London: Springer, 1989:236.
14. Schwartz D, Lellouch J. Explanatory and pragmatic attitudes in therapeutic trials. J Chronic Dis 1967;20:637.
15. Gotay CC, Korn EL, McCabe MS, Moore TD, Cheson BD. Quality-of-life assessment in cancer clinical treatment portocols: research issues in protocol development. J Natl Cancer Inst 1992;84:575.
16. Moinpour CM, Feigl P, Metch B, Hayden KA, Meyskens FL, Crowley J. Quality-of-life endpoints in cancer clinical trials: review and recommendations. J Natl Cancer Inst 1989;81:481.
17. Wyatt J. Use and sources of medical knowledge. Lancet 1991;338: 1368.
18. Wasson JH, Cushman CC, Bruskewitz RC, Littenberg B, Mulley AG, Wennberg JE. A structured literature review of treatment for localized prostate cancer. Arch Fam Med 1993;2:487.
19. Early Breast Cancer Trialists' Collaborative Group. Systemic treatment of early breast cancer by hormonal, cytotoxic, or immune therapy. Lancet 1992;339:1, 71.
20. Felson DT. Bias in meta-analytic research. J Clin Epidemiol 1992;45: 885.
21. Tversky A, Kahneman D. Judgement under uncertainty: heuristics and biases. Science 1974;185:1124.
22. Wilson TD, DePaulo BM, Mook DG, Klaaren KJ. Scientists' evaluations of research: the biasing effects of the importance of the topic. Psychol Sci 1993;4:322.
23. Lord CG, Ross L, Lepper MR. Biased assimilation and attitude polarization: the effects of prior theories on subsequently considered evidence. J Pers Soc Psychol 1979;37:2098.
24. Messick D, Asuncion AG. The Will Rogers illusion in judgements about social groups. Psychol Sci 1993;4:46.
25. Haynes RB, McKibbon KA, Fitzgerald D, Guyatt GH, Walker CJ, Sackett DL. How to keep up with the medical literature: I–VI. Ann Intern Med 1986;105:149, 309, 474, 636, 810, 978.
26. Sackett DL, Haynes, Guyatt FH, Tugwell P. Clinical epidemiology: a basic science for clinical medicine. Boston, Little, Brown, 1991.
27. RB Haynes. Clinical review articles: should be as scientific as the articles they review. Br Med J 1992;304:330.
28. Oxman AD, Guyatt GH. Guidelines for reading literature reviews. Can Med Assoc J 1988;138:697.
29. Cook DJ, Guyatt GH, Laupacis A, et al. Rules of evidence and clinical recommendations on the use of antithrombotic agents. Chest 1992; 102(Suppl 4):S305.

30. Slevin ML, Stubbs L, Plant HJ, et al. Attitudes to chemotherapy: comparing views of patients with cancer with those of doctors, nurses, and general public. Br Med J 1990;300:1458.
31. Slevin ML, Plant H, Lynch D, et al. Who should measure quality of life, the doctor or the patient? Br Med J 1988;57:109.
32. Cassileth BR, Zupkis RV, Sutton-Smith K, et al. Information and participation preferences among cancer patients. Ann Intern Med 1980; 92:832.
33. Sutherland HJ, Llewellyn-Thomas AJ, Lockwood GA, et al. Cancer patients: their desire for information and participation in treatment decisions. J R Soc Med 1989;82:260.
34. Stockler M, Butow PN, Tattersall MHN. The take-home message: doctors' views on letters and tapes after a cancer consultation. Ann Oncol 1993;4:549.
35. Struff WM, Lo B, Charles G. Do patients want to participate in medical decision making? JAMA 1984;252:2990.
36. Tannock I, Gospodarowicz M, Meakin W, et al. Treatment of metastatic prostate cancer with low-dose prednisone: evaluation of pain and quality of life as pragmatic indices of response. J Clin Oncol 1989;7:590.
37. Moore MJ, Osoba D, Murphy K, Tannock, et al. Use of palliative endpoints to evaluate the effects of mitoxantrone and low dose prednisone in patients with hormonally resistant prostate cancer. J Clin Oncol 1994;12:689.
38. Talcott JA. Complications of treatment for early prostate cancer: a prospective, multi-institutional, outcomes study. Proc Annu Meet Am Soc Clin Oncol 1994;711. Abstract
39. Fowler F Jr, Barry MJ, Lu-Yao G, et al. Patient-reported complications and follow-up treatment after radical prostatectomy. Urology 1993;42: 622.
40. Froberg DG, Kane RL. Methodology for measuring health-state preferences. J Clin Epidemiol 1989;42:345, 459, 585, 676.
41. Llewellyn-Thomas HA, Naylor CD, Cohen MM, et al. Studying patients' preferences in health care decision-making. Can Med Assoc J 1992;147:859.
42. O'Connor AMC, Boyd NF, Trichtler DL, et al. Eliciting preferences for alternative cancer drug treatments: the influence of framing, medium and rater variables. Med Decis Making 1985;5:453.
43. McNeil BJ, Pauker SG, Sox HC, et al. On the elicitation of preferences for alternative therapies. N Engl J Med 1982;306:1259.
44. O'Connor AM. Effects of framing and level of probability on patients' preferences for cancer chemotherapy. J Clin Epidemiol 1989;42:119.
45. Naylor CD, Chen E, Strauss B. Measured enthusiasm: does the method of reporting trial results alter perceptions of therapeutic effectiveness? Ann Intern Med 1992;117:916.
46. Forrow L, Taylor WC, Arnold RM. Absolutely relative: how research results are summarized can affect treatment decisions. Am J Med 1992; 92:121.
47. Weinstein MC. Time preference in the health care context. Med Decis Making 1993;13:218.
48. Krahn M, Gafni A. Discounting in the economic evaluation of health care interventions. Med Care 1993;31:403.
49. Redelmeier DA, Heller DN. Time preferences in medical decision making and cost effectiveness analysis. Med Decis Making 1993;13:212.
50. Stockler M, Coates A. What have we learned from meta-analysis? Med J Aust 1993;159:291.
51. Sox HC, Blatt MA, Higgins MC, et al. Medical decision making. Stoneham, MA: Butterworth, 1988.
52. Feinstein AR. The chagrin factor and qualitative decision analysis. Arch Intern Med 1985;145:1257.
53. Hershey JC, Baron J. Clinical reasoning and cognitive processes. Med Decis Making 1987;7:203.
54. Fleming C, Wasson JH, Albertson PC, et al. A decision analysis of alternative treatment strategies for clinically localized prostate cancer. JAMA 1993;269:2650.
55. Mold JW, Holtgrave DR, Bisonni RS, et al. The evaluation and treatment of men with asymptomatic prostate nodules in primary care: a decision analysis. J. Fam Pract 1992;34:561.
56. Krahn MD, Mahoney JE, Eckman MH, Trachtenberg J, Pauker SG, Detsky A. Screening for prostate cancer: a decision analytic view. JAMA 1994;272:773.

Principles and Practice of Genitourinary Oncology, edited by Derek Raghavan, Howard I. Scher, Steven A. Leibel, and Paul H. Lange. Lippincott-Raven Publishers, Philadelphia, © 1997.

CHAPTER 4

Radiologic Imaging of Genitourinary Neoplasms

Susan Hilton and Lawrence H. Schwartz

Historically, diagnostic radiology has contributed much to the workup of suspected genitourinary neoplasms, from the early days of urography, which began with observations of urinary tract opacification with intravenous administered iodide compounds in the 1920s, to present-day cross-sectional imaging with ultrasound, computed tomography (CT), and magnetic resonance (MR) imaging. Angiographic techniques developed in the 1950s and 1960s allowed improved visualization and characterization of renal parenchymal lesions, as well as evaluation of the renal arterial and venous system. More recent trends in radiologic imaging of the urinary system have been an increase in the safety of intravenous contrast agents for imaging of the urinary tract and the development of cross-sectional imaging techniques to allow more detailed visualization of the renal parenchyma, retroperitoneum, and pelvic structures than is possible with intravenous urography (IVU).

Although cross-sectional imaging techniques (CT, ultrasound, MR imaging) allow better visualization of parenchymal lesions in the kidneys than is possible with IVU, these diagnostic studies have not completely supplanted IVU for study of the urinary tract. IVU affords superior visualization of the urinary tract, largely because of better spatial resolution and display of the entire course of the urinary tract on a single image rather than on multiple individual sections. The capabilities of cross-sectional imaging to evaluate vascular structures have almost completely obviated the need for invasive angiography in the evaluation of renal lesions, however. The type of information provided by each imaging modality is different (Table 4-1), and therefore, the decision to request a particular imaging test should be based on careful consideration of the clinical question and consultation with the urologic radiologist.

PRIMARY RENAL NEOPLASMS

Detection

An imaging workup for a suspected primary renal neoplasm may be prompted by signs and symptoms suggesting a renal tumor (hematuria, flank pain), by discovery of a lesion distant from the kidney that suggests a metastatic renal neoplasm, or by the incidental demonstration of a renal mass on a diagnostic imaging study obtained for an unrelated indication. For a patient with hematuria, a complete imaging workup should include IVU. Given the poor sensitivity of ultrasound for detection of upper tract urothelial tumors and small renal masses,[1] ultrasound is often employed in conjunction with IVU, rather than as the sole imaging modality for diagnostic workup of a patient with hematuria. For example, ultrasound is used to confirm that a smooth mass detected on urography, a common finding in adult patients, represents a benign cyst. If urographic and ultrasound findings are negative, however, and if clinical suspicion of a renal neoplasm remains, CT has a definite role in the detection of renal masses.[2,3]

Once a renal mass with characteristics other than those of a simple cyst has been detected on initial imaging studies, a CT scan of the abdomen should be performed to define and stage the lesion. A primary renal carcinoma appears as a partially or entirely solid mass that increases in density (enhances) after intravenous contrast administration (Fig. 4-1). Renal cell carcinoma accounts for approximately 86% of all primary malignant renal parenchymal neoplasms in adults. The remainder, including Wilms' tumors and sarcomas,[4] are radiographically indistinguishable from primary renal carcinoma. Renal lymphoma and metastases may have an imaging appearance similar to that of primary renal carcinoma, although in most cases specific imaging features and the appropriate clinical setting suggest the diagnosis.

The introduction of CT and ultrasound scanning within the past 15 years has resulted in the incidental detection of renal masses, often small (<3 cm). This phenomenon has allowed the detection of a larger proportion of renal carcinomas at an early, curable stage.[5,6] Some of the renal masses demonstrated on imaging studies present a diagnostic dilemma, however, in that their appearance may not be characteristic of either a benign lesion or a malignant neoplasm. Any mass that contains a solid component (therefore, does not appear as a simple cyst) on cross-sectional imaging studies raises suspicion of a malignant lesion. If a solid or complex (solid and cystic) mass is demonstrated on ultrasound examination, CT scan of the kidneys may

Table 4-1 *Imaging modalities for evaluation of genitourinary neoplasms: renal parenchymal, adrenal, and urothelial lesions*

Modality	Information provided	Advantages	Disadvantages
Intravenous urography (IVU)	Display of entire urinary tract; outline and contour of renal parenchyma (not used to detect small adrenal lesion)	Detailed imaging of collecting structures and ureters in additon to visualizing renal parenchymal lesions	Poor sensitivity for small renal parenchymal lesions, risk of intravenous (IV) contrast complication
Ultrasound	Detection of some small renal lesions missed by IVU; characterization of lesions seen on IVU as solid or cystic; detection and evaluation of hydronephrosis (not used to detect small adrenal lesion)	Inexpensive, noninvasive	Poor sensitivity to some solid lesions, operator-dependent, limited by patient body habitus; incomplete visualization of urinary tract
Computed tomography (CT)	Detection and characterization of renal and adrenal lesions; presence of enhancement with IV contrast indicating lesion perfusion, a finding associated with neoplasm; assessment of surrounding structures, presence of adjacent organ invasion, adenopathy; assessment of patency of renal veins and inferior vena cava	Relatively noninvasive, good for staging as well as detection	Relatively expensive, risk of IV contrast complication, no display of urinary tract in continuity
Magnetic resonance imaging (MRI)	Detection and characterization of renal and adrenal lesions; enhancement with IV gadolinium indicating lesion perfusion; assessment of surrounding structures in multiple imaging planes; vessel patency shown, and extent of inferior vena cava involvement with tumor	Multiple imaging planes: good for assessment of vessels, organ invasion; useful for surgical planning	Expensive; spatial resolution lower than CT, therefore lower sensitivity to small renal and adrenal lesions
Angiography	Anatomic "road map" of lesion blood supply, patency of renal vein, inferior vena cava	Detailed assessment of arterial supply; useful if embolization considered; occasionally used for surgical planning	Invasive, expensive
Radionuclide bone scan	Detection of osseous lesions that may represent metastases	Noninvasive, more sensitive than plain film survey	Nonspecific; workup of incidental nonmetastatic lesions possibly incurring unnecessary expense

be performed to define the lesion further. In certain cases, a complex cystic lesion may be shown to contain only thin septations or high-density fluid, thereby characterizing it as a minimally complicated cyst and avoiding unnecessary surgery.[7] Some benign lesions exhibit features found in malignant renal neoplasms, however, and therefore a small percentage of patients with benign tumors undergo surgery. For detection of renal neoplasms, MR imaging is reserved for patients in whom intravenous contrast for CT is contraindicated.[8]

Staging

Abdominal CT scanning with intravenous contrast is used to assess the local extent of a renal mass, to detect tumor involvement within the renal vein and inferior vena cava, and to detect the presence of enlarged retroperitoneal lymph nodes, which may indicate metastatic disease (Fig. 4-2). A CT scan of the the chest may be useful to detect pulmonary metastases. MR imaging can more precisely define the extent of inferior vena cava involvement with tumor thrombus, important for surgical planning (Fig. 4-3). If a patient with suspected renal carcinoma complains of bone pain, plain film radiography of the affected area and radionuclide bone scanning should be performed. In the absence of symptoms, a bone scan is probably unnecessary, because about 85% of patients with bone metastases have bone pain.[9]

ADRENAL NEOPLASMS

Three common indications for radiologic evaluation of the adrenal glands exist:

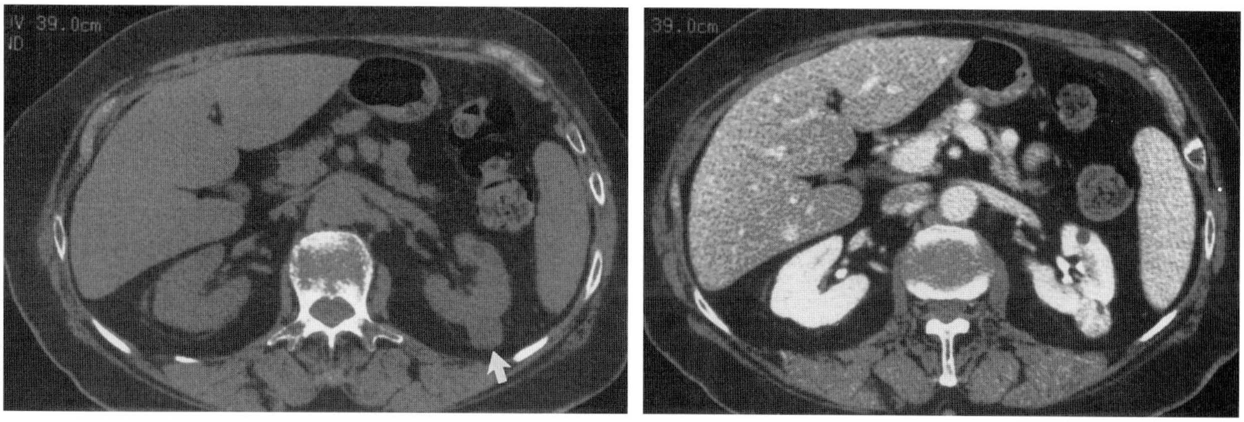

A B

FIG. 4-1. Left renal carcinoma, CT scan. (**A**) CT scan before administration of intravenous (IV) contrast shows a solid mass projecting posteriorly from left kidney (*arrow*). (**B**) Scan after IV contrast administration demonstrates dense enhancement of the mass, typical for a vascular neoplasm. An incidental small renal cyst is noted anteriorly.

1. Radiologic study is useful as a screening tool for adrenal metastases in patients with primary tumors, such as lung cancer, that have a propensity to metastasize to the adrenals. The adrenal glands are the *fourth* most common site for spread of metastatic disease.
2. Radiologic study is indicated in patients with a laboratory diagnosis of a potential hyperfunctioning adrenal gland tumor.
3. Radiologic evaluation is indicated when an adrenal mass incidentally discovered on another imaging study requires further evaluation.

Primary tumors of adrenal cortical origin include adrenal cortical carcinomas and nonhyperfunctioning adrenal adenomas. Adrenal cortical carcinomas do not have a typical CT or MR appearance. They tend to vary in size, but by the time of presentation they are usually large, measuring between 4 and 12 cm; these tumors may contain calcification, they may have central low attenuation on CT indicative of necrosis, and they may demonstrate irregular enhancement after intravenous contrast administration.[10] CT features alone cannot distinguish between these two adrenal cortical lesions, although the larger lesions and those with more irregular contrast enhancement tend to be carcinomas. Confirmation of vascular involvement or evidence of distant metastatic disease is also indicative of an adrenal cortical carcinoma.

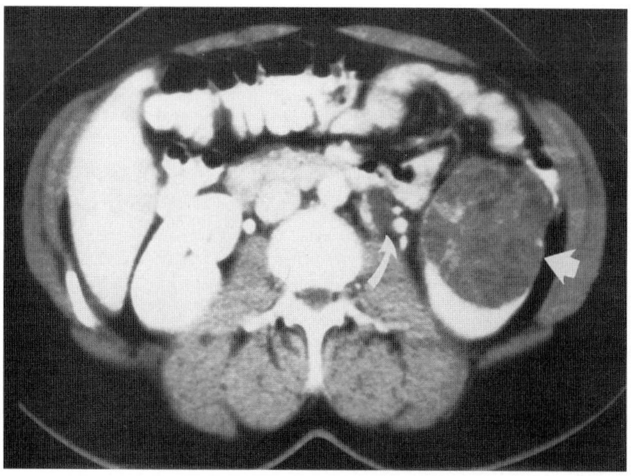

FIG. 4-2. Left renal carcinoma with paraaortic nodal metastasis. Intravenous contrast-enhanced CT scan demonstrates a heterogeneous left renal mass (*arrow*) and a left paraaortic enlarged lymph nodal metastasis (*curved arrow*). Note the appearance of similar density of the primary tumor and the metastatic lymph node.

When an adrenal mass is large, assessing the organ of origin may be difficult. This is especially true of right-sided masses, which, on routine axial CT images, may appear to arise from the liver, adrenal gland, or kidney. MR imaging, specifically in the coronal and sagittal planes, is especially helpful in this regard (Fig. 4-4), and it is also an excellent tool for evaluating vascular invasion. Irregular contrast enhancement may also be seen in adrenal cortical lesions after gadolinium administration.

Pheochromocytomas, which arise in the adrenal medulla, are usually associated with symptoms of excessive catecholamine production. Before any imaging study is performed, documentation of laboratory elevation of catecholamine is important because radiologic evaluation for pheochromocytoma in all hypertensive patients is too costly. CT is highly accurate in detecting pheochromocytomas, which are generally unilateral, homogeneous solid masses larger than 2 cm. Infrequently, they may have cystic components.[11] Pheochromocytomas intensely enhance after intravenous contrast administration.[12] CT is best at evaluating unilateral, intraadrenal tumors. Extraadrenal lesions, multicentric lesions, and recurrences of pheochromocytoma are more difficult to evaluate by CT. In these cases, radionuclide evaluation with MIBG (metaiodobenzylguanidine), a norepinephrine analog taken up by adrenal medullary tissue and tagged with iodine-131 (^{131}I), is helpful. MR imaging is also helpful both to evaluate the solitary adrenal mass suspected of being a pheochromocytoma and to detect multicentric lesions. Pheochromocytomas tend to have prolonged T2 relaxation times and therefore are bright on heavily weighted T2 images.[13] The multiplanar capability of MR imaging, including the ability to scan sagitally and coronally, allows MR imaging to image

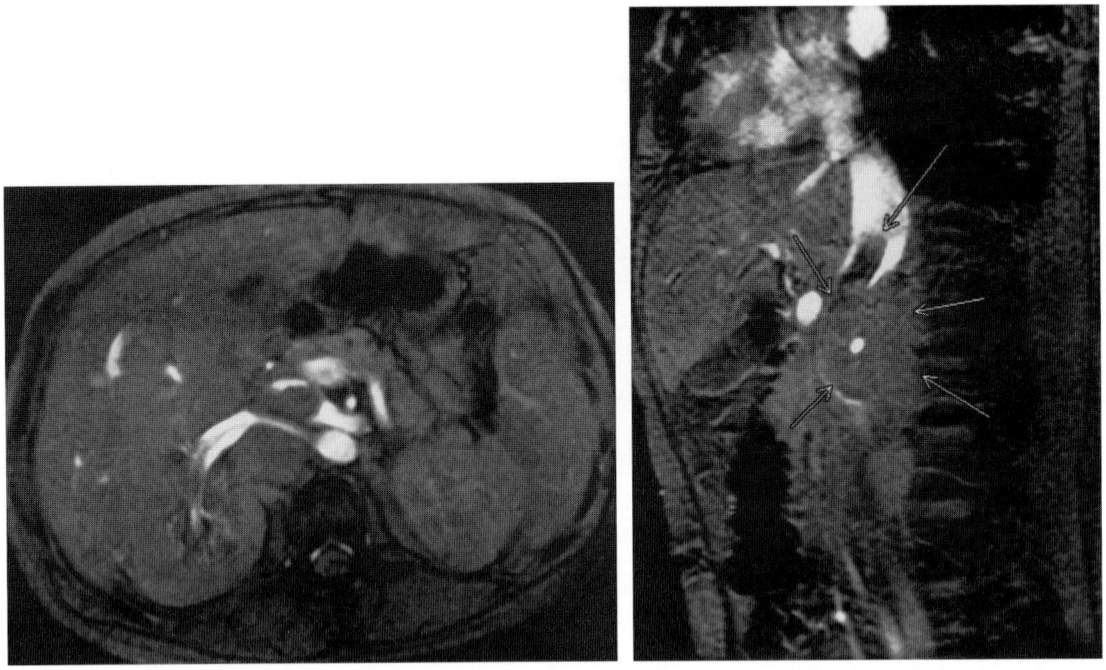

A B

FIG. 4-3. Renal carcinoma invading the inferior vena cava, MR scan. (**A**) Axial gradient echo image demonstrating bright signal intensity within the aorta, right renal artery, and portions of the inferior vena cava. Low-signal-intensity tumor mass displaces the right renal artery and extends into the inferior vena cava. (**B**) Sagittal gradient echo image with tumor and thrombus (*arrows*) encircling the right renal artery and extending into the inferior vena cava.

the entire abdomen and pelvis in a short period. Therefore, MR imaging is useful to evaluate extraadrenal lesions and suspected recurrences.

Adrenal adenomas are the most common adrenal masses. They may be nonhyperfunctioning, associated with Cushing's disease, or associated with primary aldosteronism. Most adenomas are small, ranging from 1 to 5 cm. They tend to be homogeneously low in attenuation and mildly enhance after intravenous contrast administration on CT scans. CT attenuation values (Hounsfield units) may be helpful in distinguishing adenomas from metastases (Fig. 4-5). A CT Hounsfield unit attenuation value of less than 0 is indicative of adenoma, with a sensitivity and specificity of 47% and 100%.[14] On MR imaging, adenomas are generally low in signal intensity on T2-weighted images, as compared with metastases and pheochromocytomas. Adenomas are intermediate to high in signal intensity on T1-weighted images, again because of fat. Because adenomas contain a significant quantity of fat, MR chemical shift imaging has been used to distinguish adenomas

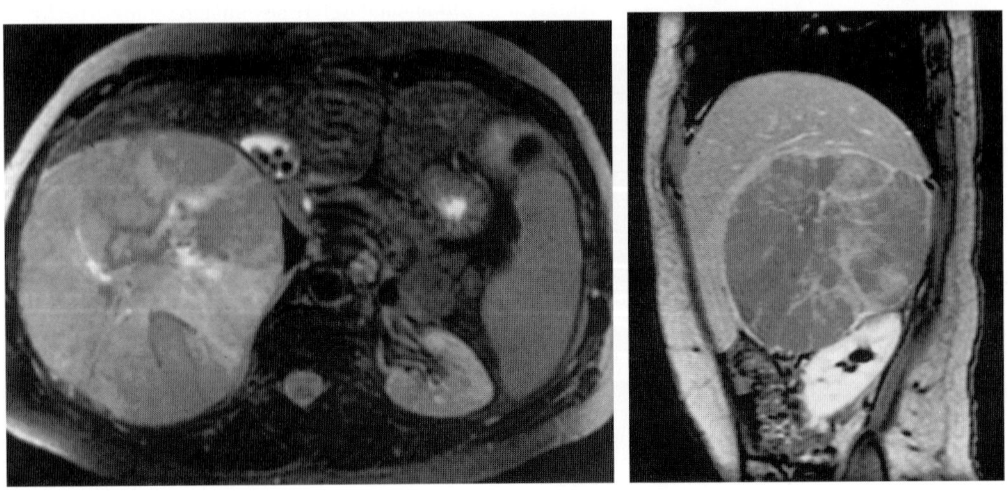

A B

FIG. 4-4. MR scan of adrenal cortical carcinoma. (**A**) Axial T2-weighted images demonstrate intermediate- to high-signal intensity within a large mass. (**B**) The sagittal postgadolinium scan demonstrates a hypervascular suprarenal mass, separate from the liver and the kidney.

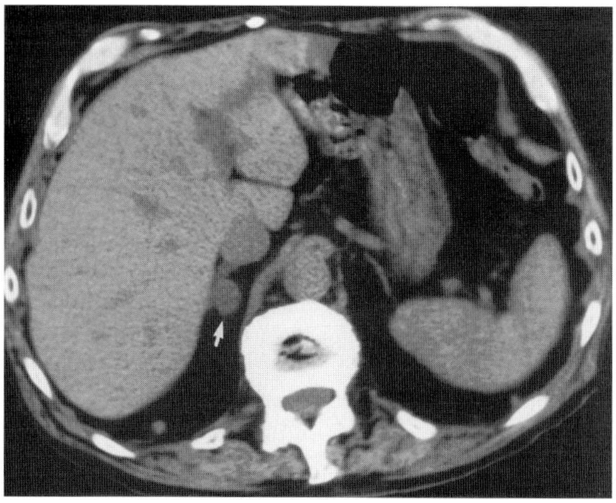

FIG. 4-5. Low-attenuation adrenal mass consistent with an adenoma, CT scan.

from other lesions (Fig. 4-6), with reported sensitivities between 80% and 95%, with 100% specificity for adenoma.[15]

Metastases are common adrenal masses as well. Lung carcinoma is the most common tumor to metastasize to the adrenal gland. Carcinomas of the breast, thyroid, and colon and melanoma are other primary tumors with a propensity to spread to the adrenal glands. The physician must differentiate the incidental benign adenoma from metastases in patients with these primary malignant tumors. Both the CT Hounsfield unit criteria and MR imaging are helpful in this regard. MR imaging, the diagnostic study of choice in this differentiation, uses fast scanning techniques and chemical shift imaging. When the features of adrenal masses are not classic for benign adrenal adenomas on CT or MR imaging, percutaneous biopsy is necessary.

Adrenal myelolipomas are uncommon benign tumors composed of lipid and myeloid tissue, so on CT they are of low attenuation with Hounsfield unit values between −30 and −140. Up to 20% of these tumors contain calcification. MR characteristics of adrenal myelolipomas are also due to the presence of fat within them. On fat-suppressed pulse sequences, such as short tau inversion recovery, these tumors tend to be low in signal intensity. On CT, adrenal cysts are also uncommon primary adrenal tumors. Adrenal cysts tend to be well circumscribed, low-attenuation masses, possibly containing a thin rim of calcification. They may be difficult to distinguish from adenomas on CT because both lesions are low in attenuation. Contrast enhancement distinguishes between these two lesions because cysts do not enhance. MR imaging also enables the physician to distinguish between these lesions because cysts are extremely bright on T2-weighted images as a result of the presence of fluid.

UROTHELIAL NEOPLASMS

Transitional carcinoma of the urinary tract has a high incidence (20% to 40%) of multicentricity, and therefore, imaging of the pelvocalyceal systems and ureters should be meticulous to maximize detection of all lesions.

Renal Pelvocalyceal Neoplasms

Detection

Patients with urothelial neoplasms of the upper urinary tract most often present with hematuria with or without flank pain. IVU is used for initial imaging examination of the urinary tract for suspected urothelial neoplasm. Lowe and Roylance described five types of abnormalities on IVU seen in transitional cell carcinoma of the kidney: (I) filling defects within the opacified renal pelvis; (II) filling defects within distended calyces; (III) calyceal obliteration; (IV) hydronephrosis with renal enlargement; and (V) reduced function without renal enlargement.[16] Although these findings are nonspecific, and a filling defect within a collecting structure may represent stone, clot, or inflammatory mass, a fixed (nonmobile, unchanging) filling defect strongly suggests neoplasm.

A

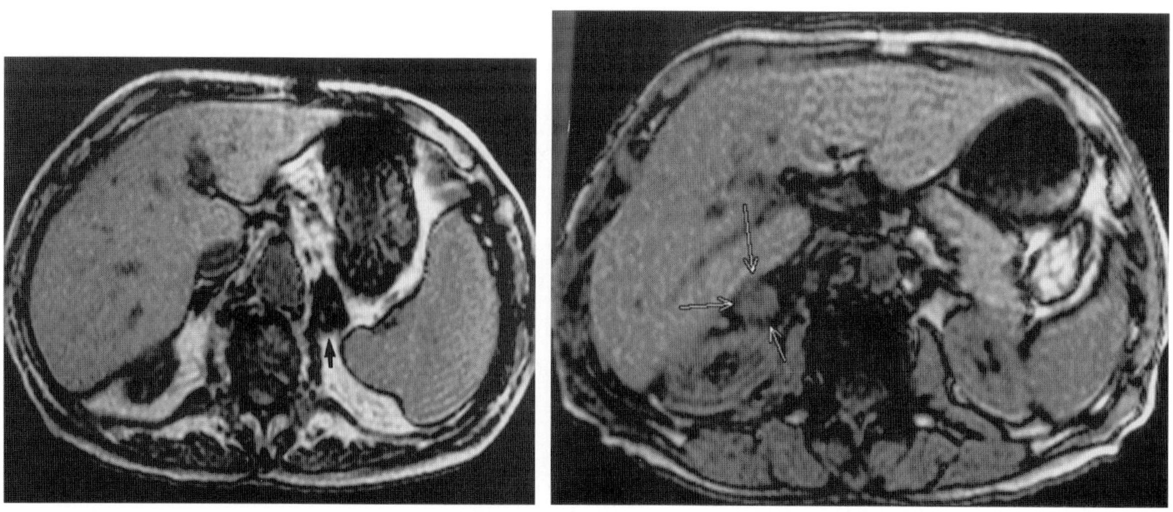

B

FIG. 4-6. (**A**) Adrenal adenoma on magnetic resonance, chemical shift images. The mass has a low signal intensity because of the presence of fat and water within it. (**B**) A classic metastasis (*arrows*) is intermediate in signal intensity.

Sonography is useful to evaluate a nonfunctioning kidney demonstrated on urography or to study further a defect within a collecting structure suspected to be a stone. Most commonly, a renal transitional cell carcinoma is a discrete mass that is as echogenic as renal parenchyma but less echogenic than the adjacent renal sinus fat.[17,18] Although a renal mass demonstrated on ultrasound may be due to other neoplasms or even infection, a centrally located mass, especially with involvement of the central renal sinus, strongly suggests the diagnosis of transitional cell carcinoma.[19] The typical sonographic appearance of a stone is easily differentiated from that of a urothelial tumor in most cases, except in the rare instance when transitional cell carcinoma contains calcification.[20] Small lesions within the proximal renal collecting system that do not produce obstruction may not be detectable on ultrasound.

Retrograde pyelography may be used to visualize upper collecting structures more clearly when the question exists of a possible abnormality due to suboptimal visualization on IVU, or the technique may be used to better define an abnormality seen on the urogram. Retrograde pyelography is especially useful to evaluate the collecting system when the kidney is nonfunctioning because of obstruction or involvement by tumor.

On CT scanning, three patterns of appearance of the primary urothelial lesion have been described. The tumor may be seen as an intraluminal mass or as a centrally located infiltrating mass, or it may appear as renal pelvic or ureteral wall thickening[21] (Fig. 4-7).

Staging

CT scanning is helpful for demonstrating the regional extent of a urothelial lesion of the upper urinary tract, as well as the presence of enlarged retroperitoneal lymph nodes. CT is a sensitive indicator of high-stage tumor when direct extension through the renal pelvic or ureteral wall is demonstrated, but it may be of limited value for staging of local disease when this finding is not present.[22,23] The demonstration of enlarged retroperitoneal lymph nodes on CT raises a strong suspicion of metastatic disease. CT scanning may also be used to detect liver and lung metastases. If clinical symptoms suggest bone metastases, plain films and radionuclide bone scanning may be useful.

Primary Ureteral Neoplasms

Detection

Most often, these patients present with hematuria or flank pain. IVU, the primary diagnostic imaging modality, may show a nonfunctioning kidney (46%), hydronephrosis with or without hydroureter (34%), or a ureteral filling defect with or without hydronephrosis or hydroureter (19%)[24] Hydronephrosis or nonvisualization is associated with invasive ureteral tumor in the majority of cases.[25] Retrograde pyelography is the major diagnostic tool for diagnosis of ureteral neoplasm.[26] The tumor may appear as a pedunculated mass, a fixed filling defect, a focal irregularity of the ureteral wall, or even a smooth stricture.[27] The "goblet sign," considered pathognomonic for ureteral tumor, refers to focal dilation of the ureter below the lesion in the shape of a champagne glass (Fig. 4-8). CT scanning may be used when retrograde pyelography cannot be done because of an inability to catheterize the ureter. On CT, ureteral neoplasms may appear as filling defects of soft tissue density within the ureter or as thickening of the ureteral wall[28] (Fig. 4-9).

Benign ureteral neoplasms may be radiographically indistinguishable from urothelial carcinoma. Metastatic disease to the ureter may also produce a similar radiographic appearance, although such patients usually have metastases at other distant sites.[29]

Staging

CT scanning is useful for demonstrating both the intraluminal ureteral mass and the degree of extraureteral tumor extension, as well as for detecting retroperitoneal nodal metastases. As with neoplasms of the upper urinary tract, additional plain film

A

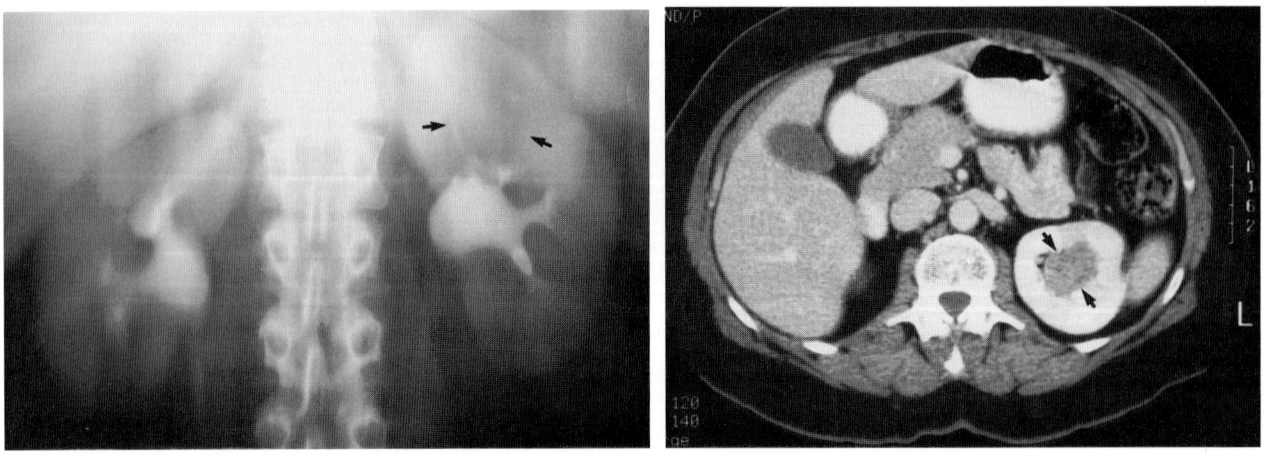

B

FIG. 4-7. Left upper renal pole transitional cell carcinoma, intravenous urographic (IVU) and CT scan. (**A**) Tomographic film from an IVU scan demonstrates obliteration and mass effect (*arrows*) involving collecting structures of the left upper pole. (**B**) IV contrast-enhanced CT scan demonstrates a central left upper pole mass (*arrows*).

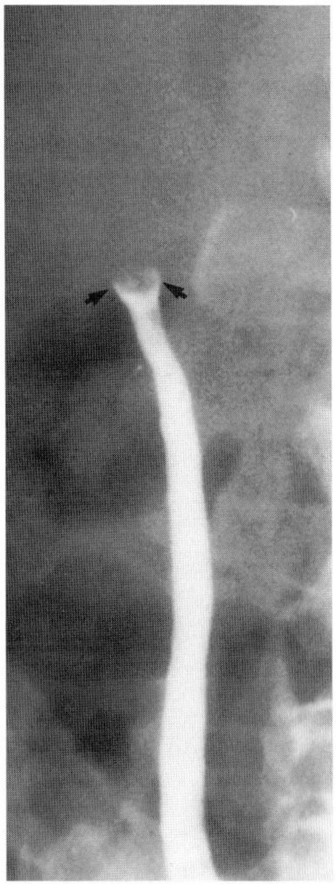

FIG. 4-8. Transitional carcinoma, proximal right ureter, "goblet sign" on retrograde pyelogram. The neoplasm is seen as a proximal right ureteral filling defect, with dilatation of the ureter immediately below the lesion (*arrows*).

radiographs, CT studies, and radionuclide bone scanning may be indicated if clinical symptoms suggest metastases at specific distant sites.

Primary Urothelial Neoplasms of the Urinary Bladder

Detection

Although bladder lesions may be recognized on IVU, cystography, CT, or ultrasound, cystoscopy remains the initial procedure for detection of bladder neoplasms.

Bladder neoplasms may be identified by IVU, in patients undergoing this examination for urinary or unrelated symptoms, but IVU is an insensitive test.[30] On IVU, the tumor appears as a fixed filling defect, outlined by contrast within the urinary bladder. Although this finding can be nonspecific, caused by blood clot, nonopaque stone, or inflammatory lesion, the trapping of contrast within the interstices of the lesion (radiographic "stipple sign"[31]) is highly suggestive of urothelial neoplasm.

CT scanning can also demonstrate neoplasms within the bladder wall, but sensitivity is insufficient to allow CT to be used for initial imaging.

Staging

IVU is useful for evaluation of the upper urothelial tract in patients with bladder carcinoma. Otherwise, IVU has limited use for staging of bladder cancer. The presence of ureteral obstruction on IVU at the time of diagnosis is associated with a 92% incidence of bladder muscle invasion and a 55% incidence of lymph node metastasis, however.[32] CT can detect transmural or extramural extension of tumor, but it cannot enable the physician to assess lesser degrees of tumor invasion within the bladder wall. Studies using gadolinium-enhanced dynamic MR imaging for local staging of bladder tumors show early promising results, which remain to be confirmed by additional investigation.[33,34] CT can detect regional pelvic or retroperitoneal nodal metastatic disease, if the involved lymph nodes are enlarged. As with neoplasms of the upper urinary tract, the necessity of additional radiographic studies should be determined by clinical symptoms.

PROSTATE CANCER

The most important recent development in the evaluation of the prostate gland has been serum prostate-specific antigen (PSA) screening. Radiology plays a small role in the actual diagnosis of prostate cancer, rather; its role is in image guidance for biopsy, staging, and evaluating response to therapy. Transrectal ultrasound (TRUS), CT, MR imaging, and nuclear bone scanning are all integral parts of the imaging strategies for patients with prostate cancer.

Most (90%) of prostate cancers occur within the peripheral zone of the prostate.[35] Most imaging modalities do not distinguish between cancer and benign prostatic hypertrophy arising in the central zone or transitional zone. Ultrasound and MR imaging are more readily able to evaluate prostate cancers arising from the peripheral zone. Prostate cancer generally spreads outside the prostate to local structures through the prostate capsule, through the neurovascular bundles, to the seminal vesicles, bladder, and lymph nodes. Prostate cancer also tends to metastasize to bone.

The use of radiology for evaluating patients with prostate cancer depends on the purpose of the evaluation. No radiologic test, including TRUS, is adequate for screening the prostate gland. TRUS is primarily used as a technique for guiding biopsies of the prostate. Prostate cancers visualized in the peripheral zone are generally of diminished echogenicity relative to the normal echotexture of the peripheral zone. A limitation of ultrasound, however, is that up to 30% of prostate cancers are isoechoic and thus are not distinguishable from normal peripheral zone.[36] Additionally, the specificity of ultrasound is relatively low; the actual incidence of cancer in a solitary hypoechoic nodule in the peripheral zone is only 20% to 25%.[37]

Ultrasound also has limited success in staging prostate cancers, with an overall accuracy of 58% in a multiinstitutional study.[38] Ultrasound is better for evaluating extracapsular extension of tumor, especially into the seminal vesicles, where up to 92% of cases of seminal vesicle invasion were correctly diagnosed.[39] Therefore, the major role of ultrasound is as an image guidance tool for TRUS biopsy. Any area of abnormality, especially hypoechoic regions in the peripheral zone, should be carefully evaluated; however, because of the relatively low sensitivity and specificity of ultrasound, the regions of the entire prostate gland are generally examined by biopsy.

MR imaging provides excellent tissue contrast between pros-

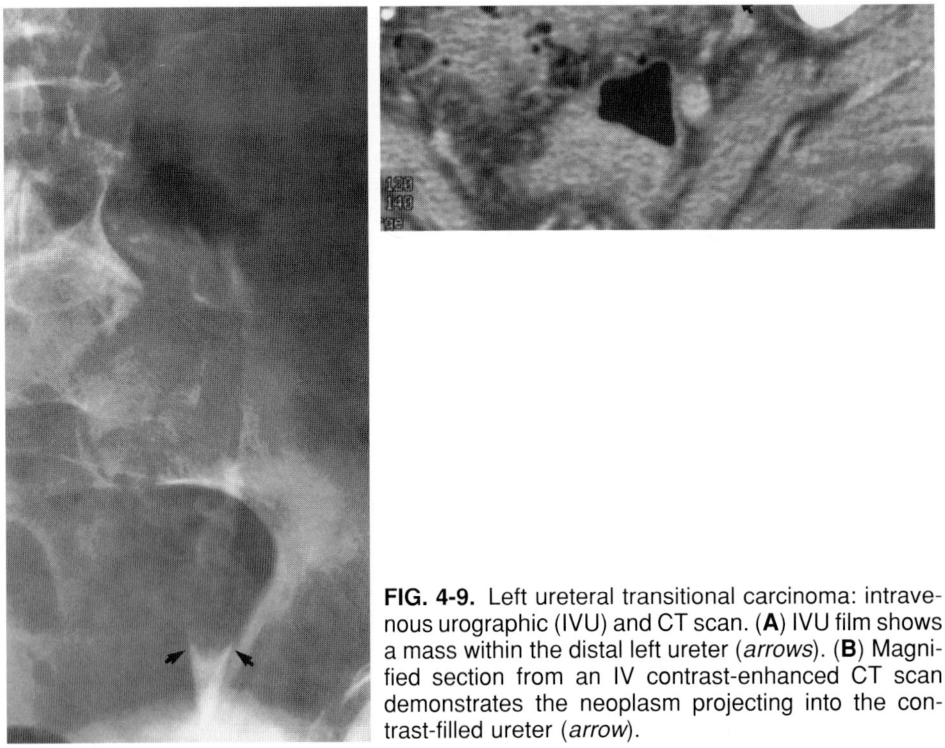

FIG. 4-9. Left ureteral transitional carcinoma: intravenous urographic (IVU) and CT scan. (**A**) IVU film shows a mass within the distal left ureter (*arrows*). (**B**) Magnified section from an IV contrast-enhanced CT scan demonstrates the neoplasm projecting into the contrast-filled ureter (*arrow*).

tate cancers in the peripheral zone and normal prostate tissue (Fig. 4-10). Staging prostate cancer with MR imaging was initally disappointing because of poor accuracy of MR imaging for evaluation of small structures such as the neurovascular bundles, using the body coil. Subsequently, specialized receiver (surface) coils to assess for extracapsular extension were designed to allow high-resolution images of the prostate to be obtained. These coils, which are placed within the rectum or wrapped around the anterior and posterior pelvic walls, provide images of better quality. Improved accuracy of 16% has been demonstrated with the endorectal coil.[40] The overall accuracy of staging prostate cancers is currently between 69% and 89%. To evaluate the prostate gland, T1- and T2-weighted images of the gland are obtained. Tl-weighted images are most useful for visualizing the neurovascular bundles. Extension of tumor into the neurovascular bundle is evident when the high-signal-intensity fat is obliterated between the prostate gland and the neurovascular bundle. Zonal architecture and the presence of prostate cancer is assessed on the T2-weighted images. Prostate cancer generally appears as areas of low signal intensity on the T2-weighted images (see Fig. 4-10). The seminal vesicles are of intermediate signal on T1-weighted images and of high signal on T2-weighted images, appearing as tubular structures. When prostate cancer invades the seminal vesicles, the normal high signal on T2-weighted images is replaced by a mass of low signal intensity (Fig 4-11).

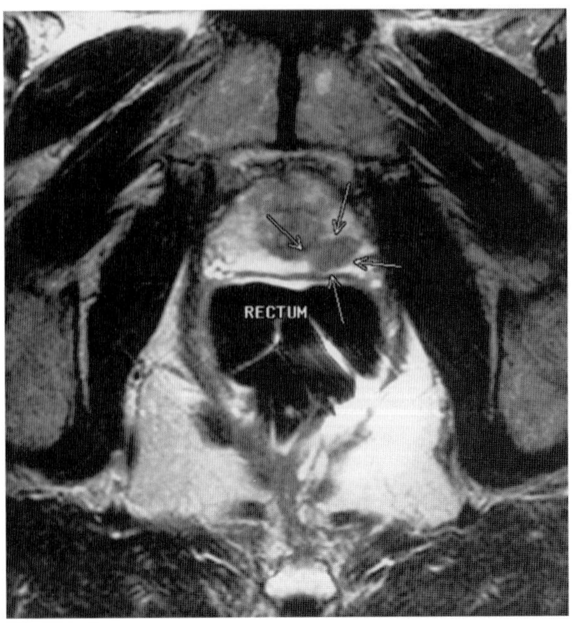

FIG. 4-10. Axial T2-weighted image demonstrating abnormal decreased signal intensity (*arrows*) in the pheripheral zone of the prostate compatible with prostate cancer.

MR imaging and CT have approximately equal accuracy in detecting lymphadenopathy, and they rely on lymph node size to assess whether metastases may be present. Lymph nodes larger than 1.0 cm are considered suspicious for metastatic disease. Tumor in normal-sized lymph nodes cannot be detected with MR imaging. MR imaging has been reported to have a sensitivity of 69% and an accuracy of 95%.[41] The advantages of MR imaging over CT are the lack of iodinated contrast use and the ability to evaluate bone marrow involvement better in the visualized bones.

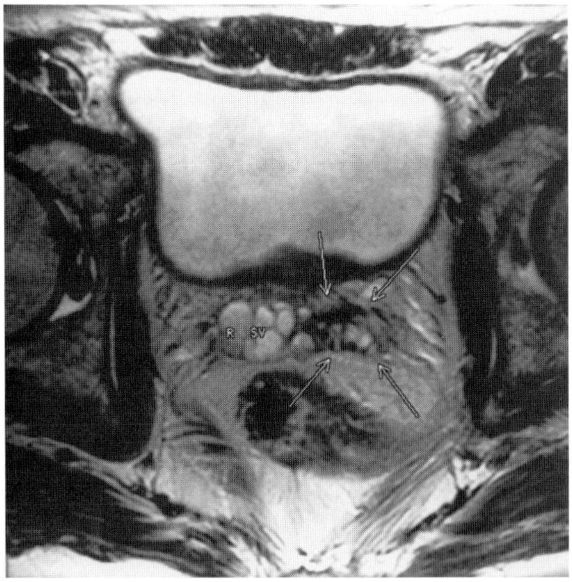

FIG. 4-11. Invasion of the left seminal vesicles by tumor (*arrows*). Note the normal high signal intensity is replaced by tumor. Right seminal vesicle (RSV) is normal.

TESTICULAR CARCINOMA

Detection

Although imaging has a limited role in the detection of testicular cancer, ultrasound may be used to clarify abnormal findings identified on physical examination of the testis. When a retroperitoneal mass or adenopathy is found in a male patient, and physical examination of the testes is negative, ultrasound should be used to exclude the presence of an occult testicular primary neoplasm,[42] because high-frequency ultrasound can detect nonpalpable testicular lesions.

Staging

Once the diagnosis of testicular cancer has been confirmed by orchiectomy, clinical staging with radiologic imaging, along with serum markers (alphafetoprotein and the beta subunit of human chorionic gonadotropin), has an important role in the assignment of patients to appropriate therapeutic regimens.

Distant spread of testicular carcinoma occurs most commonly to retroperitoneal lymph nodes, followed by lung, liver, viscera, and bone.[43] The lymphatic drainage of the testis follows predictable pathways. Lymphatic drainage from the right side tends to be midline, with primary sites of nodal involvement being the aortocaval, precaval, and preaortic regions of the retroperitoneum, in that order. Lymphatic drainage from the left side is to left paraaortic and preaortic zones, with extension to the aortocaval region in patients with more advanced disease. The right and left (renal) suprahilar nodes are rarely involved in low-stage disease.[44]

CT scanning has almost completely replaced lymphangiography as the primary imaging technique to evaluate for retroperitoneal lymphadenopathy. The accuracy of lymphangiography is comparable to that of CT. Although lymphangiography can detect disease in normal-sized nodes, the false-negative rate is similar to that with CT,[45] and the false-positive rate is significant.[46,47] Because lymphangiography is both invasive and labor intensive, many radiology departments no longer perform this procedure. For nodal disease larger than 2 cm, CT better defines the extent of disease than does lymphangiography.[46,48] For early-stage disease, however, in which lymph nodes of normal size may be involved with tumor, sensitivity of CT for retroperitoneal metastases may be as low as 58%.[49] This high false-negative rate raises special concern when evaluating patients

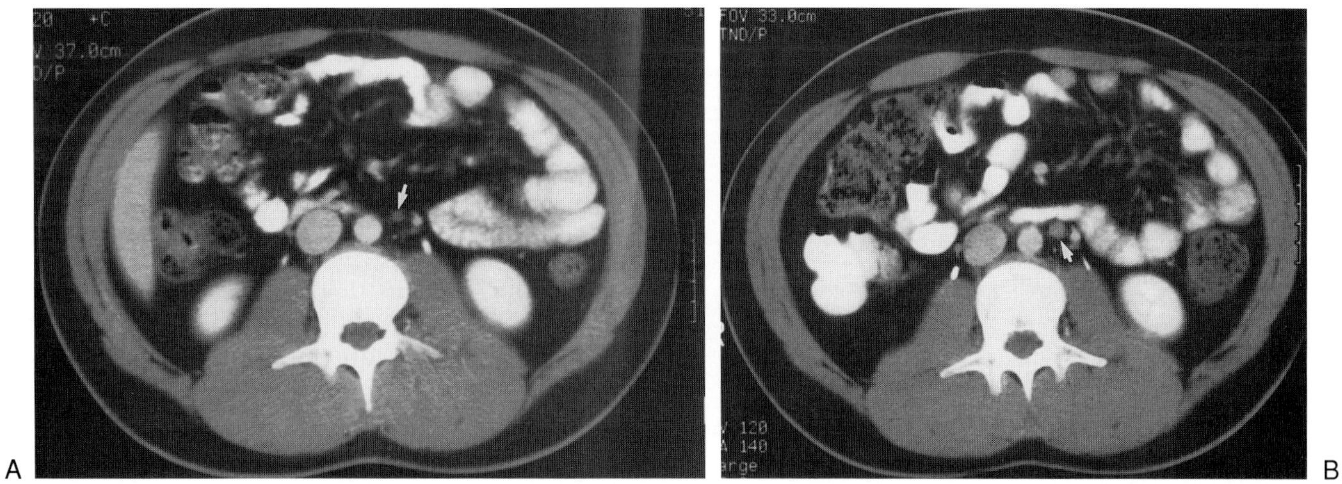

FIG. 4-12. Patient with nonseminomatous germ cell cancer of the left testis metastatic to the left paraaortic lymph nodes, with initially nonenlarged involved nodes on computed tomography (CT): serial CT studies. (**A**) Intravenous contrast-enhanced abdominal CT at presentation: small left paraaortic nodes (*arrow*) measure 5 to 6 mm. (**B**) The patient was initially reluctant to undergo staging retroperitoneal lymph node dissection. Because of suspicion raised on the first CT scan, the CT was repeated 2½ weeks later. There is definite interval enlargement of the paraaortic nodes (*arrow*), confirmed to represent metastatic disease at surgery.

considered for treatment with orchiectomy alone, without treatment with either low-dose radiotherapy to the retroperitoneum (usually patients with clinical stage I seminoma), or staging retroperitoneal lymphadenectomy (patients with clinical stage I nonseminomatous germ cell tumor) (Fig. 4-12).

For evaluation of metastatic disease in the chest, CT scanning is the most sensitive radiologic technique. CT scanning is more sensitive than plain film radiography for detection of nodal disease as well as for diagnosis of pulmonary metastases; however, the detection of nodules of nonneoplastic origin such as granulomatous disease or subpleural intrapulmonary lymph nodes renders this test nonspecific. CT scanning is also useful for detection of extranodal metastases to uncommon sites in the chest, abdomen, pelvis, and brain. Bone metastases are rare at presentation, and imaging evaluation is reserved for patients with clinical symptoms at a specific site.

REFERENCES

1. Lewis-Jones HG, Lamb GHR, Hughes PL. Can ultrasound replace the intravenous urogram in preliminary investigation of renal tract disease? A prospective study. Br J Radiol 1989;62:977.
2. Kass DA, Hricak H, Davidson AJ. Renal malignancies with normal excretory urograms. AJR Am J Roentgenol 1983;141:731.
3. Warshauer DM, McCarthy SH, Street L, et al. Detection of renal masses: sensitivities and specificities of excretory urography/linear tomography, US, and CT. Radiology 1988;169:363.
4. Levine E. Malignant renal parenchymal tumors in adults. In: Pollack HM, ed. Clinical urography. Philadelphia: WB Saunders, 1990:1216.
5. Bosniak MA. The small (≤3 cm) renal parenchymal tumor: detection, diagnosis and controversies. Radiology 1991;179:307.
6. Smith SJ, Bosniak MA, Megibow AJ, Hulnick DH, Horii SC, Raghavendra BN. Renal cell carcinoma: earlier discovery and increased detection. Radiology 1989;170:699.
7. Bosniak MA. The current radiological approach to renal cysts. Radiology 1986.
8. Rofsky NM, Weinreb JC, Bosniak MA, Libes RB, Birnbaum BA. Renal lesion characterization with gadolinium-enhanced MR imaging: efficacy and safety in patients with renal insufficiency. Radiology 1991; 180:85.
9. Levine E. Malignant renal parenchymal tumors in adults. In: Pollack HM, ed. Clinical urography. Philadelphia: WB Saunders, 1990:1262.
10. Fishman EK, Deutch DM, Hartman DS, Goldman SM, Zerhouni EA, Siegelman SS. Primary adrenocortical carcinoma: CT evaluation with clinical correlation. Am J Roentgenol 1987;148:531.
11. Glazer GM, Francis IR, Quint LE. Imaging the adrenal glands. Invest Radiol 1988;23:3.
12. Francis IR, Glazer GM, Shapiro B, Sisson JC, Gross BH. Complementary roles of CT and I^{131} MIBG scintigraphy in diagnosing pheochromocytoma. Am J Roentgenol 1983;141:719.
13. Glazer GM. MR Imaging of the liver, kidneys and adrenal glands. Radiology 1988;166:303.
14. Lee MJ, Hann PF, Papaniculaou N, et al. Benign and malignant masses: CT distinction with attenuation coefficients, size and observer analysis. Radiology 1991;179:415.
15. Mitchell DG, Cavello M, Matteucci T, Peterson RO, Miettiner MM. Benign adenocortical masses: diagnosis with chemical shift MR imaging. Radiology 1992;185:345.
16. Lowe PP, Roylance J. transitional cell carcinoma of the kidney. Clin Radiol 1976;27:503.
17. Subramanyam BR, Raghavendra BN, Madamba MR. Renal transitional cell carcinoma: sonographic and pathologic correlation. JCU J Clin Ultrasound 1982;10:203.
18. Grant DC, Dee GJ, Yoder IC, Newhouse JH. Sonography in transitional cell carcinoma of the renal pelvis. Urol Radiol 1986;8:1.
19. Ostrovsky PD, Carr L, Goodman J. Ultrasound of transitional cell carcinoma. J Clin Ultrasound 1985;13:35.
20. Janetschek G, Putz A, Feichtinger H. Renal transitional cell carcinoma mimicking stone echoes. J Ultrasound Med 1988;7:83.
21. Baron RL, McClennan BL, Lee JKT, Lawson TL. Computed tomography of transitional-cell carcinoma of the renal pelvis and ureter. Radiology 1982;144:125.
22. Badalament RA, Bennett WF, Bova JG, et al. Computed tomography of primary transitional cell carcinoma of the upper urinary tracts. Urology 1992;40:71.
23. McCoy JG, Honda H, Reznicek M, Williams RD. Computerized tomography for detection and staging of localized and pathologically defined upper tract urothelial tumors. J Urol 1991;46:1500.
24. Leder RA, Dunnick NR. Transitional cell carcinoma of the pelvicalices and ureter. Am J Roentgenol 1990;155:713.
25. Ghazi MR, Morales PA, Al-Askari S. Primary carcinoma of the ureter: report of 27 new cases. Urology 1979;14:18.
26. Goldman SM, Gatewood OMB. Neoplasms of the renal collecting system, pelvis, and ureters. In: Pollack HM, ed. Clinical urography. Philadelphia: WB Saunders, 1990:1325.
27. Yousem DM, Gatewood OMB, Goldman SM, Marshall FF. Synchronous and metachronous transitional cell carcinoma of the urinary tract: prevalence, incidence, and radiographic detection. Radiology 1988; 167:613.
28. Kenney PJ, Stanley RJ. Computed tomography of ureteral tumors. J Comput Assist Tomogr 1987;11:102.
29. Ambos MA, Bosniak MA, Megibow AJ, Raghavendra B. Ureteral involvement by metastatic disease. Urol Radiol 1979;1:105.
30. Hillman BJ, Silvert M, Cook G, et al. Recognition of bladder tumors by excretory urography. Radiology 1981;138:319.
31. McLean GK, Pollack HM, Banner MP. The "stipple sign": urographic harbinger of transitional cell neoplasms. Urol Radiol 1979;1:77.
32. Hatch TR, Barry JM. The value of excretory urography in staging bladder cancer. J Urol 1986;135:49.
33. Tanimoto A, Yuasa Y, Imai Y, et al. Bladder tumor staging: comparison of conventional and gadolinium-enhanced dynamic MR imaging and CT. Radiology 1992;185:741.
34. Narumi Y, Kadota T, Inoue E, et al. Bladder tumors: staging with gadolinium-enhanced oblique MR imaging. Radiology 1993;187:145.
35. McNeal JE, Villers AA, Redwine EA, Freika FS, Stamey TA. Capsular penetration in prostate cancer. Am J Surg Pathol 1990;14:240.
36. Hamper UM, Sheth S. Prostate ultrasonography. Semin Roentgenol 1993;28:57.
37. Danhert WF, Hamper UM, Walsh PC, et al. Prostatic evaluation by transrectal sonography with histopathologic correlation: the echopenic appearance of early carcinoma. Radiology 1986;158:97.
38. Rifkin MD, Zerhouni EA, Gatsonis CA, et al. Comparison of magnetic resonance imaging and ultrasonography in staging early prostate cancer. N Engl J Med 1990;323:621.
39. Terns MK, NcNeal JE, Stamey TA. Invasion of the seminal vesicles by prostate cancer: detection with transrectal sonography. Am J Roentgenol 1990;155:811.
40. Schnall MD, Jmai Y, Tomaszchski J. Prostate cancer local staging with endorectal surface coil MR imaging. Radiology 1991;178:797.
41. Bezzi M, Kressel HY, Allen KS, et al. Prostate carcinoma: staging with MR imaging at 1.5 T. Radiology 1988;169:339.
42. Stewart R, Carroll BA. The scrotum. In: Rumack CM, Wilson SR, Charboneau JW, eds. Diagnostic ultrasound. St. Louis: CV Mosby, 1991:573.
43. Beahrs OH, Henson DE, Hutter RVP, Kennedy BJ, eds. American Joint Committee on Cancer Manual for staging of cancer, 4th ed. Philadelphia: JB Lippincott, 1992:187.
44. Donahue JP, Zachary JM, Maynard BR. Distribution of nodal metastases in nonseminomatous testis cancer. J Urol 1982;128:315.
45. Husband J. Advances in tumour imaging. In: Horwich A, ed. Testicular cancer: investigation and management. Baltimore: Williams & Wilkins, 1991:22.
46. Thomas JL, Bernardino ME, Bracken RB. Staging of testicular carcinoma: comparison of CT and lymphangiography. Am J Roentgenol 1981;137:991.
47. Harding M, Dall B, Corbett R, Vallance R, Kaye SB. Does lymphangiography have any role in the management of early non-seminomatous germ cell tumours? Clin Radiol 1990;41:392.
48. Dunnick NR, Javadpour N. Value of CT and lymphography: distinguishing retroperitoneal metastases from nonseminomatous testicular tumors. AJR Am J Roentgenol 1981;136:1093.
49. Stomper PC, Fung CY, Socinski MA, Jochelson MS, Garnick MB, Richie JP. Detection of retroperitoneal metastases in early-stage nonseminomatous testicular cancer: analysis of different CT criteria. Am J Roentgenol 1987;149:1187.

Principles and Practice of Genitourinary Oncology, edited by Derek Raghavan, Howard I. Scher, Steven A. Leibel, and Paul H. Lange. Lippincott-Raven Publishers, Philadelphia, © 1997.

CHAPTER 5

Principles of Retroperitoneal and Pelvic Surgery

Rodney J. Taylor and Scott F. Howe

The retroperitoneum and pelvis represent the sites of origin of nearly all urologic cancers. Exceptions are cancer of the genitalia and urethra, and for these disorders, the retroperitoneum and pelvis assume importance because of lymph node drainage. Therefore, the management of urologic cancer requires an understanding of the anatomic relationships and contents of the retroperitoneum. In addition, to understand unique aspects and problems associated with management of these cancers and considerations in surgical management, we need to appreciate the decision process in choosing why, how, and when to approach the problem surgically. The purpose of this chapter is to provide an introduction of the principles of retroperitoneal and pelvic urologic cancer surgery, especially for nonurologic surgeons. Discussions of treatment options for specific cancers are provided elsewhere in this textbook.

ANATOMIC BOUNDARIES

The retroperitoneum is made up of two areas, the lumbar and iliac regions, which encompass the "surgical" retroperitoneum and pelvis. The cephalad portion of the lumbar region starts at the 12th thoracic vertebral body and follows the 12th ribs laterally. The caudal boundary is the base of the sacrum medially and follows the iliac crests to the lateral borders defined by the quadratus lumborum muscle. The floor of the lumbar region consists of the quadratus and psoas muscles. The anterior boundary is the peritoneum. Within this area, the most striking structures are the great vessels and their branches.[1–3] Investing structures around these vessels of importance in urologic oncology are the lymphatics[4,5] and the sympathetic nerves.[6,7]

Visceral structures contained in this area include the kidneys, adrenal glands, second portion of the duodenum, and ureters. Contiguous intraperitoneal structures include the liver, spleen, pancreas and bowel.[1–3]

The iliac portion of the retroperitoneum or "pelvis" extends caudally from the lumbar portion. It is bounded anteriorly by peritoneum and the abdominal wall. The inferior boundaries are the pelvic floor musculature. Within the pelvis, structures of significance include the iliac vasculature, the femoral, obturator, ilioinguinal, and genitofemoral nerves, and the lymphatics. Visceral structures include the bladder, prostate, vagina, uterus, and rectum.[8,9]

Sites of origin of urologic cancers include the penis, scrotum, testes, bladder, urethra, ureters, kidney, prostate, and adrenal gland. In all cases, the structures either lie in the retroperitoneum or have primary or secondary lymphatic drainage (testis, penis) in this region. The close proximity of the visceral structures and their lymphatics to the great vessels reinforces the concept that a majority of retroperitoneal oncologic operations are "vascular procedures," many of the more complex of which require specific expertise and experience to avoid complications and to be performed properly and safely.[6,10] In the past, these skills were primarily acquired through repeated surgical experience in the retroperitoneum and pelvis for benign diseases such as calculi and ureteropelvic junction obstructions.[11] Achieving and maintaining these skills have become more problematic as endourologic procedures and nonsurgical management strategies of stones have expanded.[12,13] Options to overcome these deficiencies include specialized fellowship training in genitourinary oncology and involvement in "nontraditional" procedures such as cadaveric multiorgan recovery,[14–16] organ transplantation,[17–18] and renal vascular surgery.[19–21] These procedures offer opportunities to hone the vascular skills and surgical awareness needed to perform many of the difficult retroperitoneal oncologic procedures safely.[11,22,23]

SURGICAL DECISION PROCESS

When a patient is diagnosed with a malignant urologic disease, a decision process is undertaken to ascertain the most appropriate course of action. This process involves a team approach, with the patient as the primary focus. Two controlling parameters must be considered in all surgical discussions; these are the quantity and the quality of life achievable for the patient. These parameters must be evaluated carefully, so appropriate decisions are reached.

The patient and family need to be informed and educated about the disease process, alternatives, and expectations. A team

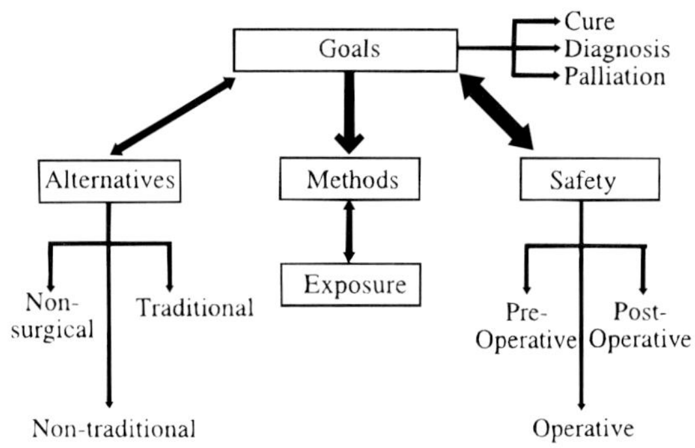

FIG. 5-1. The GAMES (goals, alternatives, methods, exposure, safety) algorithm can be used to teach patients and families about the disease process, to evaluate treatment options, and to establish goals.

approach involving the primary physician, surgical and medical oncologists, radiation oncologists, internal medicine specialists, anesthesiologists, and others may be required to meet these goals. To teach this process, we use a mnemonic we refer to as surgical GAMES, which stands for Goals, Alternatives, Methods, Exposure, and Safety. (Fig. 5-1). Using this algorithm, we evaluate each patient and help the patient select what is believed to be the best treatment option. For some patients, this may include observation, for example, a patient with clinical stage A testis cancer[24] or prostate cancer in patients over the age of 70 years.[25,26] For others with concurrent medical conditions that preclude a safe, surgical approach, alternative therapies may be indicated.[27,28]

Goals

The first step is to define the goals of surgical treatment. These goals include cure, diagnosis, and palliation. All have a role, but everyone involved must understand and agree with the intent. Examples of surgical procedures intended to cure are radical nephrectomy for renal cell cancer and radical prostatectomy for prostate cancer.[28,29] By contrast, a retroperitoneal lymph node dissection for nonseminomatous germ cell cancer may be diagnostic only, although it can result in a surgical cure.[30,31] Another example is renal exploration for a mass not diagnostic of renal cell cancer and treated with nephron-sparing surgery.[32]

Examples of palliative surgery include nephrectomy in the rare case of a patient with incurable renal cell cancer and severe local symptoms such as bleeding.[33] Another example is supravesical diversion for patients with pelvic cancer and ureteral obstruction and azotemia. These individuals often have regional metastases and tumor extension preventing surgical cure, but long-term treatment with nephrostomy tubes may have an adverse impact on their quality of life.[34] Again, these decisions need to consider the likelihood of favorably or adversely affecting the patient's survival and the quality of life.

Alternatives

At this point, it is reasonable to review alternative therapies. This may include reexamination of nonsurgical options, (e.g.,

Table 5-1. *Examples of alternative therapies available for urologic cancer*

Problem	Option
Renal cell cancer	Radical nephrectomy versus nephron-sparing surgery
Transitional cell cancer of the renal pelvis	Nephroureterectomy versus conservative surgery
Invasive bladder cancer	Radical versus partial cystectomy Radical cystectomy versus bladder-sparing therapy
Urinary diversion	Ileal loop versus continent urinary diversion
Nonseminomatous germ cell testis cancer	Retroperitoneal lymph node dissection versus observation Classic retroperitoneal lymph node dissection versus nerve sparing
Prostate cancer	Radical prostatectomy versus alternative therapies
Ureteral cancer	Nephroureterectomy versus partial ureterectomy

combination radiation and chemotherapy for invasive bladder cancer), [35] nontraditional surgical options (e.g., laparoscopic versus open surgery for lymph node dissections),[36] or open surgical alternatives (e.g., nephron-sparing surgery) available to achieve the goal.[37] Although the chapters that address specific problems cover alternative therapy in more detail, a brief listing (Table 5-1) of problems and alternative options illustrates the importance of this exercise.

The patient needs to be informed of the options available for treating the disease and should be encouraged actively to participate in the decision.

Methods

Once the goal has been determined, alternatives examined, and surgery chosen, then the timing the operation, the approach to the tumor, involvement of additional personnel, and any other special requirements need to be examined. Multiple factors (Table 5-2) can influence these decisions, especially the location for the incision and approach to the retroperitoneum.

The choice of incision is directly influenced by the site and extent of the pathologic process. For example, a small renal cell cancer in the upper pole of a kidney is easily approached by a subcostal or modified eleventh rib incision, whereas for a

Table 5-2. *Factors influencing choice of operative incision*

Goals of the operation to be performed
Pathologic and radiographic findings
Concurrent pathologic findings
Body habitus
Previous surgical procedures
Incisional morbidity
Delayed additional therapy (i.e., radiotherapy, chemotherapy, surgery)

large upper pole tumor, the best approach may be through a thoracoabdominal incision.[38] If the patient has vena caval tumor involvement below the liver, a standard approach is usually satisfactory, but if thrombus extends within the liver or above it, an approach using a median sternotomy and venous bypass or cardiopulmonary bypass may be a better alternative.[10,38–39]

If the patient has a history of significant pulmonary disease, avoidance of a thoracic incision can decrease postoperative morbidity.[38] In addition, if the patient has two unrelated lesions, for example, an aortic aneurysm and a renal cell cancer, this situation will influence the route of exposure.[40,41] In obese patients, a modified left flank incision can be superior to a subcostal incision for approaching the kidney and retroperitoneum because the positioning helps to open the retroperitoneal space and rotates the abdominal contents well away from the site of surgery, thereby dramatically improving the surgical exposure.[42] Finally, in patients with significant skeletal deformities (e.g., kyphoscoliosis, meningomyelocele) exposure to the retroperitoneum and pelvis is often severely hampered and may require significant ingenuity on the part of the operating surgeon to achieve adequate exposure.

Previous surgical procedures often make reoperation significantly more difficult because of scarring and adhesions. The choice of incision in these patients may be influenced by a desire to use a previously undisturbed site. In addition, prior retroperitoneal surgery (e.g., aortic aneurysm repair or colon resection) may ablate the usual tissues planes and landmarks and may complicate access and exposure, thereby influencing the route of exposure and operative decisions.[11,43]

In choosing an incision, the surgeon must consider the associated operative morbidity and must attempt, when possible, to balance it against the need for good surgical exposure. As examples, a thoracoabdominal incision is associated with greater morbidity in most cases than a subcostal or an 11th rib incision.[38,40,41] A perineal prostatectomy may result in less postoperative pain and quicker recovery than a radical retropubic prostatectomy, and under appropriate circumstances, it can be more acceptable to the patient.[43,44] Furthermore, the healing characteristics of an incision need to be considered in conjunction with comorbidities such as obesity, chronic obstructive pulmonary disease, and diabetes mellitus, to lessen the likelihood of postoperative wound complications.[40–42]

Finally, the choice of incision may be influenced by the potential for additional therapy. If pelvic radiation, for instance, is to be given postoperatively, an incision that compromises lymphatic drainage the least is desirable. If additional surgery is probable in the future, for example, in patients with superficial transitional cell cancer of the upper urinary tract with nephron sparing, the chosen surgical approach (endoscopic versus open) needs to be carefully weighed.[45–47] All these factors must be evaluated when deciding on the choice of incision.

Although a detailed description of each incision is beyond the intent and scope of this review (Table 5-3), the reader is referred to the specific chapters of interest or to other surgical atlases.[38,40–42] A brief description, however, of the advantages and disadvantages of each incision is appropriate.

Table 5-3. *Surgical incisions to the retroperitoneum and pelvis*

Route of exposure	Incision
Flank	Thoracoabdominal
	Flank incision
	Eleventh rib*
Anterior abdomen	Anterior subcostal/chevron*
	Midline transperitoneal*
	Midline lower abdominal* (extraperitoneal)
	Transplant incision (Gibson)
	Pfannenstiel
	Midline transpubic
Pelvis	Perineal*
	Transcoccygeal
Other	Posterior lumbodorsal

* Most common.

Flank Incisions

The usually cited primary advantage for these incisions is the avoidance of the peritoneum. When dealing with malignant disease, this situation is rarely of great concern.[40] These incisions offer exposure to the retroperitoneum and great vessels that few other approaches can match; however, a true flank incision is rarely used in urologic cancer surgery because the positioning places the vessels at risk at the least accessible portion of the wound.

A thoracoabdominal incision with proper positioning offers excellent unilateral exposure to the upper retroperitoneum, renal vessels, and great vessels above the renal vessels. This approach is primarily indicated when dealing with large adrenal and renal cancers. Its disadvantages are the associated violation of the chest, tedious closure, and postoperative morbidity.[38,40]

The modified 11th rib incision with the patient placed in a 20- to 25-degree flank position offers excellent exposure to the renal vessels and peritoneal contents.[17] This incision can be extended down to allow for a single-incision nephroureterectomy in patients with moderate body habitus.[40] Its primary advantage is the avoidance of the thoracic cavity. Its primary disadvantage is that it is not as useful; for a large upper pole or upper retroperitoneal tumor, and use of this incision in those circumstances may compromise exposure.

Anterior Incisions

A subcostal incision and its bilateral component, the chevron incision, provide good exposure to the renal vessels and good exposure to the upper abdomen and retroperitoneum, depending on the patient's build and the pathologic process.[14,15,38,40] These incisions provide the advantage of excellent strength of closure and a low likelihood of hernia formation. Their use in obese patients may be limited, and these incisions lack versatility for easy extension, especially to provide more cephalad exposure.

Midline incisions are easy to open and close. They provide the best exposure to the combined retroperitoneum and pelvis and are especially useful for retroperitoneal lymph node dissections[5,6] and radical cystectomies.[48] The disadvantages in obese patients are similar to those mentioned earlier, but none of the other surgical incisions offers a better alternative. These incisions do have a greater risk of ventral herniation than either subcostal or paramedian incisions.[40]

The Gibson, or transplant incision, with proper patient positioning, provides excellent exposure to the medial and distal ureter and can be done without incising muscle.[40] This incision can be difficult to extend in either direction for more exposure, but it offers the advantage of excellent healing and low risk of herniation. In properly chosen circumstances, it can be a useful incision.

Pelvic Incisions

The perineal incision is currently limited to radical prostatectomies. Some surgeons have suggested the possibility of doing cystectomies through this incision in combination with laparoscopic lymph node dissections, however.[43,44,49,50] The primary advantage is the significant decrease in pain and the patient's improved postoperative ambulation and recovery. Its disadvantage is lack of flexibility and access to lymphatics or pelvic vessels. The transcoccygeal approach is primarily of historical note,[51] although a series of radical prostatectomies through this approach has been reported.[52]

Finally, the posterior lumbodorsal approach has limited application in urologic oncology. It may, however, be a good choice for small adrenal lesions or for renal lesions in patients with end-stage renal disease that are incidental findings requiring surgical excision.[36,52,53] The advantage is limited postoperative morbidity.

Exposure

Once the choices of positioning and incision are made, the factors related to surgical field control need to be addressed. The three most important elements of surgical control are exposure, exposure, and exposure. Optimal exposure means limiting surgical morbidity, avoiding complications and injury of adjacent structures, being sufficiently flexible to adapt to intraoperative findings, and having uncompromised access to the area of interest (Table 5-4). Compromised exposure can mean increased risk of surgical injury, longer operative time, and possible inability to perform or to complete the operation.[42]

Different approaches may accomplish the desired goals equally well (e.g., radical retropubic prostatectomy versus perineal prostatectomy), based on the surgeon's preference or other considerations.[29,43,44] The old adage that a small incision is for a small surgeon may well hold, however. The patient does not benefit from compromised exposure if it results in an undesirable outcome and if wounds heal from side to side, not from end to end.

Visibility is a key to control in surgery, and the use of three items can dramatically improve surgical visibility, improve the precision of dissection, and decrease bleeding. These are surgical loupes (2.5 × or 3.5 ×), a surgical headlight, and a mechanical retractor.[22,54]

Finally, control of the *entire* surgical field is of paramount importance when dealing with large tumor masses that have extensive neovascularity or obscure or obliterate the normal anatomic landmarks.[11,42] This is especially true for surgery after radiotherapy, chemotherapy, or other operations.[55,56] In such instances, optimal exposure provides not only access to the tumor, but also easy vascular access in the event of vascular injury or if vascular resection is required for complete tumor excision.[11,57] In addition, good exposure provides access to and promotes awareness of adjacent structures such as bowel, spleen, pancreas, and nerves and thereby makes the manipulation of these structures much safer and decreases the likelihood of injury and postoperative complications.

Table 5-4. *Principles of surgical exposure*

Correct incision and positioning
Visualization
Surgical loupes
Headlights
Mechanical retractor
Control
Vascular access
Anatomic awareness

Safety

The GAMES mnemonic is a teaching and clinical guide, and the order of concern is not rigid. The patient's safety needs to be considered early in the decision algorithm. The best indication for an operation is not the ability to perform one, but rather, the presence of factors in the decision algorithm that support the indications for surgery. Again, the decision needs to take into account all factors, and the surgeon must carefully discern the risks to the patient versus the presumed benefits.[58]

Patients undergoing surgery for genitourinary cancer cover the entire age and health span from infants and children to the elderly. As with most solid cancers, urologic cancers most frequently occur in patients 50 years of age and older,[59] and these patients often have comorbidities that need to be evaluated before undertaking surgery[58,60] (Table 5-5). Operative mortality for comparable operations increases four to eight times for patients over the age of 70 years when compared with younger patients (Chap. 29).[61] Concurrent illnesses that decrease cardiac and pulmonary reserves or the immune response add to these risks.[58,60–63]

Table 5-5. *Surgical risk factors*

Age
Poor nutritional status
Obesity
Cardiac disease
Pulmonary disease
Vascular disease
Endocrine disease and hematologic disorder

Preoperative Assessment

Given a patient with good cardiopulmonary function, almost any operation can be performed safely and an uneventful recovery anticipated. Preoperative assessment is of paramount importance in evaluating patients for the presence of comorbidities and in stabilizing these conditions before undertaking the operation. Most operations for genitourinary cancers are elective, allowing for adequate preoperative evaluation and preparation. Most of these evaluations and treatments are performed on an outpatient basis because of cost constraints, and the operating surgeon has the responsibility to make sure these preparations are completed before undertaking surgery.[60–63]

The basis of a preoperative evaluation is a complete history and physical examination. This evaluation includes a complete list of the patient's current medications and allergies, a complete review of systems, and a social history, especially inquiring about use of alcohol and tobacco. Past medical history needs to be reviewed, and information regarding any recent treatments such as chemotherapy or radiotherapy needs to be evaluated. The surgical risks for at least 60% of patients are delineated by these steps alone.[62] Routine preoperative studies are adjusted for age and risk according to the individual patient.[58,60,63,64] Based on the results of the patient's history and physical examination and routine studies, if significant problems are discovered, further evaluation is undertaken.[61,64–73]

Preoperative nutritional status is easily overlooked, especially in patients with cancer. Patients with evidence of preoperative cachexia, defined as a loss of more 12% of body weight in the previous 6 months, need careful evaluation. Cachexia is associated with increased risk of postoperative complications, delayed wound healing, immunocompromise, and respiratory distress.[73] Such patients should have their nutritional catabolism converted to an anabolic state through the use of both parenteral and enteral hyperalimentation before they undergo surgery.[62,73]

Intraoperative Management

Operative risk factors include the type of anesthesia, the operation and inherent risks, the experience of the surgical team, and the availability of hospital resources.[64] These factors are best evaluated using clinical judgment because objective data are often lacking. A team approach involving anesthesiologists, surgeons, primary physicians, and consultants is important in increasing the operative safety. In our program, we individualize the use of invasive monitoring. Depending on the diagnosis, preoperative evaluation, co-morbidities, and operation planned and its attendant risks, we often use central venous monitoring, arterial lines, and Swan-Ganz catheters.[62,70,74,75]

As previously stated, essentially all surgery for cancer in the retroperitoneum is vascular and requires a more than cursory knowledge of vascular surgical techniques and experience in control of surgical bleeding. In all cases, surgical setups should include vascular clamps, needle holders and forceps, and appropriate vascular suture material.[11,22] The surgeon needs to be aware of the most likely sites of bleeding (i.e., lumbar vessels, hypogastric branches, spleen) and prepared to deal appropriately with them.[11,38] Although numerous methods are available, the two best are (1) prevention of bleeding by careful dissection and avoidance of injury and (2) correct surgical repair of any injury. Based on the nature of these tumors, however, vascular injury is often unavoidable, so the surgeon must quickly recognize and control bleeding to prevent intraoperative and postoperative complications.[11,55]

The use of intraoperative blood and blood products needs to be critically monitored because, in addition to the risk of transmission of disease, transfusions can decrease the postoperative immune response, and they have a significant incidence of adverse reactions. Using an intraoperative hemoglobin value of 7 g/dL as a transfusion indicator instead of 10 g/dL may decrease blood use and lessen risks.[76–78] In addition, methods such as the use of cell savers and autologous blood transfusions may be helpful in cancer operations that are expected to result in significant blood loss without identifiable increased risk of metastases.[77]

Postoperative Management

Postoperatively, patients are at increased risk during two unique periods. These are the first 48 hours, when the primary risks are related to anesthesia and the operation itself. In this period, acute myocardial infarction, stroke, respiratory failure, metabolic abnormalities, and operative or technical complications are the most likely to occur. The second period is from 3 to 30 days postoperatively. During this time, postoperative complications such as pulmonary emboli, wound sepsis, peritonitis, bacteremia, and multiorgan failure are more likely to occur.[64,79]

Postoperative management and monitoring are based on a patient's preoperative status, medical history and diagnosis, surgical procedure, and intraoperative events.[62,64,79,80] Judicious use of an intensive care unit is often indicated.[81] Invasive monitoring using a central line, Swan-Ganz catheter, arterial line, and ventilator support may also be appropriate.[62,79,80] Many patients can be treated as safely and as well in less costly settings postoperatively, however, but no compromise with safety should be made for cost savings.[82]

The surgical team's primary responsibility in the postoperative period is the prevention or early recognition of postoperative complications with appropriate therapy.[64,79,80] As we have become better able to prevent and to treat postoperative problems, operative mortality has dropped dramatically, as evidenced by the decline in operative mortality associated with radical cystectomy.[83]

Finally, if the basic principles of preoperative, intraoperative, and postoperative care are observed, and if patients are carefully evaluated and selected, then in most cases identifiable benefit will occur with limited morbidity and acceptable mortality.

REFERENCES

1. Banowsky L. Surgical anatomy. In: Novick AC, Streem SB, Pontes JE, eds. Stewart's operative urology, 2nd ed, vol 1. Baltimore, Williams & Wilkins, 1989:2.
2. Young JD. Retroperitoneal surgery. In: Glenn JF, ed. Urologic surgery, 2nd ed. Hagerstown, MD: Harper & Row, 1975:848.
3. Kabalin JN. Anatomy of the retroperitoneum and kidney. In: Walsh PC, Retik AB, Stamey TA, Vaughn ED, eds. Campbell's urology, 6th ed, vol 1. Philadelphia, WB Saunders, 1992:3.
4. Donohue JP, Zachary JM, Maynard BR. Distribution of nodal metastases in nonseminomators cancer. J Urol 1982;128:315.
5. Donahue JP, Rowland RP. Complications of retroperitoneal lymph node dissection. J Urol 1981;125:338.
6. Donahue JP, Foster RS, Rowland RG, Bihrle R, Jones J. Nerve-sparing retroperitoneal lymphadenectomy with preservation of ejaculation. J Urol 1990;144:287.
7. Richie JP. Clinical stage one testicular cancer: the role of modified retroperitoneal lymphadenectomy. J Urol 1990;144:1160.
8. Redman J. An anatomic approach to the pelvis. In: Crawford ED, Das S, eds. Current genitourinary cancer surgery. Philadelphia, Lea & Febiger, 1990:140.

9. Tanagho EA. Anatomy of the lower urinary tract. In: Walsh PC, Retik AB, Stamey TA, Vaughn ED, eds. Campbell's urology, 6th ed, vol 1. Philadelphia, WB Saunders, 1992:40.
10. Marshall FF, Dietrick KD, Baumgartner WA, Reitz BA. Surgical management of renal cell carcinoma with intracaval neoplastic extension above hepatic veins. J Urol 1988;139:1166.
11. Zinman L, Libertino JA. Control of bleeding in upper urinary tract and retroperitoneal surgery. Urol Clin North Am 1988;15:139.
12. Karlin GS, Smith AD. Endopyelotomy. Urol Clin North Am 1988;15: 439.
13. Riehle RA, Naslund E. Patient management and results after ESWL. In: Riehle RA, eds. Principles of extracorporeal shock wave lithotripsy. New York, Churchill Livingstone, 1987:121.
14. Marsh CL, Lange PH. Exposure of the upper retroperitoneum (URP): revelations from liver and pancreas transplantation and retrieval. J Urol 1992;147:434A. Abstract.
15. Marsh CL, Lange PH. Liver transplant and organ retrieval techniques for upper retroperitoneal cases in urology. J Urol 1994;151:201A. Abstract.
16. Starzl TE, Hakala TR, Shaw BW, et al. A flexible procurement of multiple cadaveric organ procurement. Surg Gynecol Obstet 1984;158: 223.
17. Lowell JA, Taylor RJ. The evaluation of the living donor, surgical techniques and results. Semin Urol 1994;12:102.
18. Khauli RB. Surgical aspects of renal transplantation: new approaches. Urol Clin North Am 1994;21:321.
19. Novick AC, Jackson CL, Straffon RA. The role of autotransplantation in complex urologic reconstruction. J Urol 1990;143:452.
20. Libertino JA, Beckmann CF. Surgery and percutaneous angioplasty in the management of renovascular hypertension. Urol Clin North Am 1994;21:235.
21. Libertino JA, Zinman L. Revascularization of the poorly functioning and non-functioning kidney. In: Novick AC, Straffon RA, eds. Vascular problems in urologic surgery. Philadelphia, WB Saunders, 1982:173.
22. Banowsky LH. Basic principles and techniques of vascular surgery. In: Novick AC, Straffon RA, eds. Vascular problems in urologic surgery. Philadelphia: WB Saunders, 1982:3.
23. Bartle EJ, Edwards WS. Vascular surgery for the urologic oncologist. In: Crawford ED, Das S, eds. Current genitourinary cancer surgery. Philadelphia, Lea & Febiger, 1990:646.
24. Sogani P. Evaluation of the management of stage I non-seminomatous germ-cell tumors of the testis. Urol Clin North Am 1991;18:561.
25. Chodak GW, Thisted RA, Gerber GS, et al. Results of conservative management of clinically localized prostate cancer. N Engl J Med 1994; 330:242.
26. Smith PH. The case for no initial treatment of localized prostate cancer. Urol Clin North Am 1990;17:827.
27. Wajsman Z, Marino R, Parsons J, Oblon D, McCarley D. Bladder-sparing approach in invasive cancer. Semin Urol 1990;8:210.
28. Robson CJ. Radical nephrectomy for renal cell carcinoma. J Urol 1963; 89:37.
29. Walsh PC. Radical retropubic prostatectomy. In: Walsh PC, Gittes RF, Perlmutter AD, Stamey TA, eds. Campbell's textbook of urology, 6th ed, vol 3. Philadelphia, WB Saunders, 1986:2754.
30. Pizzocuro G, Salvioni R, Zanoni F. Unilateral lymphadenectomy in intraoperative stage I non-seminomatous germinal testis cancer. J Urol 1985;134:485.
31. Braedel JJ, Vugrin D, Whitmore WF Jr. Selected experience with surgery and combination chemotherapy in the treatment of non-seminomatous testis tumors. J Urol 1983;129:985.
32. Montie JE. The incidental renal mass. Urol Clin North Am 1991;18: 427.
33. Couillard DR, deVere White RW. Surgery of renal cell carcinoma. Urol Clin North Am 1993;20:263.
34. Montie JE. Cutaneous urinary diversion. In: Novick AC, Streem SB, Pontes JE, eds. Stewart's operative urology, 2nd ed, vol 1. Baltimore, Williams & Wilkins, 1989:425.
35. Kaufman DS, Shipley WU, Griffin PP, Heney NM, Althausen AF, Efird JT. Selective bladder preservation by combination treatment of invasive bladder cancer. N Engl J Med 1993;329:1377.
36. Winfield HN. Laparoscopic pelvic lymph node dissection: application to genitourinary malignancies. In: Gomella LG, Kozminski M, Winfield HN, eds. Laparoscopic urologic surgery. New York, Raven, 1994: 111.
37. Taylor RJ. Case for nephron-sparing surgery in managing renal cell carcinoma. Semin Urol 1993;11:104.
38. Novick AC, Streem SB. Surgery of the kidney. In: Walsh PC, Retik AB, Stamey TA, Vaugh ED, eds. Campbell's urology, 6th ed, vol 3. Philadelphia, WB Saunders, 1992:2413.
39. Burt M. Inferior vena caval involvement by renal cell carcinoma. Urol Clin North Am 1991;18:437.
40. Montague DK. Surgical incisions. In: Novick AC, Streem SB, Pontes JE, eds. Stewart's operative urology, vol 1. Baltimore, William & Wilkins, 1989:15.
41. Grayhack JT. Renal surgery. In: Glenn JF. Urologic surgery, 2nd ed. Hagerstown MD: Harper & Row, 1975:48.
42. Montie JE. Operative approaches to pelvic structures. In: Novick AC, Streem SB, Pontes JE, eds. Stewart's operative urology, vol 2. Baltimore, Williams & Wilkins, 1989:479.
43. Lerner SE, Fleishmann J, Taub HC, Chamberlin JW, Kahan NZ, Melman A. Combined laparoscopic pelvic lymph node dissection and modified Belt radical perineal prostatectomy for localized prostate adenocarcinoma. Urology 1994;43:493.
44. Resnick MI. Editorial comment. Urology 1994;43:498.
45. Oriheula E, Smith AD. Percutaneous treatment of transitional cell carcinoma of the upper urinary tract. Urol Clin North Am 1988;15:425.
46. Murphy DM, Zincke H, Furlow WL. Primary grade I transitional cell carcinoma of the renal pelvis and ureter. J Urol 1980;123:629.
47. Seaman EK, Slavin KM, Benson MC. Treatment options for upper tract transitional-cell carcinoma. Urol Clin North Am 1993;20:349.
48. Freiha FS. Open bladder surgery. In: Walsh PC, Retik AB, Stamey TA, Vaughn ED. Campbell's urology, 6th ed. Philadelphia, WB Saunders, 1992;2:2750.
49. Crawford ED, Wolach M. Perineal cystoprostatectomy. In: Olsson CA, ed. Surgical techniques in urology, vol 6. Wilmington, DE, Medical Publications, Inc. 1993:2.
50. Williams RD. Surgery of the seminal vesicles. In: Walsh PC, Retic AB, Stamey TA, Vaughn ED, eds. Campbell's urology, 6th ed, vol 3. Philadelphia, WB Saunders, 1992:2942.
51. Rigahi P, DaPozzo L, Francesca F, Broglia L, Montorsi F, Guazzoni G. Radical transcoccygeal prostatectomy. J Urol 1994;151:202A. Abstract.
52. Novick AC. Posterior approach to the adrenal gland. In: Novick AC, Streem SB, Pontes JE., eds. Stewart's operative urology, 2nd ed, vol 1. Baltimore, Williams & Wilkins, 1989:68.
53. Schmidt NIS. Strategic management of adrenal tumors. Oncology 1994;8:73.
54. Marshall FF, Brooks JD, Schoenberg MP. Partial nephrectomy: new techniques. J Urol 1994;151:202A. Abstract V9.
55. Ritchie JP. Complications of retroperitoneal lymph node dissection. AUA Update Series 1993;12(Lesson 16):122.
56. Nabors W, Crawford ED. Salvage cystectomy after irradiation failure. In: Crawford ED, Das S, eds. Current genitourinary cancer Surgery. Philadelphia, Lea & Febiger, 1990:253.
57. Smith RB. Surgical management of retroperitoneal tumors. In: Crawford ED, Das S, eds. Current genitourinary cancer surgery. Philadelphia, Lea & Febiger, 1990:128.
58. Waters JM, McClaran JL. The elderly surgical patient. In: Wilmore DW, Brennan MF, Harken AH, Holcroft JW, Meakins JL, eds. Care of the surgical patient, vol 2. New York, Scientific American, 1989; VII:13:2.
59. Boring CC, Squires TS, Tong T. Cancer statistics, 1993. CA Cancer J Clin 1993;43:7.
60. Moon RE. Preoperative evaluation. Probl Urol 1992;6:1.
61. Cole WH. Medical differences between the young and the aged. J Am Geriatr Soc 1970;18:589.
62. Brendler CB. Perioperative care. In: Walsh PC, Retic AB, Stamey TA, Vaughn ED, eds. Campbell's urology, 6th ed, vol 3. Philadelphia, WB Saunders, 1992:2315.
63. Curreri PW, Moylan JA. Preparation for elective surgery. In: Wilmore DW, Brennan MF, Harken AH, Holcroft JW, Meakins JL, eds. Care of the surgical patient, vol 2. New York, Scientific American, 1989; 1:3.
64. Christou NV. Evaluation of operative risk. In: Wilmore DW, Brennan MF, Harken AH, Holcroft JW, Meakins JL, eds. Care of the surgical patient, vol 2. New York, Scientific American, 1989;V:2:3.
65. Eiseman B. Necessary preoperative tests. In: Wilmore DW, Brennan

MF, Harken AH, Holcroft JW, Meakins JL, eds. Care of the surgical patient, vol 5. New York: Scientific American, 1989;V:3:3.
66. Caldwell MD. Diabetes mellitus: Perioperative management of the diabetic patient. In: Wilmore DW, Brennan MF, Harken AH, Holcroft JW, Meakins JL, eds. Care of the surgical patient, vol 2. New York, Scientific American, 1989;VII:1:3.
67. Rizzo RJ, Tilney NL. Renal dysfunction: perioperative management of the patient with renal failure. In: Wilmore DW, Brennan MF, Harken AH, Holcroft JW, Meakins JL, eds. Care of the surgical patient, vol 2. New York, Scientific American, 1989:2:1.
68. Sugerman HJ. Obesity: approach to the morbidly obese patient. In: Wilmore DW, Brennan MF, Harken AH, Holcroft JW, Meakins JL, eds. Care of the surgical patient, vol 7. New York, Scientific American, 1989;VII:4:3.
69. Bartlett RH. Pulmonary insufficiency: approach to pulmonary insufficiency. In: Wilmore DW, Brennan MF, Harken AH, Holcroft JW, Meakins JL, eds. Care of the surgical patient, vol 7. New York, Scientific American, 1989;VII:6:3.
70. Fullerton DA, Harken AH. Cardiac insufficiency: preoperative cardiac assessment. In: Wilmore DW, Brennan MF, Harken AH, Holcroft JW, Meakins JL, eds. Care of the surgical patient, vol 7. New York, Scientific American, 1989;VII:7:3.
71. Addonizio VP. Thrombotic problems: approach to thrombotic complications. In: Wilmore DW, Brennan MF, Harken AH, Holcroft JW, Meakins JL, eds. Care of the surgical patient, vol 7. New York, Scientific American, 1989;VII:8:3.
72. Gann DS. Adrenal insufficiency: management of the patient with known on suspected steroid deficiency. In: Wilmore DW, Brennan MF, Harken AH, Holcroft JW, Meakins JL, eds. Care of the surgical patient, vol 7. New York, Scientific American, 1989;VII:9:3.
73. Daly J. Malnutrition: approach to nutritional management of elective surgical patients. In: Wilmore DW, Brennan MF, Harken AH, Holcroft JW, Meakins JL, eds. Care of the surgical patient, vol 7. New York, Scientific American, 1989;VII:12:3.
74. Lumb PD, Cohen IL. Non invasive monitoring. Prob Urol 1992;6:29.
75. Cohen IL, Lumb PD. Monitoring blood pressure. Prob Urol 1992;6:56.
76. Addonizio VP, Stahl RF. Bleeding. In: Wilmore DW, Brennan MF, Harken AH, Holcroft JW, Meakins JL, eds. Care of the surgical patient, vol 1. New York, Scientific American, 1989;I:7:3.
77. Greenberg AG. Indications for transfusion. In: Wilmore DW, Brennan MF, Harken AH, Holcroft JW, Meakins JL, eds. Care of the surgical patient, vol 1. New York, Scientific American, 1989;I:6:3.
78. Klimberg IW. Autotransfusion and blood conservation in urology (Lesson 16). AUA Update Series 1990;9:122.
79. Sheldon GF, Rutledge R. Postoperative management. In: Wilmore DW, Brennan MF, Harken AH, Holcroft JW, Meakins JL, eds. Care of the surgical patient, vol 2. New York, Scientific American, 1989;VI:6:3.
80. Raghavan K, Cohen IL, Lumb PD. Postoperative care. Prob Urol 1992;6:79.
81. Demling RH. Surgical patients in the ICU: administrative Issues. In: Wilmore DW, Brennan MF, Harken AH, Holcroft JW, Meakins JL, eds. Care of the surgical patient, vol 2. New York, Scientific American, 1989;X:4:2.
82. Lindenauer SM, Ashcraft ML, Lound JL, Zuidema GD. Cost containment. In: Wilmore DW, Brennan MF, Harken AH, Holcroft JW, Meakins JL, eds. Care of the surgical patient, vol 2. New York, Scientific American, 1989;V:4:3.
83. Lerner SP, Skinner E, Skinner DG. Radical cystectomy in regionally advanced bladder care. Urol Clin North Am 1992;19:713.

Principles and Practice of Genitourinary Oncology, edited by Derek Raghavan, Howard I. Scher, Steven A. Leibel, and Paul H. Lange. Lippincott-Raven Publishers, Philadelphia, © 1997.

CHAPTER 6

Principles of Endoscopic Surgery for Genitourinary Cancer

Howard N. Winfield

The emblem on the cover of the *Journal of Urology* depicts a urologist performing an endoscopic procedure. This symbolizes the important and central role endoscopy has played in the specialty of urology and why urologists have always been leaders in the use of minimally invasive procedures. The origins of endoscopy can be clearly traced to 1805, when Bozzini reported the use of the "lichtleiter" for visualization of the human urethra.[1] However, it was really Nitze[1a] in 1877 who helped develop the cystoscope by employing lenses for magnification of the operative field. A few years later, in 1890, the invention of the incandescent bulb by Edison ushered in a new generation of endoscopes. The modern era of endoscopy was introduced by Hopkins and Kapany in 1952 with the development of fiberoptics.[2] Refinements in rigid and flexible endoscopic instrumentation in conjunction with the explosion of video technology has further improved this technique. These technologic advances are being extended to the development of laparoscopic equipment that will allow the successful completion of many new and previously unimaginable urolaparoscopic procedures.

This chapter elucidates the state-of-the-art techniques in endourology and laparoscopic surgery with respect to urooncologic diseases. Indications and rationales for approaching urologic malignancies in a minimally invasive fashion are discussed. The basic techniques and instrumentation of endoscopy and laparoscopy are reviewed to allow the safe and effective completion of these surgical procedures.

ENDOUROLOGIC APPLICATIONS FOR UROLOGIC MALIGNANCIES

Transurethral Surgery of the Lower Urinary Tract

The cystoscope and resectoscope were the key instruments that allowed urology to become a separate surgical specialty, distinct from general surgery. Transurethral surgery of the lower urinary tract has undergone significant improvements and increases in applications over the past 25 years. This form of surgery plays an integral role in the management and staging of lower urinary tract malignancies.

Resection suites require, at a minimum, the following equipment:

- calibrating male sounds (grooved van Buren)
- 12- or 30-degree foroblique lens
- 24-, 26-, or 28-Fr resectoscope (Iglesias or Stern-McCarthy)
- 90-degree loops
- rollerball electrode
- biopsy forceps
- irrigating syringe or evacuator for cytology (Toomey or Ellik)
- irrigating solution—sterile water or isotonic fluid (glycine 1.5%)

In addition to the standard equipment, certain ancillary pieces are helpful in completing transurethral surgery in an effective and safe fashion.

- angled bladder wall loop
- flexible 15- or 18-Fr choledochonephroscope
- continuous flow resectoscope
- Nd:Yag laser unit and fiber
- video equipment
    - split- or full-beam CCD camera chip
    - digital imaging video monitor
    - video recorder, printer, and still camera
    - television monitor

A continuous-flow resectoscope may be helpful in individuals with a small-capacity bladder or in situations in which there is abundant tumor and time cannot be expended for repeated bladder emptying. By maintaining the amount of irrigant within the bladder at a constant volume, the risk of perforation should be diminished. The use of angled loops are ideal for tumors on the lateral, posterior, or dome regions of the bladder and should also help to reduce the risk of perforation.[3] Flexible cystoscopes are ideal not only for monitoring bladder recurrences but also in treating tiny superficial tumors with laser or electrocautery instruments within the office setting. Furthermore, the ability of the flexible cystoscope to retrovert enables the urologist to visualize the anterior bladder neck, where bladder tumors may be hidden.

With the advent of video technology, the urologist acquired the capacity to move away from the cystoscopic eyepiece and view the procedure on a large video monitor. This decreases the urologists risk of facial and ocular contamination with the patient's potentially life-threatening bodily fluids and eliminates strain on the surgeon's back and neck. Furthermore, other individuals present in the operating room may view the progress of the transurethral procedure, thus providing an important teaching tool not only for the residents but also for the nursing staff.

Bladder Cancer

Management Using Electrocautery and Lasers

Important characteristics to consider when cystoscopically evaluating a patient with cancer of the bladder are the appearance, location, size, and number of tumors. Superficial or papillary tumors generally suggest the absence of bladder muscle wall invasion and thus predict a better prognosis than tumors that appear sessile and wide-based. The amount of tumor and the degree of lateral and downward extension may obviate complete resection and necessitate a diagnostic rather than a therapeutic procedure. Complete resection may not be possible with multiple tumors or with tumors covering extensive surface areas of the bladder. Similarly, tumors located within bladder diverticula or on the anterior bladder neck region may be difficult to access, thus necessitating alternate treatment approaches. Chapter 25 discusses in detail the technique of bladder tumor resection.

The 1060-nm wavelength of the neodymium:yttrium-aluminum-garnet (Nd:Yag) laser has been found to be effective for the treatment of superficial tumors of the bladder. The power is normally set at 35 to 40 W, and the energy can be applied in a noncontact or contact mode, depending on the fiber tip employed. The 400- to 600-μm laser fiber is easily passed through the working port of a rigid or flexible cystoscope. Using the continuous mode, the surgeon applies the laser point slowly across the tumor bed until the tissue blanches.[4]

Because there is less pain and minimal to no bleeding with laser treatment, it can be performed in the office setting with the patient under local anesthesia supplemented with intravenous sedation. A Foley catheter is usually not required in the postoperative period, and intravesical chemotherapy may be started earlier than with electrocautery resection because there should be minimal disruption of the urothelium and no perforation.

Considerable debate exists regarding whether laser treatment is superior to a simple electrocautery of the tumor with a Bugbee electrode. Some investigators have reported that laser treatment of bladder tumors reduces the rate of superficial bladder tumor recurrences.[5] It is believed that bladder tumor recurrences may be the result of implantation of tumor cells at the time of earlier resection. Because of the decreased risk of perforation, laser treatment of bladder tumors located within bladder diverticuli should be considered in high-risk, poor surgical candidates. Furthermore, tumors in the region of the ureteric orifices may be effectively treated with lasers with a decreased risk of stenosis of the orifice compared with electrocautery.

In addition to the significant expense of laser equipment and need for specialized training, the major disadvantage of the use of laser technology for the treatment of bladder cancer is the absence of satisfactory pathologic material for subsequent examination. Another major concern is the risk of bowel perforation. Approximately 20% to 30% of the laser energy is transmitted as forward scatter beyond the point of impact. Laser treatment of tumors located on the dome or anterior regions of the bladder runs the risk of injuring adjacent small bowel. This concern may be accentuated in the presence of tumors within bladder diverticula. In addition to abiding by the usual recommended parameters for laser power and time duration, the concomitant use of laparoscopy has been advocated. Loops of small bowel may be mobilized away from the intraperitoneal surface of the bladder and thereby protected.[6] In poor-risk patients with invasive bladder tumors, the combined use of transurethral resection of the mucosa and muscle layers with laparoscopic laser fulguration of the serosa may be considered.

Endoscopic Management of Complications Related to Urinary Diversions

Urinary diversion following removal of the bladder has been the source of many complications requiring endoscopic management. The most significant and difficult of these is ureterointestinal anastomotic strictures. With the advent of newer types of diversions and bladder replacement (orthotopic), the complexity of managing this problem has increased.

It is critical to fully review the operative details of the ureterointestinal anastomosis to determine whether it is refluxing, nonrefluxing, direct, or conjoined, and to what portion of the bowel the ureter is attached. Antegrade studies must be obtained and the function of the involved renal unit determined before embarking on an endoscopic procedure. Recurrent tumor within or surrounding the distal ureter must be evaluated by axial computed tomography.

In most cases, access to the stricture in a retrograde fashion is not possible because of the inability to locate and then navigate the obstructed ureterointestinal region. However, attempts should be made in the office setting using a 15-Fr flexible choledochonephroscope. If success is obtained, a double-J catheter is placed temporarily until general anesthesia can be scheduled. Subsequent management is identical to that described later for the antegrade approach.

Access to the kidney follows usual percutaneous techniques via a posterior upper or middle calyx. This allows a relatively straight route down the ureter to the region of the stricture. In most cases, the upper collecting system is dilated and can be easily punctured under ultrasonographic or fluoroscopic guidance.

The patient is positioned and prepared in semiprone position on the fluoroscopic table so the surgeon has access not only to the flank but also to the stoma of the urinary diversion. If a bladder replacement with urethra is present, prone flexible urethroscopy and pouchoscopy will be required. The percutaneous tract is dilated to the size of a 24-Fr Amplatz sheath, which will easily accommodate the flexible 15-Fr choledochonephroscope or smaller ureteropyeloscope. By advancing the scope down the dilated proximal ureter, the area of narrowing is identified, and any suspicious tissue should be biopsied and sent for frozen pathologic sectioning. Cytologic washings should also be obtained.

Attempts should be made to manipulate a 0.035″ Bentson or hydrophilic guidewire through the strictured area and retrieve it from within the diversion or orthotopic bladder substitution. Having gained a through-and-through guidewire, this is exchanged for a stiffer guidewire such as an 0.038″ Amplatz stiff or superstiff. At this point in the procedure, the surgeon has excellent control over the collecting system and can feel comfortable that the tract will not be lost.

After sheathing the guidewire to prevent arcing of the electrocurrent, a 2- to 3-Fr Greenwald electrode is passed through the working port of the flexible scope, and the strictured area is incised using a low cutting current. There is no right or wrong place to incise. Obviously, the surgeon should avoid areas of pulsation (posterior), realizing that loops of bowel may be lying just anterior to the stricture. The depth of incision should be through the visualized scar tissue until supple fatty tissue or bleeding periureteral tissue is seen. In many cases, this level cannot be safely obtained, and ureteral balloon dilation is routinely performed.

To correctly position the ureteral balloon, the area of stricture must be accurately determined. The flexible scope is advanced to the proximal aspect of the stricture. Under fluoroscopic guidance, a 22-gauge spinal needle is placed into the patient's back in a subcutaneous plane so that it overlies the tip of the flexible scope. In this way, a 4-cm length of ureteral balloon dilation catheter is positioned such that the radiopaque markers are above and below the fluoroscopically positioned needle (Fig. 6-1). The balloon is inflated with contrast to a diameter of 15- to 18-Fr at 12 atmospheres of pressure. Often, the surgeon can see the waist of the stricture disappear on fluoroscopy.

The ureteral balloon catheter is removed, and the flexible scope is advanced down to the area of surgery. The strictured area is reevaluated, and further cutting and ballooning may be undertaken (Fig. 6-2). Careful injection of contrast is done to determine good flow into the diversion (bladder substitution) and to minimize contrast extravasation. The region is then stented using a suitably sized 14/7-Fr endopyelotomy catheter (Cook Urological, Spencer, IN) with the 14-Fr segment placed distally. This catheter is left in place for 4 to 6 weeks. An 8- to 10-Fr pigtail catheter is left as a percutaneous nephrostomy tube and capped after 3 to 5 days. It is my policy to leave this small nephrostomy tube in place to act as a safety valve if the endopyelotomy catheter does not drain well or if the obstruction at the ureterointestinal region persists after removal of the endopyelotomy catheter. After removal of the endopyelotomy tube by the stoma or using a transurethral route, an antegrade study through the pigtail catheter and a renal scan are performed 2 weeks later. Follow-up renal scan is repeated in 3 to 6 months.

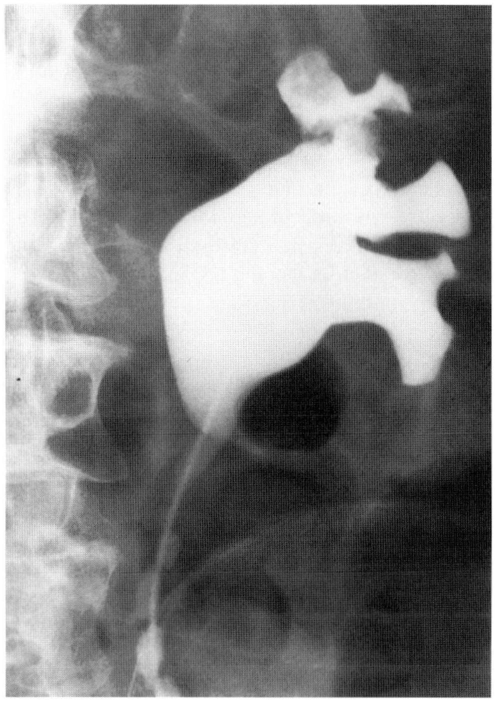

FIG. 6-2. Superficial low-grade transitional cell carcinoma involving the medial wall of the renal pelvis.

When a guidewire cannot be manipulated through the strictured region, the chances of success with the endoscopic approach are minimal. The surgeon can attempt to blindly puncture through the stricture using the stiff end of the guidewire under fluoroscopic and endoscopic visualization. Alternatively, the surgeon can cut to the light using simultaneous flexible scopes from both antegrade and retrograde approaches. Clearly,

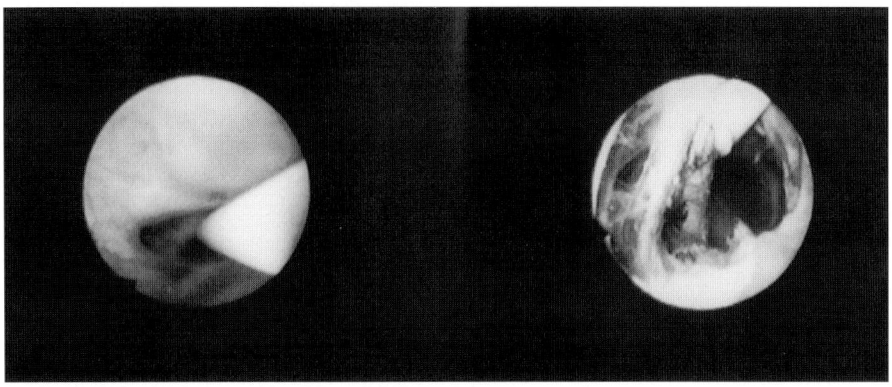

FIG. 6-1. Appearance of ureterointestinal stricture before incision and dilation. Subsequent intraoperative appearance of stricture after electroincision and dilation. (See Color Figure 6-1.)

these techniques engender the considerable risks of perforation, hemorrhage, and loss of the tract. If in fact, these procedures are successful, a through-and-through guidewire is obtained, and the procedure continues as described previously.

A fluoroscopically positioned 8-mm balloon catheter with a 100-μm electrocautery cutting wire (Acucise balloon, Applied Medical Systems, Laguna Hills, CA) has been marketed as a potential tool for incising ureteropelvic junction obstructions using a retrograde approach.[7] This balloon has been employed for ureterointestinal strictures but has met with limited success and significant complications. Its use for ureterointestinal strictures is not advised.

Up to 20% of patients with ileal conduits develop renal calculi during prolonged periods of observation.[8] These stones may result from metabolic abnormalities, but the vast majority result from colonization of the urine by urea-splitting organisms, compounded by urinary stasis leading to the formation of infection stones (i.e., struvite or calcium carbonate). With the advent of continent diversions and orthotopic bladder replacement surgery, the exuberant use of surgical staples act as a nidus for stone encrustation. This may be compounded by the need for intermittent catheterization acting as another avenue for upper tract or pouch stone formation.[9]

Renal and most upper ureteral stones smaller than 3 cm can be managed effectively with extracorporeal shockwave lithotripsy (ESWL) and careful management of urinary tract infections. Larger stones require a percutaneous approach to stone removal, using electrohydraulic or ultrasonic fragmentation. Stones within a diversion or pouch usually can be managed using a rigid cystoscope or 15-Fr flexible choledochonephroscope with a 3- to 5-Fr electrohydraulic lithotripsy probe for fragmentation and removal. Staples that have eroded through the mucosa and are exposed to urine should be grasped and removed.[10,11]

Prostate Cancer

Incidentally discovered cancer of the prostate occurs in about 10% of patients at the time of transurethral resection. When the grade of the tumor is well differentiated (Gleason score <5) and less than 5% of the submitted pathologic specimen is involved with adenocarcinoma (T1A), many series indicate that no further treatment is necessary.[12,13] This approach may not apply in the patient younger than 65 years of age. When the tumor is less well differentiated or a larger percentage of the sample contains cancer (T1B), further treatment is suggested. Transurethral surgery is not advocated as primary curative therapy for clinically known prostate cancer (see Chapters 49 and 50).

Transurethral prostate surgery is advocated in the following situations:

Primary bladder transitional cell cancer involving the prostatic urethral mucosa with carcinoma in situ but not involving the stroma.[14] This may occur in 10% to 15% of cases of associated bladder tumor. The resection may be curative, and destruction of the bladder neck (internal) sphincter mechanism allows satisfactory bathing of the prostatic fossa with intravesical chemotherapy, if prescribed.[15]

As a palliative technique in patients with hormone-refractory cancer of the prostate who have a significant obstructive component requiring catheter drainage or are not responsive to androgen ablation.

Intractable or recurrent hematuria not responsive to temporary catheter tamponade, androgen ablation, or laser fulguration.

Postprostatectomy Injection Therapy for Urinary Incontinence

Depending on the study and the authors' definition, persistent significant urinary leakage occurs in 0% to 12.5% of patients following radical prostatectomy for cancer of the prostate. The rate of significant urinary incontinence following transurethral resection of the prostate should be negligible (1% or less).

A variety of injectable agents have been employed to create a suitable mucosal seal and recreate the continence line within the intraabdominal urethra.[16] Glutaraldehyde-crosslinked bovine collagen (Contigen, Bard Urological, Covington, GA) is the agent used in men after allergy to this material has been excluded. Because of the less compliant and short male urethra, at least two injections are required to obtain satisfactory coaptation.[17] Chances of success are minimal if the patient has also had adjunctive radiotherapy. Results with autologous fat have been poor for postprostatectomy incontinence.

The technique for transurethral injection of Contigen is simple, but there is a learning curve related to understanding when sufficient material has been injected. Using a 21-Fr panendoscope, a 23-gauge flexible needle is passed through the working port and advanced into the urethra wall to gain a submucosal plane just proximal to the external sphincter and is slowly moved proximal through the anastomotic ring. In postprostatectomy patients, it is sometimes difficult to obtain the correct tissue depth with the needle. Generally, four quadrants are circumferentially injected until urethral coaptation is apparent.

Urethral Cancer

Carcinoma of the urethra is rare and occurs more frequently in women than in men. In men, 60% of urethral cancers are found within the bulbomembranous region, 35% within the pendulous urethra, and 5% within the prostatic urethra. Squamous cell carcinoma is by far the most common histology, with transitional cell cancer composing 15% and adenocarcinoma or undifferentiated tumors composing 5%.

Endoscopic techniques are primarily used for visualization and biopsy of distal and proximal urethral tumors. The location and stage of tumor dictates the extent and type of therapy. It is important to determine involvement of the corpora cavernosa and prostatic stroma. There is no role for endoscopic curative therapy other than as an aid to planned radiotherapy, chemotherapy, or both.

Endoscopic Surgery of the Upper Urinary Tract

Transitional cell cancer involving primarily the upper urinary tract is rare, accounting for 2% to 4% only of all urothelial tumors cases. It has been reported that individuals who have previously been treated for bladder cancer have a 2% to 4%

likelihood of developing an upper tract tumor.[18] In order to diminish the risk of tumor recurrence, the standard form of treatment for transitional cell cancer involving the renal pelvis and proximal two thirds of the ureter has been nephroureterectomy with excision of bladder cuff.[19] This surgical approach, although radical, is associated with a 5 year survival rate of over 80% if the tumor is low grade and does not invade into or through the muscular wall of the upper collecting system (Stage Tis, TA, T1). For patients with high grade and stage of tumor, the prognosis is poor with either conservative or radical surgery. Tumors of the distal ureter may be treated by distal ureterectomy and bladder cuff with psoas hitch, Boari's ureterovesical reimplantation, or both.[20] However, in the following select clinical situations, consideration must be given to an endoscopic treatment approach (see Chap. 32):

- solitary kidney with low-grade tumor
- bilateral synchronous low-grade transitional cell cancer of the upper urinary system
- preexisting renal insufficiency
- preoperative evidence of a single, low-grade, superficial tumor smaller than 1 cm
- severe medical problems in the presence of significant hematuria or upper tract obstruction
- patient preference after informed consent

Over the past 10 years, endoscopic approaches to transitional cell cancer of the upper collecting system have been used both diagnostically and for therapeutic intervention. Rigid and flexible ureteropyeloscopy is highly effective in the diagnosis of upper tract tumors, with success rates of 86% to 90% for renal pelvic and ureteral tumors, respectively.[21,22] Clearly, endoscopic treatment of upper tract transitional cell cancer is more controversial, and the critical question is not whether it can be done but whether this minimally invasive treatment is cancer sparing or treating. Long-term follow-up is minimal but indicates that in select cases the endoscopic approach is highly effective with minimal complications; however, it does remain a controversial approach. The inherent risks of ureteroscopy perforation with seeding of the retroperitoneal space, hypothetical pyelovenous and lymphatic backflow with spread of tumor cells, and inadequate or inaccurate staging or treatment must be weighed against the potential benefits of sparing a renal unit by the endourologic approach.

Ureteroscopic Treatment

The retrograde ureteroscopic approach is preferable to the percutaneous approach primarily because it is a closed procedure and the urinary tract is not violated. The distal ureter is easily accessed using the rigid ureteroscope, which may have an outer diameter as small as 6.9 Fr with a working channel that accepts 3-Fr instruments. Limitations include the ability to reach the proximal two thirds of the ureter, renal pelvis, and calyceal system. The actively deflectable ureteropyeloscopes that use fiberoptic bundles have outer diameters as narrow as 8.5 Fr or smaller with 2.5-Fr working channels; these have revolutionized urologists' ability to treat lesions of the upper collecting system. The actively deflectable ureteropyeloscopes have primary deflection in two directions of 100/160 degrees and additional secondary (passive) deflection, making inspection of all calyces, including the lower group, possible. Secondary deflection is obtained by initially obtaining maximum active (primary) deflection and then advancing the ureteroscope forward to allow the softer segment of the scope to passively deflect just proximal to the actively deflected segment.

Technique

The technical aspects of rigid and flexible ureteroscopy are beyond the scope of this chapter. The goal is to minimize trauma to the urothelium; therefore, placement of guidewires and ureteroscopes should be performed in a careful and atraumatic fashion. A 0.035″ Bentson safety wire is required in all cases, whereas a 0.038″ Amplatz stiff working wire is helpful for placing the flexible ureteropyeloscope. Fluoroscopic monitoring is mandatory.

The tumor is identified and may be treated using the 12.5-Fr ureteroresectoscope, which resects the tumor using a suitably sized electrocautery loop. Alternatively, the tumor may be grasped using 3-Fr or smaller grasping-cup biopsy forceps, flat-wire baskets, or spherical baskets and the residual tumor and base fulgurated using a 2- to 3-Fr Greenwald electrocautery probe or Nd:Yag 400-μm laser fiber. When using electrocautery, the surgeon must remember to shield the safety guidewire with a 5-Fr open-ended ureteral catheter to prevent arcing of the current. Alternatively, the Bentson guidewire may be exchanged for a hydrophilic coated guidewire, which will not conduct the electrocautery energy.

As described for bladder cancer, the Nd:Yag laser is a highly effective tool in the endoscopic treatment of upper tract tumors. The laser permits deep irradiation of the ureteral wall and renal pelvis without the risk of perforation and urine extravasation.[23] Furthermore, the minimal denuding of the urothelium by laser therapy is thought to decrease the number of recurrences compared with electrocautery resection. The rate of stricture is reportedly less with laser energy than with electrocautery.[24]

Follow-up of upper tract transitional cell cancer should be by urine cytology, cystoscopy, and upper tract contrast study (intravenous pyelography or retrograde ureterography) performed every 3 months. However, it has been the experience of many urologists that small recurrent tumors seen at ureteroscopy were undetected by either intravenous pyelography or retrograde ureterography.[25] Kerbl and Clayman[26] suggest that by creating a refluxing ureteric orifice at the time of initial upper tract tumor resection, subsequent ureteroscopy can be performed in the office without the need for dilation of the orifice, oral or parenteral analgesics, or postureteroscopy stent placement. In this fashion, direct upper tract surveillance can be accomplished every 3 to 6 months, as desired.[26] This technique is not recommended in the presence of associated bladder tumor, because the risk of upper tract seeding may be increased almost 22-fold.[27]

In skilled hands, the risk of complications resulting from routine ureteroscopy performed for stone disease is about 5%, and these complications consist primarily of ureteral wall perforation, urine extravasation, and postoperative stricture. When tumor biopsy, resection, and fulguration are performed, the risk of perforation and stricture formation increases.[28]

Percutaneous Treatment

The percutaneous approach to tumors involving the upper collecting system was first described in 1988. It is my opinion that percutaneous management of renal pelvic or ureteral tumors should be reserved for highly selected cases in which traditional surgical treatment (i.e., nephroureterectomy or selective ureterectomy) is not possible or practical and retrograde ureteroscopic management is not technically feasible. These situations include tumors larger than 1 cm, tumors not accessible to ureteroscopy in the proximal two thirds of the ureter or within the renal pelvis, and most tumors in the calyces. In certain cases, open surgery may not be acceptable to the patient.

Technique

Standard percutaneous equipment is employed to access and dilate a tract into the collecting system. Tumors in the upper or lower calyces should be approached from another calyx that will give reasonably straight access. Direct puncture and dilation into a calyx harboring a tumor theoretically is expected to increase the risk of tumor seeding and tract implantation.

My approach is to dilate only to the minimal size necessary. If a 24-Fr resectoscope is to be used, a tract sheath no larger than 30 Fr is all that is required. Alternatively, if a laser tumor ablation is planned, the 15-Fr flexible nephroscope will be used, requiring no more than a 24-Fr percutaneous sheath.

In addition to the risk of seeding the percutaneous tract, the thin wall of the renal pelvis and ureter as well as the small capacity of the collecting system increase the possibility of perforation. Some surgeons prefer to initially place and dilate the percutaneous tract and then allow the tract to mature and urine to clear over a 3- to 4-day interim. At this time, the nephroscope is inserted directly into the upper collecting system without the aid of an Amplatz sheath. This approach allows clear access to the tumor and allows the collecting system to be filled more effectively with irrigant without leakage through the Amplatz sheath. This has not been my practice, because it is believed that this may increase the risk of tract seeding with tumor. There is no objective data to support either approach.

If the tumor is to be resected, a 24-Fr loop is carefully used, with sterile water or 1.5% glycine solution as the irrigant (Fig. 6-3). Cautery current should be minimized so as to improve the quality of specimen submitted to the pathologist. After adequate resection, the tumor base should be lightly fulgurated with electrocautery or Nd:Yag laser energy. Cold-cup random biopsies are optional.

If the tumor is not accessible with the rigid resectoscope, it must be approached with a 15-Fr or smaller flexible nephroscope. Under these circumstances, the tumor may be biopsied using 5-Fr or smaller grasping forceps and the tumor fulgurated using electrocautery or laser energy via a flexible 2- to 3-Fr electrocautery probe or 400-μm laser fiber through the working channel of this instrument. Such tumors normally reside in the calyces, infundibuli, or ureter.

Following percutaneous treatment, a suitably sized nephrostomy tube (18-Fr Councill) is placed. The purpose is to provide initial tamponade of any bleeding that may occur from the area of resection as well as from the percutaneous tract. It also provides optimal drainage of the renal pelvis in the presence of large or small perforations and allows second-look percutaneous procedures to be performed in 3 days, if necessary. Additionally, intracavitary therapy using mitomycin C, bacillus Calmette-Guerin, or another suitable chemotherapeutic agent may be administered after antegrade nephrostogram demonstrates absence of extravasation. This therapy is normally initiated 3 to 5 days after eradication of the tumor and is administered for 3 to 5 days, as tolerated. Intrapelvic pressures are closely monitored to run below 15 cm H_2O using manometric measurements.

After removal of the nephrostomy tube, follow-up urine cy-

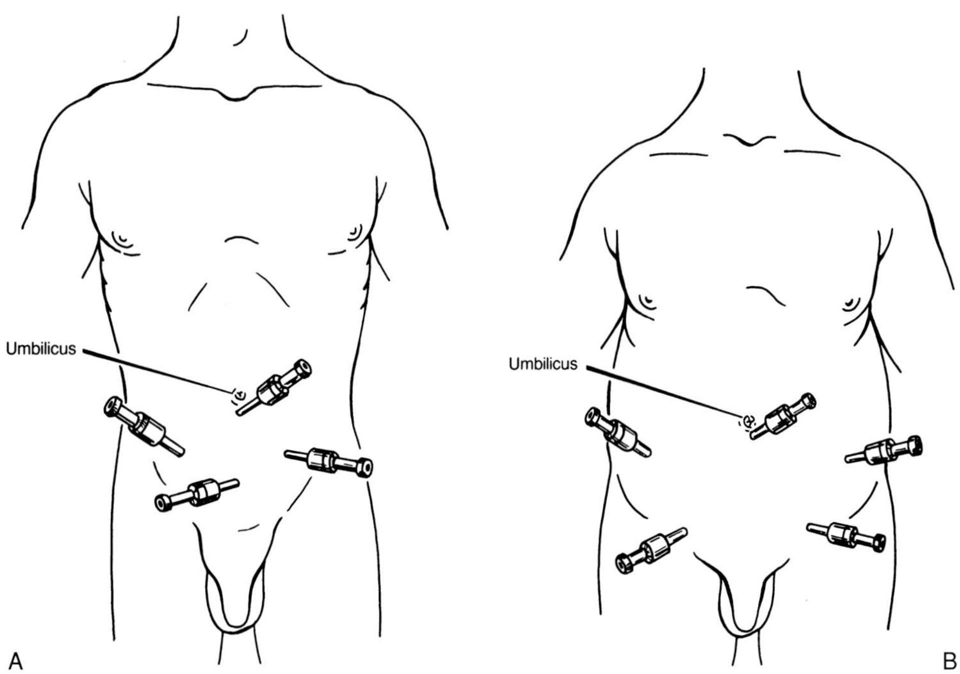

FIG. 6-3. (**A**) A diamond configuration of laparoscopic ports is used for laparoscopic pelvic lymph node dissection (PLND) in an average size patient, and (**B**) a U-shaped configuration of laparoscopic ports is used for PLND in an obese patient.

tology and upper tract contrast studies should be performed every 3 months for at least 1 year. In these highly selected patients, recurrences should be low and often occur within the bladder. Orihuela and Smith[29] have reported recurrence in 4 of 14 patients in whom the initial tumors were multifocal and high grade and had an invasive appearance. Interestingly, none of the recurrences occurred in the nephrostomy tract, and only one recurrence was reported in the retroperitoneum. Overall, the success rate at 2 years with respect to recurrence of transitional cell carcinoma following endoscopic treatment is superior for tumors in the ureter compared with those in the renal pelvis.[30]

LAPAROSCOPIC SURGERY FOR UROLOGIC MALIGNANCIES

Prior to 1990, the primary indication to perform laparoscopy in the field of urology was for the evaluation of nonpalpable testis.[31] In rare situations, laparoscopy was employed for the diagnosis and biopsy of intraabdominal masses.[32] However, with the advent of new and technically superior video and hand equipment, laparoscopy moved from a diagnostic "look-and-see" procedure to an actual surgical intervention. The major application of urolaparoscopy has been the assessment of pelvic lymph nodes, primarily as a staging technique for patients with cancer of the prostate. Laparoscopic pelvic lymph node dissection has also been applied in select cases of bladder, urethral, and penile malignancies.

With respect to the upper urinary tract, laparoscopic nephrectomy and nephroureterectomy have been performed in select medical centers for renal cell and transitional cell cancers, respectively. Laparoscopic retroperitoneal lymph node dissection for early-stage nonseminomatous testis tumors is feasible and should be undertaken by individuals with advanced laparoscopic skills. Adrenal neoplasms of a benign or malignant nature have also been removed laparoscopically. A discussion of the rationale, techniques, and results of these laparoscopic interventions are reviewed in the following sections.

General Principles

Laparoscopic intervention is very different from open surgery and requires the surgeon to become familiar with a completely new set of instruments and equipment. This technointensive procedure requires a wide variety of laparoscopic instruments with which the surgeon must become familiarized, such as CO_2 insufflator, pneumoperitoneal needles, trocars, sheaths, graspers, forceps, scissors, clip applicators, monopolar and bipolar coagulation probes, and irrigation-suction devices. The urologist has an advantage over other surgical specialists in that he or she is familiar with endoscopic and percutaneous surgery and will more rapidly master the limited two-dimensional visual field inherent with laparoscopic surgery. Similarly, the blunted tactile sensation of using long instruments to perform surgery is also not new to the endoscopic surgeon. With any new surgical procedure, it is important that the surgeon fully understand the indications and contraindications of the operation. To successfully perform laparoscopic surgery, two experienced surgeons should be capable of operating on the patient in tandem and synchrony while visualizing the procedure on a television monitor by use of a full-beam camera chip attached to the laparoscope. The nursing staff must be fully acquainted with the laparoscopic instrumentation and steps of the proposed procedure. A separate table with a laparotomy setup should be available in the operating room should emergencies arise. The arrangement of the equipment and surgical personnel should be planned in advance of the first laparoscopic procedure.

Laparoscopic Pelvic Lymph Node Dissection

Cancer of the Prostate

In a recent survey of urologist in the United States, the most common laparoscopic procedure performed is pelvic lymph node dissection (LPLND) for staging of men with prostate cancer.[33]

The importance of determining the presence or absence of metastatic lymph node involvement with cancer of the prostate, or any other urologic malignancy, is that this finding most likely will determine the extent of treatment and the feasibility of curative therapy.[34] In many urologic centers, the detection of positive nodes from cancer of the prostate would negate the possibility for curative radical prostatectomy or radiotherapy. At this point, the patient would be offered the options of immediate medical or surgical castration or observation until the malignancy became symptomatic. Absence of positive lymph nodes would allow urologists to offer a radical retropubic or perineal prostatectomy or external or interstitial radiotherapy, with curative intents.[35]

Two different approaches have been advocated regarding the extent of PLND. The earlier approach suggested an extensive PLND laterally to the genitofemoral nerve, removing all fibrolymphatic tissue from the external iliac vessels, extending proximally to the common iliac vessels and medially to skeletonize the obturator vessels and nerve as well as the hypogastric artery and branches. The dissection included the presacral and presciatic (lateral sacral) lymph nodes. The distal extent of the dissection included Cloquet's inguinal node and progressed inferiorly to the point where the circumflex vein crosses over the external iliac artery.[36]

In the past 10 to 15 years, urologic surgeons have become more apt to perform a less extensive PLND, and in more recent years to perform a modified PLND that includes primarily nodal and fibrofatty tissue within the obturator fossa surrounding the obturator vessels and nerves. The lateral and medial borders of this dissection include the external iliac vein and hypogastric artery, respectively. Cranial and caudal limits are the bifurcation of the iliac vessels and Cloquet's node or Cooper's ligament, respectively. The reasons for this modification are twofold:

Studies indicate that 86% to 94% of positive nodes will involve those within the obturator-hypogastric region, with only 6% to 14% of cases showing skip lesions involving only the presciatic or common iliac and aortic regions.

There is a significant rate of early complications (12% to 24%) associated with the more extensive dissection, especially when followed by external beam radiotherapy.[35–41]

With this background into the rationale and significance of PLND for staging cancer of the prostate, why should the surgeon consider performing this procedure by the laparoscopic route? The advantages to the patient, as initially described by Schuessler and colleagues[42] and Winfield and colleagues,[43] are decreased length of postoperative hospitalization and convalescence. Comparative studies indicate that the staging effectiveness of LPLND is comparable to that of the open procedure.[43] From a cosmetic point of view, the four or five small (5-to 11-mm) abdominal puncture sites appear to be superior to the disfigurement of the midline umbilical–to–symphysis pubis incision.

Technical Aspects

Preoperative Preparation. After having been selected a suitable candidate for this procedure, the patient is informed of the potential advantages as well as the limitations of the laparoscopic approach and the possible need for conversion to open surgery should technical problems develop. The possibility of significant hemorrhage, bowel or other visceral injury, and death is discussed.

If only LPLND is planned, the patient is admitted the day of surgery, having self-administered oral laxatives the afternoon prior to the procedure. If immediate retropubic or perineal prostatectomy is planned should the nodes be negative on frozen pathologic examination, a full-bowel preparation is administered the night prior to the procedure when the patient is admitted into the hospital. Similarly, patients suspected of having significant adhesions from previous abdominal surgery, which might increase the risk of intestinal injury, receive a full-bowel preparation the evening before surgery. All patients receive one dose of a broad-spectrum parenteral antibiotic 1 hour prior to the procedure and are typed and screened for blood products before undergoing laparoscopic surgery.

Laparoscopic Obturator Pelvic Lymph Node Dissection

Intraperitoneal Approach

After induction of general anesthesia, a Foley catheter and a nasogastric tube are positioned in the bladder and stomach, respectively. A full abdominal skin preparation is done, and all instruments and videolaparoscopic equipment are arranged around the patient.

With the patient in a 10-degree Trendelenburg position, the Veress needle is inserted at the inferior crease of the umbilicus. Entrance into the peritoneal cavity is ascertained, and carbon dioxide is insufflated to an initial pressure of 18 to 20 mm Hg. Should the peritoneal cavity not be satisfactorily entered from the inferior crease of the umbilicus, attempts from the superior crease are made. Failing this, my approach is to employ the open laparoscopy approach using a Hasson or other similar blunt-tip trocar-sheath unit.

The 10/11-mm trocar-sheath unit is inserted at the umbilicus, and the laparoscope-camera unit is inserted into the sheath. Inspection of underlying structures is performed to determine that no injury has occurred; working ports are then inserted under laparoscopic monitoring. Shining the light of the scope helps to delineate superficial epigastric vessels that should be avoided. My working port spatial arrangement is shown in Figure 6-4. Alternatively, in corpulent patients in whom abundant fatty tissue hangs in the region of the obliterated umbilical ligaments, four working ports are placed in a U-shaped configuration. After the ports are in place, the intraperitoneal pressure is lowered to 15 mm Hg.

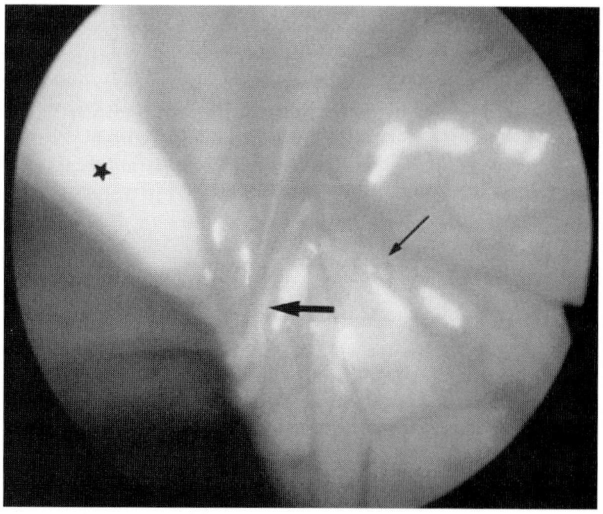

FIG. 6-4. Appearance of the obturator-iliac region before the initiation of dissection. The right obliterated umbilical artery (*star*), right testicular vessels (*narrow arrow*), and right vas deferens (*bold arrow*) are shown. (See Color Figure 6-4.)

The patient is then repositioned to a 30-degrees Trendelenburg position with lateral rotation to allow loops of small bowel to migrate under gravity away from the iliac region of dissection. It is important to identify key landmarks, as shown in Figure 6-1. Familiarity with these structures will aid in avoiding major surgical accidents. On the left side, it is often necessary to take down adhesions from the sigmoid colon by cutting along the white line of Toldt; on the right side, the cecum and appendiceal regions may be tethered down over the iliac region and require release.

The initial incision through the posterior peritoneal membrane begins just lateral to the obliterated umbilical ligament, high over the pubic bone, and is brought down just medial to the pulsating external iliac artery back toward the bifurcation of the common iliac artery, where the ureter may be identified. The vas deferens becomes apparent and is coagulated or clipped and then transected. I feel most comfortable in determining the location of the external iliac vein and clearing all fibrolymphatic tissue from its anterior and medial surfaces. This essentially creates the lateral border of the obturator lymph node packet. The tissue below the external iliac vein is swept off the pelvic side wall, which is then traced to its junction with the pubic bone. With the obliterated umbilical ligament retracted medially, a plane is created just lateral to form the medial border of the obturator nodal packet. At this point, the obturator nerve and associated vessels should be identified, and thus the inferior apex of the nodal tissue is created. Normally, there are no significant vessels in this apical tissue; therefore, electrocautery can be employed to release it away from the pubic bone. The lymph node packet is then stripped proximally from the obturator nerve back toward the bifurcation of the iliac vessels. A 10-mm vein retractor can be employed to manipulate the external iliac vein

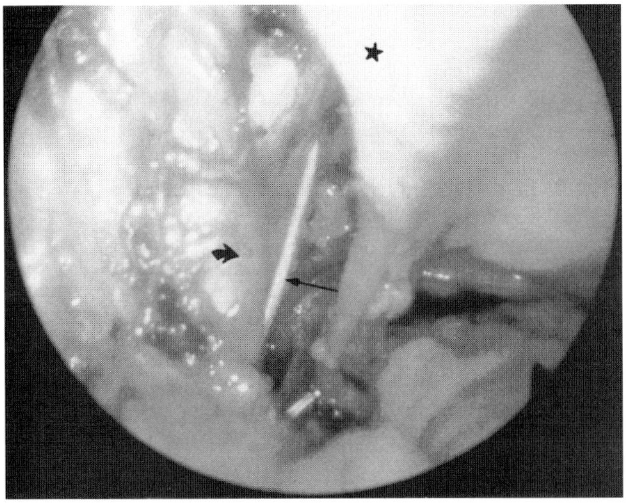

FIG. 6-5. Completed obturator lymph node dissection on left side. The left obliterated umbilical artery (*star*), left external iliac vessels (*curved arrow*), and left obturator nerve (*straight arrow*) are shown.(See Color Figure 6-5.)

laterally, allowing improved access into this difficult area. In addition, newly designed laparoscopic Russian graspers have been used to tease the nodal packet out of the obturator fossa (Fig. 6-5).

I also clear fibrolymphatic tissue from the anterior surface of the external iliac artery back toward the bifurcation of the common iliac to be certain that the margins of the obturator dissection are of satisfactory proximal extent. No attempt to remove tissue laterally to the genitofemoral nerve or over the common iliac artery is made for patients with cancer of the prostate.

The nodal packet is then removed through the 11-mm suprapubic port with spoon-shaped graspers or a ''lap sac'' (Cook Urological, Spencer, IN). Frozen pathologic specimen examination is always requested if immediate prostatectomy is being considered or if the dissected tissue is palpably hard and suspicious. Hemostasis is assured, and trocar entry points are inspected at the peritoneal surface, including the umbilical site. Sheaths are removed under laparoscopic vision, and all CO_2 is expelled from the peritoneal cavity. Punctures sites that are 10 mm or larger are closed using an absorbable suture on the fascia and subcutaneous tissues, and SteriStrips are applied on all skin incisions. The nasogastric tube is removed.

Postoperatively, most patients are allowed to begin oral feedings the night of surgery. The Foley catheter is removed when the patient is alert and ambulating. Barring any problems, the patient is discharged within 24 hours of surgery and may return to full activity in 1 week.

Extraperitoneal Approach

I have had the opportunity to perform LPLND using an extraperitoneal approach. The potential advantages and disadvantages of this procedure are being examined and evaluated.

A 2-cm incision is made at the inferior crease of the umbilicus down to the rectus abdominis fascia. The rectus abdominis fascia is split in the midline, as is the fascia of the transversus abdominis, to enter the preperitoneal space. Using finger dissection, a space is initiated, and the inflation balloon catheter device is inserted. I initially used a modified Gaar device consisting of a 16-Fr red Robinson catheter to which the middle finger of an 8½ Triflex glove is secured by 2-0 silk-free ties. The balloon device was then filled with 800 to 1000 mL of saline. Unfortunately, the latex material often ruptured, requiring the surgeon to search the preperitoneal space for glove fragments. In some cases, I used the commercially available preperitoneal balloon catheter with good results. However, these also ruptured upon occasion; therefore, I have switched to the finger cot of an O'Connor perineal transurethral resection drape. This polyethylene natural rubber seems to withstand higher pressures and the risk of rupture is diminished.

With good inflation, a large space is created in the space of Retzius to the extent that the pubic bone may be fully exposed as well as the external iliac vessels. A Hasson-type cannula is secured in place at the umbilicus, and CO_2 insufflation proceeds at 10 to 12 mm Hg. Working ports are carefully inserted into the extraperitoneal space in a diamond-shaped arrangement as described previously. Should the peritoneal membrane be traversed, the extraperitoneal space will most likely be collapsed and require conversion of the ports to an intraperitoneal position. The experienced laparoscopic surgeon should be facile with this type of conversion.

Once the ports are in place, the LPLND proceeds as described for the intraperitoneal approach. The major difference is that the vas deferens is now displaced cephalad and often apposed to the peritoneal membrane. It is not been necessary to transect the vas in many cases. The major advantages of the extraperitoneal approach appear to be the minimal need to mobilize the sigmoid colon on the left side and no interference from loops of small bowel. It has been possible to perform the extraperitoneal LPLND in patients who have undergone previous appendectomy and other forms of intraperitoneal surgery. Patients who have undergone previous inguinal hernia repair or other extraperitoneal pelvic procedures are not good candidates for the extraperitoneal approach. Similarly, if a retropubic prostatectomy is planned at a later date, this surgery will be considerably more difficult if the nodes are evaluated by the extraperitoneal route.

Results

At the University of Iowa, 26 of the initial 66 LPLNDs for the staging of cancer of the prostate were converted to an open procedure: 15 to perform a radical retropubic prostatectomy, 10 for incomplete or unsatisfactory dissections, and 1 for bleeding. These patients provided the opportunity to assess the completeness of this procedure when performed laparoscopically. In one patient, some residual tissue at the bifurcation of the iliac artery was sent for pathologic examination separately after conversion to an open operation, and proved to harbor a microscopic focus of adenocarcinoma. Thus, the false-negative rate in this initial series was at least 1 of 26 (4%), based on the patients who were converted to an open procedure. It is certainly possible that patients who were not opened or who had metastatic skip lesions were missed. Parra and associates[44] studied 24 men, 12 undergoing modified open PLND and 12 undergoing LPLND followed by open inspection. There was no significant difference in the number of nodes obtained between the two groups, and no additional nodal tissue was recovered from the dissection zones on open exploration.

Between May 1990 and March 1994, 192 patients have undergone LPLND for the staging of prostate cancer at the University of Iowa. Overall, 36 (19%) were found to have positive nodes. As would be expected, increasing stage correlated with an increased risk of positive nodes. No patients with stage A1 prostate cancer had nodal metastasis, increasing to 11% for stage A2, 20% for stage B2, 37% for stage C, and 50% for stage D0 (elevated enzymatic prostatic acid phosphatase [PAP]). Likewise, the incidence of lymph node metastasis increased with higher grade of the primary tumor. No patient with a Gleason score of less than 5 was found to have metastasis; this rate increased to 20% for those with a Gleason score of 7 and to 75% for those with a Gleason score of 9. With regard to prostate-specific antigen (PSA) level, the incidence of metastasis increased from 13% for a PSA level less than or equal to 30 ng/mL, to 36% for PSA level of 31 to 50 ng/mL, 43% for PSA level of 51 to 70 ng/mL, and to 47% if the PSA level was greater than 70 ng/mL. No patient with a normal PSA level (<4 ng/mL) was found to have positive lymph nodes.

Other authors have had considerable experience with this technique. Griffith and colleagues[45] reported their first 31 patients who underwent LPLND. The average operating time was 184 minutes, and the average length of hospitalization was 1.2 days. They concluded that this procedure is associated with less ileus, less narcotic administration, and a shorter hospital stay than open surgery. Kerbl and colleagues[46] compared their initial 30 patients who underwent LPLND with 16 patients who underwent open PLND and concluded that analgesic use, hospital stay, and interval to recovery were less after LPLND. The results of Winfield and colleagues[43] concur with these studies.

Of concern is the increased complication rate seen with LPLND. In a multiinstitutional study, Kavoussi and colleagues[47] assessed the intraoperative and postoperative complications in 372 patients who underwent LPLND. In 16 patients, the procedure could not be completed because of technical difficulties, but 14 of these occurred during the initial 8 procedures at each institution. Complications occurred in 55 patients (15%), 14 of which were noted intraoperatively and 41 of which were diagnosed postoperatively. Surgical intervention was required for complications in 13 patients. The results of this collective review emphasize that significant complications can result from LPLND. Most authors reporting their experience with laparoscopic procedures underscore the steepness of the learning curve. Kerbl and associates[46] compared the results from their initial and subsequent experience with LPLND. Major morbidity decreased from 25% in the initial 12 patients to 0% in the subsequent 12 patients, and minor morbidity decreased from 33% to 8% accordingly. Proper patient selection should maximize success and minimize complications. It appears that, as with other new procedures, as surgeons gain facility with this procedure and acquire a better working knowledge of the anatomy, many of these misadventures can be avoided.

Conclusions

LPLND is an excellent staging procedure that can be performed in a minimally invasive fashion for patients with cancer of the prostate. The steep learning curve is of concern, but by strict adherence to the basic principles of laparoscopic surgery, many complications can be avoided.

The advent of the extraperitoneal approach to laparoscopic surgery may obviate some of the intraperitoneal complications, such as bowel or major visceral injury. Conversely, this approach may lead to an increased rate of lymphocele formation or CO_2 respiratory problems related to subcutaneous and properitoneal emphysema. It is my opinion that the extraperitoneal LPLND is ideal in obese patients in whom a large space of Retzius may be created because the peritoneal membrane holds back loops of bowel. However, it is unclear whether this approach is superior to the intraperitoneal route with respect to shorter operative time, hospitalization, and convalescence and reduced need for analgesia.

Based on my results for LPLND in patients with cancer of the prostate, one or more of the following indications should be present to offer a patient this operation as a staging technique.

- stage B2-D0 (TB2-TM1) cancer of the prostate, whether surgery, radiotherapy, or hormonal manipulation is being considered
- stage A2 (TA2) cancer with a Gleason score of 6 or greater
- elevated enzymatic prostatic acid phosphatase
- PSA levels greater than 30 ng/mL using a Hybritech assay
- patient election to undergo perineal prostatectomy
- patients with A1, A2, or B1 (TA1, TA2, TB1) disease who desire radiotherapy or surgery but have moderately or poorly differentiated histopathology (i.e., Gleason score of 5 or greater)

The data of McLaughlin and colleagues[48] support the results with open PLND that the chance of discovering metastatic lymph node tissue is rare in low-stage and low-grade disease (i.e., T1A, T2A)—generally, less than a 25% chance. Therefore, if a radical retropubic prostatectomy is planned, it is best to proceed directly to open PLND. For stage T1B disease with Gleason scores of 6 or greater, the risk of positive nodes may be greater than 25%; therefore, this group should be considered for LPLND.[49]

With increasing experience, more difficult cases or cases that had relative contraindications to laparoscopy were considered. Use of the open laparoscopic approach using a Hasson or similar type cannula was employed for obese patients or for those who had previous extensive intraperitoneal operations. LPLND has been used in patients considered for salvage prostatectomy who previously received full-course external beam radiotherapy or brachytherapy. Although tissue planes are distorted, the procedure has been very successful in 10 of 12 patients.

Patients who elected to receive external beam radiotherapy or interstitial gold-198 (^{198}Au) seed percutaneous implantation were strongly encouraged to undergo preliminary LPLND. Again, the need for nodal evaluation is less likely to be of benefit for those with low-grade and low-stage disease. Patients who wished to have their prostate removed by the perineal approach were considered ideal candidates for LPLND.

Cancer of the Bladder

With the realization that careful pelvic lymphadenectomy in combination with radical cystectomy did not significantly increase the mortality or morbidity compared with cystectomy alone but also improved the clinical staging and survival of patients with micrometastases in a single or few nodes, most urologic surgeons now advocate this radical approach.[50,51]

Using modern techniques, the intraoperative detection of lymph nodes involved with transitional cell carcinoma may lead the surgeon to abort the radical cystectomy and offer neoadjuvant chemotherapy. At a later date, the urologist might consider performing a salvage cystectomy; however, results have not been overwhelmingly good. Patients showing metastatic squamous cell carcinoma or adenocarcinoma involving lymph nodes from a bladder primary have a very poor prognosis, and curative extirpative surgery is unlikely.

I would consider LPLND for patients with invasive bladder cancer in the following situations:

- Radiologic evidence of nodal enlargement that is not accessible by computed tomographic– or ultrasonographic–guided needle biopsy.
- Patients who refuse cystectomy and desire definitive radiotherapy.
- Patients being considered for partial cystectomy. The LPLND and partial cystectomy can be approached by an extraperitoneal route.
- Patients with squamous cell carcinoma or adenocarcinoma of the bladder, where, in the presence of positive nodes, radical cystectomy would not be curative. However, these patients may be considered for palliative urinary diversion, which also may be approached laparoscopically.
- Clinical evidence of lymph node involvement that cannot be visualized radiologically.

Technique

The approach for these patients is similar to those with cancer of the prostate, with minor modifications. A full-bowel preparation is administered the day before surgery, because open radical cystoprostatectomy or anterior exenteration may be performed following a negative node dissection. The limits of the dissection are wider, including the genitofemoral nerve laterally, the common iliac artery proximally, and the bladder wall medially. This dissection requires more extensive mobilization of the sigmoid colon and cecoappendiceal regions. In addition, care to identify the ureter and the bifurcation of the iliac vessels is critical.

My experience with this type of LPLND is limited to two female patients. Both had negative nodes, and a successful anterior exenteration was performed.

Cancer of the Penis

The clinical history and surgical approach to patients with cancer of the penis is well described in Section VI. The presence of positive iliac or periaortic lymph nodes portends a dismal prognosis, and the morbidity from bilateral ilioinguinal node dissection is significant (10% to 40%), with a 3% mortality rate. Therefore, in patients who have biopsy-proven carcinoma in the inguinal region and are being considered for radical inguinal dissection, my approach would be to perform preliminary extended LPLND. If the nodes are negative, I proceed to open inguinal dissection, either immediately or at a later time.

Technique

The approach to LPLND for cancer of the penis is identical to that for bladder cancer, beginning the dissection on the side of the lesion and examining frozen pathologic sections as necessary. To date, I have had no laparoscopic experience with patients with cancer of the penis. Assimos and Jarow[52] have recently reported the use of extended LPLND in three men with stage T3 (UICC staging system) squamous cell carcinoma of the penis.

Cancer of the Urethra

Primary carcinoma of the urethra is exceedingly rare but does occur more frequently in the female population. Because of its rarity and vague presenting symptoms, it often presents in an advanced stage. Regional lymphatic involvement is common, ranging from 10% to 15%. The anterior urethra initially drains to the superficial and deep inguinal nodes, whereas the posterior urethra drains primarily to the external iliac, hypogastric, and obturator nodes. The presence of palpable inguinal nodes implies metastatic involvement in about 80% of cases.[53] Because of characteristic local invasion, hematogenous spread occurs late in the course of the disease.

Because of the rarity of primary carcinoma of the urethra, treatment approaches are not well established. It has been suggested that in the presence of positive pelvic or inguinal adenopathy radical exenterative surgery is probably not indicated, because the prognosis at this stage is grim.[54,55] In the absence of palpable and radiologic inguinal adenopathy, prophylactic groin dissection is not routinely advised.

What is the suggested role of LPLND for primary cancer of the urethra? It would seem prudent to consider this dissection in the following situations:

- Ambiguous or positive-appearing lymph nodes on computed tomographic scan, magnetic resonance image, or lymphangiogram of the pelvic region that cannot be percutaneously needle biopsied.
- Performed prior to all exenterative procedures for posterior urethral cancer, because the discovery of pelvic metastatic adenopathy would abort further surgery.
- Women with distal urethral carcinoma that invades muscle or periurethral tissue.

For distal urethral tumors in the male population, inguinal and pelvic node dissection is probably not necessary, assuming the physical and radiologic examinations are negative for metastatic disease. This would also be true for noninvasive tumors of the distal female urethra.[56]

Technique

The approach of LPLND for cancer of the urethra would be similar to that for cancer of the bladder or penis. I have had experience performing this procedure on one male patient with primary cancer of the urethra.

Laparoscopic Renal Surgery

Through the pioneering work of Clayman and colleagues,[57] laparoscopic renal surgery, specifically nephrectomy, has become reality. The first laparoscopic nephrectomy was performed in 1990; since then, a limited number of these procedures have been done worldwide. Not only is this laparoscopic intervention very technically demanding, the accepted indications for this procedure are limited. Most urologists would agree that laparoscopic nephrectomy and ureterectomy for malignant disease is controversial and should be offered only in select cases. For renal cell carcinoma, there is presently only one curative option: successful en bloc removal of the tumor. Similarly, transitional cell cancer responds to adjunctive chemotherapy, but chances of cure may be compromised by inadequate surgical excision. These issues must be carefully and clearly addressed with the patient as well as among members of the urologic community when laparoscopic excision is considered.

I believe that, in skilled hands, there are certain situations in which laparoscopic nephrectomy or ureterectomy may be considered for malignancy. These would be small intraparenchymal renal tumors, preferably of the lower pole, that do not extend beyond the capsule of the kidney (clinical stage I) and transitional cell carcinoma of the upper urinary tract that is radiologically confined to the collecting system. In these cases, the difficult dissection to include the adrenal gland within the specimen is not as critical. Based on results of conservative surgery for renal cell carcinoma, not removing the adrenal glands does not seem to compromise long term results.[58,59]

The ureter and cuff of bladder can be removed laparoscopically as part of the nephroureterectomy specimen in patients with transitional cell carcinoma. It would be preferable not to morcellate a kidney or ureter containing a malignancy but to extend one of the laparoscopic port sites slightly and bring the entrapped kidney out intact.

Laparoscopic Nephrectomy

Preoperative Preparation

After selecting the appropriate patient for this procedure, a full-bowel preparation is administered. Antibiotics as part of the bowel preparation is optional. All patients receive a broad-spectrum parental antibiotic and are cross-matched for two units of packed red blood cells.

On the morning of the procedure, the patient is transported to the cystoscopy suite, where, under local sedation, a 7-Fr end-hole or occlusion balloon ureteral catheter is inserted retrograde to the renal pelvis of the diseased kidney. An Amplatz superstiff guidewire is left within the ureteral catheter; these are then fixed to a 16-Fr Foley catheter placed in the bladder. The ureteral catheter–Amplatz wire unit will be helpful in locating the ureter intraoperatively.

Intraperitoneal Approach

Within the main operating room, general anesthesia is administered and appropriate intravenous and arterial monitoring lines are established as deemed necessary by the anesthesiologist. A Foley catheter and nasogastric tubes are mandatory. Positioning the patient correctly is the key to a successful operation performed in a safe fashion. The patient is placed on an inflatable bean bag, the operating table is rotated to full flank position, and the patient is placed in the full flank position (Fig. 6-6). In this way, the table can be rotated back into the neutral or contralateral position to bring the patient into the supine position, so that the patient does not need to be physically shifted during the procedure, with the associated potential for field contamination. All pressure points are padded, and the patient is secured carefully to the operating table.

The pneumoperitoneum and telescopic trocar-sheath unit are placed with the patient in the supine and flank positions. A total of four working ports are normally required to perform laparoscopic nephrectomy. I do not become obsessed with the size and location of the laparoscopic ports, because each patient's kidney is in a different location, and a good laparoscopic surgeon should be able to vary the technique according to individual circumstances. As a general rule, the initial 10/11-mm telescopic port is placed at the superior umbilical region, and two midclavicular ports are placed: one just below the costal margin and one slightly below the level of the umbilicus. One of these ports is 10 to 11 mm and the other 12 mm for use of the endo-GIA device (US Surgical, Norwalk, CT), if required.

The table is rotated, thereby bringing the patient into the full flank position. Two 5- or 10-mm ports are positioned on the anteroaxillary line between the iliac crest and tip of the 12th rib (Fig. 6-7).

The white line of Toldt is incised using curved electrocautery scissors, allowing the colon to be mobilized medially. The incision should be extended so as to release the peritoneal reflection away from the spleen on the left and the liver on the right. In this fashion, the retroperitoneum is entered and the ureter is sought. By manipulating the ureteral catheter and wire, the area of the ureter should be identified and then carefully dissected

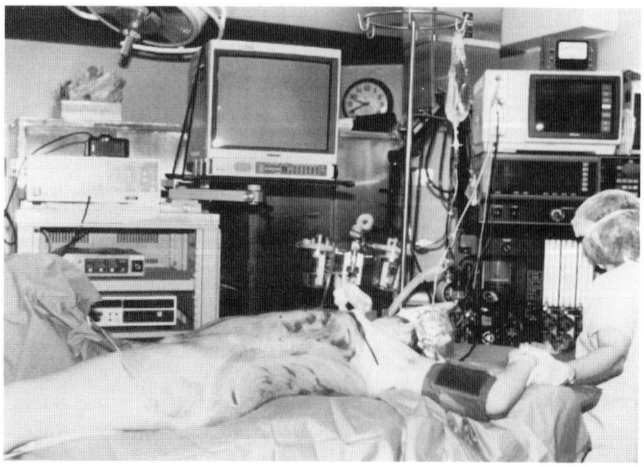

FIG. 6-6. Positioning of patient for laparoscopic nephrectomy.

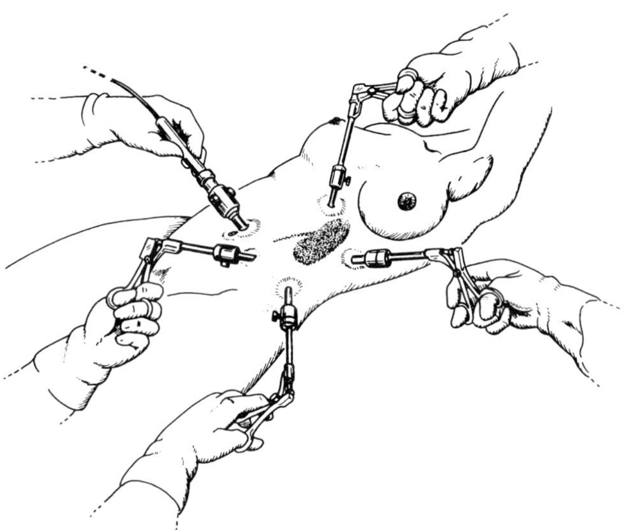

FIG. 6-7. Normal spatial arrangement of ports for intraperitoneal laparoscopic nephrectomy.

free of surrounding tissue. It has been my experience that the gonadal vessels cross anteriorly at about the point where the ureter will be first mobilized. These vessels should be clipped and transected, because they will compromise further ureteral dissection and may be avulsed from their associated great vessels. When the ureter is identified, it is grasped with an endo-Babcock (US Surgical, Norwalk, CT) or similar instrument and then traced upward toward the lower pole of the kidney and renal hilum.

Using a careful dissecting technique employing straight and curved instruments, the renal arteries and veins are individually cleared of surrounding fibrolymphatic and fatty tissue. At least two 9-mm clips are placed on the proximal or "stay" side of these vessels, and one or two clips are placed on the distal or "go" side (Fig. 6-8). It is strongly advised to first interrupt the arterial vessels so as to prevent excessive venous pressure and undesirable bleeding. It is also suggested that if the width of the renal vein, especially on the right side, is too large for a single 9-mm clip, the vascular cartridge of the endo-GIA should be employed. The remaining vein is hemostatically sealed with three rows of staples (Fig. 6-9).

With the renal hilum transected, the lateral attachments of the kidney are released. Pulling inferiorly on the ureter, the upper pole of the kidney and upper medial portion of the kidney are dissected free, being careful not to disrupt adrenal vessels or direct vascular branches from the inferior vena cava or aorta. As mentioned previously, in most cases of laparoscopic nephrectomy, Gerota's fascia is entered at the upper pole of the kidney so as to spare the adrenal gland; however, I have had the experience of removing the adrenal gland en bloc within Gerota's fascia. The final step of the dissection is removal of the catheter and wire from the ureter prior to clipping and transection of the ureter.

With the kidney fully mobilized, an impermeable sack (Lapsac-Cook Urological, Spencer, IN) is placed down the 12-mm port into the peritoneal cavity. The kidney is manipulated into the sack and the tie strings brought out of a larger port. This manipulation of the kidney into the sack can be difficult with large specimens. The periumbilical incision can be extended 1 or 2 cm further to allow the sack containing the kidney to be delivered intact. This approach is strongly suggested if laparoscopic nephrectomy is being considered for malignancy.

The periumbilical incision may be closed at this point or the 12-mm port reestablished; then a final laparoscopic inspection for hemostasis and visceral integrity is completed. Sheaths are removed as described previously for exiting the abdomen.

Extraperitoneal Approach

The extraperitoneal approach to nephrectomy has been applied primarily to benign renal disease. However, in select cases in which the kidney is small and the tumor well encapsulated, the extraperitoneal laparoscopic route may be beneficial.

The preoperative preparation is identical to that described previously. With the patient in the flank position, a 3- to 4-cm transverse incision is made in the area of Petit's (lumbar) trian-

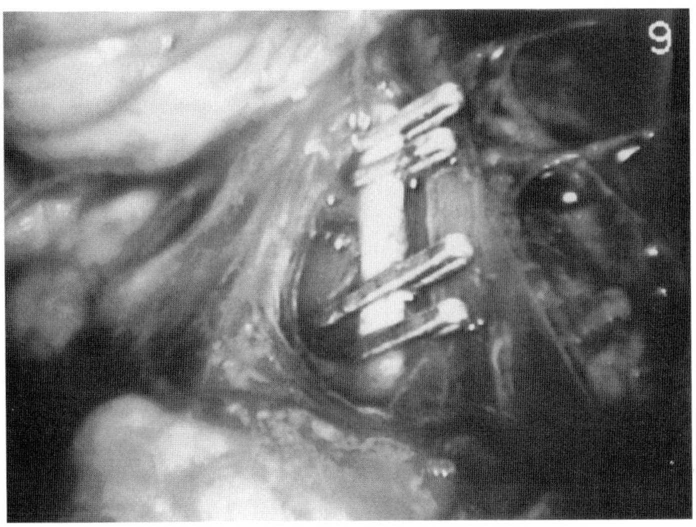

FIG. 6-8. Double-clipped and transected renal artery. (See Color Figure 6-8.)

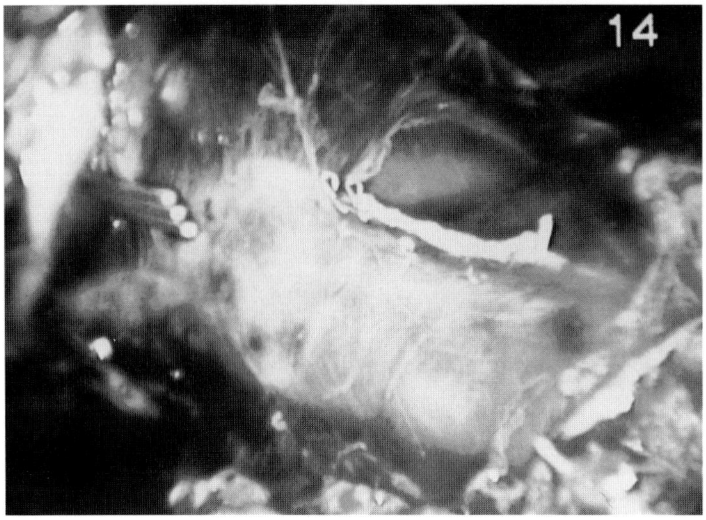

FIG. 6-9. Transection of the right renal vein with a vascular endo-GIA stapling device leaves three rows of staples at the junction with the inferior vena cava. (See Color Figure 6-9.)

gle formed by the external oblique and latissimus dorsi muscles with the posterior iliac crest. The incision is sharply and bluntly dissected down to the retroperitoneal fascia (Fig. 6-10). By observing from an intraperitoneal port, the surgeon can see the fingertip pushing against the posterior peritoneal membrane.

A space large enough to accept an inflation device is created as described previously for LPLND. As 800 to 1000 mL of saline is injected into this inflation device, the retroperitoneal gossamer fibrofatty tissues are separated away from the kidney and ureter.

A Hasson-type port is secured in place, and the pneumoperitoneum is maintained at 8 to 12 mm Hg. Three working ports are arranged in the midaxillary and anterior axillary lines to pass into this newly created extraperitoneal space (Fig. 6-11). The kidney and proximal ureter are then easily dissected and the renal vessels clipped and ligated from a posterior approach. Access to the lower ureter is difficult; this structure is more easily reached using an intraperitoneal approach.

My experience with the retroperitoneal laparoscopic approach to the kidney has been limited but very rewarding. The

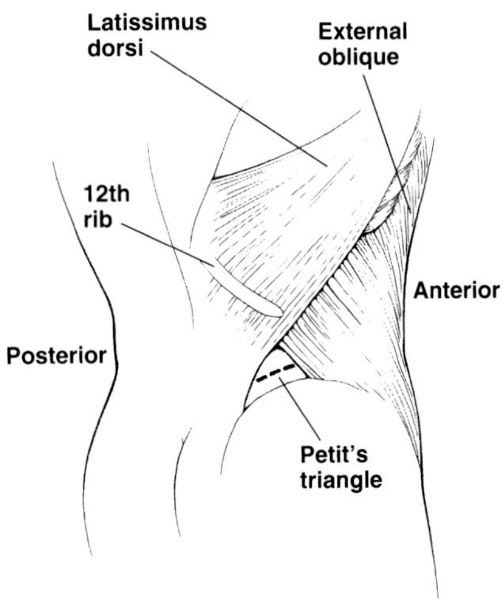

FIG. 6-10. Point of incision in Petit's triangle for extraperitoneal renal surgery.

operative time is reduced, and patients do exceedingly well in the postoperative period.

Postoperative Management

The nasogastric tube is removed in the recovery room, and oral fluids may be administered on the first postoperative day. Ambulation is encouraged the evening of surgery. Two doses of parenteral antibiotics are administered as an empirical practice. In most cases, a normal diet and hospital activity is achieved by the third postoperative day, and discharge closely follows. My patients have resumed full activity within 1 to 2 weeks following laparoscopic surgery.

Results

My laparoscopic nephrectomy series at the University of Iowa College of Medicine consists of 18 patients, one of whom had renal cell cancer and two of whom had transitional cell cancer. When approached using the intraperitoneal route, the operative times were lengthy, averaging between 5 and 6 hours. With conversion to the extraperitoneal route, the operative times diminished to an average of 3.2 hours. Despite the long operative times, the advantages of the laparoscopic procedure were realized in the postoperative period. The average hospital stay was 4.3 days, and analgesic requirements were low. Time of convalescence was 1 to 2 weeks, which is superior to the usual quoted convalescence of at least 6 weeks following open nephrectomy. As with any laparoscopic procedure, complications have and will occur. The most feared are hemorrhage and tumor spill when performing this procedure for malignancy. I have not had to abort any laparoscopic renal cases related to cancer, but the surgeon should be prepared to open the patient should significant bleeding occur. A surgical plan should be mentally prepared prior to embarking on any laparoscopic procedure. The anesthesiologist should be advised that less crystalloid is required during laparoscopic nephrectomy, because evaporation from bowel or visceral walls does not occur to the same extent as during open surgery.

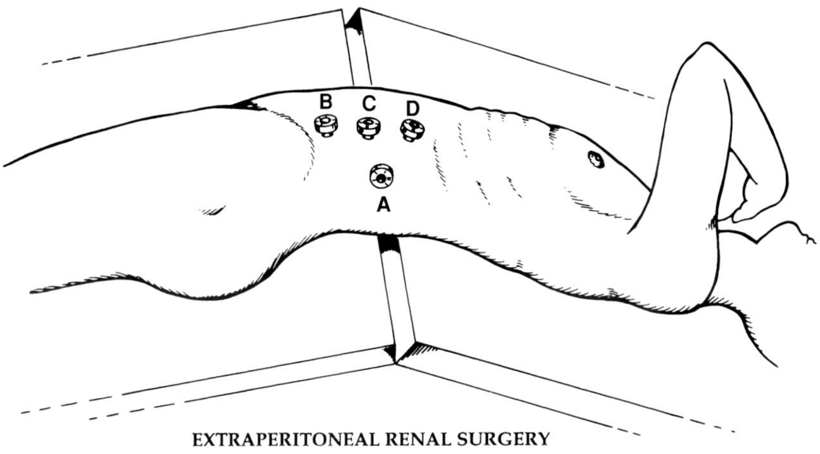

FIG. 6-11. Laparoscopic port (A) and three working ports (B, C, D) for extraperitoneal laparoscopic renal surgery.

Laparoscopic Nephroureterectomy

This procedure, as described by Clayman and colleagues,[60] is similar to that described for laparoscopic nephrectomy with the following exceptions:

The ureteric orifice is encircled transurethrally using an Orandi electrosurgical knife to incise up to the level of the ureterovesical junction. Then, using a roller electrode, the entire ureteral os and tunnel as well as a 2-cm perimeter are electrocauterized.

The kidney is dissected as described previously, but the ureter is not transected.

An additional port is placed in the midline between the symphysis pubis and the umbilicus to aid in dissecting the lower ureter down to the level of the bladder.

A laparoscopic GIA stapler (US Surgical, Norwalk, CT) is passed through the 12-mm periumbilical port and around the lower ureter and cuff of surrounding bladder. The stapler is fired, allowing the specimen and bladder cuff to be sealed and delivered. Alternatively, the bladder cuff may be excised and the opening repaired using laparoscopic suturing techniques.

The specimen is delivered either with the organ entrapment and morcellation system or by enlarging the periumbilical incision. The bladder should be cystoscopically inspected for adequacy of resection and integrity of the repair. The Foley catheter should be left indwelling for 1 week and removed after obtaining a satisfactory cystogram.[60]

Laparoscopic Retroperitoneal Lymph Node Dissection

One of the more advanced laparoscopic procedures performed in urology is the retroperitoneal lymph node dissection for stage I nonseminomatous testis cancer. Such a procedure is feasible in skilled and experienced hands, but its ultimate role in the staging and treatment of testis tumors must be defined. For clinical stage I testicular cancer, there are currently two traditional treatment options: surveillance or open RPLND using a modified unilateral template as described by Donohue and colleagues.[61] Approximately 25% to 30% of patients entering into a surveillance program will have relapse in the retroperitoneum. Conversely, a well-performed open RPLND is effective as a staging tool and is known to be curative in more than 50% of pathologic stage II cases.[62]

The largest series of laparoscopic RPLND reports a 30% complication rate, with bleeding being the most common event. Follow-up is short, and the completeness of the dissection is unknown because the patients were not opened except for surgical complications. The possibility of tumor cell spillage into the peritoneal cavity during laparoscopic dissection is a theoretical concern. Despite prolonged operative times of 4 to 6 hours, the major advantages of laparoscopic RPLND are realized in the postoperative period. In my series of two patients and in the series reported by Gerber and colleagues,[63] paralytic ileus is minimal, with most patients beginning oral feeding within 24 to 48 hours. Nursing requirements are reduced as a result of decreased postoperative pain and need for narcotics. Patients are hospitalized for 3 to 4 days, and convalescence is no more than 7 to 14 days.[63]

The ultimate role of this advanced procedure is undefined. It appears that it may be considered as an excellent staging tool in patients who are not considered ideal for surveillance but do not wish to undergo open RPLND. Laparoscopic RPLND may aid in differentiating the 70% of pathologic stage I patients from the 30% of pathologic stage II patients by employing a minimally invasive procedure with improved postoperative course. This procedure has been performed in a limited number of patients, primarily in men with stage A nonseminomatous testis cancer. The patient must be fully informed of the novelty of this procedure and be prepared to undergo an open laparotomy if technical problems arise.

Laparoscopic Adrenalectomy

The laparoscopic approach to the adrenal gland is similar to that for nephrectomy with respect to port placement. Perirenal fatty tissue must be carefully separated from the surface of the upper portion of the kidney. The adrenal vein on the left side is normally easily found emanating off the left renal vein. The right side is more treacherous because of the short adrenal veins branching from the inferior vena cava. The adrenal mass must be carefully dissected from surrounding structures with liberal use of laparoscopic clips. Attempts are made to avoid direct manipulation of the friable and highly vascular adrenal tissue. The adrenal tissue is removed from the abdominal cavity using a laparoscopic sack.

Most laparoscopic adrenalectomies have been performed for benign neoplasms.[64] The obvious risk of the laparoscopic approach for adrenal carcinoma is dissemination of malignant cells into the operative field during dissection. The advantages of the laparoscopic adrenalectomy are in the postoperative period and include short length of hospitalization and convalescence.

Laparoscopic adrenalectomy for malignant processes should be considered for very small tumors, weighing the novelty and risks of this procedure against gains in the postoperative period.

Laparoscopic Surgery and the Future of Urologic Oncology

Despite the great advances witnessed over the past 5 years, the ultimate role for urolaparoscopic surgery is still being defined. LPLND has gained overall approval within the urologic community for the staging of pelvic malignancies, primarily for prostate cancer. Extirpative en bloc procedures advocated for malignancies involving the kidney, bladder, prostate, or adrenal glands have received less enthusiasm for a number of reasons. First, there is the fear of tumor spillage and inadequate tumor margins, thus compromising the patient's prognosis. Second, the technical demands and long operative times in comparison to the open surgical approach have presented significant obstacles to the urologist. Finally, the requirement for laparoscopic reconstruction of the urinary tract with respect to bladder and prostatic cancer surgery has added another echelon of complexity to the procedure. All of these oncologic procedures have been performed and reported as single case reports or small series. It is evident that as the complexity of these procedures increases, the possibility of a minimally invasive laparoscopic surgery becoming maximally invasive also correspondingly increases.

This is not to say that laparoscopic applications to urologic malignancies are not feasible and that their use will not increase in the future. It is certain that future laparoscopic surgeons will be far more skilled with this type of surgery than what has been demonstrated to date. This, combined with significant advances in hand and reconstructive laparoscopic instrumentation, will make unimaginable oncologic procedures safe, possible, and within the capabilities of all surgeons.

However, all of this wonderful and sophisticated technology and minimally invasive surgery may be for naught. It is my belief that in the next few decades, noninvasive focused therapy, whether it be ultrasound, laser, radiotherapeutic, immunotherapeutic, or chemotherapeutic energy will supersede any form of invasion through the skin or mucous membranes.

REFERENCES

1. Bush R, Leonhardt H, Bush IM, Landers RR. Dr. Bozzini's Lichtleiter: a translation of his original article (1806). Urology 1974;3:119.

1a. Gunning J. The history of laparoscopy. J Reprod Med 1974;12:6.

2. Harrison R. Development of modern endoscopy. J Med Primat 1976; 5:73.

3. Soloway M, Patel J. Endoscopic resection of bladder cancer. Urol Clin North Am 1992;19:467.

4. Smith JA. Laser surgery for transitional-cell carcinoma: technique, advantages, and limitations. Urol Clin North Am 1992;19:473.

5. See WA, Chapman WH. Tumor cell implantation following Nd:YAG bladder injury: a comparison to electrocautery injury. J Urol 1987;137: 1266.

6. Hofstetter A, Kriegmair M, Baumgartner R. Evaluation of laser treatment of bladder cancer. In: Smith JA, Stein BS, Benson RC, eds. Lasers in urologic surgery, 3rd ed. St. Louis: Mosby-Year Book, 1994:114.

7. Chandhoke PS, Clayman RV, Stone AM, et al. Endopyelotomy and endoureterotomy with the Acucise ureteral cutting balloon device: preliminary experience. J Endourol 1993;7:45.

8. Sullivan JW, Grabstald H, Whitmore WF Jr. Complications of ureteroileal conduit with radical cystectomy: review of 336 cases. J Urol 1980;124:797.

9. Hensle TW, Dean GE. Complications of urinary tract reconstruction. Urol Clin North Am 1991;18:755.

10. Golonb J, Klutke CG, Raz S. Complications of bladder substitution and continent urinary diversion. Urology 1989;34:329.

11. Lieskovsky G, Boyd SD, Skinner DG. Management of late complications of the Kock pouch for continent urinary diversion. J Urol 1987; 137:1146.

12. Hanash KA, Utz DC, Cook EN, Taylor WF, Titus JL. Cancer of the prostate: a 15-year follow-up. J Urol 1972;107:450.

13. Smith JA, Cho YH. Management of stage A prostate cancer. Urol Clin North Am 1990;17:769.

14. Schellhammer PF, Bean MA, Whitmore WF Jr. Prostatic involvement by transitional cell carcinoma: pathogenesis, patterns, and prognosis. J Urol 1977;18:399.

15. Bretton PR, Herr HW, Whitmore WF Jr, et al. Intravesical bacillus Calmette-Guerin therapy for in situ transitional cell carcinoma involving the prostatic urethra. J Urol 1989;141:853.

16. McGuire EJ, Appell RA. Injection therapy for urinary incontinence. Urology 1994;43:413.

17. McGuire EJ, Appell RA. Collagen injection for the dysfunctional urethra. Contemp Urol 1991;3:11.

18. Catalona WJ. Urothelial tumors of the urinary tract. In: Walsh PC, Retik AB, Stamey TA, Vaughan ED, Jr., eds. Campbell's urology. Philadelphia: WB Saunders, 1992:1137.

19. Mazeman E. Tumours of the upper urinary tract calyces, renal pelvis, and ureter. Eur Urol 1976;2:120.

20. Johnson DE, Babaian RJ. Conservative surgical management for noninvasive distal ureteral carcinoma. Urology 1979;13:365.

21. Streem SB, Pontes JE, Novick AC, Montie JE. Ureteropyeloscopy in the evaluation of upper tract filling defects. J Urol 1986;136:383.

22. Blute ML, Segura JW, Patterson DE Jr, Benson RC, Zincke H. Impact of endourology on the diagnosis and management of upper urinary tract urothelial cancer. J Urol 1989;141:1298.

23. Gaboardi F, Bozzola A, Dotti E, Galli L. Conservative treatment of upper urinary tract tumors with Nd:YAG laser. J Endourol 1994;8:37.

24. Schmeller NT, Hofstetter AG. Laser treatment of ureteral tumors. J Urol 1989;141:840.

25. Bagley DH, Huffman JL, Lyon ES. Flexible ureteropyeloscopy: diagnosis and treatment in the upper urinary tract. J Urol 1987;138:280.

26. Kerbl K, Clayman RV. Incision of the ureterovesical junction for endoscopic surveillance of transitional cell cancer of the upper tract. J Urol 1993;150:1440.

27. De Torres Mateos JA, Banus Gassol JM, Palou Redorta J, Morote Robles J. Vesicorenal reflux and upper urinary tract transitional cell carcinoma after transurethral resection of recurrent superficial bladder carcinoma. J Urol 1987;138:49.

28. Grasso M. Resecting upper-tract urothelial cancer by ureteroscopy. Contemp Urol 1993;5:52.

29. Orihuela E, Smith AD. Percutaneous treatment of transitional cell carcinoma of the upper urinary tract. Urol Clin North Am 1988;15:425.

30. Clayman RV, Kavoussi LR. Endosurgical techniques for the diagnosis and treatment of noncalculous diseases of the ureter and kidney. In: Walsh PC, Retik AB, Stamey TA, Vaughan ED Jr, eds. Campbell's urology. Philadelphia: WB Saunders, 1992:2231.

31. Cortesi N, Ferrar P, Zambarda E, et al. Diagnosis of bilateral abdominal crytorchidism by laparoscopy. Endoscopy 1976;8:33.

32. Das S, Amar AD. The impact of laparoscopy on modern urologic practice. Urol Clin North Am 1988;15:537.

33. See WA, Cooper CS, Fisher RJ. Urological laparoscopic practice patterns 1 year after formal training. J Urol 1994;151:1595.
34. Whitmore WF Jr. The rationale and results of ablative surgery for prostatic cancer. Cancer 1963;16:119.
35. Grossman IC, Carpiniello V, Greenberg SH, Malloy TR, Wein AJ. Staging pelvic lymphadenectomy for carcinoma of the prostate: review of 91 cases. J Urol 1980;124:632.
36. Golimbu M, Morales P, Al-Askari S, Brown J. Extended pelvic lymphadenectomy for prostatic cancer. J Urol 1979;121:617.
37. Ray GR, Pistenma DA, Castellino RA, Kempson R, Meares E, Bagshaw MA. Operative staging of apparently localized adenocarcinoma of the prostate: results in fifty selected patients. I. Experimental design and preliminary results. Cancer 1976;38:73.
38. McLaughin AP, Saltzstein SL, McCullough DL, Gittes RF. Prostatic cancer: incidence and location of unsuspected lymphatic metastases. J Urol 1976;115:89.
39. Lieskovsky G, Skinner DG, Weisenburger T. Pelvic lymphadenectomy in the management of carcinoma of the prostate. J Urol 1980;124:635.
40. Paulson DF. The prognostic role of lymphadenectomy in adenocarcinoma of the prostate. Urol Clin North Am 1980;7:615.
41. McDowell GC, Johnson JW, Tenney DM, Johnson DE. Pelvic lymphadenectomy for staging clinically localized prostate cancer. Urology 1990;35:476.
42. Schuessler WW, Vancaillie TG, Reich H, Griffith DP. Transperitoneal endosurgical lymphadenectomy in patients with localized prostate cancer. J Urol 1991;145:988.
43. Winfield HN, Donovan JF, See WA, Loening SA, Williams RD. Laparoscopic pelvic lymph node dissection for genitourinary malignancies: indications, techniques and results. J Endourol 1992;6:103.
44. Parra RO, Andrus C, Boullier J. Staging laparoscopic pelvic lymph node dissection: comparison of results with open pelvic lymphadenectomy. J Urol 1992;147:875.
45. Griffith DP, Schuessler WW, Nickell KG, et al. Laparoscopic pelvic lymphadenectomy for prostatic adenocarcinoma. Urol Clin North Am 1992;19:407.
46. Kerbl K, Clayman RV, Petros JA, et al. Staging pelvic lymphadenectomy for prostate cancer: a comparison of laparoscopic and open techniques. J Urol 1993;150:396.
47. Kavoussi LR, Sosa E, Chandhoke P, et al. Complications of laparoscopic pelvic lymph node dissection. J Urol 1993;149:322.
48. McLaughin AP, Saltzstein SL, McCullough DL, Gittes RF. Prostatic cancer: incidence and location of unsuspected lymphatic metastases. J Urol 1976;115:89.
49. Golimbu M, Schinella R, Morales P, Kurusu S. Differences in pathological characteristics and prognosis of clinical A2 prostatic cancer from A1 and B disease. J Urol 1978;119:618.
50. Dretler SP, Ragsdale BD, Leadbetter WF. The value of pelvic lymphadenectomy in the surgical treatment of bladder cancer. J Urol 1973;109: 414.
51. Skinner DG. Management of invasive bladder cancer: a meticulous pelvic node dissection can make a difference. J Urol 1982;128:34.
52. Assimos DG, Jarow JP. Role of laparoscopic pelvic lymph node dissection in the management of patients with penile cancer and inguinal adenopathy. J Endourol 1994;8:365.
53. Grabstald H, Hilaris B, Henschke U, Whitmore WF Jr. Cancer of the female urethra. JAMA 1966;197:835.
54. Grabstald H. Tumors of the urethra in men and women. Cancer 1973; 32:1236.
55. Levine RL. Urethral cancer. Cancer 1980;45:1965.
56. Sarosdy MF. Urethral carcinoma. AUA Update Series, lesson 13, vol 6. 1987.
57. Clayman RV, Kavoussi LR, Soper NJ, et al. Laparoscopic nephrectomy. N Engl J Med 1991;324:1370.
58. Novick AC, Streem S, Montie JE, et al. Conservative surgery for renal cell carcinoma: a single-center experience with 100 patients. J Urol 1989;141:835.
59. Robey EL, Schellhammer PF. The adrenal gland and renal cell carcinoma: is ipsilateral adrenalectomy a necessary component of radical nephrectomy. J Urol 1986;135:453.
60. Clayman RV, Kavoussi LR, Figenshaw RS, Chandhoke PS, Albala DM. Laparoscopic nephroureterectomy: initial clinical case report. Lap Surg 1991;1:343.
61. Donohue JP, Foster RS, Rowland RG, Bihrle R, Jones J, Geier G. Nerve-sparing retroperitoneal lymphadenectomy with preservation of ejaculation. J Urol 1990;144:287.
62. Donohue JP, Thornhill JA, Foster RS, Bihrle R, Rowland EF, Einhorn LH. The role of retroperitoneal lymphadenectomy in clinical stage B testis cancer: the Indiana University experience (1965–1989). J Urol 1995;153:85.
63. Gerber GS, Bissada NK, Hulbert JC, et al. Laparoscopic retroperitoneal lymphadenectomy: multi-institutional analysis. J Urol 1994;152:1188.
64. Suzuki K, Kageyama S, Ueda D, et al. Laparoscopic adrenalectomy: clinical experience with 12 cases. J Urol 1993;150:1099.

Principles and Practice of Genitourinary Oncology, edited by Derek Raghavan, Howard I. Scher, Steven A. Leibel, and Paul H. Lange. Lippincott-Raven Publishers, Philadelphia, © 1997.

CHAPTER 7

Technical Innovations and the Biologic Basis for Three-Dimensional Conformal Radiotherapy

Steven A. Leibel, Gerald J. Kutcher, Radhe Mohan, Gikas S. Mageras, Chandra M. Burman, Chen-Shou Chui, Michael J. Zelefsky, C. Clifton Ling, and Zvi Fuks

The search for new radiotherapy techniques to improve local tumor control continues to represent a major challenge in the management of localized human cancer. Like surgery, radiotherapy is an approach to eradicate localized tumors while attempting to preserve maximally the surrounding normal tissue structures. Ideally, radiation dose distributions should be perfectly focused onto the entire tumor volume while avoiding the surrounding normal organs. However, the achievement of this objective with external beam techniques is fundamentally impossible, because some dose is always deposited along the path of the incidental beam. Furthermore, before computed tomography (CT) scans became available for planning of radiation treatments, tumor target volumes and the boundaries between tumor and normal organs were derived from radiographic images and other techniques and were poorly defined. To reduce the risk of local relapse as a result of tumor localization uncertainties, radiation target volumes have classically included a wide safety margin of surrounding normal tissue. Restrictions imposed by normal tissue tolerance often limited the radiation doses administered to less than optimal levels. Hence, radiation treatment dose levels have been frequently constrained by normal tissue tolerance limitations rather than responding to tumor-associated parameters. Attempts to increase tumor doses required reductions in normal tissue safety margins, often leading to inadvertent underdosing of portions of the tumor and subsequent marginal recurrences.[1,2] CT-assisted treatment planning has significantly improved the ability to define tumor target volumes for radiotherapy[3,4]; however, the problem of geographic misses has not been completely eliminated. The limitations imposed by computer technology have confined the use of CT information in conventional two-dimensional (2D) treatment planning to only one or at most a few CT slices, mostly at or near the level of the central axis of the radiation beam, whereas treatment planning at levels beyond the central axis is not based on detailed CT anatomic information. The lack of precise dose-distribution information for the entire tumor volume has resulted in the same types of treatment planning uncertainties and compensatory mechanisms as those described in the pre-CT era.[1,2,5]

Three-dimensional conformal radiotherapy (3D-CRT) is a mode of high-precision radiotherapy designed to address some of these issues. Sophisticated computer-aided systems are used to plan and deliver prescribed radiation doses, accurately conforming the desired dose distribution to the entire anatomic 3D configuration of the tumor target while excluding to the maximum extent possible the surrounding normal tissues.[6,7] This approach uses dynamic modes or large numbers of static coplanar and noncoplanar fields to improve the ability to focus high-energy external x-ray beams on the entire tumor while reducing the risk of underdosing portions of the target volume.[6,8] At the same time, a rapid decrease in the dose delivered to the surrounding normal tissue as a function of distance from the targeted tumor often permits effective exclusion of the surrounding normal tissues from the volume carried to high radiation dose levels. The resulting decrease in the risk of normal tissue complications has allowed an escalation in tumor dose to levels beyond those feasible with conventional 2D radiotherapy (see Chap. 51.1).[7–11] The improved accuracy of tumor coverage and increase in tumor dose are expected to enhance local tumor control, although such benefit from 3D-CRT remains to be demonstrated.

Although 3D-CRT was implemented in the past using protons[12] and heavy charged particles,[13] the application of this approach to high-energy external x-ray beams (i.e., photons) was not possible or practical until the highly complex software required for treatment planning and for computer-controlled radiation delivery became available.[1] The emergence of high-performance workstations for graphics and fast mathematical computations, as well as the development of new computer-controlled treatment delivery machines with multileaf collimators (MLCs) and electronic on-line portal imaging devices that monitor automated treatments and ensure their quality have made it possible to implement this improved mode of treatment as an advanced radiotherapeutic strategy in several major centers throughout the world.

Inasmuch as this new technology has been applied most frequently to the treatment of patients with carcinoma of the prostate, it represents a major advance in urologic radiation oncology. This chapter highlights the biologic rationale for 3D-CRT as well as the technologic developments designed for the application of this modality. The Memorial Sloan-Kettering Cancer Center (MSKCC) 3D treatment planning and delivery techniques, which have been in clinical use since 1988 for the treatment of prostatic carcinoma as well as other primary tumors,[6,9,14] are presented in this overview.

THE BIOLOGIC BASIS OF THREE-DIMENSIONAL CONFORMAL RADIOTHERAPY

The success of radiotherapy is related to its ability to confer permanent local tumor control. Although the causes of local relapse after radiotherapy are not completely known, variations in the sensitivity of tumor clonogenic stem cells to radiation appear to frequently underlie the failure to control the treated tumor.[15–19] The heterogeneity in the radiation sensitivity of tumor clonogens is a function of several inherent and microenvironmental factors. Anatomic and physiologic parameters, such as the size of the clonogenic stem cell pool and tumor cell kinetics during the course of radiotherapy, were shown to affect the sensitivity of tumors to irradiation. Furthermore, specific microenvironmental factors (i.e., the extent and level of tumor cell hypoxia and autocrine-paracrine effects of cytokines and growth factors that modulate the radiation response) were found to determine the proficiency for cellular radiation damage repair, and this also affects the sensitivity of tumors to radiation exposure.[16–22] Some microenvironmental parameters may vary to a significant degree even within the same tumor, leading to temporal and spatial variations in the radiation sensitivity of clonogenic cell populations.[23–25] Therefore, although many tumor clonogens may be eradicated by a certain dose level, others may survive it, eventually producing a local relapse.

The probability of permanent tumor control is dependent at each dose level on the number of surviving clonogens in the tumor stem cell population. The relation between tumor control and surviving clonogens is described by a Poisson distribution,[26,27] and tumor control probability (TCP) when plotted as a function of dose is graphically represented by a sigmoid-shaped curve.[28] Accordingly, at low radiation dose levels, TCPs are small. At higher doses there is a steep increase in control from 10% to 90% over a relatively narrow dose range, whereas at the highest dose range there is only a small incremental increase of local control with dose until a plateau is reached. A similar dose-response pattern has been observed for radiation-induced injury to normal tissue.

The few available clinical dose-response studies in human tumors generally confirm the sigmoidal nature of dose-tumor control curves.[29–33] However, the dose-response curves for early stage tumors are relatively steep, whereas the curves for locally advanced cancers tend to be shallow and to plateau at relatively low TCP levels.[34,35] The failure to more effectively control large-volume tumors is most likely associated with heterogeneities in the radiation sensitivity of clonogenic tumor cell populations.[21,25,34,35] However, inaccuracies in tumor target coverage by traditional radiotherapy treatment planning techniques also contribute in a major way to the failure to control such tumors.[1,2,6,21,25,34,35] If the precision of treatment planning was optimized, the relative resistance of some types of human tumors to radiation would decrease, and the change in TCP with dose would be steeper than that suggested by published retrospective studies.

The ability of 3D treatment planning to provide complete anatomic and dose information for the entire tumor volume and its surrounding normal tissues has resulted in a marked improvement in target coverage compared with classic 2D techniques.[36–38] However, improving the accuracy of tumor coverage by itself may not be sufficient to confer a maximum probability of local tumor control, because in many instances additional dose is required to achieve this effect.[21] The application of radiation doses required for maximal rates of local control in such tumors is not feasible without producing unacceptable toxicity to the surrounding normal tissues when classic 2D approaches are used. For example, although the actuarial 7-year local relapse rates in stage C prostate cancer patients were found to decrease when the radiation dose to the prostate increased from 60 Gy to 70 Gy or higher,[39] the rates of long-term complications also increased, doubling with doses exceeding 70 Gy.[40] 3D-CRT provides an effective approach to tumor dose-escalation because of the meticulous exclusion of normal tissues from the volume receiving high radiation doses.[6,9] Clinical studies have been designed to test the effect of dose on the probability of local tumor control using the 3D conformal photon beam approach.[2,6–11] Although the clinical application of 3D-CRT is still in the preliminary phases of implementation, the experience accumulated thus far confirms the validity of the basic principles for the design of this approach and suggests an enormous potential for improving the therapeutic ratio of localized human tumors.[8–11]

Efforts to develop 3D-CRT in this context can be justified only if enhanced local tumor control will result in a significant improvement in the survival of treated patients. However, outcome studies have shown that tumor metastasis represents the specific cause of cancer death in the majority of those who succumb to cancer.[41] Therefore, the significance and putative impact of improved local tumor control by radiotherapy is a topic of ongoing debate.[42] Although it is obvious that eradication of the primary tumor is essential for achieving cancer cure, many investigators argue that the presence of incurable micrometastases from spread before initial diagnosis still represents the determinant target for curative efforts in early-stage cancer. Concerns have been raised that attempts to improve survival by enhancement of local control alone may be futile in many types of cancer, because even if achieved, local control will be offset by the eventual development of distant metastatic disease.[43,44]

Although relapse as a result of early micrometastatic dissemination is a documented pattern of failure in a fraction of locally controlled patients, retrospective clinical studies have demonstrated that the development of metastatic disease is frequently associated with recurrences at the original site of the primary tumor.[1,2,42] Some investigators have interpreted these data as indicating that tumors that are resistant to local cure represent biologically aggressive phenotypes that also have a high propensity for metastatic dissemination. According to this hypothesis, prevention of local relapse is unlikely to affect the ultimate curative outcome.[45,46] Although this may be true in some cases, studies of the temporal relation between the appearance of a local relapse and the first detection of metastatic disease are most consistent with the hypothesis that an incremental increase in distant metastases is derived from residual tumor clonogens that acquire a metastatic potential subsequent to the failure to eradicate the primary tumor.[1,2,42] This hypothesis suggests that local failure is a critical biologic determinant in the metastatic outcome and that total eradication of the primary tumor is crucial in affecting the probability of cure.

This concept is supported by evidence from several carefully designed experimental studies in animal models.[47–50] In general, these data indicate that the relapsing tumor is more proficient than the primary tumor at producing metastases.[49,50] There have been few studies that specifically focused on the impact of local control on the occurrence of distant metastases in human tumors. However, available retrospective studies of the patterns of failure in patients undergoing curative local-regional therapy indicate that human tumors conform with the patterns of relapse observed in animal models and exhibit increased metastatic dissemination after failure to control the primary tumor.[1,2,42] These observations suggest a possible cause-effect relation between local relapse and metastatic disease.

Carcinoma of the prostate represents a particularly relevant model for examining the impact of local control on the metastatic outcome, because local failure rarely leads to patient death. Thus, locally relapsing patients survive long enough to evaluate a possible association with metastatic disease. An analysis of 733 surgically staged T2-T3, N0 prostate cancer patients treated at MSKCC with retropubic permanent ^{125}I source implants demonstrated that local failure was the most significant independent variable in predicting the development of metastatic disease (Table 7-1).[51,52] The 20-year actuarial distant metastases–free survival for locally controlled patients was 70%, compared with 13% for those who recurred locally ($P < .00001$; Fig. 7-1*A*).[52] The relation between local disease status and the development of distant metastatic dissemination was uniformly observed across the entire spectrum of biologic variants, from low-stage, low-grade tumors to locally advanced, high-grade lesions.[51] Even in the less-aggressive, stage T2a, N0, well-differentiated tumors, locally controlled patients had a 15-year distant metastases–free survival rate of 82%, compared with 22% in those with local relapse ($P < .00001$). In locally relapsing patients, local failure preceded the diagnosis of distant metastases by a median of 20 months.[51] Furthermore, distant metastases were detected a median of 17 months earlier in patients with local control than in those with local failure, presumably because the former were already preexisting as micrometastases at initial diagnosis whereas the majority of the latter originated secondary to the local recurrence.[51] These relations were, however, confined only to patients with surgically proved node-negative disease (Fig. 7-1*B*). In patients with nodal involvement, control of the primary tumor had no impact on the development of distant metastases (Table 7-2), confirming the notion that nodal involvement in prostate carcinoma is a harbinger of disseminated disease.[52] Similar observations on increased metastatic disease in patients with locally recurring prostatic carcinoma have been reported by other investigators (Table 7-3).[53–57] Associations between local failure and metastatic disease have also been reported in carcinomas of the breast,[46,58,59] lung,[60,61] rectum,[62,63] uterine cervix,[64–66] endometrium and vagina[67,68]; tumors of the head and neck[69–72]; and soft tissue sar-

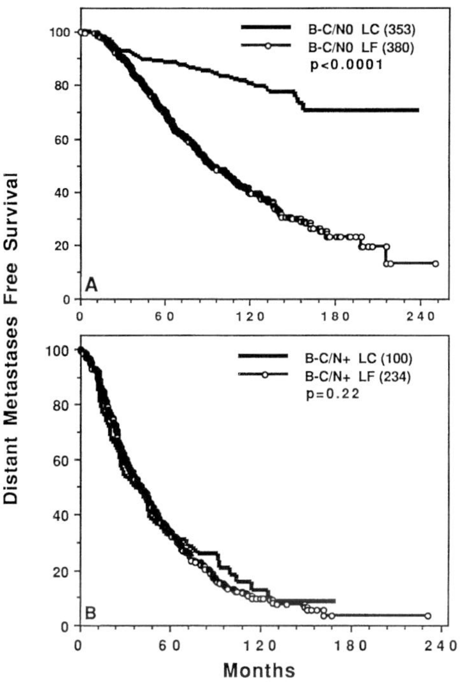

FIG. 7-1. (**A**) Time-adjusted (Kaplan-Meier) distant metastases–free survival (DMFS) by local tumor status in 733 patients with stage T2-T3, N0 prostatic carcinoma treated with pelvic lymphadenectomy and retropubic ^{125}I implantation. The DMFS for locally controlled patients (LC) was significantly improved compared with those who developed a local failure (LF; $P < .00001$). (**B**) Time-adjusted DMFS by local tumor status in 334 patients with stage T2-T3, N1-N2 prostatic carcinoma treated with pelvic lymphadenectomy and retropubic ^{125}I implantation. Control of the primary tumor had no effect on the subsequent development of distant metastases ($P = .22$). (From Leibel SA, Zelefsky MJ, Kutcher GJ, et al. The biological basis and clinical application of three-dimensional conformal external beam radiation therapy in carcinoma of the prostate. Semin Oncol 1994;21:580.)

Table 7-1. *Cox proportional hazards regression anaysis of variables affecting distant metastases–free survival in 733 stage T2-T3/N0 prostate cancer patients treated with pelvic lymphadenectomy and ^{125}I implantation*

Variable	*P* value	Regression coefficient (±SE)	Regression coefficient exponent
Local failure	<.0001	1.38 ± 0.16	4
Grade	.0002	0.31 ± 0.07	1.33
Clinical stage	.008	0.16 ± 0.06	1.11
Implant volume	.014	0.20 ± 0.08	1

SE, standard error.

Table 7-2. *Cox proportional hazards regression anaysis of variables affecting distant metastases–free survival in 334 stage T2-T3/N1-2 prostate cancer patients treated with pelvic lymphadenectomy and ^{125}I implantation*

Variable	*P* value	Regression coefficient (± SE)	Regression coefficient exponent
Nodal stage	.001	0.49 ± 0.13	1.63
Clinical stage	.004	0.35 ± 0.12	1.42
Grade	.05	0.21 ± 0.11	1.24
Local failure	.73		

SE, standard error.

coma.[73–76] These data provide evidence that local relapse exerts a dominant effect on the probability of disease spread to remote sites, even in tumors such as carcinomas of the breast and lung, which exhibit an inherent propensity for early and frequent metastatic dissemination.

Although the biologic mechanism that leads to the association between local tumor failure and metastatic dissemination is not completely understood, the current hypothesis on this relation is based on evidence that the metastatic phenotype arises through a pleiotropic, multistage process of genetic and epigenetic alterations in tumor clonogens that originally lack metastatic competence.[1,2,42,77,78] The mutational gene activity responsible for the metastatic transformation is believed to be part of the general process known as tumor progression.[77,78] Multiple mutational events in several recessive suppressor and dominant regulatory genes are associated with the transformation of nonmetastatic clonogens into cells with metastatic potential,[1,2,42,77–83] including *RB1*, *NM23*, and *P53* suppressor genes.[80–84] Furthermore, several pleiotropic alterations in normal gene function have been identified specifically in metastatic phenotypes and are not present in nonmetastatic phenotypes.[80–86] Such alterations are exemplified by the suppressed expression of the major histocompatibility complex,[86] increased expression of oncogene and regulatory protooncogene products,[87,88] and ectopic expression of enzymes involved in the metastatic cascade (i.e., collagenase type IV,[82] heparanase,[89] and cathepsin proteases[90]).

The recognition that this multistep mutational process exists may explain the mechanism by which local failure enhances the rate of metastatic disease. The fact that localized modes of treatment such as surgery and radiotherapy are capable of curing the majority of patients with early-stage cancer suggests that in many instances the metastatic conversion has not been completed by the time the initial diagnosis of cancer is made. However, tumor cell clonogens remaining in residual tumors after failure to eradicate the primary lesion may be primed with at least some of the genetic alterations required for conversion into the metastatic phenotype.[1,2,42] The enhanced mitotic activity associated with the regrowth of locally failing residual lesions[91,92] provides an apparent opportunity for an accelerated progression through the mutations required for metastatic competence, thus promoting metastatic spread and the observed increase in the incidence of metastatic disease in patients with locally failing cancers.[1,2,42]

To test the validity of this hypothesis, mathematical modeling was used in a recent study to calculate the probability of metastatic disease in relation to the growth kinetics of the primary tumor and that of the local relapse in a simulated model of prostate cancer.[92] Calculations of growth kinetics for the primary tumor, the local relapse, and metastatic tumor deposits were performed according to the Gompertzian formula,[93] whereas the probability of acquiring gene mutations associated with the generation of metastatic competence was estimated according to the algorithm proposed by Goldie and Coldman[94] for the mutagenic development of multidrug resistance. Other parameters of the model were estimated from published clinical data on prostate carcinoma. Hypothetical actuarial rates of distant metastases–free survival were generated for 700 simulated prostate cancer patients with presumed local control or local failure, using a Monte Carlo technique to randomly allocate model parameters for each patient. The computed distant metastases–free survival curves for the simulated patients were compared with the actual long-term outcome data published for 679 stage T2-T3, N0 patients treated with permanent ^{125}I implants.[51] The best agreement with the clinical data for locally relapsing patients was observed when the biologic parameters used in the model assumed that primary tumors in locally relapsing patients were inherently more aggressive and more metastasis-prone than in locally controlled patients, yielding higher rates of micrometastatic dissemination before initial diagnosis. Nonetheless, the model calculations clearly indicated that the expected overall incidence of metastatic disease in patients with local failure was significantly increased over that expected from spread occurring before initial diagnosis.[92]

Based on the model parameters, distant metastases–free survival was calculated for patients with clinical local failure had their disease been locally controlled during initial therapy. Because the model parameters assume a metastatically more ag-

Table 7-3. *Effect of local tumor status on the incidence of distant metastases in prostatic carcinoma*

Investigators	Stage	Patient number	Percent distant metastases	
			Local control	Local failure
Fuks et al, 1991[51] Leibel et al, 1994[52]	B-C/N0	733	30	83
Kuban et al, 1987[53]	A2-C	414	19	68
Zagars et al, 1991[54]	A2-C	601	40	70
Kuban et al, 1992[55*]	A2-C	94	35	71
Prestidge et al, 1992[56*]	A-C	203	41	65
Lai et al, 1992[57]	A2-C	712	24	57

* Local tumor status was determined from postirradiation biopsy specimens.

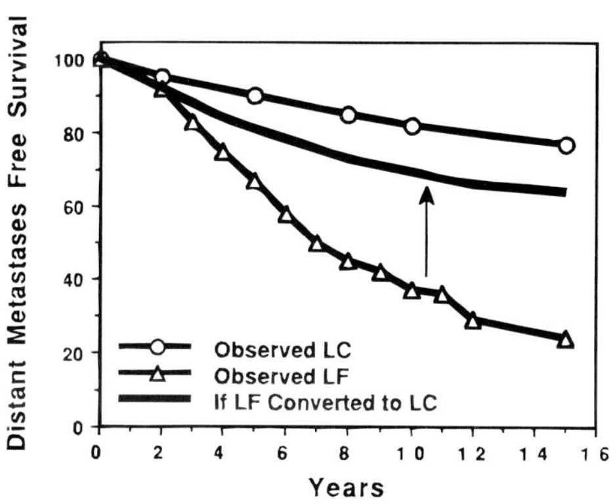

FIG. 7-2. Modeling of the probability of distant metastases–free survival (DMFS) in locally controlled (LC) and locally failing (LF) prostate cancer patients after external beam irradiation. The clinical observations on LC and LF patients were obtained from the data shown in Figure 7-1*A*. DMFS is also calculated for patients with clinical local failure if their disease would have been locally controlled during initial therapy (e.g., three-dimensional conformal radiotherapy; *solid curve*) using the tumor parameters of the model described by Yorke and colleagues.[92] The 15-year estimated DMFS is markedly improved from 23% to 64% with local control; however, because the model parameters assume a metastatically more aggressive primary tumor than is seen in primarily LC patients, DMFS would actually still be lower for patients who converted from LF to LC than for the primarily LC group. (Modified from Yorke ED, Fuks Z, Norton L, Whitmore W, Ling CC. Modeling the development of metastases from primary and locally recurrent tumors: comparison with a clinical data base for prostatic cancer. Cancer Res 1993;53:2987.)

gressive primary tumor than in primarily locally controlled patients, distant metastases–free survival would be lower for this group of patients than for those with local control. However, even after this correction, the hypothetical distant metastases–free survival for this group of patients was markedly improved compared with the clinical results for patients with local failure, demonstrating a potential gain through the avoidance of metastases by improving local control (Fig. 7-2).[92] These data support the hypothesis that improved local control in prostate cancer may significantly decrease the overall incidence of metastatic dissemination, underscoring the importance of complete eradication of the primary tumor during the initial attempt at curative therapy. The potential of improving local control with 3D-CRT provides an opportunity to test this hypothesis in prospective clinical studies. Similar modeling studies and clinical testing in other types of human tumors will be of great interest. Such clinical research will assist in identifying which tumor types will benefit from an improved probability of eradication of the primary tumor in terms of decreasing the mortality from metastatic disease in patients with clinically localized cancer.[1,2]

THREE-DIMENSIONAL TREATMENT PLANNING AND DELIVERY TECHNIQUES

Simulation Procedures

Although 3D treatment planning systems vary in several details, they are based on similar principles. The MSKCC system[1,6,14] is used as a model in this chapter. This planning system is CT-based because dose-calculation formalisms and planning algorithms require that the anatomic information be presented in terms of electron density ratios, which can be obtained only from CT images.[5] However, other imaging methods are also used for the acquisition of the necessary detailed anatomic information. These include magnetic resonance (MR) imaging, positron emission tomography, single photon emission CT, ultrasound, lymphography, and monoclonal antibody imaging. The integration of these data into the planning process requires specialized software programs for image correlation and registration to produce accurate 3D reconstruction of the anatomical configuration of the tumor and the surrounding normal organs.[36]

The simulation process comprises a combination of traditional simulation procedures and specialized CT imaging. Patients are initially fixed in individualized, custom-made immobilization devices (i.e., thermoplastic facial masks, thermoplastic body casts, and alpha cradle body molds). The customized immobilization device used in the treatment of prostate cancer patients at MSKCC[7,9,95] is illustrated in Figure 51.1-1. This cast is also used throughout the treatment course to minimize daily patient positional setup errors and to assure the reproducibility and precision of treatment. The efficacy of this device in accomplishing these goals is discussed later.

Conventional simulation is used to determine the positioning of the patient, to define a provisional isocenter, and to produce reference localization skin marks. For example, prostate cancer patients receive tattoos at the posterior center and two lateral triangulation points in a single transverse plane at the approximate level of the center of the prostate, one mark on each leg at approximately 3 to 4 cm above the popliteal fossa to reproduce leg positioning, and one mark at midback to reproduce upper body position. The patient is CT scanned in the treatment position within the immobilization device fastened to the CT couch, and radiopaque catheters are placed over the localization marks. Alignment lasers in the CT scanner room are matched to the skin marks, and the position of the isocenter and the overall alignment of the patient's bony anatomy are reconfirmed using radiographic anterior and lateral scout views. The number of CT slices obtained and the spacing between slices depends on the size, shape, and location of the region of interest and the treatment technique to be used. To produce the high-resolution 3D reconstructions necessary for the complex 3D dose-distribution calculations, the interslice spacing is generally 0.3 to 0.5 cm, and the slice thickness is chosen to avoid gaps or overlaps in the CT image data set. For example, prostate cancer patients are scanned using 0.5-cm CT slices within the target volume and 1-cm slice thickness over regions 5-cm inferior and 5-cm superior to the treatment volume.

Definition of Target Volume and Critical Organs

The clinical target volume (CTV) for treatment is defined as the volume of tissue that includes the tumor as visualized on CT (gross target volume) and the regions considered to be at risk for microscopic tumor extensions. The CTV is encompassed by a third volume, the planning target volume (PTV). The PTV is defined by adding an additional margin of tissue (0.5 to 1 cm) to the CTV to compensate for patient setup errors and organ motion.[96] Because the PTV is a fixed volume in space in which the CTV moves as a result of setup errors and organ motion, it is essential that a sufficient margin be applied to the tumor-bearing region (CTV) to ensure that these motions are contained within the PTV. Thus, one of the important aims in designing the treatment plan is to assure that the low-dose region (i.e., the region that receives doses below the prescribed value) is excluded from the PTV, thereby avoiding the potential for tumor underdosage.[97]

The contours of the target volume and the surrounding critical normal tissues are identified and drawn manually using a track ball or light pen on every CT section in which they appear. Contours of the body surface, lungs, head and neck air cavities, and bony structures can be extracted automatically using edge-detection computer algorithms. The considerable amount of time and effort required for manual extraction of anatomic features from the large CT image data set and the inaccuracies associated with distinguishing the boundaries between low-contrast tumor and normal tissue structures represent two of the more challenging problems of available 3D treatment planning systems. Artificial intelligence and new image processing techniques are under development to facilitate the anatomic extraction process; however, regardless of improved technology, human input will remain an essential component in this process. It is unlikely that the effort required for contouring the tumor and its adjacent normal tissue structures will ever be eliminated or reduced to levels typical for traditional 2D treatment planning techniques.

Following the extraction of anatomic data, the PTV and normal tissue structures required for treatment planning are reconstructed graphically on the treatment planning system in 3D and displayed using the beam's-eye view (BEV) technique.[6,98] In the BEV mode, anatomic structures are displayed as seen by the viewer if positioned at the beam's source. This enables the identification of all organs that will be included and facilitates the selection of beam shapes and directions that minimize the radiation exposure of normal tissues while simultaneously conforming the beam to the accurate anatomic details of the tumor (Fig. 7-3). To facilitate the visualization of the spatial orientation of the beam, reference images are concomitantly displayed showing the intersection of the beam on axial, sagittal, and coronal CT images through the isocenter. Furthermore, the machine configurations, including gantry, couch, collimator angles, and collimator jaw positions, are shown as a three-panel representation of the treatment machine viewed from three orthogonal perspectives.

Selection of Beams and Calculation of Dose Distributions

Most 3D-CRT plans are based on the application of multiple fields in transaxial coplanar, nonaxial coplanar, or noncoplanar (i.e., beam directions that are outside a plane perpendicular to the patient axis) static field arrangements, with each beam precisely shaped to conform to the anatomic shape of the tumor as visualized by BEV from its directional angle. Once the beam orientations for a treatment plan are selected, continuous beam apertures with an additional margin of 0.5 to 1 cm to account for beam penumbra are automatically created by the planning system. When computer-driven MLCs are used for beam shaping (discussed later), the position of each MLC leaf is automatically determined based on the continuous boundary design by the "transecting" convention.[99] According to this convention, each MLC leaf edge transects the surrogate aperture boundary such that the total area exposed is the same. The leaf arrangement parameters are eventually transferred from the treatment planning system to the treatment machine.[100] For future reference and evaluations of treatment compliance by portal images, the MLC leaf positions for each treatment field are transferred from digitally reconstructed radiographs (DRRs), generated

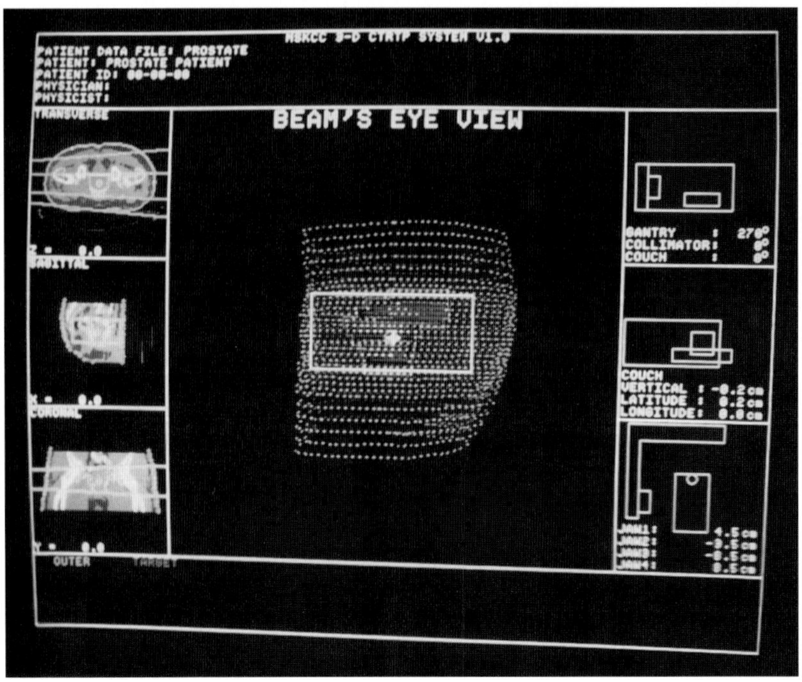

FIG. 7-3. Beam's-eye view of the prostate, seminal vesicles, and body surface contour shown as wire-frame projections. Reconstruction of the prostate and seminal vesicles (*blue*) and the body surface (*red*) are displayed in relation to the beam path of a lateral irradiation field (*yellow rectangle*). In this field, a beam aperture (*green line*) representing the leaves of a multileaf collimator is drawn around the target volume. Midplane axial, sagittal, and coronal computed tomographic images with the intersections of the displayed beam in each image are shown on the left, and treatment machine orientation parameters for this field are displayed on the right. (See Color Figure 7-3.)

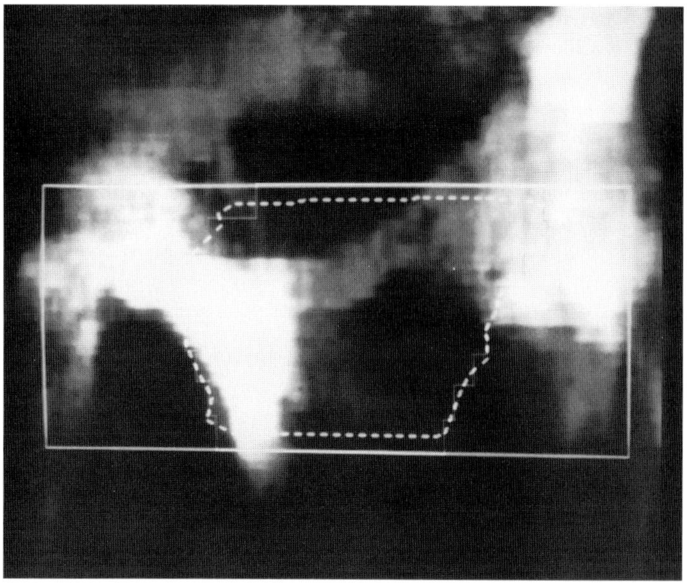

FIG. 7-4. Digitally reconstructed radiograph (DRR) produced from the planning computed tomography image set. The DRR is superimposed with a treatment field (*solid red line*) with beam aperture shapes for a conventional low melting alloy block (*broken red line*) and for a multileaf collimator field (*green line*). Radiographic simulator films are obtained for each of the treatment fields, and the beam aperture block outline for each treatment field on the DRR is transferred onto the simulator films, which are used for comparison with treatment portal and verification films. (See Color Figure 7-4.)

from the simulation CT image set, onto radiographic simulator films obtained for each of the fields (Fig. 7-4). DRRs with beam aperture block outlines can also be used as templates for traditional low melting alloy block fabrication.

Dose computations are performed for the entire 3D space. Powerful computers are required because of the enormous complexity of the dose calculation formalisms. Modern methods of 3D dose calculations are based on data of complex transport of radiation through the entire geometry of the tissues and its pleiotropic interactions with absorbing media, and they also account for variations in tissue composition and density.[101] The techniques most commonly used include the radiologic path length method,[101] the scatter integration technique,[102,103] and the more advanced delta-volume,[104] differential pencil beam (DPB),[105,106] and Fourier convolution methods.[107,108] At MSKCC, 3D dose distributions are calculated using a pencil beam convolution algorithm with pixel-by-pixel inhomogeneity corrections.[5] In this method, the broad beam is divided into a large number of narrow beams called pencils, and the dose is computed by summating the contributions from each of the individual pencil beams. The computation formalism uses the convolution of Monte Carlo–generated 2D pencil beam profiles (called pencil beam kernels) with photon fluence distributions that facilitate calculations of dose distributions for irregularly shaped fields.[105] The computing times needed to perform the convolution are minimized by using fast Fourier transforms.[107] Corrections for surface curvatures and internal inhomogeneities are performed using the conventional radiologic path length technique.[101]

The accuracy of computed dose distributions for curved patient surfaces and inhomogeneous internal structures can be further improved by the DPB method.[106] A DPB is the portion of a photon pencil beam that has collisions within an infinitesimal volume element at a specified point in the medium through which the pencil beam is propagating. This method incorporates the 3D distribution of the dose deposited by electrons ejected by primary, first-scattered, and all multiply scattered photons. The effect of the internal structure on the scattered radiation is incorporated by using the electron-density–weighted path length between the point of collision and the point of calculation instead of the actual geometric path length. This technique is especially well suited for high-energy photon beams and for regions where electronic equilibrium does not exist. The DPB method requires integrations over energy and volume and 3D ray tracing to compute path lengths, and is highly CPU time-intensive. As a result, its utility is limited to investigational projects; however, new generation computers and new highly efficient algorithms are being developed to facilitate the implementation of the DPB method for routine clinical use.

To further improve the efficiency of the 3D treatment planning, various ''autoplans'' are used to automate a variety of procedures in the treatment planning process.[109] This approach is applicable once a ''class solution'' to a planning problem has been achieved, and the same planning steps are applied repeatedly in a given situation. This approach is currently used at MSKCC for treatment planning of carcinoma of the prostate. After contouring each of the relevant structures and selecting an isocenter, the autoplan automatically applies radiation ports from the standard gantry orientations (beam directions), designs each field shape, calculates the dose distributions, displays isodose distributions in three orthogonal planes, and provides quantitative dose-volume information. Values of the various parameters (e.g., gantry angles, margins on aperture design) are user-selectable and contained in libraries that are disease site– and treatment technique–specific.

Quantitative Treatment Plan Evaluation

Traditional treatment plan evaluation methods in which isodose distributions are superimposed onto 2D axial CT displays of the tumor and surrounding tissues along the central axis of the radiation beam or at a few off-axis levels do not provide sufficient information to adequately evaluate 3D treatment plans.[110] Several different methods of spatial dose display are available, including the capability to superimpose isodose curves on 2D axial, sagittal, and coronal CT images as well as on any reconstructed oblique plane. Color wash displays in which the pixels within a given dose range are assigned a specific color are also used as CT overlays and serve as useful tools for the graphic examination of 3D dose distributions (Fig. 7-5). Similar techniques are used to generate dose-difference displays, which highlight the difference in dose distributions between rival plans (Fig. 7-6), and for images of regret in which regions of overdose to normal critical structures or of underdose to the target volume may be readily identified. Dose distributions may also be displayed as isodose surfaces superimposed or covering 3D anatomic configurations of the tumor and normal organ structures. Different surface rendering techniques are used to distinguish anatomy from isodose surfaces. For example, the anatomy may be shown as a stack of contours and the dose as a mesh of points or as a solid transparent surface. Simultaneous volumetric displays of the 3D CT data and dose distribution have also been implemented in which both the structures and the dose distributions are shown in a see-through manner with different degrees of transparency. Although these graphic presentations of spatial dose distributions are useful for rapid qualitative evaluations of treatment plans and for the identification of ''hot'' or ''cold'' spots within a given dose distribution, such methods by themselves provide only a quali-

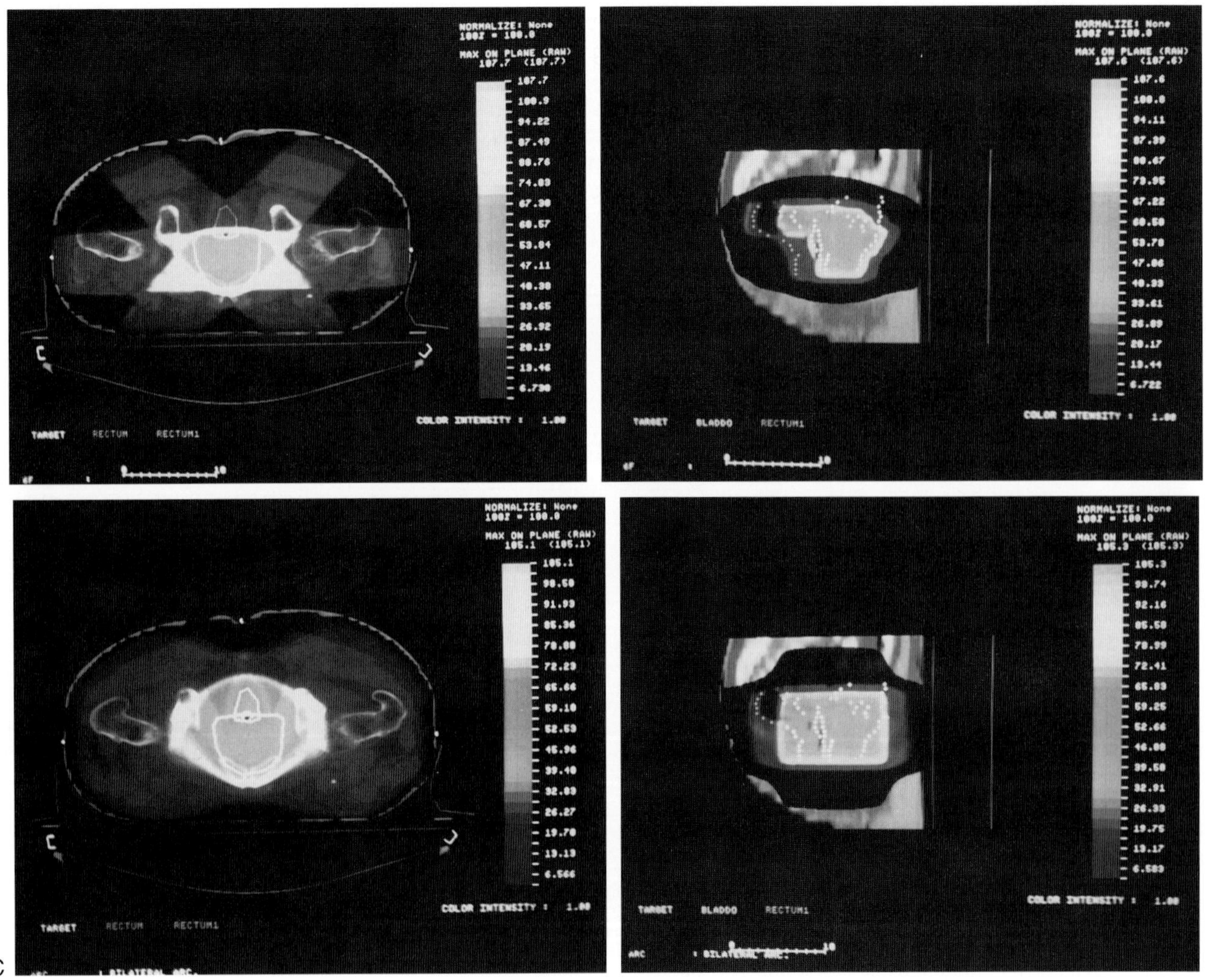

A B C D

FIG. 7-5. Comparison of dose distributions for a three-dimensional (3D) conformal six-field plan and a traditional 120-degree bilateral arc rotation plan for a patient with carcinoma of the prostate. Midplane (**A**) axial and (**B**) sagittal color-wash dose-distribution displays of the six-field coplanar 3D prostate treatment plan for 15-mV x-rays, consisting of one pair of lateral and two pairs of oblique fields. In this display, a band of the color spectrum (*right*) corresponds to a range of doses. The prescription dose is normalized to 100%. The red region corresponds to the prescription isodose distribution (100% to 107%), yellow represents approximately 75% to 95%, green represents 50% to 74%, and blue represents 49% or less. The target contour is outlined in yellow dots, and the rectum and bladder (**B** and **D**) are represented by blue and magenta dots, respectively. Midplane (**C**) axial and (**D**) sagittal color-wash dose-distribution displays for a conventional 120-degree bilateral arc rotational approach. Because this technique does not allow the use of shaped blocks to shield normal tissues, a greater volume of the rectum and bladder receive high radiation doses than with the conformal approach. (See Color Figure 7-5.)

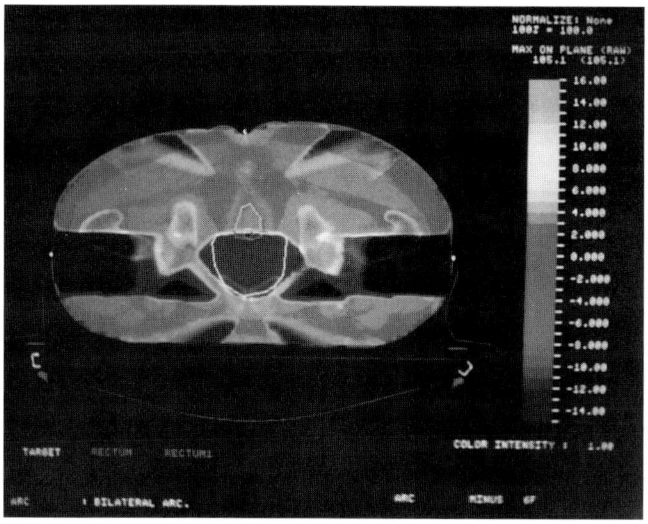

A

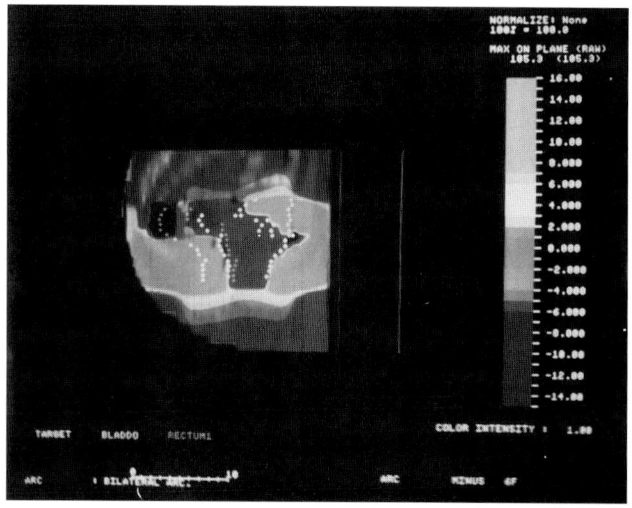

B

FIG. 7-6. Midplane (**A**) axial and (**B**) sagittal color-wash displays of the difference in dose distribution between the two treatment plans shown in Figure 7-5. The region that receives a higher radiation dose with the traditional rotational plan than with the conformal plan is shown in red, the region in which the dose is similar is shown in green, and the area in which the dose is lower in the rotational plan than in the conformal plan is shown in blue. (See Color Figure 7-6.)

tative representation of a treatment plan and are insufficient for the final selection of the most appropriate plan. Complementary information is obtained from evaluation methods based on objective numerical criteria and quantitative indices.

Cumulative dose-volume histograms (DVHs) represent the most useful numerical treatment plan evaluation method.[111,112] DVH displays condense the dose-distribution data and graphically present the cumulative volume, or the percentage of the total organ volume, receiving at least the dose D as a function of the total dose or a percentage of the total dose. One DVH is generated for the tumor and one for each organ of interest in the treatment plan. A compilation of the curves is used for evaluation of the adequacy of the proposed plan and for comparing different plans (Fig. 7-7). DVHs are also clinically useful in the treatment of prostate cancer for determining the indication for neoadjuvant hormonal therapy to reduce the size of the prostate before radiotherapy.[113] When DVHs indicate that the volume of the rectal wall, bladder wall, or small bowel receiving the prescription dose exceeds limits that place the patient at a presumed increased risk of treatment-related toxicity ($>$ 30% for rectal wall, $\geq$ 50% for bladder wall, and $\geq$ 65% for adjacent small bowel), a three-month course of androgen deprivation therapy is prescribed. Significant reductions in the respective volumes irradiated have been observed in nearly 90% of patients treated with this approach, and to date we have not observed even moderate-grade late rectal, bladder, or bowel complications by adhering to this treatment policy.[113]

There are several limitations to DVHs. If the DVHs do not cross one another, then the curve which is located furthest to the left in the case of normal organ DVHs (Fig. 7-7*B*) and furthest to the right in the case of tumor DVHs is considered the best plan; frequently, however, the histograms cross one another, and the ranking of the DVHs in rival plans is not so clear. Thus, it is not always evident which plan is better. If there are a number of rival plans and many organs, DVH comparisons can become complex and cumbersome. In addition, DVHs do not provide spatial information, so that if hot or cold regions are present, their positions cannot be obtained directly from the DVH, and spatial dose distributions must be used to complement the DVH information. Moreover, DVHs do not take into account the complex tradeoffs between tumor control and normal tissue toxicities. Therefore, although DVHs yield information complementary to spatial dose distribution displays, numerical scoring function indices that correlate with biologic endpoints have also been introduced to further improve the selection of an optimum plan.

The most frequently used quantitative indices are normal tissue complication probabilities (NTCPs)[114–121] and TCPs,[122,123] which condense structure-specific dose-distribution data to yield a single number for defined endpoints in each tissue of interest. Unfortunately, NTCP and TCP indices are based on rather rudimentary models normalized to clinical endpoints that are generally not well established.[124] New approaches to the computation of NTCP are currently in development. NTCP calculations may be classified into two general categories: empirical or statistical. Following an empirical approach of Lyman,[119] Burman and colleagues[114] fit clinically derived normal tissue tolerances for uniform whole- and partial-organ irradiation to a sigmoidal function. The input data were taken from compiled human organ tolerance doses.[124] Because normal organ dose distributions are invariably inhomogeneous, it was necessary to interpolate or extrapolate from these data. Thus, a histogram reduction scheme was developed that converts a nonuniform histogram into an equivalent uniform function.[115,125] Once an equivalent histogram is calculated, the NTCP is obtained by interpolation of the NTCPs for uniform irradiation.

The statistical NTCP calculation approach is based on the hypothesis proposed by Withers and colleagues[126] that organs consist of independent functional subunits (FSUs), and the response of an organ to irradiation depends on the radiosensitivity of the FSUs and their architectural arrangement (i.e., the manner in which the FSUs combine to provide organ function). Two

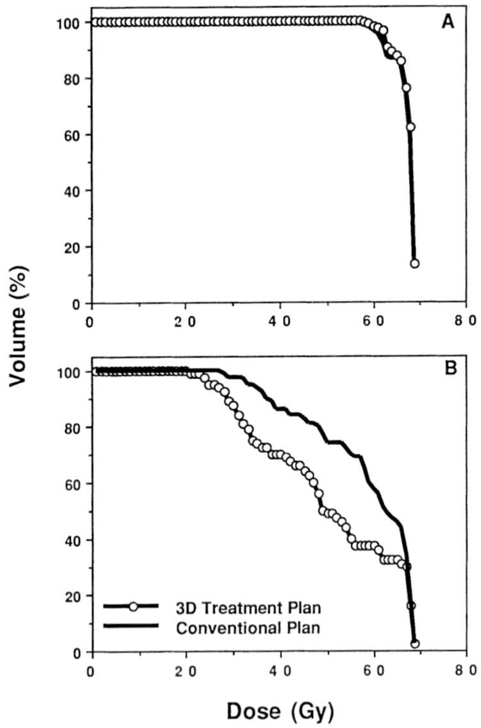

FIG. 7-7. Comparison of dose-volume histograms for (**A**) the tumor target (prostate and seminal vesicles) and (**B**) the rectal wall for a three-dimensional (3D) conformal six-field treatment plan and a traditional 120-degree bilateral arc rotational plan for a patient with carcinoma of the prostate. Although coverage of the tumor target is identical in the two treatment plans, the volume of the rectal wall receiving high radiation doses is increased with the rotational plan because this technique does not permit the use of shaped blocking to shield normal tissues. (From Leibel SA, Zelefsky MJ, Kutcher GJ, et al. The biological basis and clinical application of three-dimensional conformal external beam radiation therapy in carcinoma of the prostate. Semin Oncol 1994;21:580.)

putative arrangements exist; these are referred to as serial and parallel architectures. In the serial model it is assumed that a complication will occur if at least one FSU is eradicated. The NTCP then follows from binomial statistics. Serial models have been applied to neural tissue and to small bowel complications.[126–128] Parallel organs with integral response have received very limited attention.[121,129] Jackson and colleagues[130] and Yorke and colleagues[131] have developed an NTCP model for organs with parallel architecture that may manifest quantal behavior. The model assumes that a complication occurs if the number of FSUs eradicated exceeds a threshold value, the organ's functional reserve. Parallel quantal models may apply to the kidneys, liver, lungs, and parotid glands. Binomial statistics can again be used to derive general expressions for the NTCP. For example, when the number of FSUs is large, the NTCP is represented by an error function that depends on the mean and standard deviation of the number of irradiated FSUs as well as the functional reserve. The special cases of whole or partial uniform irradiation were studied for the kidney, lung, and liver, comparing the parallel NTCP model with clinical data. Adopting reasonable biologic and radiobiologic parameters for the FSUs (i.e., number of cells per FSU and linear and quadratic coefficients for cell inactivation), calculated results were shown to fit clinical data for whole- and partial-organ complications reasonably well.[131,132]

An important consequence of this modeling is that the volume effect (i.e., change in NTCP with volume) differs between the serial and parallel architectures, and furthermore, that the volume effect for these architectures differs from predictions based on empirical data.[131] In addition, some organs with parallel architecture may also exhibit a graded response, in which the intensity of organ response increases with dose. Because normal organ dose distributions for rival plans differ, sometimes significantly, the volume effect will not cancel out; thus, treatment plan evaluation and optimization programs are likely to be sensitive to the model used. Additional studies are required to investigate the sensitivity of ranking of rival treatment plans by using different models and by varying their parameters. It may turn out that ranking plans will be less sensitive to the model than anticipated. For example, Kutcher and colleagues[115] found that although NTCP could be changed significantly when the volume effect parameter was adjusted in the empirical model, there was little change observed in the ranking of four rival nasopharynx treatment plans. In addition, the fact that serial and parallel architecture organs have a different volume effect implies that the optimal treatment strategy for a tumor near an organ with a serial model configuration may be quite different from that for a tumor near an organ with a parallel configuration. Studies in experimental animals and clinical investigations are required to further elucidate the volume effect.

TCPs for inhomogeneously irradiated tumors are estimated using an algorithm by Goitein[122] in which the tumor is divided into voxels or "tumorlets" that are sufficiently small that the dose within each is considered to be uniform. The TCP of each tumorlet is computed by assuming a biologic response function and values of its parameters for an individual patient. The TCP of the whole tumor is the product of the TCPs of its component tumorlets. This TCP is then averaged over the entire population of patients. The parameters of the model are chosen in such a way that the population-averaged TCP for an uniformly irradiated tumor agrees with observed tumor-response data. Goitein and colleagues[133] and Niemierko and Goitein[134] have incorporated intratumoral heterogeneity, tumor size, and SF_2 (the surviving fraction of tumor cells for a dose of 2 Gy) as TCP model parameters. Knowledge of the SF_2 of a tumor may permit a prognostically more accurate, patient-specific estimate of TCP.

Currently, NTCPs, derived by the effective volume technique,[115,125] and TCPs, determined by the Goitein method,[122] are calculated for each of the conformal plans to evaluate the consistency and accuracy of the input data and the algorithms. Studies have shown that in some cases the absolute value of the calculations do not agree with clinical experience, whereas in others they appear to be clinically consistent. Nevertheless, the relative values may still prove useful for ranking rival treatment plans. It is important to emphasize that the models for quantitative treatment plan evaluation use endpoints that are based on limited clinical experience; thus, their predictions should be viewed with caution. However, their potential predictive power makes their development important. Together with DVHs and spatial dose distributions, these models may make it possible to obtain a fairly complete evaluation of 3D treatment plans to facilitate the selection of the most optimal plan.

Computer-Aided Optimization

The selection of 3D treatment plans using a trial-and-error approach is a slow, labor-intensive process. 3D treatment planning requires detailed, complex integration of graphic and numeric information on anatomy and dose distributions that may often approach the limits of human capabilities. Furthermore, the number of options to be explored, including beam energy, modality (photons or electrons), beam weights, wedge type and orientation, aperture shapes and margins, and gantry and couch angles, is large and may require tremendous effort to prioritize plans according to their predicted clinical usefulness. For example, the conformal treatment plan used in the MSKCC prostate dose-escalation study to increase the dose from 75.6 to 81 Gy required 1.5 physicist-months for exploring different treatment plan options by trial and error before an optimal class solution was reached and selected.[109] It is unlikely that the full clinical potential of 3D treatment planning can be realized without the application of computer-aided techniques. Computer-aided optimization of treatment planning exploits the high-performance capabilities of high-power computer workstations in the systematic search for an optimal plan. The criteria for search are based on the probabilities of tumor control, subject to limitations imposed by the acceptable probability of normal tissue complications. The MSKCC computer-aided optimization method incorporates biophysical models of TCP and NTCP (described previously) to quantify the predicted clinical consequences of a tested dose distribution in terms of an objective score function.[135] In this technique, all beam parameters except beam weights are preselected, and the beam weights are adjusted by the optimization process. After selection of a "domain of search" consisting of the number of beams and their characteristics, an optimization process is initiated to identify the subset of beams in the domain and the weights of these beams that will result in the maximum clinical benefit to the patient.

As a first step in this optimization approach, an arbitrary weight value is assigned to each beam, and the dose distributions are calculated for each of the beams in the domain of search. Based on the dose distribution obtained, TCP and the NTCP for each of the critical normal structures in the treatment volume are computed. The optimization algorithm subsequently adjusts the weights of these beams to balance NTCPs against each other and against TCP to maximize the score using a modified form of the simulated annealing technique.[136] Optimization approaches that do not use simulated annealing allow changes in the configuration of beams and their weights only in the direction in which the plan improves according to the specified criteria. Changes are continued until there is no further improvement in the plan. However, the best plan achieved by this approach may not necessarily be the most optimal plan feasible, because the balancing of TCP and NTCP of a number of normal may involve many maxima (hills) and minima (valleys) and may, thus, be trapped in one of the local valleys. The simulated annealing technique overcomes these difficulties and not only allows improvement in plans but also decreases the probability of accepting a "trapped" inferior plan. Given a sufficient number of trials, this method permits the objective function to avoid local traps and improves the confidence factor of optimization plans.

As noted previously, the currently available biophysical models for computing clinical indices (TCP and NTCP) are simplistic and are based on limited normal tissue–tolerance and tumor-response information. To overcome some of these weaknesses in the optimization process, strict constraints must be imposed to ensure that the results of optimization are consistent with the judgment of the physician. Only preliminary results of the application of optimization methods, mainly for evaluating treatment plans for carcinoma of the prostate, are available, but the results have been highly encouraging.[135]

Another optimization approach is the inverse planning technique.[137–139] In this method, the intensity distribution (i.e., the weights of individual rays) within each field is allowed to vary. Modulation of individual ray weights and the combination of multiple fields produces a distribution of dose that is as close to the specified desired dose distribution as physically possible (Fig. 7-8). The desired dose distribution and its uniformity throughout the target volume, as well as the upper limits of dose to critical normal organs, are initially defined. Using reconstruction techniques applied routinely for tomographic images, the desired dose distribution is mathematically inverted. A typical intensity profile resulting from the inversion process is shown in Figure 7-9. Although in image reconstruction the CT image is computed from measured transmitted intensities of x-rays, the converse is true for inverse planning in radiotherapy, in which incident intensity profiles are reconstructed from a given dose image. Because of this relation between the two problems, methods developed for image reconstruction, such as filtered back-projection, can be readily adapted for optimizing intensity modulation in radiotherapy. The dose distribution calculated using the resulting intensity distributions are as close to the prescribed dose distribution as feasible in terms of the sum of least square differences.[139]

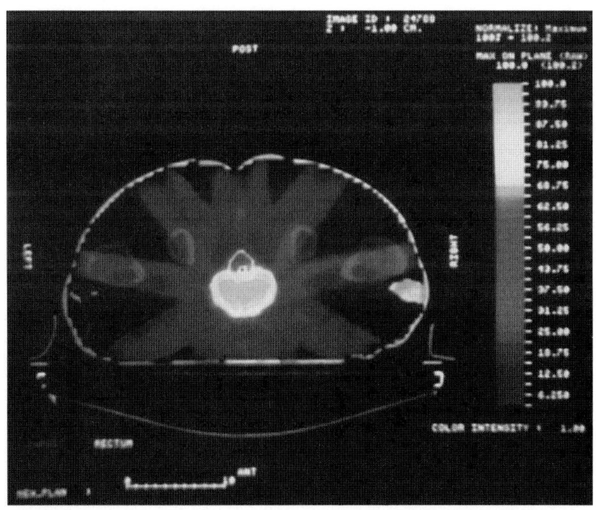

FIG. 7-8. Axial color-wash dose-distribution display of an inverse treatment plan consisting of nine equiangular intensity-modulated fields for a patient with carcinoma of the prostate. There is marked improvement in the conformality of the dose distribution to the shape of the target volume (*white dots*) compared with the six-field conformal plan shown in Figure 7-5*A*. The objective of this plan was to deliver a dose of 81 Gy to the target volume while limiting the upper dose to the rectum (*yellow dots*) to 60% of the target dose. (See Color Figure 7-8.)

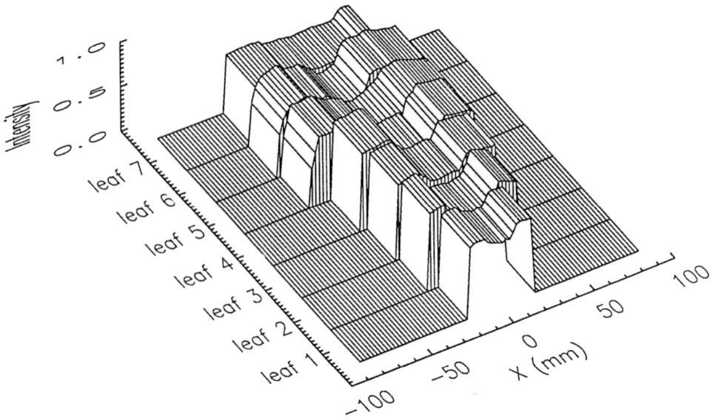

FIG. 7-9. Two-dimensional intensity profile for the anterior field of a nine-field prostate plan generated by inversion of the desired dose distribution using the Memorial Sloan-Kettering Cancer Center inverse planning algorithm. The decrease in intensity at the midbeam region is necessary to reduce the radiation dose to the rectum. (From Mohan R, Xang XH, Jackson A, et al. The potential and limitations of inverse radiotherapy technique. Radiother Oncol 1994;32:232.)

The inverse technique produces satisfactory results for some treatment sites (e.g., prostate, brain) but is a poor method for others (e.g., lung). This pattern is a consequence of the fact that the inverse planning approach specifies optimization objectives purely in terms of a desired distribution of dose but does not consider biologic indices; objective functions based on dose-volume criteria and other biologic indices are not readily invertible. A new scheme for optimizing intensity distributions that employs biologic indices has been applied.[140] The incorporation of biologic parameters produces plans that are considerably superior to those in which only dose-based objectives are used, especially in the planning of the treatment of lung tumors. In contrast, incorporation of biologic parameters produces only a marginal improvement in other organ sites, such as the prostate, indicating that there are situations in which dose limits alone are an adequate index of the value of a plan.

Because intensity distributions for each field may be nonuniform, new methods of treatment delivery that incorporate beam intensity profile modulation are required. One approach is to use computer-controlled MLCs in the dynamic mode. In this technique, gaps between pairs of opposing MLC leaves sweep across the target volume, creating a sliding window. The gap widths and leaf speeds are varied to deliver the requisite amount of radiation. The gaps are maximized as a function of monitor units to minimize the time required for treatment delivery.[141,142] Clinical testing of this approach is expected to begin in the near future.

Treatment Delivery Systems

The application of 3D treatment techniques generally requires a large number of fields administered daily to improve the ratio of tumor–to–normal tissue dose. The practical application of 3D-CRT has been facilitated by the availability of new radiation delivery machines that are capable of safely and rapidly delivering large numbers of arbitrarily shaped fields under automated computer control (i.e., the multisegment approach).[6,100,143] Automated beam shaping using MLCs is an essential component of such 3D treatment delivery systems. These developments have enabled the delivery of 3D multisegment therapy within time frames that are comparable to traditional techniques, despite the use of a large number of fields and complex treatment maneuvers.

The MLC is a secondary collimator system, which consists of independently movable slabs or leaves made of tungsten. Each leaf is independently mobile in the horizontal plane, each is operated by an individual dedicated motor, and the function of all motors is coordinated under computer control. The leaves on both sides can thus be automatically positioned to shape the treatment beam for successive multisegment fields according to a preprogrammed plan. Some MLCs can be retrofitted onto existing linear accelerators, whereas other types are designed as built-in components. The spatial resolution with currently available MLCs is usually 1 to 1.25 cm, or the projected leaf width in the patient's midplane, although narrower leaf widths

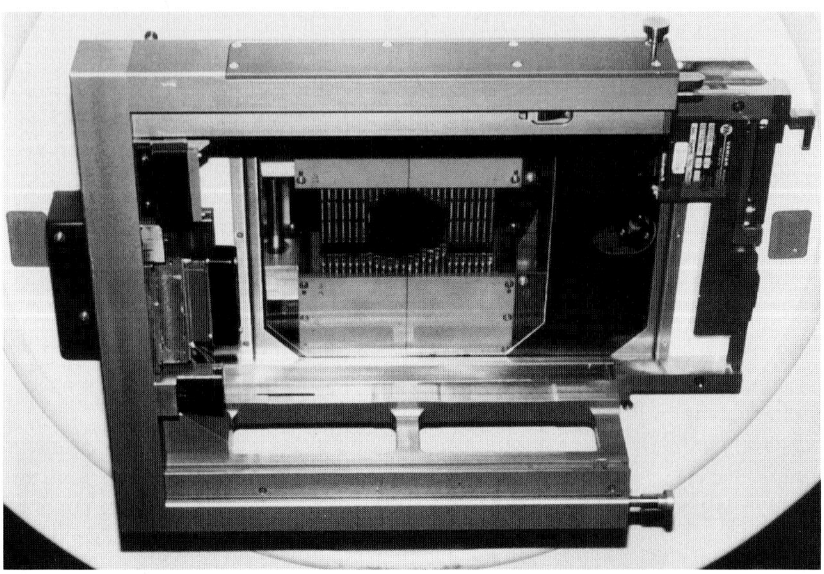

FIG. 7-10. Computer-controlled multileaf collimator for photon beam shaping on a Varian 2100C Linear Accelerator (Varian Associates, Palo Alto, CA) at the Memorial Sloan-Kettering Cancer Center. This multileaf collimator features 26 pairs of leaves, each individually driven by a dedicated motor. The function of all motors is computer coordinated according to preplanned specifications. (From Leibel SA, Kutcher GJ, Mohan R, et al. Three-dimensional conformal radiation therapy at the Memorial Sloan-Kettering Cancer Center. Semin Radiat Oncol 1992;2:274.)

may be available in the future for treatment of small target volumes. Integration of MLC beam shaping with other automated motions of the machine is currently being developed to produce the full range of static multisegment and dynamic conformal systems. One example of a MLC is shown in Figure 7-10.

The applicability of MLC as a replacement for conventional cerrobend beam-shaping blocks has been evaluated.[99] The aim of this study was to examine whether isodose distributions produced by the discontinuous field edges of the MLC would be acceptable compared with those produced by conventional cerrobend blocks. The effects of scatter within the patient, the contributions from many fields to the dose at each point in the patient, and the influence of patient setup uncertainty tended to smooth the increased penumbra inherent for the MLC such that the dose distributions and the TCPs and NTCPs for MLC-shaped fields were indistinguishable from those obtained using smooth cerrobend apertures.[99]

The accuracy and initial clinical experience of automated segmental therapy has been assessed in 31 patients with prostate cancer treated with a conformal 3D plan.[143] This study showed that computer-controlled segmental therapy can be performed reliably on a routine basis. The reproducibility of computer-controlled positioning of the gantry and MLC leaves was better than 0.5 degrees and 0.1 cm, respectively. Importantly, treatment times with the specific system tested were much shorter than those with a conventional linear accelerator. The net treatment delivery time, excluding the time required for patient setup, was 4 minutes for MLC treated patients, compared with 12 minutes for the same treatment with traditional cerrobend blocks for field shaping. Overall, the daily throughput of patients treated using automated machines is approximately doubled when MLC is used instead of cerrobend blocks. The demonstrated accuracy of computer-controlled setup is consistent with that needed for conformal therapy, permitting future developments in computerized treatment delivery, including intensity modulation and incorporation of couch motion and noncoplanar fields into treatment plans. The latter, however, will require that additional safeguards be incorporated for collision avoidance.

Treatment Verification

The enhanced technical capability associated with 3D-CRT brings with it increasing complexity in assurance and verification of radiation delivery. To assure that treatment is delivered as planned, treatment verification is performed in most 3D systems with traditional portal films, produced at least once per week. However, the conventional method of treatment verification by portal films is labor intensive for segmental therapy and would be impossible for dynamic modes of radiotherapy. To address this issue, on-line electronic portal imaging systems have been introduced that enable fluoroscopy-like real-time examination of the actual treatment fields as given daily to the patient (Fig. 7-11).[144] Although the component structure of these devices differs among manufacturers, they all have in common an imaging detector attached to the machine gantry, methods of digitizing and computer analyzing the image data, and a display system. In addition, the images can be electronically enhanced for improved visualization of details that are difficult to observe with conventional screen film systems. The major potential of these systems for conformal therapy is the ease with which each field can be verified. Thus, with on-line systems it is possible to image all segments during treatment, whereas with traditional portal verification methods this cannot be accomplished without stopping treatment and entering the treatment room.

Other advantages of on-line imaging beyond its use as replacement for port film is the potential for assessing setup errors and their dosimetric consequences and in providing potential capabilities for automated on-line correction systems of patient setup errors prior to or during treatment, using internal anatomic

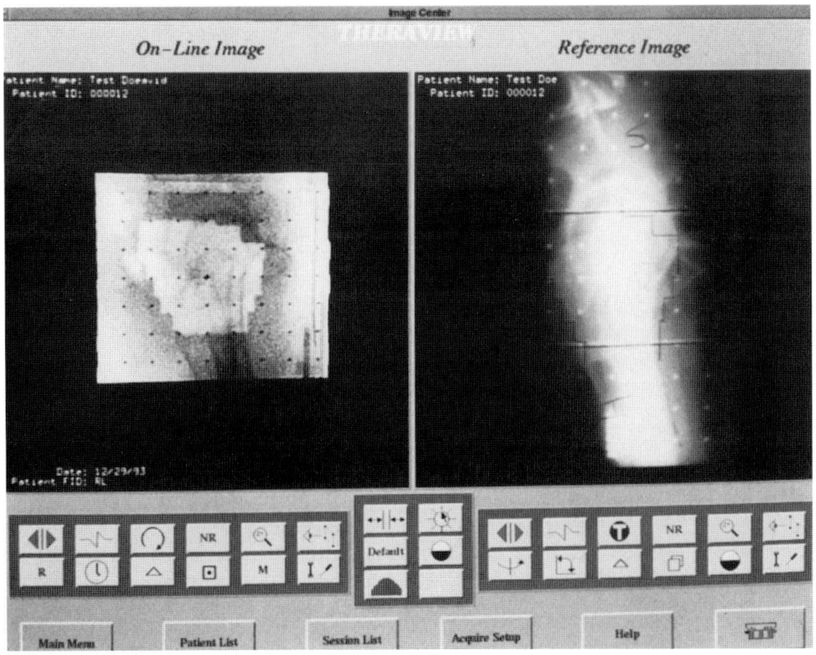

FIG. 7-11. Monitor screen of a Theraview electronic portal imaging device (Infimed, Liverpool, NY). On the left is a portal image of a treatment field obtained in real-time. A digitized reference simulator image for the same treatment field, used for comparison with the portal image, is shown on the right. Fiducial markers facilitate evaluation of the correctness of the field position in relation to bony anatomic landmarks. (From Leibel SA, Zelefsky MJ, Kutcher GJ, et al. The biological basis and clinical application of three-dimensional conformal external beam radiation therapy in carcinoma of the prostate. Semin Oncol 1994;21:580.)

structures as points of reference. Investigations are underway to assess the magnitude of setup errors with the new 3D treatment delivery systems.[145–157] In a study on uncertainties regarding the treatment of nasopharynx tumors,[145] it was shown that 3D conformal plans were more sensitive to setup errors than traditional plans. The daily reproducibility of a multifield conformal treatment technique as represented by ± 1 standard deviation of the setup varied between 1.5 and 2.8 mm from the mean. For the target volume and normal organs of each patient, a family of daily DVHs was generated. It was found that nominal treatment plans (i.e., those generated without taking setup errors into consideration) present an overly optimistic plan with respect to target coverage and normal organ dose distributions. This occurs because the conformal dose distribution that surrounds the target volume and excludes critical structures such as the brain stem and spinal cord has a horseshoe shape, and positional setup errors in almost any direction lead to a decrease in dose to the tumor target and an increased dose to the adjacent normal tissues.[145]

A partial solution for the problem of setup errors was provided by the use of immobilization devices. For example, at MSKCC, a custom-designed thermoplastic immobilization device (Aquaplast, Wycoff, NJ) is made for each patient. The device is attached to a board on the treatment couch beneath the patient using slotted plates that interlock with pegs along the lateral edges of the board (see Fig. 51.1-1).[7,9,95] To determine the efficacy of this device for prostate cancer immobilization, the sequential port films of 15 patients treated with a six-field conformal technique were analyzed.[150] The port films were digitized and compared with the ideal treatment position, represented by simulator films, using image registration software.[150] Patient positioning uncertainty was determined using port films from three projections: two oblique and one lateral. An average of 24 films, accrued for all fields on the first day of treatment and from routine weekly portal film checks during the course of treatment, were analyzed for each patient. The frequency of systematic error per patient, associated with structural machine differences between the simulator and the treatment unit, was calculated by averaging errors over the seven treatment film sessions. The frequency of random errors, associated with setup errors and patient body movement, was calculated as the deviation about the mean for systematic errors. The average systematic error between simulation and treatment isocenters was 1.6 mm. The magnitude of the setup errors was between 0.5 mm and 0.9 mm for translational errors and 0.2 degrees for rotational errors. Random setup errors were distributed in an approximately normal distribution, with standard deviations of 2.2 mm, 1.5 mm, and 1.7 mm in the left-right, superoinferior, and anteroposterior directions, respectively. The use of this immobilization device leads to random, day-to-day fluctuations, represented by the average values of the standard deviations for random errors, that are minor in comparison to the currently used margins for the PTV, demonstrating the efficacy of this device.[150]

The impact of treatment uncertainties as a result of organ motion was also evaluated in several recent studies.[97,151–156] Organ motion refers to the variation of organ position and shape relative to the skeletal anatomy. Studies of prostate motion associated with 3D-CRT have focused on measuring the intertreatment positional variability of this organ. For example, Melian and colleagues[151] performed four serial CT scans on each of 12 patients treated in the prone position at MSKCC. After an initial treatment planning CT scan, a second scan was obtained 2 to 3 weeks later (just before treatment), and the third and fourth scans were taken during the third week of treatment. In each scan and on each CT slice, the pelvic bones, PTV enclosing the prostate and seminal vesicles, and the bladder and rectal walls were outlined using an interactive graphics computer. The data from the different scans were then aligned with one another using the pelvic bones. Borders of the outlined PTV, as determined from individual CT sections, were observed to shift from 0 to 3 cm anteroposteriorly and were correlated primarily with bladder filling. The superior aspect of this target volume (i.e., the seminal vesicles) was particularly affected. The standard deviation of the shifts of the target volume adjacent to the bladder was 1.4 cm, whereas it was only 0.4 cm below the bladder. As shown in Table 7-4, there are large discrepancies in published series of the magnitude of prostate movement. These differences result from a variety of factors, including the use of different treatment and measurement protocols (e.g., frequency and intervals between CT scans, supine versus prone treatment position, amount of bladder and rectal filling), differences in the quantities measured (e.g., maximum border shift of individual contours, center-of-mass shift as determined by averaging over contours or implanted marker positions), and whether or not the seminal vesicles were included in the analysis.[97,151,153–156] Although some of the reported results are preliminary, there appears to be agreement that anteroposterior movement is largest, occurring primarily in the superior portion of the prostate and seminal vesicles, and that movement is correlated with bladder and rectal filling. Moreover, there are indications that bladder filling is more significant for prone patients and rectal filling is more significant for supine patients. Investigators who have examined the dosimetric consequences of the

Table 7-4. *Positional variations of the prostate as a result of organ motion between treatment calculated from serial three-dimensional treatment planning computed tomographic studies*

	Positional variations	
Investigators	Range	Median/average/standard deviation
Melian et al, 1993[151]	0–3 cm	Above bladder: σ = 1.4 cm AP, 0.4 cm lateral Below bladder: σ = 0.4 cm AP, 0.2 cm lateral
Beard et al, 1993[154]	0–1.6 cm	Median = 0.45 cm AP
Forman et al, 1993[155]	0–3.5	Average = 1.7 cm AP
Balter et al, 1995[156]		σ = 0.22 cm AP, 0.08 cm lateral, 0.18 SI

σ, ± 1 standard deviation; AP, anteriorposterior; SI, superiorinferior.

observed movement on conformal treatments have concluded that there can be a significant effect both on target volume coverage as well as on the irradiated volume of the bladder and rectum that receive high doses.[151,153,155]

With realistic information on setup errors, it may be possible to identify which components of setup and immobilization can be modified to reduce uncertainties. On-line images may be useful to achieve this goal. For example, an orthogonal pair of images can be obtained and compared with a reference pair. In this approach, two on-line images are obtained before daily treatment begins. The technologist identifies prespecified bony landmarks on the on-line images, and these are compared using computer techniques to a preplanned reference configuration. Based on the comparison, the setup error is calculated and evaluated relative to predetermined criteria. Errors exceeding a certain threshold may be corrected by adjusting machine parameters (e.g., couch positions, gantry angles). Another possible future benefit of on-line imaging systems is the use of automated on-line corrections via loop-feedback modes to compensate for setup errors or patient movement during treatment sessions. If deviations between the intended and measured position of the patient exceed tolerance limits, the computer will calculate the necessary corrections and carry out the gantry, collimator, and couch position changes needed to rectify the error. Such use of on-line imaging systems may lead to significant improvement in the accuracy of treatment delivery.

Despite the application of sophisticated techniques to reduce treatment uncertainties, some uncontrollable setup and organ motion errors may still remain. The conventional approach to account for these uncertainties has been to add a sufficient safety margin to the CTV to nonspecifically account for these errors. Quantitative approaches to account for these uncertainties can be achieved by incorporation of the sources of uncertainty into the dose calculation process. Kutcher and colleagues[97,157] have described methods of incorporating into treatment plans the effects of systematic setup errors, defined as the deviation of the patient's setup from the simulation position, averaged over the course of treatment. The results are presented in DVHs comparing the nominal DVH without calculation of the effect of the setup error with other DVHs specified to demonstrate the confidence limits as a result of systematic setup error. Modeling organ motion in a similar fashion is inherently more difficult, because the magnitude and direction of organ motion in general will vary for different organs in the same patient. In addition the shapes of the organs themselves may change. Because of the lack of data on organ motion until recently, there has been little development in dosimetric modeling for organ motion in treatment plans. In organ motion studies involving multiple CT scans over the patient's treatment course, the dosimetric consequences have been examined by applying the beams designed with the initial planning CT scan to the organ position on subsequent scans.[152] However, the application of this technique would necessitate multiple CT scans of all patients undergoing treatment—a costly and impractical solution. Moreover, such calculations are retrospective, whereas a prediction of what might happen to the patient is required. Kutcher and colleagues [97] and Mageras and colleagues[152] have described a method of modeling variations in organ position and shape during the treatment planning process to calculate their effect on the dose to those organs. The model is based on measured organ motion in a group of patients for the same treatment site as the patient under study[151] and is used to derive predictions of how the dose actually received may differ from the planned value. The results are given as confidence limits of DVHs or any dose-based quantity, such as dose to a given volume of organ, probability for tumor control, NTCP, or uncomplicated control. Because the model uses data from organ motion studies directly, it can account for arbitrary changes in the position and shape of each particular organ or target volume. Moreover, it can include the effects of day-to-day variations in organ motion on the dose received over the course of treatment.

CONCLUSIONS

Although full exploitation of 3D-CRT will require significant additional effort, experience with early prototypes of 3D treatment planning and delivery systems indicates that 3D-CRT offers enormous potential for improving the probability of local tumor control. More sophisticated 3D treatment planning tools are being developed, and new automated treatment delivery systems are being tested and implemented. The rate at which technical progress can be made is dependent on the availability of new, faster computers and on new approaches to treatment planning software design. A critical development is the anticipated introduction of treatment planning optimization using inverse planning and intensity modulation techniques. The implementation of this new approach offers an improvement in dose distributions and is essential if the full potential of conformal 3D radiotherapy is to be realized. However, the successful use of optimization is dependent on the availability of reliable biologic indices for prediction of TCP and NTCP from ongoing clinical investigations.

The efficacy of the treatment is also dependent on the tumor being reasonably well defined by the imaging procedures, so that a relatively small margin can be added with the expectation that the target volume has been appropriately identified and treated. There are no imaging techniques that can provide information about the existence of microscopic deposits of tumor cells. The resolution of CT and MR imaging are not sufficient to provide such information, although there is a potential for such developments in the future, especially with MR spectroscopy. In addition, MR spectroscopy may offer biologic information regarding the state of the tumor, such as tumor oxygenation, cell cycle parameters, and other biologic variables that might be used to determine appropriate time-dose-fractionation schemes.

The extraordinary increase in the complexity of treatment with conformal techniques raises issues of both quality assurance of treatments and patient safety. On-line portal imaging systems may address some of these issues. With recent advances in image correlation, it may be possible to develop a treatment verification mode that will have feedback control loops to automatically correct setup errors before or even during treatment. With noncoplanar treatment approaches, accuracy and safety of couch and gantry motions will need to assessed to overcome the increased potential for machine-patient collisions. Multisegment therapy with couch and gantry motions in separate segments, thereby eliminating the need to ensure synchronization of motions, is one approach for reducing the potential for collisions. In addition, new hardware to detect potential collisions is under development.

Studies designed to better understand and to develop methods to correct for organ motion effects on dose distribution and target coverage are in progress.[97,152] Organ motion and setup uncertainties that cannot be corrected will be incorporated into treatment plans to provide a more realistic representation of the dose distribution under daily treatment conditions.[97,152,157] These approaches may dictate the need to use margins of safety during treatment, albeit based on patient-specific data. Such an approach may improve the prospective evaluations of the risk of normal organ complications in each patient for a given treatment plan and may affect the selection of the most optimal treatment plan by computer-aided optimization systems.

The application of 3D-CRT, together with improved staging and better assessment of tumor characteristics (e.g., DNA ploidy, proliferative profiles, radiosensitivity), is expected to improve TCPs. The ultimate success of 3D-CRT depends on the ability to deliver high radiation doses to a variety of tumors without significantly increasing the toxicity to surrounding normal tissues. The results of phase I dose-escalation studies in prostate cancer demonstrate that 3D-CRT does indeed make it possible to safely escalate radiation doses to unprecedented levels in patients with prostatic cancer,[9,10] confirming the validity of the basic paradigms and suggesting enormous potential for improving the therapeutic ratio with 3D-CRT in carcinoma of the prostate.[10] However, the true clinical advantages of 3D-CRT will not be known until studies are conducted to test whether improved local control can be achieved and whether it affects the outcome in a variety of human cancers. If proven to be clinically useful, it is expected that 3D-CRT will become available for routine patient care at the community level by the turn of the century.

REFERENCES

1. Fuks Z, Leibel SA, Kutcher GE, Mohan R, Ling CC. Three dimensional conformal treatment: a new frontier in radiation therapy. In: DeVita VT Jr, Hellman S, Rosenberg SA, eds. Important advances in oncology. Philadelphia: JB Lippincott, 1991:151.
2. Leibel SA, Ling CC, Kutcher GJ, Mohan R, Cordon-Cardo C, Fuks Z. The biological basis of conformal three-dimensional radiation therapy. Int J Radiat Oncol Biol Phys 1991;21:805.
3. Munzenrider JE, Pilepich M, Rene-Ferrero JB, Tchakarova I, Carter BL. Use of body scanner in radiotherapy treatment planning. Cancer 1979;40:170.
4. Goitein M. The utility of computed tomography in radiation therapy: an estimate of outcome. Int J Radiat Oncol Biol Phys 1979;5:1799.
5. Mohan R. Three-dimensional radiation treatment planning. Aust Phys Engin Sci Med 1989;12:73.
6. Leibel SA, Kutcher GJ, Mohan R, et al. Three-dimensional conformal radiation therapy at the Memorial Sloan-Kettering Cancer Center. Semin Radiat Oncol 1992;2:274.
7. Leibel SA, Zelefsky MJ, Kutcher GJ, Burman CM, Kelson S, Fuks Z. Three-dimensional conformal radiation therapy in localized carcinoma of the prostate: interim report of a phase I dose-escalation study. J Urol 1994;152:1792.
8. Fuks Z, Hellman S. Three-dimensional conformal radiotherapy. In: DeVita VT Jr, Hellman S, Rosenberg SA, eds. Cancer: principles and practice of oncology, 4th ed. Philadelphia: JB Lippincott, 1992:2614.
9. Leibel SA, Zelefsky MJ, Kutcher GJ, et al. The biological basis and clinical application of three-dimensional conformal external beam radiation therapy in carcinoma of the prostate. Semin Oncol 1994;21: 580.
10. Zelefsky MJ, Leibel SA, Kutcher GJ, Kelson S, Ling CC, Fuks Z. The feasibility of dose-escalation with three-dimensional conformal radiotherapy in patients with prostatic carcinoma. Cancer J 1995;1: 142.
11. Robertson JK, Kessler ML, Lawrence TS. Clinical results of three-dimensional conformal irradiation. J Natl Cancer Inst 1994;86:968.
12. Suit H, Urie M. Proton beams in radiation therapy. J Natl Cancer Inst 1992;84:155.
13. Castro JR, Chen GT, Blakley EA. Current considerations in heavy charged particle radiotherapy. Radiat Res 1985;(Suppl 8):PS227.
14. Mohan R, Barest G, Brewster LJ, et al. A comprehensive three-dimensional radiation treatment planning system. Int J Radiat Oncol Biol Phys 1988;15:481.
15. Fertil B, Malaise EP. Inherent cellular radiosensitivity as a basic concept for human tumor radiotherapy. Int J Radiat Oncl Biol Phys 1981; 7:621.
16. Fertil B, Malaise EP. Intrinsic radiosensitivity of human cell lines is correlated with radioresponsiveness of human tumors analysis of 101 published survival curves. Int J Radiat Oncol Biol Phys 1985;11:1699.
17. Deacon JM, Peckham MJ, Steel GG. The radioresponsiveness of human tumours and the initial slope of the cell survival curve. Radiother Oncol 1984;2:317.
18. Suit HD, Baumann M, Skates S, et al. Clinical interest in determinations of cellular radiation sensitivity. Int J Radiat Biol 1989;56:725.
19. Weichselbaum RR, Rotmensch J, Swan SA, et al. Radiobiological characterization of 53 human tumor cell lines. Int J Radiat Biol 1989; 56:553.
20. Steel GG, McMillan TJ, Peacock JH. The picture has changed in the 1980s. Int J Radiat Biol 1989;56:525.
21. Dutreix J, Tubiana M, Dutreix A. An approach to the interpretation of clinical data on tumour control probability-dose relationship. Radiother Oncol 1988;11:239.
22. McMillan TJ. Residual DNA damage: what is left over and how does this determine cell fate? Europ J Cancer 1992;28:267.
23. Wheldon TE, Abdelaal AS, Nias AHW. Tumour curability, cellular radiosensitivity and clonogenic cell number. Br J Radiol 1977;50:843.
24. Moore JV, Hendry JH, Hunter RD. Dose-incidence curves for tumour control and normal tissue injury, in relation to the response of clonogenic cells. Radiother Oncol 1983;1:143.
25. Peters LJ, Withers HR, Thames HD, et al. Keynote address: the problem: tumor radioresistance in clinical radiotherapy. Int J Radiat Oncol Biol Phys 1981;8:101.
26. Munro TR, Gilbert CW. The relation between tumour lethal doses and the radiosensitivity of tumour cells Br J Radiol 1961;34:246.
27. Hendry JH, Moore JV. Is the steepness of dose-incidence curves for tumour control or complications due to variation before or as a result of irradiation? Br J Radiol 1984;57:1045.
28. Porter EH. The statistical dose-cure relationships for irradiated tumors Br J Radiol 1980;53:336.
29. Fischer JJ, Moulder JE. The steepness of the dose-response curve in radiation therapy. Radiology 1975;117:179.
30. Thames HD Jr, Peters LJ, Spanos WS Jr, Fletcher GF. Dose response of squamous cell carcinomas of the upper respiratory and digestive tracts. Br J Cancer 1980;41(Suppl 4):35.
31. Metz CE, Tokars RP, Kronman HB, Griem ML. Maximum likelihood estimation of dose-response parameters for therapeutic operating characteristic (TOC) analysis of carcinoma of the nasopharynx. Int J Radiat Oncol Biol Phys 1982;8:1185.
32. Peters LJ, Fletcher GH. Causes of failure of radiotherapy in head and neck cancer. Radiother Oncol 983;11:53.
33. Zagars GK, Schultheiss TE, Peters LJ. Inter-tumor heterogeneity and radiation dose-control curves. Radiother Oncol 1987;8:353.
34. Fowler JF. Potential for increasing the differential response between tumors and normal tissues: can proliferation rate be used? Int J Radiat Oncol Biol Phys 1986;12:641.
35. Thames HD, Schulthheiss TE, Hendy JH, Tucker SL, Dubray BM, Brock WA. Can modest escalations of dose be detected as increased tumor control? Int J Radiat Oncol Biol Phys 1992;22:241.
36. Photon Treatment Planning Collaborative Working Group. State of the art of external photon beam radiation treatment planning. Int J Radiat Oncol Biol Phys 1991;21:9.
37. Ten Haken RK, Perez-Tamayo C, Tesser RJ, McShan DL, Fraass BA, Lichter AS. Boost treatment of the prostate using shaped fixed beams. Int J Radiat Oncol Biol Phys 1989;16:193.
38. Leibel SA, Kutcher GJ, Harrison LB, et al. Improved dose distribu-

tions for 3D conformal boost treatments in carcinoma of the nasopharynx. Int J Radiat Oncol Biol Phys 1991;20:823.
39. Hanks GE, Martz KL, Diamond JJ. The effect of dose on local control of prostate cancer. Int J Radiat Oncol Biol Phys 1988;15:1299.
40. Hanks GE. External-beam radiation therapy for clinically localized prostate cancer: patterns of care studies in the United States. Natl Cancer Inst Monogr 1988;7:75.
41. Cancer Trends: 1950–1985. In: 1987 Annual Cancer Statistics Review, NIH Publication No. 88-2789. Washington DC: US Department of Health and Human Services, 1988:11.1.
42. Leibel SA, Fuks Z. The impact of local tumor control on the outcome in human cancer. In: Beck-Bornholdt HP, ed. Medical radiology. Current topics in clinical radiobiology of tumors. Berlin: Springer-Verlag, 1993:113.
43. Suit HD. Potential for improving survival rates for the cancer patient by increasing the efficacy of treatment of the primary lesion. Cancer 1982;50:1227.
44. DeVita VT, Lippman M, Hubbard SA, Idhe DC, Rosenberg SA. The effect of combined modality therapy on local control and survival. Int J Radiat Oncol Biol Phys 1986;12:487.
45. Walsh PC. Adjuvant radiotherapy after radical prostatectomy: is it indicated? J Urol 1987;138:1427.
46. Fisher B, Anderson S, Fisher ER, et al. Significance of ipsilateral breast tumour recurrence after lumpectomy. Lancet 1991;338:327.
47. Sheldon PW, Begg AC, Fowler JF, Lansley IF. The incidence of lung metastases in C3H mice after treatment of implanted tumors with x-rays or surgery. Br J Cancer 1974;30:342.
48. Todoroki T, Suit HD. Therapeutic advantage in preoperative single dose radiation combined with conservative and radical surgery in different size murine fibrosarcoma. J Surg Oncol 1985;29:207.
49. Ramsay J, Suit HD, Sedlacek R. Experimental studies on the incidence of metastases after failure of radiation treatment and the effect of salvage surgery. Int J Radiat Oncol Biol Phys 1983;14:1165.
50. Peters LJ. A study of the influence of various diagnostic and therapeutic procedures applied to a murine squamous carcinoma and its metastatic behaviour. Br J Cancer 1975;32:355.
51. Fuks Z, Leibel SA, Wallner KE, et al. The effect of local control on metastatic dissemination in carcinoma of the prostate: long term results in patients treated with ^{125}I implantation. Int J Radiat Oncol Biol Phys 1991;21:549.
52. Leibel SA, Fuks Z, Zelefsky MJ, Whitmore WF Jr. The effects of local and regional treatments on the metastatic outcome in prostatic carcinoma with pelvic lymph node involvement. Int J Radiat Oncol Biol Phys 1994;28:7.
53. Kuban DH, El-Mahdi AM, Schellhammer PF. Effect of local tumor control on distant metastasis and survival in prostatic adenocarcinoma. Urology 1987;30:420.
54. Zagars GK, von Eschenbach AC, Ayala AG, et al. The influence of local control on metastatic dissemination of prostate cancer treated by external beam megavoltage radiation therapy. Cancer 1991;68: 2370.
55. Kuban DA, El-Mahdi AM, Schellhammer P. The significance of post-irradiation prostate biopsy with long-term follow-up. Int J Radiat Oncol Biol Phys 1992;24:409.
56. Prestidge BR, Kaplan I, Cox RS, Bagshaw MA. The clinical significance of a positive post-irradiation biopsy without metastases. Int J Radiat Oncol Biol Phys 1992;24:403.
57. Lai PP, Perez CA, Lockett MA. Prognostic significance of pelvic recurrence and distant metastasis in prostate carcinoma following definitive radiotherapy. Int J Radiat Oncol Biol Phys 1992;24:423.
58. Chauvet B, Reynaud-Bougnoux A, Calais G, et al. Prognostic significance of breast relapse after conservative treatment in node-negative early breast cancer. Int J Radiat Oncol Biol Phys 1990;9:1125.
59. Whelan T, Clark R, Roberts R, et al. Ipsilateral breast tumor recurrence postlumpectomy is predictive of subsequent mortality: results from a randomized trial. Int J Radiat Oncol Biol Phys 1994;30:11.
60. Chung CK, Stryker JA, O'Neill M, et al. Evaluation of adjuvant postoperative radiotherapy for lung cancer. Int J Rad Oncol Biol Phys 1982;8:1877.
61. Malissard L, Nguyen TD, Jung GM, et al. Localized adenocarcinoma of the lung: a retrospective study of 186 non-metastatic patients from the French Federation of Cancer Institutes—The Radiotherapy Cooperative Group. Int J Radiat Oncol Biol Phys 1991;21:369.
62. Schild SE, Martenson JA Jr, Gunderson LL, et al. Postoperative adjuvant therapy of rectal cancer: an analysis of disease control, survival and prognostic factors. Int J Radiat Oncol Biol Phys 11989;7:55.
63. Vigliotti A, Rich TA, Romsdahl MM, et al. Postoperative adjuvant radiotherapy for adenocarcinoma of the rectum and rectosigmoid. Int J Radiat Oncol Biol Phys 1987;13:999.
64. Paunier JP, Delclos L, Fletcher GH. Cause, time of death, and sites of failure in squamous cell carcinoma of the uterine cervix on intact uterus. Radiology 1967;88:552.
65. Anderson P, Dische S. Local tumor control and subsequent incidence of distant metastatic disease. Int J Radiat Oncol Biol Phys 1981;7: 1645.
66. Fagundes H, Perez CA, Grigsby PW, Lockett MA. Distant metastases after irradiation alone in carcinoma of the uterine cervix. Int J Radiat Oncol Biol Phys 1992;24:197.
67. Stokes S, Bedwinek J, Kao MS, et al. Treatment of stage I adenocarcinoma of the endometrium by hysterectomy and adjuvant irradiation: a retrospective analysis of 304 patients. Int J Radiat Oncol Biol Phys 1986;12:339.
68. Perez CA, Camel HM, Galakatos AE, et al. Definitive irradiation in carcinoma of the vagina: long-term evaluation of results. Int J Radiat Oncol Biol Phys 1988;15:1283.
69. Merino OR, Lindberg RD, Fletcher GH. An analysis of distant metastases from squamous cell carcinoma of the upper respiratory and digestive tracts. Cancer 1977;40:145.
70. Leibel SA, Scott CB, Mohiuddin M, et al. The effect of local-regional control on distant metastatic dissemination in carcinoma of the head and neck: results of an analysis from the RTOG head and neck database. Int J Radiat Oncol Biol Phys 1991;21:549.
71. Lee AW, Sham JS, Poon YF, et al. Treatment of stage I nasopharyngeal carcinoma: analysis of the patterns of relapse and the results of withholding elective neck irradiation. Int J Radiat Oncol Biol Phys 1989;17:1183.
72. Kwong D, Sham J, Choy D. The effect of loco-regional control on distant metastatic dissemination in carcinoma of the nasopharynx: an analysis of 1301 patients. Int J Radiat Oncol Biol Phys 1994;30:1029.
73. Markhede G, Angervall L, Stener B. A multivariate analysis of the prognosis after surgical treatment of soft tissue tumors. Cancer 1982; 49:1721.
74. Suit HD, Mankin HJ, Wood WC, et al. Treatment of the patient with stage M0 soft tissue sarcoma. J Clin Oncol 1988;6:854.
75. Gustafson P, Rooser B, Rydholm A. Is local recurrence of minor importance for metastases in soft tissue sarcoma? Cancer 1991;67: 2083.
76. Gaynor JJ, Tan CC, Casper ES, et al. Refinement of clinicopathologic staging for localized soft tissue sarcoma of the extremity: a study of 423 adults. J Clin Oncol 1992;10:1317.
77. Vogelstein B, Fearon ER, Kern SE, et al. Allelotype of colorectal carcinomas. Science 1989;244:207.
78. Bishop M. Molecular themes in oncogenesis. Cell 1991;64:235.
79. Fearon ER, Vogelstein B. A genetic model for colorectal tumorigenesis. Cell 1990;61:759.
80. Hollstein M, Sidransky D, Vogelstein B, et al. p53 mutations in human cancers. Science 1991;253:49.
81. Kerbel RS. Towards an understanding of the molecular basis of the metastatic phenotype. Invasion Metastasis 1989;9:329.
82. Sobel ME. Metastasis suppressor genes. J Natl Cancer Inst 1990;82: 267.
83. Liotta LA, Steeg PS, Stettler-Stevenson WG. Cancer metastasis and angiogenesis: an imbalance of positive and negative regulation. Cell 1991;64:327.
84. Steeg PS, Bevilacqua G, Kopper L, et al. Evidence for a novel gene associated with low tumor metastatic potential. J Natl Cancer Inst 1988;89:200.
85. Cance WG, Brennan MF, Dudas ME, et al. Altered expression of the retinoblastoma gene product in human sarcomas. N Engl J Med 1990; 323:1457.
86. Cordon-Cordo C, Fuks Z, Eisenbach L, et al. Expression of HLA-A,B,C antigens on primary and metastatic tumor cell populations of human carcinomas. Cancer Res 1991;51:6327.

87. Greenberg AH, Egan SE, Wright JA. Oncogenes and metastatic progression. Invasion Metastasis 1989;9:360.
88. Muschel R, Liotta RA. Role of oncogenes in metastasis. Carcinogenesis 1988;9:705.
89. Vlodavsky I, Michaeli RI, Bar-Ner M, et al. Involvement of heparanase in tumor metastasis and angiogenesis. Isr J Med Sci 1988;24:464.
90. Sloane BF, Dunn TR, Honn KV. Lysosomal cathepsin B: correlation with metastatic potential. Science 1981;212:1151.
91. Tubiana M. Repopulation in human tumors. Acta Oncol 1988;27:83.
92. Yorke ED, Fuks Z, Norton L, Whitmore W, Ling CC. Modeling the development of metastases from primary and locally recurrent tumors: comparison with a clinical data base for prostatic cancer. Cancer Res 1993;53:2987.
93. Norton LA. Gompertzian model of human breast cancer growth. Cancer Res 1988;48:7067.
94. Goldie JH, Coldman AJA. A mathematical model for relating the drug sensitivity of tumors to their spontaneous mutation rate. Cancer Treat Rep 1979;63:1727.
95. Leibel SA, Heimann R, Kutcher GJ, et al. Three-dimensional conformal radiation therapy in locally advanced carcinoma of the prostate: preliminary results of a phase I dose-escalation study. Int J Radiat Oncol Biol Phys 1994;28:55.
96. ICRU Report 50. Prescribing, recording, and reporting photon beam therapy. Bethesda: International Commission on Radiation Units and Measurements, 1993.
97. Kutcher GJ, Mageras GS, Leibel SA. Control, correction and modeling of setup errors and organ motion. Semin Radiat Oncol 1995;5: 134.
98. Goitein M, Abrams M, Rowell D, et al. Multi-dimensional treatment planning. II. Beam's eye-view, back projection, and projection through CT sections. Int J Radiat Oncol Biol Phys 1983;9:789.
99. LoSasso TJ, Chui CS, Kutcher GJ, et al. The use of multi-leaf collimator for conformal radiotherapy in carcinomas of the prostate and nasopharynx. Int J Radiat Oncol Biol Phys 1993;25:161.
100. Mageras GS, Podmaniczky KC, Mohan R. A model for computer-controlled delivery of 3D conformal treatments. Med Phys 1992;19: 945.
101. Photon Treatment Planning Collaborative Working Group. Three-dimensional dose calculations for radiation treatment planning. Int J Radiat Oncol Biol Phys 1991;21:25.
102. Cunningham JR. Scatter-air ratios. Phys Med Biol 1972;17:42.
103. Larson KB, Prasad SC. Absorbed-dose computations for inhomogeneous media in radiation treatment planning using differential scatter-air ratios. Proceedings of the Second Annual Symposium on Computer Application in Medical Care, New York: IEEE, 1978:93.
104. Wong JW, Slessinger ED, Hermes RE, Offutt CJ, Roy T, Vannier MW. Portal dose images. I. Quantitative treatment plan verification. Int J Radiat Oncol Biol Phys 1990;18:1455.
105. Chui CS, Mohan RM. Extraction of pencil beam kernels by the deconvolution method. Med Phys 1988;15:138.
106. Mohan R, Chui C, Lidofsky L. Differential pencil beam dose computation model for photons. Med Phys 1986;13:64.
107. Mohan R, Chui CS. Use of Fourier transforms in calculating dose distributions for irregularly shaped fields for three dimensional treatment planning. Med Phys 1987;14:70.
108. Boyer AL, Mok EC. Fourier convolution incorporating inhomogeneities. Med Phys 11985;2:507.
109. Ling CC, Burman C, Chui CS, et al. Perspectives of multidimensional conformal radiation treatment. Radiother Oncol 1993;29:129.
110. Photon Treatment Planning Collaborative Working Group. Three-dimensional displays in planning radiation therapy: a clinical perspective. Int J Radiat Oncol Biol Phys 1991;21:79.
111. Shipley WU, Tepper JE, Prout GR, et al. Proton radiation as boost therapy for localized prostatic carcinoma. JAMA 1979;241:1912.
112. Drzymala RE, Mohan R, Brewster L, et al. Dose-volume histograms. Int J Radiat Oncol Biol Phys 1991;21:71.
113. Zelefsky MJ, Leibel SA, Burman CM, et al. Neoadjuvant hormonal therapy improves the therapeutic ratio in patients with bulky prostatic cancer treated with three-dimensional conformal radiation therapy. Int J Radiat Oncol Biol Phys 1994;29:755.
114. Burman C, Kutcher GJ, Emami B, et al. Fitting of normal tissue tolerance data to an analytic function. Int J Radiat Oncol Biol Phys 1991;21:123.
115. Kutcher GJ, Burman C, Brewster L, et al. Histogram reduction method for calculating complication probabilities for three-dimensional treatment planning evaluations. Int J Radiat Oncol Biol Phys 1991;21: 137.
116. Munzenrider JE, Brown AP, Chu JC, et al. Numerical scoring of treatment plans. Int J Radiat Oncol Biol Phys 1991;21:147.
117. Bush M, Rosenow U. Dose volume relationships in computer applications. In: Sternick E, ed. Radiation oncology. Hanover, NH: University Press of New England, 1976:279.
118. Dritschilo A, Chaffey JT, Bloomer WD, et al. The complication probability factor: a method of selection of treatment plans. Br J Radiol 1978;51:370.
119. Lyman JT. Complication probability as assessed from dose volume histograns. Radiat Res 1985;104:S13.
120. Lyman JT, Wolbarst AB. Optimization of radiotherapy III: a method of assessing complication probabilities from dose volume histograms. Int J Radiat Oncol Biol Phys 1987;13:103.
121. Wolbarst AB, Chin LM, Swenssen GL. Optimization of radiation therapy: integral-response of a model biological system. Int J Radiat Oncol Biol Phys 1982;8:1761.
122. Goitein M. The probability of controlling an inhomogeneously irradiated tumor. In: Zink S, ed. Evaluation of treatment planning for particle beam radiotherapy. Bethesda, MD: National Cancer Institute, 1987:5.8.1.
123. Brahme A. Dosimetric precision requirements in radiation therapy. Acta Radiol Oncol 1984;23:379.
124. Emami B, Lyman J, Brown A, et al. Tolerance of normal tissue to therapeutic irradiation. Int J Radiat Oncol Biol Phys 1991;21:109.
125. Kutcher GJ, Burman C. Calculation of complication probability factors for non-uniform normal tissue irradiation: the effective volume method. Int J Radiat Oncol Biol Phys 1989;16:1623.
126. Withers HR, Taylor JMG, Maciejewski B. Treatment volume and tissue tolerance. Int J Radiat Oncol Biol Phys 1988;14:751.
127. Niemierko A, Goitein M. Calculation of normal tissue complication probability and dose-volume histogram reduction schemes for tissues with a critical element architecture. Radiother Oncol 1991;20:166.
128. Schultheiss TE, Orton CG, Peck RA. Models in radiotherapy: volume effects. Med Phys 1983;10:410.
129. Niemierko A. Modeling of normal tissue response. [Abstract] Int J Radiat Oncol Biol Phys 1991;21(Suppl 1):143.
130. Jackson A, Kutcher GJ, Yorke ED. Probability of radiation-induced complications for normal tissues with parallel architecture subject to non-uniform irradiation. Med Phys 1993;20:613.
131. Yorke ED, Kutcher GJ, Jackson A, Ling CC. Probability of radiation-induced complications for normal tissues with parallel architecture under conditions of uniform whole or patial organ irradiation. Radiother Oncol 1993;26:226.
132. Jackson A, Ten Haken RK, Lawrence TS, Kessler ML, Kutcher GJ. Analysis of clinical complication data for radiation hepatitis using a parallel architecture model. Int J Radiat Oncol Biol Phys 1995;31: 883.
133. Goitein M, Niemierko A, Okunieff P. The probability of controlling an inhomogeneously irradiated tumor. In: Report of the working group on the evaluation of treatment planning for particle beam radiotherapy. Bethesda, MD: National Cancer Institute, 1987:5.8.1–17.
134. Niemierko A, Goitein M. Implementation of a model for estimating tumor control probability for an inhomogeneously irradiated tumor. Radiother Oncol 1993;29:140.
135. Mohan R, Mageras GS, Baldwin MS, et al. Clinical relevant optimization of 3D conformal treatments. Med Phys 1992;19:933.
136. Szu H, Hartley R. Fast simulated annealing. Phys Lett A 187;122: 157.
137. Brahme A. Optimization of stationary and moving beam radiation therapy techniques. Radiother Oncol 1988;12:129.
138. Bortfeld T, Burkelbach J, Boesecke R, Schlegel W. Methods of image reconstruction from projections applied to conformation radiotherapy. Phys Med Biol 1990;35:1423.
139. Mohan R, Xang XH, Jackson A, et al. The potential and limitations of inverse radiotherapy technique. Radiother Oncol 1994;32:232.
140. Wang X-H, Mohan R, Jackson A, Leibel SA, Fuks Z, Ling CC. Optim-

ization of intensity-modulated treatment plans based on biological indices. Radiother Oncol 1995;37:140.

141. Spirou SV, Chui CS. Generation of arbitrary intensity profiles by dynamic jaws of multileaf collimators. Med Phys 1994;21:1031.
142. Chui C-S, LoSasso T, Spirou S. Dose calculation of photon beams with intensity modulation generated by dynamic jaw or multileaf collimations. Med Phys 1994;21:1237.
143. Mageras GS, Fuks Z, O'Brien J, et al. Initial clinical experience with computer-controlled conformal radiotherapy of the prostate using a 50-MeV medical microtron. Int J Radiat Oncol Biol Phys 1994;30:971.
144. Boyer AL, Antonuk L, Fenster A, et al. A review of electronic portal imaging devices (EPIDs). Med Phys 1992;19:1.
145. Hunt MA, Kutcher GJ, Burman C, et al. The effect of positional uncertainties on the treatment of nasopharynx cancer. Int J Radiat Oncol Biol Phys 1993;27:437.
146. Rabinowitz I, Broomberg J, Goitein M, et al. Accuracy of radiation field alignment in clinical practice. Int J Radiat Oncol Biol Phys 1985;11:1857.
147. Bijhold J, van Herk M, Vijlbrief R, et al. Fast evaluation of patient setup during radiotherapy by aligning features in portal and simulator images. Phys Med Biol 1991;36:1665.
148. Meertens H, Bijhold J, Strackee J. A method for the measurement of field placement errors in digital portal images. Phys Med Biol 1990;35:299.
149. Ezz A, Munro P, Porter AT, et al. Daily monitoring and correction of radiation field placement using a video-based portal imaging system: a pilot study. Int J Radiat Oncol Biol Phys 1992;22:159.
150. Hanley J, Mageras GS, Sun J, Leibel SA, Fuks Z, Kutcher GJ. The use of port films from multiple projections to determine the spatial distribution of setup errors for prostate cancer patients. [Abstract] Int J Radiat Oncol Biol Phys 1994;30(Suppl 1):175.
151. Melian E, Kutcher G, Leibel S, Zelefsky M, Baldwin B, Fuks Z. Variation on prostate position: quantification and implications for three-dimensional conformal radiation therapy. [Abstract] Int J Radiat Oncol Biol Phys 1993;27(Suppl 1):137.
152. Mageras GS, Kutcher GJ, Melian E, et al. A method of incorporation organ motion uncertainties in 3D conformal treatment plans. Int J Radiat Oncol Biol Phys (in press).
153. Ten Haken RK, Forman JD, Heimburger DK, et al. Treatment planning issues related to prostate movement in response to differential filling of the rectum and bladder. Int J Radiat Oncol Biol Phys 1991;20:1317.
154. Beard CJ, Bussiere MR, Plunkett ME, Coleman CN, Kijewski PK. Analysis of prostate and seminal vesicle motion. [Abstract] Int J Radiat Oncol Biol Phys 1993;27(Suppl 1):136.
155. Forman JD, Mesina CF, He T, et al. Evaluation of changes in the location and shape of the prostate and rectum during a seven week course of conformal radiotherapy. [Abstract] Int J Radiat Oncol Biol Phys 1993;27(Suppl 1):222.
156. Balter J, Sandler HM, Lam K, Bree RL, Lichter AS, Ten Haken RK. Measurement of prostate motion over the course of radiotherapy using implanted markers. Int J Radiat Oncol Biol Phys 1995;31:113.
157. Kutcher GJ, Mageras G, Chui C, et al. Inclusion of systematic setup uncertainties in treatment plans. [Abstract] Int J Radiat Oncol Biol Phys 1994;30(Suppl 1):242.

Principles and Practice of Genitourinary Oncology, edited by Derek Raghavan, Howard I. Scher, Steven A. Leibel, and Paul H. Lange. Lippincott-Raven Publishers, Philadelphia, © 1997.

CHAPTER 8

Principles of Chemotherapy for Genitourinary Cancer

Implications for Development of New Anticancer Drugs

Patrick J. Creaven and Derek Raghavan

Cytotoxic chemotherapy has been in use for the management of advanced cancer for more than a century,[1] arising from concepts developed by Lissauer, Ehrlich, and many others. The initial attempts at such treatment were characterized by a lack of specificity, with a fine balance between the toxicity to the tumor and that experienced by the host. As reviewed in detail elsewhere,[1] during the past century, our application of chemotherapy to the treatment of cancer has been refined, predicated on an improved understanding of the biochemical basis of its action and a clearer insight into the cellular and molecular mechanisms underlying normal and malignant growth.

TUMOR CELL BIOLOGY IN RELATION TO CHEMOTHERAPY

The anticancer agents are a varied collection of drugs that act through a range of mechanisms, predominantly focused on interference with cell reproduction. Investigators generally agree that the differences between the growth characteristics of normal and malignant tissues form the major basis of the effective use of cytotoxic chemotherapy.[2] Differences among cellular transport characteristics, with differential uptake and efflux of cytotoxic agents, may also contribute to the difference in response to some cytotoxic agents. Moreover, important differences apparently exist among intracellular metabolic functions, such as the expression of glutathione, an intracellular scavenger, which interacts with some alkylating agents and the platinum complexes to inactivate them. More recent data suggest the possibility of subtle interactions between the expression of growth-controlling factors, such as the receptor for the epidermal growth factor, and the impact of cytotoxic agents, with resulting synergistic or antagonistic effects.

Normal tissues are composed predominantly of a static population of cells that rarely undergo cell division, an expanding population of cells that retain the ability to grow, under stringent physiologic control mechanisms, and a self-renewing population for tissues that turn over rapidly, such as bone marrow and gastrointestinal epithelium. In this situation, balance is maintained between natural attrition and replacement.

The static, or terminally differentiated, population usually includes cells that do not undergo cell division after fetal life, such as skeletal muscle and neuronal tissue. The cells of an expanding population do not normally undergo continuous growth and division, but they may respond to stress, such as injury, with a period of replacement growth. For example, hepatocytes can respond to surgical resection of liver tissue by reentering the cell cycle and replacing the lost tissue. Another example of the expanding population is the stem cells in the bone marrow; these cells normally rest in the G_0 phase, but they can reenter the cell cycle. That they are predominantly in G_0 may protect them, in part, from the effects of cytotoxic agents.

By contrast, the self-renewing cell populations, such as cells of the gastrointestinal tract, hair follicles, and bone marrow, are in a continuous proliferative state, with constant cell turnover, and are thus most commonly injured by cytotoxic chemotherapy; the static cell populations are the least vulnerable to the effects of chemotherapy.

Malignant growth is essentially uncontrolled, occurring as a result of a breakdown in the mechanisms that turn off growth. The patterns that contribute to tumor growth may include a reduction in the length of the cell cycle, a decrease in the rate of cell death, or an increase in recruitment of cells into the active cell cycle. In general, malignant growth appears to follow a Gompertzian pattern,[2] in which a period of exponential growth is followed by a slowing of the growth rate. This process may occur through the tumor's outgrowing its vascular supply, as a result of the development of toxic breakdown products associated with cellular turnover, or through other subtle cell–cell interactions.

Cellular Kinetics and Cell Cycle Control

The kinetics of tumor cell growth, both in vitro and in vivo, has been the subject of considerable study,[2] although our concepts on this topic remain fluid. Surprisingly little information is available regarding the kinetics of human tumor growth,[3] although a greater body of information is available on the growth of animal tumors.[2] Investigators generally agree that tumor cells grow through an orderly sequence of steps:

1. The initial growth phase (G_1) is characterized by synthesis of ribonucleic acid (RNA) and protein, as well as deoxyribonucleic acid (DNA) repair; this is a period of variable length, and its duration determines the length of the total cell cycle of the individual cell.
2. This phase is followed by the synthetic (S) phase, in which new DNA is synthesized.
3. The cells progress through the G_2 phase, in which the total DNA content is double that of the normal cell.
4. The mitotic (M) phase sees the division of the chromosomes and separation into two offspring cells.
5. After mitosis, the cells may spend a variable period in a resting state known as G_0: the cells are out of active cycle and appear not to be affected by chemotherapy to any major extent.

A detailed description of the molecular biology of cell cycle control is beyond the scope of this chapter, and the principles are reviewed elsewhere.[4] In brief, several candidate genes and growth factors appear to regulate the various steps of the cell cycle. For example, in different tissues, entry into G_1 appears to be regulated by a range of factors, including *MYC* and *FOS* (formerly known as c-*myc* and c-*fos*), platelet-derived growth factors, and insulin-like growth factor-1 and its receptor.

A major cell cycle controller, $p34^{cdc2}$, regulates entry into S phase; this protein appears to have been conserved during evolution from yeasts to humans, with regard to both structure and function.[5] In turn, this kinase appears to interact with its targets by association with the cyclins, a family of proteins found in different stages of the cell cycle. The G_1 cyclins are present before S phase, and they interact with p34 to cause the cells to enter S phase. Entry into S phase is the first major cell cycle control point. These cyclins appear to interact directly with oncogenes and suppressor genes, probably through a phosphorylation function of the cyclin-p34 complex.

Several oncogenes, such as *RAS* and *SRC* (formerly known as *ras* and *src*), have activity in the M phase of the cell cycle; in fact, they may actually interact in the process leading to activation of the M-phase promoting factor, which, in turn, controls entry into mitosis (the second major cell cycle control point). Tumor progression may be a function of a series of events involving progressive loss of control over entry into the S phase and loss of regulation of M phase; such progression is due to genetic instability and is central to the evolution of malignancy. These changes may be contingent on the loss of checkpoint function, a mechanism by which the cell cycle pauses transiently and allows checking of the accuracy of replication.[6]

The concept of the cell cycle is of great importance to our understanding of cytotoxic action. Most agents affect some aspect of the synthesis of DNA, RNA, or protein and act at different points within the cell cycle. This finding may be important when adding agents in a combination regimen; for example, the use of a spindle poison (such as a vinca alkaloid) may hold up cells from entry into the G_1 phase and thus may reduce the impact of an agent that acts predominantly at that point of the cell cycle. This effect is limited by the finding that many agents act at multiple points in the cell cycle. Inhibition of checkpoint function may explain the way in which tumor cells can be more vulnerable to the effects of cytotoxic agents than are normal cells; thus, the vulnerability of cancer cells to agents that target the S phase or the M phase may occur because the malignant cells proceed unchecked through the cell cycle despite a series of errors, whereas the normal cells stop at finite checkpoints while needed repairs occur.

Cell cycle characteristics can be measured in several ways, including the use of labeling of mitoses[2] and flow cytometry. When considering the biology of tumor growth as assessed by flow cytometry, the proportion of cells in the G_1 and S phases is thought to be most important, although the level of aneuploidy (proportion of cells that do not have a normal or diploid DNA content) appears to be an important prognostic determinant in some tumors. Another, more direct parameter of the cell cycle is measurement of tumor doubling time.[2]

Also of importance is the growth fraction (proportion of cells within a tumor that are in active proliferative phase), which can range from 25% to over 90% in human tumors. The rate of cell loss is also important; in most tumors, it is high, ranging from 70% to over 90%.[2] In general, the length of the G_1 phase is one of the primary determinants of proliferative behavior; thus, if G_1 is short, the duration of the cell cycle is usually rapid, whereas cells with a long G_1 or those that spend considerable time in G_0 have a much longer cell cycle and are less sensitive to the impact of chemotherapy.

Clonality of Tumor Cell Populations

In animal tumors, which tend to be clonal, first-order kinetics appears to apply in response to chemotherapy; that is, a dose of single-agent chemotherapy kills a fixed proportion of tumor cells. For example, if a tumor mass containing 10^7 cells is treated with an agent that kills 90% of the cells, 9×10^6 cells will be killed by a single dose, leaving behind 10^6 viable cells (or 10% of the original tumor mass). A second dose kills 9×10^5 cells and leaves 10^5 cells still alive. If treatment is not repeated, these cells will regrow, and the mass will rapidly return to its former size. This process is also influenced by the proportion of cells that undergo spontaneous cell death, as well as the proliferative rate of any remaining viable cells.

Clinically, the situation is much more complex, because many human tumors appear not to be purely uniclonal, but rather are composed of multiple subpopulations of cells with different characteristics.[7] Whether this phenomenon is due to the evolution from single clonal populations (stem cells) or is caused by initial evolution of multiple clones in response to an initial carcinogenic stimulus is not clear.

PHARMACOLOGY OF ANTICANCER AGENTS

The time course of the sojourn of drugs in the body is determined by the rates of drug absorption, distribution, metabolism, and excretion. The mathematic description of these rate processes is referred to as pharmacokinetics. Often, the data can be fitted to mathematic models that are simplified descriptions of the complex physiologic realities. Many of these processes are so-called first order: that is, the rate at which the process occurs is proportional to the drug concentration, although some processes that depend on enzymes or carriers follow Michaelis-Menten kinetics, in which the process is first order at low concentrations and zero order (i.e., occurring at a fixed rate) at high concentrations of the drug.

Absorption

Cytotoxic agents may be administered directly into the circulation (intravenous or intraarterial administration) or by the extravascular approach, which includes oral, intramuscular, intrathecal, intravesical, and intraperitoneal routes. The route of extravascular delivery influences absorption. Factors that determine the uptake characteristics of a drug include the structure and size of the molecule and its negative log of dissociation constant (pKa) and, thus, its solubility characteristics.

The clinical activity of specific agents may vary with the nature of the route and schedule of administration and consequent absorption. For example, cyclophosphamide can be administered orally in a dose of 100 mg/m^2/d for 14 days to patients with advanced prostate cancer and is well tolerated, causing only modest myelosuppression and gastrointestinal toxicity.[8] When the drug is administered to similar populations of patients by intravenous bolus injection (e.g., 750 to 1000 mg/m^2 every 3 weeks), the side effects may be more substantial,[9] with no apparent improvement in therapeutic outcome.

Successful intravesical chemotherapy is predicated on the desire for cytotoxic agents to be active locally *without* systemic absorption, thus protecting the patient from systemic side effects while maximizing the concentration at the tumor surface. Thus, thiotepa, a small, readily absorbed molecule, is potentially less useful in this context than larger molecules, such as doxorubicin or mitomycin C.[10] Furthermore, the level of systemic absorption of thiotepa can be increased if the agent is administered soon after transurethral tumor resection in the presence of a residual denuded bladder epithelium.

Ultimately, the key to therapeutic effectiveness of any cytotoxic agent is a function of the product of its concentration and the time available at the tumor site ($C \times t$). Most cytotoxic agents are administered by intravenous or intraarterial routes, and calculations of the actual plasma $C \times t$ equation are made accordingly.

Distribution and Transport

The amount of cytotoxic agent available at the tumor target and the length of time during which it is present determine its level of efficacy. Several factors are influential, including the lipid solubility of the drug, its binding to protein and other carriers, and the mechanisms available to allow entry into the tumor (such as passive diffusion or active transport). A major factor is the plasma level of the drug, major determinants of which are its distribution characteristics. After rapid intravenous injection, the plasma concentration of the drug initially falls rapidly. In time, the rate of decline decreases. A plot of the natural logarithm (ln) against time (semilog plot) generally shows two components of the plasma decay: an initial rapid component and a subsequent slower component, both of which have the characteristics of log-linear, that is, first-order, processes. Mathematically, such a plasma decay can be fitted to a two-compartment model in which the body is conceptualized as consisting of two compartments, a central compartment into which the drug is introduced and a peripheral or tissue compartment into which it diffuses, ultimately to equilibrium. The second component of the plasma decay consists of the elimination processes of metabolism or excretion. The rate of this second process gives the half-life of the drug in the body and is an important pharmacokinetic characteristic of all drugs ($t\frac{1}{2}\beta$). For some drugs such as the anthracyclines, a third component of the plasma decay is seen indicating a so-called deep tissue compartment usually corresponding to the binding of the drug to some tissue component such as nucleic acid from which the drug is slowly released. An even simpler model in which the body is regarded as a single compartment can sometimes be used, but for many drugs it can lead to major errors in computing the important pharmacokinetic parameters. These "compartments" are mathematic constructs that usually have little or no correspondence with actual physiologic compartments. The total area under the plasma concentration $\times$ time curve (AUC or $C \times t$) is an important measure of the total exposure of the tissues to the drug. Other important pharmacokinetic parameters that can be calculated from the indices of plasma decay are the total body clearance and the apparent volume of distribution, the theoretic volume required to dissolve the total body content of the drug if it were uniformly distributed in the concentration found in plasma.

In general, the drug is distributed in intravascular, extracellular, and intracellular water, but it must cross a membrane to pass from one of these locations to another. In addition, certain sites are protected from easy drug access. Such sanctuaries are usually characterized by lower drug concentration than other tissues.

The presence of sanctuary sites may be of real importance; for example, the blood-brain barrier appears to protect the brain against the local uptake of cytotoxic agents, and thus the brain may be the site of first relapse in tumors otherwise responsive to chemotherapy. Similarly, the testis apparently may functionally constitute a sanctuary site against the effect of chemotherapy; up to a third of patients treated for metastatic testis cancer before surgical removal of the affected testis have residual cancer within the testis at subsequent orchiectomy, despite an extratesticular complete response.

Metabolism

Two important types of metabolism of antitumor agents are known. Antitumor agents that resemble normal metabolites are often metabolized by the same mechanisms as the normal metabolites. Most purine and pyrimidine antimetabolites require activation to a nucleotide, usually the triphosphate, to be active, and these reactions are carried out by the mechanisms in the cell used to metabolize the corresponding normal preformed purines and pyrimidines (the so-called salvage pathways). Some of the antifolates undergo polyglutamation by the mechanisms used for folates. Degradative pathways are also active in the cell, such as those responsible for reducing 5-fluorouracil (5-FU) to dihydro-5-fluorouracil and converting cytosine arabinoside to the corresponding uracil arabinoside by deamination. These reactions occur in the cells of the tumor and in the cells of normal tissues. In addition to these specific metabolic reactions, compounds that do not show resemblance to physiologic substrates are metabolized primarily in the liver by the pathways used for detoxification of xenobiotics. Most important is oxidation, often followed by conjugation. Oxidation is carried out by cytochrome P450, a family of enzymes located primarily in the microsomal or smooth endoplasmic reticulum fraction of the liver. This pathway is nonspecific in terms of structural requirements and oxidizes most lipid-soluble compounds. This pathway is responsible for the initial oxidation of the oxazaphosphorine ring of the oxazaphosphorines cyclophosphamide and ifosfamide, a reaction leading to the conversion of these compounds to their active metabolites.

Knowledge of the metabolism of cytotoxic agents is important in designing treatment strategies; for example, intravesical delivery of cyclophosphamide would make no sense, because the drug requires hepatic metabolism to its active form to be effective (see later). In the patient with hepatic dysfunction or hepatic failure, impaired hepatic conjugation alters the metabolism of doxorubicin and of the vinca alkaloids, whereas the microsomal activation of cyclophosphamide may be impaired in this clinical setting.

Excretion

Excretion of cytotoxic agents occurs predominantly in the kidneys and liver, and abnormalities in the function of either or both organs may influence the pattern of toxicity.[11] Renal dysfunction particularly affects the disposition of the platinum complexes, methotrexate, and bleomycin.

Factors Modifying Pharmacokinetics

Absorption of drugs may be affected by diseases of the gastrointestinal tract, by previous surgical procedures, by compounds that change the pH of the gut, by coadministration of other drugs, and by other factors.[12,13] Distribution can be influenced by disease states, such as cardiac failure, ascites, pleural effusion, and edema, and by the coadministration of substances that can displace compounds from binding to serum albumin.[14] Age and amount of adipose tissue may have an impact on the clearance and toxic effects of cytotoxic agents. For example, obesity appears to reduce the clearance of doxorubicin in adults,[15] although the impact on toxicity of the drug is unclear. Age may alter disposition of doxorobucin; for example, Robert and Hoerni[16] demonstrated reduced clearance in older patients, compared with younger cohorts (Chap. 29). Numerous factors affect the rate at which drugs are metabolized by cytochrome P450.[17] Many compounds can induce cytochrome P450, including phenobarbitol and hydantoin, chlorinated hydrocarbon insecticides, food additives, and carcinogens present in tobacco smoke. Some antineoplastic agents may inhibit drug metabolism,[18] as may the presence of hepatic disease.[19] Excretion of compounds by the kidneys depends heavily on renal function. Coincidental administration of compounds that can compete for tubular reabsorption may affect renal clearance of certain compounds,[20] as may urinary pH if the compound is able to become ionized.[21]

MECHANISMS OF DRUG RESISTANCE

Several mechanisms of resistance to cytotoxic chemotherapy are known (Table 8-1). In general, these mechanisms can be classified on the basis of cellular distribution. Intracellular factors include those that act at the cell surface, others within the cytoplasm, and those functioning at the level of the nucleus. In addition are extracellular factors, such as those that affect the distribution and metabolism of the drugs, including competitors for cellular transport mechanisms.

Some cytotoxic agents can be exported from tumor cells through a mechanism based on the cellular surface, the so-called multidrug efflux pump, which is characterized by the expression of a specific 170-kd protein complex, P glycoprotein.[22] Investigators initially demonstrated that response to the cellular effects of agents as diverse as the vinca alkaloids, actinomycin D, and doxorubicin is reduced in normal and malignant cells that express a protein complex on the cell surface, coded by a series of multidrug resistance genes (*PGY*, formerly known as *mdr*). This occurs as a result of reduced intracellular concentrations of the agents because of increased cellular efflux.[23] Expression of the *PGY* phenotype appears to be an example of induced resistance, because previous exposure to colchicine or to one of these agents can induce *PGY*-based resistance to the entire group.

Expression of *PGY* phenotype has been identified in renal carcinoma, although its significance has been difficult to define because most renal carcinomas are resistant to the available cytotoxic agents, and the presence or absence of this phenotype does not correlate with outcome. The study of the multidrug phenotype in bladder cancer cells has also proved difficult; the expression of P glyoprotein in bladder cancer has been variable and inconstant.[24,25] Expression of P glycoprotein may be upregulated in resistant populations of bladder cancer cells after treatment with the methotrexate, vinblastine, Adriamycin (doxorubicin), cisplatin (MVAC) regimen.[26] In other tumor types, multidrug resistance can occur in the absence of expression of the 170-kd P glycoprotein, whereas other proteins may be associated with similar patterns of resistance,[27] a finding that perhaps explains this phenomenon in the absence of expression of P glycoprotein.

Ultimately, apart from its predictive function, this work is unlikely to be of great importance unless the multidrug resistance phenotype can be overcome at a functional level. For example, the calcium channel blockers, such as verapamil, have been shown to reverse multidrug resistance,[28] although the toxic side effects of this approach have precluded routine use. Although clinical trials have not yet been published in bladder cancer, work initiated in our laboratories suggests that verapamil can overcome the impact of the *PGY* phenotype, at least in bladder cancer cell lines in vitro.[29]

The mechanisms of resistance to the platinum coordination complexes have been studied in detail, particularly in relation to ovarian cancer and malignant melanoma (Chap. 9). Although several mechanisms have been identified, including factors that influence cellular accumulation, signal transduction, ionic fluxes, and intracellular enzyme function,[30] the function of the intracellular scavenger, glutathione (GSH), has been the focus of particular attention in the context of the resistance of bladder cancer to the effects of cisplatin. GSH is found in most mamma-

Table 8-1. *Targets of modulation of resistance*

Mechanism	Effector	Agent
Accumulation	Hyperthermia	Cisplatin (cDDP)
	Dipyridamole	Cisplatin
Membrane activity	Tamoxifen	Cisplatin
	Epidermal growth factor	Cisplatin
	Cyclosporin A	Cisplatin
Detoxification		
Glutathione	Buthionine sulfoximine	Cisplatin, alkylating agents
Metallothioneins	?	Cisplatin
DNA repair	Polymerase inhibitors	
	Thymidine triphosphate inhibitors	Cisplatin
Access to DNA	DFMO	Cisplatin
	Hyperthermia	Cisplatin
Gene amplification	Dihydrofolate reductase	Methotrexate
Target alteration	Tubulin	Vinca alkaloids
	Thymidylate synthase	5-Fluorouracil
Poor activation	Low uridine kinase	5-Fluorouracil
	Low polyglutamylation	Methotrexate

lian cells and has many functions, including regulation of protein and DNA synthesis and detoxification. It appears to react with cisplatin to reduce the drug's intracellular availability. Inhibitors of GSH synthesis, such as buthionine sulfoximine, have been shown to cause a decrease in intracellular levels of GSH, with a concomitant increase in the cytotoxicity of some anticancer agents, such as the alkylating agents, cisplatin,[31] and paclitaxel.[32] Although many of the experimental data regarding the significance of glutathione in cisplatin resistance have been derived from models of ovarian cancer, we have demonstrated that high levels of glutathione are present in cell lines derived from bladder cancer, and this finding may correlate with cisplatin resistance.[33]

Our understanding of these mechanisms is relatively crude, and other factors appear to influence the responsiveness of bladder cancer to cytotoxic chemotherapy. The expression of several oncogene products seems to influence resistance to cytotoxic agents. The exact nature of this interaction is not yet clear and is particularly difficult to define because several of these products code for specific aspects of cellular growth control, irrespective of exposure to cytotoxic agents. For example, the interaction of epidermal growth factor and its specific receptor (epidermal growth factor receptor [EGFR]) is involved in the regulation of growth of bladder cancer. In vitro treatment with epidermal growth factor can increase cellular sensitivity of epithelial tumors to cisplatin, however, presumably by an effect on a signal transduction pathway.[34] Investigators have also reported that specific monoclonal antibodies can block the function of the EGFR,[35] and further, treatment with these anti-EGFR monoclonal antibodies plus cisplatin can cause a synergistic antitumor effect.[36] These data are particularly difficult to interpret in view of the previously documented impact of expression of EGFR on the natural history of bladder cancer, as well as the demonstration that *ERB2* (formerly known as *erb*B-2) gene amplification and overexpression are adverse prognostic determinants in bladder cancer.

Another complex relationship has been demonstrated among the expression of P53 (a suppressor gene product), growth regulation, and cytotoxic response in bladder cancer. Alterations of the *P53* gene are among the most frequent genetic abnormalities found in human cancer and appear to have a broad range of postulated roles in cell growth control, including involvement in cellular repair and apoptosis. Apoptosis, or programmed cell death, is regarded as a form of physiologic cell death because it represents a genetically determined cellular sequence that is part of the normal tissue homeostatic mechanism. Investigators have shown that P53, which is normally present only transiently, can be induced to accumulate within the cell by exposure to cytotoxic agents, such as cisplatin and mitomycin C,[37] and conversely, P53-dependent apoptosis modulates the cytotoxicity of radiotherapy, 5-FU, and doxorubicin.[38] In our laboratory, however, we have demonstrated that cisplatin cytotoxicity appears not to be mediated by apoptosis in bladder cancer cell lines.[39] These issues may be of particular importance because investigators have already postulated that P53 expression may constitute an independent prognosticator of response to the MVAC regimen. Because P53 may be induced by cytotoxic exposure, the timing of tissue sampling may possibly be critical in determining the expression of this potential prognostic factor, especially if intravesical or systemic chemotherapy has been used previously.

Models for Overcoming Drug Resistance of Tumor Populations: Clinical Implications

Several models have been proposed to explain the varying levels of resistance to the impact of chemotherapy seen in human tumors. For example, Goldie and Coldman[40] proposed that tumors have a spontaneous mutation rate, and the larger the number of tumor cells, the greater the chance of spontaneous mutation. As a consequence, these investigators proposed that the most effective mechanism for cancer killing would be to initiate chemotherapy early (with a small cellular burden) and to introduce multiple agents in an attempt to overcome the various mechanisms of resistance. To date, this hypothesis has not been validated in clinical trials, although most of the studies reported have been flawed and have not truly evaluated the principles of this hypothesis.

Another model of resistance, proposed after a reanalysis of

the model presented by Goldie and Coldman, leads to the conclusion that cytotoxic agents can be used most effectively in sequence, rather than as combination schedules.[41] Thus, an initial series of treatments with the less effective of two drugs would eliminate a proportion of the tumor cells present, leaving behind a resistant population that may respond to several courses of treatment with the more effective drug; in this way, investigators have postulated that the impact of the less effective therapy can be maximized.

ASSESSMENT OF THE EFFICACY OF ANTICANCER TREATMENT

The efficacy of anticancer treatment can be assessed in various ways, depending on the end points under consideration. In most current studies, a reduction in tumor-related symptoms (subjective response), the development of tumor shrinkage (objective response), length of disease-free or overall survival, and improvement in quality of life are regarded as significant indices of patient benefit in response to treatment. To assess these outcomes objectively and accurately, we use the process of the clinical trial wherein a defined population of patients, who fit specified criteria, are managed according to a defined protocol with specified measurement of outcome. A clinical trial may be one of two types.[10,42]

An *explanatory* trial has the primary aim of acquisition of information; thus, it usually only requires small numbers of patients and often has a biologic end point (e.g., tumor response); a typical example is the assessment of the anticancer agent, gemcitabine, in the treatment of advanced bladder cancer, that provides the documentation of response and toxicity, but does not give comparative information versus a standard type of treatment. It is often appropriate to report only the patients who are fully treated (complete the minimum requirements of the protocol of assessment), to minimize the chance of rejecting an active new approach. This protocol may overestimate the potential benefit of the drug in the general patient population, however.

In contrast, a *pragmatic* trial is concerned with the assessment of comparative patient benefit, which can then be used as a guide to decision making in treatment. For example, the current Intergroup randomized trials that compare neoadjuvant intravenous chemotherapy plus locoregional treatment versus locoregional treatment alone for invasive bladder cancer are pragmatic trials and require large numbers of patients. Because the goal of a pragmatic trial is to determine overall benefit to all eligible patients, end points should include both quality and quantity of survival, and investigators should report the outcome for all entered patients, irrespective of treatment received.

Another classification of clinical trials is according to the descriptors *phase I*, *phase II*, *phase III*, and *phase IV*. A *phase I* trial is designed to determine the appropriate clinical dosage of a new treatment (often translated from preclinical studies) and to assess the side effects of this treatment. Such trials often incorporate pharmacologic studies that allow a clearer understanding of the distribution and metabolism of the novel agent in humans. The initial dose is usually developed from preclinical testing, in which the initial dose is that equivalent to $\frac{1}{10}$ of the dose required to cause toxic deaths in 10% of mice tested. Phase I trials should only be performed on fully informed patients who have advanced disease and for whom no standard treatment has a significant chance of controlling their disease. Although anticancer response is recorded, this is not a primary end point of a phase I trial, and patients must understand that the chance of significant tumor shrinkage is small. Patients often participate in such trials in the hope that they may secure the small percentage chance of success, or occasionally they participate for reasons of altruism.[43] Regrettably, it has become increasingly clear that patients often have a poor understanding of the true purpose of phase I trials and of the small likelihood of individual patient benefit.[44] Phase I trials are explanatory and should be designed to minimize the expenditure of patient resources, usually with only 3 to 4 patients entered at each dose level.[45] These numbers allow relatively accurate identification and description of toxicity at each dose level, without the necessity to treat unreasonably large numbers of patients at potentially subtherapeutic doses.

Unless the toxicity from a phase I trial is prohibitive or truly unpredictable and dangerous, the new agent automatically proceeds to phase II testing. In most cases, an absence of antitumor activity in phase I testing does not preclude initial phase II assessment. *Phase II* trials are also explanatory and attempt to define whether a new approach has antitumor activity. These studies usually involve treatment with a predetermined dosage of a novel agent in defined groups of patients who have a particular disease, with assessment of tumor shrinkage and toxicity as primary end points. The demonstration of tumor shrinkage does not equate with long-term patient benefit, which is assessed subsequently in a phase III trial. Detailed mathematic assessments of numbers of patients required to document true anticancer efficacy, to minimize false-positive and false-negative outcomes, are published elsewhere.[46,47] In general, phase II studies require small numbers of patients (usually fewer than 50, depending on the number of responses seen).

Phase III trials are designed to define the role of a new treatment compared with a standard approach. These studies are pragmatic and usually require randomization and large numbers of patients. The number of required patients is predicated on the level of statistical confidence (power) that is required for the outcome (Chap. 13).

A more recent term, the *phase IV* trial, is used to describe a postmarketing study, in which a pharmaceutical company attempts to develop additional information regarding the indications for a newly approved agent that is being marketed; sometimes, such studies are actually marketing (or "seeding") studies, in which the primary purpose of the trial is to increase the level of interest or familiarity among physicians.

The requirements of these clinical trials and a detailed discussion of the potential sources of error (Table 8-2) are beyond the scope of this chapter, but are reviewed elsewhere[10,48] (Chap. 13).

Table 8-2. *Potential sources of error in clinical trials*

Failure to establish uniform reporting criteria of efficacy and toxicity
Measurement error
Bias in patient sampling: selection, exclusion
Insufficient patient numbers
Use of historical controls
Stage migration
Inadequate follow-up

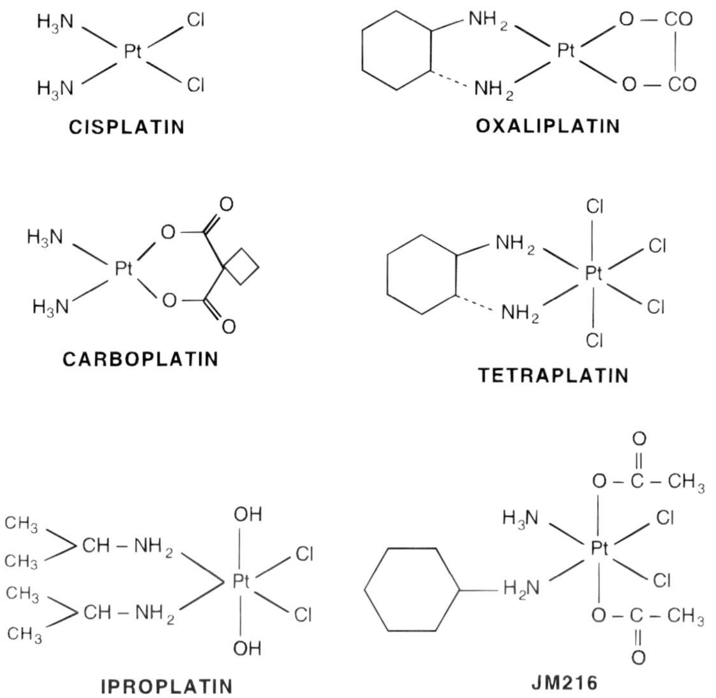

FIG. 8-1. Structures of platinum complexes.

SPECIFIC AGENTS COMMONLY USED AGAINST GENITOURINARY CANCERS

Platinum Complexes

Cisplatin (cis-diamminedichloroplatinum II) was introduced into the clinic in 1972 when observations by Rosenberg and associates[49] of its activity in interfering with the growth of *Escherichia coli* led to the demonstration of broad-spectrum antitumor activity in experimental tumors. The lead compound of the platinum antitumor drugs, cisplatin (Fig. 8-1), has contributed in a major way to the development of cure in testicular germ cell tumors (Chaps. 68 and 69) and is highly active in combination in bladder cancer (Chaps. 27 through 29).

The mode of action of the platinum complexes and the mechanisms of resistance to this group of drugs are discussed in detail in Chapter 9. In brief, leaving groups ionize to be replaced by water, forming positively charged (electron-deficient) moieties that form adducts with DNA. These adducts are primarily intrastrand crosslinks. Interstrand crosslinks also form but in much smaller amounts. They are, however, much more lethal than intrastrand crosslinks. The contribution of the two types of adducts to the overall cytotoxicity of platinum complexes is a matter of dispute. Based on the sites of action of cisplatin, its major focus of activity is in the G_1 and S phases of the cell cycle. Resistance to the platinum complexes may be due to impaired cell uptake of the drug, inactivation of the active species by intracellular thiols (primarily glutathione), and enhanced capacity of the cell to repair the damage to DNA (Chap. 9).

Cisplatin is usually administered intravenously or intraarterially, and in both instances, nephrotoxicity is markedly reduced or eliminated if a high urine output is maintained by enforced parenteral hydration before, during, and after cisplatin administration, augmented by the use of mannitol and, in some instances, small doses of furosemide. In early studies, cisplatin was administered for intravesical use by instillation through a urinary catheter, but unpredictable allergic reactions with occasional anaphylaxis were documented, and this indication is no longer under investigation.

Measurement of total plasma platinum after administration of cisplatin shows a triphasic disappearance curve with half-life values of 20 minutes, 1 hour, and 24 hours[50,51]; the terminal phase probably reflects the slow release of platinum from plasma proteins. More than 90% of excretion is by renal mechanisms (a combination of glomerular filtration and tubular secretion), with less than 10% due to biliary excretion. The plasma decay of unchanged cisplatin generally has a monophasic pattern, with a half-life of less than 1 hour.[52]

Renal failure, with acute tubular necrosis, degeneration, and interstitial edema, is the dose-limiting toxic effect, as noted earlier.[53] Additional side effects of parenteral administration include severe nausea and vomiting, diarrhea, and occasional anaphylaxis. Ototoxicity, manifest by high-frequency hearing loss, has been well documented, with a greater level of damage demonstrated by audiometry than on clinical grounds. With higher doses of cisplatin, and especially in combination regimens that include the vinca alkaloids, neurotoxicity is an important side effect. This effect may present clinically as peripheral or autonomic neuropathy and may be seen more commonly on nerve conduction testing.[54] Reported cardiovascular side effects include hypertension, myocardial infarctions, electrocardiographic (ECG) abnormalities, and an increased risk of peripheral thromboembolic phenomena and Raynaud's phenomenon.[55] In some cases, however, the relationship between cisplatin and these side effects is obscured by the impact of antecedent cigarette smoking by the population of patients under treatment. Myelosuppression may occur with standard doses of cisplatin, with anemia occurring in particular. Occasionally, Coombs-positive hemolytic anemia has been documented. Leukopenia and thrombocytopenia occur sometimes, but they are usually not dose limiting. In an attempt to overcome the substantial toxic effects of this useful agent, a range of analogs has been developed to reduce toxicity without loss of activity (see later).

Cisplatin is probably the most widely used cytotoxic agent in the management of genitourinary cancer. In addition to being a drug of choice in the management of germ cell tumors (Chaps. 66 through 68) and bladder cancer (Chaps. 27 through 29), cisplatin has activity against adenocarcinoma and small cell carcinoma of prostate, adrenal cancer, and penile cancer. It is inactive against renal carcinoma, although we have demonstrated modest activity in this setting when cisplatin is modulated by pretreatment with *N*-phosphonacetyl-L-aspartate (PALA) (Chap. 9).

Anticancer Antibiotics

Bleomycin

Bleomycin is isolated from the fungus-like bacterium *Streptomyces verticills* and consists of a complex molecule of high molecular weight. It is composed predominantly of so-called A_2 peptides, which contain a DNA-binding portion and an iron-binding component at the opposite end. The primary action of bleomycin is to produce single-strand and double-strand breaks in DNA through the action of oxygen radicals formed in association with activation of the Fe^{++}-bleomycin complex that binds to nitrogen-containing groups in the bleomycin molecule. The entire complex, consisting of Fe^{++}-bleomycin-oxygen, binds to DNA, through intercalation by the bithiazole groups of bleomycin, and DNA damage is created through the formation of superoxide or hydroxyl radicals. Tumor cells are most sensitive to the effects of bleomycin in late G_2 or the M phase,[56] although cells may also be killed in G_1.[57] The exact mechanism of resistance to bleomycin has not been delineated, although a cytosolic hydrolase appears to inactivate the drug.[58]

Bleomycin is administered either by subcutaneous bolus dosing, intravenously (bolus or continuous infusion), or by intramuscular injection. The optimal route has not been defined, although the drug is most commonly given (in combination with cisplatin and either vinblastine or etoposide) as a weekly bolus dose. Bleomycin has a biphasic clearance, with $t\frac{1}{2}\alpha$ of about 20 minutes and a $t\frac{1}{2}\beta$ of about 3 hours. Bleomycin is excreted predominantly by the kidneys, with more than 50% being excreted in the first 24 hours.[59] The dosage should be modified in a patient with impaired renal function, and caution should be used when the drug is administered after cisplatin, which can cause transient renal dysfunction.

The major toxic effect of bleomycin is interstitial pneumonitis, the pathogenesis of which is poorly understood. The syndrome may be characterized by the evolution of subtle pulmonary symptoms, including cough, dyspnea on exertion, chest pain, and fever, or occasionally it may be revealed only by changes in lung function tests. Pulmonary toxicity occurs especially in older patients, those who have previously received pulmonary or mediastinal irradiation, those with underlying lung disease, and in particular cigarette smokers. In a study of the long-term toxic effects of bleomycin, we were unable to demonstrate major pulmonary toxicity in patients who did not smoke.[54] In our experience, the acute toxicity of bleomycin can usually be ameliorated by corticosteroids, although care should be taken to avoid tapering the dose too quickly. Other side effects include mild myelosuppression, allergic reactions, fever, Raynaud's phenomenon, and cutaneous pigmentation.

The major indication for the use of bleomycin is in the management of germ cell tumors (Chaps. 68 and 69), and most attempts to delete the drug from standard protocols have resulted in reduced pulmonary toxicity, but at the expense of a reduced cure rate.[60,61] In addition, bleomycin has also been applied in some series to the management of advanced cancer of the penis (Chap. 95). The drug appears to have no indications for use in the treatment of bladder cancer (Chap. 28), renal carcinoma (Chap. 85), or prostate cancer (Chap. 58).

Mitomycin C

Mitomycin C is an anticancer and antibacterial antibiotic isolated from *Streptomyces caespitosus*.[62] The drug is unusual in that it undergoes activation in a hypoxic environment, a characteristic of solid tumors. It is activated by visible, but not ultraviolet, light, and it is unstable in acidic and extremely basic conditions. Mitomycin is activated by reduction of a quinone moiety, mediated by microsomal enzymes, such as cytochrome reductase, DT-diaphorase, xanthine oxidase, or cytochrome P450 reductase, or even by exposure to acidic pH. This activation releases a methanol side chain from the molecule and allows an aziridine ring to open. This process exposes the alkylating site. The alkylating agent crosslinks complementary DNA strands. Oxygen-derived free radicals may also participate in the cytotoxic function of mitomycin C through the production of DNA strand breaks.[63]

Mitomycin is usually administered by intravenous injection or through a urinary catheter for intravesical use. Its large molecular weight allows it to be retained within the luminal surface of the bladder, without significant systemic absorption. Because the drug is degraded at acid pH, the urinary pH must be maintained at alkaline levels for intravesical use.

Because of its ubiquitous metabolism, mitomycin is cleared rapidly after intravenous or intraarterial injection. Renal excretion is minor (10% of administered dosage), and hepatic excretion seems to play only a small role despite the importance of hepatic inactivation. Hepatic dysfunction does not appear to alter the pharmacokinetics of this drug to any great extent.[64]

The major toxic effect of mitomycin is myelosuppression, which involves platelet, leukocyte, and erythrocyte precursors.[62] This myelosuppression may be delayed and can occur 6 to 7 weeks after treatment. The level of myelosuppression correlates with dosage, and a cumulative effect appears to exist as well. Other side effects include gastrointestinal disturbances, occasional stomatitis, and renal toxicity.[65,66] Mitomycin C can occasionally induce microangiopathic hemolytic anemia with associated renal failure (the hemolytic-uremic syndrome); this syndrome can be delayed in onset.[65,66] Not infrequently, mitomycin C causes interstitial pneumonitis, especially in high cumulative doses and in patients who have had previous chest irradiation; the syndrome is characterized by progressive cough and dyspnea, accompanied by changes in pulmonary function tests, and it responds dramatically to high-dose corticosteroids.[67] Mitomycin C is a vesicant and causes extensive soft tissue reaction if extravasated; sometimes, the ulceration occurs as a delayed phenomenon.

The major indications for the use of mitomycin C include intravesical administration for superficial bladder cancer and intravenous administration for advanced bladder cancer; activity of mitomycin has also been demonstrated in the management of adenocarcinoma of the prostate (Chap. 58) and in advanced penile carcinoma (Chap. 95). This agent has no routine role in the management of renal carcinoma (Chap. 85), germ cell tumors (Chaps. 68 and 69), or adrenal carcinoma (Chap. 98).

Doxorubicin and Other Anthracyline Antibiotics

Doxorubicin (Adriamycin) is a high-molecular-weight anthracycline antibiotic isolated from *Streptomyces peucetius* var. *caesius*. Its structure includes a water-soluble basic reducing amino sugar linked by a glycosidic bond to carbon atom 7 on the D ring of the chromophore aglycone, adriamycinone. This four-ring planar structure constitutes the anthraquinone nucleus. Several analogs are in clinical use, including epirubicin, which differs in the steric configuration of the -OH group on the 4′ position of the daunosamine sugar, and idarubicin, which lacks an A ring -OCH_3 substitution. A detailed discussion of each of these agents is beyond the scope of this review, but the subject is covered elsewhere in detail.[68]

Several mechanisms of cytotoxic action of the anthracycline antibiotics appear possible,[68], including the formation of free radicals, intercalation between nucleotide pairs in the DNA molecule, and the initiation of topoisomerase II–dependent DNA fragmentation. Doxorubicin appears to be active in all phases of the cell cycle, with its maximal effect in S phase; however, it is not phase specific. For example, its topoisomerase type II function is concentrated in G_2.

Doxorubicin and epirubicin can be administered by bolus or continuous intravenous or intraarterial injection or by urinary catheter for intravesical use. Doxorubicin is extremely vesicant, and great caution should be used in its administration. After intravascular administration, the pharmacokinetics of doxorubicin and its analogs are best represented by two- or three-compartment modeling.[69] The plasma half-lives are 11 minutes, 3 hours, and 25 to 30 hours; the long terminal phase is likely due to slow dissociation from DNA. These agents are rapidly distributed (into liver, lymph nodes, muscle, bone marrow, fat, and skin, but not central nervous tissue), and more than 70% is bound to plasma proteins. These drugs are extensively metabolized and are excreted predominantly in the bile and feces. Biliary excretion accounts for more than 40% of each dose,[70] whereas less than 10% is excreted in the urine. Obstructive hepatic dysfunction interferes with the disposition of these agents and mandates dose modification, whereas hepatocellular dysfunction without impaired conjugation does not seem to require these changes in dosing.[71] One potentially attractive feature of idarubicin is its retention of antitumor activity when administered orally. Although this agent is apparently useful in the treatment of leukemia and lymphoma, its utility against the solid tumors appears more limited.

The most common dose-limiting acute toxic effect is myelosuppression, with leukopenia at 10 to 14 days after treatment. Thrombocytopenia and anemia occur, but they are less clinically important. As noted earlier, doxorubicin is a significant vesicant and can produce extensive ulceration and soft tissue necrosis after extravasation. The other dose-limiting toxic effects are found in the heart. Dose-related cardiomyopathy has been extensively described,[72] and it usually occurs with cumulative doses higher than 500 to 550 mg/m^2 in previously untreated patients. These effects are more pronounced with conventional 3-weekly bolus dosing than if weekly low-dose bolus doses or 96-hour continuous low-dose infusions are implemented. Other factors that predispose patients to cardiac toxicity include known cardiac disease, previous mediastinal or cardiac irradiation, age older than 70 years, and chronic hypertension. In addition to cardiomyopathy, other cardiac effects have been recorded, including nonspecific ECG changes, occasional rhythm disturbances, an uncommon myocarditis-pericarditis syndrome, and rarely sudden death. Some investigators have suggested that epirubicin may be less cardiotoxic than doxorubicin,[68] although the contrary view has been expressed, that equiactive doses of the two agents are equitoxic.

Doxorubicin is a radiosensitizer and has a radiomimetic function; thus, it causes recall reactions in areas previously treated with radiotherapy.[73] Other toxic effects include nausea, vomiting, stomatitis, and alopecia.

The clinical indications for the use of this group of agents against the genitourinary cancers have been defined on the basis of the activity of doxorubicin. Whether the analogs, epirubicin and idarubicin, offer any clear advantage in this context is unclear. Doxorubicin has been identified as one of the agents of choice for use against superficial and advanced bladder cancer (Chaps. 26 through 29), and it has significant activity against adenocarcinoma and small cell carcinoma of prostate (Chap. 58). In previous experience, in particular at the University of Indiana and at the Memorial Sloan-Kettering Cancer Center, New York, doxorubicin was built into combination chemotherapy regimens for germ cell tumors, but it has been omitted in more recent trials, based on randomized trials in Indiana in which the drug appeared not to add to the anticancer effect of standard cisplatin-based combination regimens (Chap. 68). Limited activity against adrenal carcinoma has been recorded (Chap. 98), but doxorubicin appears to be inactive against renal carcinoma (Chap. 85).

Vinca alkaloids

The vinca alkaloids, which occur naturally in the periwinkle (*Catharanthus roseus*), are formed from two multiple ring planar units, an indole nucleus and a dihydroindole nucleus. The two most commonly used drugs, vincristine and vinblastine, are almost identical, differing only in a single substitution on the dihydroindole nucleus.[74] They both act by binding to tubulin, and they inhibit microtubule assembly, a process that, in turn, inhibits mitotic spindle formation. This situation causes an accumulation of cells in metaphase. Although the vinca alkaloids are thought to be cell cycle-phase specific for mitosis, the cytotoxic effect probably occurs in S phase, and its effect is seen in the M phase. After intravenous administration, the vinca alkaloids are extensively bound by serum proteins and blood components and are rapidly cleared from the plasma and are concentrated in various tissues. The disposition is triphasic,[75] with a rapid initial half-life ($t^1/_2\alpha$ of less than 5 minutes), $t^1/_2\beta$ of 1 to 2 hours, and $t^1/_2\gamma$ of 1 to 3 days. The vinca alkaloids approximate total body water in their distribution. The major route of excretion is hepatic,[76] with appreciable amounts appearing in the stool, and liver disease may necessitate a change in dosage. A small component of excretion is urinary.

Although similar in structure, the vinca alkaloids have substantially different profiles of toxicity. Vincristine is predominantly associated with neurologic side effects, including a range of peripheral sensorimotor neuropathic changes, autonomic neuropathy, jaw pain, and central nervous system effects. Less commonly, vincristine causes myelosuppression, gastrointestinal effects, alopecia, and the syndrome of inappropriate antidiuretic hormone (ADH) production. By contrast, vinblastine is associated with predominant myelosuppression (in particular granulocytopenia), more marked gastrointestinal toxicity (especially paralytic ileus), and alopecia; the neurologic toxicities, although prominent, occur less frequently and less severely than with vincristine. Both agents are significant vesicants.

The vinca alkaloids have had particular application in the treatment of advanced germ cell tumors (Chaps. 68 and 69), in small cell cancer of the prostate, and in bladder cancer (vinblastine, in particular) (Chap. 28), but they appear to have less single-agent activity in the treatment of prostate adenocarcinoma (Chap. 58), adrenal carcinoma, and renal carcinoma.

Alkylating Agents

The alkylating agents are a group of chemical compounds of diverse structure that share the common property of labile, electrophilic alkyl groups that can react with most biologic molecules to form adducts. The alkyl groups can be added to oxygen, nitrogen, phosphorus, or sulfur atoms and thus can function at extremely diverse sites. Their most important reactions, however, are with the nitrogen atoms of DNA, particularly the N^7 position of guanine residues, altering the structure or function of the DNA. These drugs are all cell cycle dependent, but not cell cycle specific; that is, they exert their effects on cells throughout the cell cycle (analogous to irradiation). They appear most active against rapidly proliferating cells. Agents included in this group include cyclophosphamide, ifosfamide, thiotepa, melphalan, nitrogen mustard, busulfan, chlorambucil, and the nitrosoureas.

The alkylating agents, through their common mechanism of action, are potentially cytotoxic and carcinogenic. Although they share common functional traits, differences in their chemical structures account for the variation in their pharmacologic characteristics. This difference is of particular importance as an explanation for the failure of cross-resistance to occur in all situations.

Cyclophosphamide

Cyclophosphamide is 2-bis-(2-chloroethyl)amino-tetrahydro-2H-1,3,2-oxazaphosphorine-2-oxide monohydrate, a cyclic phosphamide ester of nornitrogen mustard. The monohydrate is not ionized and is lipid soluble. This agent is a bifunctional substituted nitrogen mustard, which must be activated in the liver before it is active. Activation is a multistep process that occurs in the hepatic microsomal P450 enzyme system.[77,78] Thus, no rationale exists for using the drug for intraarterial chemotherapy or as an intravesically administered agent. Cyclophosphamide can be usefully administered as an oral agent (90% bioavailability) or intravenously. Hepatic inactivation is the major mechanism of active drug elimination, whereas after intravenous administration, about 15% of the drug is excreted unchanged in the urine and the rest is excreted as metabolites. The plasma half-life is approximately 5 to 6 hours.[78]

Because cyclophosphamide is bifunctional, it can crosslink the two strands of DNA, yielding an interstrand crosslink, or it can produce intrastrand crosslinks or even can bind DNA to protein. The binding of the active metabolite of cyclophosphamide to DNA does not cause cell death itself; rather, the cells progress slowly through the S phase and arrest and subsequently die in the G_2 phase.

Information regarding potential drug interactions with cyclophosphamide is scant. Because the drug must be metabolized by hepatic microsomes to be active, drugs that induce this system (such as the barbiturates, phenytoin, and chloral hydrate) may increase the conversion of cyclophosphamide to its metabolites; similarly, cyclophosphamide may affect the activity of the barbiturates. Moreover, cimetidine has been reported to increase the toxicity of cyclophosphamide by a change in the concentration $\times$ time relationship of its active metabolites.[79]

Cyclophosphamide produces significant leukopenia and immunosuppression, but it is not usually associated with thrombocytopenia.[77] Nausea and vomiting may occur, although usually in association with high-dose intravenous usage. Similarly, alopecia is more commonly associated with high-dose administration. Of particular importance, excretion of acrolein, one of the metabolites particularly irritating to the bladder mucosa, can cause hemorrhagic cystitis, and this disorder can lead to bladder fibrosis or even transitional cell carcinoma of the bladder. In the context of intravenous administration, this toxic effect can be avoided by the use of sodium-2-mercaptoethane sulfonate (MESNA), which is excreted in the urine; it provides reactive thiols that bind to the acrolein and protects the bladder mucosa. Occasionally, cyclophosphamide may cause interstititial pneumonitis, testicular atrophy, anaphylaxis, and, in higher doses, the syndrome of inappropriate ADH production and cardiotoxicity (including acute cardiac necrosis when the drug is given in transplant-intense dosage).

The most common application of cyclophosphamide for genitourinary cancer is in the treatment of adenocarcinoma of the prostate,[8,9] and it was also used in the past to treat advanced germ cell tumors.[80,81] It is less frequently used for germ cell tumors in current practice because of the risks of carcinogenicity and infertility. The drug is inactive in the treatment of renal and adrenal carcinomas and has only limited activity in the treatment of bladder cancer.

Ifosfamide

Ifosfamide is a structural analog of cyclophosphamide, differing only in the position of one of the two chloroethyl groups. It is also a metabolically activated alkylating agent and must first undergo hydroxylation by hepatic microsomes.[78] The change in its structure has altered its pharmacologic features, however, and its activation within the liver occurs more slowly than for cyclophosphamide.

Ifosfamide is well absorbed orally and can also be administered intravenously. Its pharmacology is similar to that of cyclophosphamide. Its plasma half-life has been reported to be as short as 5 to 6 hours, either after oral or intravenous administration,[82] although Creaven and associates[83] documented a plasma half-life of radioactively labeled ifosfamide of nearly 14 hours. In clinical practice, the agent is most commonly administered intravenously, with schedules varying from a single infusion to multiple-day schedules, with MESNA coverage to prevent hemorrhagic cystitis. Creaven and associates have suggested that the alkylating activity ratio of ifosfamide is 1:5, when compared with that of cyclophosphamide.[83] The pattern of toxicity is similar to that of cyclophosphamide,[84] but with less myelosuppression and a greater tendency to cause cystitis. In addition, ifosfamide has a greater prevalence of central nervous system toxicity, including altered mental status, cerebellar dysfunction, seizures, and extrapyramidal effects.[84,85]

Ifosfamide is currently used in salvage and high-risk regimens for advanced germ cell tumors (see Chap. 69) and for metastatic bladder cancer (Chap. 28). In broad-based phase I-II trials, little activity has been reported in prostate cancer, although the drug has not been assessed since prostate-specific antigen has been introduced as a surrogate marker of response. Ifosfamide is inactive in renal carcinoma (Chap. 85), but single-agent activity has been identified in squamous cell carcinoma, including cancer of the penis (Chap. 95).

Thiotepa

N,N′,N″-triethylenethiophosphoramide (thiotepa) is an aziridine drug, a polyfunctional alkylating agent, which can produce interstrand cross links, DNA adducts and strand breaks, and other DNA lesions.[86] After intravenous injection, the $t\frac{1}{2}\alpha$ was 7.7 minutes, and the $t\frac{1}{2}\beta$ was 125 minutes in the study by Cohen and associates.[87]

Thiotepa is administered by intravenous or intracavitary routes, the latter including intraperitoneal, intrathecal, and intravesical delivery. It is not a vesicant and does not cause local soft tissue reactions.

In the standard dose range, thiotepa is associated with myelosuppression, both granulocytopenia and thrombocytopenia, and nausea, vomiting, headache, and occasionally alopecia. In transplant-intense doses, thiotepa may cause mucositis, cutaneous changes, and occasionally organic brain syndrome.[88] When administered intravesically, thiotepa causes little systemic toxicity unless it is used within a few days of extensive transurethral resection; thiotepa, a relatively small molecule, is absorbed significantly through an extensively denuded bladder surface.

The major clinical application for thiotepa has been in the intravesical chemotherapy of superficial bladder cancer (Chap. 26), although this agent is now used less frequently because of its risk of carcinogenicity and the development of more effective treatment options.

Epipodophyllotoxins

Podophyllotoxin, a derivative of the mandrake root, has been known to have antimitotic properties for more than half a century, and extracts of the mandrake root have been used for medicinal purposes for centuries.[89] Although the early podophyllotoxin derivatives were excessively toxic, two derivatives (etoposide and teniposide) have shown substantial clinical activity with a tolerable profile of side effects.[89–91] Although these agents were initially believed to act by binding to tubulin and inhibiting microtubule assembly, additional studies have suggested that the epipodophyllotoxins arrest cells in late S phase or early G_2 phase,[92] rather than at G_2 to M. More recent studies have shown that these agents exert their anticancer effects by impeding the function of the topoisomerase II enzyme.[93]

Each compound has a complex, multiringed structure linked to a glucopyranoside sugar. Both drugs are routinely administered intravenously, although etoposide is now formulated for oral administration. The optimal schedule of administration has not been defined, but prolonged schedules (multiple daily short infusions or continuous infusion) are most common because of the phase-specific mode of action. The pharmacokinetics is biphasic, with half-life values of 90 minutes and 3 and 11 hours.[91] After administration of radiolabeled etoposide to humans, 40% to 90% of radioactivity is recovered in the urine within 48 hours, fecal recovery is less than 20%, and biliary excretion is only minimal.[89]

The major toxicity of the epipodophyllotoxins is dose-related myelosuppression, with predominant leukopenia.[90] Gastrointestinal complications, such as nausea, vomiting, and anorexia, are usually mild. Other side effects include alopecia, headache, fever, and hypotension. Severe hypotension may occur if the drug is infused too rapidly, and this can occasionally be accompanied by bronchospasm or rarely by anaphylaxis. These allergic phenomena are believed to be due to the use of the diluent, cremophor. Etoposide phosphate, a water-soluble derivative that is rapidly hydrolysed to etoposide in the plasma, is undergoing clinical trial. Emerging information has suggested that etoposide is occasionally associated with iatrogenic acute myeloid leukemia, and such cases have now been recorded among patients cured of germ cell tumors.[55]

The indications for the use of the epipodophyllotoxins for genitourinary cancer are limited; the most common application is in the management of advanced germ cell tumors (Chaps. 66 through 69). Most studies have suggested that the drug has only limited activity against bladder cancer and prostatic adenocarcinoma, although this drug has a clear role in the treatment of small cell anaplastic prostate cancer. Etoposide is inactive in the treatment of renal carcinoma, and only scant data are available with respect to penile and adrenal cancers.

Antimetabolites

Antifolates

The role of the antimetabolites in cancer treatment was first explored 50 years ago with the investigation of aminopterin, an analog of folic acid. This early work gave rise to the development of methotrexate, the 4-amino,10-methyl analog of the parent compound, which has come to be one of the most widely used agents for the treatment of genitourinary cancers.

Methotrexate inhibits dihydrofolate reductase (DHFR), an important enzyme in folic acid metabolism, which catalyzes the reduction of dihyrofolate to tetrahydrofolate. DHFR maintains the intracellular reduced folate pool, which, in turn, is required for the synthesis of thymidine and purines and thus for the production of DNA, RNA, and protein. Methotrexate undergoes polyglutamation intracellularly to varying extents; the polyglutamated forms do not traverse cellular membranes. Polyglutamation occurs to a greater extent in tumor cells than in normal cells, and this phenomenon may explain the selective action of the drug. The polyglutamated form is retained preferentially within cells, sometimes for lengthy periods,[94] and it can directly inhibit other folate-dependent enzymes, including thymidylate synthase.[95]

Methotrexate may also cause single- and double-stranded breaks in DNA.[96] It is most active against rapidly proliferating cells and appears to exert its major effect during S phase; it is thus classified as a cell cycle phase-specific antimetabolite.

Methotrexate uses the same active transport mechanisms to enter cells as does folic acid. At least two such mechanisms have been identified, including a low-affinity carrier that transports methotrexate and reduced folates and a high-affinity system that is more avid for reduced folates than for methotrexate. The metabolic block induced by methotrexate can be circumvented by the use of calcium leucovorin, which feeds into the folic acid cycle beyond the block of DHFR. Calcium leucovorin and its metabolite, 5-methyltetrahydrofolate, share the latter common transport mechanism with methotrexate. Apparently, normal cells can be selectively rescued by calcium leucovorin, either because of differences in transport or because of differences in the rate of DNA synthesis between normal and cancer cells. The complex biochemistry of methotrexate, its reversal, and mechanisms of resistance are beyond the scope of this chapter, but these topics are discussed in detail elsewhere.[97]

Methotrexate may be given by oral, intramuscular, intravenous, intraarterial, or intrathecal routes. Optimal dosing route and schedule have not been defined. A broad range of parenteral dosing has been reported, with doses ranging between 50 mg/m^2 and 15000 mg/m^2, predicated on the ability to rescue normal tissues with calcium leucovorin. Caution must be exercised because the higher dose range is potentially lethal if sufficient leucovorin is not administered. Alkalinization of the urine, by increasing the solubility of the drug and of the 7-hydroxy metabolite, also reduces toxicity. Methotrexate levels must be monitored after high-dose treatment to determine the length of leucovorin rescue.

More than 50% of the drug is bound to plasma proteins. Methotrexate is widely distributed in the body. In standard doses, methotrexate is excreted unchanged in urine, whereas in high doses, some metabolism of the drug occurs. Plasma decay of methotrexate is either biphasic or triphasic,[98,99] with the terminal phase of excretion reported to be in the range of 10 to 26 hours. Methotrexate is highly schedule dependent, its toxicity being more a function of the time during which plasma levels are maintained above a minimum cytotoxic concentration than of the total AUC. Thus, any factor that can prolong a low level of drug increases its toxicity. Principal among such factors are impaired renal function and localization in third-space compartments, such as pleural effusion or ascites with a slow release into the circulation. In these situations, methotrexate must be used with caution and reserve, with leucovorin used as necessary.

The spectrum of toxicity of methotrexate is a function of age, dose, the use of calcium leucovorin, drug metabolism, drug interactions, and renal function.[97] Patients may experience no toxic effects at all. Hematologic side effects include leukopenia, thrombocytopenia, and anemia. Gastrointestinal toxicity includes nausea, vomiting, diarrhea, and stomatitis. Hepatotoxicity has been reported in patients receiving long-term low-dose oral therapy and high-dose parenteral administration. Occasionally, methotrexate can cause self-limited pneumonitis. One of the most dangerous toxic effects is the induction of renal failure, because adequate renal function is necessary to ensure satisfactory excretion of the drug. Methotrexate can cause skin rash, pruritis, urticaria, alopecia, and other cutaneous side effects. Less commonly, central nervous toxicity can occur, especially after intrathecal administration.

Fluoropyrimidines

5-Fluorouracil (5-FU) was synthesized to act as a false pyrimidine and thus to inhibit the formation of thymidine.[100] Several mechanisms of action have been proposed, including inhibition of thymidylate synthase by an active metabolite (FdUMP), incorporation of the triphosphate 5-FUTP into RNA, and incorporation of the 2′-deoxy triphosphate 5-FdUTP into DNA.[101] The presence of reduced folate is critical to the function of 5-FU in inhibiting thymidylate synthase.

5-FU can be administered by oral, intravenous, intraarterial, or intraperitoneal routes. Bioavailability is poor and erratic when the drug is given by mouth,[102] and this route of administration is no longer used (however, see later, under modulation). When given intravenously, the drug has an extremely short terminal-phase half-life measured in minutes.[103,104] This is due to its rapid degradation by dihydrouracil dehydrogenase (DHD) to 5,6-dihydro 5-FU, which then undergoes ring rupture and is degraded to small molecules.[101] A rare deficiency of this enzyme can lead to severe toxicity after administration of 5-FU.[101]

Because of its mode of action, 5-FU is an S-phase-specific drug, and this characteristic, combined with its extremely short half-life, would lead us to anticipate that the drug would be highly schedule dependent. Paradoxically, however, rapid infusions of 5-FU are more toxic than the same dose given over a period of several hours. This is probably because, although the drug itself has a short plasma half-life, the persistence of the active metabolite FdUMP intracellularly is measured in days.[105] The bolus injection of the drug probably temporarily exceeds the capacity of DHD, thus making drug available for conversion to active metabolites. The nucleoside derivative of 5-FU, 5-fluoro-2′-deoxyuridine (FUdR, floxuridine), is extremely schedule dependent. The dose that can be given by short-term infusion is approximately 3 orders of magnitude greater than the dose that can be given when the drug is administered by long-term continuous infusion.[106]

Some compounds have been used in conjunction with fluoropyrimidines to enhance their activity through biochemical modulation. These include interferon, PALA, and leucovorin.[107] Of these compounds, leucovorin has been the most extensively investigated and has proved the most clinically useful, and it has raised the response rate to 5-FU in colorectal cancer by a factor of about 3.[108] It acts by stabilizing the ternary complex formed between the active metabolite FdUMP, the active site of the enzyme thymidylate synthase, and a reduced folate cofactor (5,10-methylene tetrahydrofolate), which is derived from leucovorin.[109] An investigational modulator, 5-ethynyluracil, has been introduced into clinical trial.[110] This compound, which inhibits DHD, decreases the first-pass effect and enables 5-FU to be given orally.

The primary toxicities of the fluoropyrimidines are gastrointestinal toxicity, stomatitis and diarrhea, and myelosuppression. The pattern of toxicity varies with the schedule of administration and is also influenced by the presence of modulators. Weekly bolus administration of 5-FU produces mainly myelosuppression, primarily leukopenia. Loading-dose 5-FU, prolonged infusions, and 5-FU used with leucovorin produce primarily gastrointestinal toxicity; cerebellar toxicity and cardiotoxicity have been described,[111] but these effects are uncommon at standard doses.

DEVELOPMENT OF NEW ANTICANCER DRUGS

In this section, we review new chemical entities that are in clinical development and may find a place in the treatment of genitourinary cancers in the next several years. This discussion does not include every new drug or class of drugs, but it highlights those that seem to offer the most promise in this area.

New Platinum Analogs

As noted earlier, cisplatin is one of the most active and useful agents in the management of genitourinary cancer. Its substantial toxicity, however, led to the search for analogs with equivalent anticancer activity but a reduced pattern of side effects that culminated in the introduction of several second-generation compounds into clinical trials. One of these, carboplatin, is now commercially available in the United States. Although less toxic than cisplatin (it has virtually no nephrotoxicity, has less neurotoxicity and ototoxicity, and produces much less nausea and vomiting), carboplatin is highly cross-resistant with the older compound. This may be related to the finding that once the cyclobutanedicarboxylato leaving group has separated from the molecule, the structure of the active hydrated species is identical to that of cisplatin. Thus, the major difference is in the kinetics of the formation of the active species. In the structure of cisplatin, the amine groups are carrier ligands, and the chlorides are leaving ligands. In the analogs, both types of ligands may differ from those in cisplatin. Changing the carrier ligand gives rise to an active species different from that of cisplatin or carboplatin; the resulting complexes may be less cross-resistant with cisplatin than is carboplatin.

Diamino Cyclohexane Platinum Complexes

In one of the early modifications of the cisplatin molecule, the two ammine groups were replaced by 1,2-diaminocyclohexane (DACH). The molecule so formed has certain stereoisomers because each amino group may be axial or equatorial to the ring. An early example of a DACH platinum complex tested clinically was 4′-carboxyphthalato (1,2-diaminocyclohexane) Pt II.[112] It had antitumor activity in the early trials; however, it was a mixture of isomers and was not developed further. Two DACH compounds, tetraplatin and oxaliplatin, have entered clinical trial. Tetraplatin (ormaplatin) was synthesized by Anderson and coworkers and is in early clinical evaluation.[113] It is one of two complexes of quadrivalent platinum to have completed initial clinical trials (the other, iproplatin, is discussed later). It is racemic trans-tetrachloro-1,2-diaminocyclohexane Pt IV. It is active in preclinical systems and shows an increased life span of 566% against L1210 leukemia with 5 of 8 long-term survivors.[114] In vivo, it is rapidly reduced to the corresponding divalent Pt complex, which is considered to be the active drug.[115] In early clinical trials, it showed antitumor activity. Unfortunately, it produces severe neurotoxicity,[116] and its future clinical development is currently uncertain.

The second DACH compound of interest is oxaliplatin. Synthesized by Kidani and coworkers,[117] the drug is currently undergoing extensive phase II and phase III clinical trials in Europe and will be introduced into the United States in 1996. Its structure is shown in Figure 8-1. Evidence indicates that, in solutions containing high chloride content, the oxalato group is replaced by chloride, a finding that suggests that the active metabolite of both oxaliplatin and tetraplatin is the same.[118] The toxicity profile of oxaliplatin is distinct, however. The drug produces a characteristic peripheral neuropathy manifested by a cold-induced dysesthesia that tends to be cumulative.[119] The drug is being primarily evaluated in colorectal carcinoma, but it has shown evidence of activity against urothelial cancer in an early trial.[120]

As noted earlier, another variant on the platinum molecule is the use of compounds containing quadrivalent platinum. Unlike the divalent platinum compounds, which are square planar complexes, these molecules have two ligands that are at right angles to the plane and are thus octahedral. The first such compound to be introduced into clinical trial was cis-dichloro-trans-dihydroxy-bis-isopropylamine platinum IV (iproplatin), which underwent phase I and phase II testing in England and in the United States.[121–124] Biochemical studies showed that the hydroxyl groups are quickly removed, reducing the compound in vivo to cis-dichloro-bis-isopropylamine Pt II,[125] which is probably the active form.[126] In the clinic, this agent showed a high degree of activity against ovarian carcinoma[122] and against small cell carcinoma of the lung,[123] and it was active against bladder cancer.[127] A trial of the agent used against heavily pretreated testicular carcinoma was negative.[128] The compound showed a toxicity profile less favorable than that of carboplatin, however, and it is not likely to be developed further.

Of great interest is the compound with the designation JM216, a quadrivalent platinum complex with mixed ammine and cyclo hexylamine carrier ligands, which is being developed by Harrap and coworkers in the United Kingdom.[129] The structure of this compound, bis-acetato-ammine-dichloro-cyclohexylamine Pt IV, is shown in Figure 8-1. The compound is active in preclinical experimental systems against cisplatin-resistant cell lines and is undergoing phase I clinical testing.[130] This agent is lipophilic and is the first orally active platinum complex to undergo clinical trial. The potential benefits of JM216 and similar compounds are likely to be actively pursued in the future in the design and synthesis of the next generation of platinum complexes.

The pharmacokinetics of the of the new platinum complexes have been incompletely studied; the most complete studies have been carried out with iproplatin. The pharmacokinetics of platinum complexes are complicated by the finding that, soon after the administration of most of these drugs, most of the platinum metal in the plasma is covalently bound to plasma proteins and becomes biologically inactive. With carboplatin, the platinum in the plasma ultrafiltrate is composed of only unchanged drug, and thus platinum measurements in the plasma ultrafiltrate can be used to determine the pharmacokinetics of the unchanged drug.[131] With iproplatin, this is not the case, and a separate method must be used to identify the unchanged drug.[132,133] Plasma decay of the unchanged drug is biphasic with a β-phase half-life of 2.4 hours in patients with normal renal function.[134] Impaired renal function reduces the plasma clearance and prolongs the half-life.[134] As with carboplatin,[135,136] a relationship can be developed between the creatinine clearance and the total body exposure to iproplatin, as measured by the AUC, and this relationship can be correlated with toxicity, as measured by a reduction in platelet count.[134]

Camptothecins

An important group of drugs under active clinical development consists of analogs of camptothecin (Fig. 8-2). Camptothecin was isolated from extracts of the Japanese tree *Camptotheca acuminata* by Wall and colleagues and was shown to be active in experimental leukemia and some solid tumors.[137] As shown in Figure 8-2, the structure of camptothecin has five rings. The fifth, or E, ring can exist in a closed-ring lactone or an open-ring hydroxy acid form. The closed-ring form of camptothecin is highly water insoluble; however, the sodium salt of the open-ring hydroxy acid form is water soluble. In this form, the compound was introduced into early clinical trials in the late 1960s. Phase I trials showed that the compound gave rise to substantial gastrointestinal toxicity and myelosuppression and also had a tendency to produce hemorrhagic cystitis.[138,139] The agent showed antitumor activity in the phase I studies, but a subsequent phase II study in gastrointestinal cancers proved negative,[140] and development of the compound was halted. Work continued in the laboratory on the mode of action of this compound, which proved to be unique.[141–143] The compound combines with a cleavable complex formed between DNA and the enzyme topoisomerase I, an enzyme important in relieving the torsion that develops as the strands of DNA unwind for replication and transcription. The role of topoisomerase I is to cleave one of the strands of the DNA, thus allowing the supercoiled DNA to unwind. The combination of camptothecin-cleavable complex prevents the resealing of the DNA and thus causes single-strand DNA breaks. The identification of this unique mode of antitumor action stimulated the development of analogs of camptothecin that would be more soluble and more active. The closed-ring form of the E ring was shown to be essential for activity, being several orders of magnitude more active than the hydroxy acid form.[144] This phenomenon may account for the variable activity of camptothecin, which, as noted earlier, was given as a sodium salt of the open-ring hydroxy acid form. Several compounds were developed as analogs of camptothecin; to date, the two most important are irinotecan (CPT-11) and topotecan. The structures of these compounds are shown in Figure 8-2.

Irinotecan

Irinotecan is 7 ethyl 10[4-(1 pyridino)-1-pyridino] carbonoxy camptothecin. It is the most extensively evaluated of the newer

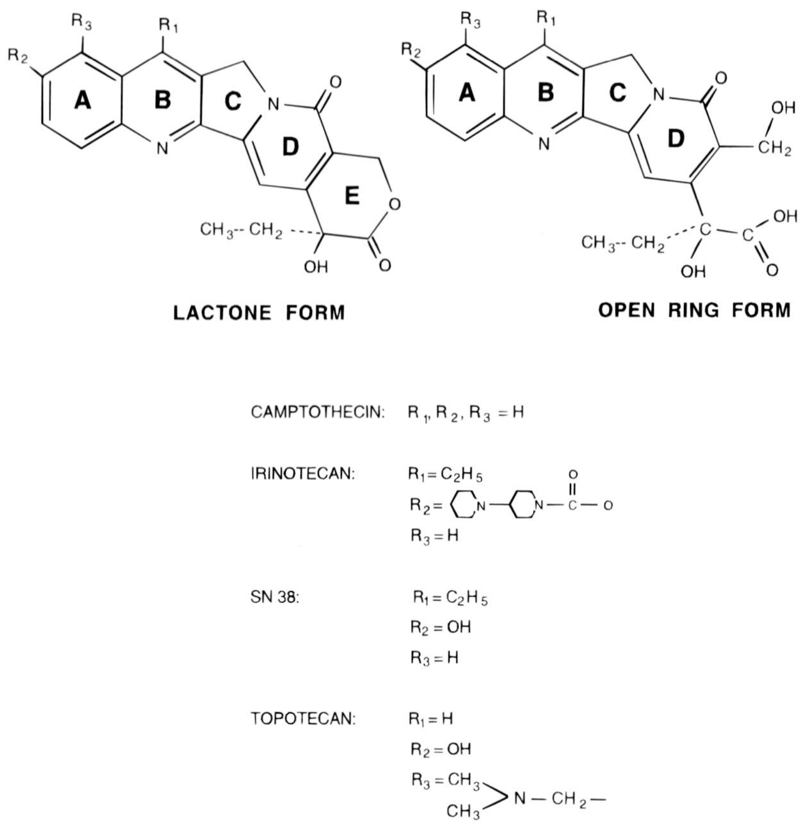

FIG. 8-2. Structure of camptothecins.

camptothecins. In phase I studies, the drug showed major toxicities of leukopenia, nausea, and vomiting and diarrhea.[145] On a weekly schedule, the recommended dose for phase II studies was 100 mg/m^2/wk.[146] When intermittent doses were administered every 3 weeks,[147] the recommended dose was 240 mg/m^2. With intensive treatment of diarrhea with loperamide, dosing up to 750 mg/m^2 every 3 weeks has been reported.[148–149] Other schedules have been reported, including a single dose every 4 weeks, 5-day continuous infusion every 3 to 4 weeks, and daily × three every 3 weeks.[145] CPT-11 is virtually inactive in vitro. To be activated, the agent must be hydrolyzed to 7-ethyl-10-hydroxy camptothecin (SN38), which is three orders of magnitude more active than the parent drug.[150] Consequently, pharmacokinetic studies of the drug require the measurement of the total and the lactone forms of both CPT-11 and SN38. No relationship between nonmyeloid toxicity and any pharmacokinetic parameter was found in the study of Rowinsky and associates.[147] A relationship between AUC of total SN38 and percentage of decrease in absolute neutrophil count (ANC) was found using a sigmoidal E_{max} model. The AUC found to give a 50% decrease in ANC was 51 μM/min. Data on the activity of CPT-11 against genitourinary tumors is scant, but evaluation is ongoing.

Topotecan

Topotecan is a semisynthetic water-soluble camptothecin analog, which, in preclinical systems, is active against experimental tumors and against human xenografts. In early phase I trials, the drug was given daily for 5 days every 3 or 4 weeks.[151,152] On this schedule, the dose-limiting toxicity was neutropenia, and the recommended dose for phase II studies was 1.25 to 1.5 mg/m^2. Subsequent studies have evaluated infusions of from 24 hours up to 21 days.[153,154] With the 24-hour infusion, a dose of 1.5 mg/m^2/wk was recommended for phase II evaluation. Thrombocytopenia was more marked than neutropenia in the 21-day infusion study (maximum tolerated dose [MTD] of 0.53 mg/m^2/d). Granulocyte colony-stimulating factor (G-CSF) did not permit dose intensification in one study because dosing was limited by fatigue and thrombocytopenia.[152]

In pharmacodynamic studies, dose, but not the AUC, of the topotecan lactone was related to mean percentage change in ANC by a sigmoidal E_{max} model. The dose required to produce a 50% decrease in ANC was 0.86 mg/m^2/d, given daily for 5 days.[151]

Taxanes

An important class of drugs that is being extensively evaluated in a broad spectrum of tumor types is the taxanes. The two drugs now under clinical evaluation are paclitaxel and docetaxel. The structures are shown in Figure 8-3. Paclitaxel is extracted from the bark of the western yew tree,[155] and, for several years, this source severely limited the supply of the drug for investigation. The slow development of the drug was compounded by the low water solubility of the drug. These difficulties were overcome, however, because of the interest generated by the high degree of activity of the drug in experimental systems and because the drug was shown to have a unique mode of action.[156–158] Paclitaxel acts on the microtubules, but unlike the vinca alkaloids, which also interact with microtubules, the taxanes stabilize the microtubule. A microtubule is in dynamic equilibrium with the tubulin heterodimers that make up its structure. These heterodimers associate at one end and dissociate at the other. The action of the vinca alkaloids is to prevent the tubulin from binding, and thus, the microtubules undergo spontaneous disassembly. The action of the taxanes is the opposite. The microtubule is stabilized, such that growth continues by association of tubulin but disassembly does not occur. Thus, the

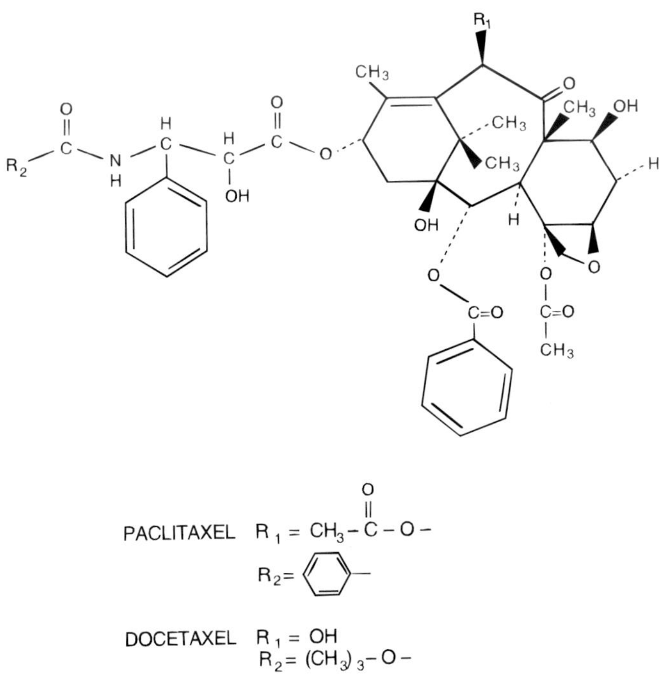

FIG. 8-3. Structures of paclitaxel and docetaxel.

cell becomes filled with a tangle of elongated but functionally useless microtubles. This process leads to cell death.

Paclitaxel has undergone extensive testing,[159] and it is approved for use in ovarian carcinoma. In phase I studies, it was initially given by short infusion. Acute allergic reactions and disturbances of cardiac rhythm, however, led to progressive lengthening of the infusion time to 24 hours, which became the standard for administration of the drug. When given by 24-hour infusion, the MTD was 200 to 275 mg/m^2 given every 3 weeks, and the dose-limiting toxicity was neutropenia, which was often profound but short lived and was seldom fatal.[160] Other toxicities, as noted earlier, included acute cardiac effects (mainly arrhythmias), hypersensitivity reactions, peripheral neuropathy, and gastrointestinal toxicity. In a phase I study in leukemia,[161] in which grade 4 myelosuppression was accepted as routine, mucositis was the dose-limiting toxicity at a dose of 390 mg/m^2. Total alopecia was another feature, and it involved the hair on the head, body hair, and eyelashes. More recently, investigators have recognized that the cardiac arrhythmias (and in particular bradycardia, the most common paclitaxel-related arrhythmia) are clinically inconsequential, and with suitable premedication with steroids and with H_1 and H_2 histamine antagonists, the drug can be safely given by 3-hour infusion. This regimen reduces the myelosuppression without apparently reducing the antitumor effect.[162,163] One-hour infusion of the drug is under evaluation. These developments are important in enabling the drug to be given on an outpatient basis. The pharmacokinetics of paclitaxel were evaluated during the early clinical studies using high-performance liquid chromatography (HPLC) assay for the drug. Both a biphasic and a triphasic plasma decay have been described, with the terminal-phase half-life in the range of approximately 4 to 7 hours for the biphasic plasma decay and in the range of approximately 10 to 50 hours when a γ phase was described.[164] The earlier studies reported linear pharmacokinetics, but more recent reports have indicated nonlinear pharmacokinetics with shorter infusions. Volumes of distribution have been variable in the reported studies and have been generally in the range of 50 to 100 L/m^2; however, large volumes of distribution have been described in the study reported by Huizing and associates.[165] Little of the drug is eliminated unchanged through the kidneys, and systemic clearance appears to result from metabolism, biliary excretion, and binding to tissue components. The main route of metabolism is by cytochrome P450-dependent hydroxylation, the principal hydroxylated metabolite in bile being 6-hydroxy paclitaxel.[166] Cisplatin given first in combination with paclitaxel is more toxic than the reverse sequence. This phenomenon appears to be related to the finding that cisplatin inhibits the metabolism of paclitaxel and causes an increase in the AUC of the latter drug.[167] For the same schedule of administration, the degree of myelosuppression is related to the total drug exposure, as measured by the AUC. That a shorter infusion gives less toxicity for the same AUC than a longer infusion suggests that the duration of exposure to a minimum cytotoxic concentration may be an important factor in the toxicity of the drug.[168] Paclitaxel has shown antitumor activity in early studies of germ cell tumors and transitional cell carcinoma of the urothelium. Patients with germ cell tumors, with previous therapy, showed a 24% response rate to paclitaxel, 250 mg/m^2 24-hour infusion with 2 complete remissions and 4 partial remissions in 25 patients.[169] Previously untreated patients with transitional cell carcinoma of the urothelium received the same dose and schedule of paclitaxel and showed a 42% response rate, with 7 of 26 complete remissions and 4 of 26 partial remissions.[170] Early studies in prostate carcinoma and renal cell carcinoma have so far been negative.[171,172]

Docetaxel (Taxotere) is a synthetic analog of paclitaxel that is prepared from 10-diacetyl baccatin III, a compound extracted from the needles of the European yew tree, *Taxus baccata*. It is thus derived from a biologically renewable source. Docetaxel is more potent in vitro than paclitaxel.[173] Although its mode of action is similar to that of paclitaxel, docetaxel is reportedly active against cells resistant to paclitaxel.[173] It has undergone phase I testing in 1-, 2-, 6-, and 24-hour infusions[174–176] and as a 1-hour infusion daily for 5 days.[177] The MTD ranged from 70 to 115 mg/m^2, and neutropenia was dose limiting in all the studies, although mucositis was also a major toxicity in the study of the 24-hour infusion.[176] Investigators have suggested that anaphylactic reactions are less common with docetaxel than with paclitaxel, but skin toxicity may be more marked. Plasma decay is triphasic, with a $t\frac{1}{2}\gamma$ of 11.8 ± 6.7 hours.[175] The potential of docetaxel in the treatment of urologic cancer has not yet been defined.

Antimetabolites

In general, the purine and pyrimidine antimetabolites have been relatively ineffective against solid tumors and have been largely used in the treatment of hematologic cancers. The exceptions are the fluorinated pyrimidines, which have been used against gastrointestinal cancers and breast carcinoma and have shown some activity in bladder cancer, especially nontransitional cell carcinoma. A newer pyrimidine antimetabolite, 2′deoxy-2′difluoro-cytidine (gemcitabine), however, has been introduced into clinical trial and in preclinical systems has shown significant activity against experimental solid tumors[178] and human tumor xenografts.[179] Its structure is shown in Figure 8-4. Like cytosine arabinoside, an antimetabolite that it resembles structurally, gemcitabine is activated intracellularly to the triphosphate, and in this form is incorporated into DNA.[180–182] The level of active metabolites achieved within the cell is much higher with gemcitabine than with cytosine arabinoside, however. Moreover, the active metabolite is more resistant to breakdown within the cell. In the initial phase I clinical trial, the drug was given over a 30-minute infusion weekly for 3 weeks every 4 weeks. The MTD was 790 mg/m^2, with myelosuppression predominantly thrombocytopenia and anemia being the dose-limiting toxicities.[183] Other toxicities have been relatively mild. Subsequent studies have shown that higher doses can be given safely, however, particularly to patients who have undergone little or no previous therapy. In patients with non–small cell lung cancer and no previous therapy, Richards and associates explored doses up to 2200 mg/m^2/week and reported an MTD of 1500 mg/m^2/wk on the same schedule.[184] Brown and associates found that 2500 mg/m^2 given over 4 hours every 2 weeks was below the MTD.[185] Initial pharmacokinetic studies showed a rapid elimination of the drug with a median half-life of 8 minutes. The drug was rapidly converted to the corresponding uracil metabolite difluoro deoxyuridine, which had a longer half-life, with a median of 14 hours. The active metabolite difluoro deoxycytidine triphosphate was analyzed in circulating mononuclear

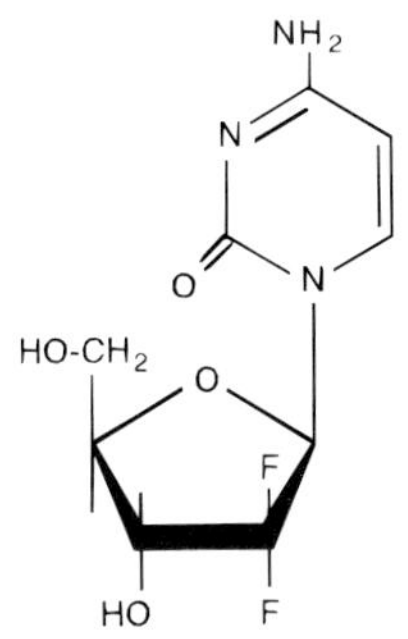

GEMCITABINE

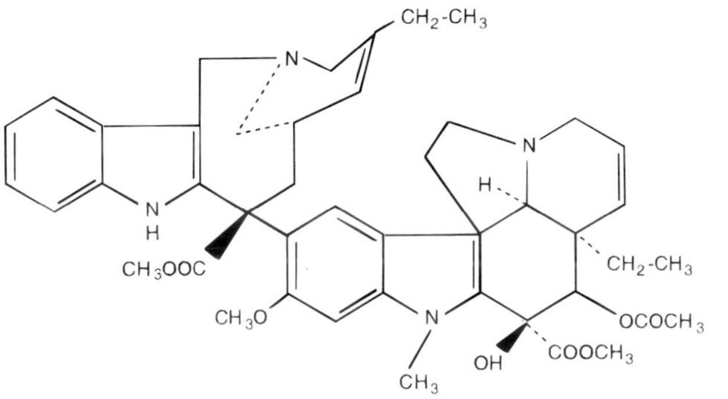

VINORELBINE

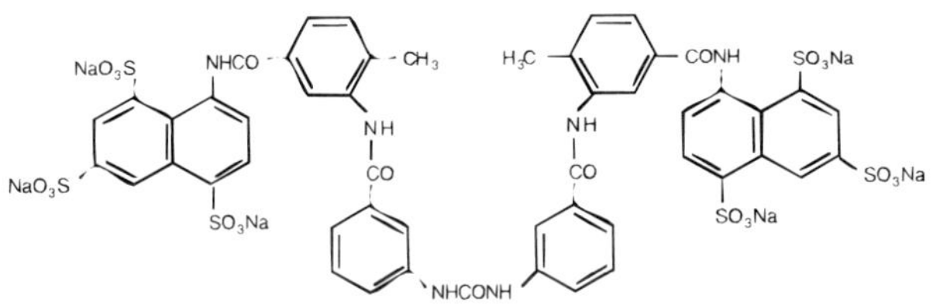

SURAMIN SODIUM

FIG. 8-4. Miscellaneous compounds.

cells. A peak was observed within 30 minutes of the end of the infusion and increased with dose up to a dose of 350 mg/m^2. Beyond this dose, there was no increase in the active metabolite, indicating saturation of the activation to the triphosphate.[180]

Antitumor activity against bladder cancer was noted in the phase I study by Pollera and colleagues in 14 patients receiving gemcitabine at doses higher than 875 mg/m^2; these investigators observed 1 complete remission and 2 partial remissions.[186] We have demonstrated a response rate of 40% in an ongoing phase II trial in previously untreated patients with bladder cancer.[187] Weisbach and associates noted 1 complete remission and 2 partial remissions in 30 evaluable patients in a phase II study of gemcitabine in renal cell carcinoma.[188] This represented a low response rate of only 10%, but 2 of the responses were durable, the complete remission lasting more than 12 months, and 1 of the partial remissions 15 months.[188] Phase II studies in prostate cancer are ongoing, and the results are not yet available.

Vinorelbine

As noted earlier, the vinca alkaloids have substantial clinical activity against urologic cancers, in particular, germ cell tumors and urothelial cancers. For this reason, the development of new vinca alkaloids with a higher degree of experimental antitumor activity is of interest. The most promising new agent in this class is vinorelbine (Navelbine), which has been under investigation in Europe and has been introduced into the United States. The compound is 5′-noranhydrovinblastine. Although it shares the mode of action of the other vinca alkaloids, discussed earlier, in experimental systems it has less affinity for axonal microtubules, compared with its affinity for the microtubules of the mitotic spindle. This characteristic indicates the possibility that it may interrupt mitosis at concentrations that would not give rise to neurotoxicity.[189] This agent has also shown a higher degree of activity than vincristine or vinblastine against some experimental tumors.[190,191]. In phase I testing, neutropenia was the dose-limiting toxicity, and the MTD was 35 mg/m^2/wk. It did give rise to peripheral neuropathy at higher doses, but this side effect was mild.[192] An initial study of the pharmacokinetics by Bore and associates,[193] using tritiated vinorelbine and also a radioimmunoassay, showed a low urinary excretion based on elimination. The primary excretion route was the feces, with 34% to 58.4% of the total dose being excreted by this route over 21 days.[193] More recently, Rowinsky and associates published the results of a bioavailability study in which the drug was given intravenously and orally to the same patients.[194] Bioavailability was $27 \pm 14\%$. The volume of distribution was large, 20.02 ± 8.55 L/kg, and the terminal-phase half-life was 18 hours. Plasma decay was triphasic.[194] Data on the activity of this drug in urologic cancers are not yet available.

Suramin

Suramin is a polysulfonated naphthylurea that has been in use for treatment of sleeping sickness, onchocerciasis, and filariasis. The compound has certain biochemical activities, which include inhibition of lysosomal enzymes leading to accumulation of glycosaminoglycan and proteoglycan, and it has a broad spectrum of activity in inhibiting growth factors. [195–199] These include fibroblast growth factor, epidermal growth factor, insulin-like growth factor, platelet-derived growth factor, and transforming growth factor. The compound is also active against viral reverse transcriptase and has been evaluated as a possible treatment for acquired immunodeficiency syndrome (AIDS).[200] Although the agent is active against many different experimental tumors in vitro,[201] its specific mode of antitumor activity is still undefined. Because its toxicity includes damage to the adrenal cortex, suramin was originally evaluated as a treatment for adrenocortical carcinoma.[202,203] Most of the clinical investigations to date have focused on its potential as a chemotherapeutic agent against prostatic carcinoma, however. Toxicity in early trials has included myelosuppression, renal and hepatic toxicity, hyperglycemia, bleeding disorders, adrenal insufficiency, and malaise.[203,204] The most important toxicity of this agent, however, appears to be a peripheral neuropathy often producing proximal muscle weakness that can progress to severe disability. Early reports suggested that the neurotoxicity was related to plasma concentrations greater than 300 μg/mL, and evidence indicated that antitumor activity required a sustained plasma concentration of 150 to 200 μg/mL.[203,205] These observations, with the combination of a narrow therapeutic range and a long half-life (40 to 50 days),[206] have led to intensive investigation of methods to monitor and predict plasma concentrations of the drug.

In one study,[207] a two- and a three-compartment open model were explored for monitoring of data from patients treated with suramin. The three-compartment open linear model was found best to fit the data. Patients received a 2-hour intravenous infusion of suramin on days 1 to 5. Subsequently, dose and dosage interval were adapted to individual patient pharmacokinetics. This so-called adaptive control with feedback strategy using a Bayesian algorithm to estimate patient pharmacokinetic parameters with a limited number of plasma samples[208,209] maintained plasma concentrations within the target range for 85% or more of the treatment duration. Toxicity was frequent in the group treated to a target plasma concentration of 200 to 300 μg/mL. Results in prostate cancer indicate that the higher plasma levels may not be necessary to achieve antitumor effect, however.[210,211] With these approaches, the compound appears active in prostate carcinoma.[204,209–212] Because of sophisticated monitoring, based on serial measurement of blood levels of prostate-specific antigen, however, investigators have suggested that the apparently high level of activity is an artifact of stage shift, and thus, suramin is likely to remain an investigational drug for some time.

CONCLUSIONS

No consensus exists on the optimal strategy for the clinical use of chemotherapy against cancers of the genitourinary tract. The most common approach has been to use combination regimens in preference to single agents, predicated largely on the success of combination chemotherapy for various other solid tumors. The introduction of the combination of cisplatin, vinblastine, and bleomycin (see Chaps. 66 through 69) revolutionized the management of advanced germ cell tumors, providing a cure rate of at least 70%, compared with a cure rate of less than 40% with single-agent treatment. Similarly, after several years of clinical development of combination regimens for bladder cancer, a seminal randomized trial revealed a survival benefit from the combination of methotrexate, vinblastine, doxorubicin, and cisplatin compared with cisplatin alone in this context (see Chap. 28).

By contrast, randomized trials have not proved a role for combination chemotherapy in renal carcinoma or for advanced adenocarcinoma of the prostate, and clinical practice in these areas is still in an early stage of evolution. In addition to the need for new treatment strategies, careful definition of end points and appropriate design of clinical trials are essential if outcomes are to improve.

REFERENCES

1. Burchenal JG. The historical development of cancer chemotherapy. Semin Oncol 1977;4:135.
2. Steel GG. Growth kinetics of tumours. Oxford, Oxford University Press, 1977:1, 185.
3. Shackney SE, McCormack GW, Cochural GJ. Growth rate patterns of solid tumors and their relation to responsiveness to therapy. Ann Intern Med 1978;89:107.
4. Baserga R. Principles of molecular cell biology of cancer: the cell cycle. In: DeVita VT Jr, Hellman S, Rosenberg SA, eds. Cancer: principles and practice of oncology, 4th ed. Philadelphia: JB Lippincott, 1993:60.
5. Lee M, Nurse P. Cell cycle control genes in fission yeast and mammalian cells. Trends Genet 1988;4:287.
6. Hartwell LH, Weinert TA. Checkpoints: controls that ensure the order of cell cycle events. Science 1989;246:629.
7. Brown JL, Russell PJ, Philips J, Wotherspoon J, Raghavan D. Clonal analysis of a bladder cancer cell line: an experimental model of tumour heterogeneity. Br J Cancer 1990;61:369.
8. Raghavan D, Cox K, Pearson B, et al. Oral cyclophosphamide for the management of hormone refractory prostate cancer. Br J Urol 1993; 72:625.
9. Beckley S, Wajsman Z, Slack N, et al. The chemotherapy of prostatic carcinoma. Scand J Urol Nephrol Suppl 1980;55:151.
10. Raghavan D, Tannock IF. Clinical trials in genitourinary oncology: what have they achieved? In: Smith PH, Chisholm GD, eds. Combination therapy in urological malignancy. London: 1989:226.
11. Powis G. Effect of human renal and hepatic disease on the pharmacokinetics of anticancer drugs. Cancer Treat Rev 1982;9:85.
12. Prescott LF. Gastrointestinal absorption of drugs. Med Clin North Am 1974;58:907.
13. Cadwallander DE. Biopharmaceutics and drug interactions. Nutley, NJ, Hoffman-LaRoche, 1971.
14. Wagner JG. Effect of normal and pathologic physiology on pharmacokinetics. In: Wagner JG, ed. Fundamentals of clinical pharmacokinetics. Chicago: Drug Intelligence, 1975:359.
15. Rodvold KA, Rushing DA, Tewksbury DA. Doxorubicin clearance in the obese. J Clin Oncol 1988;6:1321.
16. Robert J, Hoerni B. Age dependence of the early phase pharmacokinetics of doxorubicin. Cancer Res 1983;43:4467.
17. Testa B, Jenner P. Induction and inhibition of drug-metabolizing enzyme systems. In: Swarbrick J, ed. Drugs and the pharmaceutical sciences, vol 4. New York: Marcel Dekker, 1976:329.
18. Tardiff RG, Dubois KP. Inhibition of hepatic microsomal enzymes by alkylating agents. Arch Int Pharmacodyn Ther 1969;177:445.
19. Drayer DE. Pathways of drug metabolism in man. Med Clin North Am 1974;58:927.
20. Liegler DG, Henderson ES, Hahn MA, et al. The effect of organic acids on renal clearance of methotrexate in man. Clin Pharmacol Ther 1969;10:849.
21. Milne MD. Influence of acid base balance on efficacy and toxicity of drugs. Proc R Soc Med 1965;58:961.
22. Juranka PF, Zastawny RL, Ling V. P-glycoprotein: multidrug resistance and a superfamily of membrane-associated transport proteins. FASEB J 1989;3:2583.
23. Goldstein LJ, Galski H, Fojo A, et al. Expression of a multidrug resistance gene in human cancers. J Natl Cancer Inst 1989;81:116.
24. Sugawara I. Expression and functions of P-glycoprotein (mdr-1) in normal and malignant tissues. Acta Pathol Jpn 1990;40:545.
25. Shinohara N, Liebert M, Wedemeyer G, Chang JHC, Grossman HB. Evaluation of multiple drug resistance in human bladder cancer cell lines. J Urol 1993;150:505.
26. Petrylak DP, Scher HI, Reuter V, et al. P-glycoprotein (PGP) expression in invasive and metastatic urothelial tract cancer (UTC). Proc Am Soc Clin Oncol 1992;11:200.
27. Barrand MA, Heppell-Parton AC, Wright KA, Rabbitts PH, Twentyman PR. A 190-kilodalton protein overexpressed in non-p-glycoprotein-containing multidrug-resistant cells and its relationship to the MRP gene. J Natl Cancer Inst 1994;86:110.
28. Dalton WS, Grogan TM, Meltzer PS, et al. Drug resistance in mutiple myeloma and non-Hodgkins lymphoma: detection of P-glycoprotein and potential circumvention by addition of verapamil to chemotherapy. J Clin Oncol 1989;7:415.
29. Palavidis Z. Mechanisms of drug resistance in bladder cancer: the role of P-glycoprotein. Thesis for Master of Science in Medicine, University of New South Wales, Sydney, 1993.
30. Timmer-Bosscha H, Mulder NH, de Vries EGE. Modulation of cis-diamminedichloroplatinum (II) resistance: a review. Br J Cancer 1992; 66:227.
31. Hospers GAP, Mulder NH, DeJong B, et al. Characterization of a human small cell lung carcinoma cell line with acquired resistance to cis-diamminedichloroplatinum (II) in vitro. Cancer Res 1988;48: 6803.
32. Liebmann JE, Hahn SM, Cook JA, Lipschutz C, Mitchell JB, Kaufman

DC. Glutathione depletion by l-buthionine sulfoximine antagonizes Taxol cytotoxicity. Cancer Res 1993;53:2066.
33. Pendyala L, Glaves D, Russell PJ, Ciesielski M, Creaven PJ, Raghavan D. Glutathioine (GSH) in human bladder carcinoma cell lines. Proc Am Assoc Cancer Res 1994;35:376.
34. Christen RD, Hom DK, Porter DC, et al. Epidermal growth factor regulates the in vitro sensitivity of human ovarian carcinoma cells to cisplatin. J Clin Invest 1990;86:1632.
35. Fan Z, Masui H, Altas I, Mendelsohn J. Blockade of epidermal growth factor receptor function by bivalent and monovalent fragments of 225 anti-epidermal growth factor receptor monoclonal antibodies. Cancer Res 1993;53:4322.
36. Fan Z, Baselga J, Masui H, Mendelsohn J. Antitumor effect of anti-epidermal growth factor receptor monoclonal antibodies plus cis-diamminedichloroplatinum on well established A-431 cell xenografts. Cancer Res 1993;53:4637.
37. Fritsche M, Haessler C, Brandner G. Induction of nuclear accumulation of the tumor-suppressor protein p53 by DNA-damaging agents. Oncogene 1993;8:307.
38. Lowe SW, Ruley HE, Jacks T, Housman DE. p53-Dependent apoptosis modulates the cytotoxicity of anticancer agents. Cell 1993; 74:957.
39. Glaves D, Hitt S, Raghavan D. Apoptosis is not the mechanism of cisplatin-induced cell death in bladder cancer cell lines. Submitted for publication.
40. Goldie JH, Coldman AJ. A mathematic model for relating the drug sensitivity of tumors to the spontaneous mutation rate. Cancer Treat Rep 1979;63:1727.
41. Day RS. Treatment sequencing asymmetry and uncertainty: protocol strategies for combination chemotherapy. Cancer Res 1986;46:3876.
42. Schwartz D, Lelouch J. Explanatory and pragmatic attitudes in theraeputic trials. J Chronic Dis 1967;20:637.
43. Daugherty C, Ratain MJ, Grochowski E, et al. Perceptions of cancer patients and their physicians involved in phase I trials. J Clin Oncol 1995;13:1062.
44. Ratain MJ, Mick R, Schilsky RL, et al. Statistical and ethical issues in the design and conduct of phase I and II clinical trials of new anticancer agents. J Natl Cancer Inst 1993;85:1637.
45. Creaven PJ, Mihich E. The clinical toxicity of anticancer drugs and its prediction. Semin Oncol 1977;4:147.
46. Staquet M, Sylvester R. A decision theory approach to phase II clinical trials. Biomedicine 1977;26:262.
47. Lee YJ, Staquet M, Simon R, Catane R, Muggia F. Two-stage plans for patient accrual in phase II cancer clinical trials. Cancer Treat Rep 1979;63:1721.
48. Simon RF. Design and conduct of clinical trials. In: DeVita VT Jr, Hellman S, Rosenberg SA, eds. Cancer: principles and practice of oncology. Philadelphia: JB Lippincott, 1993:418.
49. Rosenberg B, Van Camp L, Trosko JE, Monsour VH. Platinum compounds: a new class of potent antitumor agents. Nature 1969;222:385.
50. DeConti RC, Toftness BR, Lange RC, Creasy WA. Clinical and pharmacological studies with cis-diamminedichloroplatinum (II). Cancer Res 1973;33:1310.
51. Gormley PE, Bull JM, LeRoy AF, Cysyk R. Kinetics of cis-dichlorodiammineplatinum. Clin Pharmacol Ther 1979;25:351.
52. Patton TF, Repta AJ, Sternson LA. Clinical pharmacology of cisplatin. In: Ames MM, Powis G, Kovach JS, eds. Pharmacokinetics of anticancer agents in humans. Amsterdam: Elsevier, 1983:155.
53. Safirstein R, Winston J, Goldstein M, et al. Cisplatin nephrotoxicity. Am J Kidney Dis 1986;8:356.
54. Boyer MJ, Raghavan D, Harris PJ, et al. Lack of late toxicity in patients treated with cisplatin containing combination chemotherapy for metastatic testicular cancer. J Clin Oncol 1990;8:27.
55. Boyer MJ, Raghavan D. Toxicity of treatment of germ cell tumors. Semin Oncol 1992;19:128.
56. Barranco SC, Humphrey RM. The effects of bleomycin on survival and cell progression in Chinese hamster cells in vitro. Cancer Res 1971;31:1218.
57. Barlogie B, Drewinko B, Schumann J, et al. Pulse cytophotometric analysis of cell cycle perturbation with bleomycin in vitro. Cancer Res 1976;36:1182.
58. Lazo JS, Boland CJ, Schwartz PE. Bleomycin hydrolase activity and cytotoxicity in human tumors. Cancer Res 1982;42:4026.
59. Alberts DS, Chen HSG, Liu R, et al. Bleomycin pharmacokinetics in man I Intravenous administration. Cancer Chemother Pharmacol 1978;1:177.
60. Levi J, Raghavan D, Harvey V, et al. The importance of bleomycin in combination chemotherapy for good prognosis germ cell carcinoma. J Clin Oncol 1993;11:1300.
61. Loehrer PJ, Johnson D, Elson P, Einhorn LH, Trump DL. Importance of bleomycin in favorable-prognosis disseminated germ cell tumors: an Eastern Cooperative Oncology Group Trial. J Clin Oncol 1995; 13:470.
62. Crooke ST, Bradner WT: Mitomycin C: a review. Cancer Treat Rep 1976;3:121.
63. Dustre L, Covey JM, Collins C, et al. DNA damage cytotoxicity and free radical formation by mitomycin C in human cells. Chem Biol Interact 1989;71:63.
64. Van Hazel GA, Scott M, Rubin J, et al. Pharmacokinetics of mitomycin C in patients receiving the drug alone or in combination. Cancer Treat Rep 1983;67:805.
65. Hanna WT, Krauss S, Regester RF, et al. Renal disease after mitomycin C therapy. Cancer 1981;48:2583.
66. Valavaara R, Nordman E. Renal complications of mitomycin C therapy with special reference to the total dose. Cancer 1985;55:47.
67. Chang AY, Kuebler JP, Pandya KJ, et al. Pulmonary toxicity induced by mitomycin C is highly responsive to glucocorticoids. Cancer 1986; 57:2285.
68. Chabner BA, Myers CE. Antitumor antibiotics. In: DeVita VT Jr, Hellman S, Rosenberg SA, eds. Cancer: principles and practice of oncology, 4th ed. Philadelphia: JB Lippincott, 1993:376.
69. Benjamin RS. Pharmacokinetics of Adriamycin in patients with sarcomas. Cancer Chemother Rep 1974;58:271.
70. Riggs CE Jr, Benjamin RS, Serpick AA, et al. Biliary disposition of Adriamycin. Clin Pharmacol Ther 1977;22:234.
71. Chan KK, Chlebowski RT, Tong M, et al. Clinical pharmacokinetics of Adriamycin in hepatoma patients with cirrhosis. Cancer Res 1980; 40:1263.
72. Von Hoff DD, Layard MW, Basa P, et al. Risk factors for doxorubicin-induced congestive heart failure. Ann Intern Med 1979;91:710.
73. Greco FA, Brereton HD, Kent H, et al. Adriamycin and enhanced radiation reaction in normal esophagus and skin. Ann Intern Med 1976;85:294.
74. Nelson RL. The comparative clinical pharmacology and pharmacokinetics of vindesine, vincristine and vinblastine in human patients with cancer. Med Pediatr Oncol 1982;10:115.
75. Owellen RJ, Harike CA, Hains FO. Pharmacokinetics and metabolism of vinblastine in humans. Cancer Res 1977;37:2597.
76. Jackson DV, Castle MC, Bender RA. Biliary excretion of vincristine. Clin Pharmacol Ther 1978;24:101.
77. Colvin M. A review of the pharmacology and clinical use of cyclophosphamide. In: Pinedo HM, ed. Clinical pharmacology of antineoplastic drugs. Amsterdam: Elsevier-North Holland, 1978:245.
78. Connors TA, Cox PJ, Farmer PB, et al. Some studies of the active metabolites formed in the microsomal metabolism of cyclophosphamide and isophosphamide. Biochem Pharmacol 1974;23:115.
79. Dorr RT Soble MJ Alberts DES. Interaction of cimetidine but not ranitidine with cyclophosphamide in mice. Cancer Res 1986;46:1795.
80. Newlands ES, Begent RHJ, Rustin GJS, Parker D, Bagshawe KD. Further advances in the management of malignant teratomas of the testis and other sites. Lancet 1983;1:948.
81. Motzer RJ, Bajorin DF, Bosl GJ. ''Poor risk'' germ cell tumors: current progress and future directions. Semin Oncol 1992;19:206.
82. Carney T, Margison JM, Thatcher N, et al. Bioavailability of ifosfamide in patients with bronchial carcinoma. Cancer Chemother Pharmacol 1986;18:261.
83. Creaven PJ, Allen LM, Alford DA, Cohen MH. Clinical pharmacology of isophosphamide. Clin Pharmacol Ther 1974;16:77.
84. Creaven PJ, Allen LM, Cohen MH, Nelson RL. Studies on the clinical pharmacology and toxicology of isophosphamide (NSC-109724). Cancer Treat Rep 1976;60:445.
85. Anderson NR, Tandon DS. Ifosfamide extrapyramidal neurotoxicity. Cancer 1991;58:72.
86. Cohen NA, Egorin MJ, Snyder SW, et al. Interaction of N,N′,N″-triethylenethiophosphoramide and NN′N″-triethylenephosphoramide with cellular DNA. Cancer Res 1991;51:4360.
87. Cohen BE, Egorin MJ, Kohlhepp EA, Aisner J, Gutierrez PL. Human

plasma pharmacokinetics and urinary excretion of thiotepa and its metabolites. Cancer Treat Rep 1986;70:859.
88. Wolff SN, Herzig RH, Fay JW, et al. High-dose NN'N"-triethylenethiophosphoramide (thiotepa) with autologous bone marrow transplantation phase I studies. Semin Oncol 1990;17:2.
89. Vogelzang NJ, Raghavan D, Kennedy BJ. VP-16-213 (etoposide): the mandrake root from Issyk-kul. Am J Med 1982;72:136.
90. Creaven PJ. The clinical pharmacology of VM-26 and VP-16-213: a brief overview. Cancer Chemother Pharmacol 1982;7:133.
91. Clarke P, Slevin M. The clinical pharmacology of etoposide and teniposide. Clin Pharm 1987;12:223.
92. Krishan A, Paika K, Frei E III. Cytofluorometric studies on the action of podophyllotoxins and epipodophyllotoxins (VM-26 and VP-16-213) on the cell cycle traverse of human lymphoblasts. J Cell Biol 1975;66:521.
93. Yang L, Rowe TC, Liu LF. Identification of DNA topoisomerase II as an intracellular target of antitumor epipodophyllotoxins in simian virus 40-infected monkey cells. Cancer Res 1985;45:5872.
94. Jolivet J, Schilsky RL, Bailey BD, et al. Synthesis retention and biological activity of methotrexate polyglutamates in cultured human breast cancer cells. J Clin Invest 1982;70:351.
95. Chu E, Drake JC, Boarman D, et al. Mechanism of thymidylate synthase inhibition by methotrexate in human neoplastic cell lines and normal human myeloid progenitor cells. J Biol Chem 1990;256:8470.
96. Borchers AH, Kennedy DA, Straw JA. Inhibition of DNA excision repair by methotrexate in Chinese hamster ovary cells following exposure to ultra-violet irradiation or ethyl-methanesulfonate. Cancer Res 1990;50:1786.
97. Allegra JC. Antifolates. In: Chabner BA, Collins JM, eds. Cancer chemotherapy: principles and practice. Philadelphia: JB Lippincott, 1990:110.
98. Huffman DH, Wan SH, Azarnoff DL, et al. Pharmacokinetics of methotrexate. Clin Pharmacol Ther 1973;14:572.
99. Stoller RG, Kaplan HG, Cummings FJ, et al. A clinical and pharmacological study of high dose methotrexate with minimal leucovorin rescue. Cancer Res 1979;39:908.
100. Heidelberger C, Chaudhuri NK, Dannenberg P, et al. Fluorinated pyrimidines: a new class of tumor inhibitory compounds. Nature 1957; 179:663.
101. Diasio RB, Harris BE. Clinical pharmacology of 5-fluorouracil. Clin Pharmacokinet 1989;16:215.
102. Bruckner HW, Creasy WA. The administration of 5-fluorouracil by mouth. Cancer 1974;33:14.
103. Cano JP, Rigault JP, Aubert C, Carcassonne Y, Seitz JF. Determination of 5-fluorouracil in plasma by GC/MS using an internal standard: application to pharmacokinetics. Bull Cancer 1979;66:67.
104. Pinedo HM, Peters GF. Fluorouracil: biochemistry and pharmacology. J Clin Oncol 1988;6:1653.
105. Myers CE, Young RC, Chabner BA. Biochemical determinants of 5-fluorouracil response in vivo: the role of deoxyuridylate pool expansion. J Clin Invest 1975;56:1231.
106. Creaven PJ, Rustum YM, Petrelli NJ, et al. Phase I and pharmacokinetic evaluation of floxuridine/leucovorin given on the Roswell Park weekly regimen. Cancer Chemother Pharmacol 1994;34:261.
107. Meropol NJ, Creaven PJ, Petrelli NJ. Metastatic colorectal cancer: advances in biochemical modulation and new drug development. Semin Oncol 1995;22:1.
108. Petrelli N, Herrera L, Rustum Y, et al. A prospective randomized trial of 5-fluorouracil and methotrexate in previously untreated patients with advanced colorectal carcinoma. J Clin Oncol 1987 5:1559.
109. Evans RM, Laskin JD, Hakala MT. Effect of excess folates and deoxyinosine on the activity and site of action of 5-fluorouracil. Cancer Res 1981;41:3288.
110. Khor SP, Lucas S, Schilsky R, et al. A phase I/pharmacokinetic study of 5-ethynyluracil plus 5-fluorouracil in cancer patients with solid tumors. Proc Am Assoc Cancer Res 1995;36:241.
111. Keefe DL, Roistacher N, Pierri MK. Clinical cardiotoxicity of 5-fluorouracil. J Clin Pharmacol 1993;33:1060.
112. Kelsen DP, Scher H, Alcock N, et al. Phase I clinical trial and pharmacokinetics of 4'-carboxyphthalato-(1,2-diaminocyclohexane) platinum (II). Cancer Res 1982;42:4831.
113. Anderson WK, Quagliato DA, Haugwitz RD, Narayanan VL, Wolpert-DeFilippes MK. Synthesis, physical properties, antitumor activity of tetraplatin and related tetrachloroplatinum (IV) stereoisomers of 1,2-diaminocyclohexane. Cancer Treat Rep 1986;70:997.
114. Rahman A, Roh JK, Wolpert-DeFilippes MK, Goldin A, Venditti JM, Woolley PV. Therapeutic and pharmacological studies of tetrachloro(d,l-trans)1,2-diaminocyclohexane platinum (IV) (tetraplatin), a new platinum analogue. Cancer Res 1988;48:1745.
115. Chaney SG, Wyrick S, Till GK. In vitro biotransformations of tetrachloro (d,l-trans)-1,2-diaminocyclohexaneplatinum (IV) (tetraplatin) in rat plasma. Cancer Res 1990;50:4539.
116. Schilder RJ, LaCreta FP, Perez RP, et al. Phase I and pharmacokinetic study of ormaplatin (tetraplatin NSC 363812) administered on a day 1 and day 8 schedule. Cancer Res 1994;54:709.
117. Kidani Y, Noji M, Tashiro T. Antitumor activity of platinum (II) complexes of 1,2-diamino-cyclohexane isomers. Jpn J Cancer Res 1980;71:637.
118. Pendyala L, Creaven PJ. In vitro cytotoxicity protein binding red blood cell partitioning and biotransformation of oxaliplatin. Cancer Res 1993;53:5970.
119. Brienza S, Fandi A, Hugret F, et al. Neurotoxicity (NTX) of long term oxaliplatin (L-OHP) therapy. Proc Am Assoc Cancer Res 1990; 25:299.
120. Extra JM, Espie M, Calvo F, Ferme C, Mignot L, Marty M. Phase I study of oxaliplatin in patients with advanced cancer. Cancer Chemother Pharmacol 1990;25:299.
121. Creaven PJ, Madajewicz S, Pendyala L, et al. Phase I clinical trial of cis-dichloro-trans-dihydroxy-bis-isopropylamine platinum (IV) (CHIP). Cancer Treat Rep 1983;67:795.
122. Bramwell VHC, Crowther D, O'Malley S, et al. Activity of JM9 in advanced ovarian cancer: a phase I-II trial. Cancer Treatment Rep 1985;69:409.
123. Madajewicz S, Takita H, Creaven PJ, Bareniewski H, Regal A-M, Cushman K. Phase II study of iproplatin (IPP) in small cell carcinoma of the lung (SCCL). Proc Am Soc Clin Oncol 1984;3:224.
124. Creaven PJ, Pendyala L, Madajewicz S. Clinical development of iproplatin (CHIP). Drugs Exp Clin Res 1986;12:287.
125. Pendyala L, Cowens JW, Chheda GB, Dutta SP, Creaven PJ. Identification of cis-dichloro-bis-isopropylamine platinum (II) as a major metabolite of iproplatin in humans. Cancer Res 1988;48:3533.
126. Pendyala L, Arakali AV, Sansone P, Cowens JW, Creaven PJ. DNA binding of iproplatin and its divalent metabolite cis-dichloro-bis-isopropylamine platinum (II). Cancer Chemother Pharmacol 1990;27: 248.
127. de Witt R, Tesselaar M, Kok TC, et al. Randomised phase II trial of carboplatin and iproplatin in advanced urothelial cancer. Eur J Cancer 1991;1383.
128. Clavel M, Monfardini S, Gundersen S, et al. Phase II study of iproplatin (CHIP JM-9) in advanced testicular cancers progressing after prior chemotherapy. Eur J Cancer Clin Oncol 1988;24:1345.
129. Kelland LR, Abel G, McKeage MJ, et al. Preclinical antitumor evaluation of bis-aceto-ammine-dichloro-cyclohexylamine platinum (IV): an orally active platinum drug. Cancer Res 1993;53:2581.
130. McKeage MJ, Raynaud F, Ward J, et al. Phase I and pharmacokinetic study of an orally administered platinum (PT) complex (JM216) using a daily × 5 administration schedule. Proc Am Soc Clin Oncol 1994; 13:136.
131. Gaver RC, Deeb G. High-performance liquid chromatographic procedures for the analysis of carboplatin in human plasma and urine. Cancer Chemother Pharmacol 1986;16:201.
132. Pendyala L, Cowens JW, Creaven PJ. Studies on the pharmacokinetics and metabolism of cis-dichloro-trans-dihydroxy-bis-isopropylamine platinum (IV) in the dog. Cancer Treat Rep 1982;66:509.
133. Pendyala L, Greco W, Cowens JW, Madajewicz S, Creaven PJ. Pharmacokinetics of cis-dichloro-trans-dihydroxy-bis-isopropylamine platinum IV (CHIP) in patients with advanced cancer. Cancer Chemother Pharmacol 1983;11:23.
134. Pendyala L, Madajewicz S, Creaven PJ. Effect of renal function impairment on iproplatin pharmacokinetics and relation to toxicity. Cancer Res 1985;45:5936.
135. Egorin MJ, van Echo DA, Tipping SJ, et al. Pharmacokinetics and dosage reduction of cis-diammine (11-cyclobutane-dicarboxylato) platinum in patients with impaired renal function. Cancer Res 1984; 44:5432.
136. Calvert AH, Newell DR, Gumbrell LA, et al. Carboplatin dosage:

prospective evaluation of a simple formula based on renal function. J Clin Oncol 1989;7:1748.
137. Wall ME, Wani MC, Cook CE, Palmer KH, McPhail AT, Sim GA. Plant antitumor agents. 1. The isolation and structure of camptothecin a novel alkaloidal leukemia and tumor inhibitor from *Camptotheca acuminata*. J Am Chem Soc 1966;83:3888.
138. Gottlieb JA, Guarino AM, Call JB, Oliverio VT, Block JB. Preliminary pharmacologic and clinical evaluation of camptothecin sodium (NSC-100880). Cancer Chemother Rep 1970;54:461.
139. Muggia FM, Creaven PJ, Hansen HH, Cohen MH, Selawry OS. Phase I clinical trial of weekly and daily oral treatment with camptothecin sodium (NSC 100880): correlation with preclinical studies. Cancer Chemother Rep 1972;56:515.
140. Moertel CG, Schutt AJ, Reitemeier RJ, Hahn RG. Phase II study of camptothecin (NSC-100880) in the treatment of advanced gastrointestinal cancer. Cancer Chemother Rep 1972;56:95.
141. Hsiang Y-H, Hertzberg R, Hecht S, Liu LF. Camptothecin induces protein-linked DNA breaks via mammalian DNA topoisomerase I. J Biol Chem 1985;260:14873.
142. Hsiang Y-H, Liu LF. Identification of mammalian DNA topoisomerase I as an intracellular target of the anticancer drug camptothecin. Cancer Res 1988;48:1722.
143. Liu LF. DNA topoisomerase poisons as antitumor drugs. Annu Rev Biochem 1989;58:351.
144. Hertzberg RP, Caranfa MJ, Holdern KG, Jakas DR, Gallagher G, Mattern MR. Modification of the hydroxy lactone ring of camptothecin: inhibition of mammalian topoisomerase I and biological activity. J Med Chem 1989;32:715.
145. Slichenmyer WJ, Rowinsky EK, Donehower RC, Kaufmann SH. The current status of camptothecin analogues as antitumor agents. J Natl Cancer Inst 1993;85:271.
146. Negoro S, Fukuoka M, Masuda N, et al. Phase I study of weekly intravenous infusions of CPT-11 a new derivative of camptothecin in the treatment of advanced non–small-cell lung cancer. J Natl Cancer Inst 1991;83:1164.
147. Rowinsky EK, Grochow LB, Ettinger DS, et al. Phase I and pharmacological study of the novel topoisomerase I inhibitor 7-ethyl-10-[4-(1-piperidino)-1-piperidino]carbonyloxy-camptothecin (CPT-11) administered as a ninety-minute infusion every 3 weeks. Cancer Res 1994;54:427.
148. Abigerges D, Armand J-P, Chabot GG, et al. Irinotecan (CPT-11) high-dose escalation using intensive high-dose loperamide to control diarrhea. J Natl Cancer Inst 1994;86:446.
149. Abigerges D, Chabot GG, Armand J-P, Herait P, Gouyette A, Gandia D. Phase I and pharmacologic studies of the camptothecin analog irinotecan administered every 3 weeks in cancer patients. J Clin Oncol 1995;13:210.
150. Kaneda N, Nagata H, Furuta T, Yokokura T. Metabolism and pharmacokinetics of the camptothecin analogue CPT-11 in the mouse. Cancer Res 1990;50:1715.
151. Rowinsky EK, Grochow LB, Hendricks CB, et al. Phase I and pharmacologic study of topotecan: a novel topoisomerase I inhibitor. J Clin Oncol 1992;10:647.
152. Saltz L, Sirott M, Young C, et al. Phase I clinical and pharmacology study of topotecan given daily for 5 consecutive days to patients with advanced solid tumors with attempt at dose intensification using recombinant granulocyte colony-stimulating factor. J Natl Cancer Inst 1993;85:1499.
153. Haas NB, LaCreta FP, Walczak J, et al. Phase I/pharmacokinetic study of topotecan by 24-hour continuous infusion weekly. Cancer Res 1994;54:1220.
154. Hochster H, Liebes L, Speyer J, et al. Phase I trial of low-dose continuous topotecan infusion in patients with cancer: an active and well-tolerated regimen. J Clin Oncol 1994;12:553.
155. Wani M, Taylor H, Wall M, Coggon P, McPhail A. Plant antitumor agents. VI. The isolation and structure of taxol a novel antileukemic and antitumor agent from Taxus brevifolia. J Am Chem Soc 1971; 93:2325.
156. Schiff P, Horowitz S. Taxol stabilizes microtubules in mouse fibroblast cells. Proc Natl Acad Sci USA 1980;77:1561.
157. Manfredi J, Horowitz S. Taxol: an antimitotic agent with a new mechanism of action. Pharmacol Ther 1984;25:83.
158. McGuire W, Rowinsky E, Rosenshien N, et al. Taxol: a novel investigational antimicrotubule agent. Ann Intern Med 1989;111:273.
159. Proceedings of the Second National Cancer Institute Workshop on Taxol and Taxus. Monogr Natl Cancer Inst 1993;15:1.
160. Rowinsky EK, Onetto N, Canetta RM, Arbuck SG. Taxol: the first of the taxanes an important new class of antitumor agents. Semin Oncol 1992;19:646.
161. Rowinsky EK, Burke PJ, Karpe JE, Tucker RW, Ettinger DS, Donehower RC. Phase I and pharmacodynamic study of taxol in refractory acute leukemias. Cancer Res 1989;49:4640.
162. Schiller JH, Storer B, Tutsch K, et al. Phase I trial of 3-hour infusion of paclitaxel with or without granulocyte colony-stimulating factor in patients with advanced cancer. J Clin Oncol 1994;12:241.
163. Eisenhauer EA, ten Bokkel Huinink WW, Swenerton KD, et al. European-Canadian randomized trial of paclitaxel in relapsed ovarian cancer: high-dose versus low-dose and long versus short infusion. J Clin Oncol 1994;12:2654.
164. Rowinsky EK, Wright M, Monsarrat B, Lesser GJ, Donehower RC. Taxol: pharmacology metabolism and clinical implications. Cancer Surv Pharmacokinet Cancer Chemother 1993;17:283.
165. Huizing MT, Keung ACF, Rosing H, et al. Pharmacokinetics of paclitaxel and metabolites in a randomized comparative study in platinum-pretreated ovarian cancer patients. J Clin Oncol 1993;11:2127.
166. Monsarrat B, Alvinerie P, Wright M, et al. Hepatic metabolism and biliary excretion of taxol in rats and humans. Monograph Natl Cancer Inst 1993;15:39.
167. Rowinsky EK, Gilbert MR, McGuire WP, et al. Sequences of taxol and cisplatin: a phase I and pharmacologic study. J Clin Oncol 1991; 9:1692.
168. Gianni L, Kearns CM, Giani A, et al. Nonlinear pharmacokinetics and metabolism of paclitaxel and its pharmacokinetic/pharmacodynamic relationships in humans. J Clin Oncol 1995;13:180.
169. Hutter H, Motzer R, Schwartz L, et al. Phase II trial of taxol in cisplatin-resistant germ cell tumor (GCT) patients (PTS). Proc Am Soc Clin Oncol 1994;13:232.
170. Roth BJ, Dreicer R, Einhorn LH, et al. Significant activity of paclitaxel in advanced transitional cell carcinoma of the urothelium: a phase II trial of the Eastern Cooperative Oncology Group. J Clin Oncol 1994; 12:2264.
171. Einzig AI, Gorowski E, Sasloff J, et al. Phase II trial of taxol in patients with renal cell carcinoma. Cancer Invest 1991;9:133.
172. Roth B, Yeap B, Wilding G, Kasimis B, McLeod D, Loehrer P. Taxol (NSC 125973) in advanced hormone-refractory prostate cancer: an ECOG phase II trial. Proc Am Soc Clin Oncol 1992;11:296.
173. Ringel I, Horowitz SB. Studies with RP56976 (Taxotere): a semisynthetic analog of Taxol. J Natl Cancer Inst 1991;83:288.
174. Tomiak E, Piccart MJ, Kerger J, et al. Phase I study of docetaxel administered as a 1-hour intravenous infusion on a weekly basis. J Clin Oncol 1994;12:1458.
175. Burris H, Irvin R, Kuhn J, et al. Phase I clinical trial of taxotere administered as either a 2-hour or 6-hour intravenous infusion. J Clin Oncol 1993;11:950.
176. Bisset D, Setanoians A, Cassidy J, et al. Phase I and pharmacokinetic study of taxotere (RP56976) administered as a 24-hour infusion. Cancer Res 1993;53:523.
177. Pazdur R, Newman RA, Newman BM, et al. Phase I trial of taxotere: five-day schedule. J Natl Cancer Inst 1992;84:1781.
178. Hertel LW, Boder GB, Kroin JS, et al. Evaluation of the antitumor activity of gemcitabine (2′2′-difluoro-2′-deoxycytidine). Cancer Res 1990;50:4417.
179. Merriman RL, Schultz RM, Hertel LW, Houghton PJ, Houghton JA, Grindey GB. Evaluation of the antitumor activity of gemcitabine against human carcinoma xenografts. Proc Am Assoc Cancer Res 1994;35:448.
180. Heinemann V, Hertel LW, Grindey GB, Plunkett W. Comparison of the cellular pharmacokinetics and toxicity of 2′2′-difluorodeoxycitidine and 1-β-D-arabinofuranosylcytosine. Cancer Res 1988;48:4024.
181. Heinemann V, Xu Y-Z, Chubb S, et al. Cellular elimination of 2′2′-difluorodeoxycytidine 5′-triphosphate: a mechanism of self-potentiation. Cancer Res 1992;52:533.
182. Ghandi V, Huang P, Xu Y-Z, Heinemann V, Plunkett W. Metabolism and action of 2′2′-difluorodeoxycitidine: self-potentiation of cytotoxicity. In: Harkness RA, et al, eds. Purine and pyrimidine metabolism in man. VII, part A. New York: Plenum Press, 1991:125.
183. Abbruzzese JL, Grunewald R, Weeks EA, et al. A phase I clinical

plasma and cellular pharmacology study of gemcitabine. J Clin Oncol 1991;9:491.
184. Richards F, White D, Muss H, et al. Phase I trial of gemcitibine (2′2′-difluorodeoxycytidine) (G) over 30 minutes in patients (PTS) with non small cell lung cancer (NSCLC). Proc Am Soc Clin Oncol 1994; 13:344.
185. Brown T, O'Rourke T, Burris H, et al. A phase I trial of gemcitabine (LY188011) administered intravenously every two weeks. Proc Am Soc Clin Oncol 1991;10:115.
186. Pollera CF, Ceribelli A, Crecco M, Sabino F, Calabresi F. Weekly gemcitabine: a phase I study with short and prolonged infusion schedules. Proc Am Soc Clin Oncol 1992;11:127.
187. Stadler W, Kuzel T, Raghavan D, et al. A phase II study of gemcitabine in the treatment of patients with advanced transitional cell carcinoma. Proc Am Soc Clin Oncol 1995 14:241.
188. Weisbach L, de Mulder P, Osieka R, Ermisch S, Jakse G. Phase II study of gemcitabine in renal cancer. Proc Am Soc Clin Oncol 1992; 11:219.
189. Fellons A, Ohayon R, Vacassin T, et al. Biochemical effects of navelbine on tubulin and associated proteins. Semin Oncol 1989;16:9.
190. Cros S, Wright M, Moromoto M, et al. Experimental antitumor activity of navelbine. Semin Oncol 1989;16:15.
191. Photiou A, Sheikh MN, Bafaloukos D, et al. Antiproliferative activity of vinorelbine against six human melanoma cell lines. J Cancer Res Clin Oncol 1992;118:249.
192. Mathe G, Reizenstein P. Phase I pharmacologic study of a new vinca-alkaloid: Navelbine. Cancer Lett 1985;27:285.
193. Bore P, Rahmani R, van Cantfort J, Focan C, Cano JP. Pharmacokinetics of a new anticancer drug navelbine in patients: comparative study of radioimmunologic and radioactive determination methods. Cancer Chemother Pharmacol 1989;23:247.
194. Rowinsky EK, Noe DA, Trump DL, et al. Pharmacokinetic bioavailability and feasibility study of oral vinorelbine in patients with solid tumors. J Clin Oncol 1994;12:1754.
195. Constantopoulos G, Rees S, Cragg B, et al. Experimental animal model for mucopolysaccharidosis: suramin-induced glycosaminoglycan and sphingolipid accumulation in the rat. Proc Natl Acad Sci USA 1980;77:3700.
196. Horne M, Stein CA, LaRocca RV, et al. Circulating glycosaminoglycan anticoagulants associated with suramin treatment. Blood 1988; 71:273.
197. Coffee RJ, Leof EB, Shipley GD, et al. Suramin inhibition of growth factor receptor binding and mitogenicity in AKR-2B cells. J Cell Physiol 1987;132:143.
198. Moscatelli D, Quarto N. Transformation of NIH 3T3 cells with basic fibroblast growth factor or the hst/K-fgf oncogene causes downregulation of the fibroblast growth factor receptor: reversal of morphological transformation and restoration of receptor number by suramin. J Cell Biol 1989;109:2519.
199. Pollak M, Richard M. Suramin blockade of insulinlike growth factor I–stimulated proliferation of human osteosarcoma cells. J Natl Cancer Inst 1990;82:1349.
200. Betsholtz C, Johnsson A, Heldin C, et al. Efficient reversion of simian sarcoma virus-transformation and inhibition of growth factor-induced mitogenesis by suramin. Proc Natl Acad Sci USA 1986;83:6440.
201. Stein CA, LaRocca R, Myers C. Suramin: an old compound with new biology. In: Principles and practice of oncology updates, vol 4. Philadelphia: JB Lippincott, 1990:1.
202. Feuillan OP, Raffeld M, Stein CA, et al. Effects of suramin on the function and structure of the adrenal cortex in the cynomolgus monkey. J Clin Endocrinol Metab 1987;65:152.
203. Stein CA, LaRocca RV, Thomas R, McAtee N, Myers CE. Suramin: an anticancer drug with a unique mechanism of action. J Clin Oncol 1989;7:499.
204. Myers C, Cooper M, Stein C, et al. Suramin: a novel growth factor antagonist with activity in hormone-refractory metastatic prostate cancer. J Clin Oncol 1992;10:881.
205. LaRocca RV, Meer J, Gilliatt RW, et al. Suramin-induced polyneuropathy. Neurology 1990;40:954.
206. Collins JM, Klecker RW, Yarchoan R, et al. Clinical pharmacokinetics of suramin in patients with HTLV-III/LAV infection. J Clin Pharmacol 1986;26:22.
207. Jodrell DI, Reyno LM, Sridhara R, et al. Suramin: development of a population pharmacokinetic model and its use with intermittent short infusions to control plasma drug concentration in patients with prostate cancer. J Clin Oncol 1994;12:166.
208. Forest A, Scher HI, Tong W, et al. Development of an adaptive control algorithm for suramin. Proc Am Soc Clin Oncol 1990;10:73.
209. Scher HI, Jodrell DI, Iversen JM, et al. Use of adaptive control with feedback to individualize suramin dosing. Cancer Res 1992;52:64.
210. Eisenberger MA, Reyno LM, Jodrell DI, et al. Suramin an active drug for prostate cancer: interim observations in a phase I trial. J Natl Cancer Inst 1993;85:611.
211. Eisenberger M, Reyno L, Sinibaldi V, et al. Phase I/II trial of suramin (SUR) in hormone-refractory prostate cancer (HRPC): evidence of anti-tumor activity over a broad range of plasma SUR concentrations. Proc Am Soc Clin Oncol 1993;12:247.
212. Petrylak DP, Yagoda A, O'Connor J, et al. Phase II trial of suramin (SUR) in hormone refractory prostate cancer (HRPC). Proc Am Soc Clin Oncol 1994;13:249.

Principles and Practice of Genitourinary Oncology, edited by Derek Raghavan, Howard I. Scher, Steven A. Leibel, and Paul H. Lange. Lippincott-Raven Publishers, Philadelphia, © 1997.

CHAPTER 9

New Strategies of Systemic Therapy: Mechanisms and Modulation of Resistance to Platinum-Containing Anticancer Drugs

Raymond P. Perez, Steven W. Johnson, and Thomas C. Hamilton

The platinum-containing anticancer drugs cisplatin and carboplatin are among the most active available agents for use against chemotherapy-sensitive genitourinary malignancies (i.e., testis and bladder carcinomas) and are key constituents of combination chemotherapy regimens used to treat these diseases.[1–3] Unfortunately, the efficacy of cisplatin and carboplatin in patients with genitourinary malignancies is limited by resistance of these tumors to chemotherapy. Prostate and renal cell carcinoma respond poorly to available chemotherapeutic agents, including platinum-containing drugs; these malignancies are considered intrinsically resistant to chemotherapy. In addition, although the majority of patients with advanced bladder carcinoma have an initial response to platinum-based chemotherapy, most patients eventually relapse and develop chemotherapy-resistant disease. Even in testis cancer, a small percentage of patients fail to respond to chemotherapy or manifest resistance to therapy at the time of relapse. It is estimated that approximately 72,000 deaths per year among patients with genital and urinary malignancies can be attributed to the resistance of these tumors to chemotherapy.[4]

The cellular mechanisms responsible for resistance to platinum compounds are incompletely defined. Few investigations have focused on genitourinary model systems; however, data accumulating from other disease types suggest that multiple mechanisms, alone or in combination, contribute to cisplatin resistance. This chapter summarizes the current understanding of the cellular and molecular mechanisms responsible for cell killing by and cellular resistance to platinum-containing drugs. Preclinical and clinical strategies to overcome resistance also are reviewed.

CELLULAR PHARMACOLOGY AND MECHANISMS OF ACTION OF PLATINUM COMPOUNDS

The precise mechanisms responsible for cisplatin accumulation have not been defined. Cisplatin accumulation is nonsaturable and cannot be inhibited by competition with structural analogs, consistent with entry into cells by diffusion.[5] However, a component of cisplatin accumulation is energy dependent, pH dependent, sodium dependent, voltage sensitive, and ouabain inhibitable.[6,7] These data are consistent with the hypothesis that cisplatin may enter cells via transmembrane channels.[5] These channels could be affected by changes in voltage or ion concentrations, while also allowing high-capacity diffusion of cisplatin into cells. Although this hypothesis is appealing, it is presently supported only by indirect evidence.

A small percentage (~1%) of the intracellular cisplatin or carboplatin reacts with genomic DNA. These chemotherapeutic drugs form an array of intrastrand and interstrand monoadducts and crosslinks. The most common lesion formed is an intrastrand crosslink between adjacent guanine residues.[8,9] Cisplatin and carboplatin form identical lesions in DNA, although the reaction kinetics for carboplatin are considerably slower than those for for cisplatin.[10] Relatively few reports have been published regarding the specific types of DNA lesions formed by other platinum compounds. Cisplatin also binds RNA and cellular protein,[11] which could also contribute to cytotoxicity.

Considerable evidence indicates that DNA is an important intracellular target for platinum compounds.[8,9,11,12] Evidence implicating DNA as an important target for cisplatin includes the following:

- Cisplatin-induced DNA damage correlates with in vitro cytotoxicity and clinical response.[13,14]
- Cell lines with known deficiencies in DNA repair, such as those derived from patients with xeroderma pigmentosum, are hypersensitive to cisplatin.[15,16]
- Enhanced DNA repair has been observed in cell lines selected for cisplatin resistance in vitro.[17–22]
- Cisplatin cytotoxicity in vitro can be potentiated by drugs that inhibit DNA repair.[17,23,24]

Which platinum-induced lesions are ultimately responsible for cellular death remain to be determined. Regardless of the specific lesions responsible, cisplatin is capable of inducing apoptosis, a form of programed cell death, in some model systems.[25,26] Internucleosomal DNA cleavage and ultrastructural changes characteristic of apoptosis have been observed following cisplatin treatment of murine L1210 leukemia and Chinese hamster ovary cell lines.[25,26] Cisplatin-induced apoptosis has also been reported in a proliferating rat hepatoma cell line but was not apparent in nonproliferating rat thymocytes.[27] These data suggest that apoptosis may be more readily triggered in proliferating cells in some model systems. Glaves-Rapp and Raghavan[*] observed apoptosis, detected by internucleosomal DNA cleavage and by in situ digoxygenin-dUTP 3′-end labeling, in three human bladder carcinoma cell lines (UCRU-BL13, -BL17, and -BL28) following treatment with relatively high concentrations of cisplatin. The relation between expression of genes that regulate cell proliferation, such as the *P53* tumor suppressor gene, and apoptosis in these and other cell lines remains an area of active investigation.

Further evidence supporting apoptosis as a mechanism of cisplatin-induced cell death comes from investigations of the effects of genes postulated to inhibit apoptosis, such as *BCL2* (formerly known as Bcl-2). Transfection of the *BCL2* gene into human neuroblastoma and leukemia cell lines produced resistance to cisplatin, and other anticancer drugs, and inhibited cisplatin-mediated apoptosis.[28,29] Similar investigations have not yet been reported in genitourinary model systems.

It is possible that mechanisms other than apoptosis also contribute to cell killing by cisplatin. The concentrations of cisplatin required to produce apoptosis in most model systems exceed the concentrations of cisplatin that can be achieved in patients. Thus, uncertainty persists regarding whether apoptosis is an important mechanism of cell death at pharmacologically relevant concentrations.

One potential mechanism of activity for cisplatin is transcription factor hijacking.[30] The rRNA transcription factor hUBF was observed to bind the cisplatin G–G intrastrand adducts and the rRNA promoter with equal affinity. The sequestration of an rRNA transcription factor by binding to cisplatin–DNA adducts could potentially decrease the expression of several critical genes. In addition, binding of the transcription factor to cisplatin–DNA adducts could interfere with the ability of cells to recognize and repair cisplatin-induced DNA damage. Further investigation of this mechanism should prove most interesting.

RESISTANCE TO PLATINUM-CONTAINING DRUGS

The available data suggest that resistance to cisplatin is multifactorial at the cellular level (Table 9-1).[31,32] Alterations in drug accumulation, glutathione metabolism, and DNA repair are the most consistently observed changes in cisplatin-resistant cell lines. Decreased accumulation is common in cell lines selected for cisplatin resistance in vitro.[5,31,32] Increased active efflux of cisplatin was recently observed in one cisplatin-resistant cell line in vitro.[33] However, decreased accumulation does not generally correlate well with the magnitude of resistance observed, which implies that additional mechanisms contribute to resistance.

[*]Glaves-Rapp D, Raghavan D, personal communication, August, 1995.

TABLE 9-1. *Mechanisms of resistance to platinum compounds*

Decreased accumulation
Decreased influx
Increased efflux
Conjugation with cellular thiols
Glutathione
Metallothioneins
Increased DNA repair
Tolerance of DNA damage
Expression of specific genes
HSPD1
P^{53}
RAS family
Mitochondrial mechanisms

Cytosolic inactivation is another cellular mechanism for reducing intracellular levels of active drug. Glutathione (GSH), the major nonprotein sulfhydryl, and the metallothionein (MT) proteins may function in this manner. GSH covalently binds cisplatin at physiologically relevant concentrations[34] and quenches platinum–DNA monoadducts prior to conversion to potentially cytotoxic crosslinks.[35] The direct interaction between GSH and cisplatin in a cellular system also has been reported, and the drug–GSH conjugate has been shown to be exported by an ATP-dependent glutathione-S-conjugate export pump.[36] The formation of a GSH–Pt complex in human ovarian cancer cell lines also has been demonstrated.[37]

Increased cellular glutathione levels have been shown to be associated with decreased cisplatin sensitivity in human renal[38], bladder[38,39], and ovarian[40–44] cancer cell lines, as well as in human ovarian tumor biopsy specimens.[45] Elevated GSH levels were also apparent in melphalan-resistant sublines derived from the DU145 prostate carcinoma cell line.[46,47] These cell lines were cross-resistant to the platinum-containing drugs cisplatin and tetraplatin. Pendyala and colleagues[39] reported that mean GSH levels in five human bladder carcinoma cell lines were significantly higher (~4.5-fold) than in a panel of 12 nonbladder malignant cell lines (ovarian, colon, glioblastoma, and melanoma). Absolute levels of GSH in two bladder carcinoma cell lines were comparable to those in a human ovarian carcinoma cell line selected for several hundred–fold resistance to cisplatin in vitro. These investigators also found that mean GSH levels in bladder carcinoma specimens ($n = 7$) were approximately twofold higher than those in normal bladder biopsies ($n = 9$; $P < .01$).[48] These data support the hypothesis that GSH is an important contributor to cisplatin resistance in general, and to cisplatin resistance in bladder carcinoma in particular.

Increased GSH levels may result from increased cellular γ-glutamylcysteine synthetase (γ-GCS) activity, γ-glutamyl transpeptidase (γ-GT) activity, or both. γ-GCS catalyzes the rate-limiting step in GSH synthesis, whereas γ-GT functions to "salvage" GSH that has been exported from the cell. Elevated GSH levels in a panel of highly cisplatin-resistant human ovarian carcinoma cell lines were associated with increased mRNA expression of both γ-GCS and γ-GT.[44] Expression of γ-GCS mRNA was also significantly increased in melphalan- and cisplatin-resistant DU145 prostate carcinoma sublines.[47] The expression of γ-GT was not analyzed in these cell lines. In contrast, elevated GSH levels in two human bladder carcinoma cell lines were associated only with increased γ-GCS activity; γ-GT activity was not detectable in these cell lines.[39] Data on γ-GCS and γ-GT mRNA expression in these bladder carcinoma cell lines are pending. Depletion of GSH levels by buthionine sulfoximine (BSO), which inhibits the activity of γ-GCS, has resulted in enhanced cisplatin sensitivity in some cell lines[40,41] but not in others.[49–51]

In addition to inactivating platinum drugs in the cytoplasm, GSH may also prevent cytotoxic lesions from forming on DNA. Using DNA incubated with cisplatin in vitro, Eastman[35] demonstrated that GSH can quench platinum–DNA monoadducts prior to conversion to potentially cytotoxic crosslinks. In addition, GSH may directly or indirectly participate in the DNA repair process. For example, the active-site cysteine residues of the HMG-1 and HMG-2 proteins must be in a reduced state to recognize cisplatin-damaged DNA.[52] Also, the depletion of GSH levels by BSO, which inhibits the activity of γ-GCS, results in the inhibition of unscheduled DNA synthesis in cisplatin-resistant human ovarian cancer cells.[53]

Metallothioneins (MTs) are a family of low-molecular-weight, cysteine-rich metalloproteins that exhibit high affinity for metal ions.[54] The reaction of cisplatin with MT has clearly been demonstrated,[55] and cells transfected with the human *MT2A* (formerly known as MT-IIA) cDNA have shown increased resistance to cisplatin and alkylating agents.[56] It is uncertain, however, whether MTs play an important role in tumor cell resistance to platinum drugs. For example, increased levels of MT were not observed in human 2008 ovarian cancer cell lines selected for primary cisplatin resistance.[57] *MT2A* gene expression also did not correlate with cisplatin sensitivity in ovarian cancer cell lines selected for cisplatin resistance in vitro nor in cell lines derived from patients who either responded or failed to respond to platinum-based combination chemotherapy.[58] Furthermore, no difference in MT content was observed in ovarian tumors between patients who were untreated and those who were treated using a platinum-based regimen.[59] In contrast, immunohistochemical analysis has shown increased MT levels in human testicular germ cell tumors[60] and human bladder cancer cell lines and tumors[61] following platinum-drug exposure.

If mechanisms such as those described previously fail to limit the formation of Pt–DNA adducts, a cell must either tolerate or repair the DNA damage. Evidence for increased DNA repair associated with cisplatin resistance has been demonstrated primarily in human ovarian cancer models using a variety of methods. Masuda and colleagues[23] initially showed a twofold enhancement of repair in A2780/CP70 cells relative to the A2780 cell line from which they were derived using unscheduled DNA synthesis (UDS). A similar study was performed in another pair of ovarian cell lines, PEO1 and PEO4, which were derived from a patient before and after the onset of clinical resistance to a platinum-based chemotherapeutic regimen, respectively. The cisplatin-resistant cell line (PEO4) exhibited a twofold to threefold increase in UDS relative to the cisplatin-sensitive PEO1 cell line.[62] A correlation between increased platinum–DNA adduct removal and cisplatin resistance has been demonstrated by atomic absorption spectrometry in subsequent studies with the A2780 cell line and variants derived from its in vitro cisplatin exposure.[17,21,22]

In some model systems it appears that the repair of certain types of DNA damage occurs preferentially in actively transcribed genes relative to the overall genome.[63] Thus, it is possible that cisplatin-resistant cells excel at gene-specific repair to increase the probability of survival. Evidence has been reported for increases in cisplatin interstrand crosslink (ICL) removal from actively transcribed genes and nontranscribed genes by cisplatin-resistant human ovarian cancer cell lines relative to removal from the overall genome.[20] Other studies that measured ICL removal from a nontranscribed, nongene sequence as well as actively transcribed regions indicated that ICL removal rates were also increased in cisplatin-resistant cells; however, the rate of removal did not vary in the DNA sequences examined.[22,64]

Further evidence supporting a role for DNA repair in cisplatin resistance has come from studies with aphidicolin glycinate, an inhibitor of DNA polymerases a, d and e. Aphidicolin inhibited UDS in A2780 and A2780/CP70 cells in a dose-dependent manner. Furthermore, aphidicolin in combination with cisplatin produced a 3.5-fold reduction in cisplatin cytotoxicity in A2780/CP70 cells, whereas the same treatment had minimal effect on cisplatin-sensitive A2780 cells.[23] In the 2008/DDP human ovarian cell line, aphidicolin exhibited strong synergism with cisplatin after short-term drug exposure, whereas the parental, cisplatin-sensitive cell line (2008) showed no change.[24] Expression of putative DNA repair genes in tumor tissues has also been measured. mRNA levels of the *ERCC1* (excision repair cross complementing) gene and the *XPA* (xeroderma pigmentosum group A) gene were elevated in malignant tissues from ovarian cancer patients who were refractory to platinum-based chemotherapy relative to levels in patients who were responsive to treatment.[65]

Despite the body of evidence supporting DNA as the cytotoxic target of platinum drugs, a significantly higher level of platinum-induced DNA damage is often required to kill resistant cells than sensitive cells.[64,66] In one report, cisplatin-sensitive and -resistant human ovarian carcinoma cell lines were treated with cisplatin under equitoxic (IC50) conditions.[21] Levels of platinum remaining in the DNA following completion of DNA repair were threefold higher in the resistant subline compared to the sensitive parental cell line. This tolerance of DNA damage may result from resistant cells having an enhanced ability to synthesize DNA past a lesion. Alternatively, DNA damage in the resistant cells may no longer serve as a signal for the cells to undergo programed cell death, or another component of the cell death pathway may be functioning improperly. Using the 2008 and A2780 human ovarian cancer models, Mamenta and colleagues[67] demonstrated a 4.5- and 2.3-fold increased Pt–DNA replicative bypass ability of the cisplatin-resistant C13 and A2780/CP70 cell lines, respectively. In both cell lines, (diaminocyclohexane)Pt–DNA adducts caused a greater inhibition of DNA synthesis than cisplatin-induced DNA lesions.

It is becoming increasingly evident that cisplatin resistance is associated with altered expression of one or more cellular genes. The frequency with which cisplatin resistance was observed in cultured A2780 human ovarian carcinoma cells was comparable to the expected spontaneous mutation frequency.[68] Moreover, the frequency with which resistant clonal sublines could be isolated was increased by pretreatment of the parental cell population with mutagens. The association between mutation and resistance suggests that changes in the expression of specific genes may contribute to resistance. The previously noted associations between resistance and increased expression of genes involved in GSH metabolism or DNA repair further support this contention.

Several lines of evidence suggest that expression of the *HSPD1* (heat shock protein 60) gene is associated with cisplatin resistance. The *HSPD1* gene encodes a 60-kd protein which participates in assembly, folding, and transport of proteins in the mitochondria. Enns and colleagues[69] observed that this gene was overexpressed in a human ovarian carcinoma cell line selected for cisplatin resistance in vitro compared with parental cells. Wilkes and colleagues[70] have similarly observed a several-fold elevation in *HSPD1* mRNA expression in another cisplatin-resistant human ovarian carcinoma cell line. Decreased survival has been reported among ovarian cancer patients with relatively high levels of *HSPD1* mRNA expression.[71] *HSPD1* expression was also associated with increased cisplatin resistance in head and neck carcinoma cell lines in vitro.[72] Finally, the human *HSPD1* gene was isolated from a cisplatin-resistant murine NIH-3T3 subline transformed by DNA-mediated gene transfer from a cisplatin-resistant human hepatoma cell line.[73†] These data suggest that *HSPD1* expression may be significantly related to cisplatin resistance.

Several lines of evidence suggest that the tumor suppressor gene *P53* is a potentially important determinant of cellular sensitivity or resistance to cisplatin. Increased levels of the wild-type P53 protein have been observed in association with cell cycle arrest in G1 phase following exposure of cells to gamma irradiation, cisplatin, or other DNA-damaging agents.[74–76] Expression of wild-type P53 is required for induction of apoptosis in some model systems[77] but not in others.[78] There are also limited data suggesting that P53 interacts with the Gadd45 and ERCC3 proteins, which may be involved in DNA repair.[79,80] Increased levels of P53 protein correlated with cisplatin resistance in a series of clonal sublines derived by single-step selection from the A2780 cell line.[81] However, transfection of the wild-type *P53* gene into human non–small cell lung[82] and cisplatin-resistant ovarian[81] carcinoma cell lines increased the sensitivity of both cell lines to cisplatin. Thus, the precise role of *P53* as a determinant of cisplatin sensitivity awaits further clarification.

Conflicting data have been published regarding the potential relation between expression of *RAS* genes and cisplatin resistance. Several investigators have reported that expression of mutationally activated *RAS* oncogenes in NIH-3T3 fibroblast cell lines was associated with increased resistance to cisplatin,[83–85] although other investigators did not observe any change in the cisplatin sensitivity of 3T3 cells following transformation with *RAS*.[86] One preliminary report suggested that sensitivity of *RAS*-transformed mammary epithelial cell lines to cisplatin was actually increased compared with that of parental controls.[87] Perez and colleagues[88] failed to observe any relation between expression of mutant *RAS* mRNA or protein expression and sensitivity to cisplatin in a series of rat ovarian epithelial and fibroblast cell lines. Because the effects of *RAS* on cisplatin sensitivity appear to be restricted to NIH-3T3 fibroblasts, there is little evidence that this gene is related to cisplatin resistance on a general level.

Resistance to cisplatin has also been associated with changes in a specific organelle, the mitochondrion. Abnormalities of mitochondrial ultrastructure, intracellular distribution, and membrane potential have been reported in a human ovarian carcinoma cell line selected for cisplatin resistance by chronic exposure to the drug (2008/C13*).[89] Analyses of cisplatin accumulation, GSH levels, and mitochondrial membrane potential in these cell lines and in a revertant mutant subline suggest that mitochondrial mechanisms accounted almost entirely for the magnitude of resistance observed.[90] Similarly, the magnitude of resistance was substantially decreased following depletion of mitochondrial DNA in 2008/C13* cells by chronic ethidium bromide treatment.[91] Precisely how mitochondria contribute to resistance and how mitochondrial mechanisms interact with other potential resistance mechanisms has not yet been defined.

The overwhelming majority of data regarding cellular mechanisms of resistance to platinum compounds relate to cisplatin. Few data are available for other compounds. Cisplatin and carboplatin demonstrate nearly complete cross-resistance in vitro and in the clinic, which implies that similar resistance mechanisms are important for both compounds. Limited data suggest that the lack of cross-resistance between tetraplatin or JM216 and cisplatin is at least partially attributable to the ability of the former compounds to circumvent decreased cisplatin accumulation.[92,93] This suggests that some platinum-containing drugs may enter cells by mechanisms different from those for cisplatin.

Data from Pendyala and colleagues[‡] suggest that GSH is an important mediator of resistance to the platinum-containing drug oxaliplatin. Levels of GSH and resistance directly correlated in human ovarian carcinoma cell lines selected for oxaliplatin resistance by chronic in vitro exposure to the drug.[94] Enzyme activity and mRNA expression of γ-GT were increased in these cell lines relative to parental cells. The activity and mRNA expression of the GSH-synthetic enzyme γ-GCS did not differ between parental cells and oxaliplatin-resistant sublines. Thus, salvage of GSH by reactions involving γ-GT is primarily responsible for elevated levels of GSH in these cell lines.

STRATEGIES TO CIRCUMVENT PLATINUM RESISTANCE

Biochemical Modulation

Enhancement of Drug Accumulation

Preclinical data suggest that numerous agents can increase or decrease cisplatin accumulation.[5] Dipyridamole and hyperthermia are among the more extensively evaluated of these agents. Dipyridamole increased the accumulation of cisplatin and synergistically enhanced in vitro cisplatin cytotoxicity by approximately fivefold in the 2008 human ovarian carcinoma cell line.[95] Similar effects were observed in a resistant subline selected for cisplatin resistance in vitro. Dipyridamole has also been reported to enhance the in vivo activity of cisplatin, alone or in combination with other anticancer drugs, in human bladder and testicular carcinoma xenograft model systems.[96,97] Combination therapy using dipyridamole and cisplatin has not yet been investigated in patients with genitourinary malignancies.

†Shen D-W, personal communication, January 1995.

‡Pendyala L, Elakawi Z, Creaven PJ, et al, personal communication, August, 1995.

Hyperthermia has also been reported to enhance the uptake and cytotoxicity of cisplatin in some in vitro model systems.[98,99] Cisplatin-based combination chemotherapy regimens have been administered with irradiation and hyperthermia to a small number of patients with locally advanced bladder cancer.[100] Although objective responses were observed, it is not clear that this approach offers any advantages over more conventional regimens.

Further attempts to modulate cisplatin accumulation will probably be facilitated by a better understanding of the precise cellular and molecular mechanisms involved in cisplatin uptake and efflux. Preclinical and clinical strategies to modulate accumulation are still in the early stages of development.

Buthionine Sulfoximine

Cellular GSH can be depleted by BSO, a specific inhibitor of the GSH synthetic enzyme γ-GCS. Depletion of GSH with BSO enhanced the cytotoxicity of cisplatin in in vitro and in vivo preclinical models.[101,102] BSO is being administered in combination with the alkylating agent melphalan in phase I trials.[102–104] Initial data from these trials indicate that BSO can safely be given in combination with melphalan. In addition, depletion of GSH in tumor samples and in peripheral lymphocytes was apparent in the majority of BSO-treated patients.[102–104] Increased γ-GCS mRNA expression was detected in peripheral lymphocytes of BSO-treated patients by reverse-transcription polymerase chain reaction, consistent with a cellular compensatory response to pharmacologic inhibition of γ-GCS.[105] Patients in these trials have generally been heavily pretreated. However, objective responses have been observed among patients with ovarian cancer and melanoma.[102,104]

BSO has not been used in combination with cisplatin because of concern about increasing the potential risk of nephrotoxicity; however, trials of BSO plus carboplatin are in progress. Available data suggest that modulation of GSH is a potentially important strategy to enhance the efficacy of platinum-containing drugs and alkylating agents. Unfortunately, BSO is in limited supply, which may impede attempts to define its usefulness as a clinical modulator of resistance. Further investigations of novel strategies for modulating GSH levels are warranted.

Aphidicolin

Aphidicolin inhibits the activity of DNA polymerases a, d, and e, and it has been shown to potentiate the in vitro cytotoxicity of cisplatin in some model systems, as noted previously. O'Dwyer and colleagues[106] reported that aphidicolin glycinate enhanced the in vivo efficacy of cisplatin against several murine tumor models and against a xenografted human ovarian carcinoma cell line from a cisplatin-refractory patient. Aphidicolin glycinate has also been evaluated in two European phase I trials.[107] Overall, the drug was well tolerated. Plasma levels (3 μg/mL) obtained following administration of drug by 24-hour infusion were comparable to those that inhibited DNA repair and enhanced cisplatin cytotoxicity in vitro. These data suggest that clinical trials to test the safety and efficacy of cisplatin or carboplatin in combination with aphidicolin are warranted. Approval for the investigational use of this drug in the United States is pending.

Platinum Analogs

Carboplatin and Analogs

Carboplatin is a second-generation diammine platinum analog that was approved for clinical use in 1989. Its activity profile in vitro is virtually identical to that of cisplatin,[108–110] and there is substantial clinical cross-resistance between the two drugs.[111,112] In patients with cisplatin-refractory ovarian cancer, defined by progressive disease during treatment or relapse within 6 months of treatment, the response rate of carboplatin is approximately 7%.[112] The efficacy of higher-than-conventional doses or intravesicular administration of carboplatin in patients with genitourinary malignancies has not yet been defined. Thus, carboplatin at conventional doses is usually not effective in patients who have not benefited from cisplatin therapy.

Carboplatin has a clinical toxicity profile that is considerably different from that of cisplatin.[113] The principal toxicity of carboplatin is myelosuppression. Unlike cisplatin, carboplatin is not neurotoxic or ototoxic, and it rarely produces clinically apparent renal toxicity. Therefore, carboplatin usually can be administered in the outpatient setting without the hydration and diuretics required with cisplatin administration. Some authors have advocated hydration prior to carboplatin administration in patients with impaired renal function or in those who are to be treated with high doses (i.e., ≥800 mg/m^2).[114]

Several derivatives of carboplatin are being evaluated in the United States. CI-973 (also known as NK-121) is a carboplatin analog with an in vitro activity profile similar to that of cisplatin, although activity has been noted in some cisplatin-resistant cell lines.[109] Its major clinical toxicity is myelosuppression.[115,116] Like carboplatin, CI-973 produces minimal nephrotoxicity, neurotoxicity, and ototoxicity.[115,116] Its overall clinical activity profile remains to be determined in phase II trials. Two other carboplatin derivatives, zeniplatin and enloplatin, are potentially nephrotoxic, and their further clinical development in the United States is uncertain.

Isopropylamine Compounds

Iproplatin (cis-dichloro-trans-dihydroxy-bis-isopropylamine platinum[IV], CHIP, JM9), the first quadrivalent platinum complex to reach clinical trials, is a nonnephrotoxic, water-soluble complex. Initial clinical evaluation in Europe and the United States demonstrated that its dose-limiting toxicity was myelosuppression, primarily thrombocytopenia.[117] However, the gastrointestinal toxicities of iproplatin (i.e., nausea, vomiting, and diarrhea) were somewhat greater than those of carboplatin.[113] Activity was observed in patients with ovarian carcinoma[118] and small cell lung cancer.[119]

Iproplatin has been evaluated in a limited number of patients with genitourinary malignancies. In one randomized phase II trial in previously untreated patients with urothelial cancer, carboplatin was inactive (0/14 patients responded), whereas iproplatin had modest activity (5/29).[120] Iproplatin had no activity in phase II trials of patients with cisplatin-refractory germ cell malignancies.[121,122] It is possible that patient selection somewhat accounts for the limited iproplatin activity observed in these trials. However, iproplatin has not shown sufficient activity or toxicity differences in comparison with cisplatin and carboplatin to support its further development.

Mixed Ammine–Amine Dicarboxylate Compounds

The ammine–amine dicarboxylates constitute a particularly interesting group of platinum compounds. Several of these compounds appear to have activity in cisplatin-resistant preclinical model systems.[123–125] In some models, these drugs are considerably more potent than cisplatin. In addition, these compounds are reliably absorbed from the gastrointestinal tract, allowing for oral administration.

The prototype for this group of compounds is amine diacetato-dichloro-(cyclohexylamine)platinum(IV), or JM-216. A phase I trial of JM-216 is underway in the United Kingdom.[126] Nausea has been the most frequent toxicity encountered thus far, and this side effect has been well-controlled with antiemetics. No renal or neural toxicity has been observed. Additional toxicities, recommended phase II doses, and the clinical activity of these compounds remain to be defined.

Diaminocyclohexane Compounds

There has been considerable interest in tetraplatin (ormaplatin), a platinum compound containing the diaminocyclohexane (DACH) ligand.[127] Tetraplatin has an octahedral geometry, with four chlorides and the DACH ligand bound to platinum. Tetraplatin is essentially a prodrug that is rapidly reduced to the biologically active DACH–dichloroplatinum(II) species.[128] Interest in this compound followed the demonstration that it retained activity in cisplatin-resistant murine and human cell lines.[108,109,127] Some investigators have reported less impressive results in ovarian carcinoma xenograft model systems.[129]

Phase I trials of tetraplatin administered in different intravenous schedules have been completed at several institutions.[130–133] Myelosuppression was dose-limiting in the National Cancer Institute trial.[132] However, neurotoxicity was observed in all phase I trials and was not clearly related to any pharmacokinetic parameter, except possibly cumulative dose. Neuropathy was predominantly sensory, although at least one patient may have developed an autonomic neuropathy. This unpredictable neurotoxicity resulted in termination of most trials without establishment of a dose for phase II testing. In addition, administration of tetraplatin on a day 1 and day 8 schedule was associated with transiently increased excretion of β_2-microglobulin in several patients, which is consistent with subclinical renal tubular toxicity.[130] Elevation of the serum creatinine level was observed in one patient, and one patient with non–small cell lung cancer had an objective response.[130] In one trial tetraplatin was administered intraperitoneally.[134] When administered by this route, abdominal pain was dose-limiting but hematologic and neurotoxicities were mild. The future development of this compound is uncertain, although intraperitoneal administration may permit phase II trials in patients with peritoneal carcinomatosis.

Oxaliplatin is a newer DACH-containing platinum drug which is in clinical trials in Europe. Like tetraplatin, oxaliplatin retains activity in several cisplatin-resistant preclinical model systems.[135] In vitro, oxiplatin was active against cisplatin-resistant L1210 murine leukemia and A2780 human ovarian carcinoma cell lines, as well as against the HT-29 colon carcinoma cell line, which is a model of intrinsic cisplatin resistance.[136,137] The cytotoxic activity profile of oxaliplatin in vitro is very similar to that of tetraplatin and differs markedly from that of cisplatin and carboplatin. DACH-dichloroplatinum(II) is one of the major biotransformation products when oxaliplatin is incubated in human plasma in vitro. Studies in vitro indicate that a significant proportion of oxaliplatin in the blood is erythrocyte bound.[137]

Oxaliplatin can produce neurotoxicity, although frequency and severity appears to be somewhat less than that observed with tetraplatin.[135] The neurotoxicity induced by oxaliplatin typically consists of noncumulative extremity paresthesias that resolve within days of discontinuing treatment. Other clinical toxicities include myelosuppression, nausea, diarrhea, and elevation of transaminases, all of which are typically mild to moderate in severity. No nephrotoxicity has been reported. Initial reports from phase II trials suggest that oxaliplatin can reduce remissions in melanoma, colon carcinoma, breast carcinoma, and ovarian carcinoma.[135] These results are particularly intriguing because cisplatin, carboplatin, and iproplatin have limited activity against melanoma and colon carcinoma. Preliminary reports suggest significant activity of combination regimens containing both cisplatin and oxaliplatin in heavily pretreated patients with ovarian cancer or germ cell tumors.[138,139] Data on the activity of this compound in patients with other genitourinary malignancies are pending. Clinical trials of oxaliplatin will be initiated in the United States in 1996.

CONCLUSION

Resistance to platinum-containing drugs is a significant and complicated problem. However, understanding of the mechanisms responsible for resistance to cisplatin and other anticancer drugs has improved remarkably in recent years. The limited available data suggest that many of the mechanisms described in better-characterized model systems also confer cisplatin resistance in genitourinary malignancies. Ongoing investigations in this area offer the potential for rational design of new treatment strategies to overcome cisplatin resistance, and ultimately to improve the survival of patients with genitourinary malignancies.

ACKNOWLEDGMENT

The authors thank Drs. Dorothy Glaves-Rapp, Derek Raghavan, Lakshmi Pendyala, and D.-W. Shen for providing unpublished data, as noted in the text. We also acknowledge the secretarial support of Lynn Duewiger, who assisted in preparation of the manuscript.

REFERENCES

1. Ozols RF, Williams SD. Testicular cancer. Curr Prob Cancer 1989; 13:285.
2. Mosset-Auselo N, Bons-Rosset F, Costa P, Louis JF, Navratil H. Carboplatin and urothelial tumors. Oncology 1993;50(Suppl 2):28.

3. Miller RS, Torti FM. Chemotherapy of advanced transitional-cell carcinoma of the bladder. Cancer Chemother Pharmacol 1992;30(Suppl): s99.
4. Young RC. Mechanisms to improve chemotherapy effectiveness. Cancer 1990;65:815.
5. Gately DP, Howell SB. Cellular accumulation of the anticancer agent cisplatin: a review. Br J Cancer 1993;67:1171.
6. Andrews P, Velury S, Mann S, Howell S. cis-diamminedichloroplatinum(II) accumulation in sensitive and resistant human ovarian carcinoma cell lines. Cancer Res 1988;48:68.
7. Andrews P, Mann S, Huynh H, Albright K. Role of Na^+,K^+-adenosine triphosphatase in the accumulation of cis-diamminedichloroplatinum(II) in human ovarian carcinoma cells. Cancer Res 1991;51:3677.
8. Eastman A. Reevaluation of the interaction of cis-dichloro(ethylenediamine)platinum(II) with DNA. Biochemistry 1986;25:3912.
9. Eastman A. Characterization of the adducts produced in DNA by cis-diamminedichloroplatinum(II) and cis-dichloro(ethylenediamine)platinum(II). Biochemistry 1983;22:3927.
10. Knox RJ, Friedlos F, Lydall DA, Roberts JJ. Mechanism of cytotoxicity of anticancer platinum drugs: evidence that cis-diamminedichloroplatinum(II) and cis-diammine-(1,1-cyclobutanedicarboxylato)platinum(II) differ only in the kinetics of their interaction with DNA. Cancer Res 1986;46:1972.
11. Douple EB. Cis-diamminedichloroplatinum(II): effects of a representative metal coordination complex on mammalian cells. Pharmacol Ther 1984;25:297.
12. Zwelling LA, Kohn KW. Mechanism of action of cis-diamminedichloroplatinum(II). Cancer Treat Rep 1979;63:1439.
13. Reed E, Parker R, Gill I, et al. Platinum-DNA adducts in leukocyte DNA of a cohort of 49 patients with 24 different types of malignancies. Cancer Res 1993;53:3649.
14. Ducore J, Erickson L, Zwelling L, Laurent G, Kohn K. Comparative studies of DNA cross-linking and cytotoxicity in Burkitt's lymphoma cell lines treated with cis-diamminedichloroplatinum(II) and l-phenylalanine mustard. Cancer Res 1982;42:897.
15. Fraval H, Rawlings C, Roberts J. Increased sensitivity of UV-repair-deficient human cells to DNA bound platinum products which unlike thymidine dimers are not recognized by an endonuclease extracted from micrococcus luteus. Mutat Res 1978;51:121.
16. Dijt F, Fitchinger-Schepman A, Berends F, Reedijk J. Formation and repair of cisplatin-induced adducts to DNA in cultured normal and repair-deficient human fibroblasts. Cancer Res 1988;48:6058.
17. Masuda M, Tanaka T, Matsuda H, Kusaba I. Increased removal of DNA-bound platinum in a human ovarian cancer cell line resistant to cis-diamminedichloroplatinum (II). Cancer Res 1990;50:1863.
18. Eastman A, Schulte N. Enhanced DNA repair as a mechanism of resistance to cis-diamminedichloroplatinum(II). Biochemistry 1988; 27:4730.
19. Sheibani N, Jennerwein M, Eastman A. DNA repair in cells sensitive and resistant to cis-diamminedichloroplatinum(II): host cell reactivation of damaged plasmid DNA. Biochemistry 1989;28:3120.
20. Zhen W, Link CJ Jr, O'Connor PM. Increased gene-specific repair of cisplatin interstrand cross-links in cisplatin-resistant human ovarian cancer cell lines. Mol Cell Biol 1992;12:3689.
21. Parker RJ, Eastman A, Bostick-Bruton F, Reed E. Acquired cisplatin resistance in human ovarian cancer cells is associated with enhanced repair of cisplatin-DNA lesions and reduced drug accumulation. J Clin Invest 1991;87:772.
22. Johnson SW, Perez RP, Godwin AK. Role of platinum-DNA adduct formation and removal in cisplatin resistance in human ovarian cancer cell lines. Biochem Pharmacol 1994;47:689.
23. Masuda H, Ozols RF, Lai G-M, Fojo A, Rothenberg M, Hamilton TC. Increased DNA repair as a mechanism of acquired resistance to cis-diamminedichloroplatinum(II) in human ovarian cancer cell lines. Cancer Res 1988;48:5713.
24. Katz EJ, Andrews PA, Howell SB. The effect of DNA polymerase inhibitors on the cytotoxicity of cisplatin in human ovarian carcinoma cells. Cancer Comm 1990;2:159.
25. Sorenson CM, Barry MA, Eastman A. Analysis of events associated with cell cycle arrest at G2 phase and cell death induced by cisplatin. J Natl Cancer Inst 1990;82:749.
26. Barry MA, Behnke CA, Eastman A. Activation of programmed cell death (apoptosis) by cisplatin, other anticancer drugs, toxins, and hyperthermia. Biochem Pharmacol 1990;40:2353.
27. Evans DE, Dive C. Effects of cisplatin on the induction of apoptosis in proliferating hepatoma cells and nonproliferating immature thymocytes. Cancer Res 1993;53:2133.
28. Dole M, Nunez G, Merchant AK, et al. Bcl-2 inhibits chemotherapy-induced apoptosis in neuroblastoma. Cancer Res 1994;54:3253.
29. Miyashita T, Reed JC. Bcl-2 oncoprotein blocks chemotherapy-induced apoptosis in a human leukemia cell line. Blood 1993;81:151.
30. Treiber DK, Zhai X, Jantzen H-M, Essigmann JM. Cisplatin-DNA adducts are molecular decoys for the ribosomal RNA transcription factor hUBF (human upstream binding factor). Proc Natl Acad Sci USA 1994;91:5672.
31. Andrews P, Howell S. Cellular pharmacology of cisplatin: perspectives on mechanisms of acquired resistance. Cancer Cells 1990;2:35.
32. Perez R, Hamilton T, Ozols R. Resistance to alkylating agents and cisplatin: insights from ovarian carcinoma model systems. Pharmacol Ther 1990;48:19.
33. Fujii R, Mutoh M, Niwa K, et al. Active efflux system for cisplatin in cisplatin-resistant human KB cells. Jpn J Cancer Res 1994;85:426.
34. Dedon PC, Borch RF. Characterization of the reactions of platinum antitumor agents with biologic and nonbiologic sulfur-containing nucleophiles. Biochem Pharmacol 1987;36:1955.
35. Eastman A. Cross-linking of glutathione to DNA by cancer chemotherapeutic platinum coordination complexes. Chem Biol Interact 1987;61:241.
36. Ishikawa T, Ali-Osman F. Glutathione-associated cis-diamminedichloroplatinum(II) metabolism and ATP-dependent efflux from leukemia cells: Molecular characterization of glutathione-platinum complex and its biological significance. J Biol Chem 1993;268:20116.
37. Mistry P, Loh SY, Kelland LR. Effect of buthionine sulfoximine on PtII and PtIV drug accumulation and the formation of glutathione conjugates in human ovarian-carcinoma cell lines. Int J Cancer 1993; 55:848.
38. Ahn H, Lee E, Kim K, Lee C. Effect of glutathione and its related enzymes on chemosensitivity of renal cell carcinoma and bladder carcinoma cell lines. J Urol 1994;151:263.
39. Pendyala L, Glaves D, Russell PJ, et al. Glutathione in human bladder carcinoma cell lines (BL). (Abstract) Proc Am Assoc Cancer Res 1994;35:2243.
40. Behrens BC, Hamilton TC, Masuda H. Characterization of a cis-diamminedichloroplatinum(II)–resistant human ovarian cancer cell line and its use in evaluation of platinum analogues. Cancer Res 1987;47: 414.
41. Mistry P, Kelland LR, Abel G, Sidhar S, Harrap KR. The relationships between glutathione, glutathione-S-transferase and cytotoxicity of platinum drugs and melphalan in eight human ovarian cancer cell lines. Br J Cancer 1991;64:215.
42. Hamilton TC, Winker MA, Louie KG. Augmentation of adriamycin, melphalan and cisplatin cytotoxicity in drug-resistant and -sensitive human ovarian cancer cell lines by buthionine sulfoximine–mediated glutathione depletion. Biochem Pharmacol 1985;34:2583.
43. Lewis AD, Hayes JD, Wolf CR. Glutathione and glutathione-dependent enzymes in ovarian adenocarcinoma cell lines derived from a patient before and after the onset of drug resistance: intrinsic differences and cell cycle effects. Carcinogenesis 1988;9:1283.
44. Godwin AK, Meister A, O'Dwyer PJ. High resistance to cisplatin in human ovarian cancer cell lines is associated with marked increase of glutathione synthesis. Proc Natl Acad Sci U S A 1992;89:3070.
45. Britten RA, Green JA, Warenius HM. Cellular glutathione (GSH) and glutathione S-transferase (GST) activity in human ovarian tumor biopsies following exposure to alkylating agents. Int J Radiat Oncol Biol Phys 1992;24:527.
46. Ripple M, Mulcahy RT, Wilding G. Characteristics of the glutathione/glutathione-S-transferase detoxification system in melphalan-resistant human prostate cancer cells. J Urology 1993;150:209.
47. Bailey HH, Gipp JJ, Ripple M, Wilding G, Mulcahy RT. Increase in gamma-glutamylcysteine synthetase activity and steady-state messenger RNA levels in melphalan-resistant DU-145 human prostate carcinoma cells expressing elevated glutathione levels. Cancer Res 1992; 52:5115.
48. Pendyala L, Creaven PJ, Zdanowicz J, Velagapudi S, Huben R, Raghavan D. Glutathione (GSH) in human bladder carcinoma (BC) and normal bladder (NB) tissue. (Abstract) Proc Am Assoc Cancer Res 1995;36:1877.
49. Teicher BA, Holden SA, Kelley MJ. Characterization of a human squamous-carcinoma cell line resistant to cis-diamminedichloroplatinum(II). Cancer Res 1987;47:388.
50. Andrews PA, Murphy MP, Howell SB. Differential potentiation of

alkylating and platinating agent cytotoxicity in human ovarian carcinoma cells by glutathione depletion. Cancer Res 1985;45:6250.

51. Richon VM, Schulte N, Eastman A. Multiple mechanisms of resistance to cis-diamminedichloroplatinum(II) in murine leukemia L1210 cells. Cancer Res 1987;47:2056.
52. Billings PC, Davis RJ, Engelsberg BN, Skov KA, Hughes EN. Characterization of high mobility group protein binding to cisplatin-damaged DNA. Biochem Biophys Res Comm 1992;188:1286.
53. Lai G-M, Ozols RF, Young RC, Hamilton TC. Effect of glutathione on DNA repair in cisplatin-resistant human ovarian cancer cell lines. Biochem Pharmacol 1989;37:4597.
54. Hamer DH. Metallothionein. Annu Rev Biochem 1986;55:913.
55. Pattanaik A, Bachowski G, Laib J. Properties of the reaction of cis-dichlorodiammineplatinum(II) with metallothionein. J Biol Chem 1992;267:16121.
56. Kelley SL, Basu A, Teicher BA, Hacker MP, Hamer DH, Lazo JS. Overexpression of metallothionein confers resistance to anticancer drugs. Science 1988;241:1813.
57. Andrews PA, Murphy MP, Howell SB. Metallothionein-mediated cisplatin resistance in human ovarian carcinoma cells. Cancer Chemother Pharmacol 1987;19:149.
58. Schilder RJ, Hall L, Monks A. Metallothionein gene expression and resistance to cisplatin in human ovarian cancer. Int J Cancer 1990; 45:416.
59. Murphy D, McGown AT, Crowther D, Mander A, Fox BW. Metallothionein levels in ovarian tumors before and after chemotherapy. Br J Cancer 1991;63:711.
60. Chin JL, Banerjee D, Kadhim SA, Kontozoglou TE, Chauvin PJ, Cherian MG. Metallothionein in testicular germ cell tumors and drug resistance. Cancer 1993;72:3029.
61. Saika T, Akebi N, Tsushima T, Matsumura Y, Ohmori H. Expression of metallothionein in bladder cancer. J Urol 1991;145:404A.
62. Lai G-M, Ozols RF, Smyth JF, Young RC, Hamilton TC. Enhanced DNA repair and resistance to cisplatin in human ovarian cancer. Biochem Pharmacol 1988;37:4597.
63. Bohr VA. Gene specific DNA repair. Carcinogenesis 1991;87:1983.
64. Johnson SW, Swiggard PA, Handel LM. Relationship between platinum-DNA adduct formation, removal, and cytotoxicity in cisplatin sensitive and resistant human ovarian cancer cells. Cancer Res 1994; 54:5911.
65. Dabholkar M, Vionnet J, Bostick-Bruton F, Yu JJ, Reed E. Messenger RNA levels of XPAC and ERCC1 in ovarian cancer tissue correlate with response to platinum-based chemotherapy. J Clin Invest 1994; 94:703.
66. Hill BT, Shellard SA, Hosking LK, Fitchinger-Shepman AMJ. Enhanced DNA repair and tolerance of DNA damage associated with resistance to cis-diamminedichloroplatinum(II) after in vitro exposure of a human teratoma cell line to fractionated x-irradiation. Int J Radiat Oncol Biol Phys 1990;19:75.
67. Mamenta EL, Poma EE, Kaufmann WK, Delmastro DA, Grady HL, Chaney SG. Enhanced replicative bypass of platinum-DNA adducts in cisplatin-resistant human ovarian cancer cell lines. Cancer Res 1994;54:3500.
68. McLaughlin K, Stephens I, McMahon N, Brown R. Single-step selection of cisplatin resistant mutants from a human ovarian carcinoma cell line. Cancer Res 1991;51:2242.
69. Enns RE, Hom DK, Thiebaut F, Howell SB. An amplified mitochondrial chaperonin gene causes resistance to cisplatin in human ovarian tumor cells. (Abstract) Proc Am Assoc Cancer Res 1991;32:2098.
70. Wilkes J, Abu-hadid M, Perez R. Relationship between heat shock protein 60 (HSP60) mRNA expression and resistance to platinum analogues in human ovarian and bladder carcinoma cell lines. (Abstract) Proc Am Assoc Cancer Res 1995;36:2396.
71. Kimura E, Enns RE, Alcaraz JE, Arboleda J, Slamon DJ, Howell SB. Correlation of the survival of ovarian cancer patients with mRNA expression of the 60-kD heat shock protein HSP-60. J Clin Oncol 1993;11:891.
72. Nakata B, Barton R, Howell SB, Los G. Association between overexpression of hsp60 and cisplatin resistance in head and neck cancer cells. (Abstract) Proc Am Assoc Cancer Res 1994;35:2778.
73. Shen D-W, Pastan I, Gottesman M. A 52 kD protein is overexpressed in cisplatin-resistant human liver carcinoma cells and in cisplatin-resistant mouse cells after DNA-mediated transformation. (Abstract) Proc Am Assoc Cancer Res 1994;35:2630.
74. Kastan MB, Onyekwere O, Sidrasky D, Vogelstein B, Craig RW. Participation of p53 protein in the cellular response to DNA damage. Cancer Res 1991;51:6304.
75. Fritsche M, Haessler C, Brandner G. Induction of nuclear accumulation of the tumor-suppressor protein p53 by DNA-damaging agents. Oncogene 1993;8:307.
76. Kuerbitz SJ, Plunkett BS, Walsh WV, Kastan MB. Wild-type p53 is a cell cycle checkpoint determinant following irradiation. Proc Natl Acad Sci U S A 1992;89:7491.
77. Lowe SW, Schmitt EM, Smith SW, Osborne BA, Jacks T. p53 is required for radiation-induced apoptosis in mouse thymocytes. Nature 1993;362:847.
78. Clarke AR, Purdie CA, Harrison DJ, et al. Thymocyte apoptosis induced by p53-dependent and independent pathways. Nature 1993; 362:849.
79. Smith ML, Chen I-T, Zhan Q, et al. Interaction of the p53-regulated protein Gadd45 with proliferating cell nuclear antigen. Science 1994; 266:1376.
80. Wang XW, Forrester K, Yeh H, Feitelson MA, Gu JR, Harris CC. Hepatitis B virus X protein inhibits p53 sequence-specific DNA binding, transcriptional activity, and association with transcription factor ERCC3. Proc Natl Acad Sci USA 1994;91:2230.
81. Brown R, Clugston C, Burns P, et al. Increased accumulation of p53 protein in cisplatin-resistant ovarian cell lines. Int J Cancer 1993;55: 678.
82. Fujiwara T, Grimm EA, Mukhopadhay T, Zhang W-W, Owen-Schaub LB, Roth JA. Induction of chemosensitivity in human lung cancer cells in vivo by adenovirus-mediated transfer of wild-type p53 gene. Cancer Res 1994;54:2287.
83. Isonishi S, Hom D, Thiebaut F, et al. Expression of the c-Ha-ras oncogene in mouse NIH 3T3 cells induces resistance to cisplatin. Cancer Res 1991;51:5903.
84. Peters G, Wets M, Keepers Y, Van Ark-Otte J, Pinedo H. The effect of transformation of mouse fibroblasts with H-ras and trk on drug sensitivity and metabolism. (Abstract) Proc Am Assoc Cancer Res 1991;32:2373.
85. Sklar M. Increased resistance to cis-diamminedichloroplatinum(II) in NIH 3T3 cells transformed by *ras* oncogenes. Cancer Res 1988;48: 793.
86. Toffoli G, Viel A, Tumiotto L, Buttazi P, Biscontin G, Boiocchi M. Sensitivity pattern of normal and Ha-ras transformed NIH3T3 fibroblasts to antineoplastic drugs. Tumori 1989;75:423.
87. Merriman R, Shackelford K, Tanzer L, Robison P, Swift R. Transformation of epithelial cells by *ras* oncogenes does not increase their resistance to anticancer drugs. (Abstract) Proc Am Assoc Cancer Res 1990;31:2647.
88. Perez RP, Hamaguchi K, Tracey PA, Handel LM, Hamilton TC, Godwin AK. Transformation of Rat ovarian epithelial and Rat-1 fibroblast cell lines by *RAS* T24 does not influence cisplatin sensitivity. Cancer Res 1993;53:3771.
89. Andrews P, Albright K. Mitochondrial defects in cis-diamminedichloroplatinum(II)-resistant human ovarian carcinoma cells. Cancer Res 1992;52:1895.
90. Zinkewich-Peotti K, Andrews P. Loss of cis-diamminedichloroplatinum(II) resistance in human ovarian carcinoma cells selected for rhodamine 123 resistance. Cancer Res 1992;52:1902.
91. Zinkewich-Peotti K, Andrews P. Mitochondrial DNA-depletion of cisplatin resistant human ovarian carcinoma cells is accompanied by loss of drug resistance. (Abstract) Proc Am Assoc Cancer Res 1992; 33:3213.
92. Kelland LR, Mistry P, Abel G, et al. Mechanism-related circumvention of acquired cis-diamminedichloroplatinum(II) resistance using two pairs of human ovarian carcinoma cell lines by ammine/amine platinum(IV) dicarboxylates. Cancer Res 1992;52:3857.
93. Parker R, Vionnet J, Bostick-Burton F, Reed E. Ormaplatin sensitivity/resistance in human ovarian cancer cells made resistant to cisplatin. Cancer Res 1993;53:242.
94. Glavy J, Pendyala L, Creaven PJ, Perez R, Zdanowicz J, Elakawi Z. Isolation and preliminary characterization of oxaliplatin resistant A2780 ovarian carcinoma sublines. (Abstract) Proc Am Assoc Cancer Res 1994;35:2590.
95. Jekunen A, Vick J, Sanga S, Chan TC, Howell SB. Synergism between dipyridamole and cisplatin in human ovarian carcinoma cells in vitro. Cancer Res 1992;52:3566.
96. Keane TE, Rosner GL, Gingrich JR, Poulton SH, Walther PJ. The therapeutic impact of dipyridamole: chemopotentiation of the cyto-

toxic combination 5-fluorouracil/cisplatin in an animal model of human bladder cancer. J Urol 1991;146:1418.
97. Keane TE, Rosner G, Donaldson JT, Norwood DL, Poulton SH, Wealther PJ. Dipyridamole-cisplatin potentiation: enhanced in vivo cytotoxicity in xenograft models of human bladder and testicular cancers. J Urol 1990;144:1004.
98. Wallner K, DeGregorio M, Li G. Hyperthermic potentiation of cis-diamminedichloroplatinum(II) cytotoxicity in Chinese hamster ovary cells resistant to the drug. Cancer Res 1986;46:6242.
99. Mansouri A, Hanle K, Benson A, Moss A, Nagle W. Characterization of a cisplatin-resistant subline of murine RIF-1 cells and reversal of drug resistance by hyperthermia. Cancer Res 1989;49:2674.
100. Noguchi S, Kubota Y, Miura T, Shuin T, Hosaka M. Use of methotrexate, vinblastine, adriamycin, and cisplatin in combination with radiation and hyperthermia as neo-adjuvant therapy for bladder cancer. Cancer Chemother Pharmacol 1992;30(Suppl):s63.
101. Chen G, Zeller W. Augmentation of cisplatin (DDP) cytotoxicity in vivo by d,l-buthionine sulfoximine (BSO) in DDP-sensitive and -resistant rat ovarian tumors and its relation to DNA interstrand cross-links. Anticancer Res 1991;11:2231.
102. O'Dwyer P, Hamilton T, Young R, et al. Depletion of glutathione in normal and malignant human cells in vivo by buthionine sulfoximine: clinical and biochemical results. J Natl Cancer Inst 1992;84:264.
103. Bailey HH, Mulcahy RT, Tutsch KD, et al. Phase I clinical trial of intravenous L-buthionine sulfoximine and melphalan: an attempt at modulation of glutathione. J Clin Oncol 1994;12:194.
104. Bailey HH, Wilding G, Tutsch KD, et al. A phase I trial of L-S,R-buthionine sulfoximine (BSO) given as a 24- to 48-hour continuous infusion (CI) with iv melphalan (L-PAM). (Abstract) Proc Am Soc Clin Oncol 1994;13:334.
105. Yao K-S, Godwin AK, Ozols RF, Hamilton TC, O'Dwyer PJ. Variable baseline γ-glutamylcysteine synthetase messenger RNA expression in peripheral mononuclear cells of cancer patients, and its induction by buthionine sulfoximine treatment. Cancer Res 1993;53:3662.
106. O'Dwyer PJ, Moyer LD, Suffness M, et al. Antitumor activity and biochemical effects of aphidicolin glycinate (NSC 303812) alone and in combination with cisplatin in vivo. Cancer Res 1994;54:724.
107. Sessa C, Zuchetti M, Davoli E, et al. Phase I and clinical evaluation of aphidicolin glycinate. J Natl Cancer Inst 1991;83:1160.
108. Hills C, Kelland L, Abel G, Siracky J, Wilson A, Harrap K. Biological properties of ten human ovarian carcinoma cell lines: calibration in vitro against four platinum complexes. Br J Cancer 1989;59:527.
109. Perez R, O'Dwyer P, Handel L, Ozols R, Hamilton T. Comparative cytotoxicity of CI-973, cisplatin, carboplatin, and tetraplatin in human ovarian carcinoma cell lines. Int J Cancer 1991;48:265.
110. Schurig JE, Rose WC, Catino JJ, et al. The pharmacologic characteristics of carboplatin: preclinical experience. In: Bunn PA, Canetta R, Ozols RF, Rozencweig M, eds. Carboplatin (JM8): current perspectives and future directions. Philadelphia: WB Saunders, 1990:3.
111. Gore ME, Fryatt I, Wiltshaw E, Dawson T, Robinson BA, Calvert AH. Cisplatin/carboplatin cross-resistance in ovarian cancer. Br J Cancer 1989;60:767.
112. Eisenhauer EA, Swenerton KD, Sturgeon JFG, Fine S, O'Reilly SE, Canetta R. Carboplatin therapy for recurrent ovarian carcinoma: a National Cancer Institute of Canada experience and a review of the literature. In: Bunn PA, Canetta R, Ozols RF, Rozencweig M, eds. Carboplatin (JM8): current perspectives and future directions. Philadelphia: WB Saunders, 1990:133.
113. Van Glabbeke M, Renard J, Pinedo HM, et al. Iproplatin and carboplatin induced toxicities: overview of phase II clinical trials conducted by the EORTC early clinical trials cooperative group (ECTG). Eur J Cancer Clin Oncol 1988;24:255.
114. Cornelison TL, Reed E. Nephrotoxicity and hydration management for cisplatin, carboplatin, and ormaplatin. Gynecol Oncol 1993;50:147.
115. Theriault RL, Cohen IA, Esparza L, Kowal C, Raber MN. Phase I clinical evaluation of [SP-4-3(R)]-[1,1-cyclo-butanedicarboxylato-(2-)](2-methyl-1,4-butanediamine-N,N^1) platinum in patients with metastatic solid tumors. Cancer Chemother Pharmacol 1993;31:333.
116. O'Dwyer PJ, Hudes GR, Walczak J, et al. Phase I and pharmacokinetic study of the novel platinum analogue CI-973 on a 5-daily dose schedule. Cancer Res 1992;52:6746.
117. Creaven PJ, Madajewicz S, Pendyala L, et al. Phase I clinical trial of cis-dichloro-trans-dihydroxy-bis-isopropylamine platinum IV (CHIP). Cancer Treat Rep 1983;67:795.
118. Bramwell VHC, Crowther D, O'Malley S, et al. Activity of JM9 in advanced ovarian cancer: a phase I-II trial. Cancer Treat Rep 1985;69:409.
119. Madajewicz S, Takita H, Creaven PJ, Bareniewski H, Regal A-M, Cushman K. Phase II study of iproplatin (IPP) in small cell carcinoma of the lung (SCL). (Abstract) Proc Am Soc Clin Oncol 1984;3:224.
120. de Wit R, Tesselaar M, Kok TC, et al. Randomised phase II trial of carboplatin and iproplatin in advanced urothelial cancer. Eur J Cancer 1991;27:1383.
121. Murphy BA, Motzer RJ, Bosl GJ. Phase II study of iproplatin (CHIP) in patients with cisplatin-refractory germ cell tumors: the need for alternative strategies in the investigation of new agents in GCT. Invest New Drugs 1992;10:327.
122. Drasga RE, Williams SD, Einhorn LH, Birch R. Phase II evaluation of iproplatin in refractory germ cell tumors: a Southeastern Cancer Study Group trial. Cancer Treat Rep 1987;71:863.
123. Harrap KR, Kelland LR, Jones M, et al. Platinum coordination complexes which circumvent cisplatin resistance. Adv Enzyme Regul 1991;31:31.
124. Kelland LR, Murrer BA, Abel G, Giandomenico CM, Mistry P, Harrap KR. Ammine/amine platinum(IV) dicarboxylates: a novel class of platinum complex exhibiting selective cytotoxicity to intrinsically cisplatin-resistant ovarian carcinoma cell lines. Cancer Res 1992;52:822.
125. Twentyman PR, Wright KA, Mistry P, Kelland LR, Murrer BA. Sensitivity to novel platinum compounds of panels of human lung cancer cell lines with acquired and inherent resistance to cisplatin. Cancer Res 1992;52:5674.
126. McKeague MJ, Mistry P, Ward J, et al. Phase I study of orally administered ammine diacetatodichloro(cyclohexylamine)platinum(pt)(IV) (PO JM216). (Abstract) Proc Am Soc Clin Oncol 1993;12:320.
127. Anderson WK, Quagliato DA, Haugwitz RD, Narayanan VL, Wolpert-Defilippes MK. Synthesis, physical properties, and antitumor activity of tetraplatin and related tetrachloroplatin(IV) stereoisomers of 1,2-diaminocyclohexane. Cancer Treat Rep 1986;70:997.
128. Chaney SG, Wyrick S, Till GK. In vitro biotransformations of tetrachloro(d,l-*trans*)-1,2-diaminocyclohexaneplatinum(IV) (tetraplatin) in rat plasma. Cancer Res 1990;50:4539.
129. Kelland LR, Jones M, Abel G, Valenti M, Gwynne J, Harrap KR. Human ovarian carcinoma cell lines and companion xenografts: a disease-oriented approach to new platinum anticancer drug discovery. Cancer Chemother Pharmacol 1992;30:43.
130. Schilder RJ, La Creta FP, Perez RP, et al. Phase I and pharmacokinetic study of ormaplatin (tetraplatin, NSC 363812) administered on a day 1 and day 8 schedule. Cancer Res 1994;54:709.
131. O'Rourke T, Rodriguez G, Eckardt J, et al. Neurotoxicity of ormaplatin (NSC 363812) in a phase I trial of a daily times five schedule. (Abstract) Proc Am Soc Clin Oncol 1993;12:348.
132. Christian MC, Kohn E, Sarosy G, et al. Phase I and pharmacokinetic study of ormaplatin (OP)/tetraplatin. (Abstract) Proc Am Soc Clin Oncol 1992;11:291.
133. Tutsch KD, Arzoomanian RZ, Alberti D, Feierabend C, Robins HI, Spriggs DR. Phase I trial and pharmacokinetic study of ormaplatin. (Abstract) Proc Am Assoc Cancer Res 1992;33:3202.
134. Plaxe SC, Braly PS, Freddo JL, et al. Phase I and pharmacokinetic study of intraperitoneal ormaplatin. Gynecol Oncol 1993;51:72.
135. Misset JL, Kidani Y, Gastiaburu J, et al. Oxaliplatin (l-OHP): experimental and clinical studies. In: Howell SB, ed. Platinum and other metal coordination compounds in cancer chemotherapy. New York: Plenum Press, 1991:369.
136. Tashiro T, Kawada Y, Sakuri Y, Kidani Y. Antitumor activity of a new platinum complex, oxalato (trans-l-1,2-diaminocyclohexane)platinum(II): new experimental data. Biomed Pharmacother 1989;43:251.
137. Pendyala L, Creaven PJ. In vitro cytotoxicity, protein binding, red blood cell partitioning, and biotransformation of oxaliplatin. Cancer Res 1993;53:5970.
138. Cvitkovic E, Fereres M, Soulie P, et al. High activity in pretreated germ cell tumors (GCT) of combined oxaliplatin (l-OHP) cisplatin (CP) based salvage regimen. (Abstract) Proc Am Assoc Cancer Res 1994;35:1389.
139. Misset JL, Soulie P, Fereres M, et al. High efficacy of combined oxaliplatin (l-OHP) cisplatin (CP) as salvage treatment in pretreated ovarian cancer (OC). (Abstract) Proc Am Assoc Cancer Res 1994;35:1398.

Principles and Practice of Genitourinary Oncology, edited by Derek Raghavan, Howard I. Scher, Steven A. Leibel, and Paul H. Lange. Lippincott-Raven Publishers, Philadelphia, © 1997.

CHAPTER 10

Gene Therapy for Genitourinary Cancer

William H. Sweatt and Jonathan W. Simons

Human gene therapy has emerged as an experimental modality of cancer therapeutics in the past few years. As a field, clinical cancer gene therapy is thus in its infancy. More reviews about gene therapy have appeared in the literature than published complete clinical responses. Nevertheless, since 1993, over 100 peer-reviewed manuscripts in human gene therapy have been published. Furthermore, 98 clinical protocols of human gene therapy have gained approval of the Recombinant DNA Advisory Committee (RAC) of the National Institutes of Health (NIH) since the treatment of the first patient with gene therapy in 1990. Seven clinical trials of therapeutic gene transfer in the treatment of urologic cancers are under way, and more are under active development or are pending approval (Fig. 10-1).

RATIONALE FOR THE CANCER GENE THERAPY RESEARCH EXPLOSION

Investigation into the potential gene therapy for cancer has exploded since the first human gene therapy experiments were performed in 1989 and 1990. Expansion in gene therapy research for cancer is notable when compared with gene therapy for other diseases, especially inherited disorders, in which gene therapy in human clinical trials first started and immediately showed promise, as described in this chapter.

Gene therapy as a field of inquiry is the natural consequence in medicine of the wider societal revolution wrought in the second half of this century by the "information age." Its ascendance coincides with the growth of telecommunications and computers. At its essence, gene therapy is simply therapy using *molecular* information. The identification of the pivotal role of DNA in the information systems of life and the subsequent emergence of molecular biology and its technologies have led to the inevitable use of the genetic code itself to treat human disease.[1–6] Human gene therapy for genitourinary cancers was made possible by concurrent advances in therapeutic gene transfer in animal models of disease and the molecular biology of recombinant vectors for therapeutic DNA transfer into human cells.

Six reasons can specifically help to explain the phenomenon of gene therapy research growth in oncology:

1. The current need for more effective cancer treatment of many high-incidence solid tumors (prostate, breast, lung, and colon cancers) has been a potent motivator.[7]
2. Of all the diseases amenable to gene therapy, the ethics of clinical trials are perhaps most compelling for metastatic cancers, with the lowest risk-to-benefit ratio.[8] So far, clinical trials for cancer therapy approved in the United States have involved metastatic malignant diseases that are incurable, with life expectancies measured in months. Thus, cancer has been considered more appropriate ethically for untested technologies of human gene transfer.[9]
3. A formidable increase in understanding the molecular origin of neoplastic disease has clearly occurred over the last 10 years. Neoplasia is not one disease resulting from the same genetic lesions, which produces similar pathologic phenotypes. Rather, neoplastic disease is generally considered to be 150 to 200 different neoplastic diseases, with different genetic lesions resulting in different phenotypic characteristics, depending on the tissue source of the neoplastic cells.[7] Many genetic lesions contributing to carcinogenesis have been identified for various neoplasms, including the expression of oncogenes, loss of function of tumor suppressor genes, and acquisition of resistance to chemotherapy through altered gene expression.[7] The success of the Human Genome Project is intercurrent with expanding gene therapy research. Identifying the diversity of genetic lesions in carcinogenesis lends itself to an ever-expanding list of human genes as potential targets for therapeutic pharmacologic agents based on DNA sequence.
4. Organized cancer research has the funding and young investigator research manpower in molecular biology to make greater headway in this field.
5. Human tumor cells can be manipulated ex vivo, whereas the affected tissues (e.g., lung, central nervous system) from individuals with other genetic diseases often cannot. Ex vivo manipulation is often much easier and more controlled than in vivo manipulation and is more acceptable to the regulatory review committees for studying effects of transduction in early clinical trials.[9]
6. Gene therapy using immunostimulatory genes or tumoricidal bystander killing may be generalizable across different types of common epithelial cancers in preclinical testing,

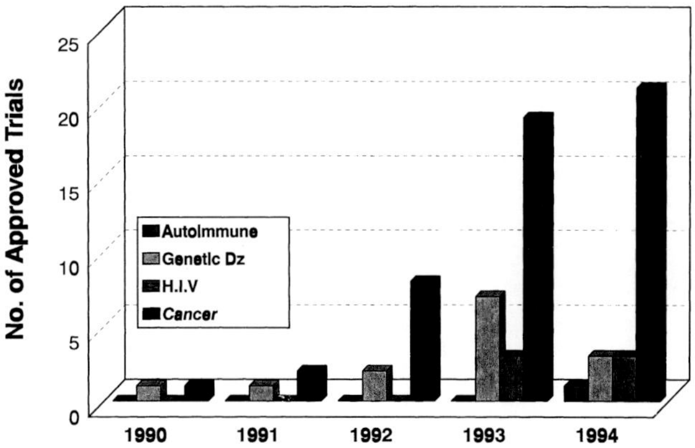

FIG. 10-1. Growth in the number of human gene therapy trials approved by the National Institutes of Health Recombinant DNA Advisory Committee (NIH RAC) between 1990 and 1994.

> whereas molecular treatment of rare inherited genetic diseases requires the isolation, cloning, and functional characterization of the appropriate gene in each disorder.[9]

Familiarity with basic principles of gene therapy can assist the thoughtful clinician to evaluate critically the expanding clinical literature in this area.

DEFINITIONS AND HISTORICAL OVERVIEW

Gene therapy can be precisely defined as the introduction of a normal or modified gene into human cells to reverse a genetic or acquired disease through the in vivo synthesis of an absent, mutant, or insufficient gene product[1] (Fig. 10-2). The strategy is to treat, cure, or prevent cancer by altering the genetic characteristics and, in most cases, the diseased phenotype of the human cell.[1] The genetic modification can be performed either ex vivo or in vivo, depending on the strategy.

Gene therapy with permanent incorporation of the therapeutic gene into the cell's chromosomes closely resembles molecular surgery. A tissue or organ is modified through anastomosis of the therapeutic gene into the DNA of human cells of the recipient. Gene therapy is also rooted in pharmacology, with the application of genetic principles to the treatment of human disease, that is, the ability to treat human disease with externally administered vectors or gene-modified human cells that have specific therapeutic actions. Aposhian, one of the first investigators to attempt recombinant viral vector usage, stated in 1969, "If one considers the purpose of a drug to be to restore the normal function of some particular process in the body, then DNA would be considered to be the ultimate drug."[10,11]

In the absence of identification of the molecules encoding heredity, theoretical biologists, such as Haldane, speculated on the possibility of gene manipulation to treat disease as early as the 1920s.[12] Much of this scientific speculation was brought on by the spectacular success in the United States in agriculture of hybrid corn during the early part of the twentieth century. Out of this rediscovery of Mendel and an expanding knowledge of Mendelian genetics came the first uses of the term *genetic engineering* in a paper of that title presented at the Sixth International Congress of Genetics held in 1932 in Ithaca, New York.[13] Genetic engineering was defined as the application of genetic principles to animal and plant breeding. The term *gene therapy* was adopted by Szybalski, who performed some of the earliest mammalian gene transfer experiments in poultry. He later wrote, " . . . when presenting our data at seminars and symposia in 1962–64, we coined the terms 'gene surgery' and 'gene therapy' to stress the clinical potential of our work . . . . "[14,15] In the interval immediately preceding the modern recombinant DNA era, key elements of current gene therapy research were clearly enumerated. In 1966, Tatum predicted that viruses could be used to introduce therapeutic genes into human cells. Tatum speculated that, because the basis of cancer is altered genes, "treatment could be achieved by modification and regulation of gene activities, or by means of gene repair or replacement."[16] By the late 1960s and early 1970s, gene therapy became the subject of an increasing number of articles and meetings.[11]

Gene therapy as a field was advanced technically by Hershey and Chase in 1952, with their work demonstrating the roles of nucleic acids in bacterial viruses; DNA was subsequently accepted as the genetic material.[17] In 1953, Watson and Crick demonstrated the double-helical structure of DNA,[2,18] allowing scientists to understand the way in which information coded by DNA could be replicated and could also accurately be turned into protein. Fundamental discoveries by geneticists, biochemists, and cell biologists led to concepts that underpin current gene therapy strategies. These concepts include (1) the determination of the genetic code for amino acids and (2) definition of the process of using DNA sequences in the generation of full-length messenger RNA. Most of these advances were made by work carried out on the bacterium *Escherichia coli*. Work on mammalian cells was subsequently done by scientists in the late 1960s and early 1970s.[19]

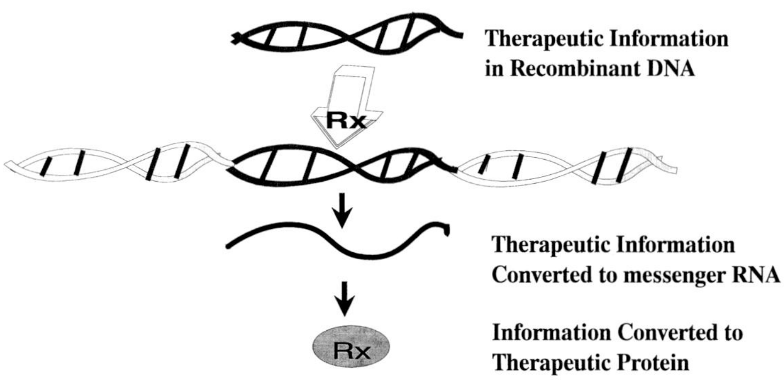

FIG. 10-2. Flow chart depicting the process of introducing therapeutic information to reverse disease with gene therapy.

Practical methods of gene transfer began to be considered after discovery in three research areas in the 1970s and early 1980s. These three areas were, respectively, (1) the achievement by tumor viruses of oncogenic transformation by integration of viral DNA stably into the DNA of target human cells, (2) development of effective ways to transfer DNA into mammalian cells, and (3) general advances in recombinant DNA technologies capable of isolating and generating large amounts of pure gene sequences in a short time.[20]

Out of the study of retroviruses in cancer pathogenesis emerged, in 1989, the first clinical research in human gene therapy, as a "proof of concept" clinical trial. The ex vivo approach to gene therapy was essential in the development of the first sanctioned gene therapy clinical protocols. The objective of this ex vivo approach was to demonstrate technical feasibility and human safety. An objective was to test the ability to monitor and control the quality of genetically modified human cells before their administration to a patient. The first clinical testing of cancer gene therapy was in the form of a clinical protocol to use retroviral vectors to introduce a gene into human lymphocytes, tumor infiltrating lymphocytes (TIL). These genetically marked TIL cells were generated to follow the fate of the cells in humans in an adoptive immunotherapy procedure.

In this first human gene transfer trial for TIL therapy of metastatic cancers, TIL cells were taken from tumor deposits, were cultured and expanded with interleukin-2 (IL-2), and were then reinjected into the patients. In a patient cohort with refractory cancers, Rosenberg and colleagues had previously reported that a significant fraction of the patients responded to therapy with IL-2 plus TIL.[21] More than 50% of the patients' cancers still failed to respond, however, and even among responders, relapse could occur within 6 to 12 months. A significant hindrance at the time to understanding these clinical results was the inability to follow or "track" the fate of autologous TIL cells, except with short half-life indium-111 labeling.[22] The gene marking protocol was therefore developed to monitor trafficking of TIL back to metastatic sites of tumors. The bacterial antibiotic resistance gene, neomycin phosphotransferase, was chosen as the marker gene. No adverse effects were noted from genetically marking the lymphocytes with a bacterial gene using a retroviral gene transfer. Genetically marked TIL were measurable by the polymerase chain reaction (PCR) in patients months after gene transfer and reinfusion. Although it was only a feasibility study, the trial showed that the biotechnology and the United States regulatory review process for clinical trials in human gene therapy were in place.

After the TIL gene marker clinical protocol was successfully and safely implemented, Anderson, Blaese, and Culver at the NIH conducted a therapeutic protocol for the genetic disease, adenosine deaminase (ADA) deficiency, which is manifested as severe combined immunodeficiency. This protocol involved the isolation of peripheral lymphocytes from patients with *ADA* gene deficiency, introduction of a human *ADA* gene by retroviral vector in vitro, expansion of the genetically modified lymphocytes making the ADA enzyme for a few days, and their subsequent reintroduction into the patient. The clinical protocol received the approval of the RAC and the Food and Drug Administration (FDA), and it was begun on a 4-year-old girl at the NIH in September 1990, followed by a second patient in January 1991.[20]

RESULTS

Data from the early cohort of human gene therapy clinical trials are limited. Most trials were phase I studies, with efficacy testing now commencing. Success in meeting the modest study objectives of safety of administration with some of these clinical trials has already occurred. Results in the care of patients with ADA deficiency have been encouraging; these patients have had significantly improved immune functions and the presence of gene-corrected T cells in the circulation. Clinical results obtained with these studies have been widely reported.[23,24]

Gene marking was originally used to prove feasibility and safety, but it has also helped solve questions in cancer chemotherapy. Subsequently, gene transfer techniques for gene marking studies have been used for acute myeloid leukemia and neuroblastoma; both have been successful.[20] Efforts are now being directed to studying other processes, including bone marrow purging techniques, which have been useful in demonstrating that the clonal source of relapse is in the harvested bone marrow, rather than in the cytoreduced host. Gene marking of bone marrow has allowed novel approaches to bone marrow purging to be studied in human patients rather than in animal models.[8,25,26]

Ethical considerations are still central to the evaluation of human gene therapy clinical trials. Somatic cell gene therapy is now successfully under way in patients and appears to have gained widespread acceptance. Germ-line and enhancement genetic engineering techniques are being implemented in laboratory and farm animals. The technical ability to attempt human application of these techniques exists.[27] Since the Holocaust, however, discussions of gene therapy research have clearly distinguished between diseased somatic cell therapy and germ cell manipulation. Human germ cell gene transfer and its eugenic implications are the province of ethical debate only. The RAC of the NIH, which oversees all United States human gene therapy research, has not sanctioned this area for clinical research.

CORRECTIVE STRATEGIES OF GENE THERAPY

Basic research in molecular biology has shown that cancer has a genetic basis, that is, a disease of altered genes in which a series of genetic abnormalities accumulates in a cell and results in a pattern of abnormal proliferation.[9] Probably, four to six genetic changes are necessary to produce most genitourinary cancers, whether by point mutations, deletions, translocations, rearrangements, or amplification.[8] These genetic changes cause a dysfunction of the growth control mechanism of the stem cells that turn over in genitourinary organ homeostasis. Enough insight into the molecular mechanisms of carcinogenesis has been gained to identify some of the genetically broken switches, such as oncogenes, tumor suppressor genes, mutator genes, transcription factors (in the nucleus), growth receptors (at the cell membrane), signaling enzymes such as G proteins, tyrosine kinase, and protein kinase C (in the cytoplasm).[28–34] From this knowledge, novel gene therapy strategies to destroy tumors are being developed.[8]

Overall, two human gene therapy strategies are under clinical or preclinical development for the treatment of genitourinary cancers. The first strategy is *corrective* gene therapy; this is the replacement or inactivation of defective copies of genes in preneoplastic or neoplastic cells with genes used to slow or reverse the loss of growth-control pathways. The second strategy is *cytoreductive* gene therapy and includes treatment strategies based on the common goal of selectively killing malignant cells.

The target genes for correction in genitourinary cancers await detection in the majority of cases. Corrective gene therapy is directed at preventing or reversing steps in the pathophysiology of the disease by insertion of a normal, wild-type gene into diseased cells in diseased tissue. For example, treatment of cystic fibrosis (CF) by insertion of wild-type *CF* genes into bronchial epithelial cells of patients with CF is under study. Several inherited urologic cancer syndromes have been identified. A growing list of potential mutated tumor suppressor genes may be "corrected" in urologic cancers by in vivo gene therapy of early neoplasia. Antisense constructs are under development to block effects of overexpressed or mutated oncogenes or genes that block cancer cell apoptosis. Mutated *P53* genes in bladder cancers, mutated retinoblastoma genes in bladder cancer, the von Hippel Lindau (*VHL*) gene on chromosome 3p in renal cancer, and two Wilms' tumor suppressor genes (*WT1* and *WT2*) are all genomic DNA lesions that are potential targets of corrective gene therapy in ongoing investigations.[28–34]

In theory, affected genitourinary tract stem cells in the setting of known inheritance of a genitourinary cancer syndrome could be treated by transfer of wild-type genes before the onset of clinical disease. Genetic testing on the horizon will clearly allow identification of patients at risk of developing familial cancer syndromes. One potentially attractive aspect of bladder cancer gene therapy in particular is the possibility of delivering corrective genes, for example wild-type retinoblastoma or *P53* genes, through intravesical instillation by the urologist of vectors to the bladder mucosa.[35] Efficient gene transfer and fidelity of expression are essential to the success of this approach. Through cystoscopy, biopsy, and PCR, efficiency of gene transfer in vivo could be easily measured and therapeutic effects monitored.

This approach has three potential limitations. First, corrective gene therapy requires ultimately that 100% of cancer cells be corrected, or inevitably malignant clones expand and metastasize. In vivo gene transfer efficiencies by intravenous administration or local administration are under 10% of cancer cells at best with a single treatment. Second, correcting one genetic defect in a multistep process of genetic hits may not be sufficient once the cancer has produced a fully invasive and metastatic clone. Corrective gene therapy may be tested as an active strategy for cancer prevention in situ in the future. Finally, some target genes for correction have not yet been identified for common genitourinary cancers such as bladder and prostate cancers.

CYTOREDUCTIVE STRATEGIES OF GENE THERAPY

In addition to reversing genetic mutations, cancer gene therapy also permits the local (paracrine) delivery of therapeutic agents to kill neoplastic cells. The tumoricidal effects can be driven from therapeutic information in the DNA molecule either through activation of antitumor T-cell killing or directly by tumoricidal proteins.

The most thoroughly evaluated form of cytoreductive cancer gene therapy involves stimulation of an antitumor immune response against a malignant process by vaccinating affected patients with genetically modified tumor cells. Tumor cells are removed surgically from the patient, are placed into tissue culture, and are genetically transduced with a gene for immunostimulatory cytokines. The gene-modified tumor vaccine is then irradiated to prevent subsequent tumor growth and is reinjected into the patient. Cells mediating an antitumor immune response are activated by the presence of immunostimulatory gene products made by the transduced tumor vaccine cells in close proximity to tumor-specific antigens present on the vaccine tumor cell surface. These immune mediator cells, including T cells, natural killer cells, and antigen-presenting cells, can then circulate and eradicate or slow the growth of distant micrometastases. Ex vivo gene transfer into the tumor cells is required because the tumor cells alone do not make sufficient immunostimulatory gene products to act as an effective vaccine. This form of cancer gene therapy, known as cytoreductive gene therapy, already shows clear promise in preclinical testing and is maturing into clinical trials.

Over 20 immunostimulatory genes that modulate the immune response have been screened for use in gene-modified tumor vaccine strategies of gene therapy (Dranoff, personal communication). The original report using this strategy showed induction of antitumor effect in nude mice by vaccination of tumor cells transduced to secrete IL-2; this study aimed to achieve nonspecific (T-cell independent) antitumor effect by producing significant systemic levels of IL-2.[36] Fearon and colleagues then demonstrated that an immune response that was tumor specific and T-cell mediated can be augmented by vaccination of tumor cells of the same origin as treated cells after transduction with IL-2[37]; such vaccination protected animals from subsequent tumor challenge.[38] Interferon gamma was shown to protect against subsequent tumor challenge as well.[39] Other cytokines, including IL-4, IL-6, and granulocyte-macrophage colony-stimulating factor (GM-CSF), were then shown to have the ability to eliminate microscopic tumor cell deposits when mouse tumor cells were transduced with the respective cytokine genes and when these cytokine-secreting tumors were then used as therapeutic vaccines.[40–52]

These preclinical gene therapy studies should be viewed in context, however. The antitumor effect seen in animal models in treating preestablished cancers has been modest, in the range of 4 log kill. In these animal models, the tumor cells may multiply faster than T cells generated by genetically engineered tumor vaccines. Only clinical trial testing will determine whether larger tumor burdens in humans can be cytoreduced using genetically modified tumor vaccines. In addition, many of the preclinical studies were performed with highly immunogenic animal tumor models (expressing high levels of class I major histocompatibility complex [MHC]) that may not necessarily reflect potentially weak immunogenicity of human cancer cells as vaccines.[35–37] The description of prostate cancer production of transforming growth factor-beta (TGF-β),[46] a potent immunosuppressant, raises further questions regarding potential limitations of any form of immunotherapy in prostate cancer specifically. In addition, defects at the molecular level in presenting cell surface antigens have been identified in prostate cancer by our laboratory and by others.

Researchers have addressed some of these potential limitations of cytokine gene-transduced tumor cell vaccines and have extended the studies to animal models of malignant urologic disease, including renal cancer, bladder cancer, and prostate cancer.[42,47–50] IL-2 and GM-CSF gene-transduced tumor vaccines induce antitumor effects that do not rely solely on the interaction of class I MHC and T cells. Furthermore, in poorly immunogenic, androgen-refractory prostate cancer models that secrete TGF-β, GM-CSF-transduced prostate cancer vaccines were more effective than nonspecific adjuvant or systemic cytokine administration.[48,51,52] Both IL-2 and GM-CSF have become ''lead compounds'' for gene therapy clinical research in the immunotherapy of renal, prostate, and bladder cancer.

Based on these studies and others, clinical trials of cytokine-gene-transduced tumor cell vaccines are either planned or ongoing at several institutions (Table 10-1). One limitation in clinical application of gene-transduced cancer cell vaccines is the small tumor burden cured by this strategy of gene therapy in preclinical models; clinical efficacy may be found in the setting of adjuvant therapy. Identification of patients at high risk of urologic cancer relapse from micrometastatic disease after surgery is a critical area for clinical trial development. The advent of new molecular markers of invasive and metastatic clones at diagnostic biopsy should clearly affect the selection of patients for adjuvant gene therapy.

All the data so far suggest that, in addition to the need for harvesting cancer cells from an individual patient for expansion of patient-specific cancer antigens, tumor burden reduction makes urologic surgery currently indispensable.[48,53,54] The resected genitourinary cancer cells serve principally as vehicles for autologous tumor antigens and are transduced for immunostimulatory gene expression. In theory, once tumor-specific antigens for urologic cancers are identified, the practical hurdle of cell culture may be replaced by direct genetic engineering of vaccines expressing DNA sequences of tumor antigens and immunostimulatory genes, bypassing the need for harvesting an individual patient's cells.

Not all patients at the time of cancer, recurrence, for instance, in prostate cancer, have surgically accessible cancer cells for direct genetic modificaton. This is particulary common in prostate cancer recurrences after hormonal therapy. An alternative strategy is to use established human cancer cell lines that have been genetically modified to secrete immunostimulatory molecules as the tumor-specific antigen source.

A second direction in cytoreductive gene therapy under clinical development is transfer of tumoricidal drug susceptibility genes.[55–63] A simple definition of cytoreductive in vivo cancer gene therapy is selective cancer cell killing by expression of a cytotoxic gene, delivered by a vector, administered by a therapist. The therapeutic DNA molecule acts as a prodrug, carrying the cytotoxic information in its sequence. The cancer cell must be transduced to express the cytotoxin gene. Selective cancer cell killing can be a consequence of (1) selective tropism of the vector for cancer versus normal cells, (2) cancer-specific transcription promoters versus normal tissue promoters to express the cytotoxin, cDNA, or (3) selective cytotoxicity of the toxin cells versus normal cells. Critical in this approach is the bystander effect. The bystander effect is the killing of cancer cells by an activated cytotoxin gene several cell diameters away from the transduced cell. This bystander effect amplifies the low efficiency of actual gene transfer into measurable shrinkage of solid tumors in rat models.

The only widely used ''suicide'' gene approach has been with the herpes simplex virus thymidine kinase (*HSV-TK1*) gene in brain tumors and other tumors.[64,65] No data have been published about this approach in preclinical prostate cancer. The most relevant animal model, an experimental rat brain tumor model, has shown efficacy when ganciclovir is administrered intraperitoneally.[64] Ganciclovir has a high affinity for HSV-tk, which phosphorylates ganciclovir to a monophosphate form. Cellular guanosine monophosphate kinase then phosphorylates

Table 10-1. *Phase I clinical trials using gene transfer in the treatment of genitourinary cancers*

Site (principal investigator)	Treatment modality	Disease (limited to urological histology)	Gene transferred	Date of NIH RAC approval
National Cancer Institute (Rosenberg)	Gene-modified tumor cell vaccine	Advanced cancer including renal cell carcinoma	TNF	7/90
National Cancer Institute (Rosenberg)	Gene-modified tumor cell vaccine	Advanced cancer including renal cell carcinoma	IL-2	7/90
University of California Los Angeles (Economou)	Adoptive antitumor lymphocyte tracking	Advanced renal cell carcinoma	Neomycin-resistant	2/92
Sloan-Kettering (Gansbacher)	Gene-modified tumor cell line vaccine	Advanced renal cell carcinoma	Il2	3/92
Johns Hopkins (Simons)	Gene-modified autologous tumor cell vaccine	Advanced renal cell carcinoma	GMCSF	3/93
University of Chicago (Vogelzang)	Direct liposome gene transfer	Metastases of renal cell carcinoma	B7	3/94
Johns Hopkins (Simons)	Gene-modified autologous tumor cell vaccine	Advanced prostate carcinoma	GMCSF	9/94
Slaon-Kettering (Gansbacher and Scher)	Gene-modified cell line vaccine	Advanced prostate carcinoma	IFNG + IL-2	3/95

Several additional protocols are currently under review. NIH RAC, National Institutes of Health Recombinant DNA Advisory Committee.

the monophosphate form of ganciclovir to a triphosphate form. This triphosphate form of ganciclovir is toxic to cancer cells through its high affinity (K_m = 1.5 μmol) for DNA polymerase. Therefore, ganciclovir triphosphate is toxic to any cell in S phase of the cell cycle. Because not all cells are cycling at the same time, some escape the immediate toxic effects of ganciclovir triphosphate.[65,66]

Introduction of the *HSV-tk* gene has been achieved by adenoviral or retroviral vectors.[66] A measurable antitumor effect occurs after exposure of the cells to ganciclovir. Apparently, not all tumor cells must incorporate the ''suicide'' gene.[58,67,68] Noninfected tumor cells can be eradicated by the bystander effect. This effect has been hypothesized to be due to (1) transfer of the HSV-tk enzyme through vesicles, (2) transfer of toxic molecules through gap junctions, (3) transfer of hydrolases or other enzymes associated with programmed cell death that may be induced to nearby cells, (4) upregulation of immune recognition secondary to killing of affected cells, and (5) tissue or tumor ischemia due to integration of *HSV-tk* gene on cell death to adjacent cells.[68] Close cell-cell contact is required for the bystander effect to work. The bystander effect is an attractive feature of cancer gene therapy because current vectors are unable to transduce all cells of a tumor.

Unfortunately, the *HSV-tk* gene for many genitourinary cancers may have limited utility clinically: the S-phase fraction of human prostate cancer is minimal, typically less than 2% of cells at any time.[69] Isaacs and associates have shown that human prostate cancer progression is due to loss of programmed cell death pathways, rather than to increased mitotic rates.[69] In this respect, the preclinical testing of American Type Culture Collection (ATCC) human cell lines for human PCA with high mitotic rates does not reflect the disease clinically. These cell lines are sensitive to S-phase-specific cytotoxic agents such as cytosine arabinoside and methotrexate, but clinical PCA is not. Thus, human PCA in particular may often be resistant to *HSV-tk* gene therapy and ganciclovir, as it is to chemotherapy specific for the S phase of the cell cycle.[70,71] In contrast, bladder cancer with its clinical sensitivity to regimens based on methotrexate, vinblastine, doxorubicin, and cisplatin (MVAC) is an obvious target for this form of gene therapy.

The pathways of cell death in the bystander effect need molecular dissection for improving efficacy. Clearly, this effect can also lead to toxicity related to bystander effect harming local, normal cells. Although this approach has been studied extensively in animal models of brain tumors and mesothelioma, it has not yet been critically tested in the treatment of preclinical models of urologic cancers or taken to clinical trials.

A modification of cytoreductive gene therapy involves *tissue-specific* expression of drug susceptibility genes or cell toxins.[72,73] Vectors being constructed contain tissue-specific promoters that restrict expression of the transferred cytotoxic gene. Prostate cancer is a potentially optimal target for such approaches. By designing a construct with a gene of interest whose expression is controlled by the prostate-specific antigen (PSA) promoter and regulatory sequences, only cells that normally express PSA would express the transferred therapeutic gene product. Pilot studies have examined this approach by evaluating expression of luciferase (a reporter gene that encodes a readily assayed gene product) transcribed downstream from a human PSA promoter sequence after transfection of prostate cancer cell lines in vitro.[73] This approach confers an element of specificity to prostate cell killing using gene therapy.

Finally, using promoters specific for tissue or cancer cells, high concentrations of tumoricidal proteins may be obtained locally by gene transfer when systemic administration would be too toxic. For example, recombinant tumor necrosis factor (rTNF) has been actively explored in gene therapy for its tumoricidal properties and its ability to engender antitumor immune responses. TNF has produced encouraging antitumor responses in mice,[74] but the maximal tolerated dose in humans is 40-fold less than the doses required to elicit this response in mice.[75] Local high concentrations by rTNF gene transfer and secretion by transduced cells appear promising.

INSTRUMENTS OF GENE TRANSFER: VECTOR SYSTEMS

Central to all forms of human gene therapy technology are vectors. Vectors are engineered DNA or RNA sequences that encode sites into which genes of interest can be inserted. The therapeutic gene of interest is generally placed downstream of a promoter sequence for RNA polymerase that allows for expression of the messenger RNA of the gene of interest after the vector enters the cell targeted for gene therapy. Promoter sequences control the expression of downstream genes and thus serve as a critical engineering element of transduction, the process of gene transfer. Indeed, in many applications of gene therapy, the target cell may already have copies of the therapeutic human gene being transferred; however, expression of the native copies of this gene may have been ''turned off'' as a consequence of differentiation, or it may have been mutated as in carcinogenesis. The therapeutic vector provides a copy of the therapeutic gene together with an appropriate promoter, so the ability to *express* the gene of interest is conferred on the target cell.

For example, all human cells have the gene for PSA; however, this gene has a specific regulatory DNA sequence that limits expression to epithelial prostate cells. A vector containing the PSA gene next to an insulin gene promoter could potentially be used to induce PSA expression by beta islet cells of the pancreas; alternately, a vector containing an insulin gene placed next to the PSA promoter could be used to induce prostate-specific expression of insulin, a gene not normally secreted by epithelial prostate cells at endocrine levels.

Both physical and viral methods are being used for vector entry with introduction of therapeutic genes. Physical methods such as bullets of DNA fired from a gene gun, direct microinjection, electroporation, calcium phosphate transfection, liposomal encapsulation, and dextran precipitation are often less efficient, but these techniques are well established in the laboratory.[19] In addition, physical methods are generally inadequate for stable DNA incorporation and cannot readily be adapted for wide in vivo use.[8] Although some physical methods such as liposomal encapsulation do have human gene therapy applications, viral methods are generally much more effective.[75]

Efficacy of vectors is is determined by the need for high-efficiency transduction. High-efficiency transduction is defined as the ability of a vector to insert the gene of interest into many target cells (1 in 2 cells, for instance). As in drug dosage, the copies of the transferred gene per treated cell can be measured by Southern blots. The therapeutic objective is to induce successful expression of the gene of interest in most of those cells. This goal is in contrast to traditional, in vitro gene transfer, which can be achieved for experimental purposes using electroporation, direct injection of DNA, or calcium phosphate precipitation and can transduce only a few cells (1 in 10,000).[72]

Under the constraint of high-efficiency transduction, three current methods for vectors to enter target cells are available for clinical applications: (1) the use of engineered viruses that are indiscriminate in target cell preference; (2) the use of engineered viruses that enter only specific tissues or cells; and (3) the physical method of DNA constructs packaged in liposomes (lipid envelopes) that biophysically fuse and deliver DNA into the cell cytoplasm.[72]

Transduction using viruses can be accomplished with various vectors that are DNA viruses or retroviruses that have been rendered replication defective by genetic engineering, to minimize their potential for causing viral infection in humans[72,76–80] The different types of such constructs available are listed in Table 10-2, and several properties define the potential limitations and advantages of each vector system.[72] First, retroviral vectors and adeno-associated virus (AAV) vectors have the property of mediating gene transfer by stable integration of the gene of interest into the chromosomal DNA of the treated cells. As the target DNA is replicated, so too is the inserted therapeutic gene imbedded in the chromosomal DNA. Thus, transduction with these vectors may be durable, with the gene of interest expressed on a long-term basis in the target cell as well as its progeny. For corrective gene therapy, this characteristic is essential to maintain the corrected cell phenotype over the lifetime of the patient. Gene transfer mediated by adenovirus, vaccinia, and liposomal constructs, in contrast, is generally *episomal:* the transferred gene is expressed without actual integration of the gene into the target cell chromosomal DNA. Until further engineering, these vector systems may not be as well suited for clinical strategies requiring durable expression of transferred therapeutic genes as are retroviral or AAV constructs. For cytoreductive gene therapy, however, transient tumoricidal gene expression may be not only sufficient but desirable in maintaining a high therapeutic index (high cancer cell kill-low normal tissue toxicity). One special family of vectors under development for clinical trials that show tissue specificity is the herpes viruses, which can infect nonreplicating neural cells.

Although retroviral vector-mediated gene transfer can be durable, the decay of viral titer when given intravenously has limited the potential for direct intravenous in vivo gene transfer to diseased cells.[74] These constructs appear better suited for ex vivo gene transfer into cells that are then returned to the patients. Retroviral vectors also require target cell proliferation for integration; gene transfer succeeds only in dividing cells.[81] The possibility of pathogenic mutagenesis during chromosomal insertion of the vector and the difficulty in isolating high titers of retrovirus for clinical use are further limitations of with this vector system.[72]

Some AAV vectors appear to mediate durable genetic transduction and are themselves sufficiently stable for potential direct in vivo gene transfer.[82,83] Integration of AAV genomes into target cell DNA appears less efficient than the best retroviral vectors, however, and it has been associated with a tendency toward inactivations by deletions or rearrangements during gene transfer. Adenovirus and vaccinia vectors can readily transfer genes directly in vivo, but expression of the transferred genes is transient. Adenoviral vectors can transfer larger DNA sequences (in the range of tens of thousands of base pairs) than other viral vector systems. In concept, several therapeutic genes can be delivered simultaneously using these vectors. Adenovirus vectors have been chosen for transmembrane regulatory gene transduction in gene therapy clinical trials in CF; these vectors are attractive because they can efficiently infect nondividing respiratory epithelial cells in vivo. The replication-defective virus particles are amenable to purification and concentration without significant loss of transduction activity. The extensive viral genomic machinery that allows transfer of large sequences of DNA in adenovirus vectors is not without potential cost: these vectors may induce antiviral vector antibodies, potentially limiting prospects for long-term intermittent therapy with this vector in sensitized individuals.[84] Similarly, vaccinia vectors also can induce antiviral vector antibodies, and these vectors are limited by their propensity to induce lysis of target cells.[85] Vaccinia viral vectors are highly immunogenic, however, and they may be excellent platforms for presenting antigen genes to a patient's immune system.

Sophisticated genetic engineering is required to render vector systems clinically safe. For example, one retroviral vector in intensive cancer clinical trials is MFG; it is derived from a mouse leukemia virus. To render this virus replication defective (thus nonpathogenic and useful as a vector), genes encoding the pathogenic viral products GAG and POL were excised. A "packaging cell line" that produces the GAG and POL products is required for final assembly of the retroviral vector for gene transfer.[78] In some adenovirus vectors, portions of the E1 onco-

Table 10-2. *Characteristics of vectors for clinical gene transfer*

Vector	Stable gene expression	Effective in vivo transfer	Current advantages	Current disadvantages
Replication defective retrovirus	+	−	High-efficiency genomic integration	Requires target cell proliferation; potential recombinant retrovirus
Adeno-associated virus	+	?	High stable titer attainable	Deletions on integration?
Replications defective adenovirus	±	+	High titer; accepts large DNA constructs	Episomal
Vaccinia	−	+	High titer	Replication in vivo
Liposomal DNA	−	+	Ease of production, safety features	Low efficiency in vivo intravenously

protein viral sequences are similarly deleted for increased likelihood of clinical safety.[77] Moreover, to engineer virus-derived vectors, mere deletion of sequences important for viral replication is not sufficient. For clinical use, the absence of potential homologous recombination events leading to replication-competent viral particles must also be tested. These issues in the molecular biology of vector construction contribute to the substantial preclinical regulatory review that is required for a vector system to be approved for human gene therapy clinical trial use by the RAC of the NIH, as well as the FDA.[86]

No single vector possesses all the desirable features of every therapeutic application of cancer gene therapy. Some clearly desirable properties of human gene therapy vectors include permanence of transduction, target tissue specificity, high efficiency of in vivo direct gene transfer, fidelity of gene expression levels over time, and capacity for transfer of large DNA sequences. In choosing a vector system for a clinical application in genitourinary cancer research, the relative importance of these performance characteristics is considered. These properties must be evaluated in the context of the therapeutic principle tested.

CONCLUSIONS

In these pioneer years of clinical investigation of human gene therapy, essential are well-designed clinical trials that test principles that inform future basic and clinical research. The simple feasibility of human gene therapy is no longer a compelling rationale for clinical study on its own. Questions of "proof of therapeutic principle" the savvy clinician should ask of future human gene therapy trials include the following:

1. How clear are the data that form the basis for a preclinical therapeutic principle translated into testing in a clinical question?
2. How efficiently was the therapeutic gene put into the targeted cells?
3. How durable and how specific were the expression of the transferred therapeutic gene; what were the pharmacokinetics of the gene therapy?
4. What intermediate end points were measured to detect a therapeutic biologic effect in patients that was predicted from preclinical testing?
5. How can each tested gene therapy approach be integrated into the multimodality treatment of patients with genitourinary cancers?

Gene therapy is unlikely to efface the need for multimodality approaches to the reduction of morbidity and mortality of urologic cancers. If past performance indicates future behavior, however, the rapid discovery in this area of molecular medicine can be predicted to have a great impact on the practice of genitourinary oncology in the twenty-first century. Current approaches, especially vector systems, will likely become outmoded prototypes of technology, like obsolescent software. Yet the new *principles* of molecular therapeutics gene therapy explores have clear potential to be applied to practice.

REFERENCES

1. Kelley WN. The impact of gene therapy on medicine and society: gene therapy for neoplastic diseases. Ann NY Acad Sci 1994;76:12.
2. Watson JD, Crick FH. Molecular structure of nucleic acids: a structure for deoxyribose nucleic acid. Nature 1953;171:737.
3. Abels RI, Rudnick SA. Erythropoietin: evolving clinical applications. Exp Hematol 1991;19:842.
4. Brandt SJ, Peters WP, Atwater SK, et al. Effect of recombinant human granulocyte-macrophage colony-stimulating factor on hematopoietic reconstruction after high-dose chemotherapy and autologous bone marrow transplantation. N Engl J Med 1988;318:869.
5. Rosenburg SA. Karnofsky Memorial Lecture: the immunotherapy and gene therapy and gene therapy of cancer. J Clin Oncol 1992;10: 180.
6. Friedmann T. Progress toward human gene therapy. Science 1989;244: 1275.
7. Huber BE. Gene therapy strategies for treating neoplastic disease. Ann NY Acad Sci 1994;716:6.
8. Sikora K. Genes, dreams, and cancer. Br Med J 1994;308:1217.
9. Culver KW, Blaese RM. Gene therapy for cancer. Trends in Genetics 1994;10:174.
10. Aposhian HV. The use of DNA for gene therapy: the need, experimental approach, and implications. Perspect Biol Med 1970;14:987.
11. Wolff JA, Lederberg J. An early history of gene transfer and therapy. Hum Gene Ther 1994;5:468.
12. Dronamraju KR. J.B.S. Haldane's (1892–1964) biological speculations. Hum Gene Ther 1993;4:303.
13. Crow JF. 60 years ago: the 1932 International Congress of Genetics. Genetics 1992;131:761.
14. Szybalski W. A forerunner of monoclonal antibodies and human gene therapy. Curr Contents 1991;34:11.
15. Szybalski W. Use of the HPRT gene and the HAT selection technique in DNA-mediated transformation of mammalian cells: first steps toward developing hybridoma techniques and gene therapy. Bioessays 1992; 14:495.
16. Tatum EL. Molecular biology, nucleic acids and the future of medicine. Perspect Biol Med 1966;10:19.
17. Hershey AD, Chase M. Independent function of viral protein on nucleic acid on growth of bacteriophage. J Gen Physiol 1952;36:39.
18. Watson JD, Crick FHC. Genetical implications of the structure of deoxyribonucleic acid. Nature 1953;171:37.
19. Harris J, Sikora K. Human genetic therapy. Mol Aspects Med 1993; 14:451.
20. Tolstoshev P. Gene therapy, concepts, current trials and future directions. Annu Rev Pharmacol Toxicol 1993;32:573.
21. Rosenberg SA, Packard BS, Aebersold PM, et al. Use of tumor infiltrating lymphocytes and interleukin-2 in the immunotherapy of patients with metastatic melanoma. N Engl J Med 1988;319:1676.
22. Fisher B, Packard BS, Read EJ, et al. Tumor localization of adoptively transferred indium-111 labeled tumor infiltrating lymphocytes in patients with metastatic melanoma. J Clin Oncol 1989;7:250.
23. Anderson WF. Human gene therapy. Science 1992;256:808.
24. Miller AD. Human gene therapy comes of age. Nature 1992;357: 455.
25. Brenner MK, Rill DR, Moen RC, et al. Gene marking to trace origin of relapse after autologous bone marrow transplantation. Lancet 1993; 341:85.
26. Anderson W. Gene therapy for genetic diseases. Hum Gene Ther 1994; 5:281. Editorial.
27. Anderson W. Uses and abuses of human gene transfer. Hum Gene Ther 1992;3:1. Editorial.
28. Friend SH, Bernards R, Rogeli S, et al. A human DNA segment with properties of the gene that predisposes to retinoblastoma and osteosarcoma. Nature 1986;323:643.
29. Latif F, Tory K, Gnarra J, et al. Identification of the von Hippel-Lindau disease tumor suppressor gene. Science 1993;260:1317.
30. Baker SJ, Fearon ER, Nigro JM, et al. Chromosome 17 deletions and p53 gene mutations in colorectal carcinomas. Science 1989;244:217.
31. Fearon ER, Vogelstein B. A genetic model for colorectal tumorigenesis. Cell 1990;61:759.
32. Rose EA, Glaser T, Jones C, et al. Complete physical map of the WAGR region of 11 p13 localizes a candidate Wilm's tumor gene. Cell 1990;60:495.
33. Carter BS, Ewing CM, Ward WS, et al. Allelic loss of chromosome

16q and 10q in human prostate cancer. Proc Natl Acad Sci USA 1990; 87:8751.

34. Presti JC Jr, Reuter VE, Galan T, Fair WR, Cordon-Cardo C. Molecular genetic alterations in superficial and locally advanced human bladder cancer. Cancer Res 1991;51:5405.
35. Werthman P, Drazan K, Csete M, et al. Adenoviral-mediated transfer of human p53 tumor suppressor gene to rat bladder in vivo. J Urol 1994;151:389A.
36. Bubenik J, Voitenok NN, Kieler J, et al. Local administration of cells containing an inserted Il-2 gene and producing IL-2 inhibits growth of human tumors in nu/nu mice. Immunol Lett 1988;19:279.
37. Fearon ER, Pardoll DM, Itaya T, et al. Interleukin-2 production by tumor cells bypasses T helper function in the generation of an antitumor response. Cell 1990;60:397.
38. Gansbacher B, Bannerji R, Daniels B, Zier K, Cronin K, Gilboa E. Retroviral vector-mediated gamma-interferon gene transfer into tumor cells generates potent and long lasting antitumor immunity. Cancer Res 1990;50:7820.
39. Gansbacher B, Zier K, Daniels B, Cronin K, Bannerji R, Gilboa E. Interleukin 2 gene transfer into tumor cells abrogates tumorigenicity and induces protective immunity. J Exp Med 1990;172:1217.
40. Golumbek PT, Lazenby AJ, Levitsky HI, et al. Treatment of established renal cancer by tumor cells engineered to secrete interleukin-4. Science 1991;254:713.
41. Porgador A, Tzehoval E, Katz A, et al. Interleukin 6 gene transfection into Lewis lung carcinoma tumor cells suppresses the malignant phenotype and confers immunotherapeutic competence against parental metastatic cells. Cancer Res 1992;52:3679.
42. Dranoff G, Jaffee E, Lazenby A, et al. Vaccination with irradiated tumor cells engineered to secrete murine granulocyte-macrophage colony-stimulating factor stimulates potent, specific, and long-lasting antitumor immunity. Proc Natl Acad Sci USA 1993;90:3539.
43. Cordon-Cardu C, Fuks Z, Drobnjak M, Moreno C, Eisenbach L, Feldman M. Expression of HLA-A,B,C antigens on primary and metastatic tumor cell populations of human carcinomas. Cancer Res 1991;51: 6372.
44. Sanda, M, Simons J, Pardol D, Restifo N. Human prostate cells escape immunity via reversible heterogeneous defects in antigen processing. J Urol 1993;149:374A.
45. Hock H, Dorsch M, Kunzendorf U, et al. Vaccinations with tumor cells genetically engineered to produce different cytokines: effectivity not superior to a classical adjuvant. Cancer Res 1993;53:714.
46. Steiner M, Barrack E. Transforming growth factor-B1 overproduction in prostate cancer: effects on growth in vivo and in vitro. Mol Endocrinol 1992;6:15.
47. Connor J, Bannerji R, Saito S, Heston W, Fair W, Gilboa E. Regression of bladder tumors in mice trated with interleukin-2 gene-modified tumor cells. J Exp Med 1993;177:1127.
48. Sanda M, Ayyagari S, Jaffee E, et al. Demonstration of a rational strategy for human prostate cancer gene therapy. J Urol 1994;151: 622.
49. Vieweg J, Rosenthal F, Bannerji R, et al. Immunotherapy for prostate cancer in the Dunning rat model: use of cytokine gene modified tumor vaccines. Cancer Res 1994;54:1760.
50. Moody B, Lazenby A, Ewing C, Isaacs W. Interleukin-2 transfected prostate cancer cells generate a local anti-tumor effect in vivo. Prostate 1994;24:244.
51. Levitsky H, Lazenby A, Hayashi R, Pardoll D. In vivo priming of 2 distinct antitumor effector populations: the role of MHC class-I expression. J Exp Med 1994;179:1215.
52. Sanda M, Carducci M, Ayyagari S, et al. Gene therapy for human prostate cancer: efficacy in animal models and feasibility for human trials. J Urol 1994;151:492A.
53. Jaffee E, Dranoff G, Cohen L, et al. High efficiency gene transfer into primary human tumor explants without cell selection. Cancer Res 1993; 53(Suppl 10):2221.
54. Belldegrun A, Tso C, Sakata T, et al. Human renal carcinoma line transfected with interleukin-2 and/or interferon alpha gene(s): implications for live cancer vaccines. J Natl Cancer Inst 1993;85:207.
55. Furman P, McGuirt P, Keller P, Fyfe J, Elion G. Inhibition by acyclovir of cell growth and DNA synthesis of cells biochemically transformed with herpes virus genetic information. Virology 1980;102:420.
56. St Clair M, Lambe C, Furman P. Inhibition by ganciclovir of cell growth and DNA synthesis of cells biochemically transformed with herped virus genetic information. Antimicrob Agents Chemother 1987;31: 844.
57. Matthews T, Boehme R. Antiviral activity and mechanism of action of ganciclovir. Rev Infect Dis 1988;10(Suppl 3):S490.
58. Freeman S, Abboud C, Whartenby K, et al. The "bystander effect": tumor regression when a fraction of the tumor mass is genetically modified. Cancer Res 1993;53:5274.
59. Culver K, Ram Z, Wallbridge, S, Ishii H, Oldfield E, Blaese R. In vivo gene transfer with retroviral vector-producer cells for treatment of experimental brain tumors. Science 1992;256:15550.
60. Moolten F, Wells J. Curability of tumors bearing herpes thymidine kinase genes transferred by retroviral vectors. J Natl Cancer Inst 1990; 82:297.
61. Smythe W, Hwang H, Amin K, et al. Use of recombinant adenovirus to transfer the herpes simplex virus thymidine kinase (HSVtk) gene to thoracic neoplasms: an effective in vitro drug sensitization system. Cancer Res 1994;54:2055.
62. Caruso M, Panis Y, Gagandeep S, Houssin D, Salzmann J, Klatzmann D. Regression of established macroscopic liver metastases after in situ transduction of a suicide gene. Proc Natl Acad Sci USA 1993;90: 7024.
63. Takamiya Y, Short M, Ezzeddine Z, Moolton F, Breakefield X, Martuza R. Gene therapy of malignant brain tumors: a rat glioma line bearing the herpes simplex virus type 1-thymidine kinase gene and wild type retrovirus kills other tumor cells. J Neurosci Res 1992;33: 493.
64. Ram Z, Culver KW, Walbridge S, Blaese RM, Oldfield EH. In situ retroviral-mediated gene transfer for the treatment of brain tumors in rats. Cancer Res 1993;53:83.
65. Culver KW, Van Gilder J, Link CJ, et al. Gene therapy for the treatment of malignant brain tumors with in vivo tumor transduction with the herpes simplex thymidine kinase gene/ganciclovir system. Hum Gene Ther 1994;5:343.
66. Chen SH, Shine HS, Goodman JC, Grossman RG, Woo SL. Gene therapy for brain tumors: regression of experimental gliomas by adenovirus mediated gene transfer in vivo. Proc Natl Acad Sci USA 1994; 91:3057.
67. Bi WL, Parysek LM, Warnick R, Stambook. In vitro evidence that metabolic cooperation is responsible for the bystander effect observed with HSV-tk retroviral gene therapy. Hum Gene Ther 1993;4:725.
68. Ram Z, Walbridge S, Shawker T, Culver KW, Blaese RM, Oldfield EH. The effect of thymidine kinase transduction and ganciclovir therapy on tumor vasculature and growth of 9L gliomas in rats. J Neurosurg 1994; 81:256.
69. Isaacs JT, Landniu PI, Berges R, Martikainen P, Kyprianou N, English HF. Androgen regulation of programmed cell death of normal and malignant prostate cells. J Androl 1992;13:455.
70. Isaacs JT. Development and characteristics of the available animal model systems for the study of prostatic cancer. In: Coffey DS, Gardner WA, Bruchovsky W, Resnick MI, Karr JP, eds. Current concepts and approaches to the study of prostate cancer. New York: Alan R Liss, 1987;513.
71. Isaacs JT, Isaacs WB, Feitz WFJ, Scheres J. Establishment and characterization of seven Dunning rat prostatic cancer cell lines and their use in developing methods for predicting metastatic abilities of prostatic cancers. Prostate 1986;9:262.
72. Mulligan R. The basic science of gene therapy. Science 1993;260:926.
73. Taneja S, Belldegrun A, Dardashti K, Cohan P, DeKernion J, Pang S. Construction of a prostate specific antigen promoter-driven gene transfer vector: a novel strategy for target specific gene therapy in prostate cancer. J Urol 1994;151:491A.
74. Cornetta K, Moen R, Culver K, et al. Amphotropic murine leukemia retrovirus is not an acute pathogen for primates. Hum Gene Ther 1990; 1:15.
75. Fujiwara T, Grimm E, Roth J. Gene therapeutics and gene therapy for cancer. Curr Opin Oncol 1994;6:96.
76. Johnson P, Miyanohara A, Levine F, Cahill T, Friedmann T. Cytotoxicity of a replication-defection mutant of herpes simplex virus type 1. J Virol 1992;66:2952.

77. Jones N, Shenk T. Isolation of adenovirus type 5 host range deletion mutants defective for transformation of rat embryo cells. Cell 1979; 17:683.
78. Danos O, Mulligan R. Safe and efficient generation of recombinant retrovirus with amphotropic and ecotropic host ranges. Proc Natl Acad Sci USA 1988;85:6460.
79. Miller A. Retrovirus packaging cells. Hum Gene Ther 1990;1:5.
80. Kozarsky K, Wilson J. Gene therapy: adenovirus vectors. Curr Opin Genet Dev 1993;3:399.
81. Roe T, Reynolds T, Yu G, Brown P. Integration of murine leukemia virus DNA depends on mitosis. EMBO J 1993;12:2099.
82. Kotin RM, Siniscalco M, Samulski R, et al. Site-specific integration fo adeno-associated virus. Proc Natl Acad Sci USA 1990;87: 2211.
83. Muzyczka N. Use of adeno-associated virus as a general transduction vector for mammalian cells. Curr Top Microbiol Immunol 1992;158: 97.
84. Anderson W. Human gene therapy. Science 1992;256:808.
85. Moss B, Flexner C. Vaccinia virus expression vectors. Annu Rev Immunol 1987;5:305.
86. Freeman S, Zwiebel J. Gene therapy of cancer. Cancer Invest 1993; 11:676.

Principles and Practice of Genitourinary Oncology, edited by Derek Raghavan, Howard I. Scher, Steven A. Leibel, and Paul H. Lange. Lippincott-Raven Publishers, Philadelphia, © 1997.

CHAPTER 11

Palliative Care and Advances in Symptom Management

Russell K. Portenoy

The complex symptoms and functional disturbances experienced by patients with genitourinary cancers demand a comprehensive approach to palliative care. Palliative medicine is becoming established as a medical subspecialty devoted to the delivery of this care. This chapter discusses the concept of palliative care and its role in the populations with genitourinary cancers. One critically important area, the treatment of prevalent physical symptoms, is emphasized.

DEFINITION OF PALLIATIVE CARE

Although the concept of palliative care is now firmly established within the broad field of oncology, its parameters are not well defined. An evolving consensus exists, however, and is exemplified in the definition of palliative care promulgated by the World Health Organization[1]:

> Palliative care is the active total care of patients whose disease is not responsive to curative treatment. Control of pain, of other symptoms, and of psychologic, social and spiritual problems is paramount. The goal of palliative care is the achievement of the best possible quality of life for patients and their families.

The goals expressed in this definition of palliative care initially found expression in the hospice movement.[2] Although the first hospice can be traced back more than 2 centuries, the organized advocacy of the hospice model in developed countries began only 3 decades ago. Impelled by the desire to improve care for the dying,, hospice legitimized the involvement of diverse health-related disciplines in the care of the terminally ill. The focus was the end of life, and the primary goal was the relief of suffering through measures that improved comfort and addressed the psychologic, social, and spiritual needs of the dying.

In the United States, the hospice movement has continued as a system for the delivery of care to patients who are imminently dying. Financial considerations and tradition have combined to limit the availability of hospice programs to patients who are no longer receiving active antineoplastic therapy and who have short life expectancies. The type of care provided by hospice programs typically emphasizes nursing and pastoral support, the goals of which are symptom control and the relief of suffering. In one sense, the basic objective is to create conditions that facilitate a ''good death.''

The broader concept of palliative care described in the definition of the World Health Organization encompasses a level of care well beyond this hospice model. Palliative care aims to address the physical, psychosocial, and spiritual concerns that contribute to both the quality of life and quality of death for patients with life-threatening diseases. Although the focus intensifies at the end of life, the core issues—comfort and function, defined broadly and evaluated within the context of the family—are salient throughout the course of the disease.

A palliative care model recognizes the need to address symptom distress, physical impairments, and psychosocial disturbances even during the period of aggressive primary therapy, the avowed goal of which may be cure or prolongation of life. For the many patients with incurable and progressive diseases who are undergoing active life-prolonging therapies and have life expectancies that potentially extend to years, palliative care must provide a mix of symptom management, function-oriented therapies, and psychologic support or interventions. In many circumstances, palliative care overlaps with the parallel discipline of cancer rehabilitation, the purview of which may range from the restoration of physical and cognitive functioning to vocational counseling.

For the dying patient, optimal palliative care addresses the traditional concerns of the hospice movement. Comfort for the patient and preparation of both patient and family for the inevitability of dying are often the overriding challenges in this setting.

The evolving perspective on palliative care has encouraged the gradual acceptance of a medical specialization in this area. Palliative medicine is a recognized subspecialty of medicine in the United Kingdom and has gained the stature of academic posts in the United Kingdom, Canada, and Australia. A major textbook devoted to palliative medicine has been published,[3] and both national and international organizations have been established to further the goals of this discipline. The largest of these organizations, the European Association of Palliative Care, has over 7000 members.

Palliative Care and Genitourinary Cancers

Although any of the diverse cancers and clinical populations in the field of genitourinary oncology could potentially be used to illustrate the clinical relevance of the palliative care concept, the lack of empiric information about symptom distress and functional disturbances in most of these groups continues to be limiting. A few studies have begun to characterize these concerns in the population with prostate cancer, and the data provide a stark indication of the need for a therapeutic model that addresses quality-of-life concerns.

A survey of 172 patients with prostate cancer and 83 of their spouses or partners is illustrative.[4] More than three quarters of these patients reported sexual dysfunction, and several symptoms, specifically fatigue, urinary problems, and pain, were extremely common. Psychologic symptoms, such as worrying, depressed mood, tension, and irritability, were also prevalent in both patients and spouses; 10% of the patients and 7% of the spouses experienced a degree of psychologic distress that was substantially heightened compared with the group as a whole. Worsening quality of life was associated with both advanced disease and treatment with hormonal therapy.

Other studies confirm the high prevalence of symptoms and functional disturbances in the population with advanced prostate cancer. In a survey of 63 patients with hormone-refractory disease,[5] the following symptoms had a prevalence rate of at least 50%: pain (68%), fatigue (67%), worrying (56%), dry mouth (56%), feeling drowsy (54%), feeling sad (52%), difficulty sleeping (51%), and feeling nervous (51%). A survey of 72 similar patients observed that 40% had decreased functional status, and 21% had reduced social activity.[6]

The diversity and prevalence of problems that may impair quality of life during and after the administration of primary antineoplastic therapies necessitate the broad perspective incorporated into the current concept of palliative care. At all stages of the disease, a compelling need exists for a comprehensive assessment of these quality-of-life concerns, the outcome of which can guide a management strategy designed to enhance comfort and function in accordance with the goals of care.

PATIENT ASSESSMENT AND PALLIATIVE CARE

The foundation of palliative care is the comprehensive assessment. The management of each symptom or functional concern depends on a detailed knowledge of its presentation, pathogenesis, and impact within the larger set of phenomena that support or undermine well-being. In contrast to the traditional medical model, which encourages an approach to the patient that focuses on the chief complaint in relative isolation, the model of palliative care requires ongoing consideration of multiple concurrent problems and their combined effect on the individual.

Construct of Suffering

This assessment process may be illuminated by the construct of suffering.[7] Although admittedly difficult to define, the construct of suffering in medical illness is intuitively understood by clinicians and patients alike. Suffering has been characterized as a perceived threat to the patient as person[8] or as "total pain."[2] From a more operational perspective, suffering has been described as the distress associated with factors that together impair quality of life.[7,9] These factors potentially involve aversive experiences in many domains, including the physical, psychologic, and social.

In addition to its specific impact on function and well-being, each of the problems presented by the patient can potentially be understood in terms of its contribution to the overall level of suffering (Fig. 11-1). This perspective encourages a clinical assessment that extends beyond the presenting complaint to a broader understanding of concurrent and anticipated problems. It potentially avoids a common error, in which narrow therapeutic goals lead to outcomes that are themselves favorable but have little positive effect on overall quality of life. Concern about this type of error is now a strong theme in oncology, underscored by the growing trend toward the use of quality-of-life instruments in clinical trials.[10,11]

Goals of Care

The issues encountered in the patient assessment may also be clarified by another construct, which may be termed the goals of care. At any point during the course of the disease, the approach to the patient and family may be guided by one (or more) overriding goal: (1) to cure or prolong life; (2) to maintain function; or (3) to provide comfort. Although clinicians are usually explicit about the immediate aims of therapy, these larger goals may not be overtly expressed, or they may be obscured by the complexity and acuity of the immediate clinical problem. This lack of clarify may skew the assessment process and may introduce additional challenges into therapeutic decision making.

Assessment of the goals of care derives from the patient's desires and from knowledge of the medical realities. Although patients or families may ascribe equal importance to each of these goals, the clinician usually comes to realize that one or another deserves emphasis in communicating about treatment options and in recommending a specific course of therapy.

In many cases, the goals of the clinician mirror those of the patient. At one end of a spectrum are patients who have a reasonable chance of cure or prolonged remission, who become highly informed about the potential risks and benefits of treatment, and who request aggressive therapy. Physicians are usually anxious to oblige this request, and palliative care is typically limited to the management of treatment-related morbidity as therapeutic efforts focus on intensive primary treatments. At the other extreme are patients with clearly refractory and progressive disease, who openly acknowledge the lack of primary treatment, and who request comfort care only. In such cases, the reality stated by the patient is usually apparent to the physician, and therapy is focused on palliative care only. Unfortunately, most patients do not typify one or the other end of this spectrum. The clinical situation is dynamic, and ample opportunity exists for misapprehension and conflicting goals. In developed countries, for example, many patients undergo aggressive, life-prolonging therapy with little realistic hope of a cure or long-term remission. The useless administration of such thera-

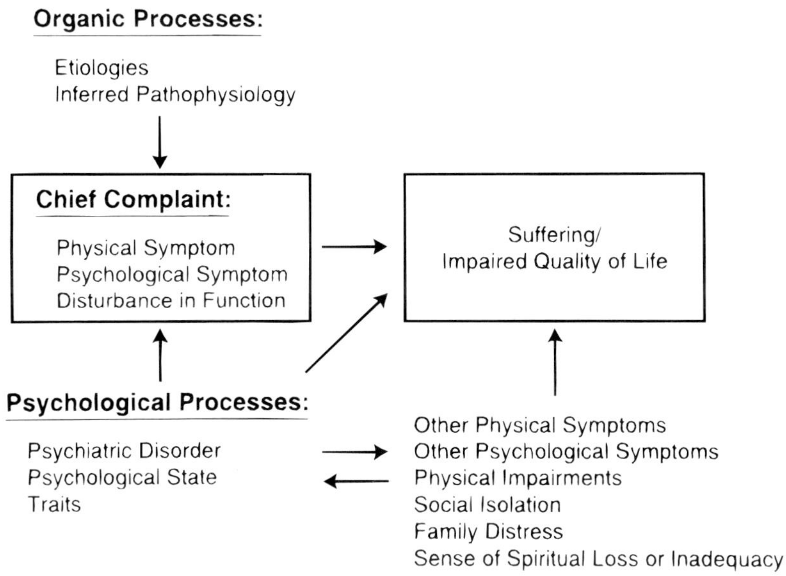

FIG. 11-1. A model that depicts the relationship between symptoms and a more global construct, suffering. The clinical assessment based on this model attempts to elucidate the factors that may sustain the symptom, or the distress associated with the symptom, while simultaneously evaluating the degree to which the symptom and other factors contribute the patient's overall suffering or impairment in quality of life.

pies, combined with the corollary process sometimes called the "medicalization" of dying, have become increasingly troubling to some medical ethicists and clinicians.[12,13] These phenomena exact a huge financial toll and may focus therapy on treatment-related issues, such as acute drug toxicity, when a more comprehensive approach to palliative care would be far more salutary. Given the stakes, assessment of the goals of care and communication with the patient and family about these goals, must be considered among the most important and challenging aspects of caring for a patient.

To clarify the goals of care over time, the clinician must undertake an ongoing evaluation of the patient's medical and psychosocial status and must maintain a broad knowledge of both the available primary therapies and the options that exist in the domain of palliative care. Clinicians must become comfortable with palliative care as an active therapeutic endeavor and must reject the unfortunate, and untrue, position that the lack of an antineoplastic treatment means that "nothing can be done." Both patient and caregivers are better served if the clinician has successfully communicated from the start that palliative care, with its focus on quality of life, functionality, and symptom control, is as central to oncologic practice as treatment for the tumor. Patients who have learned from experience that help is available to assist them in living with the disease are more likely to accept the transition to a phase without primary antineoplastic treatment. The overriding goals of care may shift, and the intensity with which palliative care is provided may increase after life-prolonging therapies are exhausted, but the patient is able to perceive a continuity characterized by the ongoing desire of the clinician to manage symptoms and to address other quality-of-life concerns.

SYMPTOM DISTRESS AND PALLIATIVE CARE

Symptom management is an essential component of palliative care. Physical and psychologic symptoms are prevalent in all patients with cancer, and most patients with active disease experience multiple symptoms concurrently.[1,4,5,14–20] Although patterns of symptoms probably vary systematically across diseases or treatment settings, some studies also indicate substantial similarities in diverse populations. Irrespective of the primary disease, a few symptoms, including pain, fatigue, psychologic distress, and gastrointestinal complaints, strongly influence global symptom distress.[5,21,22]

Expertise in the assessment and management of these common symptoms is a minimum requirement for the clinician who seeks to provide appropriate palliative care to cancer patients. Although detailed information about the specific symptoms and other quality-of-life concerns associated with genitourinary cancers is desirable, the absence of these data does not lessen the importance of effective symptom management. These patients could benefit dramatically if recent advances in the treatment of common symptoms were applied systematically. The following sections of this chapter describe some of the more important of these advances.

Pain

Surveys have demonstrated that as many as 50% of cancer patients experience chronic pain during antineoplastic therapy, and more than 75% experience pain during the advanced phase of the disease.[1,4,5,14–17,23–29] Although optimal pharmacotherapy using simple opioid regimens can provide adequate relief to 70% to 90% of these patients,[30–36] unrelieved pain continues to be prevalent. This situation can improve only if practitioners focus on the management of pain as a clinical imperative in this population.

The treatment of cancer-induced pain has been extensively reviewed in publications,[1,37–40] including an influential set of guidelines endorsed by the United States Agency for Health Care Policy and Research.[40] Chapter 59 discusses these principles with reference to selected genitourinary cancers.

Psychologic Distress

Although psychooncology is now a recognized subspecialty of psychology and psychiatry, its day-to-day practice is actually woven into the work of palliative care. Psychologic symptoms and psychiatric disorders are prevalent in patients with cancer,[19, 41–43] and therapeutic efforts intended to improve quality of life must address these problems. Hence, all clinicians should develop the ability to assess common psychologic symptoms, particularly depressed mood and anxiety states, and should fashion a plan for treatment or referral on this basis.

Information pertaining to the diagnosis and management of prevalent psychiatric disorders in the cancer population has been exhaustively reviewed in a textbook, the first of its kind for the discipline.[44] Numerous reviews discuss specific issues in psychooncology.[45,46]

Somnolence and Other Impairments of Higher Functions

An impairment in the ability to think clearly or to interact with others commonly contributes to the distress experienced by cancer patients. The phenomenology associated with these problems is diverse. Some patients experience only somnolence and can be easily aroused to normal cognition. Others experience disturbances in cognition, perception, or mood, any of which may occur without a change in arousal. In many cases, a more global syndrome occurs that fulfills criteria for a diagnosis of delirium.

The prevalence of this range of problems is unknown, but it can be presumed to be high, particularly among patients with advanced disease. Studies of delirium have documented prevalence rates in hospitalized cancer patients of 8% to 40%[41,43] and even higher rates at the end of life.[46,47] Given the evidence that delirium itself is an underrecognized problem,[48,49] the prevalence of the full range of changes in consciousness or cognition is likely to be even higher.

Diagnosis

The diagnosis of these problems may be clarified by defining the criteria for the more global syndrome, delirium.[49–51] Specific criteria for this syndrome have been developed by the American Psychiatric Association and are described in the *Diagnostic and Statistical Manual* (DSM) III-R,[52] and more recently, in DSM-IV.[53,54] The following are diagnostic elements endorsed by both versions: (1) impairment in responsiveness and alertness; (2) cognitive dysfunction of recent onset that is not explained by preexisting dementia; (3) acute onset (usually hours or days); and (4) evidence of an organic process that is etiologically related to the disturbance. DSM-III-R also specifies that at least two of the following are needed to establish the diagnosis: reduced level of consciousness, perceptual disturbances, disturbance of the sleep-wake cycle, increased or decreased psychomotor activity, disorientation, and memory impairment.

Diagnostic instruments may be useful in establishing the presence of delirium. These instruments include screening tests, diagnostic tools based on DSM criteria, rating scales, and measures of physiologic correlates.[55] Simple screening tools for cognitive impairment, which are not specific for delirium, include the Mini-Mental Status Exam[56] and the Blessed Orientation-Memory-Concentration Test.[57] The Confusion Assessment Method[58] and the Delirium Rating Scale[59] are valid tools for the diagnosis of delirium.

In the clinical setting, the assessment of delirium or related disturbances is complicated by the variability in the presenting phenomena. Altered thinking may range from mild memory impairment to frank confusion. Distorted perception may be limited to vivid dreams or nightmares or to daytime illusions or hallucinations. Affective disturbances may range from dysphoria to hypomania. The level of arousal may be predominantly hypoalert-hypoactive, hyperalert-hyperactive, or mixed.[51] Patients may demonstrate severe disturbances in one or more areas (such as affect) and may function normally in others. Although the diagnosis of delirium cannot be established in the absence of a change in arousal or cognition, isolated organic disturbances must be identified to offer an appropriate therapeutic response.

After the existence of a delirium or related disturbance has been confirmed, the assessment must focus on the identification of potentially reversible causes. Metastatic disease, drugs, metabolic disturbances, vascular complications, and paraneoplastic syndromes must all be considered.[60,61] An appropriate clinical evaluation usually reveals multiple potential factors.[61]

Management

Treatment of one or more of the potential causese often yields clinical improvement, even among patients with advanced cancer. In one study of patients admitted to a palliative care unit, for example, a clear explanation for cognitive impairment was discerned in 43% of cases, and one third improved, most after specific treatment.[62] The therapeutic strategy may include dose reduction or discontinuation of nonessential drugs, correction of metabolic disturbances, treatment for sepsis, or other specific interventions.

The approach to the underlying cause must be guided by the medical status of the patient and the goals of care. The prevalence of delirium increases as the disease progresses, and many patients experience a period of cognitive decline immediately before death. If the goal is comfort, and death is known to be imminent, the appropriate therapy may involve only control of the behavioral manifestations of the syndrome, rather than restoration of alertness and normal cognition.

These principles are well illustrated by the management of cognitive changes associated with opioid therapy. Although tolerance typically develops rapidly to the adverse cognitive effects of opioids,[63] treatment with these drugs may contribute to persistent disturbances in arousal, thinking, mood, or perception. Reduction in the opioid dose may be followed by improvement in these complaints. To test this possibility, patients with adequate pain control can undergo dose reduction of 25% to 50% as a therapeutic trial. This strategy is not appropriate, however, for patients with unrelieved pain, who must be managed in a manner that addresses both pain and adverse cognitive changes. Among the interventions that may be considered are coadministration of a nonopioid analgesic, a trial of a different opioid, or a change to an alternative route of opioid administration (specifically spinal).[39] Similarly, dose reduction is also inappropriate for patients at the end of life, for whom the risk of pain recurrence cannot be justified.

Additional interventions are often needed to address the be-

Table 11-1. *Drugs used in the management of somnolence and other impairments of higher functions*

Class	Drugs	Comments
Neuroleptics	Haloperidol Thioridazine Chlorpromazine	Most clearly indicated in the confused, agitated patient, or the hallucinating patient; haloperidol preferred because of low anticholinergic effect; side effects minimized by careful dose titration
Benzodiazepines	Lorazepam	Most clearly indicated in the confused patient with severe agitation; can worsen symptoms and must be used cautiously
Psychostimulants	Methylphenidate Pemoline Dextroamphetamine	Most clearly indicated in the patient with opioid–related somnolence; consider also for somnolence due to other causes, mild hypoactive delirium or cognitive impairment without somnolence, and depressed mood

havioral disturbances associated with delirium or related disorders.[64,65] Depending on the setting, these interventions may be nonpharmacologic or pharmacologic. If the patient is confused, the approach to the patient and the family should incorporate frequent explanations and reassurance about the nature of the problem, the likely etiologic factors, and the plans for therapy. In the institutional setting, an effort should be made to keep the environment quiet and well lit, and staff should provide supervision, maintain routine, and continually reorient and reassure the patient. "One-to-one" nursing observation may be needed, and, occasionally, mechanical restraints are necessary for the agitated patient until adequate sedation has been achieved.

If pharmacologic intervention is needed to reduce cognitive dysfunction, eliminate hallucinations, and calm agitation, then neuroleptics are generally considered to be the drugs of choice (Table 11-1). Although comparative studies are lacking, the common acceptance of haloperidol as the first-line drug is justified by its relatively low incidence of anticholinergic and cardiovascular side effects and by the availability of both oral and parenteral formulations. Other neuroleptic drugs, such as thioridazine and chlorpromazine, have also been used.

When symptoms are moderate, initial doses of haloperidol may be low (e.g., 0.5 to 1 mg orally or 0.25 to 1 mg parenterally), and the dosing interval may be long (usually 12 to 24 hours and sometimes "as needed"). The oral formulation is used if possible. When symptoms are severe, parenteral administration is used to achieve more rapid control, and escalating doses may be repeated as often as every 30 minutes until clinical improvement is observed.

The use of a benzodiazepine (such as lorazepam) in combination with the neuroleptic can be recommended for highly anxious patients and for those who manifest a hyperalert-hyperactive variant of delirium. The administration of a benzodiazepine is strongly recommended when the delirium can be ascribed, even in part, to withdrawal of alcohol or sedative-hypnotic agents.

If the most important problem is somnolence, a different therapeutic approach can be recommended. Psychostimulants are now accepted medical therapy for excessive sleepiness in the cancer patient, particularly if the symptom is related to opioid therapy. Studies have demonstrated that the psychostimulant drugs can ameliorate somnolence, fatigue, cognitive impairment, pain, and depression in patients with cancer or acquired immunodeficiency syndrome (AIDS).[66–72] Surveys of patients with advanced disease have demonstrated the safety of methylphenidate and pemoline,[66,68,70–72] and a controlled trial of methylphenidate confirmed the efficacy of this drug for opioid-related somnolence in such patients.[67] More recently, methylphenidate was also demonstrated to improve mild cognitive impairment,[69] a finding that suggests the potential utility of psychostimulants in patients with mild hypoactive delirium or cognitive change, even in the absence of somnolence.

Clinical guidelines for the use of psychostimulants in the treatment of somnolence or cognitive impairment are empiric. Experience with methylphenidate is greatest, but the use of pemoline should be considered, based on several unique characteristics, including lesser sympathomimetic effects and the availability of a chewable tablet that can deliver drug directly through the buccal mucosa. A cautious dosing regimen, such as may be administered to the elderly or those with serious medical disorders, begins with a morning dose of methylphenidate, 2.5 to 5 mg, or pemoline, 18.75 to 37.5 mg. This dose can be repeated midday, if needed, to sustain effects until evening. Doses often require escalation after therapy is begun.

Side effects of psychostimulant therapy, when they occur, usually develop soon after treatment is initiated or when the dose is raised. The clinician must monitor the patient for the development of anorexia, tremulousness, insomnia, anxiety, or cognitive change (for example, the development of subtle paranoid thinking) and for cardiovascular effects including hypertension and tachycardia. Preexisting problems with anorexia, insomnia, or anxiety, or a history of a paranoid personality, should be viewed as relative contraindications for this therapy.

Fatigue

Fatigue is among the most common symptoms experienced by patients with cancer.[5,14,15,17,28] It has been associated with various primary antineoplastic therapies, including chemotherapy and radiotherapy,[73] and is commonly reported by patients with advanced disease who are not receiving treatment. Like pain, fatique is a complex symptom that may be influenced by many disturbances and may interact with other factors that impair quality of life.

Diagnosis

The complexity inherent in the complaint of fatigue derives from both the varying phenomena to which the term is applied and the diverse pathophysiologic processes that underlie each of these phenomena.[74–76] Patients may describe the symptom in different terms and may apply it to perceptions associated with muscular weakness, lack of energy or vitality, dysphoric mood, or somnolence. An association exists between fatigue and cognitive functioning, and patients may also describe fatigue in language that suggests difficulty in concentrating or focusing attention. None of these phenomena occurs exclusive of the others, and in the clinical effort to clarify the nature of the symptom, several of these phenomena are commonly identified as coexisting.

Thus, the first step in the clinical approach to fatigue is an assessment that attempts to define the meaning of the symptom for the patient. Various multidimensional assessment instruments have been developed that could potentially assist in this process,[73,77] but none can substitute for a comprehensive clinical evaluation. None of these instruments has been widely applied in either clinical practice or investigations.

A detailed understanding of the symptom provides a basis for a second level of assessment, which seeks to identify specific, potentially reversible, etiologic factors. For example, a patient whose complaint of fatigue is related to a sense of muscular weakness and whose physical examination is suggestive may be a candidate for further neurologic assessment, such as electrodiagnostic studies. This type of evaluation is occasionally necessary to identify the rare patient whose fatigue is due to a disorder of the neuromuscular junction (such as Eaton-Lambert syndrome) or of muscle.

Similarly, lack of vitality may be related to any of a variety of medical or psychiatric disorders. The assessment should attempt to exclude factors, such as anemia or depression, that may be easily treated and to identify likely causes. A temporal relationship between the onset of fatigue and a primary antineoplastic therapy is presumptive evidence of causation, but this attribution should be questioned if the fatigue continues for months after the end of therapy. A reevaluation may then be warranted, again to seek treatable causes of the symptom.

Management

In the absence of well-defined therapies for cancer-related fatigue, treatment of primary etiologic factors, if feasible, becomes essential. Primary approaches may involve correction of anemia or other metabolic disturbances, pharmacotherapy of major depression or insomnia, or treatment of a neuromuscular disorder.

Additionally, the clinician should not underestimate the importance of reassurance and education. Patients may benefit from information about the anticipated time course of the symptom, if it is linked to a transitory phenomenon such as radiotherapy. Some patients also respond favorably to counseling about techniques that have proved anecdotally helpful to other patients. These techniques include organization of activities so essential functions can be performed in the morning, a scheduled afternoon nap, and acceptance of help (from family members or others) for some tasks that had previously been performed by the patient.

Although pharmacologic therapy for cancer-related fatigue has not been evaluated in controlled studies, evidence supports the use of several drug classes for this indication. The utility of psychostimulants has been suggested in studies of methylphenidate and pemoline.[67,69,78] A large experience with these drugs in the treatment of opioid-related somnolence has accumulated, and a favorable anecdotal experience supports a therapeutic trial for the treatment of fatigue. The use of low-dose corticosteroids, such as dexamethasone, 1 to 2 mg twice daily, or prednisone, 5 to 10 mg twice daily, has also been supported empirically[79,80] and may be particularly helpful in patients with advanced disease and multiple symptoms. Finally, a trial of an antidepressant drug is clearly appropriate if fatigue is related to clinical depression. Based on anecdotal observation, such a trial may also be considered in occasional nondepressed patients with severe fatigue that has failed to respond to other therapies. Anecdotal reports of increased energy after treatment with the newer serotonin-specific reuptake inhibitors, including fluoxetine, sertraline, paroxetine, and venlafaxine, suggest the utility of these drugs.

Constipation

Constipation may be defined as diminished frequency of defecation associated with difficulty or discomfort.[81–83] It is extremely prevalent and often becomes a major problem for patients who receive long-term opioid therapy. Symptom distress may be worsened by the abdominal pain, bloating, distention, anorexia, and nausea associated with constipation, and rare patients develop life-threatening bowel obstruction as untreated constipation progresses to obstipation. Constipation may also be a significant risk factor for intestinal perforation in patients receiving long-term corticosteroid therapy.[84]

Diagnosis

The pathophysiology of constipation is complex and may involve processes that relate primarily to central or peripheral effects of drugs, bowel dysmotility or obstruction, impaired fluid regulation, or psychologic factors. Cancer patients commonly have a combination of potential causes of constipation (Table 11-2). The assessment of constipation must clarify these contributing factors, determine their treatability, and elucidate their relationship with the underlying disease or its treatment.

Table 11-2. *Common causes of constipation in cancer patients*

PHYSIOLOGIC AND PSYCHOSOCIAL FACTORS
Advanced age, inactivity, dehydration, depression, change in diet, physical or social impediments to defecation, rectal or abdominal pain
Metabolic disturbances: hypercalcaemia, hypokalemia, or hypothyroidism
STRUCTURAL FACTORS
Intraluminal or extraluminal masses, adhesions or fibrosis
DRUGS
Opioids, drugs with anticholinergic actions, antacids, diuretics, anticonvulsants, iron, antihypertensives
NEUROLOGIC DISORDERS
Damage from any cause to sacral plexus, cauda equina, or spinal cord; autonomic neuropathy due to the cancer, concurrent disease (e.g., diabetes), or drug (e.g., vincristine)

The long-term administration of opioid drugs is often the most obvious cause. Opioids decrease peristalsis, impair the defecation reflex, and dessicate intraluminal contents through increased absorption of fluid and electrolytes. These effects are produced through both central and peripheral actions. The demonstration of the therapeutic efficacy of oral naloxone,[85,86] which is poorly absorbed systemically, has confirmed the importance of a peripheral opioid mechanism and has suggested a possible treatment approach for refractory cases.

Patients who develop constipation in close relation to the initiation of opioid therapy or some other discrete event may not need additional evaluation. In contrast, sophisticated imaging procedures may be appropriate to assess fully the patient who develops progressive constipation in the absence of a clear precipitating cause. The physician must recognize the multiplicity of potential causes and must consider further evaluation of patients with an obvious cause if the course of the symptom is atypical. As discussed previously, the extent of this clinical assessment must be guided by the goals of care.

Management

Similar to other symptoms, constipation may be ameliorated by reversal of contributing causes and by specific therapies. Any of a large group of therapeutic strategies may be selected (Table 11-3). Few controlled trials of these treatments and no comparative trials in cancer patients have been conducted. Hence, clinical decisions must be made in each case based on the evaluation of the symptom and clinical judgment.

Table 11-3. *Strategies for the management of constipation in the cancer population*

USE THESE APPROACHES FOR ALL PATIENTS
Increase fluid intake
Increase dietary fiber (unless patient is debilitated or bowel obstruction is suspected)
Ensure comfort, privacy, and convenience for defecation
Ensure that impaction has not complicated constipation
DISCUSS APPROACHES WITH THE PATIENT AND SELECT ONE OR MORE
Administer intermittent (every 2–3 days) osmotic laxative, such as magnesium hydroxide, magnesium citrate, or sodium phosphate
Try a daily softening agent (sodium docusate) alone
Use a contact cathartic, such as senna, bisacodyl, or phenolphthalein intermittently (every 2–3 days)
Use daily contact cathartic (with or without softening agent)
Use daily lactulose or sorbitol
OPTIMIZE SELECTED THERAPY
Adjust dose and dosing schedule
Consider combining approaches if the initial therapy is inadequate
Switch approaches if needed
CONSIDER ALTERNATIVE APPROACHES IN REFRACTORY CASES
Use rectal approaches, including rectal administration of contact cathartic or intermittent use of enemas
Use colonic lavage intermittently or daily with polyethylene glycol
Treat with a prokinetic drug daily, such as cisapride or metoclopramide
Treat with oral naloxone daily if patient is receiving an opioid

Routine laxative therapy should not be initiated in patients with severe constipation until serious problems, such as fecal impaction, have been excluded. Low impaction can be assessed by examination of the rectum; suspicion of a high impaction or another cause of bowel obstruction requires abdominal imaging for evaluation. The management of impaction is empiric and may require physical disimpaction, repeated enemas, and a combination of rectal and oral laxatives. Routine laxative therapy can begin after impaction is cleared.

Therapeutic interventions for constipation may be administered rectally or orally.[81–83] For most cancer patients, the use of enemas and rectal suppositories is not preferred because of the inconvenience and the potential for local trauma. Some patients do prefer rectal laxatives on a regular basis, however, and these measures should be available to patients who do not otherwise have contraindications to their use (e.g., thrombocytopenia).

Oral laxatives are the mainstay of the management of constipation. These drugs include (1) bulk agents, (2) osmotic compounds, (3) agents for colonic lavage, (4) lubricants, (5) contact cathartics, (6) prokinetic drugs, and (6) oral naloxone.

Bulk agents typically use cellulose or psyllium seeds to supplement the consumption of fiber in the food. These products are generally safe, but anecdotal experience suggests that they can worsen some symptoms, such as flatulence, distention, bloating, or abdominal pain, in patients with intraabdominal disease. They are best avoided in patients who are severely debilitated and in those with partial bowel obstruction from any cause.

Osmotic laxatives include magnesium salts (magnesium hydroxide and magnesium citrate) and sodium salts (for example, sodium phosphate). These agents draw fluid into the intestinal lumen and are most commonly used for acute bowel cleansing before medical procedures. Some patients, however, find that intermittent administration (usually every 2 to 3 days) is an effective method of long-term laxation. Although the risks associated with these agents are generally minor, rare patients develop serious electrolyte disorders or volume overload from electrolyte absorption. The use of these drugs by patients who may be predisposed to these problems, such as patients with renal insufficiency or cardiac failure, should be carefully monitored.

Lactulose and sorbitol are poorly absorbed sugars that act as osmotic laxatives, liquifying the intraluminal contents and increasing their bulk. Lactulose is used most often, but one controlled trial demonstrated that the less expensive alternative, sorbitol, was equally effective.[87] Most patients consume a dose once or twice daily after a period of dose adjustment.

Uncommon patients, usually those refractory to other types of laxative therapy, benefit from the intermittent use of an agent for colonic lavage. Consumption of a large volume of a nonabsorbable fluid such as polyethylene glycol (GoLYTELY) is used for lavage before procedures. Smaller daily volumes, such as 250 to 500 mL, can be used to reverse chronic constipation.[88]

A lubricating oil, such as mineral oil, may be an effective laxative in some patients, but the long-term use of this approach is limited by concerns related to perianal irritation, poor absorption of fat-soluble vitamins, and the potential for serious lipoid pneumonia should aspiration occur. This approach is not recommended for long-term laxation in patients with cancer.

The contact cathartics are probably the most commonly administered laxatives in cancer patients. This group of agents comprises diverse drugs in two major classes, the anthraquinones and the diphenylmethanes. The former group includes cascara, senna, and danthron, and the latter includes phenolphthalein and bisacodyl. Although these agents have some differences in modes of action, all act by increasing peristalsis and by reducing absorption of water and electrolytes.[89,90] No comparative trials of these agents have been conducted, and any may be used in the long-term management of constipation. Clinical experience suggests that these drugs do possess a dose-response relationship in the clinical setting, and doses may need to be escalated in some patients. The physician can initiate therapy using a standard dose (such as one senna tablet twice daily), then increase the dose every 2 to 3 days until constipation is relieved, the patient reports side effects, or the therapy becomes too burdensome or costly to continue. Some patients prefer to use a contact cathartic on an intermittent basis, such as every 3 to 4 days if needed.

Castor oil is the only contact cathartic with a mechanism of action mediated in the small bowel. Cramping and diarrhea are common with this agent, and it is not generally used in cancer patients.

The risks associated with short-term use of the contact cathartics are minimal. Long-term ingestion, however, may result in so-called laxative bowel, a condition characterized by dependence on laxatives for bowel function. This syndrome, which is putatively the result of drug-induced damage to the myenteric plexus, is not a contraindication to therapy in the setting of advanced cancer, but it should be considered a potential problem for patients with long life expectancies. The physician may wish to consider alternative laxatives in such patients.

At the doses used clinically, sodium docusate and related drugs produce a surfactant effect that allows water and fats to mix with feces. Docusate is commonly added to a contact carthartic, based on the presumption that a combination of laxatives that act differently increases efficacy. Although no empiric confirmation of this presumption exists, the risks of combination therapy appear to be minimal, and clinical experience has been favorable.

Two other approaches are usually considered in the setting of refractory constipation. First, some evidence indicates that the use of a prokinetic agent may improve colonic transit,[91] and, on this basis, cisapride or metoclopramide can be considered for a therapeutic trial. Second, oral naloxone can potentially reverse opioid-induced constipation without causing systemic withdrawal.[85,86] The latter approach is not without risk, however, because some patients clearly absorb sufficient naloxone to develop uncomfortable signs of abstinence.[85] This potential effect suggests that naloxone should not be used until conventional therapies have failed. A reasonable approach begins with a dose of 0.4 mg twice daily and doubles the dose every 2 or 3 days until favorable effects occur or side effects are experienced.

Finally, the value of prophylactic therapy for opioid-induced constipation must be considered. Many specialists in palliative medicine believe that the prevalence of opioid-induced constipation is high enough to warrant prophylaxis with a laxative when opioid therapy is begun.[92] Apparently, however, some patients can manage this symptom by simple dietary approaches, and others develop tolerance to the constipatory effects of these drugs. Because the use of laxatives can be burdensome, it is reasonable to limit prophylactic therapy to those patients with other predisposing factors (see Table 11-2) and to manage constipation expectantly in those, such as younger ambulatory patients with relatively early disease, who are probably at the lowest risk of this side effect.

Nausea and Vomiting

In contrast to the extensively investigated syndrome of post-chemotherapy emesis, chronic or recurrent nausea is a less recognized clinical problem, notwithstanding surveys that have yielded prevalence rates ranging from less than 15% to more than 70% among patients with solid tumors.[5,14,17,93–95] The management of chronic nausea has not been systematically studied, and treatment approaches derive from anecdote and extrapolation from other settings.

Diagnosis

The diverse potential causes of chronic or recurrent nausea include drugs, direct effects of the tumor, antineoplastic therapy, metabolic disturbances, neurologic disorders, and psychologic factors (Table 11-4). As with other symptoms, the extent

Table 11-4. *Some causes of chronic or recurrent nausea in the cancer patient*

DRUGS
Opioids
Nonsteroidal antiinflammatory drugs
Other centrally acting drugs
INTRAABDOMINAL NEOPLASM
Partial bowel obstruction
Peritoneal carcinomatosis
Retroperitoneal neoplasm
ANTINEOPLASTIC THERAPY
Abdominal radiotherapy
Chemotherapy
AUTONOMIC NEUROPATHY
Paraneoplastic
Drug-related (e.g., after chemotherapy)
Other causes (e.g., diabetes)
METABOLIC DISTURBANCES
Hepatic failure
Renal failure
Electrolyte abnormalities
CONSTIPATION
INTRACRANIAL PROCESSES
Posterior fossa neoplasm
Increased intracranial pressure
PSYCHOLOGIC PROCESSES
Conditioned responses
Anxiety disorder

of the evaluation needed to clarify the most likely contributing factors must be determined on a case-by-case basis. Although the clinician should eschew elaborate testing when a cause (such as a drug effect) is likely and efforts are better focused on treatment, to presume an etiologic role for some temporally related factor uncritically is also inappropriate. If the course or features are atypical for the predisposing factors, additional evaluation is needed.

The pathophysiology of nausea and vomiting is complex,[96,97] and the elaboration of clinical inferences about the sustaining mechanism is an important aspect of diagnosis. The subjective experience of nausea presumably results from interactions among afferent and efferent activity at multiple levels of the nervous system, all of which is coordinated in the so-called emetic center in the medulla. On the basis of the connections identified in experimental models, it may be speculated that nausea and vomiting in humans may be precipitated by input to this center from any of several regions, including the gastrointestinal tract, labyrinthine-vestibular system, other brain stem sites (the best characterized of which is the chemoreceptor trigger zone in the area postrema of the medulla), and the cerebral cortex.

On theoretic grounds, the phenomenology of nausea may be postulated to relate to the predominant mechanism. Clinical inferences about the underlying mechanism may influence the selection of therapies. Many factors, including numerous drugs, presumably cause nausea by direct activation of the chemoreceptor trigger zone or by irritation of receptors in the gastrointestinal tract. In such cases, the precipitant is often clear, and the severity of nausea is greatest at the time of maximum stimulus, such as the time of peak effect for drugs. Other factors precipitate nausea through stimulation or sensitization of the vestibular system. This mechanism can be imputed in patients with nausea that is severely increased by movement or is associated with frank vertigo. Some disturbances appear to produce nausea through an intermediary phenomenon of gastroparesis, which is suggested by the association of nausea with postprandial vomiting, early satiety, and abdominal bloating. Finally, a prominent role for conditioned nausea may be suggested by the repeated occurrence of the symptom after specific stimuli.

Management

Nausea can act as a strong conditioning stimulus. Prompt and aggressive management of nausea is necessary to minimize the development of intervening psychologic processes that can complicate further assessment and treatment.

Some patients with chronic or recurrent nausea respond to conservative measures. Simplification of drug regimens, discontinuation of nonessential drugs, dietary changes (such as smaller, more frequent meals), change in some environmental cues (such as eating in a different room), and treatment of contributing causes (such as constipation) may be sufficient. Additionally, some patients whose nausea appears to be related to opioid therapy appear to benefit from a change in the route of administration; for example, patients who become intensely nauseated at the start of opioid therapy may obtain some relief and may acclimate to the drug more easily if parenteral therapy is used as a prelude to oral treatment.

Numerous drugs in many classes may have antiemetic effects

Table 11-5. *Antiemetic drugs potentially useful for chronic nausea in the cancer population*

Class	Examples
Neuroleptics	
Phenothiazines	Prochlorperazine
	Chlorpromazine
	Methotrimeprazine
Butyrophenones	Haloperidol
	Droperidol
Anticholinergic drugs	Scopolamine
	Atropine
Antihistamines	Promethazine
	Meclizine
Prokinetic drugs	Metoclopramide
	Cisapride
Corticosteroids	Prednisone
	Methylprednisolone
	Dexamethasone
Benzodiazepines	Lorazepam
Cannabinoids	Tetrahydrocannabinol
5-HT Antagonists	Ondansetron
	Granisetron

and may be helpful to the cancer patient with chronic or recurrent nausea (Table 11-5). Patients who do not have prominent symptoms consistent with vestibular dysfunction or gastroparesis are usually administered a drug that is primarily active at the chemoreceptor trigger zone, specifically a neuroleptic or metoclopramide. The dose-response relationship of these drugs during long-term administration has not been investigated, and the safety of relatively high doses for prolonged periods is unknown. Nonetheless, escalation of the dose above the standard starting dose is reasonable if benefits are not promptly observed. Maximal doses are not known, and most clinicians assume the failure of the drug if doses two to three times the standard starting dose are ineffective. Substantial individual variation also appears to exist in the antiemetic response to drugs that presumably act through similar mechanisms, and sequential trials of these agents may be useful in those patients who do not have a rapid therapeutic response.

Patients who experience nausea associated with vertigo or dramatically worsened by movement may be considered for a trial of an antivertiginous drug. Options include anticholinergic drugs (such as scopolamine), antihistamines (such as meclizine), and benzodiazepines (such as lorazepam). Similarly, patients who report prominent abdominal distention with postprandial nausea should be considered for a pharmacologic treatment that enhances gastric emptying, specifically metoclopramide or cisapride.

Other pharmacologic approaches to the refractory patient are similarly empiric. The antiemetic efficacy of corticosteroids is unexplained, but some patients clearly benefit from these drugs. Occasional patients who have responded poorly to previous trials obtain substantial relief from the use of a cannabinoid, such as delta-9-tetrahydrocannabinol (dronabinol). Rare patients with refractory symptoms are considered for a trial of ondansetron or granisetron, 5-HT3 antagonists that are extremely effective in the short-term treatment of chemotherapy-induced emesis. No evidence indicates that the 5-HT3 antagonists have particular efficacy in chronic nausea, and the high cost of this therapy limits its utility.

Based on the observation that antiemetic drugs vary in their mechanisms of action, the use of drug combinations may be reasonable. In the absence of studies that have assessed the safety and efficacy of combination therapy, this approach must be undertaken cautiously.

Patients who experience chronic or recurrent nausea can also be considered for an approach that incorporates cognitive therapy. Cognitive approaches have established efficacy in the treatment of chemotherapy-induced emesis,[98] and the techniques developed for this setting are likely to be generalizable to other situations. Such an approach should be particularly considered for patients whose histories suggest a prominent conditioned component to the nausea.

Anorexia

Anorexia is also a prevalent symptom that may coexist with chronic nausea or may be a separate problem. Loss of appetite can occur without reduction in food intake sufficient to cause malnutrition or weight loss. In this situation, anorexia is presumably the result of processes distinct from the metabolic disturbances that underlie the anorexia-cachexia syndrome. Treatment in such patients may focus specifically on symptomatic improvement.

Many patients present a more complex syndrome in which severe anorexia associated with reduction in food intake is accompanied by progressive weight loss and other disturbances consistent with the diagnosis of cachexia. These patients may experience other related symptoms, such as asthenia, and may demonstrate severe laboratory abnormalities, including anemia and hypoglycemia. The metabolic abnormalities associated with cachexia are protean and may involve increased protein turnover, skeletal muscle catabolism, and lipolysis with loss of lipid stores.[99]

In patients with the syndrome of anorexia and cachexia, the anorexia is presumably related, at least in part, to metabolic disturbances that also produce loss of weight. Weight loss is not merely the result of reduced caloric intake. Indeed, surveys have demonstrated that repletion of calories does not produce any substantial weight gain in many affected patients.[100]

The cause of the anorexia-cachexia syndrome is unknown, but investigations have begun to clarify some of the potential processes. Earlier theories were based on the assumption that the tumor diverted calories from host functions or directly released substances that induced catabolism. More recent models accept a role for these disturbances[101] and suggest further that a change in the metabolic and immune responses of the patient is a prominent factor. The potential role of macrophage-secreted tumor necrosis factor (cachectin) has been a strong focus of this model.[102]

Diagnosis

The assessment of anorexia must both clarify its relationship with malnutrition and cachexia and evaluate the many possible contributing factors. Although the presence of cachexia in association with anorexia suggests a unifying pathophysiologic process, the physician should not assume that other, potentially treatable, causes of anorexia are absent. Appetite may be impaired by change in taste, nausea or other gastrointestinal symptoms, dysphagia, pain in the head or neck, psychologic distress (particularly depression), and other disorders. The evaluation of the anorectic patient should attempt to identify all contributing factors.

The impact of anorexia on quality of life should also be considered in this assessment. The quality-of-life impairment associated with this symptom may reflect loss of pleasure in eating or intense concern about weight loss as an indicator of disease progression. Meals are a social and familial activity, and the loss of well-being associated with anorexia may also relate to disturbances in family interactions.

Management

Some therapeutic efforts can be directed at anorexia independent of approaches for weight loss. Conservative measures may be helpful in some cases. Anorexia due to change in taste may be ameliorated by varying the diet or seasoning the food. If early satiety is a problem, smaller and more frequent meals can be helpful. These dietary changes may be facilitated by referral to a dietician.

Other contributing causes may also be amenable to treatment. Chronic nausea and other gastrointestinal symptoms should be managed, and other symptoms, such as dysphagia and pain, may require additional interventions. In some cases, nonessential drugs that may be contributing to anorexia can be discontinued.

These measures may produce increased caloric intake, but such an improvement is generally transitory.[100] They should nonetheless be continued if they yield an improved sense of well-being. Patients whose anorexia is not accompanied by significant malnutrition or weight loss have no additional need for therapy.

Pharmacologic approaches can be considered for the treatment of anorexia that is refractory to these conservative measures. Although drug therapy is most often used for patients with concurrent weight loss, cachexia should not be viewed as a precondition for a therapeutic trial. Indeed, the data extant do not provide compelling evidence that reversal of weight loss yields benefits independent of improvement in the sense of well-being. Numerous studies have evaluated oral or parenteral nutritional support in terms of survival, tumor response, and treatment-related toxicity, and, with few exceptions, intensive protein-calorie repletion has had no clear-cut advantages.[103]

Given the latter data, the role of nutritional support in cancer care is complex. Parenteral nutritional support is rarely indicated because of its cost and potential morbidity, and nutritional support by the gastrointestinal tract is best viewed as a means to provide symptom control and improved well-being, rather than maintenance or restoration of weight in itself. For some patients, the improvement in well-being associated with the maintenance or restoration of weight is substantial enough to justify an aggressive approach, including a feeding tube. For others, the quality-of-life issues surrounding anorexia and weight loss are less prominent, and the decision to proceed with nutritional support must be carefully considered.

The pharmacologic approaches for anorexia and weight loss

include corticosteroid drugs, progestational drugs, cannabinoids, and miscellaneous agents. Studies have begun to provide a scientific basis for the selection of these therapies. Although additional studies are needed to clarify the relative risks and benefits in the population with cancer-related anorexia and anorexia-cachexia syndrome, the available drugs offer several options. Sequential trials may be needed to identify the most favorable agent.

The value of low-dose corticosteroid therapy has been suggested in surveys[104] and confirmed in controlled trials of methylprednisolone and prednisolone.[80,105] These drugs may also be useful for other symptoms, such as pain, fatigue, and nausea. As noted previously, the benefits of long-term corticosteroid therapy clearly exceed the risks for many patients with advanced cancer and multiple symptoms.[106]

Controlled trials of megestrol acetate, a progesterone derivative, have demonstrated favorable effects on appetite, caloric intake, weight, and quality of life.[107–111] Although this drug has dose-related side effects, including edema, hot flashes, glucose intolerance, and coagulation disturbances, clinical experience has been generally favorable. Dose-ranging studies have suggested that a relatively low dose, 160 mg/d, may optimize the balance between favorable effects and side effects.[109,110]

The cannabinoid, delta-9-tetrahydrocannabinol (dronabinol), is also an effective appetite stimulant.[112,113] A placebo-controlled trial of 2.5 mg twice daily in patients with AIDS demonstrated improved appetite, maintenance of weight or weight gain, and reduced nausea in the treated group.[113] This drug has been approved by the United States Food and Drug Administration for the treatment of anorexia associated with AIDS.

Other drugs may also stimulate appetite. A controlled trial of the antihistamine, cyproheptadine, suggested a modest benefit for anorexia, without weight gain.[114] The potential for sedation from this drug limits its utility in patients with advanced cancer. Early controlled trials of hydrazine sulfate yielded mixed results in terms of appetite and weight,[115,116] but more recent controlled studies have clearly demonstrated no benefit from this compound.[117–119]

CONCLUSIONS

The management of common distressing symptoms is one of the foundations for effective palliative care. At all stages of the disease, effective symptom control increases the likelihood that the patient will cope adequately with the rigors of therapy and maintain a satisfying level of physical and psychosocial functioning. Clinicians must recognize, however, that symptom control may not be sufficient to address the varying quality of life concerns presented by the cancer patient. Palliative medicine offers a model for the assessment and management of the complex needs of patients who seek to maintain function and comfort during the course of a life-threatening disease. These goals complement life-prolonging therapy and are viewed as essential by the patient and family.

REFERENCES

1. World Health Organization. Technical Report Series 804. Cancer pain and palliative care. Geneva: World Health Organization, 1990:11.
2. Saunders C. The philosophy of terminal care. In: Saunders C, ed. The management of terminal malignant disease, 2nd ed. Baltimore: Arnold, 1984:232.
3. Doyle D, Hanks GWC, MacDonald N, eds. Oxford textbook of palliative medicine. Oxford, Oxford University Press, 1993.
4. Kornblith AB, Herr HW, Ofman US, Scher HI, Holland JC. Quality of life of patients with prostate cancer and their spouses: the value of a data base in clinical care. Cancer 1994;73:2791.
5. Portenoy RK, Thaler HT, Kornblith AB, et al. Symptom prevalence, characteristics and distress in a cancer population. Qual Life Res 1994; 3:183.
6. Fossa SD, Aaronson NK, Newling D, et al. Quality of life and treatment of hormone resistant metastatic prostatic cancer. Eur J Cancer 1990;26:1133.
7. Cherny NI, Coyle N, Foley KM. Suffering in the advanced cancer patient: a definition and taxonomy. J Palliat Care 1994;10:57.
8. Cassell EJ. The nature of suffering and the goals of medicine. N Engl J Med 1982;306:639.
9. Portenoy RK. Pain and quality of life: theoretical aspects. In: Osoba D, ed. Effect of cancer on quality of life. Boca Raton, FL: CRC Press, 1991:279.
10. Osoba D. Lessons learned from measuring health-related quality of life in oncology. J Clin Oncol 1994;12:608.
11. Nayfield SG, Ganz PA, Moinpour CM, et al. Report from a National Cancer Institute (USA) workshop on quality of life assessment in cancer clinical trials. Qual Life Res 1992;1:203.
12. Rodney P. A nursing perspective on life-prolonging treatment. J Palliat Care 1994;10:40.
13. Hill TP, Shirley D. A good death. Reading, MA: Addison-Wesley, 1992:19.
14. Curtis EB, Kretch R, Walsh TD. Common symptoms in patients with advanced cancer. J Palliat Care 1991;7:25.
15. Dunphy KP, Amesbury BDW. A comparison of hospice and homecare patients: patterns of referral, patient characteristics and predictors of place of death. Palliat Med 1990;4:105.
16. Reuben DB, Mor V, Hiris J. Clinical symptoms and length of survival in patients with terminal cancer. Arch Intern Med 1988;148:1586.
17. Dunlop GM. A study of the relative frequency and importance of gastrointestinal symptoms and weakness in patients with far-advanced cancer: student paper. Palliat Med 1989;4:373.
18. Derogatis LR, Morrow GR, Fetting J, et al. The prevalence of psychiatric disorders among cancer patients. JAMA 1983;249:751.
19. Craig TJ, Abeloff MD. Psychiatric symptomatology among hospitalized cancer patients. Am J Psychiatry 1974;131:1323.
20. Levine PM, Silberfarb PM, Lipowski ZJ. Mental disorders in cancer patients: a study of 100 psychiatric referrals. Cancer 1978;42:1386.
21. McCorkle R, Young K. Development of a symptom distress scale. Cancer Nurs 1978;1:373.
22. Kukull WA, McCorkle R, Driever M. Symptom distress, psychosocial variables and survival from lung cancer. J Psychosoc Oncol 1986;4: 91.
23. Portenoy RK. Cancer pain: epidemiology and syndromes. Cancer 1989;63:2298.
24. Brescia FJ, Adler D, Gray G, Ryan MA. A profile of hospitalized advanced cancer patients. J Pain Symptom Manage 1990;15:221.
25. Twycross RG, Fairfield S. Pain in far-advanced cancer. Pain 1982; 14:303.
26. Parkes CM. Home or hospital? Terminal care as seen by the surviving spouse. J Coll Gen Pract 1978;28:19.
27. Aitken-Swan J. Nursing the late cancer patient at home. Practitioner 1959;183:64.
28. Portenoy RK, Kornblith AB, Wong G, et al. Pain in ovarian cancer: prevalence, characteristics, and associated symptoms. Cancer 1994; 74:907.
29. Portenoy RK, Miransky J, Thaler HT, et al. Pain in ambulatory patients with lung or colon cancer: prevalence, characteristics and impact. Cancer 1992;7:1616.
30. Schug SA, Zech D, Dorr U. Cancer pain management according to WHO analgesic guidelines. J Pain Symptom Manage 1990;5:27.
31. Ventafridda V, Tamburini M, DeConno F. Comprehensive treatment in cancer pain. In: Fields HL, Dubner R, Cervero F, eds. Advances in pain research and therapy, vol 9. Proceedings of the Fourth World Congress on Pain. New York: Raven Press, 1985:617.
32. Moulin DE, Foley KM. A review of a hospital-based pain service.

In: Foley KM, Bonica JJ, Ventafridda V, eds. Advances in pain research and therapy, vol 16. Proceedings of the Second International Congress on Cancer Pain. New York, Raven, 1990:413.
33. Ventafridda V, Tamburini M, Caraceni A, et al. A validation study of the WHO method for cancer pain relief. Cancer 1987;59:850.
34. Walker VA, Hoskin PJ, Hanks GW, White ID. Evaluation of WHO analgesic guidlines for cancer pain in a hospital-based palliative care unit. J Pain Symptom Manage 1988;3:145.
35. Jorgensen L, Mortensen M-B, Jensen N-H, Eriksen J. Treatment of cancer pain patients in a multidisciplinary pain clinic. Pain Clin 1990; 3:83.
36. Schug SA, Zech D, Grond S, Jung H, Meurser T, Stobbe B. A long-term survey of morphine in cancer pain patients. J Pain Symptom Manage 1992;7:259.
37. American Pain Society. Principles of analgesic use in the treatment of acute pain and chronic cancer pain, 3rd ed. Skokie, IL: American Pain Society, 1992.
38. Grossman S, Staats P. Current management of pain in patients with cancer. Oncology 1994;3:93.
39. Cherny NI, Portenoy RK. The management of cancer pain. Cancer 1993;72(Suppl):3393.
40. Jacox A, Carr DB, Payne R, et al. Management of cancer pain. Clinical practice guideline no. 9. Agency for Health Care Policy and Research Publication No. 94-0592. Rockville, MD, Agency for Health Care Policy and Research, U.S. Department of Health and Human Services, Public Health Service, 1994.
41. Derogatis LR, Morrow GR, Fetting J, et al. The prevalence of psychiatric disorders among cancer patients. JAMA 1983;249:751.
42. Ahles TA, Blanchard EB, Ruckdeschel JC. The multidimensional nature of cancer-related pain. Pain 1983:17:277.
43. Levine PM, Silberfarb PM, Lipowski ZJ. Mental disorders in cancer patients: A study of 100 psychiatric referrals. Cancer 1978;42:1386.
44. Holland JC, Rowland JH. eds. Handbook of psychooncology. New York: Oxford University Press, 1989.
45. Massie MJ, Gagnon P, Holland JC. Depression and suicide in patients with cancer. J Pain Symptom Manage 1994;9:325.
46. Breitbart W, Levenson JA, Passik SD. Terminally ill cancer patients. In: Breitbart W, Holland JC, ed. Psychiatric aspects of symptom management in cancer patients. Washington, DC: American Psychiatric Press, 1993:173.
47. Massie MJ, Holland J, Glass E. Delirium in terminally ill cancer patients. Am J Psychiatry 1983;140:1048.
48. Trzepacz PT, Teague GB, Lipowski ZJ. Delirium and other organic mental disorders in a general hospital. Gen Hosp Psychiatry 1985;7: 101.
49. Johnson JC, Kerse NM, Gottlieb G, Wanich C, Sullivan E, Chen K. Prospective versus retrospective methods of identifying patients with delirium. J Am Geriatr Soc 1992;40:316.
50. Lipowski ZJ. Delirium (acute confusional states). JAMA 1987;258: 1789.
51. Liptzin B, Levkoff SE. An empirical study of delirium subtypes. Br J Psychiatry 1992;161:843.
52. American Psychiatric Association. Diagnostic and statistical manual of mental disorders, 3rd rev ed. Washington, DC, American Psychiatric Association, 1987.
53. Tucker GJ, DSM-IV Organic Disorders Work Group. DSM-IV: proposals for revision of diagnostic criteria for delirium. Int Psychogeriatr 1991;3:197.
54. American Psychiatric Association, Task Force on DSM-IV. Diagnostic and statistical manual of mental disorders: IV draft criteria. Washington, DC: American Psychiatric Association, 1993.
55. Smith MJ, Breitbart WS, Platt MM. A critique of instruments and methods to detect, diagnose, and rate delirium. J Pain Symptom Manage 1995;10:35.
56. Folstein MF, Folstein SE, McHugh PR. Mini-mental state. J Psychiatr Res 1975;12:189.
57. Katzman R, Brown T, Fuld P, Peck A, Schechter R, Schimmel H. Validation of a short orientation-memory-concentration test of cognitive impairment. Am J Psychiatry 1983;140:734.
58. Inouye SK, Van Dyck CH, Alessi CA, Balkin S, Siegal AP, Horwitz RI. Clarifying confusion: the confusion assessment method. Ann Intern Med 1990;113:941.
59. Trzepacz PT, Baker RW, Greenhouse J. A symptom rating scale for delirium. Psychiatry Res 1988;23:89.
60. Patchell RA, Posner JB. Cancer and the nervous system. In: Holland JC, Rowland JH, eds. Handbook of psychooncology. New York: Oxford University Press, 1989:327.
61. Tuma R, DeAngelis L. Acute encephalopathy in patients with systemic cancer. Ann Neurol 1992;32:288.
62. Bruera E, Miller L, McCallion J, Macmillan K, Krefting L, Hanson J. Cognitive failure in patients with terminal cancer: a prospective study. J Pain Symptom Manage 1992;7:192.
63. Bruera E, Macmillan K, Hanson J, MacDonald RN. The cognitive effects of the administration of narcotic analgesics in patients with cancer pain. Pain 1989;39:13.
64. Fainsinger RL, Tapper M, Bruera E. A perspective on the management of delirium in terminally ill patients on a palliative care unit. J Palliat Care 1993;9:4.
65. Fleishman SB, Lesko LM, Breitbart W. Treatment of organic mental disorders in cancer patients. In: Breitbart W, Holland JC, eds. Psychiatric aspects of symptom management in cancer patients. Washington, DC: American Psychiatric Press, 1993:23.
66. Bruera E, Brenneis C, Paterson AH, MacDonald RN. Use of methylphenidate as an adjuvant to narcotic analgesics in patients with advanced cancer. J Pain Symptom Manage 1989;4:3.
67. Bruera E, Chadwick S, Brenneis C, MacDonald RN. Methylphenidate associated with narcotics for the treatment of cancer pain. Cancer Treat Rep 1987;71:67.
68. Breitbart W, Mermelstein H. An alternative psychostimulant for the management of depressive disorders in cancer patients. Psychosomatics 1992;33:352.
69. Bruera E, Miller M, Macmillan K, Kuehn N. Neuropsychological effects of methylphenidate in patients receiving a continuous infusion of narcotics for cancer pain. Pain 1992;48:163.
70. Katon W, Raskind M. Treatment of depression in the medically ill elderly with methylphenidate. Am J Psychiatry 1980;137:963.
71. Kaufmann MW, Murray GB, Cassem NH. Use of psychostimulants in medically ill depressed patients. Psychosomatics 1982;23:817.
72. Fernandez F, Adams F, Levy JK. Cognitive impairment due to AIDS-related complex and its response to psychostimulants. Psychosomatics 1988;29:38.
73. Irvine DM, Vincent L, Bubela N, Thompson L, Graydon J. A critical appraisal of the research literature investigating fatigue in the individual with cancer. Cancer Nurs 1991;14:188.
74. Winningham ML, Nail LM, Burke MB, et al. Fatigue and the cancer experience: the state of the knowledge. Oncol Nurs Forum 1994;21: 23.
75. Smets EMA, Garssen B, Schuster-Uitterhoeve ALJ, de Haes JCJM. Fatigue in cancer patients. Br J Cancer 1993;68:220.
76. Piper B, Lindsey A, Dodd M. Fatigue mechanisms in cancer patients: developing nursing theory. Oncol Nurs Forum 1987;14:17.
77. Glaus A. Assessment of fatigue in cancer and non-cancer patients and in healthy individuals. Support Care Cancer 1993;1:303.
78. Krupp LB, Coyle PK, Cross AH, Scheinberg LC. Amelioration of fatigue with pemoline in patients with multiple sclerosis. Ann Neurol 1989;26:155.
79. Tannock I, et al. Treatment of metastatic prostatic cancer with low-dose prednisone: evaluation of pain and quality of life as pragmatic indices of response. J Clin Oncol 1989;7:590.
80. Bruera E, Roca E, Cedaro L, Carraro S, Chacon R. Action of oral methylprednisolone in terminal cancer patients: a prospective randomized double-blind study. Cancer Treat Rep 1985;69:751.
81. Levy MH. Constipation and diarrhea in cancer patients. Cancer Bull 1991;43:412.
82. Sykes NP. Constipation and diarrhoea. In: Doyle D, Hanks G W, MacDonald N, eds. Oxford textbook of palliative medicine. New York: Oxford University Press, 1993:299.
83. Portenoy RK. Constipation in the cancer patient: causes and management. Med Clin North Am 1987;71:303.
84. Fadul CE, Lemann W, Thaler HT, Posner JB. Perforation of the gastrointestinal tract in patients receiving steroids for neurologic disease. Neurology 1988;38:348.
85. Culpepper-Morgan JA, Inturrisi CE, Portenoy RK, et al. Treatment of opioid-induced constipation with oral naloxone: a pilot study. Clin Pharmacol Ther 1992;52:90.
86. Sykes NP. Oral naloxone in opioid associated constipation. Lancet 1991;337:1475.
87. Lederle FA, Busch DL, Mattox KM, West MJ, Aske DM. Cost-effec-

tive treatment of constipation in the elderly: a randomized double-blind comparison of sorbitol and lactulose. Am J Med 1990;89:597.
88. Androsky RI, Goldner F. Colonic lavage solution (polyethylene glycol electrolyte lavage solution) as a treatment for chronic constipation: a double-blind, placebo-controlled study. Am J Gastroenterol 1990;85: 261.
89. Binder HJ. Pharmacology of laxatives. Annu Rev Pharmacol Toxicol 1977;17:355.
90. Leng-Peschlow E. Effects of sennosides A + B and bisacodyl on rat large intestine. Pharmacology 1989;38:310.
91. Krevsky B, Maurer AH, Malmud LS, Fisher RS. Cisapride accelerates colonic transit in constipated patients with colonic inertia. Am J Gastroenterol 1989;84:882.
92. Walsh TD. Prevention of opioid side effects. J Pain Symptom Manage 1990;5:363.
93. Coyle N, Adelhardt J, Foley KM, Portenoy RK. Character of terminal illness in the advanced cancer patient: pain and other symptoms during the last 4 weeks of life. J Pain Symptom Manage 1990;4:83.
94. Fainsinger R, Bruera E, Miller MJ, Hanson J, MacEachern T. Symptom control during the last week life on a palliative care unit. J Palliat Care 1991;7:5.
95. Ventafridda V, Ripamonti C, DeConno F, Tamburini M, Cassileth BR. Symptom prevalence and control during cancer patients' last days of life. J Palliat Care 1990;6:7.
96. Allan SG. Nausea and vomiting. In: Doyle D, Hanks GW, MacDonald N, eds. Oxford textbook of palliative medicine. New York: Oxford University Press, 1993:282.
97. Naylor RJ, Rudd JA. Emesis and anti-emesis. In: Hanks GW, ed. Palliative medicine: problem areas in pain and symptom management. Plainview, NY: Cold Spring Harbor Laboratory Press, 1994:117.
98. Burish TG, Tope DM. Psychological techniques for controlling the adverse side effects of cancer chemotherapy: findings from a decade of research. J Pain Symptom Manage 1992;7:287.
99. Alexander HR, Norton JA. Pathophysiology of cancer cachexia. In: Doyle D, Hanks GW, MacDonald N, eds. Oxford textbook of palliative medicine. Oxford: Oxford University Press, 1993:316.
100. Bruera E, MacDonald N. Nutrition in patients with advanced cancer: an update and review of our experience. J Pain Symptom Manage 1988;3:133.
101. Beck S, Mulligan H, Tisdale M. Lipolytic factors associated with murine and human cancer cachexia. J Natl Cancer Inst 1990;82:1922.
102. Mahony S, Beck S, Tisdale M. Comparison of weight loss induced by recombinant tumor necrosis factor with that produced by a cachexia-induced tumor. Br J Cancer 1988;57:385.
103. Vigano A, Watanabe S, Bruera E. Anorexia and cachexia in advanced cancer patients. In: Hanks GW, ed. Palliative medicine: problem areas in pain and symptom management. Plainview, NY: Cold Spring Harbor Laboratory Press, 1994:99.
104. Schell H. Adrenal corticosteroid therapy in far-advanced cancer. Geriatrics 1972;27:131.
105. Willox J, Corr J, Shaw J, et al. Prednisolone as an appetite stimulant in patients with cancer. Br Med J 1984;200:37.
106. Ettinger AB, Portenoy RK. The use of corticosteroids in the treatmen of symptoms associated with cancer. J Pain Symptom Manage 1988; 3:99.
107. Bruera E, MacMillan K, Hanson J, Kuehn N, MacDonald RN. A controlled trial of megestrol acetate on appetite, caloric intake, nutritional status, and other symptoms in patients with advanced cancer. Cancer 1990;66:1279.
108. Loprinzi CL, Ellison NM, Schaid J, et al. A controlled trial of megestrol acetate treatment of cancer anorexia and cachexia. J Natl Cancer Inst 1990;82:1127.
109. Kornblith AB, Hollis DR, Zuckerman E, et al. Effect of megestrol acetate on quality of life in a dose-response trial in women with advanced breast cancer. J Clin Oncol 1993;11:2081.
110. Loprinzi CL, Michalak JC, Schaid DJ, et al. Phase III evaluation of four doses of megestrol acetate as therapy for patients with anorexia and/or cachexia. J Clin Oncol 1993;11:762.
111. Tchekmedyian NC, Tait N, Moody M, et al. High dose megestrol acetate: a possible treatment for cachexia. JAMA 1987;257:1195.
112. Nelson K, Walsh D, Deeter P, et al. A phase II study of delta-9-tetrahydrocannabinol for appetite stimulation in cancer-associated anorexia. J Palliat Care 1994;10:14.
113. Beal JE, Olson R, Laubenstein L, et al. Dronabinol as a treatment for anorexia associated with weight loss in patients with AIDS. J Pain Symptom Manage 1995;10:89.
114. Kardinal C, Loprinzi C, Shaw P, et al. A controlled trial of cyproheptadine in cancer patients with anorexia. Cancer 1990;65:2657.
115. Chlebowski RT, Bulcavage L, Grosvenor M, et al. Hydrazine sulfate in cancer patients with weight loss: a placebo-controlled clinical experience. Cancer 1987;59:406.
116. Chlebowski RT, Bulcavage L, Grosvenor M, et al. Hydrazine sulfate influence on nutritional status and survival in non–small cell lung cancer. J Clin Oncol 1990;8:9.
117. Loprinzi CL, Goldberg RM, Su JO, et al. Placebo-controlled trial of hydrazine sulfate in patients with newly diagnosed non–small-cell lung cancer. J Clin Oncol 1994;12:1126.
118. Loprinzi CL, Kuross SA, O'Fallon JR, et al. Randomized placebo-controlled evaluation of hydrazine sulfate in patients with advanced colorectal cancer. J Clin Oncol 1994;12:1121.
119. Kosty MP, Fleischman SB, Herndon JE, et al. Cisplatin, vinblastine and hydrazine sulfate in advanced non–small-cell lung cancer: a randomized, placebo-controlled, double-blind phase III study of the Cancer and Leukemia Group B. J Clin Oncol 1994;12:1113.

Principles and Practice of Genitourinary Oncology, edited by Derek Raghavan, Howard I. Scher, Steven A. Leibel, and Paul H. Lange. Lippincott-Raven Publishers, Philadelphia, © 1997.

CHAPTER 12

Orthopaedic Management of Metastases in Genitourinary Cancer

Robert M. Lifeso and Brian E. McGrath

Metastatic cancer is the most common malignant lesion of bone in patients older than 40 years of age. Bone is the third most common site of metastatic disease after lung and liver, and is often the first symptomatic site.[1] Five carcinomas—prostate, thyroid, breast, lung, and kidney—are responsible for 85% of skeletal metastases. The most common bones involved are the spine, pelvis, proximal femur, skull, and upper extremity, in order of decreasing frequency.

During the past 20 years, advances in the treatment of malignancy have led to significant increases in life expectancy. The 5-year survival of a patient with prostate cancer is greater than 75%.[1]

There were 122,000 new cases of prostate cancer and 25,300 new cases of renal cell carcinoma diagnosed in the United States in 1991.[1] In these malignancies of genitourinry origin it is estimated that 70% of prostate, 30% of bladder, and 25% of renal cell carcinomas will metastasize to bone.[2] Autopsy studies by Walker showed that 84% of prostate cancer and 37% of renal cell carcinoma metastasize to bone.[3] Genitourinary malignancies account for a significant percentage of clinically relevant skeletal metastases.

The morbidity of bone metastases lies in their ability to compromise the three major functions of the skeleton: structural, hemopoietic, and mineral metabolism.[1] The loss of structural support can render the patient painfully bedridden for the remaining months of his or her life.[2] Bone marrow replacement can cause severe anemia, myelosuppression, or platelet loss. The osteolytic phase and associated paraneoplastic syndrome can cause significant disruption of the calcium and phosphate metabolism, resulting in muscle, nerve, and mental status changes.

The initial complaint of patients suffering from osseous metastases is usually localized pain. Skeletal metastases are the presenting lesions in 10% to 15% of metastatic carcinomas of unknown primary lesions. Appropriate investigations should be determined after a thorough history and physical examination. Laboratory evaluation of an unknown primary lesion with an isolated bony metastasis should include at a minimum complete blood count, calcium, phosphate, alkaline phosphatase, prostate specific antigen (PSA), acid phosphatase, urinalysis, protein electrophoresis, chest radiograph, and computed tomographic (CT) scans of the chest, abdomen, and pelvis. Such a diagnostic work-up results in 85% success in identifying the primary lesion.[4]

Standard skeletal x-ray films generally reveal either an osteoblastic or osteolytic lesion. Forty to fifty percent of the involved bone cortex must be replaced before a lesion will be detectable on a standard x-ray film. Bone scintigraphy is a more sensitive indicator of a skeletal lesion and can scan the entire skeleton with a single study. Most osseous metastases from carcinomas are detectable by bone scintigraphy. A few cancer cell lines, such as myeloma and occasionally renal cell, produce little bone reaction and are difficult to identify by bone scintigraphy. Fortunately, most renal cell, prostate, and transitional cell carcinomas of the bladder are detectable on bone scans. CT and magnetic resonance (MR) scans are extremely helpful in determining the exact anatomy and possible histologic type of a lesion. A CT scan can determine the presence of residual cortical integrity or mineralization within a lesion. The MR scan can accurately delineate marrow involvement, as well as the presence or absence of a soft tissue mass.[5,6] The combination of the plain x-ray film, bone scan, CT scan, and MR imaging scan is extremely valuable to the clinician caring for the patient with metastatic carcinoma. If surgery is contemplated, it is also of tremendous value in preoperative planning.

The pathogenesis of osseous metastases is currently an area of great research interest. Metastases to bone from a primary carcinoma require the de-adhesion and passage of viable cancer cells through the endothelial membrane from the primary site. These cells must then traverse the circulatory or lymphatic system to find their way to the bone marrow. Once the tumor cells have reached the bone marrow, they must again traverse the capillary endothelium. The endothelial cells have a gap of 60 Å and do not appear to have a significant basement membrane. The cells then re-adhere to marrow cells or matrix and begin the process of proliferation.[7]

In 1889, Stephen Paget proposed the "seed-and-soil" theory of metastasis, wherein specific cancer types preferentially metastasize to specific sites. He felt that successful metastasis occurred when the "right seed found the correct soil".[8] Miyasaka's[7] theory of cell adhesion and de-adhesion further supports Paget's theory. Cadherins, transmembrane glycoproteins that mediate homotypic calcium dependent intracellular adhesions, regulate the invasiveness of certain malignant cell lines. The modulation of the expression of these cell surface binders has altered the invasiveness of certain malignant cell lines.[7]

Orr and colleagues[9] stressed the importance of the early vascular spread of cancer cells and their adhesion in the safe harbor of the bone microenvironment. The red marrow and its matrix provides excellent growth and chemotactic factors that promote tumor cell proliferation. Multiple growth factors have been identified in bone marrow: osteoblast-derived growth factor, transforming growth factor-β (TGF-β), insulin-like growth factor (IGF) I and II, fibroblast growth factor (FGF), platelet-derived growth factor (PDGF), and interleukins (IL) 1 and 6. Chemotaxis has also been shown to be increased with rising levels of bone degradation products such as type I collagen, alpha-II (α_2) glycoprotein, osteocalcin, and TGF-β.[9]

PROPERTIES OF BONE

Bone is a rather simple organ. It responds to invasive processes such as cancer in one of two ways: resorption (osteolytic phase) or proliferation (osteoblastic phase). Cancer cells can induce widespread bone destruction and hypercalcemia systemically through humoral factors or locally through local paracrine mediators. Systemic release of parathyroid hormone (PTH)-related protein by some tumor cells can cause hypercalcemia; other tumor-derived factors implicated in development of hypercalcemia include TGF-β1, IL-1, IL-6, tumor necrosis factors α and β.[9] At the local level, bone degradation and calcium release are mediated by osteoclasts, tumor-associated macrophages, and cancer cells themselves.[9] Osteolytic lesions are associated with pain, pathologic fracture, hypercalcemia, and alterations in the mechanical properties of the affected bones. Hypercalcemia may be aggravated by immobilization.

An osteoblastic response is seen primarily in prostate cancer and is mediated by cytokines with selective mitogenic activity for osteoblasts.[9] The elution of these cytokines results in an increased rate of lamellar bone resorption and woven bone formation. Although the affected bone volume is increased, the strength of the bone is decreased by the loss of the stress-oriented lamellar bone. Prostate metastases are rarely osteolytic; however, the presence of an osteolytic prostatic metastasis further weakens the bone.

IMPENDING PATHOLOGIC FRACTURES

Indications for prophylactic fixation of an impending fracture should be based on the biologic and biomechanical alterations caused by the invading process and the response of the host bone to that process. Harrington[10] developed the most well-established classification system. He studied the effect of metastatic disease on bone's structural integrity to determine the risk of pathologic fracture. He suggests that the indications for prophylactic internal fixation of a long bone is any lesion larger than 2.5 cm in diameter or more than 50% circumferential cortical destruction. Osteolytic osseous metastases that reach these critical dimensions result in a more than 70% diminution in the torsional strength of the affected bone.[10] A study using quantitative CT scanning is underway to correlate specific areas of bone destruction with their corresponding risk of fracture.[11]

Lesions of the lesser trochanter of the femur that result in either an avulsion of or fracture of the lesser trochanter are an indication for prophylactic internal fixation. Generally, metastatic deposits in large metaphyseal regions such as the proximal tibia or distal femur are less likely to fracture because of the greater diameter of the surrounding cancellous bone, which tends to buttress the lesion.

Prostatic cancer patients with bone metastases constitute the largest single group and longest survivors of osseous metastases (10% 10-year survival).[12] Although prostate cancer represents the most common carcinoma metastatic to bone in man, its osteoblastic response and its preference for the pelvis and spine results in a surprisingly low incidence of pathologic fracture. Prostate cancer metastases are responsible for only 4% of pathologic fractures.[12]

Osteoblastic, clinically active skeletal metastases present with pain and can cause pathologic fractures that can render a patient nonambulatory or bedridden. Upper extremity lesions can produce both pain and a significant limitation of function. The use of external walking aids in minimally ambulatory patients may be seriously compromised by painful upper extremity lesions.

Symptomatic skeletal metastases from prostate cancer must be addressed by the oncology team. The multitude of treatment modalities available requires a true team approach; this team should include a medical oncologist, radiation oncologist, genitourinary oncologist, and orthopaedic oncologist. Hormonal manipulation, external beam radiotherapy, systemic radiopharmaceuticals, and orthopaedic surgical intervention have all been shown to be effective in palliation. Huben[13] states that endocrine therapy can relieve pain and prevent pathologic fractures and neurologic complications secondary to prostatic metastases in 80% to 85% of patients. Douglas and colleagues[14] found that 80% of patients experienced significant pain relief from external beam radiotherapy. Strontium-89, a beta-emitting radioisotope with a long half-life (50.5 days), has also been shown to have a statistically positive correlation with complete pain relief in patients with prostatic osseous metastases.[15] Patients that suffer from impending or pathologic fractures in the preadjuvant or postadjuvant setting can experience significant relief of their pain and resume more normal activities after orthopaedic internal fixation or prosthetic replacement of the affected bone.[16]

Renal cell carcinoma, usually seen in the fifth and sixth decades of life, can run either an incredibly rapid or an indolent course.[12] The roughly 20,000 new cases of renal cell carcinoma in the United States each year translates into 4000 to 9000 cases of renal cell carcinoma with osseous metastases.[5,12] deKernion[17] estimated the overall 5-year survival rate for patients with renal cell cancer to be 45% to 50%. The median survival of patients with metastases is roughly 10 to 12 months, but an estimated 25% will survive 3 years, and some patients will survive for as long as 10 years.[17–19] The treatment of osseous metastases typically involves surgery, embolization, radiotherapy, or some combination of these. The pace of the patient's disease and the patient's overall health status should be thoroughly evaluated and discussed among the oncology team before beginning a particular treatment regimen. Swanson and colleagues[20] reviewed the clinical course of 250 patients with renal cell carcinoma metastases to bone and found improved survival after nephrectomy in patients with solitary metastases (37.5 months compared with 18 months).

Weiner and colleagues[21] reviewed 36 patients with renal cell carcinoma and found that a disease-free interval of longer than 1 year from presentation to osseous metastasis was the most important determinant of improved survival. In their group with a disease-free interval longer than 12 months, the mean survival was 27.7 months, compared with 11.9 months in the patient group with a disease-free interval shorter than 12 months. These researchers advocate more aggressive treatment for isolated renal cell osseous metastases.

Radiotherapy can be used for palliation of pain or to slow the growth of residual tumor after interlesional surgery. Halperin and Hausiadis[22] reported relief of pain in 77%, which was found to be a permanent effect in 86% of their patient population. Varma and colleagues[23] reported a small series that combined embolization and external beam radiotherapy to pelvic metastases. They found that this treatment produced improved pain relief compared with the historical control of similar lesions treated with irradiation alone.

Unlike prostate cancer, renal cell carcinoma osseous metastases are osteolytic and generally expansive (Fig. 12-1*A*). They may be the first site of metastatic involvement and can involve any bone. These lesions must be approached with great trepidation because of the risk of profuse bleeding, even from biopsy. Prior to biopsying a suspected renal cell metastasis, the oncologist should obtain a urinalysis, bone scan, and a renal ultrasound. A needle or percutaneous Tru-Cut biopsy is preferable to an open biopsy because of the highly vascular nature of these lesions.

The relatively short life expectancy of these patients has relegated much of their care to the radiation oncologist. However, because of the size of these lesions at presentation and the occasional mass that continues to grow following radiotherapy, orthopaedic intervention is often required. Internal stabilization or replacement of the destroyed periarticular segment often results in significant pain relief and tremendously improves the patient's quality of life.

Surgical intervention for internal fixation or replacement of an affected metastatic lesion in these patients should be preceded by arterial embolization of the feeding vessels, if possible (Fig. 12-1*B*). Bowers and colleagues[24] reviewed eight patients who underwent surgery for hypervascular bone metastasis from renal cell carcinoma. Embolization was successful in six patients (75%), resulting in a dramatic decrease in operative blood loss (Fig. 12-1*C, D*).

Metastatic transitional cell carcinoma frequently involves the skeletal system.[25] It can affect any bone but has a predilection for the pelvis, ribs, and spine. These metastatic deposits cause local osteolysis and therefore leave the affected bone susceptible to pathologic fracture. Treatment of these lesions should follow the principles outlined for other osteolytic metastases.

SPINAL METASTASES FROM GENITOURINARY TUMORS

Dramatic advances in the surgical management of metastatic disease of the spine have occurred over the past decade. Traditionally, surgical treatment of spinal lesions was limited to biopsy, decompression, or stabilization. The results were often unsuccessful, and in many cases patients' conditions were worsened by ill-advised surgical decompressions.

The results of surgical decompression were so poor in these patients that despite neurological status on presentation, patients did better with radiotherapy than with laminectomy or laminectomy combined with radiotherapy.[26] Interestingly enough, the results of radiotherapy appear to be similar whether or not the tumor was radiation sensitive.[27] In the decade since these results were published, there have been dramatic advances in the effectiveness of chemotherapy and radiotherapy, and these have been matched by advances in spinal instrumentation and localized tumor management in metastatic disease of the spine.

The risk of fracture of the vertebral spine is a complex concept that depends on the size and location of the metastatic lesion and the type of tumor cell of origin. For example, renal cell tumors produce large lytic lesions with minimal new bone formation that are at a much higher risk for early fracture than the osteoblastic lesions usually found in prostatic metastases.

Incidence

Approximately 18,000 new patients per year present with spinal metastases.[28] This number represents about 5% of all patients with malignancies in the United States. McLain and Weinstein[29] found that nearly 60% of tumors metastatic to the spine were related to primary cancers of the breast, lung, or prostate; myeloma; or lymphoma. Because prostatic tumor is often osteoblastic, fractures related to prostatic metastases to the spine are rare; generally, these metastases are asymptomatic and become apparent only on bone scanning. It is estimated that approximately 70% of patients who ultimately die of a primary malignancy will have evidence of vertebral metastases on careful postmortem examination.[30]

Presentation

Spinal pain as a result of neoplasm is typically progressive and is often more pronounced at night. It may not be associated with activity and may even be relieved by activity. Pain that is worsened by activity and relieved by rest is more characteristic of mechanical back pain such as arthritis or discogenic disease. The sudden onset of back pain in a patient with malignant disease is usually related to a vertebral fracture, which may follow relatively minor trauma.

Insidiously increasing back pain in patients with metastatic disease may be related to pressure developed by the tumor, to microfractures occurring within weakened cancellous bone, or possibly to compression of neural or other adjacent structures. This pain may or may not be associated with radicular pain. Approximately 50% of patients with thoracic cord involvement attributable to an expanding metastatic lesion of a thoracic vertebral body complain of a radicular-type pain before the development of symptoms of cord involvement.[30] Such pain is often described as "girdle pain" because of its radiation around the costal margin.

Most tumor involvement occurs in the anterior vertebral body, primarily because of its extremely rich blood supply and

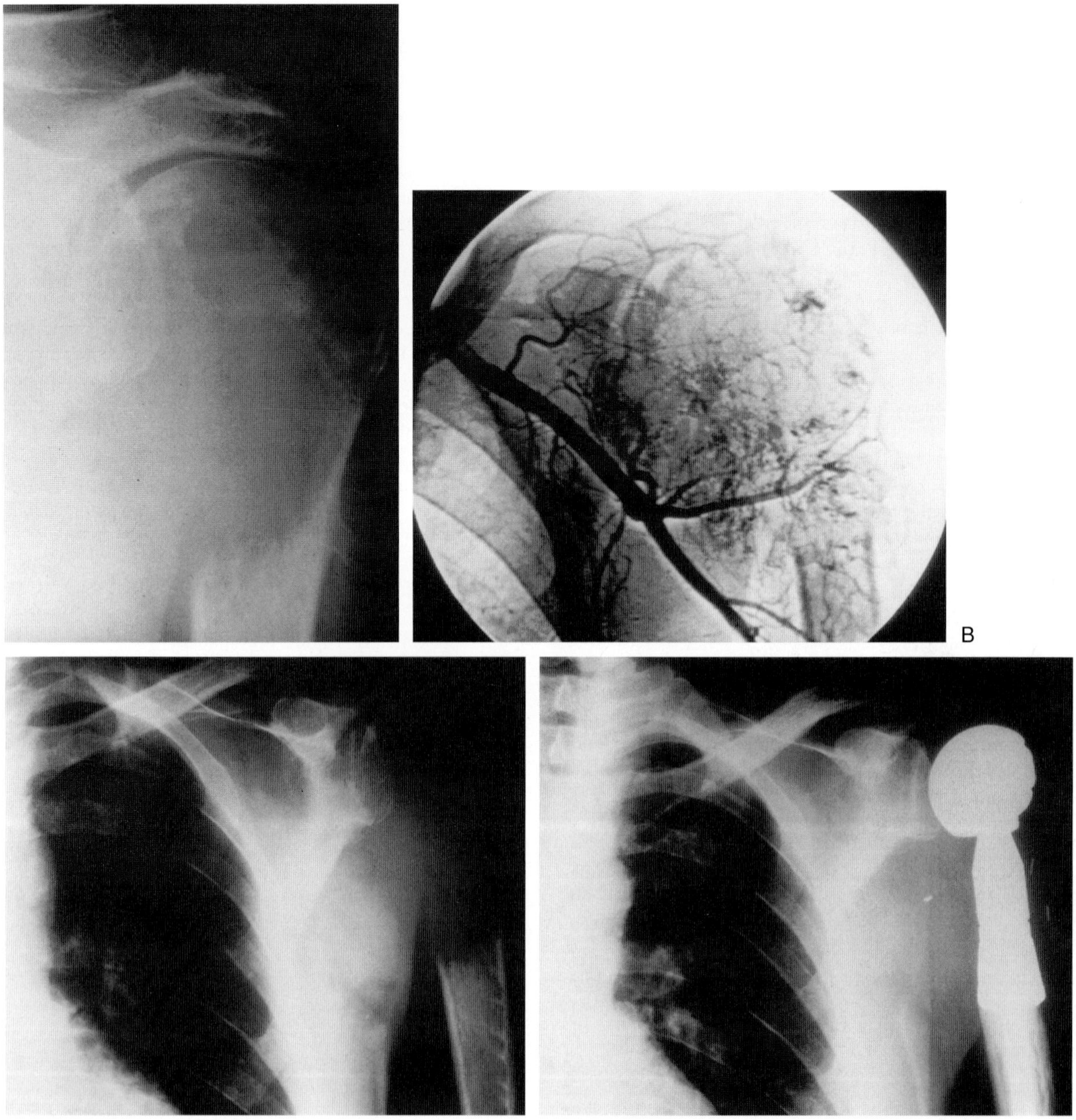

FIG. 12-1. (A) Radiograph in a 40-year-old man, 1 year after radiotherapy for a rapidly enlarging renal cell metastasis to proximal left humerus reveals almost total loss of the left humeral metaphysis. (B) Preoperative angiogram and embolization to diminish blood supply. (C) Radiographic appearance after marginal resection of the proximal humerus. (D) Radiographic appearance after surgical reconstruction of the proximal humerus (i.e., hemiarthroplasty).

the close association of Batson's plexus. The motor tracts lie in the anterior spinal cord; consequently, motor loss often precedes sensory loss in the lower extremities. The anterior portion of the spinal cord is at greatest risk for vascular insufficiency or direct tumor compression (Fig. 12-2*A*).[31]

The sensory tracts lie more posteriorly in the spinal cord; therefore, sensory loss may occur later in the course of disease and may not accurately correlate with the level of spinal compression. The sensory loss is often two or three segments distal to the actual level of cord involvement.[32] Similarly, loss of sphincter control and cauda equina involvement may occur, either acutely or subtly, and must be specifically noted by rectal examination at the time of initial presentation.

The rapidity of onset of weakness and neurologic deficit generally indicates a poor prognosis. Constans and colleagues[33] reported that 166 of 600 patients presenting with cord involvement (28%) had an acute onset, with a delay of less than 48 hours between initial symptoms and maximal neurologic compromise. These patients had the worst prognosis for recovery, regardless of treatment modality. Conversely, patients with slower development of neurologic compromise have a decidedly better prognosis. Whether this is related to anterior verte-

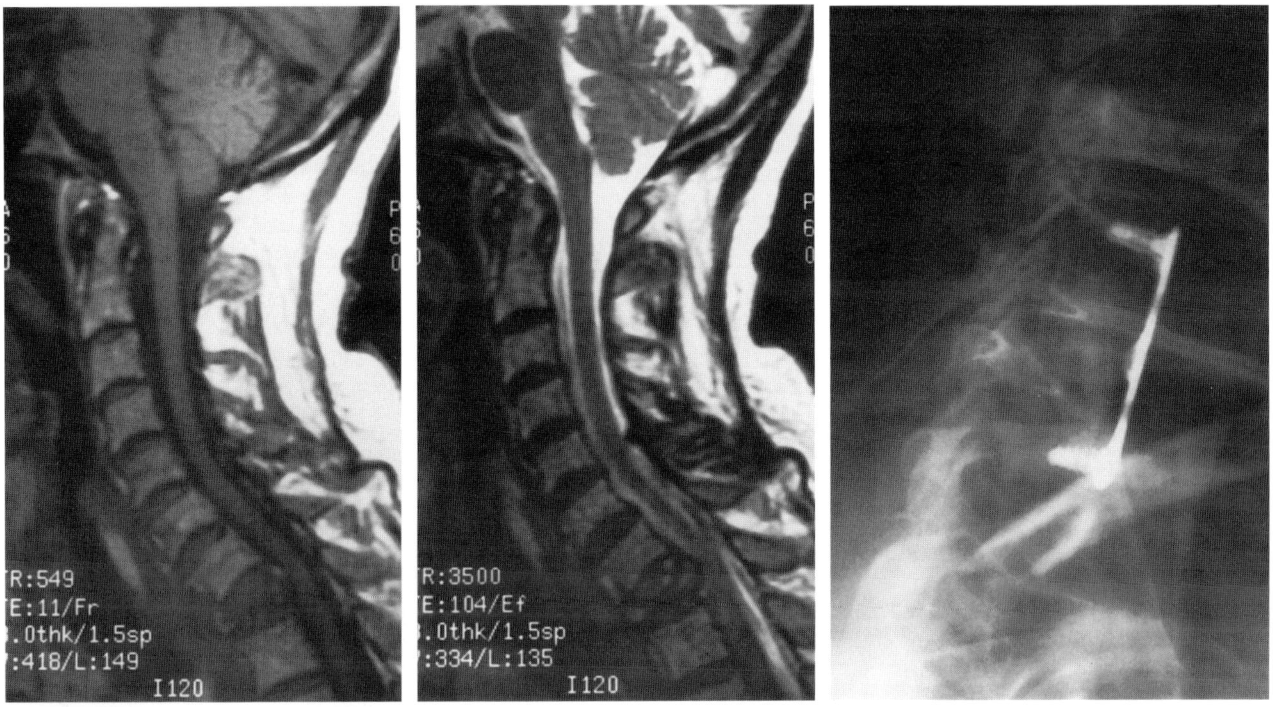

A,B C

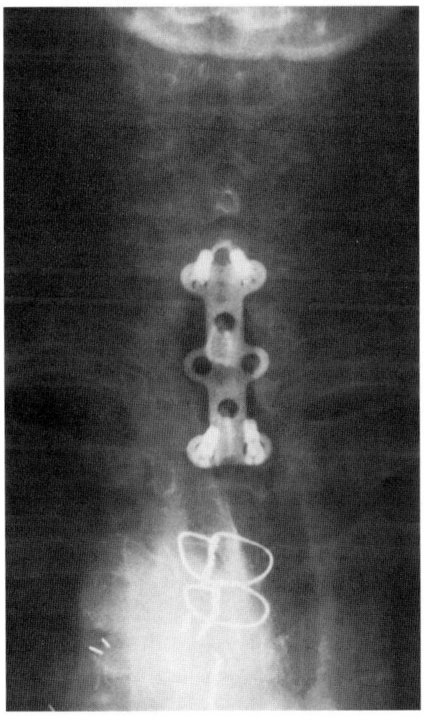

D

FIG. 12-2. A 72-year-old man, 3 years after radical prostatectomy for prostatic carcinoma. (**A, B**) T1- and T2-weighted magnetic resonance images show a destructive process at T1 with anterior vertebral collapse and posterior retropulsion into the spinal canal. Incomplete paraplegia occurred at the T1 level. (**C, D**) One year following anterior T1 vertebrectomy and iliac crest strut graft augmented with anterior titanium plate, the patient was pain-free and neurologically normal.

bral artery involvement (i.e., avascular changes in the cord) or the possibility of direct vertebral compression of the spinal cord is not definitively known. Vascular compromise probably plays a significant role in neurologic sequelae and may be the cause of a patient's failure to respond to what would appear to be adequate tumor decompression.

The majority of bony metastases originate from five visceral organs: breast, prostate, lung, kidney, and thyroid.[34] These bony metastases usually involve the spine, pelvis, ribs, skull, and proximal long bones, all of which are major sites of erythrocyte production and are exceedingly well vascularized.

In 1940, Batson[35] noted an intercommunicating network of thin-walled veins with a low intraluminal pressure lying on the anterior vertebral bodies. This system was valveless and allowed retrograde embolization of tumor cells. It is this Batson's plexus that probably accounts for the predilection of prostate and kidney embolization to the thoracic, thoracolumbar, and lumbar spines.

Investigation

Physical Examination

In patients with suspected metastatic disease of the spine, assessment of deformity and a detailed neurologic examination on first presentation are mandatory. A kyphotic deformity may indicate pathologic collapse of a vertebral body. Spasticity, clonus, and hyperreflexia indicate a lesion at cord level (i.e., at or above T12). A flaccid presentation indicates a level at or below L1. Localized tenderness over the affected area of the spine is a common finding and, if present in multiple areas, may suggest multiple levels of spinal involvement. A rectal examination must be performed, and in patients with suspicion of bladder dysfunction, the amount of postvoiding residual urine should be measured.

Radiographic Findings

Usually, the first investigations performed in a patient with a suspected spinal metastasis are plain radiographs. The radiographic features of skeletal metastases are dependent on the amount of bone destruction and corresponding new bone formation. As discussed previously, metastatic tumors usually involve the anterior vertebral body, with relative preservation of the posterior elements. The vertebral body becomes unable to withstand normal compressive forces, fractures under normal physiologic loading, and produces a kyphotic deformity because of the relative preservation of the posterior structures (Fig. 12-3*A*).

Many vertebral metastases remain asymptomatic and, especially in bone-forming tumors such as prostate metastases, may be discovered only incidentally on routine bone scintigraphy. To be identified radiographically, at least 30% to 50% of the vertebral body must be replaced by tumor; consequently, in many cases plain x-ray films of a patient with clinically suspicious metastatic tumor may appear deceptively normal.

Technetium-99 Bone Scan

Bone scanning is a nonspecific test and does not differentiate a fracture from infection, neoplasm, or even some forms of osteoarthritis. This technique is very sensitive in lesions with an osteoblastic response; that is, it is more useful in patients with prostatic carcinoma than in patients with a nonblastic response such as renal cell carcinoma.

False-negative scans can occur in patients with renal cell carcinoma or myeloma because of the rapidly destructive nature of the lesion and the lack of new bone formation. Similarly, patients receiving chemotherapy may have a false-negative scan because of the resultant suppression of osteoblastic activity.[36]

The most important use of bone scintigraphy is to identify bony metastases that may be asymptomatic. The presence of multiple metastases may prompt a change in the patient's chemotherapeutic or hormonal manipulation regimen, but if these metastases are asymptomatic, they may not require additional treatment.

Computed Tomography

CT is primarily of value in surgical planning; the detail from a CT scan shows residual bone mass and allows more accurate planning of surgical procedures, if surgery or biopsy is indicated. Although MR has generally replaced CT and CT myelography in the evaluation of the spine, cortical bone is not well demonstrated with MR scanning, and CT still has a very valuable place in the assessment of residual bone mass (Fig. 12-4*A*).

Magnetic Resonance Imaging

MR imaging offers superior visualization of metastatic deposits in the epidural space, the vertebral body, and the adjacent soft tissues. Multifocal metastatic disease, areas of epidural compression, and even the source of epidural compression may be identified on MR images. The use of gadolinium with MR increases the imaging signal from lesions and is helpful in the differential diagnosis of many other nontumorous conditions in the spine (see Fig. 12-2*A*, *B*).[37]

A benign osteoporotic compression fracture can often be differentiated from a malignant fracture by the fact that the benign fracture often has a normal marrow signal, whereas the malignant pathologic fracture reveals evidence of replacement of normal cancellous bone by tumor. Although MR imaging usually has a high level of sensitivity, its specificity may be somewhat obscured when an acute benign fracture is associated with marked edema and hemorrhage in the vertebral marrow. These marrow changes are usually reversible with fracture healing (see Fig. 12-3*B*).

Differential Diagnosis

Patients presenting with a known preexisting tumor are in many cases elderly and are often immunocompromised because of previous courses of chemotherapy or radiotherapy or because of the presence of other disease entities. Even patients with known primary tumors may develop collapse or instability as a result of nonmalignant causes; these must be ruled out before planning therapeutic intervention.

Spinal tumors and infections can be differentiated using MR. An and colleagues[38] studied 30 patients with proven spinal tumors or infections using MR. MR correctly differentiated spinal tumor from infection in 29 of 30 cases (97%). Their findings suggested that disc spaces were uninvolved in tumor cases, whereas vertebral osteomyelitis involved the disc space and adjacent vertebral bodies; contiguous vertebral involvement was seen more frequently in infections than in tumors; soft tissue changes, especially the fat planes, were diffusely obscured by the edema of infection and were intact in tumor; and cord compression was accurately diagnosed by MR in both tumors and infections (see Fig. 12-2*A*, *B*).

Similarly, osteoporotic collapse fractures may be diagnosed using MR. Although there is an overlap on MR images between metastatic tumor appearance and an acute compression fracture from osteoporosis, the clinical course helps to differentiate the two; occasionally, needle biopsy is required for this purpose (see Figs. 12-2*A*, *B* and 12-3*B*).

Arthritis can usually be differentiated from tumor as a source

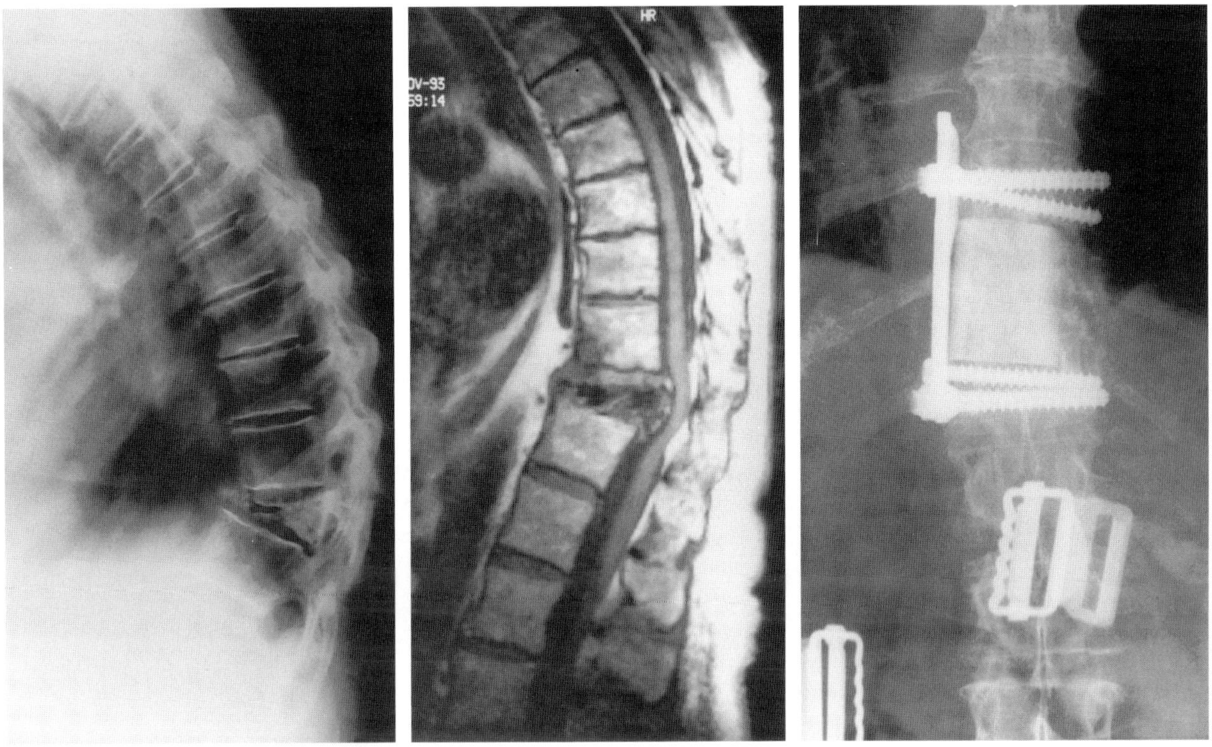

A,B C

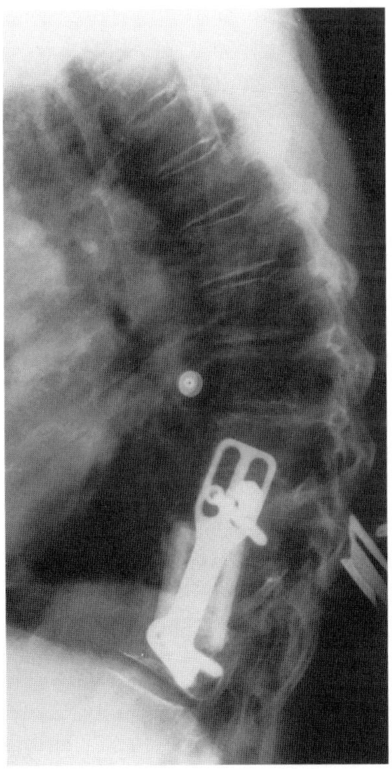

D

FIG. 12-3. A 72-year-old woman with a known history of surgically treated renal cell carcinoma presented 2 years postnephrectomy with severe thoracolumbar pain and increasing paraplegia to the T11 level. (**A**) Lateral radiograph shows collapse of the anterior vertebral body of T11 with vacuum sign in the anterior T11 body. (**B**) Magnetic resonance imaging shows marked retropulsion of the body of T11 into the spinal canal and significant cord compromise. Marrow in all visualized vertebral bodies is normal, and a vacuum sign is present in the center of T11. (**C**) Anterior and (**D**) lateral radiographs 1 year following reconstruction of the body of T11 with femoral allograft and anterior titanium plate reveal complete resolution of the neurologic deficit. Pathologic examination of the resected vertebral body shows no evidence of malignancy; this is an insufficiency fracture, probably occurring as a result of osteoporotic collapse rather than malignant tumor.

of spinal pain by its mechanical nature. Arthritic pain is generally aggravated by activity and relieved by inactivity or rest. Similarly, nonsteroidal antiinflammatory agents often effectively reduce the pain of arthritis.

Insufficiency fractures of the spine may be related to previous irradiation and may appear months or years after a course of radiotherapy. These fractures are related to avascular necrosis of bone and subsequent late collapse of the vertebral body. They can generally be differentiated from an acute metastatic process by MR. Signal intensity changes secondary to previous radiotherapy have a reasonably unique appearance that is the converse of metastatic disease.[36] These changes have been described as occurring as early as 2 months and as late as 10 years following radiotherapy.

A,B

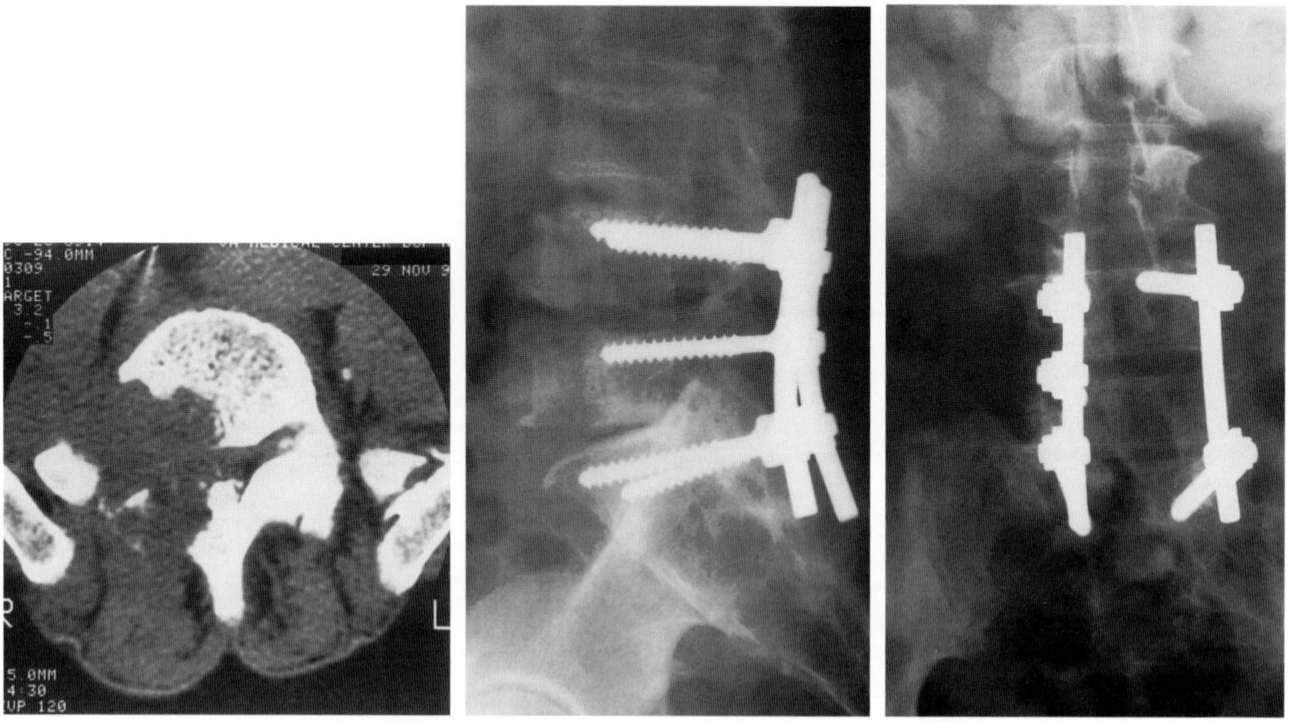

C

FIG. 12-4. A 67-year-old man presented 2 years following surgical resection of carcinoma of the bladder with significant pain in a right L5-S1 radiculopathy. (**A**) Computed tomography shows destruction of the posterior right pedicle and posterolateral corner of the right vertebral body at L5. (**B** and **C**) Radiographs after radical surgical excision and stabilization using pedicle screws and a rod construct. Two years postsurgery, the patient was neurologically normal and pain-free.

Gadolinium-enhanced MR may also be useful for assessing the effectiveness of therapy for spinal metastases. Sugimura and colleagues[37] found that before radiotherapy or chemotherapy, metastatic foci in the spine enhanced significantly more on MR than did normal vertebral bodies. After therapy, responding lesions showed diminished enhancement, and these patients remained clinically asymptomatic for 2 to 6 months. In patients in whom there was no response to radiotherapy or chemotherapy, lesion enhancement on MR did not diminish significantly.

Management

The primary goal of treatment in patients with a spinal malignancy is a rapid diagnosis and initiation of appropriate treatment modalities to maintain pain-free mobility. Many patients present with a known primary lesion with asymptomatic metastases that are noted only on routine bone scintigraphy. If these lesions are asymptomatic, their mere presence may prompt a change in chemotherapy or hormonal manipulation regimen, but no specific additional treatment measures are indicated for the spinal lesions. These patients should be followed by routine radiographic studies, but other treatment modalities are rarely indicated. If spinal pain does develop, it is essential to clarify whether it is attributed to the tumor itself or to other problems.

Harrington[39] categorized patients with metastatic disease of the spine into one of five classes based on the degree of neurologic involvement and bone destruction. Class 1 patients have asymptomatic spinal metastases. Class 2 patients have pain or minor neurologic deficit without bone collapse or instability. Class 3 patients have major sensory or motor compromise without significant bone involvement. Class 4 patients have pain from instability or mechanical causes as a result of vertebral collapse, without significant neurologic deficit. Class 5 patients have both significant neurologic deficit and vertebral collapse or instability.

Class 1 and class 2 patients generally respond to chemotherapy or hormonal manipulation. If improvement is not seen with these modalities, radiotherapy may be considered. Generally, most patients in these categories do not develop progressive spinal instability or neurologic involvement and can be treated successfully with local irradiation or temporary bracing as necessary. They should be followed on a routine basis and advised that if neurologic sequelae or severe back pain develops, they must be reassessed on an urgent basis.

Class 3 patients usually respond to radiotherapy, although tumor types vary significantly in their radiosensitivity. These patients often require a period of temporary bed rest and soft bracing, but as long as their vertebral column remains intact and the neurologic impairment is related to tumor in the epidural space, these patients usually do well with radiotherapy.

Patients in classes 4 and 5 with pathologic spinal fractures present the most significant diagnostic and therapeutic challenges. The philosophy of treatment for these patients has evolved over the years. With chemotherapy, radiotherapy, and hormonal manipulation, patients without visceral involvement may survive for many years. The primary goal of treatment in patients with a known spinal malignancy is to keep the patients mobile and pain-free for as long as possible. Generally, patients with widespread visceral and bony metastases succumb to their disease within a short time.[40] In this group, spinal surgery is necessary only when pain relief cannot be achieved by other means.

In contrast, aggressive treatment of spinal metastases is indicated in patients without significant visceral metastases and in whom the disease can be reasonably controlled by radiotherapy, chemotherapy, or hormonal manipulation. It is important to remember that most patients with spinal metastases do not develop progressive spinal instability or neurologic involvement and can be treated successfully with short periods of bed rest, temporary bracing, and systemic chemotherapy or local irradiation.

Biopsy

Whether vertebral biopsy is required when the site of a primary tumor is known remains debatable. Because of the potential for other disease entities in association with a known primary (e.g., other possible tumors, sepsis, osteonecrosis), some oncologists recommend biopsy before definitive treatment is planned.

If the only identified site of metastasis is in the spine, the lesion can be approached with a CT biopsy. CT-guided needle biopsy is efficient, has a low risk of morbidity, and generally yields sufficient histologic matter for diagnosis. If there is a high suspicion for a renal cell tumor, special care may be required because of the lesion's propensity for bleeding.

Radiotherapy

Radiotherapy is of most use in patients presenting prior to the development of significant bone collapse (i.e., Harrington class 2 or 3). Radiation complications, including myelopathic change, radiation osteitis, radiation-induced avascular necrosis, interference with wound healing, and interference with bone graft incorporation and healing, generally occur with doses above 3000 to 3500 cGy. The control of local tumor recurrence in the spine does not seem to improve with doses above 3000 cGy, and local irradiation is usually limited to this dose level.[30]

Even patients with significant neurologic impairment related to tumor in the epidural space generally respond well to radiotherapy. The most favorable responses to radiotherapy are observed in patients with the most radiosensitive malignancies.[41]

In prostatic bone metastases, a total dose of radiation of 40 to 50 Gy is the regimen of choice for bone pain, and the use of strontium-80 and -89 may be considered.[42] Prophylactic irradiation of the lumbar spine in prostatic malignancy may forestall the development of metastatic disease. Whether this prophylactic radiotherapy prevents or delays recurrence is unknown.[43]

Operative Management

The principal indications for operative intervention are progressive neurologic compromise or intractable mechanical spine pain that is unresponsive to other modalities of treatment. Relative indications include biopsy where other diagnostic techniques have failed, relatively radioinsensitive tumors, recurrence of cord compression following radiotherapy, and recurring pain and instability in patients who have received maximal conservative modalities of treatment.

Radiotherapy and chemotherapy are ineffective in the treatment of bony instability or epidural compression secondary to bony debris retropulsed into the spinal canal (see Fig. 12-3*B*).[39] Regardless, patients with involvement of multiple spinal levels, those with involvement of multiple viscera, and those whose predicted survival is less than 3 to 4 months are best treated using nonsurgical means.

Surgery for spinal stabilization has become increasingly effective with the evolution of anterior spinal decompression and stabilization techniques and the more widespread use of posterior rod-screw constructs to improve immediate stabilization following major decompressive procedures.

It is simplest to consider the problems of spinal stability and neurologic compression as separate issues when considering decompression for neurologic impairment. The surgeon must be very certain that there is neurologic compression related to either bone or disc in the spinal canal. Other causes of motor compromise may occur, including transverse myelitis related to previous irradiation, sepsis, and peripheral neurotoxic effects of certain chemotherapeutic agents. Patients with pain related to spinal instability but who remain neurologically normal do not require emergency operative intervention. These patients should be tried on a course of external bracing, and surgery can be considered on a semielective basis.

The approaches for spinal decompression are dependent on amount of bone destruction, location of neural compromise, and residual bone stock. Generally, an anterior approach in the cervical and upper thoracic spine allows rapid tumor decompression, and an anterior strut either from autogenous iliac crest or allograft will achieve immediate stabilization. Following anterior strutting, radiotherapy should be deferred for 4 to 6 weeks to allow soft tissue healing and bone ingrowth (see Fig. 12-2*C*).

At the thoracolumbar junction, combined anterior and posterior procedures are often necessary. The posterior structures can be stabilized using a segmental rod or rod-screw construct followed by a complete anterior vertebrectomy. This surgical procedure is more extensive and the blood loss is greater than for either approach alone, but immediate stabilization and decompression can be achieved in most cases (see Fig. 12-3*C*, *D*).

In the lumbar spine, decompression can usually be performed from a posterior approach. A vertebral body excision can be performed posteriorly and stabilization effected during the same operative procedure with posterior screws and rods. The immediate stability afforded these patients is such that they may be mobilized without external immobilization within days of surgery (see Fig. 12-4*A*–*C*).

Occasionally, in a patient who has had extensive anterior radiation or has preexisting pulmonary disease, a posterolateral decompression of the thoracic spine may be indicated. This allows significant neural decompression without the necessity of violating the thoracic or pleural cavity.

Unfortunately, a true cure for metastatic tumor is rarely achieved by any spinal operative procedure. It must be stressed that these procedures are primarily intralesional resections, and concomitant chemotherapy or radiotherapy is almost always required in the postoperative period to achieve tumor control.

Decompression for metastatic tumor should be performed according to Sutton's law: go where the disease is. If the lesion is in the front, use an anterior approach. If it is in the back, use a posterior approach. If it is a napkin ring–type (i.e., circumferential), approach posteriorly first for decompression and stabilization, then perform anterior resection and further stabilization.

Surgery for spinal instability without significant neurologic compromise presents a separate spectrum of diagnostic and therapeutic challenges. There is no completely accepted system for defining spinal stability or instability. Perhaps the simplest classification system was devised by Denis for traumatic fractures.[44] This system divides the spine into three columns: the anterior column, including anterior longitudinal ligament, anterior half of the vertebral body, disc, and annulus; a middle column, including the posterior half of the vertebral body, disc, and annulus and the posterior longitudinal ligament; and a posterior column, including the posterior pedicles, lamina, and associated ligaments and capsules. Generally, the spine is considered unstable if two of these three columns are disrupted.

Kostnik and Errico[45] attempted to adapt Denis' system for the classification of patients with metastatic spinal tumors. They began with Denis' three classes and split the spine into left and right halves, creating six columns: anterior left, anterior right, middle left, middle right, posterior left, and posterior right. They felt the spine was unstable if more than three of the six columns were destroyed.

Unfortunately, no system takes into account the biology of the specific tumors, the potential risks of pretreatment radiotherapy and chemotherapy, and the postoperative problems related to healing, specifically in the light of radiotherapy or chemotherapy.

METASTATIC PROSTATIC CARCINOMA TO THE SPINE

Patients with prostatic metastatic vertebral disease often survive for a prolonged period of time, even with spinal cord compression. The incidence of spinal cord compression from prostatic tumor has been quoted as being between 1% and 10%.[46] These patients often do very well with either radiotherapy or endocrine therapy, and it has been stated that the results of surgery plus radiotherapy and of radiation alone are approximately equivalent.[47]

In patients who do not respond to radiotherapy or hormonal therapy or in whom neural compression is related to bone material in the spinal canal, about 70% to 80% do well following spinal reconstruction (see Fig. 12-2*A–C*).[48]

There is a subset of patients who present with prostatic spinal metastases in whom the neurologic compromise is related to spinal epidural tumor spread alone and in whom the skeletal column is completely intact. This group responds extremely well to external beam radiotherapy with or without hormonal manipulation.[49]

METASTATIC RENAL CARCINOMA TO THE SPINE

Although hypernephroma accounts for less than 10% of all cases of metastatic carcinoma to the spine, it is the most common cancer to present with a neurologic deficit secondary to an undetected primary malignancy.[50]

Renal cell carcinoma is a chemotherapeutic and hormonally insensitive tumor, and radiotherapy and surgical decompression remain the mainstays of treatment. Unfortunately, because of the extensive blood supply to this tumor, surgery, whether performed from the anterior or posterior approach, is not without significant risk of morbidity and mortality (see Fig. 12-1*A–D*).[51]

According to King and colleagues,[51] survival following spinal decompression for metastatic renal carcinoma averaged 8 months, but recurrent cord compression developed in 49% of patients. Preoperative embolization appeared to be beneficial to diminish the amount of blood loss. Despite the complications, these researchers felt that 88% of their patients achieved significant pain relief and 60% had improved neurologic function after the primary operation.

Sundaresan and colleagues[52] treated 30 consecutive patients with renal spinal metastases using presurgical embolization and subsequent surgical resection. Median survival of these patients was 16 months, and 27 of 30 (90%) improved neurologically following surgery. These authors stressed the major surgical complication of excessive blood loss.

Surgery for metastatic renal cell carcinoma of the spine is a high-risk proposition because of the possibility of significant blood loss. Although preoperative embolization is beneficial in diminishing blood loss, embolization itself may cause ischemic cord changes, especially in thoracic metastases.

SPECIFIC OPERATIVE CONSIDERATIONS FOR APPENDICULAR SKELETAL METASTASES

Upper extremity metastases account for less than 20% of all bone metastases, and metastatic disease to the humerus constitutes 50% of all upper extremity lesions. Painful metastatic lesions of the upper extremity may render a borderline ambulatory patient bedridden or wheelchair-bound or may interfere with normal hygiene and perineal care and the ability to function in an independent setting.[53] Splinting, casting, and palliative radiotherapy are often ineffective and frequently result in a painful nonunion of a pathologic fracture.

The proximal humeral metaphysis is a common site for renal cell metastatic disease, probably as a result of its relatively large blood pooling and supply of local chemotactic and growth factors. Present or impending pathologic fractures of the proximal humerus are well treated by a proximal metaphyseal humeral replacement using a metallic prosthesis or a metallic allograft composite prosthesis (see Fig. 12-1*D*).

Diaphyseal fractures of the humerus can be treated with intramedullary rods or dynamic compression plating, supplemented if necessary with polymethylmethacrylate (PMMA; see Fig. 12-4). The incorporation of chemotherapeutic agents into the PMMA has not been shown to improve long-term implant fixation or increase local tumor control. Fractures about the elbow, forearm, wrist, or hand are unusual, and treatment must be individualized to the patient.

Most pelvic metastases from genitourinary malignancies can be treated with embolization, radiotherapy, or both. Acetabular or periacetabular lesions from prostatic cancer may be an exception to this rule. Destructive lesions of the acetabulum that cause painful hip motion or immobility should be treated aggressively with resection and reconstruction of the involved segment of acetabulum. The reconstruction of large acetabular defects, combined with a simultaneous total hip replacement, has been described by Harrington.[54] The postoperative use of either external beam radiotherapy or chemotherapy is delayed only until soft tissue healing has occurred. Patient satisfaction and rapid return to activities of daily living are very encouraging.

The femoral neck is a common site of metastatic lesions, but prior to attempts at internal fixation, these should be carefully evaluated using MR. These lesions are often much more extensive than initially appreciated and often involve the neighboring femoral head or proximal femoral shaft with metastatic deposits. Long-stem hip replacement is often required to prevent later shaft fractures. Lane and colleagues at Memorial Sloan-Kettering Cancer Center[55] reported a series of 167 patients with long-stem arthroplasties and noted that patient satisfaction was excellent and complications were low.

Femoral shaft lesions without involvement of the proximal femur should be treated with intramedullary nails, which may be locked both proximally and distally to control rotation and prevent collapse. These nails allow partial load sharing and thereby maintain the patient's ambulatory status. Supplemental PMMA is often applied to the bony defects to further enhance stability and prevent pathologic fractures.

Metastatic lesions distal to the knee are rare and generally can be treated on an individual basis. Most patients do well with cast or brace immobilization, although more aggressive treatment of tibial lesions is often necessary for earlier weight bearing. Generally, intramedullary nails or tibial lesions work well in these patients.

A painful, fungating, metastatic lesion distal to the knee can also be treated with below-knee amputation. A below-knee amputation, accompanied by early prostatic fitting, offers the patient very early ambulatory status. We recommend the placement of nerve sheath catheters with constant 0.25% effusion of bupivacaine in the perioperative period, which has been shown to significantly decrease the occurrence of phantom limb pain.

CONCLUSIONS

Patients presenting with metastatic disease of the spine and appendicular skeleton require a systemic team approach. The goal is not only to prolong survival, but also to provide an acceptable quality of life. The true oncologic team approach involves a medical oncologist, radiation oncologist, genitourinary oncologist, and surgical-orthopaedic oncologist.

In the appendicular skeleton, indications for surgery include both impending and pathologic fractures in cases in which stabilization will rapidly improve quality of life and diminish the risks of prolonged immobilization.

In metastatic disease to the spine, most patients do not require operative intervention and can be well controlled with radiotherapy, chemotherapy, or hormonal manipulation. Indications for surgery include cord compression and neurologic compromise related to bone or disc in the spinal canal and the treatment of spinal instability refractory to other modalities of treatment.

Specific contraindications to surgery of the spine or appendicular skeleton include widespread visceral and bony disease, a significantly shortened lifespan, and widespread skeletal involvement such that stabilization is not practical. Our long-term goal of prolonged pain-free survival can only be enhanced by frequent interaction of all members of the team.

REFERENCES

1. Frassica FJ, Gitelis S, Sim H. Metastatic bone disease: general principles, pathophysiology, evaluation, and biopsy. Instruct Course Lect 1992;31:293.
2. Grant TT, deKernion JB. Treatment of skeletal metastases from urologic malignancies. Urology 1978;11:563.
3. Walker RH. Pelvic reconstruction/total hip arthroplasty for metastatic acetabular insufficiency. Clin Orthop 1993;294:170.
4. Rougraff BT, Kneisl JS, Simon MA. Skeletal metastases of unknown origin. J Bone Joint Surg [Am] 1993;75:1276.
5. Heshiki A. Bone marrow MRI in prostate cancer. In: Karr JP, Yamanaka H, eds. Prostate cancer and bone metastasis. New York: Plenum Press, 1992:209.
6. Pollack HM. Magnetic resonance imaging of bone metastases. Adv Exp Med Biol 1992;324:209.
7. Miyasaka M. Cancer metastasis and adhesion molecules. Clin Orthop 1995;312:10.
8. Paget S. The distribution of secondary growths in cancer of the breast. Lancet 1889;1:571.
9. Orr FW, Sanchez-Sweatman OH, Kostenuik P, Singh G. Tumor-bone interactions in skeletal metastasis. Clin Orthop 1995;312:19.
10. Harrington KD. New trends in the management of lower extremity metastases. Clin Orthop 1982;169:53.
11. Hipp JA, Springfield DS, Hayes WC. Predicting pathologic fracture risk in the management of metastatic bone defects. Clin Orthop 1995; 312:120.
12. Brage ME, Simon MA. Evaluation, prognosis, and medical treatment considerations of metastatic bone tumors. Orthopaedics 1992;15:589.
13. Huben RP. Hormone therapy of prostatic bone metastases. Adv Exp Med Biol 1992;324:305.
14. Douglas P, Rossier R-O, Mirimanoff PA, Coucke PA. Third-body irradiation as an effective palliative treatment for painful multiple bone metastases resistant to chemo- or hormonal treatment. Radiother Oncol 1993;28:76.
15. Mertens WC, Stitt L, Porter AT. Strontium 89 therapy and relief of pain in patients with prostatic carcinoma metastatic to bone: a dose response relationship? Am J Clin Oncol 1993;16:238.
16. Douglass HO, Shukla SK, Mindell E. Treatment of pathological fractures of long bones excluding those due to breast cancer. J Bone Joint Surg [Am] 1976;58:1055.
17. deKernion JB, Ramming KP, Smith RB. The natural history of renal cell carcinoma: a computer analysis. J Urol 1988;120:148.
18. Montie JE, Steward BH, Straffon RA, et al. The role of adjunctive nephrectomy in patients with metastatic renal cell carcinoma. J Urol 1977;177:272.
19. Papac RJ, Ross SA, Levy A. Renal cell carcinoma: analysis of 31 cases with assessment of endocrine therapy. Am J Med Sci 1977;274:281.
20. Swanson DA, Orovan WL, Johnson DE, Giacco G. Osseous metastasis secondary to renal cell carcinoma. Urology 1981;18:556.
21. Weiner S, Scarborough M, Enneking WF. Osseous metastases in renal cell carcinoma. Gainseville: University of Florida, 1992.
22. Halperin EL, Hausiadis L. The role of radiation therapy in the management of metastatic renal cell carcinoma. Cancer 1982;51:614.
23. Varma J, Huben RP, Wajsman Z, Pontes E. Therapeutic embolization of pelvic metastases of renal cell carcinoma. J Urol 1984;131:647.
24. Bowers TA, Murray JA, Charnsangavej C, et al. Bone metastases from renal carcinoma. J Bone Joint Surg [Am] 1982;64:749.
25. Nicholls PJ, Jarecky TW. The value of posterior decompression by laminectomy for malignant tumors of the spine. Clin Orthop 1985;210: 210.
26. Findlay GF. Adverse effect of the management of malignant spinal cord compression. J Neurol Neurosurg Psychiatry 1984;47:761.
27. Patterson RH Jr. Metastatic disease of the spine: surgical versus radiation therapy. Clin Neurosurg 1980;27:641.
28. Black P. Spinal metastasis: current status and recommended guidelines for management. Neurosurgery 1979;5:726.

29. McLain RF, Weinstein JN. Tumors of the spine. Semin Spine Surg 1990;2:157.
30. Harrington KD. Metastatic tumors of the spine: diagnosis and treatment. J Am Acad Orthop Surg 1993;1:76.
31. Nishijima Y, Uchida K, Koiso K, Nemoto R. Clinical significance of the vertebral vein in prostate cancer metastasis. Adv Exp Med Biol 1992;324:93.
32. Gilbert RW, Kim JM, Posner JB. Epidural spinal cord compression from metastatic tumor: diagnosis and treatment. Ann Neurol 1978;3:40.
33. Constans JP, deDivitiis E, Donzelli R, et al. Spinal metastases with neurological manifestations: review of 600 cases. J Neurosurg 1983;59:111.
34. Abrams HL, Spiro R, Goldstein N. Metastases in carcinoma: an analysis of 1000 autopsied cases. Cancer 1950;3:74.
35. Batson DV. The function of the vertebral veins and their role in the spread of metastases. Ann Surg 1940;112:138.
36. Martin DS, Awwad EE, Sundaram M. The magnetic resonance appearance of spinal radiation: the converse of spinal metastases. Orthopaedics 1990;13:378.
37. Sugimura K, Kajitani A, Okizuka H, et al. Assessing response to therapy of spinal metastases with gadolinium-enhanced MR imaging. J Magn Res Imaging 1991;1:481.
38. An HS, Vaccaro AR, Dolinskas CA, Cotler JM, et al. Differentiation between spinal tumors and infections with magnetic resonance imaging. Spine 1991;16(Suppl 8):S334.
39. Harrington KD. Metastatic disease of the spine. J Bone Joint Surg [Am] 1986;68:1110.
40. Frassica FJ, Sim FH. Metastatic bone disease: general perspectives, pathogenesis, pathophysiology, and skeletal dysfunction. Orthopaedics 1992;15:599.
41. Leviov M, Dale J, Stein M, et al. The management of metastatic spinal cord compression: a radiotherapeutic success ceiling. Int J Radiat Oncol Biol Phys 1993;27:231.
42. Bagshaw MA, Kaplan ID, Valdagni R, Cox RS. Radiation treatment of prostate bone metastases and the biological considerations. Adv Exp Med Biol 1992;324:255.
43. Kaplan, ID, Valdagni R, Cox RS, Bagshaw M. Reduction of spinal metastases after preemptive irradiation in prostatic cancer. Int J Radiat Oncol Biol Phys 1990;18:1019.
44. Denis F. The three column spine and its significance in the classification of acute thoracolumbar spinal injuries. Spine 1983;58:817.
45. Kostnik JP, Errico JN. Cited by Kostnik JP, Weinstein JN. Differentiated diagnosis and surgical treatment of metastatic spine tumors. In: Frymoye JW, ed. The adult spine: principles and practice, vol 1. New York: Raven Press, 1991:861.
46. Berrettoni BA, Carter JR. Mechanisms of cancer metastases to bone: current concepts review. J Bone Joint Surg [Am] 1986;68:308.
47. Flynn DF, Shipley WU. Management of spinal cord compression secondary to metastatic prostatic carcinoma. Urol Clin North Am 1991;18:145.
48. Bridwell KH. Treatment of metastatic prostate cancer of the spine. Urol Clin North Am 1991;18:153.
49. Sasawawa I, Gotoh H, Miyabayashi H, Yamaguchi O, Shiraiwa Y. Hormonal treatment of symptomatic spinal cord compression in advanced prostatic cancer. Int J Urol Nephrol 1991;23:351.
50. Schaberg J, Gainor BJ. A profile of metastatic carcinoma of the spine. Spine 1985;10:19.
51. King GJ, Kostuik JP, McBroom RJ, Richardson W. Surgical management of metastatic renal carcinoma of the spine. Spine 1991;16:265.
52. Sundaresan N, Choi IS, Hughes JEO, Sachdev VP, Berenstein A. Treatment of spinal metastases from kidney cancer by presurgical embolization and resection. J Neurosurg 1990;73:548.
53. Rock M. Metastatic lesions of the humerus and the upper extremity. Instruct Course Lect 41:329.
54. Harrington KD. The management of acetabular insufficiency secondary to metastatic malignant disease. J Bone Joint Surg [Am] 1981;63:653.
55. Lane JM, Sculco TP, Zolan S. Treatment of pathological fractures of the hip by endoprosthetic replacement. J Bone Joint Surg [Am] 1980;62:954.

Principles and Practice of Genitourinary Oncology, edited by Derek Raghavan, Howard I. Scher, Steven A. Leibel, and Paul H. Lange. Lippincott-Raven Publishers, Philadelphia, © 1997.

CHAPTER 13

Statistical Considerations for the Use of the Literature in Health Systems Research

Brent A. Blumenstein

Today in the United States there is increased concern over what is perceived generally to be high health care costs. As a result of increased concern over high health care costs in the United States, there is intense interest in collecting data on the performance of health systems so that cost-reducing changes in health care delivery can be planned. Health systems research efforts affect every aspect of the health care delivery system—from the administration of third party payments, to finding new and less expensive ways to deliver quality care, to evaluating less expensive patient care alternatives. The greatest potential for cost reductions are in diseases which are common and costly, and such research has meaning only when there are distinct alternative treatments to evaluate. Prostate cancer meets this criteria; however, other urologic cancers are also of interest.

Published clinical research findings are used in health systems research efforts and are often the only source of data available regarding the efficacy and complication outcomes of treatment alternatives. However, any proposal to reduce health care costs must be based on accurate data; otherwise, the chances are greater of having an opposite effect on cost or adversely affecting the quality of care patients receive. Because clinical researchers are responsible for generating data used in health systems research, it is important for them to be aware of how these data are being used in health systems research and the limitations of the use of published clinical data in health systems research. Refined knowledge of the uses of clinical data in health systems research enables clinical researchers to better evaluate health systems research findings that are based on published data and to work with health systems researchers in the proper use of published data. For example, it is important for clinicians to discourage the use of clinical research data that are of poor quality or are invalid when used in the context of health systems research.

The urologic cancer clinical research community must become more aware of health care systems research methods, including outcomes research, systems modeling, and meta-analysis. This chapter focuses on the intersection between clinical research in urologic cancers and health care systems research relative to data on efficacy and complications of interventions. Although this chapter focuses on evaluating treatment alternatives, many of the principles discussed also apply to the evaluation of alternative screening or disease prevention strategies; important differences are explicitly described. The formal process of treatment guideline formulation shares many aspects of the data needs and some of the methodologies used in health systems research, particularly the often unavoidable necessity of using published data. Therefore, the applicability of many of the principles discussed in this chapter is somewhat broader than the evaluation of treatment alternatives for use in health systems research efforts.

DATA NEEDS OF HEALTH SYSTEMS RESEARCH

Health systems research has much broader goals than typical clinical research. The goal of health systems research is usually the formulation of health policy, whereas the goals of clinical research are usually targeted at evaluating the efficacy and complications of a given treatment; there might also be some biologic hypothesis. Additional areas of concern in health systems research include treatment costs, quality of life, functional status, patient satisfaction with care, lifetime impact, and societal impact.

Health systems research that is focused on interventions is a form of outcomes research, and the U.S. government has played a major role in stimulating such research. In 1989 the U.S. Congress passed the Outcomes Assessment Research Act, creating the Agency for Health Care Policy Research[1]. This agency has sponsored various research programs under a Medical Treatment Effectiveness Program (MEDTEP). The MEDTEP brought into being various Patient Outcomes Research Teams (PORTs), which conduct myriad types of health systems research.[2] One of these PORTs focuses on benign prostatic hypertrophy and localized prostate cancer.

There are two classes of data needed by health systems research efforts: data comparing interventions, and descriptive data on the treatment of urologic cancers and outcomes in the general population. In discussing health systems research, it is crucial to distinguish data comparing interventions from descriptive data, because the ideal sources for these two classes of data should be mutually exclusive. The optimal way to generate data comparing interventions (e.g., relative efficacy, complication rates, impact on the quality of life) is through randomized clinical trials. Descriptive data (e.g., estimates of stage-specific incidence rates, age distributions of men with various types of urologic cancer, rates of utilization of specific interventions, incidence rates for comorbid diseases in men with urologic cancers, costs of specific treatments) are used to study the impact of proposed changes in health care policy. To minimize errors in formulating health care policy, descriptive data must be an accurate representation of what happens in the population in which health care policy changes are to be implemented.

Ideally, descriptive data should be generated using formal statistical sampling methodologies such as those used in national health surveys, national censuses, or political polling. Unfortunately, studies based on formal statistical sampling methodologies are very difficult and expensive; therefore, such sources of descriptive data are virtually nonexistent. Thus, descriptive data must be generated from any available source and synthesized into useful estimates for the target population. However, often the component sources only address specific population segments, such as only MEDICARE patients; therefore, the synthesis of data can lead to inaccuracies.

Health systems researchers are keenly aware that randomized clinical trials are the superior method for comparing interventions. The purpose of a randomized clinical trial is to compare interventions with minimal interference from uncontrolled factors. In a randomized clinical trial, patients are assigned randomly to interventions. It is unlikely that the patient groups assigned to each intervention will differ in a substantial way; therefore the comparison of the outcomes between the groups is not confounded by extraneous between-group differences.

When possible, health systems researchers encourage the initiation of or collaborate to initiate randomized trials. However, it is often difficult to implement randomized trials because of the difficulties inherent in establishing collaborations between clinicians and health systems researchers. Such collaborations are made even more difficult when clinicians believe they already know the answer to the treatment efficacy question (even in the absence of comparative trials) and resist attempts to implement comparative studies or are passive with respect to contributing patient data to such studies. An example is early stage prostate cancer, for which a controversy between prostatectomy and expectant management exists. The Prostate Intervention Versus Observation Trial (PIVOT), a randomized trial addressing this issue, has been initiated by the Veterans Administration System Cooperative Studies with additional participation by the National Cancer Institute–sponsored cooperative groups.[3] Some urologists think that PIVOT is unethical because of a strong belief in the efficacy of the prostatectomy and therefore refuse to participate. Others believe that a randomized trial is necessary to gather the kind of data needed to resolve this controversy. The potential economic impact of the results of this trial, regardless of the outcome, are enormous, and therefore are of great interest to health systems researchers. However, this question will not be resolved for many years because of the generally long survival time of the men entering this trial.

When the disease under study requires a long follow-up to obtain data comparing interventions, there has been little or no effort to compare interventions in a randomized trial, and data comparing interventions are needed immediately for planning, health care systems researchers must use published data from nonrandomized trials, data bases, or both. The major issue associated with using data bases (e.g., registries) as a source of data comparing interventions are similar to that associated with the use of clinical series data as a source of data comparing interventions.

Clinical series data and data bases should not generally be used to compare interventions except in the crudest and most speculative ways. Because the allocation of interventions is not controlled through randomization, the comparison of the interventions will be confounded by other between-group differences and the intervention comparison will be biased in ways that are not fully ascertainable. For example, suppose outcome data for two interventions are available, but the patients were given the intervention based on patient choice, physician preference, or institutional policy. Because there has been no experimental control over which intervention a patient received in any given series, it is not possible to argue that the groups of patients receiving each of the interventions are comparable. As a result, the comparison of the outcomes for the groups is not simply a comparison of intervention differences but is also a comparison of differences between the groups. In this situation, the patient intervention comparison is said to be confounded by patient group differences. Green and Byar provide further details on the limitations of clinical series and registry data.[4]

It is possible to adjust for group differences between clinical series using advanced statistical models that include covariates. For example, the survival outcomes for a prostatectomy series might be compared to the survival outcome of a radiotherapy series using proportional hazard (Cox) regression with covariates age, race, stage, Gleason grade, performance status, and baseline prostate-specific antigen. In such a model, the intended role of the covariates is to adjust for between-sample differences in patient group. For example, the prostatectomy patients may have a lower mean age than that of the radiotherapy patients. The ability of covariate adjustments to overcome the inherent sampling differences between case series is often greatly overstated. There are three serious problems. The types of adjustments that can be made are functionally limited by the statistical model being used; for example, in linear adjustments on the logarithmic hazard scale. The data may not contain enough information in specific important subsets to allow reliable adjustments to be made, or there may be missing data on some covariates. Covariate adjustments can be made only for those variables that are available (i.e., present in the data set). Covariate adjustment does not approach the capabilities of a randomized clinical trial to minimize the effect of between-treatment sampling differences.

MODELING

Modeling methodologies are perhaps the most important tool of health systems researchers because they allow them to create simple models of portions of the health care system. These models use assumptions about rates of events (e.g., complications), duration of specific states relative to the disease under study (e.g., interval with no evidence of disease following a treatment), costs, attributions of the relative value of specific outcomes, or dependencies between various states and outcomes, among others. The structure of the model is created from a consensus of experts in health policy, urology, and modeling, and the assumptions (e.g., complication rates, state durations) come from available data. A model is evaluated by performing sensitivity analyses, in which the assumptions are varied over what are believed to be feasible ranges of values. An example of a health systems research model using published clinical data is a Markov model for prostate cancer care.[5]

Modeling is often criticized by those who claim the data on which assumptions are based are inaccurate, but the criticism of a modeling effort with the primary focus on data quality is likely to miss other important modeling features. Although it is important to have accurate data, modeling efforts are somewhat resilient to data inaccuracies because of the availability of sensitivity analyses. It is more important for clinicians to ensure that the range of feasible outcomes are well represented in the modelling sensitivity analyses. Of equal importance are model structure considerations (i.e., the interdependencies between model components). It is often difficult for clinicians to fully comprehend the structural aspects of a model because they are not trained in the complex mathematics of this methodology. Many clinicians face a similar problem regarding the use of actuarial statistical methods, with the result being a general distrust of such methods. Unfortunately, models cannot be regarded simply as "black boxes," as actuarial statistical methods can when the clinician comes to trust statistical methods, because it is the model structure that the clinician must use his or her experience to evaluate.

THE SAMPLING PROBLEM

The applicable underlying and all-important statistical principle in all inferences is sampling. Health systems researchers need estimates of effect sizes and descriptive data for the the general population of afflicted individuals, because the planning to be done using the data collected must apply to this population or some specifically defined subset of it. Any clinical research study, randomized or nonrandomized, reports data on a sample of patients from some population of patients, the definition of which is not always explicitly stated. The terms "sample" and "population" have very precise statistical meanings and are often misused in medical research writings. The purpose of almost all clinical research is to study a sample and then make inferences about the population from which the sample was drawn. To precisely understand the scope of an inference based on a sample, the population from which the sample was drawn must be precisely defined, and the method used to obtain the sample must be fully understood.

A fundamental assumption in statistical inference is that the sample is drawn from the population using a random selection process, and is therefore representative of the population. Statistical estimation procedures depend on this assumption for valid inferences. However, in much published clinical research it is rare to find a precise definition of the population, and the method used to obtain the sample is often absent as well. The following examples illustrate the application of this fundamental statistical principle to two types of clinical studies: the clinical series and the randomized trial.

Consider a single institution's clinical series of sequentially enrolled patients that includes outcome data. What is the sample and what is the population for a report of data of this type? The author could claim that the sample (i.e., patients included) are a random sample in time (i.e., more or less random start time for enrollment). Such a claim would meet the requirements for the random sample assumption, provided the author is convincing about the uniformity of the types of patients available over time. However, this sampling structure does not provide for broad inferences, because the population is the patients seen at that institution. The author could also claim that the institution from which the patients are enrolled is a random selection from institutions of the same class, in which case the inference would be to institutions of the given class; however, in this case the definition of this class must be precise, and the author must be convincing in claiming that there was no special selection with respect to his or her institution. Clinical series data are not published from all types of institutions, however; therefore it is not credible to argue that the institution publishing a clinical series is a random representative of all institutions. This is a form of publication bias that is not easy to quantify but probably has a relatively consistent direction across reports. Therefore the author must argue that the clinical series is representative of some vague class of institutions that are potential publishers of clinical series. It is not surprising that authors of clinical series data do not typically discuss population and sampling issues. The most formal statistical sampling evaluation leads to the conclusion that there is no basis for inference beyond the sample of patients included because there is no clearly defined population and the sampling methodology is ill-defined. Other forms of publication bias are related to the propensity of an author to seek publication only for interesting results, and the tendency for journals to preferentially accept interesting papers.

The statistical principle of taking a random sample from a population is not the same statistical principle as randomization in a clinical trial. Randomization between arms in a randomized clinical trial is a treatment allocation method that is designed to minimize between-arm differences for extraneous factors and provides the statistical basis for comparing the arms. Using the principle of randomized allocation between arms as the basis for deciding whether there are between-arm differences in a randomized trial does not depend on the sampling plan used to select the patients included in the trial but does limit the conclusion to the patients included. The emphasis in a clinical trial is to discover whether between-arm differences exist and estimate the magnitude of the between-arm treatment or complication effects within the context of the trial. Therefore, the reader is left to speculate about the extension of the clinical trial results beyond those patients enrolled in the trial. This speculation is usually based on the presentation of data characterizing the patients enrolled. This critical inferential step of regarding the results of the between-arm comparison from a clinical trial as being representative of a population is often done without full recognition of the applicable statistical principles, and it is at this inferential step that the quality of the patient sampling becomes important. In addition to making population inferences concerning between-arm differences in treatment effects or complications, outcome data from each arm of the randomized clinical trial are often regarded as a separate clinical series. The same fundamental statistical sampling principles applied to inferences for clinical series data also apply to population inferences based on clinical trial data. However, for randomized clinical trials it is much more difficult to be describe the population from which the sample of patients have been randomly drawn, because typically, not all patients are offered a randomized clinical trial and not all patients consent to be enrolled. Therefore, it is very difficult to identify a population from which the patients enrolled can be argued to be a random sample. In a same manner as for clinical series data, a formal statistical sampling evaluation leads to the conclusion that there is no statistical basis for inference beyond the sample included for either treatment effect differences or for arm-specific outcome data.

These two general examples illustrate that inferences from published clinical findings do not have precise sampling structures and therefore lack an inferential framework for providing outcomes estimates applicable to general populations. In contrast, consider activities such as census sampling or political polling, in which a great deal of effort is put into formal statistical sampling plans intended to allow for inferences to populations.

Most readers of published clinical research findings are at least intuitively aware of these inferential limitations, but the full impact of these inferential limitations are not well understood, especially when clinical research findings are used outside the context of research evaluation, for example, as a basis for making patient care decisions or planning changes in the health care system.

PROBLEMS EXTRACTING FAILURE TIME DATA FROM THE LITERATURE

The urologic clinical research literature is generally diverse with respect to the manner of data presentation. This diversity exists both within the types of studies (i.e., clinical series and randomized clinical trials), and between classes of studies. For example, in characterizing patients included in a study, different grading systems can be used, and there can be variability in the completeness of the reported patient characteristics. As an example of diversity in reporting outcomes, consider survival. Some articles report median survival, whereas others report survival at specific points in time (e.g., 5- or 10-year survival); few articles report the appropriate measures of uncertainty (i.e., confidence intervals or standard errors) for survival statistics.

The problems of dealing with differences in patient characterization between articles are sometimes quite difficult to solve and may be intractable in some cases, but are not discussed further in this chapter. Instead, this chapter focuses on the problems of extracting failure time data from the literature because of the importance of failure time outcome measures in urologic cancers and the complex conceptual problems associated with failure time data. The complexity of failure statistical methods often leads to mistakes in how failure time data are extracted and used in health systems research and other types of literature synthesis, such as treatment guideline formulation and meta-analysis.

Many reports of clinical series or randomized clinical trials focus on failure time outcomes, and failure time outcomes are of particular importance to health systems research because they are often the best measure of the efficacy of an intervention. Commonly used failure events are recurrence, progression, and death.

The first problem is that of the definition of a failure and how censored observations are handled. Ideally, all patients would be enrolled on the same day and followed until all have been observed to have had failure events. If this were the case, the data consisting of the failure times could be analyzed using relatively straightforward statistical methods. However, this ideal situation is rarely found. The usual situation is that of staggered entry, incomplete follow-up, and censored observations.

Patients are enrolled into a study whenever they become available; therefore, the entry times are distributed over the whole enrollment period (usually with a nearly uniform distribution), and the study entry times are said to be staggered. However, the statistical analysis of failure time data is based on making inferences about the distribution of failure times, and in these analyses each patient's date of entry becomes the base date (i.e., time zero) for that patient. Thus, failure time analyses treat all patients as if they were enrolled into the study on the same day even though they were not. The major consequence of staggered entry is that the opportunity to observe a failure diminishes for the patients entered later in the study.

Incomplete follow-up results when the data are reported before all patients have failed are a consequence of the time the data are analyzed and staggered entry into the trial. Incomplete follow-up leads to censored observations (i.e., the knowledge that a patient has not failed as of the date of last assessment for failure). Many of the statistical methods available for analyzing failure time data are designed specifically to use the information contained in censored observations along with the information about failure times in patients who have failed during the study. For example, the Kaplan-Meier plot, which is a representation of the failure time distribution, displays all data. Similarly, estimates of the failure time characteristics (e.g., median time to failure, actuarial estimate of the percent free of failure at a specific time, hazard rate) use all the available data, including censored observations. The various procedures for analyzing failure time data, such as the log rank test and proportional hazard (Cox) regression, are designed to fully utilize all data. Statistical methods using censored observations are much more efficient than methods that do not use censored observations; therefore, statistical methods that do not use censored observations should be avoided.

A given study may be analyzed for a variety of failure time outcomes, and the definition of failure is a factor in how many observations are censored in the analysis. Consider progression-free interval and progression-free survival. When using progression as the failure event, patients who die before progression is observed become censored observations, whereas when using progression-free survival, patients who die before progression are are treated as failures. A detailed discussion of the choice between these two failure definitions, as well as the myriad of other analogous choices, such as those between survival and disease-free survival, are beyond the scope of this chapter. As a general principle, it is more correct to include death as part of the definition of failure whenever there is any possibility of death being related to disease (e.g., a consequence of treatment, suicides) or there exists any degree of uncertainty in this ascertainment. Also, Kaplan-Meier plots in which deaths are censored become very complicated to interpret, because the probability of being free of failure (vertical axis) is a probability conditional on having lived long enough to have been observed to fail from disease. Because there are so many choices in the definition of failure, it can be difficult to extract a uniform outcome measure from across a collection of articles, even if the articles use rigorous statistical methods that account for censored observations.

A more insidious problem, assuming that a satisfactory uniform outcome estimate is extractable, is that of attaching a measure of uncertainty (e.g., confidence interval, standard error) to the outcome estimate extracted from each article. Suppose that the purpose of a study is to tabulate percent survival at 5 years across a collection of articles. Tabulations of outcome measures are incomplete unless each outcome estimate (e.g., 5-year survival) is accompanied by measure of uncertainty.

It is technically feasible to extract a crude estimate of 5-year survival from almost any characterization of the survival distribution in an article. For example, if the article reports median survival, an estimate of 5-year survival can be computed by assuming a mathematical shape for the survival distribution (exponential shape is generally assumed). If the article has a Kaplan-Meier plot of survival, a crude estimate of 5-year survival can be extracted from the graph. If the coefficients from a proportional hazard regression are presented, a crude estimate can computed by making mathematical assumptions. The ideal would be for each article to report an actuarial estimate of 5-year survival together with a standard error (e.g., Greenwood standard error). Measures of uncertainty are related to the sample size and number of failure events, which in turn depends on the time the data presented in each article were analyzed, and allow the results from each article to be weighted appropriately in composite estimates of outcomes. Satisfactory measures of uncertainty are not available for indirect estimates of failure time outcome measures such as those described.

In contrast, suppose that the outcome measure to be tabulated across articles is a proportion estimate, such as the proportion of patients having a specific type of adverse event. Proportion estimates are likely to be easily available from articles, and the variability of definitions as described for failure time outcomes is likely to be less of a problem. Furthermore, estimates of uncertainty for proportion estimates are easy to obtain using a standard statistical formula, provided the denominator is known. Therefore, tabulations of proportion estimates including valid measures of uncertainty are much easier to implement than are tabulations for failure event outcomes. The valid tabulation of proportion estimates does not mean the sampling issues raised earlier in this article have been overcome.

As a result of the ease with which proportion estimates are handled, there is a natural temptation to convert the failure time outcome problem to a proportion problem by attempting to extract the proportion who have failed at a specific point in time and using this proportion as auxiliary information for computing a measure of uncertainty for that failure time outcome measure. Returning to the 5-year example, this would involve extracting the estimate of the 5-year survival by whatever means is available, and then basing the computation of uncertainty on the proportion of patients who have failed at 5 years. This procedure does not yield statistically defensible measures of uncertainty, however.

Austenfield and colleagues[6] used a proportion-based measure of uncertainty for prostate cancer failure time data. This article describes the planned methodology and early results from the literature review efforts of the American Urological Association (AUA) Prostate Cancer Guideline Panel and is based on Eddy's confidence profile method.[7,8] The three panels of Figure 4 in the Austenfeld and colleagues article[6] are confidence profile graphs of prostate cancer 10-year survival for three treatments of interest. These graphs illustrate a synthesized estimate of the outcome distribution in which the width of the distribution is related to the synthesized measure of uncertainty. There are two major elements of invalidity for these graphs: the sampling problems previously discussed (primarily publication bias) have not been dealt with in any way, and therefore the location of the center of the distributions shown are likely incorrect; and the method used to compute the measures of uncertainty for the failure time outcome from each article reviewed is based on proportions; as a result, the synthesized measure of uncertainty shown as the width of distributions is probably inaccurate.

SYNTHESIS, OR META-ANALYSIS

Health systems researchers and those engaged in treatment guideline formulation often use meta-analysis methodologies as a method of synthesizing estimates of interest from multiple studies. Meta-analysis is literally an analysis of analyses and involves statistically analyzing data extracted from published research. The analysis of collections of raw data from identified studies is also regarded as a meta-analysis methodology but is often referred to as an overview analysis to distinguish it from efforts that use published data. The most important general threats to the validity of a meta-analysis are two sampling issues: whether the studies included are representative of a useful population (as discussed previously) and whether the selection of studies included in the meta-analysis is biased.

The worst-case type of meta-analysis with respect to validity is a meta-analysis of published clinical series data, because in addition to the sampling issues inherent in clinical series data (as described previously), and the study sampling issue (i.e., are the studies included representative of anything useful?), there are issues of how to effectively extract valid data from the publications (discussed previously). In addition, when meta-analyses of literature are done, it is sometimes difficult to obtain satisfactory measures of uncertainty for use as weights in the synthesis of estimates.

At the foundation of meta-analysis methodologies for combining literature data from nonrandomized studies is the assumption that each clinical series is a random datum in a sampling process that generates the entire collection of clinical series available, and that this larger sampling process somehow represents a describable population of interest. This argument is seriously flawed for clinical series data in urologic cancers, and in many other settings as well, because of publication bias (as described previously). The confidence profile method advocated by Eddy[8] is an example of a meta-analysis method based on the assumption that the published articles constitute a random sample. The confidence profile method is a mathematically sophisticated application of the Bayesian probability principles and random effects statistical models for synthesizing outcomes from published articles. When there are known but unquantifiable biases, such as publication bias, the confidence profile method and other methods based on this kind of random sampling assumption should be avoided.

The highest level of meta-analysis with respect to validity is an overview analysis of data from randomized trials with a focus on intervention comparisons.[9,10] A urologic disease example of such a meta-analysis is the treatment of advanced prostate cancer, in which there is a controversy concerning whether the addition of an antiandrogen to androgen ablation has long-term benefits. The cost of adding the antiandrogen is of major concern. This controversy exists largely because of study design and statistical issues.[11] As a result of this controversy, a meta-analysis of the randomized studies of combined therapy has been reported.[12] However, even though this meta-analysis is to use only randomized studies and has been carefully designed with respect to sampling, there are problems in its interpretation.

The overview analysis of clinical series data, in which data from each series is gathered and re-analyzed, avoids the data extraction problem that is a part of performing a meta-analysis on published clinical series, but the sampling issues discussed previously still exist and may be compounded because only those series that are willing and able to submit raw data can be used in the analysis. There has been an overview analysis of six clinical series data sets for men treated conservatively for early stage prostate cancer.[13] The authors of this effort describe very carefully and thoroughly the limitations and potential biases inherent in their analysis and their effects on interpretation. However, because of the great interest in the issue of conservative therapy and the absence of results from a randomized trial, the potentially biased data from this article will probably become a major source of data used in future health systems research modeling.

SUMMARY AND DISCUSSION

Health systems research efforts require estimates of the relative efficacy of interventions and the relevant descriptors of the system being studied. In many cases, the only source of data for these estimates are articles published in clinical journals. For urologic cancers, particularly prostate cancer, the literature is dominated by clinical series data. There are three major problems in using published data for health systems research: sampling, data extraction, and synthesis. The sampling problem is a function of how well published results represent a population. The data extraction problem is a function of how data are tabulated across a collection of publications. The synthesis problem is a function of how data extracted are summarized. The data extraction and synthesis problems are made more acute because of the necessity of using clinical series data, particularly data on the time to failure (e.g., progression, death).

Clinical series data are never the best source of data for comparing interventions because such comparisons are confounded by patient differences between groups. Clinical series data have questionable value as a source of descriptive data because of the sampling and data extraction problems described previously. The ascertainment from a published randomized trial of whether interventions differ and in what direction are valid for the patients studied, but estimates of the magnitude of treatment differences from a randomized trial are probably biased because the sample of patients included in randomized clinical are probably not representative of a useful population. Similarly, outcomes estimates from arms of randomized trials (as opposed to treatment effect difference estimates) are not representative of populations in health system research. Therefore, estimates of the magnitude of intervention differences and descriptive data from clinical trials and clinical series are not very useful in health systems research because the type of data needed by health systems researchers must be more representative of the general population.

The presentation of results of a data synthesis using a mathematically sophisticated meta-analysis methodology can potentially obscure flaws in the underlying data by distracting attention from the data. Additionally, the use of mathematically sophisticated meta-analysis methodology may require too much preprocessing of the data to prepare it for analysis, thereby further obscuring flaws in the underlying data or requiring the use of indefensible statistical procedures, as was done initially, for example, by the AUA Prostate Cancer Guideline Panel. Under these circumstances, a biased data synthesis turns into a sophisticated presentation of results that appears to have legitimacy because of the techniques used to process the data.

Data synthesis should be avoided when the data have known biases. For example, for its final report, the AUA Prostate Cancer Guideline Panel abandoned the confidence profile method of data synthesis and instead implement a much simpler and more accessible graphical approach to displaying the data gathered from the literature.[14] The data from each clinical series is a point on a graph in which all related clinical series are represented. For example, with the vertical axis of percent surviving and the horizontal axis of time with discrete values of 5, 10, and 15 years, a point represents the datum from each clinical series, with a tiny bit of horizontal noise added to avoid coincident points. In this way, the reader can see the full variability of the data gathered. This graphical approach does not include a representation of a measure of uncertainty for each series, however. I proposed, in the spirit of the exploratory data analysis methods advocated by Tukey,[15] to let the size of each point be inversely proportional to a crude measure of uncertainty (e.g., a larger point for larger sample sizes). This proposal for variable point sizes was not accepted by the Panel because it was thought perhaps with some justification to be too difficult to explain.

The synthesis of estimates of intervention differences or descriptive data for use in health systems research or treatment guideline formulation from data sources with known biases should be criticized in the same manner that inadequate study design is criticized as bad science. The use of biased estimates in the formulation of health policy or practice guidelines could have enormous consequences if implemented on a large scale.[16]

There are significant differences between science and health systems research activities. Each scientist has his or her work validated by others who repeat or extend the original work. Scientific progress consists of small steps. The manner in which health systems research efforts are validated are not as obvious as those for traditional scientific activities and are primarily centered on public debate and opinion, although there are occasional efforts to validate and extend models by researchers other than those responsible for the original publication.[17] Health system research efforts often require enormous resources and are therefore less likely to be independently replicated, yet there is usually broad interest in results, and the results may have large effects on policy.

Given the sampling problems and data extraction problems described in this chapter, should tabulations and syntheses of clinical series data be done? The tabulation of results from clinical series reports adds perhaps undeserved value to these reports. Altman[18] argues that poor research is a major problem and advocates that research using suboptimal methodology not be done. Following this reasoning, the publication of clinical series data simply for the reason of presenting outcome data for a series of patients receiving a specific intervention should be discouraged; however, clinical series reported to illustrate an exploratory look at a new intervention or the prognostic value of a new baseline diagnostic assessment has value for hypothesis generation, even though its value as a source of data for health systems research is low.

There is an ethical obligation to the patient to generate valid and useful data. The needs of the health systems researchers make it imperative that clinical researchers become more aware of clinical research data quality and validity. Although it is not possible to control all uses of published data, it is possible to focus on research activities that generate the most valid, useful, and needed types of data. Ideally, researchers in the urologic oncology community should convert the energy spent on generating clinical series data with questionable value into promoting and participating in randomized clinical trials efforts. Very few trials accrue patients so rapidly that additional accruals would be unwelcome, and there are significant advantages for any trial to accrue patients rapidly. Accruing patients to randomized clinical trials requires the researcher to be intellectually and scientifically honest in distinguishing between data and opinion and rigorous in the assessment of available data or its absence. Additionally, those researchers with the inclination and energy should attempt to become leaders in the community of clinical trialists; although such a pursuit can be frustrating because of the necessity to develop consensus, it can also be quite productive. I recommend participation in cooperative groups at any level in clinical trials.

REFERENCES

1. Raskin IE, Maklan CW. Medical treatment effectiveness research: a view from inside the Agency for Health Care Policy Research. AHCPR Program Note AHCPR Pub. No. 91-0025, 1991.
2. Maklan CW, Greene R, Cummings MA. Methodological challenges and innovations in patient outcomes research. Med Care 1994; 32(Suppl):JS13.
3. Wilt TJ, Brawer MK. The prostate cancer intervention versus observation trial: a randomized trial comparing radical prostatectomy versus expectant management for the treatment of clinically localized prostate cancer. J Urol 1994;152:1910.
4. Green S, Byar D. Using observational data from registries to compare treatments: the fallacy of omnimetrics (and discussion). Stat Med 1984; 3:361.
5. Fleming C, Wasson JH, Albertson PC, Barry MJ, Wennberg JE. A decision analysis of alternative strategies for clinically localized prostate cancer. JAMA 1993;269:2560.
6. Austenfield MS, Thompson IM, Middleton RG, for the American Urological Association Prostate Cancer Guideline Panel. Meta-analysis of the literature: guideline development for prostate cancer treatment. J Urol 1994;152:1866.
7. Eddy DM, Hasselblad V, Shachter R. A Bayesian method for synthesizing evidence: the confidence profile method. Int J Technol Assess Health Care 1990;6:31.
8. Eddy D. The confidence profile method: a Bayesian method for assessing health technologies. Oper Res 1989;37:210.
9. Antiplatelet Trialists' Collaboration. Secondary prevention of vascular disease by prolonged antiplatelet treatment. Br Med J 1988;296: 320.
10. Early Breast Cancer Trialists' Collaborative Group. Effects of adjuvant tamoxifen and of cytotoxic therapy on mortality in early breast cancer. N Engl J Med 1988;319:1681.
11. Blumenstein BA. Some statistical considerations for the interpretation of trials of combined androgen therapy. Cancer 1993;72(Suppl): 3834.
12. Prostate Cancer Trialists' Collaborative Group. Maximum androgen blockade in advanced prostate cancer: an overview of 22 randomized trials with 3283 deaths in 5710 patients. Lancet 1995;346:265.
13. Chodak GW, Thisted RA, Gerber GS, et al. Results of conservative management of clinically localized prostate cancer. N Engl J Med 1994; 330:242.
14. Middleton RG, Thompson IM, Austenfeld MS, et al. Prostate cancer clinical guidelines panel summary report on the management of clinically localized prostate cancer. J Urol 1995;154:2144.
15. Tukey JW. Exploratory data analysis. Reading, MA: Addison-Wesley, 1977:688.
16. Anderson G. Measuring what works in health care. Science 1994;263: 1080.
17. Beck JR, Kattan MW, Miles JM. Critique of the decision analysis for clinically localized prostate cancer. J Urol 1994;152:1894.
18. Altman DG. The scandal of poor medical research. Br Med J 1994; 308:283.

Principles and Practice of Genitourinary Oncology, edited by Derek Raghavan, Howard I. Scher, Steven A. Leibel, and Paul H. Lange. Lippincott-Raven Publishers, Philadelphia, © 1997.

CHAPTER 14

The Nurse Practitioner and the Organization of Support Services for the Patient with Genitourinary Cancer

Sharon Hyland and Donna Wilkinson

The optimal management of the patient with a malignant disease of the genitourinary tract requires a complex interplay of medical diagnosis and treatment, psychologic asessment and care, and the provision of an integrated network of social support for the patient and the family (the team approach). Specific concerns and fears relate to the diagnosis of cancer itself, including the potential for pain, mutilation, loss of income, change of life style, the stigma of cancer, loss of autonomy, power, and control, and the risk of premature death.[1,2]

In addition, unique problems are endemic to cancers of the genitourinary tract: the patient with testicular cancer may face problems with psychosocial and sexual connotations from the loss of his testicle(s) and the potential toxicity of aggressive chemotherapy programs; the attempt at cure of cancer of the bladder, penis, or prostate is often characterized by the loss of libido or sexual function and self-esteem and by the potential complications of treatment such as chronic diarrhea, loss of urinary continence, or the development of urinary urgency or frequency; the aftermath of treatment for renal carcinoma, with the potential for chronic renal failure or, in the case of advanced disease, the reputation of this disease for an inexorable, downhill course, can extract a substantial toll on the patient and the family.

Against this background, a successful cancer management team must provide a seamless program of care to cover the problems inherent in treatment and support for such patients and their families. Recognition of the importance of such services is emerging. A survey of National Cancer Institute-designated cancer centers has demonstrated an increased level of availability and application of cancer support services, augmented by research initiatives in this area.[3]

In a practical context, the medical team usually defines the overall plan of management, frequently designating the responsibility for aspects of ongoing medical care and the coordination of support and family services to the nurse practitioner, with structured interaction with social workers and other support staff. Although physicians or paramedical personnel may undertake the responsibility to coordinate such care, the function of the nurse practitioner in this context can provide a useful paradigm of global patient management.

EMERGING ROLE OF THE NURSE PRACTITIONER

With the changing face of medical practice and health care reimbursement, clinical nurses have assumed an evolving role in the health care system. The nurse practitioner, an advanced practice, registered nurse with additional training beyond a basic bachelor of science in nursing degree, is qualified to assume a range of roles in medical management, anesthetic practice, palliative care, and other clinical domains. The initial purpose of developing these roles was to meet the growing needs of primary care and to improve health care delivery in clinic and ambulatory settings.[4] With the emerging imbalance in physician-to-patient ratios and the success of nurse practitioners in the primary care setting, however, the range of functions has rapidly increased. State-based legislation has evolved to broaden the scope of practice and privileges of nurse practitioners,[5] and direct third-party reimbursement and narcotic prescription privileges have been ratified in many states.[6] Legislative efforts are now directed toward the promotion of national and state recognition of the provider role of the nurse practitioner.[7]

Nurse practitioners are employed in a variety of settings with an impact on the patient with genitourinary cancer, including primary care and specialty practice. In both settings, the nurse practitioner may provide various services and activities, including cancer screening and prevention, provision of diagnostic services, clinical follow-up, and patient education and counseling on health and nutrition. Because more than 80% of cancer care is delivered in the outpatient setting,[8] these functions are predominantly fulfilled in the ambulatory environment, which is characterized by different requirements for efficient communication and management from the traditional inpatient model.

In addition to the foregoing routine clinical responsibilities, the nurse practitioner is in a unique position to undertake a critically important role in coordination with paramedical and support personnel (e.g., social workers, home care workers, clinical psychologists, physical therapists, nutritional consultants), especially because the nature of the nurse practitioner-patient relationship is often different from that between the physician and the patient. In particular, patients may see the nurse as a less dominant or potentially less intimidating figure, or they may feel more comfortable with the level of verbal communication, especially in the setting of a busy clinical or academic practice. As a consequence, communication may be more effective regarding the goals and potential side effects of treatment, the psychosocial ramifications of the disease, and the available resources for treatment and support of the patient and family. In addition, repetition may be helpful in the transfer of information on complex issues, and the nurse practitioner can serve a useful role in reinforcing concepts advanced by the physician.

Another factor that might contribute to the role of the nurse practitioner is that the current organizational structure of urooncologic practice is such that a greater proportion of the working time of the nurse practitioner may be focused specifically on patient-related issues with more frequent direct patient contact, whereas many physicians are required to participate excessively in practice or hospital management, administrative functions, and extramural educational activities. In some instances, the clinical activities of the physician reduce the time available for direct communication with patients (e.g., performance of surgery or preparation and planning of radiotherapy treatment programs).

When the nurse practitioner is required to assume the foregoing responsibilities, certain features of the common genitourinary cancers may require unique patterns of intervention and the application of specific sets of data or clinical experience.

TABLE 14-1. *Factors in coping with cancer*

PATIENT
Age
Education
Race and ethnicity
Prior experience with cancer and other illnesses
Fiscal constraints
Relationship with the physician
Psychologic and psychiatric factors (illness, alcoholism, drug abuse, personality)
Level of understanding regarding the cancer and its treatment
Fear
Available level of family and social support
FAMILY
Education
Prior experiences with cancer and other illnesses
Socioeconomic and financial status
Distance from the hospital
Numbers available to help
Prior family dynamics
Race and ethnic features and attitudes about cancer
Level of understanding regarding the cancer and its treatment
Cancer families
ILLNESS
Type and site of cancer
Expectation of cure and prolonged survival
Requirements of treatment
Potential for mutilation and suffering
Presence of pain
Implications for sexuality and related factors
MEDICAL TEAM
Nature of the team
Level of resources and experience
Attitudes to global patient management
Interpersonal relationships with patient and family
Continuity of care

TESTICULAR CANCER

The results of treatment of testicular cancer have improved dramatically in the past 2 decades, largely because of improvements in the technology of diagnosis, surgery, and chemotherapy (see Chaps. 65 through 68). With these changes in management, however, a much greater level of active cooperation is required from the patient. The nurse practitioner caring for the patient with testicular cancer is often challenged to use both psychosocial and physical assessment skills. The ability of any patient to cope with the implications of the diagnosis of cancer and then to undergo the required treatment reflects several factors (Table 14-1). Because this malignant disease affects younger males, issues common to anyone in this age group need to be considered, in addition to the unique implications of the diagnosis and planned treatment. The initial reactions at the time of the diagnosis of cancer (including fear, grief, and anger) are often heightened by the youth of the patient, by the potential for the loss of life at a time when less has been achieved, and in particular by the potential loss of fertility.[9–12] Furthermore, at this time of life, autonomy has only recently been achieved, with emerging independence from the family structure, and training, establishment, and career goals are at their maximum. Self-image, body image, and sexuality are in a state of flux, and the requirements of treatment (including orchiectomy and, in some instances, chemotherapy) potentially cause major disruptions in this context.

Several studies have investigated the premorbid and posttreatment psychosocial characteristics of patients with testicular cancer, but no consensus has been achieved regarding the personality characteristics associated with testicular cancer or its treatment.[9–12] An unusual feature of some patients with testicular cancer (before treatment) is a curious, almost sociopathic, personality, characterized by rejection of authority figures and a systematic refusal to comply with the requirements of medical care. Other clinicians have reported no evidence of any difference between patients who have (or have had) testis cancer, however, as compared with age-matched controls. The discrepancies in the results of the various studies may be methodologic; for example, in the study of Riecker and associates,[10] mail surveys were used, to which a significant proportion of patients did not respond. This method may have inadevertently excluded the noncompliant patients described previously, thus biasing the outcome of the study in favor of apparent normality.

Whether or not the patient has a normal premorbid personality, the health care team must develop a support mechanism for him, especially in the context of orchiectomy, lymphadenectomy, or cytotoxic chemotherapy with their attendant complications (see Chaps. 64 through 71). The nurse practitioner and other members of the medical and support teams need to interact closely with the patient and his family. For the sociopathic patient, with an innate reluctance to cooperate with medical care, the nurse practitioner, often representing a less conservative, less authoritarian posture, can play a particularly important role in view of having knowledge of the disease and of the specifics of treatment, while having the time and the training to participate in the psychosocial support program. Such a patient must be followed with a mixture of firmness and compassion. Frequent reminders that the goal of therapy is *cure* may be helpful. Coordinating efforts with home care nurses may help to ensure the attendance of the patient for scheduled treatment, as well as adherence to follow-up and monitoring schedules.

In the management of other malignant diseases, compliance with treatment programs can be improved by reducing the symptoms of the disease and the side effects of treatment.[13] This effect is most pronounced in younger patients, the characteristic feature of men with testis cancer. The nurse practitioner, through frequent interactions with the patient, can monitor the intensity of symptoms, while following the course of treatment for the prevalence and severity of side effects. With extensive knowledge of chemotherapy and of the mechanisms to reduce these problems, the nurse practitioner is well placed to improve patient compliance with the treatment program.

In addition, early referral to the agencies that offer additional support for patients with cancer, and in some cases a specific cancer support group (Table 14-2), assists in all aspects of the overall care of the patient and may achieve a greater level of cooperation between the patient and the members of the expanded medical team.

Issues that relate to fertility are also important in many patients with germ cell tumors. Infertility is associated with the genesis of germ cell tumors.[14] In addition, orchiectomy, retroperitoneal lymph node dissection, and cytotoxic chemotherapy may each interfere with fertility. Each of these treatment modalities can have important implications for the sexuality of patients and their partners, although the extent to which these issues interfere with their lives appears to vary.[9–12] For example, in a retrospective study of survivors of testis cancer, no effect on employment, divorce, or disabling psychologic problems was identified.[15] Patients did report a high level of distress regarding infertility and sexual performance, however; in particular, patients without children at the time of diagnosis and those with lower levels of education and lower socioeconomic status had greater concerns regarding sexuality and sexual performance. In turn, men who reported sexual impairment were more likely to have a negative impact on their relationships (32%) and a negative mental outlook than the survivors without reported sexual dysfunction.

The nurse practitioner can play an essential role by counseling the relevant members of the family, by providing information, and even by referral to specific sex counselors or medical specialists in the management of infertility, including sperm banking.

Symptom control during treatment is also an important priority, especially for the patient undergoing chemotherapy. Although some young men fail to report the extent of toxicity as part of playing a role commensurate with their view of ''maleness,'' careful and sympathetic enquiry may often unmask unreported events and may facilitate more complete control of symptoms. This control, in turn, improves adherence to treatment schedules and cooperation by the patient.

In follow-up clinics, several important functions are undertaken. The nurse practitioner can provide general medical and psychologic follow-up and support. In particular, however, familiarity with the potential long-term complications (such as hypertension, iatrogenic cancers, and the dysplastic nevus syndrome)[16–18] (see Chap. 71) allows the nurse practitioner to provide a valuable screening function and to give specific advice on these issues. Similarly, in follow-up of the patient on active surveillance protocols for stage I testicular cancer (see Chap. 67), in collaboration with the managing physician, the nurse practitioner with a specific knowledge of the natural history of the disease and its pattern of metastasis can provide a mechanism for the early detection of relapse, with a specific focusing of testing protocols during the period of maximum risk. In addition, the nurse practitioner with a specific interest in such a clinic should establish a mechanism for follow-up and recall of patients who do not attend their scheduled visits.

Thus, as part of an extended team of clinical and support staff managing the patient with testicular cancer, the nurse practitioner can play a central and unique role, contributing to improved cure rates and reduced levels of morbidity and ensuring the optimal outcomes of the management programs.

PROSTATE CANCER

As discussed in detail in Chapter 36, the health care system is being challenged by the rising incidence of prostate cancer. Prostate cancer is one of the two most common cancers detected in men and is the second leading cause of cancer deaths in men.[19] This increased incidence can be attributed to several factors, including the discovery and application of prostate-specific antigen (PSA) to screening programs, more refined diagnostic imaging techniques, an increasing proportion of men aged 70 years and older in the community, and an increased level of public education and awareness of this entity.

The role of the nurse practitioner in the care of patients with prostate cancer includes contributions to prevention and detection, as well as routine management as part of a medical team. In the context of cancer prevention, the role of the nurse practitioner is predominantly educational. For example, family history, excess dietary fat intake, obesity, occupational exposure (e.g., to cadmium), and cigarette smoking are suggested contributors to the genesis of this disease. Thus, the nurse practitioner can fulfill an educative function by informing patients of these factors in screening and high-risk detection clinics, as well as by participating in such activities in community health centers and hospitals and other ambulatory services departments. Some investigators have even suggested that the risk of prostate cancer can be reduced by changes in life style and perhaps by the use of chemopreventative agents[20] (see Chap. 43), and the nurse practitioner, with a knowledge of the available clinical trials and of the current database, can participate in studies of this type by identifying and enlisting patients and by monitoring outcomes.

The issue of screening for prostate cancer is particularly controversial, and no complete concordance exists regarding its

TABLE 14-2. *Community resources for support for the patient with genitourinary cancer*

Organization	Address	Purpose
PATIENT RESOURCES		
American Cancer Society (ACS)	1599 Clifton Road, NE Atlanta, GA 30329-4251 404-320-3333 (general information) 404-329-7616 (Department of Nursing) (Phone numbers for local units and divisions are listed in the white pages of the telephone book.)	ACS is a nationwide, community-based, volunteer health agency dedicated to eliminating cancer as a major health problem.
American Foundation for Urologic Disease, Inc.	300 West Pratt Street, Suite 401 Baltimore, MD 21201-2463 410-727-2908 410-528-0550 (fax)	The American Foundation for Urologic Disease, Inc., provides printed information to both the public and professionals related to urologic problems, including cancer. It also provides information concerning the availability of scholarships for research that focuses on urologic problems.
National Black Leadership Initiative on Cancer (NBLIC)	Frank E. Jordan Program Director Executive Plaza North, Room 240-D Bethesda, MD 20892 301-496-8589 301-496-8675 (fax)	NBLIC is one of the National Cancer Institute's community outreach initiatives intended to increase cancer awareness among African-Americans. NBLIC offers individuals an opportunity to become part of a network of concerned and active African-American leaders across the United States who are bringing cancer prevention and control programs to African-American communities. Coalitions of NBLIC include national organizations, historically black colleges and universities, medical colleges, business and industry, media, and community-based programs. Chapters of national organizations and other local groups work together to mobilize community programs around the country.
National Hispanic Leadership Initiative on Cancer	En Accion Coordinating Center South Texas Health Research Center The University of Texas Health Sciences Center at San Antonio 7703 Floyd Curl Drive San Antonio, TX 78284-7791 210-614-4496 210-615-0661 (fax)	En Accion: National Hispanic Leadership Initiative on Cancer is the first comprehensive assessment of risk factors for cancer in all Hispanic and Latino populations and among both men and women. Experts in public health and in medicine, together with grass-roots community-based organizations, are forming a national network to develop programs to reduce these risk factors. Their common mission is to empower Hispanic and Latino populations with the knowledge and the resources they need to prevent and control cancer among their own people.
United Ostomy Association (UOA)	36 Executive Park, Suite 120 Irvine, CA 92714 714-660-8624 1-800-826-0826	UOA is a nonprofit organization that provides speakers, literature, and monthly information meetings for people with ostomies. Volunteers, most of whom are ostomates, may visit patients with ostomies in the hospital or at home with the consent of the patient's physician.
COUNSELING AND SUPPORT SERVICES		
Cancer Care, Inc.	1180 Avenue of the Americas New York, NY 10036 212-221-3300	Cancer Care, Inc., is a nonprofit social service agency founded to help patients with cancer and their families cope with the impact of cancer. The organization provides psychologic and financial support; counseling is available on both a group and individual basis.
Help for Incontinent People (HIP)	P.O. Box 544 Union, SC 29379 803-579-7900 803-579-7902 (fax) 1-800-BLADDER	HIP is a nonprofit organization dedicated to improving the quality life of people with incontinence. HIP is a leading source of education, advocacy, and support to the public and the health profession about the causes, prevention, diagnosis, treatments, and management alternatives for incontinence. HIP provides a wide variety of printed and audio-visual materials, including The HIP Report newsletter; the Resource Guide of Continence Products and Services; a 33-minute videotape called "Bladder Control: How to Regain It, How to Maintain It"; and an audiocassette and booklet that coaches individuals through pelvic muscle exercises. Send a long, stamped, self-

TABLE 14-2. *Continued.*

Organization	Address	Purpose
		addressed envelope for an introductory packet about incontinence and for a list of HIP's publications and member services.
Look Good, Feel Better (LGFB)	The Cosmetic, Toiletry, and Fragrance Association Foundation 1101 17th Street, NW Suite 300 Washington, DC 20036 202-331-1770 or 1-800-395-LOOK	LGFB is a free national public-service program dedicated to teaching women with cancer (through hands-on experience) beauty techniques that will help to restore their appearance and self-image during chemotherapy and radiation treatment. LGFB offers group or individual sessions conducted by trained and certified cosmetologists, complimentary make-up kits for patients participating in a group program, and free materials such as videotapes and pamphlets. In addition, LGFB materials are available in Spanish. The program is a joint venture of the Cosmetic, Toiletry, and Fragrance Association Foundation, the American Cancer Society (ACS), and the National Cosmetology Association. For information about program locations in your community, contact your local ACS office or call toll-free 1-800-395-LOOK.
Make Today Count	Connie Zimmerman, Executive Director 1235 East Cherokee Springfield, MO 65804-2263 417-885-2273 800-432-2273	Make Today Count is an international organization for people with cancer or other life-threatening illnesses. It provides support groups and educational programs as well as brochures and handouts.
National Coalition for Cancer Survivorship (NCCS)	1010 Wayne Ave., Fifth Floor Silver Springs, MD 20910 301-650-8868 301-565-9670 (fax)	NCCS is a network of independent organizations and individuals working in the areas of cancer support and survivorship. The primary goal of the coalition is to generate a nationwide awareness of cancer survivorship. NCCS facilitates communication among people involved with cancer survivorship, promotes the development of cancer support activities, serves as a clearinghouse for information and materials on survivorship, acts as an advocate for survivors of cancer, and encourages the study of survivorship.
US TOO Prostate Cancer Survivor Support Group	930 North York Road Suite 50 Hinsdale, IL 60521-2993 1-800-82-USTOO or 708-323-1002 708-323-1003 (fax)	US TOO provides various types of support for survivors of and patients with prostate cancer. The nonprofit organization offers information and counseling and conducts educational meetings to assist patients in the decision-making process. It has chapters across the United States and Canada that hold regular monthly meetings for patients with prostate cancer and their families. At these meetings, specialists in various fields provide information about prostate cancer and related surgery, radiation, medicine, nutrition, and psychology. Meetings are free of charge and open to family members, friends, and professionals in the healthcare field. US TOO is affiliated with the American Foundation for Urologic Disease and is recognized by the American Cancer Society as a national support group for survivors of prostate cancer and their families.
Women's Cancer Network	2413 West River Road Grand Island, NY 14072	The Women's Cancer Network provides support, referral, and resource services to women who have or have had cancer. Support services offered include a monthly newsletter, a support group, and a telephone network for women confined to the home. An information resource and referral system provides information to women with cancer relating to their psychosocial or physical needs and to the health care system. Public and professional programs are offered in addition to individual, institutional, or agency consultations. The Women's Cancer Network provides a vehicle through which women can share cancer experiences, receive positive energy and support, learn from each other, acquire strategies for healing, and learn ways to survive the health care system.

(continued)

TABLE 14-2. *Continued.*

Organization	Address	Purpose
PUBLIC GENERAL INFORMATION		
Cancer Information Service (CIS)	National Cancer Institute Building 31, Room 10A07 Bethesda, MD 20892 1-800-4-CANCER 1-800-422-6237 Attn: Chris Thomsen 301-496-8664	CIS can be accessed by telephone to provide answers to questions from the general public, patients and their families, and health professions. Information specialists at CIS are not physicians, but they can provide accurate, up-to-date, and understandable information about cancer causes, prevention, detection, diagnosis, treatment, rehabilitation, and research. In addition, CIS may know about cancer-related services and resources in local areas. Printed materials on many cancer-related topics are available to callers free of charge. Searches of the PDQ data base also are provided at no cost to the public and to healthcare professionals.
CancerFAX	National Cancer Institute (NCI) International Cancer Information Center Attn: Jean Baum Building 82, Room 123 Bethesda, MD 20892 301-402-5874 (on fax machine handset) 301-496-8880 (for technical assistance)	Using facsimile technology, the National Cancer Institute (NCI) has developed CancerFax. This service enables individuals to retrieve state-of-the-art cancer treatment information directly from NCI's comprehensive and current source of cancer information–PDQ data base (see PDQ). Two types of summaries are available: one that is written to meet the informational needs of healthcare professionals and one that is written in language geared toward the general public. Additionally, information is available on screening guidelines, supportive care, patient publications, and other information services provided by NCI. CancerFax statements are available in English and Spanish. There is no charge for the service itself; users pay only for the cost of the telephone call to the CancerFax computer in Bethesda, MD. The service is available 24 hours a day, 7 days a week. (Also see CancerNet.)
COPING	2019 North Carothers Franklin, TN 37064 615-790-2400	COPING magazine is the only nationally distributed consumer magazine for people whose lives have been affected by cancer. The magazine's primary purpose is to empower the readers (be they patients or professionals) by providing the knowledge that they need to cope with the many issues confronting their daily lives. COPING aims to inspire patients and survivors to assume greater responsibility for, and participation in, the many facets of the disease. The magazine is published bimonthly (six times a year). Subscriptions cost $18 for one year ($24 Canadian/foreign) and $32 for two years ($44 Canadian/foreign). To subscribe, write to COPING, 2019 North Carothers, Franklin, TN 37064 or call 615-790-2400.
National Cancer Institute (NCI) Information Associated Program	Building 82, Room 123 Bethesda, MD 20892 1-800-NCI-7890 (U.S.) 301-816-2083 (international) 301-231-6941 (fax)	NCI, the US government's top agency for cancer research, offers a variety of services and materials to patients, the public, and health professionals (see Cancer Information Service and PDQ) All NCI patient education materials are free of charge.
National Cancer Survivors Day (NCSD) Foundation, Inc.	2019 North Carothers, Suite 100 Franklin, TN 37064 615-794-3006 or 615-791-4719	NCSD is America's nationwide, annual celebration of life for cancer survivors and their families, friends, and oncology teams. Each celebration is an annual milestone in a survivor's fight against cancer, and there are 8 million cancer survivors in America. NCSD was founded by cancer survivor Richard Bloch and his wife, Annette, who serve each year as the co-chairs. NCSD is celebrated on the first Sunday in June of each year in communities throughout the United States and Canada. It is the world's largest cancer survivor event. For more information about NCSD, contact the NCSD Foundation.

TABLE 14-2. *Continued.*

Organization	Address	Purpose
Office of Minority Health Resource Center	U.S. Department of Health and Human Services P.O. Box 37337 Washington, DC 20013-7337 1-800-444-6472	The Office of Minority Health Resource Center provides information relating to health-related resources, targeting Asians, Pacific Islanders, African–Americans, Hispanics and Latinos, and Native Americans at the federal, state, and local levels. The center also provides various information services, a computerized data base of minority health-related publications/programs, and a resource persons network.
TERMINAL CARE		
Choice in Dying	200 Varick Street New York, NY 10014 212-366-5540	Choice in Dying, a nonprofit organization, provides information about living wills and durable power of attorney and advice and counseling (both legal and personal) about terminal-care decision making.
Hospice Link	Hospice Education Institute Suite 3-B, P.O. Box 713 5 Essex Square Essex, CT 06426-0713 1-800-331-1620 203-767-1620 (in Alaska and Connecticut)	Hospice Link provides information about hospice care and can refer patients with cancer and their families to local hospice programs.
National Hospice Organization	1901 North Moore Street, Suite 901 Arlington, VA 22209 703-243-5900 1-800-658-8898 (Hospice Helpline)	Hospice is care and support for terminally ill people and their loved ones. The National Hospice Organization is a nonprofit organization that provides literature and information about hospice care to patients and their families as well as referral to other local, regional, and national resources.

efficacy[21,22] (see Chaps. 46 and 47). In fact, opposite recommendations have been made by the National Institutes of Health and the American Cancer Society, a situation contributing to confusion in the general community. In centers that subscribe to a policy of screening, with a view to early detection and treatment, the nurse practitioner can function in an independent role. In accordance with advanced practice education, the nurse practitioner is able to identify appropriate candidates for screening, take a relevant history, perform and interpret a physical examination that includes digital rectal examination, and order and interpret the appropriate initial tests (including assay of PSA). Using a decision-tree method, the nurse practitioner recommends appropriate follow-up or interventions. For example, if the results of digital rectal examination and PSA assay are normal, annual follow-up may be recommended, depending on the clinical context. If they are abnormal, a referral is made to a urologist for diagnostic evaluation. The nurse practitioner can play a particularly useful role in attempting to explain to the patient the various controversies and helping to guide him through this complex area. The nurse practitioner working in a community practice setting can identify persons at high risk for prostate cancer and can individualize the approach to their management.[23]

Once the diagnosis of prostate cancer is made, the role of the nurse practitioner in the ambulatory setting focuses on the requirements and complications of treatment, and in particular on monitoring for toxicity of treatment and provision of appropriate support and care for these problems. Depending on the stage of the disease, the expectations and requirements of therapy differ.

For patients with localized prostate cancer, options of treatment may include periodic observation only, the use of radical radiotherapy, or prostatectomy (see Chaps. 49 through 52). In this situation, the aim of treatment is potentially to achieve cure, and this goal must be emphasized to the patient. Patients on observation-only protocols, based on the low risk of local tumor progression in a well-differentiated cancer, may require frequent counseling and psychologic support because of potential concerns regarding the lack of active "treatment" and the potential for progression of the tumor.

Patients who undergo radiotherapy may experience acute toxic effects, such as strangury, urinary frequency, urinary or fecal incontinence, or diarrhea during the period of treatment, and the nurse practitioner, in collaboration with the radiation oncologist, should monitor the patient for these complications and should provide appropriate care or referral. In this situation, long-term side effects may occur, including repetitive bouts of diarrhea or bowel dysfunction, as well as long-term changes in sexual function (see later).

The nurse practitioner has several potential roles for the patient who undergoes radical prostatectomy, including the provision of education and counseling regarding the management of the stoma or other continence devices, adaptation to the changed life style, and assistance in the management of the problems that arise from altered sexual function.

Sexual function may continue beyond the seventh and eighth decades of life. Sexuality and sexual health require the integration of somatic, emotional, intellectual, and social aspects of sexual being in ways that enhance personality, communication, and love, constituting an integral part of an individual's personality and life.[24] The incorporation of sexual health management into patient care can no longer be disputed as a legitimate role

TABLE 14-3. *The P-LI-SS-IT acronym: stages of intervention in sexual counselling*

Acronym	Function
P	Permission (stage I)
LI	Limited information (stage II)
SS	Specific suggestions (stage III)
IT	Intensive therapy (stage IV)

for the health professional.[25] Neurologic, endocrine, vascular, and genital abnormalities should be assessed as part of a thorough history taking and physical examination when assessing sexual function. After the diagnostic workup is complete, surgical and nonsurgical interventions for sexual dysfunction should be considered in conjunction with a physician.

Using the PLISSIT model,[25,26] the nurse practitioner can provide sexual counseling on anatomic and physiologic changes related to the disease process and its treatment and can provide coping strategies and factual information, to dispell myths and misconceptions (Table 14-3). Referral to a sex therapist is usually indicated if a requirement for the fourth stage is perceived.[25,26]

Another important problem associated with the diagnosis and management of prostate cancer is urinary incontinence. This complex anatomic and physiologic entity may relate to neurovascular complications from tumor growth or from its treatment, or it may be due simply to the anatomic disruption of the sphincter mechanism after conservative or radical prostatic surgery. Whatever the cause, the nurse practitioner can play an important role in helping to establish the diagnosis and in providing counseling, education, and support for the patient.[25,27] Many patients are embarrassed to confess to the symptoms associated with incontinence and prefer to deal with them privately by using absorptive devices. In the context of an ongoing relationship, the nurse practitioner may be able to determine the presence of the problem, especially in patients deemed to be at high risk, based on the anatomy of their disease or its treatment. Once the problem has been identified, the nurse practitioner can provide appropriate information or referral for clinical management or to a relevant support group (see Table 14-2).

When the cancer is more advanced at presentation, with locally extensive disease or the presence of metastases, hormonal manipulation is usually indicated (see Chap. 57). In this situation, the expectation of long-term success of treatment is less, and the patient is likely to suffer from impotence and other sexual problems, as well as additional symptoms, such as hot flashes, the develoment of gynecomastia, mood changes, and irregularity of bowel function. Analogous to the situations described previously, the nurse practitioner may have an important role in making the diagnosis of these complications and in providing the appropriate counseling and support, with referral for medical management as indicated.

The patient with metastatic disease, and in particular with the presence of hormone-refractory osseous metastases, is a difficult and demanding problem, requiring careful team management. Such patients illustrate many of the problems of advanced cancer: they are characteristically elderly, with multiple symptoms, including chronic pain, anorexia, weight loss, cachexia, and urinary problems, and they are faced with a progressively debilitating illness that is likely to be fatal. The nurse practitioner can provide an extension of the interaction with the physician, can assist in the identification and diagnosis of the patient's pain problem, can help to provide effective treatment and to coordinate social and support services, in liaison with a hospice team and a pain management unit (see Chaps. 11 and 59). Medical and nursing organizations have begun to address cancer pain in focused terms. The World Health Organization, the American Society of Clinical Oncology, and the Oncology Nursing Society have each issued position papers on this topic and have emphasized the importance of adequate diagnosis and effective pain management, with the use of pain scales and other objective indices, and the judicious application of psychologic support, nonsteroidal antiinflammatory agents, opioids, radiopharmaceuticals, and, where appropriate, pain-blocking techniques.

In many ways, the management of the problems associated with the various stages of prostate cancer provides a paradigm of the role of the nurse practitioner in cancer care. It spans the spectrum from early stage to advanced disease and yields opportunities for involvement in patient counseling and education, and screening activities, against a background of routine clinical care.

UROTHELIAL CANCER

As in prostate cancer, cancers of the bladder and urothelial tract are among the most common malignant diseases in Western society and tend to occur among the elderly.[28] Symptoms and signs are similar to those of prostatic cancer, with features of intrapelvic extension and urinary obstruction, and with the potential for dissemination. Frank hematuria and the symptoms of urinary frequency, urgency, and burning on micturition occur more commonly than in prostate cancer.

The nurse practitioner has various functions in the management of the patient with urothelial cancer. The most common pattern of presentation is superficial disease, comprising more than 80% of incident cases.[28] Thus, in the urologist's office or in a hospital-based practice, the nurse practitioner may be involved in the diagnostic workup, in the treatment program (using intravesical chemotherapy), or in follow-up and monitoring protocols (see Chap. 26). In an ambulatory care setting, the nurse practitioner is involved in screening programs (e.g., hematuria clinics or medical clinics provided by industries associated with a high occupational risk of bladder cancer) and can provide education regarding risk factors, the symptoms of the disease, and information regarding risk modification (smoking cessation, occupational practices).

Patients with locally extensive disease may complain of more substantial urinary tract symptoms and may even develop complete obstruction of urinary outlow, requiring the insertion of urinary stents or transcutaneous nephrostomy tubes. These tubes require ongoing advice and management, and in particular monitoring for infection, malfunction, or displacement. In this situation, the nurse practitioner can function independently or in collaboration with the physician, depending on the clinical context.

If the cancer is metastatic at presentation, many of the problems encountered are similar to those seen in patients with advanced prostate cancer. Cytotoxic chemotherapy has a greater role in metastatic disease than in advanced prostate cancer as combination cytotoxic regimens (e.g., the combination of methotrexate, vinblastine, cisplatin, and doxorubicin—the MVAC regimen) have been validated in randomized clinical trials.[29] These patients are elderly, however, and close monitoring for the complications of aggressive chemotherapy is required, especially in patients with an increased potential for urinary tract dysfunction or infection.

If the patient fails to respond to such treatment or is too frail to undergo intensive management programs, the physician, the nurse practitioner, and other members of the treatment team will have to prepare a program of palliative management, as outlined later.

RENAL CARCINOMA

As with refractory cancer of the prostate or bladder, management of the patient with renal cell carcinoma may be particularly difficult, especially in advanced disease. Occasionally, an early diagnosis is achieved, usually in association with early symptomatic presentation or through the detection of a stage I tumor during investigation for an intercurrent medical condition, and this early detection results in a high chance of surgical cure (see Chaps. 81 and 82).

Unfortunately, however, patients commonly present with advanced, even inoperable, disease or with widespread metastases, with a consequently worse prognosis.[30,31] This situation represents, for both the patient and the family, a frightening constellation of problems. The medical and nursing teams often reflect the hopelessness of the situation, for which no truly adequate treatment exists (see Chaps. 84 and 85), and thus may have few encouraging treatment options to offer. The patient must attempt to come to terms rapidly with the potential for a progressively deteriorating physical situation, the loss of income, and possibly early death.

In this situation, the full range of medical and support services must be introduced as early as possible. The physician deals with treatment-related issues and attempts to define options, their benefits, potential drawbacks, and the likelihood of success. In the management of advanced renal carcinoma, the list of available therapeutic options is dominated by investigational cytotoxic agents or new immunologic manipulations because the standards of therapy have yielded such disappointing results (see Chap. 85). As a result, the situation is even more uncertain for the patient, who senses the lower likelihood of a satisfactory outcome and the more speculative nature of the treatment program offered.

In this situation, several important roles can be assumed by the nurse practitioner, working in concert with the physicians in the treatment team:

1. Provision of clear information about the prognosis and options of treatment, with amplification, reinforcement or the updating of information as the disease process evolves; in some instances, when participation in a clinical trial is considered, the nurse practitioner may be of particular assistance in blending the role of patient advocate with that of a health professional who is familiar with the details of the proposed program.
2. After the identification of evolving problems, coordination with the required support services, including social workers, dietary consultants, clinical psychologists, and experts in pain management (see Chap. 11).
3. Provision of rational and detailed information regarding alternative medicine options; patients with renal carcinoma, for the reasons listed previously, are prone to search for alternative medicines and are in particular need of sound advice, predicated on fact, rather than emotion; in this situation, the nurse practitioner may constitute a sounding board for the patient's ideas, especially if the issue of alternative medical care is approached in a calm and nonjudgmental fashion.
4. Consultation and liaison with hospice and other supportive care services as the disease process evolves (see Chap. 11).

Patients with advanced renal carcinoma have a particular need for extensive medical and psychosocial support for themselves and their families in view of their desperate situation and the paucity of satisfactory treatment options. The nurse practitioner, working as a member of an extended support team, can fulfill an essential role in this context. Many hospice services are staffed predominantly by nurse practitioners, and ongoing care often represents the interaction between subspecialist nurse practitioners working in concert with their respective physician colleagues and members of the extended treatment teams.

AVAILABLE AGENCIES FOR SUPPORT OF PATIENTS WITH GENITOURINARY CANCER

To provide an encyclopedic list of support agencies in the context of the patient with cancer in general, or for genitourinary cancer in particular, is not possible. The provision of such a listing is no substitute for carefully considered and well-administered team management of the patient and the family as a whole.

Many patients benefit from direct interaction with nonmedical organizations or from information or support available from specific interest groups, however, and to some extent, they feel empowered by the ability to seek information for themselves. To this end, some of the available resources for patients with genitourinary cancer are listed in Table 14-2.

CONCLUSIONS

The role of the nurse practitioner is evolving rapidly, with the development of many new functions in the diagnosis, management, and support of the patient with cancer. Although nurse practitioners in some settings work only in collaboration with physicians, many new roles lend themselves particularly to the specialty interests and training of the nurse practitioner. In particular, these roles involve clinical interactions that require adequate time for communication and the application of communication skills at a different level, as well as the performance of tasks that relate to community education and illness prevention. As the community at large, and the medical profession in particular, gain a greater understanding of the potential utility of nurse practitioners and come to rely to a greater extent on their professional skills and expertise, these roles will likely evolve further. In time, medical and nursing practice will become more closely intertwined in a clinical partnership that optimizes the application of the skills of both professional groups for the welfare and comfort of patients.

REFERENCES

1. Cassileth BR, Lusk EJ, Strouse TB, et al. A psychological analysis of cancer patients and their next-of-kin. Cancer 1985;55:72.
2. Gotay CC. The experience of cancer during early and advanced stages: the views of patients and their mates. Soc Sci Med 1984;18:605.
3. Coluzzi PH, Grant M, Doroshow JH, Rhiner M, Ferrell B, Rivera L. Survey of the provision of supportive care services at National Cancer Institute-designated cancer centers. J Clin Oncol 1995;13:756.
4. McGivern DO. Evolution of primary care roles: the nurse practitioner. Nurse Pract Forum 1990;1:163.
5. Maraldo P. Politics and policy in primary care. In: Mezy MD, McGivern DO, eds. Nurses, nurse practitioner evolution to advanced practice. New York: Springer-Verlag, 1993:367.
6. Pearson LJ. 1992–93 update: How each state stands on legislative issues affecting advanced nursing practice. Nurse Pract 1993;18:23.
7. Inglis AD, Kjervik D. Empopwerment of advanced practice nurses: regulation reform needed to increase access to care. J Law Med Ethics 1993;20:199.
8. Harris M, Bean C. Changing the role of the nurse in the hematology-oncology outpatient setting. Oncol Nurs Forum 1991;18:43.
9. Tross S, Holland J, Bosl G, et al. A controlled study of psychosocial sequelae in cured survivors of testicular neoplasms. Proc Am Soc Clin Oncol 1984;3:74.
10. Riecker P, Edbril S, Garnick M. Curative testis cancer therapy: psychosocial sequelae. J Clin Oncol 1985;3:1117.
11. Schover L, von Eschenbach A. Sexual and marital relationships after treatment for nonseminomatous testicular cancer. Urology 1986;24: 251.
12. Bloom JR, Fobair P, Gritz E, et al. Psychosocial outcomes of cancer: a comparative analysis of Hodgkin's disease and testicular cancer. J Clin Oncol 1993;11:979.
13. Richardson JL, Marks G, Levine A. The influence of symptoms of disease and side effects of treatment on compliance with cancer therapy. J Clin Oncol 1988;6:1746.
14. Raghavan D, Neville AM. The biology of testicular tumours. In: Chisholm GD, Innes Williams D, eds. Scientific foundations of urology, 2nd ed. London: William Heinemann Medical Books, 1982:785.
15. Riecker P. Psychosocial factors, curative therapies, and behavioral outcomes. Cancer 1989;64:2399.
16. Boyer MJ, Raghavan D, Harris PJ, et al. Lack of late toxicity in patients treated with cisplatin containing combination chemotherapy for metastatic testicular cancer. J Clin Oncol 1990;8:21.
17. Boyer MJ, Raghavan D. Toxicity of treatment of germ cell tumors. Semin Oncol 1992;19:128.
18. Raghavan D, Zalcberg J, Grygiel JJ, et al. Multiple atypical nevi: a cutaneous marker of germ cell tumors. J Clin Oncol 1994;12:2284.
19. Boring C, Squires T, Tong T, Montgomery S. Cancer statistics, 1994. CA Cancer J Clin 1994;44:7.
20. Greco K, Kulawiak L. Prostate cancer prevention: risk reduction through life-style, diet and chemoprevention. Oncol Nurs Forum 1994; 21:1504.
21. Kramer BS, Brown ML, Prorok PC, Potosky AL, Gohagan JK. Prostate cancer screening: what we know and what we need to know. Ann Intern Med 1993;119:914.
22. Catalona WJ. Screening for prostate cancer: enthusiasm. Urology 1993; 42:113.
23. Waldman A, Osborne D. Screening for prostate cancer. Oncol Nurs Forum 1994;21:1512.
24. Held J, Osborne D, Volpe H, Waldman A. Cancer of the prostate: treatment and nursing implications. Oncol Nurs Forum 1994;21:1517.
25. Hampton B, Bryant R. Ostomies and continent diversions: nursing management. St Louis: Mosby–Year Book, 1992:15.
26. Dudas S. Altered body, image and sexuality. In: Greenwald SL, Frogge M, Goodman M, Yarbro CH, eds. Cancer nursing principles and practice: manifestations of cancer and cancer treatment, 2nd ed. Boston: Jones & Bartlett, 1992:581.
27. Whitehead E, Smith-Young S, Lang P. Urinary incontinence: types, etiologies, diagnostic evaluation. J Urol Nurs 1985;4:297.
28. Raghavan D, Shipley WU, Garnick MB, Russell PJ, Richie JP. The biology and management of bladder cancer. N Engl J Med 1990;322: 1129.
29. Loehrer PJ Sr, Einhorn LH, Elson PJ, et al. A randomized comparison of cisplatin alone or in combination with methotrexate, vinblastine, and doxorubicin in patients with metastatic urothelial carcinoma: a cooperative group study. J Clin Oncol 1992;10:1063.
30. Skinner DG, Colvin RB, Vermillion CD. Diagnosis and management of renal cell carcinoma: a clinical and pathologic study of 309 cases. Cancer 1971;28:1165.
31. Golimbu M, Joshi P, Sperber A. Renal cell carcinoma: survival and prognostic factors. Urology 1986;27:291.

Principles and Practice of Genitourinary Oncology, edited by Derek Raghavan, Howard I. Scher, Steven A. Leibel, and Paul H. Lange. Lippincott-Raven Publishers, Philadelphia, © 1997.

CHAPTER 15

Cost of Treating Genitourinary Cancer

Mark S. Litwin

The cost of urologic malignant disease may be measured in many ways. Although putting a price tag on human suffering is difficult, physicians today are asked to reduce costs, to improve quality, and to provide services for greater numbers of patients in an increasingly austere environment. This goal often requires rationing of resources, although it is seldom explicitly labeled as such. In the present era of sweeping change in health care financing and health services delivery, increased importance has been placed on efficiency in the allocation of scarce medical resources. The field of medical economics is well beyond its nascency, and broad public interest has emerged in studying the costs of medical and surgical therapies.

Oncology was once thought to be beyond the reach of those interested in reforming health care costs. When a patient developed cancer, the common perspective was that all possible resources should be spent on medical cure, and no energy should be expended on exploring ways to improve the cost-efficiency of treating the tumor. Through the courage and foresight of some early researchers, the principles of cost-effectiveness have now been successfully applied to malignant as well as benign disease. As payors, medical administrators, health care managers, and hospitals spend more administrative dollars on cost containment,[1] scrutiny is reaching all potential areas for conservation, including urologic oncology.

Urologists have long been attentive to issues of cost in managing health care. In his autobiography, Hugh Hampton Young, the father of American urology, described a patient on whom he agreed to perform a prostatectomy in the 1920s for a fixed fee of $500 with a promise of only 3 weeks in the hospital. Because the patient suffered complications and remained hospitalized for much longer than planned, Young had to spend his entire professional fee plus an additional $350 to pay off the hospital bill.[2]

Health policy decisions in the future will be based not only on biomedical research, but also on sound evaluations of health care costs, quality of care, and medical outcomes. As a surgical subspecialty with large numbers of Medicare patients, urologic oncology is a discipline in which cost-saving maneuvers may have tremendous financial impact. As clinicians treating patients with genitourinary cancer, we take on the task of understanding which policies safely conserve costs while continually improving quality.

TERMS AND METHODS OF ANALYSIS

In its pure form, research on health care costs involves counting the amount of money expended on facilities, equipment, supplies, and personnel during the provision of medical care. Many costs are hidden, however. A more extensive approach also includes the opportunity cost of the time patients spend receiving care. For example, when calculating the cost of a 30-minute office visit for interval outpatient cystoscopy after resection of a bladder tumor, one may include not only the cost of facility overhead, endoscopic equipment, disposable supplies, medications, laboratory tests, and medical personnel, but also the cost to the patient in lost wages during the time away from work for the procedure, travel, or any complications. This component is not insignificant. Employee absence from work for medical care has been estimated to cost businesses in the United States $37 million annually.[3]

Because true costs are difficult to quantify at the individual, institutional, or population level, researchers instead often report data on charges. *Charges* represent the amount billed to the patient for a service, whereas *costs* reflect what the provider expended to supply that service. Most of the available administrative databases in health care are based either on financial discharge abstracts from hospitals or on claims data from large payors, such as insurance companies or government agencies. These data sets include information primarily on charges, not costs. The major advantage of using charge data is that they are much easier to obtain. The primary disadvantage is that they may not accurately reflect the true underlying costs of individual medical services. For example, a hospital that is losing money on intravenous pyelograms may make up the deficit by increasing its charges for urine cytologic studies. This practice may help to balance the annual budget, but it corrupts the quality of the charge data. An economic analysis using charges for bladder cancer follow-up in this hospital will err by incorporating the inflated amounts charged for interval urine cytologic studies. Some analysts attempt to circumvent this problem by calculating a ratio of costs to charges for an entire facility, individual medical services, or diagnosis-based categories of care. Although imperfect, charges are frequently used to estimate the amount of money spent on health care.

To avoid the inherent problems in calculating costs and charges, some researchers instead measure *resource utilization* in terms of duration, frequency, and intensity of services. One of the most commonly reported units of comparative analysis is length of stay (LOS). Since 1983, when the prospective payment system was instituted to reimburse hospitals a predetermined amount of money based on the diagnosis related group (DRG) into which each Medicare inpatient is classified,[4] attention to LOS as an outcome variable in cost analyses has increased. In addition, cost of care may be measured as intensity or numbers of services provided. For example, rather than calculating the costs or charges for a 4-day hospitalization for radical prostatectomy, analysis may be based on the total number of complete blood counts, chest radiographs, bags of intravenous fluid, doses of antibiotic, and milligrams of narcotic ordered on any single day of the hospital stay or during the entire 4 days. By examining duration or frequency of actual medical services when studying costs, researchers can avoid the biases involved in using financial data.

Cost-effectiveness analysis is another popular technique used to evaluate new or established medical therapies. A cost-effectiveness analysis is performed by developing a probability model of the possible medical outcomes of different interventions (or a nonintervention), identifying the expenses associated with each outcome, and comparing the results, typically reported as cost per year of life saved.[5–8] Years of life saved, or *life-years (LYs),* are calculated for a population, not for individuals. Ten LYs may represent 2 patients, each of whom survives for 5 additional years, or 120 patients, each of whom survives for 1 additional month.[9] LYs are usually adjusted to account for different health states that may result from various treatments. These are called *quality-adjusted life years (QALYs).* For example, when comparing two treatments for localized prostate cancer, if both options are determined to cost $10,000 per year of life saved, then the two may seem equivalent. If one treatment yields years that are compromised by bothersome sexual dysfunction, however, whereas the other yields years that are free of such problems, then the difference in quality of the years saved must be factored into the equation. If patients appraise an impotent year as being worth less than a potent year, then quality adjustments may make the first treatment more expensive per QALY saved. *Cost-benefit analysis* differs by including not only the costs but also the equivalent monetary value of any benefits garnered during the extra years of life. Often, this entity refers to wages earned or income accrued during that time. In more sophisticated analyses, future income and expenses related to a particular health state are *discounted* to present value by incorporating a projected interest rate over time.

PATTERNS OF CARE

Much of the current research into the cost of treating urologic cancers is predicated on the observation that patterns of care differ for certain conditions. Physician demographics as well as patient age affect practice patterns.[10,11] Despite the relative sparsity of cost analyses in urologic oncology, significant variations in LOS and charges have been reported for many nonurologic medical and surgical hospitalizations.[12–14] Cost savings can be achieved by identifying variations in urologists' practice habits and targeting them for reduction in intensity and duration.[15] These changes in urologic practice have been shown not to result in poorer medical outcomes,[16] even though patients tend to dislike shorter postoperative hospital stays.[17–19] Overall, studies have been mixed. Some have described the successful use of cost-control mechanisms in urology,[20] whereas others have failed to show sustained results.[21] Analysis of both medical and surgical DRGs indicates that consistent patterns of resource use are identifiable during the course of hospitalizations, a finding suggesting that elements of utilization may be managed more effectively to yield cost savings.[22] This is particularly true in treatments for genitourinary cancer, many of which may be standardized. Urologic oncology is an fertile area for future economic analysis because so little is known about the cost-effectiveness of cancer screening and treatment interventions for even the most common genitourinary tumors.[23]

The advent of managed care has facilitated the study of practice patterns and medical outcomes. Most researchers agree that health maintenance organizations (HMOs) improve access to medical services and cost-efficiency of care without compromising quality,[24–26] although at least one study has suggested that cancer patients may wait longer for treatment in HMOs than in fee-for-service plans.[27]

In a study of over 1100 patients newly diagnosed with prostate cancer, those cared for in HMOs were almost 1.5 times more likely to receive radiotherapy than surgery for clinically localized tumors. This finding appears consistent with the general HMO emphasis on outpatient care. HMO patients had a lower overall mortality rate than did non-HMO patients. Low-income men treated in HMOs had survival times that were significantly longer than those of middle- or high-income men in HMOs or fee-for-service plans.[28]

When studying patterns of care or medical costs, the analyst must adjust for case mix. *Case mix* refers to the severity of illness and degree of comorbidity in a group of patients. For various reasons, sicker patients cost more, and it is important to control for this difference in comparative analyses. When examining the factors that lead to higher hospital charges for sicker patients, two forces must be considered: duration and intensity of care. Duration is usually quantified as inpatient LOS, whereas intensity of care may be assessed as numbers of services or charges per day. In a large DRG-based study of costs for 799 men undergoing prostatectomy at major teaching hospitals, investigators found that patients who were sicker with comorbidity at admission remained hospitalized longer after surgery but did not receive more intense care during their stays. Duration and not intensity was the primary force driving up hospital charges for sicker prostatectomy patients.[29] Physicians have been largely successful at attenuating the increases in hospital costs by eliminating unnecessary hospital days, but maximal savings may have been reaped from this strategy.[30] Nevertheless, continued tailoring of the intensity and duration of service to a patient's burden of illness may still be shown to reduce costs.

PROSTATE CANCER

Surgical procedures in the diagnosis, staging, and surgical treatment of prostate cancer among Medicare patients have in-

TABLE 15-1. *Volume of procedures related to the diagnosis, staging, and surgical treatment of prostate cancer among Medicare beneficiaries in 1989 and 1992 (CPT codes are shown in parentheses)*

Procedure	1989	1992	Percent change
Prostate biopsy (55700)	$123,319	$376,060	205%
Transrectal ultrasound (76872)	22,669	199,959	1,226%
Radical retropubic or perineal prostatectomy with or without bilateral pelvic lymphadenectomy or lymph node biopsy, with or without nerve sparing (55810, 55812, 55815, 55840, 55842, 55845)	12,833	39,157	205%

United States Government Health Care Financing Administration. Medicare claims data for numbers of allowed services.

creased dramatically in the last several years (Table 15-1), leading to increased expenditures. The aging of the population of the United States has caused a rapid expansion of prostate cancer-related services, based on sheer volume alone. The total annual cost of treating prostate cancer in the United States has been estimated at $1.72 billion, including $841 million for radical prostatectomy and $50 million for orchiectomy. When the costs of treating complications of prostate cancer therapies are also included, estimates are even higher.[31] The substantial financial burden of caring for patients with prostate cancer has been demonstrated in other countries as well.[32,33]

Costs of Screening and Early Detection

One of the most controversial areas of current debate in urology is whether to perform population-based screening for prostate cancer. The rate of prostate cancer diagnosis has increased rapidly during the last several years, largely because of the advent of widespread prostate-specific antigen (PSA) testing and media attention from several celebrated cases. In part because of this publicity, the awareness of prostate cancer in the general public has risen and has led many healthy men to seek prostate evaluation. Early detection of prostate cancer is different from population-based screening. In both, men are evaluated with digital rectal examination (DRE) and measurement of their serum PSA. With regard to early detection, individual patients seek out prostate programs, whereas in population-based screening, public health initiatives are used to seek out patients to be screened. This difference may seem subtle, but from the health policy perspective, the costs of screening entire populations are staggering.[34] The cost for screening in the United States has been projected to reach $5 billion per year in the near future.[35]

The first-year costs of treatment and treatment-related complications in a widespread screening program in the United States are predicted to range from $5.2 billion to $14.1 billion.[36] Indeed, various components of our health care delivery system may be overwhelmed if all asymptomatic cases are identified.[37] Furthermore, no study has ever demonstrated a significant decrease in mortality or morbidity from prostate cancer screening to identify early-stage disease,[38–42] although proponents of screening point to the added value of PSA in improving prostate cancer detection rates.[43,44]

When evaluating various screening approaches, analysts must consider not only the cost of the DRE, phlebotomy, and PSA measurement, but also the cost of transrectal ultrasound, prostate biopsy, specimen processing, and pathologic examination of tissue from all men with screening abnormalities. More detailed analyses also include the cost of treating complications, as well as the opportunity cost of patients' time and the human anxiety costs of false-positive test results. A Swedish analysis of the direct, indirect, and intangible costs of prostate cancer screening in that country suggested that the 2-year financial impact of complete screening would be equivalent to 131 to 174 million U.S. dollars, an enormous amount for a nation with fewer than 2 million men over the age of 40 years.[45]

To perform accurate cost-effectiveness calculations for prostate cancer screening is difficult because of the lack of reliable data showing any definitive decrease in mortality of morbidity from particular tests or procedures. In an elaborately constructed decision model of prostate cancer screening using average and marginal costs, researchers have shown that, although DRE by skilled examiners has the lowest cost of any one screening test, approaches that use both PSA and DRE together are actually less costly than DRE alone.[46] Markov modeling of a hypothetic cohort has confirmed this finding.[47] Transrectal ultrasound has been shown not to be cost-effective as a screening tool.[48,49]

Costs of Staging Evaluation

Once prostate cancer has been diagnosed, the treatment varies depending on the extent of disease. Hence, interest has developed in determining which components of the staging evaluation may be more cost-effective. Since the advent of laparoscopic surgery during the 1980s, many centers have explored the use of laparoscopic pelvic lymphadenectomy for staging in men with newly diagnosed prostate cancer. Direct patient costs in the United States (measured as hospital charges) using this technique have been shown to be similar preoperatively, higher during surgery, and lower postoperatively, compared with open lymph node dissection for men with prostate cancer. In a study of 61 patients, 50 of whom underwent laparoscopic pelvic exploration, total overall expenditures were less by $1345, and LOS was shorter (1.6 days versus 4.4 days) per patient undergoing laparoscopic surgery (Table 15-2).[50] The higher intraoperative charges were attributed to longer operating times and high-priced disposable equipment. Other investigators have shown that, in addition to decreasing LOS, laparoscopic pelvic exploration shortens the total convalescence time from 43 to 5 days.[51] Hence, the opportunity cost is lower.

In another study comparing open pelvic lymphadenectomy, standard laparoscopic pelvic lymphadenectomy, and minilapar-

TABLE 15-2. *Comparison of hospital charges for laparoscopic versus open pelvic lymphadenectomy for men with prostate cancer*

Charge category	Laparoscopic lymphadenectomy ($)	Open lymphadenectomy ($)	*P*-value
Preoperative	532	693	<0.05
Intraoperative	8,075	5,332	<0.05
Postoperative	1,461	2,698	<0.05
Overall	10,068	8,723	<0.05

Adapted from Troxel S, Winfield HN. Comparative financial analysis of laparoscopic versus open pelvic lymph node dissection for men with cancer of the prostate. J Urol 1994;151: 675.

oscopic pelvic lymphadenectomy (performed through a small lower midline incision), total hospital charges were reported to be $3685, $3330, and $1795, respectively. LOS was reported to be 7, 1.25, and 1.3 days, respectively. The investigators proposed that this modification to standard laparoscopy for pelvic lymph node staging could decrease charges by about 50% from the open or standard laparoscopic approaches.[52]

The enthusiasm for laparoscopic lymphadenectomy must be tempered with the understanding that it is most beneficial in men who are expected to have positive lymph nodes, thus saving them an unnecessary open lymphadenectomy. Conversely, men who are expected to have low-stage disease and who plan to return for definitive surgery are subjected to the costs of two surgical procedures that would otherwise have been performed during the same operation.[53]

Because of the high sensitivity of PSA in detecting metastatic disease, radionuclide bone imaging has been targeted as a potential source of cost savings in the staging workup of patients with prostate cancer. Oesterling[54] studied the financial burden of bone scans in 67 patients with biopsy-proven prostate cancer and PSA levels less than 10 ng/mL. The mean charge for both technical and professional components of the scans in the United States was $600. The average total charges for treatment of localized disease were $15,000. False-positive bone scans led to additional mean charges of $455 per patient for unnecessary radiographs and computed tomography (CT) or magnetic resonance imaging scans of the ribs, pelvis, and spine. Using these figures, Oesterling calculated that, by eliminating bone scans from the initial staging workup of all American men with prostate cancer, the United States could have annual direct savings of $39.6 million and an additional $3.6 million from unnecessary tests that follow false-positive scans, for a total of $43.2 million. False-negative scans (thought to occur in 0.5% of patients) would attenuate the savings. Based on this charge data, Oesterling recommended that radionuclide bone scans be dropped from the routine staging evaluation.

In another analysis, Forman and colleagues[55] examined the cost-effectiveness of abdominal-pelvic CT scans for men with prostate cancer. Consensus dictates that CT scans are of no use in the staging of the cancer, but these investigators wondered whether CT identification of comorbid disease would make the test worthwhile from the economic perspective. Among 273 consecutive patients who underwent CT scanning as part of their staging workup, 66 (25%) had findings suggestive of comorbid disease; only 4 (1.5%) had findings that changed the treatment plan (2 large aortic aneurysms, 1 lymphoma, and 1 renal cell carcinoma). These researchers reported that $4400 was spent to investigate false-positive CT findings in their sample, and the mean Medicare reimbursement per CT scan was $586. Hence, because only 1.5% of patients had significant findings, $40,141 was spent for each patient with significant comorbidity. These investigators concluded that CT scanning is not cost-effective in screening for comorbidity in men with newly diagnosed localized prostate cancer.

Costs of Treating Advanced Disease

Several cost analyses have compared the hormonal treatments for advanced prostate cancer, and all conclude that the most cost-effective method is surgical castration (Table 15-3). Although bilateral orchiectomy involves a concentrated set of charges for operating room time, recovery, and fees for the surgeon and anesthesiologist, the procedure is performed only once and does not oblige the patient to costly lifelong pharmacologic treatments. Modern pharmacologic castration resembles an annuity, in which patients return month after month for injections and, for some, daily oral medications. Over the years, the cumulative expenses of these charges typically exceed the one-time charges for surgical castration. Even estrogens, which are relatively inexpensive, although seldom used because of cardiovascular complications, are more expensive over time than orchiectomy.[33]

McClinton and colleagues[56] calculated direct and opportunity costs of orchiectomy versus luteinizing hormone-releasing hormone (LHRH) agonists in the United Kingdom's National Health Service and projected that the cost of surgical castration would be exceeded by the cost of medical castration 4 times over in a single year. Nicol and colleagues[57] examined the same question in Australia but used actual cost data from a patient sample to determine that medical androgen blockade cost 3.9 to 5.7 times more than orchiectomy during the first 2 years. At 5 years, the difference was even more dramatic. In Sweden, Rutqvist and Wilking[58] found that orchiectomy was 7% to 31% less expensive than the cumulative expense of medical androgen blockade. Because these figures were based on average hospital inpatient stays of 7 to 9 days in the mid-1980s, they underestimate the true difference in costs between therapies. After further analysis, these investigators proposed that the least expensive management approach would be to place all patients on monthly LHRH agonists and reserve orchiectomy for those who survived for 2 years. If these guidelines were applied to all men with advanced prostate cancer, aggregate costs would be decreased

TABLE 15-3. *Cost comparison of surgical versus medical castration for men with advance prostate cancer*

Study	Savings from surgical castration (%)
McClinton et al, 1989[56]	75
Nicol et al, 1993[57]	74–82
Rutqvist et al, 1992[58]	7–31

by 26%, compared with initial orchiectomy. Other work has also demonstrated the cost-effectiveness of orchiectomy.[59]

BLADDER CANCER

Costs of Screening and Diagnosis

Because transitional cell carcinoma of the bladder can often be diagnosed with a low-cost urine test, screening for this disease seems appealing. Because of the low prevalence of this disease, however, screening for bladder cancer has been shown not to be cost-effective, even in high-risk populations.[60] Once a tumor has been identified cystoscopically, biopsies performed using topical or injectable local anesthesia have resulted in up to 70% cost savings when compared with biopsies performed with the patient under general or spinal anesthesia.[61,62]

Costs of Superficial Disease

Definitive treatment of superficial tumors with laser ablation may result in further savings when compared with transurethral resection, primarily because of shorter LOS with the laser procedure.[63] Much of the subsequent cost is generated by numerous interval cystoscopies and treatment of recurrences. Various approaches to the long-term management of patients with superficial disease have attempted to achieve cost savings, and this area remains ripe for such efforts.[64]

Costs of Advanced Disease

The treatment of advanced bladder cancer with chemotherapy may generate huge costs in direct patient care, as well as lost wages and lost productivity. One cost model estimates the price to society at $34,000 per year of life saved.[65] Even palliative care can be cost-effective, however, if it reduces or eliminates expenditures that would otherwise be incurred by terminally ill patients.[66]

TESTIS CANCER

Costs of Clinically Localized Disease

After radical orchiectomy and survey of metastases, the standard approach to clinically localized disease in most patients includes retroperitoneal lymphadenectomy for nonseminomas or prophylactic irradiation for seminomas. Exponents of less aggressive management have supported the sole use of frequent radiologic and serologic monitoring. Because the duration of follow-up after treatment is so lengthy, a tremendous cost burden is accumulated over time. Hence, cost analyses may have a huge impact on clinical management. In histologic cell types associated with a low incidence of disease recurrence, such as early clinical stage seminomas, the cost-effectiveness of intensive long-term follow-up may be questioned. In the United Kingdom, investigators estimated the cost of surveillance after treatment to be £150,000 for each case of early seminoma relapse detected. These investigators suggested that intensive surveillance was not justified in these patients. For nonseminomas, however, the relapse rate is high enough that the cost per detected relapse is less, and intensive follow-up is warranted.[67]

The danger of measuring only direct costs and neglecting indirect savings in economic analyses is illustrated by studies that do not account for the future value to society of cured patients' productivity. In Norway, investigators contended simply that because retroperitoneal lymphadenectomy cost twice as much as 1 year of surveillance in men with clinically localized testis tumors, the latter option was preferable. This study overlooked the societal economic value of cured patients, as well as the expense of many subsequent years of follow-up required for patients on surveillance protocols.[68] A definitive cost-benefit study on the management options for clinically localized testis cancer has not yet been performed.

Costs of Advanced Disease

The introduction of platinum-based chemotherapy for men with advanced nonseminomatous testis cancer[69] revolutionized the treatment of this disease and led to dramatic results in both cure rates and cost-effectiveness. A human capital approach has been used to estimate the relevant direct and indirect costs. The national cost increases for providing the chemotherapy are offset by savings from the restored economic productivity of patients successfully treated. Because testis cancer affects young men at the outset of their professional careers, those who are cured typically make a lifetime of contribution back to society. Shibley and colleagues[70] built an economic model using actual data for direct patient care costs and inflation-adjusted estimates for indirect costs or savings from platinum-based combination chemotherapy in the United States. All figures were appropriately discounted to 1987 dollars. These investigators reported that the economic value of the lives saved in that year was approximately $166 million, more than tenfold greater than the $16 million spent that year on treatment. Comparing this net societal benefit with the cumulative $55.7 million spent by the National Cancer Institute to develop this chemotherapeutic regimen, it appears to have been a wise investment.

CONCLUSIONS

Costs for cancer care have escalated rapidly. By the mid-1980s, more than 10% of all health care expenditures in the United States were for caring for patients with malignant diseases.[71] Today, urologic cancers generate even greater expenditures, as the detection rate for prostate cancer continues to rise and care becomes more and more technically sophisticated. The latter part of the twentieth century has required physicians to treat not only individual patients, but also populations with diagnosed and undiagnosed disease. Ultimately, health policy decisions have begun to change clinical approaches to patients with cancer.[72,73] Society will have to set explicit priorities to direct physicians in the equitable distribution of scarce medical resources. This movement further emphasizes the importance of accurately projecting costs in the treatment of genitourinary cancers.

In a comprehensive review of the economics of cancer care,

Smith and colleagues[74] underscored a point that is especially germane when applying cost-effectiveness to urologic oncology. Health care cannot be rationed only by economic benchmarks such as dollars per LY saved, but it must include other valued principles such as compassion, societal equity, justice, and medical ethics.

Physicians treating patients with urologic cancers must also be more attentive to cost-effectiveness and to patient preferences. We cannot look only at 5- or 10-year survival curves. We must base decisions on both clinical effectiveness and cost-effectiveness by examining outcomes such as cost, patient satisfaction, and health-related quality of life. Our challenge now is to determine which cancer therapies achieve the simultaneous goals of high-quality medical care, positive outcomes, and reasonable costs.

REFERENCES

1. Woolhandler S, Himmelstein DU. The deteriorating administrative efficiency of the US health care system. N Engl J Med 1991;324:1253.
2. Young H. Hugh Young: a surgeon's autobiography. New York: Harcourt, Brace, 1940:210.
3. Walsh DC, Connor E, Tracey LV, Goldberg GA, Egdahl RH. Posthospital convalescence and return to work. Health Affairs 1989;8:76.
4. Kahn KL, Rubenstein LV, Draper D, et al. The effects of the DRG-based prospective payment system on quality of care for hospitalized Medicare patients. JAMA 1990;264:1953.
5. Kassirer JP, Angell M. The Journal's policy on cost-effectiveness analysis. N Engl J Med 1994;331:669.
6. Eddy DM. Cost-effectiveness analysis: is it up to the task? JAMA 1992; 267:3342.
7. Weinstein MC, Stason WB. Foundations of cost-effectiveness analysis for health and medical practices. N Engl J Med 1977;296:716.
8. Shepard DS, Thompson MS. First principles of cost-effectiveness analysis in health. Public Health Rep 1979;94:535.
9. Smith TJ, Hillner BE, Desch CE. Efficacy and cost-effectiveness of cancer treatment: rational allocation of resources based on decision analysis. J Natl Cancer Inst 1993;85:1460.
10. Bennett CL, Greenfield S, Aronow H, Ganz P, Vogelzang NJ, Elashoff RM. Patterns of care related to age of men with prostate cancer. Cancer 1991;67:2633.
11. Gaddipatti J, Ahmed T, Friedland M. Prostate and bladder cancer in the elderly. Clin Geriatr Med 1987;3:649.
12. Wennberg JE, Gittelsohn A. Variations in medical care among small areas. Sci Am 1982;246:100.
13. Wennberg JE, Freeman JL, Culp WJ. Are hospital services rationed in New Haven or over-utilised in Boston? Lancet 1987;1:1185.
14. Morgan M, Beech R. Variations in lengths of stay and rates of day case surgery: implications for the efficiency of surgical management. J Epidemiol Community Health 1990;44:90.
15. Sage WM, Kessler R, Sommers LS, Silverman JF. Physician-generated cost containment in transurethral prostatectomy. J Urol 1988;140:311.
16. Cleary PD, Greenfield S, Mulley AG, et al. Variations in length of stay and outcomes for six medical and surgical conditions in Massachusetts and California. JAMA 1991;266:73.
17. Hall RC. Short surgical stay: two hospital days for cholecystectomy. Am J Surg 1987;154:510.
18. Reder VA, Fineberg HV, Rosoff C, White LS. Shorter length of stay for simple cholecystectomy: cost-effectiveness or alternative strategies. Med Care 1983;21:754.
19. Cannon SR, Ralphs DN, Bolton JP, Wood JJ, Allen A. Early discharge following hernia repair in unselected patients. Br J Surg 1982;69:112.
20. Cuckow PM. Cost of urology: financial audit in a clinical department. Br Med J 1992;305:743.
21. Forrest JB, Ritchie WP Jr, Hudson M, Harlan JF Jr. Cost containment through cost awareness: a strategy that failed. Surgery 1981;90:154.
22. Carter GM, Melnick GA. How services and costs vary by day of stay for Medicare hospital stays. Santa Monica, CA: RAND Corporation, 1990.
23. Maynard A. Economic aspects of cancer care. Eur J Cancer 1993; 29A(Suppl):S6.
24. Luft HS. Assessing the evidence on HMO performance. Milbank Q 1980;58:501.
25. Enthoven AC. The RAND experiment and economical health care. N Engl J Med 1984;310:1528.
26. Gaus CR, Cooper BS, Hirshman CG. Contrasts in HMO and fee-for-service performance. Soc Secur Bull 1976;39:3.
27. Greenwald HP. HMO membership, copayment, and initiation of care for cancer: a study of working adults. Am J Public Health 1987;77: 461.
28. Greenwald HP, Henke CJ. HMO membership, treatment, and mortality risk among prostatic cancer patients. Am J Public Health 1992;82:1099.
29. Litwin MS, Kahn KL, Reccius N. Why do sicker patients cost more? A charge-based analysis of patients undergoing prostatectomy. J Urol 1993;149:84.
30. Schwartz WB, Mendelson DN. Hospital cost containment in the 1980s: hard lessons learned and prospects for the 1990s. N Engl J Med 1991; 324:1037.
31. Optenberg SA, Thompson IM. Economics of screening for carcinoma of the prostate. Urol Clin North Am 1990;17:719.
32. Carlsson P, Hjertberg H, Jonsson B, Varenhorst E. The cost of prostatic cancer in a defined population. Scand J Urol Nephrol 1989;23:93.
33. Henriksson P, Edhag O. Cost-effectiveness comparison of estrogen therapy and orchidectomy in patients with prostatic cancer. Int J Technol Assess Health Care 1987;3:523.
34. Schwartz MK. Screening for cancer: is it cost effective? Clin Chem 1993;39:2397.
35. Goluboff ET, Olsson CA. Urologists on a tightrope: coping with a changing economy. J Urol 1994;151:1.
36. Kramer BS, Brown ML, Prorok PC, Potosky AL, Gohagan JK. Prostate cancer screening: what we know and what we need to know. Ann Intern Med 1993;119:914.
37. Handley MR, Stuart ME. Use of prostate specific antigen for prostate cancer screening: managed care perspective. J Urol 1994;152:1689.
38. Feightner JW. Early detection and treatment of prostate cancer: perspective of Canadian Task Force on Periodic Health Examination. J Urol 1994;152:1682.
39. Woolf SH. Public health perspective: health policy implications of screening for prostate cancer. J Urol 1994;152:1685.
40. Wasson JH, Cushman CC, Bruskewitz RC, Littenberg B, Mulley AG, Wennberg JE. A structured literature review of treatment for localized prostate cancer. Arch Fam Med 1993;2:487.
41. Garnick MB. Prostate cancer: screening, diagnosis and management. Ann Intern Med 1993;118:804.
42. Chodak GW, Keller P, Schoenberg HW. Assessment of screening for prostate cancer using the digital rectal examination. J Urol 1989;141: 1136.
43. Catalona WJ, Smith PS, Ratliff TC, et al. Measurement of propstate-specific antigen in serum as a screening test for prostate cancer. N Engl J Med 1991;324:1156.
44. Lange P. The next era for prostate cancer: controlled clinical trials. JAMA 1993;269:95.
45. Carlsson P, Pedersen KV, Varenhorst E. Costs and benefits of early detection of prostatic cancer. Health Policy 1990;16:241.
46. Littrup PJ, Goodman AC, Mettlin CJ. The benefit and cost of prostate cancer early detection. CA Cancer J Clin 1993;43:134.
47. Simpson KN, Brown RE. Cost effectiveness of adding prostate specific antigen (PSA) test to digital rectal examination (DRE) for early detection of prostate cancer. J Urol 1993;149:413A.
48. Chang P, Friedland GW. The role of imaging in screening for prostate cancer: a decision analysis perspective. Invest Radiol 1990;25:591.
49. Mettlin C. The status of prostate cancer early detection. Cancer 1993; 72(Suppl):1050.
50. Troxel S, Winfield HN. Comparative financial analysis of laparoscopic versus open pelvic lymph node dissection for men with cancer of the prostate. J Urol 1994;151:675.
51. Kerbl K, Clayman RV, Petros JA, Chandhoke PS, Gill IS. Staging pelvic lymphadenectomy for prostate cancer: a comparison of laparoscopic and open techniques. J Urol 1993;150:396.
52. Perrotti M, Gentle D, Kaufman RP. Mini lap pelvic lymph node dissection (MLPLND) minimizes morbidity, costs and hospitalization of pelvic lymph node dissection (PLND). J Urol 1994;151:498A.
53. deKernion JB. J Urol 1993;150:399. Editorial.

54. Oesterling J. Using PSA to eliminate staging radionuclide bone scan: significant economic implications. Urol Clin North Am 1993;20:705.
55. Forman HP, Heiken JP, Brink JA, Glazer HS, Fox LA, McClennan BL. CT screening for comorbid disease in patients with prostatic carcinoma: is it cost-effective? AJR Am J Roentgenol 1993;162:1125.
56. McClinton S, Moffat LEF, Ludbrook A. The cost of bilateral orchiectomy as a treatment for prostatic carcinoma. Br J Urol 1989;63:309.
57. Nicol DL, Heathcote PS, Kateley GD, Lloyd S. Advanced prostate cancer: the role of high priced hormone therapy. Med J Aust 1993; 159:16.
58. Rutqvist LE, Wilking N. Analogues of LHRH versus orchidectomy: comparison of economic costs for castration in advanced prostate cancer. Br J Cancer 1992;65:927.
59. Johansen TEB, Fjaere HTF. Hospitalisation of prostatic cancer patients undergoing orchiectomy. Br J Urol 1991;68:62.
60. Hulka BS. Principles of bladder cancer screening in an interventional trial. J Occup Med 1990;32:812.
61. Holmang S, Aldenborg F, Hedelin H. Multiple bladder biopsies under intravesical lignocaine anesthesia. Br J Urol 1994;73:160.
62. Orandi A. Urological endoscopic surgery under local anesthesia: a cost-reducing idea. J Urol 1984;132:1146.
63. Cost analysis of neodymium-YAG laser versus transurethral resection treatment of superficial bladder carcinoma. Int Surg 1993;78:350.
64. Hall RR, Parmar MKB, Richards AB, Smith PH. Proposal for changes in cystoscopic follow up of patients with bladder cancer and adjuvant intravesical chemotherapy. Br Med J 1994;308:257.
65. Rees GJG. Cost-effectiveness in oncology. Lancet 1985;2:1405.
66. Jaakkimainen L, Goodwin PJ, Pater J, et al. Counting the costs of chemotherapy in a National Cancer Institute of Canada randomized trial of non–small cell lung cancer. J Clin Oncol 1990;8:1301.
67. Ellis M, Hartley L, Sikora K. Value of follow-up in testicular cancer. Br Med J 1984;289:1423.
68. Aass N, Fossa SD, Ous S, et al. Is routine primary retroperitoneal lymph node dissection still justified in patients with low stage non-seminomatous testicular cancer? Br J Urol 1990;65:385.
69. Einhorn LH, Donohue J. cis-Diamminedichloroplatinum, vinblastine, and bleomycin combination chemotherapy in disseminated testicular cancer. Ann Intern Med 1977;87:293.
70. Shibley L, Brown M, Schuttinga J, Rothenberg M, Whalen J. Cisplatin-based combination chemotherapy in the treatment of advanced-stage testicular cancer: cost-benefit analysis. J Natl Cancer Inst 1990;82:186.
71. Rice DP, Hodgson TA, Capell F. The economic burden of cancer, 1985; United States and California. In: Scheffler RM, Andrews NC, eds. Cancer care and cost: DRGs and beyond. Ann Arbor, MI: Health Administration Press, 1989.
72. Hadorn DC. Setting health care priorities in Oregon: cost-effectiveness meets the rule of rescue. JAMA 1991;265:2218.
73. Daniels D. Is the Oregon rationing plan fair? JAMA 1991;265:2232.
74. Smith TJ, Hillner BE, Desch CE. Efficacy and cost-effectiveness of cancer treatment: rational allocation of resources based on decision analysis. J Natl Cancer Inst 1993;85:1460.

SECTION II

Bladder Cancer

Principles and Practice of Genitourinary Oncology, edited by Derek Raghavan, Howard I. Scher, Steven A. Leibel, and Paul H. Lange. Lippincott-Raven Publishers, Philadelphia, © 1997.

CHAPTER 16

Surgical Anatomy of the Bladder

Michael L. Cher and Peter R. Carroll

The bladder is a hollow muscular organ with two primary functions. The first is to serve as a storage reservoir for urine. The second is to expel urine in an effective manner when socially convenient. These functions must be carried out in a manner that protects the upper urinary tract from damage that may occur due to high pressure or infection.

In adults, the empty bladder lies in the pelvis behind the pubic symphysis; in children, it occupies a higher, more abdominal position. When the bladder is full, it extends well above the pubic symphysis and can be palpated through the anterior abdominal wall. The bladder has a main body leading inferiorly to a cone-shaped bladder neck and urethra. On the posterior floor of the bladder is a triangular structure, the trigone, which receives the ureters. The left and right ureters enter the bladder posteriorly in an oblique manner at each ureteral hiatus. The ureters traverse the bladder wall and open into the bladder lumen at the two superior corners of the trigone. The ureteral orifices are approximately 2.5 cm from each other and are separated by a crescent-shaped interureteric ridge. The distal or caudal end of the trigone leads into the bladder neck and urethra. Although the bladder neck is often called the internal sphincter, it is not a true voluntary sphincter. Rather, it consists of a thickening of smooth muscle arranged in a cone shape leading to the smooth muscle of the urethra.

The bladder is lined with a transitional epithelium several layers thick. This epithelium is not a true mucosa in that it has no or limited secretory function. The epithelium consists of 3 to 7 layers of transitional cells resting on a basement membrane composed of extracellular matrix (collagen and adhesive glycoproteins). The basal epithelium is composed of actively proliferating cells. Luminal cells are larger, umbrella-like cells bound together by tight junctions. The urothelial surface is covered by sulfated polysaccharides (glycosaminoglycans). The surface glycosaminoglycans are a permeability barrier and prevent attachment or absorption of bacteria, proteins, and ions.[1] Permeability is also ensured by the presence of the luminal tight junctions. The bladder is capable of some ion exchange, however. Although the physiologic role of this process is unknown, ion exhange may allow for epithelial cell volume regulation during distention, or it may help to maintain a hypertonic urine.[2] Underlying the epithelium is a layer of loose connective and elastic tissue called the lamina propria. With the bladder is filling, the epithelium and lamina propria become thin and flattened, allowing a tremendous expansion in the capacity of the bladder lumen. This arrangement holds true for all the bladder, except for the trigone, where the epithelium is firmly adherent to the underlying musculature.

The muscular layer of the bladder wall, the detrusor, consists of smooth muscle fibers arranged in bundles. The detrusor is responsible for increasing intraluminal pressure during voiding. The muscle bundles of the detrusor are arranged in an seemingly random, interlacing weave-like pattern, except at the bladder neck, where three distinct layers can be discerned: inner and outer longitudinally oriented layers and a middle circularly oriented layer.

ANATOMIC RELATIONS

When empty, the bladder is described as having an apex, superior surface, left and right anterolateral surfaces, base, and neck. (Fig. 16-1) The base of the bladder remains fixed during filling. When distended, the superior and lateral walls become spheric; the bladder fills up the pelvis and extends cranially into the abdomen. The apex is the most superior and anterior portion of the bladder. It is the site of the urachus, which is the fetal connection between the urogenital sinus and the allantois.

Anterolaterally is the retropubic space (containing fat and a venous plexus), the transversalis or endopelvic fascia, the levator ani and obturator internus fascia and muscles, and the bones of the pelvis. Lateral to the bladder is the obturator nerve, the superior vesical, obturator, inferior vesical, and prostatic arteries, and the medial umbilical ligaments (obliterated umbilical arteries). The medial umbilical ligaments are branches of the superior vesical arteries.

The superior surface of the bladder is covered by peritoneum and is in close proximity to the ileum and sigmoid colon in the male and the uterus and ileum in the female. As the bladder fills, the superior portion rises to appose the inner surface of the anterior abdominal wall. The peritoneal reflection is more posterior and is called the vesicorectal pouch in the male and the uterovesical pouch in the female. The depth of this pouch increases with filling of the bladder. Posteriorly is the bladder base; it is in relation to the ampullae of the vasa deferentia,

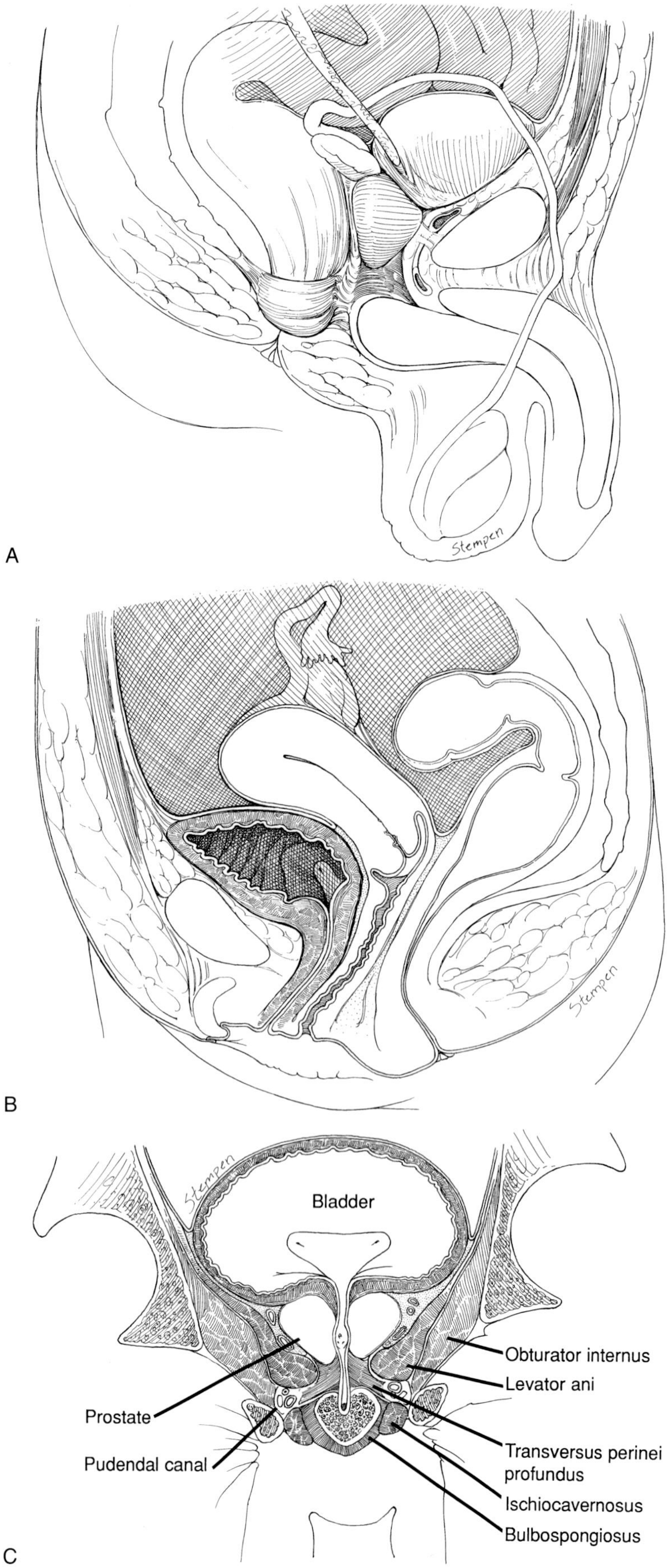

FIG. 16-1. Relationship of the bladder with adjacent structures. (**A**) Lateral view of the male pelvis with the major pelvic viscera shown intact (not sectioned). (**B**) Sagittal section of the female pelvis. (**C**) Coronal view through the male bladder and prostate. *(continued)*

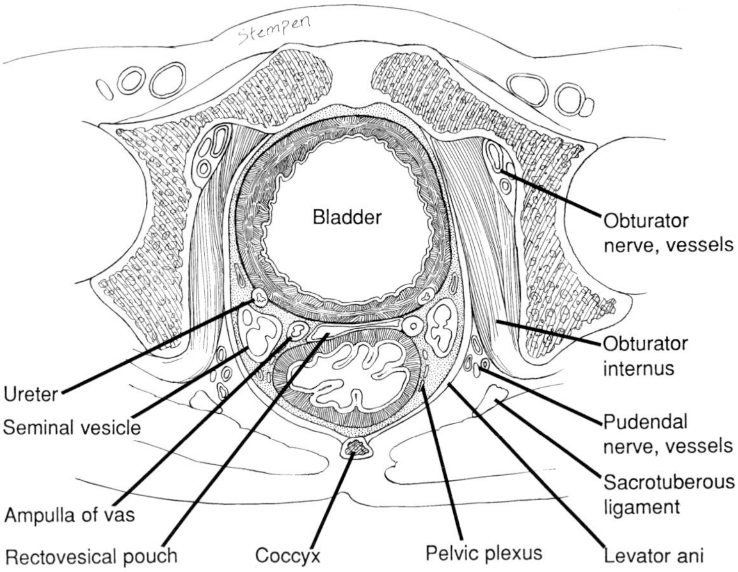

FIG. 16-1. *Continued* (**D**) Transverse section of a male pelvis.

seminal vesicles, ureters, and rectum in the male and the cervix and anterior vaginal wall in female.

In the male, the bladder base and prostate are separated from the anterior wall of the rectum by the layers of Denonvilliers' fascia. Controversy exists over whether this fascia consists of one or two layers.[3] This fascia extends from the vesicorectal pouch to the pelvic floor. Denonvilliers' fascia is thin and collagenous, with variable amounts of smooth muscle.[4] It surrounds the seminal vesicles anteriorly and posteriorly. Medially, Denonvilliers' fascia appears to fuse with the posterior capsule of the prostate. The fascia continues to the prostatic apex, where it thickens and terminates among fibers of the external striated sphincter.

In the male, the bladder neck leads to the prostate, which is supported by the puboprostatic ligaments and the funnel-shaped musculature of the pelvic floor. In the female, the bladder neck rests directly against the pelvic floor. The female urethra is inferior to the bladder, traversing the pelvic floor in a plane parallel to the vagina. The urethra and vagina share a common wall. Additionally, approximately 3.5 cm of the bladder base shares a common wall with the vagina. The posterior wall of the bladder is adjacent to the cervix. Between the bladder and the female genital organs is the vesicocervical and vesicovaginal space, which is filled with loose areolar tissue and connective tissue. This space is easily entered; it contains the pubocervical fascia, often mobilized in vaginal surgery.

URETEROVESICAL JUNCTION AND TRIGONE AND BLADDER NECK

The ureterovesical junction, trigone, and bladder neck are often considered anatomically and functionally distinct. These structures are in fact composed of several continuous layers of tissue that extend from one anatomic structure to the next, however.[5,6] These layers can be conceptualized as changing their shape from tubular in the ureter, to flat in the trigone, and back to tubular again at the bladder neck (Fig. 16-2). The innermost layer is the mucosa, which consists of a transitional epithelium and a lamina propria. External to the mucosa is a layer of smooth muscle. In the ureter, this layer is arranged in a helical fashion that propels boluses of urine toward the bladder in a peristaltic fashion. At the level of the intravesical ureter, the muscle fibers in this layer change from helical to longitudinal orientation. Thus, contraction of these fibers allows shortening

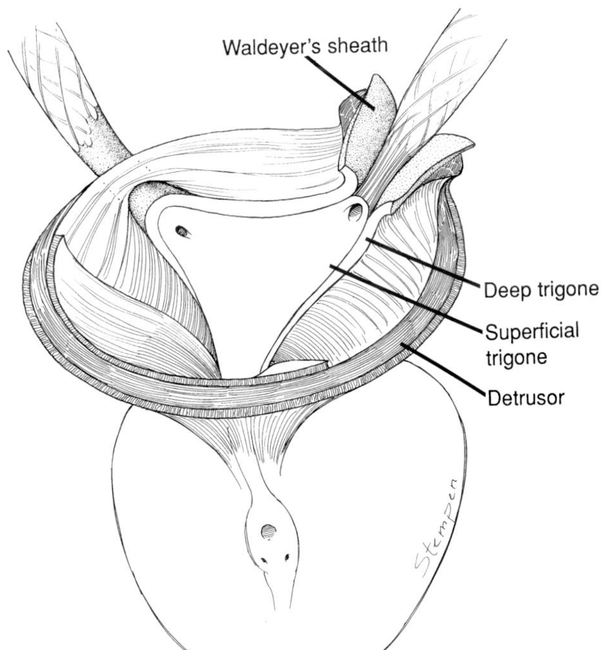

FIG. 16-2. Layers of ureterovesical junction and bladder neck.

of the ureter within the bladder wall. At the distal end of the intramural ureter, this layer of muscle fibers continues over and around the edges of the ureteral orifice and becomes the flat, relatively thin muscle of the superficial trigone. Contraction of this segment of the smooth muscle layer during voiding helps to lengthen the intramural ureter (to prevent vesicoureteral reflux) and to open the bladder neck (to allow egress of urine). The superficial trigone extends into the urethra and terminates at the verumontanum in the male (fusing with the muscle of the ejaculatory ducts) or the external meatus in the female.

Exterior to the longitudinal muscle of the ureter is a fibromuscular layer called Waldeyer's sheath. Proximally, Waldeyer's sheath is fused with the longitudinal muscle layer of the ureter, thus providing the ureter's most proximal point of fixation to the bladder. During contraction of the ureter or trigone, the intramural ureter slides within Waldeyer's sheath. At the level of the ureteral orifice, Waldeyer's sheath fans out, changes from tubular to flat, and becomes the deep trigone. The deep trigone ends as a fibrous ring at the level of the internal meatus. The deep trigone is firmly fixed to the underlying circular smooth muscle of the detrusor, which itself is backed up by a longitudinal layer. The trigone and bladder base are thus the least distensible, most fixed, and strongest parts of the bladder.

External to the trigone is the detrusor muscle. At the level of the bladder neck, the detrusor forms three distinct layers. An inner longitudinal layer extends into the urethra. A middle layer composed of circular or oblique bundles encircles the trigone and bladder neck and fuses with the deep trigone. These circular fibers do not extend into the urethra. An outer longitudinal coat sends bundles that fuse with the apex of the trigone at the internal meatus. This layer also fuses with the prostatic musculature in the male and with the vesicovaginal septum in the female. Some bundles from this layer wrap around the urethra like a sling from both ventral and dorsal sides.

FEMALE URETHRA

The vesicourethral junction lies directly behind the pubic symphysis. The adult female urethra is 4 cm in length and 6 mm in diameter and is embedded in the anterior wall of the vagina.[7,8] The innermost layer of the urethra is the epithelium. During bladder filling, the urethral walls are apposed, with the epithelium thrown into longitudinal folds. Exterior to the mucosa is the muscular wall of the urethra consisting of smooth muscle fibers embedded in collagen and elastic tissue. The muscular wall is composed of inner and outer layers. These smooth muscle layers extend throughout the entire length of the urethra. The inner layer is longitudinal; the outer layer is circular, but its extent and functional contribution to continence have been debated. The striated or skeletal component of the urethra consists of two distinct components: the intrinsic or intramural component, and the extrinsic or extramural pelvic floor component. The intrinsic component refers to skeletal muscle fibers surrounding the urethra proximal to the pelvic floor; this layer is thickest in the middle third of the female urethra but is deficient in the midline posteriorly. These striated muscle fibers are oriented obliquely with respect to the urethra and intermingle freely with the outer circular layer of smooth muscle. Distally, the intrinsic component of the striated sphincter ends at the level of the pelvic floor. The extrinsic or extramural portion of the external sphincter consists of a bulky circular muscle located in the same horizontal plane as the levator ani. The most external fibers of the extrinsic striated sphincter are contiguous with the levator ani.

MALE URETHRA

The posterior and membranous portions of the male urethra are composed of layers similar to those described for the female urethra. The preprostatic urethra is 1 to 1.5 cm in length.[7] It consists of an inner epithelium surrounded by layers of smooth muscle embedded within a collagen and elastic matrix. The smooth muscle consists of an inner longitudinal and outer circular layer. The outer circular layer of muscle fuses with the prostatic capsule. The prostatic urethra is 3 to 4 cm in length and contains both longitudinal and circular smooth muscle fibers. The smooth muscle fibers of the urethra interdigitate with the smooth muscle fibers of the prostate. The apex of the prostate sits directly on the pelvic floor, although a 1- to 1.5-cm segment of the urethra between the prostate and the pelvic diaphragm can be demonstrated after complete prostatic mobilization, as in radical prostatectomy. The membranous urethra (from the apex of the prostate to the bulb of the penis) is 2.5 to 3.0 cm long. Some longitudinal and circular smooth muscle fibers continue throughout the membranous urethra and fuse with the urethra at the level of the penile bulb. The intrinsic striated skeletal component of the urethra is circular and extends from the verumontanum to the pelvic floor. As in the female, the distal end of the intrinsic component is contiguous with the circular muscle bulk of the extrinsic or extramural striated component. This skeletal muscle lies within the pelvic floor, and its outer fibers are contiguous with the levator ani. Oelrich and Myers and associates have shown that the final configuration of the external sphincter is not ring-shaped and depends partly on upward growth of the developing prostate. The shape of the prostate also influences the final configuration of this sphincter.[9,10] The anterior urethra, from the pelvic floor to the urethral meatus, functions only as a conduit and has no bearing on continence.

URETHRAL SPHINCTER AND PELVIC FLOOR

The smooth sphincter (internal sphincter) consists of the smooth muscle of the bladder neck and urethra. As described previously, it is not a true anatomic sphincter; however, the smooth muscle fibers are arranged so to create a resting pressure that remains higher than the intraluminal pressure of the bladder during filling. This pressure depends on continuous tone provided by elastic fibers, as well as by active contraction of smooth muscle fibers. The smooth sphincter thus maintains continence during bladder filling.

The striated sphincter (external sphincter), consisting of both intrinsic and extrinsic components, is a true anatomic sphincter. The striated sphincter may not be necessary for continence when a normally functioning internal sphincter is present. The striated sphincter may be recruited during sudden rises of intra-abdominal pressure, however, and when voiding must be delayed despite a full bladder.

The pelvic organs are separated from the musculature of the

pelvic floor by the endopelvic fascia. The pelvic floor musculature consists of the levator ani, the coccygeus, the obturatorius internus, and the piriformis. The levator ani components are situated external to the endopelvic fascia and insert into the tendinous arc of the pelvis. The levator ani can be divided into two portions. The first is the pubococcygeus muscle, the more medial part of the levator ani; it surrounds the rectum and urethra, as well as the vagina in the female. Anteriorly, its insertion is into the inner aspect of the pubis. Posteriorly, it inserts into the sacrum, coccyx, and anococcygeal raphe. The second, more lateral part of the levator ani, is the iliococcygeus. It originates from the tendinous arc of the pelvis, sweeps upward posteromedially, and also inserts into the sacrum, coccyx, and anococcygeal raphe. The coccygeus muscle is a triangular muscle at the same level as the levator ani but is more posterior. It originates from the ischial spine and inserts into the sacrum and coccyx. The obturatorius internus and piriformis muscles are external to the levator ani. They are more correctly considered the lateral and posterior walls of the pelvis rather than the pelvic floor.

LIGAMENTS AND BLOOD SUPPLY

The ligaments and arterial blood supply to the bladder can be considered together because the latter is contained within the former. The ligaments of the bladder include the lateral and posterior vesical ligaments, the urachus or median umbilical ligament, the medial umbilical ligament (obliterated umbilical arteries), and the puboprostatic or pubovesical ligaments.

The bladder has a dual arterial supply defined by two pedicles, the lateral and posterior vesical ligaments (Fig. 16-3). The first source, the superior vesical artery, is a branch of the internal iliac artery and is contained within the lateral vesical pedicle. It supplies the bladder body and bladder neck. Branches of the superior vesical artery include the vesiculodeferential artery in the male, supplying the ampullae of the vas and seminal vesicles, and the uterine artery in the female. The distal ureter also receives small branches from this arterial tree. Another branch of the superior vesical or internal iliac artery is the obliterated umbilical artery. This artery courses around the anterolateral surface of the bladder toward the umbilicus and becomes the medial umbilical ligament after birth.

The second arterial supply is the inferior vesical artery, which courses to the bladder through the inferior vesical pedicle. This artery may be a branch of the internal iliac, internal pudendal, or inferior gluteal artery. The inferior vesical artery, together with smaller branches from the obturator artery, supplies the bladder base, proximal urethra, and prostate. The inferior vesical artery is also the source of the middle rectal (hemorrhoidal) artery. In the female, the uterine and vaginal arteries also provide some supply to the bladder base.

The urachus extends from the apex of the bladder to the umbilicus. After birth, the urachal remnant becomes the median umbilical ligament; it is a potential space lined with transitional or cuboidal epithelium and extends to the umbilicus between the peritoneum and the transversalis fascia.

The puboprostatic ligaments in the male and the pubovesical ligaments in the female consist of condensations of retroperitoneal connective tissue that anchor the prostate or bladder neck anteriorly to the pubis. The venous blood from the bladder collects in a rich venous plexus between the muscular wall of

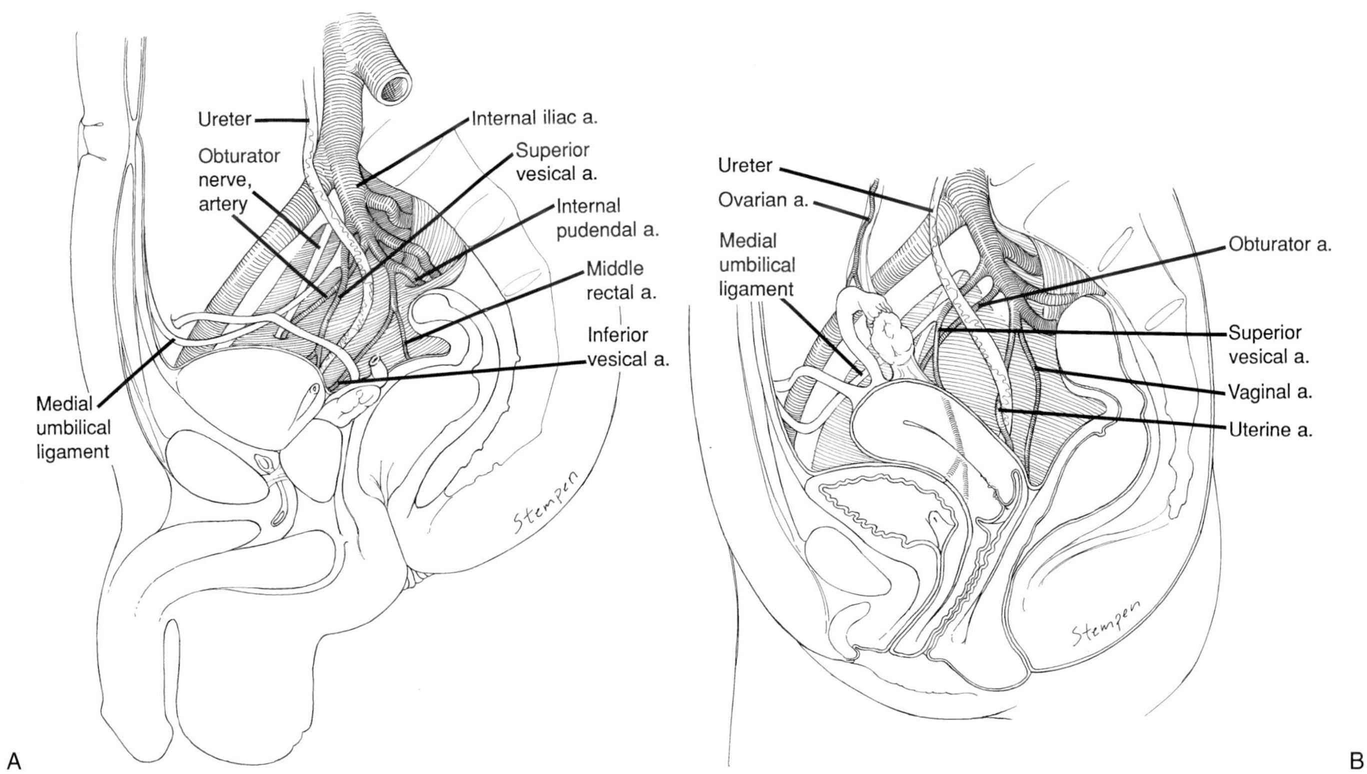

FIG. 16-3. Arterial supply of the bladder: (**A**) male; (**B**) female.

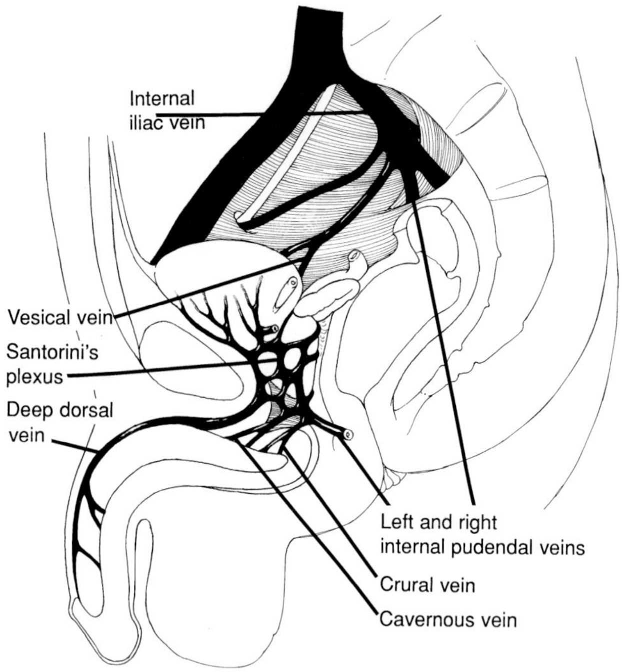

FIG. 16-4. Venous anatomy of the bladder (male).

bladder and the adventitia (Fig. 16-4). Anteriorly, this is called the retropubic venous plexus (of Santorini), and it receives contributions from the deep dorsal vein of the penis and the cavernous vein. Venous blood eventually leaves the pelvis through the internal iliac vein.

LYMPHATIC SUPPLY

Numerous anastomosing lymph channels drain the prostate and the bladder neck, base, and body. A rich lymphatic network within the bladder wall collects lymph from the mucosa. These vessels drain into larger channels in the adventitia. Small lymph nodes are often present within the adventitia of the bladder. Ultimately, these lymphatic channels lead to the obturator, internal iliac, and external iliac lymph nodes. Lymphatic metastases from transitional cell carcinoma of the bladder spread most commonly to the obturator and external iliac lymph nodes. Common iliac nodes can become involved subsequently.[11] Pelvic cancers may involve internal iliac, common iliac, sacral, and hemorrhoidal lymph nodes as well.

NERVE SUPPLY

The nerve supply to the bladder is depicted in Figure 16-5. A widening in the lower spinal cord in the lumbar region is called the lumbar intumescence. The lower half of this widening is at the T11-L1 vertebral level and contains the micturition center. This region contains the origins of nerve levels S2-S4. Trauma to this level of the spinal cord most often causes a flaccid neurogenic bladder. Trauma to higher levels tends to produce a spastic neurogenic bladder; however, mixed patterns of flaccidity and spasticity are common results of incomplete and complex lesions.

Motor innervation to the detrusor muscle is predominately parasympathetic. Parasympathetic nerves originate at sacral levels S2-S4 and travel as pelvic (splanchnic) nerves through the inferior hypogastric (pelvic) plexus and vesical plexus; then

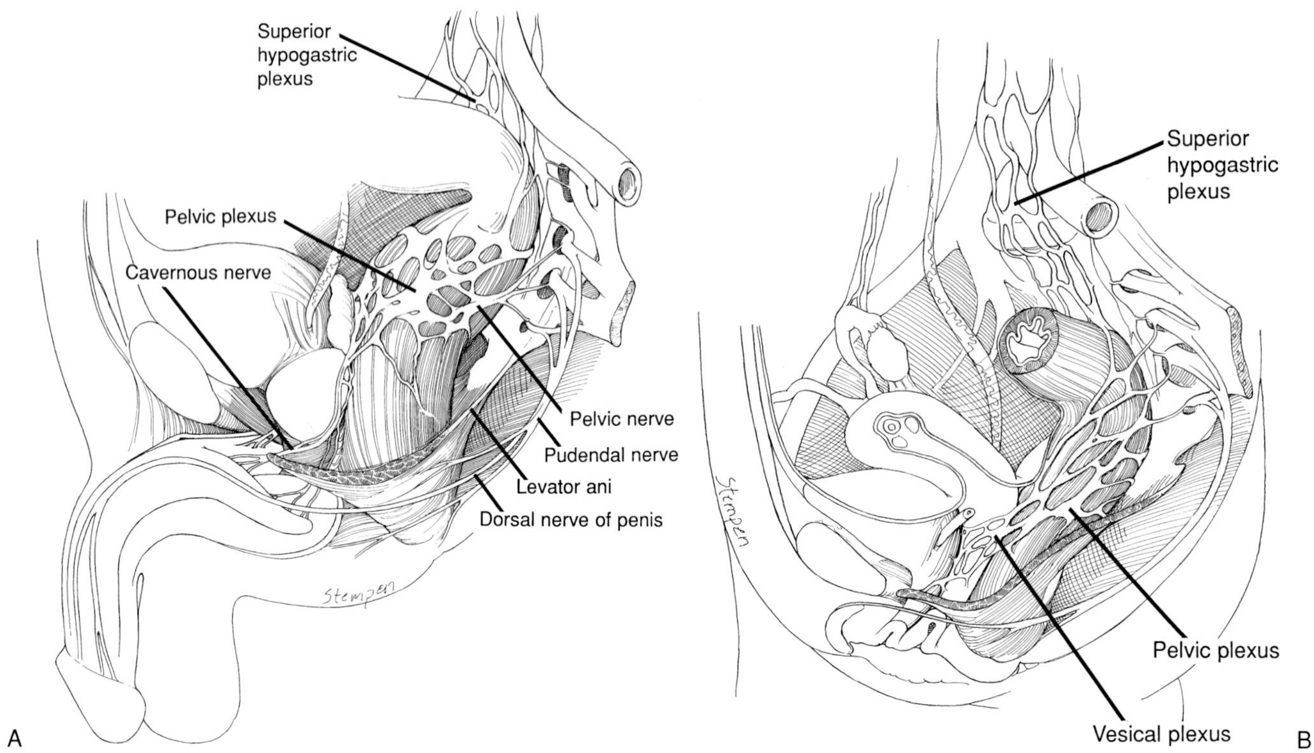

FIG. 16-5. Nerve supply to the bladder: (**A**) male; (**B**) female.

they penetrate the substance of the detrusor. Short postganglionic nerves originate at ganglia within the detrusor to innervate detrusor muscle fibers.

Motor innervation to the trigone and bladder neck is predominately sympathetic. Sympathetic nerves to the bladder begin as preganglionic fibers originating at the T11-L2 spinal level. Sympathetic fibers emerging from the spinal cord pass through the sympathetic trunk and into the superior hypogastric plexus, which is located anterior and inferior to the bifurcation of the aorta. From this point, the preganglionic fibers continue as the hypogastric nerve emerging around the side of the proximal rectum to the inferior hypogastric (pelvic) plexus, located posterolateral to the rectum and just cephalad and posterior to the tips of the seminal vesicles. After synapse, postganglionic sympathetic fibers travel through the adjacent vesical and prostatic plexus (posterolateral to the bladder and lateral to the rectum) to innervate the bladder neck, prostate, and urethra. The cavernous nerves, which supply the penis or clitoris, emerge from the prostatic or vesical plexus (lateral to the rectum) and course anteriorly and inferiorly, adjacent to the lateral surface of the prostate or vesical neck. In the male, this neurovascular bundle is found within the fascial covering of the prostate, where it can be identified and spared during nerve-sparing surgical procedures.[12]

The seminal vesicles, ampullae of the vas, and vas deferens also receive a rich sympathetic supply. Therefore, damage to the sympathetic fibers supplying the pelvic organs may result in failure of seminal emission or retrograde ejaculation because of failure of the bladder neck to close.

The striated muscle of the external sphincter and pelvic floor is supplied largely by motor nerves originating within the nucleus of Onuf (pudendal nucleus) of the spinal cord. These fibers leave the cord as spinal nerves S2-S4. These fibers coalesce into the pudendal nerve, exiting the pelvis through the pudendal (Alcock's) canal.

Sensory nerve endings in the detrusor muscle cannot distinguish well among pain, temperature, touch, and stretch. Afferents from the detrusor wall travel within the pelvic nerve and through sacral roots to many levels of the spinal cord. Afferents from the bladder neck and trigone travel to the cord through the sympathetic trunk to spinal cord segments T11-L2. Important reflex pathways involve higher centers within the central nervous system.

PHYSIOLOGY

In its function as a reservoir, the bladder must be able to distend to a capacity of 400 to 500 mL. To protect the upper urinary tract, this distention must be accomplished without a significant increase in intraluminal pressure. At or near capacity, afferent nerves provide a sensation of fullness. The detrusor muscle must then be able to sustain a contraction to empty the bladder completely. Normal sphincteric function allows this to occur in a voluntary fashion, so voiding can be delayed until socially convenient.

The sphincteric mechanism consists of two principal components: an involuntary smooth muscle sphincter at the bladder neck and a voluntary striated sphincter located along the urethra. The muscles of the pelvic floor contribute directly to the striated sphincteric function by virtue of their location adjacent to the urethra. The pelvic floor also contributes indirectly by supporting and maintaining the bladder base and proximal urethra in their normal intraabdominal position. The sphincteric components and the detrusor must be well coordinated to maintain a normal, healthy urinary tract. During filling, inhibitory pathways predominate throughout the detrusor muscle and maintain it in a relaxed state. At the same time, the internal sphincteric mechanism at the bladder neck remains closed. The striated sphincter maintains a constant tone but can be tightened in a voluntary manner during sudden increases in intraabdominal pressure or to suppress the urge to void.

During micturition, voluntary relaxation of the striated sphincter and pelvic floor musculature is coordinated with contraction of the detrusor. The bladder neck is thought to be pulled open as a result of the anatomic arrangement of the smooth muscle bundles in the detrusor and bladder neck. The bladder neck region must also be coordinated with seminal emission. Just before ejaculation, the bladder neck contracts actively to allow for normal antegrade ejaculation.

During infancy and early childhood, a reflex arc to the spinal cord governs the coordination of the sphincteric and detrusor components during filling and emptying. The bladder is considered to behave in an uninhibited fashion such that reflexive emptying occurs when capacity is reached. As the child matures, higher centers become involved in inhibiting the detrusor reflex pathway, so voiding occurs voluntarily.

The function of the ureterovesical junction is to prevent the transmission of high pressure to the upper urinary tract. This is accomplished by allowing free flow of urine into the bladder and by preventing reflux back up into the kidney. During passage of a bolus of urine into the bladder, the longitudinal muscle of the intramural ureter contracts, allowing the ureter to slide and shorten within Waldeyer's sheath. As the bladder fills, the trigone becomes stretched, and the result is an occlusive effect on the intramural ureter. During voiding, the muscle of the trigone participates in the contraction along with the rest of the trigone. Vesicoureteral reflux is prevented by the stretching and elongation of the ureter within the bladder wall.

SURGICAL RELEVANCE

Operations on the bladder are described more fully elswhere; however; some key principles of surgical technique are discussed here with reference to the anatomy of the bladder.

Radical Cystectomy

One of the first steps of cystectomy is ligation of the arterial supply within the lateral vesical pedicle. This ligation is accomplished by exposing the common and internal iliac artery and then dividing the internal iliac artery distal to its first branch, the superior gluteal artery. Alternatively, the superior vesical artery can be directly identified and ligated. If the surgeon identifies and follows the ureter caudally, then the medial umbilical ligament and superior vesical artery will be identified.

The peritoneum is divided across the rectovesical pouch posteriorly at a point where it is no longer adherent to the bladder. At this point, if the leaves of Denonvillier's fascia are left on the rectum, the dissection will lead behind the seminal vesicles, separating them from the bladder. More appropriately, a deeper plane of dissection is chosen, so Denonvillier's fascia remains attached to the bladder base and the prostate. The seminal vesicles are thus lifted out of the pelvis with the surgical specimen. The posterior pedicles of the bladder are evident laterally. In the female, the appropriate procedure for invasive cancers of the bladder is anterior pelvic exenteration. A modification of this technique whereby the urethra is preserved is discussed later in this chapter.

Preservation of Erectile Function

For preservation of potency and continence (in the case of orthotopic neobladder reconstruction or radical prostatectomy), care must be taken not to injure the nerve supply to the cavernous tissue[12,13] and urethral sphincter. After dividing the peritoneum and establishing the correct plane of dissection with respect to Denonvillier's fascia, the surgeon mobilizes the bladder anteriorly while the rectum is pushed posteriorly. This maneuver defines the left and right posterior pedicles, which contain the arterial supply to the base of the bladder and the prostate. Care is taken to divide these pedicles close to the seminal vesicles (anteriorly), to avoid injuring the plexus of nerves lateral to the rectum. Proceeding distally, the fascia overlying the prostate is divided just anterior and parallel to the neurovascular bundle containing the cavernous nerves.

Urethrectomy is often carried out along with cystoprostatectomy in patients with bladder and urethral cancer. Reported modifications to urethrectomy have resulted in the maintenance of potency.[14] In this technique, dissection is carried out in a meticulous manner to preserve pudendal arterial supply to the corpora cavernosa.

Orthotopic Bladder Replacement

A variety of surgical approaches have been developed for bladder substitution. These approaches all share common characteristics: construction of a large, compliant reservoir; maintenance of an efficient continence mechanism; and an approach for ureteral reimplanation that prevents high-pressure ureteral reflux. Segments of both large and small intestine may be used to construct the urinary reservoir, and the principles for reservoir construction are described elsewhere.[15–18]

Continence after such procedures depends on a compliant, large-volume reservoir and an intact urethral sphincter mechanism. The distal urethral sphincter mechanism is composed of urethral mucosa, longtitudinal smooth muscle of the urethral wall, striated sphincter, and the surrounding levator ani musculature of the pelvic floor. The striated urethral sphincter is innervated by branches of the pudendal nerve.[19] These nerves leave the pelvis through the ischiorectal fossa and thus are preserved during bladder and prostate surgery. Direct damage to the sphincter mechanims is most likely to occur when dissection is carried out at the prostatic apex in the male. Sphincter electromyography has shown that resection of the cavernous nerves does not compromise the distal urethral sphincter.[20] Anatomic dissections have demonstrated that a portion of the urethral sphincter's nerve supply is derived from intrapelvic nerves, however.[21] By virtue of their location, these nerve fibers are prone to injury from major pelvic surgery. They may be spared as described previously, provided surgical margins are not compromised.

If orthotopic bladder replacement is to be undertaken, the approach to apical dissection of the prostate should be meticulous, to minimize damage to the distal urethral sphincter and pelvic floor musculature. A thorough knowledge of the anatomic variations of the sphincter and prostatic apex facilitates this dissection. The urethral sphincteric unit seems to be well preserved in patients undergoing othrotopic bladder replacement because urethral pressure profiles in these patients compare favorably with those in patients undergoing radical prostatectomy.[22]

Orthotopic neobladder construction has been attempted in selected female patients. The urethra is preserved, and bilateral ureteroileal urethrostomy is performed.[23] The approach to preservation of the urethra in women is based, as in men, on a thorough understanding of pelvic anatomy. The muscle fibers of the pelvic floor insert on both the vagina and urethra, to divide the sphincter into three anatomic regions: distally, muscle fibers encircle the the urethra and vagina (urethrovaginal sphincter); in the mid-portion, they pass part way around the vagina (constrictor urethrae); and proximally, they encircle the urethra completerly (urethral sphincter). Therefore, the distal two thirds of the sphincteric mechanism in women is firmly attached to the vagina. More proximally, however, the proximal urethra and bladder base can be separated from the anterior vaginal vault easily. Within this vesicovaginal space lies smooth muscle, areolar and connective tissue, the distal ureters, and the autonomic nerve supply to the distal urethra. Preservation of these nerves is apparently unnecessary because the pudendal nerves are left intact during anterior exenteration in women. No need exists for ancillary continence procedures such as a periurethral suspension because the urethral remnant appears to be well supported after cystectomy in women by the pubourethral ligaments anteriorly, by the endopelvic fascia, by the vagina posteriorly, and by the pelvic floor musculature. These structures are not damaged when the urethra is preserved at the time of cystectomy.

REFERENCES

1. Parsons CL, Boychuk D, Jones S, Hurst R, Callahan H. Bladder surface glycosaminoglycans: an epithelial permeability barrier. J Urol 1990; 143:139.
2. Steers WD. Physiology of the urinary bladder. In: Walsh PC, Retik AB, Stamey TA, Vaughan ED, eds. Campbell's urology, 6th ed. Philadelphia: WB Saunders, 1992.
3. Myers RP. Practical pelvic anatomy pertinent to radical retropubic prostatectomy. AUA Update Series XIII(Lesson 4):26.
4. Villers A, McNeal JE, Freiha FS, Boccon GL, Stamey TA. Invasion of Denonvilliers' fascia in radical prostatectomy specimens. J Urol 1993;149:793.
5. Tanagho EA, Pugh RCB. The anatomy and function of the ureterovesical junction. Br J Urol 1963;35:151.
6. Tanagho EA, Smith DR. The anatomy and function of the bladder neck. Br J Urol 1966;38:54.
7. Carroll PR, Dixon CM. Surgical anatomy of the male and female urethra. Urol Clin North Am 1992;19:339.
8. Mostwin JL. Current concepts of female pelvic anatomy and physiology. Urol Clin North Am 1991;18:175.
9. Oelrich TM. The urethral sphincter muscle in the male. Am J Anat 1980;158:229.

10. Myers RP, Goellner JR, Cahill DR. Prostate shape, external striated urethral sphincter and radical prostatectomy: the apical dissection. J Urol 1987;138:543.
11. Smith JJ, Whitmore WJ. Regional lymph node metastasis from bladder cancer. J Urol 1981;126:591.
12. Walsh PC, Donker PJ. Impotence following radical prostatectomy: insight into etiology and prevention. J Urol 1982;128:492.
13. Walsh PC, Mostwin JL. Radical prostatectomy and cystoprostatectomy with preservation of potency: results using a new nerve-sparing technique. Br J Urol 1984;56:694.
14. Brendler CB, Schlegel PN, Walsh PC. Urethrectomy with preservation of potency. J Urol 1990;144(2 pt 1):270.
15. Hinman FJ. Selection of intestinal segments for bladder substitution: physical and physiological characteristics. J Urol 1988;139:519.
16. Hautmann RE, Miller K, Steiner U, Wenderoth U. The ileal neobladder: 6 years of experience with more than 200 patients. J Urol 1993;150:40.
17. Ghoneim MA, Shaaban AA, Mahran MR, Kock NG. Further experience with the urethral Kock pouch. J Urol 1992;147:361.
18. Rowland RG, Mitchell ME, Bihrle R, Kahnoski RJ, Piser JE. Indiana continent urinary reservoir. J Urol 1987;137:1136.
19. Juenemann KP, Lue TF, Schmidt RA, Tanagho EA. Clinical significance of sacral and pudendal nerve anatomy. J Urol 1988;139:74.
20. Liu S, Christmas TJ, Nagendran K, Kirby RS. Sphincter electromyography in patients after radical prostatectomy and cystoprostatectomy. Br J Urol 1992;69:397.
21. Zvara P, Carrier S, Kour N-W, Tanagho EA. The detailed neuroanatomy of the human striated urethral sphincter. Br J Urol (in press).
22. Gasparini ME, Hinman FJ, Presti JJ, Schmidt RA, Carroll PR. Continence after radical cystoprostatectomy and total bladder replacement: a urodynamic analysis. J Urol 1992;148:1861.
23. Stein J, Stenzl A, Esrig D, et al. Lower urinary tract reconstruction following cystectomy in the female using the Kock ileal reservoir with bilateral ureteroileal urethrostomy: initial experience. J Urol 1994;151:51a. Abstract.

Principles and Practice of Genitourinary Oncology, edited by Derek Raghavan, Howard I. Scher, Steven A. Leibel, and Paul H. Lange. Lippincott-Raven Publishers, Philadelphia, © 1997.

CHAPTER 17

Experimental Models of Bladder Cancer

Pamela J. Russell and Dorothy Glaves

Bladder cancer is a heterogeneous disease that is often multifocal and has various clinical and histopathologic appearances. Over 90% of tumors are transitional cell carcinomas (TCCs), with a minority of squamous cell carcinomas (SCCs) (5%) and adenocarcinomas (1%), although many TCCs contain squamous and adenocarcinomatous components. The majority of cancers are superficial and initially respond well to therapy, but invasive disease (20% of patients) is more difficult to treat. Moreover, 50% to 70% of bladder cancers recur, and 10% to 20% of these progress to invasive, metastatic, and fatal disease. Clinical management is based on superficial versus invasive status of disease, but we are unable to predict outcome in individual patients. Experimental model systems provide opportunities for controlled, manipulated analysis of the biologic processes in bladder tumorigenesis and progression, as well as response to therapy. This chapter summarizes the contribution of model systems to our understanding of specific aspects of these processes and the extent to which they mimic clinical disease. Available models range from carcinogen-induced bladder cancers in rodents, immortalized human ureteral cells for studying tumorigenesis, to human bladder cancer cell lines for dissection of biochemical mechanisms of tumor progression as well as response to chemotherapy, to xenografts used to reconstruct the heterogeneous, interactive microenvironment of primary bladder cancers. Cell–cell and cell–matrix recombination models emphasize the potentially significant stromal contribution to the behavior of bladder cancers.

CARCINOGENESIS

Arylamine chemicals from environmental, industrial, and other sources have played a significant role in bladder cancer since the late nineteenth century. Although some compounds are obsolete, such as 2-naphthylamine, structurally related compounds, such as 4,4′-methylenebis(2-chloroaniline) are still used and are known carcinogens.[1] Other important chemicals include pesticides such as chlordimeform, which is metabolized to the bladder carcinogen, 4-chloro-o-toluidine.[2] Animal models of chemical carcinogenesis have focussed on rodent bladder tumors induced by *N*-nitroso compounds, such as *N*-methyl-*N*-nitrosourea (MNU) and *N*-butyl-*N*-(4-hydroxybutyl) nitrosamine (BBN), and N-[4-(5-nitro-2-furyl)-2-thiazolyl] formamide (FANFT). Intravesicular MNU[3] and oral BBN and FANFT[4,5] lead to overrepresentation of SCCs, however, rather than TCCs. A combination of intravesical MNU and oral antibiotics given to Fischer, rather than Copenhagen, rats induces only TCCs with a full "clinical" spectrum of atypical hyperplasia, carcinoma in situ, and muscle-invasive tumors.[6] Similar strain-related differences occur in mice, and BBN induces SCC and TCC in C57BL/6 mice, but only TCC in C57BL/6 × DBA/2 F1 hybrids.[7]

Although progression from normal urothelium to invasive TCC is seen in autochthonous animal models, it appears to be a continuum, whereas, clinically, many bladder cancers do not progress beyond superficial papillary stages and the existence of fundamentally different invasive and noninvasive disease is debated.[8,9] Nevertheless, these models are useful for evaluation of chemotherapeutic drugs, tumorigenesis promoting factors,[10,11] including carcinogen-exposed stroma,[12] and chemopreventive agents such as antiinflammatory drugs[13] and polyamine synthesis inhibitors such as difluoromethylornithine, which has progressed to clinical trials for bladder cancer.[14]

Arylamines require metabolic activation to proximate carcinogens, with *N*-acetylation pathways playing a major role in generating DNA-reactive metabolites.[15] *N*-acetylation ability is genetically determined, and epidemiologic studies indicate an increased incidence of bladder cancer in slow acetylators exposed to carcinogens.[16] Inbred hamsters are polymorphic *N*-acetylators and provide a model for evaluating the relative contribution of genotype-dependent and genotype-independent *N*-acetyltransferases to arylamine carcinogen metabolism in the bladder cytosol.[17]

That superficial bladder cancers are often multifocal poses a persistent clinical problem and possibly explains the high recurrence rate. Investigators have suggested that these tumors arise independently because of a "field defect" induced by continuous exposure of the urothelium to carcinogens in the urine.[18] Clinical studies of allelic loss showed the same X-chromosome inactivation and loss of 9q allele in tumors from the same bladders, however, indicating a clonal origin.[19] Other chromosomal changes were not shared, prompting the hypothesis that the "uncontrolled early spread of a single cell" generates multiple tumors that then undergo independent progression. Such active invasive behavior in cancer cells at early stages appears to be at variance with the indolence of the majority of bladder cancers. Screening of *P53* mutations in clinical specimens confirms concordance of genotype among multiple primary tumors and metastases, but two tumors in one patient had different mutations, indicating that they had arisen independently.[20] Few autochthonous rodent models address the field-defect issue, although a mouse orthotopic transplantable tumor model has been used to explain multifocal recurrences on the basis of exfoliated tumor cells that are passively transported and are then reattached by fibrin clots during resection of the primary lesion.[21]

CELL-SURFACE CARBOHYDRATE MARKERS

The Thomsen-Friedenreich antigen, or T antigen, is an O-linked mucin-type structure confined to glycoproteins and characterized as Galβ 1-3GalNAcα1-0-Ser/Thr. This antigen is detectable by antibodies or peanut agglutinin (PNA) lectin.[22] Several studies have shown this structure to be sialylated in normal urothelium but demasked in urothelial tumors,[23] and monoclonal antibodies have been used for studying the presence of T antigen in serum samples as an indicator of prognosis in patients.[24] In vitro cell lines and in vivo xenografts of human bladder cancer provide models to show that other carbohydrate groups may be overexpressed in bladder cancer, compared with normal urothelium, as detected by lectin-binding studies[25] or by Western blotting of membrane proteins.[26] Data from experimental carcinogenesis models are conflicting, and rat BBN bladder tumors did not show differential PNA binding,[27] whereas binding of PNA did discriminate among normal urothelium, atypical urothelium, and invasive lesions during NMU rat bladder carcinogenesis.[28]

CYTOGENETICS

Immortalized Human Ureteral Cells

Reznikoff and colleagues[29] have immortalized human ureteral cells by expression of the SV40 virus large T antigen, or of the *E6* or *E7* genes of human papillomavirus, to construct a model to study carcinogenesis and progression in bladder cancer. Human ureteral cells exposed to bladder carcinogens became tumorigenic in nude mice after increasing passage in vitro, and these tumors have pathologic features similar to those of bladder cancers in patients, with some showing squamous differentiation or a mixed histologic pattern with TCC, squamous, and adenocarcinomatous differentiation. Karyotypic analyses of nontumorigenic and tumorigenic cell lines, as well as hybrids of the two types of cells, show that tumor formation was associated with loss of particular chromosomes thought to harbor suppressor genes important in the development of bladder cancer. The losses described as most significant were −3p, −18q, and −13q, with a less significant loss of 11p. Similar chromosomal changes have been observed in clinical bladder cancers.[30] The clinical relevance of this model is also supported by the deletion of chromosomal regions in common with other types of cancer, namely, the region on 3p containing putative *SCLC* and *RCC* suppressor genes, and the *DCC* suppressor region on 18q. Reznikoff and colleagues have used their system, and data from other investigators, to construct two working models of human bladder carcinogenesis.[29] Papillomaviruses have been implicated in urothelial carcinogenesis,[31] and one model involves early (preimmortalization) compromise of P53 and RB1 protein function by binding of DNA viruses. In the second, virus-free model, genetically inactivated P53 and RB1 are involved in the progression of superficial lesions to invasive cancers. Suppressor genes were also predicted on chromosomes 3, 18, and 13q, which could be rapidly explored in clinical materials.

Chromosome 9 aberrations have been suggested as primary events in bladder tumorigenesis,[32] and interest has focused on a putative tumor suppressor gene located on 9p, with *P16* as the prime candidate.[33] Some models may not reflect in vivo events, however. For example, mathematic models based on transformed human ureteral cells did not predict a chromosome 9 suppressor gene,[34] and controversy exists about the overrepresentation of *P16* defects by bladder cancer tissue culture models compared with primary tumors.[35] This controversy has prompted debate about both methods and location of a suppressor gene elsewhere on 9p. Clinical studies already focus on other regions of chromosome 9, and the UCRU-BL17, BL13, and BL28 model cell lines show deletions at 9p21-22.[36]

Cloned Human Bladder Cancer Cell Lines

Two models of bladder cancer progression that reflect clinical disease have been established using clonally derived bladder cancer cell lines ranging from nontumorigenic to tumorigenic and metastatic in athymic rodents. The UCRU-BL17 (BL17) heterogeneous cell line gave rise to nine cloned lines,[37] three of which were nontumorigenic. Of six tumorigenic lines, three were invasive in vivo, and the only invasive clone tested gave rise to metastatic deposits in 25% of cases when implanted orthotopically in nude rats.[38] Cloned lines derived from a rat carcinoma cell line exhibited similar behavior.[39] Karyotypic evolution of the BL17 sublines with passage through nude mice was apparent at specific chromosome regions, including 1p12, 3cen-3p21, and 6cen-6q21, thought to be hotspots for rearrangment in this tumor.[40] Several unique karyotypic features arose in the progression of two sublines that coincided with a loss of anchorage-independent growth and a change in growth in vivo from solid tumor to fluid-filled cyst.

MOLECULAR GENETICS

Oncogenes

In common with other types of cancer, bladder cancers are postulated to culminate from sequential changes in genes that control growth and proliferation.[8,41] These genes are usually protooncogenes activated by mutations or amplification and tumor suppressor genes inactivated by mutation, rearrangement, or deletion. Initial studies[42] with the archetypal human bladder cancer model, cultured T24 cells, revealed a mutation in the *HRAS* (formerly known as H-*ras*) protooncogene resulting in continual second messenger-mediated proliferation. This finding spawned identification of *RAS* activation mutants in many tumor types. Ironically, this cell line proved not to predict the *RAS* status of many other in vitro models or the clinical situation. Clinical data are conflicting, with the detection of mutations varying from less than 10%[8,43] up to 76%.[44] Two in vitro and in vivo models using *RAS*-transfected cells indicate that, if present, *RAS* activation is probably associated with invasive progression of bladder cancers.[29,45] Animal models of primary bladder cancer provide limited insight into the role of *RAS* because the rat MNU-induced TCC model[46] indicated neither amplification of total *RAS* nor mutation of *HRAS* in primary tumors, whereas activated *HRAS* was found in about half of noninvasive tumors induced by MNU in ectopically transplanted bladders of rats.[46] Overall, the experimental models support the suggestion that *RAS* aberrations are not necessary features of bladder cancer,[8,43] whereas both in vitro and in vivo models are conflicting with regard to the association of activated *RAS* with invasive disease. In general, dysregulated protooncogenes (*RAS, ERBB2* [formerly c-erbB-2]/*NEU, MYC* [formerly c-*myc*]) appear to be less common than defective tumor suppressor genes, such as the retinoblastoma and *P53* genes, in progression of bladder cancers.

Tumor Suppressor Genes

The retinoblastoma (*RB1*) gene is a prototype tumor suppressor gene located at chromosome 13q that regulates the cell cycle. The *RB1* gene is inactivated or lost in many cancers, and, in bladder tumors, most data come from clinical studies showing altered patterns of expression from undetectable levels to heterogenous expression in association with invasive, aggressive, disease[47] and decreased survival.[48] In vitro cell lines mimicked the clinical situation in one study, with inactivation of *RB1* in approximately 33% of lines,[49] and these cell lines may be useful in dissecting the role of this gene in bladder cancer. An in vitro and in vivo xenogeneic model may be also be useful in this context because transfection of *RB1* into TCC cells reduced their growth and tumorigenicity.[50]

The *P53* tumor suppressor gene located on chromosome 17p plays an important role as "guardian of the genome,"[51] regulating both cell growth and death by apoptosis.[52] Many investigators have reported that mutation or loss of *P53* occurs in many bladder cancers as a late event, correlating with invasiveness.[8] Little information is available from experimental models, but chromosomal hybridization has revealed an amplicon (Fig. 17-1) on chromosome 12 of the UCRU-BL13 human bladder cancer cell line[53] that corresponds to amplification of the *MDM2* gene (Rudduck C, et al, personal communication). The *MDM2* gene product can bind and inactivate P53 protein.[54] In contrast, the UCRU-BL17 cell line[55] has a mutation in codon 280, whereas UCRU-BL28[56] expresses wild-type P53 (Ribeiro J, et al, unpublished observations). Therefore, this series of human bladder TCCs provides a clinically relevant spectrum to explore the relative contribution of *P53* to cell survival or apoptosis in response to chemotherapy, as discussed later.

GROWTH FACTORS AND RECEPTORS

Cellular growth, differentiation, and proliferation are largely controlled by extracellular factors, including growth factors and their corresponding receptors at the cell surface. In malignant disease, alterations in growth factor pathways may release cells from regulation and may thus allow uncontrolled proliferation. Table 17-1 summarizes some of the experimental models used to evaluate growth factor pathways thought to be important in bladder cancer. In common with other malignant diseases,

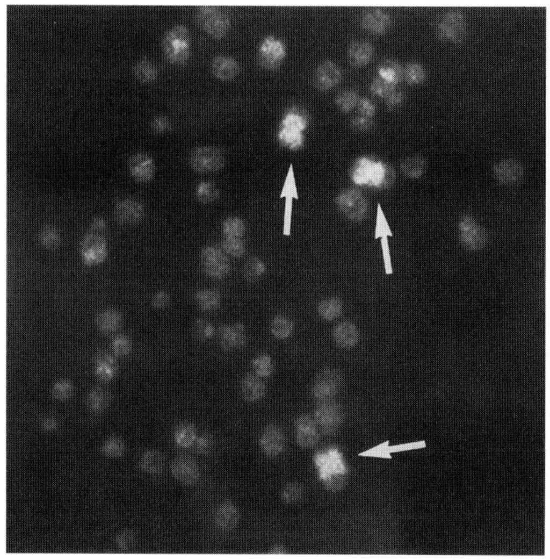

FIG. 17-1. Chromosomal hybridization of UCRU-BL13 human bladder carcinoma cells showing an amplicon on chromosome 12 (*arrows*). (Courtesy of C. Rudduck, L. Ooms, and O.M. Garson, Department of Cytogenetics, St. Vincent's Hospital, Victoria, Australia, from their unpublished results.)

invasive and poorly differentiated bladder cancers frequently overexpress epidermal growth factor receptor (EGFR),[57] and urine contains high concentrations of EGF. This combination favors a central role for EGFR and EGF in bladder tumorigenesis and progression that is validated by an in vivo ectopically transplanted rat bladder model showing that EGF can promote tumorigenesis in carcinogen-treated urothelium.[58] Cell–cell recombination models, involving TCC and urothelial mesenchymal cells, have been used to show the potential importance of stromal elements to the growth and progression of bladder cancers.[59] Moreover, transforming growth factor-α (TGF-α) production by cancer cells provides a mechanism for autocrine stimulation of tumor growth, and a cell–cell recombination model has been used to show the potential contribution of both EGFR-mediated autocrine, and stromal paracrine, stimulation in TCC growth.[60] The UCRU-BL17 clonal cell line model indicates that the insulin-like growth factor (IGF) axis may also be important, with increased IGF-1 expression correlating with aggressiveness and invasion of clones (Brown J, Russell PJ, unpublished results). The FANFT-induced rat NBT-II bladder cancer model shows that both acidic and basic fibroblast growth factors may be significant in tumor-environment interactions, because both were mitogenic.[61] Concerns have been raised about this model because of the loss of TCC morphology by the anaplastic NBT-II tumors, which may contain sarcomatous elements. Acidic fibroblast growth factor could therefore induce mesenchymal characteristics in NBT-II cells in vitro.

INVASION AND METASTASIS

In Vitro Models

Cell Lines

Various tissue culture cell lines have been developed from animal and human bladder cancers. Often, these cell lines are

Table 17-1. *Growth factors involved in bladder cancer progression*

Growth factor pathway	Model	Human studies	Observation
TGF-β_1	Rat bladder cancer clones		Expression of mRNA increases with aggressiveness[39]
	UCRU-BLU17*		High expression of mRNA in tumorigenic and invasive clones†
	5637*		Express TGFβ_1[118]
	EJ*x SW480(colon) hybrids		Nontumorigenic hybrids respond to TGF-β_1 and TGF-β_2; TGF-β_2 receptors need for inhibition by TGF-β_1[119]
TGF-α/EGF/EGFR	UCRU-BL17		EGF/TBF-α stimulate colony formation in tumorigenic clones; EGF mitogenic for clones on plastic: All clones express mRNA for TGF-α; All clones express high levels of EGFR†
	Bladder cancer cell lines*		Monoclonal antibody 425 to EGFR inhibits EGFR-induced proliferation[121]
	WH*		Urogenital mesenchyme stimulates growth and expression of TGF-α and EGFR[121]
	HT-1376, HT 1197		EGF stimulates clonal growth[122]
	Normal bladder, cancer cells	EGF low in bladder cancer patients	EGF mitogenic for cancer, not normal cells[55]
	Rat NBTII		Transfection of TGF causes invasive phenotype[123]
		EGFR expression increases with age and stage	
		EGFR on basal cells of normal; bladder[55]	
		EGFR gene not amplified in bladder cancer[125]	
		EGFR amplified in bladder cancer[126]	
c-erbB2/*neu*		Overexpressed in TCC[127,128–131]	
		Gene amplified in 1/12 bladder cancers[131]	
		Increased expression with grade[128]	
		Conflicting reports on effects of stage[129,130]	
Acidic FGF	NBTII rat bladder		"Scattering agent"; epithelial cells become motile and fibroblastic at low density[132]
			Transfection of aFGF increases invasion and metastasis[133]
		Elevated in urine of TCC; inceasing levels with stage[134]	
Basic FGF	EJ*, RT4*		Autocrine pathway in EJ (high grade/stage); EJ express high and low level receptors; no bFGF receptors on RT4[135]
		Elevated in urine of TCC[136]	
IGF	BL-17 clones*		Similar levels of mRNA for IGF-II mRNA for IGF-I increased with aggressiveness and invasion†
	T24*, 5637* J82*, TCC-SUP*		IGF-I stimulates J82 less than other cell lines due to differences in IGF-I binding site[137]

* Human bladder cancer cell lines.

† Brown JL, Russell PJ, unpublished results.

TGF, transforming growth factor; *EGF,* epidermal growth factor; *EGFR,* EGF receptor; *FGF,* fibroblast growth factor; *IGF,* insulin-like growth factor; *TCC,* transitional cell carcinoma.

held to represent the histopathologic grade or stage of the primary tumors from which they were derived, as has been confirmed in some cases by their behavior in vivo or in vitro. We discuss individual cell lines in the context of specific models within this chapter.

Recombination Models

Bladder cancers that have penetrated the basement membrane provide significant clinical risk, with a 5-year survival rate of less than 50%, and little optimism for cure of ensuing metastatic disease. The critical challenge to identify mechanisms of tumor cell dissemination in all types of cancer has led to the development of in vitro models of tumor cell invasion and interaction with extracellular matrices such as basement membrane. The most popular model involves the use of Boyden's chambers to measure the migration of tumor cells through filters, usually coated with reconstituted basement membrane matrix, in response to putative chemotactic factors. This model is versatile and permits analytic dissection of (1) the invasive phenotype or genotype of tumor cells, (2) cellular interactions with all, or individual, components of extracellular matrices by appropriate coating of filters, (3) the biochemical mechanisms of matrix penetration using enzyme inhibitors, and (4) the role of growth factors and motility factors as chemoattractants for cancer cells. For example, this model was used to show that human EJ cells, derived from an invasive TCC, penetrated reconstituted basement membrane-coated filters in response to autocrine motility factor, whereas RT4 cells from a noninvasive TCC did not, and a cysteine protease inhibitor that prevented EJ plasma membrane degradation of the basement membrane component, laminin, also inhibited chemoinvasion of EJ cells, but it did not affect their initial adhesion to the basement membrane matrix.[62]

Changes in the expression of adhesion molecules have been described in bladder cancer, and integrin expression, which is mainly at the basal surface at its junction with the lamina propria in normal bladder, appears to be altered even in early low-grade lesions. Cell lines provide models to analyze the expression of adhesion molecules,[63] and a cell-matrix confrontation model has been used to evaluate their potential role in bladder cancer progression showing that an anti-β integrin monoclonal antibody, NCC-INT-7, inhibited adhesion of cancer cells to laminin and fibronectin, as well as their invasion of an artificial basement membrane.[64]

Normal bladder tissue provides an undisturbed, readily manipulated substrate for reconstruction of the invasive milieu. Long-term organotypic coculture of rat bladder fragments with NBT-II TCC spheroids was used as a model to show that exogenous or autocrine (transfected) TGF-α and acidic fibroblast growth factor stimulated nodular outgrowths and clusters of infiltrating cells from TCC that had replaced, but otherwise not invaded, urothelial tissue.[65] A cocultivation model was used to examine the concept of a urothelial "field defect."[66] Human T24 bladder carcinoma cells showed both lateral expansion into mouse bladder explants and variable pagetoid infiltration, which was interpreted to support the unifocal origin of multiple lesions.

In Vivo Models

Autochthonous Tumors

Autochthonous animal models include the carcinogen-induced rodent bladder cancers described ealier, as well as those induced in hamsters, guinea pigs, dogs, and cattle.[9] Spontaneous urothelial cancers are less common, although up to 28% of male brown Norway rats and 45% of male DA/HAN rats develop TCC.[9] Invasive lesions have been described in all models, but little evidence suggests that these tumors are biologically distinct from localized lesions, and they have not contributed to the biologic basis for the progressional dichotomy between superficial and invasive clinical disease. Moreover, few reports exist of distant metastases in these autochthonous models.

Transplantable Tumors

Syngeneic Systems

Earlier reviews[9,67] discussed the characteristics and relative merits of transplantable animal bladder cancers. The FANFT-induced transplantable MBT-2 mouse TCC has played a significant role in the search for new therapies, but it has largely been used as a subcutaneous tumor model, and little evidence suggests that it metastasizes from this site. Other mouse systems, such as the MD-49 tumor, also appear to be overtly nonmetastatic as subcutaneous lesions. Transplantable Nb-I rat tumors are reported to generate lung and visceral metastases from subcutaneous tumors in 30% of animals,[68] but other rat tumors appear to metastasize infrequently.

Xenogeneic Systems

Athymic (nude) rodents have proved valuable for studying aspects of human tumor biology and therapy, despite concerns about differences between mouse and human physiology or stroma, and a defective host immunologic system that permits xenogeneic tumors to grow but provides a poor model for potentially major growth-modulating influences of immune responses. This is especially true for bladder cancer, which is one of the few cancers in which biologic response modifiers play a significant clinical role. In addition, attempts at xenografts of tumor cells or tissues are not always successful, a finding prompting the development of matrigel-assisted and fibroblast-assisted transplanted tumor models.[69]

Although some TCC grow and show limited invasiveness in athymic rodents, metastasis may or, more frequently, may not occur.[70] Mice with severe combined immunodeficiency have a broader immunodeficiency than nude rodents in that they lack both functional B and T lymphocytes (humoral and cell-mediated immunity). These mice support the growth of a wider range of tumor xenografts, and the incidence of metastases is generally higher.[71] Limited studies have been made with bladder cancers, but a subline of T24 cells (T24B) was among several types of human tumors that metastasized to the lungs in 100% of mice with subcutaneous tumors, whereas primary tumors grew more slowly and metastasized in only 1 of 18 nude mice.[72]

Orthotopic Tumors

The invasive and metastatic potential of tumors depends not only on their inherent properties, but also on the host microenvironment.[73] Orthotopic injection often enhances tumorigenicity and metastatic potential, and bladder cancers are no exception. Orthotopic tumors also provide excellent models for developing intravesical therapies and diagnostic imaging.[74] Soloway and colleagues[75] initially developed a syngeneic mouse model in which high-grade murine tumor cells were instilled into bladders that had been electrocauterized to damage the urothelium, a process that increased tumor take from 6% to 67%. Subsequent adaptations of the model have omitted electrocautery, to reduce the sometimes lethal trauma and to avoid tissue damage that can obscure the invasive behavior of cancer cells. For example, such a model was able to differentiate between the invasive behavior of EJ TCC cells and the noninvasive behavior of RT4 TCC in a nude mouse system, which reflected the characteristics of the original high-grade (EJ) and low-grade papillary (RT4) human tumors.[76] Tumor take rates were approximately 50%, whereas that of another ''invasive'' cell line was only 20%, and this model does not solve problems of low transplantability in every tumor system. EJ tumors generated pulmonary metastases in half the mice, but none was generated from RT4 tumors. This finding is in contrast to later studies in which a different orthotopic model was used involving ''onplant'' of *RAS*-transfected-RT4 tissue fragments onto the peritoneal surface of the bladder.[77] The take rate was improved to 100%, compared with 50% for instillation of disaggregated cells, and both lymph node metastases and peritoneal lesions were generated in almost every animal. Parental RT4 tissue fragments were also tumorigenic and metastatic to both lymph nodes and peritoneal organs.[78] The differences in RT4 spread between these studies are probably related to invasive potential of RT4 cells because intravenous injection of RT4 cells did produce pulmonary colonies in the first study, a procedure that bypasses the invasive phase of metastasis, and onplant of tissue on the peritoneal side of the bladder also circumvents local invasion. This difference between metastatic potential and organ colonization potential is frequently observed in other experimental tumor systems, and, some years ago, confusion between the two processes was part of a lively debate on the selective versus random nature of metastasis.[79]

The UCRU-BL17 xenograft model has been expanded to become an orthotopic model in athymic rats.[38] Intramural injection of a clonal cell line (2B8) produced tumors in almost 100% of rats and, in 25% of animals, metastases occurred in the peritoneal organs including the liver.

Experimental models for metastasis of bladder cancer are, at best, only partial mimics of the clinical situation. Lung and liver are common sites of metastases in patients but not in many animal systems. Some attempt to model disseminated disease can be achieved by direct intravascular dissemination of tumor cells, by the tail vein for pulmonary disease, which is already used, by the hepatic portal system for hepatic lesions, and by the left ventricle for arterial organ patterns of metastasis. Although important, possibly selective, attributes (e.g., invasive potential) of the cell are ignored, lesions are generated in anatomically relevant sites for analysis of local, organ-specific interactions and optimization of therapies for metastatic versus primary disease.

DIAGNOSTIC IMAGING

Orthotopically transplanted tumor models have provided opportunities to evaluate new imaging agents. Radioimmunoscintigraphic vizualization was achieved in nude mice with xenogeneic RT4 tumors using a monoclonal antibody against cytokeratin 8.[80] A rat model showed that fluorodeoxyglucose (FDG) uptake occurs in bladder cancer and metastatic deposits.[81] That FDG is excreted in urine thus precludes the use of FDG positron emission tomography (PET) for local bladder cancer. The clinical usefulness of the rat model was shown in FDG PET scans on a patient with recurrent bladder cancer after radiation, however, which allowed imaging of metastatic deposits in the chest, whereas scarring marred the image in the pelvis.[82] The UCRU-BL17 orthotopic xenograft model has proved useful for scintigraphic evaluation of a radiolabeled antibladder cancer monoclonal antibody,[74] and subcutaneous xenograft models have been used to explore radioimmunoscintigraphy using antibodies to growth-related cell-surface glycoproteins.[83]

CHEMOTHERAPY

In vitro models for the screening of sensitivity and resistance of bladder cancer cells to chemotherapeutic agents are not discussed in detail here, but Table 17-2 lists some of the in vitro models used to explore the biochemical mechanisms of resistance to currently used drugs, as well as the potential efficacy of new agents, therapy modulating and sensitizing agents, or alternative modalities for treating bladder cancers. Many of these studies have used standard models, such as the T24, SCaBer, and RT-4 TCC cell lines. J82, SCaBER, and HT-1197 lines model for the spectrum of inherent resistance to mitomycin C, and they have been used to evaluate the roles of defective drug activation and glutathione-glutathione transferase levels in chemoresistance. The MGH and KK47 series model classic (verapamil-reversible, p-glycoprotein-mediated) multidrug resistance, whereas the UM-UC models are useful for studying atypical multidrug resistance. Cisplatin-resistant models (RT112 and the T24DDP series) have been used to explore DNA adduct repair, topoisomerase I levels, and intracellular drug accumulation as mechanisms for resistance. Monolayer cultures may be less appropriate models for in vivo chemoresistance of bladder cancers than the same cells grown as spheroids, either alone[84] or with extracellular matrix.[85] The variety and extent of available bladder cancer models are emphasized by studies of a panel of 12 cell lines used to evaluate paclitaxel and docetaxel as potential new agents in bladder cancer. RT-4, T24, MGH-U1, and 647V models are proving useful for exploring the use of agents, such as zidovudine (formerly azidothymidine [AZT]) and thymidine analogs, to potentiate the activity of conventional drugs. Few studies include in vitro models of normal urothelial cells, but CRL-7881 cells were used in evaluation of a photosensitizer for photodynamic therapy of bladder cancers. Finally, models with inherent variability in sensitivity to heat are available for a possible reexploration of hyperthermia in the treatment of bladder cancer.

As mentioned earlier, considerable interest has been focused on the expression of *P53* in relation to apoptosis and DNA repair after exposure of cells to DNA-damaging agents. Cisplatin is commonly used to treat bladder cancers, and cisplatin resistance

Table 17-2. *In vitro human bladder cancer model systems for evaluation of sensitivity and resistance to therapy*

Model	Agent	Parameter measured
MECHANISM OF DRUG RESISTANCE		
J82;SCaBER; HT-1197	Mitomycin C	Differential sensitivity, drug activation[137,138]
UM-UC-2;UM-UC-9; UM-UC-6; UM-UC-6dox*	Doxorubicin	Multidrug resistance (atypical)[139,140]
MHG-U1; MGH-U1R*	Doxorubicin	Multidrug resistance (classic)[141]
KK47; KK47/ADM*	Doxorubicin	Multidrug resistance (classic)[142]
RT112	Cisplatin	Resistance mechanisms (DNA adducts)[143]
T24/DDP7*; T24/DDP10*	Cisplatin	Resistance mechanisms (topoisomerase I levels, drug accumulation)[144]
NEW AGENTS		
MGH-U1;CUB-2;SD;HU549;J82 A1698;HT1376;T24;COLO232 UM-UC-3; TCCSUP;SCaBER	Paclitaxel, docetaxel	Differential sensitivity[145]
CHEMOSENSITIZERS AND POTENTIATORS		
RT-4	Doxorubicin/thiotepa/ mitromycin C	Synergism[146]
MGH-UI	3′-Azido-3′-deoxythymidine/ thymidine synthase inhibitor	Potentiation[147]
647V	Bleomycin/iododeoxyuridine/ 5′amino-5′deoxythymidine	Radiosensitization[148]
647V	Cisplatin/iododeoxyuridine	Chemosensitization[149]
T24	Thiotepa/iododeoxyuridine	Potentiation[150]
ALTERNATIVE THERAPY		
CRL-7881 (normal)	Photodynamic therapy	Photosensitization
MGH-U1;A-1698, CUB-2;UM-UC-3	Hyperthermia	Differential sensitivity[152]

* Chemoresistant cell line.

has been associated with overexpression of *P53* in mutant conformation in ovarian cancer cells in vitro.[86] The UCRU-BL human bladder carcinoma lines have different profiles of constitutive and cisplatin-inducible P53 expression and, therefore, provide useful clinical models for examining the relationships among P53 expression, cisplatin sensitivity, and apoptosis in bladder cancers. UCRU-BL17 cells constitutively overexpress P53 in mutant conformation, whereas UCRU-BL13 and UCRU-BL28 cells express low levels of P53 in wild-type conformation.[87] Cisplatin-treatment induces wild-type P53 in both BL13 and BL28 cells, but with different kinetics. These differences in constitutive and inducible P53 expression in the three cell types were not correlated with differences in their sensitivities to cisplatin, which were similar, however. In addition, the kinetics of cisplatin-induced apoptosis were not correlated with cisplatin sensitivity or P53 status. Indeed, apoptosis was only detected at suprapharmacologic doses (>10 to 100 μM) of cisplatin in all three cell lines. These findings emphasize that, under clinical conditions, apoptosis may not be the major cisplatin-induced cytotoxic pathway, and overexpression of P53 may not predict cisplatin sensitivity in all cancer cell types.

In vivo models include classic subcutaneous murine tumor systems, which have provided much of the database for the drugs in clinical use for all solid cancers. These models are also used to develop treatment regimens and chemoresistance-modulating agents. For example, subcutaneous MBT-2 mouse TCCs were used to model significant clinical problems by evaluating metallothionein modulation of cisplatin nephrotoxicity and resistance.[88] The same model was used to evaluate buthionine sulfoximine sensitization of TCC to standard chemotherapeutic drugs, with cyclophosphamide as the only drug of nine showing enhanced efficacy.[89] Newer approaches to combination therapy using photodynamic therapy in conjunction with conventional drugs, as well as bacille Calmette-Guérin (BCG), rely on the MBT-2 model.[90] Synergy between photodynamic therapy and chemotherapy or immunotherapy may prompt clinical application of data from this model because photodynamic therapy is already showing promise in patients with bladder cancer.

Human TCC xenograft systems may be more clinically relevant tissue models, but all subcutaneous tumors have been criticized as anatomically inappropriate. These tumors can be measured directly, however, and permit evaluation of growth delay, partial responses, and complete responses, as well as survival. Subrenal capsule assays have been used to rapidly quantify responses to single and combination therapies (e.g., 91), but multiple measurements on the same tumors are difficult, and parameters of response are often limited to survival or final tumor volumes, although laparotomies are sometimes performed.[91]

Orthotopic models offer opportunities for exploring newer approaches to intravesical therapy. This model is especially relevant if data from a colon tumor model, indicating that tumor response to chemotherapy may be site-dependent,[92] are also applicable to bladder cancer. An orthotopic rat tumor model indicates that patients could be spared toxic side effects of photodynamic therapy if the photosensitizer were given intravesically rather than by the current intravenous route.[93]

IMMUNOTHERAPY

Intravesical Immunoconjugate Therapy of Bladder Cancer

Direct administration of immunoconjugates into the bladder may circumvent many problems associated with monoclonal antibody therapy, including localization of antibodies in normal tissues, breakdown of conjugates in blood, failure of antibodies to each avascular or necrotic metastatic deposits, and the production of human antimouse antibodies. Experimental models have been established to test this hypothesis. Antibodies administered into the bladder of nude rats carrying orthotopic human bladder cancer xenografts do not leak into the systemic circulation and show excellent tumor localization.[94] The clinical application of this model was confirmed in clinical studies in which two different indium-111–labeled monoclonal antibodies, AMA-1 and HMFG2, were administered intravesically into patients with known bladder cancers.[95,96] Although neither antibody is bladder cancer specific, higher uptake of radioactivity occurred in cancer cells than in normal cells, and antibody conjugates were not detectable in the systemic circulation of the patients. Immunotoxins require internalization to be effective, and this experimental model should prove useful for evaluation of suitable antibodies that include monoclonal antibody 48-127[97] and Fib-75 linked to ricin A chain or to α-sarcin.[98]

Bacille Calmette-Guérin Therapy

Immunotherapy with intravesical BCG is the treatment of choice for superficial bladder cancer,[99] yet its mechanism of action remains unclear, and not all patients respond. Although BCG acts as an immune stimulant, it has some direct effects on cancer cells. Both in vivo and in vitro experimental models have permitted some dissection of the complex mechanisms of BCG action, as well as the potential contribution of supplementary therapeutic agents, such as cytokines or antiinflammatory drugs. In vivo models show that, in mice with MB49 tumors, radiolabeled fibronectin localized to injured but not to intact urothelium and enhanced BCG attachment.[100] BCG treatment is accompanied by cystitis, and increased attachment was achieved by pretreating the bladder with pentosan polysulfate, a drug used to treat chronic and radiation-induced cystitis.[101] Several studies have delineated the role of inflammatory cells in BCG therapy. Intravesical BCG administered to mice with orthotopic MBT-2 tumors resulted in infiltration of the lamina propria of the bladder with macrophages and helper T cells.[102] Parallel findings in clinical studies[103] confirm the applicability of this model system. Depletion of cytotoxic, helper, or total T lymphocytes eliminated the antitumor effect of BCG and abrogated the delayed-type hypersensitivity reaction associated with intravesical BCG delivery.[104] Exogenous interleukin-2 given to induce lymphokine-activated killer cells was not able to replace depleted CD4 T-helper cells, and no induction of protective immunity was noted after BCG treatment.[105] The significant toxicity associated with BCG therapy has prompted the search for alternative biologic response modifiers. For example, a spontaneous, transplantable, rat bladder TCC, which is not complicated by squamous components, is nonimmunogenic and may provide a more clinically appropriate model than the immunogenic chemically induced rodent TCC models, especially because it responded to clinically important cytokines, tumor necrosis factor and interferon (IFN).[106]

In vitro models can be used to show direct effects of BCG on bladder cancer cells. A cell-matrix recombination model indicates that BCG can inhibit the invasion of EJ bladder cancer cells through a basement membrane, and this can be overcome by antibodies to fibronectin.[107] Human bladder cancer cell line models have shown that BCG has a direct cytotoxic effect and a dose-dependent antiproliferative effect, and it significantly enhances monocyte-macrophage and lymphocyte cytotoxicity against the UCRU-BL17 model (Pryor K, et al, unpublished results). No synergy was observed between BCG and cytokines in cell killing, but BCG plus IFN-α_{2b} had an additive antiproliferative effect. That cell lines varied in their sensitivity to each agent is reminiscent of the varied clinical responses to biologic response modifiers, and these in vitro models suggest that differences in intrinsic properties of tumors cells, in addition to host defense responses, may contribute to differences in therapeutic outcome and can be used to analyze these contributions.

EPIDERMAL GROWTH FACTOR RECEPTOR-TARGETED THERAPY

The higher expression of EGFR on bladder cancer cells compared with normal bladder has allowed targeting of bladder cancer cells through the receptor. An in vitro clonogenicity model showed that TP40, a hybrid molecule of TGF-α and a derivative of *Pseudomonas* exotoxin, PE40, was cytotoxic to human and mouse bladder cancer cells,[108] and this agent is now undergoing clinical trials for inravesical use.[109] This in vitro model is used as a screen for new constructs, including PE35/TGF-α-KDEL, which does not require intracellular proteolysis to generate the carboxy-terminal fragment of the toxin that reaches the cytosol; KDEL increases TP40 toxicity against bladder cancer cells by 10- to 700-fold.[109]

GENE THERAPY

As a means to enhance the immunologic activity of BCG, recombinant BCG organisms have been developed that actively secrete cytokine products or serve as depots for biologically relevant antigens,[110] and similar genetic techniques may eventually allow directed binding and internalization of BCG carrying toxic genes into bladder cancer cells.[111]

Experimental animal models indicate that genetic manipulation of tumor cells may offer new therapeutic modalities for bladder cancer. Tumor cells have been modified to express cytokines and have antitumor effects in vivo. For example, the MBT-2 mouse model shows that interleukin-2-secreting cells give better effects than cisplatin or than IFN-γ, and memory was established in "cured" mice.[112] These therapeutic approaches depend on in vitro propagation of individual tumors to perform gene transfections and thus have limited clinical applicability.

Exciting clinical possibilities have been raised using orthotopic mouse MBT-2 and MB49 tumor models for direct in vivo transfer of functional genes into cancer cells by intravesical instillation of recombinant *Vaccinia* virus vectors.[113]

FUTURE DIRECTIONS

New work with bladder cancer models is likely to include focus on intravesical gene therapy for recurrent tumors, as well as the preclinical evaluation of genetically engineered tumor vaccines deleveloped in vitro. Bladder cancers are prime candidates not only for exploration of EGFR-targeted therapy, but also for new combination therapies involving EGFR-targeted and standard chemotherapeutic agents. Synergy between anti-EGFR antibodies and doxorubicin or cisplatin has already been shown in experimental models of other types of cancer,[114,115] and orthotopic models should provide excellent opportunities to exploit this approach in bladder cancers. In vitro models indicate that other growth factor-receptor axes such as *NEU* and IGF-1 should also be explored as targets for therapy.

The majority of bladder cancers present as superficial disease, and orthotopic models have become a natural focus, but refractory metastatic disease receives less attention. Models are needed to evaluate the biologic basis for organ patterns of bladder cancer metastasis, for treatment of disseminated lesions, and for understanding the reasons for the different response to therapy of lymphatic versus visceral metastases. Orthotopic models and mice with severe combined immunodeficiency should provide systems for these studies.

Studies of the molecular genetics of bladder cancer, in common with all cancers, is accelerating. A genome-wide tendency to replication error, characterized by microsatellite instability, has been linked to oncogenesis of colon cancer.[116] Somatic instability at microsatellite repeats was found in 6 of 200 TCCs, with changes in (GT)n repeat lengths on chromosome 9 of 4 tumors and alterations in (CAG)n repeats of the androgen receptor gene on chromosome X in 3 tumors. These changes were in low-grade, low-stage tumors and were thought to represent an early event in bladder cancer development.[117] No studies of model tumors have yet been reported, but the spectrum of experimental models of bladder cancer, from clonal cell lines to xenograft replicates of heterogeneous primary bladder cancers, is available to address such issues central to the development of this common cancer.

REFERENCES

1. McQueen CA, Williams GM. Review of the genotoxicity and carcinogenicity of 4,4′-methylene-dianiline and 4,4′-methylene-bis-s-chloroaniline. Mutat Res 1990;239:133.
2. Stasik MJ. Carcinomas of the urinary bladder in a 4-chloro-o-toluidine cohort. Int Arch Occup Environ Health 1988;1:21.
3. Hicks RM, Wakefield JStJ. Rapid induction of bladder cancer in rats with *N*-methyl-*N*-nitrosourea. I. Histology. Chem Biol Interact 1972; 5:139.
4. Herman CJ, Vegt PDJ, Debruyne FMJ, Vooijs CP, Ramaekers FCS. Squamous and transitional elements in rat bladder carcinomas induced by N-butyl-N-4-hydroxybutyl-nitrosamine (BBN). Am J Pathol 1985; 120:419.
5. Cohen SM. Pathology of experimental bladder cancer in rodents. In: GT Bryant, SM Cohen, eds. The pathology of bladder cancer, vol 1. Boca Raton, FL, CRC Press, 1983:1.
6. Steinberg GD, Brendler CB, Ichikawa T, Squire RA, Isaacs JT. Characterization of an N-methyl-N-nitrosourea-induced autochthonous rat bladder cancer model. Cancer Res 1990;50:6668.
7. Moon RC, Detrisac CJ, Thomas CF, Kelloff GJ. Chemoprevention of experimental bladder cancer. J Cell Biochem 1992;161(Suppl):134.
8. Sidransky D, Messing EM. Molecular genetics and biochemical mechanisms in bladder cancer. Urol Clin North Am 1992;4:629.
9. Schalken JA, van Moorselaar RJA, Bringuer PP, Debruyne FMJ. Critical review of the models to study the biologic progression of bladder cancer. Semin Surg Oncol 1992;8:274.
10. Kawai K, Yamamoto M, Kameyama H, Rademaker A, Oyasu R. Enhancement of rat urinary bladder tumorigenesis by lipopolysaccharide-induced inflammation. Cancer Res 1993;53:5172.
11. Lina BAR, Hollanders VMH, Kuijpers MHM. The role of alkylizing and neutral potassium salts in urinary blader carcinogenesis in rats. Carcinogenesis 1994;15:523.
12. Uchida K, Samma S, Momose H, Kashihara N, Radenaker A, Oyasu R. Stimulation of urinary bladder tumorigenesis by carcinogen-exposed stroma. J Urol 1990;143:618.
13. Shibata M-A, Haasegawa R, Shirai T, Takesada Y, Fukushima S. Chemoprevention by indomethacin of tumor promotion in a rat urinary bladder carcinogenesis model. Int J Cancer 1993;55:1011.
14. Loprinzi CL, Messing EM. A prospective clinical trial of difluoromethylornithine (DFMO) in patients with resected superficial bladder cancer. J Cell Biochem 1992;161(Suppl):153.
15. Loer GM. Concepts in causality: chemically induced human urinary bladder cancer. Cancer 1982;49:1056.
16. Hein DW. Acetylator genotype and arylamine-induced carcinogenesis. Biochim Biophys Acta 1988;948:37.
17. Yerokun T, Kirlin WG, Trinidad A, et al. Identification and kinetic characterization of acetylator genotype dependent and independent arylamine carcinogen N-acetyltransferases in hamster bladder cytosol. Drug Metab Dispos Biol Fate Chem 1989;17:231.
18. Rao JY, Hemstreet GP, Bonner RA, et al. Mapping of multiple biochemical markers to define field disease in bladder cancer. J Urol 1992;147;507.
19. Sidransky D, Frost P, von Eschenbach A. Clonal origin of metachronous tumors of the bladder. N Engl J Med 1992;326:737.
20. Petersen I, Ohgaki H, Ludeke BI, Kleihues P. p53 mutations in phenacetin-associated human urothelial carcinomas. Carcinogenesis 1993; 14:2119.
21. See W. Plasminogen activators: regulators of tumor cell adherence to sites of lower urinary tract surgical trauma. J Urol 1993;150:1024.
22. Orntoft TF, Wolf H, Watkins WM. Activity of the human blood group ABO, Se, H, Le and X gene-encoded glycosyltransferases in normal and malignant bladder urothelium. Cancer Res 1993;48:4427.
23. Orntoft TF. Carbohydrate changes in bladder carcinomas. APMIS 1992;27:181.
24. Samuel J, Noujaim AA, MacLean GD, et al. Analysis of human tumor associated Thomsen-Friedenreich antigen. Cancer Res 1990;50:4801.
25. Russell PJ, Wotherspoon J, Jelbart M, et al. Stability of lectin binding properties expressed by human bladder carcinoma cell lines passaged *in vitro* or in nude mice. Urol Res 1988;16:407.
26. Ford SA, Russell PJ, Jelbart M, Raghavan D. Detection of tumor-associated membrane proteins in prostate and bladder carcinomas by means of protein blotting. Urol Res 1989;17:305.
27. Recker F, Otto T, Rubben. Lectins in diagnosis of bladder cancer. Urol Int 1992;48:149.
28. Langkilde NC, Wolf H, Clausen H, Orntoft TF. Localization and identification of T-(Galβ1-3GalNAcα-1-0-R) and T-like antigens in experimental rat bladder cancer. J Urol 1992;148:1279.
29. Reznikoff CA, Kao C, Messing EM, Newton, Swaminathan S. A molecular genetic model of human blader carcinogenesis. Semin Cancer Biol 1993;4:143.
30. Rodriguez E, Sreekantaiah C, Chaganti RSK. Genetic changes in epithelial solid neoplasia. Cancer Res 1994;54:3398.
31. Furihata M, Inoue K, Ohtsuki Y, et al. High-risk human papillomavirus infections and overexpression of p53 protein as prognostic indicators in transitional cell carcinoma of the urinary bladder. Cancer Res 1993;53:4823.
32. Miyao N, Tsai YL, Lerner SP, et al. Role of chromosome 9 in human bladder cancer. Cancer Res 1993;53:4066.

33. Kamb A, Gruis NA, Weaver-Feldhaus J, et al. A cell cycle regulator potentially involved in genesis of many tumor types. Science 1994; 264:436.
34. Newton MA, Wu S-Q, Reznikoff CA. Assessing the significance of chromosome-loss data: where are suppressor genes for bladder cancer? Stat Med 1994;13:839.
35. Cairns P, Mao L, Merlo A, et al. Rates of *p16* (MTS1) mutations in primary tumors with 9p loss. Science 1994;265:415.
36. Stadler WM, Sherman J, Bohlander SK, et al. Homozygous deletions within chromosomal bands 9p21–22 in bladder cancer. Cancer Res 1994;54:2060.
37. Brown JL, Russell PJ, Philips J, et al. Clonal analysis of a bladder cancer cell line: an experimental model of tumour heterogeneity. Br J Cancer 1990;61:369.
38. Russell PJ, Ho Shon I, Boniface GR, et al. Growth and metastasis of human bladder cancer xenografts in the bladder of nude rats: a model for intravesical radioimmunotherapy. Urol Res 1991;19:207.
39. Kawamata H, Azuma H, Kameyama S, et al. Effect of epidermal growth factor/transforming growth factor alpha and transforming growth factor beta 1 on growth in vitro or rat urinary bladder carcinoma cells. Cell Growth Differ 1992;3:819.
40. Brown JL, Lukeis R, Palividis Z, et al. Karyotypic analysis of a heterogeneous human transitional cell carcinoma of the bladder. Cancer Genet Cytogenet 1994;72:116.
41. Russell PJ, Brown JL, Grimmond SM, Raghavan D. Molecular biology of urological tumors. Br J Urol 1990;65:121.
42. Reddy EP, Reynolds RK, Santos E, et al. A point mutation is responsible for the acquisition of transforming properties by the T24 human bladder carcinoma oncogene. Nature 1982;300:149.
43. Knowles MA, Williamson M. Mutation of H-*ras* is infrequent in bladder cancer: confirmation by single-strand conformation polymorphism analysis, designed restriction fragment length polymorphisms, and direct sequencing. Cancer Res 1993;53:133.
44. Burchill SA, Lunec J, Mellon K, Neal DE. Analysis of H-ras mutations in primary human bladder tumours. Br J Cancer 1991;63(Suppl 3): 62.
45. Theodorescu D, Cornil I, Fernandez BJ, Kerbel RS. Overexpression of normal and mutated forms of *HRAS* induces orthotopic bladder invasion in a human transitional cell carcinoma. Proc Natl Acad Sci USA 1990;87:9047.
46. Yura Y, Azuma M, Uchida K, et al. *ras* gene alterations in invasive and non-invasive rat bladder induced by N-methyl-N-nitrosourea. Br J Cancer 1991;64:10.
47. Xu HJ, Cairns P, Hu SX, et al. Loss of RB protein expression in primary bladder cancer correlates with loss of heterozygosity at the RB locus and tumor progression. Int J Cancer 1993;53:781.
48. Cordon-Cardo C, Wartinger D, Petrylak D, et al. Altered expression of the retinoblastoma gene product: prognostic indicator in bladder cancer. J Natl Cancer Inst 1992;84:1251.
49. Horowitz JM, Park S-H, Bogenmann E, et al. Frequent inactivation of the retinoblastoma anti-oncogene is restricted to a subset of human tumor cells. Proc Natl Acad Sci USA 1990;87:2775.
50. Takahashi R, Hashimoto T, Xu H-J, et al. The retinoblastoma gene functions as a growth and tumor suppressor in human bladder carcinoma cells. Proc Natl Acad Sci USA 1991;88:5257.
51. Lane DP. Cancer: p53, guardian of the genome. Nature 1992;358:15.
52. Shaw P, Bovey R, Tardy S, et al. Induction of apoptosis by wild-type p53 in a human colon tumor derived cell line. Proc Natl Acad Sci USA 1992;89:4495.
53. Russell PJ, Wass J, Lukeis R, et al. Characterization of cell lines derived from a multiply aneuploid human bladder transitional-cell carcinoma, UCRU-BL-13. Int J Cancer 1989;44:276.
54. Momand J, Zambetti GP, Olson DC, et al. The mdm-2 oncogene forms a complex with the p53 protein and inhibits p53-mediated transactivation. Cell 1992;69:1237.
55. Messing EM. Growth factors and bladder cancer: clinical implications of the interactions between growth factors and their urothelial receptors. Semin Surg Oncol 1992;8:285.
56. Russell PJ, Palavidis Z, Rozinova E, et al. Characterization of a new human bladder cancer cell line, UCRU-BL-28. J Urol 1993;150:1038.
57. Neal DE, Mellon K. Epidermal growth factor receptor and bladder cancer: a review. Urol Int 1992;48:365.
58. Yura Y, Hayashi O, Kell M, et al. Identification of epidermal growth factor as a component of rat urinary bladder tumor-enhancing urinary fractions. Cancer Res 1989;49:1548.
59. Zhau HE, Hong S-J, Chung LWK. A fetal rat urinogenital sinus mesenchymal cell line (rUGM): accelerated growth and conferral of androgen-induced growth responsiveness upon a human bladder cancer epithelial cell line. Int J Cancer 1994;56:706.
60. Gleave ME, Hsieh J-T, Wu H-C, et al. Epidermal growth factor receptor-mediated autocrine and paracrine stimulation of human transitional cell carcinoma. Cancer Res 1993;53:5300.
61. Vailes AMN, Boyer B, Badet J, et al. Acidic fibroblast growth factor in a modulator of epithelial plasticity in a rat bladder carcinoma cell line. Proc Natl Acad Sci USA 1990;87:1124.
62. Redwood SM, Liu BC-S, Weiss RE, et al. Abrogation of the invasion of human bladder tumor cells by using protease inhibitor(s). Cancer 1992;69:1212.
63. Jackson AM, Alexandrov AB, Prescott S, James K, Chisholm GD. Expression of adhesion molecules by bladder cancer cells: modulation by interferon-gamma and tumour necrosis factor-alpha. J Urol 1992; 148:1583.
64. Fujita S, Suzuki H, Kinoshita M, Hirohashi S. Inhibition of cell attachment, invasion and metastasis of human carcinoma cells by anti-integrin beta 1 subunit antibody. Jpn J Cancer Res 1992;83:1317.
65. Tucker GC, Delouvee A, Jouanneau J, et al. Amplification of invasiveness in organotypic cultures after NBT-II rat bladder carcinoma stimulation with in vitro scattering factors. Invasion Metastasis 1991;11: 297.
66. Rebel JMJ, De Boer WI, Thijssen CDEM, et al. An in vitro model of intra-epithelial expansion of ransformed urothelial cells. Int J Cancer 1993;54:846.
67. Raghavan D, Debruyne F, Herr H, et al. Experimental models of bladder cancer: a critical review. Prog Biol Clin Res 1986;221:171.
68. Drago JR, Nesbitt JA. NB rat bladder cancer model: evaluation of the subrenal capsule assay system. J Surg Oncol 1987;36:5.
69. Kerbel RS, Cornil I, Theodorescu D. Importance of orthotopic transplantation procedures in assessing the effects of transfected genes on human tumor growth and metastasis. Cancer Metastasis Rev 1991; 10:201.
70. Russell PJ, Raghavan D, Philips J, Gregory P. Applications of the xenograft as a model of invasive transitional cell carcinoma of the bladder. Prog Clin Biol Res 1988;260:167.
71. Williams SS, Alosco TR, Croy BA, Bankert RB. The study of human neoplastic disease in severe combined immunodeficient mice. Lab Anim Sci 1993;43:139.
72. Xie X, Brunner N, Jensen G, et al. Comparative studies between nude and scid mice on the growth and metastatic behavior of xenografted human tumors. Clin Exp Metastasis 1992;10:201.
73. Fidler IJ. Critical factors in the biology of human cancer metastasis. Cancer Res 1990;50:6130.
74. Russell PJ, Shon IH, Boniface GR, et al. Growth and metastasis of human bladder cancer xenografts in the bladder of nude rats. Urol Res 1991;19:207.
75. Soloway MS, Nissenkorn I, McCallum L. Urothelial susceptibility to tumor cell, implantation: comparison of cauterization to N-methyl-N-nitroso-urea. Urology 1983;21:159.
76. Ahlering TE, Dubeau L, Jones PA. A new in vivo model to study invasion and metastasis of human bladder carcinoma. Cancer Res 1987;47:6660.
77. Fu X, Theodorescu D, Kerbel RS, Hoffman RM. Extensive multi-organ metastasis following orthotopic onplantation of histologically-intact human bladder carcinoma tissue in nude mice. Int J Cancer 1991;49;938.
78. Fu X, Hoffman RM. Human RT4 bladder carcinoma is highly metastatic in nude mice and comparable to ras-H-transformed RT4 when orthotopically onplanted as histologically intact tissue. Int J Cancer 1992,51:989.
79. Weiss L. Random and nonrandom processes in metastasis and metastatic inefficiency. Invasion Metastasis 1983;3:193.
80. Letochia H, Nilsson S, Silen A, et al. Immunotargeting with monoclonal cytokeratin 8 antibodies of human urothelial cancer transplanted to nude mice. Acta Oncol 1993;32:793.
81. Harney JV, Wahl RL, Liebert M, et al. Uptake of 2-deoxy,2-(18F)fluoro-D-glucos in bladder cancer: animal localization and initial patient positron emission tomography. J Urol 1991;145:279.
82. Harney JV, Liebert M, Wedemeyer G, et al. The expression of epider-

mal growth factor receptor on human bladder cancer: potential use in radioimmunoscintigraphy. J Urol 1991;1467:227.
83. Fradet Y, Friede J, Guertin B, et al. Radioimmunodetection of human bladder tumor xenografts in nude mice with radiolabeled monoclonal antibodies. J Urol 1992;148:418.
84. Ehrlichman C, Wu A. Resistance of MGH-U1 bladder cancer spheroids to vincristine. Anticancer Res 1992;12:1233.
85. Theodorescu D, Connors KM, Groce A, et al. Lack of influence of c-Ha-ras expression on the drug sensitivity of human bladder cancer histocultured in three-dimensions. Anticancer Res 1993;13:941.
86. Brown R, Clugston C, Burns P, et al. Increased accumulation of p53 protein in cisplatin-resistant ovarian cell lines. Int J Cancer 1993; 55678.
87. Glaves D, Hitt S, Raghavan D. Cisplatin-sensitivity does not correlate with p53 expression and apoptosis in human bladder cancer. Submitted for publication.
88. Satoh M, Kloth DM, Kadhim SA, et al. Modulation of both cisplatin nephrotoxicity and drug resistance in murine bladder tumor by controlling metallothionein synthesis. Cancer Res 1993;53:1829.
89. Lee K-E, Mayer RD, Cockett ATK. Effect of systemic glutathione depletion by buthionine sulfoximine on sensitivity of murine bladder cancer to cytotoxic agents. Urology 1989;34:376.
90. Cho Y-H, Straight RC, Smith JA. Effects of photodynamic therapy in combination with intravesical drugs in a murine bladder tumor model. J Urol 1992;147:743.
91. Keane TE, Gingrich JR, Rosner G, et al. Combination versus single agent therapy in effecting complete therapeutic response in human bladder cancer: analysis of cisplatin and/or 5-fluorouracil in an in vivo survival model. Cancer Res 1994;54:475.
92. Wilmanns C, Fan D, O'Brian CA, et al. Orthotopic and ectopic organ environments differentially influence the sensitivity of murine colon carcinoma cell to doxorubicin and 5-fluorouracil. Int J Cancer 1992; 52:98.
93. Bachor R, Flotte TJ, Scholz M, et al. Comparison of intravenous and intravesical administration of chloro-aluminum sulfated phthalocyanine for photodynamic treatment in a rat bladder cancer model. J Urol 1992;147:1404.
94. Russell PJ, Plomley J, Ho Shon I, et al. Monoclonal antibodies for intravesical radioimmunotherapy of human bladder cancer. Cell Biophys 1993;22:27.
95. Bamias A, Keane P, Krausz T, Williams G, Epenetos AA. Intravesical administration of radiolabeled antitumor monoclonal antibody in bladder carcinoma. Cancer Res 1991;51:724.
96. Bamias A, Keane P, Krausz T, et al. Intravesical administration of indium-111-labelled HMFG2 monoclonal antibody in superficiaial bladder carcinomas. Int J Cancer 1993;54:899.
97. deHarven E, Fradet Y, Connolly JG, et al. Antibody drug carrier for immunotherapy of superficial bladder cancer: ultrastructural studies. Cancer Res 1992;52:3131.
98. Wawrzynczak EJ, Henry RV, Cumber AJ, et al. Biochemical, cytotoxic and pharmacokinetic properties of an immunotoxin composed of a mouse monoclonal antibody Fib75 and the ribosome-inactivating protein alpha-sarcin from Aspergillus giganteus. Eur J Biochem 1991; 196:203.
99. Hirano A. Experimental and clinical study of intravesical BCG therapy: the role in the prevention of recurrence of superficial bladder tumor. Nippon Hinyokika Gakkai Zasshi 1992;83:1052.
100. Hudson MA, Brown EJ, Ritchey JK, Ratliff TL. Modulation of fibronectin-mediated bacillus Calmette-Guerin attachment to murine bladder mucosa by drugs influencing the coagulation pathways. Cancer Res 1991;51:3726.
101. Chung JY, Lee ES, Lee WJ, Kim HH, Min KJ, Lee C. Analysis of the immunologic mechanism of intravesical bacillus Calmette-Guerin therapy for superficial bladder tumors: distribution and function of immune cells. J Korean Med Sci 1993;8:135.
102. Schamhart DH, de Boer EC, Bevers RF, Kurth KH, Steerenberg PA. Mycobacterial adherence and BCG treatment of superficial bladder cancer. Prog Clin Biol Res 1992;378:75.
103. Prescott S, James K, Hargreave TB, et al. Intravesical Evans strain BCG therapy: quantitative immunohistochemical analysis of the immune reponse within the bladder wall. J Urol 1992;147:1636.
104. Ratliff TL. Role of the immune response in BCG for bladder cancer. Eur Urol 1992;21:17.
105. Ratliff TL, Ritchey JK, Yuan JJ, et al. T-cell subsets required for intravesical BCG immunotherapy for bladder cancer. J Urol 1993; 150:1018.
106. van Moorselaar RJA, Hendriks BTh, Borm G, et al. Inhibition of rat bladder tumor (RBT323) growth by tumor necrosis factor alpha and interferon-gamma in vivo. J Urol 1992;148:458.
107. Garden RJ, Liu BC, Redwood SM, et al. Bacillus Calmette-Guerin abrogates in vitro invasion and motility of human bladder tumor cells via fibronectin interaction. J Urol 1992;148:900.
108. Sarosdy MR, Hutzler DH, Yee D, von Hoff DD. In vitro sensitivity testing of human bladder cancers and cell lines to TP-40, a hybrid protein with selective targeting and cytotoxicity. J Urol 1993;150: 1950.
109. Theuer CP, FitzGerald DJ, Pastan I. A recombinant form of Pseudomonas exotoxin A containing transforming growth factor alpha near its carboxyl terminus for the treatment of bladder cancer. J Urol 1993; 149:1626.
110. Hara I, Sato N, Kikuchi K, Kamidono S. Immune response against BCG 65 kDa protein antigen in bladder cancer with BCG instillation therapy: analyses carried out with the gene of this protein to develop a monoclonal antibody. Nippon Hinyokika Gakkai Zasshi 1991;82: 24.
111. Connor J, Bannerji R, Saito S, Heston W, Fair W, Gilboa E. Regression of bladder tumors in mice treated with interleukin 2 gene-modified tumor cells. J Exp Med 1993;177:1127.
112. Lee SS, Eisenlohr LC, McCue PA, et al. Intravesical gene therapy: in vivo gene transfer using recombinant Vaccinia virus vectors. Cancer Res 1994;54:3325.
113. Fan Z, Baselga J, Masui, H, Mendelsohn J. Antitumor effect of anti-epidermal growth factor receptor monoclonal antibodies plus cis-diamminechloroplatinum on well-established A431 cell xenografts. Cancer Res 1993;53:4637.
114. Baselga J, Norton L, Masui H, et al. Antitumor effects of doxorubicin in combination with anti-epidermal growth factor receptor monoclonal antibodies. J Natl Cancer Inst 1993;85:1327.
115. Aaltonen LA, Peltomaki P, de la Chapelle A, et al. Clue to the pathogenesis of familial colorectal cancer. Science 1993;260:812.
116. Gonzalez-Zulueta M, Ruppert JM, Tokino K, et al. Microsatellite instability in bladder cancer. Cancer Res 1993;53:5620.
117. Bourdrel L, Lin CH, Lauren SL, et al. Recombinant human transforming growth factor-beta 1: expression by Chinese hamster ovary cells, isolation, and characterization. Protein Expr Purif 1993;4:130.
118. Geiser AG, Burmester JK, Webbink R, Roberts AB, Sporn MB. Inhibition of growth by transforming growth factor-beta following fusion of two nonresponsive human carcinoma cell lines: implication of the type II receptor in growth inhibitory responses. J Biol Chem 1992; 267:2588.
119. Rodeck U, Williams N, Murthy U, Herlyn M. Monoclonal antibody 425 inhibits growth stimulation of carcinoma cells by exogenous EGF and tumor-derived EGF/TGF-alpha. J Cell Biochem 1990;44:69.
120. Gleave ME, Hsish JT, Wu HC, et al. Epidermal growth factor receptor-mediated autocrine and paracrine stimulation of human transitional cell carcinoma. Cancer Res 1993;53:5300.
121. Kuranami M, Yamaguchi K, Fuchigami M, et al. Effects of urine on clonal growth of human bladder cancer cell lines. Cancer Res 1991; 51:4631.
122. Gavrilovic J, Moens G, Thiery JP, Jouanneau J. Expression of transfected transforming growth factor alpha induces a motile fibroblast-like phenotype with extracellular matrix-degrading potential in a rat bladder carcinoma cell line. Cell Regulation 1990;1:1003.
123. Neal DE, Mellon K. Epidermal growth factor receptor and bladder cancer: a review. Urol Int 1992;48:365.
124. Wood DP Jr, Fair WR, Chaganti RS. Evaluation of epidermal growth factor receptor DNA amplification and mRNA expression in bladder cancer. J Urol 1992;147:274.
125. Lonn U, Lonn S, Nylen U, et al. Gene amplification detected in carcinoma cells from human urinary bladder washings by the polymerase chain reaction method. Cancer 1993;71:3605.
126. Moriyama M, Akiyama T, Yamamoto T, et al. Expression of c-erbB-2 gene product in urinary bladder cancer. J Urol 1991;145:423.
127. Asamoto M, Hasegawa R, Masuko T, et al. Immunohistochemical analysis of c-erbB-2 oncogene product and epidermal growth factor receptor expression in human urinary bladder carcinomas. Acta Pathol Jpn 1990;40:322.
128. Lipponen P, Eskelinen M, Syrjanen S, Tervahauta A, Syrjanen K.

Use of immunohistochemically demonstrated c-erb B-2 oncoprotein expression as a prognostic factor in transitional cell carcinoma of the urinary bladder. Eur Urol 1991;20:238.
129. Serio G. c-erbB-2 gene product-like expression in urothelial carcinomas of the human bladder: its value as a prognostic indicator in superficial tumors. Pathologica 1991;83:413.
130. Wood DP Jr, Wartinger DD, Reuter V, Cordon-Cardo C, Fair WR, Chaganti RS. DNA, RNA and immunohistochemical characterization of the HER-2/neu oncogene in transitional cell carcinoma of the bladder. J Urol 1991;146:1398.
131. Boyer B, Thiery JP. Cyclic AMP distinguishes between two functions of acidic FGF in a rat bladder carcinoma cell line. J Cell Biol 1993; 120:767.
132. Bellusci S, Boyer B, Broders F, et al. Adhesion and mobility of embryonic and tumoral cells. Pathol Biol (Paris) 1992;40:779.
133. Chopin DK, Caruelle JP, Colombel M, et al. Increased immunodetection of acidic fibroblast growth factor in bladder cancer, detectable in urine. J Urol 1993;150:1126.
134. Allen LE, Maher PA. Expression of basic fibroblast growth factor and its receptor in an invasive bladder carcinoma cell line. J Cell Physiol 1993;155:368.
135. Nguyen M, Watanabe H, Budson AE, et al. Elevated levels of an angiogenic peptide, basic fibroblast growth factor, in the urine of patients with a wide spectrum of cancers. J Natl Cancer Inst 1994; 86:356.61.
136. Iwamura M, Ishibe M, Sluss PM, Cockett AT. Characterization of insulin-like growth factor I binding sites in human bladder cancer cell lines. Urol Res 1993;21:27.
137. Xu BH, Gupta V, Singh SV. Mechanism of differential sensitvity of human bladder cancer cells to mitomycin C and its analogue. Br J Cancer 1994;69:242.
138. Xu BH, Gupta V, Singh SV. Mitomycin C sensitivity in human bladder cancer cells: possible role of glutathione and glutathione transferase in resistance. Arch Biochem Biophys 1994;308:164.
139. Shinohara N, Liebert M, Wedemeyer G, et al. Evaluation of multiple drug resistance in human bladder cancer cell lines. J Urol 1993;150: 505.
140. Usansky JI, Liebert M, Wedemeyer G, et al. The uptake and efflux of doxorubicin by a sensitive human bladder cancer cell line and its doxorubicin-resistant subline. Sel Cancer Ther 1991;7:139.
141. Floyd JW, Lin C-W, Prout GR. Multi-drug resistance of a doxorubicin-resisitant bladder cancer cell line. J Urol 1990;144:169.
142. Kimaya K, Naito S, Naotaka T, et al. Establishment and characterization of doxorubicin-resistant human bladder cancer cell line, KK47/ ADM. J Urol 1992;148:441.
143. Bedford P, Fichtinger-Schepman MJ, Shellard SA, et al. Differential repair of platinum-DNA adducts in human bladder and testicular tumor continuous cell lines. Cancer Res 1988;48:3019.
144. Kotoh S, Naito S, Yokomizo J, et al. Increased expression of DNA topoisomerase I gene and collateral sensitivity to camptothecin in human cisplatin-resistant bladder cancer cells. Cancer Res 1994;54: 3248.
145. Rangel R, Niell H, Miller A, Cox C. Taxol and taxotere in bladder cancer: in vitro activity and urine stability. Cancer Chemother Pharmacol 1994;33:460.
146. Seraphim LA, Perrapato SD, Slocum HK, et al. In vitro study of the interaction of doxorubicin, thiotepa, and mitomycin-C, agents used for intravesical chemotherapy of superficial bladder cancer. J Urol 1991;145:613.
147. PressacoJ, Ehrlichman C. Combination studies with 3′azido-3′deoxythymidine (AZT) plus ICI D 1694. Biochem Pharmacol 1993;46:1989.
148. Kunugi KA, Lindstrom MJ, Kinsella TJ. Effects of bleomycin with iododeoxyuridine, 5′-amino-5-deoxythymidine, and radiation in a human bladder cancer cell line. Radiat Res 1993;135:262.
149. Chi K-H, Kunugi KA, Kinsella TJ. Iododeoxyuridine chemosensitization of cis-diamminechloroplatinum (II) in human bladder cancer cells. Cancer Res 1994;54:2701.
150. Fingert HJ, Pu AT, Chen Z, et al. In vivo and in vitro enhanced antitumor effects by pentoxyfylline in human cancer cells treated with thiotepa. Cancer Res 1988;48:4375.
151. Tolentino M, Okunaka T, Eckhauser ML, et al. A new porphyrin photosensitizer (PH1008) in model membranes, normal cells, and bladder cancer cells. J Urol 1992;148:1338.
152. Matzkin H, Rangel M, Soloway MS. In vitro study of the effect of hyperthermia on normal bladder cell line and on five different transitional cell carcinoma cell lines. J Urol 1992;147:1671.

Principles and Practice of Genitourinary Oncology, edited by Derek Raghavan, Howard I. Scher, Steven A. Leibel, and Paul H. Lange. Lippincott-Raven Publishers, Philadelphia, © 1997.

CHAPTER 18

Pathology of Bladder Cancer

Sonny L. Johansson and Samuel M. Cohen

The incidence of bladder cancer has steadily risen in the United States, with more than 50,000 cases diagnosed annually. At least 90% of bladder cancers are urothelial (transitional cell) carcinoma, and approximately 5% are squamous cell carcinoma (SCC), the remainder being adenocarcinoma, small cell carcinoma, undifferentiated carcinoma, and, rarely, different types of soft tissue sarcoma, especially rhabdomyosarcoma and leiomyosarcoma (Table 18-1).

PAPILLOMA

Inverted papilloma, a benign tumor that comprises less than 2% of bladder tumors, has a male-to-female ratio of 5:1 and a peak incidence in the sixth decade.[1] The major clinical symptoms include painless gross hematuria and urinary obstruction. The gross appearance is that of a 1- to 2-cm smooth, nodular, or polypoid tumor that histologically is composed of anastomosing cords of urothelial cells extending deep into the lamina propria. The cords often have palisading cells in the periphery, and small cystic spaces are commonly seen. The tumor cells are bland and lack significant anaplasia, and mitoses are virtually nonexistent (Fig. 18-1) The tumor is covered by urothelium, which can be of normal thickness, atrophic, or hyperplastic. A second variant of inverted papilloma resembles a hypertrophic tumor-like variant of cystitis glandularis with tall, mucous-containing columnar cells.[1] The clinician must distinguish inverted papilloma from carcinoma. Inverted papilloma generally has a bland cytologic appearance lacking mitotic figures. If dysplasia and mitoses are identified, especially with focal squamous features and keratinization, the lesion represents carcinoma with an inverted pattern. The treatment for inverted papilloma, transurethral resection of the tumor, results in cure.

The everted type of papilloma is defined as a papillary tumor with a central fibrovascular core lined by no more than seven layers of normal-appearing urothelial cells, including a normal umbrella cell layer[2] (Fig. 18-2.) This benign, solitary tumor is seen in younger individuals than those with bladder cancer and does not seem to be associated with recurrence or increased risk of bladder cancer.

UROTHELIAL CARCINOMA

Urothelial carcinomas may appear as single or multiple (25%) lesions. Two broad categories exist, papillary and nonpapillary. By cystoscopy, the papillary tumors have the appearance of seaweed "protruding into the lumen of the bladder." Other gross features include sessile, nodular, and ulcerated masses. Approximately 60% of bladder tumors are located in the lateral and posterior walls, whereas 20% occur in the trigone.

Papillary urothelial carcinomas comprise almost 80% of all newly diagnosed bladder cancers; they are often multiple and have a significant propensity for recurrence (57% to 85%). The role of the pathologist includes evaluation of tumor type, grading, staging, identification of vascular invasion, and associated carcinoma in situ (CIS).

The two most commonly used grading systems are the World Health Organization (WHO) system and the one originally described by Bergkvist and associates or a later modification.[3–5] The WHO system includes grades 1 to 3 and undifferentiated carcinoma. Although the system is simple, it lacks specific histologic and cytologic criteria. Grade 1 represents the most well-differentiated tumor, that is, with the least cellular atypia diagnostic of cancer, and grade 3 the worst, but still recognizable as a transitional cell carcinoma (TCC). The Bergkvist system gives more detailed criteria for malignancy grading based on deviation from the normal cellular pattern. The modified version of the Bergkvist system divides the heterogenous grade 2 group into 2A and 2B. In grade 2A, the impression of order dominates over disorder, whereas in grade 2B, the opposite is the case. The WHO system can easily be translated into the Bergkvist system. WHO grade 1 is Berkgvist grade 1 + 2A, WHO grade 2 is Bergvist grade 2B, WHO grade 3 is Bergvist grade 3, and WHO undifferentiated carcinoma is Bergvist grade 4 (Figs. 18-3 through 18-6). Grading is subjective, and reproducibility may be as low as 50% when different pathologists review the sections; intraobserver variation in grading is also common.[6–9] Promising, more objective computer-based grading methods using-object based and textural analysis are being developed, however.[10,11]

Consensus does not exist on the classification of everted pap-

Table 18-1. *Classification of urinary bladder tumors*

EPITHELIAL NEOPLASMS
TRANSITIONAL CELL (UROTHELIAL) NEOPLASMS
Papilloma
Inverted
Everted
Carcinoma
Papillary
Nonpapillary (solid)
Carcinoma in situ and possible presursor lesions
Variants of transitional cell carcinóma
Transitional cell carcinoma with gland-like lumina
Transitional cell carcinoma, nested type
Lymphoepithelial carcinoma
Micropapillary carcinoma
SQUAMOUS CELL CARCINOMA
Conventional type
Verrucous type
VILLOUS ADENOMA
ADENOCARCINOMA
Papillary, glanular, mucinous, signet ring cell and clear cell carcinoma (and mixtures)
Spindle cell carcinoma (sarcomatoid carcinoma)
SMALL CELL CARCINOMA (NEUROENDOCRINE CARCINOMA)
MIXED CARCINOMA
OTHER EPITHELIAL NEOPLASMS
Carcinosarcoma
Carcinoid tumor
SARCOMAS
LYMPHOMAS

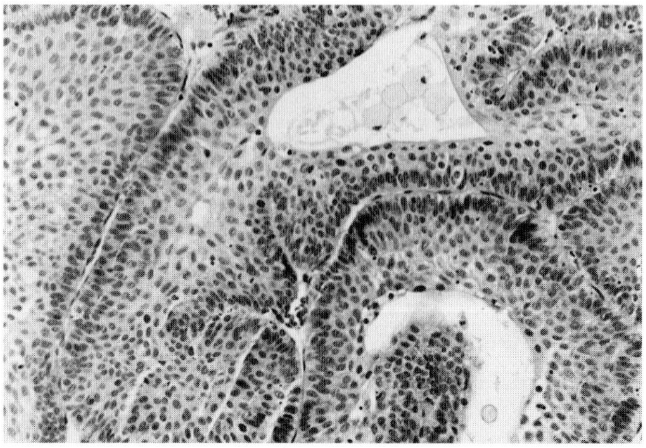

FIG. 18-1. Inverted papilloma showing cores of urothelial cells with bland nuclear features. Note the tendency to pallisading at the periphery and the presence of cystic spaces. H&E stain; original magnification × 140.

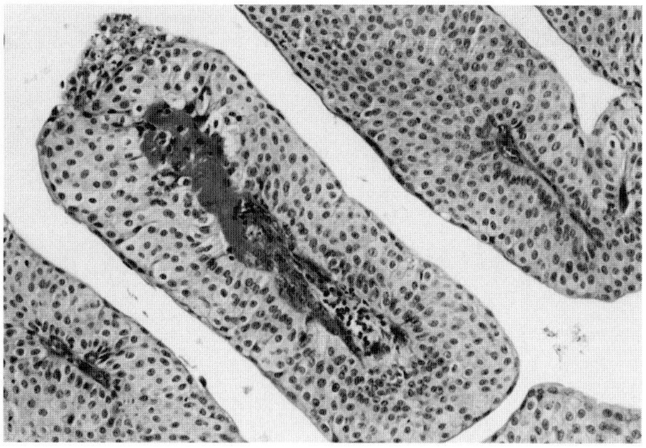

FIG. 18-2. Fragment of urothelial papilloma. The fibrovascular core is lined by normal-appearing urothelial cells less than seven layers thick. H&E stain; original magnification ×280.

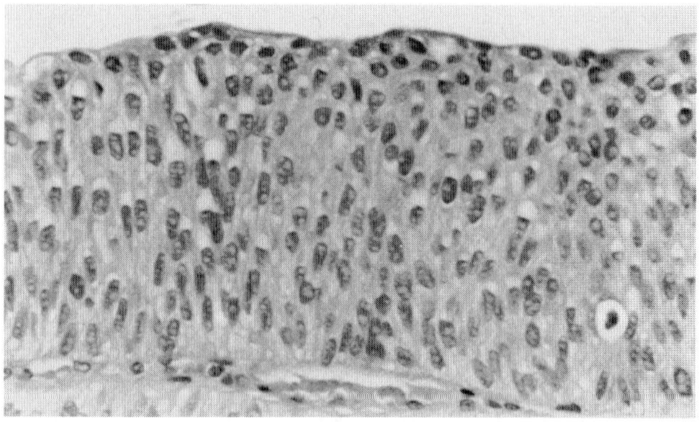

FIG. 18-3. Urothelial carcinoma grade 1. Note the preserved polarity of the bland urothelial cells with minimum nuclear atypia. H&E stain; original magnification ×280.

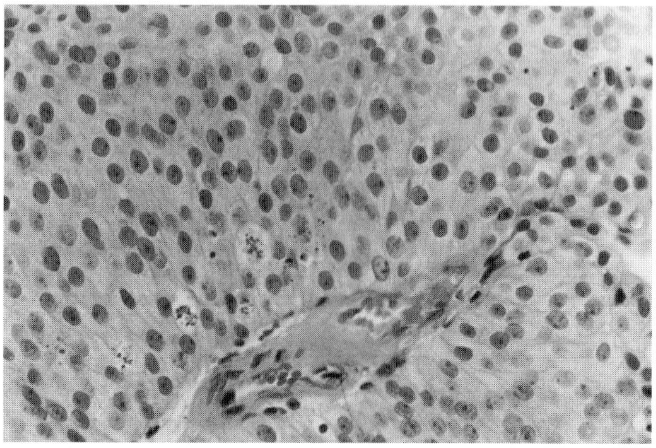

FIG. 18-4. Urothelial carcinoma grade 2A. Note the slightly increased nuclear variability and hyerchromaticity, but the impression of order is still evident. H&E stain; original magnification ×280.

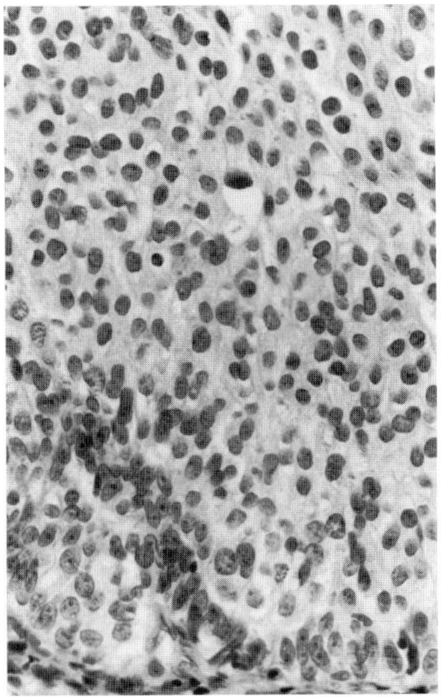

FIG. 18-5. Urothelial tumor grade 2B showing increased nuclear variability. The impression of disorder dominates. H&E stain; original magnification ×280.

illoma and papillary carcinoma grades 1 and 2A (WHO grade 1); the latter has sometimes been included in the category of papilloma or has been classified as a form of papillary hyperplasia. This issue is of limited clinical significance because, in our experience, Bergkvist grade 1 tumors do not infiltrate, and fewer than 3% of grade 2A tumors invade. All three types are treated with transurethral resection of bladder, the main difference being that papillary tumors grades 1 and 2 often recur or progress to a higher grade, whereas papillomas do not. Among patients with papillary Ta or T1 tumors, 4% to 30% progress with muscle invasion. The clinician not only must distinguish between Ta and T1 tumors because of the difference in prognosis, but also must try to determine the depth of lamina propria invasion, because invasion to the level of muscularis mucosa or deeper is associated with a worse prognosis than is superficial lamina propria invasion.[12,13] The following factors are important predictors for recurrence, progression, and prognosis of papillary urothelial tumors: (1) high grade; (2) interruption of basement membrane; (3) invasion into or below the level of the muscularis mucosa; (4) detrusor muscle involvement; (5) high mitosis density; (6) small vessel invasion (lymphatic or blood vessel); (7) tentacular invasion; (8) associated CIS; and (9) tumor size and multiplicity.

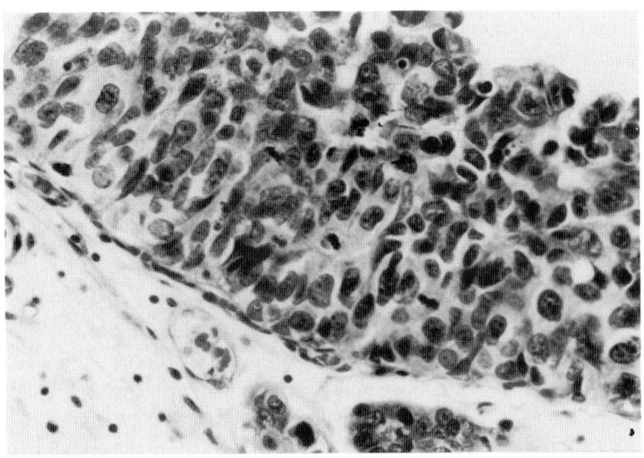

FIG. 18-6. Urothelial carcinoma grade 3. Note marked variability in size and shape of nuclei, hyperchromaticity, and markedly disturbed polarity. The impression of disorder is striking. H&E stain; original magnification ×280.

The 5-year survival is approximately 90% for patients with Ta tumors and 75% for patents with T1 tumors. Therefore, the term ''superficial tumors'' used to include both these stages should be avoided.

The nonpapillary (solid) bladder tumors that comprise approximately 20% of all bladder tumors are invasive at the time of diagnosis, with muscle invasion present in 90% of the cases. CIS is common, whereas fewer than 20% of patients have a history of papillary urothelial carcinoma. Five-year survival is reported to be between 20% and 50% in patients with muscle-invasive tumors. Local spread involves regional lymph nodes, and distant metastases are found in bone, lungs, and liver.

UROTHELIAL DYSPLASIA AND CARCINOMA IN SITU

Urothelial dysplasia is associated with nuclear abnormalities; the epithelium may be of normal thickness, or it may be hyperplastic. Up to ten morphologic criteria have been used in the

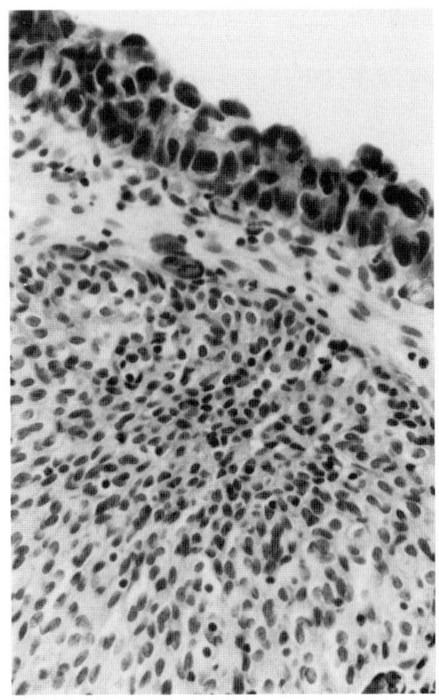

FIG. 18-7. Carcinoma in situ showing severe full-thickness dysplasia with markedly disburbed polarity and nuclear hyperchromaticity. Note adjacent von Brunn's nest with normal-appearing urothelium. H&E stain; original magnification ×280.

diagnosis of dysplasia.[14,15] These include changes in the number of cell layers, alteration of polarity, presence of mucosal denudation, cytoplasmic clearing, nuclear crowding, increased nuclear size, changes in chromatin pattern, nuclear irregularity, prominent nucleoli, and mitoses. All these criteria need not be present simultaneously.

The authors[14,15] used the terms *mild, moderate,* and *severe* dysplasia in analogy with the cervix. To achieve uniform international acceptance or reproducibility for this terminology has been difficult, however. Mostofi and Sesterhenn[16] suggested the term CIS, grades 1 and 2, for mild and moderate dysplasia, respectively, and grade 3 CIS for severe dysplasia and CIS. In a workshop on CIS, however, a panel of urologists and pathologists believed that the use of the terms CIS grades 1 and 2 should be discouraged because such terminology may result in unwarranted, aggressive treatment.[17] Furthermore, the biologic significance of dysplasia remains to be determined. In CIS, the entire thickness of the urothelium, which may be thinner than normal, of normal thickness, or hyperplastic, is replaced by a population of malignant cells (Fig. 18-7.)

The lesion is commonly seen in patients with high-grade TCC, especially of the papillary type with involvement of distal ureters, urethra, and prostatic ducts.[18,19] Primary CIS without associated urothelial tumor comprises fewer than 10% of the cases. It is characteristically diagnosed in men older than 50 years and may be associated with irritative bladder symptoms. The majority of these patients have malignant cytologic features, and the lesion is multifocal. The majority of patients develop invasive carcinoma within 3 years of diagnosis if the disease is untreated. The cystoscopic appearance shows a velvety, reddish mucosa. Because of reduced cohesiveness of the tumor cells, biopsy specimens of denuded mucosa may have only a few malignant cells, and frequently, urine cytologic examination is more accurate in determining the diagnosis.

FLOW CYTOMETRY

Many institutions use DNA analysis for determination of ploidy and proliferation function (S phase) in addition to conventional pathologic evaluation. Both flow cytometric and image analysis can be performed on exfoliated cells from bladder washings, fresh biopsy specimens, and archival, formalin-fixed, paraffin-embedded material. Voided urine specimens are less well suited because of poor cellularity and degenerative changes resulting in inadequate resolution of DNA with flow cytometry. Flow cytometry is more sensitive than cytology in the diagnosis of bladder cancer, although the value is less in the diagnosis than in the follow-up of patients with bladder carcinoma, especially in the evaluation of conservatively treated Ta and T1 tumors. Many institutions perform both DNA analysis and urine cytology. The majority of investigations evaluating DNA ploidy have shown abnormal ploidy to be associated with increased risk of recurrence, progression, and impaired prognosis.[20,21] DNA ploidy has not been shown to be a prognostic factor in muscle-invasive bladder cancer, however.[22]

TUMOR MARKERS

The blood group antigens, A, B, their precursor, H, and related antigens, such as variants of the Lewis antigens, are found on the surface of epithelial cells. Their presence depends on the secretor status. Approximately 85% of individuals are secretors, thus expressing ABH antigen in the normal urothelium. The deletion of these antigens has been reported to correlate with prognosis, but the prognostic significance is inferior to grade and stage.[23–26] Overall, ABH and Lewis antigens have not proved reliable independent prognostic factors and are not used in routine evaluations of bladder cancer.

Human chorionic gonadotropin (hCG) has been identified in bladder cancer, and increased serum levels have been found to predict metastases.[27,28] An immunohistochemical study showed increasing expression of hCG in tumors of higher grade. The expression also correlated to prognosis in one study,[29] whereas another study failed to show a correlation.[22]

With regard to proliferation markers, the antibody Ki-67, which is expressed in all phases of the cell cycle except G0, has been found to correlate to prognosis, especially within WHO grade 2 tumors.[30] A close correlation also exists with grade and stage.[31] One drawback is that the antibodies to Ki-67 only work on frozen tissue. A monoclonal antibody, Ki-S1, functions both on frozen and formalin-fixed tissue and is an independent prognostic factor in breast cancer.[32] It has yet to be tested in bladder cancer. Proliferating cell nuclear antigen (PCNA) was developed in 1978 and is synthesized especially during late G1 and S phases. The newest PCNA antibody, MO AG PC10, developed in 1991, can be used on formalin-fixed material. Lipponen and Eskelinen found it to correlate strongly with prognosis in bladder cancer.[33] Epidermal growth factor (EGF), which is present in urine, and EGF receptor (EGFR), have correlated with high tumor stage and poor patient outcome. In a multivariant analysis, however, EGFR was not found to be independent from stage.[34]

The P53 protein can stop cell proliferation, to allow repair of damaged DNA. Activation of the *P53* gene results in cell proliferation, and mutation of *P53* is involved in various human cancers. The *P53* gene is located on chromosome 17. The mutated *P53* gene has a prolonged half-life, and the mutated protein can be identified by immunohistochemistry. Lipponen found expression of P53 antigen to be prognostically significant except in superficial bladder cancer,[35] whereas Fosså and associates[22] failed to demonstrate any significant difference in prognosis between P53-positive and P53-negative muscle-invasive bladder cancer. Defects in chromosome 9, in the p arm, the q arm, or both, are frequently present in noninvasive papillary bladder tumors. In contrast, high-grade invasive TCC usually contains a defect in chromosome 17 that represents an abnormality in the *P53* gene.[36] Chromosome 9 abnormalities are uncommon in stage Ta, T1, high-grade papillary TCC or CIS. In the few examined patients with simultaneous papillary low-grade TCC and CIS, an abnormal chromosome 9 was identified in the former, and a *P53* abnormality was noted in the latter.

These differences in *P53* expression and chromosome 9 abnormality provide additional evidence that bladder cancer is two different diseases. Spruck and colleagues suggested two different pathways leading to the formation of noninvasive bladder cancer.[37] Thus, *P53* gene activation seems to occur early in CIS, a hypothesis supported by the finding that *P53* mutations were found in patients with CIS without any previous history of bladder cancer, and many of these patients did not have detectable loss of either chromosome 9 or 17. In contrast, chromosome 9 alterations may be sufficient for superficial papillary tumors to develop. Probably, progression of superficial papillary tumors or CIS requires subsequent acquisition of defects in chromosome 9 or 17.[37] Other chromosomal alterations, identified especially in high-grade invasive TCC, involve chromosomes 3, 5, 7, 8, 10, 11, and 13. Some of these abnormalities most likely represent late secondary changes related to increasing genetic instability of DNA with progression of malignancy.[38,39]

SQUAMOUS CELL CARCINOMA

SCC comprises 3% to 8% of all bladder tumors in the Western world, with an age and sex distribution similar to that of TCC. In many areas with endemic schistosomiasis, such as Egypt, SCC comprises approximately two thirds of all bladder cancer cases. Other risk factors include urinary tract infection, long-term use of an indwelling catheter, and lithiasis. The conventional type of SCC is generally an ulcerating and invasive tumor, rather than an exophytic lesion. The histologic appearance is identical to that of SCC elsewhere. The majority of tumors are grade 2 to 3. Keratinizing squamous metaplasia in other parts of the bladder has been identified in up to 25% of patients. Because the majority of patients present with high-stage disease, 5-year survival is poor, varying between 7% and 20%.[18] The verrucous type of SCC originally described in the oral cavity rarely occurs in the bladder. The gross appearance is like that of cauliflower. Histologic features include well-differentiated squamous epithelium without significant dysplasia lining "church spiral-like" fibrovascular cores. The tumor is well circumscribed, with pushing borders, and is locally aggressive but does not metastasize.

UNDIFFERENTIATED CARCINOMA

Undifferentiated carcinoma includes spindle cell (sarcomatoid) carcinoma and small cell carcinoma (neuroendocrine carcinoma). TCC, SCC, and adenocarcinoma can present as poorly differentiated spindle cell tumors with a sarcomatoid appearance. The tumors are frequently polypoid, and the carcinomatous elements may be TCC, SCC, adenocarcinoma, small cell carcinoma, or a mixture of these types. The spindle cells commonly blend with malignant epithelial cells. Flat CIS may be present. If epithelial elements and CIS are not identified by routine stains, immunohistochemical staining with antibodies against keratin and epithelial membrane antigen (EMA) may be helpful in distinguishing these tumors from true sarcomas.[40]

Small cell carcinoma of the bladder, which is identical to its pulmonary counterpart, was first reported in 1981.[41] The incidence varies between 0.5% and 1% of all bladder tumors.[42,43] Approximately 56% are pure small cell carcinomas at the time of biopsy. The remaining are combined with TCC, SCC, adenocarcinoma, or various combinations of tumor type. Both oat cell and intermediate cell variants have been described. The majority of these tumors stain positive with antibodies against neuron-specific enolase, keratin, and synaptophysin, and dense core granules can be identified by electron microscopy. Prognosis is poor, and only 10 of 115 reported patients have survived for 2 years.[43]

ADENOCARCINOMA

Adenocarcinoma comprises approximately 1% of bladder tumors and has, like other types of bladder cancer, a male predominance. Predisposing factors include bladder exstrophy, nonfunctional bladder, and schistosomiasis. Approximately one third of these cases originate in the urachus, the remainder elsewhere in the bladder. Adenocarcinomas are almost always solitary tumors. Histologically, most of these lesions are glandular, mucinous, or papillary, but signet ring cell carcinoma and clear cell carcinoma have also been reported. In approximately half the patients, more than one adenocarcinoma pattern is identified. The differential diagnosis includes secondary involvement of the bladder with colorectal, gynecologic, or prostatic carcinoma. Adenocarcinomas of the prostate almost invariably stain positive with antibodies against prostate-specific antigen and prostatic acid phosphatase, whereas bladder adenocarcinomas stain negatively for these markers. The prognosis of adenocarcinoma is related in particular to tumor size and stage as well as to tumor type, with a 5-year survival rate varying between 6% and 33%. The most recent studies have not been able to identify a difference in prognosis between urachal and nonurachal adenocarcinomas.[44]

MIXED TUMORS

Bladder tumors with mixed differentiation are common, and all possible combinations have been reported. The most common type is a mixture of TCC and SCC. If a predominant pattern exists, for example, TCC, the case should be reported as TCC with areas of SCC. The predominant pattern is likely to determine the prognosis, with the possible exception of small cell and signet ring cell carcinoma. If the components are approximately equal, the tumor should be reported as a mixed tumor of the types of differentiation present.

CARCINOSARCOMA

Carcinosarcomas are malignant neoplasms composed of both carcinomatous and malignant mesenchymal elements. In the majority of cases, mesenchymal elements are chondroid or osteosarcomatous, mixed with TCC, less frequently with SCC or adenocarcinoma. The prognosis is poor, and patients are usually dead within 2 years from local recurrence or metastatic disease.[45]

SARCOMA

Leiomyosarcoma

Although rare, with only some 100 cases reported, leiomyosarcoma is the most common mesenchymal cancer of the bladder in adults. The morphologic criteria for distinguishing leiomyoma from leiomyosarcoma in the urinary bladder remain to be established, but Walker and associates stated that, "It seems prudent to label as leiomyosarcoma any smooth muscle neoplasm demonstrating infiltrative, destructive invasion of the vesicle musculature.''[45] Leiomyomas should only be reserved for circumscribed smooth muscle neoplasms displaying minimal cytological atypia and little or no mitotic activity. Bladder leiomyosarcomas are generally large tumors displaying a polypoid intraluminal component. They either show a gelatinous cut surface or have a ''fish flesh'' appearance. The histologic appearance is no different from that of leiomyosarcoma in other locations; thus, the tumor is composed of spindle cells with cigar-shaped nuclei that tend to form fascicles crossing each other perpendicularly. The tumors are moderately cellular, with few mitotic figures, although occasional tumors show marked pleomorphism with abundant mitoses. Some tumors show marked myxoid changes. The tumor cells stain positively with antibodies against muscle-specific actin and vimentin in most cases, with occasional desmin positivity while staining against epithelial membrane antigen EMA, and keratin is negative. The tumors are generally locally aggressive, and metastases have only rarely been reported.

Rhabdomyosarcoma

Urinary bladder rhabdomyosarcoma is mainly a tumor of the pediatric population, with a peak incidence at 5 years. Often the tumor appears as polypoid multiple masses with a glistening surface or as a large solitary mass. The tumors frequently show features of embryonal rhabdomyosarcoma with a characteristic cambium layer composed of rhabdomyoblasts below the urothelium. Below this condensed cambium layer, a more dispersed cell population is present in an edematous stroma; many of the cells are rhabdomyoblasts. The large, single masses often show a solid pattern or features of alveolar rhabdomyosarcoma.

LYMPHOMA

Primary lymphoma of the bladder is rare, with about 50 cases reported in the literature. The majority are non-Hodgkin's lymphoma, and most are of low or intermediate grade (60% and 33%, respectively). Patients with primary lymphoma of the bladder have a significantly better prognosis than individuals with secondary lymphoma.[18] The main histologic differential diagnosis is small cell undifferentiated carcinoma, which, however, usually shows focal keratin positivity and often expresses neuroendocrine markers such as neuron-specific enolase and synaptophysin; staining against leukocyte common antigen is negative.

PHEOCHROMOCYTOMA

Most of the more than 100 new cases of pheochromocytoma hitherto reported have occurred in people less than 50 years of age. Clinically, hypertensive episodes are common, and most patients have increased catecholamines in the serum and urine. Typically, the tumors are composed of nests of cells separated by a thin fibrovascular core. The individual tumor cells are uniform and polygonal, displaying amphophilic pale cytoplasm and well-defined cell borders. Focally, nuclear pleomorphism with bizarre cells may be identified, but malignant behavior is seen in less than 20% of these tumors. The morphologic appearance is not useful to predict the potential malignant behavior of pheochromocytoma.[18]

TUMOR-LIKE CONDITIONS OF THE URINARY BLADDER

Polypoid cystitis is a reactive lesion involving the bladder mucosa and is associated with indwelling catheter use. The lesions are generally located in the posterior wall or the dome of the bladder as a result of irritation by the tip of the catheter. Cystoscopically, the lesions may appear as bullous, polypoid, or papillary. The papillary lesions may, when examined by cystoscopy and light microscopy, mimic low-grade urothelial tumors, but generally they lack distinct fibrovascular cores, and the urothelium is not dysplastic. The umbrella cells are preserved, and microabscesses may be present in the urothelium.[46] Polypoid cystitis is a reversible lesion; thus, if the catheter is removed, the lesions will disappear.[47]

Pseudosarcoma has also been reported as inflammatory pseudotumor, pseudomalignant spindle cell proliferation, or postoperative spindle cell nodule. The term pseudosarcoma is preferred because the lesion may develop spontaneously, subsequent to or simultaneously with mucosal damage caused by transurethral resection, chronic cystitis, and TCC. The differential diagnosis is leiomyosarcoma, spindle cell carcinoma, or undifferentiated sarcoma. The lesions are generally poorly circumscribed, composed of spindle or strap-shaped cells with mild cellular and nuclear pleomorphism. Focally, some lesions may be indistinguishable from nodular fasciitis, whereas other, more cellular areas may show tightly packed fascicles. Features of nuclear enlargement and eosinophilic nucleoli are characteristic of reactive atypia, as further emphasized by the presence of inflammatory cells, especially neutrophils and sometimes eosinophils along with myxoid matrix and thin-walled capillaries, tissue resembling granulation tissue. The spindle cells express vimentin, often smooth muscle actin, muscle specific actin, and sometimes cytokeratin; staining for EMA is negative. Transurethral resection of the lesion results in cure without local recurrence.[48]

AMYLOIDOSIS

Amyloidosis may be primary or secondary and is associated with painless gross hematuria in 85% of patients. Cystoscopically, the lesion sometimes may be indistinguishable from a bladder tumor, but histologically, deposits of amyloid can be identified in the arteries, arterioles, and veins, as well as in the lamina propria and in the muscularis propria.[18]

REFERENCES

1. Kunze E, Schauer A, Schmitt M. Histology and histogenesis of two different types of inverted urothelial papillomas. Cancer 1983;51:348.
2. Koss LG. Tumors of the urinary bladder. In: Atlas of tumor pathology, 2nd series, fascicle 11. Washington, DC: Armed Forces Institute of Pathology, 1975.
3. Mostofi FK, Sobin LH, Torloni H. Histological typing of urinary bladder tumors. In: International Histological Classification of Tumors, No. 10. Geneva: World Health Organization, 1973.

4. Bergkvist A, Ljungqvist A, Moberger D. Classification of bladder tumors based on the cellular pattern. Acta Chir Scand 1965;130:378.
5. Malmström P-U, Busch C, Norlen BJ. Recurrence, progression and survival in bladder cancer. Scand J Urol Nephrol 1987;21:185.
6. Busch C, Engberg A, Norlén BJ, Stenkvist B. Malignancy grading of epithelial bladder tumors. Scand J Urol Nephrol 1977;11:143.
7. Ooms ECM, Anderson WAD, Alons CL, Boon ME, Veldhuizen RW. Analysis of the performance of pathologists in the grading of bladder tumors. Hum Pathol 1983;14:140.
8. Sherman A, Koss LG, Adams S. Interobserver and intraobserver differences in the diagnosis of urothelial cells: comparison with classification by computer. Anal Quant Cytol 1984;6:112.
9. Abel PD, Henderson D, Bennett MK, Hall RR, Williams G. Differing interpretations by pathologists of the pT category and grade of transitional cell cancer of the bladder. Br J Urol 1988;62:339.
10. Jarkrans T, Vaskó J, Bengtsson E, et al. Grading of transitional cell bladder carcinoma by object based image analysis of histological sections. Anal Cell Pathol 1995;8:135.
11. Choi H-K, Vaskó J, Bengtsson E, et al. Grading of transitional cell bladder carcinoma by texture analysis of histological sections. Anal Cell Pathol 1994;6:327.
12. Anderström C, Johansson SL, Nilsson S. The significance of lamina propria invasion on the prognosis of patients with urinary bladder tumors. J Urol 1980;124:23.
13. Younes M, Sussman J, True LD. The usefulness of the level of muscularis mucosae in the staging of invasive transitional cell carcinoma of the urinary bladder. Cancer 1990;66:543.
14. Nagy GK, Frable WJ, Murphy WM. Classification of premalignant urothelial abnormalities: a Delphi study of the National Bladder Cancer Collaborative Group A. Pathol Annu 1982;17:219.
15. Murphy WM, Soloway MS. Developing carcinoma (dysplasia) of the urinary bladder. Pathol Annu 1982;17:197.
16. Mostofi FK, Sesterhenn IA. Pathology of epithelial tumors and carcinoma in situ of bladder. Prog Clin Biol Res 1984;162A:55.
17. Friedell GH, Soloway MS, Hilgar AG. Summary of workshop on carcinoma in situ of the bladder. J Urol 1986;136:1047.
18. Peterson RO. Urologic pathology, 2nd ed. Philadelphia, JB Lippincott, 1992.
19. Ayala AG, Ro JY. Premalignant lesions of the urothelium and transitional cell tumors. In: Young RH, ed. Pathology of the urinary bladder. New York: Churchill Livingstone, 1989.
20. Melamed MR. Flow cytometry for detection and evaluation of urinary bladder carcinoma. Semin Surg Oncol 1992;8:300.
21. Al-Abadi H, Nagel R. Deoxyribonucleic acid content and survival rates of patients with transitional cell carcinoma of the bladder. J Urol 1994; 151:37.
22. Fosså SD, Berner AA, Jacobsen A-B, et al. Clinical significance of DNA-ploidy and S-phase fraction and their relation to p:53 protein, c-erb-B-2 protein and HCG in operable muscle invasive bladder cancer. Br J Cancer 1993;68:572.
23. Cordon-Cardo C, Reuter VE, Lloyd KO, et al. Blood group-related antigens in human urothelium: enhanced expression of precursor Le^x and Le^Y determinants in urothelial carcinoma. Cancer Res 1988;48: 4113.
24. Malmström P-U, Busch C, Norlén BJ, Andersson B. Expression of ABH blood group isoantigen as a prognostic factor in transitional cell bladder carcinoma. Scand J Urol Nephrol 1988;22:265.
25. Malmström P-U, Norlén BJ, Andersson B, Busch C. Combination of blood group ABH antigen status and DNA-ploidy as an independent prognostic factor in transitional cell carcinoma of the urinary bladder. Br J Urol 1989;64:49.
26. Pauwels RPE, Schapers RFM, Smeets AWGB, Jansen LEG, Debruyne FMJ, Geraedts JPM. Blood group isoantigen deletion and chromosomal abnormalities in bladder cancer. J Urol 1988;40:959.
27. Iles RK, Jenkins BJ, Oliver RTD, Blandy JP, Chard T. Beta human chorionic gonadotrophin in serum and urine: a marker for metastatic urothelial cancer. Br J Urol 1989;64:241.
28. Iles RK, Chard T. Human chorionic gonadotropin expression by bladder cancers: biology and clinical potential. J Urol 1991;145:453.
29. Seidal T, Breborowicz J, Malmström P-U, Busch C. Immunoreactivity to human chorionic gonadotropin in urothelial carcinoma: correlation with tumor grade stage and prognosis. J Urol Pathol 1993;1:397.
30. Mulder AH, van Hootegem JCSP, Sylvester R, et al. Prognostic factors in bladder carcinoma: histologic parameters and expression of a cell cycle-related nuclear antigen Ki-67. J Pathol 1992;166:37.
31. Bush C, Price P, Norton J, et al. Proliferation in human bladder carcinoma measured by Ki-67 antibody labelling: its potential clinical importance. Br J Cancer 1991;64:357.
32. Kreipe H, Alm P, Olsson H, Hauberg M, Fischer L, Parwaresch R. Prognostic significance of a formalin-resistant nuclear proliferation antigen in mammary carcinomas as determined by the monoclonal antibody Ki-S1. Am J Pathol 1993;142:651.
33. Lipponen PK, Eskelinen MJ. Cell proliferation of transitional cell bladder tumours determined by PCNA/cyclin immunostaining and its prognostic value. Br J Cancer 1992;66:171.
34. Nguyen PL, Swanson PE, Jaszcz W, et al. Expression of epidermal growth factor receptor in invasive transitional cell carcinoma of the urinary bladder. Am J Clin Pathol 1994;101:166.
35. Lipponen PK. Over-expression of p53 nuclear oncoprotein in transitional-cell bladder cancer and its prognostic value. Int J Cancer 1993; 53:365.
36. Olumi AF, Tsai YC, Nicholas PW, et al. Allelic loss of chromosome 17p distinguishes high grade from low grade transitional cell carcinomas of the bladder. Cancer Res 1990;50:7081.
37. Spruck CH, Ohneseit F, Gonzalez-Zuleta M, et al. Two molecular pathways to transitional cell carcinoma of the bladder. Cancer Res 1994; 54:784.
38. Miyao N, Tsai YC, Lerner SP, et al. Role of chromosome 9 in human bladder cancer. Cancer Res 1993;53:4066.
39. Knowles MA, Elder PA, Williamson M, Cairus JP, Shaw ME, Law MG. Allelotype of human bladder cancer. Cancer Res 1994;54:531.
40. Young RH. Unusual variants of primary bladder carcinoma and secondary tumors of the bladder. In: Young RH ed. Pathology of the urinary bladder. New York: Churchill Livingstone, 1989.
41. Cramer SF, Aikawa M, Cebelin M. Neurosecretory granules in small cell invasive carcinoma of the urinary bladder. Cancer 1981;47:724.
42. Murphy WM, Beckwith JB, Farrow GM. Tumors of the urinary bladder, urethra, ureters, renal pelvis and kidneys. In: Atlas of tumor pathology, 3rd series. Washington, DC: Armed Forces Institute of Pathology, 1995.
43. Holmäng S, Borghede G, Johansson SL. Primary small cell carcinoma of the urinary bladder: a report of 25 cases. J Urol 1995;153:1820.
44. Johansson SL, Anderström CRK. Primary adenocarcinoma of the urinary bladder and urachus. In: Williams CJ, Krikorian JG, Green MR, Raghavan D, eds. Textbook of uncommon cancers, 1st ed. Chichester, NY: John Wiley, 1988.
45. Walker AN, Mills SE, Young RH. Mesenchymal and miscellaneous other primary turmors of the urinary bladder. In: Young RH, ed. Pathology of the urinary bladder. New York: Churchill Livingstone, 1989.
46. Ekelund P, Johansson SL. Polypoid cystitis: a catheter associated lesion of the human bladder. Acta Pathol Microbiol Scand 1979;87A:179.
47. Ekelund P, Anderström C, Johansson SL, Larsson P. The reversibility of catheter associated polypoid cystitis. J Urol 1983;13:456.
48. Lundgren L, Aldenborg F, Angervall L, Kindblom L-G, et al. Pseudosarcomatous spindle cell proliferations in the urinary bladder of adults. Hum Pathol 1994;25:181.

Principles and Practice of Genitourinary Oncology, edited by Derek Raghavan, Howard I. Scher, Steven A. Leibel, and Paul H. Lange. Lippincott-Raven Publishers, Philadelphia, © 1997.

CHAPTER 19

Epidemiology and Etiology of Bladder Cancer

Zuo-Feng Zhang and Gunnar Steineck

Bladder cancer is the 11th most frequent cancer in the world. In 1985,[1] approximately 243,100 new cases of bladder cancer (181,700 males and 61,400 females) were reported, and 112,700 patients (82,000 males and 30,700 females) died of the disease in the same year.[2] Bladder cancer accounts for 3.2% of all newly diagnosed cases of cancer and for 2.4% of cancer deaths worldwide.

DESCRIPTIVE EPIDEMIOLOGY

International Variation

The age-standardized incidence rates are high in North America and Europe and are low in developing countries in Asia. Northern Africa and Western Asia are considered high-risk areas. The ratio of the highest to the lowest incidence in the world is close to 10:1 (Fig. 19-1). In the United States, bladder cancer is the fourth most common cancer in men and the ninth in women. According to American Cancer Society (ACS) estimates, in the United States in 1996 there will be 52,900 new cases (38,300 males and 14,600 females) and 11,700 (7800 males and 3900 females) deaths.[3]

Age, Sex, and Race

The age-specific incidence of bladder cancer for both white and black males increases sharply with age and peaks at 80 years of age or older. For women, the age-specific incidence rate also increases with age, but by smaller increments (Fig. 19-2). Bladder cancer is predominantly a tumor of males, with a gender ratio of about 3:1. The excess risk of male bladder cancer cannot be explained by gender differences in smoking and occupational exposures and may be attributed to hormonal factors or environmental and dietary exposures not yet identified.[4] Experimental data show that androgenic hormones stimulate carcinogenesis in bladder tissue, and estrogenic hormones have the opposite effect.[5,6] In an epidemiologic study, parous women were at decreased risk relative to nulliparous women after adjusting for age, tobacco use, and bladder infection.[7] Survival in males is better than in females, possibly because a greater proportion of men are diagnosed with localized disease. In the United States, the incidence rate of bladder cancer is approximately twofold higher in whites than in blacks.[8] The lifetime risk of bladder cancer is less than 4% for white men, and it is 1% or less for white women, black men, and black women.[8]

Time Trends

From 1973 to 1990, the incidence of bladder cancer in the United States increased at a rate of 0.7% per year; however, mortality decreased at an annual rate of 1.8%.[8] The annual increased incidence was 1% and 1.1% for white and black males, respectively. Females experienced less of an increase as reported by the Surveillance, Epidemiology and End Results (SEER) program (Fig. 19-3). This increase may partly be an artifact attributable to the rise in diagnosis of early bladder cancer (''lead time''),[8] or it may be due to changes in the risk-factor profile of the population.

SITE AND PATHOLOGY

The transitional cell epithelium covers all the lower urinary tract: the renal pelvis, ureter, urinary bladder, and urethra. Transitional cell carcinoma (urothelial cancer) occurs in all four sites, which probably all share a common origin. Available evidence suggests, however, that the magnitude of the relative risk of transitional cell carcinoma for certain carcinogenic agents changes with site. Varying urine concentration and contact time between urine and mucosa amid the four sites as well as the metabolism of carcinogenic agents in the urine may account for the difference in risk. For simplicity, we refer to studies of ''bladder cancer'' even if other sites of the lower urinary tract are included. Additionally, if not otherwise stated, we refer to transitional cell carcinoma.

Squamous cell differentiation is frequently seen intermixed with transitional cell carcinoma, but pure squamous cell carcinomas typically comprise fewer than 3% of all cases of urinary bladder cancer in Western countries. In certain developing countries, squamous cell carcinomas are much more common,

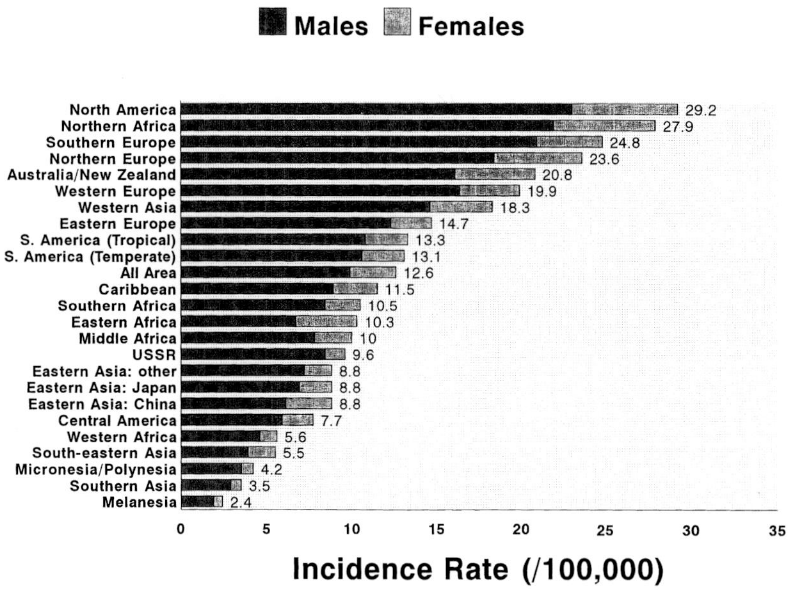

FIG. 19-1. Age-adjusted incidence rates of bladder cancer by sex and area, 1985. (Data adapted from Parkin DM, Pisani P, Ferlay J. Estimate of the world incidence of eighteen major cancers in 1985. Int J Cancer 1993; 54:594.)

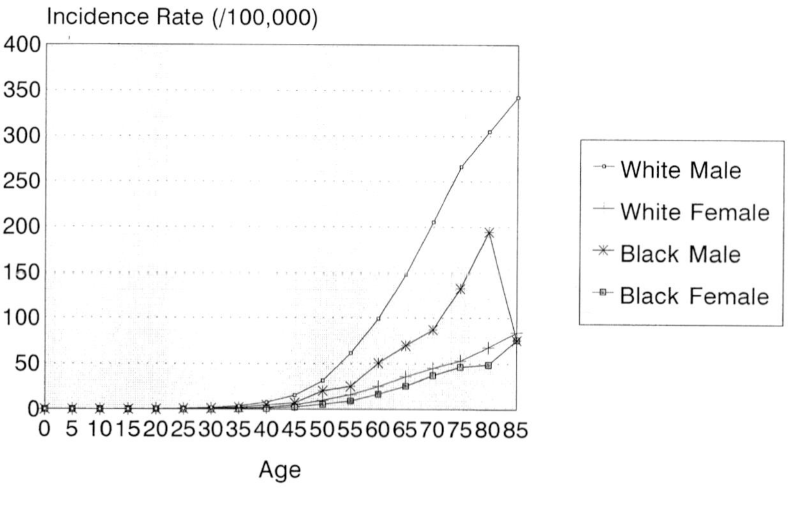

FIG. 19-2. Age distribution of bladder cancer incidence between 1986 and 1990. Note that incidence increases dramatically with age for men but less significantly for women. (Data adapted from Miller BA, Ries LAG, Hankey BF, et al. SEER cancer statistics review 1973–1990, NCI, NIH Pub. No. 93–2789, 1993.)

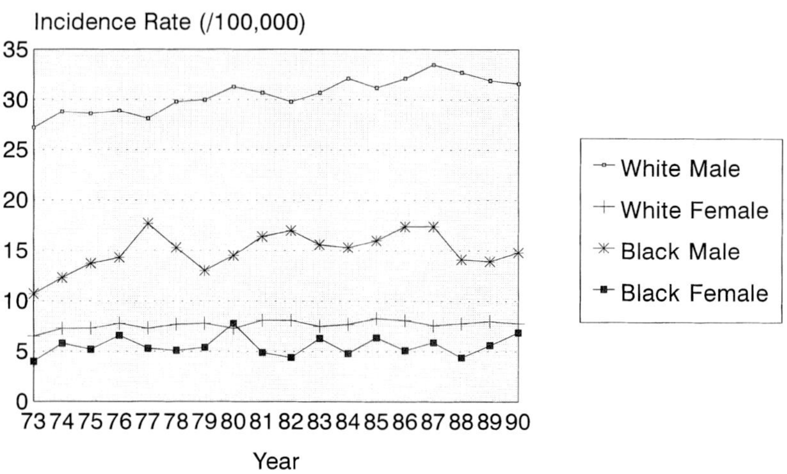

FIG. 19-3. Incidence of bladder cancer in blacks and whites by year from 1973 to 1990. Note that men experienced a higher incidence of the disease than women. (Data adapted from Miller BA, Ries LAG, Hankey BF, et al. SEER cancer statistics review 1973–1990, NCI, NIH Pub. No. 93–2789, 1993.)

as discussed later. Transitional cell cancer and squamous cell carcinoma probably share some etiologic agents. Cigarette smoking and urinary tract infections have been associated with both histopathologic subtypes, although the epidemiologic data for squamous cell carcinoma are sparse.

Pure adenocarcinomas in the urinary bladder comprise fewer than 1% of cases in Western countries. Sarcomas, lymphomas, and malignant melanomas occur infrequently. Conceivably, these histologic types are etiologically distinct from transitional cell carcinoma.[9]

ANALYTIC EPIDEMIOLOGY

Many different exposures and risk factors have been identified to increase the risk of bladder cancer. With few exceptions, however, conventional epidemiologic methods have proved insufficient to establish causality between exposure to possible carcinogenic agents and the incidence of bladder cancer. Strong associations, ''natural experiments'' with simplistic exposure patterns, or a large number of data are needed to establish causal links. Clearly, new research strategies are needed, but whether the advances in molecular biology may add to the understanding of the etiology of urinary bladder cancer is unconfirmed.

The only established exposure with a significant public health impact is tobacco smoking, but which carcinogenic agents are involved remains uncertain. The aromatic amines, including 2-naphthylamine, 4-aminobiphenyl, and benzidine, the drugs phenacetin (withdrawn from the United States market) and chlornaphazine, and external-beam radiotherapy have been causally linked to transitional cell carcinoma of the bladder. In this chapter, we mention risk groups and agents that may provide clues for the future identification of additional human bladder carcinogens and insight into the pathogenesis of the disease. Candidate carcinogens of public health importance include a dietary factor in meat (heterocyclic amines), an analgesic (acetaminophen), one or several chemicals found in exhausts and combustion gases (a polycyclic aromatic hydrocarbon) and infection with *Schistosoma haematobium*. We list agents causally linked to human bladder cancer and candidate carcinogens for the disease in Table 19-1.

Table 19-1. *Agents causally linked to human bladder cancer and candidate carcinogens for the disease*

AGENTS CAUSALLY LINKED TO HUMAN BLADDER CANCER
2-Naphthylamine
4-Aminobiphenyl
Benzidine
Chlornaphazine*
Phenacetin*
External-beam radiotherapy
CANDIDATE CARCINOGENS FOR HUMAN BLADDER CANCER
Acetaminophen
Benzene
Chlorinated aliphatic hydrocarbons
Heterocyclic amines
Nitrosamines
Polyaromatic hydrocarbons
Polychlorinated biphenyls

* No longer in use in the United States.

Tobacco Smoking

The richness of data collected in both prospective and retrospective settings supports the association between the extent of tobacco smoking and the incidence of bladder cancer.[22] In the United States, as in many other Western countries, tobacco smoking contributes to about half the bladder cancer cases among men and to about one third of those in women.[15]

Dose-Effect Relationship

Studies typically report a relative risk of 2 to 3 among current cigarette smokers, as compared with persons who have never smoked.[22] The dose-effect relationship for the amount of tobacco smoked is nonlinear. An approximation from available data indicates that an initial sharp increase in risk plateaus with a two- to threefold increase in risk for subjects smoking at least 10 cigarettes per day. This risk remains stable until the daily consumption rises to more than 40 to 60 cigarettes per day.

Type of Tobacco and Smoking Device

The two main types of tobacco are black (air-cured) tobacco, with high concentrations of aromatic amines, and blond (flue-cured) tobacco. Black tobacco is prepared differently from blond tobacco, and smokers of black tobacco have a two to three times higher risk of bladder cancer than those who smoke blond tobacco.[10–13] Smokers of low-tar and low-nicotine (''light'') cigarettes have a reduced risk, compared with smokers of high-tar and high-nicotine cigarettes.[14] Individuals who smoke unfiltered cigarettes seem to have up to 50% increased risk of bladder cancer, compared with those who smoke filtered cigarettes.[14–16] No one has been able to document that switching from unfiltered to filtered cigarettes reduces the risk, however.[15–17] This finding may imply that filters protect from early, but not late, stages of carcinogenesis. The difference in risk between pipe smokers and cigarette smokers in United States may be explained by smaller tobacco consumption and less inhalation among pipe smokers than among cigarette smokers.[18] Cigars, snuff, and chewing tobacco probably influence the risk of bladder cancer little, if any.[19]

Other Smoking Characteristics

Early age at smoking initiation probably increases the risk, as compared with a later age at initiation, after adjustment for the total amount smoked.[20] If confirmed, this finding may imply a higher susceptibility to carcinogenic agents in younger than in older age groups. Former smokers have a reduced risk compared with current smokers, but up to 10 years after smoking cessation, they still have an increased risk compared with those who have never smoked.[11,14,21–23] A possible mechanism may be that certain carcinogens in tobacco are involved in early stages of carcinogenesis, and these changes are repaired slowly, if ever. Other carcinogens are involved in later stages and a withdrawal retards the development of the malignant disease.

Tobacco-Related Carcinogens

The human bladder carcinogens 2-naphthylamine and 4-aminobiphenyl, and the suspected carcinogen *o*-toluidine, are present in tobacco.[22,24,25] In one study, DNA adducts of 4-aminobiphenyl were found in tumor samples from smokers, a finding indicating that this agent may account for some of the carcinogenicity of tobacco smoke.[26] Five years after smoking cessation, however, no such DNA-adducts were found.

Industry-Related Carcinogens

Many occupations and chemicals have been reported to increase the risk of urinary bladder cancer; however, a causal link has only been established for certain aromatic amines. The estimate that in the United States nearly 25% of bladder cancers in white males[27] and that more than 10% of cases in white females[28] can be attributed to occupational exposures is based on assumptions of causality that may or may not be justified. The agents discussed in this section, however, may be carcinogenic to the urinary bladder because increased relative risks have been reported for certain cohorts of workers exposed to these agents, and several of these chemical substances or their metabolites are excreted through the urine and are in direct contact with the lower urinary tract mucosa.

Aromatic Amines

An early observation and later comparative studies from the dyestuff and rubber manufacturing industry provide convincing evidence that 2-napthylamine, 4-aminobiphenyl, and benzidine are human bladder carcinogens. The action of 2-naphthylamine is remarkably organ-specific; all species given the carcinogen (mouse, rat, rabbit, guinea pig, dog) develop bladder tumors.[29] Moreover, the strong carcinogenic potential of 2-naphthylamine was demonstrated among 15 men who worked in distillation of the agent—all developed bladder tumors.[30] The median latency period between the initial exposure to 2-napthylamine and death from bladder cancer has been estimated at 18 years (range 12 to 41 years). Hence, 2-naphthylamine may be active in both early and late stages of carcinogenesis. Other aromatic amines that possibly are carcinogenic to the human urothelium include *o*-toluidine used in the rubber manufacturing process and 4,4-methylene bis (z-chloroaniline) used in the production of polyurethane.[31]

Polycyclic Aromatic Hydrocarbons

Aluminum industry, gas production, and chimney sweep workers are all considered high-risk groups for urinary bladder cancer. They are exposed to high levels of polycyclic aromatic hydrocarbons, but whether impurities of the foregoing aromatic amines, other impurities of, for example, nitroarenes, or unidentified polycyclic aromatic hydrocarbon are the causative agents remains to be determined. Combustion gas from coal contains polycyclic aromatic hydrocarbons, which have been associated with an increased risk of bladder cancer.[32] Diesel exhausts contain, among other things, polycyclic aromatic hydrocarbons. Truck drivers, chauffeurs, delivery workers, and garage or gas station workers and others exposed to diesel exhaust have an elevated risk of bladder cancer.[33–37]

Other Industry-Related Agents

Benzene, an organic solvent linked to leukemia, may cause bladder cancer.[37] Chlorinated aliphatic hydrocarbons, used in dry cleaning and in shoe-making and repair, may also be bladder carcinogens.[38] Creosote is a wood preservative used in telephone poles. Line workers exposed to creosote are at risk of bladder cancer.[32] Cutting fluids and oils are commonly used in the metal industry, among machinists and machine manufacturing workers. The excess risk of bladder cancer reported among these groups may be explained by the presence of aromatic amines, nitrosamines, or polycyclic aromatic hydrocarbons in cutting fluids and oils.[32,38] Polychlorinated biphenyls are used in the electrical industry for insulation as coolants, they are found in hydraulic fluids, and they have been linked to urinary bladder cancer.[32,37] Apart from the previously mentioned agents, additional carcinogens may be present in agents used by high-risk groups such as chemical workers, miners, pesticide applicators, and cooks.[39–46]

Diet

No causal factor for urinary bladder cancer has been identified in the diet. Frequent consumers of meat have an increased risk of the disease, however, and heterocyclic amines are strong candidates as causative agents. The relationship between coffee and artificial sweeteners and urinary bladder cancer is probably one of the most widely studied in the epidemiologic literature. Still, data are inconclusive, again illustrating the limitations of conventional epidemiologic methods to investigate small increases in risk in populations with complicated exposure patterns.

Meat and Heterocyclic Amines

As mentioned earlier, the increased risk of urinary bladder cancer among meat eaters may be explained by the content in meat of a group of chemicals named heterocyclic amines. Alternative explanations include the carcinogenicity of the protein itself, induction by a diet high in meat of metabolic pathways that produce carcinogens, and the presence of other dietary factors such as fat. Heterocyclic amines are mutagenic and carcinogenic to rodents and monkeys.[47,48] The amount of heterocyclic amines in fried meat depends primarily on the temperature at which the meat is cooked; the duration of cooking is of less importance. In an American diet, whether ''well-done'' meat contains more or fewer heterocyclic amines than ''rare'' meat is unknown. The latter implies cooking at high temperature, although for a short time. Only one study has investigated the relationship between fried foods and bladder cancer, and a significant association was noted. The heterocyclic amine Trp-p-2 induced tumors of the urinary bladder when given to rats.[48] Bladder carcinogens may also be found among the other 18 heterocyclic amines that have been isolated and chemically defined.

Other Dietary Constituents

Fat intake has been correlated with the risk of bladder cancer, but no mechanism for an association has been proposed. A high intake of fruits and vegetables seems to have a weak protective effect, if any. One study found a strong protective effect of vitamin A supplements, but the finding needs to be confirmed before causality can be discussed. Findings for dietary carotene are inconsistent.[49,50] Consumption of chlorinated drinking water seems to increase the risk of bladder cancer, but a carcinogenic agent must be identified before a causal association can be determined.[51,52] Although more than 30 studies have investigated coffee, whether an overall small increase in risk is spurious is still uncertain.[53] The pattern of relative risks obtained for artificial sweeteners suggests an absence of association with bladder cancer incidence, but, again, epidemiologic methods are inadequate for ruling out any risk.

Drugs and Disease

Because of simplistic exposure patterns, high exposure levels, or strong associations, certain drugs have been identified as human bladder carcinogens. Some diseases may initiate or promote bladder carcinogenesis.

Drugs

An extremely high consumption of the analgesic phenacetin among workers in a Swedish weapons factory made it possible to identify phenacetin as carcinogenic to the transitional cell mucosa of the renal pelvis.[54,55] The urinary bladder is probably also a target organ for the drug.[56] Acetaminophen is a metabolite of phenacetin, and available evidence is consistent with an increased risk of bladder cancer among frequent consumers of this drug.[57] Conversely, aspirin may be protective.[58] Chlornaphazine is closely related to 2-naphthylamine chemically and was used for a short time as a antineoplastic drug.[59] The high relative risk of bladder cancer among patients treated with chlornaphazine established the drug as a carcinogen. Similarly, cohorts of patients who have undergone external-beam radiotherapy to sites near the urinary bladder have an increased risk of bladder cancer.[60]

Diseases

Although *Schistosoma haematobium* is an accepted cause of squamous cell carcinoma of the urinary bladder, this association has not been assessed using stringent conventional epidemiologic criteria. The relationship can be explained by the concomitant occurrence of two common diseases in tropical and subtropical countries, without a causal link. Still, the mechanism for a true association may be that *Schistosoma haematobium* infection enhances formation of carcinogenic *N*-nitroso compounds or induces chromosomal instability.

Substantial evidence suggests a link between a history of urinary tract infection and squamous cell carcinoma in the urinary bladder.[9] The possible relationship with transitional cell carcinoma is less well documented.

MOLECULAR EPIDEMIOLOGY

Seemingly, the technical advances in molecular epidemiology provide many useful research strategies to define the pathogenesis and etiology of urinary bladder cancer. Although the understanding of the pathogenesis of bladder cancer has deepened, however, whether the search for etiologic factors will benefit from molecular epidemiologic methods remains to be seen. Strategies include identification of DNA adducts or an association between specific mutations in suppressor genes or oncogenes and a specific exposure.

4-Aminobiphenyl and Its DNA or Protein Adducts

DNA and protein adducts are a group of biomarkers for the study of chemical carcinogenesis, for molecular dosimetry, and for validating exposure information from external sources. In studies of bladder carcinogenesis, hemoglobin has been used as a target protein for the bladder carcinogen 4-aminobiphenyl. Metabolism of this compound is complicated, and its target organ, the bladder, is distant from the metabolic site. A high correlation between self-reported smoking history, as well as DNA adducts of 4-aminobiphenyl in exfoliated bladder cells, and hemoglobin adducts of this substance in blood has been reported.[61,62] Adducts of 4-aminobiphenyl have been used to monitor environmental tobacco smoke as well as active smoking. Levels of hemoglobin adducts of 4-aminobiphenyl are three- to fourfold higher in current smokers than in nonsmokers. Passive tobacco smokers also can be identified by measuring hemoglobin adducts of 3- and 4-aminobiphenyl. Studies on DNA adducts in both exfoliated bladder cells and biopsy specimen in humans confirm 4-aminobiphenyl as a bladder carcinogen.[63] Identification of DNA adducts may guide investigators in the disentanglement of carcinogenic agents in multichemical exposures such as polycyclic aromatic hydrocarbons.

Metabolic Polymorphisms

N-Acetyltransferase (NAT) activity in humans is coded by two distinct genes, named *NAT1* and *NAT2*. *NAT2* displayed polymorphism in humans that has resulted in the detection of individuals with slow and rapid *N*-acetylating phenotypes.[64] The increased risk of bladder cancer is modified by slow acetylation among workers occupationally exposed to arylamines. Among cigarette smokers, slow acetylators have significantly higher levels of aminobiphenyl hemoglobin adducts than fast acetylators.[63] Acetylation may modify the bladder cancer risk after smoking.[65]

Tumor Suppressor Genes and Oncogenes

Cancer arises by a multistep process.[66] Alterations in protooncogenes and in tumor suppressor genes are equally prevalent in human tumors.[67] Genetic instability leads to a sequence of events that creates phenotypic alterations, granting a selective advantage to specific tumor cells. Genetic alterations leading to inactivation of tumor suppressor genes or activation of protooncogenes are associated with the development and progression of cancer. Multiple genetic changes have been observed in the progression of colonic polyps to colon cancer.[66,68] A multistep theory of the development of bladder cancer is consistent with epidemiologic data on the association between cigarette smoking and bladder cancer, as reviewed earlier.

"Two-Hit" Model of Tumor Suppressor Genes

Knudson,[69] who reviewed the epidemiologic evidence for inherited retinoblastoma in children, first suggested the "two-hit" model. In 1971, he proposed that mutations in both alleles at the RB locus (from AA to A*A*) were needed for tumorigenesis. In his two-hit model, genetically susceptible individuals are born with every cell altered at one allele, that is, A* of locus A. These susceptible individuals will have cancer if any cell in the target tissue is altered at the other allele of A, because this cell would then be completely inactivated at A. Normal individuals may need two hits to inactivate locus A on both chromosomes. In normal individuals, cancer may occur at older ages than in those with genetically inherited susceptibility because the second hit is time dependent. The assumption was confirmed 15 years later with the isolation of the *RB* gene and the identification of alterations in both alleles of this gene in retinoblastomas. Mutations and deletions of the *TP53* gene have been suggested in a variety of inherited and sporadic forms of human cancer. The two-hit model has also been implicated in the Li-Fraumeni syndrome.[70–73]

Mutations of the *TP53* Gene and Bladder Cancer

Conceivably, most carcinogens operate through direct interaction with DNA.[74,75] Furthermore, compelling evidence indicates that specific carcinogens produce mutations in particular genes.[76] Alterations of tumor DNA may be useful markers for carcinogenic agents.

The *TP53* gene is a common target in human tumorigenesis and *TP53* mutations are the most commonly documented genetic change in human cancer. The *TP53* gene expresses proteins involved in transcriptional control. Mutations of the *TP53* gene inactivate their encoded products. Two general patterns of *TP53* mutations have been suggested[78]: "spontaneous" resulting from endogenous mutagens, and "induced" mutations, caused by exogenous carcinogens. A high proportion of spontaneous point mutations at CpGs of the *TP53* gene were found in human colon cancers, leukemias, and sarcomas. The presence of a lower proportion of spontaneous mutations at CpGs may indicate that exogenous factors such as carcinogens interact directly with DNA.[77] A high proportion of G to C transversions in codon 249 of the *TP53* gene has been found in hepatocellular carcinomas in Africa and in China, where both aflatoxin exposure[78–80] and hepatitis B virus[81] are the causative agents. In one study, 65% of *TP53* mutations in small cell lung carcinomas were transversions, a finding suggesting that lung cancer results from the direct interaction of a carcinogen, cigarette smoke, with DNA.[82] Mutations or overexpression of *TP53* have also been associated with previous exposure to ultraviolet light in squamous cell carcinoma,[83] radon in lung cancer,[84] cigarette smoking in lung cancer,[82,85,86] and in head and neck cancers.[87] Additionally, a combination of heavy smoking and drinking has been implicated in head and neck cancer,[88] as well as in squamous cell esophageal cancer.[89] The wide range of involvement of *TP53* in human tumors and the broad spectrum of mutations make this gene a good candidate for molecular epidemiologic studies.[77]

Sidransky[90] found *TP53* mutations in 61% (11 of 18) of bladder tumors. The spectrum of *TP53* mutations falls somewhere between these two general patterns, suggesting a mixture of "carcinogen-induced" and endogenous "spontaneous" mutations.[77] Spruck and associates[91] have compared the patterns of *TP53* mutations in patients with bladder cancer and found no obvious difference in the types and positions of *TP53* mutations between smokers and nonsmokers. Zhang and colleagues[92] observed a significant association between the number of cigarettes smoked per day and *P53* nuclear overexpression. The odds ratio was 2.3 for those smoking one to two packs per day and 8.4 for those smoking more than two packs per day.

Retinoblastoma Susceptibility Gene and Bladder Cancer

The retinoblastoma susceptibility gene (*RB*) encodes a 110-kd nuclear phosphoprotein (pRB). Alterations of the *RB* gene induce intraocular retinoblastoma.[69,93,94] Patients with a history of retinoblastoma are more susceptible to the development multiple malignant diseases. Mutated *RB* gene has been identified in patients with heritable retinoblastoma, and altered patterns of *RB* expression have also been reported in other forms of cancer, including soft tissue sarcomas and bladder carcinomas.[95–98]

Altered patterns of *RB* are suggested to be associated with tumor progression rather than initiation of bladder cancer. Ishikawa and associates reported loss of heterozygosity of *RB* in 3 of 18 bladder tumors and undetectable levels of pRB in 2 of 14 high-grade invasive carcinomas. In the same study, however, none of the 16 low-grade noninvasive bladder tumors showed alterations of pRB.[99] pRB plays an important role in the control of cell cycle, and in certain cancers, alterations in *RB* expression are associated with tumorigenesis and disease progression. The inactivation of the *RB* gene has been detected in tumors that have a more aggressive clinical outcome and a poor prognosis.

PREVENTION OF BLADDER CANCER

Obviously, elimination of the agents causally linked to urinary bladder cancer would prevent disease occurrence. Such measures have been taken. The proportion of smokers in Western countries has decreased, the drugs phenacetin and chlornaphazine are no longer in use, and occupational exposure to aromatic amines has been regulated. Still, the increased incidence of the disease emphasizes the need to continue searching for additional etiologic factors. When knowledge of causal factors is uncertain, whether preventive measures should be instituted is a matter of judgment. The impact of preventive action on the morbidity and mortality from all types of diseases, not only bladder cancer, should be assessed. Whether bladder cancer deaths can be avoided by screening for early disease with, for example, a cytologic examination of the urine is uncertain.

ACKNOWLEDGMENTS

This research was supported by National Institute of Environmental Health Service Grant R01 ES-06781 from the National Institutes of Health, United States Department of Health and Human Services, and by a Grant from the Swedish Cancer Society. We thank Ms. Daphna Pollack and Ms. Claudette Green for their technical support and assistance.

REFERENCES

1. Parkin DM, Pisani P, Ferlay J. Estimate of the world incidence of eighteen major cancers in 1985. Int J Cancer 1993;54:594.
2. Pisani P, Parkin DM, Ferlay J. Estimates of the world mortality from eighteen major cancers in 1985: implication and projections of future burden. Int J Cancer 1993;55:891.
3. American Cancer Society. Cancer facts and figures: 1994. Atlanta, American Cancer Society, 1996;1.
4. Hartge P, Harvey EB, Linehan WM, et al. Unexplained excess risk of bladder cancer in men. J Natl Cancer Inst 1990;82:1636.
5. Kono N, Tanahashi T, Suzawa N, Azuma C. Effects of sex hormones on oncogenesis in rat uritary bladder by N-butyl-N-(4-hydroxybutyl)-nitrosamine. Int J Clin Pharmacol 1977;15:101.
6. Reid LM, Leav I, Kwan PWL, Russell P, Merk FB. Characterization of a human sex steroid-responsive transitional cell carcinoma maintained as a tumor line (R198) in athymic nude mice. Cancer Res 1984; 44:4560.
7. Cantor KP, Lynch CF, Johnson D. Bladder cancer, parity, and age at first birth. Cancer Causes Control 1992;3:57.
8. Hankey BF, Silverman DT, Kaplan R. Urinary bladder. In: Miller BA, Ries LAG, Hankey BF, et al, eds. SEER cancer statistics review, 1973–1990. NIH pub no 93-2789. Bethesda, MD, National Cancer Institute, 1993;26.1.
9. Kantor AF, Hartge P, Hoover RN, et al. Epidemiological characteristics of squamous cell carcinoma and adenocarcinoma of the bladder. Cancer Res 1988;48:3853.
10. Clavel J, Cordier S, Boccon-Gibod L, et al. Tobacco and bladder cancer in males: increased risk for inhalers and smokers of black tobacco. Int J Cancer 1989;44:605.
11. D'Avanzo B, Negri E, LaVeccia C, et al. Cigarette smoking and bladder cancer. Eur J Cancer 1990;26:714.
12. Vineis P, Esteve J, Hartge P, et al. Effects of timing and type of tobacco in cigarette-induced bladder cancer. Cancer Res 1988;48:3849.
13. Vineis P, Esteve J, Terracini B. Bladder cancer and smoking in males: types of cigarettes, age at start, effect of stopping and interaction with occupation. Int J Cancer 1984;34:165.
14. Lopez-Abente G, Gonzalez CA, Errezola M, et al. Tobacco smoke inhalation pattern, tobacco type, and bladder cancer in Spain. Am J Epidemiol 1991;134:830.
15. Hartge P, Silverman D, Hoover R, et al. Changing cigarette habits and bladder cancer risk: a case-control study. J Natl Cancer Inst 1987;78: 1119.
16. Wynder EL, Augustine A, Kabat GC, et al. Effect of the type of cigarette smoked on bladder cancer risk. Cancer 1988;61:622.
17. Burch JD, Rohan TE, Howe GR, et al. Risk of bladder cancer by source and type of tobacco exposure: a case-control study. Int J Cancer 1989; 44:622.
18. Hartge P, Hoover R, Kantor A. Bladder cancer risk and pipes, cigars and smokeless tobacco. Cancer 1985;55:901.
19. Marrett LD, Hartge P, Meigs JW. Bladder cancer and occupational exposure to leather. Br J Ind Med 1986;43:96.
20. Vineis P. Black (air-cured) and blond (flue-cured) tobacco and cancer risk. I: bladder cancer. Eur J Cancer 1991;27:1491. Review.
21. Burch JD, Rohan TE, Howe GR, et al. Risk of bladder cancer by source and type of tobacco exposure: a case-control study. Int J Cancer 1989; 44:622.
22. IARC Working Group. Tobacco smoking. IARC Monogr Eval Carcinog Risk Hum 1986;38.
23. Augustine A, Herbert JR, Kabat GC, et al. Bladder cancer in relation to cigarette smoking. Cancer Res 1988;48:4405.
24. IARC Working Group. Overall evaluation of carcinogenicity: an updating IARC monograph Volume 1–42 (Suppl 7) 1987:359.
25. Barnes DM, Hanby AM, Gillett CE, et al. Abnormal expression of wild type p53 protein in normal cells of a cancer family patient. Lancet 1992;340:259.
26. Talaska G, Al-Juburi AZSS, Kadlubar FF. Smoking related carcinogen-DNA adducts in biopsy samples of human urinary bladder: identification of N-(deoxygauanosin-8-yl)-4-aminobiphenyl as a major adduct. Proc Natl Acad Sci USA 1991;88:5350.
27. Silverman DT, Levin LI, Hoover RN, et al. Occupational risks of bladder cancer in the United States. I. White men. J Natl Cancer Inst 1989; 81:1472.
28. Silverman DT, Levin LI, Hoover RN. Occupational risks of bladder cancer among white women in the United States. Am J Epidemiol 1990;132:453.
29. Hicks RM, Wright R, Wakefield JSJ. The induction of rat bladder cancer by 2-naphthylamine. Br J Cancer 1982;46:646.
30. Case RAM. Tumor of the urinary tract as an occupational disease in several industries. Ann R Coll Surg Engl 1966;39:213.
31. Jones RF, Debiec-Rychter M, Wang CY. Chemical carcinogenesis of the urinary bladder: a status report. J Cancer Res Clin Oncol 1992; 118:411. Editorial.
32. Steineck G, Plato N, Alfredsson L, Norell SE. Industry-related urothelial carcinogens: application of a job-exposure matrix to census data. Am J Ind Med 1989;16:209.
33. van der Werf-Messing BH, Friedell GH, Menon RS, Hop WC, Wassif SB. Carcinoma of the urinary bladder category T3 NX MO treated by preoperative irradiation followed by simple cystectomy. Prog Clin Biol Res 1988;260:453.
34. Silverman DT, Hoover RN, Albert S, Graff K. Occupation and cancer of the lower urinary tract in Detroit. J Natl Cancer Inst 1993;70:237.
35. Schoenberg JB, Stemhagen A, Mogielnicki AP, Altman R, Abe T, Mason TJ. Case-control study of bladder cancer in New Jersey. I. Occupational exposures in white males. J Natl Cancer Inst 1984;72:973.
36. Risch HA, Burch JD, Miller AB, Hill GB, Steele R, Howe GR. Dietary factors and the incidence of cancer of the urinary bladder. Am J Epidemiol 1988;127:1179.
37. Steineck G, Plato N, Gerhardsson M, Norell SE, Hogstedt C. Increased risk of urothelial cancer in Stockholm during 1985–87 after exposure to benzene and exhausts. Int J Cancer 1990;45:1012.
38. Steineck G, Plato N, Norell SE, Hogstedt C. Urothelial cancer and some industry-related chemicals: an evaluation of the epidemiologic literature. Am J Ind Med 1990;17:371. Review.
39. Claude J, Kunze E, Frentzel-Beyme R, et al. Life-style and occupational risk factors in cancer of the lower urinary tract. Am J Epidemiol 1986; 124:578.
40. Schifflers E, Jamart J, Renard V. Tobacco and occupation as risk factors in bladder cancer: a case-control study in southern Belgium. Int J Cancer 1987;39:287.
41. Brownson RC, Chang JC, Davis JR. Occupation, smoking, and alcohol in the epidemiology of bladder cancer. Am J Public Health 1987;77: 1298.
42. Claude JC, Frentzel-Beyme RR, Kunze E. Occupation and risk of cancer of the lower urinary tract among men: a case-control study. Int J Cancer 1988;41:371.
43. Zahm SH, Hartge P, Hoover R. The national bladder cancer study: employment in the chemical industry. J Natl Cancer Inst 1991;83:501.
44. Kabat GC, Dieck GS, Wynder EL. Bladder cancer in nonsmokers. Cancer 1986;57:362.
45. Blair A, Grauman DJ, Lubin JH, Fraumeni JF. Lung cancer and other causes of death among licensed pesticide applicators. J Natl Cancer Inst 1983;71:31.
46. Anton-Culver H, Lee-Feldstein A, Taylor TH. Occupation and Bladder Cancer Risk. Am J Epidemiol 1992;136:89.
47. Overvik E, Gustafsson JA. Cooked-food mutagens: current knowledge of formation and biological significance. Mutagenesis 1990;5:437.
48. Takahashi M, Toyoda K, Aze Y, et al. The rat urinary bladder as a new target of heterocyclic amine carcinogenicity: tumor induction by

3-amino-1-methyl-5H-pyridol[4,3-b]indole acetate. Jpn J Cancer Res 1994;84:852.
49. Vena JE, Graham S, Freudenheim J, et al. Diet in the epidemiology of bladder cancer in western New York. Nutr Cancer 1992 1994;18: 255.
50. Kolonel LN, Hinds MW, Nomura AM, Hankin JH, Lee J. Relationship of dietary vitamin A and ascorbic acid intake to the risk for cancer of the lung, bladder, and prostate in Hawaii. Monogr Natl Cancer Inst 1985;69:137.
51. Cantor KP, Hoover R, Hartge P, et al. Bladder cancer, drinking water source, and tap water consumption: a case-control study. J Natl Cancer Inst 1987;79:1269.
52. Vena JE, Graham S, Freudenheim J, et al. Drinking water, fluid intake, and bladder cancer in western New York. Arch Environ Health 1993 1994;48:191.
53. Viscoli CM, Lachs MS, Horwitz RI. Bladder cancer and coffee drinking: a summary of case-control research. Lancet 1993;341:1432.
54. Angerwall L, Bengtsson U, Zetterlund CG, Singmund M. Renal pelvic carcinoma in a Swedish district with abuse of a phenacetin-containing drug. Br J Urol 1969;41:401.
55. Hultengren N, Lagergren C, Ljungqvist A. Carcinoma of the renal pelvis in renal papillary necrosis. Acta Chir Scand 1965;13:314.
56. Piper JM, Matanoski GM, Tonascia J. Bladder cancer in young women. Am J Epidemiol 1986;123:1033.
57. Piper JM, Tonascia J, Mataanoski GM. Heavy phenacetin use and bladder cancer in women aged 20 to 49 years. N Engl J Med 1985;313: 292.
58. Ward E, Halperin W, Thun M, et al. Screening workers exposed to 4,4′-methylenebis(2-chloroaniline) for bladder cancer by cystoscopy. J Occup Med 1990;32:865.
59. Thiede T, Christensen BC. Bladder tumors induced by chlomaphazine: a five-year follow-up study of chlornaphazine-treated patients with polycythaemia. Acta Med Scand 1969;185:133.
60. Silverman DT, Hartge P, Morrison AS, Devesa SS. Epidemiology of bladder cancer. Hematol Oncol Clin North Am 1992;6:1.
61. Bartsch H, Caporaso N, Coda M, et al. Carcinogen hemoglobin adducts, urinary mutagenicity, and metabolic phenotype in active and passive cigarette smokers. J Natl Cancer Inst 1990;82:1826.
62. Vineis P, Caporaso N, Tannenbaum SR, et al. Acetylation phenotype, carcinogen-hemoglobin adducts, and cigarette smoking. Cancer Res 1990;50:3002.
63. Vineis P. Epidemiological models of carcinogenesis: the example of bladder cancer. Cancer Epidemiol Biomarkers Prev 1992;1:149.
64. Bartsch H, Malaveille C, Friesen M, Kadlubar FF, Vineis P. Black (air-cured) and blond (flue-cured) tobacco cancer risk. IV. Molecular dosimetry studies implicate aromatic amines as bladder carcinogens. Eur J Cancer 1993;29A:1199.
65. Vineis P, Ronco G. Interindividual variation in carcinogen metabolism and bladder cancer risk. Environ Health Perspect 1992;98:95.
66. Fearon ER, Vogelstein B. A genetic model for colorectal tumorigenesis. Cell 1990;61:759.
67. Marshall CJ. Tumor suppressor genes. Cell 1991;64:313.
68. Vogelstein B, Fearon ER, Hamilton SR, et al. Genetic alterations during colorectal tumor development. N Engl J Med 1988;319:525.
69. Knudson AG. Mutation and cancer: statistical study of retinoblastoma. Proc Natl Acad Sci USA 1971;68:820.
70. Malkin D, Li FP, Stong LC, et al. Germline p53 mutations in a familial syndrome of breast cancer, sarcomas, and other neoplasms. Science 1990;250:1233.
71. Srivastava S, Zou ZQ, Pirollo K, et al. Germline transmission of a mutated p53 gene in a cancer prone family with Li-Fraumeni syndrome. Nature 1990;348:747.
72. Malkin D, Jolly KW, Barbier N, et al. Germline mutations of the p53 tumor-suppressor gene in children and young adults with second malignant neoplasms. N Engl J Med 1992;326:1309.
73. Toguchida J, Yamaguchi T, Dayton SH, et al. Prevalence and spectrum of germline mutations of the p53 gene among patients with sarcoma (see comments). N Engl J Med 1992;326:1301.
74. Mazur M, Glickman B. Sequence specificity of mutations induced by benzo[a]pyrene-7,8-diol-9,10-epoxide at endogenous aprt gene in CHO cells. Somat Cell Mol Genet 1988;14:393.
75. Wang P, Bennett RAO, Povirk LF. Melphalan-induced mutagenesis in an SV40-based shuttle vector: predominance of A. TT. A transversions. Cancer Res 1990;50:7527.
76. Zarbl M, Sukumar S, Arthur AV, et al. Direct mutagenesis of Ha-ras-1 oncogenes by N-nitroso-N-methylurea during initiation of mammary carcinogenesis in rats. Nature 1985;315:383.
77. Jones PA, Buckley JD, Henderson BE, Ross RK, Pike MC. From gene to carcinogen: a rapidly evolving field in molecular epidemiology. Cancer Res 1991;51:3617.
78. Ozturk M, et al. p53 mutation in hepatocellular carcinoma after aflatoxin exposure. Lancet 1991;338:1356.
79. Bressac B, Kew M, Wands J, Ozturk M. Selective G to T mutations of p53 gene in hepatocellular carcinoma from southern Africa. Nature 1991;350:429.
80. Hsu IC, Metcalf RA, Sun T, Welsh JA, Wang NJ, Harris CC. Mutational hotspot in the p53 gene in human heptocellular carcinoma. Nature 1991;350:427.
81. Scorsone KA, Zhou Y, Butel JS, Slagle BL. p53 mutations cluster at codon 249 in hepatitis B virus-positive hepatocellular carcinomas from China. Cancer Res 1992;52:1635.
82. Chiba I, Takahashi T, Nau MM, et al. Mutations in the p53 gene are frequent in primary, resected non-small cell lung cancer: Lung Cancer Study Group. Oncogene 1990;5:1603.
83. Brash DE, Rudolph JA, Simon JA, et al. A role for sunlight in skin cancer: UV-induced p53 mutations in squamous cell carcinoma. Proc Natl Acad Sci USA 1991;88:10124.
84. Vahakangas KH, Samet JM, Metcalf RA, et al. Mutations of p53 and ras genes in radon-associated lung cancer from uranium miners. Lancet 1992;339:576.
85. Iggo R, Gatter K, Lane D, Harris AL. Increased expression of mutant forms of p53 oncogene in primary lung cancer. Lancet 1990;335:675.
86. Suzuki H, Takahashi T, Kuroishi T, Suyama M, Ariyoshi Y, Ueda R. p53 mutations in non-small cell lung cancer in Japan: association between mutations and smoking. Cancer Res 1992;52:734.
87. Field JK, Spandidos DA, Malliri A, Gosney JR, Yiagnisis M, Stell PM. Elevated P53 expression correlates with a history of heavy smoking in squamous cell carcinoma of the head and neck. Br J Cancer 1991;64: 573.
88. Field JK, Spandidos DA, Stell PM. Overexpression of p53 gene in head-and-neck cancer, linked with heavy smoking and drinking. Lancet 1992;339:502. Letter.
89. Hollstein MC, Peri L, Mandard AM, et al. Genetic analysis of human esophageal tumors from two high incidence geographic areas: frequent p53 base substitutions and absence of ras mutations. Cancer Res 1991; 51:4102.
90. Sidransky D, Von Eschenbach A, Tsai YC, et al. Identification of p53 gene mutations in bladder cancers and urine samples. Science 1991; 252:706.
91. Spruck CH III, Rideout WM III, Olumi AF, et al. Distinct pattern of p53 mutations in bladder cancer: relationship to tobacco usage. Cancer Res 1993;53:1162.
92. Zhang ZF, Sarkis AS, Cordon-Cardo C, et al. Tobacco smoking, occupation, and p53 nuclear overexpression in early stage bladder cancer. Cancer Epidemiol Biomarkers Prev 1994;3:19.
93. Knudson AG, Meadows AT, Nichols WW, Hill R. Chromosomal deletion and retinoblastoma. N Engl J Med 1976;295:1120.
94. Weinberg RA. The RB gene and the negative regulation of cell growth. Blood 1989;74:529.
95. Presti JC, Reuter VE, Galan T, et al. Molecular genetic alterations in superficial and locally advanced human bladder cancer. Cancer Res 1991;51:5405.
96. Cance WG, Brennan MF, Dudas ME, et al. Altered expression of the retinoblastoma gene product in human sarcomas. N Engl J Med 1990; 323:1457.
97. Cordon-Cardo C, Wartinger D, Petrylak D, et al. Altered expression of the retinoblastoma gene product is a prognostic indicator in bladder cancer. J Natl Cancer Inst 1992;84:1251.
98. Logothetis CJ, Xu H-J, Ro JY, et al. Altered retinoblastoma protein expression and known prognostic variables in locally advanced bladder cancer. J Natl Cancer Inst 1992;84:1256.
99. Ishikawa J, Xu H-J, Hu S-X, et al. Inactivation of the retinoblastoma gene in human bladder and renal cell carcinomas. Cancer Res 1991; 51:5736.

Principles and Practice of Genitourinary Oncology, edited by Derek Raghavan, Howard I. Scher, Steven A. Leibel, and Paul H. Lange. Lippincott-Raven Publishers, Philadelphia, © 1997.

CHAPTER 20

Molecular Biology of Bladder Cancer

Paul Cairns, Brian C.-S. Liu, and David Sidransky

Primary human cancers arise and progress through the accumulation of genetic changes in specific genes. These genes are divided into two broad categories, those that involve activation, called protooncogenes, and those that are inactivated, termed tumor suppressor genes. The critical hits to these genes provide a selective growth advantage that allows cells to outgrow neighboring cells and to undergo clonal expansion. Specific genetic steps in cancer progression can be correlated with morphologically defined histopathologic lesions. In colon cancer, which serves as a paradigm for molecular progression, the progression from adenoma to carcinomas has been well correlated with activation of protooncogenes and inactivation of tumor suppressor genes. This correlation has led to similar attempts at elucidation of a molecular progression model for bladder cancer.

Two well-defined pathologic lesions are recognized in bladder cancer. One type is the ''flat'' lesions of carcinoma in situ, which have a propensity to evolve into invasive carcinoma. The second type consists of papillary lesions (papillomas) with a propensity for recurrence but rarely for invasion. Molecular studies are ongoing to determine which genetic changes determine the morphologic progression of these two different presentations of bladder cancer. Some of these changes have been recognized by previous studies, and others are being elucidated by modern molecular techniques. Understanding the genetic changes in these two different lesions will aid in diagnosis and will lead to an understanding of the way in which tumors arise, invade, and metastasize. This understanding should eventually lead to improved diagnosis and therapy for the treatment of bladder cancer.

CLONAL ORIGIN OF CANCER

Clonality is a fundamental characteristic of human cancer. Clonality, based on the shared presence of advantageous genetic information among cancer cells, was first suspected based on morphologic assessment in neoplastic cells.[1,2] It was initially apparent that cancer cells from a given tumor shared common features that included shape, size, and appearance. Clonal outgrowth of progressively more ''malignant'' clones in cancer was also demonstrated by neoplastic models in animals.[3] These models demonstrated that certain clones can be selected from a tumor mass with a specific propensity for invasion and metastases. Thus, individual cells were thought to be the progenitors of subsequently more advanced and eventually metastatic tumors.

Many of these initial observations were further confirmed by cytogenetic studies.[4] The sharing of certain cytogenetic alterations among many cells within a tumor provided strong evidence for the clonality of cancer. Subsequently, X-chromosome inactivation studies based on enzyme inactivation eventually confirmed the clonal nature of human cancers at the molecular level.[5] Thus, the identification of a gene mutation or chromosomal deletion implies that most cells within a given tumor contain the identical alteration. Clonality does not exclude tumor heterogeneity. The processes that drive neoplasia allow various clones to arise with different genetic information. Each alteration is tried and tested, and those that provide a selective growth advantage become the dominant cell type within a given tumor. This heterogeneity allows the outgrowth of specifically more aggressive and invasive clones and perhaps the unstoppable clinical progression of many human neoplasms.

Thus, the initial transformation of a transitional cell leads to clonal outgrowth and the initiation of a bladder neoplasm. Subsequent genetic alterations in tumor suppressor genes and oncogenes drive the inevitable progression that eventually results in many of the common features attributable to clinical bladder cancers. In addition, molecular studies have demonstrated that multiple primary tumors may, in fact, arise from a single transformed clone.[6] These studies have shed light on a persistent clinical problem in bladder tumorigenesis related to the possible presence of a ''field defect'' secondary to continued exposure to both exogenous and endogenous compounds excreted in urine. Investigators used X-chromosome inactivation and identification of allelic loss similar to those described later to show that multiple tumors of the bladder appear to be clonal (i.e., to arise from a common progenitor cell), a finding that places the theory of a field defect in doubt. Thirteen tumors from 4 female patients were examined with a method that analyzes X-chromosome inactivation, which can determine whether tumors were derived from the same precursor cell. In each patient examined, all tumors had the same X chromosome inactivated, whereas normal bladder mucosa had random inactivation, as expected. Moreover, each of the evaluable tumors from a given patient had lost the same 9q allele (commonly found in superficial tumors). That later events in progression such as 17p and 18q loss were not shared by the different tumors from the same patient implies that multiple tumors in the same patient arose from the uncontrolled early spread of a single transformed cell. These tumors then proceeded through independent and variable genetic events during progression. If a field defect existed, one would expect multiple independent transforming events and thus a multiclonal origin of these tumors.[6]

Examples of this model of progression can be taken from chronic myelogenous leukemia, in which one stem cell initially acquires an early genetic change (*ABL1* [formerly known as c-*abl*] activation), giving rise to a chronic proliferative state in which all neoplastic cells share this genetic abnormality.[7] Subsequent events, again such as 17p loss and *P53* inactivation, lead to a further proliferative state that manifests as blast crises.[8] Thus, this model for bladder tumor progression has important implications. Because these tumors may share the same initiation event, identification of the putative tumor suppressor genes on chromosome 9, for example, may lead to novel diagnostic and therapeutic strategies. Additionally, any therapy directed against this genetic alteration would be expected to affect both clinically evident tumors and other remaining transformed cells not yet detectable.

CYTOGENETICS

Bladder tumor cells contain large numbers of structural and numeric chromosomal changes that appear to occur with some consistency.[4,9] Cytogenetic banding techniques potentially allow the identification of these numeric changes, as well as deletions and amplifications of subchromosomal segments. These chromosomal changes in tumor cells include the underrepresentation of certain chromosomes or abnormally high numbers of chromosomes (aneuploidy) and the presence of easily identifiable, structurally abnormal chromosomes that are stably inherited from one cell to another (markers). Cytogenetic analysis has been used predominantly in two ways: first, to investigate the potential use of chromosome aberrations as prognostic markers; and second, to identify nonrandom changes for further study.

Assessment of the chromosomal complement of tumors has provided a method for the determination of prognosis. In general, low-grade, noninvasive tumors are associated with a normal (diploid) number of 46 chromosomes or with numeric deviations of a few chromosomes (aneuploidy) and, in some cases, marker chromosomes. High-grade, invasive tumors are often grossly aneuploid and usually contain marker chromosomes. The presence of marker chromosomes in low-grade, noninvasive tumors has been associated with a strong tendency to recurrence or progression.[9]

Cytogenetic reports of bladder carcinomas have demonstrated the consistent gain or loss of specific chromosomes (or chromosomal regions) in a significant number of tumors.[8,9] These results strongly suggest genes located in these regions are critical for the development of the malignant cell. Any clonal (shared) change in chromosome number is likely to have either conferred a growth advantage on the original cell or to have occurred together with another event providing a growth advantage. For example, the gain of a specific chromosome region may benefit a tumor cell, or potential tumor cell, by increasing the copy number of a gene located in that region. This gene may produce higher levels of a protein involved in cell growth or differentiation (protooncogenes). According to Knudson's hypothesis, genes whose normal (wild-type) function suppresses growth are usually inactivated by a two-step mechanism; one copy is usually mutated, and the second is deleted. Thus, consistent loss of chromosome regions (deletions) implies the existence of tumor suppressor genes that are the targets of these deletions.[10] A reduction in, or loss of, function of a tumor suppressor gene may allow a cell to break out of the normal restraints on cell proliferation.

Some tumor karyotypes show neither gain nor loss of chromosomes. Either these are metaphases from normal cells, which can contaminate tumor biopsy specimens, or these tumors possess subtle mutations, perhaps detectable only at the DNA level, which do not result in cytogenetically visible chromosome alterations. Bladder tumors with only one karyotypic change have rarely been reported.[11,12] When they have been observed, the single change has not been found in other bladder tumors with any appreciable frequency. Therefore, no specific change akin to the Ph chromosome in chronic myelogenous leukemia is likely to be found.

The cytogenetic literature suggests that loss of chromosome 9 is a frequent change in bladder tumors.[13–15] Many cytogenetic studies of bladder carcinoma have described monosomy of chromosome 9 as a common karyotypic change.[15–18] These reports mention that, in some cases, monosomy 9 may be an important, or even primary, event. Smeets and associates[13] reported monosomy 9 in near-diploid bladder tumors, and a previous study[19] did not find monosomy 9 in advanced tumors, a finding suggesting that monosomy may be more prevalent in tumors of low grade and stage. Loss of chromosome 10 is also a common cytogenetic finding.[14,15,18] Berger and associates reported deletion of 10q24 as the sole abnormality in a bladder tumor,[14] and Smeets and colleagues also reported a case in which deletion of 10q was the only karyotypic abnormality.[13]

A specific chromosome abnormality in bladder carcinoma was first reported by Gibas and coworkers, namely, an isochromosome of 5p.[15] This finding appears cytogenetically as a symmetric duplication of the p arm and appears to be specific for a subset of bladder carcinomas.[14,19] Whether this abnormality activates a gene by rearrangement at the breakpoint on 5p or increases expression of a gene by the increase in copy number, or whether deletion of the q arm is actually the critical event, is unclear. Deletions and translocations of both areas of chromosome 5 are also frequently reported.[9,11]

Rearrangements of chromosome 1 and trisomy of chromosome 7 are also common in bladder tumors, as in many other tumor types. Other structural changes include deletion of 2q, 6q, 8, 11p, 13q, 16p, 17p, and 21q.[8–19] Molecular confirmation of the loss of chromosomal segments on 11p, 13q, and 17p has been provided.[20–22]

In addition to traditional cytogenetics, novel methods now allow easier identification of genomic amplifications. A method called comparative genomic hybridization (CGH) allows fluorescent identification of amplified genomic regions in human cancers.[23,24] This method entails mixing primary tumor (or cell line) DNA labeled in one color with normal DNA labeled with another color and hybridizing it with a normal metaphase spread. In the kinetic race that ensues, overabundance of specific tumor sequences favors one color, whereas deletions of tumor DNA favor another. Thus, deletion is often represented by one color, such as red, whereas amplification can be seen as increased hybridization to an area, usually as green. CGH analysis of bladder cancer has identified several areas of amplification and has confirmed other areas of deletion. Amplifications not previously seen by cytogenetics or molecular studies have been found on chromosomes 3p, 10p, 12q, 17q, 18p, and 22q.[25] Thus, CGH has become complementary to traditional cytogenetics and molecular studies.

Additionally, a related technique called fluorescent in situ hybridization (FISH) allows specific detection of small deletions or amplifications.[26] DNA probes identified and characterized from the smallest areas of deletion or amplification may be used in chromosomal hybridization to a specific tumor or cell line. Because these probes often contain the gene that is the target of deletion or amplification, small areas of alterations can be seen, as well as complex translocations and rearrangements that involve the same region. This kind of precision allows specific identification of a small alteration, such as homozygous deletion of chromosome 9p21 sequences, in primary bladder tumors usually not detected by routine cytogenetics. FISH is thus a rapid and sensitive alternative to traditional cytogenetics when the target alteration is already suspected in a given tumor type.

MOLECULAR GENETICS

Age-related cancer incidence[27] and molecular progression models[28] suggest that several critical genetic loci are involved in the progression of primary cancer. Any attempt to understand the process of carcinogenesis is necessarily concerned with identifying these genes and understanding their behavior in health and disease. In the past decade, molecular biologists have identified and characterized some of these genes, initially from studies of DNA sequences carried by some retroviruses implicated in cancer and also from searches for DNA sequences present in human cancer cells that, when introduced into noncancerous cells, provoke uncontrolled proliferation. A set of genes whose products are involved in cell proliferation were discovered and were termed protooncogenes. Mutations in these genes were discovered in human tumors, and the mutated genes were termed oncogenes.[29,30]

Protooncogenes can be made oncogenic in many ways, all involving genetic disruption. The gene may be altered by a single base change in its sequence, or it may be activated through more severe disruption by a chromosomal translocation or insertion of a mobile genetic element, such as a retrovirus. The change can occur in the protein-coding region, to yield an activated product, or it can occur in adjacent control regions, so the gene is simply overexpressed or amplified to a high copy number by an unknown process. Specific types of abnormality are characteristic of particular genes and of the responses to particular carcinogens.[31]

The central role of these genes in the creation of tumors has been underscored by the ability of each gene to evoke many of the phenotypes characteristic of cancer cells. For example, when these genes are isolated by molecular cloning and are reintroduced into normal cells, the latter take on many of the growth properties of tumor cells.[32] The roster of protooncogenes has been expanded by diverse lines of enquiry, including the dissection of chromosomal translocations and amplified DNA, the use of gene transfer, and the pursuit of phylogenetic kinships. The tally has now reached over 60, although some loci have been authenticated by weak inference only.[33] The oncogenic alleles of protooncogenes are defined often as dominant because they transform cells despite expression of their normal counterpart.

Despite the initial discovery of an *HRAS* mutation in a bladder carcinoma cell line,[34] few *RAS* gene mutations have been detected in bladder tumors. The search has concentrated on identifying mutations in codons 12, 13, and 61, which contain more than 95% of the activating mutations seen in *HRAS* and *KRAS* (formerly known as h-*ras* and k-*ras*) oncogenes. Several investigators have searched for these changes in many primary bladder tumors, and fewer than 10% appear to contain *RAS* mutations.[35,36] Viola and associates reported increased expression of RAS protein in bladder tumors,[37] but this result remains controversial because of questions about the specificity of the antibody used.

Much attention has focused on the amplification of the *ERBB2* (formerly known as c-erbB-2) protooncogene in many neoplasms, including those from the breast, in which amplification may determine prognosis.[38] Evidence indicates that the *ERBB2* gene may at times be amplified in primary bladder tumors, but amplification appears to be infrequent.[39,40] Coombs and colleagues reported that 14% of bladder tumors showed amplification of *ERBB2*, and amplification at the DNA level was associated with increased mRNA expression. Instances of overexpression at the RNA level without amplification at the DNA level have also been reported.[39] Wright and colleagues observed that the protein product of *ERBB2* is also overexpressed in some bladder tumors.[40] One study has reported a region of chromosome 11q, which includes the *BCL1/PRAD1* protooncogene, to be amplified in 20% of bladder tumors.[41] Several investigators have tried to identify alterations of *MYC* (formerly c-*myc*) in bladder tumors. Increased levels of expression[42] and alterations in the methylation status[43] have been noted in some tumors. Gross alteration or amplification of the gene have not been described. Fanning and associates have reported increased activity of the protein product of *SRC1* and elevated pp60SRC expression in some bladder tumors compared with normal mucosa.[44]

Epidermal growth factor (EGF) is found in high concentrations in urine. EGF receptors (EGFRs), normally found only on the basal layer of bladder epithelial cells, are also richly expressed on the superficial layers of malignant tissue.[45] This malignant distribution of receptors presumably allows greater access of malignant transitional cells to urinary EGF and led Messing and associates to speculate that EGF plays a role in the development and growth of bladder carcinoma.[45] Neal and colleagues reported that the *EGFR* gene is expressed mostly in high-grade invasive tumors.[46] Increased staining has been correlated with increasing stage, death from disease, and progression in patients with Ta or T1 lesions.[47] Other investigators have found no gross abnormalities at the DNA level,[48] and thus overexpression may be due to increased mRNA transcription. The *ERBB1* protooncogene, which maps to chromosome 7, encodes the *EGFR* gene. Trisomy of chromosome 7 is a frequent cytogenetic observation in bladder tumors,[4,9] and it could increase *EGFR* expression in tumor cells. Although many protooncogenes have been identified in human tumors, few have been investigated and found to be commonly altered in bladder cancer. Furthermore, alterations of several protooncogenes in bladder tumors, such as amplification of *ERBB2*,[39] *EGFR* overexpression,[48] and *RAS* point mutations,[35] are all rare in well-differentiated superficial bladder tumors.

CHROMOSOMAL DELETIONS AND TUMOR SUPPRESSOR GENES

The idea that recessive mutations may underlie the neoplastic phenotype arises from two sources. First, experimental fusion of normal and cancer cells often suppresses the neoplastic phenotype. The suppressor activity has been attributed to particular chromosomes contributed by the normal partner in fusion, and the cancer cells therefore appear to be defective in functions required for the regulation of cellular phenotype. Second, by inference from karyotypes and by the use of physical markers for chromosomal domains, evidence has been obtained for the consistent loss of chromosomal regions from cancer cells, a finding suggesting the presence of recessive genetic lesions in various human tumors. The tumors are either hemizygous or more rarely homozygous for the lesions and thus may be completely deficient in at least one gene function.[49]

In familial retinoblastoma for example, the loss of the chromosome region containing the first copy of the *RB1* gene has been visible at the cytogenetic level in a few cases.[50] More often, no visible cytogenetic abnormality has been visible, and the inherited mutation is presumably a small deletion or point mutation. The loss of the second copy of the *RB1* gene in a tumor cell, by contrast, has often involved deletion of a large piece, or all, of the chromosome.[51] This finding is of key importance because it suggests that, in the search for suppressor gene deletions, regions of chromosome loss in the tumor cells present a large target, larger than that associated with the mutation in the germline. The observation of large deletion events and the availability of DNA polymorphic markers have allowed investigators to search for chromosome losses in tumors.[52] As polymorphic DNA markers have become widely available, Southern analysis has become an alternative, or complement, to cytogenetic analysis as an approach to the screening of tumors for chromosome alterations.

Southern analysis with restriction fragment length polymorphism markers and the availability of polymorphic small repeat sequences known as microsatellites have allowed genome-wide assessment of chromosomal losses in bladder cancer.[21,22,53,54] The most common loss, and indeed genetic event, is of chromosome 9.[55] Unlike other reported losses in bladder tumors, deletion of chromosome 9 appears to be as common in superficial lesions (including papillomas and flat lesions) as in invasive tumors.[55] Inactivation of a tumor suppressor gene on chromosome 9 is therefore a candidate initiating event in bladder carcinoma. Careful mapping of chromosome 9 with microsatellites has revealed two distinct regions of loss: one on chromosome 9q and a second at chromosome 9p21.[56,57] Both Southern blot analysis and multiplex comparative polymerase chain reaction have revealed the presence of small homozygous deletions of 9p21 in primary tumors. These small deletions have also been seen in cell lines and have been implicated in the genesis of various tumor types.[58] Because this tumor suppressor locus may be so important in many types of cancers, intense research has focused on the identification of tumor suppressor genes within this area. A candidate gene termed *P16* or *MTS1* was isolated from this region[59] and was found to be mutated in familial melanoma[60] and pancreatic cancer.[61] Although a few point mutations were observed in bladder cancer cell lines, most primary tumors with loss of heterozygosity of 9p21 did not contain obvious mutations of *MTS1*.[62,63] These findings suggest an alternative mechanism for gene inactivation, or, more probably, that a second tumor suppressor locus resides nearby. Identification of the gene that is a target of 9p21 loss would be critical to understanding the initiation and progression of bladder cancer. Deletion of 9q only is also common throughout all grades and stages of bladder cancer and is another potential early event.[55] Deletion mapping of 9q has not yet finely localized the target gene.[64,65]

Perhaps the next most common area of allelic loss seen in bladder cancer is that of chromosome 17p. Loss of 17p has been correlated with mutations of a critical tumor suppressor gene called *P53* in a variety of tumor types.[66] Mutations of *P53* are probably the most common genetic change in all human cancers. Losses of 17p have correlated well with mutations of *P53* and occur predominately in invasive bladder tumors.[67,68] A subset of superficial tumors, however, especially flat lesions, contains *P53* mutations both by sequence analysis and by immunohistochemical analysis.[69,70] A large study based on immunohistochemical analysis of *P53* demonstrated a significant decrease in overall survival for *P53*-positive patients versus those with tumors that were *P53* negative. These findings implied that mutation of *P53* was an independently poor prognostic factor regardless of stage or therapy.[71]

Evidence has pointed to a role for *RB1* in bladder carcinogenesis. Inactivation of *RB1* has already been implicated in tumorigenesis of cell types other than retinal cells;[72] bladder cancer is a second malignant disease in families with retinoblastoma,[73] and RB1 protein is undetectable in a proportion of bladder tumor cell lines.[74] Southern blot analysis of primary bladder tumors with polymorphic intragenic probes and *RB1* cDNA probes has revealed frequent loss of heterozygosity and structural arrangements of the *RB1* locus.[21] Deletion of the *RB1* locus has often been associated with muscle invasive tumors,[21] and immunohistochemical studies have confirmed that *RB1* is the target of 13q deletions in these tumors.[75] The association of *RB1* loss of heterozygosity with tumors of high stage has led to further studies that examined *RB1* inactivation as a marker for progression. A worse prognosis for those tumors with negative staining has been reported.[76,77] Reintroduction of the *RB1* gene leads to slowing of cell growth and tumorigenicity in bladder carcinoma cells.[78] The normal function of the RB1 protein appears to be controlled by its phosphorylation during the G1-S phase of the cell cycle.[79] The role of *RB1* is certain to be complex, because it interacts with viral proteins and an increasing number of cellular proteins in the control of cell growth.

Other areas of allelic loss have been identified commonly in bladder cancer. Chromosome 11p losses, originally described by Southern blot analysis,[20] occur in approximately 40% of predominantly invasive tumors and have been confirmed by microsatellite analysis.[53,54] Although both Wilms tumor loci are candidate targets for the deletions of 11p observed in bladder cancer, bladder tumors are not seen in the spectrum of genitourinary abnormalities or second primary cancers associated with

Wilms tumor.[80] Losses of 3p, 5q, 14q, and 18q have also been reported.[53,54,69,81] Some of these changes are associated with invasive tumors. The deletions on these chromosomes have not been mapped, and candidate tumor suppressor genes have yet to be identified as targets of these losses.

As mentioned previously, careful characterization of the histopathologic regions at various stages with genetic alterations can allow the delineation of a molecular progression model. We previously defined a putative simple progression model for bladder cancer.[82] In this model, critical allelic losses were placed in various steps of progression. Protooncogenes were not demonstrated because they are involved in only a minority of primary bladder tumors so far. Critical steps in this model include the putative initiation of bladder cancer as a result of inactivation of a putative tumor suppressor gene on chromosome 9, the loss of *P53* function in the progression from the preinvasive to the invasive state, and other genetic alterations associated with invasion and metastases. Other investigators have tried to delineate a different progression pathway for papillomas versus flat lesions of carcinoma in situ.[69,83] These models have assumed that one locus rests on chromosome 9, however, and the identification of two distinct loci makes it difficult to delineate the role of chromosome 9 loss in these two potentially distinct pathways. The isolation and characterization of both tumor suppressor genes from chromosome 9 may be needed to understand their exact role in the varied clinical progression of bladder tumors.

FAMILIAL BLADDER CANCER

Although no common or defined form of familial bladder cancer is recognized, familial bladder tumors have been reported.[84] Often, these cases appear as a manifestation of a cancer family syndrome known as Lynch syndrome II or hereditary nonpolyposis colon cancer (HNPCC). This syndrome is inherited in an autosomal manner and is characterized by colonic and extracolonic cancer.[85] Of the extracolonic tumors, transitional cell carcinoma (TCC) is the fourth most common. Affected individuals may manifest TCC alone, TCC and colon cancer, or TCC and other carcinomas.[86,87] In Lynch syndrome, TCC appears predominantly in the upper urinary tract, in contrast to sporadic TCC.

Mutations in mismatch repair genes, including *hMSH2, hMUTL, hPMS1,* and *hPMS2,* have been found responsible for most cases.[88–90] These genes are involved in DNA mismatch repair and belong to a highly conserved family of repair proteins. Mutation results in characteristic genetic instability detected by ''shifts'' in microsatellite markers. These shifts are actually expansions or contractions of small DNA repeat elements (microsatellites). Whether mutations of mismatch repair genes occur commonly in the development of sporadic bladder tumors is not known. Approximately 2% of all sporadic tumors display characteristic, microsatellite instability associated with HNPCC and mismatch repair.[91] Patients with apparently sporadic tumors that display instability are often found to belong to Lynch kindreds on careful reexamination of family history, however. This syndrome is common and should be considered when patients have a family history of colon cancer or TCC.

MOLECULAR BIOLOGY OF INVASION AND METASTASIS

In bladder cancer, the finding of infiltration signals the capability of a tumor to behave in an aggressive manner and potentially to create a life-threatening situation. The ability to invade is carried in the tumor cell's complement of biochemical pathways, as well as in its inability to preserve or restore rather than to disrupt normal tissue architecture. What determines the activation and deployment of these biochemical activities is unclear; however, recent work is beginning to suggest possibilities.

Tumor cell invasion is facilitated by the production of degradative enzymes that can lyse basement membranes and connective tissues. Increased activities of lysosomal enzymes in tumors have been correlated with expression of the degree of malignancy in vivo.[92] These lysosomal proteases include cathepsins B, D, H, and L. In addition, several components of the extracellular matrix (proteoglycans, fibronectin, laminin, and portions of collagen types I through IV) have been found to be degraded by various families of cathepsins.[93] Weiss and associates observed that superficial, but not invasive, bladder tumors in mice were surrounded by intact laminin.[94] These investigators demonstrated that the absence of laminin was attributable to the enhanced production and the redistribution of activated protease cathepsin B to the plasma membrane fraction of the invasive cells. A cysteine protease inhibitor against cathepsin B has been shown to abrogate invasion of the EJ bladder cell line through an artificial basement membrane in a nontoxic dose-dependent manner.[95] The redistribution of cathepsin B to the plasma membrane of invasive cells thus may play an important role in the activity of the aggressive tumor cell. Cathepsin B may need to be located on the plasma membrane, where it can degrade regional basement membrane. The destruction of basement membrane components by tumor cells has particular relevance in human bladder cancers.

The activation of proplasmin or plasminogen to plasmin, a protease that is capable of degrading fibronectin and other extracellular matrix components, may account for fibrinolytic activity in human malignant tumors. Several investigators have suggested increased plasminogen activator expression in tumor samples and in the urine of patients with a greater likelihood of invasive urologic tumors.[96,97]

The characteristic of motility is necessary for tumor cells to traverse the many stages in the complex cascade of invasion and metastasis. The potential use of a cytokine, autocrine mobility factor (AMF), in determining the biologic activity of human bladder cancers has been investigated.[98] Urine samples from patients with bladder cancer were assayed for their capacity to stimulate migration of tumor cells. Comparing all cases of TCC with nonmalignant diseases, a statistically significant difference in AMF values was found. Invasive TCCs had higher AMF values than noninvasive TCCs ($P < 0.001$). Tumor cell motility is mediated in part by enzymes involved in signal transduction. A major enzyme in signal transduction is a calcium- and phospholipid-dependent serine-threonine kinase known as protein kinase C (PKC). PKC is considered a target for the inhibition of motility and, ultimately, of invasion and metastasis. Inhibition of PKC has prevented the invasion of EJ cells by interfering with cellular motility.[99]

Cell-cell and cell-matrix interactions have also been suggested as factors that may regulate tumor cell behavior. Results demonstrate that altered extracellular matrices and perhaps specific components of the these matrices can alter gene expression, cellular proliferation, and invasiveness of the overlying epithelial cells.[100] If so, altered extracellular matrices, as produced by carcinogen-exposed or transformed stroma, may play an important role in the ability of an epithelial tumor to proliferate, to recur, or to progress by providing a permissive or "fertile" environment.

CLINICAL APPLICATIONS

The molecular analysis of human bladder tumors promises to make available information that would be difficult to obtain otherwise. First, these studies may result in the localization and identification of one or more bladder carcinoma predisposition loci, involved in the initiation of the disease, allowing susceptible subgroups of the population to be screened more effectively. Identification of genes and mutations can lead to novel detection strategies in urine.[67] The detection of a *P53* mutation years before clinical diagnosis provides insight into the power of this approach.[101] Until a common lesion such as the putative tumor suppressor gene on chromosome 9 is cloned and characterized, novel markers for clonality may allow early detection.[102] In addition, an understanding of the origins and nature of bladder carcinogenesis may be gained by studying the effects of known bladder carcinogens on a gene and by elucidating the nature of its absent or mutated protein product. Second, genetic markers provide a more objective means to subclassify tumors that may appear similar histologically. Genetic analysis by karyotype, flow cytometry, and allelotyping provides information that may have prognostic significance and can direct the most appropriate choice of treatment. Any genetic marker, such as mutation of *P53*, is potentially useful to predict outcome and may have immediate application. Genetic markers may have a role in improving current histopathologic staging by molecular analysis.[103] Finally, genetic analysis of tumor-specific mutations may allow the identification of specific genetic lesions and biochemical pathways on which future therapeutic approaches may be focused.

REFERENCES

1. Nowell PC. The clonal evolution of tumor cell populations. Science 1976;94:23.
2. Fialkow PJ. Clonal origin of human tumors. Biochim Biophys Acta 1976;458:283.
3. Killion JJ, Fidler IJ. The biology of tumor metastasis. Semin Oncol 1989;16:106.
4. Sandberg AA. The chromosomes in human cancer and leukemia, 2nd ed. New York: Elsevier Science, 1990.
5. Vogelstein B, Fearon ER, Hamilton SR, et al. Clonal analysis using recombinant DNA probes from the X-chromosome. Cancer Res 1987; 47:4806.
6. Sidransky D, Frost P, Von Eschenbach A, Oyasu R, Preisinger AC, Vogelstein B. Clonal origin of bladder cancer. N Engl J Med 1992; 326:737.
7. Kurzrock R, Gutterman JU, Talpaz M, et al. The molecular genetics of Philadelphia chromosome-positive leukemias. N Engl J Med 1988; 319:990.
8. Kelman Z, Prokocimer M, Peller S, et al. Rearrangements in the p53 gene in Philadelphia chromosome positive chronic myelogenous leukemia. Blood 1989;74:2318.
9. Sandberg AA. Chromosome changes in bladder cancer: clinical and other correlations. Cancer Genet Cytogenet 1986;19:163.
10. Knudson AJ. Mutation and cancer: statistical study of retinoblastoma. Proc Natl Acad Sci USA 1971;68:820.
11. Atkin NB, Fox MF. 5q deletion: the sole chromosome change in a carcinoma of the bladder. Cancer Genet Cytogenet 1990;46:129.
12. Babu VR, Miles BJ, Cerney JC, Weiss L, Van Dyke DL. Chromosome 21q22 deletion: a specific chromosome change in a new bladder cancer subgroup. Cancer Genet Cytogenet 1989;38:127.
13. Smeets W, Pauwels R, Laarakkers L, Debruyne F, Geraedts J. Chromosomal analysis of bladder cancer. III. Nonrandom alterations. Cancer Genet Cytogenet 1987;29:29.
14. Berger CS, Sandberg AA, Todd IAD, et al. Chromosomes in kidney, ureter, and bladder cancer. Cancer Genet Cytogenet 1986;23:1.
15. Gibas Z, Prout GJ, Connolly JG, Pontes JE, Sandberg AA. Nonrandom chromosomal changes in transitional cell carcinoma of the bladder. Cancer Res 1984;44:1257.
16. Vanni R, Scarpa RM, Nieddu M, Usai E. Identification of marker chromosomes in bladder tumors. Urol Int 1986;41:403.
17. Vanni R, Scarpa RM. Nonrandom chromosomal changes in transitional cell carcinoma of the bladder. Cancer Res 1986;46:4873.
18. Atkin NB, Baker MC. Cytogenetic study of ten carcinomas of the bladder: involvement of chromosomes 1 and 11. Cancer Genet Cytogenet 1985;15:253.
19. Gibas Z, Prout GR, Pontes JE, Connolly JG, Sandberg AA. A possible specific chromosome change in transitional cell carcinoma of the bladder. Cancer Genet Cytogenet 1986;19:229.
20. Fearon ER, Feinberg AP, Hamilton SH, Vogelstein B. Loss of genes on the short arm of chromosome 11 in bladder cancer. Nature 1985; 318:377.
21. Cairns P, Proctor AJ, Knowles MA. Loss of heterozygosity at the RB locus is frequent and correlates with muscle invasion in bladder carcinoma. Oncogene 1991;6:2305.
22. Tsai YC, Nichols PW, Hiti AL, Williams Z, Skinner DG, Jones PA. Allelic losses of chromosomes 9, 11, and 17 in human bladder cancer. Cancer Res 1990;50:44.
23. Kallioniemi A, Kallioniemi OP, Sudar D, et al. Comparative genomic hybridization for molecular cytogenetic analysis of solid tumors. Science 1992;258:818.
24. du Manoir S, Speicher MR, Joos S, et al. Detection of complete and partial chromosome gains and losses by comparative genomic in situ hybridization. Hum Genet 1993;90:590.
25. Voorter C, Joos S, Vallinga M, et al. Detection of chromosomal imbalances in transitional cell carcinoma of the bladder by comparative genomic hybridization. Am J Pathol 1995;146:1341.
26. Thompson CT, Gray JW. Cytogenetic profiling using fluorescence in situ hybridization (FISH) and comparative genomic hybridization (CGH). J Cell Biochem Suppl 1993;17G:139.
27. Doll R, Peto R. Epidemiology of cancer. In: Weatherall DJ, Ledingham JGG, Warrell DA, eds. Oxford textbook of medicine, 2nd ed. Oxford: Oxford University Press, 1987:4.95.
28. Fearon ER, Vogelstein B. A genetic model for colorectal tumorigenesis. Cell 1990;61:759.
29. Bishop JM. Molecular themes in oncogenesis. Cell 1991;64:235.
30. Cantley LC, Auger KR, Carpenter C, et al. Oncogenes and signal transduction (published erratum appears in Cell 1991 May 31;65: following 914). Cell 1991;64:281.
31. Alberts B, Bray D, Lewis J, Raff M, Roberts K, Watson JD. Molecular biology of the cell, 2nd ed. New York: Garland, 1989.
32. Varmus HE. The molecular genetics of cellular oncogenes. Annu Rev Genet 1984;18:553.
33. Varmus HE. An historical overview of oncogenes. In: Weinber RA, ed. Oncogenes and the molecular origins of cancer. Cold Spring Harbor, NY: Cold Spring Harbor Laboratory Press, 1989:3.
34. Reddy EP, Reynolds RK, Santos E, Barbacid M. A point mutation is responsible for the acquisition of transforming properties by the T24 human bladder carcinoma oncogene. Nature 1982;300:149.
35. Knowles MA, Williamson M. Mutation of H-ras is infrequent in bladder cancer: confirmation by single-strand conformation polymorphism analysis, designed restriction fragment length polymorphisms, and direct sequencing. Cancer Res 1993;53:133.
36. Fujita J, Srivastava SK, Kraus MH, Rhim JS, Tronick SR, Aaronson

SA. Frequency of molecular alterations affecting ras protooncogenes in human urinary tract tumors. Proc Natl Acad Sci USA 1985;82: 3849.
37. Viola MV, Fromowitz F, Oravez S, Deb S, Schlom J. ras oncogene p21 expression is increased in premalignant lesions and high grade bladder carcinoma. J Exp Med 1985;161:1213.
38. Slamon DJ, Clark GM, Wong SG, Levin WJ, Ullrich A, McGuire WL. Human breast cancer: correlation of relapse and survival with amplification of the HER-2/neu oncogene. Science 1987;235:177.
39. Coombs LM, Pigott DA, Sweeney E, et al. Amplification and overexpression of c-erbB-2 in transitional cell carcinoma of the urinary bladder. Br J Cancer 1991;63:601.
40. Wright C, Mellon K, Neal DE, Johnston P, Corbett IP, Horne CH. Expression of c-erbB-2 protein product in bladder cancer. Br J Cancer 1990;62:764.
41. Proctor AJ, Coombs LM, Cairns JP, Knowles MA. Amplification at chromosome 11q13 in transitional cell tumours of the bladder. Oncogene 1991;6:789.
42. Masters JR, Vesey SG, Munn CF, Evan GI, Watson JV. c-myc oncoprotein levels in bladder cancer. Urol Res 1988;16:341.
43. Del-Senno L, Maestri I, Piva R, et al. Differential hypomethylation of the c-myc proto-oncogene in bladder cancers at different stages and grades. J Urol 1989;142:146.
44. Fanning P, Bulovas K, Saini KS. Elevated expression of $pp60^{c\text{-}src}$ in low grade human bladder carcinomas. Cancer Res 1992;52:1457.
45. Messing EM, Reznikoff CA. Normal and malignant urothelium: in-vitro effects of epidermal growth factor. Cancer Res 1987;47:2230.
46. Neal DE, Marsh C, Bennett MK, et al. Epidermal-growth-factor receptors in human bladder cancer: comparison of invasive and superficial tumours. Lancet 1985;1:366.
47. Neal DE, Sharples L, Smith K, Fennelly J, Hall RR, Harris AL. The epidermal growth factor receptor and the prognosis of bladder cancer. Cancer 1990;65:1619.
48. Berger MS, Greenfield C, Gullick WJ, et al. Evaluation of epidermal growth factor receptors in bladder tumours. Br J Cancer 1987;56:533.
49. Bishop JM. The molecular genetics of cancer. Science 1987;235:305.
50. Francke U. Retinoblastoma and chromosome 13. Birth Defects 1976; 12:131.
51. Hansen MF, Cavenee WK. Retinoblastoma and the progression of tumor genetics. Trends Genet 1988;4:125.
52. Ponder B. Cancer: gene losses in human tumours (news). Nature 1988; 335:400.
53. Presti JC, Reuter VW, Galan T, Fair WR, Cordon-Cardo C. Molecular genetic alterations in superficial and locally advanced human bladder cancer. Cancer Res 1991;51:5405.
54. Knowles MA, Elder PA, Williamson M, Cairns JP, Shaw ME, Law MG. Allelotype of human bladder cancer. Cancer Res 1994;54:531.
55. Cairns P, Shaw ME, Knowles MA. Initiation of bladder cancer may involve deletion of a tumor suppressor gene on chromosome 9. Oncogene 1993;8:1083.
56. Ruppert JM, Tokino K, Sidransky D. Evidence for two bladder cancer suppressor loci on human chromosome 9. Cancer Res 1993;53:5093.
57. Cairns P, Tokino K, Eby Y, Sidransky D. Homozygous deletions of 9p21 in primary human bladder tumors detected by comparative multiplex polymerase chain reaction. Cancer Res 1994;54:1422.
58. Olopade OI, Buchhagen DL, Malik K, et al. Homozygous loss of the interferon genes defines the critical region on 9p that is deleted in lung cancers. Cancer Res 1993;53:2410.
59. Kamb A, Gruis NA, Weaver-Feldhaus J, et al. A cell cycle regulator potentially involved in genesis of many tumor types. Science 1994; 264:436.
60. Hussussian CJ, Struewing JP, Goldstein AM, et al. Germline p16 mutations in familial melanoma. Nature Genet 1994;8:15.
61. Caldas C, Hahn SA, da Costa LT, et al. Frequent somatic mutations and homozygous deletions of the p16 (MTS1) gene in pancreatic adenocarcinoma. Nature Genet 1994;8:27.
62. Cairns P, Mao L, Merlo A, et al. Rates of p16 (MTS1) mutations in primary tumors with 9p loss. Science 1994;265:415.
63. Spruck CH, Gonzalez-Zulueta M, Shibata A, et al. p16 gene in uncultured tumors. Nature 1994;370;183.
64. Cairns P, Shaw ME, Knowles MA. Preliminary mapping of the deleted region of chromosome 9 in bladder cancer. Cancer Res 1993;53:1230.
65. Linnenbach AJ, Pressler LB, Seng BA, Kimmel BS, Tomaszewski JE, Malkowicz SB. Characterization of chromosome 9 deletions in transitional cell carcinoma by microsatellite assay. Hum Mol Genet 1993;2:1407.
66. Nigro JM, Baker SJ, Preisinger AC, et al. Mutations in the p53 gene occur in diverse human tumour types. Nature 1989;342:705.
67. Sidransky D, von Eschenbach A, Tsai YC, et al. Identification of p53 gene mutations in bladder cancers and urine samples. Science 1991; 252:706.
68. Habuchi T, Ogawa O, Kaheki Y, Sugiyama T, Yoshida O. Allelic loss of chromosome 17p in urothelial cancer: strong association with invasive phenotype. J Urol 1992;148:1595.
69. Dalbagni S, Presti JC, Reuter VE, Fair WR, Cordon-Cardo C. Genetic alterations in bladder cancer. Lancet 1993;342:469.
70. Fujimoto K, Yamada Y, Okajima E. Frequent association of p53 mutation in invasive bladder cancer. Cancer Res 1992;52:1393.
71. Esrig D, Elmajian D, Groshen S, et al. Accumulation of Nuclear p53 and tumor progression in bladder cancer. N Engl J Med 1994;331: 1259.
72. Friend SH, Horowitz JM, Gerber MR, et al. Deletions of a DNA sequence in retinoblastomas and mesenchymal tumors: organization of the sequence and its encoded protein (published erratum appears in Proc Natl Acad Sci USA 1988 85:2234). Proc Natl Acad Sci USA 1987;84:9059.
73. DerKinderen DJ, Koten JW, Nagelkerke NJ, Tan KE, Beemer FA, Den OW. Non-ocular cancer in patients with hereditary retinoblastoma and their relatives. Int J Cancer 1988;41:499.
74. Horowitz JM, Park SH, Bogenmann E, et al. Frequent inactivation of the retinoblastoma anti-oncogene is restricted to a subset of human tumor cells. Proc Natl Acad Sci USA 1990;87:2775.
75. Xu HJ, Cairns P, Hu SX, Knowles MA, Benedict WF. Loss of RB protein expression in primary bladder cancer correlates with loss of heterozygosity at the RB locus and tumor progression. Intl J Cancer 1993;53:781.
76. Cordon-Cardo C, Wartinger D, Petrylak D, et al. Altered expression of retinoblastoma gene product: prognostic indicator in bladder cancer. J Natl Cancer Inst 1992;84:1251.
77. Logothetis CJ, Xu HJ, Ro JY, et al. Altered expression of retinoblastoma protein and known prognostic variables in locally advanced bladder cancer. J Natl Cancer Inst 1992;84:1256.
78. Takahashi R, Hashimoto T, Hu HJ, et al. The retinoblastoma gene functions as a growth and tumor suppressor in human bladder carcinoma cells. Proc Natl Acad Sci USA 1991;88:5257.
79. Mihara K, Cao XR, Yen A, et al. Cell cycle-dependent regulation of phosphorylation of human RB gene product. Science 1989;246:1300.
80. Hawkins MM, Draper GJ, Smith RA. Cancer among 1,348 offspring of survivors of childhood cancer. Int J Cancer 1989;43:975.
81. Wu S-Q, Storer BE, Bookland EA, et al. Nonrandom chromosome losses in stepwise neoplastic transformation in vitro of human uroepithelial cells. Cancer Res 1991;51:3323.
82. Sidransky D, Messing E. Molecular genetics and biochemical mechanisms in bladder cancer: oncogenes, tumor suppressor genes, and growth factors. Urol Clin North Am 1992;19:629.
83. Spruck CH, Ohneseit PF, Gonzalez-Zulueta M, et al. Two molecular pathways to transition cell carcinoma of the bladder. Cancer Res 1994; 54:784.
84. Schulte PA. The role of genetic factors in bladder cancer. Cancer Detect Prev 1988;11:379.
85. Lynch HT. Genetics, natural history, tumor spectrum, and pathology of hereditary nonpolyposis colorectal cancer: an updated review. Gastroenterology 1993;104:1535.
86. Vasen HF, Offerhaus GJ, den Hartog Jager FC, et al. The tumour spectrum in hereditary non-polyposis colorectal cancer: a study of 24 kindreds in the Netherlands. Int J Cancer 1990;46:31.
87. Lynch HT, Ens JA, Lynch JF. The Lynch syndrome II and urological malignancies. J Urol 1990;143:24.
88. Cleaver JE. It was a very good year for DNA repair. Cell 1994;76: 1.
89. Bronner CE, Baker SM, Morrison PT, et al. Mutation in the DNA mismatch repair gene homologue hMLH1 is associated with hereditary non-polyposis colon cancer. Nature 1994;368:258.
90. Nicolaides NC, Popadopoulos N, Liu B, et al. Mutations of two PMS homologues in hereditary nonpolyposis colon cancer. Nature 1994; 371:75.
91. Gonzalez-Zulueta M, Ruppert JM, Tokino K, et al. Microsatellite instability in bladder cancer. Cancer Res 1993;53:5620.

92. Sloane BF, Rozhin J, Hatfield JS, et al. Plasma membrane-associated cysteine proteinases in human and animal tumors. Exp Cell Biol 1987; 55:209.
93. Lah TT, Buck MR, Honn KV, et al. Degradation of laminin by human tumor catepsin B. Clin Exp Metastasis 1989;7:461.
94. Weiss RE, Liu BCS, Ahlering T, et al. Mechanisms of human bladder tumor invasion: role of protease cathepsin B. J Urol 1990;144:798.
95. Redwood SM, Liu BCS, Weiss RE, et al. Abrogation of the invasion of human bladder tumor cells by using protease inhibitor(s). Cancer 1992;69:1212.
96. Hasui Y, Suzumiya J, Marutsuka K. Comparative study of plasminogen activators in cancers and normal mucosae of human urinary bladder. Cancer Res 1989;49:1067.
97. Gorelick U, Lindner A, Mayer M. Protease and plasminogen activator activity in human bladder carcinoma. Br J Urol 1990;66:170.
98. Guirguis R, Schiffman E, Liu B. Detection of autocrine motility factor in urine as a marker of bladder cancer. J Natl Cancer Inst 1988;80: 1203.
99. Schwartz GK, Redwood SM, Ohnuma T, et al. Inhibition of invasion of invasive human bladder carcinoma cells by protein kinase C inhibitor staurosporine. J Natl Cancer Inst 1990;82:1753.
100. Gordon JN, Shu W-P, Schlussel RN, Droller MJ, Liu BC-S. Altered extracellular matrices influence cellular processes and nuclear matrix organizations of overlying human urothelial cells. Cancer Res 1993; 53:4971.
101. Hruban RH, van der Riet P, Erozan YS, Sidransky D. Molecular biology and the early detection of carcinoma of the bladder: the case of Hubert Horatio Humphrey. N Engl J Med 1994;330:1276.
102. Mao L, Lee DJ, Tockman MS, Erozan YS, Askin F, Sidransky D. Microsatellite alterations as clonal markers in the detection of human cancer. Proc Natl Acad Sci USA 1994;91:9871.
103. Brennan JA, Mao L, Hruban RH, et al. Molecular assessment of histopathologic staging. N Engl J Med 1995;332:1787.

Principles and Practice of Genitourinary Oncology, edited by Derek Raghavan, Howard I. Scher, Steven A. Leibel, and Paul H. Lange. Lippincott-Raven Publishers, Philadelphia, © 1997.

CHAPTER 21

Tumor Markers in the Management of Bladder Cancer

Yves Fradet and Carlos Cordon-Cardo

The management of bladder cancer is a constant challenge due to the heterogeneous nature of this cancer type and the various therapeutic options available.[1] In papillary superficial (Ta, T1) tumors, which represent more than 75% of primary bladder cancers, pathologic information cannot accurately predict those 50% to 60% of patients who will experience tumor recurrence and thus would benefit from intravesical therapy. It also is not possible to identify which patients will respond favorably to this treatment. Progression from superficial to muscle-infiltrating cancer is observed in 10% to 20% of patients with Ta, T1 tumors. The accurate identification of high-risk patients would justify a more aggressive treatment. The diagnosis and follow-up of patients with Ta, T1 tumors is primarily based on cystoscopy, which is associated with increased costs and morbidity. The availability of sensitive, specific diagnostic tests would significantly improve the management of this disease. At the other end of the spectrum, more than 75% of muscle-invasive (T2+) bladder cancers are found at initial diagnosis. The most significant problem in the management of T2+ cancers is the identification of the metastatic potential, because more than one half of patients treated using radical cystectomy die of systemic disease. No clinical parameter currently allows the prediction of those patients who are likely to fail nor the likelihood of their response to systemic polychemotherapy.

Despite the need for prognostic and diagnostic tests and the ease of access to exfoliated cells or shed products in the urine, tumor markers have had little impact on the clinical management of bladder cancer. However, tumor biology has evolved very rapidly, resulting in the identification of numerous genes and gene products potentially involved in carcinogenesis.[2] These discoveries have been mostly driven by technologic advances in immunology, molecular biology, and genetics, which have made it possible to develop tests using a minimal amount of clinical material. Immunoassays and polymerase chain reaction (PCR) have had a tremendous impact in this regard. Although the numerous tumor markers have added complexity to the technology required for routine diagnostic testing, they have contributed significantly to the understanding of the biology of bladder cancer and the molecular pathways of carcinogenesis. A definite role for tumor markers in diagnosis and prognosis is emerging and will likely influence the management of bladder cancer patients. It is important to understand the nature of these markers, the feasibility of their measurement in clinical material, the clinical problems that such markers may help to resolve, and the extent of their clinical validation.

TUMOR MARKERS

DNA Analysis

Chromosomal anomalies are a hallmark of cancer cells. These can be grossly assessed by measuring tumor cell DNA content using flow cytometry or image analysis. Both techniques are based on the quantification of specific dyes incorporated into DNA. Tumors are defined as diploid (normal DNA content) or aneuploid when compared with normal control lymphocytes. As assessed in a consensus conference, tumor DNA cytometry provides prognostic information on the risk of progression in patients with superficial (Ta, T1, Tis) bladder cancer[3,4] but not in those with muscle-invasive cancers (T2 to T4). Moreover, aneuploidy was not predictive of a higher recurrence rate in a study of 350 newly diagnosed Ta, T1 tumors.[5] Conversely, in bladder irrigation specimens the presence of a clear, nontetraploid, aneuploid DNA population is diagnostic of recurrent tumor or carcinoma in situ. However, the sensitivity of DNA analysis of exfoliated cells to detect bladder tumors has been at best comparable and more often lower than that of urinary cytology. More recent information using image analysis systems suggests that nuclear features referred to as karyometric analysis may have increased sensitivity in screening for recurrences in patients treated for Ta, T1 tumors.[6]

Cytogenetics

Further insights into chromosomal anomalies may be gained by using fluorescent in situ hybridization. Probes for DNA sequences specific for each chromosome are hybridized to tumor nuclei obtained directly from tumor biopsy specimens or bladder irrigations. By counting fluorescent spots, numerical changes in given chromosomes or even in specific chromosomal arms can be estimated.[7,8] The loss of specific chromosome segments has also been studied by a molecular biology technique referred to as restriction fragment length polymorphism (RFLP), which exploits the difference in specific genes of the length of alleles from both parents. The power of this approach has been increased tremendously by studying microsatellite DNA using PCR techniques that essentially allow cytogenetics study of a few cells cut from a tumor or a small biopsy specimen.

Using these two techniques, several chromosomal anomalies have been consistently observed at high frequency in bladder cancer specimens.[9,10] Loss of heterozygosity on one or both arms of chromosome 9 has been observed in 60% to 77% of cases in several studies.[9,11] More refined studies on 73 primary bladder tumors showed two hot spots most frequently deleted on chromosome 9: one on 9p (9p21)[12] and one on 9q in an area more difficult to localize but most likely located on the telomeric (tail end) segment of the long chromosomal arm.[13] Furthermore, Ta lesions appear to have abnormalities mostly on 9q, whereas T1 and Tis cancers are more frequently associated with 9p deletions. These observations suggest the existence of at least two suppressor genes on chromosome 9. Deletions on the 17p chromosome were observed in approximately 60% of muscle-invasive bladder cancer, as were deletions on chromosome 3p and 5q.[14,15] Tumor suppressor genes have been identified or are suspected to be located on three chromosome regions: *P53* on 17p, suppressor genes of colon cancers on 5q, and suppressor genes of renal and lung cancers on 3p. Thus, improvements in technology have led to the identification of specific chromosomal changes associated with distinct biologic behavior of bladder tumors and may provide important clues regarding different pathways of bladder carcinogenesis.

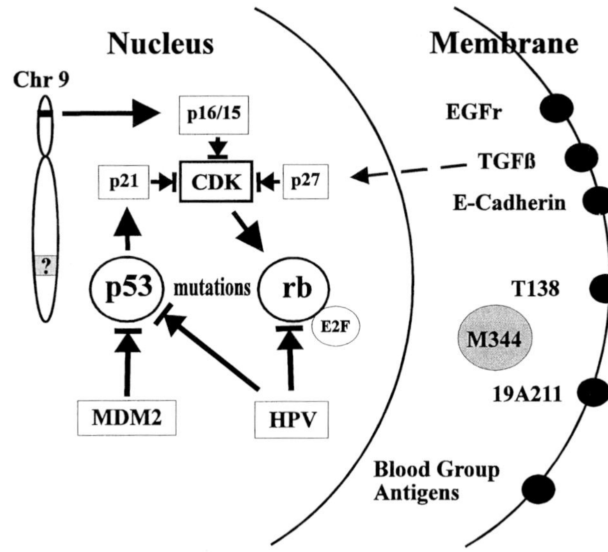

FIG. 21-1. Schematic representation of nuclear and membrane tumor markers suspected to be of clinical relevance in bladder cancer management. The RB1 protein plays a central role in controlling cell growth at the transition from G1 to S phase. RB1 phosphorylation, which releases the transcription factor E2F, is induced by cyclin-dependent kinases (CDKs) which are in turn negatively regulated by a family of proteins (i.e., P21, P16, P15, and P27). P53 is a suppressor protein induced by DNA-damage to stop cell division to allow cell repair or induce cell death. P53 exerts its inhibition on RB1 via the P21–CDK pathway. The MDM2 oncogene can inactivate P53, and both P53 and RB1 can be inactivated by gene mutations or by viral oncoproteins of the human papillomavirus (HPV). Two bladder cancer suppressor genes are suspected on chromosome 9: 9p21 appears to code for P16 inhibitory protein, and the 9q gene remains unidentified. Also represented (*right*) are phenotypic changes in membrane and cytoplasmic proteins that also have been associated with the distinct biologic behavior of bladder cancer including the epidermal growth factor receptor (EGFR), transforming growth factor beta (TGFB), and blood group antigens.

Tumor Suppressor Genes

Cancer cells are characterized by loss of differentiation, increased invasiveness and mobility, and decreased drug sensitivity. These differences arise not only from uncontrolled cellular growth but also from the unleashing of normally repressed genes. Apparently parallel lines of investigation have come together to unravel a delicate, interactive network of molecules coordinating these genes' activity to control cell cycle and to act as check point controls and repair pathways (Fig. 21-1).[16] Carcinogenesis, in part, interferes with this mechanism, thus resulting in increased genomic instability.

Of several candidate tumor suppressor genes identified, the most extensively studied are the *P53* and the *RB1* (formerly known as rb) genes. The *RB1* gene, located on chromosome 13q, encodes a phosphoprotein with a molecular weight of 110,000 kd that plays a central role in the control of the cell cycle, particularly in the progression from G1 to S phase.[17] Alterations of RB1 protein have been associated with cancer progression in different cancer types. The gene product RB1 can be studied using a monoclonal antibody that detects the protein only in frozen tissues or with a polyclonal antibody (Rb-WL-1) that is reported to work on paraffin-embedded tumors.[18,19] Antibodies detect loss of expression, which may be the result of mutations or gene deletions. However, it has become evident that the RB1 is the end result of complex protein interactions involving cyclin-dependent kinases (CDKs; see Fig. 21-1). Once activated, the CDK complexes phosphorylate the RB1 protein, which is bound to the transcription factor E2F during G1 phase. Upon phosphorylation by CDK, E2F is released and activates the transcription of genes required for transition into S phase (cell division). It is possible that a family of RB1-like molecules exists. Several proteins inhibit the activation of CDK complexes. One of them, P27, is influenced by transforming growth factor beta (TGFB). P16 and P15, which also inhibit CDK, have been identified as the likely products of the suppressor genes found on chromosome 9p21.[20,21] One study suggests that P16 is increased when RB1 is decreased, much like other cybernetic principles of retroaction observed in many biologic systems.[22] It thus appears that RB1 protein is a key element in controlling cell proliferation and may be influenced by defects in several tumor suppressor genes. In the latter case, the level of RB1 is normal, but RB1 may be phosphorylated, thus releasing E2F transcription factor. The antibodies measure only the decrease in RB1 level as a result of defects in the *RB1* gene itself, a finding observed in approximately 25% of bladder cancers.[18,19]

One of the most extensively studied tumor suppressor genes is *P53*, which is directly or indirectly involved in most human cancers.[23,24] *P53* controls a cell cycle checkpoint responsible for maintaining the integrity of the genome. It has been shown that the wild-type (normal) P53 protein mediates arrest in the G1 phase of the cell cycle when cells are exposed to DNA-damaging agents; P53 seems to exert its action on the cell cycle through P21, which inhibits CDK and in turn arrests the cell in G1 phase by preventing RB1 phosphorylation. The P53 function can be altered by the binding of viral oncoproteins or other oncogenes (as discussed below) to P53 by a deletion of the *P53* gene on chromosome 17p or by mutations in the gene itself. Mutated *P53* has a longer half-life and can be measured most precisely using an antibody, p1801, which is commonly used in many clinical studies. The high accuracy of this technique has been shown in studies comparing immunostaining, RFLP, and DNA sequencing of the *P53* gene.[25] It is thus very easy to detect the presence of *P53* mutations by a simple immunohistochemical technique. *P53* mutations are observed with increased frequency according to grade and stage of the cancer.[26–30] In a study of primary Ta, T1 tumors, it was found that 8% of Ta grade I tumors have *P53* mutations, and as many as 50% of T1 grade III tumors have abnormal P53 much like invasive bladder cancers.[31] Loss of RB1 expression is similarly not frequent in Ta tumors; its frequency increases with invasive bladder cancer.

Oncogenes

Oncogenes are normal cellular genes that may be altered by mutations or gene amplifications and result in deregulation of growth control mechanisms, leading to tumorigenesis and cancer progression. Only a few of these genes have been shown to be involved in human malignancies. *HRAS* (formerly known as H-*ras*) was the first oncogene identified and was discovered in human bladder cancer.[32] Single base-pair mutations at position 12 and 61 on the *HRAS* gene are particularly potent at inducing cancer. Although mutations were found relatively rarely in bladder cancer initially,[33] results of more recent studies suggest that using other methods may allow the detection of mutations in as many as 40% of bladder cancers.[34,35] No correlation was found, however, between *HRAS* mutation in primary Ta, T1 tumors and rate of recurrence or cancer progression. Amplification of another oncogene, *ERBB2* (formerly known as c-*erb* B2[*neu*]) has been observed in several malignancies and is correlated with a poor clinical outcome. However, results of two different studies suggest that it is a rare event in superficial bladder cancer and does not provide significant prognostic information.[31,36]

Oncogenesis may be promoted by the incorporation of viral DNA into the human genome. The family of DNA human papillomaviruses (HPV) has been found in many tumor types. Although the possible implication of HPV in human bladder cancer has been controversial, several studies have reported the detection of HPV DNA by molecular techniques in one third of bladder cancers.[37–40] In the study of LaRue and colleagues,[40] 34% of Ta, T1 tumors and 36% of T2 tumors were HPV-positive, whereas normal bladder samples were HPV-negative. The HPV 16–positive tumors tended to be of higher grade and correlated with a poorer prognosis. HPV may induce oncogenesis by the binding of its viral proteins E6 and E7 to the tumor suppressor genes *P53* and *RB1* (see Fig. 21-1).[10]

A newly described protooncogene, *MDM2*, has been shown to bind to *P53* and inactivate its physiologic role as a transcription factor and cell cycle regulator.[41,42] The *MDM2* gene is located on the long arm of chromosome 12 and encodes a 90-kd nuclear protein. In one study, *MDM2* proteins were detected at high levels in 32% of bladder cancers using the monoclonal antibody 2A10.[43] A positive nuclear reactivity, which can be studied on formalin-fixed tumors, was found more frequently in Ta, T1 tumors (62%) than in muscle-invasive cancers (24%). A detailed analysis of *MDM2*, *P53*, and chromosome 9 aberrations leads to the postulate that specific *MDM2* and *P53* phenotypes may reflect underlying biologic mechanisms of tumorigenesis in bladder cancer. *MDM2* acts as a negative regulator of *P53* and may be increased following increases in wild-type *P53* in response to minimal chromosomal changes or genetic instability. As shown in Figure 21-1, tumor suppressor genes act in a complex interactive cascade in which multiple alterations may lead to cumulative effects on genomic instability. The key anomalies identified include the chromosome 9p deletions, *RB1* and *P53* mutations, HPV infection, and probably loss of some tumor suppressor genes on 9q that may influence production of the *MDM2* oncogene.

Growth Factors

Cell cycle control mechanisms are also under the influence of external cell stimulation through growth factor receptors such as the receptor for epidermal growth factor (EGFR). Increased expression of EGFR found on subsets of bladder cancers may provide them with a growth advantage, because EGF is a potent mitogen found in large quantities in urine.[44] Studies have suggested that increased expression of EGFR on superficial bladder tumors is a good predictor of tumors prone to progress to muscle-invasive cancers.[45,46] EGFR was not of prognostic value for invasive bladder cancer, however. Several other growth factors, such as transforming growth factor (TGF) and fibroblast growth factor (FGF) have been found to be involved in the control of cancer cell behavior. They may induce the production of proteolytic enzymes capable of degrading basement membrane components in connective tissues, thus facilitating cell movements. Tissue collagenase-stimulating factor (TCSF) is one such factor that has been found in high-grade bladder cancer and may have some diagnostic value.[47,48] Many other factors, such as angiogenic factors and autocrine motility factors, are also known to be produced in high-stage bladder cancer, but their exact prognostic significance remains unknown. The mirror image of cancer cell invasion and motility is the decrease in intercellular adhesiveness mediated by E-cadherin. Recent studies have shown that loss of normal membrane E-cadherin expression correlates with increasing grade and stage of the tumor as well as shorter patient survival.[49]

Blood Group Antigens

For many years, loss of ABH blood group antigen expression was the only tumor marker in bladder cancer.[50] Monoclonal antibodies have provided better reagents allowing immunopathology studies on formalin-fixed material. The National Cancer Institute (NCI) Bladder Tumor Marker Network studied 131 patients with primary Ta, T1 tumors and long follow-up.[51] Loss of expression of ABH was observed in 40% of cases irrespective of the recurrence or progressor status of the patients, thus suggesting no benefit from the study of these antigens. Conversely, Lewis^X antigen was expressed in more than 90% of the tumors. This finding may result in increased detection of tumor cells and exfoliated cells of the urine.[52] However, Lewis^X antigen is also expressed on polymorphic nuclear cells as well as normal umbrella cells.

Tumor-Associated Antigens

Several research groups have produced monoclonal antibodies to bladder cancer.[53] However, limited data is available on the characteristics of the antigens recognized by these antibodies, and very few have been studied in a clinical setting. Some of these antibodies may have similar specificities, and several monoclonal antibodies to bladder cancer have been found to react with Lewis^X antigen.[54] Among a large group of monoclonal antibodies produced by Fradet and colleagues,[54–58] three that have been extensively characterized biochemically and on clinical material appear to have potential as diagnostic and prognostic markers. The monoclonal antibodies M344 and 19A211, which are reactive to new antigens of superficial bladder tumors, were obtained using strategies to block reactivity to normal urothelial antigens.[59] M344 reacts with a high-molecular-weight cytoplasmic-mucinous antigen expressed in 70% of Ta, T1 tumors, approximately 25% of Tis tumors, and 15% of invasive cancers.[58,60] No normal tissue, including urothelium, was found to express M344 in immunohistologic studies. Preliminary data also suggest that M344-positive tumors rarely progress. The antigen recognized by 19A211 is a sialoglycoprotein with a dominant molecular weight of 200 kd and several other lower-molecular-weight protein moieties that are clearly distinct from blood group or other known antigens.[54] 19A211 is also expressed on 70% of Ta, T1 tumors, on 60% of Tis tumors, and on 50% of invasive cancers. Overall, 90% of Ta, T1 tumors and 80% of Tis lesions express either one or both antigens. Bladder-mapping studies have also shown that M344 antigen is expressed in the preneoplastic state of normal-appearing urothelium adjacent to or at distant site from bladder tumors. Thus, M344 and 19A211 appear to be promising biomarkers for detection and monitoring of superficial bladder tumors and also as early indicators of a premalignant state.

The other antigen of interest is defined by monoclonal antibody T138.[55,56] The antigen is a 25-kd glycoprotein, although more recent studies suggest that it may be a complex of higher molecular weight. T138 is expressed in 15% to 20% Ta, T1 tumors and in 60% of invasive bladder cancers.[46,57] T138 is not expressed by normal urothelial cells or other normal tissues, with the exception of endothelial cells, blood vessels, and lymphatic vessels. The T138 antigen can be detected only in fresh or frozen cells, which limits its clinical applications. In at least three different studies, however, expression of T138 in bladder cancer was associated with high metastatic potential.[46,61,62] In a study of 68 patients, cancer death was observed in 35% of patients with diploid, T138-positive tumors, compared to 0% for diploid, T138-negative tumors and 60% for aneuploid, T138-positive tumors.[61] In addition, four of five patients with T138-positive Ta, T1 tumors later progress to invasive and metastatic cancer. In a more recent study of 57 bladder cancers, only two factors appeared to have a significant and independent prognostic value in multivariate analysis: tumor stage (P = .0001) and T138 expression (P = .006).[46]

MOLECULAR PATHWAYS OF CARCINOGENESIS

The existence of molecular pathways of carcinogenesis was initially proposed based on clinical and histopathologic characteristics and on preliminary results of tumor marker studies.[63] From genetic studies, molecular patterns are beginning to emerge that may provide fingerprints of tumors with distinct biologic potential.[14,64] As shown in Figure 21-2, distinct genetic susceptibility in addition to the influence of carcinogens may lead to papillary tumors, which are most frequently well differentiated and diploid, or to carcinoma in situ and invasive cancers, which are more commonly aneuploid. 9q deletion appears to be a common feature of noninvasive papillary bladder tumors, which also frequently express the *MDM2* oncogene and M344 and 19A211 tumor-associated antigens. These tumors are genetically more stable and thus are likely to be found clinically

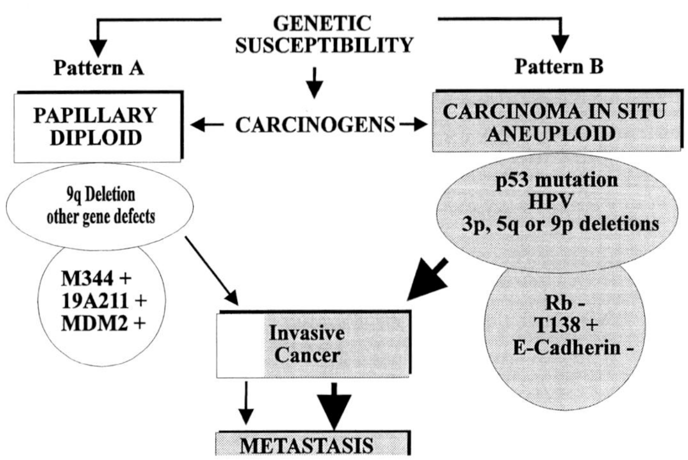

FIG. 21-2. Suspected molecular pathways of bladder carcinogenesis. The two main tumor phenotypes are represented with the suspected genetic defects and their most common protein phenotype. Papillary diploid tumors are more likely to be found at an early stage and rarely evolve toward invasive cancer. Aneuploid carcinoma in situ is rarely found at its early stage and rapidly evolves toward invasive cancers and is likely responsible for metastasis and death. HPV, human papillomavirus.

at a superficial stage. However, some of these tumors may have progressed to invasive cancer at the time of diagnosis and acquired other genetic alterations. However, these cancers are less likely to become metastatic and are rarely associated with high-grade Tis tumors. The 9q34 gene has been associated with Gorlin's syndrome,[65] and it is tempting to speculate that papillary bladder tumors may be caused by some form of genetic defect. This hypothesis may be supported by recent U.S. cancer statistics showing a comparable incidence of invasive bladder cancer but a threefold increased incidence of superficial bladder tumors in Caucasians compared to African Americans.[66]

Another molecular tumor pattern likely begins with high-grade carcinoma in situ, which has frequent *P53* mutations as well as deletions of chromosomal arms 3p and 5q. These tumors are likely to have alterations in RB1 protein, express T138 antigen, and lack E-cadherin surface expression. Because of their genetic instability, these cancers are usually diagnosed at an advanced stage and are more likely to give rise to systemic metastasis. This form of cancer may be more frequently associated with external carcinogens or HPV infection. Thus, the study of bladder tumor phenotype may provide indications about its molecular origin, as well as about its potential for rapid or slow cancer progression.

CLINICAL APPLICATIONS OF TUMOR MARKERS

From a practical point of view, the collection of available tumor markers can be used for diagnostic and prognostic purposes. It is likely that, although specific genetic or molecular changes may have a strong predictive value, cumulative anomalies of various types will provide more accurate stratification of patients. When assessing the potential application of tumor markers in clinical management, several points must be considered. Ideally, the test must be feasible on all tumor samples. If this is not the case, a selection bias may hamper interpretation of results. Additionally, tumor marker studies must be evaluated in a more rigorous way. The vast majority of published series on tumor markers have been done on selected small populations and show some correlation with grade and stage. These studies should be considered as phase I or II studies by analogy with phases of clinical trials. Promising tumor markers must undergo well-designed phase III studies to determine the independent value of any of these tests above existing clinical parameters using multivariate analysis. It is also important to determine which level of confidence is required for the clinician to modify his or her treatment plan. In the following section, the status of clinical studies is reviewed for selective applications in superficial (Table 21-1) and invasive (Table 21-2) bladder cancers.

Superficial Bladder Cancer

Prognosis of Recurrence

Several epidemiologic studies have shown that tumor stage, number of tumors, and size and grade of tumors were the most important clinical predictors of recurrence. This was further confirmed in a study of 382 newly diagnosed Ta, T1 primary tumors.[67] Expression of T138 was associated with a significantly increased risk ratio (RR, 1.6 ± 0.3) for earlier recurrence, whereas expression of M344 was associated with an increased tumor rate (RR, 1.67 ± 0.3). These two parameters were found to be independent predictors in multivariate analysis. Patients with P53-positive tumors also recurred more rapidly.[31] By combining significant clinical and tumor marker parameters, it is possible to classify patients with Ta, T1 tumors in distinct categories, with risk of recurrence ranging from less than 10% at 1 year to more than 90% at 6 months.[68] Such stratification may have important implications on follow-up cystoscopy schedule, as well as on the decision to prescribe intravesical therapy.

TABLE 21-1. *Clinical applications of tumor markers in superficial bladder cancer*

Prognostic tests	Diagnostic tests
PREDICT RECURRENCE	IMMUNOCYTOLOGY
Tests on tumors	M344,19A211[72,73]
M344, T138[67,68]	Lewis[X52,69–71]
P53[31]	TCSF(?)[48]
Tests on exfoliated cells	
Lewis[X50]	URINARY MARKERS
M344[52]	FGFA[74]
19A211[72]	FGFB[75]
	TCSF[76]
PREDICT PROGRESSION TO MUSCLE INVASION	DD23[78]
P53+[26,29,30]	
T138+[46,61]	
E-cadherin[49]	
EGFR[45]	
Aneuploidy[4]	

Prognosis of Progression

Four markers have been found to be associated with increased risk of cancer progression in superficial bladder cancer: EGFR,[45] T138,[46,61] E-cadherin,[49] and P53. All these markers were studied in select groups of patients. The presence of *P53* mutations as measured by immunostaining with pAb1801 showed a marked increase in risk of progression in a study of 43 T1 tumors,[29] 54 Ta tumors, and 33 patients with carcinoma in situ (Tis) of the bladder.[30] Similarly, in a subgroup of 45

TABLE 21-2. *Clinical applications of tumor markers in invasive bladder cancer*

PROGNOSIS OF METASTATIC POTENTIAL
RB1[18,19]
P53[26]
T138[46,61,62]
POSSIBLE NEW STAGING TOOLS
Immunolocalization of metastasis
Systemic molecular staging by reverse transcription polymerase chain reaction

patients with T1 cancer, probability of progression was 62% for patients with P53-positive tumors, compared with 7% in P53-negative tumors.[26] It is important to determine the possible relation between P53 and T138 expression and the loss of E-cadherin expression, as well as their possible additive value in predicting outcome.

Diagnostic Tests and Monitoring

Urinary cytology has been the only noninvasive diagnostic test for bladder cancer. Although it is reasonably sensitive in detecting the presence of high-grade cancers, its sensitivity may vary between 10% and 30% for the detection of low-grade, low-stage tumors, which are the most common. Thus, cystoscopy remains the main diagnostic tool for the investigation of patients with hematuria and for the follow-up of patients treated for superficial bladder tumors. The first likely improvement will occur in immunocytologic testing. Studies using antibodies to Lewis^X blood group antigen have been reported by several groups and have shown improved sensitivity over cytology alone.[52,69–71] However, careful interpretation is required, because Lewis^X antigen is also expressed on normal umbrella cells and inflammatory cells. Immunocytology studies using a monoclonal antibody to TCSF has shown results comparable to those using Lewis^X antibody.[48] Because of their high specificity, M344 and 19A211 antibodies may be particularly useful as diagnostic reagents for Ta, T1 bladder tumors. In a prospective study of 250 bladder irrigation specimens, the combination of M344 and 19A211 tests was positive for 95% of Ta or T1 tumors with positive urinary cytology, but also for 80% of tumors that gave negative urine cytology tests.[72] The combined antibody test with M344 and 19A211 antibodies was also highly sensitive and specific in predicting recurrence when found to be positive in patients with no tumor at control cystoscopy. Both antigens are well preserved on exfoliated cells of urine, and one study has shown 85% sensitivity with specificity exceeding 95% for detection of bladder cancer using M344 antibody in an immunocytology test.[73] Ongoing studies using 19A211 suggest that these results can be further improved by the combination of the two antibody tests. The NCI Bladder Tumor Marker Network is currently conducting a phase III study to determine the value of M344, 19A211, and anti-Lewis^X antibodies for the monitoring of patients after resection of a Ta or T1 bladder tumor. Results of such a study, in conjunction with results of prognostic markers on tumor specimens, should provide the level of confidence required to modify treatment strategies for superficial bladder tumors.

Other tumor markers shed as soluble antigens in the urine have also been studied. These include the bladder tumor antigen measured by latex agglutination assay named BTA, acid FGF,[74] basic FGF,[75] TCSF,[76] and the autocrine motility factor (AMF).[77] Essentially all of these markers provide results comparable to cytology in that they detect a high proportion of high-grade, high-stage cancers but a low proportion of low-grade and Ta or T1 tumors. Other new markers may perhaps be complementary in testing.[78] These tests are an important first step toward the development of noninvasive diagnostic kits for bladder cancer.

Invasive Bladder Cancer

Prognosis of Progression

Three tumor markers have been shown to stratify patients with invasive bladder cancer according to risk of distant metastasis: T138, P53, and RB1. Expression of T138 was associated with increased cancer death in three different studies of invasive bladder cancer.[46,61,62] The presence of *P53* mutation was also an independent predictor of recurrence and overall survival in a study of 243 patients, including 94 patients with T2 to T4 cancers.[26] In a study of 90 patients with muscle-invasive bladder cancer treated using neoadjuvant methotrexate, vinblastine, Adriamycin, and cis–platinum (MVAC), P53 overexpression had independent prognostic significance for survival.[28] Two studies have also reported evidence that altered RB1 expression is observed mostly in patients with invasive bladder cancer, who have a low tumor-free survival rate.[18,19] Conversely, contrary to superficial tumors, loss of E-cadherin expression or increased EGFR expression were not associated with a significant difference in survival in patients with muscle-invasive bladder cancer.[45,49] These studies are equivalent to phase II trials and strongly indicate the potential of P53, RB1, and T138 phenotypes to predict an aggressive clinical course. These tumor markers should be used as stratification factors in any treatment trial for muscle-invasive bladder cancer.

Detection of Metastases

Lymph node metastases are found at cystectomy in approximately 30% of patients with invasive bladder cancer. In approximately one half of these patients, large lymph nodes are found, which frequently contraindicate radical cystectomy. Such metastases may be detected by immunoscintigraphy with appropriate reagents. Studies are currently underway to determine the clinical potential of monoclonal antibodies found to immunolocalize well in animal studies.[79] Other approaches may be of value using techniques similar to those developed for staging of prostate cancer patients using reverse transcriptase PCR to detect rare cancer cells in circulating blood.[80,81] No such test is currently available, but ongoing research on tumor markers may provide a basis for their design.

Therapeutic Potential of Tumor Markers

The urinary bladder lends itself to easy access for intravesical therapy. As such, it provides a unique opportunity to test the tumoricidal effect of new treatments in a more or less isolated environment. Targeting EGFR with EGF coupled with TP40 toxin was shown to be effective in treating carcinoma in situ of the bladder.[82] Other studies have shown that monoclonal antibodies can be used to target radioactive agents in bladder tumors by intravesical instillation.[83,84] Other antigens may have more appropriate characteristics for successful targeting of cytotoxic agents in bladder cancer.[85]

Other possible therapies under investigation are based on gene transfer. The objective is to reintroduce into cancer cells and premalignant cells normal genes such as *P53* or *RB1* using viral vectors or liposomes. Another approach that may be of value in the future is the development of vaccines.[86] Bladder cancer is one of the most sensitive cancers to nonspecific immunotherapy. The identification of tumor-associated antigens specific for malignant and premalignant lesions of the bladder may provide a basis for the construction of vaccines using a variety of available viral vectors.[87]

CONCLUSION

Rapid progress has been made in identifying molecular pathways of bladder carcinogenesis. A constellation of new markers has been studied, and some of these markers clearly show promise for use as prognostic or diagnostic tests. Appropriately designed phase III studies should provide the information required to base treatment decisions on tumor marker tests. Moreover, new molecules identified coupled with advances in biotechnology may lead to a new generation of therapeutic products.

REFERENCES

1. Raghavan D, Shipley WU, Garnick MB, et al. Biology and management of bladder cancer. N Engl J Med 1990;322:1129.
2. Fradet Y, Cordon-Cardo C. Critical appraisal of tumor markers in bladder cancer. Semin Urol 1993;11:145.
3. Wheeless LL, Badalament RA, White RWD, Fradet Y, Tribukait B. Consensus review of the clinical utility of DNA cytometry in bladder cancer. Cytometry 1993;14:478.
4. Tributkait B. Flow cytometry in assessing the clinical aggressiveness of genito-urinary neoplasms. World J Urol 1992;5:108.
5. Têtu B, Veilleux C, Allard P, Fradet Y. Prevalence and clinical significance of Her-2/neu, p53 and Rb expression in primary superficial bladder cancer. Lab Invest 1994;84A:484.
6. van der Poel HG, Oosterhof GON, Debruyne FMJ, Schalken JA. Image analysis in superficial transitional cell carcinoma of the bladder. Semin Urol 1993;11:164.
7. Hopman AH, Moesker O, Smeets AW, Pauwels RP, Vooijs GP, Ramaekers FC. Numerical chromosome 1, 7, 9, and 11 aberrations in bladder cancer detected by in situ hybridization. Cancer Res 1991;51:644.
8. Waldman FM, Carroll PR, Kerschmann R, Cohen MB, Field FG, Mayall BH. Centromeric copy number of chromosome 7 is strongly correlated with tumor grade and labeling index in human bladder cancer. Cancer Res 1991;51:3807.
9. Mmiyao N, Tsai YC, Lerner SP. Role of chromosome 9 in human bladder cancer. Cancer Res 1993;53:4066.
10. Presti JC Jr, Reuter VE, Galan T, Fair WR, Cordon-Cardo C. Molecular genetic alterations in superficial and locally advanced human bladder cancer. Cancer Res 1991;51:5405.
11. Miyao N, Tsai YC, Lerner SP, et al. Role of chromosome 9 in human bladder cancer. Cancer Res 1993;53:4066.
12. Cairns P, Tokino K, Eby Y, Sidransky D. Homozygous deletions of 9p21 in primary human bladder tumors detected by comparative multiplex polymerase chain reaction. Cancer Res 1994;54:1422.
13. Orlow I, Lianes P, Lacombe L, Dalbagni G, Reuter VE, Cordon-Cardo C. Chromosome 9 allelic losses and microsatellite alterations in human bládder tumors. Cancer Res 1994;54:2848.
14. Dalbagni G, Presti J, Reuter V, Fair WR, Cordon-Cardo C. Genetic alterations in bladder cancer. Lancet 1993;342:469.
15. Dalbagni G, Presti JC, Reuter VE, et al. Molecular genetic alterations of chromosome 17 and p53 nuclear overexpression in human bladder cancer. Diagn Mol Pathol 1993;2:4.
16. Hartwell LH, Kastan MB. Cell cycle control and cancer. Science 1994; 266:1821.
17. Cordon-Cardo C, Dalbagni G, Richon VM. Significance of the retinoblastoma gene in human cancer. Princ Pract Oncol 1992;6:1.
18. Cordon-Cardo C, Wartinger D, Petrylak D, et al. Altered expression of the retinoblastoma gene product: prognostic indicator in bladder cancer. J Natl Cancer Inst 1992;84:1251.
19. Logothetis CJ, Xu HJ, Ro JY, et al. Altered expression of retinoblastoma protein and known prognostic variables in locally advanced bladder cancer. J Natl Cancer Inst 1992;84:1256.
20. Spruck CH, Gonzalezzulueta M, Shibata A, et al. p16 gene in uncultured tumours. Nature 1994;370:183.
21. Cairns P, Mao L, Merlo A, et al. Rates of p16(MTS1) mutations in primary tumors with 9p loss. Science 1994;265:415.
22. Yeager T, Sstaaadler W, Belair C, Puthenveettil J, Olopade O, Reznikoff C. Increased p16 levels correlate with pRb alterations in human urothelial cells. Cancer Res 1995;55:493.
23. Vogelstein B, Kinzler KW. p53 Function and dysfunction. Cell 1992; 70:523.
24. Levine AJ, Momand J, Finlay CA. The p53 tumour suppressor gene. Nature 1991;351:453.
25. Cordon-Cardo C, Dalbagni G, Saez GT, et al. P53 mutations in human bladder cancer: genotypic versus phenotypic patterns. Int J Cancer 1994;56:347.
26. Esrig D, Elmajian D, Groshen S, et al. Accumulation of nuclear p53 and tumor progression in bladder cancer. N Engl J Med 1994;331:1259.
27. Sidransky D, Von Eschenbach A, Tsai YC, et al. Identification of p53 gene mutations in bladder cancers and urine samples. Science 1991; 252:706.
28. Sarkis AS, Bajorin DF, Reuter VE, et al. The prognostic value of p53 nuclear overexpression in patients with invasive bladder cancer treated with neoadjuvant M-VAC. J Clin Oncol 1995;13:1384.
29. Sarkis AS, Dalbagni G, Cordon-Cardo C, et al. Nuclear overexpression of p53 protein in transitional cell bladder carcinoma: a marker for disease progression. J Natl Cancer Inst 1993;85:53.
30. Sarkis AS, Zhang ZF, Cordon-Cardo C, et al. p53 nuclear overexpression and disease progression in Ta-bladder carcinoma. Int J Oncol 1993; 3:355.
31. Fradet Y, Têtu B, Veilleux C, Allard P. Prevalence and clinical significance of p53, Rb and HER-2-/neu expression in newly diagnosed superficial bladder tumors. J Urol 1994;151(Suppl):390A.
32. Bos JL. Ras oncogenes in human cancer: a review. Cancer Res 1989; 49:4682.
33. Feinberg AP, Vogelstein B, Droller MJ, et al. Mutation affecting the 12th amino-acid of the c-Ha-ras oncogene product occurs infrequently in human cancer. Science 1983;220:1175.
34. Czerniak B, Deitch D, Simmons H, Etkind P, Herz F, Koss LG. Ha-ras gene codon 12 mutation and DNA ploidy in urinary bladder carcinoma. Br J Cancer 1990;62:762.
35. Ooi A, Herz F, Ii S, et al. Ha-ras codon 12 mutation in papillary tumors of the urinary bladder: a prospective study. Int J Oncol 1994;4:85.
36. Wright C, Mellon K, Johnston P, et al. Expression of mutant p53, c-erbB-2 and the epidermal growth factor receptor in transitional cell carcinoma of the human urinary bladder. Br J Cancer 1991;63:967.
37. Bryant P, Skelly J, Wilson D. Demonstration of papillomavirus structural antigen in human urinary bladder neoplasia. Br J Urol 1987;60: 405.
38. Furihata M, Inoue K, Ohtsuki Y, Hashimoto H, Terao N, Fujita Y. High-risk human papillomavirus infections and overexpression of p53 protein as prognostic indicators in transitional cell carcinoma of the urinary bladder. Cancer Res 1993;53:4823.
39. Khurshid A, Hironobu N, Kazuya N, et al. High frequency of human papillomavirus infection in carcinoma of the urinary bladder. Cancer 1992;70:1967.
40. LaRue H, Simoneau M, Fradet Y. Human papillomavirus in transitional cell carcinoma of the urinary bladder. Clin Cancer Res 1995;1:435.
41. Momand J, Zambetti GP, Olson DC, et al. The mdm-2 oncogene product forms a complex with the p-53 protein and inhibits p53-mediated transactivation. Cell 1992;69:1237.
42. Chen J, Marechal V, Levine AJ. Mapping of the p53 and mdm-2 interaction domain. Mol Cell Biol 1993;13:4107.
43. Lianes P, Orlow I, Zhang ZF, et al. Altered patterns of MDM2 and TP53 expression in human bladder cancer. J Natl Cancer Inst 1994; 86:1325.
44. Messing EM. Clinical implications of the expression of epidermal growth factor receptors in human transitional cell carcinoma. Cancer Res 1990;50:2530.

45. Neal DE, Sharples I, Smith K, et al. The epidermal growth factor receptor and the prognosis of bladder cancer. Cancer 1990;65:1619.
46. Ravery V, Colombel M, Popov Z, et al. Prognostic value of epidermal growth factor-receptor: T138 and T43 expression in bladder cancer. Br J Cancer 1995;71:196.
47. Ellis ME, Nabeshima K, Biswas C. Monoclonal antibody preparation and purification of a tumor cell collagenase-stimulatory factor. Cancer Res 1989;49:3385.
48. Muraoka K, Nabeshima K, Murayama T, Biswas C, Koono M. Enhanced expression of a tumor-cell-derived collagenase-stimulatory factor in urothelial carcinoma: its usefulness as a tumor marker for bladder cancers. Int J Cancer 1993;55:19.
49. Bringuier PP, Umbas R, Schaafsma HE, Karthaus HFM, Debruyne FMJ, Schalken JA. Decreased E-cadherin immunoreactivity correlates with poor survival in patients with bladder tumors. Cancer Res 1993; 53:3241.
50. Sheinfeld J, Reuter VE, Fair WR, Cordon-Cardo C. Expression of blood group antigens in bladder cancer: current concepts. Semin Surg Oncol 1992;8:308.
51. Sarkis AS, Charytonowicz E, Cordon-Cardo C, Fradet Y, Herz F, Mayall B. Blood group antigen expression in bladder tumors: an immunohistochemical study of low-grade bladder lesions. J Exp Clin Cancer Res 1994;13:139.
52. Sheinfeld J, Reuter VE, Melamed MR, et al. Enhanced bladder cancer detection with the Lewis X antigen as a marker of neoplastic transformation. J Urol 1990;143:285.
53. Dalbagni G, Reuter V, Sheinfeld J, Fradet Y, Fair WR, Cordon-Cardo C. Cell surface differentiation antigens of normal urothelium and bladder tumors. Semin Surg Oncol 1992;8:1.
54. Fradet Y, LaRue H, Parent-Vaugeois C, et al. Monoclonal antibody against a tumor-associated sialoglycoprotein of superficial papillary bladder tumors and cervical condylomas. Int J Cancer 1990;46:990.
55. Fradet Y. Markers of prognosis in superficial bladder cancer. Semin Urol 1992;10:28.
56. Fradet Y, Cordon-Cardo C, Thomson T, et al. Cell surface antigens of human bladder cancer defined by mouse monoclonal antibodies. Proc Natl Acad Sci USA 1984;81:224.
57. Fradet Y, Cordon-Cardo C, Whitmore WF Jr, Melamed MR, Old LJ. Cell surface antigens of human bladder tumors: definition of tumor subsets by monoclonal antibodies and correlation with growth characteristics. Cancer Res 1986;46:5183.
58. Fradet Y, Islam N, Boucher L, Parent-Vaugeois C, Tardif M. Polymorphic expression of a human superficial bladder tumor antigen defined by mouse monoclonal antibodies. Proc Natl Acad Sci U S A 1987;84: 7227.
59. Fradet Y, Lafleur L, LaRue H. Strategies of chemoprevention based on antigenic and molecular markers of early and premalignant lesions of the bladder. J Cell Biochem 1992;161:85.
60. Cordon-Cardo C, Wartinger DD, Melamed MR, Fair W, Fradet Y. Immunopathologic analysis of human urinary bladder cancer: characterization of two new antigens associated with low-grade superficial bladder tumors. Am J Pathol 1992;140:375.
61. Fradet Y, Tardif M, Bourget L, Robert J, for the Laval University Urology Group. Clinical cancer progression in urinary bladder tumors evaluated by multiparameter flow cytometry with monoclonal antibodies. Cancer Res 1990;50:432.
62. Bretton P, Cordon-Cardo C, Wartinger D, et al. Expression of the T-138 antigen and survival of patients with bladder cancer. Proc Am Cancer Res 1990;31:186.
63. Fradet Y. Molecular and immunologic approaches in the management of bladder cancer. Urol Clin North Am 1991;18:515.
64. Spruck CH, Ohneseit PF, Gonzalezzulueta M, et al. Two molecular pathways to transitional cell carcinoma of the bladder. Cancer Res 1994;54:784.
65. Gailani MR, Bale SJ, Leffell DJ, et al. Developmental defects in Gorlin syndrome related to a putative tumor suppressor gene on chromosome 9. Cell 1992;69:111.
66. Silverman DT, Hartge P, Morrison AS, Devesa SS. Epidemiology of bladder cancer. Hematol Oncol Clin North Am 1992;6:1.
67. Allard P, Fradet Y, Têtu B, et al. Tumor-associated antigens as prognostic factors for recurrence in 382 patients with primary transitional cell carcinoma of the bladder. Clin Cancer Res 1995;1:1195.
68. Fradet Y, Allard P, Têtu B. Tumor-associated antigens might help urologists determine the likelihood of bladder cancer recurrence after treatment. AUA Today 1994;7:1.
69. Chopin DK, deKernion JB, Rosenthal DL, et al. Monoclonal antibodies against transitional cell carcinoma for detection of malignant urothelial cells in bladder washing. J Urol 1985;134:260.
70. Longin A, Fontaniere B, Berger-Dutrieux N, Devonec M, Laurent JC. A useful monoclonal antibody (BL2-10D1) to identify tumor cells in urine cytology. Cancer 1990;65:1412.
71. Klan R, Huland E, Baisch H, et al. Sensitivity of urinary quantitative immunocytology with monoclonal antibody 486 P3/12 in 241 unselected patients with bladder carcinoma. J Urol 1991;145:495.
72. Fradet Y, Gauthier J, Bedard G, et al. Monitoring and prognostic determination of bladder tumors by flow cytometry with monoclonal antibodies on bladder irrigations. J Urol 1991;145:250A.
73. Bonner RB, Hemstreet GP, Fradet Y, Rao JY, Min KW, Hurst RE. Bladder cancer risk assessment with quantitative fluorescence image analysis of tumor markers in exfoliated bladder cells. Cancer 1993;72: 2461.
74. Chopin DK, Caruelle JP, Colombel M, et al. Increased immunodetection of acidic fibroblast growth factor in bladder cancer, detectable in urine. J Urol 1993;150:1126.
75. Nguyen M, Watanabe H, Budson AE, Richie JP, Folkman J. Elevated levels of the angiogenic peptide basic fibroblast growth factor in urine of bladder cancer patients. J Natl Cancer Inst 1993;85:241.
76. Guirguis R, Javadpour N, Sharareh BS, et al. A new method for evaluation of urinary autocrine motility factor and tumor-cell collagenase-stimulating factor as markers for urinary tract cancers. J Occup Med 1990;32:846.
77. Guirguis R, Schiffmann E, Liu B, et al. Detection of autocrine motility factor in urine as a marker of bladder cancer. J Natl Cancer Inst 1988; 80:1203.
78. Grossman HB, Liebert M, Sakakibara N, Wedemeyer GA, Stein JA, Washington RW Jr. Evaluation of a new bladder tumor marker. Urol Clin North Am 1991;18:509.
79. Fradet Y, Friede J, Guertin B, Leclerc J, Dufour C, Caron C. Radioimmunodetection of human bladder tumor xenografts in nude mice with radiolabeled monoclonal antibodies. J Urol 1992;148:418.
80. Katz AE, Olsson CA, Raffo AJ, et al. Molecular staging of prostate cancer with the use of an enhanced reverse transcriptase-PCR assay. Urol 1994;43:765.
81. Israeli RS, Miller WH Jr, Su SL, et al. Sensitive nested reverse transcription polymerase chain reaction detection of circulating prostatic tumor cells: comparison of prostate-specific membrane antigen and prostate-specific antigen-based assays. Cancer Res 1994;54:6306.
82. Goldberg MR, Heimbrook DC, Russo P, et al. Phase I clinical study of the recombinant oncotoxin TP40 in superficial bladder cancer. Clin Cancer Res 1995;1:57.
83. Bamias A, Bowles MJ, Krausz T, Williams G, Epenetos AA. Intravesical administration of Indium-111-labelled HMFG2 monoclonal antibody in superficial bladder carcinomas. Int J Cancer 1993;54:899.
84. Zorzos J, Skarlos DV, Epenetos AA, et al. Intravesical administration of tumor-associated monoclonal antibody Aua1 in transitional cell carcinoma of the bladder: a study of biodistribution. Urol Res 1993;21: 435.
85. de Harven E, Fradet Y, Connelly JG, et al. Antibody drug carrier for immunotherapy of superficial bladder cancer: ultrastructural studies. Cancer Res 1992;52:3131.
86. Boon T, Coulie P, Marchand M, Weynants P, Wolfel T, Brichard V. Genes coding for tumor rejection antigens: perspectives for specific immunotherapy. In: DeVita VT, Hellman S, Rosenberg SA, eds. Important advances in oncology. Philadelphia: JB Lippincott, 1994:53.
87. Saad F, Bergeron A, LaRue H, Lafleur L, Fradet Y. Biochemical characteristics and immunotherapeutic potential of a human epithelial mucin of superficial transitional cell bladder carcinoma. J Urol 1992; 147:371A.

Principles and Practice of Genitourinary Oncology, edited by Derek Raghavan, Howard I. Scher, Steven A. Leibel, and Paul H. Lange. Lippincott-Raven Publishers, Philadelphia, © 1997.

CHAPTER 22

Immunology of Bladder Cancer

Timothy L. Ratliff, Edmund C. Lattime, and Richard D. Williams

Mycobacterium bovis bacillus Calmette-Guerin (BCG) is an attenuated strain of *M bovis* that has been widely used as a vaccine against tuberculosis. In 1969, Mathe and colleagues[1] suggested that BCG immunotherapy for cancer was efficacious in the treatment of childhood leukemia, although subsequently identified limitations have restricted its use. This observation led to numerous studies testing BCG as an immunotherapy agent in animal models.[2] These investigations identified several criteria for the successful use of BCG that were summarized by Zbar and Rapp[3] as follows:

Immunocompetence of the host is required (i.e., the ability of the host to mount a delayed-type hypersensitivity response (DTH) to mycobacterial antigens is necessary). T-cell cytokines are important to the response.

Close contact between the tumor and BCG is required. As with gene therapy, local cytokine production is necessary.

Tumor size is important. Therapy is ineffective against large tumors, which may result from tumor-associated downregulation of responses.

The presence of viable bacteria is necessary. This factor may be associated with more intense or prolonged cytokine production.

Knowledge that the bladder is capable of mounting a DTH[4] and past experience with intravesical administration of chemotherapeutic agents led Morales and colleagues[5] to their landmark 1976 study. Their investigation in superficial bladder cancer led to the only clinically viable role for BCG in antitumor therapy.

Since the original observation by Morales and associates,[5] BCG has been shown in prospective randomized clinical trials to provide superior therapeutic results compared with transurethral resection alone or with various chemotherapeutic regimens.[6,7] Tumor-free responses after adjuvant BCG therapy have been reported in approximately two thirds of patients with papillary tumors, carcinoma in situ (CIS), or both, with more than 10 years of follow-up.[8–12] The clinical efficacy of BCG therapy in bladder cancer is discussed in Chapter 26. Although BCG is an extremely effective anti–bladder tumor agent, a number of patients fail to respond, and its efficacy is limited to superficial disease. Thus, alternate forms of therapy are needed, and the potential of several new immunotherapeutic regimens is discussed in this chapter.

Because BCG immunotherapy is one of the most effective forms of immunotherapy in the clinical setting, understanding its mechanisms of action may provide insights into the development of alternative forms of immunotherapy for bladder cancer. In this chapter, BCG mechanisms are discussed in the context of tumor immunity and alternate forms of immunotherapy to illustrate the interdependency of immune mechanisms for the development of new therapeutic regimens.

TUMOR IMMUNITY

Early studies by Prehn and Main[13] suggested a role for the immune response in the elimination of tumors. Subsequently, Burnett[14] popularized the immune surveillance theory, which stated that immune cells continually seek and destroy tumors. Only those tumors capable of evading the sentinel function of the immune response possess the capacity to grow. These observations led to the supposition that immunoadjuvant therapy could override tumor escape mechanisms and induce a response that would eliminate established in situ tumors. For the next decade and a half, the general promise of this hypothesis failed to materialize into clinically effective therapy, although adjuvant BCG therapy for bladder cancer emerged as an effective treatment regimen. The overall lack of success led to doubts about the ability of the immune response to effectively eliminate tumors.

Rosenberg and associates[15] revitalized interest in immunotherapy with their work on lymphokine-activated killer cells (LAK) and tumor-infiltrating lymphocytes.[16–18] These experiments demonstrated the presence of reactive immune cells that could be activated in vitro to induce tumor regression when adoptively transferred into a tumor-bearing host.[18] Again, the therapeutic efficacy of clinical trials fell short of expectations; however, these studies clearly demonstrated the ability of immunoreactive cells to respond to and eliminate tumors that previously were considered resistant to immune effector mechanisms.[15]

Implicit in these studies are the following concepts:

Most tumors, whether previously considered responsive or nonresponsive, are susceptible to immune-mediated antitumor mechanisms.

Immune cells capable of mounting an antitumor response infiltrate tumors but remain quiescent, suggesting tumor-induced downregulation takes place.

One reason for the absence of immune activation is a deficiency of immune modulators (i.e., helper factors or cytokines); provision of the helper factors in vitro are sufficient to activate cells capable of eliminating tumors after adoptive transfer.

Gene therapy studies confirmed the hypothesis that most theoretically nonresponsive tumors are indeed responsive.[19–26] These studies demonstrated that expression of a single cytokine or co-stimulatory molecule in sufficient quantities at the tumor site induces an immune response that eliminates tumors. Neither the systemic administration of cytokines nor the production of cytokines by transfected cells at sites distant from the tumor induced an antitumor response.[19–21,22] Only rarely did cytokine gene therapy induce regression of existing tumors at secondary sites, and this occurred only in the early growth stages (i.e., about 3 days after implantation) when low numbers of cells were injected.[20]

The gene therapy data reconfirmed the existence of active tumor escape mechanisms and the susceptibility of most tumors to immune destruction. Moreover, the immunotherapy data are consistent with previous reports on adjuvant BCG therapy and suggest that the modulation of tumor immunity during cytokine gene therapy occurs through pathways similar to those activated by adjuvant BCG therapy. This hypothesis is supported by the studies mentioned previously and by comparative studies demonstrating that adjuvant *Corynebacterium parvum*, a bacterial immunoadjuvant similar to BCG, was as effective as cytokine gene therapy in many tumor models.[26] Because cytokine gene therapy results in constitutive, uncontrolled cytokine production, the enhanced effects of the gene transfection studies in some tumor models may be associated with the downregulation of cytokine production in BCG therapy. Such downregulation is part of the homeostasis mechanisms that prevent unrestricted expansion of the immune response at the bacterial infection site. We have demonstrated that such regulation occurs in BCG therapy and suggest that it is a reason for reduced antitumor activity.

BACILLUS CALMETTE-GUERIN ANTITUMOR MECHANISMS

To understand the mechanisms of action of BCG, it is necessary to understand the immune response induced by BCG as a bacterial invader. It is the body's natural response to the bacterial invasion that results in the local immune response responsible for the development of an antitumor response.

T-Cell Function in Intracellular Bacterial Immunity

Protective immunity against intracellular bacteria, unlike that to pyogenic bacteria and viruses, is cellular in nature. This response is characterized by the DTH, which is associated with CD4+ T helper (Th) cells, but requires cooperation with CD8+ cytolytic T cells (CTL) in some infections.

The role of cellular immunity in protective responses to intracellular bacteria was first defined by Truitt and Mackaness[27] and further developed by other researchers.[28,29] These investigators demonstrated that cellular immune responses specific for the invading bacteria activated the macrophage that serves as the effector cell for eliminating the infection. Truitt and Mackaness[27] determined that immune specificity resided with the T-cell response to bacterial antigens but that the macrophage, once activated by the T cell, killed intracellular bacteria indiscriminately. In other words, T cells recognized specific bacterial antigens and responded by producing cytokines that activated the macrophage. The macrophage killed both the immunizing bacteria and antigenically distinct bacteria.

Subsequent studies have verified and extended these observations to include an important role for DTH in mycobacterial immunity.[28] These studies suggested that control of bacterial proliferation occurred through the activation of a macrophage. A report by Orme and associates[28] using interferon gamma (IFNG) knockout mice clearly demonstrated the requirement for IFNG in the control of mycobacterial infections. Although IFNG is known to be a necessary component in the antimycobacterial response, IFNG is not sufficient for the complete elimination of the bacteria. Kabelitz and associates[30] suggested that CD8+ CTL were necessary for the complete elimination of the infection. Subsequently, Flynn and associates[31] provided strong support for the Kabelitz hypothesis by showing that mycobacterial infections were rapidly lethal in animals that lacked CD8+ cells. These data demonstrate the requirement for both CD4+ and CD8+ T cells in mycobacterial immunity. Ratliff and colleagues[32] have observed similar requirements for the mediation of BCG-induced antitumor immunity.

In 1986, Mosmann and associates[33] defined CD4+ Th subpopulations that aided in understanding of the cellular immune response to intracellular pathogens. These investigators demonstrated that Th cells can be separated into Th1 and Th2 subsets based on their cytokine secretion profiles. These studies helped clarify the dual role of Th cells in antibody (Th2-directed) and cell-mediated (Th1-directed) immune responses and provided a framework for understanding T-cell–dependent immunoregulation. The immunoregulatory loop involves cytokines produced exclusively by each of the respective Th subsets that suppress the response of the other. For example, the production of interleukin 10 (IL10) by Th2 cells inhibits IFNG production, which results in the downregulation of the Th1 response.[34] Conversely, the activation of a Th1 response involves the induction of IL12, an IFNG inducer, which inhibits the development of a Th2 response.[35,36] Thus, intracellular bacteria, including BCG, induce a Th1-directed, cell-mediated response that was reported to be protective, whereas a Th2 response was observed to be permissive for bacterial growth.[37,38] As described later, the development of a Th1 response appears to be necessary for optimal expression of BCG-induced antitumor activity.

Bacillus Calmette-Guerin Mechanisms

The events necessary for the antitumor effects of BCG are twofold. First, BCG must attach to the bladder and be retained for induction of an immune response.[39] Data suggest that BCG binding to fibronectin is required for the initiation of BCG-mediated antitumor activity. BCG expresses receptors for fibronectin, which mediate attachment and retention of the bacteria after the instillation of a particulate bacterial suspension into the lumen of the bladder.[40] BCG attachment apparently occurs to fibronectin incorporated into the fibrin clot and is essentially irreversible. Modulation of the interaction between BCG and fibronectin has a direct effect on the expression of antitumor activity.[41] Inhibition of attachment abrogates the antitumor response, whereas augmentation of attachment enhances antitumor activity. These data suggest that BCG attachment is necessary for induction of the immune response to BCG that results in the augmentation of antitumor activity.

BCG attachment is necessary but alone is not sufficient for induction of an antitumor response. The second aspect of the antitumor effect of BCG involves induction of an immune-mediated antitumor response. This hypothesis is supported by studies in patients treated with BCG for bladder cancer that showed a correlation between urine cytokines produced after BCG instillation and a therapeutic response.[42] Furthermore, effective therapeutic results were linked to the development of a cutaneous DTH reaction to soluble antigens from mycobacteria (purified protein derivative; PPD). These studies showed a significant correlation between PPD reactivity and antitumor activity.[43] Although they are not definitive, these clinical data link BCG-induced immunity to antitumor activity and suggest that clinical responses to BCG are associated with cytokine production induced by the BCG infection.

Studies in animals also link DTH to effective BCG therapy. Bartlett and associates[44] demonstrated that BCG-induced tumor rejection is dependent on the presence of DTH to BCG. These investigators concluded that the DTH response induced by BCG results in cytokine production and macrophage activation. They suggested that the macrophages are the effector cells that mediate tumor cell killing. Further studies by Fujiwara and associates[45] showed that CD4+ T cells (the cells responsible for DTH) and the associated macrophage activation are necessary for the development of antitumor activity.

Using the orthotopic bladder tumor model, Ratliff and associates[32] showed that BCG-induced antitumor activity is associated with a T-lymphocyte response. These studies demonstrated that depletion of either CD4+ or CD8+ T-cell subsets abrogate BCG-induced antitumor activity, although no tumor-specific CD8+ CTL were observed. Similarly, other studies demonstrated that either CD4+ or CD8+ T cells are necessary for BCG-induced antitumor activity.[46–47] These results suggest that there is a collaboration between the T-cell subsets that is associated with tumor cell killing. Such a paradigm necessitates the presence of BCG-induced CD4+ cytokine-producing cells. This is consistent with previous immunotherapy studies, which suggest that helper factors in the form of cytokines are sufficient to activate antitumor effector mechanisms.[19–21]

Lattime and associates[47] demonstrated that BCG antigens are processed and presented by bladder tumor cells. These data suggest that one component in the antitumor response may be the recognition of BCG peptides expressed on bladder tumor cells. Becich and colleagues[48] have demonstrated that BCG attach to and are ingested by bladder tumor cell lines, normal epithelial cells cultured in vitro, and transitional epithelial cells obtained from patients treated with BCG. Taken together, these data suggest that bladder epithelial cells or tumor cells may modulate immunity to BCG through antigen presentation. This concept is supported by unpublished observations of Ratliff and associates demonstrating bladder tumor cell support of T-cell proliferation and lytic activity of BCG-specific T cells for bladder tumor cells expressing BCG antigens.

Several cytokines have been identified in the urine of patients treated with BCG; however, the hostile urinary environment makes thorough cytokine analysis difficult. Therefore, we used polymerase chain reaction (PCR) to evaluate the induction of cytokine mRNA after intravesical BCG treatment in an animal model. Mice were treated with BCG intravesically at weekly intervals. Bladders were harvested at varying time points after treatment, and RNA was isolated using standard isolation techniques. The RNA was reverse transcribed and amplified by the PCR reaction using cytokine-specific primers. The data show that cytokines associated with DTH (Th1 response) are induced by BCG, whereas cytokines associated with an immediate hypersensitivity response (Th2 response) are not. The modulated cytokines include IFNG, tumor necrosis factor alpha (TNFA), IL10, and IL12. Cytokines present but not modulated include IL4, IL5, and IL6. The modulation of IL10, a regulatory cytokine for DTH, provided an opportunity to investigate the role of DTH in BCG therapy. First, we determined that the IL10 protein was modulated as was observed for the mRNA. We observed an upregulation of IL10 by enzyme-linked immunosorbent assay (ELISA) analysis and determined that the in vivo administration of antibody to IL10 abrogated its induction. We then evaluated the effects of IL10 neutralization on DTH and determined that the BCG-induced DTH response was significantly prolonged when IL10 activity was abrogated. In these experiments, DTH was detected at significant levels 96 hours after challenge in the anti-IL10 treated group but was observed only for 24 hours in the control animals. Further study showed that neutralization of IL10 also enhanced antitumor activity, demonstrating that DTH and its associated cytokines are necessary for effective BCG therapy.

ALTERNATE FORMS OF THERAPY

Management studies for superficial bladder cancer generally are of two varieties: prophylaxis (i.e., prevention of recurrences) after intravesical resection or treatment of existing papillary tumors or diffuse CIS. Prophylaxis studies, although more frequently done than treatment studies, are often insufficient to make substantive conclusions. Commonly, prophylaxis studies are not randomized but instead use historical controls or the patient's prior history. Even randomized studies frequently do not compare equal numbers of patients at risk for recurrence or progression (grade and stage equivalence), and the study duration is often abbreviated; thus, only the short-term recurrence rate is examined. The important endpoint for these studies should be prevention of disease progression, but unfortunately, most studies do not extend to this level of investigation. The studies reported here tend to be phase I–II trials that suffer from many of the aforementioned concerns. An attempt has been made to select only those studies containing scientifically sound information for mention in this chapter.

Interferon

IFNs are induced cytokines with antiproliferative and immunomodulatory properties. The types of human IFN are classified

TABLE 22-1. *Systemic and intralesional IFNA treatment of bladder transitional cell carcinoma*

Investigators	Type of IFN	Route	Regimen	No. of patients	Percent and type of response
Christopherson et al, 1978[49]	A*	IM	4 million U qd × 2 mo, then 3 × w	3	100 PR
Scorticatti et al, 1982[50]	A*	IM	1 million U qod × 6 mo	7	43 PR
Grups et al, 1987[51]	A	IM	2–20 million U qd × 6 w	8	NR
Ikic et al, 1981[52]	A*	IL	4 million U qd × 21 d	8	75 CR
Distasi et al, 1993[53]	A	IL	3 million U qw × 4 w	15	7 CR 40 PR

A, recombinant IFNA; A*, natural IFNA; CR, complete response; IFNA, interferon alpha; IL, intralesional; IM, intramuscular; NR, no response; PR, partial response.

with respect to their cellular origin and mode of induction and include interferon alpha (IFNA), interferon beta (IFNB), and IFNG.

The initial studies of IFNA treatment of transitional cell carcinoma (TCC) were accomplished using natural IFNA derived from the buffy coat of centrifuged blood and administered parenterally or by direct intralesional injection (Table 22-1). Despite the limited number of patients treated, the overall conclusion is that systemic treatment of superficial TCC by IFNA is not efficacious, because no complete remissions were noted. Intralesional IFNA is more effective, although again, few patients have been treated in this manner.

Intravesical treatment of TCC, CIS, or both also has undergone only limited study (Table 22-2). The reports included in this chapter discuss only patients with unresected TCC or CIS with positive cytologies at the beginning of treatment. The initial report by Oliver and colleagues[54] used natural IFNA to treat eight patients with TCC and eight patients with CIS. Six of the TCC patients had a complete response (CR) or partial response (PR), but no patient with CIS responded. In the first study using recombinant IFNA2B, the Northern California Oncology Group[55] completed a phase I–II trial examining dose, toxicity, and efficacy in a total of 35 patients. The TCC patients had a "beacon" low-grade superficial tumor left in place after an otherwise complete transurethral resection of recurrent TCC. The escalating dose of IFNA2B began at 50 million U and progressed to 1000 million U weekly. Responses were seen at all doses. A disappointing 25% CR rate was seen for TCC. The CIS data were more encouraging in that, overall, 58% of patients had a response, and 32% obtained a CR. The responses did not appear to be dose related. Of the 10 patients who had a CR, 5 remained disease free without maintenance treatment for 18 to 37 months. Several additional findings emerged from the study[55]:

The toxicity (27%) was dose related but not dose limiting, although blood levels of IFNA were undetectable.
Systemic IFNA antibody levels were minimal, and response was unrelated.
Cytologic changes in the urine were noted late in the treatment regimen (i.e., at 7 to 8 weeks of therapy).

The toxicities recorded were primarily flu-like symptoms (i.e., headache, fever, and malaise for 24 to 48 hours). Overall, this trial suggested that IFNA had activity, particularly in CIS, similar to other intravesical agents but produced less toxicity.

Subsequently, Glashan[56] examined the efficacy of low-dose (10 million U/week) or high-dose (100 million U/week) intravesical IFNA2B for CIS in a prospectively randomized phase III trial (see Table 22-2). The high-dose regimen obtained significantly more responses than the low-dose regimen (43% CR versus 5% CR, respectively). Tumor-free status remained for more than 6 months in 90% of patients and for more than 12 months in 50% of the high-dose patients. The toxicity was higher in the high-dose group (17% versus 8%), but it was not dose limiting.

These studies support the use of intravesical IFNA, particularly in CIS patients who are not optimal candidates for intravesical BCG or perhaps in CIS patients who failed prior BCG treatment. Intravesical treatment should be avoided in BCG fail-

TABLE 22-2. *Intravesical IFNA treatment of bladder transitional cell carcinoma and carcinoma in situ*

Investigators	Type of IFN	Regimen	No. of patients	Percent and type response
Oliver et al, 1986[54]	L	50 million U qw × 8 w	8 TCC	38 CR 38 PR
			8 CIS	NR
Torti et al, 1988[55]	A	50–1000 million U qw × 8 w	16 TCC	25 CR
			17 CIS	32 CR 26 PR
Glashan, 1990[56]	A	10 million U qw × 12 w	38 CIS	5 CR 32 PR
		100 million U qw × 12 w	47 CIS	43 CR 19 PR

A, recombinant IFNA; CIS, carcinoma in situ; CR, complete response; IFNA, interferon alpha; L, lymphoblastoid IFN; NR, no response; PR, partial response; TCC, transitional cell cancer.

ure patients when the patient is at significant risk of developing regional or systemic metastasis.

There have been numerous studies using IFNA alone or in combination in the prophylaxis of superficial bladder cancer.[57–62] For the most part, these studies do not provide sufficient design or implementation to allow substantive conclusions to be drawn. Kostakopoulos and colleagues[57] and Bartoletti and associates[58] treated a total of 50 patients with 10 to 54 million U of IFNA intravesically, and suggested that lack of recurrence occurred in 63% to 79%. Patients in both groups had mixed stages and grades of tumor as well as an inconsistent history of tumor recurrence. Little can be determined from these single-arm studies.

Englemann and associates[59] evaluated IFNA alone (10 million U), mitomycin alone (40 mg), or both agents combined in a limited study (67 patients), the results of which suggest that all three regimens are equivalent with respect to frequency of recurrence but that IFNA alone caused less local symptoms. Hoeltl and colleagues[60] evaluated an even more limited group of patients (34) treated with 10 million U IFNA, 100 million U IFNA, or 1.3 g of ethoglucid. They showed an equivalent recurrence rate with high-dose IFN and ethoglucid, although ethoglucid had a higher local toxicity rate.[60] Serretta and colleagues[61] and Ferrari and associates[62] have studied intravesical IFNA with or without epirubicin; although both studies require more patients with a longer median follow-up to determine final results, they appear to indicate a reduction in recurrence rate with the combination.

The most useful prophylaxis study was reported by Boaccardo and colleagues.[63] Thier study is a randomized comparison of IFNA 50 million U/week with mitomycin 40 mg/week given to a total of 287 Ta-T1, G1-2 patients treated for a total of 8 weeks. The groups were comparable with respect to age, gender, and number, size, stage, and grade of tumor. The length of follow-up was also similar in both groups. The results showed that recurrences were noted in 52 out of 141 (37%) of the mitomycin group and 70 of 146 (48%) of the IFN group. The recurrence rates and times of recurrence both also favored the mitomycin arm; however, the local toxicity was slightly higher in the mitomycin group. The difference in efficacy was more evident in T1 tumors, whereas it was equal for the two regimens in Ta tumors, as was the percentage of patients who developed progressive disease. These data and the overall evaluation of IFNA in prophylaxis of TCC suggests that although recurrence of superficial tumors may be decreased by prophylaxis, the difference between IFNA and chemotherapeutic agents is modest; the progression rate is unaffected by any of these agents; and only patients at high risk for recurrence or progression should be treated prophylactically.

Interleukin 2

Interleukins are soluble factors whose primary function is modulation of the immune response. Many of the interleukins have been observed to mediate antitumor activity, either through direct inhibition of tumor growth or through modulation of tumor immunity. IL2 functions as an antitumor agent through its capacity to support T-cell proliferation, its ability to induce cytokine production and activate nonspecific killer cells (i.e., natural killer cells and LAK cells), or both.

The only interleukin used in bladder cancer treatment is IL2, which is a T-cell growth factor. Initial studies of systemic IL2 treatment, alone or with LAK cells, demonstrated objective tumor regression in up to 19% of patients with various types of metastatic cancer including renal cell carcinoma, but the toxicity of IL2 has been a limiting factor to high-dose systemic use. In the treatment of superficial bladder cancer, relatively few studies have been reported. Murine MBT2 experiments showed that intralesional injection of IL2 reduced tumor incidence and prolonged survival in animals. A clinical intralesional study by Pizza and colleagues[64] on 10 patients with muscle-invasive TCC showed complete remission only in those patients receiving 2000 to 4000 U of IL-2 daily over an extended period of up to 54 days (Table 22-3). In the higher-dose patients, three of six had biopsy-proven CR. None of the lower-dose patients had an objective response. Side effects were minimal. Histologic examination of bladder biopsy specimens showed a marked lymphoid infiltration in those patients who were responders.

Huland and Huland[65] used continuous intravesical infusion to treat five patients with muscle-invasive TCC using natural IL2; a complete histologic response that lasted more than 6 months was achieved in one patient. There were no adverse effects. Subsequent studies by Huland[65] have shown similar responses in bladder TCC treated by natural IL2 nasal inhalation. Tubaro and colleagues[66] used continuous arterial infusion of IL2 to treat low-stage superficial TCC in 12 patients. Two

TABLE 22-3. *IL2 treatment of bladder transitional cell carcinoma and carcinoma in situ*

Investigators	Route	Regimen	No. of patients	Percent and type response
Pizza et al, 1984[64]	IL	2000–4000 U × 7–54 d	6	50 CR 33 PR
		150–1400 U × qd 7–14 d	4	NR
Huland and Huland, 1989[65]	CI-IVScL	1000 U/mL; 2 mL/min × 24 h/d × 5d; repeat at 4–12 w	5	20 CR
Tubaro et al, 1991[66]	CI-A	18,000 to 18 million U/m²/d × 5d; repeat at 48 h	12	17 CR 25 PR
Hermann et al, 1992[67]	CI-IV	3 million U/m²/d on d 0–5 and 12–16; LAK on d 12, 13, and 15	9	NR

CI-A, Continuous arterial infusion; CI-IV, Continuous intraveneous infusion; CI-IVScL, Continuous intravesical infusion; CR, complete response; IL, intralesional; LAK, Lymphokine activated killer cells; NR, no response; PR, partial response.

5-day courses of IL1 injected into the internal iliac artery separated by 48 hours followed by repeated transurethral resection 4 days later revealed no tumor in two patients and a reduction in tumor size in three patients. Fever and hypotension caused the infusion to be discontinued in two patients. Increased number of IL2 receptor–positive lymphocytes were observed at the tumor site, indicating a local immune response had been activated. Hermann and colleagues[67] used intravenous continuous infusion of IL2 and the LAK cell regimen in 9 patients with metastatic bladder cancer. There were no tumor responses to the therapy, and the toxicity, as expected, was substantial. The use of intravesical IL2 has promise because of its low toxicity; however, the optimal dose and timing of treatment has yet to be determined.

TUMOR NECROSIS FACTOR ALPHA

TNFA is a macrophage secretory protein that can be elicited by BCG or endotoxin. TNFA is cytotoxic for numerous human tumor cells in vitro. TNFA acts synergistically with IFNG or DNA topoisomerase II–targeted drugs (VP16 or doxorubicin) and may have a role in the antitumor effect of BCG. In vitro TNFA inhibits murine MBT2 tumor growth. Clinically, a phase I–II prophylaxis trial of intravesical TNFA of up to 0.6 mg given once per week over 8 weeks was initiated in patients by Ernstoff and colleagues (Table 22-4).[68] The treatment was well tolerated, with no systemic absorption and only hematuria as a side effect. In this study, four patients relapsed at a median of 6 months and two patients with CIS had disease progression. Sternberg and associates[69] also used TNFA in a phase I–II treatment study of 18 Ta-T1-TIS patients who had a retained TCC marker lesion. Two patients had a biopsy-proven CR and two had a PR; the CRs were maintained for 8 and 18 months. No evidence of systemic absorption or toxicity was noted. Seretta and colleagues[70] similarly treated 13 patients with a Ta-T1 TCC marker lesion with intravesical TNFA at 0.5 mg once per week over 8 weeks and observed three CRs. These results provide evidence that TNFA is active intravesically and is minimally toxic.

It is not likely that TNFA will be used as a single intravesical agent; however, combination studies that take advantage of its synergistic properties with topoisomerase II–targeted drugs such as doxorubicin or other cytokines are of significant interest.

Conclusions

The use of immunotherapy alternatives to BCG have shown promise but have not yet equaled the efficiency of BCG. For the immediate future, intravesical combinations of various cytokines such as IFNA and IL2, bropirimine and IL2, or cytokines plus chemotherapy such as TNFA and doxorubicin, among others, seem most promising and are deserving of clinical treatment protocols in patients with residual TCC or CIS.

GENE THERAPY

In addition to the agents discussed previously, a number of new treatment modalities using recombinant DNA technology are being studied. Localized immunotherapeutic approaches to cancer have been particularly effective in treating bladder carcinoma and melanoma, although the mechanism of action of therapies such as intravesical or intralesional BCG and intravesical cytokines has eluded definition. Although localized mechanisms that result in tumor elimination contribute to therapeutic success, optimal antitumor effectiveness, particularly at disseminated tumor sites, requires the development of systemic immunity, which must be the goal of any new therapy. Building on an evolving understanding of the regulation of the development of systemic immunity to parasites as well as tumors, a number of laboratories have approached the treatment of bladder cancer using gene therapy strategies aimed ultimately at enhancing systemic antitumor immunity.

The underlying hypothesis of gene therapy approaches under study is that by modulating the immune milieu at the local tumor or tumor vaccination sites, systemic antitumor immunity may be induced. Treatments focus on immune enhancement via cytokine production in association with tumor immunization and use two strategies: immunization using cytokine gene–transfected tumor vaccines and in situ introduction of cytokine genes or cytokine-producing cells at the tumor site in vivo.

Studies have examined a panel of cytokines that target multiple regulatory mechanisms, including the following:

- upregulation of major histocompatibility antigens (MHC) and perhaps tumor-associated antigens (e.g., TNFA, IFNG)
- macrophage and antigen-presenting cell activation and recruitment with subsequent enhanced antigen processing and presentation (e.g., granulocyte-macrophage colony-stimulating factor [GM-CSF], IFNG)
- directing the T-cell helper response toward a TH1 response, thus enhancing the generation of DTH and cytotoxic T-lymphocyte (CTL) responses (IFNG)
- expansion of activated T cells (e.g., IL2, IL4).

In addition to induction of systemic immunity, which is the overall goal of these therapies, induction of cytokine production in tumor cells has been shown to result in tumor elimination locally via non–T-cell-mediated mechanisms. Cytokines with direct antitumor activity such as IFNG and TNFA may directly

TABLE 22-4. *Intravesical TNFA treatment of transitional cell carcinoma and carcinoma in situ*

Investigators	Regimen	No. of patients	Percent and type response
Ernstoff et al, 1991[68]	<0.6 mg qw	7	NR
Sternberg et al, 1992[69]	400–1800 mg 2 × w	18	2 CR 2 PR
Seretta et al, 1992[70]	0.5 mg qw × 8	13	3 CR

CR, complete response; NR, no response; PR, partial response.

effect tumor growth. In addition, recruitment of eosinophils by IL4 transduced tumors have been shown to result in local tumor elimination.[71]

Cytokine Gene–Transduced Tumor Vaccines

A number of laboratories[19,22,25] have taken the approach that specific antitumor immunity might be enhanced by the use of gene transfection aimed at inducing cytokine and lymphokine production at the local tumor site. Studies have primarily relied on the in vitro transfection of murine tumors with cytokine genes and the use of these resultant cytokine-producing cells as "vaccines" against nontransfected tumor. Inoculation of syngeneic mice with experimental tumors transfected with the genes for TNFA,[22] IL2,[19,72] GM-CSF,[72,73] IFNG,[23,74] and IL4,[75] among others, has resulted in rejection of the injected tumor. In some cases, mice generated a measurable systemic antitumor response, and in a limited number of cases, including bladder tumors, vaccination with such cells resulted in the elimination or reduced growth of preexisting tumor.[20,73,75]

Initial preclinical studies of this type resulting in the elimination of established tumor have been reported in murine models of renal cell carcinoma and TCC of the bladder. In the bladder, studies demonstrate that whereas the murine bladder-derived TCC MBT2 grows progressively in syngeneic mice, IL2-producing transfected lines failed to grow, and inoculation of mice with the transfectant resulted in the induction of immunity in the recipients capable of protecting the mice from further tumor challenge.[20] In addition, treatment of mice with established intravesical MBT2 tumors was effective in curing some animals. A subsequent series of studies by the same group using the same protocol has shown that GM-CSF–transfected MBT2 is also effective in curing mice with preexisting intravesical tumors.[20] These studies, taken with the original therapeutic study in a murine renal carcinoma model,[75] support the use of such strategies for the therapy of established tumors in vivo. Although the bladder studies cited previously, as well as the single report of elimination of an established renal cell carcinoma, used small tumor inocula as sentinel tumors, they show that localized cytokine and lymphokine production can result in the generation of tumor-specific immunity and may have antitumor therapeutic activity.

Although these preclinical studies support the approach of enhancing antitumor immunity via the localized production of cytokines by tumors in vivo, certain aspects of the approach limit translation to the clinic. First, current studies have focused on in vitro transfection of tumor cell lines prior to injection into mice. Although this is a reasonable approach in preclinical studies, extension of this system to clinical trials will severely limit its availability. The requirement that autologous tumor be available, removed, transfected, and cloned severely limits the number of patients that would be suitable for such a study. A modified vaccine approach using transfected HLAA2-matched allogeneic tumor as a surrogate for autologous tumor has been proposed; however, this approach requires a shared tumor antigen restricted at HLAA2. Without knowledge regarding the presence or absence of such a shared tumor antigen, the use of this approach would be at best unpredictable and would limit enthusiasm for widespread clinical use.

Another approach designed to circumvent the need for autologous tumor involves the injection of cytokine-producing fibroblasts into tumor masses. Although data from a number of laboratories varies, this approach has not demonstrated results as uniform as those with the use of transfected tumor in preclinical models. In one comparative study, the injection of IL2-transduced fibroblasts was not nearly as effective as directly transfected tumor.[76] Another problem in translating the tumor-cytokine transfectant approach to the clinic is based on the need to reinject viable tumor. Preclinical studies would suggest that the transfected tumor will be rejected; however, loss of the cytokine gene or putative suicide genes could easily result in further tumor spread in the patient, a particular hazard in healthy patients with minimal tumor burden in which immunotherapeutic approaches would seem best suited. This has been addressed at least in part by studies demonstrating that irradiated transfected tumor produces cytokines for at least several days in vitro, although the effects of such irradiation on tumor antigen expression has not been studied. Nevertheless, positive antitumor responses have been demonstrated using irradiated cytokine gene–transfected tumors in a murine model of melanoma.[72] Although the above studies suggest the usefulness of focusing lymphokine or cytokine production at the tumor site, significant limitations exist in translating these findings to the clinic.

Viral Delivery Systems

Although the gene-transfected tumor studies discussed previously validate the approach of enhancing the immune milieu via cytokine production at the tumor site, the limitations of such tumor transfection in vitro are formidable in widespread clinical use. In an attempt to capitalize on the tumor transfection studies, several laboratories have focused on the in situ introduction of cytokine genes into tumors in vivo. This approach would obviate the need for resectable tumor, in vitro manipulation, and reinjection of tumor into the patient. Toward this end, studies from one of our laboratories have examined the ability to use vaccinia virus vectors for introducing functional genes into tumors. In studies using the murine bladder tumor MB49, it was found that vaccinia vectors are highly efficient in transferring encoded genes into tumors in vitro, and that intravesical instillation of vaccinia recombinants efficiently infect or transfect TCC growing in the bladder.[77] These studies demonstrated that preexisting immunity to vaccinia virus, expected in adults immunized to smallpox, which might preclude repeated viral injections did not eliminate the ability of the virus to infect tumor in vivo. Additional studies have demonstrated that vaccinia vectors are capable of transfecting bladder tumor cell lines with genes encoding IL4, IFNG, and GM-CSF with significant levels of cytokine production.[78] Vaccinia viral recombinants expressing the gene for murine IL4 have also been shown to retard and in some cases prevent the growth of two murine tumors in vivo, giving additional support to this approach.[79]

Initial clinical studies of the use of vaccinia to transfer genes to tumor cells in vivo further support the approach with injection of vaccinia intralesionally into human melanoma metastasis resulting in efficient infection, even with repeated injections in the presence of high levels of antivaccinia immunity.[80] In addition to vaccinia, several laboratories are currently examining other viruses such as adenovirus and an array of poxviruses, as well as other experimental methods such as liposomes and native DNA insertion for their ability to transfect in vivo tumors with cytokine genes. These studies have not advanced as far as vaccinia; however, they do demonstrate the enthusiasm for this approach to therapy.

Although the direct introduction of cytokine genes into tumors in vivo using viral vectors results in a functionally similar end point as seen with cytokine gene–transfected tumor cell vaccines described above, a number of the limitations of the latter are overcome. The use of viral vectors encoding cytokine genes precludes the need to resect and engineer each patient's tumor and reinject it. In addition, the unknown presence or absence of critical shared tumor antigens when using allogeneic tumor transfectants is eliminated, because the patient's own tumor serves as the antigen source.

Recombinant Bacillus Calmette-Guerin

In a similar approach to the use of viral vectors, studies have examined the use of recombinant BCG vectors as a means of generating immune-active cytokines at the site of tumors.[81] Recombinant BCG that expresses parasite antigens as a result of genetic manipulation has been used as a vaccine,[82] and studies have shown that high levels of cytokines such as IL2 can be produced by BCG engineered to express the *IL2* gene.[81] Extensive experience with the use of intravesical BCG (discussed previously) support the feasibility of using such recombinants for localized therapy, resulting in the focusing of immune-active cytokine at the tumor site. Cytokine-producing BCG would take advantage of the proven localization and antitumor effectiveness described previously and would add the positive effects of localized cytokine production and its expected enhancements in antitumor immunity. Similar to the use of viral vectors, recombinant BCG would not require the patient's tumor to be resected, transfected, and reinjected and would thus lend itself to widespread clinical use.

CONCLUSIONS

A number of approaches are under study that use state-of-the-art molecular techniques to enhance the immunologic response to bladder and other tumors. Based in principal on a large number of studies of the regulation of immunity toward parasites and viral and protein antigens that demonstrate the ability to enhance the generation of productive cellular immune responses by augmenting or shifting the pattern of cytokines at the immunization site, such approaches have focused on the generation of cytokine-producing tumor vaccines as well as induction of in situ cytokine production. Preclinical studies using murine models of TCC have shown promise and predict the efficacy of such approaches to therapy, and it is expected that these results will support early introduction of one or more of these treatment modalities in clinical trials.

REFERENCES

1. Mathe G, Amiel J, Schwarzenberg L, et al. Active immunotherapy for acute lymphoblastic leukemia. Lancet 1969;1:697.
2. Nathanson L. Use of BCG in the treatment of human neoplasms: a review. Semin Oncol 1974;1(4):337.
3. Zbar B, Rapp HJ. Immunotherapy of guinea pig cancer with BCG: Cancer, 1974;37(Suppl 4):1532.
4. Coe JE, Feldman JD. Extracutaneous delayed hypersensitivity, particularly in the guinea pig bladder. J Immunol 1966;10:127.
5. Morales A, Eidinger D, Bruce AW. Intracavitary bacillus Calmette-Guerin in the treatment of superficial bladder tumor. J Urol 1976;116:180.
6. Herr HW, Pinsky CM, Whitmore Jr WF, Sogani PG, Oettgen TF, Melamed MR. Experience with intravesical bacillus Calmette-Guerin therapy of superficial bladder tumors. Urology 1982;25(2):119.
7. Lamm DL, Thor DE, Stogdill VD, Radwin HM. Bladder cancer immunotherapy. J Urol 1982;128:931.
8. Brosman SA. Experience with bacillus Calmette-Guerin in patients with superficial bladder carcinoma. J Urol 1982;128:27.
9. Mori K, Lamm DL, Crawford ED. A trial of bacillus Calmette-Guerin versus Adriamycin in superficial bladder cancer: a Southwest Oncology Group Study. Urol Int 1986;41:254.
10. Lamm DL, Blumenstein BA, Crawford D, et al. A randomized trial of intravesical doxorubicin and immunotherapy with bacillus Calmette-Guerin for transitional cell carcinoma of the bladder. N Engl J Med 1991;325:1205.
11. Brosman SA. The use of bacillus Calmette-Guerin in the therapy of bladder carcinoma in situ. J Urol 1985;134:36.
12. Herr H, Wartinger DD, Fair WR, Oettgen HF. Bacillus Calmette-Guerin therapy for superficial bladder cancer: a 10-year follow up. J Urol 1992;147:1020.
13. Prehn RT, Main JM. Immunity to methylcholanthrene-induced sarcomas. J Natl Cancer Inst 1957;18(6):769.
14. Burnett FM. The concept of immunological surveillance: a review. Prog Exp Tumor Res 1970;13:1.
15. Rosenberg SA, Lotze MT, Muhl LM, et al. A progress report on the treatment of 157 patients with advanced cancer using lymphokine-activated killer cells and interleukin-2 or high-dose interleukin-2 alone. N Engl J Med 1987;316:889.
16. Spiess PJ, Yang JC, Rosenberg SA. In vivo antitumor activity of tumor-infiltrating lymphocytes expanded in recombinant interleukin-q2. J Natl Cancer Inst 1987;79(5):1067.
17. Topalian S, Soloman D, Rosenberg S. Tumor-specific cytolysis by lymphocytes infiltrating human melanomas. J Immunol 1989;142(10):3714.
18. Alexander RB, Rosenberg SA. Long-term survival of adoptively transferred tumor-infiltrating lymphocytes in mice. J Immunol 1990;145(5):1615.
19. Fearon ER, Pardoll DM, Itaya T, et al. Interleukin-2 production by tumor cells bypasses T helper function in the generation of an antitumor response. Cell 1990;60(3):397.
20. Connor J, Bannerji R, Saito S, Heston W, Fair W, Gilboa E. Regression of bladder tumors in mice treated with interleukin-2 gene-modified tumor cells. J Exp Med 1993;177:1127.
21. Townsend SE, Allison JP. Tumor rejection after direct costimulation of CD8 + T cells by B7-transfected melanoma cells. Science 1993;259:368.
22. Asher AL, Mule JJ, Kasid A, et al. Murine tumor cells transduced with the gene for tumor necrosis factor-alpha. Evidence for paracrine immune effects of tumor necrosis factor against tumors. J Immunol 1991;146(9):3227.
23. Porgador A, Bannerji R, Watanabe Y, Feldman M, Gilboa E, Eisenbach L. Antimetastatic vaccination of tumor-bearing mice with two types of IFN-gamma gene-inserted tumor cells. J Immunol 1993;150(4):1458.
24. Aoki T, Tashiro K, Miyatake S, et al. Expression of murine interleukin-7 in a murine glioma cell line results in reduced tumorigenicity in vivo. Proc Natl Acad Sci U S A 1992;89(9):3850.
25. Watanabe Y, Kuribayashi K, Miyatake S, et al. Exogenous expression of mouse interferon gamma cDNA in mouse neuroblastoma C1300 cell results in reduced tumorigenicity by augmented anti-tumor immunity. Proc Natl Acad Sci U S A 1989;86(23):9456.
26. Hock H, Dorsch M, Kunzendorf U, et al. Vaccinations with tumor cells genetically engineered to produce different cytokines: effectively not superior to a classical adjuvant. Cancer Res 1993;53(4):714.
27. Truitt GL, Mackaness GL. Cell-mediated resistance to aerogenic infection of the lung. Am Rev Respir Dis 1971;104:829.

28. Orme IM. Immunity mycobacteria: a review. Curr Opin Immunol 1993; 5(4):497.
29. Cooper AM, Dalton DK, Stewart TA, Griffin JP, Russell DG, Orme IM. Disseminated tuberculosis in interferon gamma gene-disrupted mice. J Exp Med 1993;178(6):2243.
30. Kabelitz D, Bender A, Schondelmaier S, Schoel B, Kaufmann SHE. A large fraction of human peripheral blood $\gamma\delta$ + T cells is activated by *Mycobacterium tuberculosis* but not by its 65-kd heat shock protein. J Exp Med 1990;171(3):667.
31. Flynn JL, Goldstein MM, Triebold KJ, Koller B, Bloom BR. Major histocompatibility complex class I–restricted T cells are required for resistance to *Mycobacterium tuberculosis* infection. Proc Natl Acad Sci U S A 1992;89(24):12013.
32. Ratliff TL, Gillen D, Catalona WJ. Requirement of a thymus-dependent immune response for BCG-mediated antitumor activity. J Urol 1987; 137(1):155.
33. Mosmann TR, Cherwinski H, Bond MW, Giedlin MA, Coffman RL. Two types of murine helper T cell clones. I. Definition according to profiles of lymphokine activities and secreted proteins. J Immunol 1986;136:2348.
34. Moore KW, Garra AO, de Waal Malefyt R, Vierira P, Mosmann TR. Interleukin-10. Annu Rev Immunol 1986;136:2348.
35. McKnight AJ, Zimmer GJ, Fogelman I, Wolf SF, Abbas AK. Effects of IL-12 on helper T cell-dependent immune responses in vivo. J Immunol 1994;152(5):2172.
36. Heinzel FP, Schoenhaut DS, Rerko RM, Rosser LE, Gately MK. Recombinant interleukin-12 cures mice infected with *Leishmania major*. J Exp Med 1993;177(5):1505.
37. Heinzel FP, Sadick MD, Holaday BJ, Coffman RL, Locksley RM. Reciprocal expression of interferon gamma or interleukin-4 during the resolution or progression of murine leishmaniasis: evidence for expansion of distinct helper T-cell subsets. J Exp Med 1989;169(1):59.
38. Scott P. The role of TH1 and TH2 cells in experimental cutaneous leishmaniasis: a review. Exp Parasitol 1989;68(3):369.
39. Kavoussi LR, Brown EJ, Ritchey JK, Ratliff TL. Fibronectin-mediated bacille Calmette-Guerin attachment to murine bladder mucosa: requirement for the expression of an antitumor response. J Clin Invest 1990; 85:62.
40. Schorey JS, Li Q, McCourt DW, et al. A *Mycobacterium lepra* gene encoding a fibronectin binding protein is used for efficient invasion of epithelial cells and Schwann cells. Infect Immun 1995;63(7):2652.
41. Hudson MA, Ritchey JK, Ratliff TL. Modulation of BCG-fibronectin binding through use of drugs influencing the coagulation pathway. Cancer Res 1991;51:3726.
42. Haaff EO, Catalona WJ, Ratliff TL. Detection of interleukin 2 in the urine of patients with superficial bladder tumors after treatment with intravesical BCG. J Urol 1986;136:970.
43. Torrence RJ, Kavoussi LR, Catalona WJ, Ratliff TL. Prognostic factors in patients treated with bacillus Calmette-Guerin for superficial bladder cancer. J Urol 1988;139:941.
44. Bartlett GL, Zbar B, Rapp HJ. Suppression of murine tumor growth by immune reaction to the bacillus Calmette-Guerin strain of *Mycobacterium bovis*. J Natl Cancer Inst 1972;48:245.
45. Fujiwara H, Takai Y, Sakamoto K, Hamaoka T. The mechanism of tumor growth inhibition by tumor-specific Lyt-1 + 2-T cells. I. Antitumor effect of Lyt-1 + 2-T cells depends on the existence of adherent cells. J Immunol 1985;135(3):2187.
46. Townsend ARM, Rothbard J, Gotch FM, Bahadur G, Wraith D, McMichael AJ. The epitopes of influenza nucleoprotein recognized by cytotoxic T lymphocytes can be defined with short synthetic peptides. Cell 1986;44(6):959.
47. Lattime EC, Gomella LG, McCue PA. Murine bladder carcinoma cells present antigen to BCG-specific CD4 + T-cells. Cancer Res 1992;52: 4286.
48. Becich MJ, Carrol S, Ratliff TL. Internalization of bacille Calmette-Guerin by bladder tumor cells. J Urol 1991;145:1316.
49. Christopherson I, Jordel R, Osther K, et al. Interferon therapy in neoplastic disease. Acta Med Scand 1978;204:471.
50. Scorticatti C, de la Pena N, Bellora O, et al. Systemic IFN-alpha treatment of multiple bladder papilloma grade I or III patients: pilot study. J Interferon Res 1982;2:339.
51. Grups J, Frohmuller H, Ackermann R. Can recombinant human alpha-2 interferon prevent recurrence of high-grade superficial bladder tumors? Cancer Detect Prev 1987;10:405.
52. Ikic D, Nola P, Maricic Z, et al. Application of human leukocyte interferon in patients with urinary bladder papillomatosis, breast cancer, and melanoma. Lancet 1981;1:1022.
53. Distasi S, Virgili G, Vespasiani G, et al. Intralesional alpha interferon therapy in papillary superficial transitional cell carcinoma of the bladder (a pilot study). Br J Urol 1993;71:422.
54. Oliver R, Waxman J, Kwok H, et al. Alpha lymphoblastoid interferon for noninvasive bladder cancer. Br J Cancer 1986;53:432.
55. Torti F, Shortliffe L, Williams R, et al. Alpha-interferon in superficial bladder cancer: a Northern California Oncology Group study. J Clin Oncol 1988;6:476.
56. Glashan R. A randomized controlled study of intravesical alpha-2-interferon in carcinoma in situ of the bladder. J Urol 1990;144:658.
57. Kostakopoulus A, Deliveliotis Ch, Mavromanolakis E, et al. Intravesical interferon alfa-2b administration in the treatment of superficial bladder tumors. Eur Urol 1990;18:201.
58. Bartoletti R, Massimini G, Criscuolo D, et al. Interferon alpha 2 in superficial bladder cancer prophylaxis: toleration and long-term follow-up: a phase I–II study. Anticancer Res 1991;11:2167.
59. Engelmann U, Knopf H, Graff J, et al. Interferon-A2b instillation prophylaxis in superficial bladder cancer: a prospective, controlled three-armed trial. Anticancer Drugs 1992;3(1):33.
60. Hoeltl W, Hasun R, Albrecht W. Prospective, randomized trial to evaluate high versus low-dose interferon-A2b versus conventional chemotherapy in prevention of the recurrence of superficial transitional cell carcinoma of the urinary bladder. Anticancer Drugs 1992;3(1):29.
61. Serretta V, Pavone C, Corselli G, et al. A pilot study comparing different dose levels administration schedules of interferon-A2b combined with epirubicin for prevention of recurrence in bladder cancer. Anticancer Drugs 1992;3(1):19.
62. Ferrari P, Castagnetti G, Pollastri C, et al. Chemoimmunotherapy for prophylaxis of recurrence in superficial bladder cancer: interferon-A2b versus interferon-A2b with epirubicin. Anticancer Drugs 1992;3(1):25.
63. Boccardo F, Cannata D, Rubagotti A, et al. Prophylaxis of superficial bladder cancer with mitomycin or interferon alpha-2b: results of a multicentric Italian study. J Clin Oncol 1994;12(1):7.
64. Pizza G, Severini G, Menniti D, et al. Tumor regression after intralesional injection of interleukin 2 (IL-2) in bladder cancer: preliminary report. Int J Cancer 1984;34:359.
65. Huland E, Huland H. Local continuous high dose interleukin 2: a new therapeutic model for treatment of advanced bladder carcinoma. Cancer Res 1989;45:5469.
66. Tubaro A, Velotti F, Stoppacciaro A, et al. Continuous intra-arterial administration of recombinant interleukin-2 in low-stage bladder cancer. Cancer 1991;68:56.
67. Hermann G, Geertsen P, von der Maase H, et al. Recombinant interleukin-2 and lymphokine-activated killer cell treatment of advanced bladder cancer: clinical results and immunological effects. Cancer Res 1992;52:726.
68. Ernstoff M, Bahnson R, Hakala T. Tumor necrosis factor alpha: a potential anticancer agent for superficial bladder cancer. Surgical Rounds 1991;May:417.
69. Sternberg C, Arena M, Pansadoro V, et al. Recombinant tumor necrosis factor for superficial bladder tumors. Ann Oncol 1992;3:745.
70. Seretta V, Corselli G, Piazza B, et al. Intravesical therapy of superficial bladder transitional cell carcinoma with tumor necrosis factor-alpha: preliminary report of a phase I–II study. Eur Urol 1992;22:112.
71. Tepper RI, Coffman RL, Leder P. An eosinophil-dependent mechanism for the antitumor effect of interleukin-4. Science 1992;257:548.
72. Dranoff G, Jaffee E, Lazenby A, et al. Vaccination with irradiated tumor cells engineered to secrete murine granulocyte-macrophage colony stimulating factor stimulates potent, specific, and long lasting antitumor immunity. Proc Natl Acad Sci U S A 1993;90:3539.
73. Saito S, Bannerji R, Gansbacher B, et al. Immunotherapy of bladder cancer with cytokine gene-modified tumor vaccines. Cancer Res 1994; 54:3516.
74. Lattime EC, McCue PA, Ross RP, Baltish MA, Gomella LT. Cells bearing t/d receptor in human transitional cell carcinoma of the bladder. [Abstract] Proc Am Assoc Cancer Res 1992;33:334.
75. Golumbek PT, Lazenby AJ, Levitsky HI, et al. Treatment of established renal cancer by tumor cells engineered to secrete interleukin-4. Science 1991;254:713.
76. Tsai SC, Gansbacher B, Tait L, Miller FR, Heppner GG. Induction of antitumor immunity by interleukin-2 gene-transduced mouse mammary

tumor cells versus transduced mammary stromal fibroblasts. J Natl Cancer Inst 1993;85:546.

77. Lee SS, Eisenlohr LC, McCue PA, Mastrangelo MJ, Lattime EC. Intravesical gene therapy: in vivo gene transfer using vaccinia vectors. Cancer Res 1994;54:3325.
78. Lee SS, Eisenlohr LC, McCue PA, Mastrangelo MJ, Lattime EC. Vaccinia virus vector mediated cytokine gene transfer for in vivo tumor immunotherapy. [Abstract] Proc Am Assoc Cancer Res 1994;35:514.
79. Elkins KL, Ennist DL, Winegar RK, Weir JP. In vivo delivery of interleukin-4 by a recombinant vaccinia prevents tumor development in mice. Human Gene Ther 1994;5:809.
80. Lattime EC, Maguire HCJ, McCue PA, et al. Gene therapy using vaccinia vectors: repeated intratumoral injections result in tumor infection in the presence of anti-vaccinia immunity. [Abstract] Proc Am Soc Clin Oncol 1994;13:397.
81. O'Donnell MA, Aldovini A, Duda RB, et al. Recombinant Mycobacterium bovis BCG secreting functional interleukin-2 enhances gamma interferon production by splenocytes. Infect Immun 1994; 62:2508.
82. Jacobs WR Jr, Snapper SB, Lugosi L, Bloom BR. Development of BCG as a recombinant vaccine vehicle. Curr Top Microbiol Immunol 1990;155:153.

Principles and Practice of Genitourinary Oncology, edited by Derek Raghavan, Howard I. Scher, Steven A. Leibel, and Paul H. Lange. Lippincott-Raven Publishers, Philadelphia, © 1997.

CHAPTER 23

Clinical Presentation, Investigation, and Staging of Bladder Cancer

Michael J. Droller

Staging systems in cancer have been based on correlations between the pathologic extent of a particular cancer and its prognosis. Because prognosis is based on the biologic potential and natural history of a particular cancer, assignment of a cancer to a specific stage has been used as a means to assess treatment outcome. Variations in the results of treatment for a given stage of disease have contributed to the continuing evolution and refinement of staging systems. Treatment results themselves may be reinterpreted in the context of increased understanding of a particular cancer's potential behavior and its changed assignment of stage.

As technologies have advanced, the clinical staging of a cancer has achieved greater accuracy. This has permitted further assessment of the efficacy of various treatments, allowing refinements in the understanding of the biology of disease and corresponding revisions in cancer staging.

Bladder cancer constitutes a representative example of how staging systems have evolved, have factored into the selection of specific therapies, and have been used in the evaluation of treatment outcomes. Bladder cancer can also be used to demonstrate the inadequacies of staging systems when they are interpreted as more than a construct, to be indicative of the natural history of a particular cancer process and its biologic capabilities.

This chapter describes the manner in which various forms of bladder cancer present clinically and how observations of prognosis in association with the pathologic extent of the cancer have been used in the development of current staging systems. This chapter also reviews the means by which the pathologic extent of a particular bladder cancer can be assessed and factors that may be used in the future in refining estimates of the prognosis of a particular form of the disease on the basis of its potential biologic capabilities.

CLINICAL PRESENTATION

Hematuria is the most common finding in bladder cancer.[1] The degree of hematuria does not correlate with the extent of disease. It may be grossly visible to the patient or simply found on routine urinalysis. Any degree of hematuria, however, requires evaluation for bladder cancer, even if another potential cause of hematuria (e.g., renal calculus, bacterial cystitis) is found.

In addition to gross or microscopic hematuria, bladder cancer may also present with symptoms of voiding irritability. Patients may complain of urgency, dysuria, and increased urinary frequency. Although these symptoms are more commonly indicative of bacterial cystitis, negative bacterial cultures with persistence of symptoms, with or without hematuria, should prompt investigation for the possible presence of bladder cancer.

Imaging

Evaluation of hematuria includes imaging of the kidneys and ureters, cystoscopy, and urinary cytology. Intravenous pyelography (IVP) can be used to detect the presence of a renal cortical mass, filling defects in the renal pelvis and ureters, and hydronephrosis, which may indicate the presence of a ureteral cancer or a muscle-invasive bladder cancer at the ureteral orifice.[2] Although the cystogram phase of the IVP is not considered definitive in excluding the presence of small bladder cancers, larger tumors may be seen as filling defects in the bladder or may restrict symmetrical bladder wall expansion during filling.[3]

Ultrasonography has been used with increasing frequency as the initial means of urinary tract imaging, not only because it avoids the use of contrast agents, to which some patients may be allergic, but also because more sensitive transducers have allowed improved imaging of the upper urinary tract and bladder. Transabdominal ultrasound permits characterization of renal masses whether they are solid or cystic, detection of hydronephrosis, and visualization of intraluminal filling defects in the bladder.[4] Visualization of the upper tract collecting systems, however, may not be sufficiently sensitive to identify transitional cell cancers of the renal pelvis or sufficiently specific to exclude them.[5] Conversely, the sensitivity and specificity of superficial tumors in the bladder have been reported to be 91%

and 93%, respectively, and for invasive tumors as 93% and 91%, respectively.[6] In these studies, only 9% of superficial tumors were overstaged and only 7% of invasive tumors were understaged.

Transurethral ultrasonography has also been suggested to be useful in diagnosing bladder cancer, but with variable results. Reports of sensitivity for detection of superficial tumors range between 71% and 100%, and reports of specificity range between 85% and 100%, with overall levels of 76% and 90%, respectively.[7] Corresponding ranges in the diagnosis of invasive tumors are 85% to 100% sensitivity (90% overall) and 71% to 100% specificity (75% overall). The overstaging error for superficial tumors is 24%, and the understaging error for invasive tumors is 10%.[7] Of particular interest in these reports is the apparent ability to distinguish between stage T3b and stage T4a cancers (discussed later), with only 29% cumulative understaging, a sensitivity of 71%, and a specificity of 95%.[8]

Detection of disease by ultrasonography may be particularly difficult when previous therapy (e.g., irradiation, transurethral resection) has been administered. In addition, unless there is substantial enlargement of pelvic lymph nodes, the use of ultrasonography to define the nodal status of disease is not particularly productive. Conversely, transabdominal ultrasonography may be used to guide needle aspiration of enlarged lymph nodes to document regional metastatic disease.

Computed tomography (CT) generally is not a particularly useful imaging study in the diagnosis of transitional cell cancer. When a noncystic lesion has been identified in the kidney, CT scanning may allow further characterization of the lesion.[9] It is virtually diagnostic for renal cell cancer[10] and may be useful in the diagnosis of transitional cell cancer of the renal pelvis. In these instances, the use of intravenous contrast may suggest the type of tumor that is present.[10] In such instances, renal cell cancers demonstrate enhancement with contrast, whereas transitional cell cancers may not. In addition, CT scanning may permit characterization of the extent of the transitional cell cancer of the upper tract.

Although CT scanning may be useful in identifying a bladder tumor, in characterizing the thickness of the bladder wall, and in determining whether the tumor has penetrated through the bladder wall into the perivesical soft tissue, sensitivity and specificity are less than that which can be achieved with transurethral ultrasonography. For example, several studies have reported 67% overstaging for superficial disease, which correlates with 33% specificity for invasive disease.[11] Corresponding attempts to distinguish between superficial and deep muscle invasion have underestimated the depth of invasion in 30% of tumors and overestimated it in 20%. As many as 40% of stage T1 tumors have been classified as muscle invasive by CT scanning.[11]

In addition, usefulness of CT scan in characterizing extravesical extension of disease may be influenced by artifactual abnormalities in the perivesical tissues as a result of inflammatory processes or extravasation of fluids from prior resection.[12] Both the sensitivity and specificity of CT scanning in characterizing extravesical extension of disease varies widely, ranging between 60% and 90% for an overall sensitivity of 83% and between 66% and 93% for an overall specificity of 82%.[12] Approximately 17% of tumors stage T3b or higher are understaged and 18% are overstaged.[12]

CT scanning may permit evaluation of lymph node enlargement but does not provide reliable information on the microscopic aspects of disease. Thus, the sensitivity in detecting nodal metastasis has been only 48% overall, with 52% of positive nodes being understaged, whereas specificity has been 94% overall, with only 6% of enlarged nodes being overstaged as indicative of metastatic disease. On this basis, the major use of CT has been relegated to the guidance of needle aspiration of enlarged lymph nodes. CT can also be used to assess solid masses in the pelvis and guide needle aspiration for the characterization of those masses.[13]

Magnetic resonance (MR) imaging can be used with objectives similar to those of CT scanning but with the theoretical advantage of being able to provide imaging information in multiple planes. Tumors at the base or dome of the bladder may be better visualized with MR than with CT. Extravesical extension at these sites may also be assessed with greater reliability.[13] T1-weighted MR images provide definition of a primary tumor through its contrast with the low signal intensity of urine in the bladder and the high signal intensity of perivesical fat. T2-weighted MR images permit assessment of cancer invasion through its disruption of the muscle wall. However, sensitivity and specificity have been reported to be only slightly greater with MR imaging (73% and 84%, respectively) than with CT imaging (70% and 81%, respectively).[14] Gadolinium-enhanced MR has been reported to provide greater accuracy in definition of bladder cancer masses than that obtained with CT with or without contrast or transurethral ultrasonography.

Although the sensitivity and specificity of MR imaging in detecting nodal metastases has been reported to be better than that for pedal lymphangiography, microscopic metastases may remain undetected in 25% of instances.[14] However, MR may be more useful than CT in characterizing the reason for pelvic lymph node enlargement in association with the possible presence of metastatic disease. MR imaging does permit distinction between blood vessels and pelvic lymph node tissue without the need for intravenous contrast. Lymphadenopathy is best characterized on T1-weighted images, but both T1- and T2-weighted images are important in distinguishing between lymph nodes and surrounding fat.

Cytology

Examination of a voided urine specimen for exfoliated cancer cells is particularly useful when a high-grade malignancy or carcinoma in situ is present.[15,17] Even if upper tract or bladder imaging studies are negative, findings of a positive urinary cytology may indicate a source anywhere in the urinary tract, from the uppermost calyx, through the ureters, into the bladder and prostatic urethra. Moreover, a negative voided urinary cytology does not necessarily exclude the presence of a bladder tumor; it may only indicate that the bladder tumor is of low grade. In these instances, positive urinary cytology may reflect the presence of papillary clusters of low-grade cells in the urine.[18] These may be difficult to distinguish from clusters of normal cells that are dislodged by instrumentation. Voided specimens are therefore important in assessing these possibilities. Positive urinary cytology in the context of a low-grade bladder tumor may also indicate the presence of malignancy at other sites, especially if the cells are of higher grade than the histologic appearance of the resected tumor. Therefore, the entire urinary tract must be examined to determine the source of high-grade cancer cells.

Urinary specimens for cytology should not be obtained from the first-voided morning specimen.[15,16] Instead, specimens for cytology should be provided when the patient is well hydrated to optimize the appearance of the cancer cells. Because instrumentation may introduce artifacts that can interfere with accurate interpretation of a cytology specimen, use of the cystoscope or a catheter to obtain a urinary specimen for cytologic evaluation should be avoided. Conversely, if flow cytometry is to be used for diagnosis, the cellular content of a urinary specimen may need to be increased. Catheter barbotage of the bladder can increase the cellular content of the specimen, and instrumentation in these instances does not interfere with accurate analysis of cell ploidy.[19,20]

Cytoscopy

The diagnosis of bladder cancer ultimately depends on cystoscopic examination of the bladder and pathologic evaluation of the resected lesion. Cystoscopy may initially be performed without anesthesia in assessing a patient for bladder cancer. If a bladder cancer has been visualized on earlier imaging studies, or if urinary cytology has previously been found to be positive, diagnostic cystoscopy can be omitted and the patient scheduled instead for cystoscopy and biopsy or tumor resection under anesthesia.

With the patient anesthetized, a bimanual examination should be performed first to assess whether a mass is palpable in the bladder and, if so, whether it is fixed to the pelvic wall.[21] Bimanual examination may be performed both before and after transurethral resection. The presence of a palpable mass after resection implies that there is extravesical tumor to a greater extent than the residual exophytic tumor that can be visualized endoscopically.[22] Conversely, negative bimanual examination or only the impression of induration without a palpable mass implies that the invasive tumor may be more superficial and potentially associated with a better outcome.

Previous pelvic surgery, irradiation, or inflammatory disease may limit interpretation of bimanual examination. Moreover, small tumors may not be palpated, even if they extend extravesically. Obesity and areas that are inaccessible to palpation can also compromise bimanual examination.

Although the correlation between clinical and pathologic stage on the basis of bimanual examination is not good, the value of this examination is based on observations that a palpable mass is likely to be infiltrative, and that this observation can provide a significant prognostic consideration in determining whether primary or adjunctive therapy will be provided.[22] Cystoscopy can then be used to examine the gross appearance of the tumor (i.e., papillary or nodular), the extent and multiplicity of the tumor, and the presence of any other abnormal areas in the bladder or prostatic urethra.

Papillary tumors generally are more superficial, even when invasive, than nodular tumors.[23] In addition, papillary tumors that are confined to the bladder mucosa are generally associated with normal bladder wall thickness, whereas more deeply invasive nodular or papillonodular tumors are often associated with a thicker bladder wall. In addition to assisting in the assessment of the potential behavior of the cancer, these considerations may aid in determining how aggressive transurethral resection should be.

High-grade tumors are more likely to be associated with abnormal areas elsewhere in the bladder, whether these areas appear normal or abnormal endoscopically.[24] Biopsy specimens of abnormal areas in the bladder may assist in defining the diffuseness of malignant urothelial changes in these instances. Systematic biopsy of endoscopically normal areas of the bladder mucosa may also be useful in this regard. When done, it should include specimens of mucosa immediately lateral to each ureteral orifice, of the posterior bladder floor, of the lateral walls on each side posteriorly, and of the prostatic urethra.

Transurethral resection of the bladder tumor should be done so as to maximize the preservation of architectural detail and the relation of the tumor to the various layers of the bladder wall. It is primarily the extent to which the tumor involves the various layers of the bladder wall that has traditionally been used as a means of staging bladder cancer and determining prognosis.

For pathologic evaluation, the more superficial component of the tumor should be resected separately from its deeper component. Use of cautery current should be minimized to preserve pathologic detail and avoid cautery artifact.

For tumors that appear to be papillary and superficial, complete resection may require only resection into the lamina propria or possibly into the superficial muscularis to provide sufficient material for accurate staging assessment. In contrast, tumors that appear to be more nodular may require a more extensive resection that extends deeply into the muscularis and even into the perivesical fat. This will not only provide more accurate staging information but may also serve adjunctively in the treatment of this type of malignancy.

An indication of the difficulty inherent in staging by transurethral resection alone has been provided in a number of reports that suggest the presence of residual tumor in as many as 30% to 35% of patients thought to have only superficial disease.[25,26] This finding has prompted some surgeons to suggest that a second transurethral resection should be performed in patients thought to have superficial disease who are found on pathologic evaluation of the initial resection specimen to have tumor infiltration into the lamina propria.[27] In this regard, tumor grade has also been considered as an important indicator of potential understaging by initial transurethral resection. In a review of 238 cases, it was observed that more than one half of tumors that were thought to be superficial but were actually high grade were found on subsequent transurethral resection to have invaded the muscularis.[28] Moreover, 90% of tumors that were high grade and underwent cystectomy were actually found to be muscle invasive. Understaging by transurethral resection is therefore an important consideration in the overall assessment of the staging of a patient with bladder cancer, especially in the setting of high-grade, papillonodular, or nodular disease.

STAGING

The development of a staging system for bladder cancer has been based on observations of prognostic differences between various forms of tumor as represented either by the extent to which they may have penetrated the bladder wall or by their histologic grade.[29,30] The continued evolution of the staging system for bladder cancer reflects changing observations and insights through the recognition of additional features that correlate with the variable course of histologically similar cancers. These are often manifested by variable responses to similar therapies.

The earliest characteristic that was used in predicting prognosis was the degree of differentiation of the particular cancer.[30] Low-grade tumors were generally found to have little likelihood of progressing regionally or of metastasizing. High-grade cancers were often found to have extended regionally and to be associated with concurrent or subsequent metastatic disease.

In the 1940s, Jewett and Strong[31] suggested that the depth of penetration of the bladder cancer was more important than the degree of differentiation alone in predicting prognosis. Tumors that were not palpable on bimanual examination and did not infiltrate the bladder muscle appeared to be curable by transurethral resection. Tumors that were palpable and penetrated the muscularis were considered incurable by transurethral resection but possibly curable by cystectomy. Tumors that appeared to be fixed in the pelvis were nearly always incurable.

Subsequent studies refined these observations and led to modifications of this initial staging system. For example, prognostic differences became apparent between superficial tumors that were confined to the bladder mucosa and those that had invaded the lamina propria.[32] Prognostic differences were also observed between muscle-invasive tumors that had penetrated only the superficial muscle and those that had infiltrated more deeply into the muscle layer or had penetrated through the muscle into the perivesical fat.[33,34] The likelihood that metastasis to regional lymph nodes or to distant sites had already taken place appeared to correlate with the depth to which the cancer had infiltrated.

The American Joint Committee on Cancer–Union Internationale Contre le Cancre (AJCC-UICC) system is currently the most commonly used staging system (Table 23-1).[35,36] This system comprises both clinical and pathologic staging. The former is based predominantly on resection specimens, whereas the latter is based on evaluation of partial or total cystectomy specimens in which the full-thickness bladder wall specimen is available for pathologic examination.

Clinical staging provides the basis on which treatment decisions are made. For the most part, clinical staging is also the basis on which results of various types of therapy for a given stage of disease are assessed and compared. Clinical staging has therefore come to be used as a means of assigning prognosis regardless of the therapy applied and as a means of determining whether a particular treatment has altered prognosis for a particular stage of malignancy.

Staging systems for bladder cancer are traditionally based on the histologic layer to which the particular cancer has penetrated the bladder wall (Fig. 23-1). This has been found to correspond to the likelihood of progression and the possible future development of metastatic disease. Although other factors such as grade, tumor configuration, architecture of infiltration (i.e., papillary or solid, broad front or tentacular), abnormalities at sites other than the primary tumor (e.g., carcinoma in situ), and vascular and lymphatic involvement have also been found to influence prognosis, these have not been incorporated into standard staging schemata. Bladder cancer is multifocal in both space and time. Initial neoplastic changes, potential behavioral characteristics, or both therefore may either persist or change with recurrence.

The format in which staging systems such as the AJCC-UICC are presented implies a simple pattern of development according to which early cancers appear at lower stages and progress to higher stages in sequence; however, this is not necessarily what is seen clinically. Although bladder cancers begin by intraepithelial neoplastic transformation and then may progress by penetration through the various layers of the bladder wall, the various forms of bladder cancer may progress through a variety of pathways that, although possibly interrelated, do not necessarily occur in sequence, as is implied by these staging systems.

At the time that Jewett originally formulated his staging scheme,[31] carcinoma in situ was not appreciated as a clinical entity. Jewett characterized papillary, mucosally confined tumors as "stage 0," subsequently combining all "superficial" tumors in the category "stage A".[37] This stage included not only mucosally confined tumors but also those that had penetrated into the lamina propria. A number of reports subsequently used "stage 0" to indicate that there was no tumor present in a patient who previously had had superficial disease.[38]

In his initial reports, Jewett classified muscle-infiltrative tumor as "stage B."[31] Prognostic differences subsequently became apparent between tumors that had penetrated only the superficial muscularis and those that had penetrated more deeply into the bladder wall musculature.[39] This led to the subclassification of stage B into stage B1 and stage B2, respectively. In the former category, it was unclear whether tumors that simply impinged on the muscularis were considered to have actually invaded the muscle, albeit superficially, and whether such tumors were distinct in their prognosis from those that either had only infiltrated into the lamina propria but had not reached the muscle layer or from those that had actually penetrated into the superficial muscle. Of interest has been the question of whether muscle fibers in the lamina propria itself (i.e., "muscularis mucosae") may have been misinterpreted in earlier studies as representing the true detrusor muscle layer.[40] If so, reports of prognosis and results of therapy for muscle-infiltrative disease may have been inaccurate in their staging assessment, possibly producing a bias in favor of whatever treatment was used because of the overstaging that resulted.

Jewett's "stage C" disease comprised tumors that extended through the muscularis into the perivesical fat.[31] In his initial studies, tumors that could be detected as a fixed mass on bimanual examination were surgically incurable; those that were palpable but not fixed could occasionally be cured by radical cystectomy. Practically speaking, palpable disease most likely represents a cancer that is already advanced, whereas fixation indicates a greater degree of regional advancement to the pelvic sidewall. Although a bladder cancer that is not palpable may still be deeply infiltrative, bimanual examination is still considered to be of some importance in the clinical staging of disease, both at initial diagnosis and following bladder-conserving therapy.[22]

The likelihood of regional or distant metastatic disease has been found to have a direct correlation with the depth of penetration of the tumor into and through the bladder wall. Metastatic disease has traditionally been classified as stage D, with stage D1 representing either regional or pelvic lymph node metastases, and stage D2 representing metastases to distant sites.

TABLE 23-1. *AJCC-UICC TNM classification of bladder cancer*

PRIMARY TUMOR

The suffix (m) should be added to the appropriate T category to indicate multiple tumors. The suffix (is) may be added to any T category to indicate the presence of associated carcinoma in situ.

TX Primary tumor cannot be assessed
T0 No evidence of primary tumor
Ta Noninvasive papillary carcinoma
Tis Carcinoma in situ ("flat tumor")
T1 Tumor invades subepithelial connective tissue
T2 Tumor invades superficial muscle (inner half)
T3 Tumor invades deep muscle or perivesical fat
- T3a Tumor invades deep muscle (outer half)
- T3b Tumor invades perivesical fat
  - i Microscopically
  - ii Macroscopically (extravesical mass)

T4 Tumor invades any of the following: prostate, uterus, vagina, pelvic wall, or abdominal wall
- T4a Tumor invades the prostate, uterus, vagina
- T4b Tumor invades the pelvic wall, abdominal wall, or both

REGIONAL LYMPH NODES (N)

Regional lymph nodes are those within the true pelvis; all others are distant nodes.

NX Regional lymph nodes cannot be assessed
N0 No regional lymph node metastasis
N1 Metastasis in a single lymph node that is 2 cm or smaller in greatest dimension
N2 Metastasis in a single lymph node that is larger than 2 cm but not larger than 5 cm in greatest dimension or multiple lymph nodes, none of which is larger than 5 cm in greatest dimension
N3 Metastasis in a lymph node that is larger than 5 cm in greatest dimension

DISTANT METASTASIS (M)

MX Presence of distant metastasis cannot be assessed
M0 No distant metastasis
M1 Distant metastasis

STAGE GROUPING

Stage	T	N	M
0_a	Ta	N0	M0
0_{is}	Tis	N0	M0
I	T1	N0	M0
II	T2	N0	M0
	T3a	N0	M0
III	T3b	N0	M0
	T4a	N0	M0
IV	T4b	N0	M0
	Any T,	N1-3	M0
	Any T,	Any N	M1

AJCC, American Joint Committee on Cancer; UICC, Union Internationale Contre le Cancer.
Adapted from references 35 and 36.

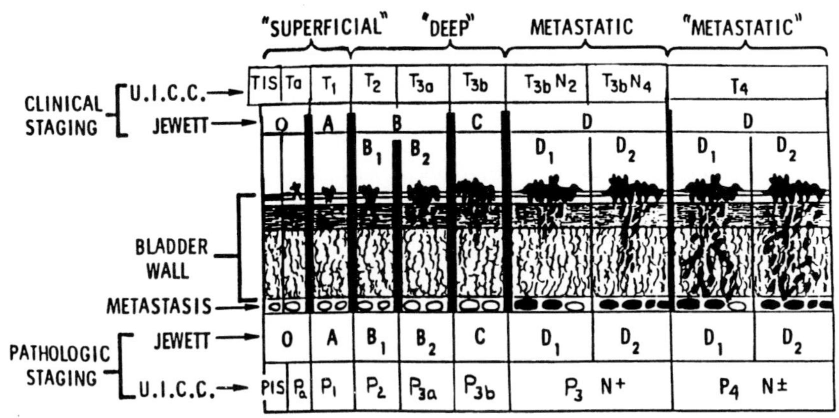

FIG. 23-1. This staging system for bladder cancer is a composite of the original staging system proposed by Jewett,[37] current staging systems based on clinical and pathologic observations, and diagrams illustrative of the configuration of tumors at a particular stage, the depth to which they penetrate the bladder wall, and the possibility that they may be associated with regional and distant metastases. UICC, Union Internationale Contre le Cancer. (From Koss LG. Tumors of the urinary bladder. In: Atlas of tumor pathology, series 2, fascicle 11. Washington, DC: AFIP, 1975.)

Current staging systems have evolved through the recognition of additional distinctions among bladder cancers and their involvement of various layers of the bladder wall. In 1953, Melicow[41] described an entity of intraepithelial malignant transformation that he called "carcinoma in situ." Although originally described in bladders that had been removed as a result of muscle-infiltrative cancer, carcinoma in situ soon became recognized as a form of bladder cancer that could be present in the absence of any other form, leading ultimately to its separate designation in the clinical staging system as Tis.[42] Although carcinoma in situ has been found in some instances to demonstrate aggressive behavior, no distinctions have been made between those forms of carcinoma in situ that are focal and may have a more indolent course and those that appear to involve the bladder mucosa more diffusely and may be more aggressive. Furthermore, a separate category has not been assigned to the forms of carcinoma in situ that, in 20% to 30% of instances, have been found to have penetrated the basement membrane and extended into the lamina propria.[43]

The other forms of superficial disease have been subclassified into those that are mucosally confined (stage Ta) and those that have penetrated the lamina propria (stage T1).[44] The former have been associated with an excellent prognosis; less than 3% of stage Ta tumors progress.[45] Stage T1 tumors may be associated with a more ominous prognosis in as many as 30% of cases.[45] Stage Ta tumors are often multiple, and recurrence may be seen in as many as 50% to 75% of cases.[46] Neither of these phenomena appear to be associated with a worse prognosis. Usually, stage Ta tumors are found to be of low grade; high-grade stage Ta tumors are rare.[47] In addition, stage Ta tumors are rarely, if ever, associated with diffuse changes in the mucosa elsewhere in the bladder.[48]

Tumors that are staged as T1 are often found to be of higher grade.[45,46] Furthermore, it is not unusual to find areas of carcinoma in situ both adjacent to the T1 tumor and at distant sites in the bladder.[48] Although the prognosis in these instances may be more ominous, no separate classification for these tumors in association with carcinoma in situ has yet been made. In addition, recent studies have suggested prognostic differences between stage T1 tumors that have penetrated only into the fibrovascular stalk or minimally into the lamina propria of the bladder wall while remaining superficial to the muscularis mucosae (stage T1a) from those that are more aggressive, having infiltrated across the muscularis mucosae layer and penetrated the lamina propria more extensively (stage T1b).[49] This potential distinction between different types of stage T1 tumors has not been incorporated into available clinical staging systems.

Muscle-infiltrative disease has been classified as stage T2 when only the superficial muscularis propria has been invaded and as stage T3a when the deeper muscularis has been invaded.[50] A number of investigators have suggested that stages T2 and T3a should be combined, because it is difficult to distinguish between the various depths of infiltration of the muscularis on the basis of transurethral resection alone.[51] Other investigators feel that some provision is necessary in considering whether invasion of only the superficial muscularis can be diagnosed with accuracy and whether its prognosis can then be shown to be truly different from that in which more extensive invasion of the muscularis has occurred. Evidence in support of maintaining this distinction remains strong on the basis of the following factors:

- the more papillary configuration of more superficially invasive tumors[52]
- involvement of the bladder wall vasculature and lymphatics only half as often in superficially invasive tumors as in deeply invasive tumors[53]
- the greater likelihood of eradication of superficially invasive tumors by transurethral resection[54]
- the apparently dramatic differences in ultimate prognosis (discussed later).

Infiltration through the muscle layer into the perivesical fat has been classified as stage T3b. It is unclear whether the prognosis of this stage of disease is sufficiently different from that of stage T3a. Conceivably, these clinical stages distinguish between masses described by Jewett as only being palpable from those found to be both palpable and fixed. In addition, some researchers have suggested distinctions between tumors that extend into the perivesical fat only microscopically and those that are more extensive in their perivesical invasion.[22] In either case, the results of a variety of treatments have not been promising, and the distinction between these two stages has therefore not been particularly useful.

The clinical staging of metastatic disease has been based on the status of regional and distant nodes and whether or not other organs, either regionally or at distant sites, are involved. The number of lymph nodes involved is designated in the UICC clinical staging system as a numerical subscript for the letter N. However, the accuracy of such staging depends on both the meticulousness with which lymph node dissection is done and the degree to which excised lymph nodes are examined pathologically.[55] Studies have suggested that it may be useful to distinguish between microscopic disease involving only one regional node from microscopic disease involving more than one node.[56] Conversely, the uniformly poor prognosis associated with gross involvement of even one lymph node does not appear to factor into these considerations.

When metastases are present in other organs, this is designated as stage T4 for adjacent organs, with the presumption that this more likely represents direct extension rather than metastatic disease, and as M for metastases at distant sites. Because distant metastases are generally present when infiltration into adjacent organs has occurred, this distinction may be moot. Conversely, different treatment decisions have been made on the basis of these distinctions, because distant metastases may not be evident when regionally extensive disease has been diagnosed. In these situations, regional treatments may be applied and distant metastases may become apparent only subsequently.

The possible exception in the staging of transitional cell cancer as stage T4 when it involves adjacent organs pertains to the question of prostatic involvement. Initially, involvement of the prostate by transitional cell cancer implied an ominous prognosis.[57] Subsequently, different patterns of involvement were identified,[58] and it became apparent that some of these patterns did not necessarily imply a high likelihood of metastatic disease whereas others did. The increased use of intravesical therapy in both the treatment and prophylaxis of different types of superficial transitional cell cancer, including carcinoma in situ,[59] as well as the discovery that bacillus Calmette-Guerin was particularly effective in treating carcinoma in situ even if it involved the prostatic urethra and extended into the prostatic ducts,[60] prompted the suggestion that substages were appropriate in considering whether involvement of the prostate should be classified as stage T4, or whether some forms of involvement actually reflected only superficial disease whereas others truly reflected more aggressive disease with the associated more ominous prognosis.[61]

Stage T4 disease in other instances (e.g., invasion of the prostate, uterus, or vaginal wall) may imply M + disease, and this may need to be considered when efforts to stage tumors are made. Patients who have metastases confined to the lungs often appear to have a better prognosis than those with metastases to other sites, with the possible exception of regional lymph nodes.[62,63] Although it may be useful to designate whether metastases are exclusive to the lung in a particular patient because of the apparently better prognosis in this setting, it is likely that such distinctions will not necessarily come into play until more effective systemic therapies become available. This distinction as part of a formal staging system has generally not been used and requires further study to become established.

The accuracy of staging for metastatic disease is dependent on the variety of imaging modalities available. Accuracy of staging also depends on the accessibility of these various sites to tissue sampling to confirm their identify as metastatic lesions. The most sensitive imaging studies for the detection of metastatic disease are CT and MR imaging. These can survey the chest, abdomen, and pelvis and identify metastatic deposits at each of these sites. A bone scan may also be done, although metastases to the bones are less common. Similarly, a CT scan of the brain may be done, but metastasis to this site is rare.

The most difficult aspect in the assessment of metastatic disease is confirmation that metastatic deposits that appear on imaging studies actually represent metastases from the primary cancer and not other pathologic processes. Needle aspirates can be performed, but this may be tedious or even impossible for each metastatic deposit. Generally, the appearance of soft tissue lesions in the context of deeply invasive transitional cell cancer is assumed to represent metastatic disease. Histologic confirmation is generally reserved for instances in which the primary cancer is only a superficial process. Under these circumstances, other sites of transitional cell cancer that may be more advanced (e.g., within the substance of the prostate, in the upper tracts with invasion of the kidney) or the possible existence of other primary cancers should be evaluated.

The construction of a staging system based on increasing involvement of the bladder wall by transitional cell cancer has prompted the impression that the progression of bladder cancer is represented by a sequence of changes manifested not only by increasing depth of penetration but also by a decreasing papillary configuration, both extending into the lumen of the bladder and infiltrating into the bladder wall, and an increasing nodular or solid appearance as higher stages are seen.[64] There have also been observations of increasing involvement of the bladder wall lymphatics and vasculature corresponding to an increasing depth of penetration and increasing solid or nodular configuration of the tumor.[64] These features have not been incorporated into the standard staging system. Similarly, various surface markers that correlate with depth of tumor penetration and a worse prognosis have not been incorporated into the AJCC-UICC staging system.[65]

In addition, the natural history of bladder cancer development has been presumed to be represented by a sequence of stages, as indicated by the AJCC-UICC staging scheme. Thus, intraepithelial neoplastic transformation has been assumed to lead to the development of a superficial transitional cell cancer, which has been presumed to infiltrate progressively into the wall of the bladder and ultimately to metastasize, first to regional lymph nodes and then to distant sites. On this basis, superficial tumors, which represent the majority of bladder cancers, could for the most part be amenable to conservative treatments, whereas deep tumors presumably require cystectomy for any chance of cure. An additional impression derivative of this staging system has been that superficial tumors represent an early manifestation of neoplastic transformation, whereas muscle-invasive tumors represent late manifestations of this process.

Neither of these presumptions as derived from the construct of a sequential staging scheme are necessarily correct. For example, tumors within each stage of this system have been found to have a variable course and a heterogeneous response to treatment. Other variables such as grade,[66] endoscopic and histologic architectural appearance (i.e., papillary or nodular),[52] pattern of invasion (i.e., broad front or tentacular),[53] and involvement of the bladder wall lymphatics or vasculature[64] have been examined as means of predicting the potential behavior of a particular stage of disease.

Thus, some cancers that have invaded only the lamina propria have also been found to involve bladder wall lymphatics and to have an aggressive course. In contrast, some cancers that have infiltrated the bladder wall muscle actually appeared to have a less aggressive course and were occasionally amenable to cure by transurethral resection. In effect, cancers thought to be of a lower stage may be a greater life-threatening risk than cancers thought to be of a higher stage.

Additional confusion resulting from suggestions of the sequential nature of cancer progression revolves around the nature of the entity called carcinoma in situ. Although by definition, carcinoma in situ indicates an intraepithelial, early form of neoplasia, it has most often been found to represent a potentially highly aggressive form of bladder cancer and to be associated with high-grade, nodular, deeply invasive transitional cell cancers.[48,67] When found in association with superficial papillary bladder cancer, the latter has generally been found to have invaded the lamina propria and to have a rapidly progressive course.[68] Carcinoma in situ has rarely been found in association with mucosally confined papillary tumors, the latter being of high grade in less than 2% of instances.[47,48]

These observations appear to be inconsistent with implications of a sequential staging system, in which carcinoma in situ is the initial form of transitional cell cancer from which papillary superficial cancers develop. Rather, carcinoma in situ may be predominantly involved as the earliest form of higher-grade cancer diathesis, in which progression to invasion may be rapid, with the gradual development of a papillonodular and finally a more solid appearance with the occurrence of deeply infiltrative bladder cancer.

The development of bladder cancer may not represent a simple sequence of events or a common pathway of tumor development and progression. Instead, the existence of a variety of developmental pathways may more accurately characterize the different patterns of bladder cancer development that are seen.[69] This could also explain the heterogeneous results that may be observed in response to similar treatments applied to a particular stage of disease.

At the same time, disparate developmental pathways must

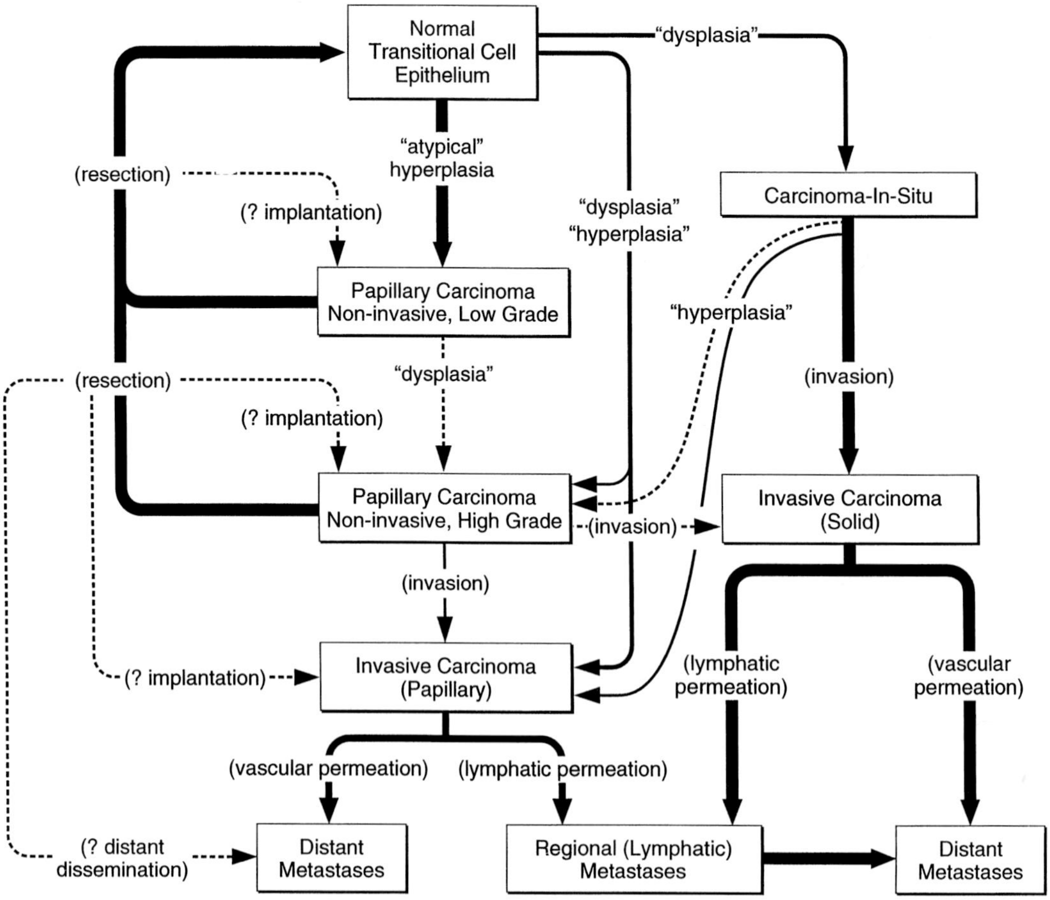

FIG. 23-2. Hypothetical pathways for the development of transitional cell cancer of the bladder. Clinical observations, cytopathologic examinations, and correlations of both with the prognosis of various forms of bladder cancer suggest that there may be a variety of pathways to explain the different types of bladder cancer and their distinctive natural histories. These hypothetically separate but interrelated pathways of cancer development and progression can be used to facilitate an understanding of the potential natural history of a particular stage, grade, and appearance of a transitional cell cancer at diagnosis or during its clinical course.

also be sufficiently interrelated to account for the divergent and concordant patterns of bladder cancer that are seen. Clinical observations, cytopathologic examinations, and correlations of both with the prognoses of various forms of bladder cancer suggest that there may be a variety of pathways to explain the different types of bladder cancer and their distinctive natural histories (Fig. 23-2). The most common form is represented by a process that can be termed atypical hyperplasia. Neoplastic transformation in these instances results in the formation of a proliferative diathesis that leads to the formation of a papillary carcinoma that is noninvasive and generally of low grade. Resection of this type of bladder cancer theoretically restores the transitional cell epithelium to normal. The presence of clonal stem cells elsewhere in the bladder that are not endoscopically visible or tumor cell implantation at the time of transurethral resection may account for the frequent recurrences that are seen. Such tumors appear to present very little risk for progression.

Higher-grade papillary transitional cell tumors may reflect a process that can be termed dysplasia, which is superimposed on the process of atypical hyperplasia. However, the rarity of high-grade tumors that are mucosally confined suggests the possibility that a different pathway in which the process of dysplasia may be primary may account for their development. The superimposition of hyperplasia may then lead to the development of either papillary high-grade carcinoma that is noninvasive or, more often, to the development of invasive high-grade papillary carcinoma.

When dysplasia is the primary process, it may lead more frequently to the development of infiltration of the epithelial basement membrane before the presence of a malignancy is clinically apparent and produce solid or nodular invasive transitional cell cancers. The risk of deep infiltration and lymphatic or vascular invasion is twice as great with solid invasive carcinomas than with papillary invasive carcinomas. These hypothetically separate but interrelated pathways of cancer development and progression can be used to facilitate an understanding of the potential natural history of a particular stage, grade, and appearance of a transitional cell cancer at diagnosis or during its clinical course.

For example, one common pathway might be characterized as reflecting atypical hyperplasia, in which cell proliferation is the primary process in accounting for the development of a bladder tumor.[70] In this instance, neoplastic transformation presumably induces the ability of a transformed stem cell to proliferate in an uncontrolled fashion, which leads to the development of a papillary, usually low-grade, transitional cell tumor that lacks the enzymatic machinery necessary to penetrate the basement membrane and underlying connective tissue matrix and therefore remains mucosally confined. Transurethral resection of the tumor presumably restores the urothelium to its normal state. However, multiple recurrences of mucosally confined tumors at different sites in the bladder is common, occurring in 50% to 75% of instances.[45,46] Persistence of transformed stem cells that participate in the same proliferative process to produce additional papillary mucosally confined tumors and implantation of tumor cells at the time of initial resection have each been suggested to explain this phenomenon.[71] In either case, repeat resection will again theoretically restore the bladder mucosa to normal. Alternatively, a variety of intravesical agents have been used to prevent tumor recurrence. This type of tumor diathesis rarely if ever leads to a life-threatening situation. Although these tumors may develop at multiple sites in the bladder, rarely is the urothelium itself diffusely involved by a neoplastic process. Indeed, flat carcinoma in situ is rarely, if ever, seen, and high-grade, papillary, mucosally confined lesions are seen in fewer than 2% of cases.[48]

A more ominous pathway, which can be termed dysplastic, may be less common than atypical hyperplasia but may lead to the development of high-grade cancer cells with a more aggressive biologic potential.[70] It may be this pathway that produces flat carcinoma in situ. This pathway may also lead, albeit less commonly, to the development of high-grade, mucosally con-

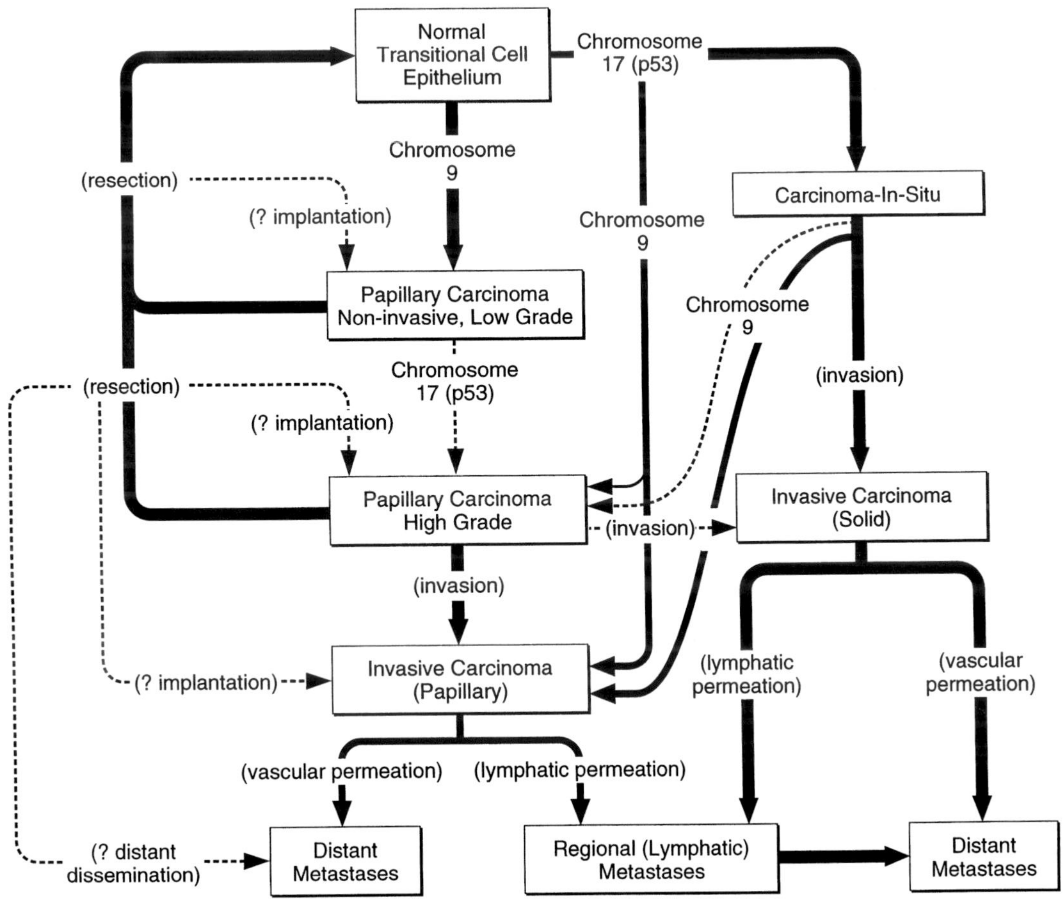

FIG. 23-3. The use of techniques in molecular biology to characterize chromosomal changes in the different types of bladder cancer have suggested that different chromosomal changes may account for different types of bladder cancer and their differences in prognosis. For example, changes in chromosome 17 with expression of *P53* are commonly observed in carcinoma in situ and in solid invasive transitional cell cancers. Such changes are not seen in low-grade, noninvasive papillary carcinoma. Conversely, changes in chromosome 9 have been seen in both types of cancers, suggesting that these changes may be associated with the proliferative activities of a particular tumor, whereas changes in chromosome 17 may account for the more dysplastic appearances and more aggressive behaviors of the more infiltrative carcinomas. Further study and understanding of these types of changes may ultimately be used to generate a molecular profile of bladder cancers that can be correlated with their histologic appearance and used to predict with greater accuracy their potential biologic behavior. This data may then translate into the design of more specific therapies to control disease recurrence and progression.

fined tumors, or more commonly, to the development of high-grade, lamina propria–invasive tumors. The latter cancers are often associated with diffuse malignant changes of the urothelium at the margin of the intraluminal tumor itself and at distant sites in the bladder.

These high-grade diatheses are also more often associated with the development of tumors that have a nodular configuration. Some researchers have suggested that deep penetration of tumor cells into the bladder wall may occur even before these tumors become clinically evident.[48] Although high-grade papillary tumors and flat carcinoma in situ may share in the commonalty of a dysplastic developmental pathway, a majority of patients with deeply invasive bladder cancer present at this stage when initially diagnosed.[72] When the dysplastic pathway combines with the proliferative pathway to generate a papillary high-grade tumor, early diagnosis may provide a window through which successful treatment may be delivered before progression takes place.

These same considerations permit the inference that more advanced tumors may actually be early tumors in the overall course of disease from initial, neoplastic transformation to clinical presentation, and that low-grade, papillary, noninvasive tumors may actually be diagnosed relatively late in the course of their natural history. In effect, highly aggressive infiltrative cancers that theoretically develop along a dysplastic pathway may actually progress rapidly from the time of initial stem cell transformation and not be diagnosed until they are advanced. The symptom history of such patients is short compared with the history of patients in whom only a proliferative diathesis (i.e., low-grade, mucosally confined papillary disease) is present.[72] Diagnosis in the latter situation may actually occur late in the course of the natural history of the diathesis because it is generally dependent on the occurrence of hematuria, which may not be grossly visible. Because the risk of progression of a low-grade, mucosally confined diathesis is small, early diagnosis is less critical than, theoretically, for cancers that develop rapidly along the dysplastic pathway.

Advances in the understanding of the molecular biology of bladder cancer have provided new information on the fundamental differences between papillary, mucosally confined, low-grade transitional cell cancers and nodular, invasive, high-grade transitional cell cancers.[73] Several studies have suggested that abnormalities of chromosome 9 are more commonly associated with a proliferative, low-grade tumor diathesis,[74] whereas abnormalities in chromosome 17, as indicated by an increased expression of protein P53 are more commonly associated with high-grade, infiltrative transitional cell cancers (Fig. 23-3).[75] Aberrations in chromosome 9 have also been found in high-grade invasive cancers[76]; it has therefore been suggested that these changes represent an initial genetic event in neoplastic transformation that may lead to a cascade of additional changes culminating in the development of an aggressive cancer. In contrast, abnormalities in chromosome 17 have not been found in low-grade, mucosally confined papillary tumors; thus, alterations in chromosome 9 may lead only to a proliferative diathesis, and only if changes in other chromosomes occur will a more aggressive cancer develop. Such differences coincide with the suggestion of the existence of varying pathways of cancer development (described previously). Abnormalities in the expression of P53 have also been found in flat carcinoma in situ, which may lead directly to the development of solid, deeply invasive cancers, whereas abnormalities in chromosome 9 have not; this fact supports the previously described theories.

These observations suggest that a variety of genetic events may lead to biochemical changes that initiate separate developmental pathways and generate a variety of bladder cancers with distinct biologic potentials. These concepts support clinical observations that the different types of bladder cancer reflect their development along a number of distinct pathways. If the role of a staging system is to classify tumors according to prognosis and to permit analysis of the efficacy of treatments of a specific stage in a particular diathesis, the concept of the existence of a variety of pathways in tumor development suggests the need for further refinement of staging systems to take into account this possibility in explaining differences in both tumor development and in the interpretation of results of various treatments for a particular cancer diathesis.

Understanding of the genetic changes that determine the biologic behavior of different types of bladder cancer is embryonic. Additional information regarding the means by which specific genetic changes contribute to the development of different types of cancer may eventually be used to create a profile of a particular bladder cancer. This profile could then be used in conjunction with the staging system to further refine the classification of different types of bladder cancer. This in turn may permit application of more individualized treatments, based on both the specific histologic type of a given tumor and its particular pathway of past and possibly future development.

REFERENCES

1. Fitzpatrick JM. Superficial bladder cancer: natural history, evaluation, and management. AUA Update Series 1989;8:82.
2. See WA, Fuller JR. Staging of advanced bladder cancer: current concepts and pitfalls. Urol Clin North Am 1992;19:663.
3. Dershaw DD, Panicek DM. Imaging of invasive bladder cancer. Semin Oncol 1990;17:544.
4. Yeh H-C. Ultrasonography. In: Droller MJ, ed. Surgical management of urologic disease: an anatomic approach. St Louis: Mosby-Yearbook, 1992:111.
5. Dinsmore BJ, Pollack HM, Banner MP. Calcified transitional cell carcinoma of the renal pelvis. Radiology 1988;167:401.
6. Denkhaus H, Crone-Munzelrock W, Huland H. Noninvasive ultrasound in detecting and staging bladder carcinoma. Urol Radiol 1985;7:121.
7. Resnick MI, Kursh E. Transurethral ultrasonography in bladder cancer. J Urol 1986;135:253.
8. Nakamura S, Niijima T. Staging of bladder cancer by ultrasonography: a new technique by transurethal intravesical scanning. J Urol 1980; 124:341.
9. Mendelson DS. Computerized tomography. In: Droller MJ, ed. Surgical management of urologic disease: an anatomic approach. St. Louis: Mosby-Yearbook, 1992:140.
10. Sandler CM, Raval B, David CL. Computed tomography of the kidney. Urol Clin North Am 1985;12:657.
11. Voges GE, Tauschke E, Stockle M, et al. Computerized tomography: an unreliable method for accurate staging of bladder tumors in patients who are candidates for cystectomy. J Urol 1989;142:1972.
12. Husband JE. Staging bladder cancer. Clin Radiol 1992;46:153.
13. Malmstrom PU, Lonnemark M, Busch C, et al. Staging of bladder carcinoma by computer tomography—guided transmural core biopsy. Scand J Urol Nephrol 1993;27:193.
14. Tanimoto A, Yuasa Y, Imai Y, et al. Bladder tumor staging: comparison of conventional and gadolinium-enhanced dynamic MR imaging and CT. Radiology 1992;185:741.
15. Badalament RA, Fair WR, Whitmore WF Jr, et al. The relative value of cytometry and cytology in the management of bladder cancer. Semin Urol 1988;6:22.
16. Carbin BE, Ekman P, Eneroth P, et al. Urine TPA (tissue polypeptide antigen), flow cytometry and cytology as markers for tumor invasiveness in urinary bladder carcinoma. Urol Res 1989;17:269.

17. Attallah AS, Tribukait B, El-Bedeiwy A, et al. Prediction of lymph node metastases in bladder carcinoma with deoxyribonucleic acid flow cytometry. J Urol 1990;144:884.
18. Gustafson H, Tribukait B, Esposti PL. DNA profile and tumor progression in patients with superficial bladder tumours. Urol Res 1982;10: 13.
19. Tachibana M, Deguchi N, Baba S, et al. Multivariate analysis of flow cytometric deoxyribonucleic acid parameters and histologic features for prognosis of bladder cancer patients. J Urol 1991;146:1530.
20. Blomjous CFM, Schipper NW, Baak JPA, et al. Retrospective study of prognostic importance of DNA flow cytometry of urinary bladder carcinoma. J Clin Pathol 1988;41:21.
21. Fossa SD, Ous S, Berner A. Clinical significance of the "palpable mass" in patients with muscle-infiltrating bladder cancer undergoing cystectomy after preoperative radiotherapy. Br J Urol 1991;67:54.
22. Gospodarowicz MK, Reder WD, Keen CW, et al. Bladder cancer: long-term followup results of patients treated with radical radiation. Clin Oncol 1991;3:155.
23. Kakizoe T, Tobisu K, Takai K, et al. Relationship between papillary and nodular transitional cell carcinoma in the human urinary bladder. Cancer Res 1988;48:2299.
24. Vicente J, Lagura MP, Duarte D, et al. Carcinoma in situ as a prognostic factor for G_3pT_1 bladder tumors. Br J Urol 1991;68:380.
25. Herr HW, Scher HI. Surgery of invasive bladder cancer: is pathologic staging necessary? Semin Oncol 1990;17:590.
26. Herr HW, Whitmore WF Jr, Morse MJ, et al. Neoadjuvant chemotherapy in invasive bladder cancer: the evolving role of surgery. J Urol 1990;144:1083.
27. Klan R, Loy V, Huland H. Residual tumor discovered in routine second transurethral resection in patients with stage T_1 transitional cell carcinoma of the bladder. J Urol 1991;146:316.
28. Varkarakis MJ, Gaeta J, Moore RH, et al. Superficial bladder tumor: aspects of clinical progression. Urology 1974;4:414.
29. Hall RR, Beynon LL, Horwich A, et al. Urology and the TNM classification. Lancet 1988;1:1145.
30. Jordan AM, Weingarten J, Murphy WM. Transitional cell neoplasms of the urinary bladder: can biologic potential be predicted from histologic grading? Cancer 1987;60:2766.
31. Jewett HJ, Strong GH. Infiltrating carcinoma of the bladder: relation of depth of penetration of the bladder wall to incidence of local extension and metastases. J Urol 1946;55:366.
32. Brown PN. The relationship between non-invasive papillary lesions and invasive bladder carcinoma. Cancer 1984;54:620.
33. Frazier HA, Robertson JE, Dodge RK, et al. The value of pathologic factors in predicting cancer specific survival among patients treated with radical cystectomy for transitional cell carcinoma of the bladder and prostate. Cancer 1993;71:3993.
34. Herr HW. A proposed simplified staging system of invasive bladder tumors. Urol Int 1993;50:17.
35. American Joint Committee on Cancer. Manual for staging of cancer, 4th ed. Philadelphia: JB Lippincott, 1992.
36. Cummings KB. Clinical versus pathologic staging and the classification of bladder cancer. Urology 1984;23:55.
37. Jewett HJ. Carcinoma of the bladder: development and evaluation of current concepts of therapy. J Urol 1959;82:92.
38. Nichols JA, Marshall VF. The treatment of bladder carcinoma by local excision and fulguration. Cancer 1956;9:559.
39. Pomerance A. Pathology and prognosis following total cystectomy for carcinoma of the bladder. Br J Urol 1972;44:451.
40. Engel P, Anagnostaki L, Braenstrup O. The muscularis mucosae of the human urinary bladder: implications for tumor staging on biopsies. Scand J Urol Nephrol 1992;26:249.
41. Melicow MM. Histological study of vesical epithelium intervening between gross neoplasms in total cystectomy. J Urol 1952;68:261.
42. Lamm DL. Carcinoma in situ. Urol Clin North Am 1992;19:499.
43. Farrow GM, Utz DC. Observations on microinvasive transitional cell carcinoma of the urinary bladder. Clin Oncol 1982;1:1609.
44. Anderstrom C, Johansson S, Nilsson S. The significance of lamina propria invasion in the prognosis of patients with bladder tumors. J Urol 1980;124:23.
45. Heney NM, Ahmed S, Flanagan MJ, et al. Superficial bladder cancer: progression and recurrence. J Urol 1983;130:1083.
46. Fitzpatrick JM, West AB, Butler MR, et al. Superficial bladder tumors (stage pTa, grade I and II): the importance of recurrence pattern following initial resection. J Urol 1986;135:920.
47. Heney NM, Nocke BN, Daly JJ, et al. Ta and T1 bladder cancer: location, recurrence and progression. Br J Urol 1982;54:152.
48. Kakizoe T, Tobisu K, Takai K, et al. Relationship between papillary and nodular transitional cell carcinoma in the human urinary bladder. Cancer Res 1988;48:2299.
49. Hasni Y, Osada Y, Kitada S, et al. Significance of invasion to the muscularis mucosae on the progression of superficial bladder cancer. Urology 1994;43:782.
50. Prout GR Jr. The surgical management of bladder carcinoma. Urol Clin North Am 1976;3:149.
51. Droller MJ, Gospodarowicz M. Current concepts in staging of bladder cancer. In: Vogelzang N, et al, eds. Comprehensive textbook of genitourinary oncology. Baltimore: Williams and Wilkins, 1996:359.
52. Friedell GN, Parija GC, Nagy K, et al. The pathology of human bladder cancer. Cancer 1980;45:1823.
53. Soto EA, Friedell GH, Tiltman AJ. Bladder cancer as seen in giant histologic sections. Cancer 1977;39:447.
54. Solsona E, Iborra J, Ricos JV, et al. Feasibility of transurethral resection for muscle-infiltrating carcinoma of the bladder: prospective study. J Urol 1982;147:1513.
55. Skinner DG, Daniels JR, Russell DA, et al. The role of adjuvant chemotherapy following cystectomy for invasive bladder cancer: a prospective comparative trial. J Urol 1991;145:459.
56. Smith JA Jr, Whitmore WF Jr. Regional lymph node metastases from bladder cancer. J Urol 1981;126:591.
57. Matzkin H, Soloway MS, Hardeman S. Transitional cell carcinoma of the prostate. J Urol 1991;146:1207.
58. Sakamoto N, Tsuneyoshi M, Naito S, et al. An adequate sampling of the prostate to identify prostatic involvement by urothelial carcinoma in bladder cancer patients. J Urol 1993;149:318.
59. Kilbridge KL, Kantoff P. Intravesical therapy for superficial bladder cancer: is it a wash? J Clin Oncol 1994;12:1.
60. Brosman SA, Lamm DL. The preparation, handling and use of intravesical bacillus Calmette-Guerin for the management of stage T_a, T_1 carcinoma in situ and transitional cell cancer. J Urol 1990;144:313.
61. Schellhammer PF, Bean MA, Whitmore WF Jr. Prostatic involvement by transitional cell carcinoma: pathogenesis, patterns and prognosis. J Urol 1977;118:399.
62. Burger MM, Folkman J. UICC study group on basic and clinical cancer research: tumor angiogenesis. Int J Cancer 1994;56:311.
63. Walther PJ. Adjunctive adjuvant or neoadjuvant chemotherapy for locally advanced bladder cancer: a critical appraisal of the present status. Semin Urol 1993;11:227.
64. Slack NH, Prout GR Jr. Heterogeneity of invasive bladder carcinoma and different responses to treatment. AUA Monographs 1908;1:213.
65. Aprikan AG, Sarkis AS, Reuter VE, et al. Biological markers of prognosis in transitional cell carcinoma of the bladder: current concepts. Semin Urol 1993;11:137.
66. Jordan AM, Weingarten T, Murphy WM. Transitional cell neoplasms of the urinary bladder: can biological potential be predicted from histologic grading? Cancer 1987;60:2761.
67. Weinstein R, Miller AW, Pauli BV. Carcinoma in situ: comments on the pathology of a paradox. Urol Clin North Am 1980;18:523.
68. Kakizoe T, Matumoto K, Nishio Y, et al. Significance of carcinoma in situ in association with bladder cancer. J Urol 1985;133:395.
69. Droller MJ. Bladder cancer. Curr Prob Surg 1980;18:209.
70. Brawn PN. The origin of invasive carcinoma of the bladder. Cancer 1982;50:515.
71. Weldon TE, Soloway MS. Susceptibility of urothelium to neoplastic cellular implantation. Urology 1975;5:824.
72. Kaye KW, Lange PH. Mode of presentation of invasive bladder cancer: reassessment of the problem. J Urol 1982;128:31.
73. Jones PA, Droller MJ. Pathways of development and progression in bladder cancer: new correlations between clinical observations and molecular mechanism. Semin Urol 1993;11:177.
74. Tsai YC, Nichols PW, Hiti AL, et al. Allelic losses of chromosomes 9, 11 and 17 in human bladder cancer. Cancer Res 1990;50:44.
75. Fujimoto K, Yamada Y, Okajima E, et al. Frequent association of *p53* gene mutation in invasive bladder cancer. Cancer Res 1992;52:1393.
76. Cairns P, Margaret ES, Margaret AK. Preliminary mapping of the deleted region of chromosome 9 in bladder cancer. Cancer Res 1993;53: 1230.

Principles and Practice of Genitourinary Oncology, edited by Derek Raghavan, Howard I. Scher, Steven A. Leibel, and Paul H. Lange. Lippincott-Raven Publishers, Philadelphia, © 1997.

CHAPTER 24

Bladder Cancer

Radiologic Investigation

Janet E. Husband

Diagnostic imaging, a cornerstone in the assessment of bladder cancer, provides information on the depth of infiltration of the primary tumor through the bladder wall, an overall assessment of tumor volume, and a statement on the presence of metastases in lymph nodes and blood-borne sites. Recent years have seen exciting developments in all aspects of imaging, so today, the information derived is far superior to that obtained only a decade ago. In ultrasound, image quality has improved, and more experience has been gained with endoscopic techniques. Computed tomography (CT), first introduced for body imaging in the mid-1970s, has also undergone important advances that have been especially related to reduction in scanning times and improvement in spatial resolution. The most recent development in CT is the introduction of helical (spiral) scanning in which a continuous scanning motion permits examination of large volumes of tissue, such as the whole pelvis, in short scan times.[1] Magnetic resonance (MR) imaging has already made an enormous impact on clinical practice, but its full potential has not yet been reached. Vigorous research and development programs promise to yield a flexible and very fast scanning modality. MR imaging is regarded as the method of choice for evaluating the central nervous system and musculoskeletal disorders, and it now challenges the use of CT in the evaluation of pelvic cancer.

PRIMARY TUMOR

Ultrasound

Although transabdominal ultrasound may be used for staging bladder tumors,[2] the technique has now been largely superseded by CT and MR imaging. Transurethral ultrasound has gained a wider following than transrectal ultrasound, but the major disadvantage of this technique is the need for the patient to be under general anesthesia at the time of cystoscopic evaluation.

Bladder tumors appear on ultrasound as echogenic masses projecting into the bladder lumen. The bladder wall has a stronger and more intense echo pattern than tumor, thus permitting distinction of early superficial lesions from tumors invading the deep layers of the bladder wall. Accurate results using intraluminal ultrasound have been obtained in the assessment of early cancers. Once the tumor has broken through the bladder wall into the perivesical fat, however, intraluminal ultrasound is less satisfactory because tumor may extend beyond the penetration depth of the ultrasound beam.[3] Furthermore, evaluation of lymph node involvement is not possible. With intravesical sonography, Schuller and associates[3] reported a 92% accuracy for correct staging, but the technique is usually only used in those departments with a special research interest in ultrasound techniques.

Computed Tomography

Computed tomography provides a reliable and effective method of staging invasive bladder cancer, and for at least 10 years, between 1975 and 1985, it remained unchallenged as the most appropriate technique for staging these tumors.

On CT, bladder tumors appear as soft tissue density lesions. Tumor may be represented as a localized area of thickening of the bladder wall or as a definite soft tissue mass arising from the bladder wall with or without perivesical extension (Figs. 24-1 and 24-2). Occasionally, the surface of the tumor may be encrusted with calcium or with blood clot.

CT should be carried out after or during a rapid injection of intravenous contrast medium to enhance both the primary tumor and the adjacent organs, as well as to opacify the pelvic blood vessels. This technique has the advantage of increasing the contrast between tumor and perivesical fat and also facilitates the diagnosis of enlarged lymph nodes.[4] As in the evaluation of other pelvic cancers, all patients should be scanned after the administration of oral and rectal contrast medium, and, in female patients, a vaginal tampon to delineate the vaginal vault is also helpful. Patients with bladder cancer may have difficulty

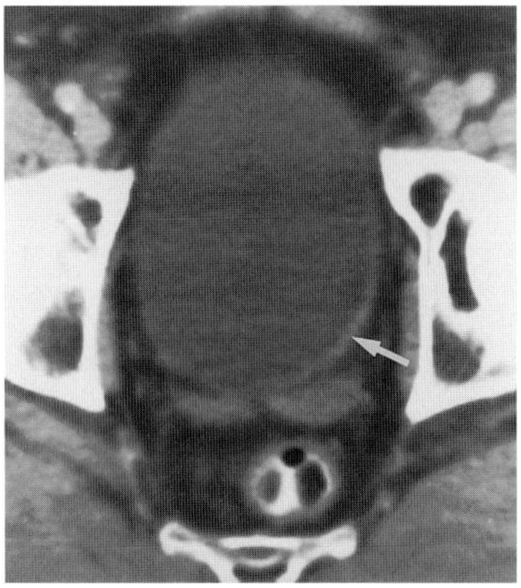

FIG. 24-1. CT scan showing localized thickening of the left bladder wall (*arrow*) in a patient with a superficial bladder tumor (stage T2).

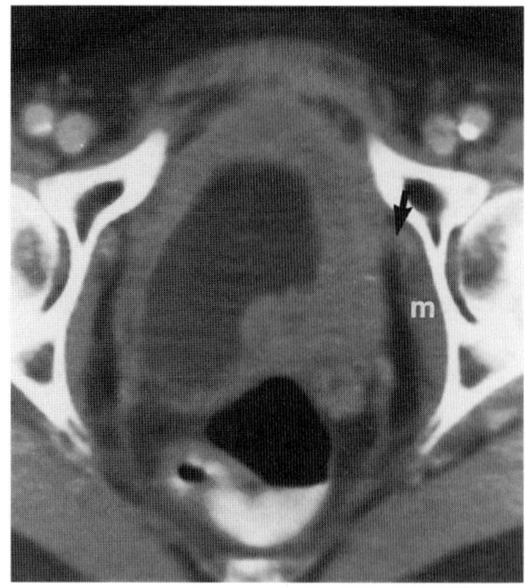

FIG. 24-3. CT scan showing advanced bladder cancer involving most of the bladder wall and extending as far as the pelvic side wall on the left (*arrow*). Note that the left internal obturator muscle (m) is enlarged.

in maintaining a full bladder, but interpretation of the scans is certainly easier if the bladder is distended as much as possible.

Using the classification of the International Union Against Cancer (UICC),[5] T1 lesions, that is, those involving the lamina propria, cannot be distinguished from those involving superficial muscle (T2) and T3A lesions on CT.[4,6–8] Thus, CT is impractical for staging early lesions, and its major advantage lies in the ability to distinguish extravesical spread from those tumors confined to the bladder wall.[6–8] Early extravesical spread is recognized as strands of soft tissue extending into the perivesical fat in direct contiguity with the primary tumor. Thin sections, 4 to 5 mm, are often helpful for evaluating doubtful cases,

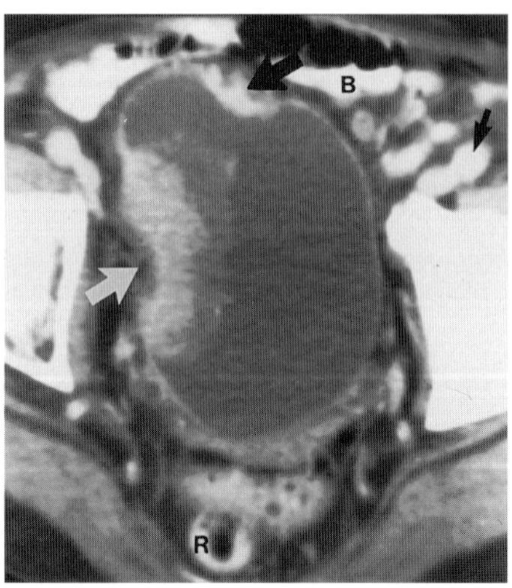

FIG. 24-2. CT scan following a bolus of intravenous contrast medium showing multifocal invasive bladder cancer (stage T3b). A large intraluminal component is visible, as well as extravesical spread (*large arrows*). Note good opacification of external iliac vessels (*small black arrow*). The rectum (R) and the small bowel (B) are also opacified with contrast medium.

but in more advanced disease, extravesical tumor extension is easily recognized (see Fig. 24-2). Spread to the pelvic side wall is diagnosed if tumor extends through the pelvic fat and is contiguous with the pelvic side wall muscles. These muscles may even be enlarged by tumor infiltration or edema (Fig. 24-3).

Early organ invasion can be difficult to detect if the only sign is loss of the fat plane between the bladder wall and an adjacent structure. Enlargement of the structure or organ and contrast enhancement of tissue within the organ in direct contiguity with the primary tumor are strong evidence of tumor invasion, however.[4] Invasion of the seminal vesicles is identified easily because the fat angle between the posterior bladder wall and the anterior surface of the seminal vesicles is lost (Fig. 24-4).[9]

CT scanning of the abdomen may reveal hydronephrosis and ureteric dilatation in patients with tumors in the region of the trigone. On occasion, the clinician may also be able to identify tumor spread from the bladder into the distal end of the ureter.

The major limitations of CT for staging bladder cancer relate to the inability to stage early tumors, to difficulties in identifying minimal extravesical tumor spread, and to difficulties encountered when attempting to identify adjacent organ invasion. Other problems occur in patients who have previously been investigated by cystoscopy or treated with radiotherapy. Thus, after endoscopy, edema and inflammation of the bladder wall may be misinterpreted as tumor, and for this reason, CT staging should be carried out either before cystoscopy or after an interval of at least 2 weeks. Patients who have previously been treated with radiotherapy present a particular problem, because irradiation fibrosis produces thickening and irregularity of the bladder wall.[10] In addition, edema and fibrosis within the perivesical fat lead to a generalized increase in perivesical density. These features frequently make the diagnosis of persistent or recurrent tumor within the bladder wall impossible, and even in patients with known tumor recurrence, to define the extent of spread accurately may be difficult.

CT is usually undertaken for staging bladder cancer in pa-

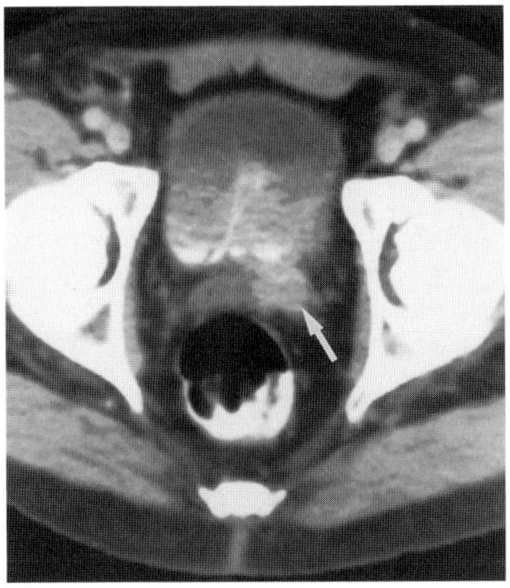

FIG. 24-4. CT scan showing invasion of the left seminal vesicle (*arrow*). Note the almost complete loss of the seminal vesicle fat angle and contrast enhancement of tumor within the seminal vesicle in direct contiguity with the bladder tumor involving the posterior bladder wall.

tients in whom the diagnosis has been proved histologically. Occasionally, however, a diagnostic problem exists in the distinction of a primary prostatic cancer from a primary bladder tumor. In this situation, CT is usually unhelpful in determining the origin of the tumor, because a large prostate cancer invading the bladder may have identical appearances to a bladder cancer invading the prostate. Other primary tumors that invade the bladder directly, such as carcinoma of the colon or cervix, can readily be distinguished from a primary bladder tumor because the major component of the mass lies outside the bladder wall. Metastases to the bladder, for example, from melanoma, or other rare tumors such as pheochromocytoma, leiomyosarcoma, or primary bladder lymphoma,[11] have similar appearances to primary bladder cancer (Fig. 24-5).

Most of the studies carried out to assess the value of CT for staging bladder cancer were undertaken in the early and mid-1980s. In these studies, the range of accuracy varied from 64% to 92%.[6–8,12] This wide diversity in results is partly due to differences in age of equipment used and partly due to differences of study design. For example, in some reports, patients with early lesions were included in the study, and their inclusion led to errors of understaging and overstaging; in some studies, patients who had undergone radiotherapy were also included, leading mainly to errors of overstaging. In the latter 1980s, CT studies were carried out to compare the results with those of MR imaging, but despite improvements in CT scanning techniques, the overall accuracy of CT has remained unchanged.[4,13]

The advent of helical-spiral CT is an exciting development, but its impact on staging bladder cancer has not yet been established. Apart from the obvious advantage of reduction in examination time, helical-spiral CT may be valuable in those patients with tumors of the bladder base or dome, because computer reconstructions in alternative imaging planes may provide useful additional information.

Magnetic Resonance Imaging

Magnetic resonance imaging is well suited to examination of the pelvic organs and has important advantages over CT. These include superior contrast resolution, the ability to obtain images in multiple planes, and images that reflect T1 or T2 relaxation times. Thus, compared with CT, MR imaging is a more flexible modality and therefore can be tailored more appropriately to a specific clinical question.

As with CT, patients should be examined when they have a full bladder. Axial images are obtained using T1- and T2-weighted sequences. The images obtained should cover the whole pelvis. Further sequences in alternative planes of imaging are then carried out, depending on the site of the primary tumor. Oral contrast agents for MR imaging are just beginning to be used routinely in clinical practice, and as with CT, they are helpful for differentiating tumor from bowel.[14,15]

On MR imaging, the normal bladder has a completely different appearance on T1-weighted images than on T2-weighted images. On T1-weighted images, the bladder wall has a low

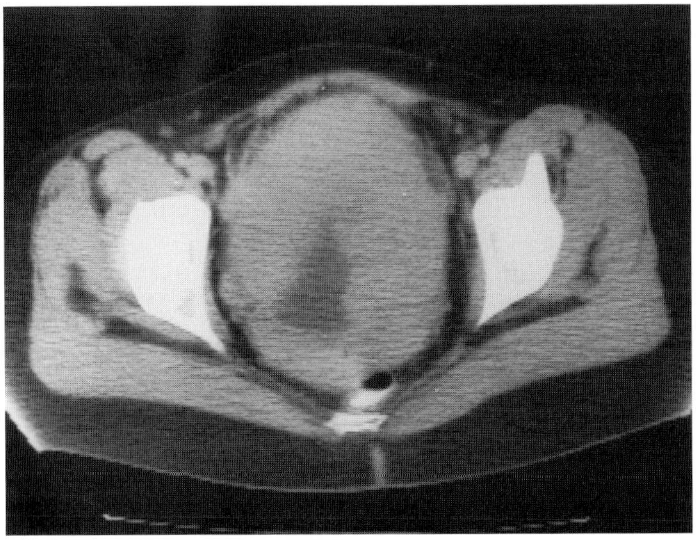

FIG. 24-5. Primary lymphoma of the bladder. CT scan demonstrating a large, homogenous soft tissue mass arising from the bladder wall.

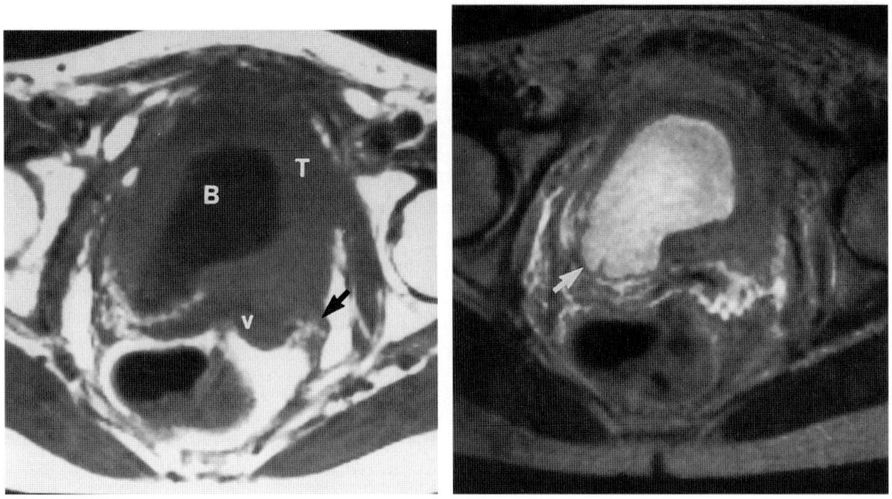

A B

FIG. 24-6. MR scans showing advanced bladder cancer in the same patient as in Figure 24-3. (**A**) T1-weighted image. Urine has a low signal intensity (SI) within the bladder (B). The tumor (T) has a relatively low SI and is well contrasted against the perivesical fat. Note extension of tumor into the perivesical fat (arrow). The vaginal vault (v) is inseparable from tumor. (**B**) T2-weighted image at the same level as (**A**). Urine has a high SI. The normal bladder wall has a low SI (*arrow*). Tumor has a relatively low SI. The vaginal vault is shown to be separate from tumor, with fat intervening between the posterior aspect of the tumor and the anterior wall of the vagina.

signal intensity, similar to that of urine within the bladder lumen. Perivesical fat has a high signal intensity (Fig. 24-6*A*). On T2-weighted sequences, the bladder lumen has a high signal intensity, whereas the bladder wall has a low signal intensity and appears as a thin line separating the bladder lumen from perivesical fat, which has an intermediate signal intensity (see Fig. 24-6*B*). Bladder tumors appear as lesions of low signal intensity on T1-weighted images and as lesions of intermediate signal intensity on T2-weighted images.[4,13] T1-weighted images are therefore the most appropriate images for detecting perivesical tumor spread, whereas T2-weighted sequences are best for evaluating the bladder wall and also for detecting tumor invasion of muscle and into adjacent organs such as the prostate, seminal vesicles, and cervix uteri.[4,13]

Studies suggest that intravenous contrast medium may be useful for staging early tumors because tumors enhance, whereas normal muscle of the bladder wall shows little enhancement. In addition, small tumors down to the size of 7 mm can be detected on contrast-enhanced scans.[16–19] In more advanced disease, however, the value of intravenous contrast medium is not substantiated because, unlike CT, contrast enhancement of extravesical tissue reduces the contrast between tumor and perivesical fat, which has a high signal intensity on T1-weighted images. Contrast enhancement may be useful for detecting organ invasion, but, at present, information is insufficient to determine whether the use of intravenous contrast medium upstages disease (Fig. 24-7).

Images in the sagittal or coronal plane may demonstrate tumor spread beyond the bladder wall that cannot readily be appreciated in the transaxial plane. This is particularly important for staging tumors of the bladder base and dome. In a study reported from the Royal Marsden Hospital in England in which CT and MR were compared in 30 patients, in several patients, sagittal or coronal MR images provided superior demonstration of tumor spread to that shown on CT[4] (Fig. 24-8). In my experience and that of my colleagues, the use of additional planes of imaging frequently increases confidence of diagnosing perivesical disease, as well as occasionally upstaging disease. MR imaging also provides superior information to CT in the demonstration of adjacent organ invasion because of the superior contrast resolution of the technique (Fig. 24-9).

As with all imaging techniques, MR imaging has important limitations with regard to the assessment of bladder cancer. It seems unlikely that edema and fibrosis can be distinguished from active tumor within the bladder wall reliably,[20] and understaging of minimal and microscopic spread beyond the bladder or into adjacent organs is likely to remain a problem with MR imaging, just as it is with CT.

Several studies have been undertaken comparing the accuracy of MR imaging with that of CT for staging bladder cancer. The results of these studies have shown that MR imaging has a similar accuracy to that of CT and ranges from 72% to 96%.[4,13] The important advantages of MR imaging are clearly seen in those studies in which both MR imaging and CT were undertaken in the same patients, however. Studies using intravenous contrast medium to assess early tumors have revealed an accuracy of 69% to 89%, and several authors have reported additional information on contrast-enhanced images in more

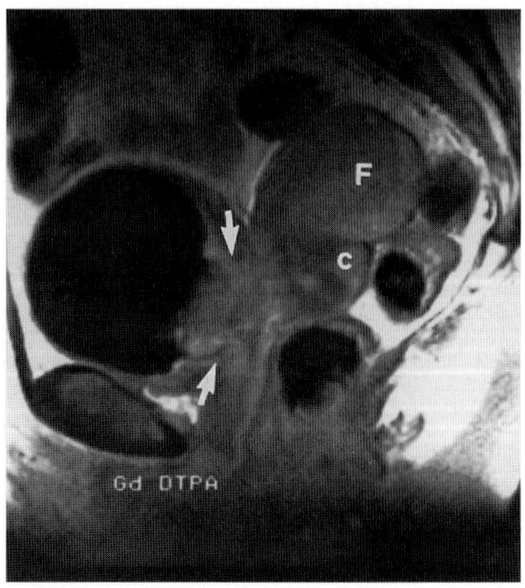

FIG. 24-7. MR scan of advanced bladder cancer, T1-weighted image following injection of intravenous contrast medium (Gd DTPA). Contrast-enhancing tumor is shown extending posteriorly into the anterior wall of the vagina (*arrows*). C, cervix; F, fundus.

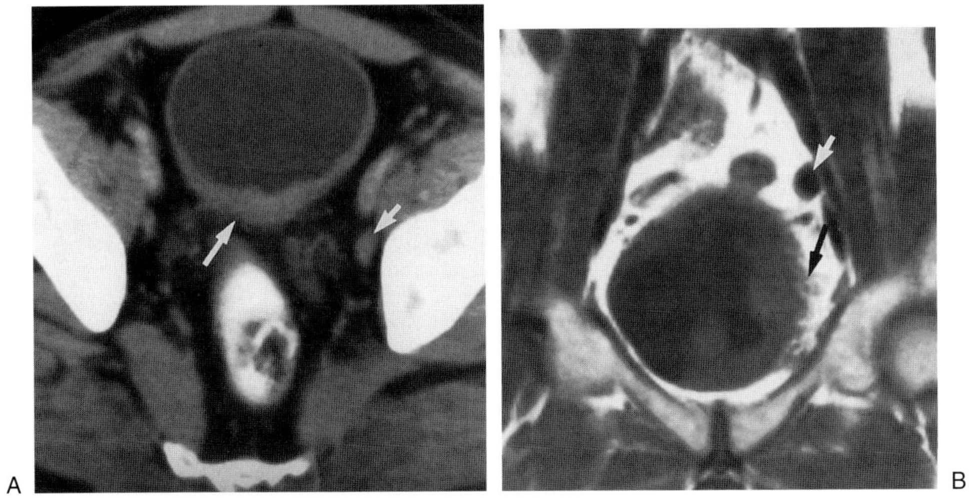

FIG. 24-8. CT and MR scans of a stage T3b bladder tumor. (**A**) CT scan. (**B**) MR scan. Although CT shows tumor arising from the posterior wall and extending into the perivesical fat (*arrows* in [**A**]), the tumor is better delineated on the coronal T1-weighted MR image. The perivesical extension is shown to best advantage on MR image (*arrows* in [**B**]) because of the superior contrast resolution of the technique.

than 10% of patients.[16,17,19,21–23] Thus, MR imaging appears to provide accurate staging of superficial bladder cancers and of invasive lesions.

MR imaging continues to evolve rapidly, and new sequences and new surface coils as well as endoscopic coils being introduced may be valuable to staging bladder cancer.[22,23] For example, selective suppression of fat and water may be helpful combined with intravenous contrast medium for evaluating early tumor spread beyond the bladder by eliminating the signal from fat. Dedicated surface coils and endorectal coils are now available, and these, together with the use of intravenous contrast medium, have led to the production of images showing exquisite anatomic detail of the bladder wall and of superficial tumors.[18]

LYMPH NODE METASTASES

Carcinoma of the bladder spreads initially to the regional pelvic lymph nodes; those first involved include the anterior and lateral perivesical nodes and the hypogastric, obturator, external iliac, and lateral sacral nodes. In more advanced disease, lymph nodes in the common iliac, paraaortic, and inguinal chains are involved. The incidence of lymph node metastases increases with advancing disease and rises to approximately 50% to 60% in patients with extravesical extension.[24]

Until the mid-1970s, bipedal lymphography was the only method of detecting metastases to the pelvic and paraaortic lymph nodes. The technique, although requiring considerable expertise, was successful, and reported series revealed a mean accuracy rate of approximately 75% for staging pelvic cancers (range 48% to 94%).[25–27] A significant disadvantage of lymphography was the inability to demonstrate internal iliac nodes and to demonstrate obturator nodes reliably. Because the obturator nodes are frequently the first nodal stations of involvement to be detected on imaging, they are particularly important. CT and MR imaging can identify enlarged lymph nodes in the external obturator and internal iliac groups within the pelvis (see Fig. 24-8), but unlike lymphography, they cannot provide any information on the internal architecture of the enlarged nodes. Thus, tumor cannot be distinguished from benign causes of nodal enlargement. Nevertheless, CT and MR imaging are considered equally effective as lymphography in the identification of nodal

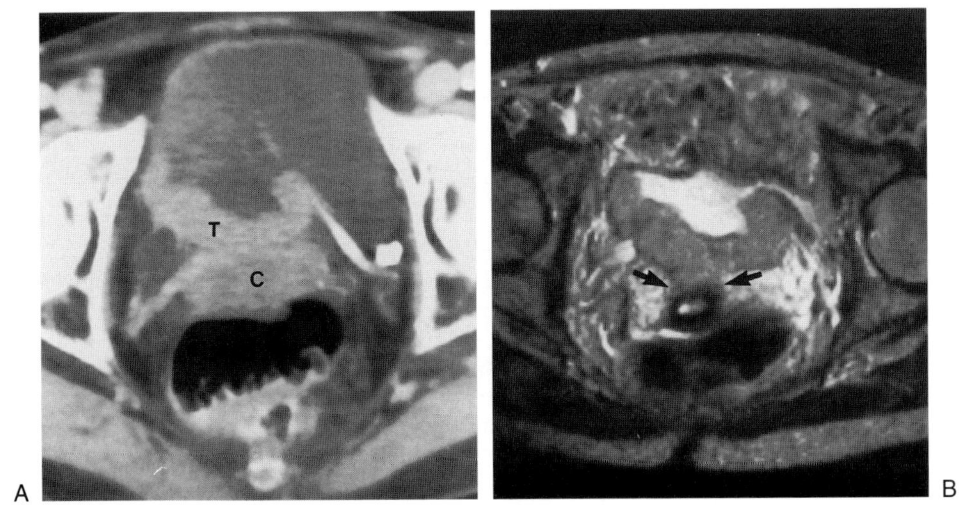

FIG. 24-9. CT scan (**A**) and MR scans (**B**) of advanced bladder cancer. (**A**) CT shows a posterior bladder tumor extending beyond the bladder wall. No fat plane exists between the bladder tumor (T) and the cervix (c). Organ invasion cannot be diagnosed with confidence. (**B**) T2-weighted MR image shows tumor extension posteriorly beyond the bladder wall. The fibrous ring of the cervix is ill-defined anteriorly, and tumor extends directly into this region (*arrows*). Information provided on these MR images is superior to that obtained with CT.

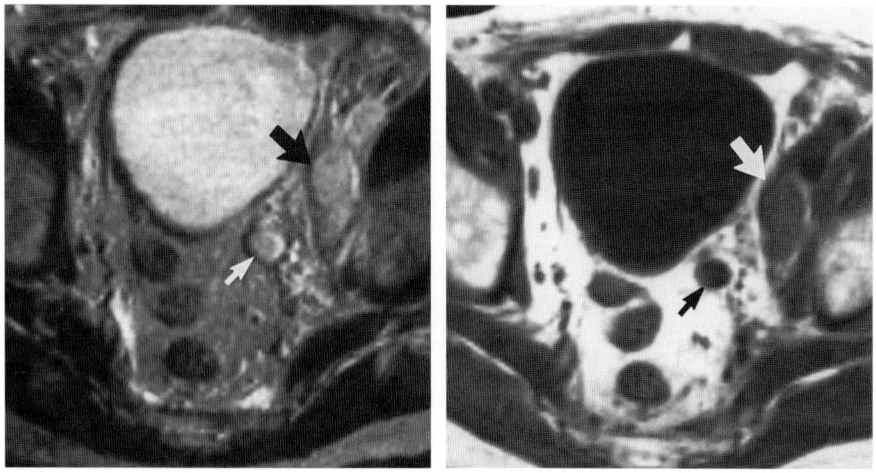

A B

FIG. 24-10. MR scan showing enlarged lymph nodes. (**A**) T1-weighted image showing a mass of involved lymph nodes of low signal intensity (SI, *white arrow*). Lymph node enlargement of the left ureter (*black arrow*) is dilated by tumor at the bladder trigone and has an identical SI to urine within the bladder. (**B**) T2-weighted image showing a mass of involved nodes (*arrows*) of intermediate SI. Note the high SI of the dilated left ureter (*white arrow*).

metastases.[4,13,18] For CT, the accuracy rates reported range from 70% to 96%, and in the few studies reported for MR imaging, similar results have also been achieved.

On CT, enlarged lymph nodes appear as soft tissue density structures. They may show uniform or heterogeneous enhancement after injection of intravenous contrast medium, and occasionally they may opacify to such an extent that they are difficult to distinguish from opacified blood vessels.[28,29] With MR, enlarged lymph nodes show a low signal on T1-weighted images and a high signal on T2-weighted sequences (Fig. 24-10). If any doubt exists regarding the presence of an enlarged lymph node on conventional sequences, then fat-suppression techniques can be particularly helpful.[18] Coronal images may also be helpful for confirming the presence of enlarged lymph nodes suspected on initial axial images.

Because enlargement is the only criterion for detecting metastases in lymph nodes with CT and MR imaging, the size taken as the upper limit of normal is of critical importance. My colleagues and I reviewed the size of normal lymph nodes in the pelvis as demonstrated by CT, both before and after lymphography. Guidelines for the upper limit of normal were then drawn, based on our findings. These guidelines are as follows: lymph nodes larger than 10 mm in the external iliac group should be considered as suspicious, and the upper limit of normal for the internal iliac group and obturator groups should be taken as 7 and 8 mm, respectively.[30] If more than one lymph node is enlarged, the likelihood that these nodes contain metastases increases, but if doubt exists, percutaneous fine-needle aspiration under CT control can readily be undertaken. Special MR scanners with easy patient access have now been developed, which now opens the way for interventional MR procedures, so lymph node sampling under MR imaging control is now a practical option.

An important question that is not completely resolved is whether a place still exists for lymphography in the management of bladder cancer. Certainly, lymph node metastases may be demonstrated using lymphography in lymph nodes of normal size, and such metastases are missed on CT and MR imaging. Furthermore, enlargement resulting from benign hyperplasia or inflammation may be misinterpreted as tumor on CT and MR imaging, leading to false-positive examinations. Thus, if CT and MR imaging are inconclusive, and if patient management relies heavily on the presence or absence of involvement of lymph nodes, then lymphography should be considered, but it should only be undertaken in those where expertise in performance of the examination and interpretation still exists.

DISTANT METASTASES

Because hematogenous spread usually occurs late in bladder cancer, investigation for metastatic disease is usually carried out when symptoms and signs develop in a particular site. Occasionally, however, bone metastases may be detected at the time of presentation. These metastases are frequently in the pelvic bones, and the CT or MR study must cover the whole of the pelvic bones including the pubic rami, so such metastases are not missed.

Lung metastases in bladder cancer are usually diagnosed on plain chest radiographs, and CT is not routinely indicated as part of the initial staging procedure unless cystectomy is being considered as a primary treatment option.

In patients with involved pelvic lymph nodes, the likelihood of paraaortic lymph node involvement and of liver metastases increases, and all patients should undergo pelvic and abdominal CT or MR examinations at the time of staging, not only to detect early hematogenous and lymphatic spread, but also to look for hydronephrosis and dilatation of the ureters. In addition, examination of the abdomen provides a baseline for future examinations, so incidental lesions such as hemangiomas of the liver or benign cysts can be documented and do not cause confusion in interpretation at a later date.

RADIOTHERAPY TREATMENT PLANNING

In those patients selected for external-beam irradiation, CT plays an important role in determining tumor extent by providing an accurate cross-sectional display of the tumor and related normal anatomy. CT-guided radiotherapy planning is only required if small-volume radical treatment is to be given. The target volume should include a 1.5- to 2-cm margin around the bladder and such tumor extension as detected by CT. The patient empties the bladder before the CT examination and also before treatment on each day, to ensure that the tumor remains within the planned treatment volume. A skin tattoo is placed over the symphysis pubis and is marked with barium paste, with two additional lateral tattoos placed over the iliac crests. The patient is scanned in the treatment position with the bladder full for diagnostic purposes. The bladder is then emptied, and the CT examination is repeated, to ensure that the whole-body contour is contained within the field of view. Using the CT-planning integrated system, the image through the center of the tumor and bladder is used to obtain the patient's body contour, treatment volume, and localization of the rectum and femoral heads. CT sections at different levels are used to check that the tumor is encompassed within the planned volume throughout its length.[31,32]

In the late 1970s and early 1980s, several studies compared conventional tumor localization with CT-integrated planning and demonstrated the superiority of CT-integrated planning over conventional techniques.[31,33] Rothwell and associates[32] demonstrated a significant improvement in survival in those patients in whom the tumor received 90% or more of the prescribed dose as delineated by CT, compared with those patients who had not undergone accurate tumor localization. The information derived from MR imaging is being investigated for radiotherapy planning purposes. Little doubt exists that the additional information derived from MR imaging in the coronal and sagittal planes, when integrated into radiotherapy planning, will increase the accuracy of radiotherapy planning still further.

MONITORING TREATMENT RESPONSE

CT and MR imaging can both be used to assess treatment response either to radiotherapy or to chemotherapy. The CT findings of radiotherapy changes within the pelvis are well established.[10] They include edema of the subcutaneous tissues and perivesical fat, thickening of the bladder wall, and reduction in bladder capacity, as well as thickening the pelvic ligaments and an increase in the amount of perirectal fat. Such findings may mask the extent of tumor response or the presence of recurrent disease. Indeed, the distinction of tumor from fibrosis is one of the most challenging issues in the radiology of treated cancer today. Some evidence indicates that MR imaging may be better than CT in the distinction of fibrosis from tumor, because fibrosis has a low signal intensity on T2-weighted sequences,[10,20] and it appears to enhance to a lesser degree after injection of intravenous contrast medium.[18] In most patients, however, detection of recurrent disease with confidence is not possible unless the patient has a soft tissue mass arising within the bladder wall or adjacent structures.

After chemotherapy, reduction in tumor volume is more readily assessed. This is partly because the majority of patients receiving chemotherapy have large-volume disease at presentation and partly because irradiation fibrosis is not an issue.

CONCLUSIONS

As imaging techniques continue to develop and become more sophisticated, their relative roles change. CT is the most widely used technique for evaluating bladder cancer, but MR imaging provides important information, and in centers where MR imaging is readily available for tumor staging, it is rapidly becoming the technique of choice. During the next few years, however, it will be interesting to monitor the impact of spiral CT on radiologic practice. In relation to pelvic cancers, its major advantage will be the ability to carry three-dimensional volume scanning and to obtain multiplanar reformatted images after rapid image acquisition. These features are likely to have important implications not only for diagnosis, but also for radiotherapy planning.

ACKNOWLEDGMENTS

The Clinical Magnetic Research Group at the Royal Marsden Hospital is funded by the Cancer Research Campaign; this support is gratefully acknowledged.

REFERENCES

1. Brink JA, Heiken JP, Wang G, et al. Helical CT: principles and technical considerations. Radiographics 1994;14:887.
2. Singer D, Itzchak Y, Fischelovitch Y. Ultrasonographic assessment of bladder tumours. II. Clinical staging. J Urol 1981;126:34.
3. Schuller J, Walther V, Schmiedt E, et al. Intravesical ultrasound tomography in staging bladder carcinoma. J Urol 1982;128:264.
4. Husband JES, Olliff JFC, Williams MP, et al. Bladder cancer: staging with CT and MR. Radiology 1989;173:435.
5. UICC (International Union Against Cancer), Spiessl B, Hermanek P, Scheibe O, Wagner G, eds. TNM-atlas: illustrated guide to the TNM/pTNM-classification of malignant tumours. Berlin: Springer, 1982;172.
6. Hodson NJ, Husband JE, Macdonald JS. The role of computed tomography in the staging of bladder cancer. Clin Radiol 1979;30:389.
7. Morgan CL, Calkins RF, Cavalcanti EJ. Computed tomography in the evaluation, staging and therapy of carcinoma of the bladder and prostate. Radiology 1981;140:751.
8. Sager EM, Talle K, Fossa S, et al. The role of CT in demonstrating perivesical tumour growth in the preoperative staging of carcinoma of the urinary bladder. Radiology 1983;146:443.
9. Seidelmann FE, Cohen WN, Bryan, et al. Accuracy of CT staging of bladder neoplasms using the gas-filled method: report of 21 patients with surgical confirmation. AJR Am J Roentgenol 1978;130:735.
10. Johnson RJ, Cartington BM. Review: Pelvic radiation disease. Clin Radiol 1992;45:4.
11. Yeoman LJ, Mason MD, Olliff JFC. Non Hodgkin's lymphoma of the bladder: CT and MRI appearances. Clin Radiol 1991;44:389.
12. Koss JC, Arger PH, Coleman BG, et al. CT staging of bladder carcinoma. AJR Am J Roentgenol 1981;137:359.
13. Buy JN, Moss AA, Guinet C, et al. MR staging of bladder carcinoma: correlation with pathologic findings. Radiology 1988;169:695.
14. MacVicar D, Jacobsen TF, Guy R, et al. Phase III trial of oral magnetic particles in MRI of abdomen and pelvis. Clin Radiol 1993;47:183.
15. Rinck PA, Smevik O, Nilsen G, et al. Oral magnetic particles in MR imaging of the abdomen and pelvis. Radiology 1991;178:775.
16. Tachibana M, Baba S, Deguchi N, et al. Efficacy of gadolinium-diethylenetriaminepentaacetic acid enhanced magnetic resonance imaging for differentiation between superficial and muscle-invasive tumour of the bladder: a comparative study with computed tomography and transurethral ultrasonography. Radiology 1991;181:910.
17. Tanimoto A, Yuasa Y, Imai Y, et al. Bladder tumour staging: comparison of conventional and gadolinium-enhanced dynamic MR imaging and CT. Radiology 1992;185:741.
18. Barentsz JO, Ruijs SHJ, Strijk SP. The role of MR imaging in carcinoma of the urinary bladder. AJR Am J Roentgenol 1993;160:937.
19. Nicolas V, Spielmann R, Maas R, et al. The diagnostic value of MR tomography following gadolinium-DTPA compared to computed tomography in bladder tumours. Fortschr Roentgenstr 1991;154:357.
20. Hawnaur JM, Johnson RJ, Read G, et al. Magnetic resonance imaging with gadolinium-DTPA for assessment of bladder carcinoma and its response to treatment. Clin Radiol 1993;47:302.
21. Neuerburg JM, Bohndorf K, Sohn M, et al. Staging of urinary bladder

neoplasms with MR imaging: is Gd-DTPA helpful? J Comput Assist Tomogr 1991;15:780.
22. Reiman TH, Heiken JP, Totty WG, et al. Clinical MR imaging with a Helmoltz-type surface coil. Radiology 1988;169:564.
23. Schnall MD, Lenkinski RE, Pollack IM, et al. MR imaging with an endorectal surface coil. Radiology 1989;172:739.
24. van der Werf-Messing B, Schroeder RH, Bush H. Bladder. In: Halnan KE ed. Textbook of cancer. London: Chapman & Hall. 1982:457.
25. Wajsman Z, Baumgertner G, Murphy GP, et al. Evaluation of lymphangiography for clinical staging of bladder tumours. J Urol 1975;114:712.
26. Loening SA, Schmidt JD, Brown RC, et al. A comparison between lymphangiography and pelvic lymph node dissection in the staging of prostatic cancer. J Urol 1977;117:752.
27. Chagnon S, Cochand-Priollet B, Gzaeil M, et al. Pelvic cancers: staging of 139 cases with lymphography and fine needle aspiration biopsy. Radiology 1989;173:103.
28. Vock P, Haertel M, Fuchs WA, et al. Computed tomography in staging of carcinoma of the urinary bladder. Br J Urol 1982;54:158.
29. Husband JE, Robinsin L, Thomas G. Contrast enhancing lymph nodes in bladder cancer: a potential pitfall on CT. Clin Radiol 1992;45:395.
30. Vinnicombe SJ, Norman AR, Nicolson V, Husband JE. Normal pelvic lymph nodes: evaluation by CT scanning after bipedal lymphangiography. Radiology 1995;194:349.
31. Dobbs HJ, Parker RP, Hodson NJ, et al. The use of CT in radiotherapy treatment planning. Radiother Oncol 1983;1:133.
32. Rothwell RI, Ash DV, Thorogood J. Analysis of the contribution of computed tomography to the treatment outcome in bladder cancer. Clin Radiol 1985;36:369.
33. Goitein M, Wittenberg J, Mendiondo M, et al. The value of CT scanning in radiation therapy treatment planning: a prospective study. Int J Radiat Oncol Biol Phys 1979;5:1787.

Principles and Practice of Genitourinary Oncology, edited by Derek Raghavan, Howard I. Scher, Steven A. Leibel, and Paul H. Lange. Lippincott-Raven Publishers, Philadelphia, © 1997.

CHAPTER 25

Surgical Staging and Surgery for Superficial Bladder Cancer

H. Barton Grossman

Bladder cancer presents predominantly as transitional cell carcinoma. Despite this common histology, the clinical presentation has long suggested that bladder cancer develops along two different pathways. Superficial bladder cancer is usually defined as encompassing all neoplasms that have not invaded the muscularis propria. This includes carcinoma in situ (Tis), noninvasive papillary cancer (Ta), and tumors that invade the lamina propria (T1). Individuals who present with superficial papillary disease, although at high risk for recurrence, are at low risk for progression to invasion of the detrusor muscle.[1] In contrast, approximately 85% of people who require cystectomy initially present with muscle-invasive disease.[2] A specific form of superficial disease, carcinoma in situ, is associated with a different pattern of presentation (urinary frequency and dysuria, in contrast to the classic sign of gross hematuria) and carries a higher risk of tumor progression.[3] Recently, molecular biologic techniques have confirmed that papillary bladder cancer and carcinoma in situ are fundamentally different. Superficial papillary bladder carcinoma is associated with a high frequency of loss of heterozygosity of chromosome 9q.[4] On the other hand, *P53* mutations are common in carcinoma in situ and muscle-invasive tumors. These data suggest that superficial papillary tumors and carcinoma in situ arise through different mechanisms and that patients presenting with invasive bladder cancer are likely to have reached this stage through the development of carcinoma in situ.

SURGICAL STAGING

The goal of surgical staging is to determine accurately the local extent of disease so that appropriate therapy can be selected. Three areas of input can be used effectively to ascertain a surgical stage: the visual appearance of the bladder obtained at the time of endoscopy, results from biopsies, and results from bimanual examination of the bladder. The algorithms for staging of superficial papillary disease and muscle-invasive disease are different. In selected patients (i.e., those at high risk for metastasis by virtue of having muscle-invasive bladder cancer), additional imaging modalities such as chest radiography and abdominal computed tomography may be helpful. The role of an experienced pathologist cannot be overestimated. Accurate pathologic categorization of minimally invasive tumors (T1) can provide prognostic information.[5] T1 tumors that invade the muscularis mucosae have a higher rate of recurrence and progression than more superficial T1 neoplasms.

Urologic surgeons are usually accurate in characterizing papillary low-grade noninvasive bladder cancer by appearance alone. Particularly if these lesions are small and unifocal, have the typical appearance of a low-grade tumor, and are accompanied by negative urine cytology results, adequate diagnosis and therapy may consist of only endoscopic visualization of the bladder, eradication of the neoplasm (by fulguration, excisional biopsy, or transurethral resection), and bimanual examination. In patients with low-grade superficial tumors, bimanual examination should not demonstrate any bladder thickening or masses.

A bladder map should be recorded to document the site or sites of gross disease and the locations at which site-directed "random" biopsies were obtained. This information may be helpful in patient follow-up. Random biopsies are not necessary in all patients with superficial bladder cancer. However, additional staging information can be obtained by site-directed random biopsy of both bladder and prostatic urethra in patients with positive cytology, multifocal disease, large solitary or sessile tumors, or an endoscopic appearance suspicious for carcinoma in situ (e.g., bladder erythema). Random biopsies should be identified by site and can be obtained adequately with a biopsy forceps. Although cystoscopy and biopsy can be performed under local anesthesia,[6] multiple biopsies and transurethral resection are usually performed under general or spinal anesthesia. A biopsy forceps adequately samples the urothelial lining of the prostatic urethra, but prostatic parenchymal biopsies are more effectively obtained by transurethral resection. In specific instances, needle biopsy of the prostate can also be helpful. Larger bladder tumors are best treated endoscopically by transurethral resection. The goal in all cases is complete excision of the neoplasm. Use of a continuous-flow resectoscope, with adjustment of the flow so that input equals output, facilitates resection by maintaining the bladder in a constant shape. This can be particularly helpful in resection of tumors that are hard to reach with a conventional resectoscope. If complete resection is not possible, accurate staging is facilitated by obtaining deep biopsies to document invasion of the detrusor muscle. With extensive disease, this can be accomplished by visually ascertaining that the level of resection is below the normal surrounding mucosa and lamina propria.

The appearance of the bladder tissue during and after resection should be carefully assessed. The observation of normal-appearing muscle suggests that the tumor is grossly, if not microscopically, resected. However, the converse is not always true. The bladder wall may be grossly abnormal in the absence of cancer if a prior resection and fulguration have been performed at that site. In cases in which the level of invasion remains in doubt, additional transurethral resection may be diagnostic and may confirm that all the T2 neoplasm has been resected.[7] Transurethral resection is usually limited to superficial disease (i.e., tumors that can be completely resected endoscopically), and some T2 tumors can be perceived to fall within this functional definition.

Bimanual examination after completion of resection is particularly important in patients with invasive neoplasms. A residual mass in the bladder suggests the presence of a T3 neoplasm. A fixed bladder mass in the absence of other confounding causes (e.g., prior radiotherapy) indicates the presence of a T4 neoplasm. If local treatment is being considered for a solitary invasive tumor (e.g., segmental resection, brachytherapy), site-directed biopsies of the bladder are indicated to rule out the presence of multifocal disease. Tumors adjacent to the vesical neck and prostate may require resection biopsy to evaluate the extent of disease in the prostate.

Although transurethral resection and extensive site-directed biopsies provide the most information regarding surgical staging, they are not necessary in many patients. Particularly with follow-up cystoscopic examination, urine or bladder washing cytology (or both) can effectively be used to confirm that high-grade lesions, including carcinoma in situ, are not present and to decrease the need for random biopsy. Although usually uneventful, bladder biopsy does carry a small risk of hemorrhage and bladder perforation.

PROBLEMS AND INACCURACIES WITH STAGING

The typical low-grade, noninvasive papillary tumor is usually correctly staged as Ta after the initial visual inspection of the bladder and subsequently confirmed to be Ta by resection and histologic evaluation. Similarly, large sessile tumors that present as a residual bladder mass on bimanual examination after the completion of an obvious incomplete resection are easily characterized as T3 tumors. The classification of intermediate stages, including carcinoma in situ, is frequently less precise. A high index of suspicion is required to detect carcinoma in situ, which can exist even in the absence of visual changes in the bladder. Extensive bladder mapping of patients with carcinoma in situ has demonstrated that occult invasion of the bladder can occur.[6] Furthermore, understaging of patients with carcinoma in situ who undergo cystectomy is common.[8]

If invasion occurs and local treatment is considered, it is important to be reasonably sure that the gross tumor has been completely excised. This is somewhat easier for T1 than for T2 tumors. Although I usually do not perform second resections for T1 tumors, if there is doubt about the adequacy of the initial resection, a repeat resection can help characterize these tumors.[9] People with T1 tumors should have additional treatment with bacille Calmette-Guérin or another agent (see Chap. 27). If another resection is not performed immediately, it can still be helpful at the next follow-up cystoscopy (after 3 months), because normal urothelium can grow over the resection site and mask residual invasive cancer. A second resection of T2 tumors can be helpful in deciding which patients are suited for local therapy.[7] The occurrence of no residual tumor in some cystectomy specimens is testimony to the fact that occasionally all disease is been resected.

Lasers, primarily the neodymium:yttrium-aluminum-garnet (Nd:YAG) laser, have also been used for the treatment of superficial bladder cancer.[10] Staging is less precise with this technique because of the lack of histologic review.

Pathologic verification of stage in patients with superficial bladder cancer by cystectomy or partial cystectomy is uncommon. If cystectomy is performed, understaging and clinically occult metastases may be found, as shown in Table 25-1. However, the results presented in Table 25-1 involve highly selected groups of patients, who usually had superficial bladder cancer refractory to endoscopic therapy or possessed clinical features associated with a poor prognosis (e.g., high-grade lesion).

SURGICAL THERAPY FOR SUPERFICIAL BLADDER CANCER

The primary goal of surgery in the treatment of superficial bladder cancer is complete excision of the tumor or tumors.

Table 25-1. *Superficial bladder cancer: staging error*

Investigators	Stage*	No. of patients	% Understaged	% Metastatic
Kenny et al, 1970[18]	O–A	25	44	0
Richie et al, 1975[19]	0	4	0	0
	A	51	14	8
Wajsman et al, 1975[20]	0	9	33	0
	A	7	57	0
Amling et al, 1994[21]	Ta	31	39	
	Tis	23	30	
	T1	166	30	7
Freeman et al, 1994[22]	Ta	16	56	12
	Tis	19	26	0
	T1	106	51	8

* Stage 0, Tis or Ta; stage A, T1.

Because clinical staging is inherently imprecise, as accurate an assessment as possible is required to achieve this goal and ensure that adequate treatment has been administered. Another goal, which is achieving greater recognition, is the preservation of quality of life, a frequently used but poorly defined term which in this context can be construed to imply maintenance of a normally functioning bladder. With the advent of newer forms of urinary reconstruction, including continent urinary diversions and neobladders fabricated out of bowel segments, some have argued that the importance of avoiding cystectomy as primary therapy for superficial bladder cancer has been overstated. Nevertheless, even the best of these diversions approximates but does not equal normal bladder function.

Transurethral Resection

Endoscopic resection has retained its pivotal role in diagnosis and treatment of superficial bladder cancer despite an increasing variety of diagnostic and therapeutic alternatives. Transurethral resection provides the visual and histologic data required for staging, excises tumors, and ensures maintenance of good bladder function. Transurethral resection is of limited efficacy for extensive multifocal disease (e.g., carcinoma in situ) or locally extensive tumor, which may not be excised adequately by this technique. In selected cases, T2 (superficial muscle-invasive) tumors can adequately be treated by endoscopic resection and may be included in the broad category of superficial disease.[7]

A significant limitation to the long-term effectiveness of transurethral resection as definitive treatment for superficial bladder cancer is the well-documented, high incidence of recurrence. Even solitary, noninvasive tumors have a recurrence rate that approaches 50% at 5 years, and the rate of recurrence of multifocal bladder cancer is 71% at 1 year.[11] If transurethral resection is used as the primary form of therapy for T1 bladder cancer, the rate of recurrence with progression in stage is 20% to 30%.[1,12,13] Because of these significant recurrence and progression rates with surgery alone, a variety of intravesical chemotherapeutic and immunotherapeutic strategies have been devised (see Chap. 27).

Lasers

An alternative method for ablation of superficial bladder tumors is the delivery of energy by laser. Two strategies have been employed: imparting of laser energy directly to the tumor and employment of laser light for photodynamic therapy. Noncontact delivery of effective therapy through the use of lasers offers the potential advantage of decreased spread of bladder cancer, which has been hypothesized to occur in some cases by physical disruption of the tumor at the time of resection and subsequent implantation of viable tumor cells. Circumstantial evidence exists to implicate bladder tumor seeding at the time of resection as a contributing factor to a poorly defined proportion of recurrent disease.[14] However, the importance of this phenomenon is uncertain. For example, patients who undergo simultaneous resection of bladder tumors and transurethral resection of the prostate are not at increased risk for recurrence in the prostatic urethra.[15] The potential advantage of decreased tumor seeding and a lower recurrence rate with laser treatment in comparison to traditional resection remains controversial.[10]

Because carcinoma in situ is often multifocal and may be difficult to detect, complete resection of this form of bladder cancer is usually not possible. Photodynamic therapy has been successfully employed for the treatment of some cases of carcinoma in situ.[16] However, a significant complication that has been noted is the occasional occurrence of bladder contracture. Newer agents and better adjustment of light intensity may enhance the effectiveness of this technique while simultaneously decreasing the morbidity.

Segmental Resection

Segmental resection (partial cystectomy) provides adequate therapy for large, solitary tumors that cannot adequately be resected endoscopically. As can be seen from Table 25-2, the results with this technique compare favorably with those of other methods of treatment. However, relatively few patients with superficial bladder cancer are candidates for this form of treatment. Local tumor recurrence is common after high-grade tumors are treated by this technique.[17]

Cystectomy

Radical cystectomy continues to be employed in the treatment of selected patients with superficial bladder cancer. Patients whose tumors are no longer adequately controlled by endoscopic and intravesical therapeutic strategies can achieve excellent disease control with cystectomy (see Table 25-2). Furthermore, the ability to create continent urinary reservoirs from bowel, although they are less than perfect substitutes for a normal bladder, decreases the major functional sacrifice historically associated with this form of treatment.

RESULTS AND CONCLUSIONS

Table 25-2 summarizes results reported in the surgical treatment of superficial bladder cancer. However, significant limitations restrain the generalization of this information to all patients with bladder cancer. First, much of this material is old. Many of these patients would currently receive intravesical therapy in addition to transurethral resection. Second, the data on cystectomy concern a highly selected patient group. These individuals were refractory to conventional therapy or had features suggesting that they were at high risk for progression. Third, patients with Ta and low-grade tumors have a better survival rate than would be expected from a cursory review of this table. The rate of progression to muscle invasion or metastasis at 3 years is 4% for Ta tumors and 30% for T1 tumors.[1]

Endoscopic treatment (i.e., cystoscopy, biopsy, and transurethral resection) continues to be the foundation of treatment of superficial bladder cancer. These procedures often are not only diagnostic but therapeutic as well. However, pure surgical therapy is associated with a high risk of recurrence and a smaller but clinically important risk of progression in stage. For this reason, patients with carcinoma in situ, multifocal tumors, recurrent tumors, and invasive tumors should receive additional treatment, usually intravesical chemotherapy or immunotherapy.

Table 25-2. *Surgical therapy for superficial bladder cancer*

Investigators	Treatment	Stage*	No. of Patients	5-year survival rate
Barnes et al, 1977[23]	Transurethral resection	A	64	73%
Resnick et al, 1973[24]	Partial cystectomy	p0	4	75%
		pA	24	71%
Novick et al, 1976[25]	Partial cystectomy	p0–A	15	67%
Cummings et al, 1978[26]	Partial cystectomy	p0	9	100%
		pA	29	79%
Richie et al, 1975[19]	Cystectomy	p0–A	49	79%
Mathur et al, 1981[27]	Cystectomy	A	11	73%
Amling et al, 1994[21]	Cystectomy	pTa	11	88%†
		pTis	19	100%†
		pT1	91	76%†
Freeman et al, 1994[22]	Cystectomy	Ta	16	71%
		Tis	19	100%
		T1	106	63%

* Stage 0, Tis or Ta; stage A, T1; *p* signifies pathologic staging (partial cystectomy or cystectomy).
† Cancer-specific survival.

REFERENCES

1. Heney NM, Ahmed S, Flanagan MJ, et al. Superficial bladder cancer: progression and recurrence. J Urol 1983;130:1083.
2. Kaye KW, Lange PH. Mode of presentation of invasive bladder cancer: reassessment of the problem. J Urol 1982;128:31.
3. Lamm DL. Carcinoma in situ. Urol Clin North Am 1992;19:499.
4. Spruck CH 3rd, Ohneseit PF, Gonzalez-Zulueta M, et al. Two molecular pathways to transitional cell carcinoma of the bladder. Cancer Res 1994;54:784.
5. Hasui Y, Osada Y, Kitada S, Nishi S. Significance of invasion to the muscularis mucosae on the progression of superficial bladder cancer. Urology 1994;43:782.
6. Utz DC, Farrow GM. Management of carcinoma in situ of the bladder: the case for surgical management. Urol Clin North Am 1980;7:533.
7. Herr HW. Conservative management of muscle-infiltrating bladder cancer: prospective experience. J Urol 1987;138:1162.
8. Soloway MS, Lopez AE, Patel J, Lu Y. Results of radical cystectomy for transitional cell carcinoma of the bladder and the effect of chemotherapy. Cancer 1994;73:1926.
9. Klan R, Loy V, Huland H. Residual tumor discovered in routine second transurethral resection in patients with stage T1 transitional cell carcinoma of the bladder. J Urol 1991;146:316.
10. Smith JA Jr. Laser surgery for transitional-cell carcinoma: technique, advantages, and limitations. Urol Clin North Am 1992;19:473.
11. Morgan JDT, Bowsher W, Griffiths DFR, Matthews PN. Rationalisation of follow-up in patients with non-invasive bladder tumours: a preliminary report. Br J Urol 1991;67:158.
12. Jacobsen F, Lundbeck F, Vaeth M, Kjaer TB. Transurethral treatment of invasive tumours of the urinary bladder (T1, T2): recurrence and progression. Scand J Urol Nephrol Suppl 1987;104:123.
13. Wolf H, Iversen H-G, Rosenkilde P, Schroder T. Transurethral surgery in the treatment of invasive bladder cancer (T1 and T2). Scand J Urol Nephrol Suppl 1987;104:127.
14. Sidransky D, Frost P, Von Eschenbach A, Oyasu R, Preisinger AC, Vogelstein B. Clonal origin bladder cancer. N Engl J Med 1992;326:737.
15. Laor E, Grabstald H, Whitmore WF. The influence of simultaneous resection of bladder tumors and prostate on the occurrence of prostatic urethral tumors. J Urol 1981;126:171.
16. D'Hallewin MA, Baert L, Marijnissen JP, Star WM. Whole bladder wall photodynamic therapy with in situ light dosimetry for carcinoma in situ of the bladder. J Urol 1992;148:1152.
17. Peress JA, Waterhouse K, Cole AT. Complications of partial cystectomy in patients with high grade bladder cancer. J Urol 1977;118:761.
18. Kenny GM, Hardner GJ, Murphy GP. Clinical staging of bladder cancer. J Urol 1970;104:720.
19. Richie JP, Skinner DG, Kaufman JJ. Carcinoma of the bladder: treatment by radical cystectomy. J Surg Res 1975;18:271.
20. Wajsman Z, Merrin C, Moore R, Murphy GP. Current results from treatment of bladder tumors with total cystectomy at Roswell Park Memorial Institute. J Urol 1975;113:806.
21. Amling CL, Thrasher JB, Frazier HA, Dodge RK, Robertson JE, Paulson DF. Radical cystectomy for stages Ta, Tis and T1 transitional cell carcinoma of the bladder. J Urol 1994;151:31.
22. Freeman JA, Esrig D, Simoneau A, et al. Radical cystectomy for patients with superficial bladder cancer. J Urol 1994;151:234A.
23. Barnes RW, Dick AL, Hadley HL, Johnston OL. Survival following transurethral resection of bladder carcinoma. Cancer Res 1977;37:2895.
24. Resnick MI, O'Çonor VJ Jr. Segmental resection for carcinoma of the bladder: review of 102 patients. J Urol 1973;109:1007.
25. Novick AC, Stewart BH. Partial cystectomy in the treatment of primary and secondary carcinoma of the bladder. J Urol 1976;116:570.
26. Cummings KB, Mason JT, Correa RJ Jr, Gibbons RP. Segmental resection in the management of bladder carcinoma. J Urol 1978;119:56.
27. Mathur VK, Krahn HP, Ramsey EW. Total cystectomy for bladder cancer. J Urol 1981;125:784.

Principles and Practice of Genitourinary Oncology, edited by Derek Raghavan, Howard I. Scher, Steven A. Leibel, and Paul H. Lange. Lippincott-Raven Publishers, Philadelphia, © 1997.

CHAPTER 26

Management of Superficial Bladder Cancer

Harry W. Herr, Donald L. Lamm, and Louis Denis

Approximately 80% of all bladder cancers occur as tumors confined to the epithelium or submucosa—the so-called superficial tumors. Morphologically, such tumors appear as either frond-like papillary tumors composed of malignant transitional cells limited to the mucosa (stage Ta) or invading the lamina propria (stage T1) or as flat carcinoma in situ (Tis) with diffuse malignant cells confined to the epithelium. These tumors represent a heterogeneous group of malignancies with differing natural histories.[1]

Transurethral endoscopic resection (TURB) is the standard initial treatment for superficial bladder tumors. Despite complete resection, most patients who undergo this procedure develop new bladder tumors (i.e., tumor recurrence). In the majority of cases, the recurrence is also superficial, but in 5% to 30% of patients a tumor recurs with invasion into the muscle layer of the bladder (i.e., tumor progression). Once the tumor has penetrated the muscle, there is a substantial risk for the development of metastases and death from bladder cancer. This grim prognosis for muscle-invasive disease has lead to a strategy of vigilant follow-up and repeat TURBs of recurrent superficial tumors.

Since TURB alone may not control all tumors and cannot prevent new tumor occurrences, intravesical (topical) therapy has been widely used both as definitive treatment and as prophylaxis against recurrent superficial bladder tumors.[2] In this chapter, we review the natural history, biology, and management of superficial bladder cancers.

NATURAL HISTORY

The natural history of superficial bladder cancer is largely unpredictable because of tumor heterogeneity. In some patients, this is evidenced by rapid progression to deeply invasive disease, and in others, by the slow growth of multiple metachronous tumors that remain confined to the urothelium.

Papillary lesions are most common at diagnosis. Approximately 70% are Ta and 30% are T1 tumors. Ta tumors are usually low grade (G1), whereas the majority of T1 tumors are high grade (G2-G3). Carcinoma in situ uncommonly presents alone and is recognized most often in patients with previous or concurrent papillary tumors. Tis is a high-grade neoplasm. It may be focal or diffuse, indolent or rapidly invasive, and symptomatic or clinically silent.

Tumor Recurrence and Progression

Factors affecting tumor recurrence or progression include tumor stage (Ta versus T1), tumor grade (G1 versus G2-G3), prior recurrence rate, number of tumors(<4 versus ≥4), size of the tumors (<3 versus ≥3 cm), tumor configuration (solid versus papillary), tumor site (dome versus base), positive or negative urine cytology, presence of Tis, and response to local therapy. Table 26-1 shows multivariate analyses of prognostic variables for recurrence and progression of superficial bladder tumors.[3] The factor most predictive of recurrence is multifocality (i.e., polychronotopism), whereas high stage, and to a lesser extent, high grade, are correlated with tumor progression and metastasis. Lesser degrees of urothelial abnormalities (i.e., atypical hyperplasia) probably contribute to new tumor occurrences.

Tumor recurrence after initial therapy varies from 30% in patients with a solitary papillary tumor to more than 90% in patients with multiple tumors. Most tumors recur in 6 to 12 months but remain noninvasive and pose little risk to the patient. Both the extent and duration of disease help define the majority of patients who will suffer tumor recurrences within 5 years. Virtually all patients, if followed long enough, will have noninvasive tumor recurrence regardless of local therapy.

Although it is obvious that tumors must recur to progress, tumor progression is rare in comparison with the high frequency of tumor recurrences. It is likely that recurrence and progression may be biologically disassociated phenomena. Findings from three different studies support this assertion. Torti and colleagues[4] reported a series of 241 patients with superficial cancer who had a total of 161 recurrences after a median follow-up of 62 months. The risk of developing muscle invasion at each subsequent recurrence of previous superficial tumor did not increase from the first to fifth recurrences, respectively. A recent series by Thompson and colleagues[5] reported 124 consecutive patients on a surveillance protocol for superficial bladder cancer. Of 20 patients who had completed 5 years of follow-up and were free of recurrence, 7 suffered a late, muscle-inva-

TABLE 26-1. *Multivariate analysis of prognostic variables for recurrence and progression* of superficial bladder tumors*

Investigators	Number of patients	Tumor characteristics: Stage (Ta vs T1)	Grade (G1 vs G2–G3)	Multifocality (Tis)
RECURRENCE				
Kurth	240	0.006	0.064	0.016
Dalesio	308	NS	0.03	0.001
Herr	247	NS	NS	0.01 N
INVASION				
Torti	252	NS	0.009	NS
Herr	221	0.03	0.06	NS
Kalish	249	0.01 N	0.07 N	

* Tumor progression is defined as development of muscle invasion or metastases.
NS; not significant. Data from Herr HW. Bladder cancer: natural history and implications for urothelial cancer prevention. J Cell Biol Chem 1992;16:112.

sive tumor as the first recurrence of their disease. Herr and Wartinger[6] reported that of 61 patients followed for more then 10 years, tumor progression occurred in 25 (41%), of whom only 8 patients had prior superficial recurrences. Paradoxically, a tumor recurrence does not necessarily herald tumor progression, and freedom from recurrence is no guarantee against developing muscle invasion.

A muscle-invasive tumor occurs in 5% to 15% of patients with Ta tumors, 15% to 30% of those with T1 tumors, and in as many as 50% of those with Tis tumors associated with papillary lesions. Factors influencing risk of muscle invasion or metastases include high stage (T1), high grade (G3), multifocal Tis, and failure to respond completely to TURB and intravesical therapy. For example, patients with refractory T1 tumors have a 50% chance of developing muscle invasion within 5 years.[7] For patients with diffuse Tis, complete responders to local therapy have an 11% chance of progression, whereas incomplete responders have a 65% probability of developing muscle-invasive cancer.[8]

BIOLOGY

Molecular analysis of bladder tumors has uncovered a possible genetic basis for the disassociation between tumor recurrence and progression. Early studies showed monosomy 9 in many tumors, and alterations in chromosome 17 were reported more commonly in advanced or poorly differentiated cancers. Later studies documented that loss of heterozygosity (LOH) occurred with the greatest frequency on 9q and 17p. Loss of 9q is the first recognizable genetic event observed in low-grade Ta tumors, and LOH of 17p, some of which may be *P53* mutations, follows as tumors increase in grade and stage.[9] Additionally, the discovery of aberrant 9p genotypes (loss of tumor suppressor gene) and *P53* mutations, as well as some dysplasia, in Tis, T1 tumors could explain their propensities to progress, because these mutations are known to destabilize the genome.[10] The disassociation between tumor recurrence and tumor progression may be explained by interrelated but unique genetic alteration pathways.[11] Additional molecular studies may help refine the distinction between low- and high-risk groups for disease progression (see Chap. 21).

Tumor Markers

The variable clinical behavior of tumors of similar stage and grade makes desirable the determination of predictors of the biologic potential of the tumor and remaining urothelium. Tumor markers that have been evaluated include DNA abnormalities (aneuploidy) and flow cytometry, blood group antigens (A, B, H, Le_x), cell surface differentiation antigens (T16, Om5, T43, T138, M344), tumor suppressor genes (*RB1*, *P53*), epidermal growth factor receptors (*EGFR*), and E-cadherin, among others. Most of these putative prognostic markers are not independent relative to tumor stage and grade, and none has been prospectively validated.

Table 26-2 shows *P53* mutation and progression among 130 patients treated by TURB alone and followed for more then 10 years.[12] *P53* nuclear overexpression was associated with tumor progression to muscle invasion and metastases, especially of T1 and Tis tumors. Of the cohort of 130 patients, 75% with *P53*-positive (≥20% expression) tumors progressed, compared with 14% with *P53*-negative (<20% expression) tumors. Relative to stage, grade, and number of tumors, *P53* mutation was an independent prognostic variable for tumor progression. Additional prospective studies of this and other tumor markers are needed.

MANAGEMENT

The treatment of superficial bladder tumors has three objectives:

1. To eradicate existing disease
2. To inhibit or delay recurrence
3. To prevent progression to muscle invasion or metastases

TURB is the primary treatment of papillary tumors and focal in situ carcinoma. TURB does not prevent the common development of new tumors arising elsewhere in the bladder, nor does it prevent progression. Intravesical therapy following TURB may be cytotoxic to residual overt or occult carcinomas and premalignant mucosal lesions.

TABLE 26-2. *P53 mutation and progression of superficial bladder cancer*

Tumor type	*P53**	Number of patients	Number of progressions	*P* value	Multivariate analysis: Relative risk	*P* value	95% CI
T1	<20%	18	3	.0002	1.0	.002	
	≥20%	25	19		11.36		2.44–52.9
Ta	<20%	42	5	.01	1.0	.001	
	≥20%	12	7		9.5		2.4–36.8
Tis	<20%	18	3	.002	1.0	.004	
	≥20%	15	13		8.6		2.0–36.7
Totals	<20%	78	11 (14%)				
	≥20%	52	39 (75%)				

* The presence of *P53* was determined by immunohistochemistry. A tumor was considered positive if more than 20% of nuclei stained for *P53* and was considered negative if less than 20% of the nuclei expressed *P53*.

CI, confidence intervals.

Intravesical Therapy

Intravesical therapy is divided into two major categories: therapeutic, designed to treat established disease, and prophylactic or adjuvant, designed to prevent recurrence. Definitive therapy aims to treat disease that cannot be resected surgically, (e.g., tumors that are too numerous or too large, inaccessible tumors, some invasive T1 cancers, and Tis that persists after TURB). Prophylactic therapy is given after a presumed "complete" TURB as an adjunct to prevent true recurrences as a result of incomplete resection of the primary tumor or tumors or new tumor occurrences resulting from multiple tumor origins. Effective therapeutic or prophylactic therapy prevents or significantly delays progression to a higher tumor stage.

Intravesical therapy brings high concentrations of drugs into contact with tumor-bearing mucosa. Tumor implantation after resection may be inhibited by reducing the number or viability of free-floating malignant cells. Residual carcinoma or precursor mucosal lesions may be destroyed, thus preventing tumor recurrence. Progression of disease requiring more intense local therapy, cystectomy, or systemic chemotherapy may be prevented or delayed. The limited systemic absorption of intravesical agents minimizes serious toxicity.

Many agents have been used for intravesical therapy. In this chapter, we consider only those drugs used in the treatment of sufficient numbers of patients in randomized protocols to permit an overall assessment of results. These include thiotepa (TT), adriamycin (ADR), mitomycin C (MMC), and bacillus Calmette-Guerin (BCG).

Individual drug doses and schedules vary widely. An induction schedule of between 4 and 8 weekly doses is usually given. This may be followed in the event of a response by monthly doses for up to 1 year, and in some cases for 2 years as maintenance therapy. Average chemotherapy doses are 30 to 60 mg for TT, 40 to 80 mg for ADR, and 20 to 40 mg for MMC. Drugs are dissolved in saline for instillation to achieve a concentration of 1 mg/mL. BCG, an attenuated strain of *Microbacterium bovis*, is a biologic response modifier and dose varies with the substrain: 120 mg (Pasteur, Frappier), 50 mg (Tice), and 40 mg (Connaught). Between 10^7 and 10^9 viable colony-forming units are required. Exceptions to these doses and schedules are common.

Prophylactic Intravesical Therapy

Results of intravesical therapy given as prophylaxis are shown in Table 26-3.[1,13] Data obtained on 3852 patients entered into 29 randomized clinical trials are included. These studies met the criteria of having a control (TURB alone) group, an end point of the number of patients with tumor recurrence, and a follow-up of at least 1 year. The results showed control patients treated with TURB had a recurrence rate of 43% over 1 year in patients presenting with their first Ta or T1 tumor and 70% in patients with a prior history of bladder cancer. Overall, intravesical chemotherapy produced a small but measurable effect on the observed recurrence rate but was less then that achieved with BCG. The net reduction in tumor recurrences among the treated patients relative to patients having TURB alone was 12% for TT, 15% for MMC, 13% for ADR, and 40% for BCG.

Table 26-4 shows randomized studies comparing prophylactic BCG with chemotherapy.[2,13] In most studies, BCG reduced the number of tumor recurrences significantly more than did TT, ADR, or MMC. The Southwestern Oncology Group study comparing BCG with MMC included 377 evaluable patients.[14] This significant study was closed early after an interim analysis showed significant reduction in tumor recurrence among the BCG group. Additional long-term (10-year) follow-up results show no reduction in the incidence of tumor recurrence among chemotherapy-treated patients, whereas approximately one third of BCG-treated patients remain tumor free.[6]

TABLE 26-3. *Prophylactic intravesical therapy*

Drug	Number of patients	Percent tumor recurrence: Control (TURB)	Percent tumor recurrence: Treatment (drug)	Net benefit (%)
TT	1007	56	44	12
MMC	1157	50	35	15
ADR	1241	47	34	13
BCG	447	70	30	40

ADR, adriomycin; BCG, bacillus Calmette-Guerin; MMC, mitomycin C; TT, thiotepa; TURB, transurethral endoscopic resection.

TABLE 26-4. *BCG versus chemotherapy*

Investigators	Percent tumor recurrence by drug BCG	TT	ADR	MMC	*P* value
Brosman '82	0	47			<.05
Netto '83	7	43			<.05
Pineiro '89	13		43		<.05
SWOG '91	57		78		<.05
Tanaka '94	24		42		<.05
Finnbl '89	28			62	<.05
Rubben '90	35			35	NS
Witjes '92	34			25	NS
Witjes '94	47			42	NS
SWOG '94	19			33	<.005

ADR, adriamycin; BCG, bacillus Calmette-Guerin; MMC, mitomycin C; NS, not significant; SWOG, Southwestern Oncology Group; TT, thiotepa. Data cited in reference 13.

Therapeutic Intravesical Therapy

The percentage of patients achieving a complete response with intravesical therapy administered as treatment of superficial bladder tumors is shown in Table 26-5.[2,15] The data are assembled from multiple studies that provide a minimum 1 year of follow-up. Results are given as the response rates of papillary tumors and carcinoma in situ combined. A complete response is indicated by no cystoscopic, biopsy, or cytologic evidence of disease after therapy. The complete-response rate to BCG is significantly greater then that achieved with any of the chemotherapeutic agents. BCG is particularly effective against Tis, often protecting against disease spread for 5 years or more.[16]

Impact on Tumor Progression

Tumor recurrence is frequently used as a surrogate end point for disease progression. However, if recurrence and tumor progression are indeed clinically and biologically disassociated, it may be incorrect to assume that by preventing recurrence, tumor progression will be avoided. Numerous agents have been tested and thousands of patients enrolled into intravesical therapy trials. Table 26-6 collates the results of 10 studies, which include progression data of patients receiving chemotherapy.[13,15] Overall, in 1612 randomized patients, progression occurred in 8.3% of those receiving intravesical chemotherapy and in 8.6% of those treated with surgery alone.

TABLE 26-5. *Response of papillary and in situ tumors to therapeutic intravesical therapy*

Drug	Number of patients	Complete response (%)*
TT	474	34
MMC	407	47
ADR	585	42
BCG	718	72

* A complete response was considered no evidence of tumor on cystoscopy, biopsy, and urine cytology for at least 1 year.

ADR, adriomycin; BCG, bacillus Calmette-Guerin; MMC, mitomycin C; TT, thiotepa.

TABLE 26-6. *Intravesical chemotherapy: stage progression*

Drug	Treatment group Number of patients	Progression (%)	Control group Number of patients	Progression (%)
TT	314	4.5	199	6.0
MMC	336	3.9	191	7.3
ADR	389	15.2	183	12.6
Totals	1039	8.3	573	8.6

ADR, adriamycin; MMC, mitomycin C: TT, thiotepa

BCG may alter the progression of superficial bladder cancer.[17] Herr and colleagues[17] conducted a randomized trial between 1978 and 1981, and after 5 years showed that intravesical BCG delayed disease progression, prolonged the period of bladder preservation, and increased survival. A 10-year follow-up of this trial revealed a 10-year progression-free rate of 62% for patients treated with BCG and of 37% for the control patients.[18] Figure 26-1 shows the median progression-free interval was not reached for the BCG group and was 46 months for the control group (P = .006). Of 18 control patients who were crossed over to the BCG arm, 15 did not show tumor progression. Figure 26-2 shows that TURB plus BCG resulted in a 10-year disease-specific survival of 75%, compared with 55% with TURB alone (P = .03). This long-term study showed that intravesical BCG therapy delayed or prevented muscle infiltration, metastases, and death from bladder cancer in high-risk patients presenting with superficial bladder tumors.

Side Effects and Toxicity

Systemic side effects of intravesical chemotherapy include myelosuppression and allergic reactions. BCG produces more intense local effects than does chemotherapy. The intravesical route allows a high concentration of a drug to be delivered to the tumor with relatively little systemic absorption. As with any drug capable of systemic absorption, the rare case of anaphylaxis can occur.

Myelosuppression occurs in 18% of patients receiving TT. Chemical cystitis occurs in as many as 50% of patients receiving ADR, and 20% require discontinuation of therapy. MMC is not absorbed from the bladder, and bone marrow depression does not occur. Local effects of MMC are mild. The most common side effect is bladder irritation, which occurs in 15% of patients. Palmar rash of the hands occurs in 5% to 15% of patients; this is a contact dermatitis and can be avoided by washing the hands and perineum after treatment. Bladder contracture has also been reported. Persistent tumor requiring repeated endoscopic resections probably contributes to bladder dysfunction.

BCG produces an intense local inflammatory reaction in most patients. This local reaction is manifested as dysuria, frequency, urgency, hematuria, and passing of tissue debris lasting from

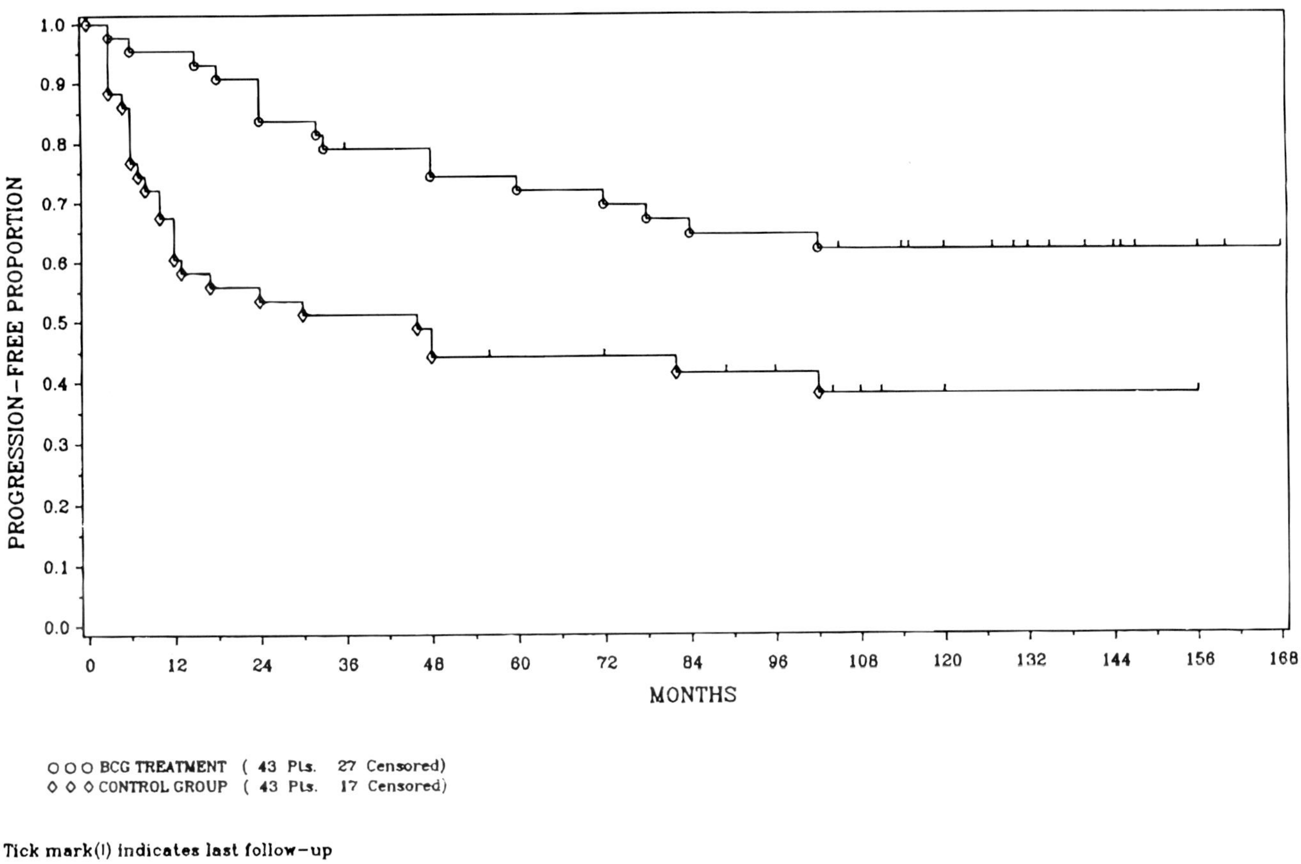

FIG. 26-1. Progression of superficial bladder cancer (BCG): 10-year results of a randomized trial. Times to muscle invasion or metastasis following transurethral resection are shown. BCG (43 patients, 27 censored) versus control (43 patients, 17 censored; $P = .006$).

6 to 24 hours after instillation. Although such local effects can be ameliorated with isoniazid, this is rarely necessary. Local symptoms generally do not require dose reduction or cessation of therapy. BCG has a cumulative effect; therefore, local side effects escalate significantly in severity and incidence with maintenance treatments. Serious systemic complications are uncommon but can occur. As many as 25% of patients have a flu-like syndrome lasting from 12 to 24 hours after instillation. Patients suspected of having systemic BCG infection or allergic reactions are treated successfully in most cases with antituberculosis medication.[19] There have been at least seven deaths attributed to intravesical BCG administration. In such cases, BCG was given after a traumatic catheterization or immediately after TURB was performed. Both situations foster systemic absorption of BCG organisms and should be avoided. Relative contraindications to BCG include active tuberculosis or immunosuppression.

Other Agents

Numerous other agents have been instilled into the bladder as definitive therapy or prophylaxis against recurrent superficial bladder tumors.[20] These include interferon, interleukin-2, keyhole limpet hemocyanin, maltose tetrapalmitate, levamisole, OK-432, transfer factor, *Corynebacterium parvum*, and the chemotherapy agents methotrexate, cisplatin, 5-fluorouracil and ethoglucid. None has proved effective relative to BCG.

One study compared intravesical interferon alfa-2b (IFN) with MMC as prophylactic treatments for superficial recurrence.[21] The median time to tumor recurrence was 36 months in the MMC arm versus 21 months in the IFN arm ($P = .048$). There was no difference between groups in tumor progression. Although MMC was more effective than IFN in reducing tumor recurrence, a multivariate analysis showed that tumor characteristics influenced disease outcome more than choice of intravesical therapy. IFN may play role in the management of carcinoma in situ.[22]

RECOMMENDATIONS FOR THERAPY

Many patients derive little benefit from intravesical therapy. Patients with Ta, G1 tumors are at such low risk of tumor progression that standard intravesical therapy is not required. Most achieve satisfactory results with outpatient cystoscopic fulguration or TURB alone.

Recurrent Ta, G1 tumors may benefit from a single postoperative instillation of chemotherapy after TURB.[23] However, long-term results of a multicenter randomized clinical trial involving 417 patients dispute this convention.[24] After TURB, patients were randomized to receive no TT, one instillation of TT at the time of resection, or one instillation at the time of resection and then at 3-month intervals for 1 year. After a median follow-up of 8 years and 9 months, there was no difference

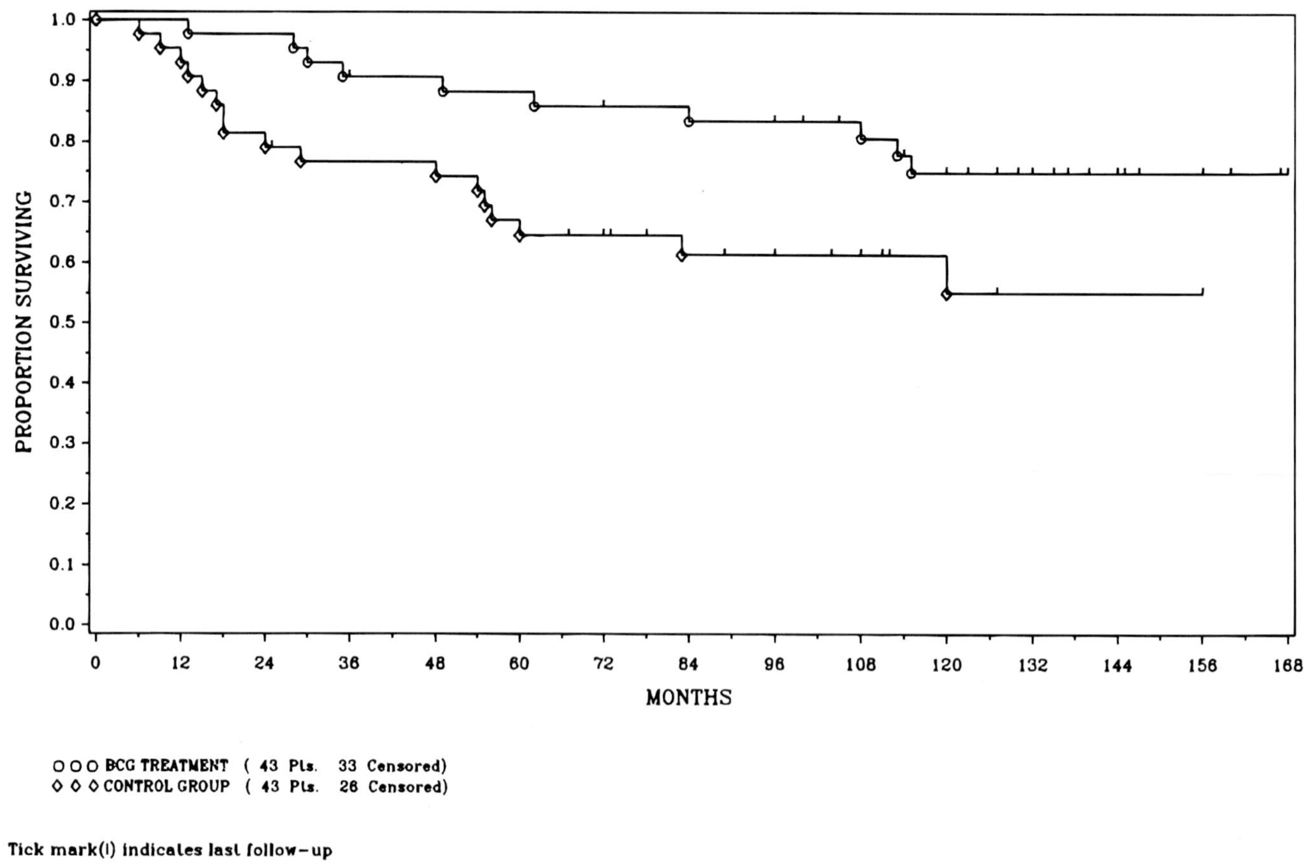

FIG. 26-2. Disease-specific survival of patients with superficial bladder cancer (BCG). This graph includes three patients in the BCG group who died of upper collecting system tumors despite absence of progression within the bladder. BCG (43 patients, 33 censored) versus control (43 patients, 26 censored; $P = .03$).

among the three groups with respect to time to first recurrence, recurrence rates, or failure-free interval rate. Additionally, this study confirmed that given enough time, noninvasive recurrences are extremely common, but they pose little risk to the patient because progression is rare.

Patients with high-grade (G3) or high-stage (T1) tumors and patients with diffuse Tis are at substantial risk for disease progression and death from bladder cancer. These patients require a complete TURB followed by adjunct intravesical therapy. The weight of the evidence favors the initial use of BCG over chemotherapy. Response rates to BCG appear to be much greater and generally more durable, especially against carcinoma in situ.[16,25] The optimal length of therapy has been studied by Badalament and colleagues.[26] Between 1981 and 1984, 93 patients were randomized to receive either nonmaintenance or maintenance BCG therapy once per month for 2 years. Both groups received the standard induction 6-week intravesical BCG regimen. There was no reduction in tumor recurrences or progression with maintenance BCG compared with the 6-week course, and long-term BCG increased cumulative local toxicity.

If long-term BCG therapy offers no additional benefit, should patients who fail to respond to an initial course be given a second course of BCG? Catalona and colleagues[27] reported that a 60% response rate after a single 6-week course increased to 80% after 12 weeks of BCG. Bretton and colleagues[28] have also observed that patients who respond to BCG for more then 1 year are likely to respond again for a similar duration to a repeat induction course given in the event of a late relapse. Traynelis and Lamm[15] reported in patients with Tis that 3-week BCG treatments at 3 months increased the complete response rate at 6 months from 73% to 87% ($P = .04$). Furthermore, 3-week BCG treatments every 6 months for 3 years resulted in an increase in long-term disease-free status from 65% in the group receiving the 6-week induction therapy to 83% in patients receiving regular retreatment.[29]

Response rates of superficial bladder tumors to BCG are independent of dose. The current recommendation is to render the patient continuously disease free as determined by repeated negative biopsy specimens and urine cytology specimens for more than 1 year. In some patients, this can be achieved with a single 1-week course of BCG; in others, it may require a repeat 6-week course consolidation with regular retreatments at 3- to 6-month intervals.

Endoscopic experience and sound clinical judgment are necessary to determine when a patient should be considered to have failed TURB and intravesical therapy. Three months after the start of a course of therapy is probably too soon to assess results, but after 6 months, a complete response to continued use of an active agent should be expected. It is unlikely that additional intravesical treatment using the same drug will convert a failure into a complete responder and puts the patient at risk of cancer progression. An occasional recurrence of a cytologically benign papillary tumor that is easily fulgurated or resected does not require a radical change in treatment. However, a positive biopsy specimen for persistent bladder cancer or a positive urine cytology specimen strongly indicates that an alternative therapeutic strategy should be tried. There are no controlled and little circumstantial data to support protracted (maintenance) intravesical therapy in nonresponding patients. Inconvenience, expense, cumulative toxicity, and most importantly, risk of disease progression outweigh any individual long-term benefit.

For persistent noninvasive disease, alternative intravesical therapy is reasonable but should not be continued beyond 1 year in nonresponding patients. Uncontrolled or recurrent T1 and Tis tumors portend an ominous prognosis. Cystectomy is currently the safest approach for these patients.

CHEMOPREVENTION

Prevention of bladder invasion exposes the extravesical urothelium as a potential site of relapse as a result of the emergence of dormant cells that have not been exposed to local therapy. Of 221 BCG-treated patients followed for as long as 10 years, 34 (15%) developed upper tract tumors and another 29 (13%) relapsed in the prostate.[30] Relapses were discovered as long as 10 years after local control of bladder tumors, and 15% of these tumors were invasive. In a separate group[30] of 75 patients who converted to a positive urine cytology specimen after disease-free intervals varying from 12 to 96 months, 48 (64%) relapsed in the bladder, 15 (20%) had supravesical disease, and 12 (16%) had prostatic urethral recurrences.

Among patients with lower urinary tract relapses, 85% were salvaged with cystectomy, whereas 65% with upper collecting system recurrences survived. These data illustrate that superficial bladder tumors represent a spectrum of panurothelial disease. In designing therapeutic strategies, a combination of intense therapy directed to the bladder early in the course of tumor evolution and systemic chemoprevention designed to protect the urothelium as a whole are required. The aim is to maintain an intact urinary tract and prevent silent tumor invasion from progressing to metastases. Chemopreventative agents should be oral and well tolerated by the patient.

Bropirimine, megadose vitamins, and retinoids have been tested in patients with superficial bladder tumors. Bropirimine stimulates endogenous interferon and has antiviral and antitumor activity, especially against carcinoma in situ.[31] A phase II trial of oral bropirimine for salvage of BCG-resistant bladder carcinoma in situ is being conducted.

Megadose vitamins have also received attention as chemoprevention agents. Lamm and colleagues[32] randomized 65 patients treated with intravesical BCG to supplemental therapy with multiple vitamins in the recommended daily allowances (RDA) or to RDA multivitamins plus 40,000 U vitamin A, 100 mg vitamin B_6, 2000 mg vitamin C, 400 U vitamin E, and 90 mg zinc. Recurrence after 10 months was markedly reduced in patients receiving the megadose vitamins. The 5-year estimated tumor recurrence rate was 91% in the RDA arm and 41% in the megadose vitamin arm. The conclusion of this small study was that megadose vitamins A, B6, C, and E plus zinc decreased bladder tumor recurrences in patients receiving BCG immunotherapy. The panurothelial effect of supplemental vitamins remains to be seen.

Fenretinide (4-HPR) is a synthetic amide derivative of all-trans retinoic acid and is among the most active and least toxic of several retinoids tested in animals. High concentrations of 4-HPR are achieved in the bladder. Earlier synthetic retinoids showed some activity in the prophylaxis of superficial bladder cancer, but the substantial toxicity precluded the use of adequate doses. A pilot trial evaluated the feasibility of a randomized trial of fenretinide and superficial bladder cancer in which DNA flow cytometry was used as the intermediary end point for response.[33] The study treatment consisted of 4-HPR at the daily oral dose of 200 mg. Conversion of a hyperdiploid fracture to diploidy by flow cytometry was observed in the group treated with fenretinide ($P = .007$), whereas no trend was evident in the control group ($P = .55$). The data suggest that retinoids might effect the tumor content by decreasing proliferative activity or by delaying DNA aneuploidy, and in some instances by reverting DNA aneuploidy of transformed urothelium to normal. A randomized trial in patients with carcinoma in situ of the bladder receiving BCG, with or without 4-HPR, is ongoing.

Antiproliferative drugs (i.e., retinoids) may decrease tumor recurrence, but they must be taken for the rest of the patient's life and may not prevent progression. Antimitotic agents may prove to be a better alternative, because they have the capacity to fundamentally alter unstable epithelium.

FUTURE INVESTIGATIONS

Additional clinical investigations into the treatment of bladder tumors will involve new agents, treatment regimens, and management strategies coupled with a better understanding of the molecular mechanisms of tumor development and progression. The challenge for the future is twofold: to identify earlier those patients at high risk for progression and to select the optimal drugs, regimens, and alternative treatment strategies for such patients.

If tumor recurrence and progression are indeed clinically and biologically disassociated, then the premise on which the management of superficial bladder cancer is based is flawed. It may be incorrect to assume that by preventing tumor recurrence, tumor progression will be avoided. In particular, the widespread use of intravesical agents as prophylactic therapy to prevent tumor progression by decreasing the rate of tumor recurrence must be reexamined. Decreased incidence of muscle invasion, reduced need for cystectomy, and improved survival should be the principle aims of therapy.

There are several important questions that remain to be answered concerning management of superficial bladder cancer. Does intravesical therapy improve overall survival? Does prophylactic therapy after successful TURB alter the ultimate course of disease? What are the optimal drugs, timing, and duration of intravesical therapy? What is appropriate therapy for patients who have failed local therapy but still have superficial tumors confined to the bladder or prostate? Can low- and high-risk patients with similar tumor types be identified before treatment? Patients at high risk for disease progression require intense local therapy and early cystectomy in the event of failure, whereas low-risk patients might be spared the burden of aggressive local treatment. Both low- and high-risk patients with superficial bladder tumors are candidates for chemoprevention.

REFERENCES

1. Herr HW, Laudone VP, Whitmore WF. An overview of intravesical therapy for superficial bladder tumors. J Urol 1987;138:1363.
2. Herr HW. Intravesical therapy. Hematol Oncol Clin North Am 1992; 6:117.
3. Herr HW. Bladder cancer: natural history and implications for urothelial cancer prevention. J Cell Biol Chem 1992;16:112.
4. Torti FM, Lum BL, Aston D, et al. Superficial bladder cancer: the primacy of grade in the development of invasive disease. J Clin Oncol 1987;5:125.
5. Thompson RA, Cambell EW, Kramer HC, et al. Late invasive recurrence despite long-term surveillance for superficial bladder cancer. J Urol 1993;149:1010.
6. Herr HW, Wartinger DD. BCG therapy for superficial bladder cancer. A 10-year follow-up. J Urol 1992;149:1020.
7. Herr HW. Progression of stage T1 bladder tumors after intravesical BCG. J Urol 1991;145:40.
8. Herr WH, Badalament RA, Amato DA, et al. Superficial bladder cancer treated with BCG: a multivariate analysis of factors effecting tumor progression. J Urol 1989;141:22.
9. Olumi AF, Tsai YC, Nichols W, et al. Allelic loss of chromosome 17p distinguishes high grade from low grade transitional cell carcinoma of the bladder. Cancer Res 1990;50:7081.
10. Orlow I, Lianes P, Lacombe L, et al. Chromosome 9 allelic losses and microsatellite alterations in human bladder tumors. Cancer Res 1994; 54:2848.
11. Spruck CH, Ohneseit PF, Jones PA, et al. Two molecular pathways to transitional cell carcinoma of the bladder. Cancer Res 1994;54:784.
12. Sarkas AS, Dalbagni G, Cordon-Cardo C, et al. Nuclear overexpression of small p53 protein in transitional cell bladder carcinoma: a marker for disease progression. J Natl Cancer Inst 1993;85:53.
13. Lamm DL, Riggs DR, Traynelis CL, et al. Apparent failure of current intravesical chemotherapy prophylaxis to influence the long term force of superficial transitional cell carcinoma of the bladder. J Urol 1995; 153:1444.
14. Lamm DL, Crawford ED, Blumenstein R, et al. A randomized comparison of BCG and MMC prophylaxis in stage Ta and T1 transitional cell carcinoma of the bladder. (Abstract) J Urol 1993;149:282.
15. Traynelis CL, Lamm DL. Current status of intravesical therapy for bladder cancer. Urol Ann 1994;8:112.
16. Herr HW, Pinsky CM, Whitmore WF, et al. Long-term effect of intravesical BCG on flat carcinoma in situ of the bladder. J Urol 1986;135: 265.
17. Herr HW, Laudone VP, Badalament RA, et al. BCG therapy alters progression of bladder cancer. J Clin Oncol 1988;6:1451.
18. Herr HW, Schwab DM, Zhang ZF, et al. Intravesical BCG therapy prevents tumor progression and death from superficial bladder cancer: 10-year follow-up of a prospective randomized trial. J Clin Oncol 1995; 13:1404.
19. Lamm DL, Vander Meijden A, Morales A, et al. Incidence and treatment of complications of BCG intravesical therapy in superficial bladder tumors. J Urol 1992;147:596.
20. Herr HW. Instillation therapy for bladder cancer. In: DeVita VT, Hellmann S, Rosenberg SA, eds. Biologic therapy of cancer. Philadelphia: JB Lippincott, 1991:643.
21. Boccardo F, Cannata D, Rubagotti A, et al. Prophylaxis of superficial bladder cancer with mitomycin or interferon alfa-2b: results of a multicenter Italian study. J Clin Oncol 1994;12:7.
22. Torti FM, Shorliffe LC, Williams RD, et al. Alfa-interferon in superficial bladder cancer. J Clin Oncol 1988;6:475.
23. Oosterlink W, Kurth KH, Schroder F, et al. A prospective randomized trial comparing transurethral resection followed by a single intravesical instillation of epirubicin or water in single stage Ta, T1 papillary carcinoma of the bladder. J Urol 1993;149:749.
24. Medical Research Council. The effect of intravesical thiotepa on tumor recurrence after endoscopic treatment of newly diagnosed superficial bladder cancer: a further report with long-term follow-up of a Medical Research Council Randomized Trial. Br J Urol 1994;73:632.
25. Nadler RB, Catalona WJ, Hudson MA, et al. Durability of the tumor-free response for intravesical BCG therapy. J Urol 1994;152:367.
26. Badalament RA, Herr HW, Wong GY, et al. A prospective randomized trial of maintenance vs non-maintenance intravesical BCG therapy of superficial bladder cancer. J Clin Oncol 1987;5:441.
27. Catalona WJ, Hudson MA, Gillen DP, et al. Risks and benefits of repeated courses of intravesical BCG. J Urol 1987;137:220.
28. Bretton P, Herr HW, Kimmel M, et al. The response of patients with superficial bladder cancer to a second course of BCG. J Urol 1990; 143:710.
29. Lamm DL, Crawford ED, Blumenstein B, et al. Maintenance BCG immunotherapy of superficial bladder cancer: a randomized prospective SWOG study. (Abstract) J Urol 1992;147:4.
30. Schwab DM, Herr HW, Sogani PC, et al. Positive urinary cytology following a complete response to intravesical BCG therapy: pattern of recurrence. J Urol 1994;15:382.
31. Sarosdy DF, Lamm DL, Williams RD, et al. Phase I trial of oral bropirimine in superficial bladder cancer. J Urol 1992;147:31.
32. Lamm DL, Riggs DR, Shriver JS, et al. Megadose vitamins in bladder cancer: a double-blind clinical trial. J Urol 1994;151:21.
33. Decensi A, Bruno S, Constantini M, et al. Phase II study of fenretinide in superficial bladder cancer, using DNA flow cytometry as an intermediary end point. J Natl Cancer Inst 1994;84:138.

Principles and Practice of Genitourinary Oncology, edited by Derek Raghavan, Howard I. Scher, Steven A. Leibel, and Paul H. Lange. Lippincott-Raven Publishers, Philadelphia, © 1997.

CHAPTER 27

Biology and Management of Invasive Bladder Cancer

Derek Raghavan, William U. Shipley, Reginald R. Hall, and Jerome P. Richie

Invasive bladder cancer constitutes only 20% to 25% of initial presentations of this disease and represents about 5 new cases per 100,000 males per year and 1 per 100,000 females. Traditionally, most cases of invasive bladder cancer have shown the features of invasion at first presentation.[1] The trend is toward bladder conservation for patients with superficial bladder cancer, however, and the emphasis is increasingly on intravesical therapy rather than cystectomy (see Chap. 26). Thus, more cases of invasive disease can be expected in the future, but because they will not be initial presentations, they will not be represented in the usual published demographic figures.

Although the approach to the investigation and staging of bladder cancer has been standard for many years (see Chaps. 23 and 24), the management of invasive disease has been particularly controversial. Issues of debate have been predicated on such factors as patient selection for treatment, heterogeneity of the disease, and stage shifts occasioned by changes in imaging and surgical techniques.[2] No clear consensus regarding optimal locoregional treatment exists, and the issue has been further complicated by the introduction of adjunctive systemic therapy in an attempt to improve outcomes of management. We do not share a common view on this issue, and we have therefore attempted to summarize and to integrate the data that are pertinent from different perspectives. We have reviewed the current concepts of the biology of invasive bladder cancer, the options for locoregional treatment, and the available data regarding the role of systemic therapy in this context.

BIOLOGY OF INVASIVE BLADDER CANCER

Differentiation and Prognostic Factors

The entity of invasive bladder cancer has been well defined histologically, consisting predominantly of tumors that have moderately to poorly differentiated morphology and that invade beyond the lamina propria into muscle and surrounding tissues.[3–5] More than 90% of invasive tumors are of transitional cell type, with or without elements of glandular or squamous cell differentiation.[4] Occasionally, invasive bladder cancer consists of pure adenocarcinoma, squamous cell carcinoma, choriocarcinoma, small cell undifferentiated cancer, or soft tissue sarcoma; the management of these uncommon patterns is covered in Chapter 30. Although the common patterns of invasive bladder cancer appear essentially to represent the uniform histologic entity of transitional cell carcinoma, they actually have a diverse collection of biologic and functional characteristics.

When physicians attempt to attribute prognostic significance to the features of invasive bladder cancer, the stage (extent of invasion) and grade (degree of differentiation) are the most important known factors.[4–6] In some early series, however, investigators did not recognize that the lamina propria is invested with a muscularis of its own (muscularis mucosae), as demonstrated by Ro and associates,[7] and some superficial tumors that merely penetrated this muscle layer were overstaged as "invasive" disease, a misconception that led to errors in the design of management programs or in the interpretation of the results of treatment.

The pattern of growth (papillary versus solid) is also of importance; the papillary type is associated with a clearly better prognosis.[4,8] The solid variant is more commonly associated with the phenomenon of invasion and thus has a worse prognosis. Other reported prognostic factors (Table 27-1),[1–6,8–31] such as size, aneuploidy, hydronephrosis, the presence of lymphatic and vascular invasion, and expression of receptors for the epidermal growth factor (EGF) and for transferrin, often exhibit univariate significance that is lost in multivariate analyses that include stage and differentiation.[2] Less clearly explained is the adverse prognostic significance of anemia, which may reflect the extent of underlying disease or may reduce the impact of radical radiotherapy on the tumor tissues.[11–13] The presence of blood group antigens[18,19] and the expression of certain oncogenes or mutations of suppressor genes appear to correlate with prognosis,[23–27,29–31] although their relationship with other prognosticators has not yet been fully defined (see Chaps. 17 and 20).

Another important biologic factor in assessing the outcome of management of metastatic uroepithelial cancer is histologic type. Clear differences exist in the outcome of treatment of metastases of transitional cell carcinoma and of the nontransi-

TABLE 27-1. *Prognostic factors in bladder cancer*

Prognostic index	Adverse impact for treatment of primary tumor	Increased risk of metastasis or relapse of primary tumor	References
Depth of invasion	Yes	Yes	1–6, 8–13
High grade	No	Yes	1–6, 8–13
Sessile morphology	No?	Yes	8, 11
Large size	Yes	Yes	11, 14
Multicentricity	No?	Yes	10, 15
Age of patient	Variable	No	10, 11
Hydronephrosis	Yes	Yes	10–13
Anemia	Yes*	No	10–13, 16
Extent of prior transurethral resection of the bladder	No	Yes?‡	11–13
Prior radiotherapy without downstaging	Yes	Yes	12–14, 16
Lymphatic/vascular invasion	Yes†	Yes	16, 17
Absence of ABO blood group antigen expression	?	Yes	18
Expression of T antigen	?	Yes	19
Aneuploidy	Yes†	Yes	20, 21
Chromosomal alterations	?	Yes	22–24 (see Chap. 20)
Amplification of oncogenes	?	Yes	24, 25 (see Chap. 20)
Expression of cytokeratin 18	?	Yes	26
Expression of epidermal growth factor receptor	?	Yes	24, 27
Expression of transferrin receptor	?	Yes	28
Abnormal expression of *P53* suppressor gene	?	Yes	23, 24, 29, 30
Lack of response to neoadjuvant chemotherapy	Yes	Yes	31

* Response to radiotherapy impaired by anemia.
† Response to intravesical chemotherapy.
‡ Inversely correlated.

tional cell types (adenocarcinoma and squamous carcinoma) of uroepithelial cancer (see Chap. 30). In addition, although the dominant histologic type of most metastatic deposits is transitional cell carcinoma, considerable occult heterogeneity exists within deposits of transitional cell cancer, with respect to grade, histologic features, growth parameters, ploidy, karyotype, gene expression, and tumor markers,[23,32–35] and provides an added source of variation in the outcomes of treatment.

Cell Lineages

The traditional view has been that separate cell lineages of the different histologic types of uroepithelial cancer exist,[4] although studies in our laboratory have suggested the existence of a common stem cell of origin of transitional cell carcinoma, squamous carcinoma, and adenocarcinoma of the bladder.[35–37] This view also appears to be supported at a molecular level[24] (see Chap. 20). This observation may explain the occasional discrepancies noted between the histologic features of primary tumors and subsequent metastatic disease, and it emphasizes the importance of reconfirming the histologic features of apparent metastatic deposits, especially because second malignant tumors are seen in up to 5% to 10% of patients with invasive bladder cancer.

Distribution of Metastases: Implications for Treatment ofInvasive Disease

The common sites of metastasis of bladder cancer and the other malignant uroepithelial diseases are regional lymph nodes, bone, lung, skin, and liver; less common sites are brain, meninges, and the organs within the peritoneal cavity.[4,38–40] The distribution of metastases is of particular importance when considering treatment, because the sites of involvement correlate with prognosis when systemic chemotherapy is administered. Improved median survival and tail of the survival curve have been documented in patients with metastases limited to the lymph nodes, skin, and perhaps lung, whereas a substantially worse prognosis has been reported in patients with liver, bone, and visceral metastases.[41,42] Because the pattern of spread of invasive bladder cancer is usually ordered, it seems reasonable to consider the use of systemic chemotherapy in the strategy of primary management, given the responsiveness of bladder cancer with clinically defined sites of involvement limited to lymph nodes and soft tissues.

Cellular Determinants of Treatment Response

When considering the use of systemic chemotherapy for the treatment of invasive bladder cancer, the physician should also review what is known regarding the cellular determinants of response to treatment with drugs commonly used for bladder cancer (see Chap. 8). Some cytotoxic agents can be exported from tumor cells through a mechanism based on the cellular surface, the so-called multidrug efflux pump, characterized by the expression of a specific 170-kd protein complex, P-glycoprotein.[43] Investigators initially demonstrated that resistance to the cellular effects of agents as diverse as the vinca alkaloids and doxorubicin is reduced in normal and malignant cells that express a protein complex on the cell surface, coded by a series of multidrug resistance (*PGY*, formerly known as *mdr*) genes. This phenomenon occurs as a result of reduced intracellular concentrations of the agents resulting from increased cellular efflux.[43] Several workers have attempted to study the expression of the multidrug phenotype in bladder cancer cells, but for reasons that are unclear, this problem has proved particularly difficult. Although many other tumors have been studied in detail, revealing correlations between the expression of the *PGY* phenotype and drug resistance, in preclinical and clinical studies, the expression of P-glyoprotein in bladder cancer has been variable and inconstant.[44–46] Nevertheless, expression of P-glycoprotein may be upregulated in resistant populations of bladder cancer cells after treatment with the methotrexate, vinblastine, doxorubicin, cisplatin (MVAC) chemotherapy regimen.[47] Moreover, in other tumor types, multidrug resistance can occur in the absence of expression of the 170-kd P-glycoprotein, whereas other proteins may be associated with similar patterns of resistance,[48] a finding that may explain this phenomenon in the absence of expression of P-glycoprotein.

Ultimately, apart from its predictive function, this work is unlikely to be of great importance unless the multidrug resistance phenotype can be overcome at a functional level. For example, the calcium channel blockers, such as verapamil, have been shown to reverse multidrug resistance,[49] although the toxic side effects of this approach have precluded routine use. Although clinical trials have not yet been published in bladder cancer, work initiated in our laboratories suggests that verapamil can overcome the impact of the *PGY* phenotype, at least in bladder cancer cell lines in vitro.[50]

The mechanisms of resistance to the platinum coordination complexes have been studied in detail, particularly in relation to ovarian cancer and malignant melanoma (see Chap. 9). Although several mechanisms have been identified, including factors that influence cellular accumulation, signal transduction, ionic fluxes, and intracellular enzyme function,[51] the function of the intracellular scavenger, glutathione (GSH), has been the focus of particular attention in the context of the resistance of bladder cancer to the effects of cisplatin. GSH is found in most mammalian cells and has many functions, including regulation of protein and DNA synthesis and detoxification. It appears to react with cisplatin, reducing cisplatin's intracellular availability. Inhibitors of GSH synthesis, such as buthionine sulfoxamine, have been shown to cause a decrease in intracellular levels of GSH, with a concomitant increase in the cytotoxicity of some anticancer agents, such as cisplatin[52] and paclitaxel.[53] Although many of the experimental data on the significance of GSH in cisplatin resistance have been derived from models of ovarian cancer, we have demonstrated that high levels of GSH are present in cell lines derived from bladder cancer, and this phenomenon may correlate with cisplatin resistance.[54]

Our understanding of these mechanisms is crude, and other factors appear to influence the responsiveness of bladder cancer to cytotoxic chemotherapy. The expression of several oncogene products appears to influence resistance to cytotoxic agents. The exact nature of this interaction is not yet clear, and it is particularly difficult to define because several of these products code for specific aspects of cellular growth control irrespective of exposure to cytotoxic agents. For example, investigators have shown that the interaction of EGF with its specific receptor (EGFR) is involved in the regulation of growth of bladder cancer.[33] In vitro treatment with EGF can increase cellular sensitivity of epithelial tumors to cisplatin, however, presumably by an effect on a signal transduction pathway.[55] Investigators have also reported that specific monoclonal antibodies can block the function of EGFR,[56] and further, treatment with these anti-EGFR monoclonal antibodies plus cisplatin can have a synergistic antitumor effect.[57] These data are particularly difficult to interpret in view of the previously documented impact of expression of EGFR on the natural history of bladder cancer,[27] as well as the demonstration that *ERBB2* gene amplification and overexpression are adverse prognostic determinants in bladder cancer.[25]

Another complex relationship has been demonstrated among the expression of P53 (a suppressor gene product), growth regulation, and cytotoxic response in bladder cancer. Alterations of the *P53* gene are among the most frequent genetic abnormalities found in human cancer and appear to have a broad range of postulated roles in cell growth control, including involvement in cellular repair and apoptosis. Apoptosis, or programmed cell death, is regarded as one of the forms of physiologic cell death because it represents a genetically determined cellular sequence that is part of the normal tissue homeostatic mechanism. Investigators have shown that P53, which is normally present only transiently, can be induced to accumulate within the cell by exposure to cytotoxic agents, such as cisplatin and mitomycin C,[58] and conversely, P53-dependent apoptosis modulates the cytotoxicity of radiotherapy, 5-fluorouracil, and doxorubicin.[59] In our laboratory, however, we have demonstrated that cisplatin-induced cytotoxicity appears not to be mediated by apoptosis in bladder cancer cell lines.[60] These issues may be of particular importance because investigators have postulated that P53 expression may constitute an independent prognosticator of response to the MVAC chemotherapy regimen.[30] Because P53 may be induced by cytotoxic exposure, the timing of tissue sampling may possibly be critical in determining the expression of this potential prognostic factor, especially if intravesical or systemic chemotherapy has been administered previously.

At the present time, the full implications of these data for patient management are unclear. These observations underscore the complexity of function of bladder cancer cells, however, and illustrate the subtleties of the interplay between prognostic determinants that affect the natural history of this disease and factors that specifically affect response to treatment.

SURGICAL MANAGEMENT OF INVASIVE BLADDER CANCER

Transurethral Resection

The least aggressive surgical approach to the management of invasive bladder cancer is the use of transurethral resection (TUR) alone, in which the aim is to resect the invasive tumor completely, while attempting to spare the bladder. For example, Barnes and coworkers[61] reported a 27% 5-year survival rate in a series of patients who underwent TUR alone for stage T2 tumors of medium and high grade.

Similarly, Herr[62] reported on a selected subgroup of 45 patients from a denominator of 217 consecutive cases referred with invasive disease, in whom repeat TUR was negative for invasion and in whom bimanual examination revealed no palpable mass. Herr elected to observe these patients, in an attempt to preserve their bladders intact, and demonstrated that 30 patients (67%) remained continuously free of tumor or required only conservative surgery or intravesical chemotherapy for recurrent superficial disease. The remainder developed invasive or metastatic disease, and 4 had died at the time of reporting. Herr concluded that a small subset of patients with limited muscle-invasive disease could be identified for whom conservative therapy was a reasonable alternative.[62]

A similar experience has also been reported from the University of Iowa, again demonstrating the great importance of careful patient selection if TUR alone is considered for stage T2 disease.[63] In this retrospective analysis, 114 patients with stage T2 tumors were seen, and 59 patients with "favorable" prognostic factors were selected for treatment by TUR with or without external beam irradiation; the 5-year survival was 46%. Of 43 patients treated by TUR alone (without radiotherapy), 10 required radical cystectomy, although no late follow-up information regarding sites of local recurrence and rate of distant metastasis was provided.[63]

More recently, Solsona and associates[64] selected 59 patients with T2 tumors who had undergone radical TUR, which was judged to be visually and palpably complete, and with negative biopsies at the base of the resection and at the periphery of the resected tumor bed, for a careful protocol of surveillance without immediate further treatment. After a mean follow-up period of 55 months, 52% of the patients remained free of recurrence, whereas 24% had developed superficial disease, 20% had recurrence of invasive tumor, and 3 had developed distant metastases. The overall survival rate of this highly selected series was 83%; 73% of these patients retained their bladders.[64] In a more recent update, presented at the 1994 meeting of the Société Internationale d'Urologie in Sydney, Australia, Solsona and colleagues reported 5-year follow-up data: no recurrence in 42.4%; disease progression in 32.2%; bladder preservation in 40.7%; and 5-year disease-free survival of 78%.[65] These authors also assessed a confirmatory series of 51 cases and confirmed their initial observations.[65]

As with all other innovative approaches, follow-up must be adequate, especially in patients with tumors that are potentially curable by more radical surgery. The key issue is the balance between the morbidity and mortality associated with the respective approaches.

Partial Cystectomy

Another option, which has potentially allowed preservation of the bladder, has been the use of surgical resection of the portion of the bladder that contains the tumor. Analogous to TUR, this approach usually preserves continence and bladder and sexual function, and it avoids the psychologic impact of a stoma or the changes in urinary function associated with a neobladder. On the other hand, the risk associated with partial cystectomy is the violation of the important surgical principle of complete tumor clearance, especially because the margins of invasive tumors (particularly if associated with carcinoma in situ) may not be macroscopically or visually evident at the time of surgery.

Sweeney and associates[66] reviewed in detail the relative risks and benefits of this approach in 10 published series, incorporating more than 500 cases. These investigators noted that fewer than 20% of patients with invasive disease were candidates for partial cystectomy, and despite careful selection, a high rate of local tumor recurrence (38% to 78%) was documented. Sweeney and associates noted no major difference in 5-year survival figures from series of radical cystectomies, although considerable selection bias in favor of the group treated by partial cystectomy is likely–for example, the inclusion of patients with favorable prognostic factors, such as smaller or less invasive tumors.[66]

At the Bladder Cancer Consensus Meeting[67] in Antwerp in 1993, investigators concluded that partial cystectomy is rarely an appropriate alternative to radical cystectomy, but in carefully chosen patients, appropriate selection criteria for partial cystectomy should include, as a minimum:

- solitary primary lesion at the dome of the bladder, well away from the bladder neck or ureteral orifices
- 2-cm margin of normal bladder surrounding the tumor
- likelihood of good bladder capacity and function after the procedure
- absence of carcinoma in situ from random biopsy samples

In some instances, partial cystectomy has been combined with radiotherapy to reduce the chance of local recurrence and to prevent pelvic tumor seeding.[66]

The other potentially attractive alternative has been to combine organ-preserving conservative surgery with systemic chemotherapy, as discussed in detail later in this chapter under combined modality therapy.

Radical Cystectomy

Surgical extirpation of the bladder for invasive cancer evolved initially through three basic stages of increasingly radical proportion: simple cystectomy, cystoprostatectomy, and radical cystectomy, with or without surgical sampling or excision of the pelvic and retroperitoneal lymph nodes.[3,9,68–73] Once the urothelial cancer has penetrated the muscularis (stage T2 or deeper), complete local control of known tumor is essential, and if surgery is to be the modality of choice, this requires radical cystoprostatectomy in men or anterior exenteration in women.[70] These techniques have ensured a greater certainty of tumor clearance, although the increased extent of dissection has been associated with only a minor increase in morbidity. At the same time, techniques of perioperative surgical and anesthetic management have improved, causing a steady reduction in surgical mortality, despite the increased vigor of surgical pursuit. Between 1955 and 1970, surgical mortality was approximately 15%,[68] compared with current series, which report a perioperative mortality of only about 1%.[70,73] In addition, modifications to the surgical approach have lessened the prospect of impotence and have reduced the need for the use of external urine-collecting devices, thus making cystectomy a more attractive procedure from the patient's perspective. Thus, the development of newer techniques for urinary diversion and bladder replacement has given greater flexibility to both the patient and the clinician in determining the optimal plan of management for invasive bladder cancer (see Chaps. 25 and 26).

The results of surgical therapy for invasive bladder cancer

TABLE 27-2. *Results of treatment of invasive bladder cancer with radical cystectomy alone*

Investigators	No. of patients	Clinical stage	Pathologic stage	Survival (%)
Jewett et al, 1964[3]	59	—	T2-4	15
Richie et al, 1975[68]	134	T0-4	T0-4	44
Pearse et al, 1978[71]	27	—	T3	30
Skinner and Lieskovsky[73]	33	—	T2-3a	50
Skinner et al, 1991[140]*	47	?	pT3, pT4, N+	40
Pagano et al, 1991[75]	261	T1-4	pT1-pT4	54
Lerner et al, 1992[76]	132	?	pTa-pT4, N+	29/29
Stockle et al, 1992[141]	23	?	pT3b, pT4a, N0, N+	<30
Martinez-Pineiro et al, 1995[121]*	60	T2-4a, NX, M0	—	37
Freiha*	25	?	pT3b-4, N0 or N1	38

* Randomized trial.

are reviewed in Table 27-2.[68–76] As can be seen, the 5- and 10-year survival rates decrease with increasing T stage, and the overall cure rate for deeply invasive disease is less than 50%. Before 1970, the surgical mortality rate compromised the survival figures to such an extent as to vitiate a comparison with current series. In all series in which follow-up has extended beyond 5 years, the traditional endpoint of 5-year survival is clearly inadequate, because relapses continue to occur beyond that point. Moreover, these data predominantly reflect classification on the basis of surgical staging.

Despite the improvements in surgical and anesthetic technique, approximately half the patients with invasive bladder cancer (in particular stages T3b-4) die of the disease, and the majority of disease recurrences are at distant sites rather than within the pelvis. Thus, modifications of local therapy alone are not likely to improve cure rates to any significant extent.

Surgical Technique

Although the approach to radical cystectomy is individualized, depending on the experience and practice of the surgeon, certain principles obtain in most centers.[9,70,76] Optimal preoperative assessment and preparation by the combined surgical and anesthetic team are essential. In the typically aged population of patients, involvement of relevant internists, with adequate assessment of cardiopulmonary and nutritional status, is essential (see Chap. 29).

Specific preoperative preparation, including the cessation of smoking, treatment of renal tract infection or dysfunction, and education of the patient and family regarding the aims, anticipated outcomes, and hazards of treatment, contributes to improved results. Similarly, a standardized and meticulous approach to bowel preparation is mandatory, analogous to the standard practice for colonic surgery. Wound sepsis is reduced by combining a preoperative regimen of mechanical bowel preparation with a system of bowel sterilization.

The best surgical approach is through an incision slightly to the left of the midline.[70] An inverted V incision is then made into the anterior peritoneum, beginning at the umbilicus and continuing to the internal inguinal ring on each side. The lateral margins of the incision are defined by the inferior epigastric vessels. The lower portion of the peritoneal envelope is incised, and the incision is carried cephalad in the posterior peritoneum, using the spermatic cord as the lateral margin of the dissection.

Pelvic lymphadenectomy is begun at the level of the bifurcation of the aorta, and it should include the node-bearing tissues that surround the common and external iliac vessels, the hypogastric vessels, and the obturator nerves. When the process of lymph node dissection has been completed, the lateral pedicles, based on the hypogastric artery, are doubly clipped and divided. The posterior peritoneum is divided at the retrovesical pouch, and the posterior layer of Denonvillier's fascia is separated from the serosa of the rectum by blunt dissection. The posterior pedicles are ligated, and the bladder and surrounding structures are removed, so the pelvic floor contains only the intact rectal serosa, external iliac vessels, obturator nerve, and urethral stump at this level.

Considerations Regarding Urinary Diversion

The complexity of normal bladder function is fully understood when the qualities of an ideal bladder substitute are considered. A reliable and permanent continence mechanism must support retention of urine in a replacement bladder, which, in turn, must have adequate capacity with low pressure at maximum volume. The bladder replacement must have unimpaired, unidirectional flow of urine from the upper tracts to preserve renal function. Furthermore, the bladder replacement must be associated with minimal alteration in lifestyle and body image.

Perhaps the main determinant of the success of a continent urinary diversion or bladder substitution procedure is careful patient selection. Among of the most important aspects are the personality and commitment of the patient. Moreover, patients should have bladder cancer with an expected "good prognosis" (see previous discussion of prognostic factors) and a reasonable life expectancy. Traditionally, continent diversions or bladder substitution procedures have not been recommended for patients older than 60 to 65 years, although the upper range of inclusion age seems to be changing with changes in surgical techniques, supportive care, and the fitness of the elderly (see Chap. 29).

Important anatomic factors must also be considered. For example, in the past, females were not considered good candidates for bladder substitution procedures because of an inadequate urethral sphincter mechanism. More recent series, however, have supported the use of neobladders in carefully selected female patients. Continent stomas may be placed below the beltline or in the vagina for optimum cosmetic effects. Similarly, men who are undergoing possible bladder substitution procedures must have adequate sphincter function and no history of incontinence before the planned procedures. Another important anatomic consideration is the widely accepted concept that transitional cell carcinoma of the bladder reflects a field change, and the upper tracts, prostatic urethra, and distal urethra are also at risk for the development of urothelial tumors. Prostatic urethral involvement with transitional cell carcinoma must be excluded when such surgery is contemplated. In most series, when the prostatic urethra is involved, the incidence of subsequent development of urethral transitional cell carcinoma has ranged from 5% to 13%,[77] and the high risk of developing urethral recurrence should preclude consideration of a bladder substitution procedure and should mandate that en bloc urethrectomy be performed at the time of radical cystoprostatectomy.

Other anatomic factors may only be evaluated at the time of surgery, such as the mobility and suitability of the relevant section of bowel. In a patient in whom a colonic segment is to be used for a bladder replacement or continent diversion, the surgeon must exclude the existence of underlying bowel disease by performing a barium enema (and possibly endoscopy) before the procedure. Patients who have received prior radiotherapy may also exhibit bowel changes that obviate certain types of continent diversion or bladder substitution procedures. The presence of a short mesentery, which precludes placement of a bowel segment deep into the pelvis (a problem more likely to be discovered in a patient who is obese), may also be detected for the first time at laparotomy.

The actual procedure selected for a particular patient or clinical situation is also important.[70,78] The enteric conduit is preferred by many surgeons because it effectively separates the urinary and fecal streams, and the ileal conduit is regarded as the standard, representing the maximum allowable complication rate, with acceptable outcomes regarding quality of life and physiologic function.

The primary consideration in the construction of an enteric conduit is to ensure that the bowel tube is created at a sufficiently short length to allow it to function as a conduit and not as a reservoir for urine, thus minimizing reabsorption of urine and avoiding electrolyte disorders.[70] The details of surgical technique vary from one institution to another. The following typical approach is practiced at the Brigham and Women's Hospital in Boston.[70] The distal ileum is often the preferred bowel segment in this context. A 15-cm ileal segment is isolated, and the continuity of the bowel is reestablished with a two-layer ileoileostomy or staples. The proximal end of the isolated segment is then closed with an inverted running absorption suture. The left ureter is led through a tunnel beneath the sigmoid mesocolon to lie in the right retroperitoneum next to the right distal ureter. The ureters are then spatulated to prevent postoperative stricture formation and are anastomosed to the proximal end of the isolated ileal segment on the antimesenteric border, by means of mucosal-to-mucosal anastomosis with an absorbable suture. The distal end of the isolated ileal segment is led out through a defect in the right lower abdominal wall, usually placed halfway between the anterior superior iliac spine and the umbilicus (mostly determined by the preoperative testing by the patient of potential sites for the apparatus). An everted mucocutaneous anastomosis is established with absorbable suture material. Surgical technique varies from one institution to another, and the preceding description is included as an example of one structured approach.

Mechanisms of Preserving Continence

Stomal Reservoirs

The choice of continence mechanisms remains controversial. The major approaches are offered by stomal reservoirs (e.g., cecoappendicostomy, cecoileostomy or Indiana pouch, and continent ileostomy or Kock pouch) or by orthotopic neobladders (e.g., hemi-Kock, W-shaped ileobladder, and detubularized colonic bladder). The right colon offers the most reliable continent stomal reservoir. It has a capacious volume in its spherical detubularized form, and it is technically easier to mobilize, as well as having an intrinsic valve mechanism for continence and dependable and easily dissected teniae for the construction of reliable urethral antirefluxing anastomoses. The right colon has a higher intraluminal contractility pressure and is thus not as suited for an orthotopic bladder because of the development of enuresis in up to 50% of patients. Careful investigation to exclude colonic cancer is mandatory before a right colonic reservoir is created.

Whichever approach is advocated, certain principles must apply:

1. An adequate length of bowel must be available.
2. Complete disruption of the cylinder is required, with proper reconfiguration to change the cylinder to a sphere.
3. A cylindrical efferent limb ileourethral anastomosis should be avoided in the construction of a neobladder because it may produce a dysfunctional, partly obstructed bladder outlet.
4. An effective antireflux mechanism should be used.

The details of the various types of urinary collection approaches are beyond the scope of this review. A brief overview of the common types is provided, however.

The construction of a continent cecal reservoir with a reversed bowel segment and an ileal stoma was introduced by Gilchrist and Merichs.[79] Subsequent experience revealed limitations, including difficulties with stomal self-catheterization, infection, and incontinence. Modifications of this approach, however, led to the evolution of the reconfigured right colon segment to achieve large-volume, low-pressure receptacles, with a tapered, imbricated short terminal ileum to provide continence.[80–83] Subsequent experience with this approach (the Indiana pouch) has shown a continence rate higher than 85%. At the Brigham and Women's Hospital in Boston, the reconfigured reservoir (including distal ileum, cecum, and ascending and transverse colon) has been associated with reservoir capacities of 600 to 1200 mL, with maximum pressures at capacity of 18 to 55 cm H_2O.[70]

Another variant of the continent stoma, the Kock pouch, was introduced in 1969 as a continent ileostomy, with a report of the first 12 cases published a decade later.[84] Skinner and associates have published the most extensive North American experience with this approach; these workers modified the efferent limb by fixing the nipple construction with staples, replacing the Marlex mesh with Dexon, discarding a short bowel segment proximal to the measured segment (to ensure a broad mesenteric vascular supply to the pouch), stripping the mesentery, and using a Dexon strip around the mesentery of the efferent loop to prevent herniation.[85] In this report, late complications occurred in 77 of 245 patients and required 85 repeat operations, including 55 revisions to achieve continence. The technique of pouch fixation with a stapling procedure has reduced the revision rate to about 15% and allows the formation of a reservoir with a capacity of 800 to 1000 mL. The catheterization interval of 6 to 8 hours offers a significant advantage over the right colon pouches. An overview of the experience with Kock pouches has concluded that they are associated with a mortality rate of 2%, a 5% incidence of serious complications, and a reoperation rate of 30% to create a continent stoma, but they have only a small prevalence of metabolic and nutritional problems.[86]

Whichever approach is considered, the ileal conduit should be regarded as the standard reference point that represents the maximum allowable complication rate, balanced against acceptable quality of life for the patient. When considering the outcomes of various innovative approaches, the reported data vary from one institution to another. At the Brigham and Women's Hospital, the tunneled appendix has yielded the greatest success rate with respect to continence mechanisms (98%), although the plicated ileocecal valve (with a 93% success rate), sphincter preservation (80%), and the intussuscepted nipple (75%) provide reasonable alternatives.[70] One problem with the tunneled appendix is its small lumen, with consequent slow emptying time.

With respect to the antirefluxing ureteral mucosal anastomosis, Richie[70] has preferred the Leadbetter tunneled anastomosis (with a success rate of 98%), although other surgeons advocate the Le Duc trough procedure (80% success) and the ileocecal or ileal nipple intussusception (80% success). The Leadbetter anastomosis may be associated with a higher incidence of delayed stricture formation.

Configuration of the Pouch. The configuration of the pouch is an important variable in the function of a continent reservoir; the radius of the pouch is the key to the balance between volume and length of cylindrical bowel segment. The segment of bowel must be detubularized, thus allowing conversion from a cylindrical shape into a sphere, with the ultimate goal of achieving a large volume capacity relative to surface area, with low maintained pressure between voiding. The process of detubularization limits the spontaneous contractions of the bowel to half its circumference and produces a disorganized pattern of contraction that results in a reduced pressure wave.

Surgical Technique

Right colon continent stomal reservoir. The cecum, ascending colon, proximal transverse colon, and terminal ileum should be detached from their attachments up to the third and fourth part of the duodenum.[70] This technique opens up the retroperitoneum for ease of transfer of the ureter. The bowel segment that will be used for the reservoir should include 35 to 45 cm of bowel, from the cecum to the transverse colon. The middle colic artery can be preserved: the colonic mesentery should be divided between the middle and right colic arteries, sacrificing the marginal vessels while preserving the right colic artery. A segment of terminal ileum approximately 10 to 12 cm in length should be included. The bowel continuity should be reestablished with a standard, end-to-end, two-layer closure. Benefits of this approach include the safety of the anastomosis and the reliable vascular supply.

The bowel lumen of the pouch should be cleaned with irrigations of saline, and the antimesenteric border should be incised by cautery between the teniae, thus detubularizing the segment effectively. The incision should be carried to the base of the cecum to eliminate the high contractile pressures of any cylindrical component. The right colon is then folded on itself and is partially closed with a two-layer closure of 3-0 Vicryl suture. The ureters are implanted in the teniae in a 5-cm tunnel, after the seromuscular coat is widely separated from the mucosa. The ureters are stented (no. 7 single J Silastic catheters) and are fixed with a fine catgut suture to the bowel wall. Because of the large mesenteric pedicle, the pathway of the left ureter can be tortuous and at times should be brought anterior to the bowel. This can be done by an intraluminal Goodwin technique, in which the spatulated tunneled ureteral wall is sutured directly to the mucosa transcolonically.

The key aspect of the Indiana pouch is the creation of a terminal ileal sphincter by imbrication (folding in) of the lumen of a short segment of attached terminal ileum. This can be done by placing a 14-gauge French catheter into the lumen of the ileum and grasping the antimesenteric border with a row of Babcock clamps.[70] A GIA stapler is placed between the Babcock clamps and the catheter, and the bowel wall is tapered by this technique. The distal 2-cm segment of ileum is imbricated with pursestring suture of 2-0 silk, brought directly onto the proximal cecal wall. The silk sutures at the base of the ileum are reinforced with a 3-0 running silk suture, and the catheter is left in situ by fixing it to the bowel mucosa. The pouch is drained with a no. 20 Malecot catheter, which is pulled through a separate stab incision on the lateral end of the pouch. Ureteral stents (no. 7) are brought out above this through two separate small stab wounds in the bowel wall. The ureteral stents are removed in 7 days, and the pouch tube is removed in 3 weeks. Starting on day 7 postoperatively, a mucolytic agent (20% urea) is used for irrigation.

By the third week, the patient is taught to self-catheterize. The frequency of this procedure depends on the final volume of the pouch. The capacity is commonly in the range of 450 to 850 mL; maximum capacity is usually attained 3 to 6 months after the operation. Mucus production usually decreases over time, but 10% to 20% of patients suffer from diurnal or nocturnal stomal leakage. Gastrointestinal and nutritional disorders are not characteristic of this approach.

Mitrofanoff Principle (Cecoappendicostomy) The most reliable continent form of urinary diversion is provided by an in situ appendiceal stomal mechanism, which requires a 4- to 6-cm appendix with a mobile mesoappendix. This technique is limited by the problems of a small-diameter lumen, however, which accommodates only a narrow-gauge catheter and requires a longer emptying time. In addition, endoscopy is difficult, and the incidence of stenosis is higher.

A reliably continent stoma is produced by cecal wall tunneling. This technique also allows the abdominal skin opening to be hidden. The umbilicus may be used for the stoma to conceal it, although this is usually more applicable to the pediatric population.

The requisite technique is similar to that for the Indiana pouch and includes the entire detubularized right colon and proximal transverse colon on an ileocolic vascular pedicle. A segment of terminal ileum about 12 cm in length is left intact and can be used as the ureteral antirefluxing device. The base of the appendix is separated from the fatty pedicle and is buried in a tight 5-cm submucosal tunnel without including any intussusception. The tip of the appendix is excised, and then the lumen is dilated with a French bougie (no. 14). The tunnel is then closed. Ureteral stents and pouch tubes are managed in the same way as for an Indiana pouch.

Orthotopic Urethroenteric Anastomosis

Perhaps the most desirable forms of diversion are those that provide sphincter preservation, with reservoirs that empty by intentional voiding through coordinated relaxation of the pelvic floor and abdominal straining: the so-called orthotopic neobladder. These techniques can only be applied to males with normal urethras and normal results of prostatic mucosal biopsy, however. Initial efforts using the intact cylindrical bowel segment generated high pressures at the lower capacities, causing the complication of enuresis in 80% to 90% of patients. Up to 20% of patients also suffered daytime incontinence.

Lilien and Camey[87] reported an uncommonly low incidence of enuresis and incontinence. These investigators used a U-shaped segment of 40 cm of the terminal ileum, brought down to the membranous urethral stump. Investigators have suggested that the meticulous dissection of the prostatic apex and urethra, with a nerve-sparing technique, contributed to its success. The experience of other surgeons has been less impressive, however, and whether the problems relate to experience of the surgeon or to the reliability and complexity of the surgical procedure is not clear. Moreover, the procedure cannot be applied if the mesentery is too short, as occurs in many obese patients.

Sigmoid and ileocecal intestinal segments have been used in similar fashion, with less enuresis, but similar incontinence rates. The lowest pressures and largest capacities are seen in patients with hemi-Kock and W-shaped Hautmann ileal bladders,[88] and segments of colon may not be appropriate in this context because the ileum has a larger capacity, less contractility, and lower pressure. The W-shaped pouch[88] involves a detubularized configuration with a W shape, offering the largest radius by the folding technique used. It is simple, involves no valves, and has perioperative complication rates identical to those of the simple conduits. These pouches have a range of capacities of 300 to 2000 mL, with an average volume of 700 mL. One advantage of this approach appears to be a reduced incidence of enuresis, although patients over 70 years of age appear to have a high incidence of incontinence. The problem appears to be a lower incidence of an effective antireflux mechanism in the ileum. In a follow-up report of 211 patients at 6 years, Hautmann and associates[89] noted that 32% of patients suffered significant problems that required rehospitalization or reoperation, and complications included ileus (2%), abscess (1%), colon-reservoir fistula (1.5%), hydronephrosis (1%), ureteral stenosis (3.6%), and transurethral incision of the urethroileal anastomosis (7%). By 3 years, 85% of the patients were continent at night, 5.5% had nocturnal incontinence, and 6% used protection for occasional episodes of nocturnal incontinence.

Preservation of Potency

Consequent on the delineation of pelvic neurovascular anatomy, including a more precise functional description of Santorini's plexus and the anatomy of the nerves supplying the corpora cavernosum and the apex of the prostate,[90] anatomic approaches described for radical prostatectomy and radical cystectomy can preserve potency in a high proportion of patients. As part of the surgical approach to cystectomy outlined earlier, a plane is developed between the bladder and the rectum by incising the peritoneum and using gentle blunt dissection to free the rectum from the prostate at Denonvillier's fascia. Dissection ceases near the pelvic fascia, before reaching the posterior pedicles of the bladder, and attention then focuses on the dorsal-venous complex and the plexus of Santorini (analogous to radical prostatectomy). After the dorsal venous complex is isolated, the membranous urethra is transected, with division of the lateral pelvic fascia and pedicles to the prostate. The seminal vesicles are then separated from the neurovascular bundle on each side, and the remainder of the posterior bladder pedicles are then ligated.

Although considerable debate exists regarding the quality of the potency that remains, up to 50% to 60% of patients (who were previously potent) regain some measure of potency between 6 and 12 months after radical cystoprostatectomy performed in this way.

CONVENTIONAL TECHNIQUES OF IRRADIATION

External Beam Irradiation

The use of radiotherapy, as an alternative to cystectomy, for the management of bladder cancer has traditionally been favored in Europe, and in the United Kingdom in particular. The approaches to irradiation of the bladder have included doses of external beam irradiation in the range of 50 to 70 Gy, with a higher level of local control achieved in series reporting dose schedules in the higher range.[10–12] The principles and techniques of pelvic irradiation are reviewed in considerable detail in Chapter 7 and are mentioned only briefly here.

A governing principle in the application of radiotherapy is that the reduced certainty of defining the extent of the tumor (because of noninvasive staging techniques) is offset by the benefits associated with bladder preservation, including urinary continence and retention of sexual function in many cases.

Technical Considerations

The techniques used to deliver curative irradiation to the bladder tumor volume while sparing normal tissue vary from one institution to another, depending on the availability of equipment and the quality of physics and computer support.[12] At the Massachusetts General Hospital, most patients have been treated with external beam irradiation using 10- to 25-MeV linear accelerators. Initially a four-field box technique is used, with contoured paired anteroposterior and lateral fields. The fields are designed to treat the entire bladder, perivesical tissues, and draining lymph nodes to a total dose of 5040 cGy, given in daily fractions of 180 cGy, five times a week. A cone-down boost of 1800 cGy is delivered to the clinically evident tumor, using the same fractionation schedule as in the original course. The boost may be delivered through paired lateral fields or through rotational fields, depending on the size of the tumor and its location within the bladder.[12]

Similarly, other studies have used a total dose of 60 to 65 cGy, in daily fractions of 180 to 200 cGy, 5 days per week, with a four-field box.[10,11]

It appears that dosimetry is critical to successful control of the primary tumor, with total dose being the key (rather than total treatment time). Parsons and Million[91] showed that doses of less than 60 Gy were ineffective in achieving local control (0%), whereas 48% of patients with advanced local tumors achieved control with doses greater than 62 Gy.

More recently, hyperfractionation, in which irradiation is delivered more than once per day in small fractions to achieve a greater therapeutic index and to overcome patterns of cellular recovery, has been assessed for the management of bladder cancer. The concern with this approach has been the risk of enhanced toxicity, with the potential for contraction of the bladder.

Careful treatment planning is critical and requires close collaboration between the urologist and the radiation oncologist. In particular, definition of the site and size of the tumor is important. Treatment planning often includes a localizing cystogram or planning computed tomography (CT) scan (in the prone, treatment position). Ideally, these investigations are most useful if implemented before extensive TUR, to allow accurate definition of the initial extent of the tumor and to avoid postresection artifacts, such as inflammation-based induration of the bladder wall; however, this is often not practicable in routine clinical practice, and the problem can be ameliorated by delaying the CT scan until the initial postresection edema has resolved.

Preservation of a well-functioning bladder is more likely if a portion of the bladder can safely be excluded from the high dose of radiation needed for the bladder cancer itself. Treatment of the entire bladder with high doses per fraction or a high total dose is more likely to result in scarring and contracture. Care must also be taken to consider known tolerance of the surrounding normal tissues, such as colorectum and femoral heads. These issues become more important in patients who have undergone several TURs of bladder tumors, in those with chronic inflammatory bowel conditions, and in those who have undergone pelvic or abdominal surgery.

Prognostic Factors

The outcomes of treatment are predicated on many of the prognostic determinants for the natural history of bladder cancer, as discussed previously. What has also become increasingly clear is that careful patient selection is essential to success. An initial complete clinical response rate of 30% to 50% is usually achieved, depending on the following prognostic features: tumor grade, size, stage, morphologic features, and the presence or absence of ureteral obstruction.[10–12] In general, patients who do not respond completely require salvage surgery for attempted cure, as do those who do achieve a clinical complete remission, but subsequently sustain a local relapse.

Moreover, the likelihood of long-term local tumor control is increased two- or threefold by visibly complete TUR before commencement of irradiation.[12,13,92] Of course, complete TUR is more likely in small papillary tumors, and the impact on prognosis may be a function of the tumor treated rather than of the resection itself.

With current staging and pathologic techniques, the exact definition of prognosis is difficult, and thus the design of bladder-preserving management programs requires judgment and some risk. Therefore, the potential benefits of bladder preservation with respect to quality of life are offset by an increased chance of treatment failure.

Survival figures from radiotherapy series are summarized in Table 27-3.[10–14,91–98] As can be seen, 5- and 10-year survival rates reflect the extent of the tumor. Case-selection biases, which emphasize the older and less physically robust patient in radiotherapy series, have a substantial impact on the results recorded. Irrespective of the extent of the tumor and the age and physical characteristics of the patient, however, the cure rate in unselected series of patients with deeply invasive bladder cancer treated by radiotherapy alone is less than 40% to 50%.

Nonetheless, when bladder preservation is desired, radiotherapy is the standard against which all innovative strategies must be compared. As a generalization, bladder-preserving therapy for malignant urothelial disease is judged reasonable only if survival is not jeopardized and if it has a high probability of achieving long-term local tumor control.

Interstitial Irradiation

In addition to the most widely practiced approach of daily single fractionated external beam irradiation, alternative approaches have been developed. One approach is brachytherapy, the implantation of radioactive sources directly into the tumor, to concentrate a greater level of radiation within the tumor.[99] In most instances, the radioactivity has only a limited depth of penetration, thus sparing the surrounding tissues, and has its most appropriate application in carefully selected, smaller tumors. Another approach is intraoperative radiation, in which surrounding tissues are retracted at operation, to allow a greater dose intensity to the bladder tumor itself. Although isolated series have suggested benefits to these approaches, they have not been uniformly applied with improved outcome, and the more traditional approaches have remained the standard of irradiation.

Comparisons of Radiotherapy Versus Cystectomy

The results obtained in surgical and radiotherapy series are not really comparable, because the selection of patients for each type of treatment usually differs, and such comparisons also reflect the difference between clinical and pathologic (surgical) staging.[100]

In general, more elderly and infirm patients are referred for radiotherapy, in particular patients deemed unfit for cystectomy because of advanced age, intercurrent disorders, consideration of surgical anatomy, or previous treatment.

TABLE 27-3. *Results of treatment of invasive bladder cancer with conventional radiotherapy*

Investigators	No. of patients	Clinical T stage	Salvage cystectomy (%)	Survival (%)	Follow-up (y)
Goffinet et al, 1975[93]	283	T2-4	<12	<20	10
Bloom et al, 1982[14]	91	T3	20	29	7
Yu et al, 1985[95]	236	T2-4	11	<25	10
Shipley et al, 1987[13]	37	T2-3	—	39	5
Shearer et al, 1988[94]	188	T3	>15	25	5
Gospodarowicz et al, 1989[11]	121	T2-4b	20	32	5
Sauer et al, 1990[92]*	29	T2-3	—	69	3
Sell et al, 1991[96]	95	T2-4a	25	30	4
Wallace et al, 1991[97]	130	T2-4	—	40	3
Dunst et al, 1994[98]*	64	T1-3	—	24	10
Mameghan et al, 1992[10]	303	T1-4	11	25	7.6

* Same series.

For patients with muscle-invading bladder cancer, three randomized trials, carried out between 1965 and 1985, compared radical cystectomy (with preoperative radiotherapy) with radical radiotherapy alone (60 Gy), which was the standard treatment approach used outside the United States. In the case of patients treated with radiotherapy, deferred salvage cystectomy was used in selected patients if local relapse occurred. Miller[101,102] reported on a small, single-institution randomized trial for patients with large T3 tumors that compared 50-Gy preoperative radiotherapy and cystectomy with full-dose radiotherapy and salvage cystectomy. Of the 35 patients randomized to receive preoperative irradiation and cystectomy, 46% survived for 5 years, compared with 13% for the 32 patients randomized to radical radiotherapy. This study has been criticized for its small sample size and the slow accrual of patients with extremely large bladder tumors, however, as well as for issues raised regarding the quality of radiation therapy in view of the poor survival figures reported. An older trial from the Veterans Administration group[103] showed no difference in outcome among patients receiving cystectomy, radiotherapy alone, and preoperative radiotherapy and cystectomy, although this also has been criticized on methodologic grounds.

Bloom and colleagues[14] compared preoperative pelvic radiotherapy (40 Gy) plus elective radical cystectomy with radical radiotherapy (40 Gy plus 20 Gy boost to the tumor, followed in selected cases by salvage cystectomy) for deeply invasive bladder cancer. A total of 189 patients were randomized, of whom 98 were allocated to combined treatment and 91 to radical radiotherapy. The analysis was carried out on the basis of "planned treatment" and "treatment actually received." Patients allocated to radiotherapy and cystectomy had a 5-year survival of 38%, compared with 29% for those who received radical radiotherapy ($P > .2$). These investigators commented that 77 patients who actually received radiotherapy or cystectomy had a 5-year survival of 44%, compared with 31% for the 85 patients who received radical radiotherapy alone, although such subset analysis is subject to significant biases of patient recruitment and of interpretation and is not considered methodologically or statistically appropriate. Also of interest, but subject to significant selection bias, a 5-year survival rate of 60% was recorded for the selected group of 18 patients who were treated by radical radiotherapy and who subsequently underwent salvage cystectomy.[14] A survival benefit from the combined treatment was demonstrated in the subset of patients aged 60 years or less, whereas a statistically insignificant benefit was noted for women who were treated by radical radiotherapy alone; in each instance, selection biases in a retrospective subset analysis could have influenced the outcome substantially.

More recently, Sell and associates[96] reported the results of a trial conducted by the Danish Vesical Cancer Group, in which 40-Gy preoperative radiotherapy plus cystectomy was compared with 60-Gy radiotherapy plus salvage cystectomy for those patients with recurrent cancer. This trial also showed no apparent survival difference between the two arms of the study, with a median follow-up of 50 months for the 183 patients. The pelvic recurrence rate of 6.8% for the group randomized to receive preoperative radiotherapy and immediate cystectomy was significantly lower than the 36% pelvic recurrence rate in the group randomized to receive radiotherapy alone. Although 27 of these 95 patients underwent salvage cystectomy for tumor recurrence, the incidence of metastatic disease was similar in both groups, that is, 32% in those randomized to receive 60 Gy of radiotherapy and 34% in those randomized to the combined therapy group. One interpretation of these data is that deferred cystectomy, in favor of radical radiotherapy, does not prejudice survival, although other investigators may question the quality of surgery in the context of the 6.8% pelvic recurrence rate.

In a separate analysis of quality of life, the Danish Vesical Study Group reported a reduction in social and sexual function among patients randomized to preoperative radiotherapy plus cystectomy,[104] although the developments in surgical technique reviewed earlier may vitiate this difference.

Lynch and colleagues[105] assessed bladder and rectal function in 69 patients treated at the Royal London Hospital whose bladder remained disease-free after 60-Gy radical radiotherapy and compared the results with those obtained in an age-matched group of controls without known bladder or bowel disease (who had never received pelvic radiotherapy). That no differences were identified illustrates that good quality of life can be anticipated in patients who remain tumor-free after radical pelvic radiotherapy. These data confirmed the results of our previous trial in which quality of life was assessed in patients who received preemptive intravenous cisplatin chemotherapy followed by radical radiotherapy.[106,107] What has emerged from these studies using contemporary techniques of planning and dosimetry of irradiation is that an acceptable quality of life can be achieved with this approach, and cure may be achieved, although it may require the use of salvage cystectomy or chemotherapy in some instances.

This issue represents one of the most extreme controversies in this area, specifically, the relative safety and efficacy of bladder-sparing approaches versus radical cystectomy. In each instance, the techniques of treatment and support have improved substantially in recent years. As outlined later, the application of systemic chemotherapy in combination with radical radiotherapy has improved response rates and local tumor control, although the issue of absolute cure has not been finally resolved. By contrast, improvements in pelvic surgery, with nerve-sparing approaches and the development of neobladders, have narrowed the gap with respect to the toxicity of treatment. We have not reached a consensus on "optimal" definitive treatment of locally advanced bladder cancer, especially in the context of the evolving balance between the indices of quality of life and ultimate cure.

COMBINED MODALITY STRATEGIES OF TREATMENT

Rationale for Combined Modality Treatment

The initial concept of combined modality treatment involved the use of radiotherapy and surgery concomitantly, with the intention of securing local tumor control with a greater level of confidence. Whitmore[108] reported that initial radiotherapy could achieve tumor downstaging, and such stage reduction was associated with improved outcome when the bladder was resected at cystectomy. Investigators postulated that this approach would reduce the likelihood of intraoperative tumor dissemination and perhaps would also secure a greater level of local tumor control if the surgical procedure itself missed a portion of the tumor.[108]

Notwithstanding the limitations of some of the randomized trials that tested this concept,[100] from the apparent improvement in treatment results from this approach it seemed logical to assess whether the combination of systemic chemotherapy with standard locoregional treatment would improve outcome. Theoretically, this hypothesis was based on the following postulates[109]:

1. Clinical and autopsy data show that micrometastases are often present at the time of presentation of invasive bladder cancer.[38,72]
2. The optimal time to treat micrometastases with systemic chemotherapy is probably when their volume is minimal,[110] favoring the application of chemotherapy around the period of treatment with radiotherapy or surgery.
3. Drug resistance to cytotoxic agents may be related to the spontaneous mutation rate of the cancer cells themselves, which, in turn, is a function of the number of cells present[111]; thus, early use of chemotherapy could overcome this obstacle.
4. Tumors may contain hypoxic regions that are resistant to treatment and in which cells progress only slowly through the cell cycle, with many held up in the G0 phase[112]; these cells may be more sensitive to the combined effects of cytotoxic agents and radiotherapy.
5. Tumors that are treated by radical radiotherapy, with doses in excess of 60 Gy, frequently exhibit substantial vascular sclerosis; the use of chemotherapy, which requires vascular access to the tumor tissue for optimal activity, before the onset of such postradiation sclerosis could increase cytotoxic responsiveness.
6. Certain cytotoxic agents, such as doxorubicin, 5-fluorouracil, cisplatin, and paclitaxel, act as radiosensitizers, which render normal and malignant tissues more sensitive to the effects of irradiation; this finding suggests that the use of these drugs before or during the period of irradiation may lead to enhanced tumor cytotoxicity, but perhaps at the expense of increased normal tissue damage.

Several strategies that combine systemic chemotherapy and definitive locoregional treatment are available for the management of invasive bladder cancer:

- concurrent chemoradiation, in which chemotherapy and irradiation are delivered synchronously in an attempt to maximize the potential for radiosensitization of tumor tissues
- preemptive or neoadjuvant chemotherapy, in which first-line systemic chemotherapy is administered, followed by assessment of response, and implementation of definitive local therapy (surgery, radiotherapy, or both)
- classic adjuvant chemotherapy, in which systemic treatment is administered after completion of locoregional treatment in an attempt to control micrometastatic disease.

The optimal approach to combination therapy has not been defined with certainty, although many randomized and nonrandomized trials have provided relevant data, as outlined later.

Chemoradiation

One of the most extensively explored strategies for the management of invasive bladder cancer has been the concomitant use of chemotherapy and irradiation (Table 27-4).[98,113–121] Given that cisplatin can be found in tissues and urine several days after administration, some of the neoadjuvant chemotherapy programs (in which chemotherapy precedes radiotherapy) may possibly represent the equivalent of concomitant chemoradiation therapy.

The most common developmental programs have used either cisplatin[113] or 5-fluorouracil,[114,115] delivered concurrently with irradiation. Although several phase I-II trials have been carried out, the short follow-up of most of these trials provides insufficient data to allow a true appraisal of durability of control.

In addition, only one randomized trial has assessed the impact of this approach. Coppin and associates[116] compared chemoradiation (using cisplatin as a single agent) with external beam irradiation alone for the management of T3-4, NX, M0 bladder cancer and demonstrated a statistically significant increase in pelvic tumor control from combined modality therapy. Combined modality treatment achieved sustained tumor control in 67%, compared with 45% from radiotherapy alone ($P = .023$). Although a trend toward improved survival was noted, it did not achieve statistical significance. This finding may have been influenced by the small numbers of cases, however.

Despite the absence of absolute proof of a survival benefit from the use of chemoradiation, most current approaches have

TABLE 27-4. *Trials of chemoradiation for invasive bladder cancer*

Investigators	No. of patients	Clinical T stage	Salvage cystectomy (%)	Overall survival (% per y)	Median follow-up (mo)
Coppin et al, 1992[116]	42	T2-4	?	61 @ 2	50
Dunst et al, 1994[98]	139	T1-3	?	40 @ 7	min 12
Housset et al, 1993[118]	54	T2-4	22	59 @ 3	18–58
Kaufmann et al, 1993[117]	53	T2-4	15	53 @ 4	48
Sauer et al, 1990[92]	67	T1-4	16	66 @ 3	
Tester et al, 1993[119]	46	T2-4	17	66 @ 3	36

extrapolated from the studies of Coppin and colleagues[116] and of the group at Massachusetts General Hospital,[113,117] to build novel approaches. For example, Housset and associates[118] have incorporated the combination of cisplatin and 5-fluorouracil as radiosensitizers in a phase II trial with a high initial objective response rate, confirmed to be 70% complete response by repeat biopsy (and shown to be pT0 at the time of elective cystectomy). The Radiation Therapy Oncology Group (RTOG) is about to study this protocol, having completed a randomized study comparing the impact of neoadjuvant cisplatin, methotrexate, vinblastine (CMV) chemotherapy followed by chemoradiation with chemoradiation alone.

In the past, the resistance of many clinicians to bladder-conserving approaches was based on the concern that survival would be compromised by retention of the bladder. Four reported studies support the case for bladder preservation.[98,117–119] Each has used combined modality chemoradiation programs, although in three of these studies, TUR was a component.[98,117–118] In three of the studies, selection of patients for bladder preservation was based on the initial bladder tumor response to induction chemotherapy.[117–119] These studies have shown overall survival figures of 45% to 52% at 4 to 5 years, with 64% to 68% for clinical T2 tumors. These figures are comparable to recent cystectomy series with patient eligibility based on clinical stage,[120,121] although the comparison with current North American series, with reporting of data restricted to pathologic staging, is much more difficult.

A key element of the success of these programs has been the importance of recognizing treatment failure in high-risk patients at the earliest opportunity, with prompt recourse to cystectomy. Thus, in these programs, cystoscopy is performed 4 to 8 weeks after the completion of chemoradiation, and radical cystectomy is advised for patients with residual cancer.

The concern that the bladder functions poorly after chemoradiation has been addressed by these studies. For example, Dunst and colleagues[98] performed only three cystectomies for bladder contraction in a series of 192 cases (1.6%). Houssett and associates,[118] using a less conventional fractionation (44 Gy in 33 fractions), also reported late complications to be uncommon. Similarly, Kachnic and associates[122] reported that 21 women had good quality of life, no compromise of bowel or bladder function, full urinary continence, and no dysuria at a median time of 56 months after completion of chemoradiation in the Massachusetts General Hospital program, although this group has an obvious selection bias (i.e., only women) in this series.

This issue remains controversial, and even we have not reached a concordance on whether chemoradiation confers a specific survival benefit, although many clinicians believe that chemoradiation does achieve greater local tumor control than radiotherapy alone. In the United Kingdom, radiotherapy alone is regarded as the standard treatment for patients for whom cystectomy is not proposed, whereas a much broader range of approaches is regarded as standard in North America.

In the view of two of us (Drs. Shipley and Hall), these studies suggest that programs of TUR and chemoradiation, with consequent bladder sparing, provide a satisfactory alternative to more radical surgical approaches, although this approach must be tempered by the importance of careful patient selection (T2-3a disease and absence of tumor-related hydronephrosis). As discussed later, Dr. Hall's preferred option is the use of TUR followed by adjuvant chemotherapy. By contrast, Drs. Richie and Raghavan remain more cautious about the role of these approaches in the absence of specific randomized trials that have compared optimal surgery or the combination of chemotherapy and optimal surgery with the current techniques of transurethral surgery and chemoradiation. Dr. Richie, in particular, regards radical cystectomy, with current techniques, as the treatment of choice for most patients with invasive bladder cancer despite the foregoing data; he cites higher cure rates in noncomparative studies, reported on the basis of pathologic staging. In Dr. Raghavan's view, the absence of a proved survival benefit from chemoradiation programs in randomized clinical trials is important, as well as the short duration of follow-up available for series of chemoradiation and radical cystectomy. Regrettably, in the current clinical climate, it is unlikely that any randomized clinical trial will be able to resolve the foregoing debate.

Neoadjuvant Chemotherapy

The other common approach to combined modality treatment is initial (neoadjuvant or preemptive) chemotherapy, in which intravenous or intraarterial cytotoxic agents are administered in an attempt to cytoreduce the primary tumor and to control occult micrometastatic disease before definitive local therapy is undertaken. As noted earlier, serum or tissue levels of the drugs sometimes persist for several days and can thus facilitate potential radiosensitization.

The initial protocols used single-agent chemotherapy (in particular cisplatin or methotrexate), given that, at the time of their design, no survival benefit had been demonstrated from combination chemotherapy. Initial reports were encouraging,[123,124] and they showed symptom reduction in nearly 80% of patients and objective tumor response in up to 60%, accompanied by only modest toxicity. Even in cohorts of older patients, this strategy of treatment was well tolerated and yielded impressive local tumor control, with sustained periods of disease-free survival.[106] Randomized trials failed to demonstrate any survival benefit from single- or dual-agent neoadjuvant chemotherapy when added to radiotherapy or cystectomy, however.[94,97,120,121] Similarly, a meta-analysis of several randomized trials, comparing single- or dual-agent neoadjuvant chemotherapy plus definitive local therapy with definitive local therapy alone, showed no benefit from the combined approach.[125]

Moreover, we have shown, in a late follow-up study conducted more than 10 years after the entry of the last patient in our original series (which entered patients between 1981 and 1983), that tumor-related deaths continue to occur well beyond the standard 5-year reporting point.[126] This study is also important in that it has revealed an unexpectedly high prevalence of cardiovascular and cerebrovascular problems; although this prevalence may be a function of the patient population (more than 80% were heavy cigarette smokers, with a range of intercurrent disorders before entry), it may also suggest that occult, late intercurrent side effects may have impact on the efficacy of treatment. Further close scrutiny of the single-arm and randomized trials for unanticipated side effects will be mandatory to assess the true impact of these novel strategies of treatment.

Several of the early neoadjuvant protocols used combination regimens, such as methotrexate-cisplatin and cyclophosphamide-doxorubicin-cisplatin, yielding higher objective response rates in early reports. These single-arm, phase II trials did not produce any obvious improvement in median or long-term survival, however, a finding that is not particularly surprising because these regimens had not shown a survival benefit, compared with single agents, in randomized trials conducted with patients who had metastatic disease.[127–129]

By contrast, early studies with the combination of methotrexate, cisplatin, and vinblastine (with or without doxorubicin), the so-called CMV and MVAC regimens, had shown particular promise for the treatment of metastatic disease.[130–131] Furthermore, an important randomized trial had demonstrated a significant survival benefit from the MVAC combination when compared with single-agent cisplatin for patients with metastatic bladder cancer.[42] This finding led to the assessment of these regimens in a neoadjuvant context.[132]

The true significance of the use of neoadjuvant MVAC or CMV is not yet clear. Early studies suggested a high local response rate,[132,133] although follow-up reports suggested a high failure rate. Schultz and coworkers[31] reviewed the results of treatment of 111 patients at a median of only 5 years, however, and documented a 5-year actuarial survival of only 52%. This study also demonstrated that significant univariate prognostic factors included initial T stage, presence of ureteral obstruction, and presence of a palpable mass. Age, initial complete resection versus no complete resection of the primary tumor, recurrent or de novo tumor, grade, and multifocality were not significant predictors in this study. Postchemotherapy variables found to be significant were the postchemotherapy clinical stage and the pathologic stage. The presence of carcinoma in situ in the pathologic specimen, delay in definitive surgery, and type of definitive surgery were not significant. Using a Cox proportional hazards model, the five univariate factors were analyzed, and only initial T stage and the pT stage remained significant prognostic determinants. This interpretation has been questioned in view of the large proportion of patients who did not undergo surgical staging initially, however, and also because of the inclusion of data from 10% of patients who agreed to undergo surgical staging only at the time of disease progression.[134]

A high response rate was also recorded in a series in Italy, in which 46 patients were treated with neoadjuvant MVAC chemotherapy, followed by radical cystectomy (17 patients), partial cystectomy (11 patients), or deep TUR of residual tumor (18 patients).[135] Of the patients who underwent deep TUR or partial cystectomy, 72% were alive with a functioning bladder at the time of reporting. This analysis was subject to substantial bias of patient accrual and short median follow-up (36 months at the time of reporting), however.

The true role of neoadjuvant MVAC or CMV chemotherapy will become clear when the results of two multicenter randomized trials, conducted by the International Intergroup and the North American Intergroup, are known. These studies are comparing the impact of three cycles of CMV or MVAC, respectively, followed by definitive local treatment, against definitive treatment alone. Although these studies will be of crucial importance in defining the role of this strategy, rigorous adherence to the complex schedules may not be as efficient or as successful as in single centers (Table 27-5). This could be one explanation if a difference in outcomes is seen between the results of single centers and those of the multicenter trial groups. For example, Fossa and coworkers[136] demonstrated the flaws and difficulties of a multicenter collaboration in a phase II assessment of neoadjuvant CMV. Whereas multicenter, randomized trials demonstrate the practical utility and problems of such regimens in the community at large, the results attained in excellent single centers are sometimes more impressive. It then becomes a philo-

TABLE 27-5. *Trials of neoadjuvant chemotherapy for invasive bladder cancer*

Investigators	No. of patients	Regimen	Clinical stage	Response rate (%)	Survival (%)	Follow-up (y)
Shearer et al, 1988[94]*	188	M	T3	?	28	5
Wallace et al, 1991[97]*	125	C	T2-4	?	39	3
McCullough	17	CDCy	T2-4	53	47 + 1 yr	1.5
Vogelzang	29	MVDC	T2-4	69	71	5
Schultz et al, 1994[31]	111	MVDC	T2-4	47	52	5
Rintala et al, 1993[120]	151	CD	T1-4	?	58	5
Martinez-Pineiro et al, 1995[121]*	62	C	T2-4, NX-2	34	35	6

M, methotrexate; *C,* cisplatin; *V,* vinblastine; *D,* doxorubicin; *Cy,* cyclophosphamide
* Randomized trial.

sophic issue as to which trial end point should be regarded as the standard.

One important observation that emerged from the phase II assessments of neoadjuvant MVAC is that only about 50% of patients have complete remissions documented at the time of cystectomy,[132] a finding clearly supporting the importance of locoregional treatment on completion of chemotherapy, with the caveat that, in some patients undergoing cystectomy, residual postchemotherapy tumor may have been the determinant of the use of surgery rather than radiotherapy or an expectant approach.

Classic Adjuvant Chemotherapy

Since the introduction of systemic chemotherapy into programs of management for bladder cancer, several nonrandomized clinical trials have been carried out with a view to improving the outcomes of treatment.[137–139] Single-agent and combination regimens have been used in a range of schedules and doses, including single agents and combination chemotherapy regimens.[137–142] Most commonly, cisplatin, doxorubicin, and 5-fluorouracil have been studied. Useful interpretation of the results has been impossible, however, because of a lack of appropriate controls and the substantial variation of the clinical population treated with these adjuvant schedules.

More recently, important randomized trials have been completed and cast some light on this issue. Skinner and associates[140] reported the results of the first randomized trial intended to compare a series of patients treated by radical cystectomy for pathologically staged invasive bladder cancer with a randomized cohort in whom adjuvant cisplatin, doxorubicin, and cyclophosphamide were administered after cystectomy. Although the trial was important and visionary, major flaws of execution, including small patient numbers, the failure of patients to receive planned treatment, and other protocol deviations, as well as possible selection biases, marred the interpretation of the data. Although Skinner and colleagues concluded that a significant survival benefit was achieved from the use of chemotherapy, other investigators have questioned the validity of this interpretation of the data.[143,144] Given the limited utility of single-agent chemotherapy for advanced bladder cancer,[42] as well as the observation in randomized trials that the combination of cisplatin, doxorubicin, and cyclophosphamide does not yield a survival benefit when compared with single-agent cisplatin in the treatment of metastatic disease,[127,128] it still seems reasonable to question whether this approach has any useful role.

By contrast, another important trial has assessed the impact of adjuvant MVAC chemotherapy after radical cystectomy.[141] Once again, the impact of this study was reduced by a major flaw in trial design, specifically, that patients were randomly allocated either to undergo cystectomy followed by three cycles of adjuvant MVAC or to undergo cystectomy alone, without chemotherapy at any time. Thus, patients who had relapses after cystectomy were not offered salvage chemotherapy and suffered an unacceptably high death rate; the trial was terminated early. Thus, although the data are provocative and suggest the possibility of major disease-free survival benefit, this study really has only addressed the issue of the use of chemotherapy at some time after cystectomy and has demonstrated that chemotherapy offers a benefit in that context. A second study, in which 54 patients with pathologic stage P3-4, N0-2, M0 disease were randomly allocated to receive four cycles of adjuvant CMV chemotherapy or observation (with CMV chemotherapy at the time of relapse), has been carried out at Stanford University.[142] Although reported only at a preliminary level, this study showed freedom from relapse in 44% of those treated with adjuvant chemotherapy and 21% for the delayed chemotherapy group. A survival benefit was not reported, although to demonstrate a difference in such a small group would be difficult, given that the patients with disease relapses in the control group were then treated with adjuvant CMV chemotherapy. Furthermore, this was only a small study, with wide confidence intervals for the statistics.

Deep Transurethral Resection and Adjuvant Chemotherapy

An important alternative approach to the management of invasive bladder cancer has been advocated in the United Kingdom. Based on the early observation that high-dose intravenous methotrexate is active against primary bladder cancer,[145] Hall and colleagues effected a series of trials in which meticulous TUR of the primary tumor was completed as thoroughly as possible, followed by adjuvant systemic chemotherapy.[146,147] In the initial trial, methotrexate was used at a dose of up to 2 g/m^2 every 3 weeks; 54 patients with T3 tumors were treated, of whom 31 (57%) were free of invasive bladder cancer at 3 years. In an attempt to improve these results, a successor trial was completed in which methotrexate and cisplatin were combined as adjunctive therapy.[147] In the initial report, 36 patients with clinical stage T3 tumors underwent TUR, followed by adjuvant chemotherapy, and 25 (60%) were alive and free of disease at a median follow-up time of 32 months.[147] A more recent report, incorporating data from 47 patients, showed that 13 patients were alive without cancer in the bladder (T0) and 4 had died, from a denominator of 23 cases at risk at 5 years.[148]

PROBLEMS OF CLINICAL TRIALS

The most significant barrier to progress is the extent to which invasive bladder cancer is managed outside the context of structured clinical trials. Whether this approach is due solely to fiscal considerations or whether it is a function of the prejudices on the part of clinicians regarding ''optimal'' care is unclear. In a provocative series of studies of medical decision making, Moore and coworkers,[149,150] using the physician-surrogate model, showed that some surpising factors influence decision making in the management of invasive bladder cancer. Clinicians appear to exhibit a significant influence from their country of origin and from the specialty in which they practice when their management decisions are made. These studies also suggest that knowledge of the results of structured trials may not, in fact, influence medical decision making to the extent that would be expected.[150] Although the physician-surrogate model has significant limitations,[151] these results must be taken into consideration when attempting to deal with the problems of patient recruitment for clinical trials.

The Intergroup international trial of neoadjuvant chemotherapy, described previously, has been less beset by these problems than has the Intergroup study in the United States. This difference presumably reflects a greater commitment to participation in randomized clinical trials by urooncologists in Europe, Canada, and Australia, or perhaps it reflects different perceptions on the part of the patient community with regard to participation in clinical trials.

In addition to the foregoing perceptions, such factors as time availability, the complexity of trial design, and increasing stringency of entry requirements for putative trial subjects are contributing to the problems of case accrual to clinical trials.

Patients themselves appear to be increasingly resistant to such participation, either because of their interpretation of available medical information regarding their illness or because of the constraints of medical insurance and reimbursement. Many patients have considerable difficulty in dealing with the issues raised by the process of randomization, suffering from a lack of confidence or certainty when the relevant clinician proposes treatment allocated by random chance.

These problems have no simple solutions, and a detailed discussion of these issues is beyond the scope of this work. To identify the problem and to encourage increasing education of clinicians and their patients in this context are appropriate, however (see Chap. 13).

THE FUTURE: OVERCOMING THE BARRIERS TO CURE

As mentioned, control of the tumor in the pelvis does not really constitute the major barrier to cure. Even for large, invasive, high-grade lesions, local control is expected from radical surgery[70,73,75,76] and in many instances from the newer programs of combined modality treatment.[116–119] Thus, the process of fine tuning the techniques of surgery or of the delivery of radiotherapy itself is unlikely to have a large impact, although the development of strategies of surgery that may minimize the process of dissemination of cancer cells could be important.

The patterns of treatment failure seen in contemporary practice reflect predominantly metastatic disease. Whether the treatment failure rate is higher in salvage chemotherapy of patients who have previously had neoadjuvant, concurrent, or classic adjuvant chemotherapy, which would imply the outgrowth of resistant clones of cells, is unclear. If the response rate to chemotherapy were equivalent at the time of relapse and at the time of first presentation, it would imply that established metastatic cells had been dormant in the G0 phase of the cell cycle and hence inaccessible to chemotherapy at the time of initial treatment. Similarly, the exact timing of the establishment of metastases remains unknown, despite abundant speculation, hypotheses, and experimental data (see Chap. 3).

Thus, the highest priority for research into the management of invasive disease should be an attempt to overcome spontaneous or induced resistance to cytotoxic agents or to develop alternative strategies for the control or prevention of metastatic disease. As discussed previously, the mechanisms of drug resistance are being elucidated, and the investigation of biochemical modulation, to overcome the functions of multidrug resistance and expression of GSH, dihydrofolate reductase, thymidilate synthase, and a range of other putative targets of chemotherapy, may be a productive avenue of research.

REFERENCES

1. Kaye KW, Lange PH. Mode of presentation of invasive bladder cancer: reassessment of the problem. J Urol 1982;128:31.
2. Raghavan D, Shipley WU, Garnick MB, Russell PJ, Richie JP. Biology and management of bladder cancer. N Engl J Med 1990;322: 1129.
3. Jewett HJ, King LR, Shelley WM. A study of 365 cases of infiltrating bladder cancer: relation of certain pathological characteristics to prognosis after extirpation. J Urol 1964;92:668.
4. Koss LG. Tumors of the urinary bladder. In: Atlas of tumor pathology, 2nd series, fascicle 11. Washington, DC, Armed Forces Institute of Pathology, 1975.
5. Reuter VE. Pathology of bladder cancer: assessment of prognostic variables and response to therapy. Semin Oncol 1990;17:524.
6. Friedell GH, Parija GC, Nagy GK, et al. The pathology of human bladder cancer. Cancer 1980;45:1823.
7. Ro JY, Ayala AG, El-Naggar A. Muscularis mucosa of urinary bladder: importance for staging and treatment. Am J Surg Pathol 1987; 11:668.
8. Slack NH, Prout GR Jr. The heterogeneity of invasive bladder carcinoma and different responses to treatment. J Urol 1980;123:644.
9. Hendry WF. Diagnosis and management of primary bladder cancer: a British perspective. In: Raghavan D, ed. The management of bladder cancer. London, Edward Arnold, 1988:69.
10. Mameghan H, Fisher RJ, Watt WH, et al. The management of invasive transitional cell carcinoma of the bladder: results of definitive and preoperative radiation therapy in 390 patients treated at the Prince of Wales Hospital, Sydney, Australia. Cancer 1992;69:2771.
11. Gospodarowicz MK, Hawkins NV, Rawlings GA, et al. Radical radiotherapy for muscle invasive transitional cell carcinoma of the bladder: failure analysis. J Urol 1989;142:1448.
12. Rose MA, Shipley WU. Radiation therapy in invasive bladder cancer: principles, results, patient selection and innovations. In: Raghavan D, ed. The management of bladder cancer. London, Edward Arnold, 1988:154.
13. Shipley WU, Prout GR Jr, Kaufman DS, Peronne TL. Invasive bladder carcinoma: the importance of initial transurethral surgery and other significant prognostic factors for improved survival with full-dose irradiation. Cancer 1987;60:514.
14. Bloom HJG, Hendry WF, Wallace DM, Skeet RG. Treatment of T3 bladder cancer: controlled trial of preoperative radiotherapy and radical cystectomy versus radical radiotherapy. Second report and review. Br J Urol 1982;54:136.
15. Lerman RI, Hutter RV, Whitmore WF Jr. Papilloma of the urinary bladder. Cancer 1970;25:333.
16. Van der Werf Messing B. Preoperative irradiation followed by cystectomy to treat carcinoma of the urinary bladder category T3NX,0-4M0. Int J Radiat Oncol Biol Phys 1979;5:394.
17. Batata MA, Chu FC, Hilaris BS, et al. Factors of prognostic and therapeutic significance in patients with bladder cancer. Int J Radiat Oncol Biol Phys 1981;7:575.
18. Limas C, Lange P, Fraley EE, Vessella RL. A,B,H antigens in transitional cell tumors of the urinary bladder: correlation with the clinical course. Cancer 1979;44:2099.
19. Coon JS, Weinstein RS, Summers JL. Blood group precursor T-antigen expression in human urinary bladder carcinoma. Am J Clin Pathol 1982;77:692.
20. Gustafson H, Tribukait B, Esposti PL. DNA profile and tumour progression in patients with superficial bladder tumours. Urol Res 1982; 10:13.
21. Bretton PR, Herr HW, Kimmel M, Fair WR, Whitmore WF Jr, Melamed MR. Flow cytometry as a predictor of response and progression in patients with superficial bladder cancer treated with bacillus Calmette-Guerin. J Urol 1989;141:1332.
22. Falor WH, Ward RM. Cytogenetic analysis: a potential index for recurrence of early carcinoma of the bladder. J Urol 1976;115:49.
23. Miyao N, Tsai YC, Lerner SP, et al. Role of chromosome 9 in human bladder cancer. Cancer Res 1993;53:4066.
24. Sidransky D, Messing E. Molecular genetics and biochemical mechanisms in bladder cancer. Urol Clin North Am 1992;19:629.
25. Sauter G, Moch H, Moore D, et al. Heterogeneity of *erb*B-2 gene amplification in bladder cancer. Cancer Res 1993;53:2199.
26. Ramaekers F, Huysmans A, Moesker O, Schaart G, Herman C, Vooijs

P. Cytokeratin expression during neoplastic progression of human transitional cell carcinomas as detected by a monoclonal and a polyclonal antibody. Lab Invest 1985;52:31.
27. Neal DE, Marsh C, Bennett MK, et al. Epidermal-growth-factor receptors in human bladder cancer: comparison of invasive and superficial tumours. Lancet 1985;1:366.
28. Seymour GJ, Walsh MD, Levin MR, Strutton G, Gardiner RA. Transferrin receptor expression by human bladder transitional cell carcinoma. Urol Res 1987;15:341.
29. Spruck CH III, Ohneseit PF, Gonzalez-Zulueta M, et al. Two molecular pathways to transitional cell carcinoma of the bladder. Cancer Res 1994;54:784.
30. Bajorin D, Sarkis A, Reuter V, et al. Invasive bladder cancer treated with neoadjuvant MVAC: the relationship of p53 nuclear overexpression with survival. Proc Am Soc Clin Oncol 1994;13:232.
31. Schultz PK, Herr HW, Zhang Z-F, et al. Neoadjuvant chemotherapy for invasive bladder cancer: prognostic factors for survival of patients treated with M-VAC with 5 year follow-up. J Clin Oncol 1994;12:1394.
32. Russell PJ, Brown JL, Grimmond SM, Raghavan D. The molecular biology of urological tumours. Br J Urol 1990;65:121.
33. Brown JL. The clonal analysis of a human bladder cancer cell line. Thesis awarded Doctorate of Philosophy, Faculty of Medicine, University of Sydney, 1990.
34. Brown JL, Russell PJ, Philips J, Wotherspoon J, Raghavan D. Clonal analysis of a bladder cancer cell line: an experimental model of tumour heterogeneity. Br J Cancer 1990;61:369.
35. Raghavan D, Russell PJ, Brown JL. Experimental models of histogenesis and tumor cell heterogeneity. Semin Surg Oncol 1992;8:279.
36. Russell PJ, Wills EJ, Philips J, Raghavan D. Features of squamous and adenocarcinoma in the same cell in a xenografted human transitional cell carcinoma: evidence of a common histogenesis? Urol Res 1988;16:79.
37. Russell PJ, Jelbart M, Wills E, Raghavan D. Establishment and characterization of a new human bladder cancer cell line showing features of squamous and glandular differentiation. Int J Cancer 1988;41:74.
38. Cooling CI. Review of 150 post-mortems of carcinoma of the urinary bladder. In: Wallace DM, ed. Tumours of the bladder. Edinburgh, E & S Livingstone, 1959:171.
39. Babaian RJ, Johnson DE, Llamas L, et al. Metastases from transitional cell carcinoma of the urinary bladder. Urology 1980;16:142.
40. Raghavan D, Chye RWM. Treatment of carcinomatous meningitis from transitional cell carcinoma of the bladder. Br J Urol 1991;67:438.
41. Geller NL, Sternberg CN, Penenberg D, Scher H, Yagoda A. Prognostic factors for survival of patients with advanced urothelial tumors treated with methotrexate, vinblastine, doxorubicin, and cisplatin chemotherapy. Cancer 1991;67:1525.
42. Loehrer PJ, Einhorn LH, Elson PJ, et al. A randomized comparison of cisplatin alone or in combination with methotrexate, vinblastine, and doxorubicin in patients with metastatic urothelial carcinoma: a cooperative group study. J Clin Oncol 1992;10:1066.
43. Juranka PF, Zastawny RL, Ling V. P-glycoprotein: multidrug resistance and a superfamily of membrane-associated transport proteins. FASEB J 1989;3:2583.
44. Goldstein LJ, Galski H, Fojo A, et al. Expression of a multidrug resistance gene in human cancers. J Natl Cancer Inst 1989;81:116.
45. Sugawara I. Expression and functions of P-glycoprotein (mdr-1) in normal and malignant tissues. Acta Pathol Jpn 1990;40:545.
46. Shinohara N, Liebert M, Wedemeyer G, Chang JHC, Grossman HB. Evaluation of multiple drug resistance in human bladder cancer cell lines. J Urol 1993;150:505.
47. Petrylak DP, Scher HI, Reuter V, et al. P-glycoprotein (PGP) expression in invasive and metastatic urothelial tract cancer (UTC). Proc Am Soc Clin Oncol 1992;11:200.
48. Barrand MA, Heppell-Parton AC, Wright KA, Rabbitts PH, Twentyman PR. A 190-kilodalton protein overexpressed in non-P-glycoprotein-containing multidrug-resistant cells and its relationship to the MRP gene. J Natl Cancer Inst 1994;86:110.
49. Dalton WS, Grogan TM, Meltzer PS, et al. Drug resistance in mutiple myeloma and non-Hodgkins lymphoma: detection of P-glycoprotein and potential circumvention by addition of verapamil to chemotherapy. J Clin Oncol 1989;7:415.
50. Palavidis Z. Mechanisms of drug resistance in bladder cancer: the role of P-glycoprotein. Thesis for Master of Science in Medicine, University of New South Wales, Sydney, 1993.
51. Timmer-Bosscha H, Mulder NH, de Vries EGE. Modulation of cis-diamminedichloroplatinum (II) resistance: a review. Br J Cancer 1992;66:227.
52. Hospers GAP, Mulder NH, DeJong B, et al. Characterization of a human small cell lung carcinoma cell line with acquired resistance to cis-diamminedichloroplatinum (II) in vitro. Cancer Res 1988;48:6803.
53. Liebmann JE, Hahn SM, Cook JA, Lipschutz C, Mitchell JB, Kaufman DC. Glutathione depletion by l-buthionine sulfoximine antagonizes taxol cytotoxicity. Cancer Res 1993;53:2066.
54. Pendyala L, Glaves D, Russell PJ, Ciesielski M, Creaven PJ, Raghavan D. Glutathioine (GSH) in human bladder carcinoma cell lines. Proc Am Assoc Cancer Res 1994;35:376.
55. Christen RD, Hom DK, Porter DC, et al. Epidermal growth factor regulates the in vitro sensitivity of human ovarian carcinoma cells to cisplatin. J Clin Invest 1990;86:1632.
56. Fan Z, Masui H, Altas I, Mendelsohn J. Blockade of epidermal growth factor receptor function by bivalent and monovalent fragments of 225 anti-epidermal growth factor receptor monoclonal antibodies. Cancer Res 1993;53:4322.
57. Fan Z, Baselga J, Masui H, Mendelsohn J. Antitumor effect of anti-epidermal growth factor receptor monoclonal antibodies plus cis-diamminedichloroplatinum on well established A-431 cell xenografts. Cancer Res 1993;53:4637.
58. Fritsche M, Haessler C, Brandner G. Induction of nuclear accumulation of the tumor-suppressor protein p53 by DNA-damaging agents. Oncogene 1993;8:307.
59. Lowe SW, Ruley HE, Jacks T, Housman DE. p53-Dependent apoptosis modulates the cytotoxicity of anticancer agents. Cell 1993;74:957.
60. Glaves D, Hitt S, Ciesielski M, Raghavan D. Cisplatin sensitivity does not correlate with p53 expression and apoptosis in human bladder cancer cells. Proc Am Assoc Cancer Res 1995;36:437.
61. Barnes RW, Dick AL, Hadley HL, et al. Survival following transurethral resection of bladder carcinoma. Cancer Res 1977;37:2895.
62. Herr HW. Conservative management of muscle-infiltrating bladder cancer: prospective experience. J Urol 1987;138:1162.
63. Henry K, Miller J, Mori M, et al. Comparison of trans-urethral resection to radical therapies for stage B bladder tumors. J Urol 1988;140:964.
64. Solsona E, Iborra I, Ricos JV, et al. Feasibility of transurethral resection for muscle-infiltrating carcinoma of the bladder: prospective study. J Urol 1992;147:1513.
65. Solsona E, Iborra I, Ricos JV, et al. Feasibility of transurethral resection for muscle-infiltrating carcinoma of the bladder: prospective study after 5 years of minimum follow-up. In: Proceddings of the Société Internationale d'Urologie, Sydney, Australia, 1994. Abstract 217.
66. Sweeney P, Kursh ED, Resnick MI. Partial cystectomy. Urol Clin North Am 1992;19:701.
67. Koiso K, Shipley W, Keuppens F, et al. The status of bladder preserving therapeutic strategies in the management of patients with muscle invasive bladder cancer: proceedings of 4th International Consensus Meeting on Bladder Cancer, Antwerp. Int J Urol 1995;2(Suppl 2):49.
68. Richie JP, Skinner DG, Kaufman JJ. Radical cystectomy for carcinoma of the bladder. 16 years of experience. J Urol 1975;113:186.
69. Richie JP. Radical cystectomy: innovations and results. In: Raghavan D, ed. The management of bladder cancer. London, Edward Arnold, 1988:140.
70. Richie JP. Surgery for invasive bladder cancer. Hematol Oncol Clin North Am 1992;6:129.
71. Pearse HD, Reed RR, Hodges CV. Radical cystectomy for bladder cancer. J Urol 1978;119:216.
72. Skinner DG. Current perspectives in the management of high-grade invasive bladder cancer. Cancer 1980;45(Suppl):1866.
73. Skinner DG, Lieskovsky G. Contemporary cystectomy with pelvic node dissection compared to preoperative radiation therapy plus cystectomy in management of invasive bladder cancer. J Urol 1984;131:1069.
74. Mathur VK, Krahn HP, Ramsey EW. Total cystectomy for bladder cancer. J Urol 1981;125:784.
75. Pagano F, Bassi P, Galetti TP, et al. Results of contemporary radical

cystectomy for invasive bladder cancer: a clinicopathological study with an emphasis on the inadequacy of the tumor, nodes, and metastases classification. J Urol 1991;145:45.

76. Lerner SP, Skinner E, Skinner DG. Radical cystectomy in regionally advanced bladder cancer. Urol Clin North Am 1992;19:713.
77. Lopez-Almanza M, Molina R, Huben RP. Transitional cell carcinoma of the urethra in men after radical cystectomy for bladder cancer: is prophylatic urethrectomy indicated? Br J Urol 1988;61:507.
78. Raghavan D, Huben R. The management of bladder cancer. Curr Probl Cancer 1995;19:5.
79. Gilchrist RK, Merichs JW. Construction of a substitute bladder and urethra. Surg Clin North Am 1956;36:1131.
80. Mitchell ME. Urinary tract diversion and undiversion in the pediatric age group. Surg Clin North Am 1981;61:1147.
81. Thuroff JW, Alken P, Riedmiller H, et al. The Mainz pouch (mixed augmentation ileum and cecum) for bladder augmentation and continent diversion. J Urol 1986;136:17.
82. Rowland RG, Mitchell ME, Bihrle R, et al. Indiana continent urinary reservoir. J Urol 1987;137:1136.
83. Mansson W, Colleen S, Sundin T. Continent caecal reservoir in urinary diversion. Br J Urol 1989;56:359.
84. Kock NG, Nilson AE, Nilsson LO. Urinary diversion via a continent ileal reservoir: clinical results in 12 patients. J Urol 1982;128:469.
85. Skinner DG, Lieskovsky G, Boyd SD. Continent urinary diversion: a 5-1/2 year experience. Ann Surg 1988;208:337.
86. McDougal WS. Mechanics and neurophysiology of intestinal segments as bowel substitutes: an editorial comment. J Urol 1987;138: 1438.
87. Lilien OM, Camey M. 25-year experience with replacement of the human bladder (Camey procedure). J Urol 1984;132;886.
88. Hautmann RE, Egghart G, Grohneberg D, Miller K. The ileal neobladder. J Urol 1988;139:39.
89. Hautmann RE, Miller K, Steiner U, Wenderoth U. The ileal neobladder: 6 years of experience with more than 200 patients. J Urol 1993; 150:40.
90. Walsh PC, Donker PJ. Impotence following radical prostatectomy: insight into etiology and prevention. J Urol 1982;128:492.
91. Parsons JT, Million RR. The role of radiation therapy alone or as an adjunct to surgery in bladder carcinoma. Semin Oncol 1990;17:566.
92. Sauer R, Dunst J, Altendorf-Hofmann A, et al. Radiotherapy with and without cisplatin in bladder cancer. Int J Radiat Oncol Biol Phys 1990; 19:687.
93. Goffinet DR, Schneider MJ, Glatstein EJ, et al. Bladder cancer: results of radiation therapy in 384 patients. Radiology 1975;117:149.
94. Shearer RJ, Chilvers CED, Bloom HJG, et al. Adjuvant chemotherapy in T3 carcinoma of the bladder. A prospective trial: preliminary report. Br J Urol 1988;62:558.
95. Yu WS, Sagerman RH, Chung CT, et al. Bladder carcinoma: experience with radical and preoperative radiotherapy in 421 patients. Cancer, 1985;56:1293.
96. Sell A, Jakobsen A, Norstrom B. Treatment of advanced bladder cancer category T2, T3, T4a. Scand J Urol Nephrol Suppl 1991;138:193.
97. Wallace DMA, Raghavan D, Kelly K, et al. Neo-adjuvant (pre-emptive) cisplatin therapy in invasive transitional cell carcinoma of the bladder. Br J Urol 1991;67:608.
98. Dunst J, Sauer R, Schrott KM, et al. Organ-sparing treatment of advanced bladder cancer: a ten-year experience. Int J Radiat Oncol Biol Phys 1994;30:261.
99. Rozan R, Albuisson E, Donnarieix D, et al. Interstitial iridium-192 for bladder cancer (a multicentric survey of 205 patients). Int J Radiat Oncol 1992;24:469.
100. Raghavan D, Tannock IF. Clinical trials in genitoruinary cancer: what have they achieved? In: Smith PH, ed. Berlin, Springer-Verlag, 1989: 225.
101. Miller LS. Bladder cancer: superiority of pre-operative radiation and cystectomy in clinical stage B2 and C. Cancer 1977;39:973.
102. Miller LS. T3 bladder cancer: the case for higher radiation dosage. Cancer 1980;45:1875.
103. Blackard DE, Byar DP, Veterans Administration Cooperative Urological Research Group. Results of a clinical trial of surgery and radiation in stages II and III carcinoma of the bladder. J Urol 1972;108:875.
104. Mommsen S, Jakobsen A, Sell A. Quality of life in patients with advanced bladder cancer. Scand J Urol Nephrol Suppl 1989;125:115.
105. Lynch WJ, Jenkins BJ, Fowler CG, Hope-Stone HF, Blandy JP. The quality of life after radical radiotherapy for bladder cancer. Br J Urol 1992;70:519.
106. Raghavan D, Grundy R, Greenaway TM, et al. Preemptive (neoadjuvant) chemotherapy prior to radical radiotherapy for fit septuagenarians with bladder cancer: age itself is not a contraindication. Br J Urol 1988;62:154.
107. Raghavan D, Grundy R, Lancaster L. Assessment of quality of life in long-term survivors treated by first-line intravenous cisplatin for invasive bladder cancer. Prog Clin Biol Res 1988;260:625.
108. Whitmore WF Jr. Integrated irradiation and cystectomy for bladder cancer. Br J Urol 1980;52:1.
109. Raghavan D. Review: pre-emptive (neoadjuvant) intravenous chemotherapy for invasive bladder cancer. Br J Urol 1988;61:1.
110. Steel GG. Growth kinetics of tumours. Oxford, Oxford University Press, 1977:5.
111. Goldie J, Coldman AJ. A mathematical model for relating the drug sensitivity of tumors to their spontaneous mutation rate. Cancer Treat Rep 1979;63:1727.
112. Kennedy AK, Teicher BA, Rockwell S, Sartorelli AC. The hypoxic tumor cell: a target for selective cancer chemotherapy. Biochem Pharmacol 1980;29:1.
113. Prout GR Jr, Shipley WU, Kaufman D, et al. Preliminary results in invasive bladder cancer with transurethral resection, neoadjuvant chemotherapy and combined pelvic irradiation plus cisplatin chemotherapy. J Urol 1990;144:1128.
114. Rotman M, Macchia R, Silverstein R, et al. Treatment of advanced bladder cancer with irradiation and concomitant 5-fluorouracil infusion. Cancer 1987;59:710.
115. Russell KJ, Boileau MA, Higano C, et al. Combined 5-fluorouracil and irradiation for transitional cell carcinoma of the urinary bladder. Int J Radiat Oncol Biol Phys 1990;19:693.
116. Coppin C, Gospodarowicz M, Dixon P, et al. Improved local of invasive bladder cancer by concurrent cisplatin and preoperative or radical radiation. Proc Am Soc Clin Oncol 1992;11:198.
117. Kaufman DS, Shipley WU, Griffin PP, et al. Selective bladder preservation by combined modality treatment of invasive bladder cancer. N Engl J Med 1993;329:1377.
118. Houssett M, Maulard C, Chretien Y, et al. Combined radiation and chemotherapy for invasive transitional-cell carcinoma of the bladder: a prospective study. J Clin Oncol 1993;11:2150.
119. Tester W, Porter A, Asbel S, et al. Combined modality program with possible organ preservation for invasive bladder carcinoma: results of RTOG protocol 85-12. Int J Radiat Oncol Biol Phys 1993;25:783.
120. Rintala E, Hannisdahl E, Fossa SD, Hellsten S, Sander S. Neo-adjuvant chemotherapy in bladder cancer: a randomized study, Nordic Cystectomy Trial 1. Scand J Urol Nephrol 1993;27:355.
121. Martinez-Pineiro JA, Martin MG, Arocenta F, et al. Neo-adjuvant cisplatin chemotherapy before radical cystectomy in invasive transitional cell carcinoma of the bladder: a prospective randomized phase III study. J Urol 1995;153:964.
122. Kachnic LA, Shipley WU, Griffin PP, et al. Quality of life assessment in women after combined modality therapy with bladder conservation for invasive cancer. Int J Radiat Oncol Biol Phys 1994;30(Suppl 1): 192. Abstract.
123. Herr HW. Pre-operative irradiation with and without chemotherapy as adjunct to radical cystectomy. Urology 1985;25:127.
124. Raghavan D, Pearson BS, Duval P, et al. Initial intravenous cisplatinum therapy: improved management for high risk bladder cancer? J Urol 1985;133:399.
125. Ghersi D, Stewart LA, Parmar MKB, et al. Does neoadjuvant cisplatin-based chemotherapy improve the survival of patients with locally advanced bladder cancer: a meta-analysis of individual patient data from randomized clinical trials. Br J Urol 1995;75:206.
126. Raghavan D, Boyer M, Rogers J, et al. Initial intravenous cisplatin therapy for invasive bladder cancer: minimum follow-up of 10 years. J Urol 1997 (in press).
127. Khandekar JD, Elson PJ, DeWys WD, Slayton RE, Harris DT. Comparative activity and toxicity of cis-diammine dichloroplatinum (DDP) and a combination of doxorubicin, cyclophosphamide, and DDP in disseminated transitional cell carcinoma of the urinary tract. J Clin Oncol 1985;3:539.
128. Troner M, Birch R, Omura GA, et al. Phase III comparison of cisplatin alone versus cisplatin, doxorubicin and cyclophosphamide in the treat-

ment of bladder (urothelial) cancer: a Southeastern Cancer Study Group trial. J Urol 1987;137:660.
129. Hillcoat BL, Raghavan D, Matthews J, et al. A randomised trial of cisplatin versus cisplatin plus methotrexate in advanced cancer of the urothelial tract. J Clin Oncol 1989;7:706.
130. Harker WG, Meyers FJ, Freiha FS, et al. Cisplatin, methotrexate, and vinblastine (CMV): an effective chemotherapy regimen for metastatic transitional cell carcinoma of the urinary tract. A Northern California Oncology Group Study. J Clin Oncol 1985;3:1463.
131. Sternberg CN, Yagoda A, Scher HI, et al. Preliminary results of M-VAC (methotrexate, vinblastine, doxorubicin and cisplatin) for transitional cell carcinoma of the urothelium. J Urol 1985;133:403.
132. Scher H, Herr H, Sternberg C, et al. Neo-adjuvant chemotherapy for invasive bladder cancer: experience with the M-VAC regimen. Br J Urol 1989;64:250.
133. Zincke H, Sen SE, Hahn RG, Keating JP. Neoadjuvant chemotherapy for locally advanced transitional cell carcinoma of the bladder: do local findings suggest a potential for salvage of the bladder. Mayo Clin Proc 1988;63:16.
134. Paz-Ares L, Paul J, Kaye S. Prognostic factors in bladder cancer after primary M-VAC. J Clin Oncol 1995;13:300.
135. Sternberg CN, Arena MG, Calabresi F, et al. Neoadjuvant M-VAC (methotrexate, vinblastine, doxorubicin, and cisplatin) for infiltrating transitional cell carcinoma of the bladder. Cancer 1993;72:1975.
136. Fossa SD, Harland SJ, Kaye SB, et al. Initial combination chemotherapy with cisplatin, methotrexate, and vinblastine in locally advanced transitional cell carcinoma: response rate and pitfalls. Br J Urol 1992; 70:161.
137. Clyne CAC, Jenkins JD, Smart CJ, Guthrie J, Buchanan RB. A trial of adjuvant chemotherapy for stage T3 bladder tumors. J Urol 1983; 129:736.
138. Richards B, Bastable JRG, Freedman L, et al. Adjuvant chemotherapy with doxorubicin (Adriamycin) and 5-fluorouracil in T3,Nx, Mo bladder cancer treated with radiotherapy. Br J Urol 1983;55:386.
139. Logothetis CJ. Postoperative adjuvant CISCA chemotherapy for high-risk invasive bladder cancer. In: Johnson DE, Logothetis CJ, Von Eschenbach AC, eds. Systemic therapy for genitourinary cancers. Chicago, Year Book, 1989:73.
140. Skinner DG, Daniels JR, Russell CA, et al. The role of adjuvant chemotherapy following cystectomy for invasive bladder cancer: a prospective comparative trial. J Urol 1991;145:459.
141. Stockle M, Meyenburg W, Wellek S, et al. Advanced bladder cancer (stages pT3b, pT4a, pN1 and pN2): improved survival after radical cystectomy and 3 adjuvant cycles of chemotherapy. Results of a controlled prospective study. J Urol 1992;148:302.
142. Freiha FS, Reese J, Torti F. A randomized trial of radical cystectomy versus radical cystectomy plus cisplatin, vinblastine, and methotrexate chemotherapy for muscle invasive bladder cancer. J Urol 1996;155: 495.
143. Droller MJ. Adjuvant chemotherapy following cystectomy for invasive bladder cancer. J Urol 1991;145:465. Editorial.
144. Raghavan D. Adjuvant chemotherapy following cystectomy for invasive bladder cancer. J Urol 1991;145:465. Editorial.
145. Soquet Y. Combined surgery and adjuvant chemotherapy with high dose methotrexate and folinic acid rescue (HDMTX-CF) for infiltrating tumours of the bladder. Br J Urol 1981;53:439.
146. Hall RR, Newling DWW, Ramsden PD, et al. Treatment of invasive bladder cancer by local resection and high dose methotrexate. Br J Urol 1984;56:668.
147. Hall RR, Roberts JT, Marsh MM. Radical transurethral surgery in chemotherapy aiming at bladder preservation. In: Splinter T, Scher HI, eds. Neoadjuvant chemotherapy in invasive bladder cancer. New York, Wiley Liss, 1990:163.
148. Roberts JT, Hall RR. The role of chemotherapy in the treatment of bladder cancer. In: Neal DE, ed. Tumours in urology. London, Springer-Verlag, 1994:80.
149. Moore MJ, O'Sullivan B, Tannock IF. How expert physicians would wish to be treated if they had genitourinary cancer. J Clin Oncol 1988; 6:1736.
150. Moore MJ, O'Sullivan B, Tannock IF. Are treatment strategies of urologic oncologists influenced by the opinions of their colleagues? Br J Cancer 1990;62:988.
151. Raghavan D. Clinician surrogates and equipoise: an analogy to lawyers who represent themselves? Eur J Cancer 1991;27:1072.

Principles and Practice of Genitourinary Oncology, edited by Derek Raghavan, Howard I. Scher, Steven A. Leibel, and Paul H. Lange. Lippincott-Raven Publishers, Philadelphia, © 1997.

CHAPTER 28

Management of Metastatic Bladder Cancer

Patrick J. Loehrer and Pieter H. M. De Mulder

The incidence of bladder cancer is rising in most populations. Its mortality, however, has begun to fall in a number of countries, including the United States, Japan, Australia, and Finland, but not in Europe as a whole. This divergence in some areas between incidence and mortality rate may be the result of improved surveillance, more successful treatment, or both.[1] Only about one in five patients who are diagnosed with bladder cancer are destined to die from this disease because most present with superficial or minimally invasive disease, which is associated with an excellent prognosis with the use of local therapies. For those patients with advanced disease, systemic therapy is warranted. During the past decade, substantial progress has been made in the treatment of patients with advanced disease. This chapter highlights these advances.

Approximately 90% of the carcinomas arising in the bladder are transitional cell carcinoma, with the remaining 5% to 10% consisting of squamous cell carcinoma (6% to 7%) and adenocarcinoma (1% to 2%). These tumors arise in the urothelial lining of the bladder but also in the linings of the renal pelvis, ureter, prostatic ducts, and urethra. Transitional cell carcinoma of the bladder clearly remains the most typical urothelial malignancy reported in most clinical trials, but some treatment trials have included urothelial tumors of nontransitional histology and of primary sites outside the bladder.

The presenting symptom of the vast majority of patients with urothelial carcinoma is hematuria, with or without dysuria. Patients with locally advanced disease may have symptoms of pelvic discomfort or pain, which may lead to sciatica from nerve root entrapment. Flank pain may be observed in patients with tumors originating within the kidney or ureter, but in general, reflects hydronephrosis associated with ureteral outlet obstruction. Patients with urothelial carcinoma arising in the prostatic ducts or urethra present with bladder outlet obstructions that may mimic typical symptoms seen in patients seen with benign prostatic hypertrophy or adenocarcinoma of the prostate. Sites of distant metastases may include liver, bone, lung, and with the improvement of the treatment of metastatic disease, brain.

CHEMOTHERAPY

Numerous single agents have been investigated in patients with advanced carcinoma of the urothelium. Those single agents with activity in 15% or more of patients with advanced urothelial cancer are as follows:

- cisplatin
- methotrexate
- doxorubicin
- vinblastine
- gallium nitrate
- ifosfamide
- piritrexim
- paclitaxel
- 5-fluorouracil
- carboplatin

Originally, cisplatin and methotrexate were felt to be the most active single agents in treating this disease, with other agents such as doxorubicin, vinblastine, 5-fluorouracil, and gallium nitrate also demonstrating activity. Ifosfamide and paclitaxel have since been added to this list of active drugs. Numerous published studies with varying response rates in part reflect the small numbers of patients in each of the respective series.

Cisplatin and Analogs

Cisplatin is thought to be one of the most active drugs in the treatment of advanced bladder cancer. Accumulated data from phase II trials give this drug a 35% response rate in more than 400 patients.[2] These trials included patients treated with dosages ranging from 40 mg/m^2 to 120 mg/m^2 in each treatment cycle. Although no prospective randomized trial evaluated the impact of dose intensity of cisplatin, most investigators have used dosages of 70 mg/m^2 or greater every 3 to 4 weeks. In one study, a direct relation between increasing planned dose and response proportion was suggested for cisplatin. The proportion of responders increased with dosages of up to 35 mg/m^2/week.[3] No data were available above this dose level. The delivered dose of cisplatin in a retrospective analysis in patients treated with MVAC revealed a dose intensity for the first cycle of 14.6 mg/m^2/week, which is on the lower end of the dose-response curve. The initial trial of cisplatin in advanced urothelial carcinoma reported a 50% objective response rate in 24 patients.[4] With further patient entry into this trial, however, the overall response

TABLE 28-1. *Effectiveness of cisplatin in bladder cancer: cooperative group results*

Investigators	Number of patients	Dose (mg/m^2)	Responses (%)
National Bladder Cancer Cooperative Group A, 1983[6]	50	70	10 (20)
Eastern Cooperative Oncology Group, 1985[7]	48	60	8 (17)
Southeastern Cancer Study Group, 1987[8]	45	60	7 (16)
Cooperative Group Study, 1992[9]	120	70	14 (12)
Australian Bladder Cancer Study Group, 1989[10]	55	70	17 (31)
Total	318		56 (17.6)

rate fell to 30% in 56 patients (11% in previously treated patients; 40% in previously untreated patients).[5] Remission duration in these studies ranged from 5 to 8 months, with a median survival time of 30 to 45 weeks for responders.

Perhaps more representative are the results of single-agent cisplatin therapy in prospective randomized trials for patients with advanced disease (Table 28-1).[6–10] In total, a 17% response rate has been observed in 321 patients entered in multiinstitutional trials. In only one of these trials did the response rate for single-agent platinum exceed 20%. The largest of these trials demonstrated only a 12% objective response rate with this drug.

Carboplatin has less nephrotoxicity, neurotoxicity, and ototoxicity than cisplatin, but it is associated with greater myelosuppression. Carboplatin seems to have less single-agent activity than its parent compound, cisplatin. Using dosages of 400 mg/m^2, carboplatin produced only a 10% response rate in 20 previously untreated patients with advanced disease.[11] In a study performed by the Medical Research Council of 48 patients with metastatic disease of whom 30 were chemotherapy naive, only three partial remissions were observed.[12] In another trial using 320 mg/m^2 as a continuous infusion, however, four partial responses in 19 (24%) patients were observed, but these responses were of brief duration.[13] The Eastern Cooperative Oncology Group (ECOG) performed a randomized phase II trial evaluating carboplatin and another platinum analog, iproplatin, with response rates of 14% and 16%, respectively.[14] Bone marrow toxicity, especially thrombocytopenia, was the most prominent side effect. In two patients treated with iproplatin, an allergic reaction consisting of erythema and hypotension was observed. Compiled data of the effectiveness of carboplatin therapy indicate a response rate of 12% (20 of 174 patients; range, 0% to 21%).[11–16] Large prospective randomized trials with direct comparison of carboplatin and cisplatin in advanced bladder cancer have not been performed.

Methotrexate and Analogs

As with cisplatin, early trials with methotrexate suggested a response rate of approximately 30% in patients with advanced disease. In most of the studies performed, dosages of methotrexate range from 30 to 40 mg/m^2 weekly.[2] The dose-response relation has been evaluated by several investigators. Escalated dosages of methotrexate from 50 mg/m^2 to 200 mg/m^2 with Leucovorin rescue have been evaluated. Although a slightly higher objective response rate was reported with increased dosages, the 95% confidence intervals overlap with the lower dosage schedules. No prospective randomized trial has been performed to address this issue. The administration schedule (i.e., weekly versus every other week or longer) has never been formally tested but might be relevant for this drug. A number of methotrexate analogs have been tested. 10-Deaza-aminopterin, a folate analog with a transport mechanism different from that of methotrexate, was evaluated in 14 patients. In three patients, a partial response was seen, but all of these had a history of a prior response to methotrexate.[17] Piritrexim, a lipid-soluble inhibitor of dihydrofolate reductase, was tested in an oral formulation in 33 patients. In 29 evaluable patients, one complete response and 10 partial responses were observed. Myelosuppression was the major side effect.[18] None of these compounds have been used in combination with other active drugs.

Trimetrexate is an antifol analog of methotrexate. In 48 evaluable patients treated with trimetrexate at a dosage of 8 mg/m^2 days 1 through 5 every 3 weeks (with dose modification for renal function), one complete response and seven partial responses were noted, producing an overall response rate of 17%. The primary toxicity was myelosuppression.[19]

Vinca Alkaloids

Data regarding the role of vinca alkaloids in metastatic urothelial carcinoma is sparse. In one study, vinblastine (0.1 to 0.15 mg/kg) produced five partial responses in 28 (18%) evaluable patients, but only nine of these patients were chemotherapy naive.[20] In the latter group of patients, the response rate was 22%. Vincristine has only minimal activity in transitional cell carcinoma. Only one of 23 patients with metastatic disease responded to single-agent vincristine therapy in a trial conducted by the European Organization for the Research and Treatment of Cancer (EORTC).[21] In nine patients with transitional cell carcinoma, four patients had objective responses, two of which were complete responses. Vincristine produced 11 complete and partial responses in 25 patients (44%) with bilharzial bladder cancer.[22]

Doxorubicin and Analogs

Doxorubicin also has modest activity in the treatment of advanced bladder cancer, with response rates of 15% to 20%. Dosages commonly used ranged from 30 to 60 mg/m^2 every 3 weeks. In trials conducted at Memorial Sloan-Kettering Cancer Center (MSKCC), the EORTC, and the Southwest Oncology Group (SWOG), 18 objective responses in 118 (15%) patients have been observed.[23–25] In another trial evaluating dosages of 60 mg/m^2 (or 40 mg/m^2 in patients with prior radiotherapy), no obvious differences were observed between the two treatment arms, with an overall response rate of 15%. In a prospective randomized trial comparing single-agent adriamycin (50 mg/m^2) with cisplatin (50 mg/m^2) plus adriamycin (50 mg/m^2), a significant improvement in the response rate (16 of 37 patients [43%] versus 8 of 41 patients [19%]; $P = .02$) was observed in the combination arm.[26] No differences, however, were noted between the arms with respect to the median duration of response or survival.

In Europe, the anthracyclin derivative epirubicin has been developed because of suggestions that this agent has comparable antitumor activity and less overall toxicity than doxorubicin. Data obtained in tumor types other than bladder cancer show that epirubicin has activity similar to doxorubicin with fewer cardiac and noncardiac toxicities.[27] Phase II data in metastatic bladder cancer are limited. In one multicenter study, an objective response rate was found in 28% of 36 patients (1 complete responder and 9 partial responders). Epirubicin was given at a dose of 100 mg/m^2 every 3 weeks, and this study confirms the activity of this compound in the treatment of this disease.[28] Another new anthracycline with a more favorable toxicity profile, pirarubicin, was tested in 20 patients with metastatic bladder cancer. All previously treated patients (n = 5) progressed. The overall response rate was 10%.[29]

Cyclophosphamide and Ifosfamide

Little modern data exists regarding the role of single-agent cyclophosphamide therapy in the treatment of metastatic bladder cancer. In a review by Yagoda,[30] the response rates ranged from 0% to 50%, with most trials averaging an approximately 20% response rate. In one of the largest phase II trials with cyclophosphamide, only 7% of 26 evaluable patients demonstrated a partial response.[31] The response rates were somewhat higher for patients with bilharzial bladder cancer (4 of 21 patients; 19%).[32]

Ifosfamide, an analog of cyclophosphamide, has an improved therapeutic index over its parent compound in preclinical trials. Few direct comparisons have been made in clinical trials, but at least one trial suggested superiority of ifosfamide over cyclophosphamide in soft tissue sarcomas.[33] In bilharzial bladder cancer, ifosfamide at a dose of 1 g/m^2 on days 1 through 5 failed to produce an objective response in 15 patients.[32] At a higher dosage of 1800 mg/m^2 on days 2 through 5, responses were seen in both bilharzial bladder cancer (4 of 9 patients) and transitional cell histologies (4 of 8 patients).

Recently, ECOG conducted a phase II trial of ifosfamide (7.5 g/m^2 total dose over 2 to 5 days).[34] In 55 previously treated patients, five complete and six partial responses were observed, producing an overall response rate of 20%. This level of activity in previously treated patients is superior to a contemporary series of patients treated with single-agent cisplatin for previously untreated advanced bladder cancer.

Gallium Nitrate

Gallium nitrate is another heavy metal–based compound that has an interesting array of activity. Early trials with this drug demonstrated activity in lymphoma and other tumor types; dose-limiting toxicities were hypocalcemia, nephrotoxicity, and visual disturbances, including blindness. These toxicities limited the therapeutic usage of gallium nitrate to the treatment of malignant hypercalcemia. More recently, infusion therapy over 5 to 7 days has been demonstrated to decrease the incidence and severity of the nephrotoxicity.

In bladder cancer, several phase II trials have been conducted using gallium nitrate, including a trial conducted by SWOG using 700 to 1000 mg/m^2 over 30 minutes with cycles repeated every 3 weeks.[35] Nine of 21 (43%) patients demonstrated an objective response to therapy, but because of severe nephrotoxicity, therapy had to be discontinued in these responding patients. Part of this toxicity was a consequence of prior cisplatin therapy.

In another trial reported by Seligman and Crawford,[36] patients were treated with continuous-infusion gallium nitrate at a dose of 300 mg/m^2 on days 1 through 7. In eight evaluable patients who were previously treated with cisplatin, five of which had also been previously treated with MVAC, four objective responses were observed, and the other four patients had stabilization of disease, reduction of bone pain, or both. Nephrotoxicity, which was limited to two patients, was apparently lessened by this method of continuous infusion.

Seidman and colleagues[37] conducted a much larger phase I/II trial of 40 patients previously treated with MVAC. A dose response (i.e., threshold) was observed when 4 of 17 (17%) patients receiving gallium nitrate at 350 mg/m^2 or greater for 5 or more days by continuous infusion responded to therapy, compared with 0 of 17 patients treated at lower dosages. The most severe toxicity was optic neuropathy, which occurred in 3 of 11 patients who received a dosage of 400 mg/m^2.

Taxanes

The taxanes, paclitaxel and taxotere, display a novel mechanism of action by preferentially binding to microtubules that promote their assembly and stabilization. A phase II trial by ECOG demonstrated marked activity for paclitaxel at a dosage of 250 mg/m^2 every 3 weeks in 26 previously treated patients with advanced transitional carcinoma of the urothelium. Seven complete and four partial responses were observed, producing an overall response rate of 42% (95% confidence interval; 23% and 63%, respectively). The primary toxicities were myelosuppression and mucositis.[38] Although clinical results regarding the activity of taxotere in bladder cancer patients are not yet available, in vitro data suggest high activity in a panel of bladder tumor cell lines, and on a molar basis, taxotere may be more active than paclitaxel.[39]

Combination Regimens

Based on the numerous single agents that have modest activity in advanced urothelial carcinoma, combination chemotherapy was a logical avenue to pursue. In the past two decades, the most commonly used regimens have been cisplatin based. Early trials evaluated cisplatin combined with cyclophosphamide, doxorubicin, or both. Cisplatin plus cyclophosphamide produced objective responses in 28 of 113 (25%) patients from various series that fall well within the confidence intervals for response rates for single-agent cisplatin.[2] The National Bladder Cooperative Group conducted a prospective randomized trial comparing single-agent cisplatin to cisplatin plus cyclophosphamide. Only 20% of patients treated with cisplatin alone demonstrated an objective response, compared with 11% of patients treated with the combination regimen.

When doxorubicin was added to these two drugs (i.e., CAP

or CISCA), slightly higher objective response rates occurred. In 351 patients treated with these three drugs, 51% (range, 43% to 68%) had a complete or partial remission.[2] The Southeastern Cancer Study Group conducted a prospective randomized trial comparing the combination regimen of cisplatin, doxorubicin, and cyclophosphamide to single-agent cisplatin. Of 87 evaluable patients, the response rates of 21% versus 17% in the two arms, respectively, were significantly different.[40]

Cisplatin plus methotrexate combination regimens have also been explored, resulting in response rates of 45% to 50%.[11,41,42] These combinations also produced higher response rates than those observed with historic controls of cisplatin or other single-agent regimens, but with greater toxicity. Because of the toxicity observed in an EORTC study in which methotrexate was given on days 8 and 15, the study was repeated with the same dose of methotrexate given on days 1 and 15. In the first study, a 46% response rate was obtained; in the second, the response rate dropped to 26%. No difference in patient characteristics could be found, suggesting the possible relevance of the scheduling of methotrexate administration. Furthermore, methotrexate excretion is influenced by prior cisplatin therapy; this factor may affect both toxicity and efficacy.[43] A prospective trial reported by Hillcoat and colleagues[44] randomized patients to receive either single-agent cisplatin (n = 55) or cisplatin plus methotrexate (n = 53). Although a slightly higher overall objective response rate was observed for the combination arm (43% versus 33%), this difference was not statistically significant. In addition, the median survival time of approximately 8 months was observed in both treatment arms. It is important to realize that the number of patients treated in this study provided a power of only 80% to detect a difference of 30% (60% versus 30%) in response rate because the trial was not designed as an equivalence study.

Two of the most commonly used combination regimens include cisplatin, methotrexate, and vinblastine (CMV) or these three drugs plus doxorubicin (MVAC). In the Northern California Oncology Group study of a CMV regimen, 26% complete and 26% partial objective response rates were observed.[45] The CMV regimen has never been evaluated in a randomized fashion, which makes true comparisons with other combination therapies such as MVAC difficult.

Investigators at MSKCC devised the MVAC combination regimen, which incorporates those drugs with the highest levels of single-agent activity.[46] This regimen includes methotrexate (30 mg/m^2, days 1, 15, 22), vinblastine (3 mg/m^2, days 2, 15, 22), doxorubicin (30 mg/m^2 day 2), and cisplatin (70 mg/m^2 day 2). In 1983, trials were initiated at MSKCC using this four-drug combination; a 72% objective response rate was achieved in 121 evaluable patients, including a 36% complete response rate. The latter group included patients rendered surgically free of disease following partial remission after chemotherapy. An update of this patient population with a 6-year follow-up demonstrated a median survival time of patients with advanced nodal disease and metastatic disease to be 32.9 months and 12 months, respectively. Although these results from the MVAC combination regimen seemed impressive, it remained uncertain whether results from a single institution would actually translate into improved survival when evaluated on a multiinstitutional scale.

Because of this uncertainty, a prospective randomized intergroup trial was conducted that compared single-agent cisplatin (70 mg/m^2) to the standard MVAC regimen.[9] Of 246 fully evaluable patients entered in this trial, 126 were randomized to single-agent cisplatin, and 120 received the MVAC regimen. As would be anticipated, toxicities were greater in the combination arm and included leukopenia, mucositis, and fever associated with leukopenia. These toxicities prevented full-dose administration of the methotrexate and vinblastine components of the MVAC regimen on days 15 and 22 in approximately 50% of treated patients. Despite this factor, a significant improvement in overall response rate was seen in MVAC compared with single-agent cisplatin (37% versus 12%, respectively; $P < .0001$). Similarly, the progression-free and overall survival rates were superior for the combination regimen.

Another trial also proved the superiority of MVAC over cisplatin, doxorubicin, and cyclophosphamide (CISCA).[47] The overall response rate for MVAC (65%) was statistically significantly greater than the 46% response rate observed with CISCA ($P < .05$). Similarly, the median survival time was higher with MVAC: 48 weeks versus 36 weeks for MVAC and CISCA, respectively ($P = .003$). In total, these two trials support the current usage of MVAC as standard therapy for patients with metastatic carcinoma of the urothelium.[9,47]

In patients with advanced urothelial carcinoma treated with MVAC, a number of characteristics correlate with both response and survival. Those associated with an adverse outcome include low performance status, weight loss during the previous 6 months, or visceral (i.e., hepatic, pulmonary, or osseous) metastasis. When examined with a proportional hazards model, each of these characteristics reach statistical significance. The differences between the response rates of single institutions (e.g., MSKCC, MD Anderson) and the intergroup trial may reflect differences in these characteristics, but the median survival times of 12 to 13 months for patients treated with MVAC are virtually identical in the reported series. For example, patients receiving treatment for local regional adenopathy alone fare better than those with more advanced cancer, and patients with nontransitional carcinoma (e.g., adenocarcinoma, squamous cell carcinoma) respond less frequently and have a shorter survival time, although these factors did not reach statistical significance.[9]

Some investigators have tried to ameliorate the toxicity of MVAC by replacing doxorubicin with epirubicin (MVEC).[48] Only phase II data is available, and indicates activity in the range that might be expected for MVAC. However, nonrandomized trials are inadequate tools to provide comparative data on efficacy and toxicity.

Dose-Escalation Studies

Despite improvements in the overall survival noted with MVAC combination chemotherapy, few patients receive full dosages of chemotherapy without dose modifications or delays because of toxicities. In an analysis of dose intensity in patients treated with MVAC at MSKCC, only modest dose escalations were achieved before reaching dose-limiting toxicities (doxorubicin, 4.5 to 5.1 mg/m^2/week; cisplatin, 12.6 to 14 mg/m^2/week). The principal reason for this is myelosuppression. With the advent of hematopoietic colony–stimulating growth factors, it is logical to evaluate improved methods of drug delivery or perhaps intensified therapy. The feasibility of recombinant humam granulocyte–macrophage colony–stimulating factor (GM-CSF) administration with MVAC was first reported by Gabrilove and colleagues.[49] Data from this study did not include

TABLE 28-2. *Dose intensities of MVAC regimens investigated in vanous studies*

Drug	Sternberg et al, 1989[46]	Moore et al, 1992[51]	Seidman et al, 1993[56]	Loehrer et al, 1994[54]	Logothetis et al, 1990[52]	Logothetis et al, 1992[53]	Sternberg et al, 1993[55]
MTX	1	1.25	1.25	1.66	1.00	1.11	0.83
VBL	1	1.27	1.27	1.66	1.66	0.72	0.83
ADM	1	1.25	1.83–3.33	1.66	2.5	3.33	2.5–2.9
CDDP	1	1.24	1.64–2.35	1.78	1.78	2.37	2.5–2.9

The Memorial Sloan-Kettering Cancer Center MVAC dose, given every 4 weeks, was considered standard.

CDDP, cisplatin; DOX, doxorubicine; MTX, methotrexate; VBL, vinblastine.

results from consecutive cycles of therapy. A study from Japan confirmed the observations of Gabrilove and colleagues.[50] Based on this rationale, several phase I/II trials have been initiated.

Investigators in Toronto treated 21 patients with multiple cycles of MVAC plus rh GM-CSF.[51] Unfortunately, the administration of rh GM-CSF did not have a significant impact on the ability to administer chemotherapy on days 15 and 22. Substantial toxicity related to rh GM-CSF administration including hypotension, syncope, swelling at the injection site, and fatigue. Fewer than one half of the patients received day-15 chemotherapy, and cumulative myelosuppression was noted on successive cycles.

Several other investigators have examined modified MVAC regimens with the goal of increasing dose intensity. When applying the concept of dose escalation, several concerns must be addressed. First, scheduling of the cytotoxic agents is considered of minor relevance for the antitumor efficacy, although this may not be true for methotrexate. The second supposition is that the relative contribution of all drugs is equivalent, implying a similar dose-response curve for all drugs. Furthermore, eventual synergy is excluded as well. As can be seen in Table 28-1, this concept is applied differently in the various studies. In previously treated patients, an escalated MVAC regimen plus rh GM-CSF was evaluated by Logothetis and colleagues.[52] The dosages of doxorubicin (60 mg/m^2), cisplatin (100 mg/m^2), and vinblastine (40 mg/m^2) were increased, whereas the "standard" dose of methotrexate (30 mg/m^2) was maintained. Quite remarkably, 8 of 15 heavily pretreated patients responded to this regimen. These authors continued their efforts in a small randomized trial that compared MVAC with or without rh GM-CSF.[53] Interestingly, the complete response rate (39% versus 16%, respectively) and overall response rate (83% versus 77%, respectively) favored the treatment arm that did not include rh GM-CSF.

ECOG conducted a phase II trial with an escalated MVAC regimen in 35 patients with advanced urothelial carcinoma.[54] The dosages for the component drugs were as follows: methotrexate (40 mg/m^2, days 1, 15, 22), vinblastine (4 mg/m^2, days 2, 15, 22), doxorubicin (40 mg/m^2, day 2), and cisplatin (100 mg/m^2, day 2). G-CSF was administered at a dose of 300 μg on days 4 through 11. Although six complete and 15 partial responses were noted, producing an overall response rate of 60%, eight early deaths also occurred. The median duration of response (4.6 months) and a median survival time (9.4 months) were inferior to those observed in the intergroup trial with MVAC.

These trials seem to exemplify the limitations of further escalation of component drugs within MVAC. In a European study, the dose schedule of MVAC administration was altered in a regimen that cycled every 2 weeks.[55] The relative dose intensity compared with other dose-intensified studies is depicted in Table 28-2. Only cisplatin and doxorubicin were increased in this schedule. In 23 patients treated at two dose levels, a 70.5% overall response rate was observed (7 complete responders and 9 partial responders). The dose-limiting toxicity was thrombocytopenia. Seidman and colleagues[56] at MSKCC performed a phase I/II trial using gradually escalated incremental dosages of drugs within the MVAC combination regimens. They found that only relatively minor dose escalations were achieved before reaching dose-limiting toxicity. This is not surprising because of the overlapping toxicity of the component drugs with respect to mucositis (caused by methotrexate and doxorubicin and to lesser degree, vinblastine), myelosuppression (caused by doxorubicin, vinblastine, and methotrexate), and nephrotoxicity (caused by methotrexate and cisplatin). The phase I/II trials for MVAC do not suggest a major breakthrough in the treatment of advanced bladder cancer; however, any possible eventual advantages cannot be drawn from nonrandomized studies. It is clear from the previously discussed data that escalation of all drugs in the MVAC regimen causes significant toxicity, and only limited dosage escalation is possible. One ongoing randomized trial is evaluating dose escalation of cisplatin and doxorubicin. New combination regimens will probably be more successful using novel drugs with nonoverlapping toxicities than using further variations on dosage with the MVAC regimens.

FUTURE INVESTIGATIONS

Cisplatin has been the cornerstone of systemic therapy for metastatic bladder cancer for more than two decades. The early results of a 35% to 40% response rate for this drug as a single agent has fallen to 15% to 20% in more recent multiinstitutional phase III trials. As mentioned previously, several single-agent drugs appear to be as active or more active than cisplatin. These include gallium nitrate, ifosfamide, gemcitabine*, and piritrexim. Alternative combination chemotherapies that exclude cisplatin have already emerged. Logothetis and colleagues[57] reported a 30% response rate in 30 patients with refractory bladder cancer treated with 5-fluorouracil plus interferon alfa-

* Since this chapter was written, gemcitabine (a fluorinated derivative of cytosine arabinoside) has been shown to have substantial antitumor activity against bladder cancer. A collaborative group from The University of Chicago, the Roswell Park Cancer Institute (Buffalo), and Northwestern University have shown an objective response rate of ≥40% in patients with advanced and metastatic transitional cell carcinoma.

2a. In 28 evaluable patients, including 26 who failed prior CMV or MVAC therapy, a 57% response rate was observed. They are now exploring a combination regimen of 5-fluorouracil, interferon-α, methotrexate, and cisplatin in a phase III trial.[58]

Trials incorporating gallium nitrate are also underway. Investigators at MSKCC are currently conducting a randomized phase II trial of gallium nitrate plus 5-fluorouracil versus MVAC. A pilot trial conducted at Indiana University and Iowa (Einhorn and colleagues, personal communication, August 1995) demonstrated a 67% objective response rate in 27 patients treated with vinblastine, ifosfamide, and gallium nitrate (VIG). This regimen was associated with significant myelosuppression and nephrotoxicity in patients whom the researchers deemed poor risk as a result of prior MVAC chemotherapy, prior nephrectomy, prior radiotherapy, or age older than 70 years. A similar remission rate with lessened toxicity has also been observed in a multiinstitutional phase II trial conducted by ECOG using a modified schedule for patients with poor-risk disease.[59] The impact of this regimen on survival will need to be examined in a trial comparing VIG to the MVAC regimen.

The treatment of advanced urothelial carcinoma has undergone steady progress in the past two decades. It is clear that combination chemotherapy produces a modest but definite improvement in overall survival compared with single-agent therapy. Moreover, several new drugs are being evaluated that suggest opportunities to evaluate novel treatment approaches in this disease. When possible, patients should be entered in these prospective clinical trials.

REFERENCES

1. McCredie M. Bladder and kidney cancers. Cancer Surv 1994;19:343.
2. Yagoda A. Chemotherapy for advanced bladder cancer. In: Yagoda A, ed. Bladder cancer: future directions for treatment. Park Row Publishers, 1986:87.
3. Scher HI, Geller NLO, Curley T, Tao Y. The effect of relative cumulative dose intensity on survival of patients with urothelial cancer treated with M-VAC. J Clin 1993;11:400.
4. Yagoda A, Watson RC, Gonzales-Vitale JC, et al. Cis-dichlorodiammineplatinum II in advanced bladder cancer. Cancer Treat Rep 1976; 60:917.
5. Yagoda A. Phase II trials in patients with urothelial tumors: Memorial Sloan-Kettering Cancer Center. Cancer Chemother Pharmacol 1983; 11:9.
6. Soloway MS, Einstein A, Corder MP, et al. A comparison of cisplatin and cyclophosphamide in advanced urothelial cancer. A National Bladder Cancer Cooperative Group A Study. Cancer 1983;52:767.
7. Khandekar JD, Elson PJ, DeWys WD, et al. Comparative activity and toxicity of cisdiamminedichloroplatinum (DDP) and a combination of doxorubicin, cyclophosphamide and DDP in disseminated transitional cell carcinoma of the urinary tract. J Clin Oncol 1985;3:539.
8. Troner M, Birch R, Omura GA, et al. Phase III comparison of cisplatin alone versus cisplatin, doxorubicin and cyclophosphamide in the treatment of bladder (urothelial) cancer: a Southeastern Cancer Study Group Trial. J Urol 1987;137:660.
9. Loehrer PJ, Einhorn LH, Elson PJ, et al. A randomized comparison of cisplatin alone or in combination with methotrexate, vinblastine, and doxorubicin in patients with metastatic urothelial carcinoma: a Cooperative Group Study. J Clin Oncol 1992;10:1066.
10. Hillcoat BL, Raghavan D, Matthews J, et al. A randomized trial of cisplatin versus cisplatin plus methotrexate in advanced cancer of the urothelial tract. J Clin Oncol 1989;7:706.
11. Oliver RTD, Kwo KHK, Highman WJ, Waxman J. Methotrexate, cisplatin, and carboplatinum as single agents and in combination for metastatic bladder cancer. Br J Urol 1986;58:1.
12. Medical Research Council Working Party on Urological Cancers. A phase II study of carboplatin in metastatic transitional cell carcinoma of the bladder. Eur J Cancer Clin Oncol 1987;23:375.
13. Creekmore SP, Waters WB, Vogelzang NJ, et al. Antitumor activity of 24-hour CBDCA infusions in metastatic transitional cell carcinoma. Proc Am Soc Clin Oncol 1986;5:101.
14. Trump DL, Elson P, Madajewicz S, et al. Randomized phase II evaluation of carboplatin and CHIP in advanced transitional cell carcinoma of the urothelium. J Urol 1990;144:1119.
15. de Wit R, Tesselaar M, Kok TC, et al. Randomized phase II trial of carboplatin and iproplatin in advanced urothelial cancer.
16. Marcuello E, Izquierdo MA, Germ JR, et al. Carboplatin for advanced bladder cancer. Eur J Cancer 1990;26:849.
17. Ahmed T, Yagoda A, Scherr HI, et al. Phase II trial of 10-deazaaminopterin in patients with bladder cancer. Invest New Drugs 1986; 4:171.
18. de Wit, Kaye BS, Roberts JT, et al. Oral piritrexim, an effective treatment for metastatic urothelial cancer. Br J Cancer 1993;67:388.
19. Wittes RS, Elson P, Khandakar J, Trump DL. An Eastern Cooperative Oncology Group phase II trial of trimetrexate in the treatment of advanced urothelial carcinoma. Cancer 1994;73:688.
20. Blumenreich MS, Yagoda A, Natale RB, et al. Phase II trials of vinblastine sulfate for metastatic urothelial tract tumors. Cancer 1982;50:435.
21. Richards R, Newling D, Fossa S, et al. EORTC Genitourinary Tract Cancer Cooperative Group: vincristine in advanced bladder cancer: an EORTC phase II trial. Cancer Treat Rep 1983;67:575.
22. Gad-el-Mawla N, Ziegler J, Hamza R, et al. Phase II chemotherapy trials of 5-FU, cyclophosphamide, ifosfamide and vincristine in carcinoma of the bilharzial bladder. Cancer Treat Rep 1984;68:419.
23. Yagoda A, Watson RC, Whitmore WF, et al. Adriamycin in advanced urinary tract cancer; experience in 42 patients and review of the literature. Cancer 1977;39:279.
24. O'Bryan RM, Baker LH, Gottlieb JE, et al. Dose response evaluation of adriamycin in human neoplasm. Cancer 1977;39:1940.
25. Pavone-Macaluso M, EORTC Genitourinary Tract Cooperative Group A. Single drug chemotherapy of bladder cancer with adriamycin, VM-26, or bleomycin. Eur Urol 1976;2:138.
26. Gagliano R, Levin H, El-Bolkainy MN, et al. Adriamycin versus adriamycin plus cis-dichlorodiammineplatinum (II) in advanced transitional cell bladder carcinoma: a Southwest Oncology Group study. Am J Clin Oncol 1983;6:215.
27. Brown TD, Havlin KA, Koeller JM, et al. New anticancer agents. In: Pinedo HM, Longo DL, Chabner BA, eds. Cancer chemotherapy and biological response modifiers. Annual 11. Amsterdam: Elsevier, 1990: 155.
28. Jones WG, Sokal MP, Ostrowski MJ, Newling DW. A phase II study of epirubicin in advanced transitional cell bladder cancer. Clin Oncol R Coll Radiol 1993;5:25.
29. Mahjoubi M, Kattan J, Ghosn M, et al. Phase II trial of pirarubicin in the treatment of advanced bladder cancer. Invest New Drugs 1992;10: 317.
30. Yagoda A. Chemotherapy of metastatic bladder cancer. Cancer 1980; 45:1879.
31. Yagoda A, Watson RC, Grabstald H, et al. Adriamycin and cyclophosphamide in bladder cancer. Cancer Treat Rep 1977;61:97.
32. Gad-el-Mawla N, Ziegler J, Hamza R, et al. Phase II chemotherapy trials of 5-FU, cyclophosphamide, ifosphamide, and vincristine in carcinoma of the bilharzial bladder. Cancer Treat Rep 1984;68:419.
33. Bramwell VHC, Mouridsen JT, Santozo A, et al. Cyclophosphamide versus ifosfamide: final report of a randomized phase II trial in adult soft tissue sarcoma. Eur J Cancer Clin Oncol 1987;23:311.
34. Witte R, Loehrer P, Dreicer R, et al. Ifosfamide in advanced urothelial carcinoma: an ECOG trial. Proc Am Soc Clin Oncol 1993;12:230.
35. Saiers JH, Baker LH, Costanzi JH, et al. Treatment of metastatic bladder cancer with gallium nitrate. Presented at the Thirteenth International Congress of Chemotherapy. Vienna, Austria, 1983.
36. Seligman PA, Crawford ED. Treatment of advanced transitional cell carcinoma of the bladder with continuous infusion gallium nitrate. J Natl Cancer Inst 1991;83:1582.
37. Seidman AD, Scher HI, Heinemann MH, et al. Continuous infusion gallium nitrate for patients with advanced refractory urothelial tract tumors. Cancer 1991;68:2561.
38. Roth BJ, Dreicer R, Einhorn LH, et al. Significant activity of paclitaxel in advanced transitional-cell carcinoma of the urothelium: a phase II trial of the Eastern Cooperative Oncology Group. J Clin Oncol 1994; 12:2264.
39. Rangel C, Niell H, Miller A, Cox C. Taxol and taxotere in bladder

cancer: in vitro activity and urine stability. Cancer Chemother Pharmacol 1994;33:460.

40. Troner M, Birch R, Omura GA, et al. Phase III comparison of cisplatin alone versus cisplatin, doxorubicin and cyclophosphamide in the treatment of bladder (urothelial) cancer: a Southeastern Cancer Study Group Trial. J Urol 1987;137:660.
41. Stoter G, Splinter TWA, Child JA, et al. Combination chemotherapy with cisplatin and methotrexate in advanced transitional cell cancer of the bladder. J Urol 1987;137:663.
42. Carmichael J, Cornbleet MA, MacDougall RH, et al. Cisplatinum and methotrexate in the treatment of transitional cell carcinoma of the urinary tract. Br J Urol 1985;57:299.
43. Goren MP, Wright RK, Horowitz ME, Meyer WH. Enhancement of methotrexate nephrotoxicity after cisplatin therapy. Cancer 1986;58:2617.
44. Hillcoat BL, Raghavan D, Matthews J, et al. A randomized trial of cisplatin versus cisplatin plus methotrexate in advanced cancer of the urothelial tract. J Clin Oncol 1989;7:706.
45. Harker WG, Meyers FJ, Freiha FS, et al. Cisplatin, methotrexate, and vinblastine (CMV): an effective chemotherapy regimen for metastatic transitional cell carcinoma of the urinary tract: a Northern California Oncology Group study. J Clin Oncol 1985;3:1463.
46. Sternberg CM, Yagoda A, Scher HI, et al. Methotrexate, vinblastine, doxorubicin, and cisplatin for advanced transitional cell carcinoma of the urothelium: efficacy and patterns of response and relapse. Cancer 1989;64:2448.
47. Logothetis CJ, Dexeus FH, Finn L, et al. A prospective randomized trial comparing M-VAC and CISCA chemotherapy for patients with metastatic urothelial tumors. J Clin Oncol 1990;8:1050.
48. Rassweiler J, Ruther U, Bauerle K. Epirubicin combination treatment (M-VEC) in advanced bladder cancer. Urologe 1988;28:25.
49. Gabrilove JL, Jakobowski A, Scher H, et al. Effect of granulocyte colony-stimulating factor on neutropenia and associated morbidity due to chemotherapy for transitional-cell carcinoma of the urothelium. N Engl J Med 1988;318:1414.
50. Akaza H, Kotake T, Miyanaga N, et al. Effect of recombinant human granulocyte colony-stimulating factor in patients receiving methotrexate/vinblastine/doxorubicin/cisplatin for the treatment of transitional cell carcinoma of the urinary tract. Semin Oncol 1994;21:70.
51. Moore MJ, Tannock IF, Iscoe N, et al. A phase II study of methotrexate, vinblastine, doxorubicin and cisplatin (MVAC) + GM-CSF in patients (pts) with advanced transitional cell carcinoma. Proc Am Soc Clin Oncol (Abstract) 1992;11:199.
52. Logothetis CJ, Dexeus FH, Sella A, et al. Escalated therapy for refractory urothelial tumors: methotrexate-vinblastine-doxorubicin-cisplatin plus unglycosylated recombinant human granulocyte-macrophase colony-stimulating factor. J Natl Cancer Inst 1990;82:667.
53. Logothetis CJ, Finn L, Amato R, et al. Escalated (ESC) MVAC ± rh GM-CSF (Schering-Plough) in metastatic transitional cell carcinoma (TCC): preliminary results of a randomized trial. (Abstract) Proc Am Soc Clin Oncol 1992;11:202.
54. Loehrer PJ, Elson P, Dreicer R, et al. Escalated dosages of methotrexate, vinblastine, doxorubicin, and cisplatin plus recombinant human granulocyte colony-stimulating factor in advanced urothelial carcinoma: an Eastern Cooperative Oncology Group trial. J Clin Oncol 1994;12:483.
55. Sternberg CN, de Mulder PHM, van Oosterom AT, et al. Escalated M-VAC chemotherapy and recombinant human granulocyte-macrophage colony stimulating factor (GM-CSF) in patients with advanced urothelial tract tumors. Ann Oncol 1993;4:403.
56. Seidman AD, Scher HI, Gabrilove JL, et al. Dose-intensification of MVAC with recombinant granulocyte colony-stimulating factor as initial therapy in advanced urothelial cancer. J Clin Oncol 1993;11:408.
57. Logothetis CJ, Hossan E, Sella A, et al. Fluorouracil and recombinant human interferon alfa-2a in the treatment of metastatic chemotherapy-refractory urothelial tumors. J Natl Cancer Inst 1991;83:285.
58. Philip P, Galinos E, Robinson E, et al. 5-Fluorouracil, alpha-interferon, cisplatin and methotrexate in patients with transitional cell carcinoma: results of a phase I trial. Proc Am Soc Clin Oncol 1994;13:253.
59. Einhorn LH, Roth BJ, Ansari R, et al. Phase II trial of vinblastine, ifosfamide, and gallium combination chemotherapy in metastatic urothelial carcinoma. J Clin Oncol 1994;12:2271.

Principles and Practice of Genitourinary Oncology, edited by Derek Raghavan, Howard I. Scher, Steven A. Leibel, and Paul H. Lange. Lippincott-Raven Publishers, Philadelphia, © 1997.

CHAPTER 29

Management of Bladder Cancer in the Elderly

Eila Skinner, Derek Raghavan, Susan Kim, and Donald G. Skinner

INTRODUCTION

Bladder cancer is predominantly a disease of aged populations in Western society, with most patients being aged 60 years or greater. In the community, the median age of presentation is 65 to 70 years of age, and in clinical trials, the median age of registered patients is in the range of 60 to 65 years.[1–3] In this context, the management of this cancer is governed particularly by the constraints imposed by the pathophysiology of the elderly, especially because the genesis of bladder cancer is heavily associated with cigarette smoking and industrial exposure, both of which cause significant intercurrent medical disorders in this population.[4]

The traditional view has been that treatment by radiation, surgery, or chemotherapy must necessarily be compromised in the elderly patient with bladder cancer. However, increasing experience in the management of these patients has shown this philosophy to be incorrect in most cases, especially in the context of the growing awareness of physical fitness among and improvements in medical care for the elderly.[4]

PATHOPHYSIOLOGY OF AGING AND OF CANCER IN THE AGED

A detailed discussion of the pathophysiology of aging is beyond the scope of this chapter, and has been reviewed elsewhere.[4,5] Nevertheless, a brief overview is necessary to set the discussion regarding management of bladder cancer in the elderly into a context.

Age-related changes in the physiology of patients over the age of 70 may alter their tolerance to cancer and to the requirements of relevant treatment programs. There is a progressive reduction of physiologic reserves, with a general decline in the ability of the aging body to respond to physiological and pharmacological stresses.[6]

Specific age-related changes occur in different bodily functions. For example, cardiac output decreases by approximately 1% each year from the mid-twenties, with a consequent reduction in perfusion of the liver, kidneys, lungs, and gastrointestinal tract.[7] In patients with bladder cancer, a smoking-related disorder, cardiovascular function can be further impaired.[1] Pulmonary function is also affected by aging. There is a reduction in pulmonary compliance, as well as alveolar septal loss and a reduction in pulmonary diffusing capacity;[8] these changes will be exacerbated in patients with a history of smoking.

Age-related changes in renal pathophysiology include a reduction in weight, number of functioning nephrons, cortical volume, renal blood flow, and glomerular filtration rate.[9,10] Of particular importance when defining drug dosage, creatinine clearance may be an unreliable marker of renal function in the elderly patient; because there is less lean muscle mass, there is a concomitant reduction in creatinine clearance. Furthermore, patients with chronic analgesic nephropathy, usually predicated on excess ingestion of phenacetin, have an increased risk of urothelial malignancy[11]; such patients certainly comprise a subset of patients treated in clinical trials of bladder cancer management.[1]

Neurologic function also alters with aging, primarily due to a loss of functioning neuronal tissue. Changes in cognitive and behavioral function have been demonstrated in the central nervous system, accompanied by reductions in peripheral nerve function. These can be compounded by changes in cardiorespiratory function as noted above, as well as by intercurrent disorders, such as diabetes, alcoholism, and a range of iatrogenic situations.

In the gastrointestinal tract, changes in function with advancing age include: impaired peristalsis, slowed gastric emptying,[12] reduction in hepatic blood flow and liver mass, with unpredictable changes in hepatic function.[10] Gastrointestinal changes are frequently compounded by the ingestion of antacids, analgesics, laxatives, or by the reduction in cardiac output associated with aging. Similarly, bone marrow involutes progressively with increasing age and there is an apparent reduction in stem cell function.[13] In addition, a reduction in peripheral lymphocyte count, which may contribute to changes in immune function, has also been recorded with aging.[14] A wide range of other changes in the pathophysiology of the healthy body occur with aging,[4,5] and these may be compounded in the elderly patient with intercurrent diseases.

These issues must be taken into consideration when planning treatment for the patient with bladder cancer, whether the program will involve surgery, radiation, chemotherapy, or combinations of each of these. Although the otherwise healthy elderly patient may tolerate active treatment programs without undue difficulty, consideration must be given to the possibility of reduced tolerance to stress or to the alterations in drug metabolism outlined above.

The other relevant issue is whether bladder cancer behaves differently in elderly populations. For example, it has been reported that bladder cancer is more advanced at presentation among the elderly in large epidemiologic series.[15,16] Similarly, in some surgical series, bladder cancer is more advanced at first presentation among elderly patients,[17,18] although this may simply reflect delayed presentation due to social factors (poverty, fear, delayed diagnosis). Nevertheless, Blandy and colleagues[17] did report a 12% 5-year survival rate among patients aged 75 to 91 years, compared to 57% for patients younger than 55 years. The reduced apparent cure rates in elderly patients reported in surgical series,[17,18] compared to younger cohorts, may reflect case selection, choice or timing of active management, or a range of other factors. By contrast, at the University of Southern California (USC), where an aggressive management approach has applied in recent years, no difference in 5-year survival was noted in a series of 108 patients, aged 70 years or older, compared with 373 younger patients (52% versus 55%) (Skinner and Skinner, unpublished data, 1994). However, this contrasts somewhat with the initial reported experience, in which patients aged 65 to 69 years had a 3-year disease-free survival of 58%, compared with 39% for patients older than 75 years.[19]

Holmes[16] has reported reduced differentiation of bladder cancer with increasing age, implying increased tumor aggressiveness. In autopsy series, the converse has been reported, with an apparent reduction in metastatic rate among the elderly.[20] If survival is used as the primary index of tumor aggression, outcome can be influenced by many factors, including patient selection, pattern of intercurrent disease, accuracy of death certificate data, and the biases contributing to selection of therapy. The Surveillance, Epidemiology and End Results (SEER) data show a decline in the observed 5-year survival rate for all tumors and stages with increasing age, but the situation changes if deaths from intercurrent disease are excluded.[21]

SURGICAL CONSIDERATIONS

The urologist is involved in the diagnostic evaluation and surgical treatment of elderly patients with bladder cancer. The diagnostic techniques used in the office to determine the cause of hematuria or voiding complaints, including intravenous urography, ultrasound, and cystoscopy, are all easily performed on even the most debilitated and aged patient. After a bladder tumor is diagnosed, the management of the very elderly patient is more of a challenge.

Transurethral resection (TUR) is usually required to establish the histologic and staging criteria necessary for making further treatment decisions. A complete TUR is also the only treatment necessary for solitary, low-grade, superficial lesions (grade 1 or 2, stage Ta). TUR can be safely performed under spinal or epidural anesthesia, and apart from the general medical considerations for this type of anesthesia, no increase in surgical complications should be encountered in older patients. In fact, most simple elective procedures can be performed safely in elderly patients, provided that care is taken to manage their specific physiological problems.[22,23]

TABLE 29-1. *Indications for radical cystectomy*

1. Muscle invasive transitional cell carcinoma (TCC) of any grade
2. High grade TCC or carcinoma in situ refractory to intravesical therapy
3. Squamous cell or adenocarcinoma of the bladder
4. Low grade superficial TCC not controlled by transurethral resection and intravesical pharmacotherapy (rare)

Similarly, intravesical therapies (see Chap. 26), including bacillus Calmette-Guerin vaccine (BCG), thiotepa, mitomycin C, and doxorubicin, are all quite well tolerated in the elderly patient without specific age-related problems. The indications for use of intravesical therapies are identical for older and younger patients.

The management of high-grade, invasive cancer in elderly patients is much more difficult. When left untreated or undertreated, the tumor rapidly progresses, and death, from metastatic disease, occurs within 2 to 3 years. Few patients with metastatic bladder cancer die of intercurrent illness rather than the cancer itself. Furthermore, there may also be considerable morbidity from the primary tumor itself if the bladder is left in situ, including hemorrhage, pain, and urinary tract obstruction. Because of these factors, elderly patients with localized disease who are thought to have a 1 to 2 year life expectancy are best treated with an aggressive surgical approach, provided that anesthesiologic and medical considerations permit such an approach.[19,24]

The indications for radical cystectomy are listed in Table 29-1. Most patients undergo cystectomy for muscle-invasive, high-grade transitional cell carcinoma (TCC) or refractory carcinoma in situ (CIS). The surgical technique has been described elsewhere.[25] Meticulous lymph node dissection adds little to the surgery in the way of morbidity, but does contribute significant staging information and is curative for up to 20% of patients with microscopic nodal disease.[26] At USC, a complete bilateral pelvic lymph node dissection is routinely performed at the time of cystectomy.

Although partial cystectomy has been portrayed as an attractive alternative in a frail patient, the results are often disappointing. Tumor spillage is inevitable during partial cystectomy, and thus pelvic recurrence is a significant concern. More importantly, partial cystectomy does not address the multifocal nature of bladder cancer, and thus 40% to 70% of patients treated in this fashion have recurrences in the retained bladder segment.[27] At USC, partial cystectomy is reserved for the rare patient with squamous cell carcinoma or adenocarcinoma of the dome, or a tumor in an isolated bladder diverticulum.

The key to successful major surgery in the elderly patient is a team approach, including anesthesiologists and intensive care specialists with experience in the management of the elderly surgical patient. A short but effective 1-day antibiotic and mechanical bowel preparation with intravenous hydration the night before surgery minimizes potential electrolyte imbalance. Prophylactic use of digitalis is applied routinely at USC in all patients over 65 years of age. The fluid shifts attendant with major pelvic surgery are not well-tolerated by elderly patients with impaired renal and cardiac function, and invasive cardiopulmonary monitoring is very helpful during the perioperative period.

Controlled hypotensive anesthesia minimizes blood loss but must be applied very carefully in the patient with significant coronary or cerebrovascular disease. Prophylaxis against venous thrombosis is crucial because pulmonary embolism is one of the most common causes of operative mortality with this operation. At USC, postoperative anticoagulation with warfarin sulfate is used routinely until the patient is fully ambulatory. Of great importance, nutritional status must be monitored carefully, and parenteral or enteral supplementation is used as needed to avoid a prolonged catabolic state.

Surgical mortality from radical cystectomy in elderly patients ranges from 3% to 6% in modern series, compared to 1% to 3% in younger patients—a modest increase considering the range of intercurrent medical disorders present in most elderly patients. Reported complication rates are also somewhat higher in older patients, ranging from 30% to 50%.[19,24,28,29]

Preoperative medical problems do not always predict postoperative complications. Although 26 patients in the early USC series had preexisting cardiac disease, only 8 of them had postoperative cardiopulmonary complications, most of which were minor arrhythmias.[19] A total of 141 patients aged 75 years or older have now been treated at USC by radical cystectomy or anterior exenteration. Sixty-nine of them were aged 80 years or older. The male to female ratio was 2 : 1, compared to approximately 5 : 1 for younger patients. The operative mortality rate was 3%, and the early complication rate 32%, with an average hospital stay of only 14 days.

Continent urinary diversion has become a widely accepted alternative to the ileal conduit in many parts of the world. However, a bias persists in many centers, where this option is offered only to younger patients. At USC, continent diversion has been performed in 84 patients aged 75 years and older, including 41 cutaneous Kock pouches, 41 Kock neobladders, and two ileoanal reservoirs. There was no difference in the early complication rate for these patients compared with those who had ileal conduits. This finding has been confirmed by several other groups performing continent diversion who have not routinely excluded older patients.[30,31]

The orthotopic neobladder is also a viable alternative for older men, and it is being assessed for women as well. AT USC, Kock pouch neobladders have been constructed in 41 males with bladder cancer, aged 75 years or older, including 8 older than 80 years of age. Continence seems to be achieved more slowly in the elderly, but most attain satisfactory results regardless of age.

For patients severely debilitated by intercurrent medical diseases, such as cardiac dysfunction, chronic airflow limitation or cirrhosis, a high operative mortality may be unavoidable. In these patients, treatment with radiotherapy or combined chemotherapy and irradiation may offer a useful alternative. However, patients should not be discouraged from surgical consideration based purely on age criteria. For example, many patients referred to the Department of Urologic Surgery at USC for consideration of salvage cystectomy for pelvic relapse, 1 to 2 years after radiotherapy, had been advised against surgery at their initial presentation because they were "too old."

RADIOTHERAPY FOR BLADDER CANCER IN THE ELDERLY

There has been considerable debate regarding the optimal treatment of invasive bladder cancer, and whether radical radiotherapy yields equivalent outcomes to radical surgery.[32] In the United States, there has been a clear bias in the selection of patients for radiotherapy, with the emphasis being on its use in patients of more advanced age, especially those deemed medically unsuitable for radical cystectomy. By contrast, in Great Britain and in some regions in Europe, more equivalent age distributions have been reported, reflecting a greater predelection for the use of radiotherapy as a standard treatment for bladder cancer.

Radiation therapy has been applied to the treatment of bladder cancer in several ways (see Chap. 27), including external beam therapy alone in a definitive or palliative setting, as preoperative or postoperative adjuvant therapy, sequentially or concurrently with chemotherapy, as interstitial brachytherapy, and as intraoperative radiation therapy. Initial complete response rates with radiotherapy alone have ranged from 40% to 50%. However, 30% to 50% of patients subsequently relapse locally, yielding an ultimate local control rate of only 25% to 30%.[33–36]

The application of radiotherapy to the treatment of bladder cancer in elderly patients requires meticulous preparation.[37] A balance must be achieved between the optimal dosage required for tumor control and the potential for iatrogenic morbidity. Several factors must be considered: the altered potential for normal tissue toxicity; the difficulty of treating an elderly patient experiencing borderline dementia or confusion in the isolation of a radiation treatment room; and the potential physical difficulties for the unfit patient undergoing planning and treatment, including the need for the patient to assume a prone position for treatment (particularly difficult for patients with severe airways disease or arthritis).

Once a patient is deemed eligible for radiation therapy, a treatment technique must be defined; many are feasible for elderly patients. Initially, simulation or treatment planning is performed to define the treatment volume. The patient is placed in either a supine or prone position, depending upon the preferred treatment technique. A 4-field box, 3-field technique with wedges, rotational arcs or even parallel opposed fields with high energy x-rays are acceptable, depending upon dose homogeneity. A Foley catheter is inserted and 30 mL of contrast medium and 10 mL of air are placed into the bladder. A rectal tube, with or without barium, is inserted to localize the rectum. At Roswell Park Cancer Institute, locoregional lymphatics, including the external and internal iliac chains, are included in the initial target volume, with a superior border at the L5-S1 region or the sacroiliac joints and the lateral border 1.5 cm beyond the pelvic brim. The inferior margin is placed at the ischial tuberosity if the bladder neck or prostatic urethra are involved, but otherwise at the obturator foramen. At 45 Gy to 50 Gy, the treatment fields are reduced to include only the tumor encompassed by a 1.5–2.0 cm margin of normal tissue. The large pelvic fields are treated while the patient has an empty bladder to ensure that the entire bladder is included, but with the boost volume, the treatment may be delivered with the bladder full to ensure that only the tumor volume with margin receives the additional treatment. The total recommended dose ranges from 64.8 Gy to 68.4 Gy, with fraction sizes of 1.8 Gy to 2.0 Gy. For elderly patients unable to tolerate a large treatment volume, it may be necessary to restrict treatment to the bladder only with a small margin, the justification being that isolated regional failure is an uncommon occurrence. If radical doses of radiotherapy are contraindicated, a typical palliative schedule can be employed, for example, 30 Gy in 10 fractions, using anterior-posterior/posterior-anterior fields. If the patient cannot tolerate 2 weeks of consecutive daily radiation treatments, single-fraction high-dose treatments (6.0 Gy to 10 Gy) delivered each month for 3 to 4 doses may be another option.

Several factors which may contraindicate definitive radiation therapy in any patient should also be considered in the elderly population. For example, patients who already have compromised bladder function due to contracture probably will not benefit, and will often deteriorate, after radiotherapy. Palliative irradiation may also be more appropriate for patients with T4 tumors, tumor size greater than 7 cm, and tumors with significant ulceration, because definitive treatment in these settings is associated with poor survival and greater morbidity.[34] In addition, patients with inflammatory bowel disease and those who have previously undergone extensive pelvic or bowel surgery may have prohibitive side effects when high radiation doses are administered.

Even in the otherwise healthy elderly patient, morbidity rates from radiotherapy can be significant. Acute side effects include diarrhea and cystitis; these can be controlled with conservative measures, such as the use of antispasmodics and antidiarrheals, as well as a change to a low-residue diet. Some patients will complain of nausea, and others will suffer nonspecific problems, such as severe fatigue or lethargy, and occasionally anorexia.

Long-term side effects such as bladder contraction, hemorrhagic cystitis, bowel obstruction, or gastrointestinal hemorrhage, have been recorded in as many as 14% of cases,[34] although the rate has been lower in series with lower fraction sizes, and more sophisticated treatment planning and more stringent case selection.[38–40] Similarly, treatment-related mortality, as high as 1.2%,[34] may be reduced by decreasing the daily fraction size, improvements in treatment planning, and by case selection.

Consideration of the use of radiation therapy in the elderly is complicated somewhat by the lack of consensus regarding the prognostic implication of advanced age on the outcome of radiotherapy for bladder cancer.[33–36,41] For example, in the Edinburgh series, 917 patients with T1 to T4 TCC were treated definitively with radiation alone; 44 were aged 79 years or older. A dose of 55 Gy to 57.5 Gy was delivered in 20 fractions, using a 10 cm by 10 cm field size over 4 weeks.[34] A complete response was achieved in 45% of patients, but approximately 50% relapsed locally, and only 30% were alive at 5 years. When analyzed by age, the survival rate for patients younger than 65 years was about 50%, compared to less than 30% for those aged 70 to 79 years, and only 11.6% for patients older than 79 years. Even when the series was corrected for intercurrent disease, the most elderly patients suffered the poorest outcomes. Similarly, at the London Hospital, where 704 patients with T1 to T4 tumors were treated with radical radiotherapy, only 12% of patients aged 75 years or older were alive at 5 years.[17] However, in this series, patients only received doses less than 50 Gy.

Because age has not been an independent prognostic factor in other studies,[35,42] it may be that dose modifications might have been the basis of impaired outcomes in the series from Edinburgh and London, especially since a dose of less than 55 Gy has been reported as an important adverse prognostic determinant.[40] Other prognostic determinants for response to irradiation, such as T stage, grade, size, presence of ureteral obstruction, anemia, and prior transurethral resection, have been identified,[35,36,42,43] but do not consistently appear to be associated with advanced age per se.

CHEMOTHERAPY

One important application of cytotoxic chemotherapy is in the context of intravesical administration for treatment of superficial bladder cancer, or as prophylaxis after transurethral resection (see Chap. 26). However, there are no major age-related issues in the latter context, apart from the fact that the elderly male patient may have an enlarged prostate, making repeated urinary catherization more difficult, or may have greater problems with the retention of intravesical solutions for the requisite period of 1 to 3 hours.

There are two major situations in which systemic cytotoxic chemotherapy is employed for elderly patients with bladder cancer, and in both instances, considerable data are available regarding the age-related issues that arise: (1) the initial management of invasive disease as part of a program of multimodality treatment (neo-adjuvant, concurrent, or classical adjuvant chemotherapy); and (2) the treatment of metastatic or locoregionally relapsed bladder cancer.

Many of the physiologic and pathologic changes associated with the aging process may alter the pharmacology of cytotoxic agents, influencing such parameters as gastrointestinal absorption, renal or hepatic excretion, drug distribution, and dose-response relationships.[4] It is important to note that the elderly have a greater propensity to receive multiple medications,[44] are at risk for poor compliance with complicated schedules of oral medication, and have increased potential for adverse drug interactions.

There is considerable controversy about whether the toxicity of chemotherapy is increased in the elderly. It appears that this varies both with the disease being treated and the nature of the treatment. Although early data suggested that methotrexate and bleomycin cause greater side effects in aged patients,[45,46] studies from the Eastern Cooperative Oncology Group have shown that toxicity in the elderly is a function of the agent and the dose employed, rather than being attributable specifically to age.[47] These studies confirmed the age-related toxicity of methotrexate, but did not show similar effects for doxorubicin, cyclophosphamide, the vinca alkaloids or mitomycin. Furthermore, cisplatin toxicity is not age-related.[48,49]

Several metabolic functions may be influenced by the underlying disease and its etiology. In the case of bladder cancer, with a strong smoking-related etiology, the cardiac toxicity of doxorubicin and the pulmonary side effects of mitomycin may be unpredictable; similarly, with the potential for renal dysfunction associated with bladder cancer, the toxicity of methotrexate or cisplatin can be severe. Attention to dosage, the use of folinic acid rescue, and meticulous use of hydration schedules are key.

There has been disagreement with regard to dose reductions in elderly patients, with the consequent reduction in dose intensity. Although data have been published for a range of malignancies, as reviewed previously,[4,23] little information is available regarding the issue of dose modification in the treatment of bladder cancer in elderly populations. Scher and coworkers[50] analyzed retrospectively their experience with dosing of the MVAC regimen in the full Memorial Sloan-Kettering Cancer

Institute series of 132 cases, and compared outcomes for patients treated with full-dose therapy, including all day 15 and day 22 booster injections, versus the situation when boosters were omitted. In this study, there was no evidence of impaired survival in the group receiving dose reductions, although the numbers of cases in each group were relatively small, and a small survival difference could have been neglected. This suggests that there may be little benefit in emphasizing dose intensity, at least in the more aged subgroup of such patients.

Invasive Bladder Cancer

The role of systemic chemotherapy for invasive, clinically nonmetastatic bladder cancer is discussed in Chapter 28. Although most of the published data with respect to the integration of systemic cytotoxics into combined modality strategies for invasive bladder cancer have reported patients of all age groups, a few published reports have addressed specifically the use of chemotherapy for the management of invasive bladder cancer in elderly populations. For example, as part of a broader study of patients treated with single-agent cisplatin (100 mg/m^2 IV) as neoadjuvant therapy before definitive radiotherapy or cystectomy, we assessed the impact of this strategy in the treatment of patients aged 70 to 79 years.[49] Although they had a broad range of smoking-related disorders, characteristic of elderly patients with bladder cancer, subjectively and objectively, these patients tolerated the treatment program remarkably well, and 33% survived 3 years or longer (Table 29-2). These observations were tested further in a randomized trial in Great Britain and Australia, comparing cisplatin plus radiotherapy versus radiotherapy alone.[51] Although no significant survival benefit was shown from the use of neoadjuvant cisplatin, it was clear that age was not an independent adverse prognostic determinant. Similarly, Shearer and colleagues[52] showed that single-agent methotrexate did not confer an improved survival when used as neoadjuvant therapy, but also confirmed that age was not an independent prognosticator of survival. However, they did demonstrate that advance age was associated with greater methotrexate-related toxicity.

Combination chemotherapy has also been used without excessive toxicity in the treatment of elderly patients with invasive bladder cancer, although the specific age-related toxicities have not always been dissected out for the older patients.[53,54] Sella

TABLE 29-2. *Neoadjuvant cisplatin for septuagenarians with locally advanced bladder cancer*

Sex	Age	ECOG performance status	Other disorders	Stage	Grade	Acute toxicity	Objective response (CR or PR)	Survival (Months)
F	71	0	Uterine fibroids	T3	III	NV grade 2	Yes	35
M	76	0	—	T4a	III	NV grade 2	Yes	63+
F	72	1	Hypertension, cataracts	T3	III	NV grade 3, renal grade 2, high tone deafness, dehydration	No	6
M	70	0	NIDDM, AAA, old TB	T3	III	NV grade 2, diarrhea grade 2	Yes	50+
M	78	0	—	T3	III	NV grade 2, renal grade 2	Yes	8
M	70	0	Hypertension, inguinal hernias	T3	III	NV grade 2, renal grade 2	Yes	13
M	79	0	Atrial-fibrillation, CCF	T4a	III	NV grade 2, confusion, incontinence	Yes	13
M	71	0	—	T2+	III	NV grade 2, diarrhea	Yes	36
M	70	0	COAD, right inguinal hernia, essential tremor	T2	III	NV, neutropenia grade 1	Yes	48+
M	71	0–1	Peptic ulcer disease, renal calculi, thromboasthenia	T2	III	NV grade 3, neutropenia grade 2, dehydration	Yes	22
M	75	0	Glaucoma	T2+	III	NV grade 2	Yes	36+
M	70	1	Hypertension, COAD, renal calculi	T3	III	NV grade 3	Yes	17
F	76	0	Hypertension, atrial fibrillation	T2+	II	NV grade 3, atrial fibrillation, femoral embolus	Yes	14
M	77	0	Esophageal stricture, reflux, renal calculi, ischemic heart disease	T4a	III	Sedation, neutropenia grade 1	Yes	14
F	70	0	Varicose veins	T3	III	NV grade 2–3	Yes	29

AAA, abdominal aortic aneurysm; CCF, congestive cardiac failure; COAD, chronic obstructive airways disease; ECOG, Eastern Cooperative Oncology Group; NIDDM, non—insulin-dependent diabetes mellitus; NV, nausea and vomiting; TB, tuberculosis; T2+, at least stage 2.

From Raghavan D. Management of advanced bladder cancer in the elderly. Urol Clin North Amer 1992;19:797.

TABLE 29-3. *Age as prognostic factor in patients treated with chemotherapy for advanced bladder cancer*

Age (years)					
Median	Range	No. of patients	Regimen	Age as adverse prognostic factor	Reference
62	23–77	132	M-VAC	No	57
66	30–79	126	M-VAC	No	3
64	35–82	120	C	No	3
65	35–75	55	C	?	2
63	40–74	53	MC	?	2
78	76–84	36	M-VAC, CMV, CyAC	No?	55
71	70–79	15	C & RT	No	49

A, doxorubicin (Adriamycin); C, cisplatin; Cy, cyclophosphamide; M, methotrexate; RT, radiotherapy; V, vinblastine.

From Raghavan D. Management of advanced bladder cancer in the elderly. Urol Clin North Amer 1992;19:797.

and coworkers[55] treated 18 patients with high-grade, locally extensive bladder cancer, aged 75 years or older, using cisplatin-based combination therapy after control of the primary tumor. These patients were carefully selected on the basis of good performance status and renal function. Nevertheless, more than 20% withdrew from therapy because of toxicity, and 33% had significant infectious complications. The median survival of this group, despite the aggressive therapy, was only 23 months, not greatly different from the figures obtained from series of patients treated with single agent cisplatin or methotrexate as neoadjuvant therapy.[49,52] In addition, it should not be forgotten that randomized trials have not yet proven the role of neoadjuvant or classical adjuvant chemotherapy in this context (see Chap. 27). Of interest, a study of the role of adjuvant chemotherapy with cisplatin, doxorubicin and cyclophosphamide at the University of Southern California, which has caused some controversy in interpretation, demonstrated that patients aged more than 65 years constituted a subgroup with a better outcome, irrespective of the use of chemotherapy.[56] This observation will bear further study.

Recurrent and Metastatic Disease

The management of recurrent invasive bladder cancer or metastatic disease constitutes a complex problem, irrespective of the age of the patient, and median survival times are usually less than 3 years, irrespective of the age of the patient.[32] Radiotherapy or salvage cystectomy will occasionally yield long-term survivors, but the relative lack of success in the treatment of younger patients has led to significant nihilism in the management of older patients. In addition, most trials of chemotherapy for metastatic or recurrent disease have yielded median survival times of only 12 to 18 months, with 5-year survival rates of only 10% to 20%.[32]

Few studies have specifically addressed the role of chemotherapy for aged patients with metastatic bladder cancer (Table 29-3). In a retrospective study of prognostic factors among the patients treated with the combination of methotrexate, vinblastine, doxorobucin, and cisplatin (MVAC) for metastatic bladder cancer at Memorial Sloan-Kettering Cancer Center, Geller and colleagues[57] showed improved survival among patient aged 60 years or older. Using the Cox proportional hazards model, normal alkaline phosphatase, high Karnofsky performance status, and age of 60 years or more were shown to predict improved survival. However, the possibility that selection factors could have influenced outcome was not excluded.

Similarly, in an international randomized trial carried out by the Eastern Cooperative Oncology Group, Southwest Oncology Group, National Cancer Institute of Canada and Australian Bladder Cancer Study Group, we showed equivalent survival figures among the elderly patients and younger cohorts.[3] In this study, the first to demonstrate a survival benefit from MVAC chemotherapy compared to single agents, nearly 45% of the 269 patients were 64 years or older.[3]

Sella and coworkers[55] reported 18 patients, aged 76 years or older, with metastatic bladder cancer, who received a range of cisplatin-containing combination regimens, including MVAC. Seven patients (39%) had objective responses, including two with complete remissions. However, the median survival in this study was only 10 months, the treatment was clearly toxic, and dose intensity was not predictive of outcome. In this context, one could question whether such intensive treatment was appropriate for metastatic bladder cancer in this elderly population group.

SUMMARY

Patients in their eighth decade are becoming an increasingly important group numerically in the practice of uro-oncology, and it will be necessary to develop more sophisticated and flexible approaches for their management. Provided that care is taken to plan for their altered physiologic requirements, it is clear that comparable (or better) outcomes can be anticipated from well-designed treatment programs that involve surgery, radiation or chemotherapy, applied as single modalities or in combination. Given the potential for successful outcomes of treatment, we must place greater emphasis on educating the elderly about the symptoms of bladder cancer, encouraging them to present as early as possible, thus facilitating the best possible results of treatment. Advanced age alone should not preclude the provision of active and effective strategies of treatment.

REFERENCES

1. Raghavan D, Pearson B, Duval P, et al. Initial intravenous cisplatinum therapy: improved management for high risk bladder cancer? J Urol 1985;133:399.
2. Hillcoat BL, Raghavan D, Matthews J, et al. A randomised trial of cisplatin versus cisplatin plus methotrexate in advanced cancer of the urothelial tract. J Clin Oncol 1989;7:706.

3. Loehrer PJ, Sr, Einhorn LH, Elson PJ, et al. A randomized comparison of cisplatin alone or in combination with methotrexate, vinblastine and doxorubicin in patients with metastatic urothelial carcioma: a cooperative group study. J Clin Oncol 1992;10:1066.
4. Raghavan D, Findlay M, McNeil E. Cancer in the elderly. In: Peckham MJ, Pindedo H, Veronesi U (eds). Oxford Textbook of Oncology, Oxford, Oxford University Press, 1995;2169.
5. Crawford J, Cohen HJ. Relationship of cancer and aging. Clin Geriatr Med 1987;3:419.
6. Leventhal EA. The dilemma of cancer in the elderly. In: Vaeth JM, Meyer J (eds). Cancer and the Elderly. Basel, S. Karger, 1986;1.
7. Bender AD. The effects of increasing age on the distribution of peripheral blood flow in man. J Am Geriatr Soc 1965;13:192.
8. Brandsteller RD, Kazemi H. Aging and the respiratory system. Med Clin North Am 1983;67:419.
9. Hollenberg NK, Adams DF, Solomon HS, et al. Senescence and the renal vasculature in normal man. Circ Res 1974;34:309.
10. Greenblatt DJ, Sellers EM, Shader RI. Drug disposition in old age. N Engl J Med 1982;306:1081.
11. McCredie M, Stewart JH, Ford JM, et al. Phenacetin-containing analgesics and cancer of the bladder or renal pelvis in women. Br J Urol 1983;55:220.
12. Evans MA, Triggs EJ, Cheung M, et al. Gastric emptying rate in the elderly: implications for drug therapy. J Am Geriatr Soc 1981;29:201.
13. Lipschitz DA, Udupa KB. Age and the hematopoietic system. J Am Geriatr Soc 1986;34:448.
14. Bender BS, Nagel JE, Adler WH, et al. Absolute peripheral blood lymphocyte count and subsequent mortality of elderly men. J Am Geriatr Soc 1986;34:649.
15. Goodwin JS, Samet JM, Key CR, et al. Stage at diagnosis of cancer varies with the age of the patient. J Am Geriatr Soc 1986;34:20.
16. Holmes FF. Clinical evidence for a change in tumor aggressiveness with age. Semin Oncol 1989;16:34.
17. Blandy JP, England HR, Evans SJW, et al. T3 bladder cancer: the case for salvage cystectomy. Br J Urol 1980;52:506.
18. Thrasher HB, Frazier HA, Robertson JE, Dodge RK, Paulson DF. Clinical variables which serve as predictors of cancer-specific survival among patients treated with radical cystectomy for transitional cell carcinoma of the bladder and prostate. Cancer 1994;73:1926.
19. Skinner EC, Lieskovsky G, Skinner DG. Radical cystectomy in the elderly patient. J Urol 1984;131:1065.
20. Suen KC, Lau LL, Yermakov V. Cancer and old age: an autopsy study of 3,535 patients over 65 years old. Cancer 1974;33:1164.
21. Ries LG, Pollack ES, Young JL. Cancer patient survival: surveillance, epidemiology, and end results. J Natl Cancer Inst 1983;70:693.
22. Patterson WB. Surgical issues in geriatric oncology. Semin Oncol 1989; 16:57.
23. Raghavan D. Management of advanced bladder cancer in the elderly. Urol Clin North Amer 1992;19:797.
24. Leibovich I, Avigad I, Ben-Chaim J, Nativ O, Goldwasser B. Is it justified to avoid radical cystoprostatectomy in elderly patients with invasive transitional cell carcinoma of the bladder? Cancer 1993;71: 3098.
25. Skinner DG. Technique of radical cystectomy. Urol Clin North Amer 1981;8:353.
26. Lerner SP, Skinner DG, Lieskovsky G, et al. The rationale for en bloc pelvic lymph node dissection for bladder cancer patients with nodal metastases: long-term resuls. J Urol 1993;149:758.
27. Sweeney P, Kursh ED, Resnick MI. Partial cystectomy. Urol Clin North Amer 1992;19:701.
28. Drago JR, Rohner TJ, Jr. Cystectomy and urinary diversion: a safe procedure for elderly patients. Urology 1983;21:17.
29. Wood DP, Jr. Radical cystectomy for carcinoma of the bladder in the elderly patient. J Urol 1987;138:46.
30. Navon J, Ahlering T. A comparative study of postoperative complications with modified Indiana pouch in elderly vs. younger patients. J Urol 1994;141:243A.
31. Tannenbaum A, Helal M, Persky L, Binard J, Pow-Sang J, Lockhart J. Continent urinary diversions in the elderly: is it safe? J Urol 1994; 141:242A.
32. Raghavan D, Shipley WU, Garnick MB, et al. Biology and management of bladder cancer. N Engl J Med 1990;322:1129.
33. Bloom HJG, Hendry WF, Wallace DM, et al. Treatment of T3 bladder cancer: controlled trial of preoperative radiotherapy and radical cystectomy versus radical radiotherapy. Second report and review. Br J Urol 1982;54:136.
34. Duncan W, Quilty PM. The results of a series of 963 patients with transitional cell carcinoma of the bladder primarily treated by radical megavoltage X-ray therapy. Radiother Oncol 1986;7:299.
35. Gospodarowicz MK, Hawkins NV, Rawlings GA, et al. Radical radiotherapy for muscle invasive transitional cell carcinoma of the bladder: failure analysis. J Urol 1989;142:1448.
36. Mameghan H, Sandeman TF. The management of invasive bladder cancer: a review of selected Australasian studies in radiotherapy, chemotherapy and cystectomy. Aust NZ J Surg 1991;61:173.
37. Crocker I, Prosnitz L. Radiation therapy of the elderly. Clin Geriatr Med 1987;3:473.
38. Morrison R. The results of treatment of cancer of the bladder—a clinical contribution to radiobiology. Clin Radiol 1975;26:67.
39. Greven K, Solin L, Hanks G. Prognostic factors in patients with bladder carcinoma treated with definitive irradiation. Cancer 1990;65:908.
40. Smaaland R, Akslen L, Tonder B, Mehus A. Radical radiation treatment of invasive and locally advanced bladder carcinoma in elderly patients. Br J Urol 1991;67:61.
41. Batata MA, Chu FCH, Hilaris BS, et al. Factors of prognostic and therapeutic significance in patients with bladder cancer. Int J Radiat Oncol Biol Phys 1981;7:575.
42. Shipley WU, Rose M, Perrone T, Mannix C, Heney N, Prout G. Full dose irradiation for patients with invasive bladder carcinoma: clinical and histological factors prognostic of improved survival. J Urol 1985; 134:679.
43. Quilty P, Kerr G, Duncan W. Prognostic indices for bladder cancer: an analysis of patients with transitional cell carcinoma of bladder primarily treated by radical megavoltage X-ray therapy. Radiother Oncol 1986; 7:311.
44. Shaw PG. Common pitfalls in geriatric drug prescribing. Drugs 1982; 23:324.
45. Hansen HH, Selawry OS, Holland JF, et al. The variability of individual tolerance to methotrexate in cancer patients. Br J Cancer 1971;25:298.
46. Ginsberg SL, Comis RL. The pulmonary toxicity of antineoplastic agents. Semin Oncol 1982;9:34.
47. Begg CB, Carbone PP. Clinical trials and drug toxicity in the elderly: the experience of Eastern Cooperative Oncology Group. Cancer 1982; 52:1986.
48. Hrushesky WJ, Shimp W, Kennedy BJ. Lack of age-dependent cisplatin nephrotoxicity. Am J Med 1984;76:579.
49. Raghavan D, Grundy R, Greenaway TM, et al. Preemptive (neo-adjuvant) chemotherapy prior to radical radiotherapy for fit septuagenarians with bladder cancer: age itself is not a contra-indication. Br J Urol 1988;62:154.
50. Scher HI, Geller NL, Curley T, Tao Y. Effect of relative cumulative dose-intensity on survival of patients with urothelial cancer treated with MVAC. J Clin Oncol 1993;11:400.
51. Wallace DMA, Raghavan D, Kelly KA, et al. Neoadjuvant (pre-emptive) cisplatin therapy in invasive transitional cell carcinoma of the bladder. Br J Urol 1991;67:608.
52. Shearer RJ, Chilvers CED, Bloom HJG, et al. Adjuvant chemotherapy in T3 carcinoma of the bladder. A prospective trial: preliminary report. Br J Urol 1988;62:558.
53. Zincke H, Sen SE, Hahn RG, et al. Neoadjuvant chemotherapy for locally advanced transitional cell carcinoma of the bladder: do local findings suggest a potential for salvage of the bladder? Mayo Clin Proc 1988;63:16.
54. Scher HI, Herr H, Sternberg C, et al. Neo-adjuvant chemotherapy for invasive bladder cancer: experience with the M-VAC regimen. Br J Urol 1989;64:250.
55. Sella A, Logothetis CJ, Dexeus FH, et al. Cisplatin combination chemotherapy for elderly patients with urothelial tumours. Br J Urol 1991; 67:603.
56. Skinner DG, Daniels JR, Russell CA, et al. The role of adjuvant chemotherapy following cystectomy for invasive bladder cancer: a prospective comparative trial. J Urol 1991;145:459.
57. Geller NL, Sternberg CN, Penenberg D, et al. Prognostic factors for survival of patients with advanced urothelial tumors treated with methotrexate, vinblastine, doxorubicin, and cisplatin chemotherapy. Cancer 1991;67:1525.

Principles and Practice of Genitourinary Oncology, edited by Derek Raghavan, Howard I. Scher, Steven A. Leibel, and Paul H. Lange. Lippincott-Raven Publishers, Philadelphia, © 1997.

CHAPTER 30

Non–Transitional Cell Bladder Cancer

Cora N. Sternberg and David A. Swanson

The incidence of transitional cell carcinoma (TCC) of the urinary bladder in the United States is second only to that of prostate cancer among genitourinary cancers. It can occur in combination with other histologic types, particularly squamous cell carcinoma (SCC) and adenocarcinoma, but in such cases TCC is almost always predominant. In distinct contrast, pure non-TCC malignancies of the bladder or histologic admixtures that exclude TCC occur infrequently, particularly in the United States and Europe. Optimal treatment for non-TCC malignancies has not yet been defined, at least in part because of the small number of patients and the wide variety of treatment regimens without the benefit of controlled trials. Nonetheless, despite the biologic differences between non-TCC and TCC, which we will try to delineate, it is possible to make recommendations for management of these malignancies using available techniques; however, for some tumors, theses recommendations may reflect only modern oncologic principles and knowledge of what has not been successful in treating these tumors in the past.

SQUAMOUS CELL CARCINOMA

SCC is a malignant epithelial neoplasm with distinct histologic squamous features: squamous pearls, intercellular bridges, and keratohyalin granules. Tumors may be purely SCC, but extensive areas of squamous differentiation can also be found in high-grade invasive TCC. Data from several series have linked SCC and squamous metaplasia, or leukoplakia,[1–5] which refers to replacement of the urothelium by mature stratified squamous epithelium (Table 30-1). The role of squamous metaplasia in the evolution of SCC has not been resolved, but long-term follow-up reveals a 16% to 28% incidence of carcinoma, most often SCC, in patients with vesical leukoplakia.[6,7] It is believed that there are two forms of histogenesis of pure SCC: malignant transformation related to squamous metaplasia of the bladder mucosa and extensive squamous differentiation in a preexisting TCC.[8] Typical squamous metaplasia must not, however, be considered premalignant. Both the squamous metaplasia and the malignancy may be related to an underlying, unidentified, causally related stimulus.[9]

Bilharzial cancer of the bladder, which is seen in the Middle East, differs significantly from the bladder cancer seen in Europe and the United States, primarily in that 75% of bilharzial cancers are pure SCC compared with fewer than 10% of Western, nonbilharzial cancers. Nonbilharzial cancers are distinct variants of SCC, perhaps with distinct etiology and biology, and merit separate discussion.

NONBILHARZIAL SQUAMOUS CELL CARCINOMA

Clinical and Diagnostic Features

In Western populations, the incidence of nonbilharzial SCC is between 3% and 6.7% of all bladder carcinomas.[1,4,10–13] Most studies report a male predominance, ranging from 56% to 65% of cases.[1,10,11,14,15] A few series report a similar female predominance, 58% of 64 patients in three series.[3,16,17] SCC has been reported to occur more frequently in blacks (17.5%) than in whites (5.4%).[18] The mean age at diagnosis for men is slightly lower (64.8 to 65.2 years) than for women (68.2 to 71.7 years).[1,10] Epidemiologists have reported an increased risk of SCC in association with cigarette smoking, with a relative risk of 6.1 among smokers of 40 or more cigarettes per day.[19] Additionally, in patients with a history of three or more urinary tract infections, the relative risk of nonbilharzial SCC was 5.7. Employment as a welder or cook was also associated with an increased risk of SCC. Despite a strong association between oncogenic human papillomaviruses and SCC of the genital tract, these viruses do not appear to play a significant role in squamous cell carcinogenesis of the bladder.[20]

SCC has been associated with exstrophy, defunctionalized bladders, and chronic irritative factors such as parasites, chronic bacterial urinary tract infection, vesical calculi, and chronic outlet obstruction. Foreign bodies have also been implicated, and paraplegic patients with indwelling catheters have a higher incidence of squamous metaplasia and SCC of the urothelium. Kaufman and colleagues[21] reported SCC in six spinal cord injury patients, including four who had no visible tumor endoscopically. There was a 10% incidence in paraplegics who had indwelling catheters for longer than 10 years (average, 21 years).[22] Intermittent self-catheterization may also lead to SCC.[23,24] SCC has been reported in patients with cyclophosphamide-induced hemorrhagic cystitis.[25] One case of SCC occur-

TABLE 30-1. *Stage, histology, treatment and 5-year survival of patients with nonbilharzial squamous cell carcinoma of the bladder*

Investigators	No. of patients	Clinical stage	Invasion presentation (%)	Squamous metaplasia (%)	Treatment	5-Year survival (%)
Daehlin, 1991	13	T3-T4	100	NI	RT, preop RT + cyst	17
Swanson et al, 1990[28]	25	T2-T3	100	NI	Preop RT + cyst	50
Winkler et al, 1989[30]	73*	Tis-T4	93	NI	No, TUR, RT, p cyst, preop RT + p cyst, cyst, preop RT + cyst	32
Quilty and Anen, 1986[35]	35	T3	100	NI	RT	18†
Prempree and Amarnmarry, 1984[33]	15	B_2-C	100	NI	Preop RT + cyst	40
	19	B_2-C	100	NI	RT	16
Rundle et al, 1982[10]	12	T2	100	NI	RT	17
	21	T3	100	NI	RT	5
Faysal, 1981[11]	33	A-C	88	NI	TUR, p cyst, p cyst + RT, RT, cyst, preop RT + cyst	27
Rous, 1978[15]	17	B_1-D	100	NI	No, TUR + RT, RT, p cyst + RT, cyst, cyst + RT	12
Richie et al, 1976[3]	33	B_1-C	100	25	Cyst, preop RT + cyst	48
Johnson et al, 1976[1]	90	B_1-D_2	100	17	No, TUR ± RT, p cyst ± RT, cyst ± RT	11
Johnson et al, 1976[1]	17	B_2-C	100	NI	RT	18
	7	B_2-C	100	NI	Preop RT + cyst	34
Bessette et al, 1974[2]	75	NI	98	17	No, TUR, p cyst, cyst	7
Utz et al, 1973[32]	20	NI	NI	NI	P cyst	35
Sarma, 1970[4]	72	T1-T4	100	‡	No, IRT, RT, p cyst, cyst	25‖
Newman et al, 1968[31]	63	A-D	96	NI	TUR ± RT, p cyst, cyst	15
Sakkas, 1966[201]	47	T1-T4	6	NI	TUR, RT, IRT, p cyst, cyst	NI
Jones et al, 1980[14]	51	T1-T4	100	NI	RT, IRT, preop RT + cyst, RT + p cyst, cyst, RT + salv cyst	16

* Includes N+ and M+ patients.
† Three-year survival rate.
‡ Present but not quantified.
‖ Patients with T3 tumors.
cyst, cystectomy; IRT, interstitial radiotherapy; NI, not indicated; no, no therapy; p cyst, partial cystectomy; preop, preoperative; RT, radiotherapy; salv cyst, salvage cystectomy; TUR, transurethral resection.

ring years after bacillus Calmette-Guérin (BCG) therapy for TCC has been reported.[26]

The most common presenting symptoms of SCC are hematuria and irritative bladder symptoms.[1,2,10] Urinary tract infection is present in as many as 93% of patients at the time of diagnosis.[1] There have been reports of an associated paraneoplastic syndrome with hypercalcemia.[27] SCC is usually an aggressive tumor. Tumors are often bulky and already locally invasive at the time of diagnosis. Distant metastatic disease is generally infrequent, occurring in only 8% to 9% in three series with a total of 190 patients.[10,14,28] A large, solitary neoplasm is typical, and ureteral obstruction is often found at cystoscopy.[1] These tumors can occur at any location in the bladder but most often are seen in the trigone and lateral walls.[10] Histologic analysis reveals squamous pearl formation. An abnormal karyotype determined by chromosome banding has been reported in one case; the abnormalities were similar to those seen in TCC.[29] Nuclear DNA ploidy, measured by flow cytometry, is a potentially important objective prognostic variable in patients with SCC.[30]

Treatment

Because SCC is usually muscle invasive at diagnosis and tends to be large, virtually no tumors are amenable to definitive management by transurethral resection. Treatment options most commonly recommended include partial or radical cystectomy including bilateral pelvic lymph node dissection, with or without preoperative radiotherapy. Radiotherapy alone is used less frequently. Survival varies according to grade and stage of the tumor and treatment, as reported in several series (see Table 30-1).

Partial Cystectomy

Newman and colleagues[31] reviewed 84 patients, of whom 75% were reported to have pure SCC, who underwent transurethral resection with or without radiotherapy, partial cystectomy, or cystectomy. The cumulative 5-year survival rate was 15%. Of those who died, 59% were dead within 1 year of diagnosis. Twenty-five percent of the tumors were not pure SCC. Partial cystectomy in 17 patients produced the best results in this series, with a 44% 5-year survival rate. Both Sarma[4] and Utz and colleagues[32] obtained good results with partial cystectomy in patients with lesions amenable to a conservative approach. Sarma[4] reported a 50% 5-year survival rate in eight patients. Utz and colleagues[32] operated on 24 patients, 2 of whom were lost to follow-up and 2 of whom died in the hospital postoperatively; 7 (35%) of these patients survived at least 5 years.

Radical Cystectomy With or Without Preoperative Irradiation

In the largest series of pure SCC of the bladder treated by radical cystectomy, Richie and colleagues[3] reported a 48% 5-year survival rate in 33 patients that correlated closely with grade of tumor and pathologic stage. Five-year survival was 100% for patients with stage A and B1 (T1 and T2) tumors, 67% for patients with stage B2 (T3a) tumors, 33% for patients with stage C (T3b) tumors, and 20% for patients with stage D tumors; for patients with grade IV SCC, only 28% survived 5 years. Preoperative radiotherapy (15 to 45 cGy) was used in only one third of patients. The authors noted that survival was better with SCC than with each corresponding stage of TCC, but the series was heavily weighted to low-stage patients: stage B1 (T2) in 13 patients, stage B2 (T3a) in 15 patients, and stage C (T3b) in only 5 patients.

Johnson and colleagues[1] reported an overall 5-year survival rate of 11% in 90 patients with SCC, but only 43 had tumors that were no more advanced than stage C (T3b). Of 17 patients who received no therapy, all died within 2 years. Of seven patients with stage B_2 (T3a) and C (T3b) disease who underwent preoperative radiotherapy and cystectomy, survival was 34%. These data were updated in the largest reported series of patients treated with this combined modality and suggest that irradiation before cystectomy may protect against pelvic recurrence.[28] Twenty-five patients with pure T2 and T3 SCC of the bladder were treated with external beam irradiation (50 Gy in 5 weeks in 24 patients, 40 Gy in 4 weeks in one patient) prior to radical cystectomy. The tumors in 10 patients (40%) were downstaged as a result of radiotherapy; 3 of 5 were downstaged from stage T2, 3 of 4 were downstaged from stage T3a, and 4 of 16 were downstaged from stage T3b. Six patients (24%) had no residual tumor (pT0). No patient who was downstaged by radiotherapy had a recurrence or died of tumor, but disease recurred in the pelvis in seven patients who had not been downstaged. Actuarial 5-year survival for all patients was 50%. For those who did not have recurrences, median survival was 87%. Only two patients (8%) had distant metastases in this series, emphasizing the importance of pelvic control in this disease.

Other studies have had similar results in smaller numbers of patients. In one study, preoperative radiotherapy plus cystectomy produced a 40% 5-year survival in 15 patients with stages B_2-C (T3a,b) SCC, whereas radiotherapy alone resulted in only a 16% 5-year survival in 19 patients.[33] In one report, a patient with a massive filling defect shown by excretory urogram and confirmed by cystoscopy to be a large, grade IV SCC was found to have an inoperable mass fixed to the pelvic wall.[34] He underwent ureteroileal urinary diversion and then received 65 Gy of radiation to the pelvis. Subsequent to irradiation, bimanual examination revealed a mobile mass, and he underwent successful cystectomy; he was alive more than 4 years after surgery.

Jones and associates,[14] however, gave irradiation prior to elective cystectomy to only 7 of 25 patients with stage T2 and T3 tumors; none survived beyond 1 year. There were two postoperative deaths in this group.

Radiotherapy

Rundle and colleagues[10] reported 5-year survival rates of only 16.7% for 12 patients with stage T2 tumors and 4.8% in 21 patients with stage T3 tumors after treatment with radical radiotherapy alone. In another study, 3-year survival was 18% in 35 patients with stage T3 tumors treated with irradiation alone.[35]

Chemotherapy

There is no truly effective chemotherapeutic regimen for treatment of SCC of the bladder; however, apart from isolated case reports, few trials have been published, all of which had extremely small patient numbers.[36–42] Patterson and colleagues[36] treated five patients who had invasive SCC with the Nigro regimen (i.e., preoperative mitomycin and 5-fluorouracil combined with external beam radiotherapy) based on its successful use in treating those with SCC of the anal canal or esophagus. Two patients underwent a subsequent partial cystectomy, and one had a transurethral biopsy of the bladder. No residual tumor was seen in these three patients, and none had clinical evidence of tumor after 18 to 48 months. The Medical Research Council in England is currently evaluating the cisplatin-methotrexate-vinblastine (CMV) regimen for the treatment of SCC of the bladder.[43] However, in a recent Intergroup study comparing the combination of methotrexate, vinblastine, doxorubicin (Adriamycin), and cisplatin (MVAC) with cisplatin alone, there was a low response rate to either regimen in patients with non–transitional cell bladder cancers.[44]

It appears that SCC of the bladder is chemotherapeutically resistant but moderately radiosensitive. The natural history predicts a high risk for pelvic relapse, but the risk of distant metastasis appears to be lower than that for TCC of the bladder. Therefore, cystectomy alone or radiotherapy followed by cystectomy is the treatment of choice for this disease. Partial cystectomy may substitute for cystectomy only in the rare and highly selected patient who has a small lesion amenable to complete extirpation with generous (≥2 cm) margins of normal bladder. There is no proven role for neoadjuvant or adjuvant chemotherapy in this disease, except, perhaps, as part of a protocol.

Annual screening for SCC of the bladder should be performed in spinal cord injury patients. If hematuria is found, patients should undergo cystoscopy and bladder biopsy, even if no tumor is seen.

BILHARZIAL SQUAMOUS CELL CARCINOMA

Clinical and Diagnostic Features

The incidence of SCC is much higher in the Middle East than in Western populations because of the prevalence of endemic schistosomiasis in the former. Bilharzial SCC is most frequently found in men, with a 4 : 1 to 5 : 1 ratio, because of their exposure while working in the fields. The histology of this tumor is typically 75% SCC, 20% TCC, and 5% adenocarcinoma or undifferentiated.[45] Bilharzial SCC is usually a well differentiated tumor. It occurs at a younger age than does SCC in Europe and the United States; the mean age at diagnosis is 47 years.[46] In Egypt, carcinoma of the bladder is the most common solid tumor in adults, responsible for 28% of all cancers in Cairo.[45] SCC of the bladder is also common in Iraq, Yemen, Saudi Arabia, and several African countries. Squamous metaplasia and dysplasia are extremely common in bladders with bilharzial infestation.[47] Chronic bacterial infection has been implicated in the production of nitrosamines, which are potent carcinogens. Mechanical irritation of the urothelium by the erupting bilharzial eggs may encourage tumor growth, although other etiologic factors may also be important.[48]

Patients most often present with symptoms of cystitis, frequency, and painful urination; they commonly pass keratinized fragments of necrotic tissue. The symptoms of bilharzial cystitis and malignant cystitis are often confused. In both cases, the bladder, distal ureters, and occasionally seminal vesicles may be outlined by calcium on x-ray films. However, in patients who have developed bladder carcinoma, the radiographs may show interruption of this regular outline by irregular calcific densities.[45] The stage of disease is usually advanced at presentation; 25% of cases are inoperable when the diagnosis is made. Tumors are most often nodular and fungating and occupy the vault (i.e., dome) or posterior or lateral walls of the bladder; however, multicentric lesions are present in 22% of patients, and squamous metaplasia is found in 65%.[47,49] Lymphatic spread is delayed as a result of fibrosis.[50] The frequency of lymph node metastasis is low. After radical cystectomy, lymph nodes are positive in only about 17% of patients.[51] The rate of distant metastasis is low (~3%); bilharzial SCC of the urinary bladder may therefore have a better prognosis than other types of bladder cancer. The low incidence of metastatic disease may be the result of the characteristically low grade of these tumors, although nonbilharzial SCC also has a low rate of distant metastasis (~8%).

The immunologic response of the host appears to play an important role in bilharzial SCC.[52] Patients with schistosomiasis of the bladder have a variety of immunologic abnormalities, including the presence of HLA-DR+ and interleukin-2 receptor-positive T lymphocytes in circulating blood.[53] In one study, DNA was studied by flow cytometric analysis in 46 patients with bilharzial bladder cancer. The most significant prognostic indicators were the DNA index and the status of the pelvic lymph nodes at operation. Diploid tumors had a low metastatic potential (7.7%) and an associated 5-year patient survival of 54% in contrast to aneuploid tumors, which had a high metastatic potential (45.5%) and an associated 5-year patient survival of only 21%.[54] Skin testing with 2,4-dinitrochlorobenzene as a measure of cell-mediated immunity may predict clinical outcome.[52] Loss of suppressor genes may also play an important role in SCC of the bilharzial bladder. In an Egyptian study, mutation of the *P53* suppressor gene was detected in six of seven bladder cancers.[55]

Treatment

Partial Cystectomy

Partial resection is feasible only when there is a small, solitary tumor that does not involve the trigone, thereby permitting an adequate surgical margin. The remainder of the bladder must be free of associated carcinoma in situ or metaplasia. In a 1975 series, El-Hammady and colleagues[56] reported that only 19 (10%) of 190 patients were eligible for partial cystectomy. Augmentation cystoplasty was required in five of these patients. Five-year survival was 27%. Patients with low-grade tumors survived twice as long as those with high-grade tumors. In 1969, Omar[57] reported less favorable results in 14 of 22 patients available for follow-up. Thirteen (59%) had a recurrence within 2 years. Patient selection almost certainly accounts for the different results among these studies.

Radical Cystectomy With or Without Preoperative Irradiation

As in the case of nonbilharzial SCC, radical cystectomy plus bilateral lymphadenectomy is usually required for local control of these locally invasive tumors. In a series of 138 cases, Ghoneim and colleagues[58] reported a postoperative mortality rate of 14%, primarily as a result of peritonitis and intestinal obstruction. Five-year survival was related to tumor stage and grade. Survival was 43% for patients with pT1 and pT2 tumors, compared with 30% for patients with pT3 and pT4 disease. Patients with low-grade tumors had a 46% 5-year survival, compared with 21% for high-grade tumors. Patients with positive lymph nodes had only a 20% 5-year survival rate. Most treatment failures were manifested by local recurrence in the pelvis within 2 years after cystectomy. For this reason, Ghoneim and colleagues[51] considered whether radiotherapy should be added to radical cystectomy.

Because most treatment failures after radical cystectomy were the result of local recurrence, several Egyptian surgeons began to use preoperative radiotherapy. Awaad and colleagues[59] compared cystectomy alone to cystectomy after preoperative 40-Gy irradiation. The reported 2-year disease-free survival rate was better for irradiated patients (53% ± 9% versus 19% ± 10%). A prospective randomized trial in 92 patients compared 20-Gy irradiation prior to cystectomy with cystectomy alone.[60] With follow-up of 60 months, irradiated patients appeared to survive longer; however, the difference was not statistically significant and was limited to patients with high-grade and high-stage tumors. In another randomized study, the addition of the radiosensitizer misonidazole did not improve results.[61] Improvement in survival seen in later trials appears to be due to elimination of postoperative morbidity and mortality when compared to earlier trials.

Chemotherapy

In a series of phase II studies at the National Cancer Institute, Cairo, 10 drugs induced overall response rates between 18% and 60%: epidoxorubicin (60%), vindesine (41%), vincristine (44%), ifosfamide (40%), hexamethylmelamine (38%), etoposide (36%), pentamethylmelamine (32%), cyclophosphamide (19%), and dibromodulcitol (18%; Table 30-2).[62] Chemotherapy appeared to be more efficacious in metastatic than in local lesions.

A randomized study evaluating neoadjuvant epirubicin in patients with T2-T3 SCC was conducted in Egypt.[63] Seventy-one

TABLE 30-2. *Chemotherapy in bilharzial squamous cell carcinoma of the bladder*

Drug	Number of patients: Evaluable	CR	PR	CR + PR	MR	SD	PD
Bleomycin	21	0	0	0 (0%)	2	6	13
Doxorubicin	27	0	0	0 (0%)	2	4	21
Tenoposide	26	0	1	1 (4%)	2	6	17
5-Fluorouracil	32	0	2	2 (6%)	3	17	10
Methotrexate	14	0	1	1 (7%)	0	2	11
Cisplatin	18	1	2	3 (16%)	0	3	12
Dibromodulcitol	22	1	3	4 (18%)	0	6	12
Cyclophosphamide	21	1	3	4 (19%)	2	9	6
Pentamethylmelamine	25	1	7	8 (32%)	2	9	6
Etoposide	19	0	7	7 (36%)	3	5	4
Mexamethylmelamine	26	0	10	10 (38%)	12	0	4
Ifosfamide	20	0	8	8 (40%)	2	2	8
Vincristine	25	2	9	11 (44%)	0	8	6
Vindesine	32	3	10	13 (41%)	0	9	10
Epidoxorubicin							
Every wk	18	0	9	9 (50%)	0	7	2
Every 3 wk	18	0	11	11 (60%)	0	7	0
Neoadjuvant	21		20	20 (95%)*			

* Twenty of 21 patients with squamous cell carcinoma treated neoadjuvantly and adjuvantly had grade 1-3 "chemotherapeutic" effects.[63]

CR, complete response; MR, minor response; PD, progressive disease; PR, partial response; SD, stable disease.

Adapted from Gad-el-Mawla N, Hamza R, Zikri Z, et al. Chemotherapy in invasive carcinoma of the bladder: a review of phase II trials in Egypt. Acta Oncol 1989;28(1):73.

patients with T2-T3 bladder cancer were randomized to receive either two courses of epirubicin (120 mg/m^2 every 21 days) preoperatively and four additional courses after radical cystectomy or radical cystectomy alone. In the neoadjuvant chemotherapy arm, necrosis was found in 95% of patients with SCC and in 57% of patients with TCC. The estimated disease-free survival rates for epirubicin-treated patients versus cystectomy-alone patients were 74% and 38%, respectively. Thus, epirubicin may be useful in the treatment of bilharzial bladder cancer.

Conclusions

Radical cystectomy with urinary diversion is the treatment of choice for patients with bilharzial SCC. It appears that patients with high-grade, high-stage bilharzial cancer may benefit from preoperative radiotherapy. The role of chemotherapy has not been definitively established, although it does appear that this disease is more sensitive to chemotherapy than is nonbilharzial pure squamous carcinoma.

VERRUCOUS CARCINOMA

Clinical and Diagnostic Features

Verrucous carcinoma (VC) is an extremely rare variant of SCC, characterized by a locally invasive, warty, exophytic gross appearance. VC invades underlying tissues with a pushing margin, has a slow growth rate, and has a low incidence of lymph node and distant metastases. VC also occurs in the penis, cervix, and vagina.[64] VC of the bladder is almost always associated with schistosomal cystitis. In the series of El Sebai's and colleagues[65] consisting of 655 bladder cancer cases, 483 were SCC, and only 22 (3.4%) were considered VC. In the series of El Bolkainy and colleagues[48] consisting of 1095 bladder cancer patients, 902 had schistosomiasis, 798 had SCC, and 33 (3%) had VC. Only a few cases of VC not associated with schistosomiasis have been reported in North America and Denmark. These tumors probably have a different epidemiology and may be associated with condyloma acuminata.[66–69] Most investigators consider Buschke-Löwenstein tumor, described as a giant condyloma, to be the same as VC.[70]

Treatment

Partial and Radical Cystectomy

Standard treatment of VC is complete surgical excision by radical cystectomy, unless adequate surgical margins are possible with partial cystectomy. Because of the low incidence of lymph node metastases, lymph node dissection may be confined to the immediately adjacent lymph node groups.[64] In the series of El Bolkainy and colleagues,[48] all patients were treated with radical cystectomy and lymph node dissection. None had lymphatic or visceral metastases.

Radiotherapy

Some investigators believe that radiotherapy may be contraindicated in the treatment of VC.[64] In a literature review,

Demian and colleagues[71] reported anaplastic transformation of the typically low-grade VC within 6 months of radiotherapy in 33 of 111 patients (30%). However, other authors have observed that the risk of transformation is substantially less than is generally believed.[72] Because the possibility of an adverse effect of radiotherapy in these patients remains controversial, and because the value of radiotherapy has not been demonstrated in this low-grade malignancy, its routine use should be avoided in this patient population.

Prognosis

Because VC is typically a low-grade tumor with low incidence of lymph node or other metastases, the prognosis is excellent. Complete surgical removal should be curative. However, in one series of 37 cases of histologically proven VC of the bilharzial bladder, 22 (59%) showed at least focal transformation to invasive SCC.[73] Sixteen were stage P2 or P3 tumors, and six were P4 tumors, three of which had spread to the lymph nodes. Among patients with invasive disease, the 5-year survival rate was 27%, but 10 patients died of locally recurrent or metastatic disease, and one patient was alive with disease. Even in the noninvasive group, one patient died of recurrent disease.

ADENOCARCINOMA

Clinical and Diagnostic Features

Primary adenocarcinoma of the bladder is the third most frequent type of bladder carcinoma after TCC and SCC. It comprises from 0.5% to 2% of all epithelial malignant bladder tumors[74,75] and is the most common type of cancer arising in patients with bladder exstrophy.[76] Adenocarcinoma may arise in bladder diverticula and occurs most frequently in areas of endemic schistosomiasis[76–79]; it may also occur after long-term catheterization.[80] In the literature, patients range in age from 6 to 92 years, with a peak frequency in the sixth decade. About 70% of reported cases occur in males. The presenting symptoms are not specific for adenocarcinoma. Most patients have gross hematuria with or without dysuria.[73] In one study, based on small patient numbers, coffee intake was associated with adenocarcinoma.[19]

Primary vesical adenocarcinomas are most frequently single lesions with a predilection for the trigone and bladder dome. These lesions are muscle invasive at presentation; only rarely are superficial lesions reported.[80–83] The lesions may be extensive, but most are localized and smaller than 5 cm.[84] Adenocarcinoma may originate in urachal remnants or the bladder itself[85]; urachal carcinoma should be suspected if adenocarcinoma in the dome or the anterior wall is mostly intramural and has deep ramifications in the bladder wall. Some authors have suggested that the urachus is a modified part of the urinary bladder and not a separate organ.[79] The urothelium of the urachus differs somewhat from that of the bladder; thus, urachal carcinoma is discussed in Chapter 31.

It is important to recognize direct extension of an extravesical tumor through the bladder wall and metastases from a distant adenocarcinoma, both of which are more common than primary adenocarcinoma of the bladder. Adenocarcinomas that originate in the kidney, prostate, colon, uterus, ovary, stomach, pancreas, breast, thyroid, or lung may involve the bladder.[86–93] Although prostate-specific antigen (PSA) is usually very useful in diagnosing prostatic adenocarcinomas metastatic to the bladder, prostatic acid phosphatase may not be; some primary bladder adenocarcinomas stain positively for prostatic acid phosphatase.[94] One group did report focal positive staining for PSA with a polyclonal antibody in 4 of 25 patients (1 male, 3 females) in whom urachal remnants had been obtained at autopsy.[95] Another group also found immunoreactivity to a polyclonal PSA antibody in 3 of 22 cases of adenocarcinoma of the bladder (7 urachal, 15 nonurachal) but no reactivity to a monoclonal PSA antibody.[96] Immunohistochemical evaluation of adenocarcinomas of the bladder with both prostatic acid phosphatase and PSA permit accurate diagnosis because most prostatic adenocarcinomas, but not primary bladder adenocarcinomas, are positive for both[94,96] (Chap. 17).

Adenocarcinoma of the bladder may occur in pure form, in combination with TCC or SCC, or as the epithelial component of a carcinosarcoma.[97–99] Tumors may appear ulcerative, papillary, or nodular. In a group of patients who underwent cystectomy, most had invasion of the bladder, and 17% to 81% of the tumors were at least pathologic stage C (T3b).[9] The histologic pattern of vesical adenocarcinomas may be glandular not otherwise specified (NOS), colonic, papillary, mucinous (colloid), signet-ring cell (linitis plastica), or mesonephric (clear cell) types, in order of decreasing frequency.[9] These patterns are described briefly in the following section.

The prevailing theory of pathogenesis is that adenocarcinomas of the urinary bladder arise from urothelium that retains the potential to undergo metaplastic change to a mucinous and glandular epithelium after stimulation by chronic irritation[97] (Chap. 17).Cystitis and cystitis cystica have been found in 10% to 50% of patients in several series, and some reports have described progression of cystitis glandularis associated with vesical adenocarcinoma.[100–103] Progressive invagination of hyperplastic epithelial buds into the lamina propria (i.e., von Brunn's nests) forms cystitis cystica, which may by further metaplasia develop mucin-producing cells to form an associated entity, cystitis glandularis.[104] Another pattern of metaplasia may result in cuboidal or columnar cells without downward invagination. Table 30-3 lists the series in which metaplasia was indicated to be present in the histologic specimen. Pelvic lipomatosis may also be associated with adenocarcinomas.[105,106]

Pure forms of the various histologic subtypes occur, but mixtures of two or more are common.[79] The most common pure patterns are colonic and glandular NOS. Most adenocarcinomas are mucin-producing, but only rarely is mucus passed while voiding. In glandular or glandular papillary adenocarcinoma this mucin production may be minimal, but in mucinous (i.e., colloid) adenocarcinomas there may be lakes or pools of mucin in which the tumor cells appear to be floating. Mucin-containing goblet cells are predominant in these lesions.[85,107,108] Anderström and colleagues[79] included pure colloid tumors in their purely differentiated group, which had worse survival rates than groups of patients with moderately or well differentiated tumors.

The signet-ring pattern is an unusual variant of adenocarcinoma. It is distinctive but rarely occurs in pure form. Its apparent aggressive course may be the result of silent local progression and delayed diagnosis.[82] There are about 50 cases reported

TABLE 30-3. *Stage, histology, treatment and 5-year survival of patients with nonurachal adenocarcinoma of the bladder*

Investigators	No. of patients	Clinical stage	Invasion at presentation (%)	Metaplasia (%)	Treatment	5-Year survival (%)
Burnett et al, 1991[202]	9	NI	NI	44 (G)	Cyst, RT, preop RT + cyst	50
Wilson et al, 1991[203]	10	T1-T4	60	NI	Cyst	48*
Grignon et al, 1991[115]	48	A-D	NI	54 (C) 24 (G) 32 (I)	No, TUR, RT, p cyst ± RT, cyst ± RT	31
Abenoza et al, 1987[204]	16†	A-D	94	50 (GM)	No, TUR, RT, p cyst, cyst	21 mo‡
Bennett et al, 1984[104]	28‖	B-D	100	NI	No, TUR ± RT, cyst ± RT p cyst	21 mo‡
Anderström et al, 1983[79]	64†	A-D	91	NI	No, TUR, RT, p cyst ± RT, cyst	18
Nocks et al, 1983[205]	12‖	Ta-T3b	71	NI	TUR, p cyst, cyst	17
Malek et al, 1983[121]	25†	A-D	88	NI	TUR ± RT, p cyst, cyst	48
Jones et al, 1980[206]	10	A-D	80	10 (G)	Cyst, p cyst ± RT, RT	36 mo‡
Kramer et al, 1979[120]	34	A-D	91	24 (GM) 18 (C) 3 (G)	No, cyst ± RT, TUR ± RT, Preop RT + cyst, p cyst ± RT, Chemo	19
Jacobo et al, 1977[207]	20	B-D	100	NI	TUR, p cyst, cyst, RT chemo	1 Patient#
Johnson et al, 1972[81]	17	A-D	88	53 (C) 18 (I)	TUR ± chemo, RT, p cyst ± RT, cyst, preop RT + cyst, pros + p cyst	18
Thomas et al, 1971[74]	28	T1-T4	96	Many (C) 14 (G)	No, RT, p cyst ± RT, cyst	7
Mostofi, 1955[97]	27‖	NI	80	Yes	No, TUR ± RT, res ± RT, RT, cyst	33

* Three-year survival rate.
† Includes patients with urachal cancer.
‡ Mean survival.
‖ Includes mixed adenocarcinoma and transitional cell carcinoma.
\# One patient with stage B disease alive without disease 24 months after partial cystectomy.
C, cystitis cystica; chemo, chemotherapy; cyst, cystectomy; G, cystitis glandularis; GM, glandular metaplasia; I, intestinal metaplasia; NI, not indicated; no, no therapy; p cyst, partial cystectomy; preop, preoperative; pros, radical prostatectomy; res, open resection and fulguration; RT, radiotherapy; salv cyst, salvage cystectomy after prior radiotherapy; TUR, transurethral resection.

in the literature; 87% of these patients were males.[80,82,83,109–112] These tumors are characterized by extensive submucosal and muscular infiltration, which may produce a thickened bladder wall, decreased volume, and loss of contractility. Linitis plastica may develop in about 30% of cases of signet-ring cell carcinoma. These tumors are often not resectable, and they progress rapidly.[113,114] The prognosis for patients with pure linitis plastica is much worse than for those in whom this pattern is part of a mixture.[115] There are few reports of long-term survivors.[83]

Clear cell, or mesonephric, carcinoma is found most commonly in the female genital tract and the urethra.[84] These tumors may resemble nephrogenic adenomas in a superficial bladder biopsy specimen but can be identified by a deeper biopsy specimen. These tumors grow in sheets as well as in papillae of anaplastic cells. Muscular invasion may indicate a more aggressive tumor, which requires radical cystectomy.[116,117]

Flow cytometric DNA analysis was performed on 38 primary adenocarcinomas of the bladder. At 5 and 10 years after diagnosis, 80% and 70%, respectively, of the patients with diploid tumors were free of disease, compared with 20% and 12% of the patients with nondiploid tumors.[118] Other investigators, however, have reported that DNA ploidy pattern is not a significant predictor of outcome for primary nonurachal adenocarcinoma of the bladder.[119]

Treatment

Partial and Radical Cystectomy

Most patients with adenocarcinoma of the bladder have been treated with either radical cystectomy or partial cystectomy in carefully selected patients with amenable lesions. Radiotherapy appears to have very little effect on these lesions.

Anderström[79] retrospectively reviewed 64 patients with primary adenocarcinoma of the urinary bladder (35 patients) and urachus (29 patients) who were seen over a 15-year period at 20 hospitals in Sweden. These tumors invaded muscle in 58 of 64 (91%) patients. Ten percent of patients had multiple tumors. Stage, size, grade, and treatment were important prognostic factors. Partial resection appeared to be adequate therapy in patients with moderately well differentiated tumors <5 cm. Five-year survival was 54% in 15 patients treated by partial cystectomy and only 21% in 7 patients treated by radical cystectomy.

The authors concluded that the difference in survival rates probably reflected selection biases rather than differences in therapeutic efficacy.

At Duke University, 34 patients with adenocarcinoma were seen over a 47-year period, 31 (91%) of whom had stage B (T2) or higher disease.[120] Radical cystectomy with or without irradiation was performed in 15 patients; 19 received various therapies that included transurethral resection, irradiation, chemotherapy, and combination therapy. The overall 5-year survival was 19%; only one patient, who presented with a stage A (T1) tumor, was free of disease. Compared with nonsurgical treatment, radical cystectomy increased survival rates only minimally.

In a series from the Mayo Clinic, 19 patients with adenocarcinoma and 6 patients with urachal cancer were found in 4500 patients (0.56%) over a 15-year period.[121] Fourteen underwent partial cystectomy, with 5-year survival of 43%. Five patients had radical cystectomy, with 5-year survival of 80%. In six patients who had transurethral resection (three with radiotherapy), 5-year survival was 33%.

At Emory University, 28 patients with adenocarcinoma of the bladder, all stage B (T2) or higher, were managed over 10 years with a variety of therapeutic modalities.[104] Overall survival averaged only 21 months, and the authors suggested that an aggressive approach be used in patients with adenocarcinoma of the bladder.

Chemotherapy

Intraarterial 5-fluorouracil infusion has been shown to be effective in stage C (T3b) and D (T4) and recurrent adenocarcinoma.[122,123] Logothetis and colleagues[124] treated eight patients with locally unresectable adenocarcinoma of the bladder or urachus, two of whom also had distant metastases; four patients had failed prior cisplatin-doxorubicin-cyclophosphamide (CISCA) therapy. All eight patients received intravenous or intraarterial 5-fluorouracil, doxorubicin, and mitomycin. Five of eight patients (63%) had an objective response, but three of the five responses were of short duration. The carcinoembryonic antigen level fell in three responding patients in whom it was elevated at presentation. Bavendam and colleagues[125] have reported that a patient who had a high-grade tumor and a mass fixed to the pelvic side wall became operable after CMV therapy. The patient received two additional courses of adjuvant chemotherapy after removal of a stage D_1 (pT4) tumor. The patient showed no disease recurrence at 1 year posttherapy.

Conclusions

For the rare superficial adenocarcinoma, transurethral resection may be adequate therapy. For invasive disease without evidence of metastases, radical cystectomy with bilateral lymphadenectomy is the preferred treatment. Partial cystectomy can be considered if multicentric disease can be excluded and the tumor is located on the mobile bladder wall. There are a few reports of tumor response to radiotherapy.[74,108] The efficacy of neoadjuvant or adjuvant chemotherapy has not been established, but because several chemotherapeutic regimens have been reported to produce responses, it may be appropriate to give initial chemotherapy to a patient with advanced adenocarcinoma of the bladder to assess the response, then restage the patient and consider surgery, more chemotherapy, or both. Based on the reports to date, a 5-fluorouracil–based chemotherapy regimen should probably be tried first.

CARCINOMA WITH MIXED DIFFERENTIATION

Clinical and Diagnostic Features

Urothelial tumors in the urinary bladder commonly exhibit mixed patterns of differentiation. Many different combinations have been reported, especially in large series of bladder cancer patients. Among the cases of small cell undifferentiated carcinoma in the literature, almost one half have been mixtures of TCC, SCC, and adenocarcinoma. Rare examples of mixtures of TCC and adenocarcinoma have also been reported.[126] The percentage of each component should be accurately assessed and reported. Prognosis reflects the predominant histologic type.

Treatment

Treatment should be directed to the predominant histologic component while considering those components that may be less responsive to therapy.

CARCINOID

Clinical and Diagnostic Features

Primary carcinoid of the urinary bladder has been reported in few patients,[9] none of whom have shown clinical features of the carcinoid syndrome. Only five cases have been well documented in the literature. Four of the cases occurred in men, who were 30 to 75 years of age. All patients presented with hematuria. Tumor behavior was indolent in three of the cases; however, one patient developed distant metastases and died within 2 years of cystectomy.[9] Analysis of tumor tissue and urine may show elevated levels of 5-hydroxyindoleacetic acid, with normal levels of vanillylmandelic acid.[127]

Treatment

As in carcinoid tumors in other locations, carcinoids may be benign or malignant.[127–131] Benign tumors can be treated with transurethral resection or partial cystectomy.[132] Malignant lesions should probably be treated with radical cystectomy and bilateral lymphadenectomy, but because so few cases have been reported, it is not possible to be certain about the optimal treatment.

SMALL CELL UNDIFFERENTIATED CARCINOMA (OAT CELL CARCINOMA)

Clinical and Diagnostic Features

Undifferentiated carcinomas have no mature tissue pattern recognizable by light microscopy.[132] Small cell carcinoma of the bladder is a subtype of undifferentiated carcinoma with pathologic features similar to those of oat cell carcinoma of the lung. It is a disease of the neuroendocrine system and a member of the amine precursor uptake and decarboxylation tumor system.[133] Diagnosis may be made by identification of dense-core neurosecretory granules on electron microscopy or by immunohistochemical staining for epithelial markers such as neuron-specific enolase (NSE) and chromogranin.[134] High-grade TCC may on occasion produce NSE.[135] Small cell carcinoma of the genitourinary tract is heterogeneous in appearance and may arise from a multipotential cell, which may be organ specific. Small cell carcinoma of the bladder may have a better prognosis than small cell carcinoma of the prostate if diagnosed at an early stage.[136]

Small cell carcinoma of the bladder is rare, occurring in only 0.5% of 3778 bladder malignancies in one multiinstitutional review.[134] Patients usually present with hematuria. Serum calcium has occasionally been reported to be elevated at presentation.[136] The median age at diagnosis is 76 years, and there is a male predominance.[132] The tumors are usually large and are often associated with other types of malignancy, such as TCC, SCC, and adenocarcinoma.[137] This neuroendocrine neoplasm has a highly malignant biologic potential. Patients present with either locally advanced or distant metastatic disease. The metastatic pattern is similar to that of TCC; the iliac and paraaortic lymph nodes, liver, bone, and abdominal cavity are the most frequent sites, but one series reported the lungs to be involved in only 2 of 18 patients (11%).[134] Survival appears to depend on tumor stage at diagnosis.[138] In most reported series, the prognosis is uniformly poor, and patients succumb to disease within 1 year of diagnosis[134,139,140]; however, there are scattered reports of long-term survivors in the literature. One review noted that patients whose tumors were confined to the bladder (stages B_1, B_2, and C [T2-T3b]) had an overall survival rate of 75% at 1 year.[138]

Treatment

Radical Cystectomy

Despite the aggressive nature of small cell undifferentiated carcinoma, if metastases cannot be demonstrated, radical cystectomy with bilateral lymphadenectomy is recommended.

Chemotherapy

Neoadjuvant or adjuvant chemotherapy may be efficacious in small cell undifferentiated carcinoma. Metastatic disease has been reported to respond to radiotherapy and cisplatin plus etoposide.[141] Two patients with advanced small cell carcinoma who were $PT_{3b}N+$ at radical cystoprostatectomy were treated with four to five courses of adjuvant MVAC.[133] Despite positive nodes, the patients were alive and disease-free at 1 and 2.5 years. In a large series of 22 patients, 26% of patients were alive and free of disease after 10 to 51 months.[96] In another reported case, combination chemotherapy with CMV followed by external beam irradiation to the bladder gave a durable continuous complete remission for more than 4.5 years.[142] In another study, two of five patients who received chemotherapy died at 5 and 15 months, but the other three patients were still alive at 22 to 38 months.[134] These patients initially responded to methotrexate and cisplatin (MP), cyclophosphamide and doxorubicin (CA), and cyclophosphamide, doxorubicin, vincristine, methotrexate, and cisplatin (CAVMP). Chemotherapy may affect the extremely aggressive course of small cell undifferentiated carcinoma, and radiotherapy may help achieve local control.

PRIMARY MALIGNANT LYMPHOMA

Clinical and Diagnostic Features

Primary lymphoid malignancies of the urinary bladder are rare.[143–146] Through 1990, only 56 cases had been reported, and only 34 of these had adequate follow-up.[143] However, in patients with widely disseminated disease, these tumors can be observed in the bladder: 13% of 599 cases in Sufrin's autopsy series.[147] Primary lymphomas of the bladder are most often discovered during evaluation for nonspecific urinary complaints such as hematuria and dysuria. One case was suspected after urinary cytology showed undifferentiated malignant cells, probably lymphoma.[148] The clinical presentation has been summarized by Garber and Prestipino[132]; 80% of patients have hematuria, and 47% have concomitant urinary tract infection. Most patients are 50 to 80 years of age, and the male-to-female ratio is 1 : 2.7. Tumors are generally polypoid submucosal masses, which are sometimes focally ulcerated. At diagnosis, lymphoid tumors are usually large and deeply invasive, typically arising from the trigone or bladder base. Many histologic types have been described, including plasmacytoma, immunoblastic sarcoma, and granulocytic sarcoma. Immunoblastic sarcoma is an unusual form of lymphoma that arises from B lymphocytes.[149] It is important to distinguish lymphomas from primary sarcomas, which are treated differently and usually have a worse prognosis.

Treatment

Primary lymphomas have a good prognosis when treated aggressively. In one of the largest series (11 patients), survival was 73% at 1 year and 64% at 5 years.[143] In an earlier review of 22 cases in the literature, survival was 68% at 1 year and 27% at 5 years, but only 1 of 19 patients who received surgery, radiotherapy, or both died of lymphoma.[150] Cures have been obtained with transurethral resection and radiotherapy or partial cystectomy with or without radiotherapy and chemotherapy.[143,145,151,152] Malignant lymphomas are radiosensitive, and radiotherapy is the treatment of choice for extramedullary plasmacytoma; Yang and colleagues[127] have demonstrated an excellent response in the bladder as well.

MALIGNANT MELANOMA

Clinical and Diagnostic Features

Primary malignant melanoma of the urinary bladder is distinctly rare, with no more than 11 well documented cases in the literature.[137,153–157] Metastatic lesions to the bladder are more frequent, but such lesions frequently remain asymptomatic and are discovered only at autopsy.[155] Criteria for the diagnosis of primary urinary bladder melanoma include the following[9,154,155]:

- no history of cutaneous melanoma
- negative physical examination using a Wood's light that excludes a concurrent cutaneous melanoma
- appropriate studies to exclude a concurrent visceral melanoma
- no apparent development of an alternative primary melanoma during the course of follow-up
- pattern of recurrences consistent with a primary tumor
- tumor associated with intramural atypical melanocytes at the tumor margin

Symptoms are nonspecific and include hematuria and vesical irritability. Cystoscopy may reveal a darkly pigmented, exophytic bladder lesion.[155] The brown-black pigment present in tumor cells can be identified as melanin by Fontana-Masson staining, and cytoplasmic melanosomes can be revealed by ultrastructural studies[9]; however, immunohistochemical staining with markers such as the mouse monoclonal antibody HMB-45 is more sensitive and specific.[158]

Treatment

Radical Cystectomy

Radical cystectomy and bilateral lymphadenectomy are generally recommended for localized bladder melanoma. However, if the lesion can be completely excised with appropriate margins of normal mucosa, partial cystectomy with bilateral pelvic lymphadenectomy may be more rational, considering how likely the lesion is to be a metastasis, or if it is a mucosal primary melanoma, how likely it is that metastases will subsequently develop. For example, a 34-year-old man seen in our practice had a pigmented tumor 3 cm in diameter located on the posterior bladder wall, shown by transurethral biopsy before referral to be malignant melanoma. Careful examination revealed no other melanoma as a potential primary site. Partial cystectomy with bilateral pelvic lymphadenectomy was performed and revealed a melanoma that infiltrated to a depth of 1 cm (i.e., the full thickness of the muscularis propria) but with margins of resection negative for tumor and 1 of 25 lymph nodes positive for tumor. The patient subsequently developed metastatic disease in the lungs and liver which was unresponsive to chemotherapy, but his bladder remained free of tumor during periodic cystoscopic evaluations. He died 27 months after partial cystectomy with a functioning bladder and remained without evidence of an alternate primary melanoma outside the bladder.

Immunotherapy

The most successful immunotherapy for skin lesions is BCG. There is one case report of a bladder lesion that responded to intralesional BCG.[159]

Chemotherapy

Although dacarbazine (DTIC) is considered the gold standard for treating malignant melanoma, with response rates of 23% to 25%, most investigators do not consider single-agent DTIC very efficacious. Combination regimens such as that developed at Dartmouth University (i.e., carmustine-cisplatin-tamoxifen) may be helpful in alleviating symptoms.[160]

MIXED CELL–TYPE NEOPLASMS

Germ Cell Neoplasms

Primary germ cell tumors of the bladder are extremely rare; only about 25 cases have been reported in the literature,[132] including choriocarcinoma, malignant teratoma, dermoid cyst, and yolk sac tumor.[135,159,161–163] Most patients are males.

The most common germ cell tumor is choriocarcinoma. Choriocarcinoma may be associated with undifferentiated, glandular, or TCC elements. This tumor is most likely the result of epithelial heterogeneity rather than abnormal embryonic development.[163] Light microscopy reveals syncytiotrophoblastic and cytotrophoblastic cells. Beta-human chorionic gonadotropin (β-HCG) is positive in both serum and tumor; however, serum β-HCG may also be elevated in high-grade TCC,[135,164,165] in bilharzial SCC,[166] and in renal and prostatic malignancies.[167] Gynecomastia may be present. Most patients have widespread metastases at presentation. Despite the progress in combination chemotherapy for patients with testicular germ cell tumors, patients with primary germ cell tumors of the bladder have a poor prognosis regardless of treatment given.[132]

Carcinosarcoma

Carcinosarcomas, also called malignant mixed mesodermal tumors, are tumors composed of malignant epithelial and stromal (i.e., mesenchymal or sarcomatous) elements. These tumors are found rarely in the bladder; fewer than 100 cases have been well documented.[9,84,98,168–174] Carcinosarcomas are thought to be admixtures of neoplastic cells that arise from a single multipotential stem cell (i.e., combination tumors) or from the simultaneous development of two distinct clones (i.e., composition tumors). They occur at a mean age of 62 years (range, 33 to 82 years) with a male-to-female ratio of 3 : 1.[174] At cystoscopy, tumors are most frequently found at the base of the bladder and trigone protruding into the lumen, where they may appear deceptively circumscribed and polypoid. The epithelial component is most commonly TCC, although adenocarcinoma, SCC, and undifferentiated carcinoma have been reported. The sarcomatous component is most frequently poorly differentiated and spindled, although cartilaginous, osseous, and skeletal muscle differentiation may be present.[84] Electron microscopy may be necessary for definitive diagnosis.[170]

Stage at presentation may be the most important prognostic factor; most carcinosarcomas are deeply infiltrative. These tumors tend to be highly aggressive; few patients survive longer than 1 year. The composition of the metastases may be pure sarcoma, pure carcinoma, or both and may help dictate therapeutic management.[175] There have been few long-term survivors after transurethral resection alone and after partial cystectomy.[169,176] Usually, radical cystectomy and bilateral lymphadenectomy are required for these aggressive lesions. The roles of adjuvant radiotherapy and chemotherapy have not been established.[98]

Collision Tumors

Collision tumors are actually two separate tumors, one of mesenchymal and one of epithelial origin. Although they are independent, they occur closely together. The bladder is the most frequent site in the urinary tract for these types of tumors.[9] It is often difficult to distinguish these tumors from carcinosarcomas.[177–179] Treatment should attempt to surgically extirpate all tumor, which usually requires a cystectomy and should include bilateral lymphadenectomy. If metastases are noted, the tissue type of the metastatic lesion should be determined so that optimal systemic therapy can be selected. Regardless of treatment, overall prognosis is poor.[132]

MESENCHYMAL TUMORS

Benign Mesenchymal Tumors

A number of benign and malignant tumors can develop from or differentiate toward mesenchyme. These lesions may occur in pure or mixed form. These tumors account for less than 1% of bladder tumors. Benign mesenchymal tumors include hemangioma, lymphangioma, granular cell tumor, neurofibroma, fibrous histiocytoma, leiomyoma, fibroma, fibromyxoma, osteoma, fibroepithelial polyp, and pseudosarcomatous reactions.

Malignant Mesenchymal Tumors

Malignant mesenchymal tumors comprise less than 0.5% of all bladder cancers. They may present as bulky pelvic masses composed of primitive mesenchymal elements mixed with cells differentiating toward soft tissue structures. It appears that prognosis is more dependent on the patient's age and extent of cancer than on the specific cell type. Most of these tumors have muscle differentiation and can be considered myosarcomas.[84,180] Malignant mesenchymal tumors are most often found in infants and children. The ratio of males to females affected is 3 : 1. Patients present with large pelvic masses that obstruct the ureters, urethra, or both.[181]

Rhabdomyosarcoma

Rhabdomyosarcoma is the most common soft tissue sarcoma in children. These tumors are most frequently found at the base of the bladder. When they resemble a bunch of grapes, they may be referred to as botryoid sarcoma. Standard therapy consists of a combined modality approach with surgery, chemotherapy, and radiotherapy.[182] Chemotherapeutic regimens commonly used are vincristine, dactinomycin, and cyclophosphamide (VAC), and VAC plus doxorubicin (Adriamycin; Adria-VAC).

Leiomyosarcoma

Few cases of childhood leiomyosarcoma have been reported.[183] Myosarcomas in the adult present with hematuria more often than with obstruction. These tumors are usually located at the base of the bladder. The male-to-female ratio is 2 : 1, and patients are usually between the ages of 40 and 60 years. The most common histologic type is leiomyosarcoma. There have been case reports of bladder myosarcomas following cyclophosphamide therapy for Hodgkin's disease and lupus nephritis.[184–186] Compared with the myosarcomas of childhood, these tumors are smaller, more localized, and more differentiated. They may be amenable to partial cystectomy.[180,181,187,188] Patients with positive surgical margins can be treated with adjuvant radiotherapy and chemotherapy. Patients with bulky disease may be treated with preoperative chemotherapy using cisplatin or doxorubicin with or without radiotherapy, followed by an exenterative operation.[189] Although these tumors tend to grow locally, they have a higher probability of metastasizing than do their childhood counterparts. Most series suggest a poor prognosis[85]; however in one series, none of the leiomyosarcomas metastasized to lymph nodes, and in selected patients excellent survival was achieved with aggressive combination chemotherapy and radiotherapy.[189]

Osteogenic Sarcoma

Osteogenic sarcoma of the urinary bladder is extremely rare; there are few well documented case reports in the literature. These tumors tend to grow locally rather than metastasize. Treatments have included chemotherapy with doxorubicin and cisplatin, and high-dose methotrexate with leucovorin rescue. Radiotherapy and surgical resection also have been recommended.[189a] Pure osteogenic sarcomas have a poor prognosis, with a 1-year survival of approximately 14%. Osteogenic sarcoma should be distinguished from bladder tumors that may have associated bone formation, such as carcinosarcoma and TCC with osseous metaplasia of the stroma, which may have a better prognosis.[190]

Miscellaneous Primary Bladder Sarcomas

There have been isolated reports of other primary bladder sarcomas, including malignant fibrous histiocytoma, hemangiopericytoma after exposure to polyvinyl alcohol, myxoid liposarcoma, malignant mesenchymoma, ganglioneuroma, and malignant varieties of benign lesions such as granular cell tumor.[85] An attempt should be made to surgically excise all tumor if no metastases can be demonstrated. Because this category of tumors is so heterogeneous, it is difficult to comment on prognosis.

PHEOCHROMOCYTOMA

Clinical and Diagnostic Features

Extraadrenal pheochromocytoma, or paraganglioma of the urinary bladder, may present with the unique symptom complex of micturitional attacks related to increased catecholamine secretion during detrusor activity.[191,192] This tumor probably arises from embryonic nests of chromaffin cells in the detrusor sympathetic plexus.[191,193] Pheochromocytomas account for 0.06% of bladder tumors. In adults, 10% of pheochromocytomas are extraadrenal, and in children, 31% are extraadrenal.[176] Vesical pheochromocytoma accounts for 10% of extraadrenal paragangliomas.[194] These lesions are slightly more common in females than in males (1.5 : 1), and the mean patient age is 41 years (range, 11 to 78 years).[192,193] There have been anecdotal associations with renal cell carcinoma, TCC, and neurofibromatosis.[195–197]

Most patients (58%) present with gross hematuria, but almost 50% have peculiar symptoms as a result of catecholamine release.[112] These symptoms may include bursting headache, blurred vision, diaphoresis, anxiety, tremulousness, a pounding sensation, and occasionally syncope. Hypertension occurs in 65% of patients.[192] Serum and urinary catecholamine levels are elevated in 50% of patients. Cystoscopy reveals a solitary, solid, poorly circumscribed, submucosal or intramural lesion.[84,193] Pheochromocytomas can occur anywhere in the bladder wall but most commonly are located in the dome or trigone.[192]

Treatment

To prevent hypertensive crisis, hormonally active patients should be treated with phenoxybenzamine hydrochloride and receive cautious hemodynamic monitoring during endoscopic or angiographic procedures.[198] About 5% to 15% of tumors have malignant behavior with hematogenous metastases. Whether tumors are benign or malignant is not resolved by histologic examination but rather by clinical behavior. In the absence of unequivocal proof of malignancy, these tumors are primarily treated with partial cystectomy with lymph node dissection.[199] Transurethral resection is inadequate, because most pheochromocytomas involve the entire bladder wall. Radical cystectomy and lymphadenectomy are performed when the lesion is large or when there is unequivocal evidence of metastases in the lymph nodes. The ipsilateral hypogastric vein should be temporarily occluded or ligated before tumor manipulation to avoid paroxysmal hypertensive episodes.[199]

METASTATIC BLADDER TUMORS

Secondary bladder adenocarcinomas can occur as a result of local extension from adjacent tumors (discussed previously; see Adenocarcinoma) or as a result of metastatic spread. In a series of 5200 autopsies, melanoma was the tumor most likely to have spread to the bladder.[200] Lymphoma also frequently metastasizes to the bladder. These two tumors are followed in order of frequency by tumors of the stomach, breast, kidney (including Wilms' tumor), lung, pancreas, testis, ovary, endometrium, and gallbladder.[84] Treatment should be guided by the type and status of the primary tumor. Therapy of metastases in the bladder is often only palliative unless the primary tumor is concurrently controlled or can be definitively managed.

CONCLUSIONS

Non–transitional cell bladder cancer comprises a diverse collection of tumors that are rare compared with TCC, except for SCC in the bilharzial bladder in areas where schistosomiasis is endemic. Many of these tumors (e.g., pure adenocarcinomas, small cell carcinomas) are typically aggressive and usually present at an advanced stage. They seem to have a poor prognosis regardless of choice of treatment.

The challenge when confronted with one of these tumors is to plan effective therapy. Because optimal treatment is not known, the oncologist must begin with a plan based on current oncologic principles, the cornerstones of which are careful staging and wide surgical extirpation when the tumor is still locoregional. This therapeutic plan must be modified when even limited prior experience suggests that there may be an alternative effective therapy or adjunctive therapy, particularly irradiation and chemotherapy.

When the efficacy of chemotherapy is unproved for a particular tumor and potential alternative regimens are available, it may be optimal to treat with initial chemotherapy before surgery and use the tumor as its own in vivo sensitivity assay. Radical surgery will still be possible after chemotherapy if there has been a response. If there has been no response, however, the clinician can select alternative therapy that might be more effective. Additionally, if extravesical tumor fails to respond, this approach may spare some patients surgery that is not worthwhile.

REFERENCES

1. Johnson DE, Schoenwald MB, Ayala AG, Miller LS. Squamous cell carcinoma of the bladder. J Urol 1976;115:542.
2. Bessette PL, Abell MR, Herwig KR. A clinicopathologic study of squamous cell carcinoma of the bladder. J Urol 1974;112:66.
3. Richie JP, Waisman J, Skinner DG, Dretler SP. Squamous carcinoma of the bladder: treatment by radical cystectomy. J Urol 1976;115:670.
4. Sarma KP. On the nature of cystitis follicularis. J Urol 1970;104:709.
5. Yoshida K, Hattori T, Abe H, Akimoto M. Squamous cell carcinoma coexisting vesical leukoplakia: case study and its clinicopathological analysis of the pathogenesis. Hinyokika Kiyo 1989;35:885.
6. Connery DB. Leukoplakia of the urinary bladder and its association with carcinoma. J Urol 1953;69:121.
7. Morgan RJ, Cameron KM. Vesical leukoplakia. Br J Urol 1980;52:96.
8. Sakamoto N, Tsuneyoshi M, Enjoji M. Urinary bladder carcinoma with a neoplastic squamous component: a mapping study of 31 cases. Histopathology 1992;21:135.
9. Petersen RO. Urinary bladder. In: Petersen RO, ed. Urologic pathology. Philadelphia: JB Lippincott, 1986:279.
10. Rundle JSH, Hart AJL, McGeorge A, Smith JS, Malcolm AJ, Smith PM. Squamous cell carcinoma of bladder: a review of 114 patients. Br J Urol 1982;54:522.
11. Faysal MH. Squamous cell carcinoma of the bladder. J Urol 1981;126:598.
12. Fetter TR, Bogaev JH, McCuskey B, Sere JL. Carcinoma of the bladder: sites of metastases. J Urol 1959;81:746.
13. Francis RR. Carcinoma of the bladder. J Urol 1961;85:552.
14. Jones MA, Bloom HJG, Williams G, Trott PA, Wallace DM. The management of squamous cell carcinoma of the bladder. Br J Urol 1980;52:511.
15. Rous SN. Squamous cell carcinoma of the bladder. J Urol 1978;120:561.
16. Hickey D, Soloway MS. Does invasive bladder cancer differ between women and men? Urology 1988;32:183.
17. Costello AJ, Tiptaft RC, England HR, Blandy JP. Squamous cell carcinoma of bladder. Urology 1984;23:234.
18. Schroder LE, Weiss MA, Hughes C. Squamous cell carcinoma of bladder: an increased incidence in blacks. Urology 1986;28:288.
19. Kantor AF, Hartge P, Hoover RN, Fraumeni JF Jr. Epidemiological characteristics of squamous cell carcinoma and adenocarcinoma of the bladder. Cancer Res 1988;48:3853.

20. Maloney KE, Wiener JS, Walther PJ. Oncogenic human papillomaviruses are rarely associated with squamous cell carcinoma of the bladder: evaluation by differential polymerase chain reaction. J Urol 1994; 154:360.
21. Kaufman JM, Fam B, Jacobs SC, et al. Bladder cancer and squamous metaplasia in spinal cord injury patients. J Urol 1977;118:967.
22. Locke JR, Hill DE, Walzer Y. Incidence of squamous cell carcinoma in patients with long-term catheter drainage. J Urol 1985;133:1034.
23. Kaye MC, Levin HS, Montague DK, Pontes JE. Squamous cell carcinoma of the bladder in a patient on intermittent self-catheterization. Cleve Clin J Med 1975;59:645.
24. Sene AP, Massey JA, McMahon RT, Carroll RN. Squamous cell carcinoma in a patient on clean intermittent self-catheterisation. Br J Urol 1990;65:213.
25. Wall RL, Clausen KP. Carcinoma of the urinary bladder in patients receiving cyclophosphamide. N Engl J Med 1975;293:271.
26. Brenner DW, Yore LM, Schellhammer PF. Squamous cell carcinoma of bladder after successful intravesical therapy with bacillus Calmette-Guérin. Urology 1989;34:93.
27. Desai PG, Khan SA, Jayachandran S, Ilardi C. Paraneoplastic syndrome in squamous cell carcinoma of urinary bladder. Urology 1987; 30:262.
28. Swanson DA, Liles A, Zagars GK. Preoperative irradiation and radical cystectomy for stages T2 and T3 squamous cell carcinoma of the bladder. J Urol 1990;143:37.
29. Lundgren R, Elfving P, Heim S, Kristoffersson U, Mandahl N, Mitelman F. A squamous cell bladder carcinoma with karyotypic abnormalities reminiscent of transitional cell carcinoma. J Urol 1989;142:374.
30. Winkler HZ, Nativ O, Hosaka Y, Farrow GM, Lieber MM. Nuclear deoxyribonucleic acid ploidy in squamous cell bladder cancer. J Urol 1989;141:297.
31. Newman DM, Brown JR, Jay AC, Pontius EE. Squamous cell carcinoma of the bladder. J Urol 1968;100:470.
32. Utz DC, Schmitz SE, Fugelso PD, Farrow GM. A clinicopathologic evaluation of partial cystectomy for carcinoma of the urinary bladder. Cancer 1973;32:1075.
33. Prempree T, Amornmarn R. Radiation management of squamous cell carcinoma of the bladder. Acta Radiol Oncol 1984;23:37.
34. Maruf NJ, Godec CJ, Strom RL, Cass AS. Unusual therapeutic response of massive squamous cell carcinoma of the bladder to aggressive radiation and surgery. J Urol 1982;128:1313.
35. Quilty PM, Duncan W. Radiotherapy for squamous carcinoma of the urinary bladder. Int J Radiat Oncol Biol Phys 1986;12:861.
36. Patterson JM, Ray EH Jr, Mendiondo OA, Medina WD, Gee WF. A new treatment for invasive squamous cell bladder cancer: the Nigro regimen: preoperative chemotherapy and radiation therapy. J Urol 1988;140:379.
37. Confer DJ, Smith RB, Gillespie L. Dramatic palliation for painful, fixed bladder squamous cell carcinoma with 5-fluorouracil infusion. J Urol 1977;118:483.
38. Gohji K, Higuchi A, Maruyama S, et al. Adjuvant chemotherapy for invasive urothelial cancer: experience with a methotrexate, vincristine, cisplatin, cyclophosphamide, Adriamycin and bleomycin (MVP-CAB) regimen: a preliminary report. Jpn J Clin Oncol 1993;23:291.
39. Harker WG, Meyers FJ, Freiha FS, et al. Cisplatin, methotrexate, and vinblastine (CMV): an effective chemotherapy regimen for metastatic transitional cell carcinoma of the urinary tract: a Northern California oncology group study. J Clin Oncol 1985;3:1463.
40. Logothetis CJ, Samuels ML, Ogden S, et al. Cyclophosphamide, doxorubicin and cisplatin chemotherapy for patients with locally advanced urothelial tumors with or without nodal metastases. J Urol 1985;134:460.
41. Sternberg CN, Yagoda A, Scher HI, et al. M-VAC (methotrexate, vinblastine, doxorubicin and cisplatin) for advanced transitional cell carcinoma of the urothelium. J Urol 1988;139:461.
42. Wishahi M. Intra-arterial cisplatin in advanced squamous cell carcinoma of the bladder letter. Eur J Cancer 1992;28:612.
43. Medical Research Council (England). CMV chemotherapy for pure squamous cell cancer of the urinary tract. Protocol BA08, 1993.
44. Loehrer PJ Sr, Einhorn LH, Elson PJ, et al. A randomized comparison of cisplatin alone or in combination with methotrexate, vinblastine and doxorubicin in patients with metastatic urothelial carcinoma: a cooperative group study. J Clin Oncol 1992;10:1066.
45. Elsebai I. Cancer of the bilharzial bladder. Urol Res 1978;6:233.
46. Sharfi ARA, El Sir S, Beleil O. Squamous cell carcinoma of the urinary bladder. Br J Urol 1992;69:369.
47. Khafagy MM, El-Bolkainy MN, Mansour MA. Carcinoma of the bilharzial urinary bladder: a study of the associated mucosal lesions in 86 cases. Cancer 1972;30:150.
48. El-Bolkainy MN, Mokhtar NM, Ghoneim MA, Hussein MH. The impact of schistosomiasis on the pathology of bladder carcinoma. Cancer 1981;48:2643.
49. El-Boulkany MN, Ghoneim MA, Mansour MA. Carcinoma of the bilharzial bladder in Egypt: clinical and pathological features. Br J Urol 1972;44:561.
50. Eissa SS, El-Said A, Omar S, Mebed H. A study of the possible limiting factors against the spread of bilharzial bladder cancer. Med J Cairo Univ 1978;46:205.
51. Ghoneim MA, El-Bolkainy MN, Mansour MA, El-Hamady SM, Ashamallah AG, Soliman ESH. Radical cystectomy for carcinoma of bilharzial bladder: technique and results. Urology 1976;8:547.
52. El-Mahrouky AS, Dawson DV, Paulson DF, Sanfilippo F. The predictive value of 2,4,-dinitrochlorobenzene skin testing in patients with bilharzial bladder cancer. J Urol 1983;129:499.
53. Raziuddin S, Sherry S, Ibrahim A, Patil K. Activated CD4-positive T-lymphocytes and impaired cell-mediated immunity in patients with carcinoma of the urinary bladder with schistosomiasis. Cancer 1990; 65:931.
54. Shaaban AA, Javadpour N, Tribukait B, Ghoneim MA. Prognostic significance of flow-DNA analysis and cell surface isoantigens in carcinoma of bilharzial bladder. Urology 1992;39:207.
55. Habuchi T, Takahashi R, Yamada H, et al. Influence of cigarette smoking and schistosomiasis on p53 gene mutation in urothelial cancer. Cancer Res 1993;53;3795.
56. El-Hammady SM, Ghoneim MA, Hussein ES, Ashamalla AC, El-Bolkainey MN. Segmental resection for carcinoma of the bladder. Mansoura Med Bull 1973;3:191.
57. Omar SM. Segmental resection for carcinoma of the bladder. Egypt Med Assoc 1969;52:975.
58. Ghoneim MA, Ashamallah AG, El-Hammady S, Gaballah MA, Soliman ESH. Cystectomy for carcinoma of the bilharzial bladder: 138 cases 5 years later. Br J Urol 1979;51:541.
59. Awaad H, El-Baki HA, El-Bolkainy N, et al. Pre-operative irradiation of T3-carcinoma in bilharzial bladder: a comparison between hyperfractionation and conventional fractionation. Int J Radiat Oncol Biol Phys 1979;5:787.
60. Ghoneim MA, Ashamallah AK, Awaad HK, Whitmore WF Jr. Randomized trial of cystectomy with or without preoperative radiotherapy for carcinoma of the bilharzial bladder. J Urol 1985;134:266.
61. Awaad HK, Barsoum M, El Merzabani M, et al. The use of misonidazole in association with a three-fractions per day regimen in advanced head and neck epidermoid cancer: a pilot study. Am J Clin Oncol 1983;6:91.
62. Gad-El-Mawla N, Hamza MR, Zikri ZK, et al. Chemotherapy in invasive carcinoma of the bladder: a review of phase II trials in Egypt. Acta Oncol 1989;28:73.
63. Gad-El-Mawla N, Mansour MA, Eissa S, et al. A randomized pilot study of high-dose epirubicin as neoadjuvant chemotherapy in the treatment of cancer of the bilharzial bladder. Ann Oncol 1991;2:137.
64. Kraus FT, Perez-Mesa C. Verrucous carcinoma: clinical and pathologic study of 105 cases involving oral cavity, larynx and genitalia. Cancer 1966;19:26.
65. El Sebai I, Sherif M, El Bolkainy MN, Mansour MA, Ghoneim MA. Verrucous squamous carcinoma of bladder. Urology 1974;4:407.
66. Walther M, O'Brien DP III, Birch HW. Condylomata acuminata and verrucous carcinoma of the bladder: case report and literature review. J Urol 1986;135:362.
67. Wyatt JK, Craig I. Verrucous carcinoma of urinary bladder. Urology 1980;16:97.
68. Holck S, Jorgensen L. Verrucous carcinoma of urinary bladder. Urology 1983;22:435.
69. Horner SA, Fisher HAG, Barada JH, Eastman AY, Migliozzi J, Ross JS. Verrucous carcinoma of the bladder. J Urol 1991;145:1261.
70. Lowe D, McKee PH. Verrucous carcinoma of the penis (Buschke-Lowenstein tumour): a clinicopathological study. Br J Urol 1983;55: 427.
71. Demian SDE, Bushkin FL, Echevarria RA. Perineural invasion and

anaplastic transformation of verrucous carcinoma. Cancer 1973;32: 395.
72. Boileau M, Hui KKS, Cowan DF. Invasive verrucous carcinoma of urinary bladder treated by irradiation. Urology 1986;27:56.
73. Mahran MR, el-Baz M. Verrucous carcinoma of the bilharzial bladder: impact of invasiveness on survival. Scand J Urol Nephrol 1993;27: 189.
74. Thomas DG, Ward AM, Williams JL. A study of 52 cases of adenocarcinoma of the bladder. Br J Urol 1971;43:4.
75. Friedell GH, Bell JR, Burney SW, Soto EA, Tiltman AJ. Histopathology and classification of urinary bladder carcinoma. Urol Clin North Am 1976;3:53.
76. Nielsen K, Nielsen KK. Adenocarcinoma in exstrophy of the bladder: the last case in Scandinavia? A case report and review of literature. J Urol 1983;130:1180.
77. Mortensen PB, Jensen KEJ, Nielsen K. Adenocarcinoma development in the trigone 34 years after trigonocolonic urinary diversion for exstrophy of the bladder. J Urol 1990;144:980.
78. Lam KY, Ma L, Nicholls J. Case report: adenocarcinoma arising in a diverticulum of the urinary bladder. Pathology 1992;24:40.
79. Anderström C, Johansson SL, von Schultz L. Primary adenocarcinoma of the urinary bladder: a clinicopathologic and prognostic study. Cancer 1983;52:1273.
80. Goble NM, Clarke TJ, Teasdale C. Signet ring cell adenocarcinoma of bladder secondary to long-term catheterization. Urology 1990;35: 279.
81. Johnson DE, Hogan JM, Ayala AG. Primary adenocarcinoma of the urinary bladder. South Med J 1972;65:527.
82. Blute ML, Engen DE, Travis WD, Kvols LK. Primary signet ring cell adenocarcinoma of the bladder. J Urol 1989;141:17.
83. Sagalowsky A, Donohue JP. Sixteen-year survival with metastatic signet ring cell bladder carcinoma. Urology 1980;15:501.
84. Murphy WM. Diseases of the urinary bladder, urethra, ureters and renal pelves. In: Murphy WM, ed. Urological pathology. Philadelphia: WB Saunders, 1989:34.
85. Mostofi FK, Thomson RV, Dean AL Jr. Mucous adenocarcinoma of the urinary bladder. Cancer 1955;8:741.
86. Remis RE, Halverstadt DB. Metastatic renal cell carcinoma to the bladder: case report and review of the literature. J Urol 1986;136: 1294.
87. Raitanen MP, Hellstrom PA, Kyllonen AP, Leisti EL, Kontturi MJ. Diagnostic and therapeutic aspects of adenocarcinoma of the urinary bladder. Ann Chir Gynaecol 1993;206:43.
88. Silver SA, Epstein JI. Adenocarcinoma of the colon simulating primary urinary bladder neoplasia: a report of nine cases. Am J Surg Pathol 1993;17:171.
89. Young RH, Johnston WH. Serous adenocarcinoma of the uterus metastatic to the urinary bladder mimicking primary bladder neoplasia: a report of a case. Am J Surg Pathol 1990;14:877.
90. Leddy FF, Peterson NE, Ning TC. Urogenital linitis plastica metastatic from stomach. Urology 1992;39:464.
91. Gill HS, Dhillon HK, Woodhouse CRJ. Adenocarcinoma of the urinary bladder. Br J Urol 1989;64:138.
92. Ganem EJ, Batal JT. Secondary malignant tumors of the urinary bladder metastatic from primary foci in distant organs. J Urol 1956;75: 965.
93. Chiang KS, Lamki N, Athey PA. Metastasis to the bladder from pancreatic adenocarcinoma presenting with hematuria. Urol Radiol 1992; 13:187.
94. Epstein JI, Kuhajda FP, Lieberman PH. Prostate-specific acid phosphatase immunoreactivity in adenocarcinomas of the urinary bladder. Hum Pathol 1986;17:939.
95. Golz R, Schubert GE. Prostatic specific antigen: immunoreactivity in urachal remnants. J Urol 1989;141:1480.
96. Grignon DJ, Ro JY, Ayala AG, et al. Small cell carcinoma of the urinary bladder: a clinicopathologic analysis of 22 cases. Cancer 1992; 69:527.
97. Mostofi FK. Potentialities of bladder epithelium. J Urol 1954;71:705.
98. Schoborg TW, Saffos RO, Rodriquez AP, Scott C Jr. Carcinosarcoma of the bladder. J Urol 1980;124:724.
99. Gregoire M, Kantoff P, DeWolf WC. Synchronous adenocarcinoma and transitional cell carcinoma of the bladder associated with augmentation: case report and review of the literature. J Urol 1993;149:115.
100. Patch FS, Rhea LJ. The genesis and development of Brunn's nests and their relation to cystitis cystica, cystitis glandularis, and primary adenocarcinoma of the bladder. Can Med Assoc J 1935;33:597.
101. Shaw JL, Gislason GJ, Imbriglia JE. Transition of cystitis glandularis to primary adenocarcinoma of the bladder. J Urol 1958;79:815.
102. Susmano D, Rubenstein AB, Dakin AR, Lloyd FA. Cystitis glandularis and adenocarcinoma of the bladder. J Urol 1971;105:671.
103. Kittredge WE, Collett AJ, Morgan C Jr. Adenocarcinoma of the bladder associated with cystitis glandularis: a case report. J Urol 1964; 91:145.
104. Bennett JK, Wheatley JK, Walton KN. 10-Year experience with adenocarcinoma of the bladder. J Urol 1984;131:262.
105. Gordon NSI, Sinclair RA, Snow RM. Pelvic lipomatosis cystitis cystica, cystitis glandularis and adenocarcinoma of the bladder: first reported case. Aust N Z J Surg 1990;60:229.
106. Heyns CF, DeKock MLS, Kirsten PH, van Velden DJJ. Pelvic lipomatosis associated with cystitis glandularis and adenocarcinoma of the bladder. J Urol 1991;145:364.
107. Young RH, Parkhurst EC. Mucinous adenocarcinoma of bladder: case associated with extensive intestinal metaplasia of urothelium in patient with nonfunctioning bladder for twelve years. Urology 1984;24:192.
108. Aygun C, Patanaphan V, Whitley NO, et al. Mucin-producing adenocarcinoma of bladder: clinicopathologic report. Urology 1983;21:135.
109. Fiter L, Gimeno F, Martin L, Tejeda LG. Signet-ring cell adenocarcinoma of bladder. Urology 1993;41:30.
110. Horne DW, Fauver HE. Primary signet-ring cell carcinoma of bladder. Urology 1987;30:574.
111. Yoshida H, Iwata H, Ochi K, Yoshida A, Fukunishi R. Primary signet-ring cell carcinoma of urinary bladder. Urology 1981;17:481.
112. Austin GE, Safford J. Signet ring cell carcinoma of bladder. Urology 1978;12:458.
113. Gonzalez E, Fowler MR, Venable DD. Primary signet ring cell adenocarcinoma of the bladder (linitis plastica of the bladder): report of a case and review of the literature. J Urol 1982;128:1027.
114. Reading LC, D'Onofrio GMD, Tulloch AGS, Knight DE, Walters MNI, Ojeda VJ. Primary linitis plastica carcinoma of urinary bladder. Urology 1983;22:310.
115. Grignon DJ, Ro JY, Ayala AG, Johnson DE, Ordóñez NG. Primary adenocarcinoma of the urinary bladder: a clinicopathologic analysis of 72 cases. Cancer 1991;67:2165.
116. Schultz RE, Bloch MJ, Tomaszewski JE, Brooks JSJ, Hanno PM. Mesonephric adenocarcinoma of the bladder. J Urol 1984;132:263.
117. Young RH, Scully RE. Clear cell adenocarcinoma of the bladder and urethra: a report of three cases and review of the literature. Am J Surg Pathol 1985;9:816.
118. Song J, Farrow GM, Lieber MM. Primary adenocarcinoma of the bladder: favorable prognostic significance of deoxyribonucleic acid diploidy measured by flow cytometry. J Urol 1990;144:1115.
119. Grignon DJ, El-Naggar A, Ro JY, Johnson DE, Ayala AG. Deoxyribonucleic acid flow cytometry on primary adenocarcinoma of the bladder: an analysis of 36 cases. J Urol 1989;142:1206.
120. Kramer SA, Bredael J, Croker BP, Paulson DF, Glenn JF. Primary non-urachal adenocarcinoma of the bladder. J Urol 1979;121:278.
121. Malek RS, Rosen JS, O'Dea MJ. Adenocarcinoma of bladder. Urology 1983;21:357.
122. Hatch TR, Fuchs EF. Intra-arterial infusion of 5-fluorouracil for recurrent adenocarcinoma of bladder. Urology 1989;33:311.
123. Nevin JE III, Melnick I, Baggerly JT, Easley CA Jr, Landes R. Advanced carcinoma of bladder: treatment using hypogastric artery infusion with 5-fluorouracil, either as a single agent or in combination with bleomycin or Adriamycin and supervoltage radiation. J Urol 1974;112:752.
124. Logothetis CJ, Samuels ML, Ogden S. Chemotherapy for adenocarcinomas of bladder and urachal origin: 5-fluorouracil, doxorubicin, and mitomycin-C. Urology 1985;26:252.
125. Bavendam TG, Kramolowsky EV, Mitros FA. Invasive adenocarcinoma of bladder response to cisplatinum, methotrexate, and vinblastine chemotherapy. Urology 1989;33:53.
126. Wiener DP, Koss LG, Sablay B, Freed SZ. The prevalence and significance of Brunn's nests, cystitis cystica and squamous metaplasia in normal bladders. J Urol 1979;122:317.
127. Yang CH, Krzyzaniak K, Brown WJ, Kurtz SM. Primary carcinoid tumor of urinary bladder. Urology 1985;26:594.
128. Walker BF, Someren A, Kennedy JC, Nicholas EM. Primary carcinoid tumor of the urinary bladder. Arch Pathol Lab Med 1992;116:1217.

129. Colby TV. Carcinoid tumor of the bladder: a case report. Arch Pathol Lab Med 1980;104:199.
130. Anichkov NM, Nikonov AA, Veresh I. Malignant carcinoid tumor of the bladder. Arkhiv Patologii 1979;41:46.
131. Aozasa K, Yokoyama M, Uda H, Nakamori S, Kishimoto S, Yano H. Primary carcinoid tumor in the urinary bladder: a case report. Med J Osaka Univ 1979;30:1.
132. Garber BB, Prestipino AJ. Non-transitional cell bladder malignancies, part II. AUA Update Series 1992;11:8.
133. Oesterling JE, Brendler CB, Burgers JK, Marshall FF, Epstein JI. Advanced small cell carcinoma of the bladder: successful treatment with combined radical cystoprostatectomy and adjuvant methotrexate, vinblastine, doxorubicin, and cisplatin chemotherapy. Cancer 1990; 65:1928.
134. Blomjous CEM, Vos W, De Voogt HJ, Van Der Valk P, Meijer CJLM. Small cell carcinoma of the urinary bladder: a clinicopathologic, morphometric, immunohistochemical, and ultrastructural study of 18 cases. Cancer 1989;64:1347.
135. Jacobsen AB, Nesland JM, Fossa SD, Pettersen EO. Human chorionic gonadotropin, neuron specific enolase and deoxyribonucleic acid flow cytometry in patients with high grade bladder carcinoma. J Urol 1990; 143:706.
136. Christopher ME, Seftel AD, Sorenson K, Resnick MI. Small cell carcinoma of the genitourinary tract: an immunohistochemical, electron microscopic and clinicopathological study. J Urol 1991;146:382.
137. Mourad WA, Mackay B, Ordonez NG, Ro JY, Swanson DA. Clear cell melanoma of the bladder. Ultrastruct Pathol 1993;17:463.
138. Podesta AH, True LD. Small cell carcinoma of the bladder: report of five cases with immunohistochemistry and review of the literature with evaluation of prognosis according to stage. Cancer 1989;64:710.
139. Swanson PE, Brooks R, Pearse H, Stenzel P. Small cell carcinoma of urinary bladder. Urology 1988;32:558.
140. Mills SE, Wolfe JT III, Weiss MA, et al. Small cell undifferentiated carcinoma of the urinary bladder: a light-microscopic, immunocytochemical, and ultrastructural study of 12 cases. Am J Surg Pathol 1987;11:606.
141. Davis MP, Murthy MSN, Simon J, Wise H, Minton JP. Successful management of small cell carcinoma of the bladder with cisplatin and etoposide. J Urol 1989;142:817.
142. Oblon DJ, Parsons JT, Zander DS, Wajsman Z. Bladder preservation and durable complete remission of small cell carcinoma of the bladder with systemic chemotherapy and adjuvant radiation therapy. Cancer 1993;71:2581.
143. Guthman DA, Malek RS, Chapman WR, Farrow GM. Primary malignant lymphoma of the bladder. J Urol 1990;144:1367.
144. Bhansali SK, Cameron KM. Primary malignant lymphoma of the bladder. Proceedings of the Sixteenth Annual Meeting of the British Association of Urological Surgeons, London, June 1960:440.
145. Aquilina JN, Bugeja TJ. Primary malignant lymphoma of the bladder: case report and review of the literature. J Urol 1974;112:64.
146. Aigen AB, Phillips M. Primary malignant lymphoma of urinary bladder. Urology 1986;28:235.
147. Sufrin G, Keogh B, Moore RH, Murphy GP. Secondary involvement of the bladder in malignant lymphoma. J Urol 1977;118:251.
148. Mincione GP. Primary malignant lymphoma of the urinary bladder with a positive cytologic report. Acta Cytol 1982;26:69.
149. Forrest JB, Saypol DC, Mills SE, Gillenwater JY. Immunoblastic sarcoma of the bladder. J Urol 1983;130:350.
150. Parton I. Primary lymphosarcoma of the bladder. Br J Urol 1962;34: 221.
151. Santino AM, Schumaker EJ, Garces J. Primary malignant lymphoma of the bladder. J Urol 1970;103:310.
152. Mäkinen J, Alfthan O, Vuori J. Malignant lymphoma of the urinary bladder: a report of 2 cases. Eur Urol 1979;5:45.
153. Anichkov NM, Nikonov AA. Primary malignant melanomas of the bladder. J Urol 1982;128:813.
154. Ainsworth AM, Clark WH Jr, Mastrangelo M, Conger KB. Primary malignant melanoma of the urinary bladder. Cancer 1976;37:1928.
155. Stein BS, Kendall AR. Malignant melanoma of the genitourinary tract. J Urol 1984;132:859.
156. Willis AJ, Huang AH, Carroll P. Primary melanoma of the bladder: a case report and review. J Urol 1980;123:278.
157. Kojima T, Tanaka T, Yoshimi N, Mori H. Primary malignant melanoma of the urinary bladder. Arch Pathol Lab Med 1992;116:1213.
158. Ordóñez NG, Xiaolong J, Hickey RC. Comparison of HMB-45 monoclonal antibody and S-100 protein in the immunohistochemical diagnosis of melanoma. Am J Clin Pathol 1988;90:385.
159. Dennis PM, Turner AG. Primary choriocarcinoma of the bladder evolving from a transitional cell carcinoma. J Clin Pathol 1984;37: 503.
160. Del Prete SA, Maurer LH, O'Donnell J, Forcier RJ, LeMarbre P. Combination chemotherapy with cisplatin, carmustine, decarbazine, and tamoxifen in metastatic melanoma. Cancer Treat Rep 1984;68: 1403.
161. Gallagher L, Lind R, Oyasu R. Primary choriocarcinoma of the urinary bladder in association with undifferentiated carcinoma. Hum Pathol 1984;15:793.161.
162. Kawamura J, Rhinsho K, Taki Y, et al. Choriocarcinoma and undifferentiated cell carcinoma of the bladder with gonadotropin secretion. J Urol 1979;121:684.
163. Obe JA, Rosen N, Koss LG. Primary choriocarcinoma of the urinary bladder: report of a case with probable epithelial origin. Cancer 1983; 52:1405.
164. McManus LM, Naughton MA, Martinez-Hernandez A. Human chorionic gonadotropin in human neoplastic cells. Cancer Res 1976;36: 3476.
165. Shah VM, Newman J, Crocker J, et al. Ectopic β-human chorionic gonadotropin production by bladder urothelial neoplasia. Arch Pathol Lab Med 1986;110:107.
166. Tungekar MF, Abdul-Sattar S, Adnani MS. Expression of chorionic gonadotropin by schistosomiasis-associated squamous carcinomas of bladder. Eur Urol 1988;14:30.
167. Dexeus F, Logothetis C, Hossan E, Samuels ML. Carcinoembryonic antigen and beta-human chorionic gonadotropin as serum markers for advanced urothelial malignancies. J Urol 1986;136:403.
168. Cross PA, Eyden BP, Joglekar VM. Carcinosarcoma of the urinary bladder: a light, immunohistochemical and electron microscopic case report. Virchows Arch A Pathol Anat Histopathol 1989;415:91.
169. Fromowitz FB, Bard RH, Koss LG. The epithelial origin of a malignant mesodermal mixed tumor of the bladder report of a case with long-term survival. J Urol 1984;132:978.
170. Grossman HB, Sonda LP III, Lloyd RV, Gikas PW. Carcinosarcoma of bladder: evaluation by electron microscopy and immunohistochemistry. Urology 1984;24:387.
171. Mazzucchelli L, Kraft R, Gerber H, Egger C, Studer UE, Zimmermann A. Carcinosarcoma of the urinary bladder: a distinct variant characterized by small cell undifferentiated carcinoma with neuroendocrine features. Virchows Archiv A Pathol Anat 1992;421:477.
172. Sen SE, Malek RS, Farrow GM, Lieber MM. Sarcoma and carcinosarcoma of the bladder in adults. J Urol 1985;133:29.
173. Smith JA Jr, Herr HW, Middleton RG. Bladder carcinosarcoma: histologic variation in metastatic lesions. J Urol 1983;129:829.
174. Young RH. Carcinosarcoma of the urinary bladder. Cancer 1987;59: 1333.
175. Smith AR, Parr PC. Squamous carcinoma. (letter) Eur J Surg Oncol 1992;18:202.
176. Huebner GD, Reed PA. Secreting tumors of chromaffin tissue. Ann Surg 1963;158:216.
177. Kishi H, Komatsu H, Kitagawa R, Ogawa A. Carcinosarcoma (collision tumor) of the urinary bladder: a case report. Nippon Hinyokika Gakkai Zasshi 1977;68:495.
178. Hejtmancik JH, Klatt WW. Co-existing carcinoma and sarcoma of the bladder. J Urol 1960;84:320.
179. Powers JH, Hawn CVZ, Carter RD. Osteogenic sarcoma and transitional cell carcinoma occurring simultaneously in the urinary bladder: report of a case. J Urol 1956;76:263.
180. Mackenzie AR, Whitmore WF Jr, Melamed MR. Myosarcomas of the bladder and prostate. Cancer 1968;22:833.
181. Ray B, Grabstald H, Exelby PR, Whitmore WJ Jr. Bladder tumors in children. Urology 1973;2:426.
182. Loughlin KR, Retik AB, Weinstein HJ, et al. Genitourinary rhabdomyosarcoma in children. Cancer 1989;63:1600.
183. Weitzner S. Leiomyosarcoma of urinary bladder in children. Urology 1978;12:450.
184. Thrasher JB, Miller GJ, Wettlaufer JN. Bladder leiomyosarcoma following cyclophosphamide therapy for lupus nephritis. J Urol 1990; 143:119.

185. Rowland RG, Eble JN. Bladder leiomyosarcoma and pelvic fibroblastic tumor following cyclophosphamide therapy. J Urol 1983;130:344.
186. Seo S, Clark SA, McGovern FD, Clark DL, Johnson EH. Leimyosarcoma of the urinary bladder: 13 years after cyclophosphamide therapy for Hodgkin's disease. Cancer 1985;55:1597.
187. Patterson DE, Barrett DM. Leiomyosarcoma of urinary bladder. Urology 1983;21:367.
188. Swartz DA, Johnson DE, Ayala AG, Watkins DL. Bladder leiomyosarcoma: a review of 10 cases with 5-year followup. J Urol 1985; 133:200.
189. Ahlering TE, Weintraub P, Skinner DG. Management of adult sarcomas of the bladder and prostate. J Urol 1988;140:1397.
189a. Berenson RJ, Flynn S, Freiha FS, et al. Primary osteogenic sarcoma of the bladder: case report and review of the literature. Cancer 1986; 57:350.
190. Young RH, Eble JN. Unusual forms of carcinoma of the urinary bladder. Hum Pathol 1991;22:948.
191. Zimmerman IJ, Biron RE, MacMahon HE. Pheochromocytoma of the urinary bladder. N Engl J Med 1953;249:25.
192. Das S, Bulusu NV, Lowe P. Primary vesical pheochromocytoma. Urology 1983;21:20.
193. Leestma JE, Price EB Jr. Paraganglioma of the urinary bladder. Cancer 1971;28:1063.
194. Fries JG, Chamberlin JA. Extra-adrenal pheochromocytoma: literature review and report of a cervical pheochromocytoma. Surgery 1968; 63:268.
195. Deklerk DP, Catalona WJ, Nime FA, Freeman C. Malignant pheochromocytoma of the bladder: the late development of renal cell carcinoma. J Urol 1975;113:864.
196. Kalff V, Shapiro B, Lloyd R, et al. The spectrum of pheochromocytoma in hypertensive patients with neurofibromatosis. Arch Intern Med 1982;142:2092.
197. Leong CH, Wong KK, Saw D. Asymptomatic phaeochromocytoma of the bladder co-existing with carcinoma. Br J Urol 1976;48:123.
198. Samaan NA, Hickey RC, Shutts PE. Diagnosis, localization, and management of pheochromocytoma: pitfalls and follow-up in 41 patients. Cancer 1988;62:2451.
199. Heyman J, Cheung Y, Ghali V, Leiter E. Bladder pheochromocytoma: evaluation with magnetic resonance imaging. J Urol 1989;141:1424.
200. Sheehan EE, Greenberg SD, Scott R Jr. Metastatic neoplasms of the bladder. J Urol 1963;90:281.
201. Burnett AL, Epstein JI, Marshall FF. Adenocarcinoma of urinary bladder: classification and management. Urology 1991;37:315.
202. Wilson TG, Pritchett TR, Lieskovsky G, Warner NE, Skinner DG. Primary adenocarcinoma of bladder. Urology 1991;38:223.
203. Abenoza P, Manivel C, Fraley EE. Primary adenocarcinoma of the urinary bladder: clinicopathologic study of 16 cases. Urology 1987; 24:9.
204. Nocks BN, Heney NM, Daly JJ. Primary adenocarcinoma of urinary bladder. Urology 1983;21:26.
205. Jones WA, Gibbons RP, Correa RJ Jr, Cummings KB, Mason JT. Primary adenocarcinoma of bladder. Urology 1980;15:119.
206. Jacobo E, Leoning S, Schmidt JD, Culp DA. Primary adenocarcinoma of the bladder: a retrospective study of 20 patients. J Urol 1977;117: 54.
207. Daehlin L, Arslen LA, Haakaa S. Squamous cell carcinoma of the urinary bladder. Scand J Urol Nephrol 1991;25:275.

Principles and Practice of Genitourinary Oncology, edited by Derek Raghavan, Howard I. Scher, Steven A. Leibel, and Paul H. Lange. Lippincott-Raven Publishers, Philadelphia, © 1997.

CHAPTER 31

Urachal Carcinoma

Richard A. Santucci and Paul H. Lange

PREVALENCE

Urachal carcinoma is a uncommon neoplasm. There are fewer than 150 well-documented cases in the literature since 1863.[1] Estimates of the incidence of urachal cancer range from .07[2] to .34[3] of all bladder tumors. However, urachal cancer makes up 36% of all reported bladder adenocarcinoma.[4] There is approximately one case of urachal carcinoma per 600 treated bladder cancers,[5] or one case for every 5 million people.[5–6]

EMBRYOLOGY

The urachus is formed in early embryonic life and is obliterated by birth in most people. The first incarnation of the urachus is the cloaca, which forms by the fourth embryonic week, when the allantois (a diverticulum of yolk sac which plays no role in the developing human but is important in lower animals) connects to the primitive hindgut (Fig. 31-1*A*). Subsequently, the cloaca divides into the anorectal canal, which becomes the rectum, and the primitive urogenital sinus, which develops into the bladder, sex organs, and (in males) the prostate (Fig. 31-1*B*). At this point in embryonic development, this primitive urogenital sinus is made up of the allantois superiorly, the urinary bladder medially, and the pelvic and definitive urogenital sinus inferiorly. Finally, the lumen of the allantois is obliterated to form the urachus (Fig. 31-1*C*). In the adult, the urachus coalesces with the obliterated umbilical arteries to form the median umbilical ligament,[7] which is also called the ligamentum commune.[8–10]

Understanding the embryology of the urachus is important because of the controversies regarding the cellular origin of urachal cancers, which can contain elements of adenocarcinoma, sarcoma, or transitional cell carcinoma.[1] Many authors believe that the urachus must derive from cloacal material[8,11–12] because of its tendency to form adenocarcinoma just as the rectum does.[13] According to this view, urothelial adenocarcinoma occurs when rests of cuboidal epithelium transform into glandular intestinal epithelium and then degenerate further into cancer.[14–16] However, other authors postulate that urachal cancer need not form from intestinal-type glands but rather is metaplastic in origin.[4,17–18] Support for the metaplastic degeneration argument is found in the existence of rare, mixed-type urachal cancers, in which inflammation, transitional cell cancer, and adenocarcinoma exist side by side.[19] Further support for this argument is found in experimental models in which bladder tissue in the rat was induced to form glandular epithelium.[20–21]

ANATOMY

Urachal cancers should be distinguished from primary bladder cancers that occur at the dome of the urinary bladder. Criteria for this distinction were first proposed by Wheeler and Hill in 1954.[22] These are:

1. Location in the dome of the bladder
2. Absence of cystitis cystica or cystitis glandularis
3. Predominant involvement of the muscularis rather than the submucosa
4. Demonstration of a urachal remnant connected to the neoplasm
5. Presence of a suprapubic mass

These criteria were modified later by Mostofi and colleagues[4] to include the following additional elements:

6. Sharp demarcation between tumor and normal surface epithelium
7. Tumor growth in the bladder wall branching into the space of Retzius

Some researchers have suggested, however, that these criteria are too restrictive, arguing that not all urachal cancers occur in association with urachal remnants and that some indeed do occur in the presence of cystitis cystica.[23–24] Modern authors have suggested that the most important consideration for diagnosis are criteria 1 and 6, as listed previously. In addition, primary adenocarcinoma located elsewhere that has spread to the bladder (e.g., breast, colon) must be excluded.[23] The search for primary adenocarcinoma of extraurachal origin may be aided by pathologic stains for sulfated acid mucopolysaccharides,

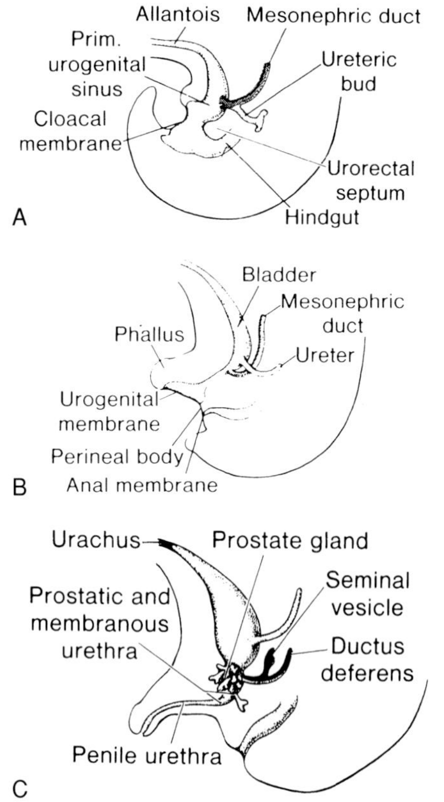

FIG. 31-1. Gestational development of the urachus. (**A**) End of fifth week. (**B**) End of eighth week. (**C**) End of twelfth week. (From Sadler TW. Langman's medical embryology, 5th ed. Baltimore: Williams & Wilkins, 1985:255.)

which are present in mucinous cells of colonic origin but not in those of urachal origin.[25]

PRESENTATION

Because so few patients are seen at any one institution, the reported presenting characteristics of patients with urachal cancers have wide variability. Most patients present with hematuria (71%) or a palpable mass (64%).[1] Other presenting symptoms include pain (21% to 42%), irritative voiding symptoms (40%), mucosuria (16% to 21%), palpable mass (3%), or umbilical discharge (3%).[1,26] In older studies, a palpable mass was common, whereas in more recent series, a palpable mass is rarely the presenting sign. Because of the mucin-producing nature of most urachal tumors, rare patients have presented with pseudomyxoma peritonaei.[27–29] Although these tumors arise in the urachus, more than 90% of such patients have a cystoscopically evident lesion at the time of presentation.[1]

Although urachal cancer is rare, the urachus exists as a small bud or a closed epithelial canal in about one third of the population,[30–31] making it a structure that is frequently present, although seldom symptomatic.

DIAGNOSIS

The diagnosis of urachal cancer ultimately must be made by biopsy, most often during cystoscopy; however, imaging can help in diagnosis. Simple x-ray films (e.g., plain films, cystograms, and intravenous pyelograms [IVP]) were historically important in diagnosing urachal cancer and are still useful today. In some patients, supravesical calcifications may indicate the existence of a urachal tumor.[32–35] Some researchers have suggested that patients with calcified tumors should be evaluated with plain films after treatment.[35] IVP may allow diagnosis of a urachal tumor when it is very large, because the urachal mass may displace ureters medially[36] or cause hydroureter.[37] Additionally, during a formal cystogram or the cystogram phase of an IVP, compression of the bladder from a superior urachal mass may be seen.[37–40] Such compression has been found in 5%[33] to 10%[41] of cases.

Although ultrasonography is not commonly used in cases of urachal tumor, a calcified[35–36,42] or uncalcified[43] suprapubic mass may be seen using this imaging modality. Ultrasonography is especially suited for urachal study, because the area is not generally obstructed by loops of bowel and the urachus can easily be seen.[36,44] The use of endovesical ultrasonography has also been reported to be useful in discovering a urachal tumor.[45] However, just as with ultrasonographic determinations of renal masses, most patients with urachal tumors will undergo staging computed tomographic (CT) scans even if ultrasonography reveals urachal pathology.

CT scanning is extremely useful in differentiating urachal carcinoma from bladder dome tumor. CT evidence of extravesical growth along the course of the urachus was found exclusively in urachal cancers, whereas bladder tumors exhibited only intravesical growth.[46] A review of literature corroborates this finding in nine of nine patients.[33]

As with other mucinous adenocarcinomas, urachal cancers may have "typical psammomatous calcification" on CT scans in some cases.[21,43,46–51] Stippled calcification, which is thought to be pathognomonic for urachal cancers when associated with a supravesicular mass, can also be seen in some urachal tumors.[26,42,52–53] Three of six patients in a recent series had such calcifications,[46] whereas only three of nine patients in a review of the literature had these calcifications. All three patients had calcifications which could be seen on plain films, making CT diagnosis unnecessary.

CT is always useful as a staging tool in the workup of a known or suspected urachal carcinoma, especially in more advanced tumors.[42,54] CT scanning also allows CT-guided biopsy of urachal tumors, which may prove useful in some nonoperative situations.[42]

Magnetic resonance (MR) imaging is increasingly being used to diagnose many types of cancer, and preliminary reports about this modality in urachal cancer are surfacing. In one case, urachal adenocarcinoma was easily seen on the T2-weighted image, although perhaps no better than on CT scans.[55] Although further study is needed, other authors feel that MR offers the benefit over CT scans of multiple-plane views of the urachus and may prove more useful than CT in determining bladder wall invasion from urachal cancers.[56]

Regardless of how the urachal cancer is found, before definitive treatment, cystoscopy and biopsy should be performed. In most cases the biopsy is conducted at the time of cystoscopy. Rarely, in a mass that is seen to be stage I on imaging and cystoscopy, biopsy might be conducted by open surgery. In our opinion, percutaneous needle biopsy should be avoided. For the majority of cases in which biopsy is performed at cystoscopy, it should be conducted in such a way as to avoid bladder perforation. Usually a loop resection is appropriate, although at other times cold cup biopsy may be more prudent to avoid perforation. In cases in which a supravesical mass is apparent but the bladder mucosa is not involved, a transcystoscopic long needle biopsy, such as is performed in transendoscopic biopsy of pancreas transplants, is appropriate.

STAGING

There is no staging system for urachal cancer that is universally accepted or verified by survival data. In the early literature, staging systems of urachal cancer were based on detailed designations of anatomic location (i.e., supravesical, intramuscular, intramucosal),[57] but these systems were probably too complex and not clinically useful.[24] The staging system proposed by Sheldon and colleagues[1] seems to be the best and is the most commonly used (Table 31-1).

HISTOLOGY

Urachal cancers consist of mucin-positive adenocarcinoma in 69% of cases, mucin-negative adenocarcinoma in 15%, sarcoma in 8%, and transitional cell carcinoma in 3%.[1] The mucin-positive cancers can be further classified into several subgroups, as is adenocarcinoma in other anatomic sites: ''colonic'' type in 50%, goblet cell type in 36%, colloid type in 36%, and the rare signet-ring type in 7% (1 in 14 patients).[23]

Urachal cancers can also present as mixed cancers of different cell types. Recent analysis of the Mayo Clinic experience revealed that 2 of 38 urachal tumors contained more than one cell type—in these cases, adenocarcinoma plus transitional cell carcinoma, and adenocarcinoma plus transitional cell carcinoma plus small cell types.[26] Little data exists regarding the ploidy of urachal cancers; however, in a small series from the Mayo Clinic, 10 of 10 urachal cancers were aneuploid, a correlate of aggressive tumors.[26]

PROGNOSIS

Historically, patients with urachal carcinoma have a poor prognosis. For example, in 1969, Gillenwater and Sandusky[58] deemed adenocarcinoma ''usually fatal.'' Old series estimate 5-year survival at about 6.5%[10]; more recent series estimate 5-year survival at 43%. The median time to death is about 5 years.[26] Even with surgery—either radical cystectomy and urachectomy or a more limited partial cystectomy and urachectomy—50% of patients die of the disease (n = 75).[59] The sites and incidences of first postoperative recurrence were as follows: local (51%), lymph nodes (31%), lung (28%), peritoneum (19%), omentum (18%), mesentery (15%), liver (14%), bone (13%), small bowel (11%), and other (13%).[60] Sheldon and colleagues[1] found that the specific location of local recurrence varied between adenocarcinoma and squamous cell cancers and sarcomas; the former commonly invade down into the bladder, whereas the latter usually invade the overlying peritoneum, abdominal wall, and umbilicus.

Debate continues about the relative lethality of each of the different urachal cell types. After a review of most of the world's urachal tumor literature in 1984, Sheldon and colleagues[1] concluded that ''There are insufficient data in the literature to make an correlation between histologic grade or differentiation and diagnosis. However, we assume that this cancer behaves like most other similar neoplasms and that prognosis is related to differentiation.'' In contrast, Rubell and Porges[9] concluded that ''the prognosis is uniformly poor'' for all cell types. Others have found no survival differences between the colloid and the colonic cell types.[23]

TABLE 31-1. *Staging of urachal carcinoma*

Stage	Description
I	No invasion beyond urachal mucosa
II	Invasion confined to urachus
III	Local extension
A	Into bladder
B	Into abdominal wall
C	Into peritoneum
D	Into viscera other than bladder
IV	Metastases
A	To regional lymph nodes
B	To distant sites

From Sheldon C, Clayman RV, Gonzales R, Williams RD, Fraley EE. Malignant urachal lesions. J Urol 1984;131:1.

TREATMENT

Chemotherapy

Chemotherapy has little success against urothelial adenocarcinoma in general and urachal adenocarcinoma specifically. For example, regimens such as 5-fluorouracil; doxorubicin and mitomycin[23,60–61]; or cisplatin, cyclophosphamide, and doxorubicin[23] have been tried in patients with urachal adenocarcinoma with little success.

Radiotherapy

Although tried many times, radiotherapy also fails against urachal tumors.[1,6,27,62–64] Rarely, urachal tumors may be radiosensitive; there are sporadic case reports relating survival of 6, 10, and 14 years after radiotherapy alone.[4,37,65] In any case, radiotherapy seems to be well tolerated by patients, whether given as primary or adjuvant therapy.[66]

Surgery

Although the literature supports the conclusion that surgery is the best initial treatment for urachal cancer, there is controversy about exactly which surgery is best. What is not debated is that in every surgery a total urachectomy is required. This entails removal of the umbilicus and the urachus together with a generous strip of peritoneum, and the median umbilical ligaments down to their origin at the internal iliac artery. Accordingly, the accompanying lymphadenectomy should include the tissue around the bifurcation of the common iliac artery where the median umbilical ligament inserts.

Many authors have recommended that radical cystectomy be performed in most cases of urachal cancer.[1,10,31,67–68] Although most of these reports recommend this radical surgery in all cases, Sheldon and colleagues[1] tempered their preference for radical surgery by suggesting that a urachectomy and partial cystectomy could suffice in those rare cases of stage I, low-grade urachal cancers and in sarcomas.

An equally large number of authors have concluded that urachectomy and partial cystectomy is sufficient in patients with urachal cancer, except when tumor size obviates such an organ-sparing approach.[23,26,59,69–70] In general, the reasoning is that the prognosis is equally dismal with either approach; about 50% of patients are cured in either case. Whitehead and Tessler[59] reported a slightly *better* 5-year survival with partial cystectomy rather than radical cystectomy; however, as with most of the reports, the number of the patients in this series was small. Herr[70] reported very good survival in urachal cancer patients treated with partial cystectomy—only 2 of 12 patients experienced a recurrence after a long follow-up. Accordingly, Herr also recommends organ-sparing surgery, although it is difficult to know whether his excellent results were because of careful patient selection. One exception to the partial cystectomy stance that would probably be advocated by all experts is signet ring adenocarcinoma. These tumors are extremely aggressive in the bladder, and are probably similarly so in the urachus.[69] With signet ring tumors, if cure appears anatomically possible, total cystectomy seems most prudent.

In a review of our own cases and the world's literature,[71] it appears that in at least one clinical setting, partial cystectomy is appropriate for urachal carcinoma. This is the situation in which the tumor is appropriately small and, as confirmed by biopsy, is composed of well-differentiated urachal adenocarcinoma reminiscent of low-grade colonic neoplasm. In these cases, 15 of 17 patients were cured with organ-sparing surgery.[18,22–23,37,41,72–75] The two that were not cured were nearly the oldest reports.[8,16]

CONCLUSIONS

Except for rare, well-differentiated cancers and sarcomas, it is not possible to determine which is the best surgical approach from the accumulated reported experience. We believe that because the cure rate of urachal cancer is so poor, and because local recurrence is the most common form of failure, that wide excision with a thorough pelvic lymphadenectomy, especially around the iliac bifurcation, is the best approach. In most cases, this approach will entail a total cystectomy. In men, a cystoprostatectomy is advised, although excision of the prostate can be less aggressive, and a potency-sparing approach is often possible. In our opinion, the price for the most organ-ablative approach is no longer as severe because of the availability of continent urinary reservoirs and neobladders. Improved methods for early diagnosis and the development of improved systemic therapy will be the most important factors for improving cure rates in the future.

REFERENCES

1. Sheldon C, Clayman RV, Gonzales R, Williams RD, Fraley EE. Malignant urachal lesions. J Urol 1984;131:1.
2. Miller A, Mitchell JP, Brown NJ. The Bristol bladder tumour registry. Br J Urol 1969;41:25.
3. Yu HHY, Leong CH. Carcinoma of the urachus: report of one case and a review of the literature. Surgery 1975;77:726.
4. Mostofi FK, Thomson RV, Dean AL Jr. Mucinous adenocarcinoma of the urinary bladder. Cancer 1955;8:741.
5. Ohman U, von Garrelts B, Moberg A. Carcinoma of the urachus. Scand J Urol Nephrol 1971;5:91.
6. Cornil C, Reynolds CT, Kickham CJE. Carcinoma of the urachus. J Urol 1967;98:93.
7. Sadler TW. Langman's medical embryology. 5th ed. Baltimore: Williams & Wilkins, 1985:254.
8. Dreyfuss ML. Benign and malignant lesions of the urachus: with special reference to the colloid carcinoma of the bladder. VA Med Monthly 1943;70:200.
9. Rubell D, Porges RF. Carcinoma of the urachus: a case report and review. Obstet Gynecol 1972;39:753.
10. Nadjmi B, Whitehead ED, McKiel CF Jr, Gray EC, Callahan DH. Carcinoma of the urachus: report of two cases and review of the literature. J Urol 1968;100:738.
11. Arey LB. The urinary system. In: Developmental anatomy: a textbook and laboratory manual of embryology. 6th ed. Philadelphia: WB Saunders, 1965:310.
12. Orr TGJ, Hardin CA. Mucinous adenocarcinoma of the urachus. Am Surg 1953;19:458.
13. Schaffarzick WR. Mucinous adenocarcinoma of the urachus: report of a case. Am Surg 1954;20:887.
14. Bandler CG, Roen PR. Mucinous adenocarcinoma in urachal cyst and involving bladder. J Urol 1950;64:504.
15. Patch FS, Pritchard JE. Mucinous adenocarcinoma of the bladder. J Urol 1947;57:126.
16. Saphir O, Kurland SK. Adenocarcinoma of the urinary bladder. Urol Cutan Rev 1939;43:709.
17. Kretschmer HL. Primary mucus secreting adenocarcinoma of the bladder. J Urol 1949;61:754.
18. Bourne CW, May JE. Urachal remnants: benign or malignant? J Urol 1977;118:743.
19. Abeshouse BS. Exstrophy of the bladder complicated by adenocarcinoma of the bladder and renal calculi. J Urol 1943;49:259.
20. Cunha GR, Chung LWK, Shannon JM, Taguchi O, Fujii H. Hormone-induced morphogenesis and growth: role of mesenchymal-epithelial interactions. Rec Prog Horm Res 1983;39:559.
21. Fujii H, Cunha GR, Norman JT. The induction of adenocarcinomatous differentiation in neoplastic bladder epithelium by an embryonic prostatic inductor. J Urol 1982;128:858.
22. Wheeler JD, Hill WT. Adenocarcinoma involving the urinary bladder. Cancer 1954;7:119.
23. Johnson DE, Hodge GB, Abdul-Karim FW, Ayala AG. Urachal carcinoma. Urology 1985;26:218.
24. Hayman J. Carcinoma of the urachus. Pathology 1984;16:167.
25. Tiltman AJ, Maytom PAN. Adenocarcinoma of the urinary bladder: histochemical distinctions between urachal and metastatic carcinomas. S Afr Med J 1977;51:74.
26. Henly DR, Farrow GM, Zincke H. Urachal cancer: role of conservative surgery. Urology 1993;42:635.
27. Ferrier PA, Craig LG, Foord AG. Tumors of the bladder of urachal origin. Urol Cutan Rev 1936;40:457.
28. Faulkner JW, Greene LF, McDonald JR. Mucinous adenocarcinoma in a urachal cyst producing pseudomyxoma peritonaei. J Urol 1954;72:217.
29. Mendeloff J, McSwain NEJ. Pseudomyxoma peritonei due to mucinous adenocarcinoma of the urachus. South Med J 1971;64:497.
30. Begg RC. The urachus: its anatomy, histology and development. J Anat 1930;64:170.
31. Schubert GE, Pavkovic MB, Bethke-Bedurftig BA. Tubular urachal remnants in adult bladders. J Urol 1982;127:40.
32. Pollock AB. A case of adenocarcinoma of the urachus showing extensive calcification. Br J Surg 1952;40:187.
33. Korobkin M, Cambier L, Drake J. Computed tomography of urachal carcinoma. J Comput Assist Tomogr 1988;12:981.
34. Spencer H. Mucoid adenocarcinoma of the urinary bladder. Br J Surg 1941;29:400.
35. Cooperman LR. Carcinoma of urachus with extensive abdominal calcification. Urology 1978;12:614.

36. Han SY, Witten DM. Carcinoma of the urachus. Am J Roentgenol 1976;127:351.
37. Prentiss RJ, Mullenix RB, Whisenand JM, Feeney MJ. Tumors of the urachus: report of five cases. Calif Med 1956;84:24.
38. Swersie AK, Solomon C, Rayos BOJ. Urachal adenocarcinoma of the urinary bladder. J Int Coll Surg 1959;31:169.
39. Jakse G, Schneider HM, Jacobi GH. Urachal signet-ring cell carcinoma, a rare variant of vesical adenocarcinoma: incidence and pathological criteria. J Urol 1978;120:764.
40. Tripathi VNP, Pandey AP, Rastogi BL. Urachus cyst with carcinoma. Int J Cancer 1976;13:183.
41. Beck AD, Gaudin HJ, Bonham DG. Carcinoma of the urachus. Br J Urol 1970;42:555.
42. Fitzgerald EJ, Pirani M. Computed tomography and ultrasound of urachal cancer. Br J Radiol 1985;58:88.
43. Spataro RF, Davis RS, McLachlan MSF, Barbaric ZL. Urachal abnormalities in the adult. Radiology 1983;149:659.
44. Williams BD, Fisk JD. Sonographic diagnosis of giant urachal cyst in the adult. Am J Roentgenol 1981;136:417.
45. Wishnow KI. Endovesical ultrasonography of urachal carcinoma. Urol Radiol 1989;11:53.
46. Narumi Y, Sato T, Kuriyama K, et al. Vesical dome tumors: significance of extravesical extension on CT. Radiology 1988;169:383.
47. Sarno RC, Klauber G, Carter BL. Computer assisted tomography of urachal abnormalities. J Comput Assist Tomogr 1983;7:674.
48. Kwok-Liu JP, Zikman JM, Cockshott WP. Carcinoma of the urachus: the role of computed tomography. Radiology 1980;137:731.
49. Mekras GD, Block NOL, Carrion HM, Ishikoff M. Urachal carcinoma: diagnosis by computerized axial tomography. J Urol 1980;123:275.
50. Nesbitt JA, Walther PJ. Computed tomographic imaging of microscopic dystrophic calcification in urachal adenocarcinoma. Urology 1986;17:184.
51. Lee SH, Kitchens HH, Kim BS. Adenocarcinoma of the urachus: CT features. J Comput Assist Tomogr 1990;14:232.
52. Ravi R, Shrivastava BR, Chandrasekhar GM, Prahlad S, Balasubramanian KV, Mallikarjuna VS. Adenocarcinoma of the urachus. J Surg Oncol 1992;50:201.
53. Garber BB, Pollack HM. Hematuria is the chief complaint: what is your diagnosis? Contemp Urol 1992;4:11.
54. Jemni M, El Mansouri F, Belhassine L, Njeh M, El Ouakdi M, Ayed M. Le cancer de l'ouraque. J Urol (Paris) 1992;98:173.
55. Brick SH, Friedman AC, Pollack HOM, et al. Urachal carcinoma: CT findings. Radiology 1988;169:377.
56. Rafal R b, Markisz JA. Urachal carcinoma: the role of magnetic resonance imaging. Urol Radiol 1991;12:184.
57. Begg RC. The colloid adenocarcinomata of the bladder vault arising from the epithelium of the urachal canal: with a critical survey of the tumours of the urachus. Br J Surg 1931;18:422.
58. Gillenwater JY, Sandusky WR. Mucinous adenocarcinoma of the urachus. Am Surg 1969;35:267.
59. Whitehead ED, Tessler AN. Carcinoma of the urachus. Br J Urol 1971; 43:468.
60. Kakizoe T, Matsumoto K, Andoh M, Nishio Y, Kishi K. Adenocarcinoma of the urachus: report of 7 cases and review of literature. Urology 1983;21:360.
61. Logothetis CJ, Samuels ML, Ogden S. Chemotherapy for adenocarcinomas of bladder and urachal origin: 5-fluorouracil, doxorubicin, and mitomycin-C. Urology 1985;26:252.
62. Franksson C. Tumours of the urinary bladder. Acta Chir Scand 1950; 151(Suppl):127.
63. Thomas DG, Ward AM, Williams JL. A study of 52 cases of adenocarcinoma of the bladder. Br J Urol 1971;43:4.
64. Taylor GD, McRae CU. Carcinoma of the urachus: Report of four cases and review of the literature. N Z Med J 1978;87:384.
65. Grogono JL, Shepheard BGF. Carcinoma of the urachus. Br J Urol 1969;41:222.
66. Ojeda L, Johnson DE. Partial cystectomy: can it be incorporated into integrated therapy program? Urology 1983;22:115.
67. Satpathy RS. Carcinoma of the urachus. J Ind Med Assoc 1966;46:38.
68. Hurwitz SP, Jacobson EB, Ottenstein HH. Mucoid adenocarcinoma of the urachus invading bladder. J Urol 1951;65:87.
69. Burnett AL, Epstein JI, Marchall FF. Adenocarcinoma of the urinary bladder: classification and management. Urology 1991;37:315.
70. Herr HW. Urachal carcinoma: The case for extended partial cystectomy. J Urol 1994;151:365.
71. Santucci RA, True L, Lange PH. Is partial cystectomy the treatment of choice for mucinous adenocarcinoma of the urachus? Report of a case. Urology 1995 (in press).
72. DeWaard T. Two rare cases of bladder tumor (urachus tumor). J Urol 1939;42:554.
73. Cawker CA. Mucinous adenocarcinoma of the urachus, invading the urinary bladder. Can Med Assoc J 1947;57:58.
74. Bobrow ML. Mucoid carcinoma of the urachus. Am J Obstet Gynecol 1953;65:909.
75. Howell MGJ, Diddle AW. Mucinous adenocarcinoma of the urachus in women. Am J Obstet Gynecol 1967;98:585.

Principles and Practice of Genitourinary Oncology, edited by Derek Raghavan, Howard I. Scher, Steven A. Leibel, and Paul H. Lange. Lippincott-Raven Publishers, Philadelphia, © 1997.

CHAPTER 32

Transitional Cell Carcinoma of the Upper Urinary Tract

James D. Brooks and Fray F. Marshall

Carcinomas of the renal pelvis and ureter account for fewer than 1% of all genitourinary neoplasms and an estimated 5% to 7% of all renal neoplasms.[1,2] Carcinoma of the upper urinary tract is two to three times more common in men than in women, and twice as common in whites as in blacks.[3] The frequency of this tumor increases with age, with a peak incidence in the sixth and seventh decades of life.[1–6]

Several retrospective studies have suggested that the incidence of upper tract tumors is increasing in industrialized countries.[4,6] The increases have been attributed to improvements in diagnostic methods and a heightened awareness of these tumors. A recent review of the Danish Cancer Registry has demonstrated a tenfold increase in upper tract tumors between 1943 and 1988.[7] During the same time period, the incidence of other tumors increased only modestly or not at all, implying that the increased incidence of upper tract tumors does not merely reflect improvements in diagnosis.

ETIOLOGY

The causes of upper tract transitional cell carcinoma remain obscure. It is likely that inherited and environmentally induced genetic changes, similar or identical to those involved in bladder cancer, combine to generate the malignant phenotype. Heritable forms of upper tract transitional cell carcinoma, occurring in association with the cancer family syndrome (Lynch syndrome II) or in isolation, have been described.[8–10] Although heritable forms of these tumors account for a small fraction of upper tract tumors, it is likely that heritable factors, such as differences in the metabolism of carcinogens, act in concert with environmental factors to generate these neoplasms.[11,12]

Several environmental risk factors have been identified for upper tract transitional carcinoma. Cigarette smoking confers a 2.6- to 4.5-fold increased risk for development of upper tract tumors.[13,14] A strong dose-effect relation has been documented, with long-term smokers having a sevenfold to eightfold risk.[15] It is estimated that 70% of cancers of the renal pelvis and ureter among men and 40% among women are caused by smoking. Cessation of smoking decreases risk with passage of time.

Analgesic abuse, particularly abuse of phenacetin (now withdrawn form the market in the United States), has been associated with transitional cell carcinoma of the upper tract.[16–24] Excessive consumption of phenacetin is known to cause chronic interstitial nephritis, capillary sclerosis, and renal papillary necrosis. In addition, phenacetin metabolites have been identified as potential carcinogens.[17] Tumors derived from phenacetin abusers often harbor *P53* mutations.[20] It is unclear whether these mutations result directly from phenacetin metabolites or from oxygen free radicals released by macrophages in response to phenacetin-induced nephritis. A case-controlled study by McCredie and associates found phenacetin consumption and renal papillary necrosis to be independent risk factors for the development of upper tract transitional cell carcinoma, suggesting that both mechanisms may be operative.[21] Tumors are associated with consumption of high doses (5 kg) of phenacetin and have a mean latency of 25 years.[18] Phenacetin abuse confers a 2.6-fold to sevenfold risk for development of upper tract tumors, and in patients with renal papillary necrosis the risk jumps to 20-fold.[21,22] In some series, up to 20% of patients with upper tract tumors gave a history of phenacetin abuse, and it is estimated that 10% of phenacetin abusers develop a urothelial neoplasm.[18] Excessive use of other analgesics, notably acetaminophen and aspirin, has also been associated with increased risk of upper tract tumors.[23]

Occupational exposure to coal, coke, asphalt, or tar and employment in the chemical, petrochemical, or plastics industries have also been associated with increased risk of upper tract tumors in several case-controlled studies.[13,25,26] Cyclophosphamide has been implicated in transitional cell carcinoma of the bladder and has been related to upper tract malignancies.[27] The contrast agent Thorotrast, used for retrograde pyelography in the early 1930s, has been associated with metaplasia and aggressive tumors of the upper urinary tracts.[28]

Individuals affected by Balkan endemic nephropathy have a markedly elevated risk of developing upper tract transitional cell carcinoma.[29–36] Balkan endemic nephropathy is a chronic tubulointerstitial renal disease that occurs almost exclusively among farm workers living in geographically discrete areas of

Romania, Bulgaria, and the former Yugoslavia.[32] Men and women are affected equally. There is strong evidence for an environmental cause of this disease. Individuals from endemic regions who emigrate before age 17 or 18 appear to be spared, whereas immigrants from nonendemic to endemic regions are liable to become affected. The latency period is approximately 20 years, and most individuals are affected during the fifth or sixth decade of life. The risk of upper tract transitional cell carcinoma is 100-fold higher in endemic regions.[29] Approximately 40% of persons with Balkan endemic nephropathy develop upper tract tumors.[35] On the other hand, 40% of persons with upper tract tumors in these regions go on to renal failure, presumably secondary to endemic nephropathy.[29] Most tumors are low grade, and 10% are bilateral. Because of the high recurrence rate and high incidence of bilateral disease, conservative surgery is advocated for patients affected by this disease.[30] In endemic regions, familial clustering of upper tract tumors, bladder tumors, and nongenitourinary tumors has been observed. This observation argues for a genetic contribution to the genesis of these neoplasms.[33,36] Continued study of this disease is likely to provide significant insights into the cause of upper tract tumors.

TABLE 32-1. *Staging systems of upper tract tumors*

AJCC Stage	UICC Stage*	Description
0	Tis	Carcinoma in situ
	Ta	Noninvasive papillary carcinoma
I	T1	Tumor involves subepithelial connective tissue
II	T2	Tumor invades muscularis
III	T3	Tumor invades peripelvic or periureteral or renal parenchyma
IV	T4	Tumor invades adjacent organs
	Any T N1	Lymph node metastasis <2 cm diameter
	Any T N2	Single lymph node 2–5 cm diameter
	Any T N3	Lymph node >5 cm diameter
	Any T, any N, M1	Distant metastases

AJCC, American Joint Committee on Cancer; UICC, International Union Against Cancer.

* T0, N0, M0 denote no primary tumor, no nodal metastasis, no distant metastasis. TX, NX, MX signifies that the presence of tumor at that site cannot be assessed.

PATHOLOGY

About 90% of renal pelvic tumors and 99% of ureteral tumors are transitional cell carcinomas[4,37,38] (see Chap. 18). The grading system for these tumors is identical to that for bladder cancer. At presentation, approximately 20% of tumors are low grade, 40% are intermediate grade, and 30% are high grade.[1–6,37] Two thirds of tumors are located in the renal pelvis. Fifteen percent of ureteral tumors are in the proximal ureter, 15% in the midureter, and 70% in the distal ureter.[24,39–41]

Squamous cell carcinoma comprises approximately 5% to 10% of renal pelvic tumors, although it rarely occurs in the ureter.[4,37,42,43] It is usually associated with renal pelvic stones, infection, and chronic inflammation. Squamous cell carcinoma is more common in men than in women and usually presents at high stage. These tumors are rarely resectable, have poor response to radiotherapy and chemotherapy, and are associated with a poor prognosis and short survival time. Adenocarcinoma of the renal pelvis and ureter accounts for a small fraction of urothelial neoplasms.

Two staging systems are primarily used to classify upper tract tumors (Table 32-1). The American Joint Committee on Cancer (AJCC) system is based on the Grabstald and Cummings modification of the Jewett classification of bladder tumors.[2,6,44] The system classifies tumors according to their depth of penetration. Stage 0 tumors are confined to the mucosa; stage I tumors demonstrate lamina propria invasion; stage II tumors invade the muscularis; stage III tumors invade the periureteric, peripelvic, or renal parenchyma; and stage IV tumors invade adjacent organs, extend through the kidney, have lymph node metastases, or have metastases to distant organs. The most common sites of metastasis are lymph nodes, lung, liver, and bone.[39,41,45] Lymph node metastases are present in the periaortic, paracaval, or pelvic nodes in 20% to 40% of cases at the time of diagnosis, depending on tumor grade, stage, and size.[39,44,46] The TNM system of the International Union Against Cancer (UICC) allows further classification of metastatic disease. In this system, stage 0 tumors are broken down into in situ (Tis) and papillary (Ta) tumors. UICC categories T1, T2, and T3 correspond to AJCC stages I, II, and III, respectively. The T4 classification implies invasion of contiguous organs. Lymph node metastases are classified as N0 for no metastases and N1 through N3 for metastases of increasing size. M0 denotes the absence and M1 the presence of metastases to distant sites.

CLINICOPATHOLOGIC CORRELATIONS

In a number of studies of upper tract transitional cell carcinoma, the most important prognostic factors have been found to be the grade and stage of the tumor.[1–6,24,39,40,44–60] Regardless of the method of treatment, patients with grade 1 transitional cell carcinoma of the upper tract have a long-term survival rate comparable to that of age- and sex-matched controls.[56] Patients with intermediate-grade tumors have 5-year survival rates that range from 40% to 80%, but those with high-grade tumors have very poor survival rates, in the range of 0% to 33% at 5 years (Table 32-2). Patients with noninvasive or minimally invasive tumors also have survival rates approaching those of the general population. Those with muscle-invasive tumors have 5-year survival rates of 30% to 80%, and those with invasion through the ureter have 5-year survival rates of less than 30%. Almost all patients with metastatic disease die within 2 years (Table 32-3). Grade and stage are closely correlated: low-grade tumors tend to be superficial, and high-grade tumors usually present as invasive or metastatic disease. Patients with ureteral or renal pelvic tumors, if matched for stage and grade, have similar survival rates; however, those with stage 3 (T3) tumors that invade the renal parenchyma appear to fare better than those with same-stage lesions that invade the peripelvic or periureteral fat.

TABLE 32-2. *Five-year survival rates after upper tract transitional cell carcinoma by histologic grade**

Investigators	Grade 1	Grade 2	Grade 3	Grade 4
Babaian and Johnson, 1980[4]	100	75	33	N/A
Cummings et al, 1974[44]	100	80	20	0
Batatu et al, 1975[39]	78	50	0	0
Matsuoka et al, 1991[51]	92.3	71	23.3	N/A
Heney et al, 1981[54]	100	81	29	N/A
Reitelman et al, 1987[55]	100	87	67	20
Davis et al, 1987[45]	100	67	5	N/A
Corrado et al, 1991[65]	83	75	52	0

N/A, Not applicable.
* Histologic grade by World Health Organization guidelines in references 4, 45, 51, and 54 and by Broder's classification in references 39, 44, 55, and 65. All figures are percentages.

Several additional prognostic factors have been identified. Patients younger than 60 years of age have higher survival rates than older patients.[51] The morphology of the tumor also has some prognostic significance. Patients with papillary tumors of all grades and stages have a 5-year survival rate of approximately 70%, compared with 25% for nonpapillary forms.[51,52] Vascular invasion on the pathologic specimen is correlated with diminished survival independent of tumor stage and grade.[61] Seventy-three percent of patients with vascular invasion develop metastases postoperatively, compared with 21% of those without vascular invasion. DNA ploidy, as measured by flow cytometry, has been reported to offer prognostic information on tumors of the upper tract.[62–68] The majority of low-grade, low-stage tumors are diploid and are associated with a favorable outcome. High-grade, high-stage tumors are predominantly aneuploid and are associated with a poor survival rate. Although the ploidy status of high- and low-grade tumors offers little new prognostic information, several groups have reported that the ploidy status of intermediate-grade tumors offers unique prognostic information. Measurement of the mitotic index of upper tract transitional cell carcinomas with bromodeoxyuridine has also been reported to offer prognostic significance for upper tract tumors.[69,70] Other techniques, such as evaluation of nuclear morphometry or analysis of mutations of tumor suppressor genes (e.g., *P53, RB1*), that have been used in bladder cancer research may also have a role in the study of upper tract tumors. Currently, the role of these techniques in determining the prognosis of upper tract tumors remains to be defined.

Transitional cell carcinoma is truly a disease of the entire urothelium. Patients with upper tract transitional cell carcinoma have a 2% to 4% chance of developing a tumor in the contralateral upper urinary tract.[39,40,71] Approximately 50% of patients with an upper tract tumor develop bladder cancer at some point in their lives.[3,72] Bladder tumors most commonly form in the ipsilateral wall of the affected upper tract. Detailed mapping studies have shown that 20% to 50% of upper tract tumors are multifocal.[24,52,73–75] There is a high rate of recurrence (30% to 75%) of transitional cell carcinoma in the ureteral stump if nephrectomy alone is performed for upper tract tumors.[72,76,77] In addition, upper tract tumors have been documented in patients with recurrent bladder tumors and vesicoureteral reflux.[78,79] These patterns of recurrence, as well as several molecular biologic studies, suggest that urothelial cancers are spread by intraluminal seeding, although seeding may not account for all tumors.[80,81]

The advent of effective topical intravesical therapies for bladder cancer may result in changes in the patterns of occurrence of upper tract tumors.[82–85] Normally, only 2% to 4% of patients with transitional cell carcinoma of the bladder develop upper tract tumors.[26,79,86] Patients treated with intravesical bacille Calmette-Guérin (BCG) are likely live longer with functioning bladders. Incidences of 13.4% and 29% have been reported for upper tract transitional cell carcinoma, particularly of the distal ureter, after treatment with BCG.[82,83] Of patients who have recurrence with positive cytology results after BCG treatment, 18% are found to have upper tract disease.[85] Periodic surveillance with radiographic and cytologic studies of the upper tracts is essential in patients treated for bladder tumors with topical

TABLE 32-3. *Five-year survival rates after upper tract transitional cell carcinoma by AJCC pathologic stage**

Investigators	Stage 0	Stage I	Stage II	Stage III	Stage IV
Cummings et al, 1974[44]	100	75	30	0	0
Bututa et al, 1975[39]	91†	—	43	23	0
Mills and Vaughn, 1983[47]	100	80	50	33.3	6
Matsuoka et al, 1991[51]	92.3	74.8	58	22.2‡	—
Heney et al, 1981[54]	100	95	82	29	0
Reitelmann et al, 1987[55]	100	89	86	33	0
Davis et al, 1987[45]	88†	—	88	33	5
Corrado et al, 1991[65]	80	83	72	51	15

AJCC, American Joint Committee on Cancer.
* All figures are percentages.
† Combined stage 0 and stage I lesions.
‡ Combined stage III and stage IV lesions.

therapy, particularly patients with carcinoma in situ, multiple tumors, T1 tumors, or failed intravesical therapy.

DIAGNOSIS

Approximately 80% of patients with upper tract transitional cell carcinoma present with gross total painless hematuria.[1–6,24,39,40,44–60] A small fraction of patients show microscopic hematuria only. The passage of vermiform clots is suggestive of upper tract bleeding. Flank pain, described as dull, aching, and nonradiating, occurs in 25% of patients and is thought be caused by local invasion and gradual ureteral obstruction. Acute colicky flank pain can occur with passage of blood clots. Constitutional symptoms, such as weight loss and anorexia, are found in fewer than 10% of patients and signal the presence of advanced disease. Physical examination is likely to be unrevealing, although up to 15% of patients have a palpable abdominal mass.[1,59] Almost 10% of patients are asymptomatic on presentation. Their lesions are discovered on intravenous pyelogram done for other reasons, such as follow-up for transitional cell carcinoma of the bladder. Although the need for routine upper tract monitoring after the diagnosis of bladder cancer is debated, interval pyelograms are prudent in patients at high risk for subsequent development of upper tract tumors. Risk factors include previous upper tract tumor, upper urinary tract symptoms, multiple recurrent bladder tumors, bladder tumors involving the ureteral orifices, previous cystectomy, Balkan nephropathy, phenacetin nephropathy, history of industrial exposure, and presence of vesicoureteral reflux.[26,86,78,79]

The evaluation of patients should include determination of serum creatinine, because the presence of azotemia may dictate a conservative procedure for the treatment of upper tract tumors. Liver function tests can provide a clue to the presence of metastatic disease. Urine culture and urine analysis are necessary because up to 15% of patients present with urinary tract infection or urosepsis.[1]

Intravenous urography is the test most commonly used to diagnose upper tract tumors; it is abnormal in 75% to 100% of cases.[1–6,24,25,37–40,42–60,87,88] A filling defect of the pelvis or ureter, the most common finding, occurs in 20% to 80% of patients. Other causes of a filling defect include a radiolucent stone, blood clot, fungus ball, extrinsic compression by a crossing vessel, overlying bowel gas, sloughed renal papilla, fibroepithelial polyp, air bubble, leukoplakia, malacoplakia, renal tuberculosis, cholesteatoma, leiomyoma, and hemangioma.[87] Nonvisualization of the involved kidney and ureter (silent kidney) occurs in one third to one half of patients. Hydronephrosis is found in approximately one third of studies, and ureteral narrowing or waisting is seen in approximately 10%. Mass effect or splaying of the calyces may be seen with renal involvement. Careful inspection of the entire collecting system and comparison with the contralateral kidney is helpful because occasionally one calyx or infundibulum does not fill. Function of

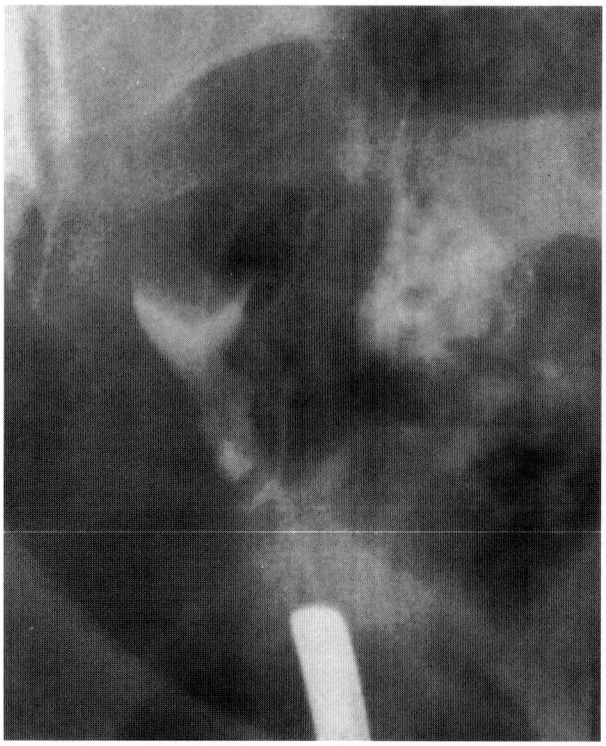

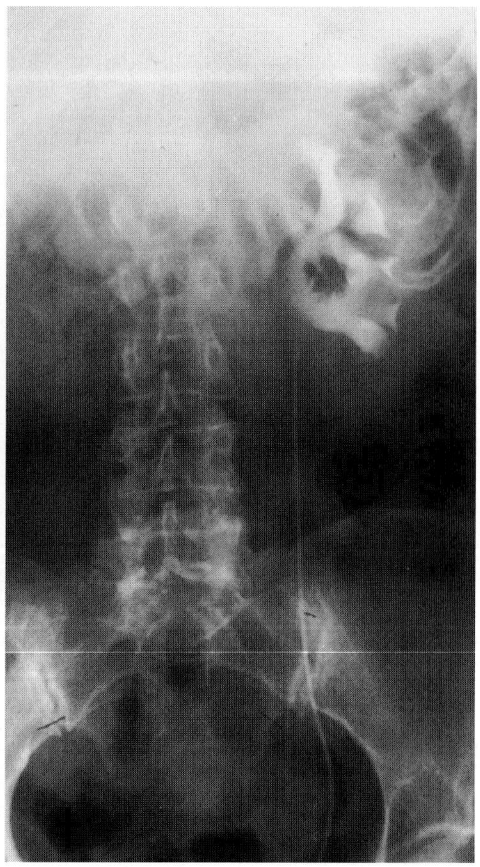

A B

FIG. 32-1. (**A**) Retrograde pyelogram demonstrates a filling defect, the wine goblet sign, that is typical of a distal ureteral tumor. (**B**) Retrograde pyelogram shows a left renal pelvic tumor.

the contralateral kidney should be assessed on the intravenous urogram to aid in planning future surgery. Radionuclide studies may be necessary to quantitate differential renal function.

Retrograde urography is useful to define abnormalities seen on excretory urography (Fig. 32-1). Approximately 75% of retrograde urograms demonstrate a filling defect. Ureteral dilatation below a filling defect, the wine goblet sign, is highly suggestive of a ureteral neoplasm. Bergman's sign, the coiling of a ureteral catheter below a filling defect, is virtually pathognomonic for ureteral tumor. At the time of retrograde urography, barbotaged urine samples can be obtained for cytology, and suspicious lesions can be sampled by ureteral brushing. Cytology specimens should be collected before a pyelogram is obtained, because the hyperosmolar contrast agents can make cytologic results difficult to interpret.

Cystoscopy is mandatory in evaluation of a patient with an upper tract tumor. Approximately 10% of patients have a concurrent bladder tumor.[88] In 21% of patients, blood can be seen effluxing from the ureteral orifice of the affected side. Tumor is seen extruding from the ureteral orifice in 6% of cases.[1] After treatment of the upper tract tumor, cystoscopy should be performed every 3 months because of the high incidence of bladder cancer recurrence in the first 2 years. Beyond 2 years, cystoscopy may be done at intervals of 6 months to 1 year.

Ultrasound has limited utility in evaluation of upper tract tumors (Fig. 32-2*A*). Slightly more than 50% of studies are abnormal.[88,89] Because of the absence of shadowing, tumors can reliably be distinguished from stones with ultrasonography.

Computed tomography (CT) and magnetic resonance (MR) imaging have definite utility for evaluation of upper tract tumors.[71,90,91] Both enhanced and nonenhanced CT should be performed, because stones may be obscured by the administration of contrast material (see Fig. 32-2). CT can reliably differentiate stones from tumors, can demonstrate metastatic disease, and many times can distinguish between transitional cell carcinoma of the renal pelvis and renal cell carcinoma. CT sensitivity for renal parenchyma invasion is approximately 75%, and for periureteral fat invasion it is 67%.[90] Almost 50% of papillary

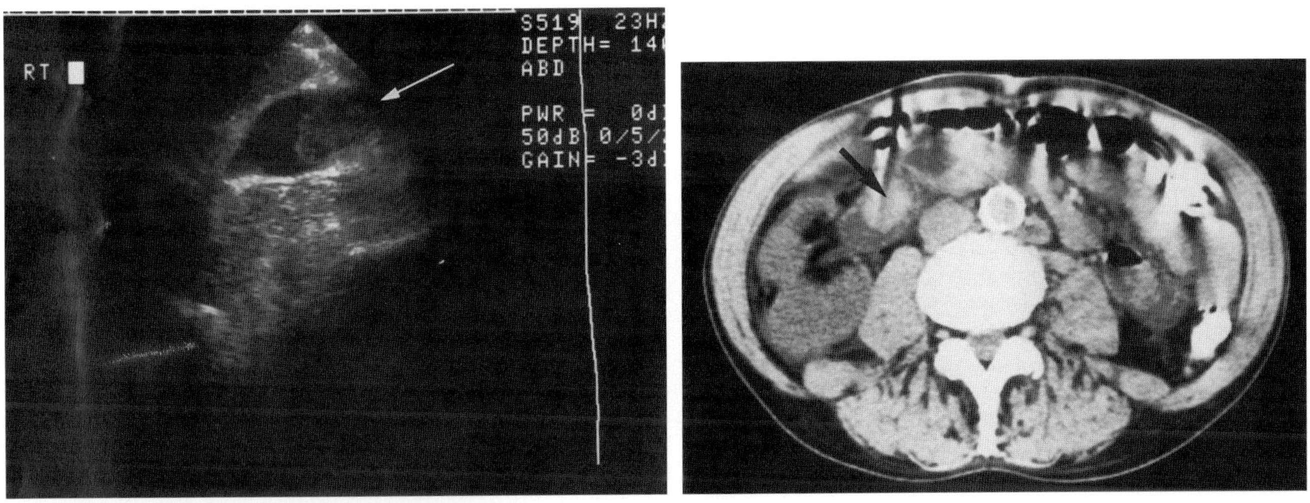

A B

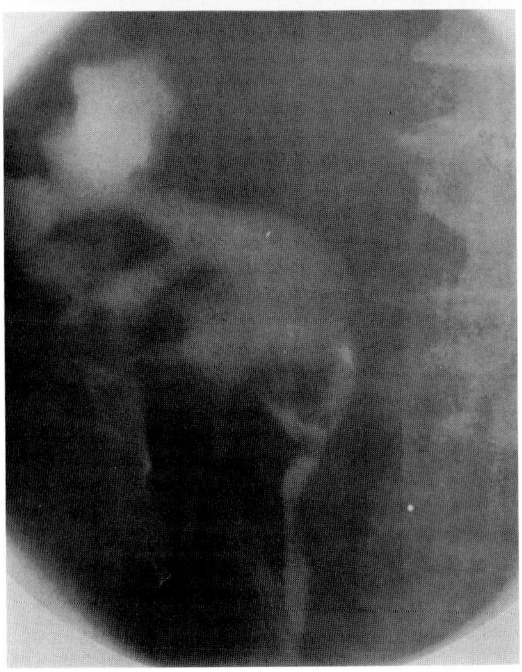

C

FIG. 32-2. (**A**) Ultrasound of a patient with a solitary kidney, hematuria, and azotemia shows a nonshadowing mass in the renal pelvis (*arrow*). (**B**) Nonenhanced CT scan confirms a right renal pelvic tumor (*arrow*). (**C**) Retrograde pyelogram delineates a carcinoma at the ureteropelvic junction. The patient underwent a segmental resection of the renal pelvis with postoperative instillation of mitomycin C. He was tumor-free with normal renal function 18 months after surgery.

tumors are missed on CT, and it is not possible to differentiate superficial from muscle-invasive disease. Spiral CT may offer improved sensitivity. MR imaging adds little to information gathered by CT except in the evaluation of patients with caval thrombus.

Urinary cytology aids in the diagnosis of upper tract tumors. Voided cytology samples are positive in only one third of patients.[46,91,92] Collection of cytology samples with a ureteral catheter increases the number of positive results to slightly more than 60%.[93] This technique also eliminates contamination from concomitant bladder tumors. The use of barbotage washing of the upper urinary tract can increase the detection rate to 80%.[94] As with bladder tumors, the likelihood of a positive urinary cytology result increases with higher-grade tumors.[95] Retrograde brush biopsy under fluoroscopic guidance may be performed at the time of retrograde studies and has a diagnostic accuracy of 78% to 89%.[96,97,98] However, brush biopsy offers no staging information, and up to 50% of tumors may be undergraded.[99] Although complications are uncommon, massive hemorrhage from ureteral perforation has been reported.[97] Brush biopsy should be reserved for situations in which a certain diagnosis is needed to plan future management.

Ureteroscopy has been used in small groups of patients to aid in the diagnosis of upper tract transitional cell carcinoma.[89,99–102] In two major referral centers, standard evaluation for upper tract tumors resulted in a definite diagnosis in slightly more than half of patients evaluated, but with ureteroscopy, biopsy, and barbotage, 80% to 90% of upper tract tumors were accurately diagnosed.[101,102] However, ureteroscopy has limited utility in staging of upper tract tumors. Approximately 60% of renal units removed after ureteroscopy have been found to be understaged.[99] Even in experienced hands, ureteroscopy is associated with significant complications, which may limit its use in the diagnostic evaluation of upper tract tumors. Ureteral perforation can occur in 7% of patients and can cause extravasation of tumor cells into the retroperitoneum.[102] Pyelovenous lymphatic migration of renal pelvic transitional carcinoma has been demonstrated after flexible ureteroscopy and probably resulted from the high pressure necessary to distend the collecting system.[103] Several case reports suggest that the exfoliation of normal mucosal cells during ureteroscopy may provide a bed for implantation of tumor cells and thereby disseminate the disease.[104] Diagnostic ureteroscopy therefore should have limited application.

TREATMENT OF LOCALIZED DISEASE

Nephroureterectomy with excision of a cuff of bladder is the standard therapy for clinically localized upper tract transitional cell carcinoma.[6,40,46,105] This procedure results in overall 5-year survival rates of 50% to 65%, although prognosis is principally related to tumor grade and stage (described previously). Surgical approaches include the thoracoabdominal retroperitoneal incision, the midline transabdominal approach, and the two-incision approach. The choice of incision is dictated mainly by patient anatomy and by the experience and preference of the surgeon. Regardless of the approach, surgery entails en bloc removal of the kidney, the ureter, and a cuff of bladder. Intravesical dissection of the ureter is necessary to ensure complete removal of its intramural portion. Extravesical approaches have been associated with retention of the ureteral stump and a 30% rate of recurrence of tumor in that stump.[106] Johansson and Wahlqvist have reported that nephroureterectomy with removal of Gerota's fascia and the ipsilateral adrenal resulted in a 5-year survival rate of 74% for patients with stage III and IV tumors, compared with 37% for patients who underwent intrafascial nephrectomy.[107] However, most patients in the latter group had nephrectomy without removal of the distal ureter. It therefore remains to be proved whether more extensive surgery is warranted in patients with high-grade, high-stage tumors.

Conservative, nephron-sparing surgical approaches have been described in the management of patients with upper tract tumors.[5,24,108–114] These approaches are most appropriate in patients with tumor in a solitary kidney, renal insufficiency, bilateral tumors, or endemic nephropathy. It is currently debatable whether conservative surgery can be applied to patients with a unilateral tumor and normal renal function. Advocates point out that the most important determinants of survival are anatomic stage and histologic grade of the cancer, regardless of the surgical approach used. However, such conclusions are hampered by the limited follow-up and small numbers of patients in published reports. To date, no prospective, randomized trial has compared conservative techniques to nephroureterectomy.

Surgeons contemplating conservative resection of upper tract tumors in any patient must consider several points. First, current techniques of preoperative grading and staging of upper tract tumors are inaccurate. Second, one third to one half of patients have multifocal disease, which many times is not detected on preoperative studies. Third, the anatomic location of the tumor dictates the appropriateness of conservative surgery. Tumors of the distal ureter treated by distal ureterectomy and reimplantation have a long-term ipsilateral recurrence rate of only 11%. However, segmental resection of upper tract tumors is associated with a 50% recurrent rate in the distal ureter.[99] Finally, patients with high-grade or high-stage disease fare worse with segmental resection than with nephroureterectomy.[59,115] McCarron and colleagues reported that 90% of patients with high-grade, high-stage tumors of the renal pelvis treated with local resection ultimately succumbed to the disease, whereas only 30% of a comparable group treated with nephroureterectomy died of cancer.[115] Appropriate patients for segmental resection are those with low-grade, low-stage disease confined to a discrete location in the upper urinary tract—ideally, the distal ureter. In this group, the 5-year survival rate among those treated with segmental resection is comparable the rate in patients treated with nephroureterectomy.

Endourologic techniques have recently been employed in the conservative management of upper tract tumors.[104,116–124] The indications for endoscopic approaches are identical to those for open conservative techniques and include patients who are unable or unwilling to undergo an open procedure. Both percutaneous and ureteroscopic approaches have been used for upper tract tumors. Several reports document the feasibility of endoscopic approaches; however, limited numbers of patients and inadequate follow-up make it difficult to assess the advisability of this treatment modality. The impact of endourology on the management of upper tract tumors is yet to be determined. Tumors are managed with either fulguration, electroresection, or neodymium-yttrium-aluminum-garnet (Nd:YAG) laser treatment. Electroresection risks perforation of the thin muscular wall of the upper urinary tract and may result in higher rates of stricture formation; therefore, the Nd:YAG laser may be the preferred modality for the treatment of upper tract tumors.[116,123] From published series, several shortcomings of endourologic techniques have become apparent. The local recurrence rate ranges from 20% to 50% within 2 years. There is a theoretic risk of dissemination of tumor cells because of the high pressures needed for visualization with endoscopic procedures and the violations of the urinary tract that are necessary in percutaneous approaches. Tomera and associates reported two renal fossa recurrences among 18 patients who underwent pyeloscopy.[125] Both patients had low-grade, low-stage tumors at initial diagnosis. Follow-up of patients undergoing endoscopic procedures can also be problematic. Given the uncertain efficacy of these approaches, strict follow-up with cytologic examination, radiographic imaging, and possibly ureteroscopy is necessary every 3 months. Several patients reported in the literature have required multiple endoscopic procedures under general anesthesia with its attendant risks. To facilitate follow-up endoscopy, Kerbl and Clayman have described incision of the ureterovesical junction, which allows office-based flexible ureteroscopy without analgesia or fluoroscopy.[126]

Topical therapy has been used as an adjunct to both open and endoscopic conservative surgery. BCG and mitomycin C are the agents used most commonly, and they appear to be relatively safe.[127–132] Although several case reports attest to the efficacy of these treatments, no controlled studies have been undertaken. Orihuela and Smith reported lower recurrence rates (29% versus 75%) in patients with upper tract tumors treated with adjuvant BCG after percutaneous tumor resection, versus those who received no treatment after resection.[120] If the ureterovesical junction is rendered incompetent, intravesical instillations may be used to treat upper tract tumors.[131]

Laparoscopic nephroureterectomy has recently been described in the management of upper tract tumors.[133,134] This procedure combines the potential high cure rates of nephroureterectomy with the low morbidity of endoscopic techniques. Variations on the procedure include (1) laparoscopic dissection of the kidney followed by a low midline incision for an intravesical resection of the distal ureter with a cuff of bladder and extraction of the kidney, (2) cystoscopic resection of the distal ureter accompanied by extravesical laparoscopic nephroureterectomy, and (3) extravesical removal of the distal ureter and a cuff of bladder with a laparoscopic GIA tissue stapler. Excellent patient tolerance has made this an attractive procedure, but extravesical ureteral dissection, tumor seeding, and poor pathology staging with morcellation are all potential negative features of laparoscopic nephroureterectomy. Greater experience and follow-up are necessary to fully evaluate this procedure.

MANAGEMENT OF ADVANCED DISEASE

The role of surgery in advanced upper tract transitional cell carcinoma is limited. Rare instances of renal pelvic transitional carcinoma with inferior vena caval thrombus have successfully been managed with surgical treatment.[135,136] Some authors have advocated lymph node dissection as being curative in patients with positive lymph nodes.[25] However, almost all patients with positive lymph nodes succumb to their disease within 2 years.[45,88] Rarely, palliative nephrectomy may be necessary in patients with intractable bleeding or pain. Every effort should be made to manage these gravely ill patients nonoperatively because of their high morbidity and mortality.

The role of radiotherapy in the management of upper tract tumors is currently uncertain because no data from randomized phase III trials are available. There are several case reports of successful use of radiotherapy in patients with residual tumor, unresectable disease, or local recurrence.[39,41] Brookland and Richter gave total doses of 4000 to 6000 cGy to 11 patients after surgical resection of advanced tumors. The local recurrence rate was 9%, compared with 41% in 12 patients not receiving radiotherapy. Median survival time of the irradiated and nonirradiated patients was 35 and 26 months, respectively.[137] Cozad and associates reported similar results in a group of 9 patients treated with postoperative radiotherapy. Irradiation appeared to decrease local recurrence and to improve the 5-year survival rate, although it had no impact on the development of distant disease.[138] Others have argued that radiotherapy should be limited to palliation of metastatic disease.[1,46,57] Radiotherapy to the renal bed carries significant gastrointestinal tract and solid organ toxicity. Further study of adjuvant radiotherapy, possibly in combination with adjuvant cisplatin-containing regimens, are necessary to define its role in the management of upper tract tumors.

The MVAC (methotrexate, vinblastine, doxorubicin, and cisplatin) regimen used for metastatic transitional carcinoma of the bladder has been applied with equal efficacy to tumors of the upper tract.[139–142] Although numbers are small, objective responses have been documented in several patients with upper tract tumors. Tumors with non–transitional cell phenotype have a low likelihood of response to this regimen.[142] Das and colleagues demonstrated prolonged survival times in patients with advanced upper tract tumors treated with platinum-based chemotherapy, or with a combination of irradiation and platinum-based chemotherapy, compared with an historical control group receiving no therapy (median survival times, 22.5 months, 22.2 months, and 6.4 months, respectively).[41] Significant complications of chemotherapy, including a 20% rate of nadir sepsis, may limit the delivery of these regimens.[140] Further discussion of chemotherapy for transitional cell carcinoma is found in Chapters 28, 29, and 31.

REFERENCES

1. Bloom NA, Vidone RA, Lytton B. Primary carcinoma of the ureter: a report of 102 new cases. J Urol 1970;103:590.
2. Say CS, Hori JM. Transitional cell carcinoma of the renal pelvis: experience from 1940 to 1972 and literature review. J Urol 1974;112:438.
3. Catalona WJ. Urothelial tumors of the renal pelvis and ureter. In: Walsh PC, Retik AB, Stamey TA, Vaughan ED, eds. Campbell's urology, 6th ed. Philadelphia: WB Saunders, 1992:1137.
4. Babaian RJ, Johnson DE. Primary carcinoma of the ureter. J Urol 1980;123:357.
5. Zoretic S, Gonzales J. Primary carcinoma of ureters. Urology 1983;21:354.
6. Grabstald H, Whitmore WF, Melamed MR. Renal pelvic tumors. JAMA 1971;218:845.
7. Mellemgaard A, Carstensen B, Norgaard N, Knudsen JB, Olsen JH. Trends in the incidence of cancer of the kidney, pelvis, ureter and bladder in Denmark. Scand J Urol Nephrol 1993;27:327.
8. Lynch HT, Ens JA, Lynch JF. The Lynch syndrome II and urological malignancies. J Urol 1990;143:24.
9. Frischer Z, Waltzer WC, Gonder MJ. Bilateral transitional cell carci-

noma of the renal pelvis in the cancer family syndrome. J Urol 1985; 134:1197.
10. Orphali SLJ, Shols GW, Hagewood J, Tesluk H, Palmer J. Familial transitional cell carcinoma of renal pelvis and upper ureter. Urology 1986;27:394.
11. Seidergard J, Vorachek WR, Pero RW, Pearson WR. Hereditary differences in the expression of the human glutathione transferase active on trans-stilbene oxide are due to a gene deletion. Proc Natl Acad Sci U S A 1988;85:7293.
12. Seidergard J, Pero RW, Markowitz MM, Roush G, Miller DG, Beattie EJ. Isoenzyme(s) of glutathione transferase (class Mu) as a marker for the susceptibility to lung cancer: a follow up study. Carcinogenesis 1992;11:33.
13. Jensen OM, Knudsen JB, McLaughlin JK, Sorensen BL. The Copenhagen case-control study of renal pelvis and ureter cancer: role of smoking and occupational exposures. Int J Cancer 1988;41:557.
14. Ross RK, Paganini-Hill A, Landolph J, Gerkins V, Henderson BE. Analgesics, cigarette smoking and other risk factors for cancer of the renal pelvis and ureter. Cancer Res 1989;49:1045.
15. McLaughlin JK, Silverman DT, Hsing AW, et al. Cigarette smoking and cancers of the renal pelvis and ureter. Cancer Res 1992;52:254.
16. Bengtsson U, Angervall L, Ekman H, Lehmann L. Transitional cell tumors of the renal pelvis in analgesic abusers. Scand J Urol Nephrol 1968;2:145.
17. Rathert P, Melchior H, Lutzeyer W. Phenacetin: a carcinogen for the urinary tract? J Urol 1975;113:653.
18. Steffens J, Nagel R. Tumours of the renal pelvis and ureter. Br J Urol 1988;61:277.
19. Gaakeer HA, DeRuiter HJ. Carcinoma of the renal pelvis following the abuse of phenacetin-containing analgesic drugs. Br J Urol 1979; 51:188.
20. Petersen I, Ohgaki H, Ludeke BI, Kleihues P. P53 mutations in phenacetin-associated human urothelial carcinomas. Carcinogenesis 1993; 14:2119.
21. McCredie M, Stewart JH, Carter JJ, Turner J, Mahony JF. Phenacetin and papillary necrosis: independent risk factors for renal pelvic cancer. Kidney Int 1986;30:81.
22. Jensen OM, Knudsen JB, Tomasson H, Sorensen BL. The Copenhagen case-control study of renal pelvis and ureter cancer: role of analgesics. Int J Cancer 1989;44:965.
23. Patierno SR, Lehman NL, Henderson BE, Landolph JR. Study of the ability of phenacetin, acetaminophen, and aspirin to induce cytotoxicity, mutation, and morphological transformation in C3H/10T1/2 Clone 8 mouse embryo cells. Cancer Res 1989;49:1038.
24. Anderstrom C, Johansson SL, Pettersson S, Wahlqvist L. Carcinoma of the ureter: a clinocopathologic study of 49 cases. J Urol 1989;142: 280.
25. Richie JP. Carcinoma of the renal pelvis and ureter. In: Skinner DG, Lieskovsky G, eds. Diagnosis and management of genitourinary cancer. Philadelphia: WB Saunders, 1988:323.
26. Shinka T, Uekado Y, Aoshi H, Hirano A, Ohkawa T. Occurrence of uroepithelial tumors of the upper urinary tract after the initial diagnosis of bladder cancer. J Urol 1988;140:745.
27. Brenner DW, Schellhammer PF. Upper tract urothelial malignancy after cyclophosphamide therapy: a case report and literature review. J Urol 1987;137:1226.
28. Verhaak RLOM, Harmsen AE, van Unnik AJM. On the frequency of tumor induction in a Thorotrast kidney. Cancer 1974;34:2061.
29. Markovic B. Endemic nephritis and urinary tract cancer in Yugoslavia, Bulgaria and Rumania. J Urol 1972;107:212.
30. Petkovic SD. A plea for conservative operation for ureteral tumors. J Urol 1972;107:220.
31. Petkovic SD. Epidemiology and treatment of renal pelvic and ureteral tumors. J Urol 1975;114:858.
32. Hall PW, Batuman V. Balkan endemic nephropathy. Kidney Int 1991; 40:S1.
33. Cukuranovic R, Ignjatovic M, Stefanovic V. Urinary tract tumors and Balkan nephropathy in the South Morava River basin. Kidney Int 1991;40:S80.
34. Radovanovic Z, Jankovic S, Jevremovic I. Incidence of tumors of urinary organs in a focus of Balkan endemic nephropathy. Kidney Int 1991;40:S75.
35. Petronic VJ, Bukurov NS, Djokic MR, et al. Balkan endemic nephropathy and papillary transitional cell tumors of the renal pelvis and ureters. Kidney Int 1991;40:S77.
36. Radovanovic Z, Krajinovic S, Jankovic S, Hall PW, Petkovic S. Family history of cancer among cases of upper urothelia tumours in a Balkan nephropathy area. J Cancer Res Clin Oncol 1985;110:181.
37. Melamed MR, Reuter VE. Pathology and staging of urothelial tumors of the kidney and ureter. Urol Clin North Am 1993;20:333.
38. Droller M. Transitional cell cancer: upper tracts and bladder. In: Walsh PC, Gittes RE, Perlmutter AD, Stamey TA, eds. Campbell's urology, 5th ed. Philadelphia: WB Saunders, 1986:1408.
39. Batata MA, Whitmore WF, Hilaris BS, Tokita N, Grabstald H. Primary carcinoma of the ureter: a prognostic study. Cancer 1975;35: 1626.
40. Auld CD, Grigor KM, Fowler JW. Histopathological review of transitional cell carcinoma of the upper urinary tract. Br J Urol 1984;56: 485.
41. Das AK, Carson CC, Bolick D, Paulson DF. Primary carcinoma of the upper urinary tract. Cancer 1990;66:1919.
42. Li MK, Cheung WL. Squamous cell carcinoma of the renal pelvis. J Urol 1987;138:269.
43. Blacher EJ, Johnson DE, Abdul-Karim FW, Ayala AG. Squamous cell carcinoma of renal pelvis. Urology 1985;25:124.
44. Cummings KB, Correa RJ, Gibbons RP, Stoll HM, Wheelis RF, Mason JT. Renal pelvic tumors. J Urol 1975;113:158.
45. Davis BW, Hough AJ, Gardner WA. Renal pelvic carcinoma: morphological correlates of metastatic behavior. J Urol 1987;137:857.
46. Wagle DG, Moore RH, Murphy GP. Primary carcinoma of the renal pelvis. Cancer 1974;33:1642.
47. Mills C, Vaughn ED. Carcinoma of the ureter: natural history, management and 5-year survival. J Urol 1983;129:275.
48. Hawtrey CE. Fifty-two cases of primary ureteral carcinoma: a clinical-pathologic study. J Urol 1971;105:188.
49. Batata M, Grabstald H. Upper urinary tract urothelial tumors. Urol Clin North Am 1976;3:79.
50. Huben RP, Mounzer AM, Murphy GP. Tumor grade and stage as prognostic variables in upper tract urothelial tumors. Cancer 1988; 62:2016.
51. Matsuoka K, Ueda S, Yamashita T, Eto K. Analysis of prognostic factors in patients with pyeloureteral carcinoma. Am J Clin Oncol 1991;14:146.
52. Nocks BN, Heney NM, Daly JJ, Perrone TA, Griffin PP, Prout GR. Transitional cell carcinoma of renal pelvis. Urology 1982;19:472.
53. Krogh J, Kvist E, Rye B. Transitional cell carcinoma of the upper urinary tract: prognostic variables and post-operative recurrences. Br J Urol 1991;67:32.
54. Heney NM, Nocks BN, Daly JJ, Blitzer PH, Parkhurst EC. Prognostic factors in carcinoma of the ureter. J Urol 1981;125:632.
55. Reitelman C, Sawczuk IS, Olsson CA, Puchner PJ, Benson MC. Prognostic variables in patients with transitional cell carcinoma of the renal pelvis and proximal ureter. J Urol 1987;138:1144.
56. Murphy DM, Zincke H, Furlow WL. Primary grade 1 transitional cell carcinoma of the renal pelvis and ureter. J Urol 1980;123:629.
57. Grace DA, Taylor WN, Taylor JN, Winter CC. Carcinoma of the renal pelvis: a 15-year review. J Urol 1968;98:566.
58. Nielsen K, Ostri P. Primary tumors of the renal pelvis: evaluation of clinical and pathological features in a consecutive series of 10 years. J Urol 1988;140:19.
59. Booth CM, Cameron KM, Pugh RCB. Urothelial carcinoma of the kidney and ureter. Br J Urol 1980;52:430.
60. Werth DD, Weigel JW, Mebust WK. Primary neoplasms of the ureter. J Urol 1981;125:628.
61. Hasui Y, Nishi S, Kitada S, Osada Y, Asada Y. The prognostic significance of vascular invasion in upper urinary tract transitional cell carcinoma. J Urol 1992;148:1783.
62. Blute ML, Tsushima K, Farrow GM, Therneau TM, Lieber MM. Transitional cell carcinoma of the renal pelvis: nuclear deoxyribonucleic acid ploidy studied by flow cytometry. J Urol 1988;140:944.
63. Oldbring J, Hellsten S, Lindholm K, Mikulowski P, Tribukait B. Flow DNA analysis in the characterization of carcinoma of the renal pelvis and ureter. Cancer 1989;64:2141.
64. Badalament RA, O'Toole RV, Kenworthy P, et al. Prognostic factors in patients with primary transitional cell carcinoma of the upper urinary tract. J Urol 1990;144:859.
65. Corrado F, Ferri C, Mannini D, et al. Transitional cell carcinoma of the upper urinary tract: evaluation of prognostic factors by histopathology and flow cytometric analysis. J Urol 1991;145:1159.

66. Al-Abadi H, Nagel R. Transitional cell carcinoma of the renal pelvis and ureter: prognostic relevance of nuclear deoxyribonucleic acid ploidy studied by slide cytometry: an 8-year survival time study. J Urol 1992;148:31.
67. Chiang PH, Huang MS, Tsai CJ, Tsai EM, Huang CH, Chiang CP. Transitional cell carcinoma of the renal pelvis and ureter in Taiwan. Cancer 1993;71:3988.
68. Corrado F, Mannini D, Ferri C, et al. The prognostic significance of DNA ploidy pattern in transitional cell cancer of the renal pelvis and ureter: continuing follow-up. Eur Urol 1992;21(Suppl 1):48.
69. Nemoto R, Hattori K, Sasaki A, Miyanaga N, Koiso K, Harada M. Estimations of the S phase fraction in situ in transitional cell carcinoma of the renal pelvis and ureter with bromodeoxyuridine labelling. Br J Urol 1989;64:339.
70. Miyakawa A, Tachibana M, Nakashima J, Deguchi N, Baba S, Tazaki H. Flow cytometric bromodeoxyuridine/deoxyribonucleic acid bivariate analysis for predicting tumor invasiveness of upper tract urothelial cancer. J Urol 1994;152:76.
71. Gatewood OM, Goldman SM, Marshall FF, Siegelman SS. Computerized tomography in the diagnosis of transitional cell carcinoma of the kidney. J Urol 1982;127:876.
72. Kakizoe T, Fujita J, Murase T, Matsumoto K, Kishi K. Transitional cell carcinoma of the bladder in patients with renal pelvic and ureteral cancer. J Urol 1980;124:17.
73. Mahadevia P, Karwa GL, Koss LG. Mapping of urothelium in carcinomas of the renal pelvis and ureter. Cancer 1983;51:890.
74. McCarron JP, Chasko SB, Gray GF. Systematic mapping of nephroureterectomy specimens removed for urothelial cancer: pathological findings and clinical correlations. J Urol 1982;128:243.
75. Fujimoto H, Tobisu K, Mizutani T, Sakamoto M, Kakizoe T. Transitional cell carcinoma of the upper urinary tract: analysis of morphology and distribution for surgical management. Jpn J Clin Oncol 1993; 23:303.
76. Williams CB, Mitchell JP. Carcinoma of the ureter: a review of 54 cases. Br J Urol 1973;45:377.
77. Williams CB, Mitchell JP. Carcinoma of the renal pelvis: a review of 43 cases. Br J Urol 1973;45:370.
78. DeTorres Mateos JA, Banus Gassol JM, Palou Redorta J, Morote Robles J. Vesicorenal reflux and upper urinary tract transitional cell carcinoma after transurethral resection of recurrent superficial bladder carcinoma. J Urol 1987;138:49.
79. Palou J, Farina LA, Villavicencio H, Vicente J. Upper tract urothelial tumor after transurethral resection for bladder tumor. Eur Urol 1992; 21:110.
80. Sidransky D, Frost P, Von Eschenbach A, Ryoichi O, Preisinger A, Vogelstein B. Clonal origin of bladder cancer. N Engl J Med 1992; 326:737.
81. Habuchi T, Takahashi R, Yamada H, Kakehi Y, Sugiyama T, Yoshida O. Metachronous multifocal development of urothelial cancers by intraluminal seeding. Lancet 1993;342:1087.
82. Herr HW, Whitmore WF. Ureteral carcinoma in situ after successful intravesical therapy for superficial bladder tumors: incidence, possible pathogenesis and management. J Urol 1987;138:292.
83. Miller EB, Eure GR, Schellhammer PF. Upper tract transitional cell carcinoma following treatment of superficial bladder cancer with BCG. Urology 1993;42:26.
84. Ward JN, Pitts WF, Bard RH. The dangerous ureter. Urology 1992; 39:322.
85. Schwalb MD, Herr HW, Sogani PC, Russo P, Sheinfeld J, Fair WR. Positive urinary cytology following a complete response to intravesical bacillus Calmette-Guérin therapy: pattern of recurrence. J Urol 1994;152:382.
86. Oldbring J, Glifberg I, Mikulowski P, Hellsten S. Carcinoma of the renal pelvis and ureter following bladder carcinoma: frequency, risk factors and clinicopathological findings. J Urol 1989;141:1311.
87. Fein AB, McClennan BL. Solitary filling defects of the ureter. Semin Roentgenol 1986;21:201.
88. Charbit L, Gendreau MC, Mee S, Cukier J. Tumors of the upper urinary tract: 10 years of experience. J Urol 1991;146:1243.
89. Bagley DH, Rivas D. Upper urinary tract filling defects: flexible ureteroscopic diagnosis. J Urol 1990;143:1196.
90. McCoy JG, Honda H, Reznicek M, Williams RD. Computerized tomography for detection and staging of localized and pathologically defined upper tract urothelial tumors. J Urol 1991;146:1500.
91. Milestone B, Friedman AC, Seidman EJ, Radecki PD, Lev-Toaff AS, Caroline DF. Staging of ureteral transitional cell carcinoma by CT and MRI?. Urology 1990;36:346.
92. Murphy DM, Zincke H, Furlow SL. Management of high grade transitional cell cancer of the upper urinary tract. J Urol 1981;125:25.
93. Sarnacki CT, McCormack LJ, Kiser WS, Hazard JB, McLaughlin TC, Belovich DM. Urinary cytology and the clinical diagnosis of urinary tract malignancy: a clinicopathologic study of 1,400 patients. J Urol 1971;106:761.
94. Leistenschneider W, Nagel R. Lavage cytology of the renal pelvis and ureter with special reference to tumors. J Urol 1980;124:597.
95. Eriksson O, Johansson S. Urothelial neoplasms of the upper tract: a correlation between cytologic and histologic findings in 43 patients with urothelial neoplasms of the renal pelvis or ureter. Acta Cytol 1976;20:20.
96. Gill WB, Lu CT, Thomsen S. Retrograde brushing: a new technique for obtaining histologic and cytologic material from ureteral renal pelvic and renal caliceal lesions. J Urol 1973;109:573.
97. Blute RD, Gittes RR, Gittes RF. Renal brush biopsy: survey of indications, techniques and results. J Urol 1981;126:146.
98. Sheline M, Amendola MA, Pollack HM, Banner MP, de las Morenas A, Wein AJ. Fluoroscopically guided retrograde brush biopsy in the diagnosis of transitional cell carcinoma of the upper urinary tract: results in 45 patients. AJR Am J Roentgenol 1989;153:313.
99. Seaman EK, Slawin KM, Benson MC. Treatment options for upper tract transitional-cell carcinoma. Urol Clin North Am 1993;20:349.
100. Huffman JL, Bagley DH, Lyon ES, Morse MJ, Herr HW, Whitmore WF. Endoscopic diagnosis and treatment of upper-tract urothelial tumors. Cancer 1984;55:1422.
101. Streem SB, Pontes JE, Novick AC, Montie JE. Ureteropyeloscopy in the evaluation of upper tract filling defects. J Urol 1986;136:383.
102. Blute ML, Segura JW, Patterson DE, Benson RC, Zincke H. Impact of endourology on diagnosis and management of upper urinary tract urothelial cancer. J Urol 1989;141:1298.
103. Lim DJ, Shattuck MC, Cook WA. Pyelovenous lymphatic migration of transitional cell carcinoma following flexible ureteroendoscopy. J Urol 1993;149:109.
104. Clayman RV, Kavoussi LR. Endosurgical techniques for the diagnosis and treatment of noncalculous disease of the ureter and kidney. In: Walsh PC, Retik AB, Stamey TA, Vaughan ED, eds. Campbell's urology, 6th ed. Philadelphia: WB Saunders, 1992:2298.
105. Cummings KB. Nephroureterectomy: rationale in the management of transitional cell carcinoma of the upper urinary tract. Urol Clin North Am 1980;7:569.
106. Strong DW, Pearse HD, Tank ES, Hodges CV. The ureteral stump after nephroureterectomy. J Urol 1976;115:654.
107. Johansson S, Wahlqvist L. A prognostic study of urothelial renal pelvic tumors. Cancer 1979;43:2525.
108. Vest SA. Conservative surgery in certain benign tumors of the ureter. J Urol 1945;53:97.
109. Brown HE, Roumani GK. Conservative surgical management of transitional cell carcinoma of the upper urinary tract. J Urol 1974;112: 184.
110. Gittes RF. Management of transitional cell carcinoma of the upper tract: case for conservative local excision. Urol Clin North Am 1980; 7:559.
111. Wallace DMA, Wallace DM, Whitfield HN, Hendry WF, Wickham JEA. The late results of conservative surgery for upper tract urothelial carcinomas. Br J Urol 1981;53:537.
112. Marshall FF, Walsh PC. In situ management of renal tumors: renal cell carcinoma and transitional cell carcinoma. J Urol 1984;131:1045.
113. Johnson DE, Babaian RJ. Conservative surgical management for noninvasive distal ureteral carcinoma. Urology 1979;13:365.
114. Ziegelbaum M, Novick AC, Streem SB, Montie JE, Pontes JE, Straffon RA. Conservative surgery for transitional cell carcinoma of the renal pelvis. J Urol 1987;138:1146.
115. McCarron JP, Mills C, Vaughan ED. Tumors of the renal pelvis and ureter: current concepts and management. Semin Urol 1983;1:75.
116. Gerber GS, Lyon ES. Endourological management of upper tract urothelial tumors. J Urol 1993;150:2.
117. Huffman JL. Ureteroscopic management of transitional cell carcinoma of the upper urinary tract. Urol Clin North Am 1988;15:419.
118. Schoenberg MP, Van Arsdalen KN, Wein AJ. The management of

transitional cell carcinoma in solitary renal units. J Urol 1991;146: 700.
119. Grossman HB, Schwartz SL, Konnak JW. Ureteroscopic treatment of urothelial carcinoma of the ureter and renal pelvis. J Urol 1992;148: 275.
120. Orihuela E, Smith AD. Percutaneous treatment of transitional cell carcinoma of the upper urinary tract. Urol Clin North Am 1988;15: 425.
121. Smith AD, Orihuela E, Crowley AR. Percutaneous management of renal pelvic tumors: a treatment option in selected cases. J Urol 1987; 137:852.
122. Tasca A, Zattoni F. The case for a percutaneous approach to transitional cell carcinoma of the renal pelvis. J Urol 1990;143:902.
123. Schmeller NT, Hofstetter AG. Laser treatment of ureteral tumors. J Urol 1989;141:840.
124. Kaufman RP, Carson CC. Ureteroscopic management of transitional cell carcinoma of the ureter using the neodymium:YAG laser. Lasers Surg Med 1993;13:625.
125. Tomera KM, Leary FJ, Zincke H. Pyeloscopy in urothelial tumors. J Urol 1982;127:1088.
126. Kerbl K, Clayman RV. Incision of the ureterovesical junction for endoscopic surveillance of transitional cell cancer of the upper urinary tract. J Urol 1993;150:1440.
127. Studer UE, Casanova G, Kraft R, Zingg EJ. Percutaneous bacillus Calmette-Guérin perfusion of the upper urinary tract for carcinoma in situ. J Urol 1989;142:975.
128. Mukamel E, Vilkovsky E, Engelstein HD, Nussbaum B, Servadio C. The effect of intravesical bacillus Calmette-Guérin therapy on the upper urinary tract. J Urol 1991;146:980.
129. Bellman GC, Sweetser P, Smith AD. Complications of intracavitary bacillus Calmette-Guérin after percutaneous resection of upper tract transitional cell carcinoma. J Urol 1994;151:13.
130. Ramsey JC, Soloway MS. Instillation of bacillus Calmette-Guérin into the renal pelvis of a solitary kidney for the treatment of transitional cell carcinoma. J Urol 1990;143:1220.
131. Smith AY, Vitale J, Lowe BA, Woodside JR. Treatment of superficial papillary transitional cell carcinoma of the ureter by vesicoureteral reflux of mitomycin C. J Urol 1987;138:1231.
132. Eastham JA, Huffman JL. Technique of mitomycin C instillation in the treatment of upper urinary tract urothelial tumors. J Urol 1993; 150:324.
133. Kerbl K, Clayman RV, McDougall EM, Urban DA, Gill I, Kavoussi LR. Laparoscopic nephroureterectomy: evaluation of first clinical series. Eur Urol 1993;23:431.
134. Chandhoke PS, Clayman RV, Kerbl K, et al. Laparoscopic ureterectomy: initial clinical experience. J Urol 1993;149:992.
135. Concepcion RS, Koch MO, McDougal WS, Stewart JR, Merrill WH. Management of primary nonrenal parenchymal malignancies with vena caval thrombus. J Urol 1991;145:243.
136. Leo ME, Petrou SP, Barrett DM. Transitional cell carcinoma of the kidney with vena caval involvement: report of 3 cases and a review of the literature. J Urol 1992;148:398.
137. Brookland RK, Richter MP. The postoperative irradiation of transitional cell carcinoma of the renal pelvis and ureter. J Urol 1985;133: 952.
138. Cozad SC, Smalley SR, Austenfeld M, Noble M, Jennings S, Reymond R. Adjuvant radiotherapy in high stage transitional cell carcinoma of the renal pelvis and ureter. Int J Radiat Oncol Biol Phys 1992;24:743.
139. Sternberg CN, Yagoda A, Scher HI, et al. M-VAC (methotrexate, vinblastine, doxorubicin and cisplatin) for advanced transitional cell carcinoma of the urothelium. J Urol 1988;139:461.
140. Trindade A, Samuels ML, Logothetis CJ. Chemotherapy of carcinoma of renal pelvis. Urology 1981;18:54.
141. Logothetis CJ, Samuels ML, Selig DE, Wallace S, Johnson DE. Combined intravenous and intra-arterial cyclophosphamide, doxorubicin, and cisplatin (CISCA) in the management of select patients with invasive urothelial tumors. Cancer Treat Rep 1985;69:33.
142. Scher HI, Yagoda A, Herr HW, et al. Neoadjuvant M-VAC (methotrexate, vinblastine, doxorubicin and cisplatin) for extravesical urinary tract tumors. J Urol 1988;139:475.

Principles and Practice of Genitourinary Oncology, edited by Derek Raghavan, Howard I. Scher, Steven A. Leibel, and Paul H. Lange. Lippincott-Raven Publishers, Philadelphia, © 1997.

CHAPTER 33

Carcinoma of the Urethra and Scrotum

Patricia J. Terry, Michael S. Cookson, and Michael F. Sarosdy

CARCINOMA OF THE URETHRA

Urethral carcinoma is rare, constituting only 0.01% to 0.02% of all genitourinary malignancies.[1] It is the only urologic cancer that occurs more frequently in women than in men, with a 3:1 ratio.[2] An estimated 1200 cases have been reported in women and 600 cases in men since urethral cancer was first described in 1834. Most patients are diagnosed after the age of 50, and about 85% are white.[3]

Etiology

The precise cause of urethral carcinoma has not been identified, although several factors have been implicated. Chronic inflammation and infection have been associated with urethral cancer in both sexes.[1,4] In women, chronic irritation secondary to sexual activity or childbirth as well as infection, urethral caruncles, and diverticula have been implicated as possible causes. A recent review revealed that 5% of all female urethral carcinomas occur in diverticula.[5] Stricture disease has not been strongly associated with urethral carcinoma in women, but up to 76% of male patients have such a history, with the site of stricture being the most frequent site of cancer.[6,7] Smoking and occupational exposure to known carcinogens have been implicated but not proven as causes of urethral carcinoma.[8]

Anatomy and Histology

Female

The proximal third of the female urethra is lined with transitional cell epithelium, the distal two thirds with stratified squamous epithelium (Fig. 33-1). Submucosal glands lined by pseudostratified and stratified columnar epithelium are also located in the dorsolateral portion of the distal third of the urethra.[9] The lamina propria consists of loose fibroconnective tissue with many elastic fibers arranged in a slightly circular but principally longitudinal direction. The muscular wall is composed of inner longitudinal and outer semicircular layers contiguous with the detrusor muscle.[9]

Lymphatic drainage also differs along the length of the urethra. The female urethra is divided into anterior (distal) and posterior (proximal) segments.[9] Lymphatics from the posterior urethra drain into the external and internal iliac and obturator chains. From the anterior urethra, lymph is carried to the superficial and deep inguinal lymph nodes.

Female urethral cancer can present initially as a small lesion prolapsing through the meatus ulcerating as the tumor progresses to the skin and vulvar region. Proximal urethral tumors tend to invade the bladder and vagina. Lymphatic spread is uncommon in the early stages but is present in half of patients with more advanced or proximal tumors.[6] Hematogenous spread can occur to the lung, liver, bone, and brain, in order of frequency.[8]

Male

The male urethra is approximately 21 cm long and is divided into three segments: prostatic, membranous, and penile (see Fig. 33-1). The prostatic portion is surrounded by prostate, with the posterior wall of the urethra forming the verumontanum. In the midline is the prostatic utricle, which is a müllerian duct remnant. The ejaculatory ducts and prostatic ducts are located lateral to the verumontanum.

The second portion of the male urethra is the membranous urethra, which extends from the prostatic apex to the bulb of the corpus spongiosum. The third portion, the penile urethra, is the longest segment (± 15 cm) and extends from the membranous urethra to the external meatus. The proximal portion of the penile urethra, which enters the corpus spongiosum and expands in a fusiform fashion, is called the bulbar urethra. The midpenile urethra expands as it enters the glans penis to form the fossa navicularis, then narrows at the external meatus.

The epithelium of the male urethra varies along its length. The prostatic urethra is lined with transitional epithelium; the membranous, bulbar, and penile segments with stratified or pseudostratified columnar epithelium; and the fossa navicularis with stratified squamous epithelium. The mucosal surface includes openings to ejaculatory and prostatic ducts, bulbourethral or Cowper's glands, and the glands of Littre in the penile urethra.[9]

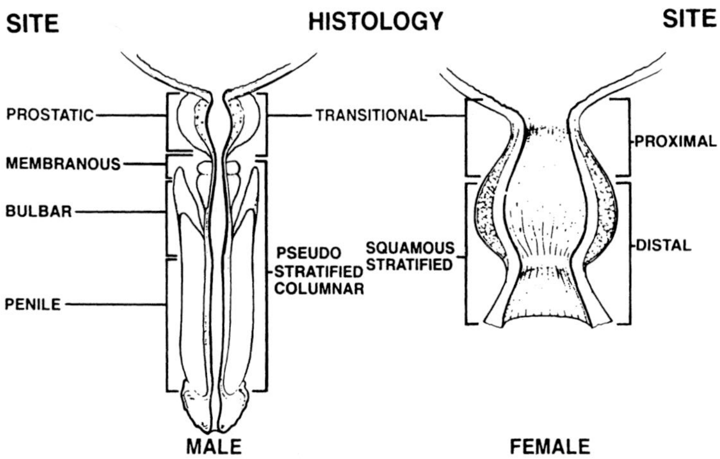

FIG. 33-1. Schematic drawing of the anatomy and histology of the male and female urethra.

The male urethra is supported by the complex perineal and pelvic musculature of the urogenital and anal triangles. The perineal membrane separates the superficial space, containing the bulbospongiosus, ischiocavernosus, and transversus perinei superficialis muscles, from the deep space structures, including the transversus perinei profundi, the striated component of the external sphincter, and the Cowper's glands.[9]

Lymphatic drainage of the male urethra also varies with each segment of its length. The glans penis and penile urethra are drained by lymphatics that empty into a plexus of superficial inguinal nodes. Lymph is then channeled into the deep inguinal or the external iliac chains, or both. The bulbar, membranous, and prostatic urethra drain into three lymphatic channels, respectively: along the dorsal vein to the external iliac nodes, along the pudendal artery to the obturator and internal iliac nodes, and to the presacral lymphatic chain.[10] A distal tumor would be expected to involve the inguinal nodes and a proximal lesion to spread to the deep pelvic nodes, but crossover is not unusual, depending on the location and extent of the tumor.[11]

Carcinoma of the distal male urethra is usually low grade and progresses regionally rather than to distant sites. Invasion into vascular spaces of the surrounding tissues is common. Tumors arising in the bulbomembranous urethra often invade into the deep structures of the perineum, and those arising from prostatic ducts or acini are frequently high grade and invasive at the time of diagnosis.[11] As in the female, hematogenous spread is uncommon unless the disease is regionally advanced.

Tumor Histology

Tumor histology reflects the anatomic site of origin in both sexes. In women, roughly one half of urethral cancers originate in the distal urethra. Squamous epithelium lines the distal two thirds of the urethra, and it follows that squamous cell cancer is seen in 50% to 70% of cases.[6,8,12] Transitional cell carcinoma and adenocarcinoma are the next most common tumors in women, and 1% to 2% of urethral cancers (in either sex) are undifferentiated, sarcoma, or melanoma.[13]

In men, the most frequent site of cancer is the bulbomembranous urethra (56% to 59%); about one third of male urethral cancers occur in the penile urethra, and about 10% arise in the prostatic urethra.[1,11] Consistent with this distribution, 70% to 80% of male urethral cancers are squamous cell carcinomas, 20% are transitional cell carcinomas, and approximately 5% are adenocarcinomas.[3]

Clinical Presentation

Patients with urethral carcinoma tend to present with locally advanced disease, with an average delay of 6 months from the onset of symptoms to diagnosis.[4] In women, the most common presenting symptom is urethral or vaginal bleeding.[14,15] Other signs and symptoms include irritative and obstructive voiding, a palpable urethral mass, incontinence, retention, perineal pain, and dyspareunia.[5]

In men, most common signs and symptoms are those of urinary irritation and obstruction. A history of urethral infection, stricture, dilatation, urethral mass, discharge, pain, or hematuria is also common.[16] Diagnosis may be delayed because symptoms are insidious and are frequently confused with those of more common conditions such as prostatism or stricture. In general, men with more distal lesions tend to present earlier than those with proximal lesions, because penile urethral symptoms are likely to be more significant at an earlier stage.[4,17]

The physical examination in the female often yields more information than in the male patient. An area of urethral induration or ulceration may be revealed, or a lesion may be seen protruding from the meatus. More invasive tumors may erode into the anterior vaginal wall, appearing similar to primary neoplasms of the vagina, vulva, or clitoris. The presentation may be confused with that of benign lesions, including urethral caruncle, diverticulum, periurethral abscess, or condyloma acuminata. Twenty percent to 30% of female patients present with palpable inguinal adenopathy, 5% with distant metastases.

Physical examination in men with anterior lesions may reveal a nodule, ventral periurethral mass, or fistula. Bulbar or bulbomembranous tumors may present with a fluctuant or solid perineal mass. Penile, scrotal, and perineal edema or induration are also common presenting symptoms.[16] Patients of either sex with advanced stages of disease may present with anorexia, weight loss, and malaise.

Diagnosis and Staging

The diagnosis of urethral carcinoma is often delayed for the reasons mentioned previously. The urologist must maintain a high index of suspicion in patients who present with urethral bleeding, obstruction, a stricture that is difficult to dilate, or appearance of a spontaneous fistula.

Visual examination is helpful only in the diagnosis of very distal tumors, although palpation may reveal the length of urethral involvement and invasion. Examination of surrounding tissues, including bimanual examination, offers valuable information regarding involvement of the anus, rectum, urogenital diaphragm, and vagina in female patients. Palpation of inguinal lymph nodes is imperative for clinical staging.[3]

Pathologic diagnosis is confirmed by biopsy of the suspected lesion. Because extensive periurethral inflammation is likely, deep biopsy specimens should be obtained to appropriately stage the tumor.[18] Cytology specimens or washings, or both, may be helpful in establishing a diagnosis, but biopsies are essential.[3]

After the pathologic diagnosis has been confirmed, potential metastatic spread must be evaluated by chest radiography, serum liver enzyme studies, and computed tomographic (CT) scan of the abdomen and pelvis to identify adenopathy.[19] Pelvic magnetic resonance imaging has shown great promise as the most accurate technique for determining local clinical stage.[20]

Although there is no universally accepted staging system, one that is frequently used for urethral cancer in women is described by Grabstald and associates[6] (Table 33-1). The most commonly used staging system for men is that proposed by Ray and associates[21] (see Table 33-1). The TNM system of the International Union Against Cancer is based on invasiveness of the tumor, presence or absence of regional lymph node involvement, and metastatic dissemination (Table 33-2).[22]

TABLE 33-2. *International union against cancer TNM staging system for female and male urethral carcinoma*

PRIMARY TUMOR (T)	
Tx	Primary tumor cannot be assessed
T0	No evidence of primary tumor
Tis	Carcinoma in situ
Ta	Noninvasive papillary, polypoid, or verrucous carcinoma
T1	Invades subepithelial connective tissue
T2	Invades periurethral musculature (corpus spongiosum or prostate)
T3	Invades anterior vagina or bladder neck (corpus cavernosum or beyond prostate or bladder neck)
T4	Invades other adjacent organs
REGIONAL LYMPH NODES (N)	
Nx	Regional lymph nodes cannot be assessed
N0	No regional lymph node metastasis
N1	Metastasis to a single lymph node, 2 cm or less in greatest dimension
N2	Metastasis to a single lymph node, >2 cm but <5 cm in greatest dimension; or multiple nodes involved, with none >5 cm in greatest dimension
N3	Metastasis to a lymph node >5 cm in greatest dimension
DISTANT METASTASIS (M)	
Mx	Presence of distant metastasis cannot be assessed
M0	No distant metastasis
M1	Distant metastasis

Adapted from Beahrs OH, et al, eds. Manual for staging of cancer, 3rd ed. Philadelphia, JP Lippincott, 1988;210.

Prognosis and Survival

For both sexes, tumor location is an important prognostic factor. In women, distal and meatal cancers have a more favorable prognosis than proximal lesions, primarily because of earlier detection. The histologic subtype is less significant than location in determining prognosis in the female.[14] Patients with anterior lesions can be expected to have a 5-year survival rate of about 50%, and those with posterior or entire urethral lesions, 13%. Overall, a 5-year survival rate of 29% can be expected for any woman presenting with urethral cancer.[1,3,23,24]

Distal lesions in men also carry a more favorable prognosis than bulbomembranous tumors, because the latter tend to be more extensive at the time of diagnosis.[25] Superficial transi-

TABLE 33-1. *Staging systems for carcinoma of the urethra*

Female		Male	
Stage	Grabstald	Stage	Ray
0	In situ (limited to mucosa)	0	Tumor confined to mucosa
A	Submucosal	A	Extension into, not beyond lamina propria
B	Infiltrating periurethral muscle	B	Extension into, not beyond corpus spongiosum; or into, not beyond prostate
C	Periurethral C1 Infiltrating muscular wall of vagina C2 Infiltrating muscular wall of vagina with invasion of vaginal mucosa C3 Infiltrating other adjacent structures such as bladder, labia, and clitoris	C	Direct extension into tissues beyond corpus spongiosum (corpora cavernosa, muscle, fat, fascia, skin, direct skeletal involvement) or beyond prostate capsule
D	Metastasis D1 Inguinal lymph nodes D2 Pelvic nodes below the aortic bifurcation D3 Lymph nodes above aortic bifurcation D4 Distant metastasis	D	Metastasis D1 Inguinal or pelvic lymph nodes D2 Distant metastasis

Adapted from Ray B, Canto SR, Whitmore WF Jr. Experience with primary carcinoma of the male urethra. J Urol 1977; 117:591, and Grabstald H, Hilaris B, Henschke U, Whitmore WF Jr. Cancer of the female urethra. JAMA 1966;197:835.

tional carcinoma of the prostatic urethra behaves similarly to cancer of the bladder and can be managed with transurethral resection, whereas invasive prostatic tumors tend to disseminate widely.[7] For men with anterior tumors and no clinical evidence of metastasis, the reported 5-year survival rate is about 50%.[1,4] The comparable rate for men with lesions of the bulbomembranous urethra plummets to 5%, whereas for prostatic urethral cancer it is 23%, probably because of the inclusion in this category of transitional cell carcinoma that is managed with transurethral resection.[3,26] Ray and associates reported survival by stage (see Table 33-1) and found a 100% 5-year survival rate for stage A, 80% for stage B, 17% for stage C, and 20% for stage D male urethral carcinoma.[1]

Treatment

Treatment recommendations for urethral cancer are primarily dependent on tumor location and clinical stage. For the female, treatment options have been formulated by distinguishing between tumors of the anterior urethra (distal third) and those of the posterior urethra (proximal two thirds).[27] This distinction has also been useful in predicting lymphatic spread. Because this disease is rare, no well-controlled prospective studies have been implemented to compare therapies.[13] Various treatment modalities have been proposed, including surgery or irradiation alone and surgery in combination with irradiation or chemotherapy, or both.

Female Anterior Urethral Carcinoma

Tumors of the anterior female urethra have been managed surgically by a variety of techniques. For small lesions confined to the mucosa, wide surgical excision, transurethral resection, or laser ablation may suffice. The carbon dioxide laser and the neodymium-yttrium-aluminum-garnet (Nd:YAG) laser have been used successfully.[14,28] Advantages of laser surgery over conventional surgical excision include the absence of bleeding, quick healing, and avoidance of hypertrophic scar formation.[28] The carbon dioxide laser has the advantage of evaporating target tissue with little penetration of deeper tissues, but it can be used only on external lesions. The Nd:YAG laser is effective at complete eradication of tumor, but it can cause damage to deeper tissues, resulting in stricture. Laser resection, unlike electrocautery, relies on vaporization of tissue. For this reason, initial deep biopsies are required for pathologic documentation of histology and depth of invasion before a decision to use laser therapy is made.[13]

Partial urethrectomy may be feasible for anterior female carcinomas of TNM stage Tis, T1, and T2 (Grabstald stage 0, A, and B), using a circumferential incision with surgical margins of 0.5 to 1.0 cm. Frozen sections of the proximal urethra should be obtained to ensure a clear margin.[13] In selected patients with stage T2 or T3 cancer, total urethrectomy with preservation of the bladder may be an option if the tumor is anterior, but clear margins cannot be ensured. The urethrectomy may be followed by construction of a continent conduit using a Mitrofanoff procedure or an ileocecal segment.[29,30]

In addition to surgery, radiotherapy has proved effective in treatment of low-stage disease. Interstitial radiotherapy with radium-226 or iridium-192 needles has resulted in local control rates of 50% to 60% in selected patients.[31–33] Intracavitary or external-beam irradiation can also be used to supplement interstitial irradiation.[8,34] Garden and associates reported that local control rates appeared to be directly related to the extent of disease, with 5-year local control rates of 74% if only a part of the urethra was involved, compared with 55% if the entire urethra was involved.[31] As with surgery, tumor histology did not affect outcome, nor did type of radiation or total dosage.[31]

One of the advantages of radiotherapy is organ preservation, but complication rates as high as 40% have been reported.[14,31] The most common complication is incontinence; others are local necrosis, fistula, stricture, cellulitis, cystitis, and vulvar abscess. Recent advances, such as dose limitation for external-beam irradiation and use of small fields, have led to fewer complications.[31]

Anterior urethral cancer tends to spread to deep inguinal lymph nodes, and if the vulva is involved, superficial inguinal nodes can also harbor metastases. Inguinal lymphadenectomy is recommended for clinically palpable nodes because they more often represent metastases than infection. Prophylactic lymphadenectomy is not currently recommended because of high morbidity and lack of proven efficacy.[13]

Despite aggressive therapy for anterior urethral tumors, local recurrence rates are high, and mortality is significant. In patients with recurrence or radioresistant tumors, neoadjuvant radiotherapy followed by local excision has resulted in a survival advantage over radiotherapy alone.[35,36] Further studies with multimodality approaches are necessary to delineate appropriate treatment recommendations.

Female Proximal Urethral Carcinoma

Most tumors of the proximal urethra are high stage, often with extension to the bladder and vagina. Radical surgery or radiotherapy alone fails to control disease in such patients, so combination therapy usually is recommended.

The initial surgical approach is anterior exenteration, which includes removal of the pelvic lymph nodes, the entire urethra and bladder, the uterus and adnexa, and the anterior and lateral vaginal walls, as well as en bloc resection of the pubic symphysis and inferior pubic rami.[13] Vaginal reconstruction with gracilis myocutaneous flaps has been recommended.[37] Supravesical diversion with an ileal or colon conduit is then performed, with the option of a continent diversion for selected patients. Results with anterior exenteration alone for high-stage urethral cancer are poor, with local recurrence rates of about 67% and 5-year survival rates of 10% to 17%.[14,38] Complications of anterior exenteration include rectovaginal fistula, pelvic abscess, osteitis pubis, adductor muscle spasm, perineal herniation, and sacroiliac instability.

Radiotherapy alone for invasive urethral cancer has resulted in poor local control, with survival rates of 0% to 57% at 5 years.[13,6,23,33,34] Preoperative radiation has been used in an effort to "downsize" advanced tumors.[26] The combination of radiation and surgery for high-stage disease has resulted in improved survival, with a mean survival rate of 55% at 5 years.[13,27,39] The addition of chemotherapy to the combination of irradiation and surgery is being investigated, with reports of antitumor activity with various combinations of mitomycin C,

5-fluorouracil, cisplatin, bleomycin, and methotrexate.[40,41] Further multiinstitutional cooperative studies are necessary in this area because of the low incidence of urethral carcinoma.

Patients with metastatic disease may be treated palliatively for extensive local invasion, using radiotherapy, surgical excision, pain management, and, occasionally, urinary diversion.

Male Urethral Carcinoma

As in the female, management of male urethral cancer is based on location and extent of the primary tumor. Although there are many reports in the literature claiming success with local excision (i.e., combinations of excision, fulguration, and transurethral resection), such cases are rare, and only carefully selected patients can benefit from such an approach.[7,21,25,42,43] Lesions considered for local excision must be of low stage and grade and preferably should be solitary tumors, but the location of the lesion should not be a factor if resection is complete.[7]

Male Distal Urethral Carcinoma

Partial penectomy is a well-established treatment for both penile and urethral carcinoma. A lesion of the distal urethra is treated with amputation of the penis 2 cm proximal to the visible tumor, palpable induration, or inflammation.[1,44] The ideal patient for partial penectomy has a low-stage distal tumor with normal biopsies of the proximal urethra. This procedure has provided the most consistent disease control, with 5-year survival of at least 50% in the absence of lymph node invasion.[26] It is not unusual for these patients to require perineal urethrostomy because of inadequate penile length for voiding while standing. Intraoperative complications are uncommon, although later problems include meatal stenosis and, more seriously, local recurrence.[18] Although preservation of sufficient penile length for intercourse is frequently possible, a review by Hoppman and Fraley disclosed that fewer than half of their patients had satisfactory function after partial penectomy for penile carcinoma.[45]

Male Proximal or High-Stage Urethral Carcinoma

Radical or total penectomy has been performed for proximal male urethral carcinoma not amenable to partial penectomy, but radical penectomy alone may not be adequate treatment for patients with locally extensive proximal disease.[4] The patient with T1 or T2 (stage 0, A, or B) disease is an ideal candidate for radical penectomy if the tumor does not extend proximal to the midbulb or if the lesion is distal, but partial penectomy results in an inadequate penile stump.[18]

Radical penectomy involves removal of the same tissue as in partial penectomy along with the root of the penis and more of the urethra, with the creation of a perineal urethrostomy. Complications include scrotal hematoma or wound infection, and, later, perineal urethrostomy stenosis and local recurrence of disease.[18] Several reports in the literature indicate poor survival after radical penectomy, but it is possible that these results represent failure in patient selection, not surgical technique.[45–47]

Although the prognosis for a patient with advanced posterior urethral cancer is grave, en bloc excision with cystoprostatectomy can be life-saving.[38] Patients considered for en bloc resection of the penis, pubis, prostate, and bladder are those presenting with stage C or higher proximal urethral tumor. Lymphadenopathy and rectal wall invasion should be ruled out by CT and physical examination to avoid morbid procedures in the face of metastatic disease. This extensive operation has the potential to produce a variety of complications, including pelvic abscess, wound dehiscence, bowel fistulae, and adductor weakness.[38,48]

For the patient with confirmed inguinal node disease, the best management remains unknown. Although most patients succumb to their disease, several series have shown that lymphadenectomy results in a survival benefit for patients with confirmed nodal disease.[43,49] It has therefore been accepted that any patient with palpable inguinal adenopathy should undergo formal lymphadenectomy, although prophylactic lymphadenectomy is not recommended.

Management of the Urethra in Patients Undergoing Radical Cystoprostatectomy

All male patients with invasive transitional cell carcinoma of the bladder being considered for cystectomy should undergo evaluation of the prostatic urethra with biopsies before surgery. This is especially important for those in whom orthotopic placement of a continent reservoir or neobladder to the urethra is being considered. Certain patients are at higher risk for development of subsequent urethral cancer, including those with carcinoma in situ, multifocal disease, or pathologic involvement of the prostatic urethra.[50,51] Urethrectomy at the time of cystectomy prevents recurrence in these patients and avoids the necessity of frequent surveillance visits. Another option is delayed urethrectomy after cystoprostatectomy and cutaneous diversion.

For the patient who develops positive urethral cytology results or a gross recurrence, clinical staging is necessary, and in the absence of metastatic spread, urethrectomy with wide margins is recommended.[52] In the face of periurethral extension, staging inguinal node dissection must be considered, because chemotherapy and radiotherapy have shown limited activity against transitional cell carcinoma.[52] Early identification of patients who are at risk for development of urethral recurrence should significantly reduce the morbidity and mortality of this disease.

CARCINOMA OF THE SCROTUM

Scrotal carcinoma is rare. Although it is 8 to 10 times more common (per capita) in the United Kingdom, fewer than 10 cases were reported in the United States in 1976.[53,54] The World Health Organization reported an incidence of only 0.2 to 0.3 cases per 100,000 men older than 35 years of age worldwide in the late 1960s.[55] The most common scrotal cancer is squamous cell carcinoma, followed by basal cell carcinoma, malignant melanoma, Paget's disease, and sarcoma, including leiomyosarcoma, liposarcoma, rhabdomyosarcoma, and fibrosarcoma.[56] Nonmalignant skin lesions in the differential diagnosis include secondary and tertiary syphilis, tuberculous epididymitis, periurethral abscess, hemangioma, and sclerosing lipogranuloma.[56]

Epidemiology

Squamous cell carcinoma of the scrotum historically has been associated with occupational exposure to industrial carcinogens, including soot and oil. Bassius first described this lesion in 1731, and Pott presented the classic description linking carcinoma of the scrotum to chimney sweeps in 1775, from which came the terms Pott's cancer and chimney sweep's cancer.[57,58] Other occupations have been investigated as causes of scrotal cancer, and associations have been established with tar, paraffin, and shale oil workers, machine and lathe operators, petroleum wax pressmen, screw makers, and cotton mule spinners.[55,57–60] More recently, studies have demonstrated the association of squamous carcinoma of the scrotum with psoralens and ultraviolet radiation (PUVA) used for the treatment of psoriasis.[61] Human papillomavirus infection has been investigated as another possible risk factor, with 45% of patients in one series having evidence of human papillomavirus infection.[62]

Clinical Presentation

Scrotal carcinoma usually presents during the sixth decade of life, most commonly as a solitary lesion on the anterolateral aspect of the scrotum.[63] It begins as a painless nodule that later becomes indurated or ulcerated. Self-treatment with topical agents is common, and most patients do not seek medical care until 8 to 12 months after development of the initial lesion.[21,57]

About 40% to 50% of patients present with palpable inguinal adenopathy. Of these, about half have nodal metastases, and the other half have inflammatory adenopathy, similar to what is seen in penile cancer.[64] Evaluation must include careful examination of the genitalia and regional and distant lymph nodes. CT scan of the abdomen and pelvis is not likely to be helpful in the evaluation of the patient with minimal or no inguinal adenopathy but may provide additional information in the presence of bulky disease. Lymphangiography has been reported to be accurate in differentiating nodal metastases from inflammatory nodes, but it is not recommended for evaluation of patients with scrotal cancer because micrometastases cannot accurately be identified by this procedure.[56]

Staging

Ray and Whitmore proposed the first staging system for scrotal carcinoma in 1977, identifying four stages (Table 33-3).[65] In general, patients with stage A or B disease have a 5-year survival rate of 70% to 75%, whereas those with stage C or D disease have little chance for long-term survival.[21,65]

TABLE 33-3. *Staging system for scrotal carcinoma*

Stage	Description
A1	Tumor localized to scrotal wall
A2	Locally extensive tumor invading adjacent structures (testis, spermatic cord, penis, pubis, perineum)
B	Metastatic disease involving inguinal lymph nodes only
C	Metastatic disease involving pelvic lymph nodes without evidence of distant spread
D	Metastatic disease beyond the pelvic lymph nodes involving distant organs

Data from Lowe FC. Squamous cell carcinoma of the Scrotum. J Urol 1983;130:423.

Treatment

Wide local excision of the primary lesion with 2 cm margins is the initial treatment for scrotal carcinoma. Removal of the scrotal contents is not recommended unless the structures are directly involved by tumor.[56] Skin grafts or thigh flaps may be required to cover large defects resulting from extensive excision.[62]

Patients presenting with palpable inguinal adenopathy should undergo local excision of the primary lesion, followed by 4 to 6 weeks of treatment with broad-spectrum antibiotics.[56] If palpable nodes remain after an appropriate trial of antibiotics, a modified inguinal node dissection should be performed to rule out metastatic disease. This approach is supported by Morley's work in 1911, which demonstrated free communication between the superficial lymphatic channels of both sides of the scrotum, with virtually all trunks from the scrotum draining first to the inguinal nodes.[66,67]

In the face of biopsy-proven metastatic disease, most authors have advocated ilioinguinal lymphadenectomy instead of inguinal lymphadenectomy.[21,57,68,69] The issue of unilateral versus bilateral dissection is not quite as clear-cut. Bilateral modified inguinal node dissection with pelvic lymphadenectomy may be warranted, although most recent experience argues for ipsilateral ilioinguinal node dissection with a contralateral sentinel node biopsy. If the contralateral sentinel node is also positive, bilateral ilioinguinal dissection is recommended.[56,62]

Irradiation is not considered effective therapy for scrotal carcinoma, although a few successes have been reported.[57,70] Radiotherapy is usually reserved for patients who are not surgical candidates or who have unresectable disease. Several chemotherapeutic agents, including bleomycin, cyclophosphamide, vincristine, methotrexate, and 5-fluorouracil, have been investigated in scrotal carcinoma, but results have been dismal.[71,72]

Scrotal carcinoma is a rare but aggressive and devastating tumor. Because of the nature of the primary lesion, diagnosis tends to be delayed, leading to a poor prognosis despite ilioinguinal lymphadenectomy. Emphasis should be on earlier detection and intervention, based on risk factors and careful examination, and on improving treatment options for patients with nodal disease.

REFERENCES

1. Ray B, Guinan PD. Primary carcinoma of the urethra. In: Javadpour N, ed. Principles and management of urologic cancer. Baltimore: William & Wilkins, 1979:445.
2. Levine RL. Urethral cancer. Cancer 1980;45:1965.

3. Sarosdy MF. Urethral carcinoma. AUA Update Series 1987;13(VI).
4. Kaplan GW, Bulkley GJ, Grayhack JT. Carcinoma of the male urethra. J Urol 1967;98:365.
5. Rajan N, Tucci P, Mallouh C, Choudhury M. Carcinoma in female urethral diverticulum: case reports and review of management. J Urol 1993;150:1911.
6. Grabstald H, Hilaris B, Henschke U, Whitmore WF Jr. Cancer of the female urethra. JAMA 1966;197:835.
7. Konnak JR. Conservative management of low grade neoplasms of the male urethra: a preliminary report. J Urol 1980;123:175.
8. Forman JD, Lichter AS. The role of radiation therapy in the management of carcinoma of the male and female urethra. Urol Clin North Am 1992;19:383.
9. Carroll PR, Dixon CM. Surgical anatomy of the male and female urethra. Urol Clin North Am 1992;19:339.
10. Johnson DE, Ames FC. Surgical anatomy and lymphatic drainage of the ilioinguinal region. In: Johnson DE, Ames FC, eds. Groin dissection. Chicago: Year Book Medical Publishers, 1985:1.
11. Hopkins SC, Grabstald H. Benign and malignant tumors of the male and female urethra. In: Walsh P, Gittes RF, Perlimutter AD, et al, eds. Campbell's urology, 5th ed. Philadelphia: WB Saunders, 1986:4441.
12. Johnson DE. Cancer of the female urethra: overview. In: Johnson DE, Boileau MA, eds. Genitourinary tumors: fundamental principles and surgical techniques. New York: Grune & Stratton, 1982:267.
13. Narayan P, Korety B. Surgical techniques of female urethral cancer. Urol Clin North Am 1992;19:373.
14. Bracken RB, Johnson DE, Miller LS, et al. Primary carcinoma of the female urethra. J Urol 1976;116:188.
15. Desai S, Libertino JA, Zinman L. Primary carcinoma of the male urethra. J Urol 1973;110:693.
16. Mostofi FK, Davis CJ Jr, Sesterhenn IA. Cancer of male and female urethra. Urol Clin North Am 1992;19:347.
17. Winkler HZ, Lieber MM. Primary squamous cell carcinoma of the male urethra: nuclear deoxyribonucleic acid ploidy studied by flow cytometry. J Urol 1988;139:298.
18. Zeidman EJ, Desmond P, Thompson IM. Surgical techniques of carcinoma of the male urethra. Urol Clin North Am 1992;19:359.
19. Carroll PR. Surgical management of urethral carcinoma. In: Crawford ED, Das S, eds. Current genitourinary surgery. Philadelphia: Lea & Febiger, 1990.
20. Vapnek JM, Hricak H, Carroll PR. Recent advances in imaging studies for staging penile and urethral cancer. Urol Clin North Am 1992;19: 259.
21. Ray B, Canto SR, Whitmore WF Jr. Experience with primary carcinoma of the male urethra. J Urol 1977;117:591.
22. Beahrs OH, et al, eds. Manual for staging cancer, 3rd ed. Philadelphia: JB Lippincott, 1988:210.
23. Prempree T, Amormain R, Patanaphan V. Radiation therapy in primary carcinoma of the female urethra. Cancer 1984;54:729.
24. Hopkins SC, Vider M, Nag SK, et al. Carcinoma of the female urethra: reassessment of modes of therapy. J Urol 1982;129:958.
25. Hopkins SC, Nag SK, Soloway MS. Primary carcinoma of the male urethra. Urology 1984;23:128.
26. Sullivan J, Grabstald H. Management of carcinoma of the urethra. In: Skinner DC, deKernion JB, eds. Genitourinary cancer. Philadelphia: WB Saunders, 1978:419.
27. Ali MM, Klein FA, Hazra TA. Primary female urethral carcinoma: a retrospective comparison of different treatment techniques. Cancer 1988;62:54.
28. Staehler G, Chaussy C, Jochan D, et al. The use of neodymium-YAG lasers in urology: indications, techniques and critical assessment. J Urol 1985;134:1555.
29. Mitrofanof P. Cystotomie continente transappendiculaire dans le traitement des vessies neurologiques. Chir Pediatr 1980;21:297.
30. Libertino JA, Zinman L. Ileocecal segment for temporary and permanent urinary diversion. Urol Clin North Am 1986;13:2.
31. Garden AS, Zagars GK, Delclos L. Primary carcinoma of the female urethra: results of radiation therapy. Cancer 1993;71:3102.
32. Sailer SL, Shipley VW, Wang CC. Carcinoma of the female urethra: a review of results with radiation therapy. J Urol 1988;140:1.
33. Delclos L, Wharton JT, Rutledge FN. Tumors of the vagina and female urethra. In: Fletcher GH, ed. Textbook of radiotherapy, 3rd ed. Philadelphia: Lea & Febiger, 1980:812.
34. Johnson DE, O'Connell JR. Primary carcinoma of the female urethra. Urology 1983;21:42.
35. Peterson DT, Dockert MB, Utz DC, et al. The peril of primary carcinoma of the urethra in women. J Urol 1973;110:72.
36. Allen R, Nelson RP. Primary urethral malignancy; review of 22 cases. South Med J 1978;71:547.
37. Lesavoy MA. Vaginal reconstruction. Urol Clin North Am 1985;12: 369.
38. Klein FA, Whitmore WF Jr, Herr HW, et al. Inferior pubic rami resection with an en bloc radical resection of invasive proximal urethral carcinoma. Cancer 1983;51:1238.
39. Johnson DW, Kessler JF, Ferrigni RG. Low-dose combined chemo/radiotherapy in the management of locally advanced urethral squamous cell carcinoma. J Urol 1989;141:615.
40. Baskin LS, Tuzan C. Carcinoma of male urethra, management of locally advanced disease with combined chemo/radiotherapy and penile preserving surgery. Urology 1992;39:21.
41. Hussein AM, Benedetto P, Sridhar KS. Chemotherapy with cisplatin and 5-fluorouracil for penile and urethral squamous cell carcinomas. Cancer 1990;65:433.
42. Stewart PAH, Anderson CK, Williams RE, et al. Urethral tumors. Br J Urol 1978;50:583.
43. Bracken RB, Henry R, Ordonez N. Primary carcinoma of the male urethra. South Med J 1980;73:1003.
44. Leiber MM, Malek RS, Farrow GM, McMurtry J. Villous adenocarcinoma of the male urethra. J Urol 1983;130:1191.
45. Hoppman HJ, Fraley EE. Squamous cell carcinoma of the penis. J Urol 1978;120:393.
46. Mandler JI, Pool TL. Primary carcinoma of the small urethra. J Urol 1966;96:67.
47. King LR. Carcinoma of the urethra in male patients. J Urol 1964;91: 555.
48. Bracken RB. Radical exenterative surgery. In: Johnson DE, Boileau MA, eds. Genitourinary tumors: fundamental principles and surgical techniques. New York: Grune and Stratton, 1982:249.
49. Marshall VF. Radical excision of locally extensive carcinoma of the deep male urethra. J Urol 1957;78:252.
50. Raz S, McLorie G, Johnson S, Skinner DG. Management of the urethra in patients undergoing radical cystectomy for bladder carcinoma. J Urol 1978;120:298.
51. Richie JP, Skinner DG. Carcinoma in situ of the urethra associated with bladder carcinoma: the role of urethrectomy. J Urol 1978;119:80.
52. Sarosdy MF. Management of the male urethra after cystectomy for bladder cancer. Urol Clin North Am 1992;19:391.
53. Doll R, Payne P, Waterhouse J. Cancer incidence in five continents. Lyon, France: International Agency for Research on Cancer, 1976.
54. Kennaway EL, Kennaway NM. The social distribution of cancer of the scrotum and cancer of the penis. Cancer Res 1946;6:49.
55. Lee WR, McCann JK. Mule spinner's cancer and the wool industry. Br J Ind Med 1967;24:148.
56. Lowe FC. Squamous-cell carcinoma of the scrotum. Urol Clin North Am 1992;19:397.
57. Graves RC, Flo S. Carcinoma of the scrotum. J Urol 1940;43:309.
58. Pott P. Cancer scroti. In: Hawes L, Clarke W, Collins R, eds. Chirurgical works. London: Longman, 1775;5:63.
59. Cruickshank CND, Squine JR. Skin cancer in the engineering industry from the use of mineral oil. Br J Ind Med 1950;7:1.
60. Passey RD. Experimental soot cancer. BMJ 1922;2:1112.
61. de la Brassinne M, Richert B. Genital squamous-cell carcinoma after PUVA therapy. Dermatology 1992;185:316.
62. Andrews PE, Farrow GM, Oesterling JE. Squamous cell carcinoma of the scrotum: long-term follow-up of 14 patients. J Urol 1991;146:1299.
63. Southam AH, Wilson SR. Cancer of the scrotum: the etiology, clinical features, and treatment of the disease. Br Med J 1922;2:971.
64. Catalona WJ. Role of lymphadenectomy in carcinoma of the penis. Urol Clin North Am 1980;7:785.
65. Lowe FC. Squamous cell carcinoma of the scrotum. J Urol 1983;130: 423.
66. Rouviere H; Tobias MJ, trans. Anatomy of the human lymphatic system. Ann Arbor: Edward Bros, 1938.

67. Daseler E, Anson BJ, Reimann AF. Radical excision of inguinal and iliac lymph glands, a study based upon 450 anatomical dissections and upon supportive clinical observations. Surg Gynecol Obstet 1948;87: 679.
68. Kickham CJE, Dufresne M. An assessment of carcinoma of the scrotum. J Urol 1967;98:108.
69. Coleman MW, Joyce R, Graves RS. Carcinoma of the scrotum, new approach to inguinal gland dissection. J Urol 1952;68:534.
70. Dean AL. Epithelioma of scrotum. J Urol 1948;60:508.
71. McDonald MW. Carcinoma of the scrotum. Urology 1982;19:269.
72. Ichikawa T, Nakano I, Hirokawa I. Bleomycin treatment of the tumors of the penis and scrotum. J Urol 1969;102:699.

PART III

Prostate Cancer

Principles and Practice of Genitourinary Oncology, edited by Derek Raghavan, Howard I. Scher, Steven A. Leibel, and Paul H. Lange. Lippincott-Raven Publishers, Philadelphia, © 1997.

CHAPTER 34

Anatomy of the Prostate

Surgical Implications

Robert P. Myers

Even though the prostate gland could be considered at the heart of the human male pelvis, its true role has not been determined.[1] By its very form, position, and ductal structure, the prostate is a gateway organ for egress of urine from bladder to urethra and for the discharge of semen, to which it contributes a prostate fraction. From a surgical standpoint, the prostate cannot be understood without keen appreciation of the pelvic floor and perineum. If the anatomy of the prostate and its environs are not clearly understood by the surgeon, patients suffer the consequences. Medicare end results for patients who have undergone radical prostatectomy reveal morbidity at an unnecessarily high level.[2] Thirty percent of these patients must wear "pads or clamps to deal with wetness."[2] Because of the poor results reported, more training is necessary; this training must include a keener appreciation of anatomy and possibly the introduction of optical loupe magnification for more precise dissection. The "establishment of guidelines for the selection of surgical candidates" also may be important.[3] Results of radical prostatectomy are consistently superior at top-ranked facilities.[4]

GENERAL ANATOMY

The prostate gland, which is unique to males and homologous to Skene's ducts in females,[5] is intimately associated with the urethra and is situated at and inferior to the bladder neck. Its size and configuration depend to a large degree on the person's age and the presence or absence of benign prostatic hyperplasia (BPH), although differences in shape (i.e., phenotypic variation) are seen in the nonhyperplastic prostates of boys during puberty.

McNeal[6] has defined the histologic architecture of the normal, nonlobar, nonhyperplastic prostate gland, as well as deviations from normal. He established "zonal anatomy of the prostate" by delineating the ductal or acinar structure of the prostate in transverse, coronal, oblique coronal, and sagittal sections and devised "regional morphology" of parenchymal and stromal elements with introduction in normal males of peripheral, central, and transition zones (Fig. 34-1).[7–9] McNeal's peripheral zone, located inferior, posterior, and lateral to the ejaculatory ducts in the coronal plane, encompasses approximately 70% of the prostate and has a fine acinar histology. The central zone, composing about 25% of prostate tissue, lies superior, posterior, and medial to the ejaculatory ducts in the coronal plane and has notably larger acini than the peripheral zone. Pathologic processes are remarkable rare in the central zone. The transition zone, which constitutes 5% to 10% of the nonhyperplastic prostate, is found in two small lobes, each flanking the anterolateral aspect of the urethra, with ducts that enter the urethra close to the verumontanum and at the distal extent of the preprostatic sphincter. The transition zone is a major location of BPH in middle-aged and elderly men. Prostates with and without hyperplasia stand in sharp contrast to each other in transverse section (Fig. 34-2*A*, *B*).

Before McNeal's description,[6] there was widespread acceptance of a lobular or lobar architecture in normal glands; reviews of these descriptions in the literature are provided by Blacklock[10] and McNeal.[11] The lobe concept has been generated or enhanced by the nodular adenomatous nature of BPH. When symmetrical, the process of hyperplasia typically produces left and right lateral lobes and a median lobe from periurethral glandular elements and the transition zone. The digitally enucleated trilobar specimen of suprapubic adenectomy is always a dramatic demonstration of lobes. Rarely, an anterior lobe develops. Asymmetry is not uncommon. Endoscopically, the surgeon may see only a right lobe or an enlarged median lobe with no lateral lobe hyperplasia. As periurethral lateral lobe hyperplasia progresses, normal parenchyma and stroma of the peripheral zone become increasingly attenuated against the periprostatic fascia by expanding hyperplastic tissue. On digital rectal examination of the patient with moderate BPH, the left and right lobes of the prostate, separated by the depression of a central sulcus, can be easily palpated. As the hyperplastic process becomes more extensive, the lobar impression on digital rectal examination often disappears completely, resulting in a

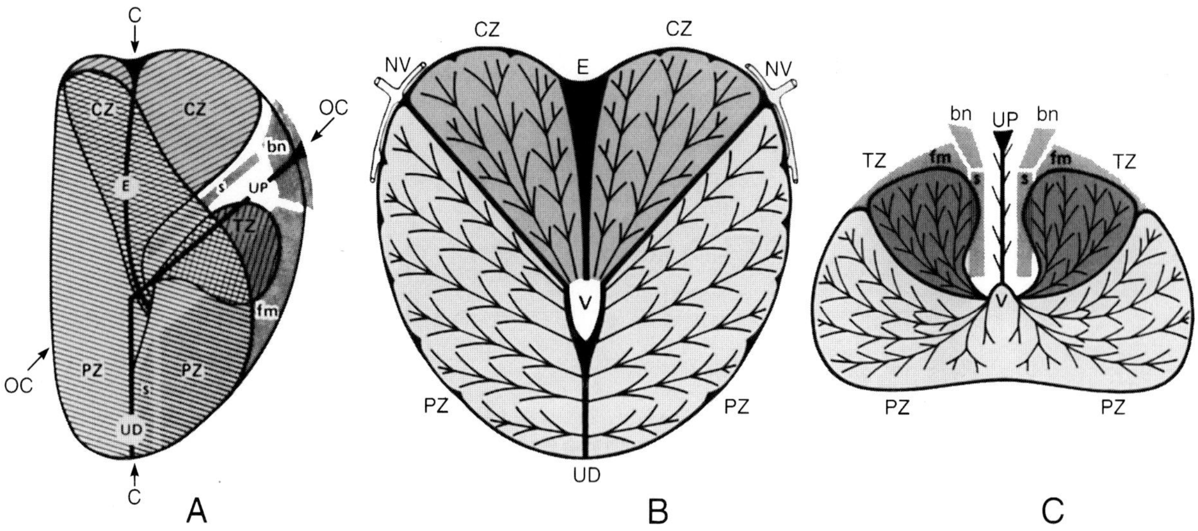

FIG. 34-1. Zonal architecture of the prostate in 3 planes: (**A**) sagittal, (**B**) coronal (C), and (**C**) oblique coronal (OC). Arrows denote the directions of planes OC and C. bn, bladder neck; CZ, central zone; E, ejaculatory duct; fm, fibromuscular stroma; NV, neurovascular tissue; PZ, peripheral zone; s, preprostatic sphincter (proximal to veru) or striated sphincter (distal to veru); TZ, transition zone; UD, distal prostatic urethra; UP, proximal prostatic urethra; V, veru. (From McNeal JE. Zonal distribution of prostatic adenocarcinoma: correlation with histologic pattern and direction of spread. Am J Surg Path 1988;12:897; and McNeal JE. The prostate gland: morphology and pathobiology. Monogr Urol 1988;9:36.)

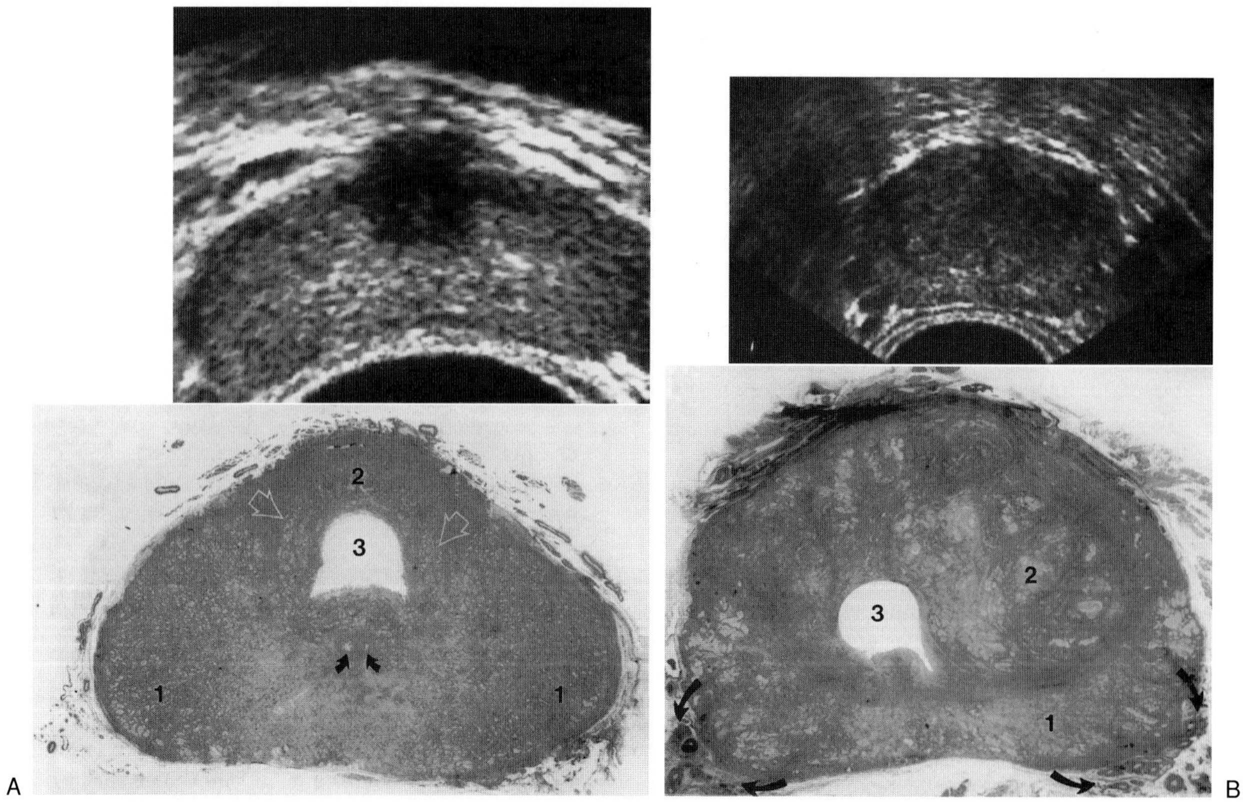

FIG. 34-2. Transverse sections of cadaveric prostates fixed with a catheter in the urethral lumen. (Masson trichrome stain.) (**A**) Normal adult prostate without hyperplasia. *Large arrows,* transition zone; *small arrows,* ejaculatory ducts; 1, peripheral zone; 2, fibromuscular stroma of anterior commissure; 3, urethral lumen. *Above:* comparable transrectal ultrasonographic image. (**B**) Adult prostate with prominent nodular hyperplasia. *Arrows,* neurovascular tissue; 1, peripheral zone (note compression); 2, nodular hyperplastic transition zone. *Above:* comparable transrectal ultrasound image. (Courtesy of Dr. Torrence Wilson.)

A 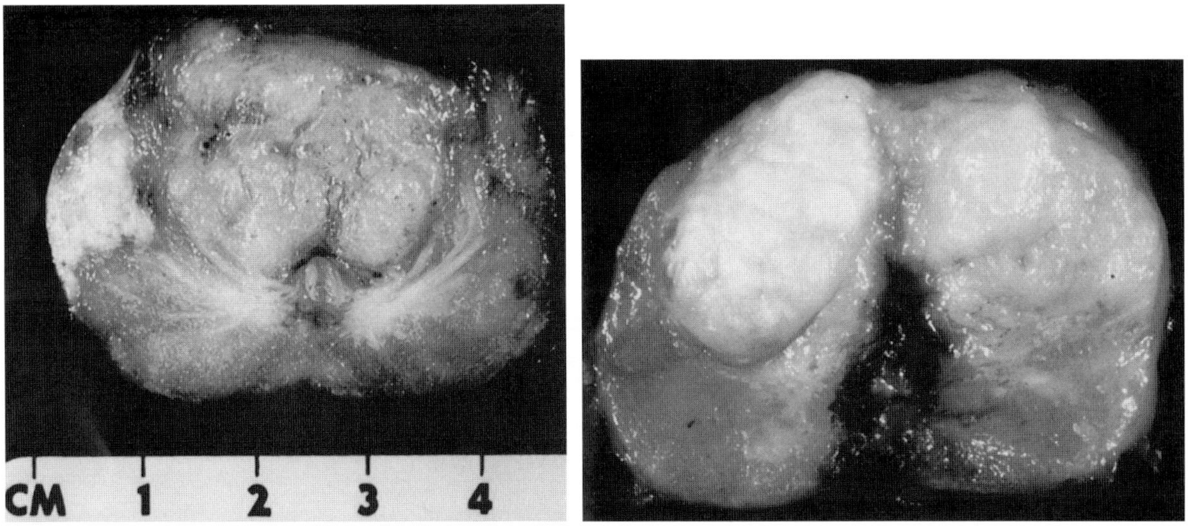 B

FIG. 34-3. Prostate glands cut transversely, showing prostatic adenocarcinoma circumscribed in starkly yellow cholesterol-laden tissue. (**A**) Cancer infiltrates the peripheral zone (*left*) and is confined by the transition zone barrier. The hyperplastic transition zone is not involved. (**B**) Cancer infiltrates the nodular transition zone (*left*) and is confined by the transition zone barrier. The peripheral zone is not involved. (Courtesy of Dr. David G. Bostwick.)

uniform benign texture. Extensive nodular hyperplasia may result in soft, asymmetrically placed, benign nodules that protrude against and can be palpated through the compressed peripheral zone tissue. These soft nodules should not be confused with nodules that are palpably suspicious for cancer, which require biopsy. Adenocarcinoma, which most often involves the peripheral zone, may be isolated in this region but also may be isolated exclusively in the transition zone. In either case, it sometimes appears that cancer does not cross what appears to be a transition zone barrier (Fig. 34-3*A*, *B*).[12] The fibromuscular transition zone barrier explains why patients with prostate cancer of peripheral zone origin who undergo transurethral resection of the prostate for significant infravesical obstructive uropathy often have BPH only in the resected specimens.

The circular smooth muscle of the bladder neck continues distally uninterrupted to envelop the proximal prostatic urethra as the ''preprostatic sphincter,'' which extends to the verumontanum (seminal colliculus) in the nonhyperplastic prostate.[10,13] Radical retropubic prostatectomy can sometimes be accomplished with complete preservation of the preprostatic sphincter in patients with no BPH, but I have never encountered an intact preprostatic sphincter in patients with significant concomitant BPH, because the hyperplasia appears to obliterate the integrity of the preprostatic sphincter. After radical removal of a hyperplastic prostate because of cancer, the bladder neck usually gapes widely and needs extensive suture plication. When sufficiently intact, the preprostatic sphincter has an obvious potential role in maintaining urinary continence, but the preprostatic sphincter is almost never preserved in the course of routine radical prostatectomy.

From the verumontanum distally, the smooth muscle sphincteric apparatus that constitutes the functional membranous urethra begins.[14] Gil Vernet stressed the ''anatomical and functional solidarity between the inframontanal prostatic urethra and the membranous urethra.''[15] Complementing this distal sphincter mechanism with its smooth muscle and elastic tissue components,[16] striated muscle envelops the urethra to form an external sphincter distal to the apex of the prostate (Fig. 34-4*A*, *B*). This muscle, although striated, is much more finely textured and of different unique tonic characteristics than ordinary striated muscle of skeletal origin, which has a much coarser composition.[17] Oelrich[18] firmly established how developmental growth of both prostate stroma and parenchyma destroys to variable degrees the upper aspect of the striated urethral sphincter. This results in disposition of striated muscle fibers across the surface of or embedded within the anterior prostate; surgical pathologists can identify the anterior prostate by the presence of striated muscle. This phenomenon, which sometimes produces an imperceptible transition from prostate to urethra, has significant implications in the conduct of urethral transection with respect to resection of cancer in radical prostatectomy.[19,20] Without appreciation of this phenomenon, the urethra may be transected too proximally, increasing the risk of incising the prostate and leaving a preventable positive margin at the apex or too far distally, leading to inordinate and preventable urinary incontinence.

The course of the urethra through the prostate from the base of prostate at the bladder neck to its exit at the prostate apex is variable. McNeal[11] emphasized anterior angulation of the urethra in the sagittal plane superior to the verumontanum, occurring in about 35% of patients, but noted the possibility of great variation. In fact, some prostates have no angulation; in some patients the angulation approaches 90 degrees, depending on the shape of the prostate and the presence or absence of BPH. When angulation is particularly acute, endoscopy with a rigid cystoscope is more difficult because the endoscopist runs into a median bar; use of a flexible instrument is preferable for patient comfort in this situation. Angulation or lack of angulation is associated with a variable length of the anterior midline prostate from base to apex, the region of the prostate known as the anterior commissure, or tissue that comprises the fibro-

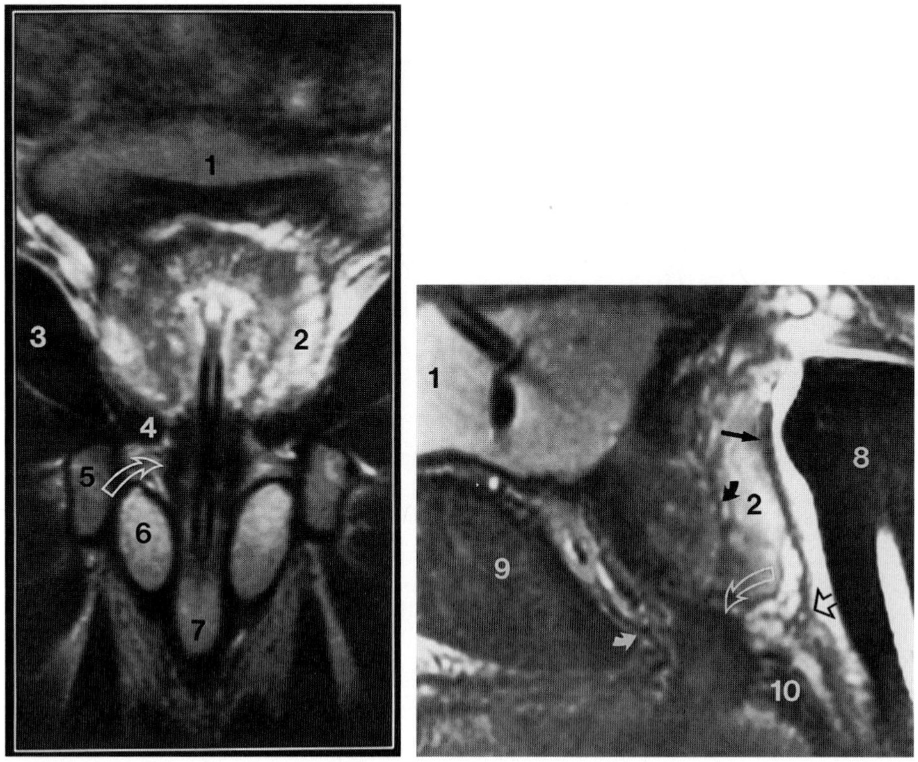

FIG. 34-4. Magnetic resonance images in two planes of the prostate and membranous urethra of a 52-year-old man. Curved open white arrows indicate the external striated urethral sphincter. (**A**) Coronal view. Note the membranous urethra within the urogenital hiatus. A Foley catheter is in place. (**B**) Sagittal view through the striated sphincter. Note the dorsal vein complex (*curved solid white arrows*), ejaculatory duct (*curved black arrows*), Denonvilliers' fascia (*straight solid black arrows*), and dimple in the anterior rectal wall created by the rectourethralis muscle (*open straight black arrows*). A Foley catheter balloon is in the bladder lumen. 1, urinary bladder; 2, prostate; 3, obturator internus muscle; 4, puborectalis muscle; 5, pubic ramus; 6, corpus cavernosum; 7, corpus spongiosum; 8, rectum with indwelling endorectal coil; 9, symphysis pubis; 10, perineal body.

muscular stroma bridging the left and right halves of the prostate anterior to the urethra.

The McNeal unifying model depicts only one of many possible prostate shapes and one with an exceptionally long anterior commissure (fibromuscular stroma).[21] Pronounced variation in prostate shape including fibromuscular stroma can be seen in radical prostatectomy specimens that have the contiguous bladder and membranous urethra removed (Fig. 34-5).[14,19] The degree of development and the periurethral placement of hyperplastic elements central to the normal peripheral zone are strong determinants of the external shape of the prostate. The gross specimen on which McNeal's model is based is attached to both the bladder and urethra; therefore, the true length of the anterior commissure is obscured by the nature of the specimen. Furthermore, the fibromuscular stroma of this model is not of uniform composition, as sometimes illustrated for the sake of simplicity,[21] but contains several histologic subdivisions, including bladder neck, smooth muscle, and striated sphincter.[13]

Many radical prostatectomy specimens with bladder and urethra removed reveal prostates with short anterior commissures. This finding is especially common in patients without BPH. The anterior commissure may be no more than 1 cm in length in the nonhyperplastic gland and 4 cm or longer in prostates with massive hyperplasia.[14,19] Formation of the anterior commissure influences the exit of the urethra at the apex. If the anterior commissure is short and extends not as far distally as the posterior midline peripheral zone, an anterior parenchymal notch is formed and is associated with a posterior lip.[19,20,22] The pres-

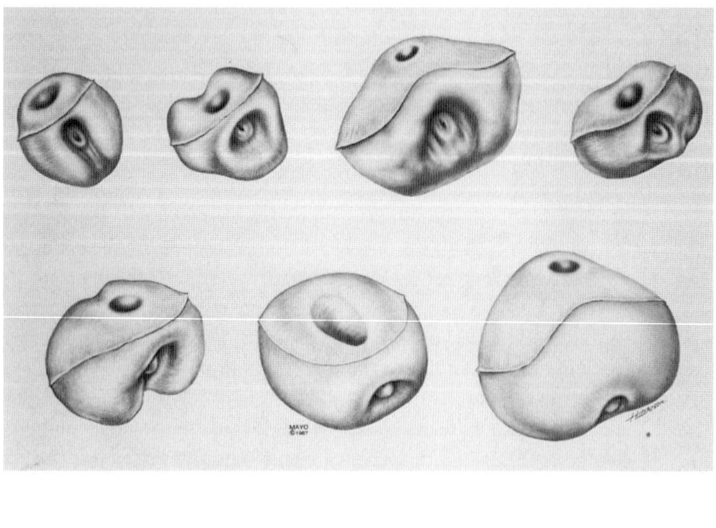

FIG. 34-5. The diversity of prostate size and shape can be seen in radical prostatectomy specimens. The bladder, membranous urethra, and seminal vesicles are absent. The prostatovesical junction is delineated on each prostate. (From Myers RP, Goellner JR, Cahill DR. Prostate shape, external striated urethral sphincter and radical prostatectomy: the apical dissection. J Urol 1987;138:543.)

ence of a notch becomes important in defining the proper line of transection of the prostate from the urethra during radical retropubic prostatectomy. If the line of transection is carried too proximally, the posterior lip may be transected, leaving unresected the lip, the verumontanum, and in some cases, cancer. In some prostates, the verumontanum is situated in the floor of the urethra at the most distal posterior extent of prostate parenchyma and may be left in situ only to be discovered at cystoscopy in the postoperative period. One advantage of radical perineal prostatectomy is the ability to easily recognize the posterior extent of the prostate.

ARTERIES

The primary arterial blood vessels to the prostate are branches of the inferior hypogastric artery that first enter the prostate base posterolaterally at its junction with the bladder (Fig. 34-6).[23] Within the prostate, the arterial distribution is twofold: capsular and urethral. The urethral group primarily supplies BPH when present, and when BPH is trilobar, the main sites of arterial entry lie between the two clefts at the bladder neck flanking the median lobe and on either side of the midline anterior cleft between the two lateral lobes. Thus, in transurethral resection of the prostate and open enucleation of adenoma, the 5-, 7-, 11-, and 1-o'clock positions at the bladder neck are important sites for hemostasis. The minor capsular arterial contribution to BPH can be quickly controlled after enucleation procedures if the previously distended capsule is allowed to contract. Packing with gauze or attempts to use a balloon pulled down into the prostatic fossa may be counterproductive and actually exacerbate troublesome capsular bleeding.

Arteries, veins, and the supporting fascia that envelop these vascular tributaries form what are known as the prostate vascular pedicles. These pedicles are routinely isolated, cross-clamped, and transected during the course of radical prostatectomy by retropubic or perineal routes and must be sectioned close to the prostate for successful preservation of potency.

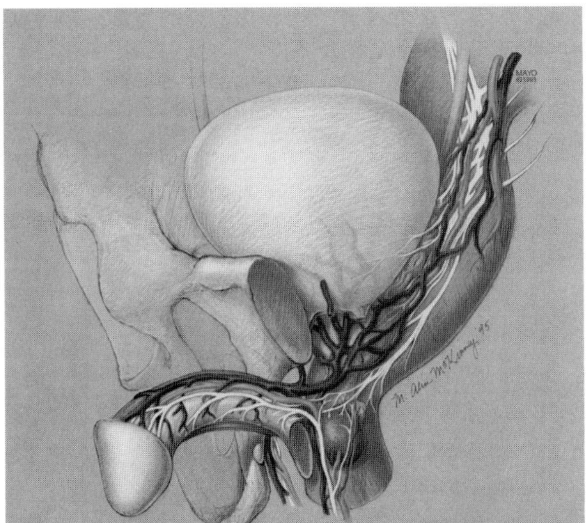

FIG. 34-6. Frontal view of a portion of the right half of the male pelvis with fascia and pelvic and perineal striated muscle absent, except for the striated urethral sphincter (SUS). Branches of the left internal iliac arteries with pelvic plexus nerves to the ureter, bladder, seminal vesicle, prostate, rectum, and cavernous tissue are shown. Dorsal veins of the penis enter the dorsal vein complex anterior to the SUS, with anastomosis to the prostatic venous plexus, the vesicovenous plexus, and finally, the internal iliac veins. The pudendal neurovascular supply enters close to disarticulated left crus of the penis. The left bulbourethral gland is located on the bulb at the posterolateral base of the membranous urethra.

VEINS

One of the most significant impediments to operating on the prostate is the dorsal vein complex, which is virtually synonymous with the prostatic venous plexus, with the exception of the veins that cover the anterolateral membranous urethra but not the prostate. This system of veins covers the prostate but represents major venous effluent of blood from the penis, not the prostate (see Fig. 34-6). The dorsal vein complex has its primary origin from the deep dorsal vein of the penis after it passes beneath the pubic arch, but it also receives direct venous input from veins that emerge from the penile crura (crural veins). Furthermore, the dorsal vein complex is in direct communication with the internal pudendal veins. In a network, veins course superiorly to cover the anterolateral surfaces of the prostate in remarkably variable distribution but finally join vesical veins, which in turn anastomose freely with the internal iliac veins. Significant advances in control of the dorsal vein complex or prostatic venous plexus during radical retropubic prostatectomy have greatly reduced associated blood loss.[24] Further control and improved exposure of the prostate can be gained by bunching the anterior portion of the plexus with suture material.[25] Bunching can be facilitated by using a clamp.[26,27] Before controlling the anterolateral portion of the prostatic venous plexus that lies beneath the prostatic fascia, care should be taken to secure superficial branches of the plexus that lie above the fascia within the retropubic fat.[28]

In radical perineal prostatectomy, the dorsal vein complex and the prostatic venous plexus can be avoided by finding a subfascial plane that allows the venous plexus to remain out of the surgical field. Blood transfusion should rarely, if ever, be necessary in a properly executed perineal approach to the prostate.

Preparations of the cadaveric pelvis in transverse section at the level of the lowest aspect of the striated sphincter show the urethra and the thick, striated urethral sphincter, with multiple veins located anterolateral to the sphincter.[14] These veins emerge from in front of a thick horizontal band of fibrous tissue called the transverse ligament of the perineum, which in certain cases is in continuity with a web of fibrous tissue across the pubic arch known as the arcuate ligament of the pubis. Notable features are the fascial and ligamentous continuity in this region and the absence of discrete ligaments, even though there are structures named ligaments such as the arcuate ligament of the pubis and the transverse ligament of the perineum. This region where the dorsal vein complex originates is also known as the penile hilum.[29] It is this region in which a pubourethral space[16] can be developed for the purpose of urethroplasty.

NERVES

In 1982, Walsh and Donker[30] demonstrated the possibility of maintaining erectile function after radical prostatectomy if the vascular pedicles to the prostate could be sectioned close enough to the prostate so that the cavernous nerves, running posterolaterally with blood vessels along the prostate, could be spared (see Fig. 34-6). At the junction of the prostate and bladder base in association with the pedicles, a neural plexus of ganglia called the prostatic plexus can be identified in association with the neurovascular tissue.[31] For the highest probability of preservation of potency after radical prostatectomy, the entire neural network of cavernous nerves and ganglia should be preserved. In general, ideal candidates for bilateral potency-preserving technique with the greatest success rates are patients who are younger than 60 years of age, are in excellent cardiovascular shape, and have nonpalpable clinical stage T1c disease with well to moderately differentiated cancer and low levels of serum prostate-specific antigen. When malignancy produces palpable parenchymal involvement, the nerve preservation option usually should not be considered on the side of palpable involvement because of the risk of direct periprostatic infiltration of the neurovascular bundle by cancer, especially if the cancer is high grade. Wide resection with inclusion of the bundle tissue to obtain a cancer-free margin is appropriate. This approach requires sacrifice of the closely applied nerve bundles in the interest of capturing the largest possible margin of soft tissue over the site of obvious tumor involvement. Unilateral preservation may be appropriate on the uninvolved side.

In cancer surgery, obtaining cancer-negative margins is often a matter of millimeters and, in some cases, micrometers. The prostate, even with its fascial coats, has little periprostatic tissue along its external surface to contain the spread of cancer that has perforated the surgical capsule. The wider the resection to include neurovascular tissue, urethra, and bladder neck to obtain negative margins, the possibly poorer functional result in terms of not only impotence but also preservation of urinary continence.

THE PROSTATE WITH RESPECT TO THE PELVIC FLOOR AND PERINEUM

Knowledge of how the prostate meets the pelvic floor is of concern for the proper execution of surgical operations. Proper exposure of the prostate requires an understanding of fascia and muscle of the pelvic diaphragm and perineum. The larger the prostate, the greater the distortion of contiguous fascia, muscle, and urinary bladder. With large prostates, functional recovery is at stake. Simple retropubic prostatectomy with an anterior capsulotomy becomes easier the larger the prostate and the higher it protrudes into the bladder and the developed retropubic space. With respect to radical prostatectomy, glands in the 100-g range may be too large to be approached easily perineally because of pubic arch limitation. Using the retropubic approach, large prostates become "knuckle grinders" for the surgeon's hands during prostate mobilization. Furthermore, the apical dissection is more complicated as a result of the sheer mass of glandular tissue anteriorly that sometimes hangs over the membranous urethra. Adherent levator ani muscle, particularly the thin, proximal pubococcygeus, may be more prone to injury when prostates are large.

A true and clear understanding of the male pelvis and perineum from the standpoint of performing any urologic surgery including the prostate is often difficult. Problems include misleading, imprecise, inadequate, and alternative nomenclature that fuels debate over correct terminology; medical drawings that create fictitious anatomy; prosector-induced artifacts in both formalin- and nonformalin-fixed pelves; and individual variation. Terminology that reflects artifact includes the following:

1. Spaces
   a. Retropubic
   b. Superficial and deep perineal
   c. Pubourethral
   d. Retrobulbar
   e. Retroprostatic
2. Urogenital diaphragm

With respect to nomenclature, His in 1895 spoke of "anarchy, under which teachers and students suffered" and that "things got even more confused" after efforts to simplify terminology by such notable anatomists as Henle, who created "many more new names."[32]

Erroneous drawings by medical artists were well characterized by Colapinto, who said, "Urologists see what they think they should see based on . . . anatomic drawings."[33] What they think they should see may translate into "inappropriate surgical procedures"[16] and in some cases disastrous surgical results. Fortunately, magnetic resonance imaging has come to the rescue in demonstrating clearly the correct anatomic relations of the various pelvic structures.

Conclusions concerning anatomy cannot be based on the study of one prostate, one pelvis, or one magnetic resonance image, and no single illustration can capture all possible variations. The more pelves a surgeon dissects, the more he or she becomes cognizant of the variations in skeletal size, relative width of the pubic arch, access to the prostate once the retropubic space has been developed, distribution of fat and fascia, development of levator ani muscle, size and placement of ligaments, and developmental differences in the prostate, the striated urethral sphincter, and the transverse muscles of the pelvic floor. Extension of the scrotal skin along the perineal and penile dermal raphes is strikingly variable; therefore, the distribution of the underlying dartos muscle is similarly variable. Placement of the anus with respect to the tip of the coccyx and the ischial tuberosities within the anal triangle is notably variable to surgeons who perform radical perineal prostatectomies.

The view into the pelvis from above in the medical drawings of many textbooks provides the illusion that the pelvic floor is relatively flat with respect to distribution of the levator ani. Gross dissection and magnetic resonance images, however, provide a completely different view: the pelvic floor is a cone, especially from the pubococcygeus distally, with the puborectalis closely embracing the prostate distally and the pubococcygeus proximally. As Hinman so aptly put it, "the prostate . . . lies wedged between the levators."[34] Sitting within the pelvic floor cone are the two major pelvic viscera: the bladder anteriorly and the rectum posteriorly, separated by the peritoneal cul-de-sac.

The rectum is separated from the seminal vesicles and prostate by an inverted sheet of triangular fascia (i.e., the septum rectovesicale, or Denonvilliers' fascia), which is continuous with the central tendon of the perineum. The central tendon of the perineum, also called the perineal body, forms a raphe of fibrous tissue posterior to the urethra and anterior to the anal canal. In examining 52 embryos "covering the period from the end of the first month to term," Silver in 1956 repudiated the popular hypothesis that the peritoneum by embryologic fusion in any way contributes to the formation of the rectovesical septum (Denonvilliers' fascia).[35] Specifically, Silver found that the septum contains smooth muscle fibers continuous with the longitudinal smooth muscle fibers of the rectum, and he concluded that the septum "appears to be formed simply by the condensation of loose areolar tissue."[35]

From superior to inferior, the levator ani muscle is a continuous mass containing recognizable subdivisions of iliococcygeus, pubococcygeus, and puborectalis; the puborectalis is continuous with the deep external anal sphincter.[36] The pubococcygeus is much thinner and is situated lateral and superior to the puborectalis, which is thicker and is located more medial and distal compared with the puborectalis. Both muscles embrace the prostate. The pubococcygeus is located approximately at the level of the vesicoprostatic junction, and its fibers can be seen during radical retropubic prostatectomy to be heading straight posteriorly toward the coccyx and anococcygeal ligament. Posterolaterally, the pubococcygeus bulges inward in response to the underlying fat of the ischiorectal fossa. More distally, medially, and anteriorly, fibers of the puborectalis embrace the prostate as well as the rectum at the anorectal flexure. Contraction of the puborectalis lifts both the anorectal flexure and the prostate, giving the puborectalis a role in seminal ejaculation. Because of the presence of complete separation by Denonvilliers' fascia between the rectum and prostate, no levator muscle other than the puborectalis can lift the prostate. In describing what he called the levator of the prostate, Santorini[37] could only have been describing the puborectalis. The term levator prostatae as a subdivision of the levator ani has no realistic basis, and its presence and illustration in the anatomic literature can be safely ignored.

The deep anal sphincter is a posterior extension of the levator ani that adds to the tip of the pelvic floor cone. Fibers of the superficial anal sphincter are in direct contact with fibers of the deep anal sphincter. The combined levator ani and anal sphincters thus form a continuous, conical sleeve of muscle.

Anteriorly, in contact with and distal to the puborectalis, are levator fibers that embrace the fascia covering the membranous urethra but insert into the superior extension of the central tendon of the perineum. These fibers are readily visualized when performing radical retropubic prostatectomy. They have been called, appropriately, the pubourethralis muscle by Turner-Warwick,[16] who has regularly observed this portion of the levator muscle during urethroplasty. Also appropriately, Krause[38] named these slips of muscle the levator urethrae. Unfortunately, this levator urethrae component of the levator ani, well recognized by urologic surgeons, appears neither in current textbooks of anatomy nor in compendia of anatomic nomenclature such as the *Nomina Anatomica*.[39]

The ultimate termination of the conical end of the levator ani consists of both a posterior extension in the external anal sphincter components, with which it is in continuity, and an anterior extension, the levator urethrae, which embraces the membranous urethra. These two most distal posterior and anterior extensions are separated by the fibrous tissue of the central tendon of the perineum, or perineal body.

FASCIA AND THE PROSTATE

With respect to the pelvic fascia, Smith made a pertinent observation concerning "traditional and stereotyped" description and how "every conscientious demonstrator must have realized the difficulty of harmonizing the facts observed in the actual body with the description."[40] Understanding the pelvic fascia is aided by realizing that every striated muscle has an external fascial surface (i.e., epimysium); that the blood vessels have their own associated fascia; that bone has its fascia-like periosteum; that the prostate gland, bladder, urethra, and rectum have their own visceral fascia (not that the prostate is a viscus); and that the fasciae of muscle, blood vessels, viscera, prostate, and the periosteum fuse as they envelop their respective structures. The levator ani has a superior or inner fascia that constitutes the pelvic or endopelvic fascia, but there is also an inferior or outer fascia that by artifact can be made to appear as the superior fascia of a urogenital diaphragm.[40] This is accomplished by stripping away levator muscle while leaving its inferior fascia in situ (discussed later). The pudendal vessels that course along the medial aspect of each inferior pubic ramus and superior ischial ramus are encompassed in a thick fascia that is continuous with the laterally adjacent periosteum and the perineal membrane medially. The thick fascia surrounding the pudendal vessels defines the pudendal canal, a portion of which, confined to the anal triangle, is called Alcock's canal. This same perivascular pudendal fascia or lunate fascia[40] limits the lateral extension of the deep transversus perineus muscle fibers.[15] The puboprostatic ligaments are really pubovesical ligaments[41]; their direct connection to the visceral fascia of the anterior bladder wall and their smooth muscle component form the adult remnant of the pubovesical fascia and muscle of infancy.

UROGENITAL DIAPHRAGM

A source of enormous confusion is the "urogenital diaphragm," the presence of which, although it lives on in medical illustrations, is supported neither by precise anatomic dissection nor by magnetic resonance imaging (Fig. 34-7*A–C*).

The term urogenital diaphragm was concocted by Henle[42]; his preparation was artifact and consisted of two horizontal fasciae with intervening muscle. His superior fascia had to be created from levator fascia left in situ after removal of the puborectalis.[40] The inferior fascia in this specimen is the current perineal membrane. The muscle sandwiched between the two fasciae was derived by transecting his mentor Müller's[31] (Fig. 34-8) vertically oriented striated urethral sphincter (musculus sphincter urethrae) flush with the inferior or outer puborectalis fascia. This maneuver left an upper, vertically oriented, cylindrical portion of the external urethral sphincter attached to the prostate and severed membranous urethra, to which a new name was given: "sphincter vesicae externus."[42] This maneuver also left within the urogenital diaphragm a dissociated, transversely oriented, distal portion of the striated urethral sphincter, which

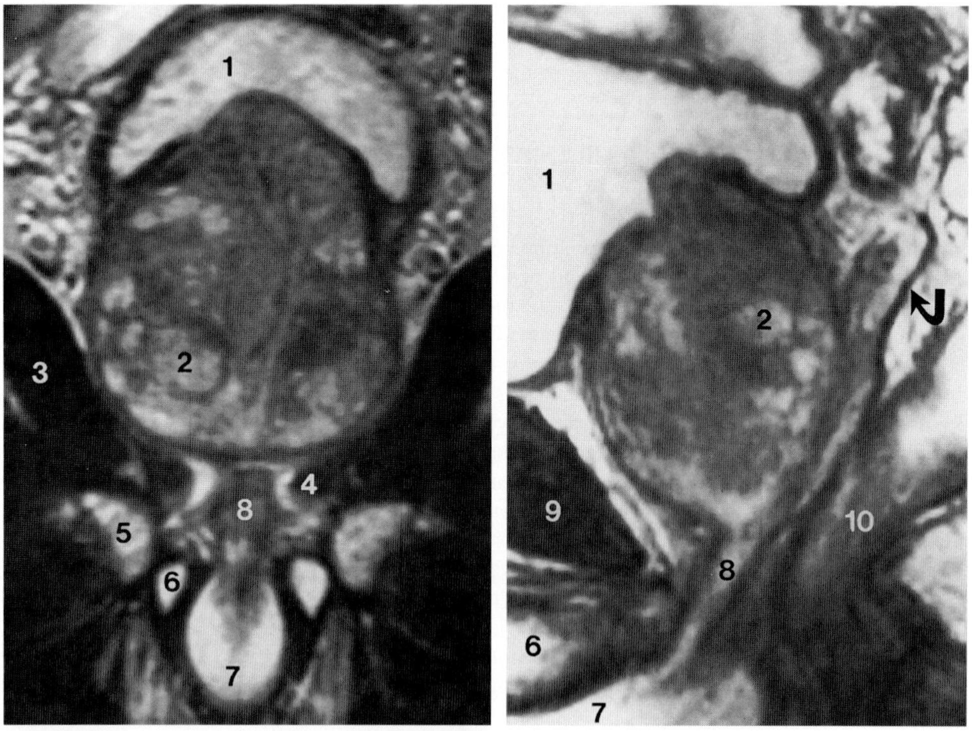

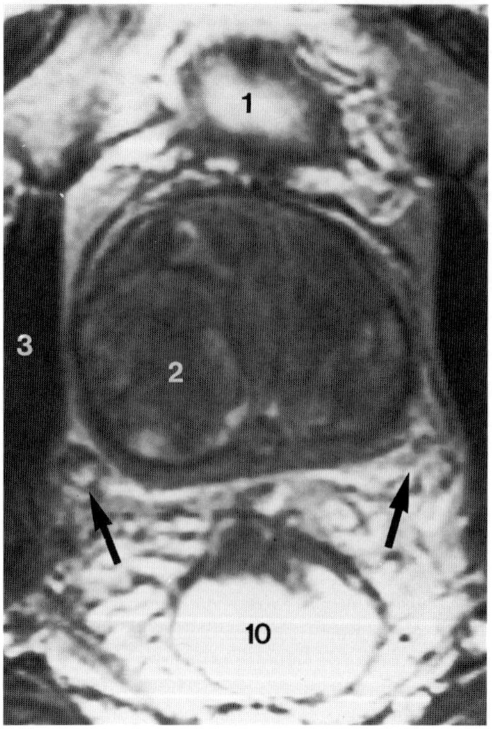

FIG. 34-7. Magnetic resonance images in three planes of a huge, nodular, hyperplastic prostate from a 63-year-old man. (**A**) Coronal view. The membranous urethra is located in the urogenital hiatus between the flanking puborectalis muscles. (**B**) Sagittal view, close to midline. The long membranous urethra and Denonvilliers' fascia (*arrow*) are shown. No evidence for a urogenital diaphragm is seen. (**C**) Transverse view reveals marked compression of peripheral zone by nodular hyperplasia. Arrows indicate the neurovascular bundles. 1, urinary bladder; 2, prostate; 3, obturator internus muscle; 4, puborectalis muscle; 5, pubic ramus; 6, corpus cavernosum; 7, corpus spongiosum; 8, membranous urethra with striated urethral sphincter; 9, symphysis pubis; 10, rectum.

Henle surprisingly called ''musculus transversus perineus profundus,'' not to be confused with the current deep transverse perineus muscle.[42] From one muscle mass of striated urethral sphincter, Henle created two muscles and provided his own new names. With Henle's urogenital diaphragm, the striated urethral sphincter as a vertical entity for the most part disappeared until brought back and reemphasized with particular clarity by Oelrich.[18]

Oelrich found no support for the urogenital diaphragm as distinct structure; rather, the correct concept is to consider the membranous urethra as passing through a ''urogenital hiatus'' and plunging directly into the substance of the corpus spongiosum (see Figs. 34-4 and 34-7).[18] The urogenital hiatus is defined by the opening through which urethra, with its striated sphincter, passes between the laterally adjacent bundles of puborectalis muscle and more distal levator urethrae. No superior fascia

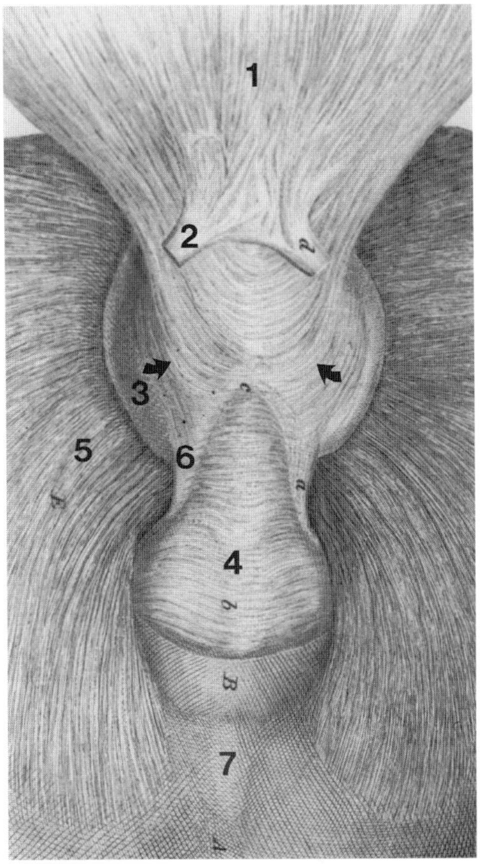

FIG. 34-8. Müller's striated urethral sphincter. Note the semicircular loop of longitudinal smooth muscle detrusor fibers of the urinary bladder sweeping onto the anterior surface of the prostate (*arrows*). 1, urinary bladder; 2, pubovesical ligament; 3, prostate; 4, striated urethral sphincter; 5, levator ani; 6, ischioprostatic ligament; 7, symphysis pubis. (From Müller J. Über die organischen Nerven der erectilen männlichen Geschlectsorgane des Menschen und der Säugethiere. [Concerning the autonomic nerves of the male erectile genital organs of man and mammals.] Berlin: F Dummler, 1836.)

of a urogenital diaphragm exists; rather the ''fascia of the sphincter muscle is inseparable from the prostatic sheath.''[18] This is precisely what the surgeon encounters during radical retropubic prostatectomy. As the lateral prostatic fascia extends distally and continuously to embrace the striated urethral sphincter and the membranous urethra, the prostate cannot be freed at its apex until a line of transection in the lateral fascia is chosen. This lateral fascia enjoys many designations.[21] The outermost layer of this multilayered fascia is the inner levator fascia, and the more medial layers are visceral layers that coat the prostate and extend distally around the urethra. Unfortunately, the concept of a urogenital diaphragm lives on in the fantasy of medical illustrators, atlases of anatomy, the *Nomina Anatomica*,[39] lay media advertisements, and the minds of urologists. The result is a victory for Henle but an abomination with respect to understanding the anatomy of the pelvic floor and perineum; a seriously flawed concept continues to plague the urologic and anatomic communities. In a sense, Henle was both right and wrong; he was correct in the subsection of his work entitled ''Prostate''[42] showing the vertical orientation of the urethral sphincter about the membranous urethra and then subsequently was incorrect in the following subsection that established the fictitious sandwich concept. What he did is captured in his statement, ''With the entrance of the urethra into the urogenital septum, the fibers of the striated sphincter (Sve) terminate without distinct demarcation with the fibers of the inner half of the urogenital diaphragm of adjacent muscle which I will be handling with the perineal muscle under the name of m. transversus perinei profundus.''[42]

DEEP TRANSVERSE PERINEUS MUSCLE

Santorini noted tremendous variation in the ''transverse muscles.''[37] Although identified as a discrete muscle, the deep transverse perineus muscle, which has no lateral osseous attachment,[15] is often continuous with the striated urethral sphincter mass of muscle, with which it appears to share the same color and fine-caliber fiber type in gross dissection specimens. In some preparations, the deep transversus consists simply of posterior fibers of the urethral sphincter that are left to encompass the bulbourethral (i.e., Cowper's) glands as they lie on the anterosuperior surface of the penile bulb.[14,15] The distribution of deep transversus fibers in such preparations appears in part to be at the mercy of bulbourethral gland growth and displacement of muscle. In other gross preparations, fibers distinct and separate from the urethral sphincter can be seen to arise in the midline and extend transversely to end in the fascia surrounding each pudendal canal. Müller used the term ''transversus of the bulb'' when describing the deep transverse perineus muscle.[31]

When tissue is grabbed with the needle posterior to the urethra to set posterior anastomotic sutures during radical prostatectomy in an attempt to improve urinary continence, these sutures must, from an anatomic standpoint, be grabbing deep transverse perineus muscle. Occasionally, this can be confirmed visually with optical loupe magnification when the rectourethralis muscle has been completely detached during radical retropubic prostatectomy.

CONCLUSIONS

From a surgical standpoint, the prostate cannot be understood without a keen appreciation of the pelvic floor and perineum. The larger the prostate, the greater the distortion of contiguous fascia, muscle, and urinary bladder.

Diversity of prostate shape and size is significant. Although varying degrees and distribution of BPH provide the major reason for such diversity, there exist recognizably different configurations of normal, nonlobar, nonhyperplastic prostates. Consequently, the fibromuscular union of the membranous urethra and prostatic urethra is variable. The limits of transurethral resection of the prostate and the technique of urethral transection during radical prostatectomy are both affected.

Fibromuscular tissue between BPH and peripheral normal prostate gland provides both a plane of surgical dissection (the capsule with respect to transurethral resection and digital enucleation of adenoma) and, as emphasized by McNeal,[12] in some cases a barrier that appears to restrict the local growth of adenocarcinoma either centrally or peripherally, depending on the site of origin of the cancer.

Urogenital diaphragm as a term and concept is misleading and should be abandoned; its presence during gross anatomic dissection can be established only by artifact. Magnetic resonance images showing undisturbed anatomy support only Oelrich's "urogenital hiatus" between flanking puborectalis muscle.[18]

ACKNOWLEDGMENTS

Donald R. Cahill, Ph.D., John McNeal, M.D., and Thomas Oelrich, Ph.D., for helpful commentary with respect to anatomy. Bernard F. King, M.D., magnetic resonance imaging. LeAnn M. Stee, editorial review. Debra A. Jacobson, typing.

REFERENCES

1. Blandy JP, Lytton B. The prostate. London: Butterworth, 1986:1.
2. Fowler FJ, Barry MJ, Lu-Yao G, Roman A, Wasson J, Wennberg JE. Patient-reported complications and follow-up treatment after radical prostatectomy. Urology 1993;42:622.
3. Walsh PC. Editorial comment. J Urol 1994;152:256.
4. Garnick MB. The dilemmas of prostate cancer. Sci Am 1994;270(4):72.
5. Campbell MF. Urology. 2nd ed. Philadelphia: WB Saunders, 1963:1516.
6. McNeal JE. Normal histology of the prostate. Am J Surg Pathol 1988;12:619.
7. McNeal JE. Regional morphology and pathology of the prostate. Am J Clin Pathol 1968;49:347.
8. McNeal JE. The zonal anatomy of the prostate. Prostate 1981;2:35.
9. McNeal JE. Prostate. In: Sternberg SS, ed. Histology for pathologists. New York: Raven Press, 1992:749.
10. Blacklock NJ. Surgical anatomy of the prostate. In: Williams DI, Chisholm GD, eds. Scientific foundations of urology, vol 2, sect 2. London: William Heineman, 1976:113.
11. McNeal JE. Anatomy of the prostate: an historical survey of divergent views. Prostate 1980;1:3.
12. McNeal JE. Zonal distribution of prostatic adenocarcinoma: correlation with histologic pattern and direction of spread. Am J Surg Pathol 1988;12:897.
13. McNeal JE. The prostate and prostatic urethra: a morphologic synthesis. J Urol 1972;107:1008.
14. Myers RP. Practical pelvic anatomy pertinent to radical retropubic prostatectomy. AUA Update Series 1994;13(4):26.
15. Gil Vernet S. Morphology and function of vesico-prostato-urethral musculature. Treviso: Canova, 1968:1.
16. Turner-Warwick R. The sphincter mechanisms of the male and the prevention of postprostatectomy incontinence. In: Debruyne FMJ, van Kerrebroek PEVA, eds. Practical aspects of urinary incontinence, vol 6. Dordrecht: Nijhoff, 1986:230.
17. Gosling JA, Dixon JS, Critchley HOD, et al. A comparative study of the human external sphincter and periurethral levator ani muscles. Br J Urol 1981;53:35.
18. Oelrich TM. The urethral sphincter muscle in the male. Am J Anat 1980;58:229.
19. Myers RP, Goellner JR, Cahill DR. Prostate shape, external striated urethral sphincter and radical prostatectomy: the apical dissection. J Urol 1987;138:543.
20. Myers RP. Male urethral sphincteric anatomy and radical prostatectomy. Urol Clin North Am 1991;18:211.
21. McNeal JE. The prostate gland: morphology and pathobiology. Monogr Urol 1988;9:36.
22. Myers RP. Radical prostatectomy: pertinent surgical anatomy. Atlas Urol Clin North Am 1994:22.
23. Flocks RH. The arterial distribution within the prostate gland: its role in transurethral prostatic resection. J Urol 1937;37:524.
24. Reiner WG, Walsh PC. An anatomical approach to the surgical management of the dorsal vein and Santorini's plexus during radical retropubic surgery. J Urol 1979;121:198.
25. Myers RP. Improving the exposure of the prostate in radical retropubic prostatectomy: longitudinal bunching of the deep venous plexus. J Urol 1989;142:1282.
26. Tobisu K. Retropubic total prostatectomy. In: Suemasu K, Kakizoe T, eds. Surgical oncology operative techniques 3: urologic cancer. Tokyo: Medical View, 1992:64.
27. Myers RP. Radical retropubic prostatectomy: techniques for early postoperative urinary continence. J Urol 1993;149:199A; AUA videotape V-47, presented at the Annual Meeting of the American Urological Association, San Antonio, May 16–20, 1993.
28. Myers RP. Anatomical variation of the superficial preprostatic veins with respect to radical retropubic prostatectomy. J Urol 1991;145:992.
29. Devine CJ, Angermeier KW. Anatomy of the penis and male perineum: part I. AUA Update Series 1994;13(2):9.
30. Walsh PC, Donker PJ. Impotence following radical prostatectomy: insight into etiology and prevention. J Urol 1982;128:492.
31. Müller J. Über die organischen Nerven der erectilen männlichen Geschlectsorgane des Menschen und der Säugethiere. (Concerning the autonomic nerves of the male erectile genital organs of man and mammals.) Berlin: F Dummler, 1836.
32. His W. Einleitung. In: Die anatomische Nomenclatur. Leipzig: Von Veit, 1895:1.
33. Colapinto V. The anatomy of the distal urethral sphincters and the myth of the urogenital sandwich: part 2. J Urol 1984;131:164A.
34. Hinman F Jr. Atlas of urosurgical anatomy. Philadelphia: WB Saunders, 1993.
35. Silver PHS. The role of peritoneum in the formation of the septum rectovesicale. J Anat 1956;90:538.
36. Courtney H. Anatomy of the pelvic diaphragm and anorectal musculature as related to sphincter preservation in anorectal surgery. Am J Surg 1950;79:155.
37. Santorini GD. De virorum naturalibus. (Concerning the male genitalia.) In: Observationes anatomicae. Venetiis: Baptistam Recurti, 1724:182.
38. Krause W. Handbuch der menschlichen Anatomie. Hannover: Hahn'sche Buchhandlung, 1879.
39. Nomina anatomica, 6th ed. London: Churchill Livingstone, 1989.
40. Smith GE. Studies in the anatomy of the pelvis, with special reference to the fascial and visceral supports. part I. J Anat 1907–1908;42:198.
41. Albers DD, Faulkner KK, Cheatham WN, et al. Surgical anatomy of the pubovesical (puboprostatic) ligaments. J Urol 1973;109:388.
42. Henle J. Handbuch der systematischen Anatomie des Menschen, vol 2. Braunschweig: F Vieweg & Sons, 1866.

Principles and Practice of Genitourinary Oncology, edited by Derek Raghavan, Howard I. Scher, Steven A. Leibel, and Paul H. Lange. Lippincott-Raven Publishers, Philadelphia, © 1997.

CHAPTER 35

Animal Models in Prostate Cancer

Martin E. Gleave and Jer-Tsong Hsieh

Although prostate cancer is the most frequent nonskin malignancy in men, it remains poorly characterized in terms of its biologic and molecular basis. Because most tissues obtained through surgery are required for pathologic staging and grading, limited tissues are available for biochemical research. Although it occurs frequently in humans, prostate cancer rarely arises spontaneously in most other animals, which hinders research study on its origin, pathogenesis, tumor biology, and therapy.

An ideal animal model for the study of human prostate cancer does not exist. The ideal animal model would closely mimic the human situation: the tumor would be of human origin, have a reasonably slow doubling time, be androgen-dependent (AD) or androgen-responsive, produce prostate-specific antigen (PSA), metastasize to lymph nodes and bone, and progress to an androgen-independent (AI) state after castration.[1] However, prostate cancer in humans varies widely in its biologic aggressiveness, androgen sensitivity, and histologic appearance, and it is neither realistic nor possible to create an animal model for prostate cancer that perfectly mimics or reflects the diverse human condition. Insights and understanding into the nature of human prostate cancer will come with the development of useful concepts through careful extrapolation from appropriate types of animal models.

Researchers have at their disposal several good animal models that mimic various aspects of the clinical disease. Although none is perfect, similarities are more common than differences. This chapter reviews tumor systems of murine, rodent, and human origin (Table 35-1). Many aspects of human prostate cancer can be investigated only by the use of suitable animal model systems, some of which have already provided valuable insights into the disease.

RODENT MODELS

Dunning R-3327 Rat Prostatic Adenocarcinoma Model

The Dunning rat model originated at the University of Miami after serial passage in syngenic hosts of a spontaneous prostate tumor discovered at autopsy in a Copenhagen rat.[2] Subcutaneously implanted tumors (denoted as R-3327) become palpable 60 days after transplantation; histologically, the tumors are well-differentiated adenocarcinomas composed of glandular and stromal elements.

Multiple sublines of the parental R-3327 tumor have been developed over the years, each with distinct biologic characteristics. A complete outline of the derivation of Dunning R-3327 nomenclature was presented by Isaacs.[3] However, an understanding of the early history of the R-3327 tumor and its various sublines is important for comparison of studies involving the Dunning model from various centers. Investigators at the Johns Hopkins University,[4] the University of Iowa,[5,6] and elsewhere[7,8] helped characterize these sublines during the late 1970s and early 1980s. Smolev and colleagues denoted the R-3327 subline characterized at Johns Hopkins as the H subline.[4] This AD subline randomly undergoes AI progression after castration, which makes it a useful system for study of the mechanisms of progression to the AI state.[9,10]

The growth rate of R-3327 and H-subline tumors is slow; they become palpable 60 to 90 days after injection of 1.5×10^6 cells, have a doubling time of approximately 21 days, and rarely metastasize.[4,10] The androgen-sensitive growth of R-3327 tumors was reported in 1974[11]; in vitro studies identified 5α-reductase activity and androgen receptors, and tumors grew faster in intact than in castrated males. After castration of tumor-bearing mice, tumor growth rates decrease and some tumors may partially regress; after 60 to 90 days, tumor growth resumes with a doubling time similar to that present before castration. Relapsing AI tumors grow equally well in intact or castrated male hosts. Ongoing serial passage of parental R-3327 tumors led to the spontaneous development of an AI squamous cell carcinoma, termed the R-3327 A subline, which lacked both 5α-reductase activity and androgen receptors and grew 10 times faster than parental tumors.[12]

Decreases in tumor growth rate after castration are also observed in the R-3327-PAP[12] and Lubaroff R-3327/130 sublines,[5] but less so than that reported for the R-3327-H sublines. The mechanism of AI progression in this model appears to be clonal selection. Genetic instability over time leads to tumor heterogeneity and a spectrum of androgen sensitivity, with subpopulations of androgen-sensitive, AD, and AI cells. After castration, AD cells die, but androgen-sensitive and AI clones survive and grow to form AI recurrent tumors.[9,10]

Serial passage of the recurrent, anaplastic, AI tumor (termed

TABLE 35-1. *Animal models for the study of prostate cancer*

Designation	Derivation/origin	Host/model system	Androgen sensitivity	Tumor marker	Metastasis	Mechanistic studies
RODENT MODELS						
Dunning R-3327[2]	Spontaneous ? Prostate origin	Copenhagen rat (in vitro + SC transplant)	AS & AI tumors; positive AR, 5αR	None	Rare R3327-H + +MAT-LyLu + +MAT-Lu	AI progression[9,10,100] Metastasis[13,15–19,66] Androgen action[4,11]
Noble[23]	Hormone-induced Prostate gland	Noble rat (SC transplant)	AD, AI, & ED; positive AR	Acid phosphatase	AI tumor 55% AD tumor 20%	Etiology[23–26] Metastasis[23,24] Cell interactions[27,28]
Pollard[30]	Spontaneous Induced: T, fats Seminal vesicle	L-W rat (in vitro + SC transplant)	AI tumor growth	None	Viscera + LN	Etiology[33,34] Metastasis[30–32]
ACI[36]	Spontaneous Prostate ventral lobe	ACI rat (in vitro + transplant)	AD & AI; positive AR, 5aR	None	None	Etiology[37] Androgen action[38]
Shionogi[39]	Spontaneous Breast	DD/S mouse (SC transplant)	AD & AI tumors; positive AR, 5αR	None	Rare	Androgen action[40,41] AI progression[41,49,50] Therapy[50]
HUMAN CELL LINES						
PC-3[57]	AI bone metastasis	Athymic mice; SC, IV, orthotopic	AI	None	Orthotopic-LN, IV-osseous	Metastasis[63–65,68]
DU-145[58]	AI brain metastasis	Athymic mice; SC	AI	Acid phosphatase	None	
LNCaP[69]	AI LN metastasis	Athymic mice; SC coinoculation, orthotopic	AS & AI tumors; positive AR, 5αR	PSA Acid phosphatase	Orthotopic-LN C4-2–bone	Androgen/GFs[53,70–74] PSA regulation[76–81,86] Cell interaction[63,70–72] Metastasis[63,70–72,88] AI progression[77,84–88] Therapy[54,56,72]
EB-33[59]	AD primary tumor	Athymic mice; SC	AI	+/− Acid phosphatase	None	
PC-93[60]	AD primary tumor	Athymic mice; SC	AI/AS; positive AR	None	None	
TSU-PR1[61]	AI LN metastasis	Athymic mice; SC	AI	None	None	
HUMAN XENOGRAFTS						
PC-82[92]	AD primary tumor	Athymic mice; SC	AD; positive AR	PSA, PAP	None	Androgen action[93–96] Therapy[48,93,99]
PC-EW[97]	AD pelic LN	Athymic mice; SC	AD; positive AR	PSA, PAP	None	Androgen action[95,97]
Honda[102]	AI testis metastasis	Athymic mice; SC	AD; positive AR	PAP	None	Androgen action[103]
LuCaP[104]	AI LN metastasis	Athymic mice; SC	AD; positive AR, 5αR	PSA, PAP	None	PSA regulation
GENE TRANSFER AND TRANSGENIC MODELS						
Transgenic[105–107]	Organ-specific transcription factors + *cis*-acting DNA promoter			Characterization in proces		Carcinogenesis[105–107]
MPR[110]	*RAS*+ *MYC* cotransfection	Fetal urogenital sinus Renal subcapsule	AS & AI cell lines	None	None	Carcinogenesis[110–114]

5αR, 5α-reductase; *AD*, androgen-dependent; *AI*, androgen-independent; *AR*, androgen receptor; *AS*, androgen-sensitive; *ED*, estrogen-dependent; *GF*, growth factor; *IV*, intravenous; *LN*, lymph node; *L-W*, Lobund-Wister; *MPR*, mouse reconstitution model; *PAP*, prostatic acid phosphatase; *SC*, subcutaneous; T, testosterone.

AT-1) has produced two distinct and highly metastatic sublines, one subline metastasized to both lung and lymph nodes (MAT-LyLu) and the other to lung only (MAT-Lu subline).[13] The development of sublines of Dunning tumor cells with high (MAT-LyLu, MAT-Lu, AT-3) and low (G, AT-1, AT-2) metastatic potential permits study of the acquisition of metastatic ability.

Metastasis is a multistep process involving protease production, increased invasiveness and motility, and decreased cell adhesion with cell migration into the circulation. Tumor embolus formation enhances survival in circulation, and, with arrest at distant sites, angioneogenesis is initiated and tumor cell growth is regulated by autocrine and paracrine mechanisms.[14] Flow cytometric and electrophoretic measurements of cell surface charge suggest that an increase in negativity at the cell surface is associated with increased metastatic potential[15,16]; these changes may reflect changes in cell surface glycoproteins and cell adhesion molecules. For example, Bussemakers and associates demonstrated that E-cadherin, a calcium-dependent cell adhesion molecule, is downregulated in highly metastatic Dunning lines.[17] Tumor cells of high and low metastatic ability also differed in their motility, with the metastatic lines exhibiting a higher degree of motility.[18] The genetic mechanisms regulating the metastatic phenotype remain poorly understood but probably involve increased expression of oncogenes or loss of tumor suppressor genes, or both. For example, if a poorly metastatic Dunning tumor subline is transplanted with the *HRAS* oncogene (formerly known as v-Harvey-ras), it demonstrates an increase in cell motility and metastatic ability.[19]

Some authors argue against the prostatic origin of the R-3327-H subline because of the presence of morphologic features that are incompatible with prostatic tissue.[20–22] Some features of the electrophoretic protein pattern of Dunning tumor extracts are more similar to those of the mammary gland than to those of the dorsal lateral prostate. Furthermore, secretory proteins typical of the lateral prostate (SVS II) and dorsal prostate (transglutaminase) are not detectable in the Dunning tumors.[21,22] The absence of a secretory form of transglutaminase and the presence of mammary gland proteins such as milk fat globule membrane proteins, lactoperoxidase, and lactalbumin in R-3327-H tumors (all of which are absent in the dorsal lateral prostate) suggest that the prostate may not be the origin of the R-3327-H subline. Nevertheless, this model has provided valuable insights into the biology of androgen-regulated tumor growth and metastasis.

Noble Rat Prostatic Adenocarcinoma Model

An inbred strain of rat susceptible to the development of prostatic adenocarcinoma by administration of exogenous sex hormone was described by Dr. R.L. Noble at the British Columbia Cancer Agency in Vancouver.[23,24] After chronic exposure to androgens and estrogens, Noble (Nb) male rats developed grossly evident prostatic tumors that were subsequently serially passaged to establish the Nb sublines, some of which were androgen-sensitive, AI, or estrogen-responsive.[23–26] Microscopic cancers were evident in 88% of animals treated for 18 months or longer, and gross tumors were evident in 21%. These tumors arose within the dorsal lobe of the prostate, and half the animals with gross tumors had evidence of metastatic disease of the viscera and lungs. The incidence of metastases was higher in AI than in AD tumors (55% versus 20%).[24,25] To establish cell lines in vitro, Chang and Chung separated and cultured epithelial (NbE) and fibroblast (NbF) cell lines from the ventral prostate of the Nb rat to study stromal-epithelial interactions.[27] Neither cell line is tumorigenic if inoculated alone into syngeneic or athymic mice; however, coinoculation of NbE with NbF results in formation of carcinosarcoma, demonstrating bidirectional paracrine-stimulating pathways between the two cell compartments.[28]

Spontaneous, clinically apparent prostate tumors in rodents are rare occurrences, and models like the Nb rat permit investigation of possible initiators and promoters of prostatic carcinogenesis. The experimental induction of prostate tumors in Nb[24] and Lobund-Wister (L-W)[29] rats after chronic administration of testosterone illustrates the critical role of androgens as promoters in the pathogenesis of prostate cancer and supports clinical observations that prostate cancer rarely, if ever, develops in men castrated before or shortly after puberty.

Pollard Rat Model

The spontaneous development of prostatic adenocarcinoma in L-W male rats was reported by Dr. Pollard,[30] who subsequently transplanted and propagated four prostatic carcinomas in random-bred L-W rats.[29] Each of these in vivo tumor sublines (denoted PA-I, PA-II, PA-III, and PA-IV) was used to establish an in vitro cell subline that produces carcinomas similar to those of the original subline if inoculated back into either male or female L-W rats. The sublines are highly metastatic if inoculated subcutaneously[30,31] or intravenously.[32]

In addition to these sublines produced through spontaneous tumors, Pollard and colleagues have also described chemically induced carcinomas in L-W male rats after long-term exposure to high levels of testosterone.[33] Grossly apparent tumors developed spontaneously in 26% of aged L-W rats and, by induction (with *N*-methyl-*N*-nitrosurea and testosterone), in approximately 90% of younger rats. Diets high in vegetable fats also had a promoting effect on the development of prostate cancers induced by chronic androgen exposure.[34] Spontaneous, induced, and inoculated tumors are highly metastatic, making this a good model for study of the metastatic phenotype. Spontaneous prostatic adenocarcinomas are prevented by lifelong moderate dietary fat restriction, and by castration, while the incidence of testosterone-induced prostatic adenocarcinoma is reduced by early treatment with retinoids. Tumorigenesis in L-W rats is therefore regulated by genetic, hormonal, and age-related mechanisms. Although premalignant stages of induced tumorigenesis are susceptible to intervention, the overtly malignant stage resists therapeutic trials with the same agents and procedures. However, the histiogenic origin of the chemically induced Pollard tumor model has recently come under question. The majority of tumors appear to arise within the seminal vesicle and are not of prostatic origin.[35]

ACI RAT MODEL

The inbred ACI strain derived its name from the crossbreeding of inbred August and Copenhagen (AXC strain with an Irish marker) rats. A high incidence of spontaneous prostatic adenocarcinoma in inbred ACI rats has been reported by a number of investigators.[36] This genetic susceptibility of aging male ACI/Seg rats produces both gross and microscopic cancers in the ventral lobe of the prostate. Transplantation in androgen-treated ACI rats has produced established, transplantable tumor lines. As in humans, the development of prostate cancers is age-associated. Microscopic lesions appear earlier and in much higher incidence than do grossly manifest prostate cancers, suggesting that, as in humans, only a minority of microscopic cancers progress to become grossly evident clinical tumors. This progression is a multistep process involving, in part, alternations in the ratio of serum testosterone to serum estrogen that are associated with aging. However, other factors in addition to alterations in serum testosterone levels are required for prostatic carcinogenesis in the ACI/Seg rat.[37] Although the ACI rats develop prostate cancers with age, they rarely die from them; this model therefore provides a system for investigating the earliest (initiation) events in prostate carcinogenesis. A number of in vitro cell lines have been established from ACI tumors and contain nuclear and cytosolic androgen receptors and 5α-reductase.[38]

Shionogi Mouse Mammary Carcinoma Model

The Shionogi mouse mammary carcinoma (SC-115) was established in 1961 from a female mouse with a spontaneously arising, hormone-independent mammary adenocarcinoma (AST-115).[39] After passage of the AST-115 tumor in male DD/S mice, the tumor was found to be AD. After injection of 5×10^6 parent tumor cells into adult male mice, tumors become palpable in 10 to 14 days and grow rapidly, with a doubling time of approximately 24 hours. The parent Shionogi mouse mammary carcinoma grows rapidly in the presence of androgens and regresses after androgens are withdrawn[38–40]; thus, the wild-type tumors are both androgen-sensitive and AD. Serial transplantation of the carcinoma over generations has yielded several variants, some of which are androgen-sensitive but AI, both androgen-insensitive and AI (i.e., autonomous), or sensitive to estrogens and glucocorticoids in addition to androgens.[41]

Because of its AD behavior, the Shionogi tumor model is particularly useful for study of the mechanisms of androgen action, the phenotypic changes associated with apoptosis and AI progression, and therapeutic approaches to delay or avert tumor progression.

Androgen Action

Apoptosis, or programmed cell death, can be induced in normal, benign hyperplastic, or malignant prostatic epithelial cells by any procedure that reduces the intracellular concentration of dihydrotestosterone by 80% or more. Androgen withdrawal in the Shionogi tumor model precipitates apoptosis and tumor regression in a highly reproducible manner.[40] Apoptotic cell death is different from necrotic cell death and is associated with a sequence of distinct molecular events characterized morphologically by shrunken cells with condensed and fragmented nuclei (apoptotic bodies) and biochemically by preferential intranucleosomal digestion of DNA that results in DNA laddering patterns.

Apoptosis appears to be a ''genetic suicide'' process that requires activation of a series of genes along with calcium (Ca^{2+})-dependent endonucleases, and it can be prevented by RNA and protein synthesis inhibitors and calcium-channel blockers. Numerous androgen-repressed genes are activated shortly after castration that are involved in either initiation or inhibition of apoptosis. These genes include the *FOS* and *MYC* protooncogenes, transforming growth factor-β (*TGFB*), and glutathione transferase.[42–44] One particular gene, testosterone-repressed prostatic message (*TRPM2*), is not expressed in either Shionogi tumors or normal prostate glands but is upregulated dramatically after castration in a temporal pattern reflecting the period of maximal apoptosis. Clusterin, the product of *TRPM2*, was initially identified and isolated as a major gene product of the regressing rat ventral prostate and was believed to help mediate apoptosis.[45] However, expression of *TRPM2* is induced in many regressing or dying systems, and it may represent an adaptive or protective mechanism by a dying cell to help abort apoptosis.

Another gene upregulated after castration is *BCL2*, a protooncogene believed to inhibit apoptosis and promote AI progression.[44,46] McDonnell and associates demonstrated that *BCL2* expression is absent in most AD prostate cancers but is present in almost all AI cancers.[46] Other genes, such as the tumor suppressor gene *P53*, may help promote apoptosis. There is evidence that *P53* is involved in initiating apoptotic deletion of cells that have sustained DNA damage.[44] Future therapeutic interventions aiming at maximization of apoptotic cell death with androgen ablation may employ drug combinations to inhibit the expression of *TRPM2* or *BCL2* or enhance expression of *P53*.

Androgen-Independent Progression

In the normal prostate, the sequence of androgen-induced cell growth and castration-induced apoptosis and regression can be continued through many cycles of androgen replacement and withdrawal.[47] Data from animal studies and observations from the long-term follow-up of Chinese eunuchs demonstrate that normal prostatic epithelial cells undergo apoptotic regression and do not develop the ability to regenerate and grow in an androgen-depleted environment. In contrast, AI progression almost always occurs after androgen ablation therapy for patients with prostatic carcinoma.

Four hypotheses have been proposed to explain why AI cell growth occurs in malignant but not benign prostatic epithelial cells. The clonal selection theory emphasizes tumor cell heterogeneity (i.e., mixtures of AD and AI cells); after castration, AD cells undergo apoptosis, but AI cells survive and ultimately progress. The adaptation theory assumes the presence of AD stem cells with a capacity for adaptation and self-renewal in an androgen-depleted environment. A third hypothesis emphasizes the importance of small amounts of residual androgens that selectively stimulate clones of androgen-sensitive cells. However, animal data using the PC-82 model[48] (see Human Xenograft Models) does not support this third hypothesis, because low levels of androgens still produce maximal tumor involution and do not stimulate tumor cell growth. Furthermore, although clinical studies show some benefit to maximal androgen blockade, AI progression remains inevitable, implying that nonandrogen growth regulatory factors are responsible for mediating AI progression. A fourth theory postulates the production of a mutant, constitutively active androgen receptor capable of binding to and activating androgen response elements (see Chap. 42) in the absence of androgen activation of their steroid-binding regions; however, little direct evidence exists to substantiate this theory.

The inability of androgen withdrawal therapy to be curative may therefore result from the preexistence of clones of AI cells in which the apoptotic process does not begin, or from upregulation of androgen-repressed adaptive mechanisms capable of aborting the apoptotic process and promoting growth in subpopulations of cells. These two possible mechanisms share an important characteristic: they assume that prostate cancers are heterogenous tumors composed of various subpopulations of cells that respond differently to androgen withdrawal therapy. Most cancers are heterogenous with respect to grade, ploidy, immunologic marker production, androgen receptor content, metastatic ability, and hormone and drug sensitivity. Tumor heterogeneity could reflect a multifocal origin, adaptation to environmental stimuli, genetic instability of the initial cancer, or a combination of these conditions; this heterogeneity, in turn, would provide the basis for AI progression by clonal expansion or adaptive mechanisms in subpopulations of cells.

Genetic instability and clonal selection, rather than adaptation, appears to be the mechanism that mediates AI progression in the Dunning rat model.[9,10] Genetic instability increases tumor heterogeneity by increasing the number of distinctly different clones of cells. Selective outgrowth of one or more of these clones can occur after androgen ablation, resulting in a less heterogenous tumor better suited for growth in an androgen-depleted environment.

Investigations by Bruchovsky and associates at the British Columbia Cancer Agency, using the AD Shionogi tumor model, stress the critical importance of adaptive mechanisms in AI progression.[43,49,50] After castration of mice bearing Shionogi's tumors, time-dependent progression from an AD to an AI state occurs, as reflected by coordinated changes in the expression of genes and proteins that regulate tumor cell proliferation and differentiation. Androgen withdrawal precipitates apoptosis and tumor regression in a highly reproducible manner. Despite complete remissions, however, castration fails to result in cure, and AI progression invariably occurs within 60 days after castration. Using an in vivo limiting dilution assay to determine the proportions of AD and AI tumorigenic stem cells in parent and recurrent tumors, Bruchovsky and colleagues[41,49] demonstrated that parent tumors are composed of both tumorigenic stem cells and differentiated AD daughter cells, in a ratio of 1:4000. After castration, most daughter and stem cells are eliminated. However, no enrichment of AI stem cells was evident in regressing parent tumors; rather, the proportion of AD stem cells decreased. The proportion of AI stem cells is increased 500-fold in AI recurrent tumors; therefore, castration culminates in a more aggressive and poorly differentiating tumor because of a massive increase in the proportion of AI stem cells. This finding implies that the survival of AI cells after androgen withdrawal may result from the ability of a small number of initially AD stem cells to adapt to an androgen-depleted environment. The expression of *TRPM2* is directly related to both tumor regression and progression. *TRPM2* encodes for the anticytolytic protein, clusterin, which becomes constitutively overexpressed in cells after androgen deprivation, even in the absence of morphologic signs of apoptosis. Overexpression of *TRPM2* and increased nuclear localization of clusterin may represent an adaptive or protective response to prevent apoptosis and thereby enhance the survival of stem cells.[51]

Autocrine and paracrine growth factors can replace androgens as primary growth stimulatory factors in AI prostate cancer progression. Progression of Shionogi tumor cells to an AI state is accompanied by increased production of a factor similar to basic fibroblastic growth factor (bFGF) that stimulates the growth of AD and AI cells, suggesting that bFGF may act as an autocrine growth factor during AI progression.[52] As discussed in the section on the LNCaP model, bFGF, epidermal growth factor (EGF), and transforming growth factor-alpha (TGF-α) stimulate LNCaP cell growth in vitro[53] and in vivo[54]; both EGF and TGF-α bind to the EGF receptor, which is expressed in increased amounts in LNCaP tumors with AI progression.[55] Taken together, these observations imply that upregulation of growth factor production may represent an adaptive response to androgen ablation in order to replace androgens in the growth regulation of AI tumors.

In summary, mechanisms mediating AI progression remain incompletely understood. The critical issue of whether dormant tumor cells are already AI from origin or progress because of adaptive responses to an androgen-depleted environment remains undecided, but both basic mechanisms are probably operative within heterogenous tumors.

Therapy

Improved understanding of the molecular processes involved in castration-induced apoptosis may lead to a therapeutic means of thwarting the stem cells' adaptive efforts to inhibit apoptosis, or a means of initiating the process in AI cells. Such therapies would attempt to increase cell death after androgen withdrawal above 2 to 3 logarithms by inhibiting compensatory adaptive mechanisms. If obliteration of all stem cells by enhancement of the apoptotic process is not possible, then therapies can be directed at inhibition or downregulation of growth regulatory pathways through intermittent androgen suppression (IAS), gene therapy, or adjuvant administration of agents capable of inducing stem cell differentiation.

If AI progression does result from adaptive cell survival mechanisms in response to androgen withdrawal with upregulation of alternative growth regulatory pathways, then reexposure or application of low levels of androgens may prevent or downregulate these mechanisms. This concept was proposed by Dr. Noble 20 years ago for the Nb rat model. He stated, "A reduction in hormone levels sufficient to prevent advancing tumor growth, but adequate to reduce the extent of regression, could possibly reduce the frequency or prevent the development of autonomous change."[24] More recent studies of the Shionogi and LNCaP tumor models lend support to this concept by demonstrating that IAS delays the time to AI progression threefold.[50,56] The parent AD Shionogi's tumor was transplanted into a succession of male mice, each of which was castrated after the estimated tumor weight became about 3 g. After the tumor had regressed to 30% of the original weight, it was transplanted into another intact male. This cycle of transplantation and castration-induced apoptosis was repeated successfully three times before AI progression occurred during the fourth cycle. The time to AI progression with IAS was about 150 days, threefold longer than in controls treated with continuous androgen suppression (CAS).[50] Similarly, in LNCaP tumors, 4 to 5 cycles of IAS were achieved before development of progression, and IAS delayed the time to AI progression threefold (26 versus 77 days). Serum PSA levels remained below precastration levels after 60 days in 75% of the IAS group but exceeded precastration levels after 28 days in 100% of the CAS group. By 15 weeks after castration, PSA levels in the CAS group had increased sevenfold above precastration levels, compared with a 1.9-fold increase in the IAS therapy group.[56] The success of IAS in these animal models suggests that delay of AI progression may be possible through androgen-induced differentiation of stem cells or downregulation of androgen-repressed growth regulatory pathways, or both.

HUMAN PROSTATE CANCER MODELS

Androgen-Independent Cell Lines

PC-3[57] and DU-145[58] are two commonly used human prostate cancer cell lines. The PC-3 cell line was established from a vertebral metastasis taken at warm autopsy from a 62-year-old man with AI disease. The DU-145 cell line was derived from a brain metastasis of a 60-year-old man taken 3 weeks after estrogen therapy was initiated. Less well known cell lines include EB-33,[59] PC-93,[60] and TSU-PR1.[61] All of these cell lines are easily maintained in vitro and produce poorly differentiated carcinomas if inoculated subcutaneously into athymic mice. None of the cell lines responds to androgens; all lack androgen receptors (except possibly PC-93), 5α-reductase, and PSA. Prostatic acid phosphatase is produced in small amounts by DU-145.[62] Because these cell lines lack prostate-specific features, extrapolation of experimentally derived information back to the clinical situation is limited.

Various models have been established to study the metastatic patterns of PC-3 cells.[63–65] Osseous metastases occur after intravenous injection with inferior vena caval occlusion in both the PC-3[64] and Dunning[66] models, supporting the hypothesis by Batson that prostate cancer cells selectively spread to the axial skeleton by means of a paravertebral venous plexus.[67] Lymph node metastases are commonly observed after orthotopic injection of PC-3 cells but are less common with subcutaneous injection.[65] Also, various PC-3 cell sublines have been isolated and partially characterized that preferentially metastasize to selected organs in mice with severe combined immunodeficiency disease (SCID mice) after intravenous inoculation.[63,68]

LNCaP TUMOR MODEL

The LNCaP cell line was established from a metastatic supraclavicular lymph node of a 50-year-old man treated for 6 months with estrogen and 1 month with methyl CCNU and estramustine.[69] This is a useful and important cell line because it is the only established human prostate cell line with functional androgen receptors and PSA expression. Horoszewicz and associates reported that subcutaneous inoculation of 1×10^7 LNCaP cells in athymic mice produced a nonmetastasizing adenocarcinoma that grew progressively and resulted in death after 4 months.[69] However, other laboratories, using later passages, were unsuccessful in inducing LNCaP tumor growth with subcutaneous inoculation. The low tumorigenicity of LNCaP cells allows investigation of tumor-stromal cell interactions by study of the inductive properties of different tissue-specific fibroblasts. The LNCaP tumor model is also valuable in the investigation of PSA pharmacokinetics, androgen-regulated gene expression, and mechanisms of AI progression.

Tumor-Stromal Cell Interactions

Using a cell-cell recombination technique, Gleave and colleagues observed that tissue-specific mesenchymal or stromal cells were potent inducers capable of stimulating LNCaP tumor growth in vivo.[70] Coinoculation of 1×10^6 LNCaP cells with various organ-specific fibroblasts demonstrated that both prostate and bone, but not lung or kidney, stromal cells were capable of inducing LNCaP tumor growth in vivo. The induced human prostate LNCaP tumors are poorly differentiated adenocarcinomas that secrete PSA. The critical importance of organ-specific mesenchymal cells in the regulation of prostate tumor cell growth is further supported by the observation that LNCaP cells form PSA-secreting prostate tumors if injected directly into the host dorsal prostate gland of athymic mice but not if injected beneath the renal capsule or subcutaneously, even in higher doses.[71] These results suggest that normal prostate stromal cells are also capable of inducing LNCaP tumors in situ. Stephenson and colleagues demonstrated enhanced growth of PC-3M and LNCaP cells after intraprostatic injection, compared with ectopic implantation, and found that orthotopic injection increases the metastatic potential of these cell lines.[65] These observations illustrate the importance of tumor-stromal cell interaction in prostate cancer growth and suggest that extracellular matrix and paracrine-mediated growth factors play a role in prostate cancer growth and site-specific metastasis.[72]

LNCaP cell growth rates in vitro are stimulated by low levels of testosterone and by various autocrine and paracrine growth factors.[70,73,74] Androgens may regulate cell growth by stimulating the production of autocrine growth factors; androgens upregulate EGF receptor expression in LNCaP cells, which binds EGF and TGF-α,[53,73] and androgens stimulate production of a bFGF-like factor in Shionogi tumor cells.[52,75] LNCaP cells express bFGF, EGF, and TGF-α, all of which are stimulatory both in vitro and in vivo,[71] but none of these potential autocrine growth factors has been shown to be directly regulated by androgen. LNCaP cell growth is also stimulated by paracrine growth factors produced by tissue-specific fibroblasts, most notably bone and prostate stromal cells. Bone stromal cells produce bFGF, and it is possible that bFGF and other growth factors act in a paracrine fashion to stimulate metastatic cancer cell growth and influence the pattern of site-specific metastasis that is characteristic of prostate cancer.[54,70–72]

Pharmacokinetics of Prostate-Specific Antigen

Because of its unique ability to produce PSA both in vivo and in vitro, the LNCaP tumor model serves as a novel and powerful tool to define aspects of the regulation of PSA. PSA production by LNCaP cells in vitro and in vivo is regulated by androgens and by various growth factors.[76,77] The promoter region of the PSA gene contains a functional androgen response element, and it is one of several genes identified thus far that are directly regulated by androgen.[78] PSA synthesis is stimulated by vitamin D,[79] and phorbol esters downregulate the androgen induction of PSA.[80] EGF and FGF may decrease the production of PSA, and both EGF and TGF-α can interfere with the androgen regulation of PSA.[77,81]

The fact that PSA is a proteolytic enzyme raises the possibility that it is either directly or indirectly active in stimulating the growth of prostate cancer and is not just a passive marker of tumor cell activity. The proteolytic activity of PSA reduces the affinity of insulin-like growth factor (IGF) for IGF-binding protein-3 and increases the availability of mitogenic IGF.[82] Also, PSA itself may increase the growth of primary tissue cultures of prostatic epithelial cells.[82] However, other in vitro experiments have failed to demonstrate a correlation between expression of PSA mRNA and tumor cell growth rates.[77] In addition, the human prostate cancer cell lines PC-3 and DU-145, which do not produce PSA, are more tumorigenic and more invasive than the PSA-producing LNCaP cell line. Such conflicting evidence makes it unclear whether PSA has an active biologic role in promoting the growth or progression of prostate cancer.

The LNCaP tumor model system provides accurate correlation between tumor volume and serum PSA level in vivo.[77] Both androgens and tumor volume are important codeterminants of circulating PSA level. Serum PSA increases by 0.24 ng/mL per cubic millimeter of tumor, which is approximately five times less than the increase estimated for humans. This lower PSA density (i.e., reduced ratio of PSA to tumor volume) probably results from a sevenfold faster clearance of PSA in athymic mice than in humans; other than this shorter halflife, PSA elimination in the murine model appears to be similar to elimination in humans, with both systems following the first-order kinetics characteristic of a two-compartment model.[83]

Immediately after castration, the serum PSA level rapidly decreases by 80%, and it increases up to 20-fold after androgen supplementation; these changes in serum PSA occur without castration-induced tumor cell death or concomitant changes in tumor volume and reflect changes in androgen-regulated PSA gene expression. Despite decreasing by 80% after castration, the expression of mRNA PSA in LNCaP tumor cells gradually returns to precastration levels in the absence of testicular androgens, in as soon as 4 weeks after castration, heralding the onset of AI PSA gene regulation.[55,77,82]

Androgen-Independent Progression

Increases in serum PSA after androgen ablation therapy are the earliest sign of AI prostate cancer progression and are also associated with reduced survival time.[84] The LNCaP tumor model has also been used to determine whether changes in serum PSA after castration can predict the duration of time to AI progression.[85] Although time to AI progression is variable, ranging from 14 to more than 100 days (mean, 28 days), progression invariably occurs. Neither precastration PSA level, nor precastration tumor volume, nor earlier versus later castration predicts the time to AI progression. PSA nadir does not predict the time to progression; low precastration levels reach low nadirs, but time to progression is not prolonged. The PSA nadir fraction, defined as the percent decrease in PSA after castration, is the only factor identified that directly correlates with time to progression ($r = 0.905$). Time to AI progression ranges from 14 days with a PSA nadir fraction of 1.2 to 90 days with a PSA nadir faction of 19.8. LNCaP tumor volume stabilizes but does not decrease after castration; hence, higher PSA nadir fractions may reflect more diffuse decreases in PSA production in more intrinsically androgen-sensitive tumors. These observations suggest that the PSA nadir fraction may be useful to identify good and poor responders to androgen ablation therapy.

The apparent transition from the AD to the AI state after castration in the LNCaP model permits rapid assessment of the molecular events that mediate or accompany this transition as well as evaluation of therapeutic agents capable of delaying it. Studies suggest that escape from AD PSA production occurs and that LNCaP cells may adapt to an androgen-deprived environment through the upregulation of alternative nonandrogenic pathways of signal transduction.[55,85,86] To permit more detailed mechanistic studies, LNCaP tumors grown in castrated mice that had progressed to the AI state were cultured to obtain cell lines.[87] A cell line was obtained from a tumor-bearing animal 4 weeks after castration and termed the C-4 LNCaP cell subline. The spontaneous recovery of PSA synthesis in AI LNCaP cells appears to be an acquired stable phenotype, because the C-4 LNCaP cell line continues to overexpress PSA in the absence of androgen stimulation. Furthermore, if the conditioned medium of the C-4 LNCaP cell line is incubated with parental LNCaP cells, PSA production in the parental LNCaP cell line is stimulated fourfold. These observations suggest that AI C-4 LNCaP cells produce a soluble, nonandrogenic factor that stimulates PSA production in an autocrine fashion and is probably partly responsible for increases in PSA with AI progression. Production of this factor may represent an adaptive response to changes in the tumor cells' hormonal milieu. Further characterization of AI LNCaP cell lines has produced a subline (C4-2) that metastasizes to lymph nodes and bone after subcutaneous or orthotopic inoculation.[86,88] The incidence of osseous metastases appears to be higher in castrated than in intact male hosts, suggesting that CAS may facilitate development of osseous metastases.

The molecular basis for the increased production of PSA in the AI state has received little attention. Although factors that down-regulate PSA production have been identified, nonandrogenic factors that increase PSA production during AI progression have not been characterized. How prostate cancer cells regain their ability to synthesize PSA in quantities similar to precastration levels in the absence of androgens is unknown, yet it can be safely assumed that greater understanding of this process is necessary before strategies for delaying or averting AI progression can be developed.

The AI progression of PSA production occurs without castration-induced cell death and suggests that subpopulations of LNCaP cells adapt to an androgen-depleted environment through the upregulation of various androgen-repressed genes. Observations from the Shionogi and LNCaP tumor models suggest that AI tumor recurrences represent an altered state of differentiation, one better adapted to survive in a hostile (i.e., androgen-depleted) environment (Fig. 35-1). AI progression may involve induction of a new, resistant phenotype that develops from previously rare AD stem cells scattered throughout the tumor and expansion of these stem cells to form an AI tumor. The adaptive process is scattered and constitutive, rather than diffuse and readily reversible. Hence, clonal expansion of stem cells may represent a normal physiologic response in abnormal (malignant) cells that is genetically programmed and precipitated or directed by epigenetic factors. This process occurs in benign tissues in other organs and has been termed *clonal constitutive adaptation* by Farber with respect to toxin-induced hepatocyte regeneration.[89] Such a process suggests the possibility that androgen resistance may be a primary but quiescent property of some prostate cancer cells that is activated in response to androgen withdrawal. Intermittent re-exposure to androgens may delay or suppress the activation of molecular processes that lead to development of the AI[50,56] and metastatic[88] phenotype.

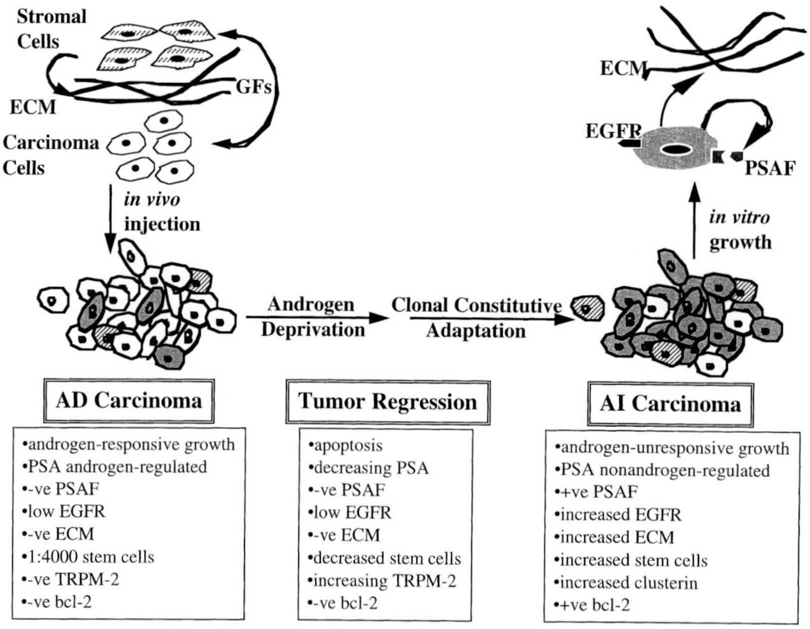

FIG. 35-1. Schematic representation of prostate cancer growth and hormone-independent progression in LNCaP and Shionogi models. Androgen-dependent (AD) carcinoma growth is regulated by genetic and epigenetic factors mediated by autocrine and paracrine growth factors (GFs), extracellular matrix (ECM), and androgens. Serum prostate-specific antigen (PSA) levels are proportional to tumor volume and are androgen regulated. Androgen deprivation results in apoptosis and tumor regression with dramatic decreases in stem cell population and PSA production and upregulation of expression of *TRPM2* and other androgen-repressed genes. With continuous androgen deprivation, adaptive changes within scattered subpopulations of stem cells lead to clonal expansion of resistant cells, characterized by androgen-independent (AI) growth and PSA production and by constitutive expression of epidermal growth factor receptor (EGFR), clusterin, ECM, and BCL2. Increases in PSA with AI progression may be partly mediated by production of PSA autocrine factor (PSAF) by AI cells. −ve, negative; +ve, positive.

Human Xenograft Models

Xenograft models rely on successful establishment and continued growth of heterotransplanted human neoplastic tissue into immunodeficient (i.e., athymic or SCID) mice. Reports documenting improved tumor growth after coinoculation with Matrigel or other artificial matrices[71,90,91] will probably lead to increasing numbers of human xenografts.

The PC-82 tumor model was the first transplantable human prostate carcinoma reported in the literature. It was initiated in 1977 by, and has since been well characterized by, investigators at Erasmus University in Rotterdam.[92] PC-82 tumors are moderately differentiated carcinomas with cribriform patterns similar to those of the original primary tumor. Subcutaneous xenografts grow relatively slowly (doubling time, >10 days), are dependent on the presence of testicular androgens, and produce prostatic acid phosphatase and PSA. After castration, tumor cell apoptosis occurs, and PC-82 tumors regress slowly; AI tumor progression does not occur in this model. However, tumor growth rates can be stimulated by administration of exogenous androgen. The PC-82 model is very useful for studying the mechanisms of androgen-regulated tumor cell growth,[93] apoptosis,[94,95] and androgen receptor regulation.[96] A second AD xenograft, denoted PC-EW, was also established in Rotterdam and shares some characteristics with PC-82.[95,97] Several more AD and also AI human prostate tumor xenografts have been established by this group and are currently being characterized biochemically to provide insights into apoptosis and AI progression.[98]

To test whether maximal androgen blockade is more effective therapy than castration alone, van Weerden and colleagues studied the effects of various levels of androgens on PC-82 tumor growth to determine whether low residual androgens after castration are capable of stimulating tumor growth.[48,99] In contrast to human adrenal glands, murine glands do not synthesize androgens, and castration in mice can therefore be regarded as maximal androgen blockade.[100] These investigators demonstrated that PC-82 (and PC-EW) tumors have an androgen threshold level for growth stimulation that is two to three times above the level produced after castration, suggesting that maximal androgen blockade is not needed to induce maximal regression of these tumors. PC-82 tumors were not stimulated by physiologic concentrations of dehydroepiandrosterone; however, administration of androstenedione prevented maximal PC-82 tumor involution after castration, primarily because of peripheral conversion of androstenedione to testosterone.[48] The authors concluded that normal levels of adrenal androgens do not induce growth of PC-82 tumors after castration; this contrasts with the findings of Schiller and associates using the Dunning R-3327 model.[101] As in humans, the importance of adrenal androgens in prostate tumor growth and progression in animal models remains debatable and contradictory.

The Honda xenograft tumor model was established in Gunma, Japan, from testicular metastatic deposits after orchiectomy of a 46-year-old man who had been treated with estrogens for 2 years.[102] Tumors are poorly differentiated carcinomas grown subcutaneously in athymic mice; no immortalized in vitro cell line has been established. The tumors are AD, involute after castration, produce PSA and prostatic acid phosphatase, and contain androgen receptors.[103] AI progression has not been reported, which limits the usefulness of this model for the study of this process.

The LuCaP xenograft model has recently been established at the University of Washington and is being characterized by Ellis and colleagues.[104] Tumors are poorly differentiated adenocarcinomas that produce PSA and contain androgen receptors and 5α-reductase type 1; growth rates are androgen sensitive, and tumors partially regress after castration.

TRANSGENIC MODELS

The rodent and human prostate cancer models reviewed in this chapter have provided valuable understanding of the tumor cell and molecular biology of human prostate cancer. However, because naturally occurring prostate cancer in nonhuman animal species is rare, animal models have not provided appropriate systems for study of the molecular mechanisms related to early development and progression of human prostate cancer. Transgenic animal models provide a potential basis for testing biologic effects of various oncogenes, tumor suppressor genes, and growth factor genes to evaluate the processes of initiation and promotion of prostate cancer. Transgenic technology offers a new generation of animal models that promise insight into key genetic events in progression and new methods of therapy. The temporal sequence of molecular and cellular interactions during the early stages of prostate carcinogenesis can be studied in reproducible fashion with the use of these model systems.

Transgenic Mouse Models

The most common approach to transgenic models involves direct alteration of gene expression within the prostate of an intact developing transgenic animal. Recent advances in molecular biology have enabled direct incorporation of exogenous transgenes into the mouse germline, with subsequent propagation of stable transgenic mouse lines. If the gene encodes for an oncogenic protein, tumors may develop in any organ in which the transgene is expressed. Tissue specificity of transgene expression is determined by the presence of tissue-specific transcription factors (e.g., steroid receptor plus ligand) that bind to and activate a corresponding *cis*-acting DNA promoter element on the transgene (e.g., androgen response element). The *cis*-acting DNA promotor element is the most important determinant for tissue-specific transgenic targeting. Through recombinant DNA technology, it is possible to genetically fuse tissue-specific DNA promotor elements with various oncogenes to create chimeric transgenes that allow targeted expression of the oncoprotein to a specific organ.

The targeted expression of growth factors and oncogenes to the prostate has produced both benign and malignant prostatic conditions. With the use of a recombinant mouse mammary tumor virus promotor element fused to the *INT2* gene, a member of the fibroblast growth factor family, transgenic mice developed benign hyperplastic prostatic epithelial growth; this illustrates the importance of fibroblast growth factors in the pathogenesis of benign prostatic hyperplasia.[105] In another transgenic mouse line, introduction of TGF-α cDNA under transcriptional regulation of an inducible metallothioneine-1 enhancer promoter produced prostate epithelial hyperplasia and focal dysplastic changes resembling carcinoma in situ.[106] This induction of dysplasia by TGF-α overexpression, along with high expression of TGF-α mRNA in human prostate cancer cell lines,[53,54] suggests that TGF-α may be involved in pathogenesis and progression of prostate cancer.

A transgenic animal model that uses a prostate-specific transgene expression system based on the regulatory elements of the rat probasin (*RPB*) gene targets heterologous genes specifically to the prostate in transgenic mice.[107] The rPB promoter appears to be unique in its ability to specifically target developmentally and hormonally regulated expression of heterologous genes in the prostates of transgenic mice. Recently, Dr. N.M. Greenberg at Baylor College of Medicine in Houston has generated lines of transgenic mice that develop prostatic epithelial hyperplasia and adenocarcinoma using a rPB promoter–SV40 T antigen fusion transgene (personal communication, 1994). Expression of tumor antigen is restricted to the prostatic epithelium, and those lines of mice expressing higher levels of the transgene developed adenocarcinomas histologically similar to those seen in human disease. The ability to induce prostate cancer in a transgenic mouse as a consequence of specifically targeted oncogene expression provides a novel animal model system to evaluate genetic events in prostate carcinogenesis and prostate cancer gene therapy strategies. Transmission of the oncogenic transgene to progeny may lead to development of lines of mice with high incidence of spontaneously occurring prostate cancers that will permit larger-scale studies of the early events of carcinogenesis and experimental therapeutics.

Transgenic Gland Models

Accumulating data from many laboratories indicate that cancer progression is not merely determined by the cancer cell itself but is also influenced by the surrounding microenvironment.[70,108,109] Future investigations regarding the molecular mechanisms associated with the initiation and progression of prostate cancer must consider both the somatic mutation (genetic alteration) and the paracrine interaction between different cell types (epigenetic alteration). Thompson and colleagues[110] developed a mouse prostate reconstitution (MPR) model that exploits the ability of fetal urogenital sinus (UGS) to form a mature prostate gland if it is transplanted into the renal subcapsular space of adult mice.[111] The MPR model allows further study of paracrine interactions between cell compartments by introduction of candidate genes of various growth factors, oncogenes, and suppressor genes into either epithelial or fibroblast compartments derived from the fetal prostate gland. After isolation from 16-day-old fetal mice, fetal prostate UGS can be separated into urogenital mesenchyme (UGM) and urogenital epithelium (UGE). If the UGM and UGE are recombined and grafted under the renal subcapsule of syngeneic male mice, the grafts are capable of undergoing morphogenesis and differentiation into mature prostate.

The introduction of candidate genes into separate stromal and

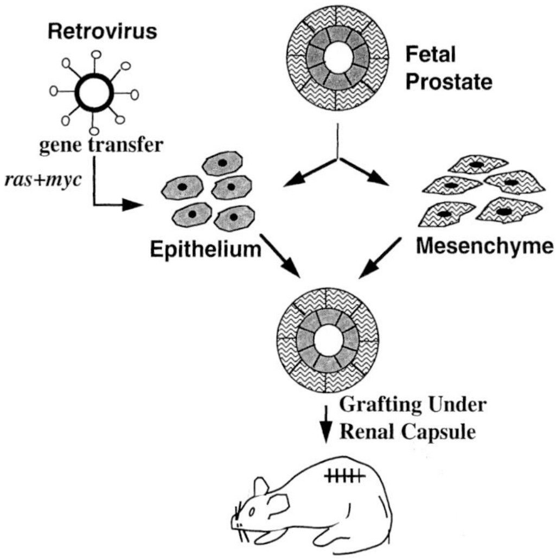

FIG. 35-2. Schematic representation of mouse prostate reconstitution model. Fetal prostate gland is separated into urogenital epithelial (UGE) and mesenchymal (UGM) cells. Separated compartments can then be genetically manipulated with candidate genes to analyze the effects of paracrine interaction between abnormal epithelial and mesenchymal compartments. If UGE is transfected with *RAS* + *MYC* oncogenes through infection with replication-defective retrovirus and then recombined with normal UGM, focal hyperplasia develops in 88% of reconstituted mouse prostates and carcinoma in 20%. In contrast, if UGM is infected with *RAS* + *MYC* oncogenes and then recombined with normal UGE, stromal dysplasia develops. (Modified from Thompson TC, Southgate J, Kitchener, Land H. Multistage carcinogenesis induced by ras and myc oncogenes in a reconstituted organ. Cell 1989;56:917, with permission.)

epithelial compartments with subsequent reconstitution provides a unique tool for the study of paracrine interactions between these two compartments and their roles in benign or malignant prostatic epithelial cell growth (Fig. 35-2). With the use of retrovirus-mediated transfer of *HRAS* and *MYC* genes into dissociated fetal UGS, the reconstituted prostate is prone to the development of dysplasia (*RAS* alone), focal epithelial hyperplasia (*MYC* alone), or adenocarcinoma (*RAS* + *MYC*).[110] In further studies, UGE and UGM cells were separated from UGS and infected with oncogenic virus to analyze the effects of paracrine interaction between abnormal epithelial and mesenchymal compartments. After *RAS* + *MYC*-infected UGE was combined with normal UGM, 88% of reconstituted mouse prostates developed focal hyperplasia and 20% developed carcinomas within 4 weeks.[112] After 8 weeks, however, more than 80% developed carcinomas.[113] In contrast, if only UGM was infected with *RAS* + *MYC*-carrying viruses, stromal dysplasia developed in all cases. These data suggest that the site of genetic alteration and subsequent paracrine interactions between epithelial and mesenchymal compartments plays a critical role in prostate tumorigenesis. Tumor suppressor *P53* gene mutation was detected in *RAS*-induced hyperplastic epithelial cells; in contrast, no *P53* mutation was detected in *RAS* + *MYC*-induced carcinoma cells, and tumor growth was not inhibited by transfection with wild-type human *P53* plasmid.[114] These data suggest that the presence of activated *RAS* and *MYC* may allow neoplastic cells to bypass *P53* suppression. Additional studies using the MPR model demonstrated that TGF-β is elevated in all carcinomas examined, which suggests that TGF-β may play an important role in mediation of paracrine interaction during prostate tumorigenesis.[115] Recombinant retrovirus transduction before organ reconstitution allows direct genetic manipulation of cells in the prostate gland to determine their potential significance in prostatic carcinogenesis.

ACKNOWLEDGMENTS

The authors would like to thank Dr. G.J. van Steenbrugge, Dr. Norman Greenberg, and Dr. Tim Thompson for generously providing information on the PC-82 human xenograft, transgenic mouse, and MPR models, respectively.

REFERENCES

1. Coffey DS, Isaacs JT. Requirement for an idealized animal model of prostatic cancer. Prog Clin Biol Res 1980;37:379.
2. Dunning WF. Prostate cancer in the rat. Monogr Natl Cancer Inst 1963;12:351.
3. Isaacs JT. Development and characteristics of the available animal models for the study of prostate cancer. In: Coffey DS, Bruchovsky N, Gardner WH, et al, eds. Current approaches to the study of prostate cancer. New York: Alan R Liss, 1987:513.
4. Smolev J, Heston WDW, Scott WW, Coffey DS. Characterization of the Dunning R-3327-H prostatic adenocarcinoma: an appropriate animal model for prostatic cancer. Cancer Treat Rep 1977;61:273.
5. Lubaroff DM, Canfield L, Reynolds CW. The Dunning tumors. In: Murphy G, ed. Models for prostate cancer. Prog Clin Biol Res 1980; 37:243.
6. Thompson SA, Johnson MP, Heidger PM Jr, Lubaroff DM. Characterization of the heterogeneity of R3327 rat prostatic tumors derived from single-cell clones. Prostate 1985;6:369.
7. Markland FS, Chopp RT, Cosgrove MD, Howard EB. Characterization of steroid hormone receptors in the Dunning R-3327 rat prostatic adenocarcinoma. Cancer Res 1978;38:2818.
8. Buttyan R, Tomashefsky R, Deitch AD, Olsson CA, deVere White R. Alterations of physical and biochemical parameters of the R-3327-CP rat prostatic adenocarcinoma following hormonal manipulations of the host. J Urol 1984;131:1218.
9. Isaacs JT, Coffey DS. Adaptation versus selection as the mechanism responsible for the relapse of prostatic cancer to androgen ablation therapy as studied in the Dunning R-3327-H adenocarcinoma. Cancer Res 1981;41:5070.
10. Isaacs JT, Wake N, Coffey DS, Sandberg AA. Genetic instability coupled to clonal selection as a mechanism for progression in prostatic cancer. Cancer Res 1982;42:2353.
11. Voigt W, Dunning WF. In vivo metabolism of testosterone-^{3}H in R-3327, an androgen-sensitive rat prostatic adenocarcinoma. Cancer Res 1974;34:1447.
12. Voigt W, Feldman M, Dunning WF. 5α-Dihydrotestosterone–binding proteins and androgen sensitivity in prostatic cancer of Copenhagen rats. Cancer Res 1975;35:1840.
13. Isaacs JT, Isaacs WB, Feitz WFJ, Scheres J. Establishment and characterization of seven Dunning rat prostatic cancer cell lines and their use in developing methods for predicting metastatic abilities of prostatic cancers. Prostate 1986;9:261.
14. Killion JJ, Fidler IJ. The biology of tumor metastasis. Semin Oncol 1989;16:106.
15. Carter HB, Coffey DS. Cell surface charge in predicting metastatic potential of aspirated cells from the Dunning rat prostatic adenocarcinoma model. J Urol 1988;140:173.
16. Carter HB, Partin AW, Coffey DS. Prediction of metastatic potential in an animal model of prostate cancer: flow cytometric quantification of cell surface charge. J Urol 1989;142:1338.

17. Bussemakers MJG, van Moorselar RJA, Giroldi LA, et al. Decreased expression of E-cadherin in the progression of rat prostatic cancer. Cancer Res 1992;52:2916.
18. Mohler JL, Partin AW, Isaacs JT, Coffey DS. Metastatic potential prediction by a visual grading system of cell motility: prospective validation in the Dunning R-3327 prostatic adenocarcinoma model. Cancer Res 1988;48:4312.
19. Partin AW, Schieninger JS, Mohler JL, Coffey DS. Fourier analysis of cell motility: correlation of motility with metastatic potential. Proc Natl Acad Sci U S A 1989;86:1254.
20. Aumuller G, Groschel-Stewart U, Altmannsberger M, Mannherz HG, Steinhoff M. Basal cells of H-Dunning tumor are myoepithelial cells. Biochemistry 1991;95:341.
21. Goebel HW, Rausch U, Steinhoff M, et al. Arguments against the prostatic origin of the R-3327 Dunning H tumor. Virchows Arch B Cell Pathol 1992;62:9.
22. Wunsch A, Rausch U, Seitz J, et al. Tissue-specific transglutaminase expression in the Dunning tumor. Urol Res 1993;21:9.
23. Noble RL, Hoover L. The classification of transplantable tumors in Nb rats controlled by estrogen from dormancy to autonomy. Cancer Res 1975;35:2935.
24. Noble RL. The development of prostatic adenocarcinoma in the Nb rat following prolonged sex hormone administration. Cancer Res 1977;37:1929.
25. Drago JR, Goldman LB, Gershwin ME. Chemotherapeutic and hormonal considerations of the Nb rat prostatic adenocarcinoma model. In: Murphy G, ed. Models for prostate cancer. Prog Clin Biol Res 1980;37:325.
26. Drago JR, Curley RM, Sipio J. Nb rat prostatic adenocarcinoma model: metastasis. Anticancer Res 1985;5:193.
27. Chang SM, Chung LWK. Interaction between prostate fibroblast and epithelial cells in culture: role of androgen. Endocrinology 1989;125: 2719.
28. Chung LWK, Chang SM, Bell C, Zhau HE, Ro JY, von Eschenbach AC. Co-inoculation of tumorigenic rat prostate mesenchymal cells with nontumorigenic epithelial cells results in the development of carcinosarcoma in syngeneic and athymic animals. Int J Cancer 1989; 43:1179.
29. Pollard M. The Pollard tumors. In: Murphy G, ed. Models for prostate cancer. Prog Clin Biol Res 1980;37:293.
30. Pollard M. Spontaneous prostate adenocarcinomas in aged germfree Wistar rats. J Natl Cancer Inst 1973;51:1235.
31. Pollard M, Luckert PH. Animal models and treatment of prostate cancer. Prostate 1984;5:661.
32. Neubauar B, Berris K, Best K, et al. Metastatic spread of the PA-III prostatic adenocarcinoma after implantation in the tail of the rat. Prostate 1986;8:165.
33. Pollard M, Luckert PH, Schmidt MA. Introduction of prostatic adenocarcinomas in Lobund-Wister rats by testosterone. Prostate 1982;3: 563.
34. Pollard M, Luckert P. Prostate cancer in a Sprague-Dawley rat. Prostate 1985;6:389.
35. Cohen MB, Heidger PM, Lubaroff DM. Gross and microscopic pathology of induced prostatic complex tumors arising in Lobund-Wister rats. Cancer Res 1994;54:626.
36. Shain SA, McCullough B, Segaloff A. Spontaneous adenocarcinomas of the ventral prostate of aged AXC rats. J Natl Cancer Inst 1975;55: 177.
37. Isaacs JT. The aging ACI/Seg versus Copenhagen male rats as a model system for the study of prostatic carcinogenesis. Cancer Res 1984; 44:5785.
38. Shain SA, Boesel RW, Kalter SS, Heberling RL. AXC rat prostatic adenocarcinoma: initial characterization of testosterone regulation of hormone receptors of cultured cancer cells and derived tumors. J Natl Cancer Inst 1981;66:565.
39. Minesita T, Yamaguchi K. An androgen-dependent mouse mammary tumor. Cancer Res 1964;25:1168.
40. Bruchovsky N. The metabolism of testosterone and dihydrotestosterone in an androgen-dependent tumor: a possible correlation between dihydrotestosterone and tumor growth in vivo. Biochem J 1972;127: 561.
41. Bruchovsky N, Rennine PS, Coldman AJ, Goldenberg SL, To M, Lawson D. Effects of androgen withdrawal on the stem cell population of the Shionogi carcinoma. Cancer Res 1990;50:2275.
42. Buttyan R, Zakeri Z, Lockshin R, Wolgemuth D. Cascade induction of c-fos, c-myc, and heat shock 70K transcripts during regression of the rat ventral prostate gland. Mol Endocrinol 1988;2:650.
43. Rennie PS, Bruchovsky N, Buttyan R, Benson M, Cheng H. Gene expression during the early phases of regression of the androgen-dependent Shionogi mouse mammary carcinoma. Cancer Res 1988; 48:6309.
44. Kerr JFR, Winterford CR, Harmon BV. Apoptosis: its significance in cancer and cancer therapy. Cancer 1994;73:2013.
45. Monpetit ML, Lawless KR, Tewnniswood M. Androgen-repressed messages in the rat ventral prostate. Prostate 1986;8:25.
46. McDonnell TJ, Troncoso P, Brisbay SM, et al. Expression of the protooncogene bcl-2 in the prostate and its association with emergence of androgen-independent prostate cancer. Cancer Res 1992;52:6940.
47. Sanford NL, Searle JW, Kerr JFR. Successive waves of apoptosis in the rat prostate after repeated withdrawal of testosterone stimulation. Pathology 1984;16:406.
48. van Weerden WM, van Kreuningen A, Elissen NMJ, et al. Effects of adrenal androgens on the transplantable human prostate tumor PC-82. Endocrinology 1992;131:2909.
49. Rennie PS, Bruchovsky N, Coldman AJ. Loss of androgen-dependence is associated with an increase in tumorigenic stem cells and resistance to cell-death genes. J Steroid Biochem Mol Biol 1990;37: 843.
50. Akakura K, Bruchovsky M, Goldenberg SL, Rennie PS, Buckley AR, Sullivan LD. Effects of intermittent androgen suppression on androgen-dependent tumors: apoptosis and serum prostate specific antigen. Cancer 1993;71:2782.
51. French LE, Wohlwend A, Sappino A-P, Tschopp J, Schifferli JA. Human clusterin gene expression is confined to surviving cells during in vitro programmed cell death. J Clin Invest 1994;93:877.
52. Sato N, Watabe Y, Suzuki H, Shimazaki J. Progression of androgen-sensitive mouse tumor (Shionogi carcinoma 115) to androgen-insensitive tumor after long-term removal of testosterone. Jpn J Cancer Res 1993;84:1300.
53. Schuurmans ALG, Bolt J, Mulder E. Androgen receptor-mediated growth and epidermal growth factor receptor induction in human prostate cell line LNCaP. Urol Int 1989;44:71.
54. Chung LW, Li W, Gleave ME, et al. Human prostate cancer model: roles of growth factors and extracellular matrices. J Cell Biochem Suppl 1992;16:99.
55. Wu H-C, Hsieh JT, Gleave ME, Chung LWK. Characterization of growth and differentiation-associated gene activities during the progression of prostate cancer from androgen-responsive to androgen-refractory status. Cancer Res 1992;33:1651. Abstract.
56. Gleave ME, Bruchovsky N, Goldenberg SL, Bowden M, Sullivan LD. Intermittent androgen suppression prolongs time to androgen-independent progression in the LNCaP prostate tumor model. J Urol 1994;151:241. Abstract.
57. Kaighn M, Shakar Narayan K, Ohnuki Y, Lechner J, Jones L. Establishment and characterization of a human prostatic carcinoma cell line (PC-3). Invest Urol 1979;17:16.
58. Mickey D, Stone K, Wunderli H, Mickey G, Vollmer R, Paulson D. Heterotransplantation of a human prostatic adenocarcinoma cell line in nude mice. Cancer Res 1977;37:4049.
59. Okada K, Schoeder FH. Human prostatic carcinoma in cell culture: preliminary report on the development and characterization of an epithelial cell line (EB-33). Urol Res 1974;2:111.
60. Claas FHJ, van Steenburgge GJ. Expression of HLA-like structures on a permanent human tumor line PC-93. Tissue Antigens 1983;21: 227.
61. Iizumi T, Yazaki T, Kanoh S, Kondo I, Koiso K. Establishment of a new prostatic carcinoma cell (TSU-PR1). J Urol 1987;137:1304.
62. Pontes J, Choe B, Rose N, Pierce J. Immunochemical identification of prostatic epithelial cells in culture. Invest Urol 1979;16:483.
63. Wang M, Stearns MM. Isolation and characterization of PC-3 human prostatic tumor sublines which preferentially metastasize to select organs in SCID mice. Differentiation 1991;48:115.
64. Shevrin DH, Kukreja SC, Ghosh L, Lad TE. Development of skeletal metastasis by human prostate cancer in athymic nude mice. Clin Exp Metastasis 1988;6:401.
65. Stephenson RA, Dinney CP, Gohji K, et al. Metastatic model for human prostate cancer using orthotopic implantation in nude mice. J Natl Cancer Inst 1992;84:951.
66. Geldof AA, Rao BR. Factors in prostate cancer metastasis. Anticancer Res 1990;10:1303.
67. Batson OV. The function of the vertebral veins and their role in the spread of metastasis. Ann Surg 1940;112:138.
68. Ware JL, Paulson DF, Mickey GH, Webb KS. Spontaneous metastasis of cells of the human prostate carcinoma cell line PC-3 in athymic nude mice. J Urol 1982;128:1064.
69. Horoszewicz J, Leong S, Chu T, Wajsman Z, et al. The LNCaP cell

line: a new model for studies on human prostatic carcinoma. Prog Clin Biol Res 1980;37:115.
70. Gleave ME, Hsieh JT, Gao CA, von Eschenbach AC, Chung LWK. Acceleration of human prostate cancer growth in vivo by factors produced by prostate and bone fibroblasts. Cancer Res 1991;51:3753.
71. Gleave ME, Hsieh JT, von Eschenbach AC, Chung LWK. Prostate and bone fibroblasts induce human prostate cancer growth in vivo: implications for bidirectional stromal-epithelial interaction in prostate carcinoma growth and metastasis. J Urol 1992;147:1151.
72. Chung LWK, Gleave ME, Hsieh JT, Hong SJ, Zhau HE. Reciprocal mesenchymal-epithelial interaction affecting prostate cancer growth and hormonal responsiveness. Cancer Surv 1991;11:91.
73. Schuurmans ALG, Bolt J, Mulder E. Androgens stimulate both growth rate and epidermal growth factor receptor activity of the human prostate tumor cell LNCaP. Prostate 1988;12:55.
74. Wilding G, Valverius E, Knabbe C, Gelmann EP. Role of transforming growth factor-alpha in human prostate cancer cell growth. Prostate 1989;15:1.
75. Sato B, Kouhara H, Koga M, et al. Androgen-induced growth factor and its receptor: demonstration of the androgen-induced autocrine loop in mouse mammary carcinoma cells. J Steroid Biochem Mol Biol 1993;47:91.
76. Young CY-F, Andrews PE, Montgomery BT, Tindall DJ. Tissue-specific and hormonal regulation of human prostate-specific glandular kallikrein. Biochemistry 1992;31:818.
77. Gleave ME, Hsieh JT, Wu H-C, et al. Serum PSA levels in mice bearing human prostate LNCaP tumors are determined by tumor volume and endocrine and growth factors. Cancer Res 1992;52:1598.
78. Riegman PHJ, Vlietstra RJ, van der Korput JAGM, Brinkmann AO, Trapman J. The promoter of the prostate-specific antigen gene contains a functional androgen responsive element. Mol Endocrinol 1991; 5:1921.
79. Miller GJ, Stapleton GE, Ferrara JA, et al. The human prostatic carcinoma cell line LNCaP expresses biologically active, specific receptors for 1, 25-dihydroxyvitamin D_3. Cancer Res 1992;52:515.
80. Andrews PE, Young CY-F, Montgomery BT, Tindall DJ. Tumor-promoting phorbol ester down-regulates the androgen induction of prostate-specific antigen in a human prostatic adenocarcinoma cell line. Cancer Res 1992;52:1525.
81. Henttu P, Liao S, Vihko P. Androgens up-regulate the human prostate-specific antigen messenger ribonucleic acid (mRNA), but down-regulate the prostatic acid phosphatase mRNA in the LNCaP cell line. Endocrinology 1992;130:766.
82. Cohen P, Graves HCB, Peehl DM, Kamarei M, Giudice LC, Rosenfeld RG. Prostate-specific antigen (PSA) is an insulin-like growth factor binding protein-3 protease found in seminal plasma. J Clin Endocrinol Metab 1992;75:1046.
83. Gleave ME, Hsieh JT, Wu H-C, von Eschenbach AC, Chung LWK. Evaluation of the pharmacokinetics of PSA using the LNCaP tumor model. J Urol 1992;147:386. Abstract.
84. Miller JI, Ahmann FR, Drach GW, Emerson SS, Bottaccini MR. The clinical usefulness of serum prostate specific antigen after hormonal therapy of metastatic prostate cancer. J Urol 1992;147:956.
85. Gleave ME, Bowden M, Bruchovsky N, Goldenberg SL, Sullivan LD. Predictors of time to androgen-independent progression in the LNCaP prostate tumor model. J Urol 1994;151:458A. Abstract.
86. Wu H-C, Hsieh JT, Gleave ME, et al. Derivation of androgen-independent human LNCaP prostate cancer sublines: role of bone stromal cells. Int J Cancer 1994;57:406.
87. Hsieh JT, Wu H-C, Gleave ME, et al. Autocrine regulation of PSA gene expression in a human prostatic cancer (LNCaP) subline. Cancer Res 1993;53:2852.
88. Thalmann GN, Anezinis PE, Chang SH, et al. Androgen-independent cancer progression and bone metastasis in the LNCaP Model of human prostate cancer. Cancer Res 1994;54:2577.
89. Farber E. Clonal adaptation during carcinogenesis. Biochem Pharmacol 1990;39:1837.
90. Thiede K, Momburg F, Zangemeister U, Schlag P, Schirrmacher V. Growth and metastasis of human tumors in nude mice following tumor-cell inoculation into a vascularized polyurethane sponge matrix. Int J Cancer 1988;42:939.
91. Pretlow TG, Delmoro CM, Dilley GG, Spadafora CG, Pretlow TP. Transplantation of human prostatic carcinoma into nude mice in Matrigel. Cancer Res 1991;51:3814.
92. Hoehn W, Schroeder F, Riemann J, Joebsis A, Hermanek P. Human prostatic adenocarcinoma: some characteristics of a serially transplantable line in nude mice (PC-82). Prostate 1980;1:95.
93. Van Steenbrugge G, Groen M, Romijn J, Schroeder F. Biological effects of hormonal treatment regimens on a transplantable human prostatic tumor line (PC-82). J Urol 1984;131:812.
94. Kyprianou N, English HF, Isaacs JT. Programmed cell death during regression of PC-82 human prostate cancer following androgen ablation. Cancer Res 1990;50:3748.
95. van Weerden WM, van Kreuningen A, Elissen NMJ, et al. Castration induced changes in morphology, androgen levels, and proliferation activity of human prostate tissue grown in athymic nude mice. Prostate 1993;23:149.
96. Ruizeveld de Winter JA, van Weerden WM, Faber PW, et al. Regulation of androgen receptor expression in the human heterotransplantable prostate carcinoma PC-82. Endocrinology 1992;131:3045.
97. Hoehn W, Wagner M, Riemann J, et al. Prostatic adenocarcinoma PC-EW: a new human tumor line transplantable in nude mice. Prostate 1984;5:445.
98. Van Steenbrugge G, van Weerden WM, de Ridder CMA, et al. Development and application of prostatic xenograft models for the study of human prostate cancer. In: Motta M, Serio M, eds. Sex hormones and antihormones in endocrine dependent pathology: basic and clinical aspects. 1994:1.
99. van Weerden WM, Van Steenbrugge GJ, Van Kreuningen A, et al. Assessment of the critical level of androgen for growth response of transplantable human prostatic carcinoma (PC-82) in nude mice. J Urol 1991;145:631.
100. van Weerden WM, Bierings GJ, van Steenbrugge GJ, de Jong FH, Schroder FH. Adrenal glands of mouse and rat do not synthesize androgens. Life Sci 1992;50:857.
101. Schiller CD, Schneider MR, Hartmann, et al. Growth-stimulating effect of adrenal androgens on the R3327 Dunning prostatic carcinoma. Urol Res 1991;19:7.
102. Ito Y, Nakazato Y. A new serially transplantable human prostatic cancer (Honda) in nude mice. J Urol 1984;132:384.
103. Ito Y, Mashimo S, Natazato Y, Takikawa H. Hormone dependency of a serially transplantable human prostatic cancer (Honda) in nude mice. Cancer Res 1985;45:5058
104. Ellis WJ, Lange PH, Bigler SA, et al. Characterization of a new prostate cancer xenograft: LuCAP 23. J Urol 1993;150:220. Abstract.
105. Muller WJ, Lee FS, Dickson C, Peters G, Pattengale P, Leder P. The int-2 gene product acts as an epithelial growth factor in transgenic mice. EMBO J 1990;9:907.
106. Sandgren EP, Leutteke NC, Palmiter RD, Brinster RL, Lee DD. Overexpression of TGFa in transgenic mice: induction of epithelial hyperplasia, pancreatic metaplasia, and carcinoma of the breast. Cell 1990; 61:1121.
107. Greenberg NM, DeMayo F, Shepard PC, et al. The rat probascin gene promoter directs hormonally and developmentally regulated expression of a heterologous gene specifically to the prostate in transgenic mice. Mol Endocrinol 1994;8:230.
108. Fukamachi H, Mizuno T, Kim YS. Morphogenesis of human colon cancer cells with fetal rat mesenchymes in organ culture. Experientia 1986;42:312.
109. Hayashi N, Cunha GR, Wong YC. Influence of male genital tract mesenchymes on differentiation of Dunning prostatic adenocarcinoma. Cancer Res 1989;50:4747.
110. Thompson TC, Southgate J, Kitchener G, Land H. Multistage carcinogenesis induced by ras and myc oncogenes in a reconstituted organ. Cell 1989;56:917.
111. Cunha GR, Fujii H, Neubauer BL, Shannon JM, Sawyer L, Reese BA. Epithelial-mesenchymal interactions in prostate development. I. Morphological observations of prostatic induction by urogenital sinus mesenchyme in epithelium of adult rodent urinary bladder. J Cell Biol 1983;96:1662.
112. Merze VW, Miller GJ, Krebs T, et al. Elevated transforming growth factor $\beta 1$ and $\beta 3$ mRNA levels are associated with ras + myc–induced carcinoma in reconstituted mouse prostate: evidence for a paracrine role during progression. Mol Endocrinol 1991;5:503.
113. Slawin K, Kadmon D, Park SH, et al. Dietary fenretinide, a synthetic retinoid, decreases the tumor incidence and the tumor mass of ras + myc–induced carcinomas in the mouse prostate reconstitution model system. Cancer Res 1991;53:4461.
114. Lu X, Park SH, Thompson TC, Lane DP. Ras-induced hyperplasia occurs with mutation of p53, but activated ras and myc together can induce carcinoma without p53 mutation. Cell 1992;70:153.
115. Thompson TC, Truong LD, Timme TL, et al. Transgenic models for the study of prostate cancer. Cancer 1993;71:1165.

Principles and Practice of Genitourinary Oncology, edited by Derek Raghavan, Howard I. Scher, Steven A. Leibel, and Paul H. Lange. Lippincott-Raven Publishers, Philadelphia, © 1997.

CHAPTER 36

Epidemiology and Etiology of Prostate Cancer

Kenneth J. Pienta

Prostate cancer is a major health problem in the United States and is now the most commonly diagnosed cancer in men as well as the second leading cause of male cancer deaths.[1,2] In 1996, there will be an estimated 317,000 new cases of prostate cancer diagnosed and 41,400 deaths from prostate cancer, and these numbers are expected to continue to rise as the population ages.[1–4] The clinical significance that prostate cancer poses today was probably best summarized by Kahler in 1939[5]:

> The morbid anatomist, finding an increasingly higher incidence of clinically undiagnosed tumors of a given organ, is apt to remind the clinician of the need for more accurate study of individual cases. He cannot more than postulate what might have happened had the absence of a lethal lesion permitted the continued growth of the early neoplasm he has discovered. The increasing life expectancy of the human race may eventually raise these tumors from the realm of purely academic to one of vital economic interest, just as increased curiosity has apparently changed the lesion of prostatic carcinoma from one of uncommon occurrence to one of alarmingly increased incidence in the glands of individuals past middle life.

Kahler recognized that the prevalence of prostate cancer increased with age and that as people continued to live longer, the incidence of this disease would increase dramatically. Autopsy study data from around the world demonstrate that 15% to 30% of men older than 50 years of age have histologic evidence of prostate cancer.[6–10] The presence of this histologic or latent cancer increases with age, so that by 80 years of age approximately 60% to 70% of men have evidence of histologic carcinoma at autopsy.[1,6–10] It is now generally accepted that the development of a fully malignant cancer cell requires multiple malignant genetic events.[11,12] If histologic cancer represents a step in the development of clinically evident prostate cancer, then the events that lead to the development of prostate cancer appear to occur at approximately the same rate regardless of race or place of birth of the individual.[1] This concept is best demonstrated by the data of Carter and colleagues, which show that the age-specific prevalence of histologic prostate cancer is similar in Japan and the United States (Fig. 36-1*A*). There is, however, a marked difference in the age-specific prevalence of clinical prostate cancer between Japanese and American men (see Fig. 36-1*B*).[1] In fact, the age-adjusted incidence rates and also the death rates for clinical prostate cancer vary dramatically from country to country, even after adjusting for differences in screening techniques (Fig. 36-2).[6] For example, Waterhouse and colleagues found a 25-fold difference between the incidence rate in Japanese men and that in American black men living in San Francisco.[13] In 1988, the age-adjusted death rates per 100,000 population were 15.7 for men in the United States and 3.5 for men in Japan.[14]

These data suggest that although the initiation rate of prostate cancer may be the same around the world, there are vast differences in the rates of progression to clinically evident prostate cancer. These data are further supported by the observation that migrants who move from low-risk areas to the United States gradually assume the higher risk of the U.S. population.[15–17] Clues to the cause of these promotional events in the multistage carcinogenesis of prostate cancer can be found in epidemiologic studies and are divided into three broad groups: genetic, endogenous, and environmental.

GENETIC FACTORS

Suggestion of a familial, genetic basis for prostate cancer derives from observed clustering of clinical cases within families. However, no consistent chromosomal markers or deletions have been reported.[18–20] In 1960, Woolf, studying familial aggregation in prostate cancer, demonstrated an approximately threefold increase in risk among the first-degree relatives of patients with prostate cancer ($0.02 < P < 0.05$).[21] Steinberg and associates, in a case-controlled study designed to estimate the relative risk (RR) of developing prostate cancer in men with a positive family history, found that 15% of patients with prostate cancer had a father or brother who was also affected, compared with 8% of controls ($P < 0.001$), and there was a trend of increasing risk with increasing number of affected family members.[22] Ghadirian and colleagues showed an eightfold difference in prostate cancer incidence for patients who gave a strong family history compared with population-based controls.[23] Spitz and associates also showed increased risk for men with first-degree relatives with prostate cancer (odds ratio = 2.41). Having a second-degree relative with prostate cancer con-

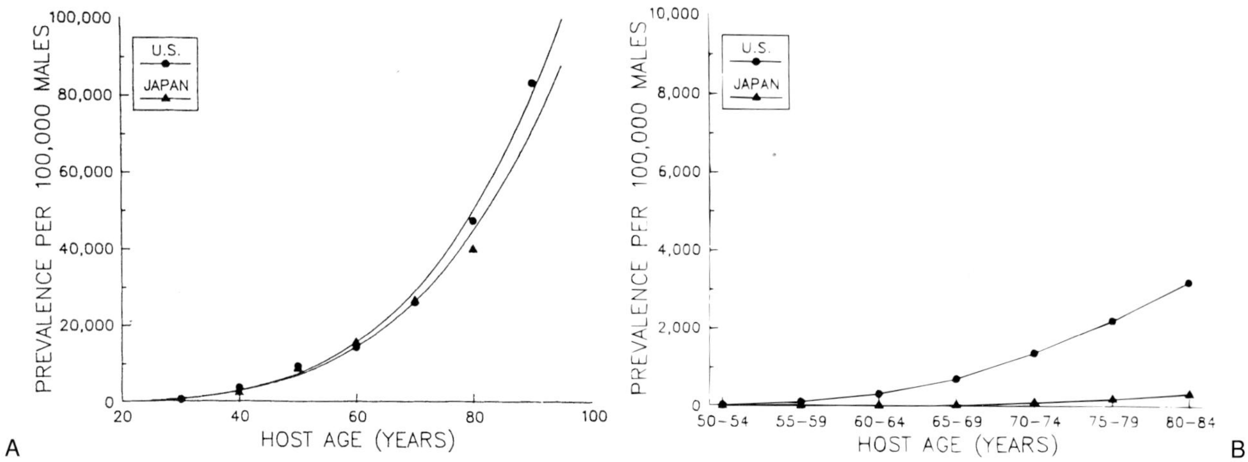

FIG. 36-1. (**A**) Age-specific prevalence of histologic prostate cancer in the United States and Japan. (**B**) Age-specific prevalence of clinical prostate cancer in the United States and Japan. (Carter HB, Piantadosi S, Isaacs JT. Clinical evidence for and implications of the multistep development of prostate cancer. J Urol 1990;143:742.)

ferred elevated risk, but the difference was not statistically significant.[24]

Carter and coworkers reviewed the evidence for familial prostate cancer by complex segregation analysis of 691 affected families and were able to demonstrate that prostate cancer in a subset of families can be explained by mendelian inheritance of a rare autosomal gene that contributes to the development of prostate cancer at an early age.[25] This rare genetic marker appears to have a frequency of 0.003 and a high degree of penetrance (88%) by 85 years of age in both homozygous and heterozygous carriers.[26]

Other investigators have demonstrated an increased risk of prostate cancer along with other malignancies in some families. Tulinius and colleagues, investigating the risk of prostate, ovarian, and endometrial cancers among relatives of patients with breast cancer in Iceland, found that the RR of prostate cancer was significantly raised (1.5) for all relatives.[27] Ghadirian and colleagues reported familial aggregations of cancers of the pancreas, breast, colon, and prostate among French Canadians with a positive family history of prostate cancer; the prevalence was 12.1%, versus 4.1% for controls without a positive family history of prostate cancer, and the difference was statistically significant (RR = 3.3; P = 0.007).[28]

Kirkali and associates studied the association of human leukocyte antigens (HLAs) and the frequency of adenocarcinoma of the prostate in 20 patients and 200 healthy kidney donors.[29]

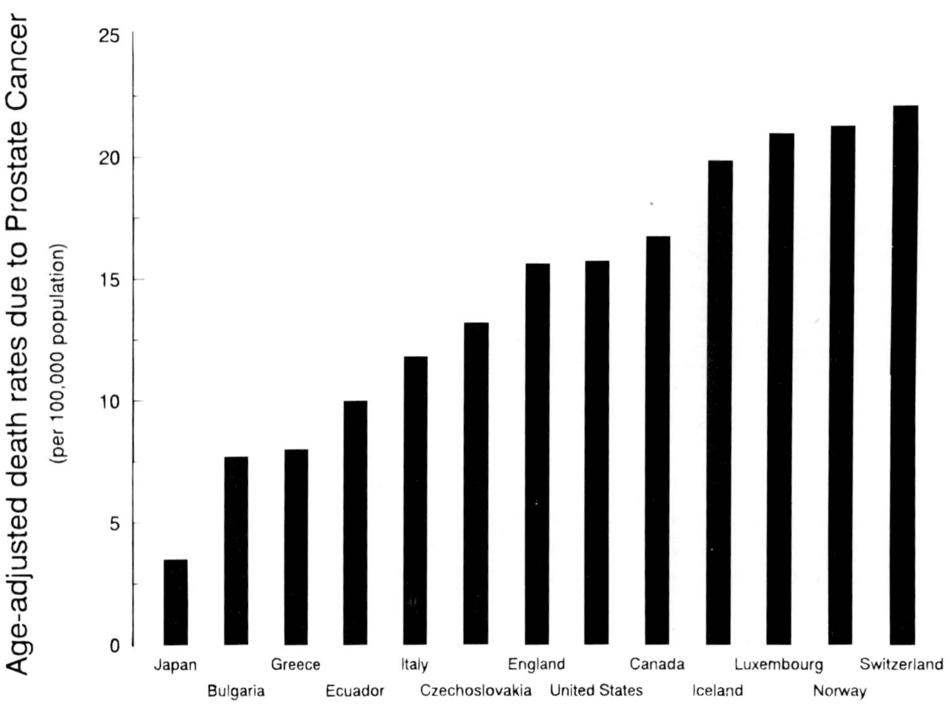

FIG. 36-2. Age-adjusted death rates from prostate cancer per 100,000 population. (Boring CC, Squires TS, Tong T. Cancer statistics, 1992. CA Cancer J Clin 1992;42:19.)

They were able to show that individuals bearing certain HLAs appeared to have a higher incidence of prostate cancer. For example, for HLA-B14 the RR was 7.78 in this study.

It should be noted that in familial aggregation studies, common environmental factors may contribute to development of the same or different cancers among family members. It is very difficult to separate genetic predisposing factors from similar environmental influences.

ENDOGENOUS FACTORS

The endogenous factors that confer increased risk for the development of prostate cancer may result from genetic or environmental predispositions or through complex interactions among genetic and environmental factors.

Age

Prostate cancer has long been associated with advanced age, and there continues to be a steady increase in the incidence and mortality rate of prostate cancer on an age-adjusted basis.[6] The prevalence of both histologic (latent) and clinical prostate cancer increases with age faster than that of any other cancer (Fig. 36-3; see Fig. 36-1). The factors contributing to this disproportionate rise in prostate cancer compared with other solid tumors are completely undefined.

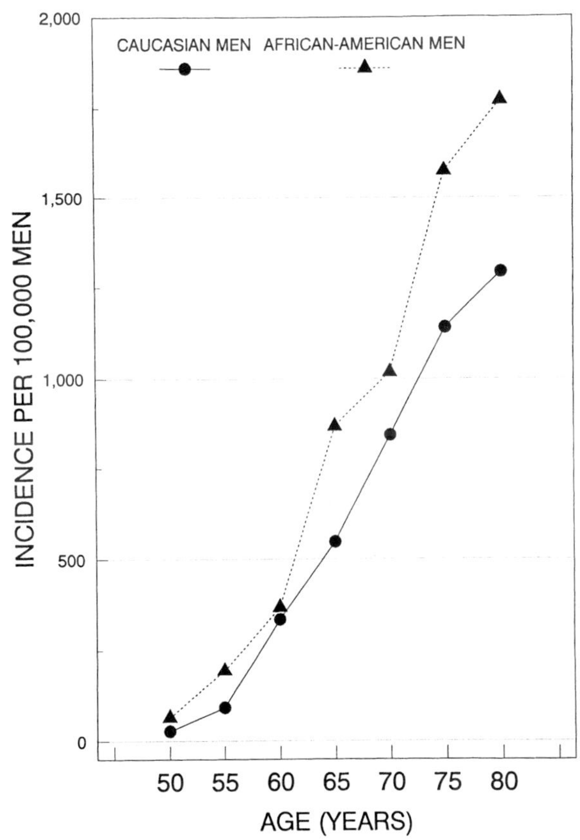

FIG. 36-3. Incidence rates for invasive prostate cancer for metropolitan Detroit tricounty residents, 1989, by age and race, as reported by the Surveillance, Epidemiology, and End Result database. Rates are age-adjusted to the 1970 US standard population. (Pienta KJ, Esper PS. Risk factors for prostate cancer. Ann Intern Med 1993;118:793.)

Race

The difference in prevalence of clinical prostate cancer between men of African, Caucasian, and Asian descent is striking (see Figs. 36-2 and 36-3). Although environmental factors may account for some of these differences, endogenous factors probably also contribute to this phenomenon. Ross and colleagues demonstrated that young African-American men had serum testosterone levels that were approximately 15% higher than those of their white counterparts and have suggested that this difference is enough to explain the increased risk of prostate cancer in African-American men.[30] In a related study comparing American and Japanese men, the same group of investigators found that American men had higher levels of sex hormone–binding globulin than their Japanese counterparts.[31] Furthermore, both African-American and white men in the United States had higher levels of 3-α,17-β-androstenediol glucuronide and androsterone glucuronide. These two androgens are indices of the activity of 5α-reductase, the enzyme in the prostate that converts testosterone to its active metabolite, dihydrotestosterone (DHT). Because DHT is responsible for the mitotic activity of the prostate, this lower enzyme level may contribute to the lower incidence of clinical prostate cancer observed in Japanese men.

The complex interplay between environmental and endogenous factors is demonstrated by studies comparing American and Nigerian blacks. Although the rate of latent carcinoma at autopsy is similar in these populations, American blacks had a higher rate of invasive cancer, and Nigerian men had lower serum levels of testosterone and estradiol.[32] Hill and colleagues found lower levels of urinary androsterone and testosterone but similar urinary androgen levels in black South African men compared with North American black and white men.[33] Black South African men fed a Western diet demonstrated an increased excretion of both androgens and estrogens, whereas the opposite trend was true for black North American men fed a vegetarian diet.

Hormones

Animal studies provide definitive evidence of a role for sex hormones in the development of prostate cancer.[34,35] Short-term treatment of rats with chemical carcinogens produces a low incidence (5% to 15%) of prostate cancer; however, a high incidence of carcinomas can be induced by chronic treatment with testosterone after administration of carcinogens, with testosterone markedly enhancing prostate carcinogenesis even at doses that do not measurably increase circulating testosterone.[36] Despite this data in animals, the precise role of sex hormones in the genesis of human prostate cancer remains largely unknown.

Indirect and direct clinical evidence suggests a role for sex hormones in humans. For example, prostate cancer is rare in androgen-deprived men (e.g., eunuchs, prisoners who have been castrated for sexual offenses). Furthermore, clinical evidence of tumor regression with surgical or medical castration suggests a hormonal dependence for prostate tumors.[37] Epidemiologic studies evaluating the role of sex hormones in prostate cancer have been of three main types: (1) those comparing sex hormone levels in patients at high and low risk; (2) those comparing levels before and at the time of diagnosis in cohort studies; and (3) those comparing hormone levels in patients at the time of diagnosis with levels in control subjects.

Hsing and colleagues, in a population-based study with 13 years of follow-up, found no significant differences in prediagnostic serum levels of testosterone, DHT, prolactin, follicle-stimulating hormone, luteinizing hormone (LH), estrone, or estradiol in patients with prostate cancer compared with control subjects.[38] Elevated levels of LH, DHT, and testosterone were associated with mildly increased risk of prostate cancer. Another study of prediagnostic samples demonstrated lower DHT levels and higher ratios of testosterone to DHT (with no difference in testosterone levels) in 98 patients subsequently found to have prostate cancer, compared with 98 matched controls.[39] Meikle and associates demonstrated higher levels of sex hormone–binding globulin in men with prostate cancer compared with a control group and also noted a higher testosterone conversion rate in patients with prostate cancer.[40] Other investigators have not been able to document consistently the presence of higher levels of testosterone and sex hormone–binding globulin when comparing persons at high risk for prostate cancer with persons considered at lower risk.[41] Barrett-Connor and colleagues, in a prospective population-based study of androstenedione, estrogens, and prostate cancer, concluded that levels of total testosterone, estrone, estradiol, and sex hormone–binding globulin were not related to the development of prostate cancer, but plasma androstenedione showed a positive dose-response gradient.[42] Some studies investigating prolactin levels have shown positive correlations with an increased risk of prostate cancer, but others have not.[43–45]

The enzyme 5α-reductase is responsible for the production of DHT from testosterone, with DHT being responsible for prostatic mitotic activity. Liang and associates studied the serum of patients with prostate cancer for anti–5α-reductase autoantibodies.[46] They were able to show the presence of such antibodies in some patients with prostate cancer.

Although the sex hormones are strongly suspected of playing a role in the development of prostate cancer, the evaluation of that role is compounded by both intrinsic factors (e.g., metabolism, circadian cycle) and extrinsic factors (e.g., diet and environment). It is unclear which sex hormones are most important and whether circulating hormone levels are related to tissue hormone levels.[47] Because normal prostate epithelium requires testosterone to grow, the specific effects of sex hormones on the development of cancer remain undefined.

Benign Prostatic Hyperplasia

Some investigators have shown an elevated risk for prostate cancer among patients with benign prostatic hyperplasia (BPH).[48,49] BPH and prostate cancer commonly coexist with increasing frequency as age increases, and both diseases demonstrate androgen dependency for growth. It therefore becomes difficult to determine whether one process leads to the other and, if so, with what frequency. Virtually all men develop BPH to some extent in their lifetime. BPH is anatomically found in the central or transitional zone of the prostate, and cancer is usually found in the peripheral zone. It has been suggested by some investigators that these two diseases are unrelated, but others believe that BPH is on the multistep pathway to prostate cancer development.

ENVIRONMENTAL FACTORS

The most striking evidence implicating environmental factors as playing a role in the development of prostate cancer comes from migration studies. Japanese immigrants to the United States develop a higher prevalence of clinical prostate cancer than that seen in Japan, one that approaches that of the general American population.[50,51] Shimizu and colleagues, studying three racial and ethnic groups (Spanish-surnamed whites, other whites, and Japanese immigrants to Los Angeles), showed that the rate of prostate cancer in each immigrant group was much higher than in the group's homeland but similar to the rate among U.S.-born persons of the same ethnic heritage, regardless of age at immigration.[15] Similar changes in rates of clinical prostate cancer have been described in studies of Polish and black African immigrants to the United States; however, the causes of these increased rates remain undefined.[52,53]

Dietary Factors

Three main dietary components have been studied extensively with regard to risk of development of prostate cancer: dietary fats, β-carotenes and vitamin A, and other nonfat dietary components. Laboratory studies have shown that n-6 fatty acids stimulate and n-3 fatty acids inhibit human prostate cancer cells in culture.[54] In athymic mice, diets rich in marine oil suppress growth of human prostate cancer cells.[55] Furthermore, international comparisons suggest a relation between the incidence of prostate cancer and dietary fat intake, an inference also supported by migration studies and by the increasing incidence of prostate cancer in Japan, where consumption of animal fats has been increasing.[56] Specifically, Armstrong and Doll found that prostate cancer deaths from 32 countries were highly correlated with total fat consumption, a finding similar to that for breast cancer.[57] Many retrospective studies and a few prospective studies report an association between dietary fat (mainly of animal origin) and prostate cancer, although a few report no association.[58–60] Postulated mechanisms by which fat intake could affect the development of prostate cancer have included altered patterns of production of sex hormones and altered levels of serum and tissue androgens. Another possible mechanism involves the stimulation of prostaglandins by polyunsaturated fatty acids, which interconnect in an autocrine manner with epidermal growth factor–related polypeptides.[61]

Reichman and colleagues reported on the relation between baseline levels of vitamin A and subsequent development of prostate cancer in 2440 men older than 50 years of age. They demonstrated a significantly lower mean level of vitamin A among men who subsequently developed prostate cancer compared with those who did not ($P = 0.01$).[62] Bravo and associates, in a case-controlled study, reported a high association between diets rich in animal fats and risk of prostate cancer, but found no association of low levels of vitamin A or vitamin C with the disease.[63] Hsing and colleagues, investigating the serum retinols, β-carotene, lycopene, and tocopherol (vitamin E), found no association between these factors and the risk of prostate cancer; however, the data did suggest an inverse relation between serum retinol and risk of prostate cancer.[64]

West and associates found little association between prostate cancer and dietary intake of zinc, cadmium, selenium, vitamin C, or β-carotene while demonstrating that dietary fat was a risk factor.[65] Ohno and coworkers found no association between prostate cancer risk and consumption of protein, carbohydrate, water, fiber, ash, retinol, vitamin B_1, vitamin B_2, vitamin C, niacin, calcium, potassium, sodium, phosphorous, or iron.[66] Mills and colleagues, in a cohort study of diet and lifestyle and prostate cancer in 14,000 Adventist men, observed a relation between increasing animal product consumption and increasing risk of prostate cancer which, however, did not persist after accounting for the influence of fruit and vegetable consumption.[67] Consumption of beans, lentils, peas, tomatoes, raisins, dates, and other dried fruits was associated with a significantly decreased risk of prostate cancer.

The true risks associated with diet are unclear.[68–70] Dietary research is challenging from the standpoint of methodology, being hampered by difficulties in quantification of true dietary intake over a long period of time, bias regarding dietary intake in retrospective studies, intraperson and interperson variability in serum nutrient levels, long latent period to development of clinical cancer, and changing dietary habits of populations. The relation between dietary factors and prostate cancer is complex. It is difficult to separate the effect of a given nutrient from that of other aspects of the diet and to ascertain association with a given cancer. In general, the data from dietary intake studies support the concept that a high-fiber, low-fat diet may be protective against the development of prostate cancer.

Other Environmental Factors

A vast literature exists concerning the many environmental factors that may contribute to prostate cancer.[6,9,17] However, no definitive links have yet been established between the risk of developing prostate cancer and smoking, socioeconomic status, occupation, drugs, infectious agents, sexual behavior, physical activity, body mass, or sunlight exposure.[71–82] The studies involving cadmium and those involving vasectomy, however, deserve special mention.

Cadmium

Cadmium is a metal most commonly found in cigarette smoke, nickel-cadmium batteries, and cadmium recovery plant smelters. Early observations suggested an increased mortality rate from prostate cancer in workers with past heavy exposure to cadmium oxide dust and fumes. Garcia Sanchez and associates reported a high incidence of prostate cancer in the Salamanca province of Spain.[83] After the most common etiologic factors were excluded, there was a suggestion that cadmium was a risk factor for prostate cancer. Elghany and associates reported, in a population-based study in Utah, that cadmium exposure appeared to result in a small increased RR for prostate cancer, which was most apparent for aggressive tumors.[84] Numerous studies with conflicting results exist in the literature, with earlier studies being positive and later studies tending to show no association between cadmium and prostate cancer.[85–87] The results are probably best summarized by Boffetta, who attributed inconsistencies to difficulties with assessment of exposure, dose response, and other concomitant occupational exposures; effects of nonoccupational risk factors (e.g., smoking, diet); and interactions between cadmium and other etiologic factors.[88]

Vasectomy

Proposed mechanisms by which vasectomy may increase the risk of prostate cancer include diminished secretory rate of prostate fluid, postvasectomy immune response, and increased circulating testosterone levels after vasectomy.[89] Sidney and colleagues, in a study of 5119 vasectomized men with a mean of 6.8 years of follow-up, was unable to show any increased RR with vasectomy nor any relation between prostate cancer and time since vasectomy.[90] Hayes and associates, in their study of vasectomy in U.S. blacks and whites, showed no statistically significant excess risk of prostate cancer with vasectomy.[91] However, they did demonstrate an increased risk among white men who had undergone vasectomy 20 years or more before the study or at less than 35 years of age. Giovannucci and colleagues, in a 13-year retrospective cohort study of 14,607 vasectomized men, demonstrated an RR of 1.56 ($P = 0.04$), with risk increasing with time since vasectomy.[92] In a prospective study by the same investigators, an RR of 1.85 was reported among vasectomized men.[93] DerSimonian and colleagues, in a critical methodology review of six major epidemiologic studies relating to vasectomy and prostate cancer, concluded that all studies were deficient in avoiding detection bias and in obtaining accurate vasectomy histories.[94] The evidence thus far is conflicting, and it remains unclear whether vasectomy increases the risk of developing prostate cancer.

CONCLUSIONS

The effective, efficient, and successful implementation of measures to prevent prostate cancer is aided by knowledge of the natural history and the associated risk factors of the disease. The incidence of latent disease is similar in every population studied around the world, regardless of country or race. The differences in the prevalence of clinical prostate cancer in these same populations, however, suggest that promotional events vary. There is no risk factor that can be implicated as the sole cause of progression to clinical prostate cancer. The definite identification of risk factors, either singly or in combination, for the development of prostate cancer, coupled with timely intervention, can be expected to result in a positive clinical impact in the future.

REFERENCES

1. Carter HB, Piantadosi S, Isaacs JT. Clinical evidence for and implications of the multistep development of prostate cancer. J Urol 1990; 143:742.
2. Parker SL, Tong T, Bolden S, Wingo PA. Cancer statistics. CA Cancer J Clin 1996;65:5.

3. Meikle AW, Smith JA. Epidemiology of prostate cancer. Urol Clin North Am 1990;17:709.
4. Carter HB, Coffey DS. The prostate: an increasing medical problem. Prostate 1990;16:39.
5. Kahler JE. Carcinoma of the prostate gland: a pathologic study. J Urol 1939;11:557.
6. Pienta KJ, Esper PS. Risk factors for prostate cancer. Ann Intern Med 1993;118:793.
7. Guileyardo J, Johnson W, Welsh R, Akazaki K, Correa P. Prevalence of latent prostatic carcinoma in two U.S. populations. J Natl Cancer Inst 1980;65:311.
8. Haas GP, Sakr W, Cassin B, Crissman J, Pontes JE. The prevalence of prostate cancer in young black and white males. J Urol 1992;147: 290A.
9. Wynder EL, Mabuchi K, Whitmore W. Epidemiology of cancer of the prostate. Cancer 1971;28:344.
10. Franks LM, Durh MB. Latency and progression in tumours: the natural history of prostate cancer. Lancet 1956;17:1037.
11. Feinberg AP, Coffey DS. The concept of DNA rearrangement in carcinogenesis and development of tumor cell heterogeneity. In: Owens AH Jr, Coffey DS, Baylin SB, eds. Tumor cell heterogeneity: origins and implications. New York: Academic Press, 1982:469.
12. Vogelstein B, Fearon ER, Hamilton SR, et al. Genetic alterations during colorectal tumor development. N Engl J Med 1988;319:525.
13. Waterhouse J, Muir C, Shanmugaratnam K, et al. Cancer incidence in five continents. In: Cancer incidence. Publication 42, vol 6. Lyon, France: International Agency for Research in Cancer, 1982.
14. Boring CC, Squires TS, Tong T. Cancer statistics, 1992. CA Cancer J Clin 1992;42:19.
15. Shimizu H, Ross RK, Bernstein L, Yatani R, Henderson BE, Mack TM. Cancers of the prostate and breast among Japanese and white immigrants in Los Angeles County. Br J Cancer 1991;63:963.
16. Muir CS, Nectoux J, Staszewski J. The epidemiology of prostate cancer: geographical distribution and time-trends. Acta Oncol 1991;30: 133.
17. Flanders WD. Review: Prostate cancer epidemiology. Prostate 1984; 5:621.
18. Henke RP, Kruger E, Ayhan M, Hubner D, Hammener P. Numerical chromosomal aberrations in prostate cancer: correlation with morphology and cell kinetics. Virchows Arch A Pathol Anat Histopathol 1993; 422:61.
19. Isaacs WB, Carter BS. Genetic changes associated with prostate cancer in humans. Cancer Surv 1991;11:15.
20. Van Veld Hulzen PJ, Saasivan R, Garcia F, Austenfeld MS, Stephens RL. Mutant P53 expression in prostate cancer. Prostate 1993;22:23.
21. Woolf C. An investigation of the familial aspects of carcinoma of the prostate. Cancer 1960;13:739.
22. Steinberg GD, Carter BS, Beaty TH, Childs B, Walsh PC. Family history and the risk of prostate cancer. Prostate 1990;17:337.
23. Ghadirian P, Cadotte M, Lacroix A, Perret C. Family aggregation of cancer of the prostate in Quebec: the tip of the iceberg. Prostate 1991; 19:43.
24. Spitz MR, Currier KD, Fueger JJ, Babaian RJ, Newell GK. Familial patterns of prostate cancer: a case control analysis. J Urol 1991;146: 1305.
25. Carter BS, Steinberg GD, Beaty TH, Childs B, Walsh PC. Familial risk factors for prostate cancer. Cancer Surv 1991;11:5.
26. Carter BS, Steinberg GD, Beaty TH, Childs B, Walsh PC. Mendelian inheritance of familial prostate cancer. Proc Natl Acad Sci U S A 1992; 89:3567.
27. Tulinius H, Egilsson V, Olafsdottir GH, Sigvaldason H. Risk of prostate, ovarian and endometrial cancer among relatives of women with breast cancer. Br Med J 1992;305:855.
28. Ghadirian P, Lacriox A, Perret C, Pavent ME. Familial aggregation of cancer of the pancreas breast, colon, and prostate in French Canadian case control studies. Proc Annu Meet Assoc Cancer Res 1992;33: A1726.
29. Kirkali Z, Eryigit M. Carcinoma of the prostate and HLA antigens. Int Urol Nephrol 1991;23:573.
30. Ross RK, Bernstein L, Judd H, Hanisch R, Pike M, Henderson B. Serum testosterone levels in healthy young black and white men. J Natl Cancer Inst 1986;76:45.
31. Ross RK, Bernstein L, Lobo RA, et al. 5-Alpha-reductase activity and risk of prostate cancer among Japanese and US white and black males. Lancet 1992;339:887.
32. Jackson M, Kovi J, Heshmat M, Jones G, Rao M, Ahlwalia B. Characterization of prostatic carcinoma among blacks: a comparison between a low incidence area, Ibadan, Nigeria, and a high incidence area, Washington, DC. Prostate 1980;1:185.
33. Hill P, Wynder EL, Garbaczewski L, Garnes H, Walker ARP. Diet and urinary steroids in black and white North American men and black South African men. Cancer Res 1979;39:5101.
34. Isaacs JT. Hormonal balance and the risk of prostate cancer. J Cell Biochem 1992;16H:107.
35. Coffey DS, Pienta KJ. New concepts in studying the control of normal and cancer growth of the prostate. In: Current concepts and approaches to the study of prostate cancer. New York: Alan R Liss, 1987:1.
36. Bosland MC, Dreef Van Der Meulen HC, Sukumar S, et al. Multistage prostate carcinogenesis: the role of hormones. International Symposium of the Princess Takamatsu Cancer Research Fund 1991;22:109.
37. Huggins C, Hodges CV. Studies on prostate cancer: the effects of castration, of estrogen and of androgen injection on serum phosphatases in metastatic carcinoma of the prostate. Cancer Res 1941;1:293.
38. Hsing AW, Comstock GW. Serological precursors of cancer: sex hormones and risk of subsequent prostate cancer. Cancer Epidemiol Biomarkers Prev 1993;2:27.
39. Nomura A, Heilburn L, Stemmerman G, Judd H. Prediagnostic serum hormones and the risk of prostate cancer. Cancer Res 1988;48:3515.
40. Meikle AW, Smith JA, Stringham JD. Production, clearance, and metabolism of testosterone in men with prostatic cancer. Prostate 1987; 10:25.
41. Ghanadian R, Puah C, O'Donoghue E. Serum testosterone and dihydrotestosterone in carcinoma of the prostate. Br J Cancer 1979;39:696.
42. Barrett-Connor E, Garland C, McPhillips JB, Khaw KT, Wingard DL. A prospective population based study of androstenedione, estrogens and prostatic cancer. Cancer Res 1990;50:169.
43. Saroff J, Kirdani Y, Ming Chu T, Wajsman Z, Murphy G. Measurements of prolactin and androgens in patients with prostatic diseases. Oncology 1980;37:46.
44. Jacobi G, Rathgen G, Altwein J. Serum prolactin and tumors of the prostate: unchanged basal levels and lack of correlation to serum testosterone. J Endocrinol Invest 1980;3:15.
45. Hammond G, Kontturi M, Maattala P, Puukka M, Vhiko R. Serum FSH, LH, and prolactin in normal males and patients with prostatic diseases. Clin Endocrinol (Oxf) 1977;7:129.
46. Liang T, Hiipakkara T, Stebbins J, Liau S. Anti 5 alpha reductase autoantibodies in the serum of patients with prostatic cancer. J Clin Endocrinol Metab 1990;71:1666.
47. Key TJ. Studies in the epidemiology of sex hormones and cancer. Diss Abstr Int 1991;51:3789.
48. Armenian HK, Lilienfeld AM, Diamond EL, Bross ID. Relation between benign prostatic hyperplasia and cancer of the prostate. Lancet 1974;115.
49. Greenwald P, Kirmiss V, Polan AK, et al. Cancer of the prostate among men with benign prostatic hyperplasia. J Natl Cancer Inst 1974;53:335.
50. Dunn JE. Cancer epidemiology in populations of the United States. Cancer Res 1975;35:3240.
51. Yu H, Harris RE, Gao Y, Gao R, Wynder EL. Comparative epidemiology of cancers of the colon, rectum, prostate and breast in Shanghai, China versus the United States. Int J Epidemiol 1991;20:76.
52. Staszewski J, Haenzel W. Cancer mortality among the Polish born in the United States. J Natl Cancer Inst 1961;26:37.
53. Isaacson C, Selzer G, Kaye V, et al. Cancer in the urban blacks in South Africa. S Afr Cancer Bull 1978;22:49.
54. Rose DP, Connolly JM. Effects of fatty acids and eicosanoid synthesis inhibitors on the growth of two human prostate cancer cell lines. Prostate 1991;18:243.
55. Rose DP, Cohen LA. Effects of dietary menhaden oil and retinyl acetate on the growth of DU 145 human prostatic adenocarcinoma cells transplanted into athymic nude mice. Carcinogenesis 1988;9:603.
56. Rose DP, Boyar AP, Wynder EL. International comparisons of mortality rates for cancer of the breast, ovary, prostate, and colon, and per capita food consumption. Cancer 1986;58:2363.
57. Armstrong B, Doll R. Environmental factors and cancer incidence and mortality in different countries with special reference to dietary practices. Int J Cancer 1975;15:617.
58. Mettlin C, Selenskas S, Natorajan N, Huben R. Beta carotene and

animal fats and their relationship to prostate cancer risk: a case control study. Cancer 1989;64:605.

59. Rose DP, Connolly JM. Dietary fat, fatty acids and prostate cancer. Lipids 1992;27:798.
60. Talamini R, Franceschi S, LeVecchia C, Serraino D, Barra S, Negri E. Diet and prostatic cancer: a case control study in Northern Italy. Nutr Cancer 1992;18:277.
61. McKeehan WL. Growth factor receptors and prostate cell growth. Cancer Surv 1991;11:165.
62. Reichman ME, Hayes RB, Ziegler RG, et al. Serum vitamin A and subsequent development of prostate cancer in the first national health and nutrition examination survey epidemiologic follow up study. Cancer Res 1990;50:2311.
63. Bravo MP, Castellanos E, del Rey Calero J. Dietary factors and prostate cancer. Urol Int 1991;46:163.
64. Hsing AW, Comstock GW, Abber H, Polk BF. Serological precursors of cancer: retinol, carotenoids and tocopherol and risk of prostate cancer. J Natl Cancer Inst 1990;82:941.
65. West DW, Slattery ML, Robinson LM, French JK, Mahoney AW. Adult dietary intake and prostate cancer risk in Utah: a case control study with special emphasis on aggressive tumors. Cancer Causes Control 1991;2:85.
66. Ohno Y, Yoshida O, Oishi K, Okada K, Yamabe H, Schroeder F. Dietary beta-carotene and cancer of the prostate: a case-control study in Kyoto, Japan. Cancer Res 1988;48:1331.
67. Mills PK, Beeson WL, Phillips RL, Fraser GE. Cohort study of diet, lifestyle and prostate cancer in adventist men. Cancer 1989;64:598.
68. Slattery ML, Schumacher ML, West DW, Robison LM, French JK. Food consumption trends between adolescent and adult years and subsequent risk of prostate cancer. Am J Clin Nutr 1990;52:752.
69. Virtamo J, Huttunen JK. Beta carotene, vitamin A and prostatic cancer. Ann Med 1992;24:143.
70. Kolonel LN, Nomura AM. Dietary intervention trials on prostate cancer micronutrients: investigating their role in cancer. In: Micozzi MS, Moon TE, eds. New York, Marcel Dekker, 1992:423.
71. Fincham SM, Hill GB, Hanson J, Wijayasinghe C. Epidemiology of prostatic cancer: a case control study. Prostate 1990;17:189.
72. Honda GD, Bernstein L, Ross RK, Greenland S, Gerkins V, Henderson BE. Vasectomy, cigarette smoking, and age at first sexual intercourse as risk factors for prostate cancer in middle-aged men. Br J Cancer 1988;57:326.
73. Sarkar FH, Sakr WA, Li YW, Sreepathi P, Crissman JD. Detection of human papilloma virus (HPV) DNA in human prostatic tissue by polymerase chain reaction (PCR). Prostate 1993;22:171.
74. Ross RK, Deapen DM, Casagrande JT, Paganini-Hill A, Henderson BE. A cohort study of mortality from cancer of the prostate in catholic priests. Br J Cancer 1981;43:233.
75. Checkoway H, DiFerdinando G, Hulka BS, Mickey DD. Medical, lifestyle, and occupational risk factors for prostate cancer. Prostate 1987; 10:79.
76. Mller H, Mellemgaard A. Prostate cancer incidence in cimetidine users. J Natl Cancer Inst 1992;84:359.
77. Mortensen PB. Neuroleptic medication and reduced risk of prostate cancer in schizophrenic patients. Acta Psychiatr Scand 1992;85:390.
78. Whelan P, Walker BE, Kelleher J. Zinc, vitamin A, and prostatic cancer. Br J Urol 1983;55:525.
79. Gyorkey F, Min K-W, Huff J, Gyorkey P. Zinc and magnesium in human prostate gland: normal, hyperplastic, and neoplastic. Cancer Res 1967;27:1348.
80. Severson RK, Grove JS, Noruma AM, Stemmermann GH. Body mass and prostatic cancer: a prospective study. BMJ 1988;297:713.
81. Hanchette CL, Schwartz GG. Geographic patterns of prostate cancer: evidence for a protective effect of ultraviolet radiation. Cancer 1992; 70:2861.
82. Baquet CR, Horm JW, Gibbs T, Greenwald P. Socioeconomic factors and cancer incidence among blacks and whites. J Natl Cancer Inst 1991;83:551.
83. Garcia Sanchez A, Antona JF, Urrutia M. Geochemical prospection of cadmium in a high incidence area of prostate cancer, Sierra de Gata, Salamanca, Spain. Sci Total Environ 1992;116:243.
84. Elghany NA, Schumacher MC, Slatlery ML, West DW, Lee JS. Occupation, cadmium exposure and prostate cancer. Epidemiology 1990;1: 107.
85. Potts CL. Cadmium proteinuria: the health of battery workers exposed to cadmium oxide dust. Ann N Y Acad Sci 1976;271:273.
86. Kipling MD, Waterhouse JAH. Cadmium and prostatic carcinoma. Lancet 1967;730.
87. Kolonel L, Winkelstein W. Cadmium and prostatic carcinoma. Lancet 1977;566.
88. Boffetta P. Methodological aspects of the epidemiologic association between cadmium and cancer in humans. Cadmium in the human environment. Toxicity and carcinogenicity. Gargnano, Italy, 1991;Sept 25.
89. Anderson DJ, Alexander NJ, Fulgham DL, Vandenbark AA, Burger DR. Immunity to tumor-associated antigens in vasectomized men. J Natl Cancer Inst 1982;69:551.
90. Sidney S, Quesenberry CP Jr, Sadler MC, Guess HA, Lydick EG, Cattolica EV. Vasectomy and the risk of prostate cancer in a cohort of multiphasic health check up examinees: second report. Cancer Causes Control 1991;2:113.
91. Hayes RB, Pattern LM, Greenberg R, et al. Vasectomy and prostate cancer in US blacks and white. Am J Epidemiol 1993;137:263.
92. Giovannucci E, Tosteson TD, Speizer FR, Ascherio A, Vessey MP, Colditz GA. A retrospective cohort study of vasectomy and prostate cancer in US men. JAMA 1993;269:878.
93. Giovannucci E, Ascherio A, Rimm EB, Colditz GA, Stampfer MJ, Willett WC. A prospective cohort study of vasectomy and prostate cancer in US men. JAMA 1993;269:873.
94. DerSimonian R, Clemmens J, Spirtas R, Perlman J. Vasectomy and prostate cancer risks: methodological review of the evidence. J Clin Epidemiol 1993;46:163.

Principles and Practice of Genitourinary Oncology, edited by Derek Raghavan, Howard I. Scher, Steven A. Leibel, and Paul H. Lange. Lippincott-Raven Publishers, Philadelphia, © 1997.

CHAPTER 37

Nonpalpable Preneoplastic Lesions of the Prostate

Jonathan I. Epstein

ATYPICAL HYPERPLASIA: A CONCEPTUAL FRAMEWORK, NOT A SPECIFIC DIAGNOSIS

"Atypical hyperplasia" is a vague term that has been used to denote various lesions depending on the author. Some of the different entities that have been referred to as atypical hyperplasia are (1) lesions that are borderline between normal and early preneoplasia, (2) preneoplastic lesions of all grades, (3) lesions that mimic cancer based on architectural grounds without cytologic atypia, and (4) small foci of atypical glands that are suspicious for but not diagnostic of carcinoma. These entities vary greatly in histology, association with carcinoma, and clinical implications. Consequently, the term atypical hyperplasia should not be used in diagnostic reports but only conceptually for lesions that resemble adenocarcinoma either cytologically or architecturally. As shown in this chapter, subcategorization of lesions of atypical hyperplasia into those with and without cytologic atypia is based not only on histologic differences but on differences in their relation to carcinoma.

LESIONS WITH CYTOLOGIC ATYPIA: PROSTATIC INTRAEPITHELIAL NEOPLASIA

Definition and Terminology

Although various atypical lesions of the prostate had been described previously, the first article to better characterize cytologically atypical lesions within the prostate and suggest a relation to adenocarcinoma was that by McNeal in 1965.[1] Between 1965 and 1986, articles written on this subject suffered from vague definitions, the inclusion of cases without cytologic atypia along with cases having cytologic atypia, and the inclusion of examples that most authorities would now consider to represent infiltrating carcinoma.

In 1986, McNeal and Bostwick coined the term intraductal dysplasia of the prostate and provided clear criteria for this lesion and a grading system for mild, moderate, and severe dysplasia.[2] This lesion consists of architecturally benign prostatic acini or ducts lined by cytologically atypical cells. Intraductal dysplasia was subcategorized into three grades. Grade 1 (mild) dysplasia was characterized by increased nuclear size with increased variability of nuclear size, along with irregular focal crowding and multilayering. Grade 2 (moderate) dysplasia represented the additional finding of hyperchromatism and occasional small prominent nucleoli. The hallmark of grade 3 (severe) intraductal dysplasia was the finding of numerous large prominent nucleoli.

Over the ensuing years, the diagnostic criteria proposed by McNeal and Bostwick have generally been adopted as the accepted method for cytologic grading of atypical lesions within the prostate. However, various criticisms of the term intraductal dysplasia have been raised, and other nomenclature has been championed. Some authors dislike the term dysplasia for description of cytologically atypical lesions. One argument against its use is that the term dysplasia is often used to describe abnormalities in embryogenesis (e.g., dysplastic kidney). Other authors note that the atypical lesions within the prostate often do not occur within large ducts but within acini. Furthermore, it is often difficult to distinguish between ducts and acini. To circumvent these criticisms, other terms (e.g., large acinar atypical hyperplasia, hyperplasia with malignant change) have been proposed, although none has gained widespread acceptance.

In 1989, the term prostatic intraepithelial neoplasia (PIN) was proposed as a synonym for intraductal dysplasia.[3] This term has some advantages, given that it is relatively recent and has not been used by different authors to denote different lesions, but it is also not without deficiencies. Throughout this chapter, the term PIN1 is used to indicate mild dysplasia, PIN2 to signify moderate dysplasia, and PIN3 to denote severe dysplasia. In addition, the term high-grade PIN encompasses both PIN2 and PIN3, whereas low-grade PIN refers to PIN1 only.[3] However, within the literature there are some reports in which PIN1 and PIN2 are considered low-grade PIN and the term high-grade PIN is reserved for PIN3.[4–6]

Histologic Appearance of PIN

Although PIN is characterized by nuclear atypia, there are often accompanying architectural abnormalities.[7,8] At low mag-

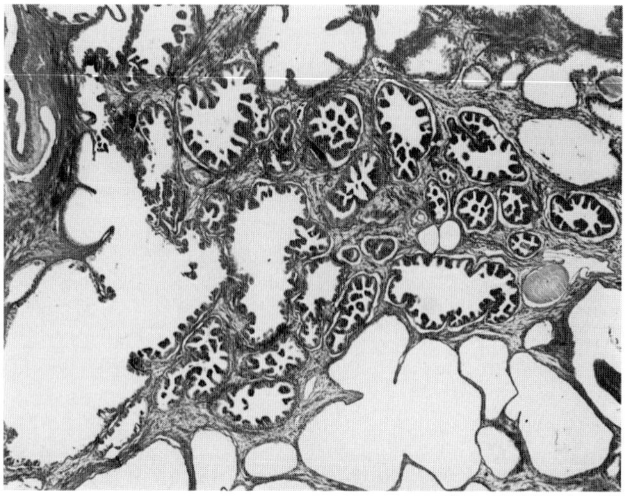

FIG. 37-1. High-grade prostatic intraepithelial neoplasia with basophilic glands preserving the normal architectural pattern of the prostate. Original magnification ×30. (Epstein JI. Interpretation of prostate biopsies. New York, Raven Press, 1995: 38.)

nification, high-grade PIN is characterized by glands that are separated by a modest amount of stroma and have a normal overall architectural pattern. These glands resemble benign glands in that they are large, exhibit branching, and have papillary and undulating luminal surfaces. At low magnification, glands with high-grade PIN have a basophilic appearance (Fig. 37-1). This basophilic appearance is caused by a combination of features, including enlarged nuclei, hyperchromatism, overlapping nuclei, and epithelial hyperplasia (Fig. 37-2). The earliest form of high grade PIN is characterized by nuclear atypia without significant epithelial hyperplasia. Often, the basal cell layer is still visible, and the demarcation between atypical and normal nuclei is often abrupt. With more pronounced forms of high-grade PIN, micropapillary projections and cribriform patterns emerge. Within these epithelial projections, nuclei toward the center of the gland tend to have a more bland cytologic appearance than do nuclei peripherally located against the basement membrane. The grade of PIN is assigned according to assessment of the peripherally located nuclei.

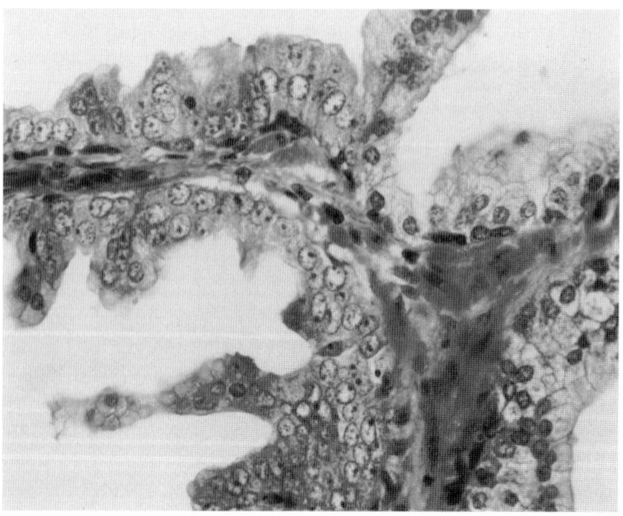

FIG. 37-2. High magnification of severe prostatic intraepithelial neoplasia (PIN3) shows large vesicular nuclei with prominent nucleoli that have become crowded and overlapping. Note the abrupt transition between benign-appearing nuclei and PIN nuclei. Original magnification × 220. (Epstein JI. Interpretation of prostate biopsies. New York, Raven Press, 1995:39.)

Incidence of PIN in Prostates With and Without Infiltrating Cancer

Much of the indirect evidence associating PIN with carcinoma of the prostate has come from studies examining differences between prostate glands with carcinoma and prostate glands without carcinoma.[2,9–12]

PIN1

The exact incidence of PIN1 in glands with and without carcinoma is difficult to determine from the literature. Studies by McNeal and Bostwick[2] and by Troncoso and colleagues[12] report only the dominant grade of PIN or the worst grade of PIN, so the number of cases with PIN1 is often obscured by the occurrence of higher-grade PIN. Nevertheless, in McNeal and Bostwick's study, PIN1 was the predominant grade of PIN in 35% of benign prostates. In the study by Kovi and associates, 22% of benign prostates had PIN1, and 40% of glands with carcinoma had PIN1.[10] Another explanation for underrepresentation of the incidence of PIN1 in benign glands is that most of these studies used autopsy specimens, in which subtle and focal degrees of PIN1 would not be identifiable.

Histologic identification of the mildest forms of atypia in almost any organ system is extremely subjective and carries a low clinical significance. McNeal summarized his consideration of PIN1 in a later work: "There is not a sharp line of demarcation between grade 1 dysplasia and mild degrees of deviation from normal histology."[13] For this reason, I do not comment on PIN1 in diagnostic reports. When reading articles concerning PIN, it is important to separately analyze cases of PIN1 from cases of high-grade PIN, even if the authors have not done so.

PIN2

As with PIN1, it is difficult to determine the incidence of PIN2 in glands with and without carcinoma because several of the larger studies have reported only the worst grade of PIN found in a gland (i.e., glands with PIN3 and PIN2 are reported as PIN3). The frequency of PIN2 in benign prostates ranges from 11% to 68% (Table 37-1). These widely differing incidences may be explained by several factors, including (1) different types of specimens (autopsy versus radical prostatectomy versus cystoprostatectomy); (2) interobserver variability as to where to draw the boundary between PIN1, PIN2, and PIN3; (3) differences in patient populations studied; and (4) different tissue sampling methods. I believe the most credible figure is that 68% of benign glands without infiltrating cancer contain PIN2.[12] This figure was derived from examination of well-fixed cystoprostatectomy specimens. Given the autolysis that occurs in even well-preserved prostates removed at autopsy, cases with

TABLE 37-1. *Incidence of PIN2 in benign prostates*

Investigators	Incidence in benign glands	Type of specimen
McNeal and Bostwick, 1986[2]	22% (worst grade)	Autopsy
Kovi et al, 1988[10]	11%	Autopsy + RP
Troncoso et al, 1989[12]	68% (worst grade)	Cysto

Cysto, cystoprostatectomy for transitional cell carcinoma of bladder, *RP*, radical prostatectomy for prostate carcinoma.

isolated foci of PIN have a high likelihood of being underestimated in such samples. There are no data reporting the incidence of PIN2 in prostates with cancer that are not confounded by the incidence of PIN3, which is often the worst grade of PIN seen in these glands.

PIN3

The most intensely investigated form of PIN is PIN3. It is with PIN3 that there is the greatest discrepancy in incidence between prostates with and without carcinoma (Table 37-2). The same potential explanations for the differences between reported incidences of PIN2 in benign and malignant glands also apply for PIN3. Based on the studies mentioned, it appears that 15% to 18% of glands without carcinoma may have foci of PIN3. The incidence of PIN3 in prostates with carcinoma varies to a greater extent, ranging from approximately 33% in autopsy studies, to 72% in surgical specimens obtained from patients with transitional cell carcinoma, to 100% in radical prostatectomy specimens from patients diagnosed as having carcinoma of the prostate.

Relation of PIN to Carcinoma of the Prostate

Histologic and Morphometric Evidence

In addition to an increased incidence of higher-grade PIN, the number and size of PIN foci are increased in prostate glands with carcinoma compared with those without carcinoma. Also, with increasing amounts of PIN there are a greater number of multifocal carcinomas. This observation follows if PIN is a precursor to some carcinomas, because more early carcinomas would be expected with more precursor lesions. The finding of zones of high-grade PIN from which carcinomatous glands appear to be budding is further histologic evidence that PIN is a precursor to some prostate carcinomas. McNeal has designated these foci as transitive glands, although most other investigators prefer to call them PIN with microinvasive carcinoma.[14] Several studies have also noted an increase of PIN in the peripheral zone of the prostate, relative to the transition zone, corresponding to the site of origin for most adenocarcinomas of the prostate.[11] All these findings would be expected if PIN were a precursor lesion to prostate carcinoma.

Montironi and colleagues have studied the histologic features of PIN more rigorously with computer-assisted morphometric measurements.[5,15,16] The following features were intermediate in PIN, as compared with epithelial cells in benign prostate glands and in cancer: nuclear size, nuclear size variability, nucleolar size, nucleolar number, and nucleolar eccentricity. Other parameters investigated included nuclear stratification and nuclear crowding. Petein has also demonstrated with an image analysis system similarities in nuclear size and chromatin measurements in PIN and in carcinoma.[17]

Histochemical and Immunohistochemical Evidence

A growing body of data demonstrates that the expression of various biomarkers is either the same in PIN and in carcinoma, as opposed to benign prostate glands, or intermediate between benign glands and carcinoma (Table 37-3).

In many cases, ploidy results for high-grade PIN also parallel those seen in carcinomas. Studies that have used image analysis techniques rather than flow cytometry have in general demonstrated ploidy patterns in PIN that are intermediate between those of benign glands and cancers.[5,6,17,21,27,28] The few flow cytometric studies that have not found ploidy abnormalities in PIN have been criticized for their lack of sensitivity and inability to directly correlate DNA measurements with histology.[29,30] In general, diploid high-grade PIN may be associated with adjacent tumors that are either diploid or aneuploid. In contrast, carcinomas adjacent to aneuploid foci of high-grade PIN are almost invariably aneuploid as well.

Relation of PIN to Cancer: Influence of Location and Tumor Grade

In a series of stage T2 (palpable) carcinomas, my colleagues and I found 66% of small multifocal cancers to have adjacent

TABLE 37-2. *Incidence of PIN3 in prostate glands with and without cancer*

Investigators	Incidence in benign glands*	Incidence in malignant glands*	Type of specimen
McNeal and Bostwick, 1986[2]	4%	33%	Autopsy
Kovi et al, 1988[10]	15%	33%	Autopsy + RP
Troncoso et al, 1989[12]	18%	72%	Cysto
Quinn et al, 1990[11]	—	100%	RP (stage T2)
Epstein et al, 1990[9]	—	100%	RP (stages T1a & T1b)

* Benign glands are prostate without infiltrating cancer; malignant glands are prostates with infiltrating cancer.

Cysto, cystoprostatectomy for transitional cell carcinoma of bladder; RP, radical prostatectomy for prostate cancer.

TABLE 37-3. *Immunohistochemical and histochemical evidence relating PIN to carcinoma*

Biomarkers	Investigators
INCREASED IN PIN AND CARCINOMA RELATIVE TO BENIGN PROSTATE	
AgNORs	Sakr et al, 1983[21]; Sesterhan et al, 1991[22]
PCNA	Montironi et al, 1994[15]
Cytokeratins 14,15,16,19	Nagle et al, 1991[19]
Acid mucin	Humphrey, 1991[20]
Ulex europaeus	Perlman and Epstein, 1990[18]
DECREASED IN PIN AND CARCINOMA RELATIVE TO BENIGN PROSTATE	
Blood group A + B	Perlman and Epstein, 1990[18]
Basal cell–specific antibodies	Bostwick and Brawer, 1987[23]
Various lectins	McNeal et al, 1988a[24]
Prostate-specific antigen	McNeal et al, 1988b[25]; Mostofi et al, 1989[26]
Vimentin	Nagle et al, 1991[19]

PIN3.[11] When these multifocal cancers were subcategorized by location and grade of carcinoma, we found that centrally located, intermediate-grade multifocal carcinomas and peripherally located, low- or intermediate-grade carcinomas were associated with adjacent PIN in 80% of cases. In contrast, only 39% of low-grade centrally located adenocarcinomas had adjacent PIN. Because the tumors that are incidentally found on transurethral resection of prostate (TURP) performed for presumed BPH tend to be low-grade, centrally located adenocarcinomas, this finding raised the question as to whether these tumors are less closely linked with PIN than peripherally located, palpable carcinomas are. Further evidence in support of this concept is that PIN3 is much more frequently seen in the periphery of the gland than in the central region, even accounting for the greater area of the peripheral region.[11]

We pursued this question in a study of radical prostatectomies performed for stage T1A and T1B carcinomas found on TURP.[9] Although all of these samples contained some PIN3, the extent of PIN3 was much less than that seen in palpable peripheral carcinomas. This weaker association of PIN3 with incidental, centrally located, low-grade carcinomas is also supported by the histologic differences between PIN and these tumors. Centrally located, low-grade adenocarcinomas tend to have bland cytologic features and often lack nuclear enlargement or nucleoli. In contrast, the cytologic features of peripherally located, intermediate-grade infiltrating carcinomas are often identical to those of PIN3. Other investigators have also noted differences in the incidence of high-grade PIN between the peripheral zone and the transition zone (periurethral region).[31,32]

Intraductal Spread Versus In Situ Growth

There are several arguments that PIN3 does not represent merely an extension of carcinoma into adjacent glands.[33] First, it is not uncommon to find areas of PIN3 away from infiltrating carcinoma. Second, the various complex architectural patterns seen with PIN3, such as micropapillary tufts and cribriform formation, would seem to be less likely a manifestation of intraductal extension from an invasive carcinoma than a primary intraductal growth. Similarly, the finding of scattered clusters of cells with PIN3 interspersed among areas of normal epithelium would be harder to explain as an extension of carcinoma into ducts than as a primary neoplastic process. Furthermore, large areas of PIN3 have been found with associated microinvasive carcinoma.[11,14] In these foci, there are numerous PIN glands which, on careful examination, show several small infiltrating glands, apparently budding off from the PIN glands. Despite these arguments, there are some cases in which the histology suggests the possibility of intraductal spread of cancer. Currently, in these cases there are no means to differentiate these two processes with certainty.

Mimickers of PIN

PIN must be differentiated on the one hand from several benign entities and on the other from variants of infiltrating carcinoma. Benign mimickers of PIN include a variant of normal histology with abnormal architecture seen at the base of the prostate toward the bladder[34] and clear cell cribriform hyperplasia.[35] Both are differentiated from PIN by their lack of nuclear atypia. Another benign entity that can be confused with PIN is cytologically atypical basal cell hyperplasia.[36,37] Although occasionally the distinction between these two entities can be difficult, usually they may be differentiated based on their architecture and, if necessary, on immunohistochemical stains with basal cell–specific antibodies to high-molecular-weight cytokeratin.

In some cases, it is impossible to differentiate a focus of cribriform PIN from cribriform Gleason pattern 3 adenocarcinoma.[34] The finding of cribriform glands with this morphology infiltrating out of the prostate demonstrates that this pattern does not always represent PIN. Although the differentiation of cribriform Gleason pattern 3 from cribriform PIN may be difficult, from a diagnostic standpoint it is usually not critical. Almost always when cribriform Gleason pattern 3 is present, the cribriform glands are accompanied by small infiltrating glands of cancer for which the diagnosis of infiltrating tumor can be made. Only if cribriform glands are so large or back-to-back that they are inconsistent with cribriform PIN should infiltrating cribriform carcinoma be diagnosed on hematoxylin and eosin–stained sections in the absence of small infiltrating glands. Immunohistochemical analysis with antibodies to high-molecular-weight keratin can be used in difficult cases to differentiate these two entities.[38] If only one or a few small cribriform glands are seen on needle biopsy material and no small glands of infiltrating carcinoma are present, the diagnosis should be not infiltrating carcinoma but "focus of atypical cribriform glands," with a comment that the distinction between cribriform PIN and cribriform carcinoma cannot be made with certainty and a recommendation for rebiopsy.

A more difficult distinction is that between cribriform PIN and the rarer ductal (endometrioid) adenocarcinoma of the prostate.[39–41] Ductal adenocarcinomas are aggressive tumors, often of advanced pathologic stage, and are associated with a poor prognosis. Consequently, their differentiation from cribriform PIN is critical. In addition to histologic differences between these two lesions, their locations within the prostate may differ.[34] Ductal adenocarcinomas are often centrally located in the periurethral region and are often sampled on TURP. In contrast, PIN is uncommonly found within the periurethral region and infrequently seen on TURP.

Significance of PIN in Biopsy Material

As discussed previously, the finding of PIN1 is both subjective and common in entirely benign prostates, and PIN1 is difficult to differentiate from normal or slightly reactive epithelium. Consequently, I do not comment on PIN1 in biopsy material. Furthermore, if PIN1 is diagnosed on needle biopsy, the likelihood of cancer being detected on rebiopsy is no higher than if the initial biopsy revealed benign prostate tissue.[42,43]

Several studies have demonstrated that the finding of high-grade PIN on needle biopsy is of greater significance.[42–45] In men with high-grade PIN on biopsy, the reported likelihood of cancer being detected on subsequent biopsy is between 33% and 50%. In the study by my group, the following features did not identify patients who were likely to have carcinoma on follow-up biopsy: the finding of PIN3 versus PIN2 on biopsy; abnormal results on rectal examination; abnormal results on ultrasound.[45] Although the finding of PIN3 could be expected to be more closely associated with the subsequent finding of carcinoma, it appears that the presence of PIN2 in such a small sample of the prostate is of equal significance. This equivalence is further support for the use of the term high-grade PIN to encompass both PIN2 and PIN3. Ultrasound does not differentiate between cases with only PIN and those with PIN and carcinoma, because high-grade PIN may appear indistinguishable from cancer as a hypoechoic lesion.[46]

In men with high-grade PIN on needle biopsy, the one finding that increases the likelihood that there is an unsampled carcinoma is disproportionate elevation of serum prostate-specific antigen (PSA) in comparison with the size of the gland.[45] This empiric finding is expected based on another study from our institution in which PIN by itself was not found to give rise to elevated serum PSA values.[47]

The significance of a finding of high-grade PIN on TURP is not as clear. First, follow-up studies are more difficult because many patients are elderly and do not undergo rebiopsy. It could be argued that this finding is of less significance because PIN is identified in the context of a greater amount of tissue sampled. On the other hand, because PIN uncommonly occurs in the periurethral region, the finding of PIN on TURP may indicate more widespread PIN and a greater risk of concomitant cancer. The management of a patient with high-grade PIN on TURP is in large part determined by the patient's age. In an elderly patient, after clinically significant tumor is ruled out by rectal examination, probably no further management would be instigated. In a younger man, the finding of high-grade PIN on TURP would trigger a more aggressive workup to rule out clinically significant tumor. This workup may include, in addition to rectal examination, transrectal ultrasonography with or without biopsies and close follow-up. If high-grade PIN is found on TURP and the specimen was not put through in its entirety, the remainder of the specimen should be processed in order to look for an infiltrating component.

PIN Versus Carcinoma In Situ (Intraductal Carcinoma)

According to the data presented herein, high-grade PIN appears to be a precursor to some forms of carcinoma of the prostate. For these reasons, some researchers believe that PIN3 should be termed carcinoma in situ or intraductal carcinoma. The one piece of evidence that we do have for premalignant lesions in other organs that is lacking in the prostate is the natural history of PIN3. For example, cases of severe cervical intraepithelial neoplasia have been monitored, and a higher than expected number of these lesions develop into infiltrating carcinoma at the site of the precursor lesion over a defined period of time. With the prostate, there is currently no such capability of monitoring a PIN focus to determine whether there is already infiltrating carcinoma at the site or whether infiltrating carcinoma that evolves has done so in the immediate vicinity of the PIN focus. There are a few reports in which prostatic lesions were seen on ultrasound and PIN was found on biopsy, after which the patient was observed for a relatively short period of time and subsequently shown to have infiltrating carcinoma.[48] In another report, PIN3 was found on fine-needle aspiration biopsy and the patient was monitored and later demonstrated to have infiltrating carcinoma.[49] Although these cases were interpreted as showing evolution from PIN to carcinoma, more likely the infiltrating component was already present at the time of the initial biopsy or aspiration but was not sampled. Because we do not know what percentage of patients with PIN3 on biopsy go on to develop infiltrating carcinoma over a given follow-up interval, most authorities do not use the terms carcinoma in situ or intraductal carcinoma of the prostate for PIN3.

It has also been suggested that the more advanced forms of PIN, those characterized by micropapillary and cribriform patterns, be called carcinoma in situ or intraductal carcinoma, with the term PIN retained for the less proliferative lesions. However, there is no greater risk of associated carcinoma with the more proliferative forms of PIN.[8] Use of the term carcinoma in situ of the prostate or intraductal carcinoma implies a relatively high frequency of development into infiltrating carcinoma and may lead some aggressive clinicians to treat these lesions in a radical fashion. Given that there is still controversy as to whether even infiltrating adenocarcinoma of the prostate should always be treated aggressively, it is doubtful that these potential precursor lesions should be treated by aggressive therapy until their natural history is better understood.

These arguments against the use of the terms carcinoma in situ and intraductal carcinoma reflect the one negative aspect of the term PIN: its relation to carcinoma is usually assumed to parallel that seen in cervical intraepithelial neoplasia by virtue of their similar terminology. However, the natural history of cytologically atypical lesions within the prostate is much less well understood than that of lesions in the cervix.

PIN as a Precursor to Prostate Cancer

Given the information presented in this chapter, it could be assumed that PIN is a universal precursor lesion to prostatic adenocarcinomas. However, some data raise questions regarding the relation of PIN to carcinoma. A recent study by Sakr and associates from Wayne State University noted that the onset of high-grade PIN occurs later than the onset of carcinoma.[50] Furthermore, 70% of prostates with early carcinomas lacked any high-grade PIN within the entirely embedded prostate gland. Even in those prostate glands in which both early cancer and high-grade PIN existed, the PIN was adjacent to cancer in only one third of cases. Other evidence against PIN as a universal precursor to prostatic carcinomas is that transition zone cancers uncommonly show adjacent PIN.[9,11,31] In conclusion, it appears that high-grade PIN is a precursor lesion to many peripheral intermediate- to high-grade adenocarcinomas of the prostate, but PIN is not always present adjacent to these early carcinomas. Low-grade tumors, especially those present within the transition zone, appear to have a different precursor lesion. It may be that the precursor lesions to some carcinomas of the prostate are individual stem cells that progress to invasive carcinoma without going through an intermediate, histologically identifiable precursor state.

Treatment of PIN

In a recent study, 10 patients who were treated with leuprovelin, flutamide, or both before surgery were compared with 10 patients who had received no therapy; the treated patients had a decrease in the mean prostatic area involved by high-grade PIN.[51] Based on this study and the theoretic prediction that high-grade PIN may regress after hormonal therapy, the National Institutes of Health has launched a prospective study to determine whether finasteride, a weaker form of hormonal therapy, can be used as a chemoprevention agent to decrease PIN and potentially decrease or delay the onset of prostatic adenocarcinoma.

LESIONS WITHOUT CYTOLOGIC ATYPIA: ADENOSIS

Adenosis of the prostate is the most common benign glandular proliferation without cytologic atypia that can be confused histologically with low-grade adenocarcinoma of the prostate.[7,34,52–53] Synonyms for adenosis include atypical adenomatous hyperplasia,[54] atypical adenosis,[55] small acinar atypical hyperplasia,[56] and small gland hyperplasia.[57] Although many of these descriptions include lesions that are identical to those we refer to as adenosis, others include lesions that many pathologists now agree are in fact low-grade adenocarcinoma or basal cell hyperplasia.[58,59] This has led to confusion, not only in definition of histologic features of adenosis, but also in attempts to determine the biologic significance of adenosis (i.e., its relation to low-grade adenocarcinoma of the prostate).

Adenosis is characteristically found in the transition zone of the prostate, is frequently multifocal, and most often is an incidental finding on TURP performed for urinary obstruction. In my experience, adenosis of the prostate is a relatively uncommon lesion; nevertheless, it is one of the most frequently encountered mimickers of low-grade adenocarcinoma in TURP specimens. In the spectrum of architectural atypia that ranges from somewhat crowded but obviously benign glands to foci that are difficult to distinguish from cancer, the diagnosis of adenosis should be restricted to cases that are sufficiently atypical in their growth pattern to require serious consideration of a diagnosis of low-grade adenocarcinoma. The variation in thresholds for diagnosing adenosis is reflected in the wide range of its reported incidence in TURP specimens, from 2.2% to 19.6%.[60,61] In TURP specimens examined at Johns Hopkins Hospital that show no cancer, 1.6% are diagnosed as containing adenosis.

The differentiation of adenosis from low-grade adenocarcinoma in TURP specimens is based on a constellation of histologic features rather than on any one histologic feature.[7,34,52,53] There are two critical points of differentiation between adenosis and low-grade adenocarcinoma. First, although there may be minimal infiltration, adenosis has in general a lobular pattern; in contrast, most adenocarcinomas have a haphazard, infiltrative appearance. Second, in adenosis an admixture of small and large glands occurs within a particular focus and, more importantly, these glands are cytologically similar. Although the smaller glands within a focus of adenosis may superficially resemble adenocarcinoma for a number of reasons (e.g., small size, crowded appearance), they are identical in their cytoplasmic and nuclear features to the admixed and adjacent larger glands that are more easily recognizable as benign based on their luminal branching and papillary infolding. Although adenosis and low-grade adenocarcinoma superficially share several histologic features, it is possible to reliably distinguish between these two lesions on histologic grounds.[52,53] The use of high-molecular-weight cytokeratin is helpful to differentiate adenosis from low-grade adenocarcinoma in difficult cases[38,62] (Fig. 37-3). In contrast to the glands in foci of adenocarcinoma, glands in foci of adenosis contain a basal cell layer that can be demonstrated with the use of antibodies to high-molecular-weight cytokeratin.

The relation of adenosis to low-grade adenocarcinoma remains controversial. An argument that has been raised to suggest that adenosis is a precursor to prostate cancer is that the two entities share certain morphologic features. Adenosis may contain acid mucin, crystalloids, nucleoli, and a patchy basal cell layer. Rather than proving a relation between adenosis and carcinoma, these findings demonstrate that any one of these features, by itself, is not specific for carcinoma. For example,

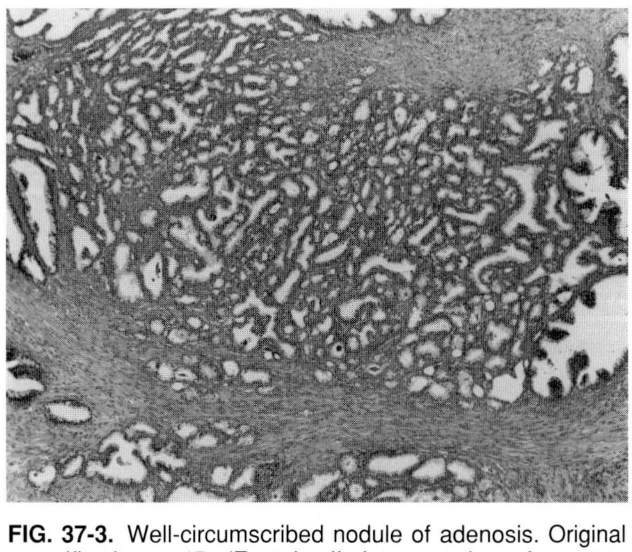

FIG. 37-3. Well-circumscribed nodule of adenosis. Original magnification ×45. (Epstein JI. Interpretation of prostate biopsies. New York, Raven Press, 1995:148.)

acid mucin may be seen in atrophy,[63] a patchy basal cell layer is seen in clear cell cribriform hyperplasia,[35] and nucleoli can be seen in basal cell hyperplasia,[36,37] but none of these lesions is considered to be a precursor to prostate cancer.

To date, no conclusive evidence has been presented to establish an etiologic link between adenosis and low-grade adenocarcinoma. Certain studies suggesting a higher risk of subsequent carcinoma in men diagnosed with adenosis have defined adenosis differently, encompassing many examples of what most authorities would call carcinoma.[58,59] In the series of cases at my institution, 14% of the TURP specimens examined contained incidental foci of adenocarcinoma of the prostate.[52] This is similar to the reported frequency of incidental adenocarcinomas found in TURP performed for clinically benign disease (range, 13% to 22%; mean, 16%).[64] In another recent study, there was no topographic association between adenosis and cancer and no difference in the prevalence of adenosis in prostates with and without cancer.[65] The authors of that study concluded that their findings did not support association between adenosis and cancer. Clearly, long-term follow-up studies are necessary to determine whether there is an association of adenosis with adenocarcinoma of the prostate. Until these studies are completed, adenosis is best considered as representing a benign lesion, distinct from low-grade adenocarcinoma.

SUMMARY

In recent years, great strides have been made in the understanding of various atypical lesions within the prostate. This clarity originated with the recognition that lesions of atypical hyperplasia of the prostate (lesions that in some manner resemble carcinoma) are diverse both in their histology and in their potential relation to adenocarcinoma. A growing body of histologic, histochemical, and immunohistologic evidence demonstrates that PIN is closely linked to some forms of adenocarcinoma of the prostate. Further studies on all forms of atypical hyperplasia are still required to determine the relative risk of developing carcinoma. These studies would be similar to those that have recently been published on various atypical hyperplastic lesions within the breast. In order for these studies to be successful, better imaging techniques of the prostate must become available to rule out the preexistence of invasive carcinoma when one of the forms of atypical hyperplasia is identified on biopsy. Additional directions of research will probe the molecular biology of various forms of atypical hyperplasia, in particular PIN, and its relation to carcinoma.

REFERENCES

1. McNeal JE. Morphogenesis of prostatic carcinoma. Cancer 1965;18:1659.
2. McNeal JE, Bostwick DG. Intraductal dysplasia: a pre-malignant lesion of the prostate. Hum Pathol 1986;17:64.
3. Drago JR, Mostofi FK, Lee F. Introductory remarks and workshop summary. Urology 1989;34(Suppl):2.
4. Jones EC, Young RH. The differential diagnosis of prostatic carcinoma: its distinction from premalignant and pseudocarcinomatous lesions of the prostate gland. Am J Clin Pathol 1994;101:48.
5. Montironi R, Scarpelli M, Sisti S, et al. Quantitative analysis of prostatic intraepithelial neoplasia on tissue sections. Anal Quant Cytol Histol 1990;12:366.
6. Crissman JD, Sakr WA, Hussein ME, Pontes JE. DNA quantification of intraepithelial neoplasia and invasive carcinoma of the prostate. Prostate 1993;22:155.
7. Epstein JI. Interpretation of prostate biopsies. Raven Press, New York 1995.
8. Bostwick DG, Amin MB, Dundore P, Marsh W, Schultz DS. Architectural patterns of high-grade prostatic intraepithelial neoplasia. Hum Pathol 1993;24:298.
9. Epstein JI, Cho KR, Quinn BD. Relationship of severe dysplasia to stage A (incidental) adenocarcinoma of the prostate. Cancer 1990;65:2321.
10. Kovi J, Mostofi FK, Heshmat MY, Enterline JP. Large acinar atypical hyperplasia and carcinoma of the prostate. Cancer 1988;61:555.
11. Quinn BD, Cho KR, Epstein JI. Relationship of severe dysplasia to stage B adenocarcinoma of the prostate. Cancer 1990;65:2328.
12. Troncoso P, Babaian RJ, Ro JY, Grignon DJ, von Eschenbach AC, Ayala AG. Prostatic intra-epithelial neoplasia and invasive prostatic adenocarcinoma in cystoprostatectomy specimens. Urology 1989;34(Suppl):52.
13. McNeal JE. Significance of duct-acinar dysplasia in prostatic carcinogenesis. Urology 1989;34(Suppl):9.
14. McNeal JE, Villers A, Redwine EA, Freiha FS, Stamey TA. Microcarcinoma in the prostate: its association with duct-acinar dysplasia. Hum Pathol 1991;22:644.
15. Montironi R, Galluzzi CM, Diamanti L, Giannulis I, Pisani E, Scarpelli M. Prostatic intra-epithelial neoplasia: expression and location of proliferating cell nuclear antigen in epithelial, endothelial and stromal nuclei. Virchows Arch A Pathol Anat Histopathol 1993;422:185.
16. Montironi R, Braccischi A, Matera G, Scarpelli PE. Quantitation of the prostatic intra-epithelial neoplasia: analysis of the nuclear size, number and location. Pathol Res Pract 1991;187:307.
17. Petein M, Michel P, Van Velthoven R, et al. Morphonuclear relationship between prostatic intraepithelial neoplasia and cancers as assessed by digital cell image analysis. Am J Clin Pathol 1991;96:628.
18. Perlman EJ, Epstein JI. Blood group antigen expression in dysplasia and adenocarcinoma of the prostate. Am J Surg Pathol 1990;14:810.
19. Nagle RB, Brawer MK, Kittelson J, Clark V. Phenotypic relationships of prostatic intraepithelial neoplasia to invasive prostatic carcinoma. Am J Pathol 1991;138:119.
20. Humphrey PA. Mucin in severe dysplasia in the prostate. Surg Pathol 1991;4:137.
21. Sakr WA, Sarkar FH, Sreepathi P, Drozdowics S, Crissman JD. Measurement of cellular proliferation in human prostate by AgNOR, PCNA, and SPF. Prostate 1983;22:147.
22. Sesterhan IA, Becker RL, Avallone FA, Mostofi FK, Lin TE, Davis CJ. Image analysis of nucleoli and nucleolar organizer regions in prostatic hyperplasia, intraepithelial neoplasia, and prostatic carcinoma. J Urogen Pathol 1991;1:61.
23. Bostwick DG, Brawer MK. Prostatic intraepithelial neoplasia and early invasion in prostate cancer. Cancer 1987;59:788.
24. McNeal JE, Leav I, Alroy J, Skutelsky E. Differential lectin staining of central and peripheral zones of the prostate and alterations in dysplasia. Am J Clin Pathol 1988;89:41.
25. McNeal JE, Alroy J, Leav I, Redwine EA, Freiha FS, Stamey TA. Immunohistochemical evidence of impaired cell differentiation in the pre-malignant phase of prostate carcinogenesis. Am J Clin Pathol 1988;90:23.
26. Mostofi FK, Sesterhenn IA, Davis CJ Jr. Malignant change in hyperplastic prostate glands: the AFIP experience. Urology 1989;34(Suppl):49.
27. Weinberg DS, Weidner N. Concordance of DNA content between prostatic intraepithelial neoplasia and concomitant invasive carcinoma. Arch Pathol Lab Med 1993;117:1132.
28. Amin MB, Schultz DS, Zarbo RJ, Kubus J, Shaheen C. Computerized static DNA ploidy analysis of prostatic intraepithelial neoplasia. Arch Pathol Lab Med 1993;117:794.
29. de la Torre M, Haggman M, Brandstedt S, Busch C. Prostatic intraepithelial neoplasia and invasive carcinoma in total prostatectomy specimens: distribution, volumes, and DNA ploidy. Br J Urol 1993;72:207.
30. O'Malley F, Grignon D, Keeney M, Kerkvliet N, McLean C. DNA flow cytometric studies of prostatic intraepithelial neoplasia. Mod Pathol 1991;4:50A.
31. Greene DR, Wheeler TM, Egawa S, Dunn JK, Scardino PT. A compari-

son of the morphological features of cancer arising in the transition zone and in the peripheral zone of the prostate. J Urol 1991;146:1069.
32. NcNeal JE, Price HN, Redwine EA, et al. Stage A versus stage B adenocarcinoma of the prostate: morphological comparison and biological significance. J Urol 1988;139:61.
33. Kovi J, Jackson MA, Heshmat MY. Ductal spread in prostatic carcinoma. Cancer 1985;56:1566.
34. Epstein JI. Differential diagnoses in pathology: urologic disorders. New York, Igaku-Shoin, 1992.
35. Ayala AG, Srigley JR, Ro JY, Abdul-Karim FW, Johnson DE. Clear cell cribriform hyperplasia of prostate: report of 10 cases. Am J Surg Pathol 1986;10:665.
36. Devaraj LT, Bostwick DG. Atypical basal cell hyperplasia of the prostate: immunophenotypic profile and proposed classification of basal cell proliferations. Am J Surg Pathol 1993;17:645.
37. Epstein JI, Armas OA. Atypical basal cell hyperplasia of the prostate. Am J Surg Pathol 1992;16:1205.
38. Hedrick L, Epstein JI. Use of keratin 903 as an adjunct in the diagnosis of prostate carcinoma. Am J Surg Pathol 1989;13:389.
39. Bostwick DG, Kindrachuk RW, Rouse RV. Prostatic adenocarcinoma with endometrioid features: clinical, pathologic, and ultrastructural findings. Am J Surg Pathol 1985;9:595.
40. Epstein JI, Woodruff J. Prostatic carcinomas with endometrioid features: a light microscopic and immunohistochemical study of ten cases. Cancer 1986;57:111.
41. Christensen W, Walsh PC, Epstein JI. Prostatic duct adenocarcinoma: findings at radical prostatectomy. Cancer 1991;67:2118.
42. Brawer MK, Bigler SA, Sohlberg OE, Nagle RB, Lange PH. Significance of prostatic intraepithelial neoplasia on prostate needle biopsy. Urology 1991;38:103.
43. Keetch DW, Humphrey P, Stahl D, Smith DB, Catalona WJ. Morphometric analysis and clinical followup of isolated prostatic intraepithelial neoplasia in needle biopsy of the prostate. J Urol 1995;154:347.
44. Davidson D, Siroky M, Rudders R, et al. Prostatic intraepithelial neoplasia is predictive of adenocarcinoma: retrospective study of 100 cases. Mod Pathol 1994;72A.
45. Weinstein MH, Epstein JI. Significance of high grade prostatic intraepithelial neoplasia (PIN) on needle biopsy. Hum Pathol 1993;24:624.
46. Hamper UM, Sheth S, Walsh PC, Holtz PM, Epstein JI. Stage B adenocarcinoma of the prostate: transrectal US and pathologic correlation of non-malignant hypoechoic peripheral zone lesions. Radiology 1991; 180:101.
47. Ronnette BM, CarMichael MJ, Carter HB, Epstein JI. Does prostatic intraepithelial neoplasia result in elevated serum prostate specific antigen levels? J Urol 1993;150:386.
48. Lee F, Torp-Pedersen ST, Carroll JT, Siders DB, Christensen-Day C, Mitchell AE. Use of transrectal ultrasound and prostate-specific antigen in diagnosis of prostatic intra-epithelial neoplasia. Urology 1989; 34(Suppl):4.
49. Markham CW. Prostatic intra-epithelial neoplasia: detection and correlation with invasive cancer and fine-needle biopsy. Urology 1989; 34(Suppl):57.
50. Sakr WA, Haas GP, Cassin BF, Pontes JE, Crissman JD. The frequency of carcinoma and intraepithelial neoplasia of the prostate in young male patients. J Urol 1993;150:379.
51. Bascham KL, Austenfeld MS, Garcia FU. Quantitative effects of antiandrogen drugs on high grade prostatic intraepithelial neoplasia in radical prostatectomy specimens. Mod Pathol 1992;6:55A.
52. Gaudin PB, Epstein JI. Adenosis of the prostate: histologic features in transurethral resection specimens. Am J Surg Pathol. 1994;18:863.
53. Kramer CE, Epstein JI. Nucleoli in low-grade prostate adenocarcinoma and adenosis. Hum Pathol 1993;24:618.
54. Bostwick DG, Srigley J, Grignon D, et al. Atypical adenomatous hyperplasia of the prostate: morphologic criteria for its distinction from well-differentiated carcinoma. Hum Pathol 1993;24:819.
55. Epstein JI. Disorders of the prostate gland. In: Sternberg, SS, ed. Diagnosis in surgical pathology. New York, Raven Press, 1989:1293.
56. Petersen RO. Urologic pathology. Philadelphia, JB Lippincott, 1992.
57. Ayala AG, Troncos P, Ro JY. Prostate gland. In: Henson DE, Albores-Saavedra J, eds. Pathology of incipient neoplasia. Philadelphia, WB Saunders, 1993:363.
58. Brawn PN. Adenosis of the prostate: a dysplastic lesion that can be confused with prostate adenocarcinoma. Cancer 1982;49:826.
59. Brawn PN. Interpretation of prostate biopsies. New York, Raven Press, 1983:48.
60. Mittal BV, Amin MD, Kinare SG. Spectrum of histological lesions in 185 consecutive prostatic specimen. J Postgrad Med 1989;35:157.
61. Srigley JR. Small acinar patterns in the prostate gland with emphasis on atypical adenomatous hyperplasia and small acinar carcinoma. Semin Diagn Pathol 1988;5:254.
62. O'Malley FP, Grignon DJ, Shum DT. Usefulness of immunoperoxidase staining with high-molecular-weight cytokeratin in the differential diagnosis of small-acinar lesions of the prostate. Virchows Arch A Pathol Anat Histopathol 1990;417:292.
63. Epstein JI, Fynheer J. Acidic mucin in the prostate: can it differentiate adenosis from adenocarcinoma? Hum Pathol 1992;23:1321.
64. Eble JN, Epstein JI. Stage A carcinoma of the prostate. In: Bostwick DG, consultant ed. Pathology of the prostate, seminal vesicles, and male urethra. In: Roth LM, ed. Contemporary issues in surgical pathology. New York, Churchill Livingstone, 1990:61.
65. Troncoso P, Ayala AG. Atypical small glandular proliferations of the transition zone in cystoprostatectomy specimens. Mod Pathol 1994;7: 85A.

Principles and Practice of Genitourinary Oncology, edited by Derek Raghavan, Howard I. Scher, Steven A. Leibel, and Paul H. Lange. Lippincott-Raven Publishers, Philadelphia, © 1997.

CHAPTER 38

Pathology of Palpable Prostate Cancer

Gary J. Miller

Historically, prostate cancer was most often detected by clinicians using digital rectal examination. The last 15 years have witnessed the introduction of a variety of body imaging techniques and serum assays that have improved our ability to identify prostate cancers. Stage migration, the detection of the disease at earlier points in its natural history, has undoubtedly occurred.[1] However, the disease we detect today with combined modalities remains largely the same histopathologically as was detected previously. This chapter focuses on the pathologic features of clinically detectable prostate cancer as it affects the prostate itself; clinically unsuspected carcinomas and metastatic carcinoma are covered elsewhere.

EVALUATION TECHNIQUES

The evaluation of clinically palpable disease usually takes place in two phases: confirmation of the presence of disease by biopsy and evaluation of radical surgical specimens. Although the diagnostic characteristics of carcinoma and histologic grading are essentially the same in both of these processes, other aspects, such as the estimation of tumor volume and pathologic stage, vary greatly.

Biopsy

The most widely used biopsy technique in the United States is the combination of the spring-loaded biopsy device with digital or ultrasound guidance. This technique has largely replaced fine-needle aspiration as a mode of primary diagnosis, although in some European countries, fine-needle aspiration is still widely used. Despite a resurgence of interest in fine-needle aspiration in the United States during the 1980s,[2,3] the technique has been largely abandoned because of the preferences and training of pathologists who are more comfortable making tissue diagnoses and because of the possibility of false-positive results caused by the cytologic similarities between carcinoma and high-grade prostatic dysplasia, such as prostatic intraepithelial neoplasia II or III.

The technique of six systematic, random core or "sextant" biopsies has become widely used in clinical practice. This technique was based on information obtained from ultrasound images and the known locations of carcinomas.[4] Hodge and colleagues[5] were the first to suggest that ultrasonographic visualization of the prostate was a better method for systematic placement of biopsy needles than for identification of carcinomas. They suggested that biopsies taken in predetermined anatomic sites, regardless of ultrasound findings, would detect a greater number of carcinomas that biopsies directed at ultrasonographic abnormalities. Concern has been raised about the possibility that this technique might detect clinically insignificant carcinomas. However, Terris and coworkers[6] determined that only 4% of 816 patients were found to have a carcinomas smaller than 0.5 cm^3 after radical prostatectomy. What volume of carcinoma is clinically "insignificant" remains controversial, because the definition probably depends more on the patient's age than on the volume of carcinoma.

Because of the potential need to obtain a second biopsy of a specific site if the initial biopsy yielded suspicious findings, it is important to identify each of the sextant biopsy samples according to the site of origin. This can be accomplished by color-coded inking of each biopsy or submission in separate cassettes.

Pathologic interpretation of needle biopsies has become somewhat difficult because of the small amounts of tissue that are available from spring-loaded devices. This limitation has made it even more important for the pathologist to be familiar with the range of benign lesions that can mimic carcinomas (Table 38-1). The differential diagnosis of these lesions has been reviewed elsewhere.[7–9] Areas of small gland atrophy, sclerosing adenosis, and atypical adenomatous hyperplasia are the most problematic. Fortunately, all of the benign lesions contain basal cells that can be identified by immunohistochemical detection of high-molecular-weight cytokeratins.[10,11] In suspicious lesions, confirmed basal cells can be taken as evidence of benignity.

After a lesion has been positively identified as carcinoma, it should be assigned a histologic grade using the Gleason system.[12] Several other systems that have been specifically developed for use in classifying prostatic cancer[13] probably give prognostically meaningful information, but the Gleason system has become so widely accepted in U.S. literature that it serves as a standard against which other techniques should be mea-

TABLE 38-1. *Benign lesions commonly confused with prostatic carcinoma*

Adenosis
Atypical adenomatous hyperplasia
Basal cell hyperplasia
Chronic prostatitis
Reserve cell hyperplasia
Sclerosing adenosis
Simple atrophy
Transitional cell metaplasia

sured. The Gleason system is based on the concept that prostatic carcinomas are inherently heterogeneous, and various patterns of malignant growth are recognized and graded (Fig. 38-1). A composite Gleason sum, ranging from 2 to 10, is based on the two most predominant patterns found in a given lesion or patient.

The suitability of the Gleason system for classifying needle biopsy samples has been questioned. However, this system was developed using needle biopsies and is therefore totally appropriate for this application. Concerns regarding reproducibility have also appeared perennially in the literature.[14,15] Gleason addressed many of the perceived problems associated with the use of this technique.[16] The major pitfalls include a failure to recognize selected patterns of high malignant potential (e.g., fused glands, comedo carcinoma, signet ring cells); a tendency to undergrade pattern 3; and clumping grades together to facilitate the interpretation of small series. In response to questions about reproducibility and accuracy, Gleason recognized that grading is "a part of the art of histopathology" that "undoubtedly will not be performed equally well by all those who attempt it."[16]

In addition to histologic grade, pathologic stage information can often be obtained from needle biopsies. Perineural infiltration has long been recognized as an indicator of invasive potential. In view of the location of nerve branches immediately within the prostatic capsule, it is not surprising that perineural invasion also correlates with an increased risk for extracapsular extension of disease.[17] Another, more reliable indication of capsule perforation is finding malignant cells within fat. Because fat does not occur within the prostatic capsule, tumor cells associated with fat provide a reliable indicator of pathologic T3 disease (i.e., stage C). One often incorrectly interpreted finding is the presence of malignant cells juxtaposed to skeletal muscle fibers. Although this can indicate extracapsular disease, skeletal muscle fibers penetrate from the pelvic diaphragm into the anterior fibromuscular band of the prostate, and carcinoma adjacent to skeletal muscle is therefore not absolute proof of pathologic T3 disease.

It has been proposed that the amount of carcinoma in needle biopsies can be used as an indicator of tumor volume and pathologic stage. Terris and colleagues[6] suggested that patients with less than 3 mm^3 of carcinoma in one of six sextant biopsies should have a second biopsy to determine whether more significant disease exists. For a series of 124 patients, Terris and coworkers[18] showed that the combination of planimetric transrectal ultrasonography carcinoma volume, preoperative prostate-specific antigen (PSA) value, and the total length of carcinoma in the biopsies provide the best estimate of the total volume of carcinomas. However, the researcher's formula is apparently insufficient to predict tumor volume in an individual patient. Combining grade with percentage of involvement, Epstein and associates[19] suggested that a Gleason pattern 4 or 5 carcinoma in any biopsy, involvement of three or more cores, or any biopsy fragment with more than 50% involvement predicts finding a significant carcinoma in the subsequent radical prostatectomy specimen. However, such studies are severely limited by the sampling error that results from the fact that patients can have only a limited number of biopsies. In practice, biopsy quality can vary widely and can greatly influence the accuracy of answers obtained in this fashion.

Radical Prostatectomy

The evaluation of radical prostatectomy specimens has been reviewed, and recommendations for reporting results have been made.[20–22] Three major pieces of diagnostic information can be obtained from radical prostatectomy specimens. The first, the histologic grade, is no different from that previously described for needle biopsies, but the grade obtained from the radical prostatectomy specimen is often different from that determined by the needle biopsy. Several researchers have investigated this phenomenon[23–25] and have concluded that the Gleason grade from a needle biopsy is more likely to be a modest underestimate of the final grade. Studies by Kojima and colleagues[1] suggested that undergrading is highest for patients with high PSA or PSA density values. They suggested that the ability to predict tumor grade can be enhanced by considering the serum PSA value.

The second feature, pathologic stage, is also best assessed in the prostatectomy specimen. Pathologic stage (Table 38-2) includes extension through the prostatic capsule and involvement of the seminal vesicles. The prostatic capsule is a somewhat vague structure that is better defined along the posterior surface of the gland than along the anterior one.[27] On the posterior aspect, the capsule is composed of a relatively compact band of smooth muscle cells that separates the prostatic parenchyma from the surrounding loose areolar connective tissue. However, on the anterior aspect, the capsule is less well demarcated, and the smooth muscle of the prostate blends with skeletal muscle elements from the pelvic diaphragm. When prostatic carcinomas perforate the prostatic capsule and spread into the surrounding connective tissue, the 5-year survival is adversely affected.[28,29] Precise quantitation of prostatic capsule perforation has not been correlated with clinical end points. However, evaluation of the capsule for possible penetration should be performed with care.

After radical prostatectomy, there are several choices of methods for processing the specimen. Although perhaps most widely used, the least desirable approach is the use of "representative sections." It is often difficult to detect carcinoma in prostatectomy specimens by gross inspection. This makes the choice of areas to be sampled problematic. For example, eight optimal representative sections would sample only 20% of the capsule of a 40-cm^3 prostate.[30] This limitation probably explains the characteristic upstaging that occurs when the entire prostate is examined compared with representative sections.[31] If the goal of the pathologic inspection is to detect capsule perforation for accurate pathologic staging, most or all of the prostatic capsule should be examined.

The method chosen to examine the prostate depends on the

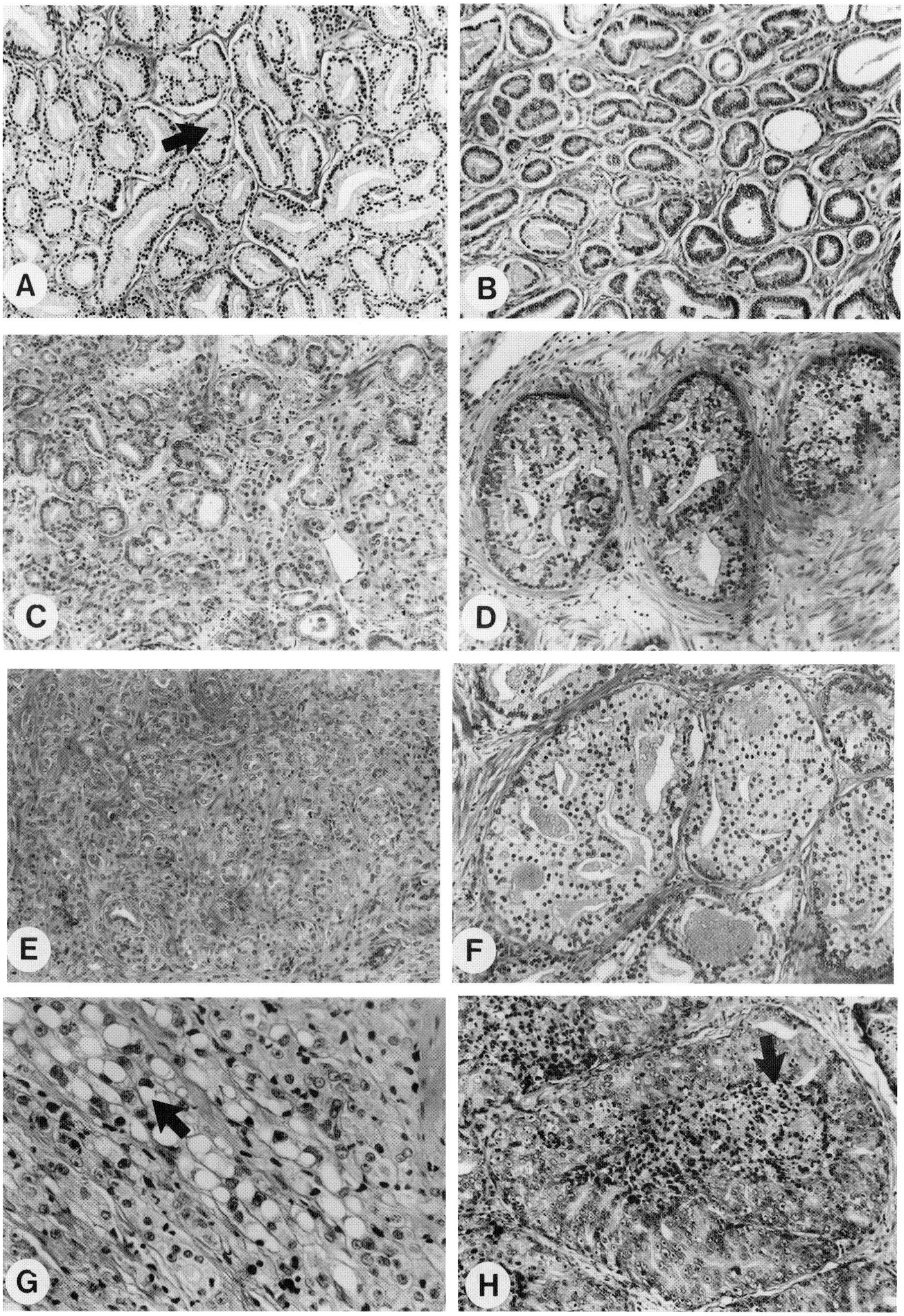

FIG. 38-1. Gleason architectural patterns of carcinoma. (**A**) Pattern 1, large, well-formed acini contain occasional prostatic crystalloids (arrow). (**B**) Pattern 2, medium-sized acini separated by prostatic stroma. (**C**) Pattern 3, small-packed acini. (**D**) Pattern 3, cribriform glands. (**E**) Pattern 4, fused glands. (**F**) Pattern 4, hypernephroid cells. (**G**) Pattern 5, anaplastic and signet ring (*arrow*) cells. (**H**) Pattern 5, comedocarcinoma with central necrosis (*arrow*).

TABLE 38-2. *Pathologic staging system*

Pathologic stage	Description
A1	Tumor involving <5% of specimen, well differentiated
A2	Tumor involving >5%, moderately or poorly differentiated
B	Capsule-confined tumor, negative margins
C1	Tumor through capsule, negative margins
C2	Margin(s) positive
C3	Involvement of seminal vesicle(s)
D1	Microscopic pelvic lymph node involvement
D2	Disease outside pelvis or distant involvement

specific needs and interests of those involved. As a research tool, the preparation of transverse whole-mount sections offers several advantages, including the ability to examine the entire capsule in a sequential fashion, which facilitates decisions regarding questionable perforation on the anterior side. We previously have described our techniques for preparing whole-mount sections.[30,32] Briefly, the specimen should be fixed for a minimum of 3 days before slicing. This allows the capsule to fix in situ and prevents capsule shrinkage artifacts that occur if the gland is sliced in the fresh state. After fixation, the gland is inked with different colors on each side to provide unequivocal orientation. India ink is used to indicate the surgical margin. The gland is then sliced in the transverse plane at 3- to 4-mm intervals. Thinner sections allow more precise estimates of tumor volume, and thicker slices result in less tissue loss from block "facing." The slices are embedded in paraffin using vacuum processing to ensure adequate infiltration. Each of the slices are then cast into single blocks for microtomy. The proximal surface of each block is used to prepare 5-μm sections.

As an alternative to whole-mount preparations, each transverse slice can be further divided into small portions (i.e., halves or quarters) such that the resulting pieces can fit into conventional embedding cassettes. Difficulty in orienting these pieces can be avoided by preparing photocopy "maps."[33] After the transverse slices are divided, they are reassembled on transparent acetate sheets. These can be photocopied to prepare an inexpensive and rapid representation of shapes and surfaces that can later be matched to the shapes of sections on glass slides. In this way, the features of each section can be recorded on the map to provide spatial orientation information.

The levels of local invasion that can be defined include invasion into but not through the capsule, invasion through the capsule (i.e., perforation) but without malignancy at the surgical margin, and involvement of the surgical margin. The latter aspect has raised controversy, because some think that different types of margin positivity exist. For example, it has been suggested that minimal involvement of the margin may not indicate that residual tumor exists in the patient.[34] In a study of 40 prostatectomy specimens, 6 of 10 cases in which the surgical margins were unequivocally positive also had involvement of the neurovascular bundle. However, malignant cells were not found in the neurovascular bundles in 11 cases in which only minimal amounts of tumor extended near or to the inked margin. Although this suggests that significant margin involvement is necessary to suggest that residual tumor cells may be present, such studies cannot examine the extraprostatic soft tissue with the same degree of scrutiny that is used to examine the prostatic capsule. In a study of 507 patients who underwent radical prostatectomy, approximately 50% experienced disease progression during 5 years of follow-up.[35] These included patients who had focally positive margins and patients with extensive margin involvement. For this reason, local recurrence must serve as the true measure of failure to completely excise prostatic carcinomas.

An important concept that has arisen from the use of whole-mount studies is the multifocality of prostate cancer. As early as 1933, Moore recognized that prostate carcinomas could be multifocal.[36] Only recently has the extent and significance of multifocality become apparent. In a study of 151 prostates prepared by whole-mount sections,[37] less than one half of the glands contained a single carcinoma (Table 38-3), and the tumors found to be single carcinomas were the largest-volume tumors. This raises the possibility that many of the single carcinomas may have represented collisions between two smaller tumors that originated independently. It is likely that we continue to underestimate the degree of multifocality that exists.

The third piece of information that is best obtained from radical prostatectomy specimens is tumor volume, which is another valuable indicator of prostate carcinoma biology. Using planimetry, McNeal and collaborators examined the morphometry of prostate carcinoma.[38] This group determined that tumor volume could be correlated with Gleason grade,[38,39] capsule perforation,[40] seminal vesicle involvement,[40] and lymph node metastasis.[41] These studies dealt almost exclusively with the largest tumor (i.e., the index tumor) in each case. McNeal has concluded that "biologically aggressive behavior in adenocarcinoma of the prostate is proposed to be a direct function of cancer volume."[40] Stamey and coworkers[42] made explicit recommendations regarding the necessity to treat clinically localized carcinomas based on tumor volume alone. However, Epstein and colleagues[43] were unable to demonstrate that tumor volume was an independent predictor of disease progression after radical prostatectomy. We have examined the relation of tumor volume to Gleason grade and pathologic stage in all of the 293 carcinomas found in 151 radical prostatectomy specimens.[37] Our results indicate that prostatic carcinomas need not reach large volumes before they attain high histologic grades. Moreover, carcinomas do not have to be high-volume or high-grade tumors before they can become locally invasive. These findings underscore the need for additional prognostic markers that can guide the clinical management of individual patients.

TABLE 38-3. *Multifocality of 293 carcinomas from 151 prostates*

Tumors/ patient	Number of patients (%)	Number of tumors	Mean tumor volume
1	66 (43.7)	66	6.52
2	47 (31.1)	94	1.48
3	25 (16.6)	75	1.01
4	8 (5.3)	32	0.59
5	4 (2.6)	20	0.40
6	1 (0.7)	6	0.22
Total	151 (100)	293	

Other Techniques

In an attempt to provide more objective measures of prognosis, a variety of techniques, including flow and static cytometry, immunohistochemistry, and in situ hybridization, have been applied to prostate carcinomas. The technique that is most widely used is the evaluation of DNA ploidy using flow cytometry. The clinical utility of this technique for studying prostate carcinoma has been extensively reviewed and summarized.[44] In univariate analyses, DNA aneuploidy has been associated with a poor prognosis, regardless of stage or therapy. The best correlations have been made with stages C and D.[45,46] Stages A and B, however, remain controversial.[47,48] In studies employing multivariate analysis, DNA ploidy has not always proved to be an independent predictor.[46,49] DNA ploidy does correlate with grade, and it has been suggested that ploidy provides additional prognostic information for intermediate-grade tumors. This may reflect an association between tumor volume and DNA ploidy.[50] Several studies have suggested that DNA ploidy may change with time,[47,51] but these results may be influenced by including multifocal carcinomas or second primaries. One correlation that maintains significance is the lack of response to hormone therapy by DNA aneuploid tumors.[46]

DNA ploidy determination by image analysis is of somewhat questionable value, in large part because of the lack of uniform standards for image histogram interpretations and because of technical issues about instrumentation.[44] Image analysis does appear to be more capable of detecting small numbers of abnormal cells than flow cytometry,[52] but the clinical significance of such findings remains uncertain. Objective markers of proliferation such as Ki-67[53] or BrdU labeling index,[54] measured by image analysis, have only been examined in a few cases; these samples do not allow for thorough evaluation of the potential clinical utility.

The presence of genes within cells that directly induce malignant transformation has been of prognostic value in a number of malignancies from sites other than the prostate. These include genes for a number of proteins that typically function as growth factors, growth factor receptors, or intermediates in intracellular signal transduction. In prostatic cancer, the picture is not quite as clear. The conclusion of a review[55] of this topic is that oncogene mutations are of little clinical utility in assessing patients with prostatic cancer. A few points, however, deserve further attention because they indicate that molecular analysis eventually may provide useful clinical information.

Mutations of the *RAS* oncogene were first detected in occasional prostatic carcinomas in the United States.[56–58] Later, *RAS* mutations were found to be relatively common in the prostatic carcinomas of Japanese.[59] These differences have persisted in newer studies.[60] Why this is the case remains unknown, but it suggests that major differences in etiologic factors may exist between races. Other oncogenes such as *MYC* were originally found to be of no clinical significance in prostatic cancer,[56] but this may reflect artifacts of specimen preparation.[61] Overexpression of *NEU* (formerly *HER2*) is not uncommon in prostatic cancers,[62] but it has not been shown to be of prognostic significance independent of tumor grade or DNA ploidy.[63] Expression of the anti-apoptosis oncogene, *BCL2,* is related to the emergence of hormone-refractory prostate cancer. Two reports[64,65] support this finding and suggest that this may be an important marker for predicting the impending failure of hormonal therapy.

Genes that suppress the malignant phenotype become clinically significant when they are deleted from the genome or mutated in such a way as to make their protein products inactive. The best studied examples of these are the retinoblastoma *(RB1)* gene and the *P53* gene. The *RB1* gene has been studied in a relatively limited number of prostatic carcinomas, but some studies[66,67] have indicated that allelic loss of this gene is a frequent and early event in prostatic tumorigenesis.

Numerous workers have used immunocytochemistry or DNA mutational analysis to examine prostatic carcinomas for *P53* abnormalities. The studies using immunohistochemistry[68] have consistently reported more abnormalities than those using direct analysis of DNA mutation.[69] In general, it appears that *P53* mutations are associated with advanced stage and increased proliferation of prostatic tumors.[70,71] It has been proposed that *P53* may provide more prognostic information from biopsies,[72] although this idea remains to be validated in a prospective study. It has been shown that *P53* mutations occur in a focal manner in prostatic carcinomas. Mirchandani and associates[73] found that, among multifocal prostatic carcinomas, only single foci are likely to be affected by this genetic mutation. The mutations occur in selected areas of carcinomas and are not always associated with the highest-grade areas. These findings suggest that *P53* mutations area relatively late events in prostatic tumorigenesis.

Although conventional biochemical assays of androgen receptors have failed to predict responses to hormone withdrawal therapy, histologic techniques may offer an alternative. Using immunohistochemistry, Sadi and Barrack[74] showed that it is the heterogeneity of expression among tumor cells, not the absolute number of androgen receptors, that predicts therapeutic response. Such findings suggest that therapies eventually may be more closely tailored to meet the specific needs of individual patients.

LIMITATIONS OF PATHOLOGIC ANALYSIS

Although the prognostic indicators of histologic grade, pathologic stage, tumor volume, and DNA ploidy are significant and at least partially effective, the course of an individual patient's disease still may appear unpredictable. In part, this deficiency results from the limitations of sampling and of our ability to accurately assess these variables. For example, significant pathologic upstaging occurs when more of the prostatic capsule is examined.[31]

A more profound problem is the difference between the information we obtain by observation and our ability to make use of the information as a prognostic indicator. Surgical pathology specimens are by necessity snapshots of disease processes, and we often confuse prediction with observation. In so doing, we ignore the element of time and its contribution to the process we are attempting to evaluate.[75] For example, in view of the long doubling times associated with carcinoma of the prostate,[76], it can be calculated that a 4-cm^3 tumor associated with lymph node metastases may have been only 0.25 cm^3 at the time that metastasis began. It is not surprising, therefore, that 10% of patients thought to have organ-confined disease at the time of prostatectomy develop distant metastases within 5 years.[77]

The precise point at which metastasis begins in a given patient remains to be determined. The early entrance of prostatic carcinoma cells into the circulation has been documented. Using the reverse-transcription polymerase chain reaction, Wood and colleagues[78] showed that 44% of patients with no clinical evidence of metastasis had metastatic prostatic carcinoma cells in their bone marrow. This was even true for 20% of patients with pathologically confined tumors after radical prostatectomy. Although the expression of cell-surface adhesion molecules such as E-cadherin correlates with the metastatic potential of prostatic carcinomas,[79], other factors are undoubtedly required. Until the point at which metastasis begins is precisely determined, the exact features of carcinomas that are necessary to support this process will remain largely unknown.

REFERENCES

1. Murphy GP, Mettlin C, Menck H, Winchester DP, Davidson AM. National patterns of prostate cancer treatment by radical prostatectomy: results of a survey by the American College of Surgeons Commission on Cancer. J Urol 1994;152:1817.
2. Kline TS, Kohler FP, Kelsey DM. Aspiration biopsy cytology (ABC): its use in diagnosis of lesions of the prostate gland. Arch Pathol Lab Med 1982;106:136.
3. Chodak GW, Bibbo M, Straus FH 2d, Wied GL, Straus FH. Transrectal aspiration biopsy versus transperineal core biopsy for the diagnosis of carcinoma of the prostate. J Urol 1984;132:480.
4. Hodge KK, McNeal JE, Stamey TA. Ultrasound guided transrectal core biopsies of the palpably abnormal prostate. J Urol 1989;142:66.
5. Hodge KK, McNeal JE, Terris MK, Stamey TA. Random systematic versus directed ultrasound guided transrectal core biopsies of the prostate. J Urol 1989;142:71.
6. Terris MK, McNeal JE, Stamey TA. Detection of clinically significant prostate cancer by transrectal ultrasound-guided systematic biopsies. J Urol 1992;148:829.
7. Miller GJ. An atlas of prostatic biopsies: dilemmas of morphologic variance. Prog Surg Pathol 1988;8:81.
8. Mostofi FK, Sesterhenn IA, Davis CJ Jr. A pathologist's view of prostatic carcinoma. Cancer 1993;71:906.
9. Jones EC, Young RH. The differential diagnosis of prostatic carcinoma. Its distinction from premalignant and pseudocarcinomatous lesions of the prostate gland. Am J Clin Pathol 1994;101:48.
10. Hedrick L, Epstein JI. Use of keratin 903 as an adjunct in the diagnosis of prostate carcinoma. Am J Surg Pathol 1989;13:389.
11. Wojno KJ, Epstein JI. The utility of basal cell-specific anti-cytokeratin antibody (34 beta E12) in the diagnosis of prostate cancer: a review of 228 cases. Am J Surg Pathol 1995;19:251.
12. Gleason DF and the Veterans Administration Cooperative Urologic Research Group. Histologic grading and clinical staging of prostatic carcinoma. In: Tannenbaum M, ed. Urologic pathology: the prostate. Philadelphia: Lea & Febiger, 1977:171.
13. Miller GJ. New developments in grading prostate cancer. Semin Urol 1990;8:9.
14. Gallee MP, ten Kate FJ, Mulder PG, Blom JH, van der Heul RO. Histologic grading of prostatic carcinoma in prostatectomy specimens. Comparison of prognostic accuracy of five grading systems. Br J Urol 1990;65:368.
15. Cintra ML, Billis A. Histologic grading of prostatic adenocarcinoma: intraobserver reproducibility of the Mostofi, Gleason and Bocking grading systems. Int Urol Nephrol 1991;23:449.
16. Gleason DF. Histologic grading of prostatic cancer: a perspective. Hum Pathol 1992;23:273.
17. Villers A, McNeal JE, Redwine EA, Freiha FS, Stamey TA. The role of perineural space invasion in the local spread of prostatic carcinoma. J Urol 1989;142:763.
18. Terris MK, Haney DJ, Johnstone IM, McNeal JE, Stamey TA. Prediction of prostate cancer volume using prostate-specific antigen levels, transrectal ultrasound, and systematic sextant biopsies. Urology 1995; 45:75.
19. Epstein JI, Walsh PC, Carmichael M, Brendler CB. Pathologic and clinical findings to predict tumor extent of nonpalpable (stage T1c) prostate cancer. JAMA 1994;271:368.
20. Henson DE, Hutter RV, Farrow G. Practice protocol for the examination of specimens removed from patients with carcinoma of the prostate gland. Arch Pathol Lab Med 1994;118:779.
21. Murphy GP, Busch C, Abrahamsson PA, et al. Histopathology of localized prostate cancer. Consensus conference on diagnosis and prognostic parameters in localized prostate cancer. Scan J Urol Nephrol Suppl 1994;162:7.
22. True LD. Surgical pathology examination of the prostate gland. Practice survey by the American society of clinical pathologists. Am J Clin Pathol 1994;102:572.
23. Catalona WJ, Stein AJ, Fair WR. Grading errors in prostatic needle biopsies: relation to the accuracy of tumor grade in predicting pelvic lymph node metastases. J Urol 1982;127:919.
24. Spires SE, Cibull ML, Wood DP Jr, Miller S, Spires SM, Banks ER. Gleason histologic grading in prostatic carcinoma. Correlation of 18-gauge core biopsy with prostatectomy. Arch Pathol Lab Med 1994; 118:705.
25. Bostwick DG. Gleason grading of prostatic needle biopsies. Correlation with grade in 316 matched prostatectomies. Am J Surg Pathol 1994; 18:796.
26. Kojima M, Troncoso P, Babaian RJ. Use of prostate-specific antigen and tumor volume in predicting needle biopsy grading error. Urology 1995;45:807.
27. Ayala AG, Ro JY, Babaian R, Troncoso P, Grignon DJ. The prostatic capsule: does it exist? Its importance in the staging and treatment of prostatic carcinoma. Am J Surg Pathol 1989;13:21.
28. Byar DP, Mostofi FK. Carcinoma of the prostate: prognostic evaluation of certain pathologic features in 208 radical prostatectomies examined by the step section technique. Cancer 1972;30:5.
29. Epstein JI, Carmichael MJ, Pizov G, Walsh PC. Influence of capsular penetration on progression following radical prostatectomy: a study of 196 cases with long-term follow up. J Urol 1993;150:135.
30. Miller GJ, Cygan J. Diagnostic correlations with whole mounts of radical prostatectomy specimens. Monogr Pathol 1992;34:183.
31. Donohue RE, Miller GJ. Adenocarcinoma of the prostate: biopsy to whole mount. Denver VA experience. Urol Clin North Am 1991;18: 449.
32. Deitch AD, Miller GJ, deVere White RW. Significance of abnormal diploid DNA histograms in localized prostate cancer and adjacent benign prostatic tissue. Cancer 1993;72:1692.
33. Rosai J. Gross techniques in surgical pathology. In: Rosai J, ed. Ackerman's surgical pathology, vol I. St Louis: CV Mosby, 1989:13.
34. Epstein JI. The evaluation of radical prostatectomy capsular margins of resection: the significance of margins designated as negative closely approaching and positive. Am J Surg Pathol 1990;14:626.
35. Epstein JI, Pizov G, Walsh PC. Correlation of pathologic findings with progression after radical retropubic prostatectomy. Cancer 1993;71: 3582.
36. Moore RA. The morphology of small prostatic carcinoma. J Urol 1935; 33:224.
37. Miller GJ, Cygan JM. Morphology of prostate cancer: the effects of multifocality on histologic grade, tumor volume and capsule penetration. J Urol 1994;152:1709.
38. McNeal JE, Bostwick DG, Kindrachuk RA, Redwine EA, Freiha FS, Stamey TA. Patterns of progression in prostate cancer. Lancet 1986; 1:60.
39. Stamey TA, McNeal JE, Freiha FS, Redwine E. Morphometric and clinical studies on 68 consecutive radical prostatectomies. J Urol 1988; 139:1235.
40. McNeal JE. Cancer volume and site of origin of adenocarcinoma in the prostate: relationship to local and distant spread. Hum Pathol 1992; 23:258.
41. McNeal JE, Villers AA, Redwine EA, Freiha FS, Stamey TA. Histologic differentiation cancer volume, and pelvic lymph node metastasis in adenocarcinoma of the prostate. Cancer 1990;66:1225.
42. Stamey TA, Freiha FS, McNeal JE, Redwine EA, Whittemore AS, Schmid H-P. Localized prostate cancer: relationship of tumor volume to clinical significance for treatment of prostate cancer. Cancer 1993; 71:933.

43. Epstein JI, Carmichael M, Partin AW, Walsh PC. Is tumor volume an independent predictor of progression following radical prostatectomy? A multivariate analysis of 185 clinical stage B adenocarcinomas of the prostate with 5 years of follow-up. J Urol 1993;149:1478.
44. Shankey TV, Kallioniemi OP, Koslowski JM, et al. Consensus review of the clinical utility of DNA content cytometry in prostate cancer. Cytometry 1993;14:497.
45. Lee SE, Currin SM, Paulson DF, Walther P. Flow cytometric determination of ploidy in prostatic adenocarcinoma: a comparison with seminal vesicle involvement and histopathological grading as a predictor of clinical recurrence. J Urol 1988;140:769.
46. Zincke H, Bergstrahl EJ, Larson-Keller JJ, et al. Stage D1 prostate cancer treated by radical prostatectomy and adjuvant hormonal treatment: evidence for favorable survival in patients with DNA diploid tumors. Cancer 1992;70(Suppl 1):311.
47. Tribukait B. DNA flow cytometry in carcinoma of the prostate for diagnosis, prognosis and study of tumor biology. Acta Oncol 1991;30: 187.
48. Mohler JL, Partin AW, Epstein JI, et al. Prediction of prognosis in untreated stage A2 prostatic carcinoma. Cancer 1992;69:511.
49. Humphrey PA, Walther PJ, Currin SM, Vollmer RT. Histologic grade, DNA ploidy and intraglandular tumor extent as indicators of tumor progression of clinical stage B prostatic carcinoma: a direct comparison. Am J Surg Pathol 1991;15:1165.
50. Deitch AD, deVere White RW. Flow cytometry as a predictive modality in prostate cancer. Hum Pathol 1992;23:352.
51. Tribukait B. Tumor biology in diagnostic cytology: DNA cytometry in carcinomas of the bladder and prostate. Recent Results Cancer Res 1993;133:23.
52. Hardt NS, Hendricks JB, Sapi Z, et al. Ploidy results in prostatic carcinoma vary with sampling method and with cytometric technique. Mod Pathol 1994;7:44.
53. Oomens EH, van Steenbrugge GJ, van der Kwast TH, Schroder FH. Application of the monoclonal antibody Ki-67 on prostate biopsies to assess the fraction of human prostatic carcinoma. J Urol 1991;145:81.
54. Scrivner DL, Meyer JS, Rujanavech N, Fathman A, Scully T. Cell kinetic by bromodeoxyuridine labeling and deoxy ribonucleic acid ploidy in prostatic carcinoma needle biopsies. J Urol 1991;146:1034.
55. Peehl DM. Oncogenes in prostate cancer. An update. Cancer 1993; 17(Suppl):1159.
56. Peehl DM, Wehner N, Stamey TA. Activated Ki-ras oncogene in human prostatic adenocarcinoma. Prostate 1987;10:281.
57. Carter BS, Epstein JI, Isaac WB. Ras gene mutations in human prostate cancer. Cancer Res 1990;50:6830.
58. Gumerlock PH, Poonamallee UR, Meyers FJ, devere White RW. Activated ras alleles in human carcinoma of the prostate are rare. Cancer Res 1991;51:1632.
59. Konishi N, Enomoto T, Buzarel G, Ohshima M, Ward JM, Rice JM. K-ras activation and ras p21 expression in latent prostatic carcinoma in Japanese men. Cancer 1992;69:2293.
60. Watanabe M, Shiraishi T, Yatani R, Nomura AM, Stemmerman GN. International comparison on ras gene mutations in latent prostate carcinoma. Int J Cancer 1994;58:174.
61. Buttyan R, Sawczuk IS, Benson MC, Siegal JD, Olsson CA. Enhanced expression of the c-myc protooncogene in high-grade human prostate cancers. Prostate 1987;11:327.
62. Zhau HE, Wan DS, Zhou J, Miller GJ, von Eschenback AC. Expression of c-erb B-2/neu protooncogene in human prostatic cancer tissues and cell lines. Mol Carcinog 1992;5:320.
63. Ross JS, Nazeer T, Church K, et al. Contribution of HER-2/neu oncogene expression to tumor grade and DNA content analysis in the prediction of prostatic carcinoma metastasis. Cancer 1993;72:3020.
64. McDonnell TJ, Troncoso P, Brisbay SM, et al. Expression of the protooncogene bcl-2 in the prostate and its association with emergence of androgen-independent prostate cancer. Cancer Res 1992;52:6940.
65. Colombel M, Colombel M, Symmans F, et al. Detection of the apoptosis-suppressing oncoprotein bcl-2 in hormone-refractory human prostate cancers. Am J Pathol 1993;143:390.
66. Phillips SM, Barton CM, Lee SJ, et al. Loss of the retinoblastoma susceptibility gene (RB1) is a frequent and early event in prostatic tumorigenesis. Br J Cancer 1994;70:1252.
67. Brooks JD, Bova GS, Isaacs WB. Allelic loss of the retinoblastoma gene in primary human prostatic adenocarcinomas. Prostate 1995;26: 35.
68. van Veldhuizen PJ, Sadasivan R, Garcia F, Austenfeld MS, Stephens RL. Mutant p53 expression in prostate carcinoma. Prostate 1993;22: 23.
69. Voeller HJ, Sugars LY, Pretlow T, Gelman EP. P53 oncogene mutations in human prostate cancer specimens. J Urol 1994;151:492.
70. Visakorpi T, Kallioniemi OP, Heikkinen A, Koivula T, Isola J. Small subgroup of high aggressive, highly proliferative prostatic carcinomas defined by p53 accumulation. J Natl Cancer Inst 1992;84:883.
71. Bookstein R, MacGrogan D, Hilsenbeck SG, Sharkey F, Allred DC. P53 is mutated in a subset of advanced-stage prostate cancers. Cancer Res 1993;53:3369.
72. Navone NM, Troncoso P, Pisters LL, et al. P53 protein accumulation and gene mutation in the progression of human prostate carcinoma. J Natl Cancer Inst 1993;85:1657.
73. Mirchandani D, Zheng J, Miller GJ, Shibata DK, Cote RJ, Roy-Burman P. Heterogeneity in intratumor distribution of p53 mutations in human prostate cancer. Am J Pathol 1995;147:92.
74. Sadi MV, Barrack ER. Image analysis of androgen receptor immunostaining in metastatic prostate cancer: heterogeneity as a predictor of response to hormonal therapy. Cancer 1993;71:2574.
75. Miller GJ. Pathology in prostate cancer: limitations with current techniques. Cancer Control 1995;2:27.
76. Schmid HP, McNeal JE, Stamey TA. Observations on the doubling time of prostate cancer: the use of serial prostate-specific antigen in patients with untreated disease as a measure of increasing cancer volume. Cancer 1993;71:2031.
77. Stein A, deKernion JB, Smith RB, et al. Prostate specific antigen levels after radical prostatectomy in patients with organ confined and locally extensive prostate cancer. J Urol 1992;147:942.
78. Wood DP Jr, Banks ER, Humphryes S, et al. Identification of bone marrow micrometastases in patients with prostate cancer. Cancer 1994; 74:2533.
79. Giroldi LA, Schalken JA. Decreased expression of the intercellular adhesion molecule E-cadherin in prostate cancer: biological significance and clinical implications. Cancer Metastasis Rev 1993;12:29.

Principles and Practice of Genitourinary Oncology, edited by Derek Raghavan, Howard I. Scher, Steven A. Leibel, and Paul H. Lange. Lippincott-Raven Publishers, Philadelphia, © 1997.

CHAPTER 39

Molecular Genetics of Prostate Cancer Progression

William B. Isaacs and John T. Isaacs

The growth pattern of the prostate gland is somewhat unique. It is probably the only organ that continues to grows throughout life, such that the size of a prostate gland from a 65-year-old man is, on the average, twofold to threefold larger than that of a 20-year-old man. The factors responsible for this characteristic growth are essentially unknown. Although most of this age-related increase in prostatic mass frequently is the result of hyperplasia of the periurethral or transition zone of the prostate, lesions that are histologically identifiable as prostate cancer can be found with a frequency of similar magnitude. Fortunately, few of these cancerous lesions progress to clinically manifest disease; however, these features of the prostatic natural history emphasize the tremendous predilection of the prostate to undergo abnormal growth. Understanding this characteristic of the prostate in molecular terms is an important goal in the study of the molecular biology of the prostate.

With respect to prostate cancer, particularly important questions from a clinical point of view include "What are the molecular events responsible for the progression of prostate cancer?" or in other words "Why and how does prostate cancer evolve from an indolent to a life-threatening disease?" "Is this evolution inevitable or are some prostate cancers destined never to progress to life-threatening disease, let alone clinically detectable disease, regardless of the time frame provided?" Although understanding of the carcinogenic process has not been completely resolved for any of the common human malignancies, it is well established that the development of a fully malignant cancer from a normal cell requires multiple transformation events. These transformation events involve genetic alterations in two general classes of cellular genes: oncogenes and tumor suppressor genes. This chapter reviews the present knowledge concerning molecular genetic changes associated with prostatic carcinogenesis. Chapter 1 provides more information about molecular biology techniques. Figure 39-1 summarizes the present understanding of the molecular biology of prostate cancer.

ROLE OF ONCOGENES

Oncogenes are genes that function to enhance the net accumulation of cells. Normally, the expression of oncogenes is tightly regulated within a particular cell type so that the net accumulation of cells does not continuously increase nor decrease over time. Adult tissues are normally self-renewing but do not grow because the rate of cell proliferation is balanced by an equal rate of cell death. Any gene that either increases the rate of cell proliferation or decreases the rate of cell death, thus favoring the continuous net accumulation of cells, can be an oncogene. Any alteration in the tightly regulated control of the expression of an oncogene can enhance the malignant phenotype of the cell. Qualitative changes involve genetic mutations in the oncogenes resulting in an altered oncogenic protein with a deregulated function. The best example of this type of genetic change is the mutation in the *RAS* family of oncogenes (i.e., *HRAS, KRAS,* and *NRAS*).[1]

RAS mutations have been identified in prostatic cancer; however, these occur at a relatively low frequency, at least in localized prostatic cancer.[2,3] Experimentally, expression of a mutated *HRAS* oncogene in prostatic cancer cells results in an enhanced genetic instability and acquisition of high metastatic ability. In addition to qualitative mutations that result in the expression of an altered RAS protein, there can be genetic changes in the noncoding region of oncogenes, resulting in an inappropriate enhancement of the qualitative levels of expression of the protein encoded by the oncogene. Such quantitative derangements result in the continuous inappropriate overexpression of the oncogene. A quantitative overexpression in the *HRAS* oncogenes appears to be more common in metastatic prostatic cancer.[5,6] Experimentally, this overexpression can greatly enhance the motility of prostatic cancer, an effect which can directly affect the metastatic potential of these cells.[7] These results suggest that enhanced expression, not mutation, of RAS P21 protein is involved in the progression of prostatic cancer. Overexpression of HRAS P21 does not appear to be an early event in initiation of prostatic carcinogenesis but is involved in the subsequent progression of the cancer to a highly metastatic state via enhancement of genetic instability of the cancer cells overexpressing HRAS proteins.[8]

The *BCL2* gene is located on chromosome 18q21 and was identified as a result of its involvement at the breakpoint of the

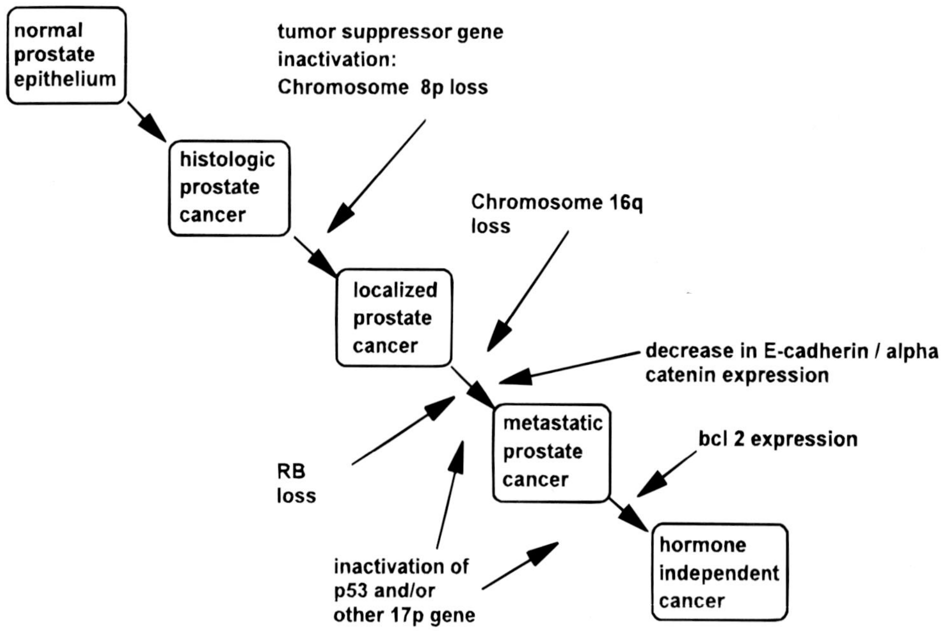

FIG. 39-1. Genetic alterations associated with progression of prostate cancer.

t(14;18) interchromosomal translocation occurring in human follicular B-cell lymphomas.[9] This translocation results in enhanced expression of the *BCL2* gene.[10,11] The *BCL2* gene encodes for a membrane-bound 26-kd protein.[10] *BCL2* has been demonstrated to be an oncogene in that its induced overexpression can lead to malignant transformation.[11] *BCL2* is unique among the oncogenes, however, in that its expression does not enhance the rate of cell proliferation, but instead decreases the rate of cell death.[9–11] The role of *BCL2* in the development and progression of carcinoma of the prostate has been examined by McDonnell and colleagues.[12] Using immunohistochemical techniques, *BCL2* is not usually expressed in androgen-dependent prostatic cancer cells, whereas it was expressed in androgen-independent prostatic cancer cells.[12] This observation has been confirmed by Colombel and colleagues.[13] These findings suggest that enhanced expression of BCL2 protein in carcinomas of the prostate is associated with the transition to androgen independence.

ROLE OF TUMOR SUPPRESSOR GENES

In contrast to oncogenes whose derangement leads to an increase in net growth rate of the affected cell, tumor suppressor genes are constitutively expressed and function to prevent the continuous net accumulation of cells. A partial list of previously identified tumor suppressor genes includes the retinoblastoma gene (*RB1*), *P53*, Wilms' tumor gene (*WT1*), deleted in colorectal carcinoma gene (*DCC*), adenomatous polyposis coli (*APC*) genes, and von Hippel-Lindau disease gene (*VHL*). The list of identified tumor suppressor genes continues to increase. Within a particular cell type (e.g., prostatic glandular cells) not all of these tumor suppressor genes are constitutively expressed. The particular tumor suppressor genes involved in regulating a particular cell type is cell differentiation–specific. It appears that for each differentiated cell type there is more than one tumor suppressor gene preventing its malignancy.

For the malignant phenotype to be expressed, the function of the particular cell type–specific tumor suppressor genes must be abrogated. This frequently occurs by the physical loss of chromosomal regions containing the tumor suppressor gene. The loss can be detected either cytogenetically or by using a molecular biology approach known as allelotyping. Using this technique, DNA is isolated from both normal and tumor tissue from the same patient. Matched DNAs are analyzed for the presence of the maternal and paternal alleles for particular DNA regions or loci chosen on the basis of their high degree of polymorphism and the fact that their chromosomal locations are known. If the analysis of normal tissue DNA from the patient at a given polymorphic locus reveals a difference between the two parental alleles, the patient is said to be heterozygous or informative at this locus. If the analysis of the matched DNA from the patient's cancer retains both polymorphic alleles for the informative locus, then no loss of heterozygosity (LOH) at the particular chromosomal region has occurred. In contrast, if one or both of the alleles are missing, then heterozygous or homozygous deletion, respectively, has occurred in the DNA of the cancer cell at this particular locus. Using this LOH method, approximately 60% of the clinically localized and 100% of the metastatic prostatic cancers show deletions on at least one chromosome.[14,15] The results of such studies and incidence rates for LOH on other chromosomes demonstrate that allelic loss is a common event in prostatic cancer and suggest that chromosomes 8p, 10q, 13q, 16q, 17p, and 18q may contain the sites for tumor suppressor genes important in the progression of human prostatic cancer. The highest frequency of LOH is seen on chromosomes 8p, 16q, and 10q (Fig. 39-2).

Additional evidence for the correlation of allelic loss with prostatic cancer progression has been demonstrated by Macoska and colleagues.[16] Using a combination of polymerase chain reaction (PCR) and fluorescent in situ hybridization (FISH) to analyze microdissected prostatic tissues, they detected higher frequencies of genetic aberrations than would be expected by using either method alone. The most common molecular altera-

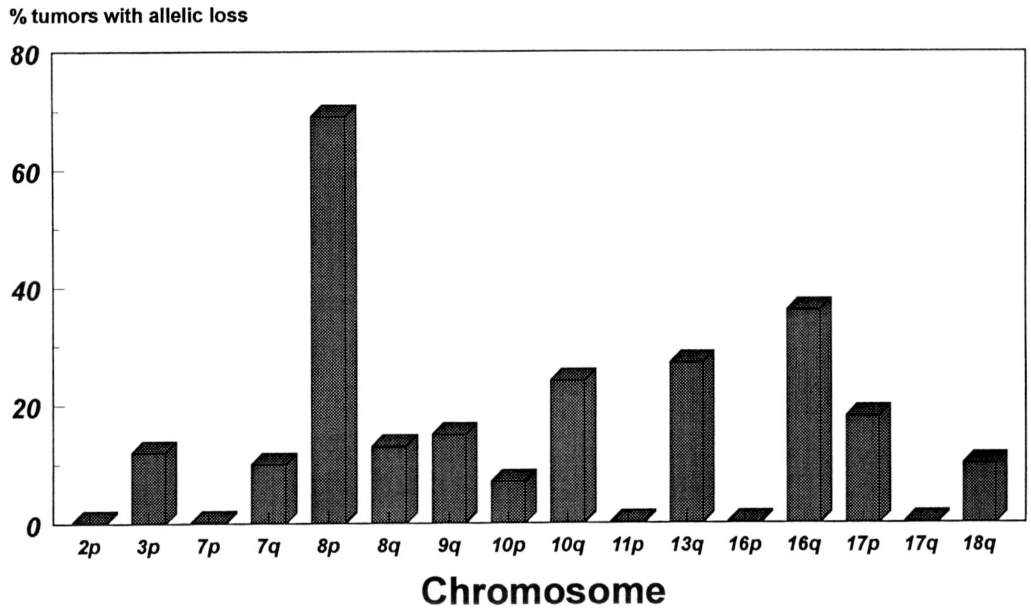

FIG. 39-2. Summary of allelic loss in prostate cancer. Results were obtained from an analysis of 60 stage B primary prostate cancers. (Bova GS, Isaacs WB, unpublished data.)

tions detected by PCR analysis involved changes in normal dosage for sequences on 10q or 8q (35% and 27%, respectively). FISH analysis revealed a gain of chromosome 8 in 54% of the tumors examined and a gain or loss of chromosome 10 in 18% of the tumors examined. The work of these researchers also demonstrated genetic heterogeneity within individual tumor lesions and within different lesions from the same patient.

Bova and colleagues[17] reported evidence that strongly indicates the presence of a tumor suppressor gene on chromosome 8, specifically in the region of 8p22. Using eight polymorphic markers for 8p, these researchers found that 32 of 51 (63%) informative tumors showed loss of at least one locus. The most frequently deleted region was observed at chromosome 8p22-8p21.2. This study confirms the earlier findings of Bergenheim and colleagues[15] of the frequent loss of 8p loci in human prostate cancer; furthermore, it defines the most likely region for tumor suppressor genes on 8p to a 14-cM area around the MSR locus at 8p22. These results demonstrated the highest rate of LOH observed for any chromosome involved with prostate cancer progression and may therefore represent a relatively early event in prostatic carcinogenesis.

E-CADHERIN AND α-CATENIN IN PROSTATE CANCER

The finding of allelic loss on chromosome 16q has led to an examination of putative candidate genes in this region. The E-cadherin gene, mapped to chromosome 16q22.1,[18] is of particular interest. The product of this gene, originally termed uvomorulin by Peyrieras and colleagues,[19] Arc-1 by Berhrens and colleagues,[20] and E-cadherin by Takeichi,[21] was demonstrated to play a critical role in embryogenesis and organogenesis by mediating epithelial cell-cell recognition and adhesion processes. The appearance of E-cadherin protein on the surface of cells of the early mouse embryo has been shown to be required for normal development. The cadherin family of proteins has been determined to be large, with expression found in numerous cell types. The role of E-cadherin in maintaining various aspects of cell differentiation led several investigators to examine E-cadherin in adenocarcinoma cells. These studies found that E-cadherin protein levels were frequently reduced or absent in cancer cell lines, and such lines were often more fibroblastic in morphology and invasive in experimental assays.[22,23] Vleminckx and colleagues[24] demonstrated that experimental inactivation of E-cadherin with either antibodies or antisense RNA resulted in the acquisition of invasive potential and that transfection of invasive adenocarcinoma cells with E-cadherin cDNA rendered the expressing cells noninvasive.

The first studies to examine E-cadherin in prostate cancer were carried out by Bussemakers and colleagues[25] in the Dunning rat model. These studies found a strong correlation between the lack of E-cadherin and metastatic potential, invasive potential, or both. This correlation was strengthened by the direct observation of the progression of a noninvasive, E-cadherin–positive tumor to a E-cadherin–negative, highly metastatic tumor. These observations have been extended to human prostate cancer in a series of more than 90 samples of prostate cancer examined for E-cadherin protein levels using immunohistochemistry.[26] Whereas all benign samples stained with uniform, strong intensity at cell-cell borders, about one half of the tumors examined showed reduced or absent E-cadherin protein staining. When compared with Gleason grade, there was a strong association between high-grade and aberrant E-cadherin staining. No Gleason grade 9 and 10 tumors had normal staining, whereas all tumors with a Gleason score of less than 6 had normal staining patterns. Aberrant E-cadherin staining is a powerful predictor of poor outcome, both in terms of disease progression and overall survival.[26]

To extend understanding of the role of E-cadherin–mediated

cell-cell adhesion in prostate cancer, the synthesis and organization of this protein and its associated proteins in prostate cancer cell lines have been examined.[27] Using immunoprecipitation experiments, cultured normal prostatic epithelial cells make abundant E-cadherin, which can be observed to form complexes with a series of cytoplasmic proteins termed catenins (α and β). These proteins, in particular α-catenin, are thought to link E-cadherin to the microfilament cytoskeleton, and the interaction of E-cadherin with these proteins has been shown to be required for induction of cell-cell adhesion.[28] In cultured prostatic cancer cell lines, E-cadherin levels are frequently reduced or absent, as in surgical specimens of prostate cancer. Furthermore, this study provided the unexpected finding that the levels of the E-cadherin–associated protein α-catenin are also frequently reduced in prostate cancer cells. Loss of this protein in human PC-3 prostate cancer cells is associated with their decreased ability to aggregate compared with cells expressing normal levels of E-cadherin and α-catenin. Thus, the E-cadherin–mediated pathway of cell-cell adhesion may become inactivated in a variety of ways. The lack of α-catenin expression in PC-3 cells is the result of a homozygous deletion within the α-catenin gene.[27] The α-catenin gene has been mapped to chromosome 5q22,[29] and preliminary results suggest that LOH in this region occurs in about 25% of prostate cancers analyzed.

RB1, P53, AND DCC IN PROSTATIC CANCER

Acquisition of metastatic ability by prostatic cancer cells represents the most lethal aspect of prostatic cancer progression. It is clear that malignant progression involves not only gains in critical transforming function but also requires the loss of regulatory function that normally suppress tumorigenesis and metastasis. The involvement of such suppressor genes is supported by the correlation of chromosomal deletions with prostatic cancer progression. Specifically, deletions on chromosomes 13, 17, and 18 may affect the expression of the known tumor suppressor genes *RB1*, *P53*, and *DCC*, respectively, and may alter the expression of unidentified suppressor functions.[30] Recent studies support a role for *P53* in the suppression of human prostatic cancer progression.[31] DNA sequence analysis shows that in three of five human prostatic cancer cell lines, the most highly conserved region of *P53* had mutations that altered the normal amino acid sequence. One of two primary prostatic cancer specimens examined also contained a mutation in this region. Accumulation of mutant *P53* has been found in histologically poorly differentiated and metastatic prostatic cancers.[32] Such accumulation was not detected in hormone-dependent lesions. These results support a role for *P53* mutation in the progression from hormone-dependent to hormone-independent metastatic disease. Additional evidence for this role has been found in in vitro experiments. Transfection of the wild-type *P53* gene versus a mutated *P53* gene into two cell lines with *P53* mutations resulted in reduced colony formation.[31] Revertants that overcame the growth suppressor activity of wild-type *P53* no longer retained wild-type *P53* sequences. Immunocytochemical data indicate that prostatic cancer cells expressing the transfected wild-type *P53* gene are growth arrested. These results suggest a functional role for *P53* gene in suppressing prostatic tumorigenesis.

Alterations in the RB1 gene product have also been suggested as an event in prostate cancer tumorigenesis. Bookstein and colleagues[33] found that the RB1 gene product is truncated in the human prostate cancer cell line DU-145. A functional role for *RB1* is suggested by the finding that when an intact copy of cloned *RB1* gene was introduced into these cells, their tumorigenicity was suppressed.[33] Two other human prostate cell lines examined in this study apparently have normal RB1 gene products, indicating that *RB1* mutation is not a universal event in prostate cancer tumorigenesis. Allelic loss of chromosome 13q (i.e., the location of the *RB1* gene) has been detected in approximately 25% of localized human prostate cancers.[14] In addition, decreased levels of RB1 protein have been observed in approximately 50% of surgical specimens obtained from metastatic sites of human prostatic cancers.[34]

The putative tumor suppressor gene *DCC*, which is located on chromosome 18q, was identified by its frequent deletion in human colorectal carcinoma.[35] The role of reduced *DCC* expression and LOH in prostatic cancer is under study. Carter and colleagues[14] reported that the frequency of LOH at the *DCC* locus was approximately 17%. Gao and colleagues[36] reported that the *DCC* gene was present and expressed in normal prostate cells. In patient samples, 12 of 14 prostate cancer cases (86%) showed reduced expression of *DCC* RNA, and 5 of 11 informative cases (45%) showed LOH of the *DCC* locus.[36] These results indicate that downregulation of the *DCC* gene, by either reduced expression or LOH at the *DCC* locus, is a common feature of prostatic cancer. The discrepancy between the two reports may be a factor of the regions of the *DCC* gene examined. Carter and colleagues[14] examined the M2 and M3 sites for LOH, while Gao and colleagues[36] examined the VNTR region in addition to M2 and M3. Both groups found approximately the same rate of loss at the M2 locus (17%). Although these data indicate a correlation between LOH of the *DCC* locus and prostatic cancer, a functional role for *DCC* in the initiation or progression of prostatic cancer has not yet been identified.

ROLE OF METASTASIS SUPPRESSOR GENES

In addition to tumor suppressor genes, which normally inhibit the tumorigenicity of cells, there are genes that suppress the metastatic ability of cancer cells without affecting the tumorigenicity of these cancer cells.[37] Efforts to identify the specific chromosomal regions and genes involved in such metastasis suppression are underway. Initially, these studies consisted of fusing nonmetastatic and highly metastatic rat prostatic cells. The hypothesis was that if the loss or inactivation of metastasis suppressor genes is involved in malignant progression, then the somatic cell hybrids from such a fusion would be nonmetastatic, because chromosomes from the nonmetastatic parental cell would supply the lost suppressor gene functions. Ichikawa and colleagues[37] found that the tumorigenicity and in vivo growth rates of the hybrid clones, which contained a full complement of parental chromosomes, were not affected. In contrast, none of the animals bearing hybrid tumors developed distant metastases. When these nonmetastatic primary tumors were passaged in vivo, animals occasionally developed distant metastases. Cytogenetic analysis of either of these metastatic revertants showed a consistent loss of a specific copy of normal rat chromosome 2.[37] This study demonstrated that prostatic cancer metastasis is associated with the loss of specific chromosomes that do not affect the growth rate or tumorigenicity, only metastatic ability.[37]

These results indicate that expression of genes located on certain chromosomes can suppress the metastatic ability of rat prostatic cancer cells. The location of homologous metastatic suppressor genes in the human is unknown. One such gene, *NM23*, has been identified.[38] *NM23* encodes a nucleoside diphosphate kinase whose expression is decreased in metastatic melanoma and breast cancer cells. Preliminary studies, which quantitated the level of NM23 protein in the Dunning system, showed that the level of *NM23* is not correlated with the metastatic ability of the cell lines.[39] This indicates that decreased expression of *NM23* is not involved in progression within this rodent system. The role of *NM23* expression in human model systems is not fully resolved. Igawa and colleagues[40] demonstrated that the levels of NM23 RNA and protein are more commonly increased in prostatic cancer cells from patients with clinically metastatic disease than in cells from patients with clinically localized disease. Jensen and colleagues[41] found that the level of NM23-H1 mRNA was increased twofold or more in prostatic tumor tissues compared with normal tissues in 13 of 27 (48%) patients, with a mean increase of 5.4-fold. These samples also showed an increase in the level of NM23 protein. Unlike the Igawa and colleagues study,[40] the Jensen and colleagues study[41] found no statistical correlation between the pathologic staging of the tumors and the fold increase in *NM23-H1* expression. As is indicated by these reports, the potential role of NM23-H1 RNA or NM23 protein overexpression in prostate tumorigenesis has yet to be resolved.

In an attempt to identify other genes involved in the suppression of prostatic cancer metastasis, a panel of cells containing defined portions of human chromosomes has been constructed. The general construction scheme employs microcell-mediated chromosome transfer to specifically transfer individual human chromosomes to the recipient cells of interest.[42] Mouse fibrosarcoma cells containing normal human chromosomes tagged with an exogenous gene encoding resistance to the neomycin antibiotic G418 are sequentially treated with colcemid to depolymerize microtubules and cytochalasin-B to depolymerize actin bundles. The treated cells are then centrifuged, and the resulting pellet contains the microcells. Microcells are, in effect, micelles that contain single or multiple chromosomes. To enrich for those containing single chromosomes, the microcells are sized by sequential filtration through polycarbonate membranes of decreasing pore size. The purified microcells are attached to recipient cells via incubation with phytohemagglutinin and finally fused by incubation with polyethylene glycol. Recipient cells containing human chromosomes are selected in G418-containing media and then characterized by FISH and other classic cytogenetic and molecular biology methods.

Using this method, specific human chromosomes have been introduced into highly metastatic rat prostatic cancer and breast cancer cell lines. By comparing the results in prostate and breast systems, both general and specific mediators of metastasis can be identified. Introduction of human chromosome 11 or 17 into highly metastatic, androgen-independent, rat prostatic cancer cells results in suppression of metastatic ability without suppression of in vivo growth rate or tumorigenicity.[39,43] In contrast, only introduction of human chromosome 17, not chromosome 11, into highly metastatic rat breast cancer cells results in suppression of metastatic ability without suppressing tumorigenicity of the cell.[39] These results demonstrate that there are genetic alterations that are uniquely required for acquisition of metastatic ability of tumorigenic prostatic versus breast cancer cells. Furthermore, these findings support a model in which tumorigenicity and metastatic ability are distinct properties of cancer cells requiring both common and unique genetic alterations.

Spontaneous deletion of portions of human chromosome 11 in some of these clones showed that the minimal portion of this chromosome capable of suppressing prostatic cancer metastasis involves a region between 11p11.2-13 and does not include the *WT1* locus.[43] In contrast, transfer of human chromosome 11 into highly metastatic, estrogen-independent, rat mammary cancer cells had no effect on the tumor growth rate or metastatic ability.[39] This result indicates that the metastatic suppressor genes in human chromosome 11p11.2-13 are prostate cancer–specific. This prostatic specificity could be the result of differences in the metastatic pathways of mammary and prostatic cancer cells or to tissue-specific transcription factors that allow expression of only the metastasis suppressor genes in cancers of prostatic origin. By combining studies of these cell panels, a molecular map of chromosomes specifically involved in prostatic cancer metastasis is constructed and used for positional cloning of genes involved in this process.

FUTURE DIRECTIONS

This chapter focuses on the characterization of consistent genetic alterations in human prostate cancer. The mutations described are somatic: that is, they are restricted to the cancer cell DNA and are not found in the germ line DNA. Evidence has been obtained for an hereditary form of prostate cancer in which a mutation is inherited in the germ line that predisposes the carriers to develop prostate cancer. Carter and colleagues[44,45] have demonstrated that familial aggregation of prostate cancer can be best explained by the Mendelian inheritance of a rare autosomal dominant allele that predisposes men to develop this disease. From the study population examined, it was estimated that the gene responsible for this predisposition accounts for approximately 9% of the total cases of prostate cancer and 45% of the cases observed in men younger than 55 years of age. In predisposed individuals, presumably a key step necessary for tumor development is inherited such that the majority of men with this inherited defect accumulate the additional genetic alterations required for the development of prostate cancer. This can be manifest as early onset and high penetrance of disease in these susceptible individuals. In other people, sporadic cases of disease may occur as the *same* genes are altered at the tissue level through random or environmentally induced errors in cellular processes. Numerous examples exist in which the identification of genes that play critical roles in solid organ carcinogenesis has been accomplished directly as a result of the study of inherited cancers, the two most recent examples being the *APC*[46,47] and *MUT*[48,49] genes in familial adenomatous polyposis and hereditary nonpolyposis colon cancer, respectively, and the *VHL* gene in renal cancer.[50,51] In these cases, genes that predispose individuals to develop these cancers when inherited in a mutated form are also genes that are frequently, if not universally, mutated in the sporadic forms of these cancers as well. Thus, the identification of prostate cancer susceptibility alleles will be an important area for future effort and should provide unique insight into the pathogenesis of prostate cancer.

REFERENCES

1. Bos JL. *ras* oncogenes in human cancer: a review. Cancer Res 1989; 49:4682.
2. Carter BS, Epstein JI, Isaacs WB. *ras* gene mutations in human prostate cancer. Cancer Res 1990;60:6830.
3. Gumerlock PH, Poonamallee UR, Meyers FJ, de Vere White RW. Activated *ras* alleles in human carcinoma of the prostate are rare. Cancer Res 1991;51:1632.
4. Treiger B, Isaacs JT. Expression of a transfected v-Harvey-*ras* oncogene in a Dunning rat prostate adenocarcinoma and the development of high metastatic ability. J Urol 1988;140:1580.
5. Viola M, Fromowitz F, Oravez S, et al. Expression of *ras* oncogene p21 in prostate cancer. N Engl J Med 1986;314:133.
6. Sumiya H, Masai M, Akimoto S, Yatani R, Schimazaki J. Histochemical examination of the expression of *ras* p21 protein and R-1881-binding protein in human prostatic cancers. Eur J Cancer 1990;26:786.
7. Partin AW, Isaacs JT, Treiger B, Coffey DS. Early cell motility changes associated with an increase in metastatic ability in rat prostatic cancer cells transfected with v-Harvey-*ras* oncogene. Cancer Res 1988;48: 6050.
8. Ichikawa T, Schalken JA, Ichikawa Y, Steinberg GD, Isaacs JT. H-*ras* expression, genetic instability, and acquisition of metastatic ability by rat prostatic cancer cells following v-H-*ras* oncogene transfection. Prostate 1991;18:163.
9. Tsujimoto Y, Finger LR, Yunis J, Nowell PC, Croce CM. Cloning of the chromosome breakpoint of neoplastic B cells with the T(14;18) chromosome translocation. Science 1984;226:1099.
10. Hockenberry DM, Nunez G, Millman C, Schreiber RD, Korsmeyer SJ. Bcl-2 protein is topographically restricted in tissues characterized by apoptotic cell death. Nature 1990;348:334.
11. Reed JC, Cuddy M, Slabiak T, Croce CM, Nowell PC. Oncogenic potential of bcl-2 demonstrated by gene transfer. Nature 1988;336:259.
12. McDonnell TJ, Troncosco P, Brisbay SM, et al. Expression of protooncogene *bcl*-2 in the prostate and its association with emergence of androgen-independent prostate cancer. Cancer Res 1992;52:6940.
13. Colombel M, Symmons F, Gil S, et al. Detection of the apoptosis-suppressing oncoprotein *bcl*-2 in hormone-refractory human prostate cancers. Am J Pathol 1993;143:390.
14. Carter BS, Ewing CM, Ward WS, et al. Allelic loss of chromosomes 16q and 10q in human prostate cancer. Proc Natl Acad Sci U S A 1990;87:8751.
15. Bergerheim USR, Kunimi K, Collins VP, Ekman P. Deletion mapping of chromosomes 8, 10, and 16 in human prostatic carcinoma. Genes Chromosom Cancer 1991;3:215.
16. Macoska JA, Micale MA, Sakr WA, Benson PD, Wolman SR. Extensive genetic alterations in prostate cancer revealed by dual PCR and FISH analysis. Genes Chromosom Cancer 1993;8:88.
17. Bova GS, Carter BS, Bussemakers MJG, et al. Homozygous deletion and frequent loss of chromosome 8p22 loci in human prostate cancer. Cancer Res 1993;53:3869.
18. Natt E, Magenis RE, Zimmer J, Mansouri A, Scherer G. Regional assignment of the human loci for uvomorulin and chymotrypsinogen B with the help of two overlapping deletions on the long arm of chromosome 16. Cytogenet Cell Genet 1989;50:145.
19. Peyrieras N, Hyafil F, Louvard D, Ploegh HL, Jacob F. Uvomorulin: a nonintegral membrane protein of early mouse embryo. Proc Natl Acad Sci U S A 1983;80:6274.
20. Behrens J, Birchmeier W, Goodman SL, Imhof BA. Dissociation of Madin-Darby canine kidney epithelial cells by the monoclonal antibody anti-Arc1: mechanistic aspects and identification of the antigen as a component related to uvomorulin. J Cell Biol 1985;101:1307.
21. Takeichi M. Cadherin cell adhesion receptors as a morphogenetic regulator. Science 1991;251:1451.
22. Frixen UH, Behrens J, Sachs M, et al. E-cadherin-mediated cell-cell adhesion prevents invasiveness of human carcinoma cells. J Cell Biol 1991;113:173.
23. Sommers CL, Thompson EW, Torri JA, Kemler R, Gelmann EP, Byers SW. Cell adhesion molecular uvomorulin expression in human breast cancer cell lines: relationship to morphology and invasive capacities. Cell Growth Differ 1991;2:365.
24. Vleminckx K, Vakaet L, Mareel M, Fiers W, Van Roy F. Genetic manipulation of E-cadherin expression by epithelial tumor cells reveals an invasion suppressor role. Cell 1991;66:107.
25. Bussemakers MJG, Van Moorselaar RJA, Giroldi LA, et al. Decreased expression of E-cadherin in the progression of rat prostatic cancer. Cancer Res 1992;52:2916.
26. Umbas R, Isaacs WB, Bringuier PP, et al. Decreased E-cadherin expression is associated with poor prognosis in patients with prostate cancer. Cancer Res 1994;54:3929.
27. Morton RA, Ewing CM, Nagafuchi A, Tsukita S, Isaacs WB. Reduction of E-cadherin levels and deletion of the α catenin gene in human prostate cancer cells. Cancer Res 1993;53:3585.
28. Ozawa M, Baribault H, Kemler R. The cytoplasmic domain of the cell adhesion molecule uvomorulin associates with three independent proteins structurally related in different species. Eur Mol Biol Organ J 1989;8:1711.
29. McPherson JD, Morton RA, Ewing CM, et al. Assignment of the human α catenin gene to chromosome 5q21-q22. Genomics 1994;19:188.
30. Isaacs WB, Carter BS. Genetic changes associated with prostate cancer in humans. Cancer Surv 1991;11:15.
31. Isaacs WB, Carter BS, Ewing CM. Wild-type p53 suppresses growth of human prostatic cancer cells containing mutant p53 alleles. Cancer Res 1991;51:4716.
32. Navone N, Troncoso P, Pisters LL, Palmer JL, von Eschenbach AC, Sand Conte CJ. P53 protein accumulation in the progression of human prostate carcinoma. J Natl Cancer Inst 1993;85:1657.
33. Bookstein R, Shew J, Chen P, Scully P, Lee W-H. Suppression of tumorigenicity of human prostate carcinoma cells by replacing a mutated *Rb* gene. Science 1990;247:712.
34. Bookstein R, Rio P, Madrepela SA, et al. Promoter deletion and loss of retinoblastoma gene expression in human prostate carcinoma. Proc Natl Acad Sci U S A 1990;87:7762.
35. Fearon ER, Cho KR, Nigro JM, et al. Identification of a chromosome 18q gene that is altered in colorectal carcinoma. Science 1990;247:49.
36. Gao X, Honn KV, Grignon D, Sakr W, Chan YQ. Frequent loss of expression and loss of heterozygosity of the putative tumor suppressor gene DCC in prostatic carcinomas. Cancer Res 1993;53:2723.
37. Ichikawa T, Ichikawa Y, Isaacs JT. Genetic factors and suppression of metastatic ability of prostate cancer. Cancer Res 1991;51:3788.
38. Steeg PS, Bevilacqua G, Kopper L, et al. Evidence for a novel gene associated with low tumor metastatic potential. J Natl Cancer Inst 1988; 80:200.
39. Rinker-Schaeffer CW, Hawkins AL, Ning R, et al. Differential suppression of mammary and prostate cancer metastasis by human chromosomes 17 and 11. Cancer Res (in press).
40. Igawa M, Rukstalis DB, Tanabe T, Chodak GW. High levels of NM23-H1 expression are related to cell proliferation in prostatic cancer. Cancer Res 1994;54:1313.
41. Jensen SL, Wood DP, Banks ER, McRoberts W, Rangnekar VM. Increased levels of NM23-H1 mRNA associated with adenocarcinoma of the prostate. Society for Basic Urological Research Abstracts, 1993.
42. Koi M, Morita H, Yamada HY, Satoh H, Barrett JC, Oshimura M. Normal human chromosome 11 suppresses tumorigenicity of human cervical tumor cell line SiHa. Mol Carcinog 1989;2:12.
43. Ichikawa T, Ichikawa Y, Dong JT, et al. Localization of metastasis suppressor genes(s) for prostatic cancer to the short arm of chromosome 11. Cancer Res 1992;52:3486.
44. Carter BS, Beaty TH, Steinberg GD, Childs B, Walsh PC. Mendelian inheritance of familial prostate cancer. Proc Natl Acad Sci U S A 1992; 89:3367.
45. Carter BS, Bova GS, Beaty TH, et al. Hereditary prostate cancer: epidemiologic and clinical features. J Urol 1993;150:797.
46. Kinzler KW, Nigbert MC, Su LK, et al. Identification of FAP locus genes from chromosome 5q21. Science 1991;256:661.
47. Groden J, Thliveris A, Samowitz W, et al. Identification and characterization of the familial adenomatous polyposis coli gene. Cell 1991;66: 589.
48. Fishel R, Lescoe MK, Rao MRS, et al. The human mutator gene homolog MSH2 and its association with hereditary nonpolyposis colon cancer. Cell 1993;75:1027.
49. Leach FS, Papadopoulos N, Liu B, et al. Mutations of a *mut*S homolog in hereditary nonpolyposis colorectal cancer. Cell 1993;75:1215.
50. Latif F, Tory K, Gnarra J, et al. Identification of the von Hippel-Lindau disease tumor suppressor gene. Science 1993;260:1317.
51. Shuin T, Kondo K, Torigoe S, et al. Frequent somatic mutations and loss of heterozygosity of the von Hippel-Lindau tumor suppressor gene in primary human renal cell carcinomas. Cancer Res 1994;54:2852.

Principles and Practice of Genitourinary Oncology, edited by Derek Raghavan, Howard I. Scher, Steven A. Leibel, and Paul H. Lange. Lippincott-Raven Publishers, Philadelphia, © 1997.

CHAPTER 40

Experimental Approaches to Skeletal Metastasis of Human Prostate Cancer

George Thalmann, Ploutarchos Anezinis, Robert Devoll, Cindy Farach-Carson, and Leland W. K. Chung

In the past several years, prostate cancer research has received increasing attention worldwide. Much of the interest has focused on understanding the cause of early disease, the genetic loci that may be associated with cancer occurrence, and the strategies that can prevent cancer development and progression. In this chapter, we discuss approaches that can delineate the molecular and cellular mechanisms that regulate the progression of advanced prostate cancer, with emphasis on the interaction between prostate cancer and bone stroma. This area of investigation of advanced states of prostate cancer progression has not been extensively evaluated in experimental models of prostate carcinogenesis. One crucial step of this progression is the acquisition of a lethal androgen-independent and metastatic phenotype after androgen ablation therapy.

Three areas of investigation are highlighted. First, we review the literature on the natural history of prostate cancer metastasis. Second, we examine the role of normal bone physiology, composition of bone matrices, and pathways that lead to prostate cancer metastasis to the bone. Third, we focus on experimental approaches to understand the molecular and cellular bases of prostate cancer and bone stroma interaction, which may be critical in determining prostate cancer growth and metastasis. We describe a novel animal model of osseous metastasis of human prostate cancer and identify potential bone-derived matrix proteins that may contribute to prostate cancer growth and progression.

NATURAL HISTORY OF OSSEOUS METASTATIC PROSTATE CANCER

Adenocarcinoma of the prostâte is rarely recognized before the age of 50, and the incidence progressively increases in the subsequent decades.[78,79] Observations at autopsy indicate that early prostate cancer evolves multifocally within the gland. Disease progression tends to follow several pathways: periprostatic and perivesicular penetration and perforation of the prostatic capsule and invasion along the perineural spaces; metastasis to pelvic lymph nodes; and metastasis to bones of the pelvis, lumbar spine, and thorax. Involvement of the axial skeleton is a common event, and at autopsy, 43% to 85% of those with prostatic adenocarcinoma have skeletal metastasis.[49,1,18,22,64,67,48] Failure to achieve a disease-free state by surgical or radiation treatment of the primary prostate cancer has provided increasing evidence that incidence of dissemination to bone at diagnosis or subsequently might be far more common than initially thought.[28]

The incidence of clinical stage D prostate cancer reported in the 1982 American College of Surgeons in short-term survey[51] can be summarized as follows. Of 20,000 new cases of prostate cancer, 21.5% of patients presented with clinical stage D prostate cancer. At 5 years from the initial diagnosis, 23% of patients with clinical stage D disease survived. Throughout this study, black patients fared poorer than white patients. Of 573 patients with prostate cancer presenting at a comprehensive cancer center, 43% had clinical stage D2.[66] In their follow-up series, Corriere and colleagues[14] found a considerably higher proportion of cancers in clinical stages C and D prostate cancers in men younger than 55 years of age than in men between 55 and 64 (70% versus 43%). Johnson and coworkers[42] studied 26 cases of men with prostatic cancer younger than 50 (mean age, 46.2 years) and compared the outcomes with those for 599 other patients older than 50 years (mean age, 66.5 years). Of the 26 patients diagnosed and treated at the M.D. Anderson Cancer Center, 16 (62%) presented with widespread metastatic disease (stage D). Of the 599 patients older than 50, 34% had stage D disease, and the difference is statistically highly significant.

The prognosis for D2 prostate cancer is generally poor, but few large surveys exist. In 1926, Bumpus[8] observed that approximately two thirds of patients with clinical stage D prostate cancer died within 9 months of the diagnosis. In a study of 260 patients with metastatic disease, Nesbit and colleagues[54] reported an average survival from diagnosis to death of 16.9 months, with a median of 9.6 months and a range of 1 to 176 months. In another study, the 1-, 3- and 5-year survival rates for 231 patients with metastatic disease receiving no hormonal therapy was 47%, 11%, and 6%, respectively.[55] Although 22%

of 599 patients older than 50 with widespread disease survived 5 years in the M.D. Anderson study, no patient younger than 50 survived that long. The actuarial survival 5 years from diagnosis by histologic grade for clinical stage D prostate cancer in 11,924 patients with prostate cancer from the long-term survey of the American College of Surgeons was 32.7% for well-differentiated tumors, 25.4% for moderately differentiated tumors, 20% for poorly differentiated tumors, and 11.8% for undifferentiated tumors.[52] In Clain's large series of 2001 cases of bone metastasis, metastasis from prostate cancer was most common, occuring in 32.4% of these cases.[11] In these series, patients with prostate disease had the longest survival after the bone metastasis was diagnosed (16.8 months). Four-hundred twenty-nine patients with bony metastasis were reviewed retrospectively by Conroy and coworkers,[13] and they recorded 2- and 5-year survival rates of 33.2% and 15.2%, respectively.

In a retrospective study of 137 autopsy cases, Harada and colleagues[30] examined the metastatic frequency of various organ sites and found bone metastases in 81% of the cases. In 83.2% of the cases with lymph node metastases, osseous involvement was also observed. In the study of the Veterans Administration Cooperative Urological Research Group, 83% men recorded with prostate cancer had the following types of bone metastasis: ischium (78%), lumbosacral spine (71%), thoracic spine (60%), ribs (53%), femur (48%), and shoulder (39%).[10] Cumming and coworkers[16] found the spine to be involved in 96.4% of patients with positive bone scans. In study of 169 men with D2 disease, Rana and associates[57] reported that the pelvis was the most frequent site (76%) of metastasis, followed by the dorsal (73%) and the lumbar vertebrae (63%).

Bone metastases are almost always multiple, and the axial skeleton is more commonly involved than the appendicular skeleton; this is thought to reflect the distribution of persistent hematopoietic active red bone marrow in the cancerous part of the bone.[79] In a collected review of radioactive technetium scans for 1355 cases from 16 institutions, Tofe[75] showed a broadly similar distribution for suspected bone metastases for all tumors, except that cancers of the prostate, bladder, cervix, uterus, and rectum demonstrated a propensity to involve the bone of the pelvis. Within the spine, the vertebral body is more commonly involved by metastases than the pedicles. A computed tomographic (CT) study of skeletal metastasis in the vertebral column by Suzuki and colleagues[73] indicates that the most affected part of the vertebral body is the peripheral region. In the spine, the lumbar and dorsal spine has a higher incidence of metastasis than the cervical spine and the sacrum. This suggests that the venous pathway first proposed by Batson and later demonstrated in human cadavers by Franks may play a role in the dissemination of prostate cancer to the vertebral column.[3,23] This system comprises a paravertebral network of thin-walled veins that communicate freely with the pelvic and intercostal veins. Subperiostal tumors form mainly where blood vessels cross the hard cortical bone. Cortical bone involvement, as well as that of the vertebral arches and processes, primarily results from invasion or expansion from bone metastases.

When tumor infiltration of the bone marrow is extensive or bone marrow has been irradiated, secondary sites of hematopoiesis may be stimulated; prostatic cancer cells can then metastasize to atypical sites, such as distal limb bones, suggesting that local factors (e.g., growth factors, chemoattractants) are necessary for site-specific growth. After invasion of the surrounding tissue, the cells of the primary tumor gain access to blood or lymphatic vessels, tumor cells or clumps are released into circulation (e.g., paravertebral venous plexus), and emboli are arrested in blood vessels in the bone marrow. The extravasation (chemotactic factors?) and subsequent multiplication of clonogenic tumor cells that survive these various steps prompt growth of vascularized stroma into the new tumor focus in the bone. Eighty to ninety percent of bone lesions due to prostate cancer are osteoblastic; 12% are mixed, and 40% are lytic.[18,40] An earlier autopsy study by Elkins and Mueller[19] reported pure osteoblastic bone metastases in more than 50% of cases, with a mixture of osteoblastic and osteolytic lesions in approximately one third of the patients and pure osteolytic metastases in fewer than 10% of patients dying of prostate cancer. The least common lytic lesion is most likely to occur in older patients.

Bone metastases demonstrate a proliferation of osteoblasts with new, often incompletely calcified bone formation within the bone marrow in the vicinity of metastatic prostate cancer cells, suggesting that vascular anatomy alone does not account for the pattern of prostate cancer metastasis and that local factors produced by mesenchymal or epithelial cells or as a consequence of mesenchymal-epithelial interactions are indispensable for metastatic implication and growth. A growing body of evidence supports these findings.

Clinical manifestations of advanced prostate cancer are ureteral obstruction, bladder outlet obstruction, rectal obstruction, hematologic dysfunction, and metabolic abnormalities. Because of prostate cancer affinity to the bone, stage D2 disease manifests itself by bone pain, pathologic fractures, and spinal cord compression by epidural lesions. Pain usually is the dominant initial symptom. Weakness, peripheral sensory deficit, and autonomic dysfunction are symptoms that usually occur late.[21] However, in as many as 37% of patients, spinal cord compression is the first presentation of malignancy. In a series reported by Smith and coworkers,[67] 5 (19%) of 26 patients had spinal cord compression as the first indication of prostate cancer. The average survival of patients with paraplegia in this study was 3.9 months, compared with 18 months for the group as a whole. Kuban and associates[46] observed a median interval of 15.5 months between the appearance of vertebral metastases and the development of spinal cord compression. Sorenson and colleagues[70] reported that, of 345 patients with metastatic epidural spinal cord compression, 18% had primary prostate cancer.[70] Myelography is usually required to evaluate the level of compression. CT scan and magnetic resonance imaging are helpful to delineate the extent of the lesion. Plain x-ray film diagnosis is not very sensitive; it successfully made only for 42% of spines with extensive osteoblastic metastatic carcinoma in a postmortem study by Bachman and Sproul.[2] In Iacovou's study,[37] roentgenographic studies of the spine revealed abnormalities in as many as 90% of these patients.

Clinically, the increase metabolic activity of these osseous lesions can be monitored by bone scans. Soloway and colleagues[69] established a grading system of bone scans with the intention to quantitate and correlate the extent of disease with treatment impact and survival. They concluded that patients with extensive disease have a particularly poor prognosis, even when treated by androgen deprivation. In 1981, Pollen and coworkers[56] reported serial bone scanning to be an appropriate method to monitor treatment response in patients with prostate cancer. In their series, patients determined to have progression at 6 months had a 41% 1-year survival rate, compared with 81% for those who had improvement or stability demonstrated on their scans. Only 7% of patients showing progression on serial scans were alive at 1 year, compared with 60% of those who improved or were stable. Deterioration of the bone scan findings indicated disease progression and poor prognosis, and improvement of the scan reflected regression of metastatic disease and implied favorable survival. However, qualitative interpretations and assessment of clinical therapeutic response by sequential bone scans may not be reliable when concomitant regions of improvement and disease progression are observed in the same patient.[65,68] This is partially because radiolabeled bone scanning agents accumulate best when the immature osteoid is being formed or is only partially calcified. There is little uptake in the preexisting normal cortex or trabeculae of lamellar bone and no uptake by the tumor cells. The intensity of radionucleotide uptake may vary and is influenced by a variety of factors, such as complete and stable mineralization, active healing in response to chemotherapy, and hormonal treatment.

To improve early recognition and treatment of patients with metastatic prostate cancer, markers and prognostic factors are needed. Pretreatment testosterone levels have been correlated with treatment response and survival. Robinson and Thomas[60] found that patients with metastatic disease who had normal or high pretreatment (i.e., hormonal ablation) testosterone levels survived longer.[60] Harper and associates[31] observed that patients who died within 1 year of treatment had significantly lower pretreatment testosterone levels than those who survived longer than 1 year. This was confirmed by a study by Ishikawa and colleagues,[38] which also indicated that only patients with less than six metastatic sites on the bone scan had a better prognosis and a longer interval free of progression after androgen deprivation therapy. In an analysis of prognostic factors by the Dutch Southeastern Urological Cooperative Group of 175 hormonally treated patients with disseminated prostate cancer, had performance status, anemia, and high alkaline phosphate levels that were significantly related to shorter survival.[50] Other molecular and cellular markers under evaluation include DNA ploidy, nonrandom cytogenetic changes and loss of heterozygosity, *p*53 gene and protein expression, E-cadherin, and C-CAM.[58,6,34] Osteocalcin, a noncollagenous bone matrix protein believed to be involved in mineralization and expressed by osteoblasts, is less sensitive than prostate-specific antigen (PSA) or prostate acid phosphatase (PAP) measurements.[64]

The treatment of choice for metastatic bone pain is androgen deprivation.[36] Hormonal treatment produces rapid results, with relief beginning within 24 hours. Bone pain in patients with hormone-refractory disease is a challenging problem for clinicians. Analgesics used vary from nonsteroidal inhibitors of prostaglandin synthesis, effective for their ability to diminish inflammatory reaction, to morphine and its derivatives. For palliation, localized external beam radiation therapy with 2000 to 3000 cGy in divided doses is the most common method used.[5] In patients with spinal cord compression not previously treated by hormones, orchiectomy offers the best and fastest response.[41] Initial high-dose dexamethasone treatment may be added. Ketoconazole also can be used. Good results have been reported with radiation therapy, laminectomy, or a combination of both.[21] Generally, previously undiagnosed and therefore untreated patients fare well. Those with paraparesis do better than those with paraplegia. Sphincter involvement and rapid onset of symptoms are unfavorable prognostic factors. The overall success rate for the different treatment modalities is approximately 30%. The results of a meta-analysis of 26 drug trials indicate that hormone-resistant adenocarcinoma of the prostate still fails to respond to most cytotoxic agents. Distant metastases create problems affecting the patient's quality of life. Further research and randomized clinical trials are necessary to improve treatment and palliation in these patients.

BONE PHYSIOLOGY AND BONE CELLS

Fewer than 2% of the total volume of bone is accounted for by living cells, with most consisting of a cellular organic material and inorganic mineral, principally hydroxyapatite $[Ca_{10}(P0_4)_6(0H)_2]$.[74] The growth, form, and density of bone is controlled by the relative activities of two distinct cell types of unique cell lineage: the bone-forming osteoblasts and the bone-resorbing osteoclasts. Osteoblasts are mesenchymal cells derived from the same family of stem cells that give rise to muscle, cartilage, and fat. Osteoblasts produce the mineralizing organic matrix, including type I collagen, and are under exquisite metabolic and endocrine control. Osteocytes are mature osteoblasts that have become isolated in the mineralized matrix and that develop a specialized phenotype, including formation of long processes, creating a cellular communication network extending throughout bone matrix. Numerous cytokines, including the bone morphogenetic proteins, transforming growth factors, and insulin-like growth factors; many steroid hormones, including estrogen, testosterone, and glucocorticoids; and vitamin D can alter net osteoblastic activity.[82] The osteoclasts represent a separate cell type, derived from the same hematopoietic cellular precursors that give rise to monocytes and macrophages. Mature osteoclasts are multinucleated cells whose overall activity is modulated at two separate and distinct steps: the rate and extent of formation of mature, bone-resorbing osteoclasts by fusion of precursors and the ability of such formed cells to migrate across mineralized matrices to form resorption pits at specific sites. The activity of osteoclastic cells is regulated by various agents, including cytokines and steroid hormones. A partial list consists of tumor necrosis factor, several interleukins, colony-stimulating factors, platelet-derived growth factors, leukemia-inhibitory factor, vitamin D, and estrogen.[33] In general, increased osteoblastic activity leads to matrix production, mineral deposition, and removal of ions such as calcium and phosphate from blood. Increased osteoclastic activity produces thinning of bone, loss of matrix and mineral, and release of sequestered ions to the fluid systems, where they must be handled. Local communication between osteoblasts and osteoclasts is essential to the growth and maintenance of skeletal structure and systemic mineral homeostasis.

Under normal physiologic conditions, bone cells along with the cells in the kidney, intestine, parathyroid, sex glands, and neuroendocrine system, act in concerted fashion to maintain normal bone density, ion homeostasis, and overall endocrine balance. Numerous pathologic conditions can disrupt the physiologic balance of these highly regulated activities and lead to functional disruption of multiple organ systems. These disruptions can result from genetic diseases, organ failure, endocrine malfunction, inactivity, or malignancy. For example, the hypercalcemia often accompanying certain malignancies can usually be traced to the ectopic production of parathyroid hormone–related protein by tumor cells, which affects multiple organ systems and results in net calcium increases in tissue fluids and serum. Tumor cells, when translocated to the rich environment of bone matrix, can disrupt the local balance of bone remodeling by secretion of various cytokines and growth factors that modify the balance between osteoblastic and osteoclastic activity. This local secretion by tumor cells and the effect this has on tumor cell–mesenchymal cell interactions are responsible for the osteoblastic and osteolytic responses seen after bone metastasis of prostate and breast cancer cells, respectively.

INTERACTIONS BETWEEN BONE MATRIX AND HUMAN PROSTATE CANCER

The composition and architecture of bone provides a uniquely rich environment to support the proliferation of prostatic metastases. The molecular scaffold of bone consists of fibrils of type I collagen, which on a protein basis constitutes approximately 90% of the organic matrix. Collagen fibrils may be found arranged in a highly ordered array, as in lamellar bone, or in a more haphazard form, as in woven bone. In the human adult, except in certain sites such as those of tendon or tooth insertion, the detection of randomly ordered woven bone generally indicates a pathologic condition.[74] It is precisely this randomly ordered type of bone that appears during the osteoblastic response characterizing prostate cancer cell invasion of bone.

The remainder of the organic phase of bone consists of noncollagenous matrix proteins, serum-derived globular proteins, and sequestered growth factors. The impact of this diverse milieu of proteins on prostatic cancer cell growth and differentiation at sites of skeletal metastases is under study.

Our laboratories have begun to evaluate the properties of individual components of bone matrix on prostatic cancer growth in vitro. As shown in Figure 40-1, two subfractions obtained from demineralized long bone by ion-exchange column chromatography,[20] called ES1-D3 and ES1-D4, increased growth of prostatic cells cultured in soft agar (Fig. 40-2); fractions ES2, ES1-D1, ES1-D2, and ES1-D5 did not have this effect. Analysis of the molecular composition of these demineralized bone fractions indicates that the primary components of the active fractions are the noncollagenous matrix proteins osteonectin and bone sialoprotein. The strongest activity is associated with osteopontin (ESI-D3 and D4), and antibodies specifically directed against osteopontin significantly block the activity of ES1-D4 in human bone stromal cell–conditioned medium (Fig. 40-3). Inactive fractions contain, among other proteins, the matrix proteins osteocalcin (ES2), soluble collagen (ES1-D1), serum-derived α_2-HS-glycoprotein (ES1-D2), and the small bone proteoglycans decorin and biglycan (ES1-D5). These results suggest that specific bone matrix proteins may be responsible for inducing prostate cancer growth and progression when cancer cells are disseminated to the bone.

The relevance of osteopontin to human prostate cancer is an exciting area for further study. The demonstration that osteopontin is expressed at low levels by androgen-dependent prostate cancer cells and at higher levels by androgen-independent lines (Thalmann and colleagues, unpublished observation) hints that this noncollagenous matrix protein may play a facilitory role in prostate cancer progression. The regulation of osteopontin expression by the steroid hormone, 1,25-dihydroxyvitamin D_3, provides the opportunity of developing therapeutic compounds that alter the course of cancer progression by interfering with cellular proliferation. Analogs of 1,25-dihydroxyvitamin D_3 that regulate the genome without producing hypercalcemia are available[19] and are being rigorously evaluated for cancer therapy alone and in combination with tumoricidal drugs. Gene therapies that target osteopontin or other autocrine or paracrine growth factors may soon provide useful therapeutic, alternatives to current therapies.

The noncollagenous components of bone and what is known of their structures and functions were reviewed by Young and colleagues.[83] Osteonectin, also called SPARC or BM-40, coisolates in our fractionation protocol in fraction ES1-D3 with a number of other uncharacterized components, although some evidence exists that vitronectin is in this fraction (unpublished results). Osteonectin is a calcium-binding, acidic, cysteine-rich protein expressed in several normal tissues, including bone, endothelium, platelets, tendon, cartilage, placenta, ovary, testis, lung, and adrenal gland. It demonstrates a highly variable distribution in tumor cell lines, and the message encoding osteonectin is generally absent in transformed cells. Osteonectin complexes with thrombospondin[12] and may alone or in complex be involved in regulating tumor angiogenesis. It remains to be investigated whether osteonectin is the active component in ES1-D3 that stimulates prostatic cancer cell growth.

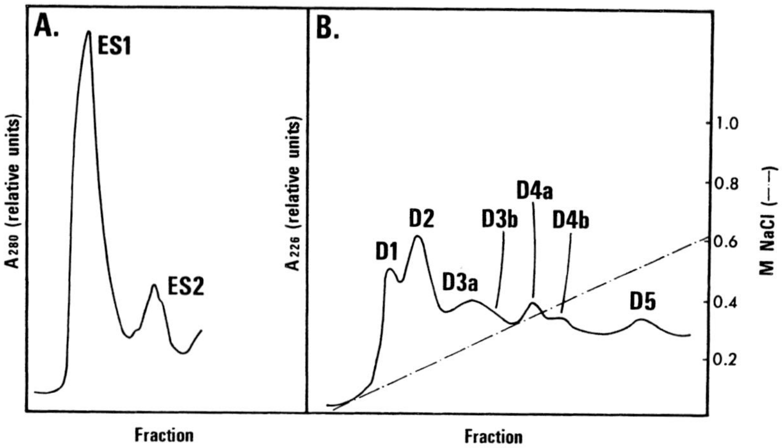

FIG. 40-1. (A) Ion-exchange column chromatography separation of bone protein fractions. **(B)** The ES1 fraction from a molecular sieving column was further eluted by a NaCl gradient, which produced the fractions designated as D1 to D5.

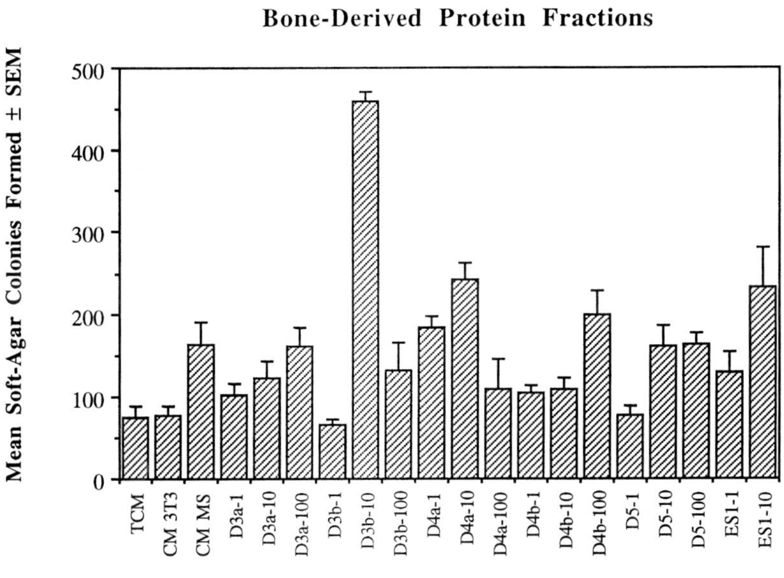

FIG. 40-2. Protein fractions isolated from the demineralized rat long bone stimulated prostatic anchorage-independent growth (AIG). Fraction D3 and D4, but not ES2, ES1-D1, D2, and D5, stimulated prostatic AIG, an activity that parallels prostatic cancer growth in vivo.

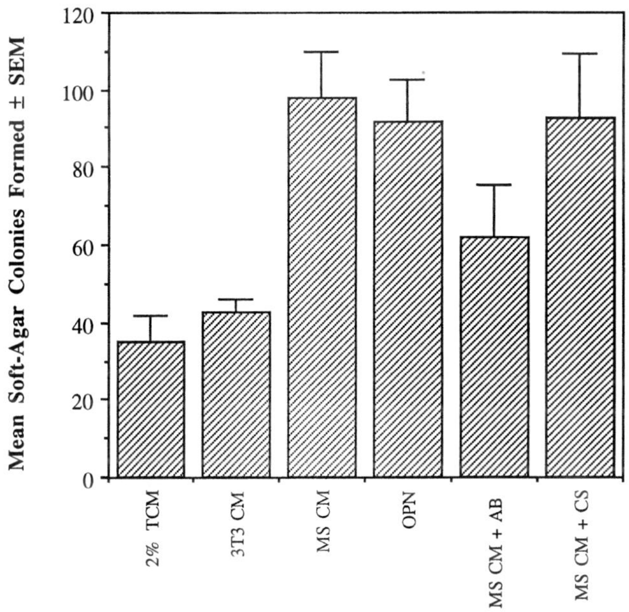

FIG. 40-3. Osteopontin (OPN)–antibody inhibition of paracrine activity derived from bone stroma (MS) conditioned medium. OPN serves as a paracrine factor for the growth of prostate cancer cells. Bone stromal cell–conditioned medium contains prostate cancer cell anchorage-independent growth-stimulating activity, which can be mimicked by OPN and blocked by an OPN antibody.

Osteopontin and bone sialoprotein are cell attachment proteins that contain an Arg-Gly-Asp (RGD) motif, through which they interact with the integrin $\alpha v \beta_3$ on osteoclasts and other cell types.[61] These proteins, however, have dissimilar structures, genes, and regulatory mechanisms controlling their transcription.[9] In our fractionation protocol, osteopontin elutes ahead of bone sialoprotein in the fraction ES1-D4, and we have found rechromatography using a shallow gradient to be a useful means of resolving the two proteins into two distinct subfractions D4a (i.e., osteopontin) and D4b (i.e., bone sialoprotein). Because D4a has significantly higher activity in stimulating prostate cancer cell growth and because antibodies to osteopontin block most of the growth-stimulating activity (see Figs. 40-2, 40-3), we think that osteopontin and not bone sialoprotein is the active component.

Osteopontin is an acidic, phosphorylated glycoprotein with a limited distribution in normal tissues. The primary sites of synthesis appear to be bone cells, including osteoblasts and some osteoclasts. Additional sites of apparently normal expression include kidney cells, trophoblast cells, and odontoblasts.[9] An interesting feature of the expression of osteopontin is its appearance in numerous cells and cell lines after transformation or treatment with tumor-promoting agents. Several laboratories have hypothesized that osteopontin expression is correlated with and may even serve as a molecular marker of tumorigenicity.[63,15] We have performed several immunohistochemical studies using antibodies specific for osteopontin and determined that osteopontin is expressed in prostate cancer cells at the site of the primary tumor and at sites of skeletal metastases.[17] Combined with our findings that ES1-D4 (i.e., osteopontin) stimulates the growth of prostate cancer cells in vitro, we hypothesize that osteopontin plays a role in neoplasia of the prostate. We are vigorously pursing studies to determine whether osteopontin in bone matrix is involved in the adhesion of prostate cancer cells to bone, acts as a local regulator of prostate cancer cell growth and differentiation, or serves as an angiogenic and immune modulator during tumor growth and metastasis.

ANIMAL MODELS FOR HUMAN PROSTATE CANCER OSSEOUS METASTASIS

Unlike other forms of solid tumors, human prostate cancer synthesizes and secretes a tissue specific marker, PSA, that can be detected conveniently in serum. Unfortunately, most of the human prostate cancer cell lines, once established from solid tumors in vitro, failed to synthesize and secrete PSA. Although several transplantable human prostate cancer xenographs have been established in vivo[47,32,39] and some of the tumors synthesize and secrete PSA.[32] These tumor xenographs appear unstable and have difficulty maintaining their differentiated state (e.g., expression of PSA) as cell culture lines.

In 1983, Horozewicz and colleagues[32a] established a prostate cancer cell line from a man with lymph node metastasis. This cell line, LNCaP, synthesizes and secretes PSA in cell culture and responds positively to androgen-induced growth and PSA production. Initially, the LNCaP cell line was capable of forming tumors in vivo. However, after serial passage of this cell line in culture, LNCaP cells failed to form tumors when inoculated subcutaneously. The tumor-forming activity of LNCaP cells can be promoted by coinoculating LNCaP cells with specific soluble growth factors,[29] Matrigel,[56a] or prostate or bone fibroblasts,[29] or by injecting them orthotopically.[29a,70a] After LNCaP cells form a tumor in vivo, the tumor progresses in a castrated host and eventually escapes androgen regulation, becomes progressively androgen independent, and acquires the ability to metastasize.

We observed that an androgen-independent LNCaP subline, C4-2, forms tumors in the primary site, invades seminal vesicles, metastasizes to the lymph nodes and the bone, and elicits marked osteoblastic reaction in the bone (Fig. 40-4). Scheme 1 indicates the effort made by our laboratory in generating LNCaP sublines, which progress from androgen-dependent to androgen-independent and acquire metastatic potential. These sublines were derived through cell-cell interactions, with LNCaP cells interacting with a human bone stromal cell line. We began with a nontumorigenic parental LNCaP cell line that can form tumors when coinoculated with a human bone stromal cell line, MS. The chimeric tumors formed in the castrated hosts are predominantly angiogenic carcinomas. The tumors, when maintained in castrated host initially, have decreased PSA synthesis and secretion. Tumors, maintained in the castrated host for several weeks begin to synthesize and secrete PSA in the absence of testicular androgen. From tumors maintained in the castrated host, we establish LNCaP sublines, C4 and C5, which acquire the ability to grow in the castrated host provided the sublines are coinoculated with the bone stromal cell line, MS.

From the chimeric C4 tumors grown in the castrated host, we generated another LNCaP subline, C4-2 (indicating the passages of parental LNCaP cell line in vivo in the castrated host twice), which acquired the ability to grow in the castrated host and to metastasize to osseous sites when administered alone orthotopically or subcutaneously to intact and castrated hosts.[74a] This observation demonstrated for the first time that a nontumorigenic LNCaP cell line can be promoted through in vivo cellular interaction with bone stromal cells and in vitro subculture to acquire the ability to metastasize to the bone. Subsequently, we[74a] generated additional bone-derived C4-2 cell lines (i.e., derived from C4-2 bony metastases) that acquired additional behavioral changes, forming tumor more efficiently and metastasizing to bone faster on subcutaneous administration. This series of C4-2 bone metastasis–derived LNCaP sublines

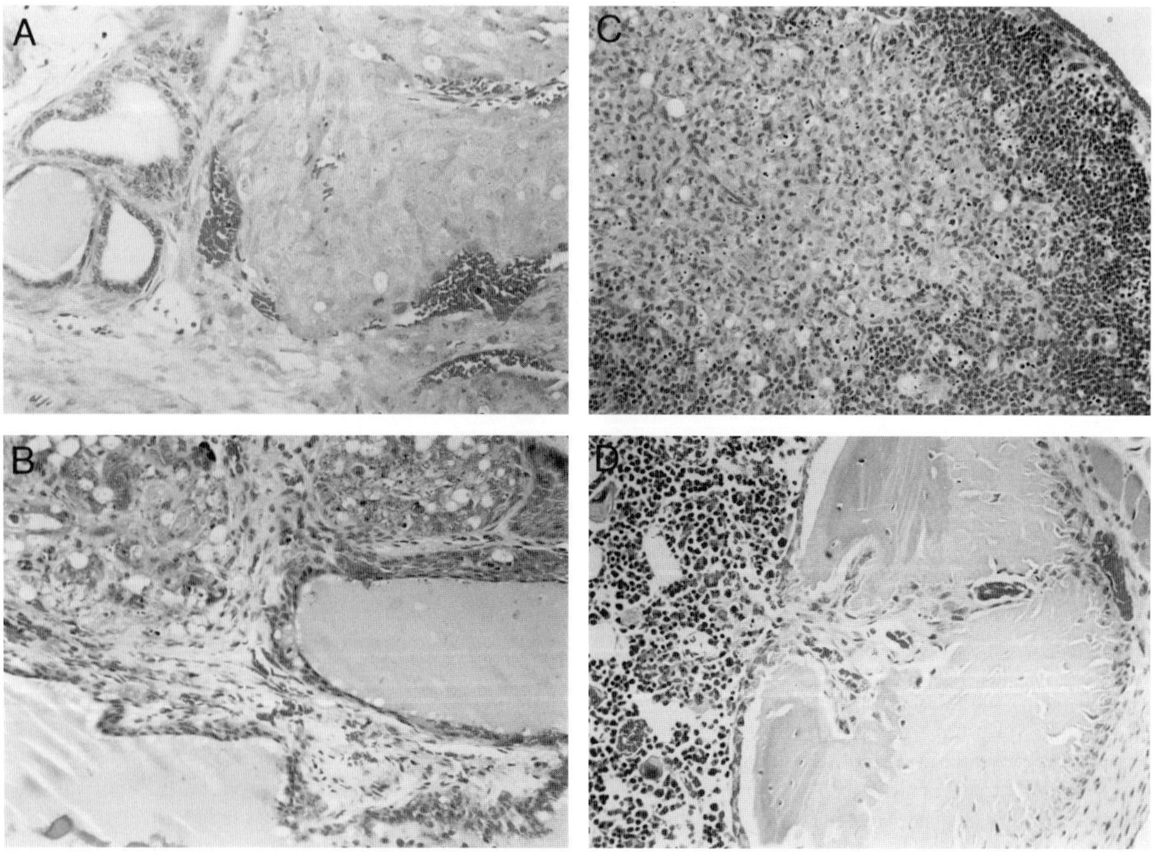

FIG. 40-4. LNCaP C4-2 human prostate cancer metastatic model. **(A)** The C4-2 cells formed an angiogenic tumor at the primary site. **(B)** The tumor invaded seminal vesicles, and **(C)** it metastasized to the lymph node and **(D)** the bone, where a marked osteoblastic response was observed.

apparently acquired further invasive and malignant potential under the experimental conditions.

These findings have important implications. First, cancer may not be a single-cell disease. Genetic alterations in cancer epithelial cells alone may be necessary but not sufficient to form solid tumors in the host without appropriate intercellular interactions with organ-specific fibroblasts. Second, cancer epithelial cells may acquire additional genetic changes through cell-cell interactions with the host organ microenvironment, including cancer-stromal interaction at the primary and metastatic sites. The resultant genetic and epigenetic alterations of the cancer epithelial cells and host microenvironment interaction with the cancer epithelium may account for the acquisition of additional malignant and metastatic potential. These behavioral changes probably are the acquired phenotype rather than preexisting in the parental LNCaP population. Third, chimeric tumors maintained in the castrated host facilitates the progression to androgen independence. C4-2 cells, when administered to a castrated host, produces more bone metastasis than cells administered to the intact host, suggesting that the castrated microenvironment may allow the selection of or the adaptive response for more aggressive androgen-independent cell clones.[74a] The adaptive microenvironment of the host may allow cancer epithelial cells to express androgen-repressed genes that may be associated with increasing malignant status of the cancer cells.

The cell-cell interaction model described by our study may be applicable to other solid tumors in which it is conceivable that organ-specific fibroblasts may also be capable of promoting tumor progression. The resulting cell lines generated through cell-cell interactions could have practical utility as models for studying mechanisms of cancer invasion and metastasis and could be attractive models for determining the efficacy of chemotherapy agents. In our osseous metastatic human prostate cancer model, we observed that bone fibroblasts can induce a human prostate cancer cell line, LNCaP, to acquire additional malignant and metastatic potential, suggesting that bone-prostate interactions may be responsible for an acquired androgen-independent phenotype of prostate cancer cells. This model system may allow the study of mechanisms of acquisition of androgen independence and increased malignant and metastatic potential of human prostate cancer cells. A strength of the model is that it permits the evaluation of specific matrix-bound or soluble factors in cancer progression and metastasis. This model may also allow the development of novel therapeutics and further molecular approaches for prevention and treatment of human prostate cancer.

ACKNOWLEDGMENTS

Dr. Anezinis was the first to make the observation that the C4-2 cell line, when administered subcutaneously or orthotopically to athymic mice, acquired the ability to metastasize to the bone. This model system of human prostate cancer osseous metastasis was characterized in detail by Dr. Thalmann. Drs. Devoll and Thalmann made significant contributions in defining the bone components that support prostate cancer growth. Drs. Anezinis, Thallmann, and Devoll are considered the first authors of this chapter. Dr. William T. Butler has developed the methodology for fractionation and characterization of the bone fractions. The authors wish to acknowledge Carolyn Davis for typing this manuscript and the financial support from NIH grant CA64863 and a grant from CaP CURE Foundation to Dr. Chung.

REFERENCES

1. Arnheim FK. Carcinoma of the prostate: a study of postmortem findings on one hundred and seventy-six cases. J Urol 1948;60:599.
2. Bachman AL, Sproul EE. Correlation of radiographic and autopsy findings in suspected metastases in the spine. Bull NY Acad Med 1955; 31:146.
3. Batson OV. The function of the vertebral veins and their role in the spread of metastases. Ann Surg 1940;112:138.
4. Belliveau RE, Spencer RP. Incidence and site of bone lesions detected by ^{99m}Tc polyphosphate scans in patients with tumors. Cancer 1975; 36:359.
5. Benson RC Jr, et al. External beam radiotherapy for palliation of pain from metastatic carcinoma of the prostate. J Urol 1982;127:69.
6. Berner A, Nesland JM, Awaehre H, Silde J, Fossa SD. Hormone resistant prostatic adenocarcinoma: an evaluation of prognostic factors in pre- and posttreatment specimens. Br J Urol 1993;68:380.
7. Boskey AL. Noncollagenous matrix proteins and their roles in mineralization. Bone Miner 1989;6:111.
8. Bumpus HC. Carcinoma of the prostate. Surg Gynecol Obstet 1926; 43:150.
9. Butler WT. The nature and significance of osteopontin Connec Tissue Res 1989;23:123.
10. Byar DP. VACURG studies on prostatic cancer and its treatment. In: Tannenbaum M, ed. Urologic pathology; the prostate. New York; Lea & Febiger, 1977:241.
11. Clain A. Secondary malignant disease of bone. Br J Cancer 1965;19: 15.
12. Clezardin P, et al. Complex formation of human thrombospondin with osteonectin. Eur J Biochem 1988;175:275.
13. Conroy T, Malissard L, Dartois D, Luporsi E, Stines J, Chardot C. Histoire naturelle et evolution des metastases osseuses; a propos de 429 observations. Bull Cancer 1988;75:845.
14. Corriere JN, Cornag JL, Murphy JJ. Prognosis in patients with carcinoma of the prostate. Cancer 1970;25:911.
15. Craig AM, Nemir M, Mukherjee BB, Chambers AF, Denhardt DT. Identification of the major phosphoprotein secreted by many rodent cell lines as 2AR/osteopontin: enhanced expression in H-ras transformed 3T3 cells. Biochem Biophys Res Commun 1988;157:166.
16. Cumming J, Hacking N, Fairhurst J, Ackery D, Jenkins JD. Distribution of bony metastasis in prostatic carcinoma. Br J Urol 1990;66:411.
17. Devoll RE, Pinero GJ, Appelbaum ER, et al. Improved immunohistochemical staining of Osteopontin in paraffin embedded archival bone specimens following antigen retrieval: anti–human OPN antibody recognizes multiple molecular forms. Calcified Tissue Int (in press).
18. Elkins M, Mueller HP. Metastases from cancer of the prostate: autopsy and roentgenological findings. Cancer 1954;7:1246.
19. Farach-Carson MC, Sergeev I, Norman AW. Nongenomic actions of 1,25-dihydroxyvitamin D_3 in rat osteosarcoma cells: structure-function studies using ligand analogs. Endocrinology 1991;129:1876.
20. Farach-Carson MC, Wright GC, Butler WT. Improved binding of acidic bone matrix proteins to cationized filters during solid phase assays. Bone Miner 1992;16:1.
21. Flynn DF, et al. Management of spinal cord compression secondary to metastatic prostatic carcinoma. Urol Clin North Am 1991;18:145.
22. Franks LM. The spread of prostatic cancer. J Pathol Bacteriol 1956; 72:603.
23. Franks LM. The spread of prostatic carcinoma to the bones. J Pathol Bacteriol 1953;66:91.
24. Galasko CSB. Mechanisms of bone destruction in the development of skeletal metastases. Nature 1976;263:507.
25. Galasko CSB. The mechanisms of uptake of bone-seeking isotopes by skeletal metastases. In: Medical radionmucleotide imaging. Vienna: International Atomic Energy Agency 1977:125.
26. Galasko CSB. The pathophysiological basis for skeletal scintigraphy. In: Galasko CSB, Weber DA, eds. Radionuclide scintigraphy in orthopedics. Edinburgh: Churchill Livingstone, 1984:34.
27. George NJR. Natural history of localized prostatic cancer managed by conservative therapy alone. Lancet 1988;1:494.

28. Gervasi LA, Mata J, Easley JD, et al. Prognostic significance of lymph node metastases in prostatic cancer. J Urol 1989;142:332.
29. Gleave ME, et al. Acceleration of human prostate cancer growth in vivo by prostate and bone fibroblasts. Cancer Res 1991;51:3753.
29a. Gleave ME, et al. Prostate and bone fibroblasts induce human prostate cancer growth in vivo: implications for bidirectional stromal-epithelial interactions in prostate carcinoma growth and metastasis. J Urol 1992; 147:1151.
30. Harada M, Iida MI, Yamaguchi M, Shida K. Analysis of bone metastasis of prostatic adenocarcinoma in 137 autopsy cases. Adv Exp Med Biol 1992;324:173.
31. Harper ME, Pierrepoint CG, Griffiths K. Carcinoma of the prostate: relationship of pretreatment hormone levels and survival. Eur J Cancer Clin Oncol 1984;20:477.
32. Hoehn W, Schroeder FH, Rieman JF, Joebis AC, Hermanek P. Human prostatic adenocarcinoma: some characteristics of a serially transplanted line in nude mice (PC-82). Prostate 1980;1:95.
32a. Horoszewicz JS, et al. LNCaP model of human prostate carcinoma. Cancer Res 1983;43:1809.
33. Hruska KA, Rolnick F, Duncan RL, Medhora M, Yamakawa K. Signal transduction in osteoblasts and osteoblasts. In Noda M, ed. Cellular and molecular biology of bone, New York: Academic Press, 1993.
34. Hsieh JT, Lin SW. Androgen regulation of cell adhesion molecule gene expression on rat prostate during organ degeneration. J Biol Chem 1994;269:3711.
35. Huggins CB. Influence of urinary tract mucosa on the experimental formation of bone. Proc Soc Exp Biol Med 1930;27:349.
36. Huggins S. Prostatic cancer treated by orchiectomy: the five year results. JAMA 1946;131:576.
37. Iacovou JW, et al. Cord compression and carcinoma of the prostate: is laminectomy justified? Br J Urol 1985;57:733.
38. Ishikawa S, Soloway MS, van der Zwaag R, Todd B. Prognostic factors in survival free of progression after androgen deprivation therapy for treatment of prostate cancer. J Urol 1989;141:1139.
39. Ito YZ, Nakazato Y. A new serially transplantable human prostate cancer (HONDA) in nude mice. J Urol 1984;132:384.
40. Jacobs SC. Spread of prostatic cancer to bone. Urology 1983;21:337.
41. Jameson RM. Paraplegia and prostatic cancer. Eur Urol 1983;9:267.
42. Johnson DE, Lanieri JP, Ayala AG. Prostatic adenocarcinoma occurring in men under 50 years of age. J Surg Oncol 1972;4:207.
43. Jorgens J. The radiographic characteristics of carcinoma of the prostate. Surg Clin North Am 1965;45:1427.
44. Kelley JM, Chung LWK, Devoll RE, et al. OPN expression in prostate cancer cell lines. J Dent Res 1995;74:180.
45. Krishmamurthy GT, et al. Distribution patterns of metastatic bone disease: a need for total body skeletal imaging. JAMA 1977;237:2504.
46. Kuban DA, et al. Characteristics of spinal cord compression in adenocarcinoma of prostate. Urology 1986;28:364.
47. Loop SM, Rozanski TA, Ostenson RC. Human primary prostate tumor cell line, ALVA-31: a new model for studying the hormonal regulation of prostate tumor cell growth. Prostate 1993;22:93.
48. McCrea LE, Karafin L. Carcinoma of the prostate: metastasis, therapy, and survival. A statistical analysis of 500 cases. Int Coll Surg J 1958; 29:723.
49. Mintz ER, Smith GG. Autopsy findings in 100 cases of prostatic cancer. N Engl J Med 1934;211:479.
50. Mulders PFA, et al. Analysis of prognostic factors in disseminated prostatic cancer. Cancer 1990;65:2758.
51. Murphy GP, et al. The national survey of prostate cancer in the United States by the American College of Surgeons. J Urol 1982;127:928.
52. Murray RO, et al. The radiology of skeletal disorders: exercises in diagnosis, 2nd ed, vol 1. Edinburgh: Churchill Livingstone, 1977:536.
53. Nade S. Bone-graft surgery reappraised: the contribution of the cell to ultimate success. Br J Surg 1970;57:752.
54. Nesbit RM, Baum WC. Endocrine control of prostatic carcinoma. JAMA 1950;143:1317.
55. Nesbit RM, Plumb RT. Prostatic carcinoma: a follow-up of 795 patients treated prior to the endocrine era and a comparison of survival rates between these and patients treated by endocrine therapy. Surgery 1946; 20:263.
56. Pollen JJ, Gerber K, Ashburn WL, Schmidt JD. Nuclear bone imaging in metastatic cancer of the prostate. Cancer 1981;47:2585.
56a. Pretlow TG, et al. Transplantation of human prostate carcinoma into nude mice in matrigel. Cancer Res 1991;51:3814.
57. Rana A, Chisholm GD, Khan M et al. Patterns of bone metastasis and their prognostic significance in patients with carcinoma or the prostate. Br J Urol 1993;72:933.
58. Rinker-Schaeffer CW, et al. Molecular and cellular markers for metastatic prostate cancer. Cancer Metastasis Rev 1993;12:3.
59. Robinson MRG, Thomas BS. Effect of hormonal therapy on plasma testosterone levels in prostatic carcinoma. Br Med J 1971;4:391.
60. Robinson MRG, Thomas BS. Effect of hormonal therapy on plasma testosterone levels in prostatic carcinoma. Br Med J 1971;4:391.
61. Ross FP, Chappel J, Alvarez JI, et al. Interactions between the bone matrix proteins osteopontin and bone sialoprotein and the osteoclast integrin $\alpha v\beta_3$ potentiate bone resorption. J Biol Chem 1993;268:9901.
62. Saitoh H, Hida M, Shimbo T, Makamura K, Yamagata J, Satoh H. Metastatic patterns of prostatic cancer. 1984;54:3078.
63. Senger DR, Perruzzi CA, Papadopoulos. Elevated expression of secreted phosphoprotein I (osteopontin, 2dr) as a consequence of neoplastic transformation. Anticancer Res 1989.
64. Shih WJ, Wierzbinski B, Collins J, et al. Serum osteocalcin measurements in prostate carcinoma patients with skeletal deposits shown by bone scintigram: comparison with serum PSA/PAP measurements. J Nucl Med 1989;31:1486.
65. Slack NH, Kan JP, Chu TM, Murphy GP, and Investigators on the National Prostatic Cancer Project. An assessment of bone scans for monitoring osseous metastases in patients being treated for prostate carcinoma. Prostate 1980;1:259.
66. Slack NH, Lane WW, Priore RL, Murphy GP. Prostatic cancer treated at a categorical center, 1980–1983. Urology 1986;27:205.
67. Smith EM, Hampel N, Ruff RL, Bodner DR, Resnick MI. Spinal cord compression secondary to prostate carcinoma: treatment and prognosis. J Urol 1993;149:330.
68. Smith PH, Bono FA, da Silva FC, et al. Some limitation of the radioisotope bone scan in patients with metastatic prostatic cancer. Cancer 1990;66:1009.
69. Soloway MS, Hardeman SW, Hickey D, et al. Stratification of patients with metastatic prostate cancer based on extent of disease on initial bone scan. Cancer 1988;61:195.
70. Sorenson PS, Borgesen SE, Rohde K, et al. Metastatic epidural spinal cord compression. Cancer 1990;65:1502.
70a. Stephenson RA, et al. Metastatic model for human prostate cancer using orthotopic implantation in nude mice. J Natl Cancer Inst 1992; 52:987.
71. Stewler GJ, Nissenson RA. Parathyroid hormone–related protein. In: Farus MJ, ed. Primer on the metabolic bone diseases and disorders of mineral metabolism. New York: Raven Press, 1993:61.
72. Surya BV, Provet JA. Manifestations of advanced prostate cancer: prognosis and treatment. J Urol 1989;142:921.
73. Suzuki T, Shimizu T, Kurokawa K, et al. Pattern of prostate cancer metastasis to the vertebral column. Prostate 1994;25:141.
74. Teitelbaum SL. Skeletal growth and development. In: Favus MJ, ed. Primer on the metabolic bone diseases and disorders of mineral metabolism. Richmond, VA: William Byrd Press, 1990.
74a. Thalmann GN, et al. Androgen-independent cancer progression and bone metastasis in the LNCaP model of human prostate cancer. Cancer Res 1994;54:2577.
75. Tofe AJ, et al. Correlation of neoplasms with incidence and localization of skeletal metastases. J Nucl Med 1975;16:986.
76. Urist MR, Iwata H, Ceccotti PL, et al. Bone morphogenesis in implants of insoluble bone gelatin. Proc Natl Acad Sci U S A 1973;70:3511.
77. Whitmore WF Jr. Natural history and staging of prostate cancer. Urol Clin North Am 1984;11:205.
78. Whitmore WF Jr. Natural history of low-stage prostatic cancer and the impact of early detection. Urol Clin North Am 1990;17:689.
79. Willis RA. Secondary tumors of bones. In: The spread of tumors in the human body, 3rd ed. London: Butterworth, 1973:229.
80. Wright RL. Malignant tumors in the spinal extradural space: results of surgical treatment. Ann Surg 1963;157:227.
81. Yagoda A, Petrylak D. Cytotoxic chemotherapy for advanced hormone-resistant prostate cancer. Cancer 1993;71(Suppl 3):1098.
82. Yoneda T. Cytokines in bone: local translators in cell-to-cell communications. In: Noda M, ed. Cellular and molecular biology of bone. New York: Academic Press, 1993:376.
83. Young MF, et al. Molecular and cellular biology of the major noncollagenous proteins in the bone. In: Noda M, ed. Cellular and molecular biology of bone. New York: Academic Press, 1993:192.

Principles and Practice of Genitourinary Oncology, edited by Derek Raghavan, Howard I. Scher, Steven A. Leibel, and Paul H. Lange. Lippincott-Raven Publishers, Philadelphia, © 1997.

CHAPTER 41

Tumor Markers in Prostate Cancer

Paul H. Lange

The tumor markers of prostate cancer are the most important in all of genitourinary cancer. This is because acid phosphatase was one of the earliest tumor markers in oncology, and for half a century prostatic acid phosphatase was the gold standard as a tumor marker for prostate cancer. However, for many reasons, there were too many false-positive and false-negative results, and the use of this marker was limited. Acid phosphatase has now been all but replaced by another prostatic enzyme, prostatic-specific antigen (PSA), which is much more exclusively produced by prostatic tissue. During the past 10 years, PSA has become indispensable for management of prostate cancer, and it is probably the best tumor marker in all of human oncology.

This chapter briefly describes (1) the principles of tumor markers and their nomenclature; (2) the biology and clinical application of PSA, acid phosphatase, and other tumor markers; and (3) the future of tumor markers in prostate cancer. Additional information about prostate cancer tumor markers, especially PSA, is contained in the other chapters on prostate cancer.

PRINCIPLES OF TUMOR MARKERS

The performance of tumor markers, especially prostate cancer markers, is evaluated by measuring sensitivity, specificity, positive predictive value, and, in rare cases, negative predictive value. Sensitivity is the number of patients designated positive by the test among all men who have the disease (i.e., prostate cancer). Specificity is the number designated negative by the test among all men without the disease. Positive predictive value is the probability that the patient actually has the disease if the test is positive, and the negative predictive value is the probability that the patient does not have the disease if the test is negative. The equations for these terms are given in Table 41-1. The letters a, b, c, and d represent true-positive, false-positive, true-negative, and false-negative results, respectively.[1,2]

The terms just defined are not applied in strictly proper fashion in all studies of markers in prostate cancer. For example, the predictive value of a test is greatly influenced by the prevalence (the rate of occurrence of the disease in the population at a given time). If the study sample is not representative of the population as a whole, the value will not be accurate. However, predictive values can be calculated from sensitivities and specificities that are obtained from populations that are already known clinically to have or not have the disease. The following formula is used:

$$\frac{SP}{SP + (1 - S)(1 - P)}$$

where S is the sensitivity and P is the prevalence.

Also, in prostate cancer the prevalence of the disease (and thus the denominator in calculations of sensitivity and specificity) is usually arbitrarily defined. Autopsy studies show the actual prevalence of prostate cancer to be about 30%, but most of these lesions are innocuous and should not and usually cannot be detected clinically because they are so small. Operationally, almost all studies define patients with prostate cancer as those who have a positive biopsy result and patients without the disease as those who have a negative biopsy result or who do not appear to have the disease on digital rectal examination or serum PSA determination. However, these tests are not totally accurate. Assuming that transrectal ultrasonography (TRUS) and biopsy are at least somewhat reliable (see later discussion), the most meaningful parameter in most large-scale prostate cancer tumor marker studies is the positive predictive value.[3]

The ideal tumor marker would be produced reliably by a specific malignancy, be 100% sensitive in its detection, and be 100% specific for that disease. (In prostate cancer, this last ideal would actually be undesirable, because most prostate cancers discovered at autopsy cause no harm.) Also, an ideal marker would be measurable by an easy, reproducible, and inexpensive test. It measurable extent or intensity would be detectable at early stages of the disease and would increase linearly with tumor volume, thereby allowing for direct correlation with the disease course. Finally, the ideal tumor marker would have a relatively short halflife, so that therapeutic interventions could be assessed accurately and quickly. Obviously, the ideal tumor marker does not exist, although PSA in prostate cancer may be as close to the ideal as has been achieved in human oncology.[3]

PROSTATE-SPECIFIC ANTIGEN

PSA was discovered by many people independently and was initially given a variety of names. In 1971, Hara identified a

TABLE 41-1. *Equations for sensitivity, specificity, positive and negative predictive values, and overall accuracy*

Test outcome	Disease-present	Disease-absent
Positive	a	b
Negative	c	d
Total	(a + c)	(b + d)

Sensitivity $= \frac{a}{a + c}$

Specificity $= \frac{d}{b + d}$

Positive predictive value $= \frac{a}{a + b}$

Negative predictive value $= \frac{d}{d + c}$

Overall accuracy $= \frac{a + d}{a + b + c + d}$

substance in human seminal plasma and called it gamma seminal protein. In 1993, Li and Beling characterized the substance and called it protein E[1] antigen. In 1970, Sensabaugh further characterized a semen-specific substance of molecular weight 30,000 and called it P30; later, both he and Graves showed it to be an excellent marker for semen identification and therefore useful in rape cases. Finally, in a series of studies from the laboratory of Chung and associates, this protein was further characterized and was found to be exclusive to prostatic tissue, distinct from acid phosphatase, and present in human sera. They called this protein prostate-specific antigen and presented preliminary evidence that its measurement in serum was useful clinically.[4,5]

A great deal of information about the biology and biochemistry of PSA has accumulated. It is a single-chain glycoprotein of 237 amino acids, with an overall molecular weight of 34,000. The antigenic domain and its three-dimensional structure have been characterized. The gene encoding PSA has been sequenced and localizes to chromosome 19. The PSA gene and protein structure are similar to those of other kallikreins, most notably human glandular kallikrein-2, which is a substance also preferentially located in prostate tissue. Unlike the glandular kallikreins, which are trypsin-like proteases, the enzymatic activity of PSA is chymotrypsin-like; that is, it slowly hydrolyzes peptide bonds behind certain tyrosines and leucine residues. PSA is a proteolytic enzyme belonging to the group of extracellular serine proteases and, like most such enzymes, has a precursor form (or zymogen), whose identity is still unknown. The inactivation of PSA in the prostate is also not yet fully understood, but in the serum it is inactivated by a variety of substances (see later discussion).[5,6]

Physiologically, PSA is secreted into the lumen of the prostate ducts and is present in high concentrations (approximately 2 mg/mL) in the seminal plasma. PSA enzymatically cleaves the major sperm-entrapping gel proteins produced by the seminal vesicle (semenogelin I and II and fibronectin), thereby liquefying the seminal coagulum. Somewhat similar biochemical and functional proteins are found within the semen of other species, but their exact characterization is incomplete.[6]

Histologically, PSA is produced by the epithelial cells that line the acini and ducts of the prostate gland. Immunohistochemical studies have shown PSA to be present in normal prostatic tissue, in benign prostatic hypertrophy (BPH), and in prostate cancer, both within the prostate and in metastases. It appears that the concentration of PSA within the cells is greatest in normal prostate, less in BPH, and significantly reduced in prostate cancer. The content of PSA in prostate cancer seems inversely proportional to histologic grade.[7] Formally, it was thought that PSA was produced exclusively by prostate tissue; now it is known that PSA is also produced by periurethral glands and probably by other glands of cloacal origin, including residual glands in females.[7–9] In addition, PSA seems to be produced under certain conditions by other tissues in very small amounts, most notably by some breast cancers.[10] To date, production of PSA by nonprostatic sources has not interfered with its value as a serum marker. For practical purposes, PSA can be considered to be histologically exclusive to the prostate.

PSA is present in the serum of all postpubescent men who have a prostate. In general, the serum concentration is greater in patients who have BPH and even higher in patients with prostate cancer although, as previously stated, the PSA concentration within the cell seems to be less in both cancer and BPH than it is in normal prostate. The reason for this difference in serum levels is not known but may be related to perturbations of the basement membrane. For practical purposes PSA can be conceived to ''leak'' out of the prostate cell more in BPH than in normal tissue, and more in cancer than in BPH. Of course, there is great variability in this process.[4,10,11]

Once PSA is in the serum, it, like all serine proteases, is inactivated and complexed. Two of the major complexing proteins are α_2-macroglobulin and α_1-antichymotrypsin. The PSA bound by α_2-macroglobulin is so enveloped that there are no PSA epitopes detectable by current antibodies. About 40% of PSA is so bound. The remaining PSA is either bound to α_1-antichymotrypsin or exists in a free but inactivated form. Because the complex with antichymotrypsin still allows PSA to expose a limited number of antigenic sites, both the complex and the free form are measured by the antibodies in commercial PSA assays, although in somewhat different ways.[5,6] The ratio of antichymotrypsin-bound PSA to free PSA in serum is about 4 : 1, but this may vary significantly between patients with BPH and those with prostate cancer (see later discussion).

As the measurement of serum PSA has increased in popularity, more commercial assays have appeared. Today in the United States, a majority of the information about PSA has been accumulated by three assays: the Tandem-R and Tandem-E monoclonal (MAb) antibody–based PSA assay (Hybritech Inc., San Diego, CA), the Pros-Check polyclonal antibody–based PSA assay (Yang Laboratories, Bellview, WA), and the IMX PSA assay (Abbott Laboratories, Abbott Park, IL), which is based on both polyclonal antibodies and MAbs. Controversy surrounds comparisons of equivalency between these assays. This issue is especially important in a variety of clinical trials, including those concerned with screening and chemoprophylaxis. because changes in serum PSA levels become important as patients are observed over time. A resolution to the problem of equivalency between assays awaits the establishment of an international standard. This development has been hindered by the problem of PSA complexation in the sera (i.e., the variation in the ratio of PSA subtypes, especially among men with BPH), because the various PSA commercial assays differ in how they measure these subtypes.[5] New information about PSA complexation has now emerged, and it seems that experts are coming closer to agreeing on an international standard (T.A. Stamey, M.D., personal communication, February, 1996). Until a standard is developed, the characteristics of the PSA assay being used must be understood, and care must be taken in interchanging results from different assays.

The definition of the normal reference range for PSA is somewhat arbitrary, because all normal mature men have some detectable level of PSA in the serum. Moreover, BPH exists to a varying degree in all aging men, and prostate cancer is found in up to 40% of older men, although it is often unrecognized. The upper limit for the normal range in most studies is 4 ng/mL, as determined by the Tandem-R PSA assay. This value encompasses the 95% confidence levels (two standard deviations) for mean serum PSA measured in a large group of men older than 40 years of age who had no apparent BPH or cancer by clinical criteria.[4] Subsequent studies have shown that, besides being elevated in cancer, serum PSA is minimally elevated (4 to 10 ng/mL) in up to 20% of patients with BPH and is higher than 10 ng/mL in 3% of patients with BPH. Elevated serum PSA levels are also seen in patients with other nonmalignant perturbations of the prostate, including prostatitis, infarction, and inflammation, and, temporarily, in patients who undergo needle biopsies of the prostate, cystoscopy, or prostatectomy. It is rarely elevated by a routine digital rectal examination, but it can be, and, if possible, phlebotomy for PSA should be performed before digital rectal examination.[12] The halflife of PSA is about 3 days.[4]

PSA does not seem to have the diurnal variation that prostatic acid phosphatase does, and most early studies indicated that serum PSA was fairly stable over time, normally rising only slowly with age, presumably because of the progression of BPH.[13] Yet it is known that the PSA concentration does change with ambulatory status,[14] and recently it was observed that the serum PSA level temporarily changes after ejaculation.[15] Many experts now believe that serum PSA can normally vary somewhat in an individual, in ways that are imperfectly understood. The degree and range of variation require further study but are probably not more than 20%.

Recently, age-adjusted references ranges were determined by taking the 95th percentile for serum PSA levels measured in men who had no evidence of prostate cancer by digital rectal examination or ultrasound.[11] The lower limit in each age group was zero; the upper limit of the range for men in the fifth, sixth, seventh, and eighth decades of life was 2.5, 3.5, 4.5, and 6.5 ng/mL, respectively. The use of these new reference ranges should lead to an increase in cancer detection (increased sensitivity) among young men, who are those most likely to benefit from treatment, and a decrease in unnecessary evaluations (increased specificity) among older men.[11] Other investigators question the wisdom of these new standards, believing that too many curable cancers in older men will be missed and that an increased number of unnecessary evaluations will occur in younger men.[16,17] Until this debate is settled, these new reference standards could at least be useful, along with knowledge about a patient's comorbidity and prostate cancer family history, for determining a course of management.

PSA in Diagnosis

Serum PSA is very useful for diagnosis of prostate cancer, but this fact was not appreciated initially. The reason is that false-positive test results are very common in a screened population, because about 20% of patients with asymptomatic BPH have PSA levels higher than 4 ng/mL. In addition, 20% to 30% of patients with clinical localized prostate cancer who are candidates for radical prostatectomy have so-called normal PSA levels.

Despite the fact that PSA is not cancer-specific, many studies have now shown the utility of PSA for diagnosis. In general, the positive predictive value for prostate cancer in otherwise asymptomatic men is approximately 30%; it is 20% in patients with low-level elevations (i.e., 4 to 10 ng/mL) and 60% in those with PSA levels greater than 10 ng/mL. The positive predictive value in patients with unremarkable digital rectal examination results is also significant, as high as 15% in some series.

PSA is best used with digital rectal examination for optimal diagnosis, both in screened populations and in men referred to urologic practices. In several large series that investigated the use of both PSA and digital rectal examination for diagnosis, about 18% of the cancers would have been missed if digital rectal examination had not been used, and 45% would have been missed if PSA had not been used.[12] Many studies have shown that TRUS adds very little (<5%) unique diagnostic information to that gained when digital rectal examination and PSA are used together. TRUS and biopsy should be used for diagnosis only if there is an abnormality in either PSA or digital rectal examination.[12,18,19]

Results have been promising with PSA alone as well as with PSA and digital rectal examination for diagnosis in both screened and unscreened populations. It would appear that more early (i.e., organ-confined) cancers are discovered with either PSA alone or PSA and DRE than if digital rectal examination is used alone. Catalona and associates[19] found, in their screening trials using PSA, that if cancer was detected in initial screening, the tumor was pathologically organ confined in about 65% of patients, and if it was detected on serial evaluation, it was organ confined in 75%. This is significantly better than the 50% or less that are organ confined if screening is performed with digital rectal examination alone. In addition, there is increasing evidence that the cancers detected by modern diagnostic methods (i.e., PSA with or without digital rectal examination initially and TRUS and biopsy if either is abnormal) are most often significant lesions, as we currently conceptualize that term pathologically. In one example, Epstein and associates[20] defined insignificant tumors as organ-confined tumors in radical prostatectomy specimens that were smaller than 0.5 cc and contained no high-grade disease. Using that definition, more than 75% of even T1C patients (normal digital rectal examination results but elevated PSA results) had significant tumors. Other investigators, using similar criteria, have generally found that more than 85% of the tumors discovered are significant.[21,22]

The success of PSA for diagnosis has increased the controversy about prostate cancer screening (see chapters 46 and 47 on prostate cancer). What can be said here is that the use of PSA in diagnosis makes it evident that the digital rectal examination is not a good single test for diagnosis of prostate cancer, and the addition of PSA increases the number of detected cancers and the proportion that are curable. Proof of the effectiveness of early diagnosis by PSA in improving quality and length of life requires randomized studies, the results of which will take many years. For now, if the object is to detect prostate cancer when it is truly organ confined, the most thorough and yet cost-effective method for achieving this goal is the combined initial use of PSA and digital rectal examination.[23]

Methods to Improve PSA as a Diagnostic Test

Because of the significant overlap in concentration of serum PSA between men with BPH and men with prostate cancer, especially in the low abnormal range of 4 to 10 ng/mL, many investigators have sought ways to enhance the usefulness of PSA for diagnosis. The four main methods are age-specific PSA reference ranges (previously discussed), PSA density (PSAD), PSA velocity (PSAV), and serum PSA binding ratios.

PSAD is the ratio between serum PSA and the volume of all or part of the prostate, as calculated by TRUS (see Chap. 49). Seaman and associates[24] proposed that PSAD is better than serum PSA alone for differentiating BPH from cancer, even among those men with PSA levels between 4 and 10 ng/mL. They proposed that a PSAD greater than 0.15 should be an indication for biopsy in a man with an otherwise normal digital rectal examination and TRUS examination whose serum PSA concentration is between 4 to 10 ng/mL. Others have also demonstrated the applicability of the relation between serum PSA and prostatic size using similar ratios (e.g., PSA to prostate transitional zone volume only) or more complicated formulas.[11]

However, other investigators have not been able to show that PSAD is better than PSA alone in distinguishing between cancer and BPH, even in men with normal digital rectal examination results.[25,26] The reasons are not known, but many theoretic factors limit PSAD as a discriminating tool, including (1) an error margin of at least 10% in determining true prostate volume by TRUS, (2) the variability in normal cellular PSA content with age and between BPH and cancer, and (3) the wide and variable difference (as much as 10%) in PSA content between the stroma and the epithelium of the prostate. Clearly, further studies on the value of PSAD ratios are needed. (PSAD has also been proposed as a better parameter than PSA alone for staging or monitoring response to therapy, but the data to date are not very convincing.)

Another method proposed to increase the usefulness of PSA for diagnosis (and staging) is to determine the rate of change of PSA over time; that is, PSAV. Carter and his colleagues first introduced this concept in a study of 54 men monitored for 7 to 25 years during the Baltimore longitudinal study of aging. They showed that PSAV was greater in men who developed cancer than in those who did not, and that velocity changes were apparent as much as 9 years before diagnosis, even if the PSA values at that time were not abnormal. They proposed that a PSAV of more than 0.75 ng/mL per year (by Tandem-R or IMX PSA assay) is suggestive of prostate cancer. Subsequently, other investigators, using data from screening studies, have verified that a cutoff point of 0.8 ng/mL per year can be used to discriminate between BPH and cancer. Further inquiry by several investigators suggests that for PSAV to be used to predict the presence of cancer, at least three measurements, separated by at least 6 to 12 months, are essential. If serum levels PSA1, PSA2, and PSA3 are measured at Time1, Time2, and Time3 (in years), respectively, an appropriate equation to calculate PSAV would be the following[12]:

$$0.5\left[\left(\text{PSA2} - \frac{\text{PSA1}}{\text{Time1}}\right) + \left(\text{PSA3} - \frac{\text{PSA2}}{\text{Time2}}\right)\right]$$

It seems that, because more men are receiving yearly PSA values, PSAV may further optimize cancer detection. Yet many issues require resolution. More PSAV information must be accumulated prospectively. Also, more studies are needed on the normal variability in PSA serum levels with daily activity and on the differences in measurements over time between the various commercial assays. For now, it would seem wise to use PSAV information only to help make management decisions in men with serial PSA levels in the normal range or in men with low abnormal PSA levels who already have had a biopsy that did not reveal cancer.

A comparison of serum PSA binding ratios may be useful for diagnosis by better differentiating men with BPH from those with prostate cancer who have mildly elevated PSA levels. As previously discussed, PSA is present in serum in three general forms. Approximately half of the PSA (termed PSA-MG) is bound to α_2-macroglobulin, a serine protease inhibitor almost 30 times the size of PSA, in a complex form that renders the bound PSA undetectable by immunoassay. A predominant portion (approximately 85%) of the remaining PSA is bound to another serine protease inhibitor, α_1-antichymotrypsin, which is slightly more than double the size of PSA; the resulting moiety (termed PSA-ACT) allows the bound PSA to react in immunoassays. Finally, a small amount of unbound or free PSA (f-PSA) is enzymatically inactive. What is detected by PSA immunoassays is the total amount of the two immunoreactive forms of PSA (PSA-ACT and f-PSA), termed t-PSA. Several groups have now observed that the relative proportions f-PSA and PSA-ACT differ in BPH and cancer: patients with prostate cancer show lower ratios of f-PSA to t-PSA. Use of these ratios would appear to improve the positive predictive value for cancer over that of PSA alone, even for patients with PSA levels in the 4- to 10-ng/mL range.[6,27,28]

Use of PSA for Staging

PSA is an important tool for staging of prostate cancer and therefore for making decisions about therapy. In large prostate cancer series, serum PSA levels have been shown to correlate well with increasing clinical stage, with tumor volume, with DNA ploidy, and with pathologic stage.[11,12] On the average, serum PSA increases at a rate of 0.57 ng/mL per gram of involved prostate in BPH, and at 5.7 ng/mL per gram in cancer (by Tandem-R PSA assay). Several series have shown that 70% to 80% of men with serum PSA concentrations lower than 4 ng/mL have organ-confined disease, 50% of those with levels higher than 10 ng/mL have extracapsular extension, and most men with levels higher than 50 ng/mL have positive pelvic lymph nodes at surgery.[11,12]

However, except at the extreme values, PSA is not accurate enough to be used for staging in the individual patient. The reasons for this inaccuracy include the following facts: (1) PSA is produced by prostate epithelial cells, but the ratio of stromal to epithelial PSA in BPH can vary by as much as threefold; (2) perturbations of the basement membrane (and therefore presumably of the propensity to "leak" PSA) occurs with prostate inflammation and possibly with prostatic intraepithelial neoplasia; and (3) in prostate cancer, the decreasing concentration of cellular PSA with increasing grade combines with the increasing volume (and presumably increasing "leak") that occurs with increasing grade to influence serum PSA levels in unpredictable ways.[12]

The value of PSA determination can be considerably enhanced by combining it with other preoperative variables such as tumor grade and clinical stage, although multivariate analysis has shown that PSA is the strongest predictor. Probability tables and nomograms, based on the parameters of preoperative clinical stage, serum PSA level, and Gleason grade, have been constructed from data on large numbers of men who have undergone radical prostatectomy. Examples of such graphs are illustrated in Figure 41-1. With a preoperative serum PSA level of 4 ng/mL, there is a 73% predicted probability that the tumor will be organ confined if the clinical stage is T1, T2A, or T2B and the grade is low, but only a 23% probability if the clinical stage is T3 and the grade is high. This kind of information can be used to counsel patients on the advisability of surgical therapy. If surgery is selected, nomograms can be used to decide whether it is worthwhile to perform a pelvic lymphadenectomy.[12]

Combinations of PSA and other preoperative parameters are being analyzed to provide probabilities that can be used to advise either radical prostatectomy or a "watch-and-wait" strategy, especially for older men. For example, Epstein and colleagues[20] defined insignificant disease as the presence of less than 0.5 cc of organ-confined cancer in a radical prostatectomy specimen and determined those preoperative parameters that best predicted this cancer. They found that the best combination of preoperative variables for predicting insignificant cancer was as follows: a PSAD lower than 0.1, biopsies with fewer than three cores involved with cancer and no more than 50% of any one core involved, and no cores with Gleason grade greater than 4 or 5. In the retrospective experience of these authors, men who fulfill these preoperative criteria have a 65% chance of having insignificant cancer in the radical prostatectomy specimen, and those who do not meet these criteria have a 92% chance that the cancer is significant.

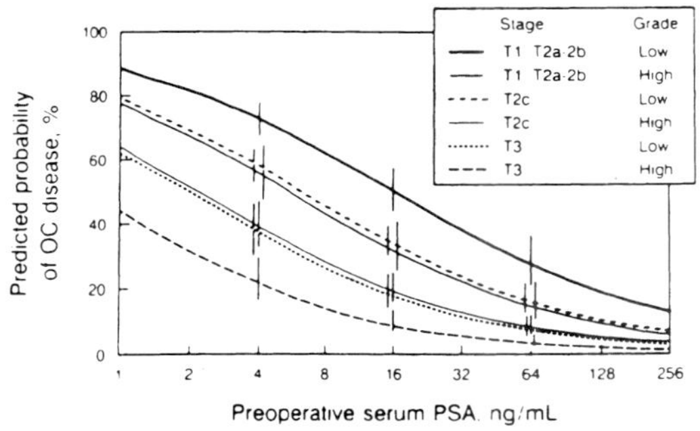

FIG. 41-1. The predicted probability of organ-confined (OC) disease as a function of preoperative serum prostate-specific antigen (PSA, ng/mL), clinical stage, and clinical grade; 95% confidence intervals are included for PSA values at 4, 16, and 64 ng/mL. Low grade includes clinical Mayo grades 1 and 2. High grade includes clinical Mayo grades 3 and 4. (Kleer E, Larson-Keller JJ, Zincke H, et al. Ability of preoperative serum prostate specific antigen value to predict pathologic stage and DNA ploidy: influence of clinical stage and tumor grade. Urology 1993;41:207, with permission.)

The probability tables for staging by PSA and other preoperative parameters are already clinically useful, but they need to be improved. In the middle ranges, where the results for most patients fall, the confidence intervals are still unacceptably wide. More of the same types of data need to be accumulated, but also additional parameters should be added, including those that are already available (e.g., biopsy volume of cancer, DNA ploidy) or those that may be newly revealed from the laboratory (e.g., degree of angiogenesis).[29] Finally, PSA and other preoperative parameters have heretofore been correlated with pathologic findings. A more appropriate end point would be clinical outcome or its surrogate, posttherapy PSA level (discussed in the next section). For radiotherapy, use of these end points for staging is essential. Some studies of patients receiving radiotherapy have combined preoperative PSA level, clinical stage, and grade to yield probabilities for outcome after irradiation[30–32]; however, many more such studies are needed.

As expected, the powerful predictive value of preoperative PSA with additional parameters has lessened the role of other staging modalities, including serum acid phosphatase (see Acid Phosphatase) and imaging tools. Magnetic resonance imaging and computed tomography rarely add additional information, except possibly when the predicted probability for extracapsular disease is high. Previous studies have shown that if the preoperative PSA is lower than 10 ng/mL and there is no bone pain, the chances of a positive bone scan are almost zero. However, because a bone scan provides a baseline and reveals information about the upper urinary tract, the decision as to whether to eliminate bone scans for preoperative staging—and thereby reap considerable national cost savings—is still controversial.[12] Certainly, if the Gleason score, clinical stage, or biopsy volume is high, a bone scan is prudent even if the PSA is below 10 ng/mL.

PSA After Radical Prostatectomy

Theoretically, no PSA should exist in the sera after radical prostatectomy if all prostate tissue, malignant or benign, has been removed. In practice, this capacity is limited by the sensitivity of the assay and possibly by biologic phenomena.

Determination of the lower detection limit of a particular PSA assay is a complex problem that has been extensively discussed elsewhere.[5] Here, it is sufficient to state that the clinical cancer detection limit for the most popular PSA assays (Tandem-R and IMX) is between 0.1 and 0.2 ng/mL. Using these limits, many studies have shown that persistently abnormal or rising PSA levels are a reliable and almost invariable sign of persistent disease after radical prostatectomy and that this sign usually occurs months to years before clinical signs of recurrence. Of course, no one laboratory value should dictate therapy, and a PSA level that seems elevated after radical prostatectomy should be validated, usually by the documentation of progressively rising levels.

Most large radical prostatectomy series are now using posttherapy PSA levels as a surrogate end point for effectiveness. Although the time to clinical recurrence can be as much as 5 years, if the PSA is unequivocally elevated recurrence is inevitable. The ultimate PSA results after radical prostatectomy are presented in detail in the other chapters on prostate cancer in this book. In general, 25% to 45% of men have PSA elevations after surgery. For example, the overall freedom from PSA relapse at 5 and 10 years was 61% and 71%, respectively, in a series from the University of California at Los Angeles, and 87% and 70% in a more recent series from the Johns Hopkins Medical Institutions.[11] Moreover, approximately 30% to 50% of those with elevated PSA levels after radical prostatectomy have cancer in biopsies from the prostate fossa, even though the digital rectal examination results are often normal.[33]

The pattern of PSA elevation after radical prostatectomy, together with other pathologic parameters, has significance with regard to the speed and site of recurrence. Usually, if the PSA does not return to normal low levels after surgery, systemic recurrence (with or without local recurrence) is likely. Among those patients whose PSA value falls to undetectable levels initially, the rate of rise (i.e., PSAV) has clinical significance, particularly if it is coupled with other pathologic parameters. For example, the rate of freedom from clinical disease at 5 years is 48% if the PSA increase is initially detected in the first year, and 85% if it is detected in the third year.[34] Also, men who initially had only local disease were found to have a PSA doubling time of 11 months, whereas those who presented with systemic disease had a doubling time of 4 months.[35]

The value of adjuvant radiation therapy cannot definitely be proven until randomized studies are completed. Until that time, PSA determination seems useful to evaluate the effects of adjuvant radiotherapy. In general, most men with elevated PSA levels after radical prostatectomy have a dramatic decline in PSA levels with adjuvant radiotherapy, and in about 50% the levels become undetectable. However, the durability of PSA suppression is not high (10% to 20% overall) and is related to the pattern of PSA relapse. Those men whose PSA values never descend to undetectable levels after surgery, or whose PSA values rise from undetectable levels very quickly, rarely have durable suppression after adjuvant radiotherapy and probably should not receive it. However, patients with slow PSA doubling times from undetectable levels may well benefit from adjuvant radiotherapy.[33]

The significance of PSA levels after radical prostatectomy has prompted the development of more sensitive PSA assays in order to detect recurrence earlier and also to shorten the time to cure (i.e., the time after which, if the PSA remains normal, the patient can be reassured that he is cured). With current assays, this time is not well known, but few patients develop PSA elevations after 5 years. Several investigators have shown that these more sensitive PSA assays can reveal clinically unique information.[5]

As more sensitive PSA assays become available, the worry increases that elevated PSA levels could result from factors other than persistent disease. These factors include normal prostate or BPH remnants, other sources of PSA, and cross-reacting substances in the sera. Briefly, normal prostate remnants (as may occur if a ''button'' of prostate apex is purposely or inadvertently left behind) have been documented to occur by needle biopsy of the prostatic fossa. Usually, the PSA level does not progressively rise in such cases. In some, subsequent biopsies do reveal cancer. Usually, normal prostate remnants are not a cause of persistently elevated PSA levels. Other sources of PSA exist outside the prostate, however. For example, there are periurethral glands that make PSA and secrete it into the urethral lumen (thereby making urethral PSA determinations not very useful as a method of detecting persistent disease). So far, these sources of PSA have not been considered to be significant as contaminants in the sera, but this situation could change with the ultrasensitive assays. Finally, cross-reacting substances have not yet proved to be a factor, although a background of unexplained ''noise'' remains in ultrasensitive assays. One important potential cross-reacting substance that is a substantial worry is human glandular kallikrein-2.[5]

In summary, PSA determinations after radical prostatectomy are a powerful tool in the management of patients with prostate cancer. It is likely that more sensitive assays will further increase this value, as will the evolving applications of polymerase chain reaction methods to detect circulating prostate cells (see Future Use of Tumor Markers in Prostate Cancer). Soon we may be able to detect persistent disease in real time, thus increasing our ability to improve existing therapies and develop newer ones.

PSA After Primary Radiotherapy

The changes in PSA levels after primary radiotherapy are less well studied than after radical prostatectomy. In contrast to radical prostatectomy, detectable serum PSA concentrations after radiotherapy could originate from either persistent cancer or normal prostate. During radiotherapy, the PSA level usually rises initially and then falls dramatically. The rate of decline is probably a result of many factors; a significant fall occurs in 95% of patients, and in about 80% PSA levels fall to normal ranges. The nadir value of PSA is related to the likelihood of subsequent PSA rise and ultimate clinical recurrence. It is not known what the nadir should be, but most studies now indicate that it is about 1 ng/mL, and this level should occur within 3 years. Increased PSA levels after that time portend disease recurrence. The ultimate percentage of durable undetectable levels of PSA after radiotherapy is reported to be between 20% and 60% and is proportional to preoperative parameters. Preoperative PSA concentration seems to be a powerful predictor of response to radiotherapy.[11,30–32,36]

PSA After Androgen Ablation Therapy

Ninety-eight percent of men with metastatic disease have increased PSA levels. Because prostate cancer is androgen-sensitive, PSA decreases significantly in most patients who receive androgen ablation therapy, but because prostate cancer is heterogeneous and some cells are not androgen-dependent, a low or undetectable PSA does not indicate cure or even significant destruction of cancer cells. Most studies have observed a rapid decline of PSA after androgen ablation therapy, sometimes to undetectable levels within the first 6 months after therapy. In one large series, 55%, 43%, and 13% of patients reached their PSA nadir within 3 months, within 6 months, and after 6 months, respectively. However, this nadir is not stable for very long. After 2 years, 9% of patients still have undetectable levels of PSA and 22% are within normal limits, but 72% (many of whom had good PSA responses during the first 6 months) have rising PSA levels. Finally, several studies have shown that the rate of decline and the absolute nadir of PSA levels after androgen therapy have prognostic value. In one example, if the nadir was lower than 4 ng/mL, the survival time was longer (average, 42 months) than if the nadir was less than 4 ng/mL (average, 10 months).[12]

The PSA level in about 92% of men who have had androgen ablation therapy begins to rise before or, less frequently, simultaneously with the development of clinical signs of progression. If the PSA level does rise again, usually the absolute levels are lower than before, and the relation between symptoms and PSA level is less linear. Although effective therapy is very limited in androgen-unresponsive disease, if a response is seen, PSA usually reflects or predicts it. Indeed, PSA levels are now a response criteria for many experimental therapy trials in androgen–unresponsive D3 disease.[4,12,37]

ACID PHOSPHATASE

The acid phosphatases are a group of enzymes that hydrolyze esters of orthophosphoric acid in an acid medium. In the period from 1936 to 1942, various investigators, most notably Gutman and associates, Higgins and Hodges, and Sullivan and colleagues, established that acid phosphatase is highly concentrated in the prostate, is under androgenic control, and, if measured in serum, is a useful marker to monitor patients, especially in the period surrounding androgen ablation therapy.[38]

Although the highest concentration of acid phosphatase is in the prostate, the enzyme is present in many other tissues and has many isoenzymes, thereby restricting its value as a serum marker. Many efforts were made to increase specificity for the prostate by using different substrates or inhibitors. The best enzymatic substrate is thymolphthalein monophosphate (the Roy enzymatic method), and the best prostate-related inhibitor is tartrate. However, these improvements did not make serum acid phosphatase prostate specific. Later, antibodies were developed that seemed to measure a more prostate-specific acid phosphatase, and immune assays initially were claimed to be better for reflecting the behavior of prostate cancer. However, eventually it was realized that the immune assays for acid phosphatase, although possibly more sensitive, were less specific and therefore no better than or even inferior to the Roy enzymatic method.[38]

By whatever assay, there are several inherent problems with the use of serum acid phosphatase as a marker for prostate cancer that do not exist with PSA. First, acid phosphatases are present in many other tissues, which is untrue for PSA. Second, even apparently prostate-specific acid phosphatase serum levels fluctuate significantly over a 24-hour period, whereas PSA varies little. Third, the enzyme is much more unstable than PSA, and there are special handling requirements; for example, with the enzymatic assays, the blood must be quickly chilled until serum separation and pH-buffered afterward. Fourth, false elevations of acid phosphatase occur more readily after digital rectal examination than is the case with PSA. Finally, serum acid phosphatase is not elevated as commonly in prostate cancer as is PSA (i.e., sensitivity not as high).[38]

Increased serum acid phosphatase levels (by the Roy assay) occur in 12% of those with T1 disease, 5% to 20% with T2, 30% to 40% with T3, and 60% to 80% with metastatic disease. Therefore, acid phosphatase is of little value in diagnosis. Its value in staging is also limited. Although studies show that an increased acid phosphatase usually means local disease extending beyond the prostatic capsule or involvement of the pelvic lymph nodes (i.e., high positive predictive value for extracapsular disease), the sensitivity for extracapsular disease is only about 10%. Some investigators claim that even this distinction for acid phosphatase rarely produces unique information, because usually digital rectal examination or PSA provides the same information regarding the likelihood of extracapsular extension. However, in patients with apparently localized cancer who have several high-risk factors for extracapsular disease (e.g., high grade, digital rectal examination suggestive of extracapsular extension), acid phosphatase determinations by the Roy method can help in management. If serum acid phosphatase is significantly elevated (more than two times the normal level), it is strong confirmatory evidence for the presence of extracapsular disease.[39] Finally, acid phosphatase has little place in the monitoring of patients after initial therapy, because PSA is much better for this purpose. After radical prostatectomy, for example, acid phosphatase is always detectable because of other nonprostatic sources of the enzyme.[39]

In summary, serum acid phosphatase was one of the first useful tumor markers, but its value is now limited. Antibodies to acid phosphatase are valuable, along with those to PSA, for immunohistochemical analysis of difficult pathologic diagnoses. Serum measurement of acid phosphatase by the Roy enzymatic method is occasionally helpful in deciding whether a patient has significant extracapsular disease.

NEW PROSTATE CANCER MARKERS

New prostate cancer tumor markers are needed for several reasons. In diagnosis, serum PSA results are either falsely positive or falsely negative in 20% to 30% of determinations. Also, serum or tissue PSA determinations cannot satisfactorily distinguish between important and unimportant local cancers. Finally, additional unique prostate cancer biomarkers would be desirable for development of antibody or gene therapies.

To date, most new prostate cancer markers have been discovered by the use of MAbs, and most have been glycoproteins. Some of these markers were discovered in other cancers and later applied to prostate cancer; examples include the pancarcinoma glycoprotein TAG-721 and the mucin protein MUC1. These markers have not yet demonstrated clinical usefulness.[40] Many of the neuroendocrine markers (e.g., neuroendocrine endolase, chromogranin-A) are found in some aggressive prostate cancers, and there is some evidence that evaluation of these markers in tissue or serum can be useful in selecting the rare patient ($<$10%) with advanced disease who may benefit from chemotherapy effective against neuroendocrine tumors.[7,41,42]

MAbs have also been developed against prostate carcinomas to help identify other unique prostate antigens. Two such antigens are prostate-associated glycoprotein (identified by the MAb TUR-27) and prostate mucin antigen (identified by the MAb PD41). Both of these antigens appear to be relatively prostate specific, although their clinical utility is still uncertain. The antigen revealed by the MAb 7E11-C5, called prostate-specific membrane antigen (PSM), is the most interesting new marker. This antigen is a membrane-spanning glycoprotein and seems to be highly restricted to prostate tissue; it is maximally expressed in poorly differentiated and metastatic cancers, and its expression does not seem to be decreased by androgen ablation. The gene that encodes for PSM has been cloned and sequenced and its amino acid sequence predicted. MAbs to PSM are currently being tested for their clinical efficacy in radioimmunoscintigraphy. The value of PSM as a serum marker is still uncertain.[40,43,44]

FUTURE USE OF TUMOR MARKERS IN PROSTATE CANCER

The fertile field of tumor markers in prostate cancer has only recently been opened. Without question, even more sensitive assays for serum PSA will soon be available and prove useful. Analysis of serum PSA binding may well increase the accuracy of PSA for diagnosis. Also, the explosion in DNA technology is continually revealing a plethora of markers in other cancers, including growth factors, nuclear matrix peptides, oncogenes, and tumor suppressor genes. Many of these substances are now being evaluated in prostate cancer, and some will undoubtedly be useful as tumor markers, especially for revealing tumor phenotypes in tissue. Finally, polymerase chain reaction techniques have allowed the amplification of tumor marker RNAs in tumor cells, so that cancer cells can be detected in ratios of $1:10^4$ to $1:10^7$ with hemopoietic cells in blood or bone marrow. Already, the approach has been applied to determinations of PSA and PSM,[45–47] and studies are underway to see whether this extremely sensitive method of detecting circulating prostate cancer tumor cells will have value for staging and judging response to therapy. In the foreseeable future, it may be that the consequences of therapies can accurately be evaluated almost in real time. Once this is achieved, the application of new treatments will be greatly enhanced.

REFERENCES

1. Bates SE. Clinical applications of serum tumor markers. Ann Intern Med 1991;115:623.
2. Crawford DE, DeAntoni EP. PSA as a screening test for prostate cancer. Urol Clin North Am 1993;20:637.
3. Cooner WH. Definition of the ideal tumor marker. Urol Clin North Am 1993;20:575.
4. Oesterling JE. Prostate specific antigen: a critical assessment of the most useful tumor marker for adenocarcinoma of the prostate. J Urol 1991;145:907.
5. Vessella RL, Lange PH. Issues in the assessment of PSA immunoassays. Urol Clin North Am 1993;20:607.
6. Lilja H. Significance of different molecular forms of serum PSA: the free, nonplexed form of PSA versus that complexed to alpha-1-antichymotrypsin. Urol Clin North Am 1993;20:681.
7. Epstein JI. PSA and PAP as immunohistochemical markers in prostate cancer. Urol Clin North Am 1993;20:757.
8. Iwakiri J, Grandbois K, Wehner N, Graves HC, Stamey T. An analysis of urinary prostate specific antigen before and after radical prostatectomy: evidence for secretion of prostate specific antigen by periurethral glands. J Urol 1993;149:783.
9. Takayama TK, Vessella RL, Brawer MK, True LD, Noteboom J, Lange PH. Urinary prostate specific antigen levels after radical prostatectomy. J Urol 1994;151:82.
10. Yu H, Diamandis EP, Sutherland DJ. Immunoreactive prostate-specific antigen levels in female and male breast tumors and its association with steroid hormone receptors and patient age. Clin Biochem 1994; 27:75.
11. Partin AW, Oesterling JE. The clinical usefulness of prostate specific antigen: update 1994. J Urol 1994;152:1358.
12. Partin AW, Carter HB. Prostate-specific antigen: use in clinical practice. In: Walsh PC, Redik AB, Stamey TA, Vaughan ED Jr, eds. Campbell's urology, 6th ed, update 10. Philadelphia: WB Saunders, 1994: 1.
13. Carter HB, Pearson JD. PSA velocity for the diagnosis of early prostate cancer: a new concept. Urol Clin North Am 1993;20:665.
14. Stamey TA, et al. Prostate-specific antigen as a serum marker for adenocarcinoma of the prostate. N Engl J Med 1987;317:909.
15. Simak R, Madersbacher S, Zhang ZF, Maier U. Impact of ejaculation on serum prostate specific antigen. J Urol 1993;150:895.
16. Etzioni R, Shen Y, Petteway J, Brawer M. Age specific PSA: A Reassessment. J Urol. In press.
17. Dalkin BL, Ahmann FR, Kopp J, et al. Derivation and application of upper limits for prostate specific antigen in men aged 50–74 years with no clinical evidence of prostatic carcinoma. Br J. Urol 1995;76:346.
18. Brawer MK. Screening for prostate cancer. Monogr Urol 1994;15:1.
19. Catalona W, Smith D, Ratliff T, Basler J. Detection of organ-confined prostate cancer is increased through prostate specific antigen-based screening. JAMA 1993;270:948.
20. Epstein JI, Walsh PC, Carmichael M, Brendler CB. Pathological and clinical findings to predict tumor extent of nonpalpable (stage T1C) prostate cancer. JAMA 1994;271:368.
21. Smith DS, Catalona WJ. Nature of prostate cancer detected through prostate specific antigen based screening. J Urol 1994;152:1732.
22. Ohori M, Wheeler TM, Dunn JK, Stamey TA, Scardino PT. Pathological features and prognosis of prostate cancer detectable with current diagnostic tests. J Urol 1994;152:1714.
23. Lange PH. Future studies in localized prostate cancer: what should we do? what should we think? J Urol 1994;152:1932.
24. Seaman E, Whang M, Olsson CA, Katz A, Cooner WH, Benson MC. PSA density (PSAD): role in patient evaluation and management. Urol Clin North Am 1993;20:653.
25. Brawer MK, Aramburu EAG, Chen GL, Preston SD, Ellis WJ. The inability of prostate specific antigen index to enhance the predictive value of prostate specific antigen in the diagnosis of prostate carcinoma. J Urol 1993;150:369.
26. McMurtry J, Keetch DW, Smith DS, Andriole GL, Catalona WJ. PSA density vs. PSA slope as predictors of prostate cancer in patients with initially negative prostatic biopsies. J Urol 1994;151:401A.
27. Christensson A, Bjork T, Nilsson O, et al. Serum prostate-specific antigen complexed to 1-antichymotrypsin as an indicator of prostate cancer. J Urol 1993;150:100.
28. Catalona WJ, Smith DS, Wolfert RL, Wang TJ, Rittenhouse HG, Ratliff TL. Evaluation of percentage of free serum prostate-specific antigen to improve specificity of prostate cancer screening. JAMA 1995;274: 1214.
29. Bigler S, Deering RE, Brawer MK. A quantitative morphometric analysis of the microcirculation in prostate carcinoma. Hum Pathol 1993; 24:220.
30. Schellhammer PF, El-Mahdi AM, Wright JGL, et al. Prostate-specific antigen to determine progressive-free survival after radiation therapy for localized carcinoma of the prostate. Urology 1993;42:21.
31. Zagars GK. Serum PSA as a tumor marker for patients undergoing definitive radiation therapy. Urol Clin North Am 1993;20:737.
32. Zagars GK. Prostate specific antigen as an outcome variable for T1 and T2 prostate cancer treated by radiation therapy. J Urol 1994;152: 17861.
33. Takayama TK, Lange PH. Radiation therapy for local recurrence of prostate cancer after radical prostatectomy. Urol Clin North Am 1994; 21:687.
34. Partin A, Pearson J, Landis P, et al. Evaluation of serum prostatic specific antigen velocity after radical prostatectomy to distinguish local recurrence versus distance metastases. Urology 1994;43:649.
35. Danella J, Steckel J, Dorey F, Smith RB, deKernion JB. Detectable prostate specific antigen levels following radical prostatectomy: relationship of doubling time to clinical outcome. J Urol 1993;149:447A.
36. Stamey TA, Ferrari MK, Schmid HP. Value of serial prostate specific antigen determinations 5 years after radiotherapy: steeply increasing values characterize 80% of patients. J Urol 1993;150:1856.
37. Petros JA, Andriole GL. Serum PSA after antiandrogen therapy. Urol Clin North Am 1993;20:749.
38. Romas NA, Kwan DJ. Prostatic acid phosphatase. Urol Clin North Am 1993;20:581.
39. Lowe FC, Trauzzi SJ. Prostatic acid phosphatase in 1993: its limited clinical utility. Urol Clin North Am 1993;20:589.

40. Schellhammer PF, Wright GL. Biomolecular and clinical characteristics of PSA and other candidate prostate tumor markers. Urol Clin North Am 1993;20:597.
41. Kadmon D, Thompson TC, Lynch GR, Scardino PT. Elevated plasma chromogranin-A concentrations in prostatic carcinoma. J Urol 1991; 146:358.
42. di Sant Agnese P, Cockett T. The prostatic endocrine-paracrine (neuroendocrine) regulatory system and neuroendocrine differentiation in prostatic carcinoma: a review and future directions in basic research. J Urol 1994;152:1927.
43. Israeli RS, Powell CT, Fair WR, Heston DW. Molecular cloning of a complementary DNA encoding a prostate-specific membrane antigen. Cancer Res 1993;53:227.
44. Kahn D, Williams RD, Seldin DW, et al. Radioimmunoscintigraphy with 111 indium labeled CYT-356 for the detection of occult prostate cancer recurrence. J Urol 1994;152:1490.
45. Vessella RL, Blouke KA, Stray JE, et al. The use of the polymerase chain reaction to detect metastatic prostate cancer cells in lymph nodes and bone marrow. Proc Am Assoc Cancer Res 1992;33:2367.
46. Moreno JG, Croce CM, Fischer R, et al. Detection of hematogenous micrometastasis in patients with prostate cancer. Cancer Res 1992;52: 6110.
47. Katz AE, Olsson CA, Raffo AJ, et al. Molecular staging of prostate cancer with the use of an enhanced reverse transcriptase PCR assay. Urology 1994;43:765.

Principles and Practice of Genitourinary Oncology, edited by Derek Raghavan, Howard I. Scher, Steven A. Leibel, and Paul H. Lange. Lippincott-Raven Publishers, Philadelphia, © 1997.

CHAPTER 42

Hormone Receptors

Roger L. Miesfeld

OVERVIEW OF HORMONE ACTION

There are two broad classes of hormone receptors. One type is exemplified by the membrane-bound growth factor receptors, which transmit extracellular signals to the nucleus through phosphorylation cascades that require specific kinases and phosphorylation-dependent transcription factors.[1] The epidermal growth factor receptor is a member of this class. The second class of hormone receptors are ligand-activated transcription factors that reside either in the cytoplasm or the nucleus and function as direct signal transducers to control the expression of cell-specific target genes.[2] Steroid hormone receptors (e.g., for estrogen or androgen) and nuclear receptors (e.g., for retinoic acid or vitamin D) belong to this group of hormone receptors, and they are the subject of this chapter. Figure 42-1 depicts the signal transduction pathways of these two distinct classes of hormone receptors. In the example shown, the activation of either pathway leads to the transcriptional induction of similar growth-promoting genes as a result of DNA binding and transactivation by discrete transcription factors. The recent finding that multiple signal transduction pathways can impinge on the steroid- or nuclear-receptor–regulated gene network through a process termed crosstalk is discussed in the last section of this chapter.

The importance of steroid and nuclear receptors in genitourinary cancers is related to their ability to transcriptionally regulate genes that play a role in growth promotion. In the classic initiation and promotion model of carcinogenesis, steroid hormones such as androgens and estrogens could contribute to tumor promotion by stimulating the proliferation of steroid-responsive cell types.[3,4] This could occur through the activation of growth-stimulating genes or, alternatively, by the transcriptional repression of genes encoding cell cycle inhibitory proteins. One explanation as to how hormonal functions may contribute to tumor progression is that the cancer cell may contain mutations that alter its appropriate responsiveness to hormones.

SUPERFAMILY OF STEROID AND NUCLEAR RECEPTORS

Although biochemists had known for more than a decade that steroid hormones bound with high affinity and specificity to cellular proteins, it was not until the mid-1980s that it became clear from molecular cloning studies that steroid receptors are members of a large superfamily of transcription factors. The isolation and characterization of the glucocorticoid (GR), progesterone (PR), estrogen (ER), androgen (AR), and mineralocorticoid (MR) receptor coding sequences revealed that they all retain a significant amino acid homology over a stretch of about 80 residues that encodes the DNA-binding domain (DBD).[5] Sequence comparisons in this region of GR, PR, AR, and MR, along with functional binding studies,[2] indicated that they were capable of interacting with similar DNA sequences. Studies with ER, however, revealed that this receptor binds to a distinct high-affinity site on DNA.[6]

Classification of Steroid and Nuclear Receptors Based on Amino Acid Homologies

Because of the high sequence homology between the DBDs of the steroid receptors, several research groups set out to isolate related coding sequences using low-stringency hybridization and degenerate polymerase chain reaction (PCR) techniques aimed at identifying cDNA clones with sequences related to those of the steroid receptor DBDs. A large number of protein coding sequences were identified,[7] and through a combination of biochemical and molecular analyses, it was discovered that some of the encoded proteins had previously been purified as receptors for thyroid hormone (TR),[8] vitamin D (VDR),[9] and retinoic acid (RAR).[10] Functional studies using the cloned TR, VDR, and RAR cDNA sequences in various prokaryotic and eukaryotic expression systems confirmed that the encoded proteins corresponded to the previously identified receptors.[2] Because TR, VDR, and RAR are localized to the nucleus in the absence of ligand, these receptors are often referred to as nuclear receptors.[11] Although the search for cDNA clones containing sequences related to those of the steroid receptor DBDs turned up several genes with known function, most of the coding sequences that were isolated corresponded to novel proteins that had very little in common with steroid and nuclear receptors outside of the putative DBD region. These proteins have been termed orphan receptors to denote that even though they are related to the steroid and nuclear receptor family by amino acid

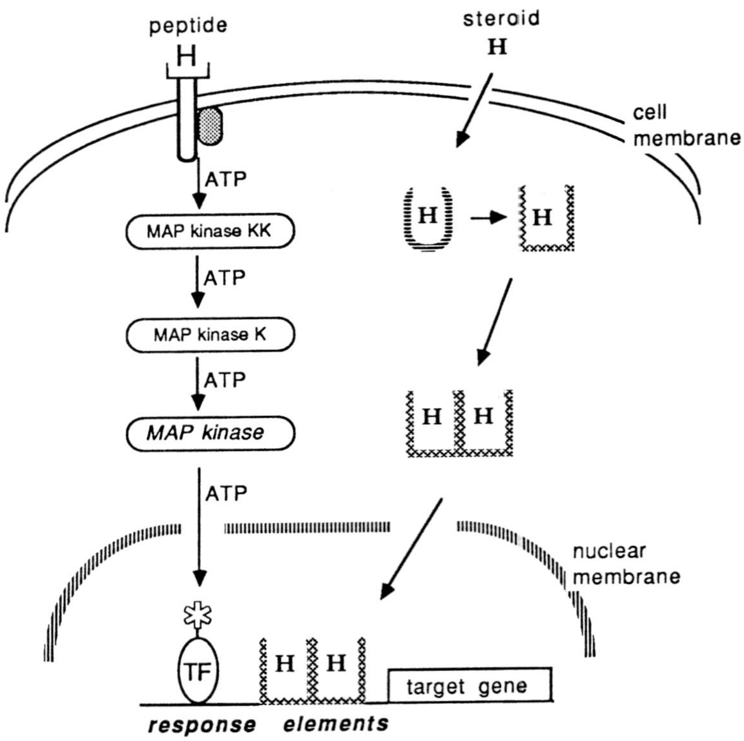

FIG. 42-1. Intracellular signaling by peptide and steroid hormones. Peptide hormones such as growth factors modulate gene expression through a complex phosphorylation cascade involving hormone binding to a membrane receptor and subsequent activation of numerous substrate-specific kinases (MAP kinases) and nuclear transcription factors (TF). In contrast, hormones that activate steroid or nuclear receptors, such as androgens and vitamin D analogs, passively diffuse through the cell membrane and bind to ligand-activated transcription factors, which bind to DNA as protein dimers and directly regulate gene expression. Some target genes involved in cell proliferation may be regulated by both signal transduction pathways by virtue of shared *cis*-acting DNA response elements.

homology, their biologic role as transcription factors and their putative ligands are unknown.[12]

Structure and Function of Steroid and Nuclear Receptor Proteins

Figure 42-2 is a functional map of a prototypic steroid or nuclear receptor that depicts the linear relation of several protein domains along the length of the receptor, from the amino-terminal end (NH_2) to the carboxyl-terminal end (COOH) The region of highest amino acid homology between various members of the superfamily is in the DBD (the C region), and evolutionary relations among the receptors can be derived by comparing these sequences.[13] Also shown in Figure 42-2 is a list of many of the receptor types in the three subgroups that have been described (steroid, nuclear, and orphan receptors). The nature of the ligand for ER (estradiol) traditionally places it in the steroid receptor group, and ER binds to DNA as a homodimer complex, just as other steroid receptors do. However, amino acid differences in the ER DBD result in a DNA binding specificity that is more similar to that of the nuclear receptors; therefore, ER is somewhat of a hybrid steroid-nuclear receptor.

Molecular genetic studies of steroid and nuclear receptor function not only have confirmed the location of the DBD (subregion C) but also have identified at least three additional subregions, as shown in Figure 42-2. The highly divergent A/B region is found at the NH_2-terminal end of the receptor, and it has been found to encode a transcriptional activation function (AF-1) in many members of the family.[14–18] Among the steroid receptors, the A/B region has been shown to encode a ligand-independent transcriptional transactivation function that may

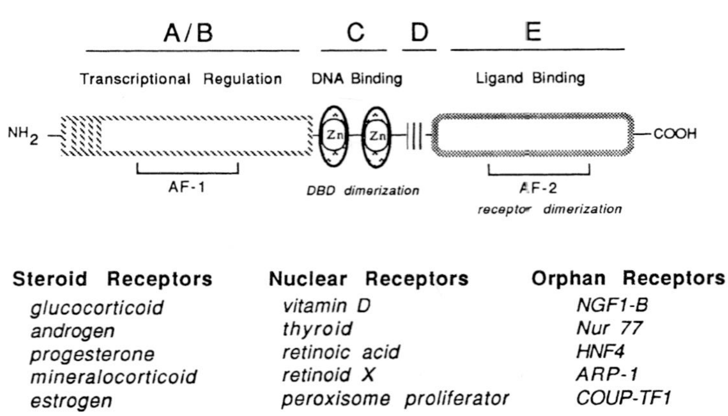

FIG. 42-2. Functional map of a prototypical steroid or nuclear receptor. The three major functional domains, which encode for transcriptional regulation, DNA binding, and ligand binding, are shown above the schematized drawing of a receptor, and the approximate location of transcriptional activation functions (AF-1 and AF-2) and dimerization functions are shown below. The hinge region (conserved region D) is depicted by vertical lines. The best characterized members from each of the three classes of receptor proteins are listed at the bottom. DBD, DNA-binding domain; Zn, zinc finger regions.

modulate cell- and promoter-specific responses.[19] This NH_2-terminal domain is variable in length and sequence. For example, in AR, the A/B region is almost half the length of the entire protein (about 500 amino acids) and is encoded within a single exon.[20] In contrast, this portion of VDR is less than 50 residues long and has little, if any, intrinsic activity.[21]

Another major functional region in the steroid and nuclear receptors is the ligand-binding domain (region E). There is much less conservation in the E region than in the DBD, which reflects the diversity of ligands that bind to these receptors. The fact that it has been more difficult to functionally dissect the ligand-binding domain is often interpreted to mean that a large portion of the COOH-terminus is required for the formation of a structurally complex "binding pocket."[22] In addition to encoding the ligand binding activity, the COOH-terminal E region is also required for receptor dimerization (both homodimerization of steroid receptors and heterodimerization of nuclear receptors).[23] A short region near the COOH end of the E region contains hydrophobic heptad repeats that have the potential to form a "leucine zipper" dimerization interface.[24] There may be an interdependent relation between ligand binding and receptor dimerization; some studies show that ligand-bound activated receptors are capable of dimerization, whereas unbound receptors exist as monomers in the cell.[25,26] The E region also encodes a ligand-dependent transcriptional regulatory function called AF-2.[27] AF-2 is the dominant transcriptional regulatory activity in the nuclear receptors but only a secondary activation function in the AR, GR, and PR steroid receptors (in which the ligand-independent AF-1 function in the A/B region is the dominant activity). The fourth receptor subregion is referred to as region D (see Fig. 42-2). This segment is sometimes called the hinge region to denote a proposed flexible protein structure.[2] Chimeric steroid and nuclear receptor DNA- and hormone-binding domains can be joined through sequences present in region D and still retain receptor-specific functions.[28]

STEROID AND NUCLEAR RECEPTORS BIND TO SPECIFIC DNA SEQUENCES AS PROTEIN DIMERS

Early studies using two-dimensional protein gels,[29,30] and more recent analyses of mRNA transcript populations,[31,32] have indicated that the number of steroid-regulated target genes in any given cell type is relatively small (10 to 50 genes). This conclusion was based on the finding that the abundance of very few RNA or protein products was altered by short-term hormone treatment (8 to 12 hours). This high specificity of steroid hormone action was predicted in the mid-1970s by Yamamoto and Alberts,[33] who used prokaryotic gene regulation as a paradigm for steroid receptor action. We now know that the mechanistic basis for this gene selectivity is a result of sequence-specific DNA binding by the steroid and nuclear receptors. Both in vitro DNA binding studies of purified proteins and functional deletion mapping by transient transfection assays in tissue culture cell lines have led to the identification of hormone response elements (HREs).[34] These are short DNA sequences (~15 to 20 base pairs long) that serve as binding sites for the steroid and nuclear receptors. HREs are found within the regulatory regions of primary target genes, and although they are usually localized to the 5′ end of the gene,[34] they have also been found within the first intron[35,36] and downstream of the last exon[37] of some genes.[105]

Figure 42-3*A* shows the genomic organization of several hormone-regulated genes and the relative positions of the HREs. In most cases, the gene contains several HREs, and their distance from the transcriptional start site is varied. The rat calbin-

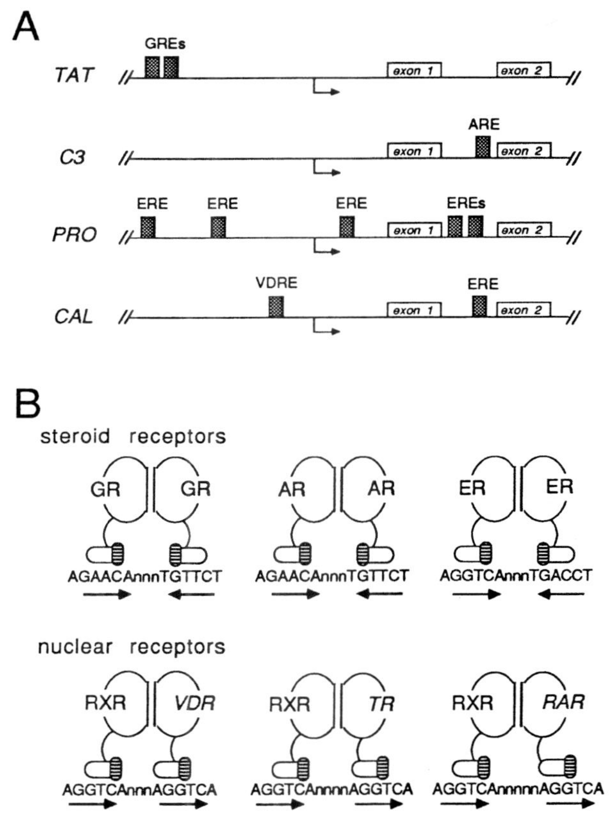

FIG. 42-3. Target gene selectivity and DNA-binding properties of steroid and nuclear receptors. (**A**) Hormone response elements for glucocorticoids (GRE), androgens (ARE), estrogens (ERE), and vitamin D analogs (VDRE) are shown as stippled boxes in their approximate genomic locations relative to the start site of transcription (*arrow*) in the rat tyrosine aminotransferase (*TAT*), rat C3 prostatein (*C3*), rat progesterone receptor (*PRO*), and rat calbindin D-9K (*CAL*) genes (see ref. 105). (**B**) Steroid receptors for glucocorticoid, androgen, and estrogen (GR, AR, and ER) bind to palindromic response elements as homodimers; GR and AR bind with high affinity to the same half-site response element (AGAACA), whereas ER binds to a palindrome containing the same half-site sequence (AGGTCA) as the nuclear receptor response elements. The nuclear receptors for vitamin D analogs (VDR), thyroid hormone (TR), and retinoic acid (RAR) bind as heterodimers with a nuclear protein factor (RXR) to direct repeats containing half-site spacings of 3, 4, or 5 nucleotides, respectively. Dimerization regions in the ligand-binding domain specify receptor interactions in solution (shown by parallel lines); however, head-to-head (steroid receptor) or head-to-tail (nuclear receptor) dimerization interfaces localized to the DNA-binding domain (*striped ovals*) require receptor DNA binding and may involve flexible protein structures in the hinge region.

din D-9K gene contains response element binding sites for both VDR (VDRE in the 5′ regulatory region)[38] and ER (ERE in the first intron),[39] consistent with its dual regulation by both vitamin D and estrogen. A number of studies have shown that HREs function as classic enhancer elements in that their ability to modulate transcription, by means of the proteins that bind to them, is position- and orientation-insensitive.[34]

Steroid Receptors Bind to Inverted Repeat Sequences as Homodimers

The AR, GR, PR, and MR subgroup of steroid receptors bind with high affinity to a palindromic sequence containing the half-site sequence AGAACA (TGTTCT on the complementary strand), as shown in Figure 42-3*B*. Two such inverted repeat half-sites, separated by a three base-pair nucleotide spacer, together form the HRE binding site for homodimers of these four steroid receptors.[40] This binding specificity is understood in detail based on protein structural data of GR_2:HRE complexes obtained by x-ray crystallography with the use of purified GR DBD polypeptides consisting of an 86–amino acid core domain.[41] Although the initial data set used a perfect palindrome with a half-site spacing of four nucleotides (rather than the optimal spacing of three nucleotides), the results from these analyses revealed the specific protein-DNA interactions between any of the steroid or nuclear receptors and their cognate DNA binding site.[42]

First, it was found that the two zinc finger modules of the GR DBD form a compact structure containing two prominent alpha-helical regions, one in each finger. The "recognition helix," located near the first zinc coordination site in the GR DBD, lies perpendicular to the DNA helix and makes direct contacts with HRE nucleotide bases within the DNA major groove. The second DBD alpha helix makes several contacts with the phosphate backbone, and it may also provide structural integrity for the DBD.[41]

The second important observation from the x-ray crystallography data was the finding that the two GR DBD monomer units make contacts with each other through a dimer interface that involves amino acids located in a region between the two alpha helices. This protein-protein interaction helps to position the GR DBDs relative to the palindromic HRE sequence and, more importantly, appears to provide cooperative interactions that enhance DNA binding affinity.[41] Molecular genetic studies using point mutations in the GR DBD confirmed the functional role of the recognition helix in modulation of DBD binding specificity in experiments that identified amino acids in the first zinc finger called the "P box."[43,44] Likewise, similar mutational studies identified amino acids in the "D box" that are required for receptor dimerization.[45,46]

By comparison of the amino acid sequences in the recognition helix (P box) of GR, AR, PR, and MR, in vitro DNA binding experiments and transient transfection studies identified the same HRE half-site sequence (AGAACA) as a high-affinity binding site for all four steroid receptors.[40] Cellular target genes for these receptors often contain functionally defined HREs that share significant similarity to the canonical GRE (glucocorticoid response element) shown in Figure 42-3*B*. However, there are also a number of in vivo factors that contribute to steroid receptor–selective gene expression under normal physiologic conditions, such as cell-specific steroid receptor expression levels[47,48] and ligand bioavailability.[49]

The structure of an ER_2:HRE complex was recently studied by x-ray crystallography with the use of an 84–amino acid ER DBD.[50] As shown in Figure 42-3*B*, the sequence of the ER binding site (called the ERE, or estrogen response element) differs at two positions (AG*GT*CA) from that of the GRE. However, like GRE, the ERE is a palindrome (an inverted repeat sequence) with an optimal spacing of three nucleotide base pairs between two half-sites.[40] Moreover, ER homodimers bind with high affinity to the ERE sequence in a ligand-dependent manner, just as the GR subgroup receptors do.[51] Based on both the x-ray crystallography data from studies of ER_2:HRE complexes[50] and molecular genetic studies of full-length ER in transient transfection assays,[44] it was demonstrated that amino acid sequence differences in the P box of the ER recognition helix confer the predicted DNA binding specificity for the ERE half-site AGGTCA. In a comparison of the ER_2:HRE and GR_2:HRE complexes, it was demonstrated that the ER P box amino acid sequence of C*EG*CK*A* specifies binding to the ERE nucleotide sequence AG*GT*CA, whereas the GR (which is the same in AR, PR, and MR) P box sequence of C*GS*CK*V* specifies GRE binding at AG*AA*CA (see Fig. 42-3*B*).

Nuclear Receptors Bind to Direct Repeat Sequences as Heterodimers

Identification of the high-affinity binding sites for VDR, TR, and RAR revealed four common themes. First, it was found that all three nuclear receptors were capable of binding to DNA sequences containing the ERE half-site AGGTCA, consistent with similarities in the critical P-box residues of these receptors (CEGCKG) with that of ER.[2] Second, DNA binding affinities of VDR, TR, and RAR were greatly enhanced by the presence of a nuclear protein factor called RXR, which had originally been cloned as one of the orphan receptors.[52] RXR is closely related to RAR in amino acid sequence and can bind the ligand 9-*cis*-retinoic acid.[53] In the presence of RXR, the heterodimers RXR-VDR, RXR-TR, and RXR-RAR are readily formed and bind to DNA sequences containing AGGTCA half-sites. The third common feature among these nuclear receptors is that the preferred DNA binding site is a direct repeat rather than a palindrome,[11] as was found for the steroid receptors. Fourth, nuclear receptors can bind to DNA in the absence of ligand, but transcriptional activation functions are ligand-dependent.[2]

It is now known that stable heterodimeric complexes between RXR and VDR, TR, or RAR bind to two DNA direct repeat (DR) half-sites with spacing of three (DR + 3), four (DR + 4), or five (DR + 5) nucleotides, respectively (see Fig. 42-3*B*). It has been found that RXR binds to the 5′ half-site, and the nuclear receptor partner binds to the 3′ half-site of the response element.[54,55] When this relation between the half-site spacing and a preferential affinity for particular RXR–nuclear receptor heterodimers was first described, it was termed the "3-4-5 rule" to denote that VDR, TR, and RAR heterodimers with RXR bind to half-sites spaced by 3, 4, and 5 nucleotides, respectively.[56] It is now known that spacing differences of one and two nucleotides are also recognized by these receptors. For example, it has been shown that RXR-RAR heterodimers can also bind to DR + 2 half-sites,[57] and RXR-RXR homodimers can bind with high affinity to DR + 1 half-sites.[58] Moreover, many of the heterodimer pairs bind promiscuously, albeit with lower affinity, to half-site spacings other than those shown in Figure 42-3*B*, and heterodimers between two nuclear receptors can also be formed (TR-RAR,[59] TR-VDR,[60] and VDR-RAR).[61] In addition, *naturally*-occurring nuclear receptor response elements have been found that have palindromic and inverted palindromic repeat structures that can be bound by homodimers.[11]

What are the implications for transcriptional regulation of nuclear receptor target genes if there is the potential for so much overlap in DNA binding specificity? How does the binding of ligand affect the activity of these nuclear receptor heterodimers? Based primarily on data obtained from in vitro DNA binding experiments and transient transfection assays showing that RXR-RXR homodimers can be formed in the presence 9-*cis*-retinoic acid,[58] a model has been proposed for ligand modulation of nuclear receptor gene networks.[62] This model postulates that, in the absence of 9-*cis*-retinoic acid, RXR-RAR heterodimers form, and target genes having DR + 2 or DR + 5 half-sites are preferentially induced if the level of all-trans retinoic acid (a ligand for RAR) is elevated. Furthermore, if 9-*cis*-retinoic acid is present, RXR-RXR homodimers are formed; in this case, genes with DR + 1 half-sites are potential targets for transcriptional regulation, and transcription of the RXR-RAR target genes is decreased. Thus, different sets of genes are regulated depending on the relative concentrations of RAR, RXR, and all-trans and 9-*cis*-retinoic acid.

Cheskis and Freedman[26] have recently proposed a similar model based on their observation that unliganded VDR-VDR homodimers are destabilized by binding of 1,25-dihydroxyvitamin D_3. The role of ligand, therefore, is to promote the formation of transcriptionally active RXR-VDR heterodimers that can induce target genes containing DR + 3.[63] However, the model predicts that if 9-*cis*-retinoic acid is present, RXR-RXR homodimers are formed, and target genes with DR + 1 response elements are preferentially regulated. Under these circumstances, the RXR-VDR complexes are destabilized, and target genes containing DR + 3 are deinduced. Because both retinoids[64] and vitamin D derivatives[65] have been shown to affect prostate cell growth in culture, there may ways to develop new therapeutic approaches to prostate cancer based on administration of these compounds.

TRANSCRIPTIONAL INDUCTION AND REPRESSION BY STEROID AND NUCLEAR RECEPTORS

One of the central questions in hormone action has been to determine how DNA-bound hormone-receptor complexes are able to modulate the transcriptional initiation rates of target gene promoters. For the steroid and nuclear receptors, it has been fairly straightforward to identify regions within the receptor proteins that are required specifically for transcriptional regulation.[2] As shown in Figure 42-2, these activation functions (AFs) can be independent of (AF-1), or dependent on (AF-2), ligand binding. Based on the finding that large, multiprotein complexes are formed between various eukaryotic transcription factors and proteins in the transcriptional initiation complex,[66,67] the emphasis in recent years has now shifted toward identifying nonreceptor proteins that functionally interact with the steroid and nuclear receptor AF sequences. Several candidate auxiliary proteins have been described that may be important to steroid receptor functions.[68–70] In this section, transcriptional control by steroid and nuclear receptors is described in terms of transcriptional induction, transcriptional repression, and combinatorial control (integrated signals). Although post-transcriptional regulation of transcript processing and mRNA stability are also possible control steps, these mechanisms probably represent secondary effects of hormone action and are not described here.

Transcriptional Induction

Activated steroid and nuclear receptor complexes are capable of inducing transcription from response element binding sites located both near and far from the target promoter, as is shown for several natural genes in Figure 42-3*A*. This property is very similar to that of other eukaryotic transcription factors that function as regulatory proteins.[71] To understand how this class of transcriptional regulators work, it is useful to consider that promoter activity can operate at two levels: basal and regulated (either induced or repressed). For genes that are transcriptionally induced, the basal level of transcription is usually low and the induced level is often 5 to 20 times higher (steady-state levels of hormone-induced transcripts may be much higher still, depending on the mRNA halflife). In the case of ligand-activated transcription by steroid and nuclear receptors, this means that DNA bound hormone-receptor complexes must be able to alter the efficiency of the transcriptional initiation process.

A large, multiprotein complex is thought to occupy a promoter under conditions of basal expression. The three basic functional units in this complex are the RNA polymerase II holoenzyme, the TATA binding protein (TBP) with its associated proteins (TAFs),[67] and a variety of auxiliary proteins (TFIIB, TFIIA, TFIIH, and TFIIE/F).[66] In the absence of a bound hormone-receptor complex at an HRE, or an activator bound to its respective response element, such a promoter would be transcribed at a low rate. One explanation for the submaximal rate of initiation at basal promoter complexes is that the complex itself may be relatively unstable.[72] However, if an activated hormone-receptor complex is bound to an HRE (for example, a homodimer of AR-dihydrotestosterone or a heterodimer of RXR–VDR–1,25-dihydroxyvitamin D_3), the basal promoter complex may be stabilized through additional protein-protein interactions.[2] Regulatory factors (and presumably hormone-receptor complexes) appear to functionally interact both with proteins in the basal promoter complex (e.g., TFIIB),[73,74] and with coactivator proteins (which are not required for basal promoter activity).[75,76] The phosphorylation state of a transcriptional regulator can modulate these protein interactions,[77] and this may also be true for some hormone-receptor complexes.[78,79]

Transcriptional Repression

There are a variety of genes in which steroid and nuclear receptors function by repressing transcriptional initiation rates.[2] Three basic mechanisms have been proposed to account for transcriptional repression by regulatory factors; competition, interference, and quenching.[80,81] A competition mechanism between the hormone-receptor complex and another activator protein would lead to reduced transcription under conditions in which the transcriptional regulatory activity of the DNA-bound steroid or nuclear receptor is less than that of the DNA-bound activator protein. In this context, unliganded nuclear receptors such as TR have been shown to bind to DNA and function as repressors,[82,83] and ligand-bound steroid receptors have been shown to bind DNA without activating transcription.[84] A second potential mechanism of receptor-mediated repression is interference, which would involve direct or indirect disruption of the basal promoter complex, leading to its disassembly.[85] Like the activation domain–protein contacts that occur between steroid or nuclear receptors and either TFII proteins in the initiation complex or a coactivator protein, it is also thought that repressor domains may function by interacting directly (TFIIB?) or indirectly (corepressor protein?) with the basal promoter complex.[2] Finally, in a third proposed mechanism of transcriptional repression called quenching,[81] the steroid or nuclear receptor would act as a repressor by inhibiting the activation function of another DNA-bound transcription factor. The distinction between quenching and a related repression mechanism called squelching[86] is that both the steroid or nuclear receptor and the transcriptional activator would have to be bound to the DNA for the quenching effect to be mediated.

Combinatorial Control of Transcription

Steroid and nuclear receptors modulate transcription (through induction or repression) in the context of many other protein factors that associate with gene regulatory regions. A typical eukaryotic promoter contains the binding sites for a variety of ubiquitous and cell-specific transcription factors.[87] Moreover, nucleosomes and chromatin structure can also affect receptor-mediated target gene expression.[72] In this context, it has been shown that GR transcriptional regulatory activity in a yeast cell system requires the activity of chromatin-modifying factors belonging to the SWI/SNF family of proteins.[88] Therefore, to understand the molecular basis for cell- and promoter-specific gene regulation by steroid and nuclear receptors, especially considering the overlap the receptors share in DNA binding specificity (see Fig. 42-3*B*), one must consider how other proteins influence steroid and nuclear receptor transcriptional regulatory activity. One one model, for example, the combined effect of multiple protein-protein interactions between steroid or nuclear receptors and regulatory factors (both repressors and activators) could result in a highly sensitive ''thermostat'' that could lead to either increased or decreased rates of transcription for the target gene promoter, depending on the concentration of each rate-limiting protein.

Although most studies aimed at understanding the effects of other factors on steroid and nuclear receptor function have used GR, the general conclusions probably hold true for other members of the superfamily. One of the best characterized examples of signal transduction crosstalk between GR and another signaling pathway involves the interaction of GR with the AP-1 transcription complex.[89] AP-1 is a heterodimer of the proteins FOS and JUN, and two examples of crosstalk between AP-1 and GR are the transcriptional repression of collagenase[90,91] and the expression of the alphafetoprotein gene.[92] Another example is the effect of elevated levels FOS and JUN proteins in the cell. Depending on the steady-state levels of FOS-JUN heterodimers and JUN-JUN homodimers, ligand-bound GR can either transcriptionally induce or repress expression of the proliferin gene.[93] This result is especially interesting because there are a variety of signaling pathways that control the intranuclear levels of activated FOS and JUN through phosphorylation cascades.[94]

Additional examples of GR crosstalk include CREB-mediated regulation of the glycoprotein hormone gene,[95] the effects of C/EBP[96] and NF-IL6[97] on GR-induction of α1-acid glycoprotein gene expression, and functional associations between GR and NF-kB that may influence transcription of the interleukin-6 gene.[98] A possible role for protein kinase A stimulation of GR DNA binding activity has also been reported.[99] One of the most striking examples of crosstalk between steroid receptors and membrane receptor-mediated pathways is the activation of PR- and ER-regulated genes by dopamine.[100,101] Recent data suggest that dopamine D_1 receptor agonists activate rat PR through a steroid-independent mechanism in the brain, resulting in altered female sexual behavior.[102] It has been postulated that phosphorylation of PR or of some other cellular transcription factor may be the mechanistic basis of ligand-independent activation of PR.[103] Based on these results, there are likely to be other examples of effects mediated by steroid and nuclear receptors that are caused by receptor-dependent transcriptional regulation even in the absence of hormonal ligands.

SUMMARY AND PERSPECTIVES

Hormones have long been implicated as contributing factors in carcinogenesis. The mechanism of action of steroid and nuclear hormone receptors is now known to be production of a direct effect on the regulated gene expression of a select set of cell-specific target genes. Connecting these two processes to better understand the role of hormones in human cancer requires further study in at least two areas.

First, it is critical to isolate and characterize primary steroid and nuclear receptor target genes from cell types that are prone to neoplastic transformation. Some of these genes may have been discovered in other systems as a result of investigations of normal cell growth and differentiation, or possibly as mediators of cell proliferation in cell types not affected by hormones. Such genes may include growth factors, growth factor receptors, and mediators of signal transduction. Other genes identified as primary targets will undoubtedly be novel, and the challenge will then be to identify the function of their gene products in order to understand how they contribute to cancer cell growth. Identification of target genes could lead to better cancer treatments, perhaps through nucleic acid–based strategies,[104] by altering the expression of these genes in a way that inhibits cell growth.

A second area of needed research is the question of how combinatorial control mechanisms and signal transduction crosstalk interface with the transcriptional regulatory activity of steroid and nuclear receptors in normal and transformed cells. This will include identification of specific cases in which deregulated control results from aberrations in one or more signaling pathways. For example, activation of the FOS-JUN AP-1 complex can proceed either by protein kinase C pathways through

G protein–coupled receptors and phospholipase C or by growth factor receptor stimulation of the mitogen–activated protein (MAP) kinase pathway. Because AP-1 activity can be modulated by protein-protein interactions with several steroid receptors, and steroid receptor function can be altered by AP-1 interactions, mutations in any number of kinase pathways leading to constitutively active AP-1 could alter the transcription of a variety of genes. Through a more molecular-based approach, it may be possible to develop new therapies using pharmacologic compounds that modify phosphorylation- and ligand-dependent signal transduction pathways.

REFERENCES

1. Strader CD, Fong TM, Tota MR, Underwood D, Dixon RAF. Structure and function of G protein–coupled receptors. Annu Rev Biochem 1994;63:101.
2. Tsai M-J, O'Malley BW. Molecular mechanisms of action of steroid/thyroid receptor superfamily members. Annu Rev Biochem 1994;63:451.
3. Waxman J. A new understanding of the hormonal regulation of endocrine dependent cancer. Br Med Bull 1991;47:197.
4. Labrie F. Endocrine therapy for prostate cancer. Endocrinol Metabol Clin North Am 1991;20:845.
5. Miesfeld RL. The structure and function of steroid receptor proteins. Crit Rev Biochem Mol Biol 1989;24:101.
6. Mader S, Kumar V, De Verneuil H, Chambon P. Three amino acids of the oestrogen receptor are essential to its ability to distinguish an oestrogen from a glucocorticoid-responsive element. Nature 1989;338:271.
7. Giguère V, Evans RM. Identification of receptors for retinoids as members of the steroid and thyroid hormone receptor family. Methods Enzymol 1990;189:223.
8. Weinberger C, Thompson CC, Ong ES, Lebo R, Gruol DJ, Evans RM. The c-erb-A gene encodes a thyroid hormone receptor. Nature 1986;324:641.
9. Baker AR, McDonnell DP, Hughes M, et al. Cloning and expression of full-length cDNA encoding human vitamin D receptor. Proc Natl Acad Sci U S A 1988;85:3294.
10. Petkovich M, Brand N, Krust A, Chambon P. A human retinoic acid receptor which belongs to the family of nuclear receptors. Nature 1987;330:444.
11. Glass CK. Differential recognition of target genes by nuclear receptor monomers, dimers and heterodimers. Endocr Rev 1994;15:391.
12. O'Malley BW, Conneely OM. Orphan receptors: in search of a unifying hypothesis for activation. Mol Endocrinol 1992;6:1359.
13. Amero SA, Kretsinger RH, Moncrief ND, Yamamoto KR, Pearson WR. The origin of nuclear receptor proteins: a single precursor distinct from other transcription factors. Mol Endocrinol 1992;6:3.
14. Hollenberg SM, Evans RM. Multiple and cooperative trans-activation domains of the human glucocorticoid receptor. Cell 1988;55:899.
15. Tora L, Gronemeyer H, Turcotte B, Gaub M-P, Chambon P. The N-terminal region of the chicken progesterone receptor specifies target gene activation. Nature 1988;333:185.
16. Miesfeld RL, Sakai D, Inoue A, Schena M, Godowski PJ, Yamamoto KR. Glucocorticoid receptor sequences that confer positive and negative transcriptional regulation. UCLA Symp Steroid Hormone Action 1988;32:193.
17. Rundlett S, Wu X-P, Miesfeld RL. Functional characterizations of the androgen receptor confirm that the molecular basis of androgen action is transcriptional regulation. Mol Endocrinol 1990;4:708.
18. Simental JA, Sar M, Lane MV, French FS, Wilson EM. Transcriptional activation and nuclear targeting signals of the human androgen receptor. J Biol Chem 1991;266:510.
19. Gronemeyer H. Transcription activation by estrogen and progesterone receptors. Annu Rev Genet 1991;25:89.
20. Faber PW, Kuiper GGJM, Van Rooij HCJ, Van der Korput JAGM, Brinkmann AO, Trapman J. The N-terminal domain of the human androgen receptor is encoded by one, large exon. Mol Cell Endocrinol 1989;61:257.
21. Jurutka PW, Hsieh J-C, MacDonald PN, et al. Phosphorylation of serine 208 in the human vitamin D receptor: the predominant amino acid phosphorylated by casein kinase II, in vitro, and identification as a significant phosphorylation site in intact cells. J Biol Chem 1993;268:6791.
22. Reese JC, Wooge CH, Katzenellenbogen BS. Identification of two cysteines closely positioned in the ligand-binding pocket of the human estrogen receptor: roles in ligand binding and transcriptional activation. Mol Endocrinol 1992;6:2160.
23. Forman BM, Yang CR, Au M, Casanova J, Ghysdael J, Samuels HH. A domain containing leucine-zipper like motifs mediates novel in vivo interactions between the thyroid hormone and retinoic receptors. Mol Endocrinol 1989;3:1610.
24. Forman BM, Samuels HH. Interactions among a subfamily of nuclear hormone receptors: the regulatory zipper model. Mol Endocrinol 1990;4:1293.
25. Fawell SE, Lees JA, White R, Parker MG. Characterization and colocalization of steroid binding and dimerization activities in the mouse estrogen receptor. Cell 1990;60:953.
26. Cheskis B, Freedman LP. Ligand modulates the conversion of DNA-bound vitamin D_3 receptor (VDR) homodimers into VDR-retinoid X receptor heterodimers. Mol Cell Biol 1994;14:3329.
27. Bocquel MT, Kumar V, Stricker C, Chambon P, Gronemeyer H. The contribution of the N- and C-terminal regions of steroid receptors to activation of transcription is both receptor- and cell-specific. Nucleic Acids Res 1989;17:2581.
28. Green S, Chambon P. Nuclear receptors enhance our understanding of transcription regulation. Trends Genet 1988;4:309.
29. Nordeen SK, Young DA. Glucocorticoid action on rat thymic lymphocytes. J Biol Chem 1976;251:7295.
30. Ivarie RD, O'Farrell PH. The glucocorticoid domain: steroid mediated changes in the rate of synthesis of rat hepatoma proteins. Cell 1978;13:41.
31. Briehl MM, Flomerfelt FA, Wu XP, Miesfeld RL. Transcriptional analyses of steroid-regulated gene networks. Mol Endocrinol 1990;4:287.
32. Briehl MM, Miesfeld RL. Isolation and characterization of transcripts induced by androgen withdrawal and apoptotic cell death in the rat ventral prostate. Mol Endocrinol 1991;5:1381.
33. Yamamoto KR, Alberts BM. Steroid receptors: elements for modulation of eukaryotic transcription. Annu Rev Biochem 1976;45:721.
34. Yamamoto KR. Steroid receptor regulated transcription of specific genes and gene networks. Annu Rev Genet 1985;19:209.
35. Claessens F, Rushmere NK, Davies P, Celis L, Peeters B, Rombauts WA. Sequence-specific binding of androgen-receptor complexes to prostatic binding protein genes. Mol Cell Endocrinol 1990;74:203.
36. Ho K-C, Marschke KB, Tan J, Power SGA, Wilson EM, French FS. A complex response element in intron 1 of the androgen-regulated 20-kDa protein gene displays cell type–dependent androgen receptor specificity. J Biol Chem 1993;268:27226.
37. Langston AW, Gudas LJ. Identification of a retinoic acid responsive enhancer 3′ of the murine homeobox gene Hox-l.6. Mech Dev 1992;38:217.
38. Oliveira IC, Sciavolino PJ, Lee TH, Vilcek J. Downregulation of interleukin 8 gene expression in human fibroblasts: unique mechanism of transcriptional inhibition by interferon. Proc Natl Acad Sci U S A 1992;89:9049.
39. Darwish H, Krisinger J, Furlow JD, Smith C, Murdoch F, DeLuca HF. An estrogen-responsive element mediates the transcriptional regulation of calbindin D-9K gene in rat uterus. J Biol Chem 1991;266:551.
40. Beato M. Gene regulation by steroid hormones. Cell 1989;56:335.
41. Luisi BF, Xu WX, Otwinowski Z, Freedman LP, Yamamoto KR, Sigler PB. Crystallographic analysis of the interaction of the glucocorticoid receptor with DNA. Nature 1991;352:497.
42. Freedman LP, Luisi BF. On the mechanism of DNA binding by nuclear hormone receptors: a structural and functional perspective. J Cell Biochem 1993;51:140.
43. Danielsen M, Hinck L, Ringold G. Two amino acids within the knuckle of the first zinc finger specify DNA response element activation by the glucocorticoid receptor. Cell 1988;57:1131.
44. Umesono K, Evans R. Determinants of target gene specificity for steroid/thyroid hormone receptors. Cell 1989;57:1139.
45. Dahlman-Wright K, Wright A, Gustafsson J-Å, Carlstedt-Duke J. In-

teraction of the glucocorticoid receptor DNA-binding domain with DNA as a dimer is mediated by a short segment of five amino acids. J Biol Chem 1991;266:3107.
46. Freedman LP, Towers TL. DNA binding properties of the vitamin D_3 receptor zinc finger region. Mol Endocrinol 1991;5:1815.
47. Vanderbilt JN, Miesfeld RL, Maler BA, Yamamoto KR. Intracellular receptor concentration limits glucocorticoid-dependent enhancer activity. Mol Endocrinol 1987;1:68.
48. Webb P, Lopez GN, Greene GL, Baxter JD, Kushner PJ. The limits of the cellular capacity to mediate an estrogen response. Mol Endocrinol 1992;6:157.
49. Russell DW, Wilson JD. Steroid 5α-reductase: two genes/two enzymes. Annu Rev Biochem 1994;63:25.
50. Schwabe JWR, Chapman L, Finch JT, Rhodes D. The crystal structure of the estrogen receptor DNA-binding domain bound to DNA: how receptors discriminate between their response elements. Cell 1993;75:567.
51. Kumar V, Chambon P. The estrogen receptor binds tightly to its responsive element as a ligand-induced homodimer. Cell 1988;55:145.
52. Mangelsdorf DJ, Ong ES, Dyck JA, Evans RM. Nuclear receptor that identifies a novel retinoic acid response pathway. Nature 1990;345:224.
53. Heyman RA, Mangelsdorf DJ, Dyck JA, et al. 9-Cis retinoic acid is a high affinity ligand for the retinoid X receptor. Cell 1992;68:397.
54. Mader S, Chen J-Y, Chen Z, White J, Chambon P, Gronemeyer H. The patterns of binding of RAR, RXR and TR homo- and heterodimers to direct repeats are dictated by the binding specificities of the DNA binding domains. EMBO J 1993;12:5029.
55. Predki PF, Zamble D, Sarkar B, Giguère V. Ordered binding of retinoic acid and retinoid-x receptors to asymmetric response elements involves determinants adjacent to the DNA-binding domain. Mol Endocrinol 1994;8:31.
56. Umesono K, Murakami KK, Thompson CC, Evans RM. Direct repeats as selective response elements for the thyroid hormone, retinoic acid, and vitamin D_3 receptors. Cell 1991;65:1255.
57. Durand B, Saunders M, Leroy P, Leid M, Chambon P. All-trans and 9-cis retinoic acid induction of CRABPII transcription is mediated by RAR-RXR heterodimers bound to DR1 and DR2 repeated motifs. Cell 1992;71:73.
58. Zhang X, Lehmann J, Hoffmann B, et al. Homodimer formation of retinoid X receptor induced by 9-*cis* retinoic acid. Nature 1992;358:587.
59. Glass CK, Lipkin SM, Devary OV, Rosenfeld MG. Positive and negative regulation of gene transcription by a retinoic acid–thyroid hormone receptor heterodimer. Cell 1989;59:697.
60. Schräder M, Müller KM, Nayeri S, Kahlen J-P, Carlberg C. Vitamin D_3–thyroid hormone receptor heterodimer polarity directs ligand sensitivity of transactivation. Nature 1994;370:382.
61. Carlberg C, Bendik I, Wyss A, et al. Two nuclear signalling pathways for vitamin D. Nature 1993;361:657.
62. Lehmann JM, Jong L, Fanjul A, et al. Retinoids selective for retinoid X receptor response pathways. Science 1992;258:1944.
63. Freedman LP, Arce V, Perez Fernandez R. DNA sequences that act as high affinity targets for the vitamin D_3 receptor in the absence of the retinoid X receptor. Mol Endocrinol 1994;8:265.
64. Peehl DM, Wong ST, Stamey TA. Vitamin A regulates proliferation and differentiation of human prostatic epithelial cells. Prostate 1993;23:69.
65. Skowronski RJ, Peehl DM, Feldman D. Vitamin D and prostate cancer: 1,25 dihydroxyvitamin D_3 receptors and actions in human prostate cancer cell lines. Endocrinology 1993;132:1952.
66. Conaway RC, Conaway JW. General initiation factors for RNA polymerase II. Annu Rev Biochem 1993;62:161.
67. Goodrich JA, Tjian R. TBP-TAF complexes: selectivity factors for eukaryotic transcription. Curr Biol 1994;6:403.
68. Meyer M-E, Quirin-Stricker C, Lerouge T, Bocquel M-T, Gronemeyer H. A limiting factor mediates the differential activation of promoters by the human progesterone receptor isoforms. J Biol Chem 1992;267:10882.
69. Kupfer SR, Marschke KB, Wilson EM, French FS. Receptor accessory factor enhances specific DNA binding of androgen and glucocorticoid receptors. J Biol Chem 1993;268:17519.
70. Halachmi S, Marden E, Martin G, MacKay H, Abbondanza C, Brown M. Estrogen receptor-associated proteins: possible mediators of hormone-induced transcription. Science 1994;264:1455.
71. Thompson CC, McKnight SL. Anatomy of an enhancer. Trends Genet 1992;8:232.
72. Kingston RE, Green MR. Modeling eukaryotic transcriptional activation. Curr Biol 1994;4:325.
73. Roberts SGE, Ha I, Maldonado E, Reinberg D, Green MR. Interaction between an acidic activator and transcription factor TFIIB is required for transcriptional activation. Nature 1993;363:741.
74. Kim TK, Roeder RG. Proline-rich activator CTF1 targets the TFIIB assembly step during transcriptional activation. Proc Natl Acad Sci U S A 1994;91:4170.
75. Tanese N, Tjian R. Coactivators and TAFs: a new class of eukaryotic transcription factors that connect activators to the basal machinery. Cold Spring Harb Symp Quant Biol 1993;58:179.
76. Ge H, Roeder RG. Purification, cloning, and characterization of a human coactivator, PC4, that mediates transcriptional activation of class II genes. Cell 1994;78:513.
77. Kwok RPS, Lundblad JR, Chrivia JC, et al. Nuclear protein CBP is a coactivator for the transcription factor CREB. Nature 1994;370:223.
78. Ali S, Metzger D, Bornert J-M, Chambon P. Modulation of transcriptional activation by ligand-dependent phosphorylation of the human oestrogen receptor A/B region. EMBO J 1993;12:1153.
79. Mason SA, Housley PR. Site-directed mutagenesis of the phosphorylation sites in the mouse glucocorticoid receptor. J Biol Chem 1993;268:21501.
80. Saha S, Brickman JM, Lehming N, Ptashne M. New eukaryotic transcriptional repressors. Nature 1993;363:648.
81. Gray S, Szymanski P, Levine M. Short-range repression permits multiple enhancers to function autonomously within a complex promoter. Genes Dev 1994;8:1829.
82. Fondell JD, Roy AL, Roeder RG. Unliganded thyroid hormone receptor inhibits formation of a functional preinitiation complex: implications for active repression. Genes Dev 1993;7:1400.
83. Baniahmad A, Ha I, Reinberg D, Tsai S, Tsai M-J, O'Malley BW. Interaction of human thyroid hormone receptor b with transcription factor TFIIB may mediate target gene derepression and activation by thyroid hormone. Proc Natl Acad Sci U S A 1993;90:8832.
84. Sakai DD, Helms S, Carlstedt-Duke J, Gustafsson J-Å, Rottman FM, Yamamoto KR. Hormone-mediated repression: a negative glucocorticoid response element from the bovine prolactin gene. Genes Dev 1988;2:1144.
85. Margolin JF, Friedman JR, Meyer WK-H, Vissing H, Thiesen H-J, Rauscher FJ III. Krüppel-associated boxes are potent transcriptional repression domains. Proc Natl Acad Sci U S A 1994;91:4509.
86. Ptashne M. How eukaryotic transcriptional activators work. Nature 1988;335:683.
87. Johnson PF, McKnight SL. Eukaryotic transcriptional regulatory proteins. Annu Rev Biochem 1989;58:799.
88. Yoshinaga SK, Peterson CL, Herskowitz I, Yamamoto KR. Roles of SWI1, SWI2, and SWI3 proteins for transcriptional enhancement by steroid receptors. Science 1992;258:1598.
89. Miner JN, Diamond MI, Yamamoto KR. Joints in the regulatory lattice: composite regulation by steroid receptor-AP1 complexes. Cell Growth Differ 1991;2:525.
90. Jonat C, Rahmsdorf HJ, Park K-K, et al. Antitumor promotion and antiinflammation: down-modulation of AP-1 (Fos/Jun) activity by glucocorticoid hormone. Cell 1990;62:1189.
91. Yang-Yen H-F, Chambard J-C, Sun Y-L, et al. Transcriptional interference between c-Jun and the glucocorticoid receptor: mutual inhibition of DNA binding due to direct protein-protein interaction. Cell 1990;62:1205.
92. Zhang X-K, Dong J-M, Chiu J-F. Regulation of α-fetoprotein gene expression by antagonism between AP-1 and the glucocorticoid receptor at their overlapping binding site. J Biol Chem 1991;266:8248.
93. Diamond MI, Miner JN, Yoshinaga SK, Yamamoto KR. Transcription factor interactions: selectors of positive or negative regulation from a single DNA element. Science 1990;249:1266.
94. Ransone LJ, Verma IM. Nuclear proto-oncogenes fos and jun. Annu Rev Cell Biol 1990;6:539.
95. Gurr JA, Kourides IA. Regulation of the transfected human glycoprotein hormone α-subunit gene by dexamethasone and thyroid hormone. DNA Cell Biol 1989;8:473.
96. Baumann H, Jahreis GP, Morella KK, et al. Transcriptional regulation

through cytokine and glucocorticoid response elements of rat acute phase plasma protein genes by C/EBP and JunB. J Biol Chem 1991; 266:20390.

97. Nishio Y, Isshiki H, Kishimoto T, Akira S. A nuclear factor for interleukin-6 expression (NF-IL6) and the glucocorticoid receptor synergistically activate transcription of the rat α1-acid glycoprotein gene via direct protein-protein interaction. Mol Cell Biol 1993;13:1854.
98. Ray A, Prefontaine KE. Physical association and functional antagonism between the p65 subunit of transcription factor NF-kappaB and the glucocorticoid receptor. Proc Natl Acad Sci U S A 1994;91:752.
99. Rangarajan PN, Umesono K, Evans RM. Modulation of glucocorticoid receptor function by protein kinase A. Mol Endocrinol 1992;6: 1451.
100. Power RF, Mani SK, Codina J, Conneely OM, O'Malley BW. Dopaminergic and ligand-independent activation of steroid hormone receptors. Science 1991;254:1636.
101. Smith CL, Conneely OM, O'Malley BW. Modulation of the ligand-independent activation of the human estrogen receptor by hormone and antihormone. Proc Natl Acad Sci U S A 1993;90:6120.
102. Mani SK, Allen JMC, Clark JH, Blaustein JD, O'Malley BW. Convergent pathways for steroid hormone- and neurotransmitter-induced rat sexual behavior. Science 1994;265:1246.
103. Denner LA, Weigel NL, Maxwell BL, Schrader WT, O'Malley BW. Regulation of progesterone receptor-mediated transcription by phosphorylation. Science 1990;250:1740.
104. Persaud SJ, Jones PM. Antisense oligonucleotide inhibition of gene expression: application to endocrine systems. J Mol Endocrinol 1994; 12:127.
105. Kraus WL, Montano MM, Katzenellenbogen BS. Identification of multiple, widely spaced estrogen-responsive regions in the rat progesterone receptor gene. Mol Endocrinol 1994;8:952.

Principles and Practice of Genitourinary Oncology, edited by Derek Raghavan, Howard I. Scher, Steven A. Leibel, and Paul H. Lange. Lippincott-Raven Publishers, Philadelphia, © 1997.

CHAPTER 43

Prostate Cancer

Chemoprevention Strategies

William J. Ellis and Michael K. Brawer

The number of new cases of prostate cancer diagnosed annually has nearly doubled over the past 10 years. Prostatic carcinoma is now the most commonly diagnosed malignancy and the second leading cause of cancer mortality in men. In 1996, it is estimated that 317,100 men will be diagnosed with prostate cancer and 41,400 men will die of the disease.[1] Despite aggressive detection and treatment efforts, the number of prostate cancer deaths continues to slowly rise. In many tumor systems, a growing emphasis is being placed on prevention. This chapter highlights the rationale behind chemoprevention activities for prostate cancer.

RISK FACTORS FOR PROSTATE CANCER

Age and family history are among the strongest risk factors for prostate cancer.[2–4] Racial and ethnic background also plays a role, with African Americans having the highest incidence of prostate cancer in the world.[5] Dietary fat consumption also is associated with prostate cancer.[6,7] Vasectomy, environmental toxin exposure, and smoking have not consistently been associated with this disease.[8–14] Chapters 36 and 39 contain more information on risk factors for prostate cancer.

Prostatic intraepithelial neoplasia (PIN) is a lesion characterized by proliferation and dysplasia of the glandular epithelium within the prostatic acini.[15] The basal cell layer, although present, is often disrupted. We have previously shown most high-grade PIN (G1-G2) is associated with invasive cancer in the prostate.[16,17] Low-grade (G1) PIN may be an isolated finding. The natural history of PIN (i.e., progression into invasive carcinoma) has not been documented; however, PIN fulfills the majority of requirements for a premalignant lesion. Men with PIN are considered at risk for the development of invasive disease. Chapter 37 contains further discussion of preneoplastic diseases of the prostate.

STRATEGIES TO DECREASE CANCER MORTALITY

Strategies to prevent death from any malignancy focus on three approaches. The first is improved treatment of established disease. This may entail any form of treatment that results in decreased mortality in patients diagnosed with the disease. The second strategy is to provide improved early detection. The ideal detection program would detect all clinically significant cancers at a point at which they are curable by one of the available treatment modalities. The third strategy of reducing cancer mortality is prevention, which may be accomplished by reducing risk factors or by the administration of agents designed to prevent the disease. Treatment and screening strategies are discussed in detail elsewhere in this book. Although radical prostatectomy and radiotherapy, the primary therapies of localized prostate cancer, have been modified over the years, they remain fundamentally unchanged. Similarly, although prostate screening holds great promise, the efficacy of early detection remains unproven.

Because prostate cancer mortality continues to increase despite aggressive detection and treatment, there has been added emphasis on the implementation of prostate cancer prevention strategies. Such approaches would be particularly suitable for men identified to be at high risk of developing the disease. As described previously, three cohorts with the highest risk of developing prostate carcinoma are men with a family history of the disease, African American men, and men with documented PIN.

CANCER PREVENTION STRATEGIES

There are three strategies that can be pursued in preventing cancer. The first is to reduce exposure to environmental toxins. An example of this strategy is the avoidance of asbestos expo-

TABLE 43-1. *Chemoprevention trials*

BREAST	COLON
Retinoids	NSAIDs
Tamoxifen	Calcium
	Betacarotene
LUNG	HEAD AND NECK
Retinoids	Retinoids
Betacarotene	Betacarotene
	Calcium
CERVICAL	SKIN (NONMELANOMA)
Betacarotene	Selenium
Interferon	
PROSTATE	
Finasteride	

Adapted from Lippman SM, Bennet SE, Waon KH. Cancer chemoprevention. J Clin Oncol 1994;12:851.

sure to reduce the incidence of mesotheliomas. No environmental toxins have clearly been implicated as a cause of prostate carcinoma; therefore, no environmental toxin policy exists that would reduce the incidence of this disease. A second strategy is modification of risk-taking behaviors. The classic example of a risk-taking behavior is cigarette smoking. As previously discussed, however, prostate carcinoma is one of the few neoplasms not associated with smoking. One potential behavior that can be modified to decrease prostate cancer risk is diet. The adoption of a low-fat diet may decrease the risk of developing prostate carcinoma.[18]

The third cancer prevention strategy is to administer chemopreventive agents to patients thought to be at risk of developing the disease. Table 43-1 lists several National Cancer Institute chemoprevention trials currently in progress.

CHEMOPREVENTION

The chemoprevention hypothesis makes two assumptions regarding carcinogenesis. The first is that carcinogenesis is a multistep process consisting of initiation, promotion, and progression, as diagramed in Figure 43-1.[19–21] The second assumption is that carcinogenesis is a field effect.[21] The field effect theory proposes that the entire epithelium of an organ is equally at risk of developing carcinoma because each of the cells comprising an epithelium has inherited the same genetic background and is exposed to the same toxins and products of metabolism that predispose that epithelium to carcinoma.[22–24] Field effect therefore predicts multifocal carcinogenesis. In most organs, even when the primary tumor has been removed, the remaining epithelium is at high risk for tumorigenesis. For example, following partial colectomy for colon carcinoma, the remaining colonic epithelium is at high risk for developing a metachronous malignancy.

Tumor initiation is the first step in carcinogenesis. Initiation is caused by direct damage to DNA, generally by direct carcinogen binding but also potentially by electromagnetic radiation. This change in the cellular genome is both rapid and irreversible.

The second step in carcinogenesis is tumor promotion. Promotion describes the transition from a transformed cell with a normal phenotype to premalignancy and is commonly caused by nongenetic factors that increase cell proliferation. Typically, such agents are epithelial irritants that increase cell proliferation, such as asbestos or cigarette smoke. Tumor-promoting substances exert their effect on the epithelium over long periods of time. These effects are generally considered reversible.

One potential promotor of prostatic carcinoma is dietary fat. Several studies have implicated high-fat diets in the pathogenesis of this disease, yet most of the data is circumstantial. A correlation between geographic per capita fat intake and prostate cancer incidence has been demonstrated.[6,7] Rose and colleagues[7] reported that the incidence of prostate cancer correlated with animal, but not vegetable, fat consumption. In the laboratory Rose and Connolly[18] have demonstrated that n-6 fatty acids stimulate prostate cancer growth, whereas n-3 fatty acids inhibit prostate cancer growth in vitro. Thus, dietary animal fat may serve as a prostate tumor promoter by increasing epithelial cell proliferation.

Tumor progression describes the evolution of an epithelium from premalignancy to malignancy. This transition is predominantly the result of genetic events such as loss of suppressor genes, which are associated with increased cellular proliferation. Although the proliferative events leading to the change from premalignancy to malignancy occur over a long period of time, because they have a genetic basis, these changes are generally irreversible.

The multistep theory of carcinogenesis has been well documented in colon carcinoma. Vogelstein and colleagues[20] have mapped the changes associated with the progression from adenoma to adenocarcinoma in the colon. Animal models have also validated this theory.[23,25] In particular, the rate of progression after initiation has been shown to be related to both the rate of gene mutation and the rate of cellular proliferation.

Two systems are available for the classification of chemoprevention agents.[21] Agents may be classified by the step at which they are active (i.e., initiation inhibitors, promotion inhibitors, or progression inhibitors). Alternatively, chemopreventive agents may be classified as either blockers of mutagenic carcinogens or blockers of hyperproliferation. In reality, the classification of chemoprevention agents is not this clear, because many of the agents act at multiple steps or may inhibit both mutagenesis and hyperproliferation.

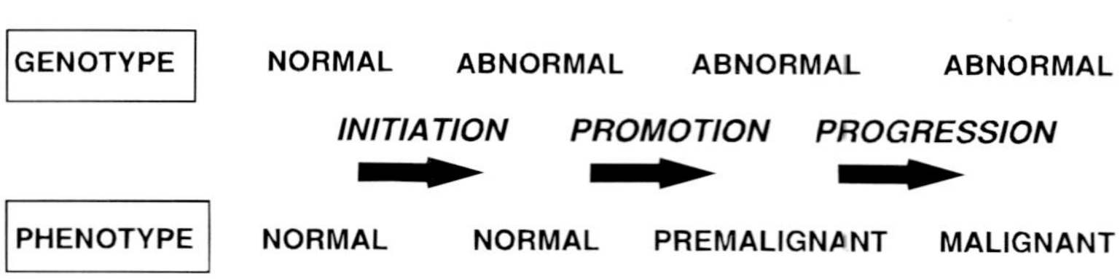

FIG. 43-1. Multistep process of carcinogenesis.

In any chemoprevention study, there are multiple end points that can be evaluated. The definitive end points are disease incidence or disease-specific survival. However, the identification of intermediate markers that can be monitored is important in the development of clinical trials. Such intermediate markers permit earlier evaluation of chemotherapeutic responses. One such intermediate marker is the presence of premalignant lesions such as PIN, carcinoma in situ, or dysplasia. A second class of markers includes biochemical or molecular markers. For example, serum prostate-specific antigen (PSA), the expression of oncogenes, the loss of normal receptors, or the presence of aneuploidy on flow cytometry may serve as intermediate markers of malignancy.

The ideal chemoprevention agent should have four characteristics. First, the agent must have proven efficacy in preventing the development of a malignancy. Secondly, the agent must have low toxicity. In some cases, the toxicity of a chemotherapeutic agent may result in an increased risk of other carcinomas. For example, tamoxifen is being studied as a possible chemoprevention agent in women at high risk for the development of breast carcinoma. However, the potential chemopreventive effect on breast carcinoma is in part offset by the increased risk of endometrial carcinoma in women on long-term tamoxifen therapy.[26] In women at high risk of developing breast carcinoma, the risk-benefit ratio may lean toward taking the drug. In women with average or low risk of developing breast carcinoma, such benefit may not accrue. The third requirement for a chemoprevention agent is that the drug should be easy to administer. Preferably, this means that the medication may be taken orally. Finally, the agent should be inexpensive, because lifetime therapy may be required.

Retinoids

In the prostate and other organ systems, retinoids have been explored as potential cancer chemoprevention agents. The retinoids promote differentiation and regulate proliferation of epithelial cells. The synthetic retinoid fenretinide (4-HPR) reduced the incidence of metastatic PA-III prostate carcinoma in Lobund-Wistar rats.[27] The development of adenocarcinoma also appears to be inhibited by the administration of 4-HPR in this model.[28] In the Dunning R3327 model, 4-HPR was demonstrated to inhibit angiogenesis, a critical event in tumor growth and development.[29] There is some variability in the effect of retinoids on cell behavior in cell lines. Fong and colleagues[30] observed a biphasic response on cell proliferation in the LNCaP model, with low levels of trans-retinoic acid increasing proliferation and higher levels inhibiting proliferation. They also noted increased PSA secretion by the LNCaP cells at all levels of trans-retinoic acid tested. In contrast, Dahiya and colleagues[31] noted a decrease in the proliferation of DU-145 cells in response to 13-cis-retinoic acid. Thus, responses to retinoids appear to be dose related. In theory, the differentiating properties of retinoids may stabilize or induce the regression of PIN and low-grade carcinomas. One advantage of retinoids is that they do not significantly alter PSA; therefore, serum PSA levels can be used as an intermediate end point. Small trials to evaluate the potential chemopreventive efficacy of retinoids in humans are underway.[32] There are dose-related side effects with retinoid therapy including dry skin and mucous membranes, hepatotoxicity, and central nervous system changes; these side effects may limit the widespread introduction of these agents, even if their efficacy is proven.[33]

Difluoromethylornithine

Ornithine decarboxylase (ODC) is an enzyme that catalyzes the synthesis of polyamines, which are involved in normal cell proliferation.[34] There is evidence that polyamines may be involved in neoplastic prostate growth as well. The prostatic concentrations of polyamines are among the highest in the body.[35] Heston and colleagues[36] found a correlation between ODC activity and tumor growth rates in the Dunning rat prostate cancer model. They also observed that administration of difluoromethylornithine (DFMO), a potent inhibitor of ODC activity, led to a reduction of tumor growth in the Dunning R3327 Mat-Ly-Lu tumor system in vivo and in vitro. Unfortunately, a phase I study of DFMO found significant gastrointestinal toxicities and audiotoxicities in addition to dose-limiting thrombocytopenia associated with this agent.[37] Thus, this particular inhibitor of ODC activity is unlikely to be suitable for a chemoprevention program.

Hormonal Therapy

The major chemoprevention efforts in prostate cancer center on the hormonal regulation of the prostatic epithelium. The androgen responsiveness of prostatic epithelium has long been used to treat clinical and prostate carcinoma. A growing body of evidence suggests that androgen manipulation may also be effective in modulating the development of prostate carcinoma. For example, prostate carcinoma is not known to develop in eunuchs who were castrated before puberty.[38] Furthermore, men with cirrhosis, who have a low testosterone-to-estrogen ratio, have lower rates of occult prostatic carcinoma.[39] Finally, the higher incidence of prostate carcinoma in African Americans is postulated to be secondary to the higher testosterone levels present in these men than in the general population.[40]

The role of androgens in prostate carcinoma pathogenesis is probably the result of the stimulatory effect androgens have on prostatic epithelial proliferation. Androgens may serve as promoting or progression agents in prostate carcinoma. Proliferation is known to increase the chance of genetic errors developing through repeated cell division. Translocation, deletion, and amplification of protooncogenes also require cell division. Damage to cellular DNA may be repaired by that cell up until the time of cell division. Following cell division, any residual defects in the cell's genome become fixed and are passed on to future generations.

The previous discussion suggests that hormonal ablation may prevent the development of prostate cancer. Such an approach is unlikely to be adopted, however, because the potential side effects of such therapy (e.g., impotence) outweigh the benefits for most people. However, experience with a group of male pseudohermaphrodites has suggested an alternative method of hormonal chemoprevention of prostate carcinoma in men.

Within the Dominican Republic, a form of familial male pseudohermaphrodism exists in which males are born with various degrees of ambiguous genitalia.[41] This ambiguous genitalia consists of undescended testes and mild to severe hypospadias.

Many boys with severe ambiguous genitalia are initially raised as females. However, at puberty, virilization occurs. These males have a normal libido and, depending on the degree of hypospadias, are perfectly capable of fathering children. Of particular note is that these males have a rudimentary prostate and do not develop benign prostatic hyperplasia (BPH) or prostate carcinoma.

Biochemical studies in these individuals have revealed that these males lack the enzyme 5α-reductase.[41,42] This enzyme is responsible for the conversion of testosterone to dihydrotestosterone (DHT) within the prostate. Both testosterone and DHT can bind to the androgen receptor. However, DHT has a greater affinity for the androgen receptor than does testosterone and is found in higher intracellular levels within the prostate. Once testosterone or DHT are bound to the androgen receptor, this androgen-receptor complex is translocated from the cytoplasm to the nucleus, where the androgenic effects are mediated.

The prostate and external genitalia are embryologically of urogenital sinus origin and require DHT for their development. Conversely, the epididymis and vas deferens are of wolffian duct origin and can develop normally with testosterone alone. Because the urogenital sinus is not exposed to DHT during development, an incomplete male phenotype is produced. At puberty, a large increase in serum testosterone occurs. Although testosterone binds weakly to the androgen receptor, because of the great excess of this hormone at puberty, an androgenic effect is exhibited on the urogenital sinus structures. As a result, at puberty these males with congenital 5α-reductase deficiency begin to show virilization of their external genitalia.

Finasteride is an oral 5α-reductase inhibitor. This drug inhibits serum DHT levels by approximately 70%.[43] Initial studies of this drug have focused on treatment of bladder outlet obstructions secondary to BPH. Over a period of 6 to 12 months, regular use of this medication results in a 20% to 25% decrease in the prostate volume; this is primarily the result of involution of the prostatic epithelium.[44] PSA, a major product of prostatic epithelial cells, is also regulated by DHT, and finasteride therapy results in a lowering of serum PSA levels by approximately 50%. On the basis of the decreased prostatic size and associated improvement in urinary symptoms, finasteride has been approved for the treatment of BPH by the U.S. Food and Drug Administration. This drug has a remarkable safety and side effect profile. The only side effects, which are clinically significant, are a decrease in ejaculatory volume and impotence (2% over placebo control).[44] This low side effect profile makes finasteride an excellent candidate for chemoprevention studies.

Circumstantial evidence exists suggesting that finasteride has a chemopreventive effect. As previously noted, males with familial 5α-reductase deficiency do not appear to develop prostate carcinoma. In addition, epidemiologic data suggests that ethnic groups with higher serum DHT levels have a higher tendency to develop prostate carcinoma, whereas ethnic groups with lower serum DHT levels have a lower tendency to develop prostate carcinoma.[45] Both animal and human prostate cancer models show that treatment with 5α-reductase inhibitors decreases tumor growth.[46–48]

In human studies, Presti and colleagues[49] have shown that finasteride therapy can decrease serum PSA levels in men with stage D2 adenocarcinoma of the prostate. Others have shown that in men with residual prostate carcinoma after radical prostatectomy as determined by persistently elevated postoperative serum PSA levels, progression as evidenced by increases in serum PSA is delayed by the initiation of finasteride therapy.[50,51]

The ability of finasteride to hormonally suppress the prostate with minimal side effects has led to the incorporation of this drug in the Prostate Cancer Prevention Trial (PCPT). This trial seeks to randomize 18,000 men to either finasteride or placebo for a 7-year period. All men with be followed yearly with serum PSA determinations and DREs. At the end of the 7-year study, all men will undergo prostate needle biopsy.

Monitoring patients in the finasteride treatment arm is somewhat problematic. Because finasteride causes shrinkage of the prostate gland and potentially of prostate tumors, the digital rectal examination (DRE) may be altered. If prostate tumors shrink, the tumors could potentially become nondetectable by DRE. Conversely, if the benign prostate tissue shrinks to a greater extent than does the tumor, the tumors may become more easily palpable. Data from the clinical trial of finasteride in the treatment of bladder outlet obstruction suggests that masking of prostate cancer detection through DRE does not occur.[52] In this study, detection of prostate carcinoma in the placebo, 1-mg finasteride, and 5-mg finasteride treatment groups were similar.[52] However, the cancer detection rates were lower than would be expected based on screening studies.[53] Interestingly, 29 of the 33 patients found to have carcinoma over the 4 years of the study had entry serum PSA levels greater than or equal to 4 ng/mL, a level that today would likely prompt biopsy before the initiation of hormone-based BPH treatment.

Because finasteride decreases serum PSA by approximately 50%, the use of this analyte to select patients for biopsy in the finasteride group in the PCPT will also be modified. Clearly, a strategy of performing biopsy only in those patients with serum PSA levels greater than 4 ng/mL is inappropriate in the finasteride treatment group. Patients with the highest serum PSA levels in the finasteride treatment group will be selected for biopsy so that the biopsy rate in the finasteride group is equal to the biopsy rate in the placebo control group.

SUMMARY

New diagnoses of and deaths attributable to prostate cancer continue to increase on a yearly basis. Thus far, new diagnostic strategies and aggressive implementation of therapies have not demonstrated a decrease in the death rate from prostate carcinoma. Implementation of strategies to prevent carcinoma is clearly in order. Because no modifiable risk factors for prostate carcinoma have yet been definitively identified, the best avenue for prostate cancer prevention at this time appears to be chemoprevention. Finasteride, a 5α-reductase inhibitor, allows hormonal modulation of the prostate with minimal side effects. This drug appears to be an good candidate for prostate cancer chemoprevention. The PCPT is in progress to evaluated finasteride as a prostate cancer chemoprevention agent.

REFERENCES

1. Parker SL, Tong T, Bolden S, Wingo PA. Cancer statistics, 1996. CA Cancer J Clin 1996;46:5.
2. Carter HB, Piantados S, Isaacs JT. Clinical evidence for the implica-

tions of the multistep development of prostate cancer. J Urol 1990; 143:742.
3. Spitz MR, Currier RD, Fueger JJ, Babaian RJ, Newell GR. Familial patterns of prostate cancer: a case-control analysis. J Urol 1991;146: 1305.
4. Carter BS, Bova SG, Beaty TH, et al. Hereditary prostate cancer: epidemiologic and clinical features. J Urol 1993;150:797.
5. Ross R, Paganini-Hill A. Epidemiology of prostate cancer. In: Skinner D, Leskovsky F, eds. Diagnosis and management of genitourinary cancer. Philadelphia: WB Saunders, 1988:40.
6. Armstrong B, Doll R. Environmental factors and cancer incidence and mortality in different countries with special reference to dietary practices. Int J Cancer 1975;15:617.
7. Rose DP, Boyar AP, Wynder EL. International comparisons of mortality for cancer of the breast, ovary, prostate, and colon, and per capita food consumption. Cancer 1986;58:2363.
8. Giovannucci E, Ascherio A, Rimm EB, Colditz GA, Stampfer MJ, Willett WC. A prospective cohort study of vasectomy and prostate cancer in US men. JAMA 1993;269:873.
9. Ross RK, Paganini-Hill A, Henderson BE. The etiology of prostate cancer: what does the epidemiology suggest? Prostate 1983;4:333.
10. Rosenberg L, Palmer JR, Zauber AG, et al. Vasectomy and the risk of prostate cancer. Am J Epidemiol 1990;132:1051.
11. Mettlin C, Natarajan N, Huben R. Vasectomy and prostate cancer risk. Am J Epidemiol 1990;132:1056.
12. Begun FP. Epidemiology and natural history of prostate cancer. In: Lepor H, Lawson RK, eds. Prostatic diseases. Philadelphia: WB Saunders, 1993:257.
13. Hsing AW, McLaughlin JK, Schuman LM, et al. Diet, tobacco use, and fatal prostate cancer: results from the Lutheran Brotherhood Cohort Study. Cancer Res 1990;50:6836.
14. Fincham SM, Hill GB, Hanson J, et al. Epidemiology of prostatic cancer: a case-control study. Prostate 1990;17:189.
15. Brawer MK. PIN: a premalignant lesion. Hum Pathol 1992;23:242.
16. Brawer MK, Nagle RB, Bigler SA, Lange PH, Sohlberg OE. Significance of PIN on prostate needle biopsy. Urology 1991;38:103.
17. Ellis WJ, Brawer MK. Repeat needle biopsy: who needs it? J Urol 1995;153:1496.
18. Rose DP, Connolly JM. Dietary fat, fatty acids and prostate cancer. Lipids 1992;27:798.
19. DiGiovanni J. Modification of multi-stage skin carcinogenesis in mice. Prog Exp Tumor Res 1991;33:192.
20. Vogelstein B, Fearson ER, Hamilton SR. Genetic alterations during colorectal tumor development. N Engl J Med 1988;319:525.
21. Lippman SM, Benner SE, Waun KH. Cancer chemoprevention. J Clin Oncol 1994;12:851.
22. Slaughter DP, Southwick HW, Smejkal W. Field cancerization in oral stratified squamous epithelium: clinical implications of multicentric origin. Cancer 1953;6:963.
23. Boone CW, Keloff GJ, Steele VE. Natural history of intraepithelial neoplasia in humans with implications for cancer chemoprevention strategy. Cancer Res 1991;52:1651.
24. Sidransky D, Frost P, Von Exchensbach A, et al. Clonal origin of bladder cancer. N Engl J Med 1992;326:737.
25. Wattenberg LW. Chemoprevention of cancer. Cancer Res 1985;45:1.
26. Arrigada R, Rutqvist LE, Group SBC. Adjuvant systemic therapy in early breast cancer and incidence of new primary malignancies. 1992; 11:522.
27. Pollard M, Luckert PH. The inhibitory effect of 4-hydroxyphenyl retinamide (4-HPR) on metastasis of prostate adenocarcinoma-III cells in Lobund-Wistar rats. Cancer Lett 1991;59:159.
28. Pollard M, Luckert PH, Sporn MB. Prevention of primary prostate cancer in Lobund-Wistar rats by N-(4-hydroxyphenyl) retinamide. Cancer Res 1991;51:3610.
29. Pienta KJ, Hguyen NM, Lehr JE. Treatment of prostate cancer in the rat with the synthetic retinoid fenretinide. Cancer Res 1993;53:224.
30. Fong CJ, Sutkowski DM, Braun EJ, et al. Effect of retinoic acid on the proliferation and secretory activity of androgen-response prostatic carcinoma cells. J Urol 1993;149:1190.
31. Dahiya R, Boyle B, Park HD, Kurhanewicz J, Macdonald JM, Narayan P. 13-Cis-retinoic acid-mediated growth inhibition of DU-145 human prostate cancer cells. Biochem Mol Biol Int 1994;32:1.
32. Kadmon D. Chemoprevention in prostate cancer: the role of difluoromethylornithine (DFMO). J Cell Biochem 1992;16H(Suppl):122.
33. Costa A, Malone W, Perloff M, et al. Tolerability of the synthetic retinoid Fenretinide (4-HPR). Exp J Cancer Clin Oncol 1989;25:805.
34. Heby O. Role of polyamines in the control of cell proliferation and differentiation. Differentiation 1981;19:1.
35. Danzin C, Jung MJ, Grove J. Effect of alpha-difluoro-methylornithine, and enzyme-activated irreversible inhibitor of ornithine decarboxylase, on polyamine levels in rat tissues. Life Sci 1979;24:519.
36. Heston WDW, Kadmon D, Lazan DW, et al. Copenhagen rat prostatic tumor ornithine decarboxylase activity (ODC) and the effect of the ODC inhibitor alpha-defluoromethylornithine. Prostate 1982;3:383.
37. Love RR, Carbone PP, Verna AK, et al. Randomized phase I chemoprevention dose-seeking study of alpha-difluoromethylorinthine. J Natl Cancer Inst 1993;85:732.
38. Deaver JB. Etiology and predetermining factors of BPH. In: Enlargement of the prostate: its history, anatomy, etiology, pathology, clinical causes, symptoms, diagnosis, prognosis, treatment, technique of operations and after-treatment. Philadelphia: Blakiston, p. 1922.
39. Lloyd CW, Williams RH. Endocrine changes associated with Laennec's cirrhosis of the liver. Am J Med 1948;4:315.
40. Ross RK, Bernstein L, Judd H, et al. Serum testosterone levels in young black and white men. J Natl Cancer Inst 1976;76:45.
41. Imperato-McGinley J, Guerrero L, Gautier T, et al. Steroid 5-alpha reductase deficiency in man: an inherited form of male pseudohermaphroditism. Science 1974;186:1212.
42. Walsh PC, Madden JD, Harrod MJ, et al. Familial incomplete male pseudohermaphroditism, type 2. Decreased dihydrotestosterone formation in pseudovaginal perineoscrotal hypospadias. New Engl J Med 1974;291:944.
43. Gormley GJ, Stoner E, Rittmaster RS. Effects of finasteride (MK-906), a 5-alpha reductase inhibitor on circulatory androgens in male volunteers. J Clin Endocrinol Metab 1990;70:1136.
44. Gormley GJ, Stoner E, Bruskewitz RC, et al. The effect of finasteride in men with benign prostatic hyperplasia. N Engl J Med 1992;327: 1185.
45. Ross RK, Bernstein L, Lobo RA, et al. Evidence for reduced 5-alpha reductase activity in Japanese compared to U.S. white and black males: implications for prostate cancer risk. Lancet 1992;339:887.
46. Lamb JC, Levy MA, Johnson RK, et al. Response of rat and human prostatic cancers to the novel 5 alpha-reductase inhibitor, SK&F 105657. Prostate 1992;20:15.
47. Damber JE, Bergh A, Daehlin L, et al. Effects of 6-methylene progesterone on growth, morphology, and blood flow of the Dunning R3327 prostatic adenocarcinoma. Prostate 1992;20:187.
48. Bologna M, Muzi P, Biordi L, et al. Antiandrogens and 5-alpha reductase inhibition of the proliferation rate in PC3 and DU145 human prostatic cancer cell lines. Curr Ther Res 1992;51:799.
49. Presti JC Jr, Fair WR, Andriole G, et al. Multicenter, randomized, double-blind, placebo-controlled study to investigate the effect of finasteride (MK-906) on stage D prostate cancer. J Urol 1992;148:1201.
50. Gormley G, Ferguson D, Lieber M, et al. Effect of finasteride on patients with elevated PSA following radical prostatectomy for prostate cancer. J Urol 1993;149:225A.
51. Andriole GL. Finasteride induced PSA reduction in patients with early stage prostate cancer. J Urol 1994;151:450A.
52. Stoner E, Round E, Ferguson D, Gormley GJ, et al. Clinical experience of the detection of prostate cancer in patients with BPH treated with finasteride. J Urol 1994;151:1296.
53. Brawer MK. Prostate cancer detection. (Editorial) J Urol 1994;151: 1308.

Principles and Practice of Genitourinary Oncology, edited by Derek Raghavan, Howard I. Scher, Steven A. Leibel, and Paul H. Lange. Lippincott-Raven Publishers, Philadelphia, © 1997.

CHAPTER 44

The Natural History of Human Prostate Cancer

Robert C. Flanigan and T. Vincent Shankey

The natural history of prostate cancer remains an enigma. We have progressed only minimally toward our goal of understanding what factors initiate this disease, cause it to proliferate or remain indolent, create the milieu for invasion beyond the prostatic capsule, facilitate metastasis, and eventually cause the death of the host. On the other hand, a great deal of information is now available regarding the natural history of some stages of localized prostate cancer from reports that have detailed the experience of centers with the expectant management of this disease. In this chapter, we review the extent of our knowledge regarding the epidemiology, presenting symptoms and clinical signs, mechanisms of metastasis, and natural history of this disease.

EPIDEMIOLOGY

An understanding of the natural history of prostate cancer would not be complete without an understanding of its epidemiology. This subject is covered in Chapter 37. Epidemiologic research may be especially important given the disparate ethnic and racial makeup of various study populations, such as the experience in Scandinavian men, as described by Iversen and colleagues, compared with the experience in American men, including African-Americans.[1,2]

PRESENTING SIGNS AND SYMPTOMS

Although there has been significant recent enthusiasm for the practice of screening men for prostate cancer or including a blood test for prostate-specific antigen (PSA) as part of a routine physical examination, most men who require treatment for their prostate cancer still seek medical attention only after they experience symptoms of their disease. The most common symptoms encountered are those of outlet obstruction or vesical irritability, but many patients present with symptoms of advanced disease, including bone pain and weight loss (Table 44-1).

Most studies done before the routine use of PSA testing demonstrated large numbers of patients with significant symptomatology. Several studies suggested that 20% to 25% of patients presenting with urinary retention harbored an identifiable prostate cancer.[3,4] In the pre-PSA era, regional symptoms, including back, leg, and perineal pain, were present in 20% to 40% of patients at diagnosis. Hematuria and constitutional symptoms such as weight loss, fatigue, and generalized weakness were found in 10% to 15% of patients. These facts led to the general axiom that symptomatic patients deserved careful consideration of the possibility of underlying prostate cancer.

The most important clinical sign of prostate cancer is abnormality on digital rectal examination. Although a palpable nodule is the most specific clinical sign of disease, the examiner must pay close attention to more subtle findings in the physical examination, including asymmetry and difference in gland texture from one location to another.

Unfortunately, reliance on the presence of symptoms or an abnormal digital rectal examination in the pre-PSA era yielded a disturbingly high percentage (40% to 50%) of patients who were found to have locally advanced disease (lack of organ confinement) after radical prostatectomy and careful pathologic evaluation of the specimen.[5,6] It has been strongly suggested by multiple studies that the addition of PSA testing to digital rectal examination increases the incidence of organ-confined disease at initial diagnosis.[7] However, even in populations of men submitting to a screening trial, most describe some symptoms of their disease. For example, in a screening trial of 6431 men at five institutions, we found that 38.4% reported increased frequency, 23.3% a weak stream, 9.3% urgency, 5.4% dysuria, 1.4% hematuria, 1.0% hematospermia, and 7% bone pain; only 47.6% of patients in this trial were asymptomatic.[7]

Other series have confirmed these findings and suggested a variability of symptomatology by patient age in men diagnosed with prostate cancer. In a study comparing younger patients (aged 50 to 64 years) with older patients, Bennett and associates found that although 25% of younger patients presented without symptoms, older patients were significantly more likely to present with severe local symptoms.[8] Not all studies have agreed

TABLE 44-1. *Presenting symptoms of prostate cancer*

Lower tract obstruction
Urinary frequency
Nocturia
Decrease in force of stream
Retention
Vesical irritability (dysuria)
Hematuria
Pain
Low back
Leg
Perineal
Weight loss
Generalized weakness

with the finding of an age-dependent variability in presentation. Aprikian and colleagues, for example, found that men younger than 50 years of age with prostate cancer presented with similar symptomatology, histologic grade, and disease stage as did older patients.[9]

NATURAL HISTORY

Prostate cancer is rarely diagnosed in patients younger than 40 years of age and is uncommonly diagnosed before age 50. After 50 years of age, there is an increase in incidence that roughly parallels a linear relation on a natural (base 2) logarithmic scale.[10] At autopsy, the majority of small carcinomas are found at the periphery of the gland.[11] McNeal and associates have shown that most TNM–UICC small stage T1a and T1b cancers in radical prostatectomy specimens occur in the anteromedial gland, adjacent to the fibromuscular stroma and to foci of benign prostatic hyperplasia; in contrast, stage T2a, T2b, and T2c cancers are usually located near the prostatic capsule at the posterior surface.[12]

It is increasingly evident that most prostatic cancers at the time they are first diagnosed are multifocal in nature and may be genetically heterogenous. Greene and associates have demonstrated that most lesions arising in the transition zone of the prostate are DNA diploid, whereas most peripheral zone lesions are DNA aneuploid (tetraploid).[13] In our laboratory, analysis on multiple tissue samples has shown that as many as 50% of patients with stage T1b cancer display both DNA diploid and DNA aneuploid tumor populations.[14] In addition, image analysis has demonstrated that areas of DNA aneuploid tumor can be found directly adjacent to areas of DNA diploid tumor. This multifocality and DNA ploidy heterogeneity give rise to speculation that prostate cancer is a field-change disease, a concept that is further strengthened by the presence of significant areas of high-grade prostatic intraepithelial neoplasia in many men in whom prostate cancer is diagnosed.[15] An analysis of the literature suggests significant disparity in the numbers of patients at various stages of disease whose tumor contains a nondiploid component. This disparity is probably a result of differences in techniques used to determine ploidy status and, to date, significantly limits the use of DNA ploidy in comparing data from center to center.

Intraprostatic Growth

Prostate cancers may be divided into two groups: transition zone cancers and peripheral zone cancers. Because of their anatomic fibromuscular boundaries, transition zone cancers tend to remain spherical until they are relatively large (>10 cc).[16] The fibromuscular structures that restrict their local spread are the urethra medially, the fibromuscular stroma anteriorly, and the "surgical capsule" posteriorly. These cancers are relatively distant from the rectal surface of the prostate but close to the anterolateral surface of the gland and to the bladder neck. These two areas are the sites of periprostatic extension in 22% and 25% of transitional zone cancers, respectively.[17,18] These factors serve to explain why many transition zone cancers remained confined to the gland despite their significant size.

Peripheral zone cancers, on the other hand, spread along the capsular surface of the gland. Early contact of these cancers with the thin posterolateral capsule, involvement of the apical prostate, and extension along the ejaculatory ducts into the seminal vesicles explains why they are likely to demonstrate extraprostatic extension even at small tumor volumes.[16,18]

Pathways for Extraprostatic Extension

The ability of a prostate cancer to escape the confines of the gland is an important aspect of its clinical behavior. Most evidence from radical prostatectomy specimens suggests that early prostatic growth occurs solely within the gland. Progression of disease tends to follow normal tissue planes within the gland and tends to be centrally oriented.[19] Penetration of the capsule is a relatively late event and occurs along perineural and vascular spaces.[16] Because there are no lymphatics within the perineural space, tumor growth within this space is by direct extension of the cancer along planes of least resistance.[20] Cephalad extension of prostate cancer often occurs, with resultant bladder neck or ureteral obstruction. Bladder neck obstruction is noted in 35% of advanced cases,[21] and ureteral obstruction has been reported in 8% to 35% of advanced cases.[21,22] Direct rectal invasion is a relatively late event, probably owing to the barrier effect of Denonvilliers' fascia. At autopsy after death from prostate cancer, rectal involvement has been noted in up to 10% of cases[21] (Fig. 44-1).

Mechanisms of Distant Metastasis

The mechanisms responsible for metastatic disease in prostate cancer remain poorly defined. Like most human malignancies, prostate cancer metastasizes in a characteristic and predictable fashion.[23] Early metastasis to bone suggests that the metastatic process in prostate cancer is not a random one, but rather is directed by specific mechanisms. Two major theories are used to explain prostatic cancer dissemination: the mechanical theory and the "seed and soil" theory.[24,25] The mechanical theory, attractive in its simplicity, states that the secondary sites of tumor growth are passively determined by the lymphatic and venous drainage of the primary disease site. In this regard, the preponderance of lower spinal metastases seen in prostate cancer may be explained by the fact that the prevertebral venous plexus (Batson's plexus) lacks valves and presumably provides

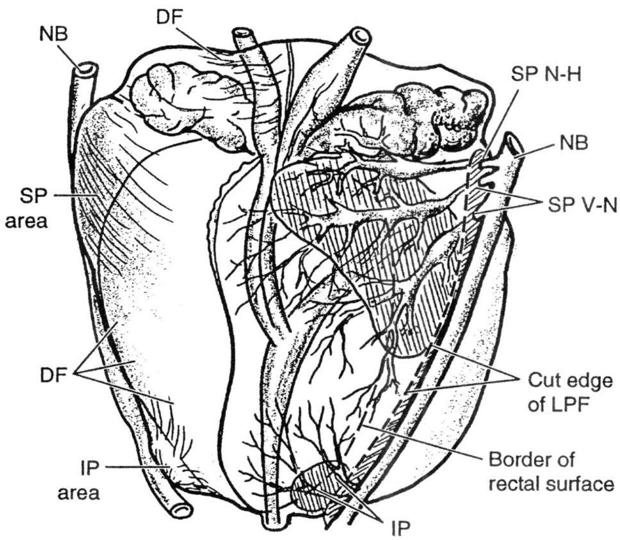

FIG. 44-1. Innervation of the prostate, showing extension from the neurovascular bundle (NB) of the superior pedicle (SP) at the prostate base and inferior pedicle (IP) at the prostate apex. The large vertical division of the superior pedicle (SP V-N) spreads over the prostate surface, with branches penetrating the capsule within the large nerve penetration area (*dotted line*). The small horizontal division (SP H-N) crosses the prostate base at midline. Denonvilliers' fascia (DF) is shown here cut away from the right half of the prostate. (Villers A. Extracapsular tumor extension in prostatic cancer: pathways of spread and implications for radical prostatectomy. In: Thomas Stamey, ed. 1994 Monographs in urology. Medical Directions, with permission.)

ready access to the vertebral system for prostate cancer cells that escape the primary lesion.[19] On the other hand, relatively large numbers of prostate cancer patients present with bone metastases that are found randomly throughout the bony skeleton. The ''seed and soil'' hypothesis recognizes the tissue-specific preferences exhibited by metastatic prostate cancer cells and attributes the predisposition for certain organ systems to combined influences of the tumor cells and target tissue. Metastasizing tumor cells may recognize local cell or tissue factors (e.g., cellular growth factors or growth-promoting components of matrix and basement membrane) that provide a suitable milieu for growth.[26] Conversely, other tissues may contain factors that inhibit tumor colonization.[27] Recent evidence suggesting that occult prostate cancer cells may be found with increasing frequency in peripheral blood of individuals with stage C and D disease[28,29] further supports the ''seed and soil'' hypothesis.

Late in the course of metastatic disease, prostate cancer metastasizes to visceral organs. Visceral metastases are often not clinically apparent and are usually noted at the time of postmortem examination. Autopsy findings, however, suggest widespread tumor involvement of the lungs (49.1%), liver (35.6%), adrenals (17.3%), and kidneys (10.6%).[30]

The overall sequence by which metastasis occurs in prostate cancer has not been fully established. Furthermore, the relation between lymphatic metastasis and metastasis to distant sites such as bone remains unclear. Although it is true that 50% of patients with involvement of the regional lymphatics also

TABLE 44-2. *Natural history of advanced prostate cancer*

Stage	Treatment	Result
C	Untreated	60% progression to D2 within 5 years
D1	Untreated	80% to 85% progression to D2 within 5 years
D2	Treated	Median survival time, 24–30 months, 5-year survival rate, 20%

demonstrate metastases to distant sites within a 2 years, and 80% within 5 years,[22] some patients do not display this pattern of progression (Table 44-2). A hypothetic schema of modes of progression of prostate cancer is shown in Figure 44-2.

After distant metastasis has occurred, the natural history of prostate cancer, despite hormonal therapy, is almost universally progressive and suggests a median survival time of 24 to 30 months[31] (see Table 44-2). One of the major contributions to our understanding of the natural history of advanced prostate cancer was provided by the finding of the National Prostate Cancer Project that several prognostic variables, including degree of bone pain, performance status, and acid and alkaline phosphatase levels, correlate strongly with patient survival time after metastasis has occurred.[32] Recent trials of maximal hormonal deprivation also appear to confirm the importance of prognostic factors, including performance status and the volume and location of bony metastases, in determining the natural history (survival time) in patients with advanced disease.[30]

NATURAL HISTORY BY CLINICAL STAGE

Prostatic cancer has often been characterized as a slow-growing tumor. In its early stages, tumor doubling time has been

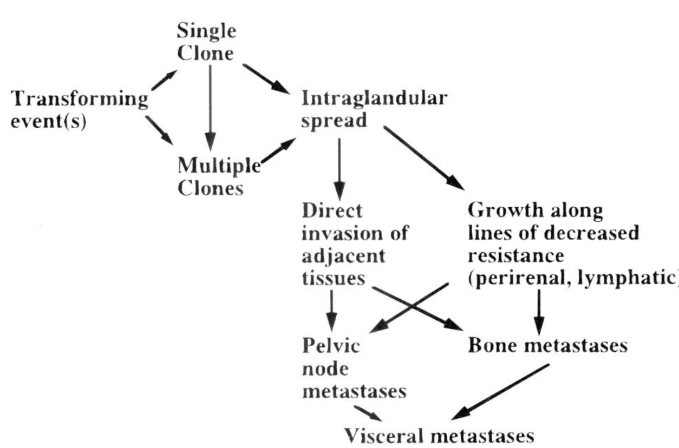

FIG. 44-2. Hypothetical model for local growth and dissemination of prostate cancers. Prostate cancers arise as a result of transforming events and progress through the preneoplastic lesion (prostatic intraepithelial neoplasia) to adenocarcinoma. The spread of tumor to sites outside the prostate may proceed by invasion of adjacent tissues or by growth along tissue planes that offer limited resistance to tumor extension. Subsequent spread to metastatic sites (e.g., pelvic nodes, bone) proceeds from extraprostatic sites.

estimated to be 2 to 4 years.[33] As it grows in volume, however, a prostate cancer is also apt to become more biologically aggressive (see Table 44-2). This is evident clinically by the relation of tumor volume to Gleason's histologic pattern, the likelihood of capsule penetration, and the presence of lymph node metastases.[17,33] A number of studies have also established a correlation between ploidy and Gleason score, showing an increasing frequency of DNA aneuploidy with higher Gleason score.[34,35] However, much evidence suggest that DNA ploidy is an independent predictor of disease course. The relation of these histopathologic criteria with newer genetic and cell proliferation markers and other measurements of tumor growth is less well established (see Fig. 44-2).

Stage T1a

Stage T1a disease is defined as a cancer that is found incidentally on removal of prostatic tissue to relieve bladder neck obstruction. It must be focal (<5% of the tissue removed) and must be well differentiated (Gleason sum <5). If other signs of more advanced disease are absent, progression of this disease over a follow-up period of 10 years is uncommon.[34,36]

Stage T1b

Stage T1b also represents an unsuspected histologic diagnosis, but one in which the prostate cancer is more widespread (>5% of the tissue removed) and less well differentiated (Gleason sum >4). Stage T1b cancers usually have a biologic potential equal to that of palpable prostatic cancers (stage T2). Lowe and Barry have correlated the biologic behavior of these tumors with patient age, Gleason score, and percent of tissue involvement as predictors of disease course.[37] In studies from our laboratory, the presence of a DNA aneuploid population also correlated significantly with progression and death in untreated stage T1b patients.[38] The relative risk ratio for patients with aneuploid versus diploid tumors was 5.25 by dichotomized factor analysis. Before the routine use of serum PSA testing, 15% to 25% of patients with T1b disease could be expected to have lymph node metastases at the time of presentation. Untreated patients are uncommonly described in the literature. Our data, from a single institution with small numbers of patients (n = 42) indicates a 10% rate of tumor-related deaths (with a 20% rate of non-prostate-cancer deaths) during a follow-up period of 10 years.[38]

Stage T1c

Stage T1c prostate cancer is defined as disease that is diagnosed only because an elevated serum PSA level led to further study and biopsy. Early conjecture that such patients may represent a population with indolent, nonsignificant disease has largely been disproved. Ohori and associates have estimated that 84% to 97% of such cancers represent clinically significant disease, based on the finding of a tumor volume greater than 0.5 cc at radical prostatectomy.[39] In addition, screening trials in which a number of such patients were identified and subsequently underwent radical prostatectomy have confirmed that as many as 20% to 25% of such cancers extend microscopically beyond the prostatic capsule.[40] Because this stage of disease has only recently been defined, long-term follow-up data are not yet available. It has been suggested that the natural history of this stage of disease approximates that of stage T2 prostate cancer, given similarities in findings from histopathologic analysis of radical prostatectomy specimens.

Stage T2

The natural history of untreated stage T2 prostate cancer has recently received considerable attention. In general, trials that have considered the question of conservative treatment (observation combined with hormonal therapy at progression) have been uncontrolled and nonrandomized. Chodak and colleagues recently compiled the pooled data from 828 case records from six nonrandomized trials published since 1985 of men treated conservatively (i.e., without radical surgery or radiotherapy at presentation).[41] In this group, factors that had significant impact on disease-free survival time included the presence of grade 3 tumors (risk ratio, 10.04) and age less than 61 years (risk ratio, 0.32). Ten years after diagnosis, the disease-specific survival rate (deaths from all other causes censored) was 8.7% for men with grade 1 or 2 cancer and 34% for men with grade 3 cancer. The rate of metastasis-free survival among men who did not die of other causes was 81% for grade 1, 58% for grade 2, and 26% for grade 3 tumors after 10 years.[41]

Stage T3

Stage T3 disease is defined as disease that has extended beyond the prostate to extraprostatic tissues, including the seminal vesicles. The incidence of associated lymphatic metastases in patients with clinical stage T3 disease is approximately 50%. The natural history of these patients is one of progressive local extension associated with urinary obstruction (Table 44-3). The natural history of prostate cancer metastatic to lymph nodes (N +) or to distant sites (M +) is described in Chapter 52. DNA ploidy status may be an extremely important predictor of natural history in metastatic prostate cancer. In addition, stage T3/T4 patients who have DNA diploid cancers display a significantly greater response to hormonal therapy as well as a significantly longer mean survival time.[42,43]

TABLE 44-3. *Cancer-specific survival after 10 years and estimated lifelong freedom from disease by clinical stage for prostatic cancer*

Stage	Cancer-specific survival rate (%)	Estimated rate of lifelong disease-free survival (%)
T1a	98	95
T1b	90	80
T1c	90	80
T2 grade 1–2	91	65
T2 grade 3	66	65
T3	60	25
N+	40	>5
M+	10	>1

MOLECULAR AND CELLULAR BIOLOGY OF PROSTATE CANCER

Autopsy studies have documented that roughly 30% of men older than 50 years of age who have no clinical evidence of disease have foci of pathologic prostate cancer.[44,45] Because the incidence of histologically defined prostate cancer is four times greater than the incidence of clinical disease in age-matched groups, it is likely that in many individuals the disease progresses at a very slow rate. However, disease progression becomes significantly more rapid in some men, and tumor cell growth probably plays an important role in prostate cancers that become clinically symptomatic. The underlying question is whether prostate cancers maintain roughly the same rate of growth throughout their existence, or whether some tumors progress from lower to higher rates of tumor cell growth.

Tumor Cell Growth

The overall rate of tumor growth is determined by the percentage of tumor cells in the cell cycle, the cell cycle transit time, and the rate of cell loss from either cell death (apoptosis or necrosis) or cell differentiation. Most studies of prostate cancers, as with other types of tumors, have focused on measurements of single aspects of tumor growth and thus failed to give an accurate determination of actual population doubling rates. Measurements using in vivo thymidine labeling have indicated very low cell proliferation for normal prostate (0.12% labeling index) and hyperplastic prostate (0.32% labeling index).[46] In vitro labeling measurements of prostatic cancers indicates a mean labeling index of 1.6%, with a range of 0.1% to 29%.[47] Although DNA content measurements using flow cytometry have been widely reported in prostatic carcinoma, these studies have only rarely included measurement of the fraction of tumor cells in the S phase of the cell cycle. Although technical factors are sometimes cited as limiting the utility of flow cytometric measurements of tumor proliferation, particularly from paraffin-embedded tissues, comparisons have shown good correlation between ^{3}H-TdR (thymidine) labeling index and flow cytometric S-phase fraction.[48]

Determination of prostate tumor proliferation, as measured by flow cytometric S-phase fraction, has demonstrated a positive predictive value for tumor progression[49] or overall survival time.[50] In these studies, individuals with high S-phase tumors have significantly higher probabilities of disease progression and death from prostate cancer. These studies suggest that tumors that demonstrate a higher proliferation rate are more likely to grow to and beyond the prostatic capsule and are likely to grow successfully in lymph nodes and other metastatic sites. In addition, tumors with high proliferative rates are less likely to respond to antiandrogen therapy, indicating that tumor proliferation is somehow related to the generation of hormone-independent (and generally DNA aneuploid) tumors.[43,50]

Genetic Changes in Prostate Cancers

The genetic basis of human cancers is now well established. Our current level of understanding is based on several seminal observations. First, as originally speculated by Boveri in 1914, chromosomal abnormalities are centrally involved in neoplasia. Second, cancer begins with the mutation of a gene within a single cell, and evolution of this clone through further mutations is a characteristic of cancer progression and metastasis.[51] Third, based on molecular genetic studies, recessive mutations in growth-suppressing genes occur early in the course of evolution of many cancers,[52] and dominant-acting mutations in growth-promoting factors occur during progression.[53] The most frequently cited model for tumor progression at this time suggests that genetic alterations (suppressor gene and dominant-acting gene mutations) occur in a stepwise fashion during tumor progression and metastasis.[54]

In contrast to other cancers (e.g., colon, bladder), the molecular genetic changes involved in human prostate cancers remain poorly understood. Classic genetic analyses using chromosome banding techniques (karyotyping) have provided limited insight. Such cytogenetic studies in prostate cancer have suggested a frequent involvement of chromosomes 2, 7, 8, 10, and 16.[55] More recent molecular genetic studies have demonstrated a number of changes in prostate cancers, including loss of loci on chromosome 8p,[56] 8q,[57] and 16q[58]; point mutations or deletions in the retinoblastoma gene[59] found on chromosome 13 and the *P53* gene[60] found on chromosome 17; and aneusomy of chromosomes 7[61] and 8.[56,62] Localization of amplified loci found on chromosome 8 by fluorescent in situ hybridization and comparative genomic hybridization to 8q24.1–24.2[63] provides one potential target locus in this chromosomal region, the *MYC* gene. This gene is well established as being involved in cellular proliferation.[64] Although these results are very preliminary and do not, as yet, provide a complete picture of the target genes involved in prostate cancer evolution (from the precursor lesion, to primary cancer, to local extension into the lymph nodes, and finally to distant metastatic disease), it is clear that these molecular genetic techniques will probably provide a model for prostate cancer related to the model proposed for colon cancer.[54]

Studies using flow and image cytometry have provided clinically important information regarding genetic changes in prostate cancers. Although these measurements of the genetics of prostate and other cancers are relatively gross, detecting only gains or losses of total genetic material or changes in DNA ploidy, they nonetheless have demonstrated that prostate cancers with the same amount of total DNA as diploid cells show a lower rate of progression, a higher patient survival rate, and a greater response to antiandrogen therapy than do DNA aneuploid prostate cancers.[65] These results would suggest that DNA diploid tumors, which probably contain fewer genetic alterations, have a different natural history than DNA aneuploid tumors. This concept is strongly supported by studies using flow cytometric DNA content analysis (DNA ploidy and S-phase fraction) of repeated fine-needle aspiration samples taken from men with clinically low-stage disease. In one study of untreated individuals, most had DNA diploid tumors initially, and a few of these individuals demonstrated progression to DNA aneuploidy in conjunction with changes in cytologic differentiation.[66] Although follow-up of these patients is incomplete, the early results suggest that those with DNA diploid tumors had significantly lower rates of metastasis and death from prostate cancer.[67] Together with a number of independent studies of progression and death rates in relation to DNA ploidy,[65] these results support the concept that tumors that remain DNA diploid have a lower rate of progression. Furthermore, they suggest that a sizable percentage of DNA diploid tumors may evolve to DNA aneuploidy, with subsequent progression at a faster rate.

Studies from our laboratory have demonstrated that DNA diploid prostate cancers have a statistically lower proliferation rate (S-phase fraction) than DNA aneuploid cancers.[14,38] These studies have included the analysis of multiple tumor-containing areas within individual prostates, demonstrating that in some individuals both DNA diploid and DNA aneuploid tumor foci are seen. In most of these cases, the DNA aneuploid tumor had significantly a higher S-phase fraction than the DNA diploid tumor in the same prostate. Studies of multiple whole-mount sections using flow and image cytometry have shown that the majority of large-volume tumors (mostly stage T3/T4) contain only DNA aneuploid tumors (unpublished data). In contrast, studies of T1a samples have demonstrated that 90% of these tumors contain only DNA diploid foci and that the few T1a tumors that contain DNA aneuploid prostate cancer have proliferation rates that are statistically the same as those of DNA diploid tumors in this group.[68]

These studies have provided us with a hypothetic model for prostate cancer evolution, presented in Figure 44-3. As indicated in the figure, the majority of preneoplastic lesions of the prostate (most likely prostatic intraepithelial neoplasia) are DNA diploid,[69] and these lesions probably progress to DNA diploid tumors that have low proliferation rates. Because most DNA aneuploid tumors seen in low-stage prostate cancer are DNA tetraploid, the probable evolutionary pathway for many prostate cancers involves a tetraploidization of the genetically abnormal DNA diploid tumors. Because most of these tumors have a low to intermediate S-phase fraction, changes in tumor proliferation probably follow the tetraploidization step. This pathway is identical to one derived by Shackney and coworkers[70] using computer simulation of model tumor cell systems. Shackney has hypothesized, using mathematical modeling for tumor evolution, that the genetic evolutionary step of tetraploidization is followed by an increase in tumor growth rate, probably because of further mutation in dominant-acting growth-promoting gene products (MYC?). As shown in Figure 44-3, DNA diploid tumors can also evolve (presumably directly) from low to high S-phase fraction, and high S-phase tumors are likely to progress at a rate similar to those of DNA aneuploid, high S-phase tumors.[50] DNA aneuploid tumors (other than DNA tetraploid tumors) are seen with increasing frequency in grade T2 to T4 lesions[14,42,43,65] and have significantly higher S-phase numbers than DNA tetraploid tumors found in lower grades.[14,50,65] Therefore, they probably reflect genetic evolutionary steps proceeding from low S-phase DNA tetraploid tumors.

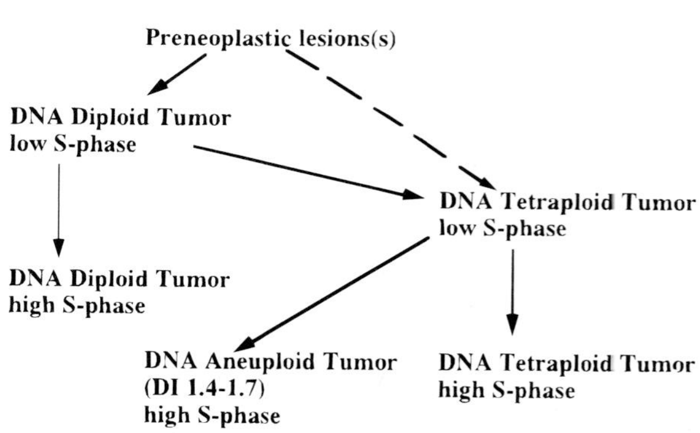

FIG. 44-3. Hypothetical model for the genetic evolution of prostate cancers. Preneoplastic lesion (prostatic intraepithelial neoplasia, or PIN) probably proceeds (with gene mutations that are undetectable by DNA content analysis) to DNA diploid low S-phase adenocarcinomas. An alternative is progression from DNA tetraploid PIN to DNA tetraploid adenocarcinoma. Overall, increase in tumor growth rate probably occurs after tetraploidization (duplication of all chromosomes in DNA diploid tumor), with subsequent chromosomal losses in some tumors evolving to a DNA index (DI) of 1.4 to 1.7.

Returning to the concept raised at the beginning of this section, the underlying question is whether all prostate cancers progress at the same rates throughout their history, or whether all tumors start with a low growth rate and some continue with the same rate while others evolve to more rapidly growing tumors. These proliferation groups correlate roughly with the "turtles and birds" paradigm attributed to Hinman by Lange.[71] Here, the slower-proliferating tumors that fail to evolve genetically are to be found in patients who will probably die of other causes than prostate cancer, and these represent the significant numbers of men who had, in the pre-PSA past, pathologic and not clinically apparent prostate cancer. At the other genetic evolutionary extreme are the high S-phase DNA aneuploid tumors, which have a high probability of local and metastatic spread.

CONCLUSIONS

Although our understanding of the natural history of human prostate cancer remains only partially elucidated at this time, advances in the ability to detect early disease probably will provide unique opportunities for further understanding this cancer. However, these advances also present an additional and sizable problem. A number of studies have provided strong evidence that not all individuals with prostate cancer, particularly at early clinical stage, are at significant risk for death from prostate cancer. The development of improved techniques to detect prostate cancer will prove beneficial only if the ability to predict disease course for individual patients is similarly developed. Although classic histopathologic techniques are useful, they have significant limitations. Clearly, there is a need for new technologies that can allow predictions of disease course for individual patients on the basis of small biopsy samples. Although molecular genetic techniques provide great promise, they are at present still in their infancy and will prove clinically useful only if they can predict the natural history of the disease for each patient.

ACKNOWLEDGMENTS

Research in the authors' laboratory was supported by a VA Merit Review Grant from the National Institutes of Health (1R55CA57910) and by the Retirement Research Foundation (RRF #93-49). The authors gratefully acknowledge the technical expertise and support of laboratory technicians Tina Lubrano and Sharon Graham. Image analysis studies of prostate cancers performed by Dr. Jia-Juan Jin in the authors' laboratory are gratefully acknowledged.

REFERENCES

1. Iversen P, Adolfsson J, Johansson J-E, Torp-Pedersen S. Localized prostate cancer: a Scandinavian view. Monogr Urol 1994;15:93.
2. Silverberg E, Lubera JA. A review of American Cancer Society estimates of cancer cases and deaths. CA Cancer J Clin 1986;36:9.
3. Catalona WJ, Scott WW. Carcinoma of the prostate. In: Walsh PC, Gittes RF, Perlmutter AD, et al, eds. Campbell's urology, 5th ed, vol 2. Philadelphia: WB Saunders, 1986;1477.
4. Moul JW, Davis R, Vaccaro JA, et al. Acute urinary retention associated with prostatic cancer. J Urol 1989;141:1375.
5. Stamey TA, Villers A, McNeal JE, Link PC, Freiha FS. Positive surgical margins at radical prostatectomy: importance of the apical dissection. J Urol 1990;143:1166.
6. Catalona WJ, Biggs W. Nerve-sparing radical prostatectomy: evaluation of results after 250 patients. J Urol 1990;143:538.
7. Catalona WJ, Richie JP, Ahmann R, et al. Comparison of digital rectal examination and serum prostate specific antigen in the early detection of prostate cancer: results of a multicenter clinical trial of 6,630 men. J Urol 1994;15:1283.
8. Bennett CL, Ganz P, Aronow HU, et al. Patterns of care in the presentation and evaluation of patients with prostate cancer. Proc Ann Mtg Am Soc Clin Oncol 1988;7:A496.
9. Aprikian AG, Zhang ZF, Fair WR. Prostate adenocarcinoma in men younger than 50 years: a retrospective review of 151 patients. Cancer 1994;74:1768.
10. Franks LM. Etiology, epidemiology, and pathology of prostatic cancer. Cancer 1973;32:1092.
11. McNeal JE. Origin and development of carcinoma of the prostate. Cancer 1969;23:24.
12. McNeal JE, Price HM, Redwine EA, et al. Stage A versus stage B adenocarcinoma of the prostate: morphological comparison and biological significance. J Urol 1988;139:61.
13. Greene DR, Taylor SR, Wheeler TM, et al. DNA ploidy by image analysis of individual foci of prostate cancer: a preliminary report. Cancer Res 1991;51:4084.
14. Dougherty S, Manion S, Jin J-K, et al. Intra-tumor heterogeneity of stage A2 (T1b) prostatic adenocarcinoma. I. Evaluation of archival tumors by flow cytometry. Cytometry. In press.
15. Oyasu R, Bahnson RR, Nowels K, et al. Cytological atypia in the prostate gland: frequency, distribution, and possible relevance to carcinoma. J Urol 1986;959.
16. McNeal JE, Redwine EA, Freiha FS, Stamey TS. Zonal distribution of prostatic adenocarcinoma with histologic pattern and direction of spread. Am J Surg Pathol 1988;12:897.
17. McNeal JE, Villers A, Redwine EA, Freiha FS, Stamey TA. Capsular penetration in prostate cancer: significance for natural history and treatment. Am J Surg Pathol 1990;14:240.
18. Rosen MA, Goldstone L, Lapin S, Wheeler T, Scardino PT. Frequency and location of extracapsular extension and positive surgical margins in radical prostatectomy specimens. J Urol 1992;148:331.
19. Kozlowski JM, Grayhack JT: carcinoma of the prostate. In: Gillenwater JY, Grayhack JT, Howards SS, Duckett JW, eds. Adult and pediatric urology. St Louis: Mosby–Year Book 1991;1277.
20. Rodin AE, Larson DL, Roberts DK. Nature of the perineal space invaded by prostatic carcinoma. Cancer 1967;20:1772.
21. Michigan S, Catalona WJ. Ureteral obstruction from prostatic carcinoma: response to endocrine and radiation therapy. J Urol 1977;118:733.
22. Barzell W, Bean MA, Hilaris BS, et al. Prostatic adenocarcinoma: relationship of grade and local extent to pattern of metastases. J Urol 1977;118:278.
23. Morgan TR, Heston WDW. The biology of solid tumor metastases. In: Chisholm GD, Fair WR, eds. Scientific foundations of urology. Chicago: Year Book Medical Publishers, 1990;474.
24. Hart IR. ''Seed and soil'' revisited: mechanism of site-specific metastasis. Cancer Metastasis Rev 1982;1:5.
25. Paget S. The distribution of secondary growths in cancer of the breast. Lancet 1989;1:571.
26. Hujanen FS, Terranova VP. Migration of tumor cells to the organ-derived chemoattractants. Cancer Res 1985;45:3517.
27. Nicholson GL, Dulski KM. Organ specificity of metastatic tumor colonization is related to organ-selective growth properties of malignant cells. Int J Cancer 1986;38:289.
28. Moreno JG, Croce CM, Fischer R, et al. Detection of hematogenous micrometastasis in patients with prostate cancer. Cancer Res 1992;52:6110.
29. Katz A, Olsson C, Eaffo A, et al. Molecular staging of prostate cancer with the use of an enhanced reverse transcriptase-PCR assay. Urology 1994;43:765.
30. Saitoh H, Hida M, Shimbo T, et al. Metastatic patterns of prostate cancer correlation between sites and number of organs involved. Cancer 1984;54:3078.
31. Crawford ED, Eisenberger MA, Investigators INT-0036. A controlled trial of leuprolide with and without flutamide in prostate cancer. N Engl J Med 1989;321:419.
32. Murphy GP. Management of disseminated prostatic carcinoma in prostate cancer. New York, PSG Publishing, New York 1979;213.
33. Schmie HP. Natural follow-up of prostate cancer and consequences for early detection. Schweiz Rundsch Med Prax 1993;82:1239.
34. Sharkey FE, Dusenbery DM, Moyer JE, et al. Correlation between stage and grade in prostatic adenocarcinoma: a morphometric study. J Urol 1984;132:602.
35. Frankfurt OS, Slocum HK, Rustum YM, et al. Flow cytometric analysis of DNA aneuploidy in primary and metastatic human solid tumors. Cytometry 1983;5:71.
36. Blute ML, Zincke H, Farrow GM. Long-term follow-up of young patients with stage A adenocarcinoma of the prostate. J Urol 1986;136:840.
37. Lowe BA, Barry JM. The predictive accuracy of staging transurethral resection of the prostate in the management of stage A cancer of the prostate: a comparative evaluation. J Urol 1990;143:1142.
38. Flanigan RC, Dougherty S, Jin J-K, et al. Prognostic factors in treated and untreated stage T1b prostate cancer. Submitted for publication.
39. Ohori M, Wheeler TM, Dunn JK, Stamey TA, Scardino PT. The pathological features and prognosis of prostate cancer detectable with current diagnostic tests. J Urol 1994;152:1714.
40. Epstein JI, Walsh PC, Carmichael M, Brendler CB. Pathologic and clinical findings to predict tumor extent of nonpalpable (stage T1c) prostate cancer. JAMA 1994;271:192.
41. Chodak GW, Thisted RA, Gerber GS, et al. Results of conservative management of clinically localized prostate cancer. N Engl J Med 1994;330:242.
42. Nativ O, Winkler HZ, Raz Y, et al. Stage C prostatic adenocarcinoma: flow cytometric nuclear DNA ploidy analysis. Mayo Clin Proc 1989;64:911.
43. Zincke H, Bergstralh EJ, Larson-Keller JJ, et al. Stage D1 prostate cancer treated by radical prostatectomy and adjuvant hormonal treatment: evidence of favorable survival in patients with DNA diploid tumors. Cancer 1992;70(Suppl):311.
44. Franks LM. Latency and progression in tumors: the natural history of prostatic cancer. Lancet 1956;2:1037.
45. Scott R, Mutchnik DL, Laskowski TZ, et al. Carcinoma of the prostate in elderly men: incidence, growth characteristics and clinical significance. J Urol 1969;101:602.
46. Meyer JS, Sufrin G, Martin SA. Proliferative activity of benign human prostate, prostatic adenocarcinoma and seminal vesicle evaluated by thymidine labeling. J Urol 1982;128:1353.
47. Scrivner DL, Meyer JS, Rujanavech N, et al. Cell kinetics by bromodeoxyuridine labeling and deoxyribonucleic acid ploidy in prostatic carcinoma needle biopsies. J Urol 1991;146:1034.
48. McDivitt RW, Stone KR, Craig RB, et al. A proposed classification of breast cancer based on kinetic information. Cancer 1986;57:269.
49. Eskelin M, Lipponen P, Majapuro R, et al. DNA ploidy, S-phase fraction and G2 fraction as prognostic determinants in prostatic adenocarcinomas. Eur Urol 1991;20:62.
50. Visakorpi T, Kallioniemi OP, Paronen IY, et al. Flow cytometric analysis of DNA ploidy and S-phase fraction from prostatic adenocarcinomas: implications for prognosis and response to endocrine therapy. Br J Cancer 1991;64:578.
51. Nowell PC. The clonal evolution of tumor cell population: acquired genetic lability permits stepwise selection of variant sublines and underlies tumor progression. Science 1976;194:23.
52. Knudson AG. Retinoblastoma: a prototypic hereditary neoplasm. Semin Oncol 1978;5:57.
53. Bishop JM. Molecular themes in oncogenesis. Cell 1991;64:235.
54. Vogelstein, B, Fearon ER, Hamilton SR, et al. Genetic alterations during colorectal-tumor development. N Engl J Med 1988;319:525.

55. Sandberg AA. Chromosomal abnormalities and related events in prostate cancer. Human Pathol 1992;23:368.
56. Macoska JA, Trybus TM, Sakr WA, et al. Fluorescence in situ hybridization analysis of 8p allelic loss and chromosome 8 instability in human prostate cancer. Cancer Res 1994;54:3824.
57. Bova GS, Carter BS, Bussemakers MJG, et al. Homozygous deletion and frequent allelic loss of chromosome 8q22 loci in human prostate cancer. Cancer Res 1993;53:3869.
58. Carter BS, Ewing CM, Ward WST, et al. Allelic loss of chromosomes 16q and 10q in human prostate cancer. Proc Natl Acad Sci U S A 1990;87:8751.
59. Bookstein R, Rio P, Madreperla S, et al. Promoter deletion and loss of retinoblastoma gene expression in human prostate carcinoma. Proc Natl Acad Sci U S A 1990;87:7762.
60. Isaacs WB, Carter BS, Ewing CM. Wild-type p53 suppresses growth of human prostate cancer cells containing mutant p53 alleles. Cancer Res 1991;51:4716.
61. Alcaraz A, Takahashi S, Brown JA, et al. Aneuploidy and aneusomy of chromosome 7 detected by fluorescence in situ hybridization are markers of poor prognosis in prostate cancer. Cancer Res 1994;55:3998.
62. Brown JA, Alcaraz A, Takahashi, et al. Chromosomal aneusomies detected by fluorescent in situ hybridization analysis in clinically localized prostate carcinoma. J Urol 1994;152:1157.
63. van den Berg C, Guan X-Y, Von Hoff D, et al. DNA sequence amplification in human prostate cancer identified by chromosome microdissection: potential prognostic implications. Clin Cancer Res 1995;1:11.
64. Kelly K, Cochran BH, Stiles CD, Leder P. The regulation of c-myc by growth signals. Curr Top Microbiol Immunol 1984;113:117.
65. Shankey TV, Kallioniemi O-P, Kozlowski JM, et al. Consensus review of the clinical utility of DNA content cytometry in prostate cancer. Cytometry 1993;14:497.
66. Adolfsson J, Tribukait B. Evaluation of tumor progression by repeated fine needle biopsies in prostate adenocarcinoma: modal deoxyribonucleic acid value and cytological differentiation. J Urol 1990;144:1408.
67. Adolfsson J, Ronstrom L, Hedlund PO, et al. The prognostic value of modal deoxyribonucleic acid in low grade, low stage untreated prostate cancer. J Urol 1990;144:1404.
68. Shankey TV, Jin J-Q, Dougherty S, et al. DNA ploidy and proliferation: heterogeneity in human prostate carcinomas. Cytometry 1995;21:30.
69. Weinberg DS, Weidner N. Concordance of DNA content between prostatic intraepithelial neoplasia and concomitant invasive carcinoma. Arch Pathol Lab Med 1993;117:1132.
70. Shackney SE, Smith CA, Miller BW, et al. Model for genetic evolution of human solid tumors. Cancer Res 1989;49:3344.
71. Lange PH. Future studies in localized prostate cancer. What should we think? What can we do? J Urol 1994;152:1932–1938.

Principles and Practice of Genitourinary Oncology, edited by Derek Raghavan, Howard I. Scher, Steven A. Leibel, and Paul H. Lange. Lippincott-Raven Publishers, Philadelphia, © 1997.

CHAPTER 45

Prostate Cancer

Diagnostic Approaches

W. Holt Sanders and William H. Cooner

Digital rectal examination (DRE), measurement of serum prostate-specific antigen (PSA), and transrectal ultrasonography (TRUS) are the three basic tools used in the detection of adenocarcinoma of the prostate. The exact role of each test in detection and screening for prostate cancer has been the subject of intense scrutiny during the past decade, a decade in which the detection of prostate cancer has increased dramatically. Although recommendations for screening and detection continue to evolve, a reasonable algorithm for the use of these tests has been developed.

DIGITAL RECTAL EXAMINATION

The detection rate of prostate cancer by DRE and digitally guided prostate biopsy is between 1.3% and 1.7% in the general population.[1,2] This detection rate is far below the reported 30% prevalence of disease in males older than 50 years of age. Although many of the tumors missed by DRE are microscopic and clinically insignificant, some lead to significant morbidity and mortality. Several independent factors contribute to the low detection rate with DRE. First, this diagnostic test is highly subjective, with considerable variations in reported findings among experienced urologists examining the same patient and also for sequential examinations of one patient by a single urologist. Second, approximately half of prostate carcinomas originate in the anterior portion of the gland.[3] These cancers are not detectable as palpable indurations until they have reached a locally advanced stage. Third, there is evidence that digitally guided biopsies miss one third to one half of tumors in the prostate.[4,5]

The DRE should be performed with the patient either standing and leaning forward so that his abdomen rests on the examining table or alternatively, with the patient in the knee-chest position. These positions allow for examination of the base of the prostate and seminal vesicles in many cases. The buttocks limit the examination to a greater extent if the patient is in the lateral decubitus or lithotomy position. The gloved, lubricated index finger is gently inserted into the anus. The entire rectal vault should be examined for masses. The prostate should then be evaluated for asymmetry and for nodules. The normal prostate feels similar to the thenar eminence when the thumb and fifth finger of the examiner are opposed. A carcinoma feels more like the bent knuckle of the thumb, and it is nontender. The shape of the prostate on DRE is variable. Some glands have a completely smooth, rounded surface. Other normal glands have well-defined lateral ridges with a central depression (Fig. 45-1). The seminal vesicles can frequently be palpated in this latter type of gland. The location and distinct boundaries of a nodule or induration should be noted, as well as effacement of the distinct sulcus that marks the lateral edge of the prostate.

PROSTATE-SPECIFIC ANTIGEN

PSA is the most useful tumor marker for adenocarcinoma of the prostate. PSA is a highly immunogenic serine protease that is primarily bound in the serum to either α_1-antichymotrypsin or α_2-macroglobulin, both protease inhibitors.[6] The immunoassays for PSA use monoclonal antibodies, either in pairs or in conjunction with polyclonal antibodies. Three assays have been approved by the U.S. Food and Drug Administration: the Ciba Corning ACS and the Abbott IMX PSA assays each employ a monoclonal antibody in conjunction with a polyclonal antibody, and the Hybritech assay uses two monoclonal antibodies. Many other assays exist that are not yet approved. Because the assays use differing techniques, standardization among them has proved an elusive goal. The issue of PSA assays is discussed in detail in Chapter 41.

TRANSRECTAL ULTRASONOGRAPHY

Theory

Early in its development, TRUS appeared to provide an ideal screening tool, but further experience has revealed its limita-

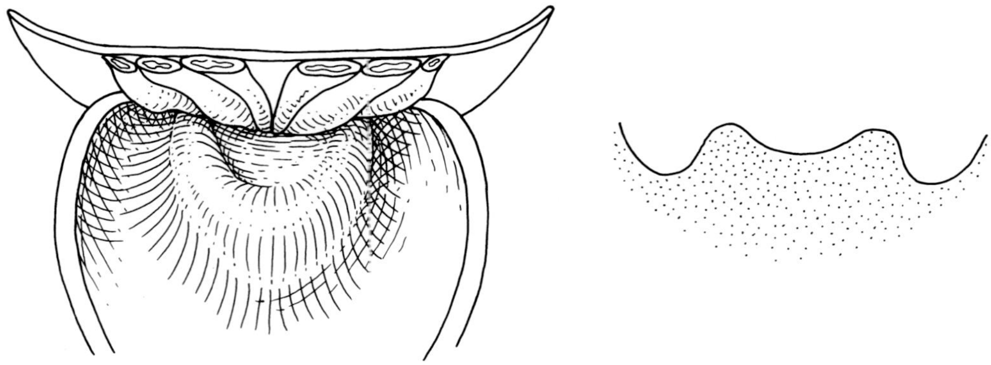

FIG. 45-1. Depiction of palpable landmarks on digital rectal examination. Although some prostates are completely smooth on palpation, others, such as the one depicted here, have well-defined lateral ridges and a central depression.

tions. A detection rate for prostate cancer of 2.6% in a solicited population is possible with TRUS alone.[1] Although its detection rate is double that of DRE, its low sensitivity and specificity, its time-consuming nature, and its reliance on a subjective interpretation limit its utility as a primary screening method. TRUS appears to be most valuable in its ability to direct with precision prostate biopsy. The reason that many tumors in the prostate are missed on digitally guided biopsies has been clarified by performing biopsies with real-time ultrasound. Many tumors remain confined to the peripheral zone, that part of the prostate between the surgical capsule and the true capsule, for most of their early evolution. They tend to spread cranially and caudally and from side to side, remaining very thin.[3] The point of the biopsy needle can tent up the capsule before it enters the prostate. It is easy, therefore, to pass the biopsy needle completely through the tumor so that only normal prostate tissue is in the sample. TRUS-guided biopsy allows confirmation that abnormal tissue is being sampled precisely.

An understanding of the physical principles of ultrasound is critical to the optimal examination of the prostate by TRUS. Most of these precepts are intuitive, and familiarity with them allows the examiner to use the ultrasound machine to its best advantage.

Sound Frequency

The frequency of a sound wave is measured in cycles per second. One hertz (Hz) is equal to 1 cycle per second; 1 kilohertz (kHz) is 1000 cycles per second; 1 megahertz (MHz) is 1,000,000 cycles per second. Sound waves whose frequencies fall between 20 Hz and 20 kHz are audible. Ultrasound comprises sound waves with frequencies higher than 20 KHz and is inaudible.[7] A dog whistle is a simple ultrasound device that emits an inaudible sound wave higher than 20 kHz. Frequencies of ultrasound between 3 and 15 MHz are useful for medical applications.

The choice of frequency to use for medical ultrasonography reflects a balance between adequate penetration of the sound waves and adequate resolution of the image. Low frequencies penetrate tissues to a greater extent than do high frequencies. High frequencies achieve a much better picture quality than do low frequencies. It is important to choose a frequency that is low enough to penetrate the tissue to be imaged yet high enough to provide good resolution of the image. The optimal frequency depends on the character of the tissue to be examined. The ideal frequency for the prostate is approximately 7 MHz.[8] A 3-MHz transmission would penetrate well beyond the prostate, displaying areas that are irrelevant, and the picture quality would be poor. A 10-MHz transmission would display only that portion of the prostate closest to the rectal wall.

Transducer

The sound wave is generated by the transducer, a crystal that operates on the principle of piezoelectricity, which enables mechanical energy to be converted to electrical energy, and vice-versa. If a crystal is attached to a volt meter and the crystal is physically bent, a voltage potential registers on the volt meter. If this crystal is attached to a battery and a voltage is applied, the crystal vibrates. The quartz watch is a common example of the piezoelectric effect: a battery stimulates a quartz crystal to vibrate, and the specific rate of vibration serves as a precise time standard. The ultrasound transducer works on this same principle.

The transducer can both transmit and receive sound waves, but it cannot do both at the same time. A pulsed-wave transducer cycles on and off, transmitting sound waves for only 0.1% of each cycle, and receiving sound waves for 99.9% of each cycle. Most transducers cycle at about 2000 times per second, transmitting only two waves of sound during each cycle.

Acoustic Interface

Although sound passes through tissue at an average of 1540 m/second, there is a slight variability in speed as it traverses different tissues. Sound is reflected at an acoustic interface, which is a boundary between two tissues that transmit sound at different speeds.[9] The discrepancy in the speed of sound transmission between the two tissues determines the magnitude of the reflected sound. It does not matter whether the wave speeds up or slows down as it crosses the interface; the difference between the two speeds is the only significant factor. Fatty tissue and stones are of completely different densities, yet both reflect a lot of sound and appear as hyperechoic areas on ultrasound. It is the number and magnitude of acoustic interfaces in tissue, not its density, that determines its echogenicity.

Early prostate ultrasound images represented reflected sound in either black or white. This provided a clear outline of the prostate, but a poor picture of its internal anatomy. The application of gray-scale technology allowed various amplitudes of reflected sound to be represented as shades of gray.[10] The technique of displaying the magnitude of sound reflection as a degree of brightness is known as B-mode scanning. The greater the number of reflectors, or the greater the acoustic mismatch, the greater the proportion of sound reflected, and the brighter the gray representation on the monitor. The equipment also measures the time (in microseconds) that it takes for the sound wave to travel from the transducer to a reflector and then back to the transducer again. Sound waves returning from distant reflectors take longer to make this round trip than sound waves that hit nearby reflectors. The software in the ultrasound instrument is programmed to convert the amount of time taken for a round trip into a specific measurement of distance from the transducer. The reflector is displayed on the monitor at a distance that corresponds to the amount of time that the sound wave required to make the round trip. This process is called the time-space conversion.

As a sound wave encounters a reflector, part of the wave is reflected and part passes through. The more reflectors through which the wave passes and the farther away from the transducer the wave travels, the weaker the wave becomes. If a weak wave encounters a distant reflector, only a weak signal is returned to the transducer, regardless of the magnitude of the acoustic mismatch. If the equipment did not compensate for this phenomenon, the monitor would display a picture that was very bright at the bottom (close to the transducer) and very dark at the top (far from the transducer). The equipment therefore performs a time-gain compensation; that is, it amplifies signals according to the length of the round trip from transducer to reflector and back to transducer again. The farther away a reflector is from the transducer, the greater the amplification of the signal. The amount of amplification per unit of distance traveled is called the *slope*. Tissue with many reflectors requires a steep slope in order to portray the distant portion of the tissue with a brightness similar to that of the near portion of the tissue. The prostate has many reflectors, and the default setting for slope is 9 dB/cm. The slope can easily be adjusted for optimal visualization of a prostate that has more or fewer reflectors.

Resolution

The clarity of an ultrasound picture is referred to as the resolution, formally defined as the ability to display two adjacent reflectors in the tissue as two separate points on the monitor. Lateral resolution is the ability to distinguish two separate reflectors that are the same distance from the transducer but are separated from each other by a short distance. The ultrasound transmission is focused by the transducer, but that focus is optimal only within a specific range. As an analogy, if a camera is focused on a specific subject at 10 feet, a secondary subject at 5 feet and a background at 15 feet will be more poorly defined in the photograph. The ultrasound instrument is like a camera without an automatic focus feature: only tissues within the focal range are sharply defined. Lateral resolution therefore depends on placing the tissue of interest within the focal range. On many ultrasound machines, the focal range is written on the probe; on others, it is found only in the operator's manual. Transducer focal range is the most important piece of information to learn from the manual.

Axial resolution is the ability to discriminate between two reflectors that lie along the path of a single sound wave but at different distances from the transducer. A signal with a long wavelength (i.e., a low-frequency signal) displays the first of two reflectors that are close together, but as it passes between the two reflectors, the tail of the sound wave drags along the first reflector, and the monitor continues to display it. The head of the wave hits the second reflector before the tail snaps free of the first. As a result, the two reflectors are displayed as a long smear on the monitor. In contrast, a short-wavelength (high-frequency) signal moves completely clear of the first reflector before it hits the second reflector and therefore displays the space between the two reflectors as a space. Axial resolution depends on the sound frequency: the lower the frequency, the better the axial resolution.

Technique

Before TRUS is performed, the patient is given a Fleet enema and prophylactic antibiotics. The enema not only eliminates the gas in the rectum, which frequently interferes with optimal visualization of the prostate gland, but also reduces the amount of fecal contamination of the biopsy needle. Because almost everyone examined by TRUS has a prostate biopsy performed at the same time, most patients receive a fluoroquinolone beginning 1 day before the procedure and continuing for 3 days. More aggressive antibiotic coverage is given to patients who have a prosthesis, a cardiac murmur, or a history of recent clinical prostatitis.

TRUS with prostate biopsy is done in an outpatient setting in the clinic and is usually well tolerated without local anesthesia. The sudden and dramatic click of the biopsy gun is more annoying to the patient than the pressure of the biopsy needle. After the DRE is performed, the patient lies down on the examining table in the left lateral decubitus position. The well-lubricated ultrasound probe is introduced very gently into the rectum, and the balloon is inflated (Fig. 45-2). The prostate is examined in a systematic fashion, beginning with the seminal vesicles in the transaxial view and moving distally through the base, midregion, and apex of the prostate. The prostate is then reexamined in the longitudinal view, beginning in the midsaggital plane and moving laterally, first to the right side and then to the left side of the gland (Fig. 45-3).

The volume of the prostate, which must be known to calculate PSA density (the ratio of serum PSA to prostate volume, or PSAD), is measured during every TRUS procedure. As a predictor of carcinoma, PSAD suffers from the difficulty of obtaining a precise, reproducible measurement of the volume of the prostate. Although measurements of width on the transaxial view and of length on the longitudinal view are reproducible, the height of the gland is especially variable if measured on the transaxial view. Although it is easy to position the probe

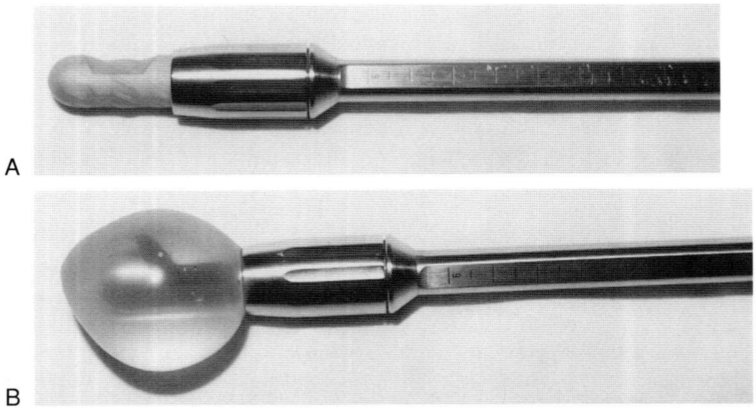

FIG. 45-2. The ultrasound probe with the balloon deflated (**A**) and inflated (**B**).

so that the entire gland is displayed on transaxial view, it is difficult in this view to avoid an inclination along the long axis, and so a somewhat oblique cut of the prostate is produced. The more oblique the cut, the greater the height that appears on the monitor. The height of the prostate gland measured on the transaxial view therefore depends not only on the size of the prostate but also on the oblique angle at which the sound passes through the prostate. Measurement of prostate height in the longitudinal view completely eliminates the artifactual component of this measurement. The height can be measured exactly perpendicular to the axis along which the length is measured in the longitudinal view.

PROSTATE BIOPSY

The ultrasound monitor displays a dotted line on the image of the prostate, which represents the projected course of the

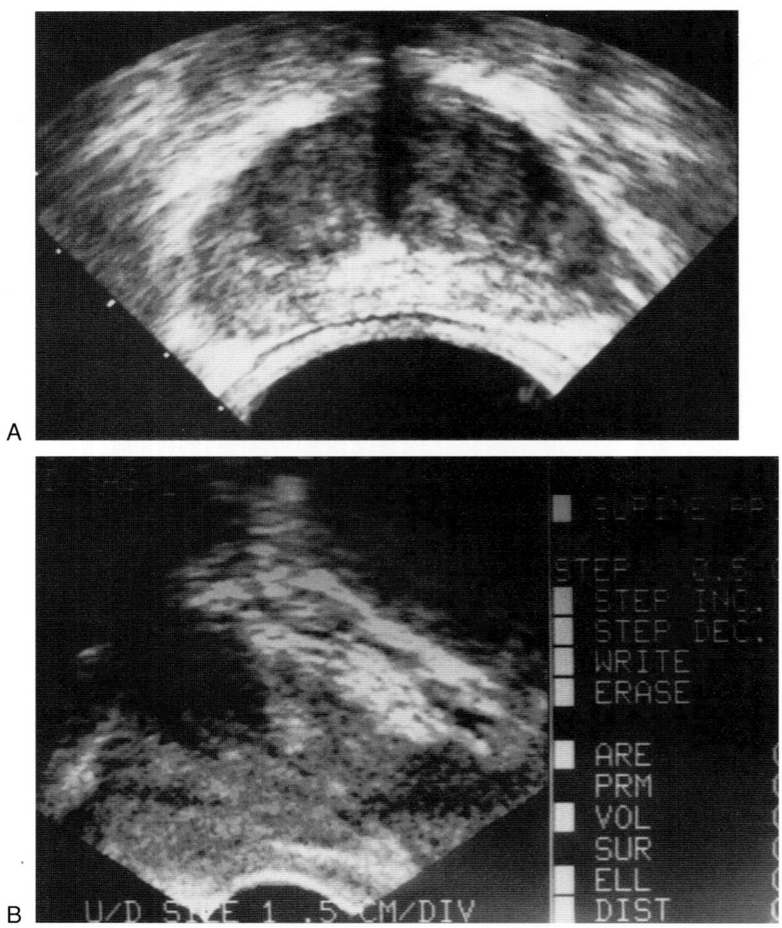

FIG. 45-3. An ultrasound image of the prostate in (**A**) the transaxial view and (**B**) the longitudinal view.

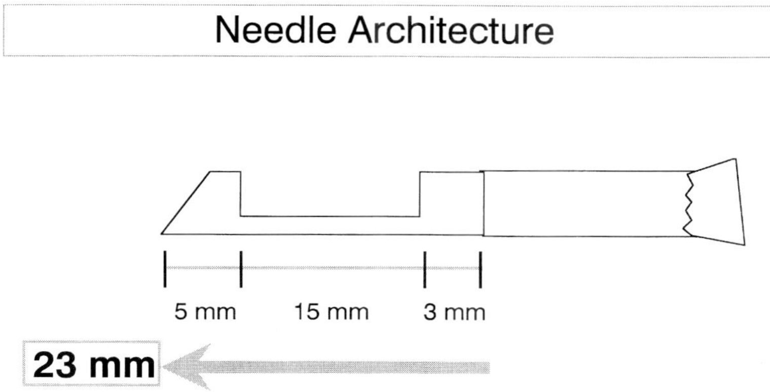

FIG. 45-4. Architecture of the biopsy needle.

biopsy needle. The biopsy needle is inserted through the needle guide until it is visible on the monitor. The needle springs forward 23 mm when it is fired and captures a core of tissue 15 mm in length (Fig. 45-4). The exact position of the needle and of the tissue-collection notch can be controlled with precision. The tissue of interest must lie within the 15-mm range. Because the needle protrudes for about 1.0 cm from the probe before it is visible on the monitor, it is important not to reposition the ultrasound probe after the needle has been inserted into the biopsy guide.

Four maneuvers performed at the end of every biopsy procedure ensure detection of any hemorrhage. First, the entire prostate is inspected for expanding hyperechoic areas, which would reflect bleeding within the gland. Second, the balloon is deflated, and the posterior margin of the prostate and the rectal wall are placed within the focal range to look for bleeding, which in this location is often hypoechoic. Third, the probe is removed, and the sheath is inspected for excessive blood. Fourth, a DRE is performed to detect thickening or hematoma formation between the rectal wall and the prostate. If any of these maneuvers detects bleeding, direct digital pressure for 5 minutes controls the bleeding in most cases.

All patients can return to work and to their activities of daily living immediately after TRUS with biopsy. Many patients have transient hematuria and notice blood in the first stool after the biopsy. The main complications of prostate biopsy are bleeding and sepsis. The rate of fever after biopsy is approximately 1% in those who receive no antibiotic prophylaxis, and less than 0.1% in those who receive prophylaxis. If a patient develops fever after a biopsy, blood and urine cultures are performed, and intravenous antibiotics are given pending results of the cultures. A few patients report hematospermia lasting for several weeks.

TABLE 45-1. *Number of sonograms required to detect one cancer, according to PSA and DRE results*

PSA (ng/mL)	No. of sonograms: DRE Normal	No. of sonograms: DRE Abnormal
≤4.0	9.7	40.8
4.1–10.0	2.6	18.0
>10.0	1.5	3.2

DRE, digital rectal examination; PSA, prostate-specific antigen.

Adapted from Cooner WH. Prostate-specific antigen, digital rectal examination, and transrectal ultrasound examination of the prostate in prostate cancer detection. Monogr Urol 1991;12:3.

APPROACHES TO THE CLINICAL DETECTION OF PROSTATE CANCER

In order to determine the precise roles of DRE, PSA, and TRUS in the diagnosis of prostate cancer and to see whether it was possible to increase the rate of detection over that of DRE alone, a study of 1807 men presenting to a urology practice was conducted.[11] All men underwent DRE and TRUS and had serum drawn for PSA. Only biopsies of hypoechoic lesions were included in the data analysis. The overall cancer detection rate for this group was 14.6%. The study was subsequently expanded to include a total of 2634 men.[12] Reanalysis of the data revealed a detection rate of 14.5%. This detection rate is a large improvement over that of DRE with digitally guided biopsy. Nevertheless, patients with an abnormal DRE result had an incidence of cancer that was six times the incidence in patients with a normal DRE.

If both the PSA and DRE results were normal, 41 sonograms were required to detect one cancer (Table 45-1).[12] Far fewer sonograms were required to detect one cancer if the DRE was abnormal or if the PSA was greater than 10 ng/mL. TRUS is

TABLE 45-2. *Unique contribution of PSA and DRE to detection of cancer in 383 patients with biopsy-proven carcinoma*

	No. of tumors found: PSA ≥ 4.0 ng/mL	No. of tumors found: PSA < 4.0 ng/mL	Total
DRE Normal	242	46	288
DRE Abnormal	64	31	95
Total	306	77	383

DRE, digital rectal examination; PSA, prostate-specific antigen.

Adapted from Cooner WH. Prostate-specific antigen, digital rectal examination, and transrectal ultrasound examination of the prostate in prostate cancer detection. Monogr Urol 1991;12:3.

most useful, then, in patients who have either an abnormal DRE or an elevated PSA. As a result of this study, TRUS is no longer recommended as a primary screening tool. Although PSA detected 64 cancers that were not detected by DRE alone, DRE picked up 46 tumors in patients who had normal PSA values (Table 45-2). Each test detected some cancers missed by the other. DRE and PSA are used as preliminary studies, and TRUS is performed only if at least one of the preliminary studies is abnormal. The optimal strategy for prostate cancer screening is discussed in more detail in Chapter 46.

REFERENCES

1. Lee F, Littrup PJ, Torp-Pedersen ST, et al. Prostate cancer: comparison of transrectal US and digital rectal examination for screening. Radiology 1988;168:389.
2. Chodak GW, Schoenberg HW. Early detection of prostate cancer by routine screening. JAMA 1984;252:3261.
3. McNeal JE, Price HM, Redwine EA, Freiha FS, Stamey TA. Stage A versus stage B adenocarcinoma of the prostate: morphological comparison and biological significance. J Urol 1988;139:61.
4. Weaver RP, Noble MJ, Weigel JW. Correlation of ultrasound guided and digitally directed transrectal biopsies of palpable prostatic abnormalities. J Urol 1991;145:516.
5. Hodge KK, McNeal JE, Stamey TA. Ultrasound guided transrectal core biopsies of the palpable abnormal prostate. J Urol 1989;142:66.
6. Christensson A, Laurell C-B, Lilja H. Enzymatic activity of prostate-specific antigen and its reactions with extracellular serine protease inhibitors. Eur J Biochem 1990;194:755.
7. Goldstein A. Physical principles of ultrasound imaging. In: Rifkin MD, ed. Ultrasound of the prostate. New York, Raven Press, 1988:15.
8. Cooner WH. Physical principles of prostate ultrasonography. Monogr Urol 1990;11:18.
9. Hykes D, Hedrick WR, Starchman DE. Ultrasound physics and instrumentation. New York: Churchill Livingstone, 1985.
10. Harada K, Tanahashi Y, Igari D, Numata I, Orikasa S. Clinical evaluation of inside echo patterns in gray scale prostatic echography. J Urol 1980;124:216.
11. Cooner WH, Mosley BR, Rutherford CL Jr, et al. Prostate cancer detection in a clinical urological practice by ultrasonography, digital rectal examination and prostate specific antigen. J Urol 1990;143:1146.
12. Cooner WH. Prostate-specific antigen, digital rectal examination, and transrectal ultrasonic examination of the prostate in prostate cancer detection. Monogr Urol 1991;12:3.

Principles and Practice of Genitourinary Oncology, edited by Derek Raghavan, Howard I. Scher, Steven A. Leibel, and Paul H. Lange. Lippincott-Raven Publishers, Philadelphia, © 1997.

CHAPTER 46

The Case for Aggressive Diagnosis and Therapy of Localized Prostate Cancer

Gerald L. Andriole and William J. Catalona

RATIONALE FOR PROSTATE CANCER SCREENING

Prostate cancer poses a significant public health problem in the United States. It is now the most common nonskin cancer affecting men in this country, and it is estimated to be the second leading cause of cancer death.[1] In 1996, an estimated 317,100 new cases of prostate cancer will be diagnosed. This represents almost 30% of all new cancers, excluding basal and squamous cell cancers of the skin. It is estimated that more than 41,400 American men died of prostate cancer in 1996. The incidence and the mortality rates of prostate cancer have risen consistently for decades and are anticipated to continue to rise as the American population ages and individual life expectancy increases.

Traditionally, prostate cancer was detected through abnormal findings on digital rectal examination (DRE) or patient symptoms, or both. If these symptoms or findings are used as indications to perform prostate biopsy, only about one half to two thirds of newly diagnosed cases of prostate cancer are found to be clinically localized to the prostate at the time of detection. Moreover, if patients judged to have clinically localized prostate cancer found in this manner undergo surgical staging with pelvic lymphadenectomy and radical retropubic prostatectomy, fewer than half are found to have pathologically organ-confined disease. Overall, therefore, only about one third of newly diagnosed cases of prostate cancer are detected by these methods before the cancer has spread beyond the prostate. Because pathologically organ-confined prostate cancer is currently the only stage of this disease that can be consistently cured, the only practical means of decreasing the mortality and morbidity rates from prostate cancer is to strive to detect pathologically organ-confined tumors more frequently. Recent innovations, such as serologic testing for prostate-specific antigen (PSA) and prostatic biopsy techniques guided by transrectal ultrasonography (TRUS) have now made the detection of pathologically organ-confined prostate cancer feasible in the great majority of patients.

Beyond a valid rationale for screening, successful screening programs for any disease should fulfill additional criteria that have been enumerated by the World Health Organization[2]: (1) the disease should be common and have serious consequences for the population; (2) the screening tools should have acceptable sensitivity and specificity; (3) detection of the disease at a preclinical, early stage should be possible; and (4) treatment of the disease at this early stage should be possible to alter its natural course. The past 5 years' experience with PSA-based screening and aggressive treatment programs suggests that prostate cancer screening fulfills each of these criteria.

CONSIDERATIONS AGAINST IMPLEMENTING PROSTATE CANCER SCREENING

There are two main arguments that are frequently cited as reasons to urge caution in implementing widespread prostate cancer screening. First, screening programs may detect prostate cancer that is not pathologically organ-confined and, therefore, not potentially curable. Second, the cancers that are pathologically organ-confined at the time of detection may be slow-growing, biologically insignificant cancers for which treatment is unnecessary. These concerns often are referred to as lead-time and length-time bias, respectively. In the former circumstance, earlier detection of cancers for which therapy is not effective may give the appearance of improved survival from the time of detection but without any change in the overall length of the individual's life. However, contemporary experience suggests that 65% to 75% of tumors detected through screening are pathologically organ-confined and can effectively be eradicated by radical prostatectomy, as evidenced by persistently undetectable postoperative serum PSA levels for 5 to 10 years after surgery.

The second concern is potentially more problematic. Because slowly growing, latent tumors have a longer preclinical course than biologically significant tumors, they may be more likely to be detected by screening. This may especially be true if repetitive examinations are performed over several years. Because slowly growing tumors are those least likely to cause symptoms or be fatal, detection of these tumors can actually result in increased treatment-related morbidity and mortality over that expected from the natural history of the disease. In this regard, prostate cancer may be especially prone to screening-induced length-time bias. Although approximately 30% of men older than 50 years of age have at least histologic evidence of prostate cancer (even if it is too small to be detected clinically), fewer than 5% can be expected to die of the disease. If every prostate cancer were detected by screening and treated, a significant proportion of patients would undergo unnecessary treatment as a consequence. However, findings during the first few years of repetitive PSA- and DRE-based screening programs have done much to quell this concern. Cancer detection rates during the first few years of screening have ranged from 3% to 7%, implying that only one out of every 6 to 10 prostate cancers is being detected. Most (80% to 95%) of these tumors appear to be medically important, as defined by histologic criteria (e.g., Gleason score, tumor volume). Moreover, not every cancer diagnosed in a screening program is treated aggressively, and there is emerging evidence that analysis of multiple clinical variables such as tumor grade, tumor volume, clinical stage, and biopsy findings can help clinicians to differentiate aggressive tumors from insignificant ones. Therefore, it appears unlikely that a large proportion of screening-detected cancers will be unnecessarily overtreated.

There are other theoretic issues that favor caution before implementation of widespread screening for prostate cancer. These include the morbidity of screening; the unnecessary anxiety induced by screening, especially if a high proportion of men are found to have a falsely positive initial result; the false sense of security if the initial result is falsely negative but prostate cancer is truly present; the economic costs of screening; and the morbidity and mortality of treatment for tumors detected by screening.[3] The actual risk and clinical impact of these potential adverse occurrences have not been quantitated with much certainty.

Decision analytic models addressing these issues have suggested there is little benefit to screening in terms of prolongation of life and that screening may actually decrease quality of life.[4,5] These reports must be interpreted cautiously, however, because they have usually underestimated the potential mortality and morbidity of untreated prostate cancer and the ability of therapy to eliminate the disease and overestimated the morbidity of therapy and its impact on reducing qualify of life.

THE PROSTATE PORT MODEL

The Prostate PORT[4] used a Markov model to analyze the problem of early-stage prostate cancer. In Markov modeling,[6] a patient is considered to be in one of a number of finite health states at any given time. Patients are assigned a probability of undergoing transformation from one health state to another. Different Markov states may be assigned different qualities, with the dead state having a quality value of 0 and the asymptomatic state a quality value of 1. In the prostate cancer Markov model, patients with clinically localized prostate cancer were considered to be in one of four health states: (1) no clinical evidence of metastatic disease, (2) hormone-controlled metastatic disease, (3) hormone-refractory metastatic disease, and (4) dead. The state of death was further subdivided into dead from prostate cancer and dead from other causes. Structuring of the problem of early-stage prostate cancer in this manner means that the most important probability in determining outcome of therapy is the projected rate of progression of asymptomatic localized disease to metastatic disease. This occurs because metastatic disease is incurable, invariably leading to hormone-refractory disease and death in a relatively short, predictable period of time. Therefore, the sole benefit of treatment for early-stage prostate cancer in this model is the prevention (or the delay) of the appearance of metastatic disease.

Analysis of this model has indicated five significant areas of concern: (1) the rate of development of metastatic disease from localized cancer, (2) the disease-control capabilities of radical prostatectomy, (3) the complications, morbidity, and mortality of radical prostatectomy, (4) the assigned quality adjustments, and (5) estimates of the utility of therapy beyond preventing or delaying metastatic disease.

Rate of Development of Metastatic Disease

In the PORT model, 2.7% of patients with grade 1 prostate cancer, 13% of those with grade 2 disease, and 41% of those with grade 3 disease are estimated to develop metastatic disease at 10 years. These metastatic rates were derived from a structured review of the literature that the authors had previously performed.[7]

Three lines of evidence suggest that the metastatic rates employed in this model significantly underestimate the probability of progression to metastatic disease in patients with localized prostate cancer managed with watchful waiting. The first is derived from evaluation of patients with localized prostate cancer who were treated with ineffective forms of radiotherapy—that is, with interstitial radioactive iodine[8] or radioactive gold seeds.[9] Patients with surgically staged localized prostate cancer treated with these forms of radiotherapy experienced the rates of metastasis shown in Table 46-1. In general, the rates of development of metastatic disease in these series were more than 10 times higher than the PORT estimates for patients with grade 1 lesions, about four times higher for patients with grade 2 lesions, and almost twice as high for patients with grade 3 lesions. The difference between these rates and those used in the PORT analysis is especially impressive considering that the radiation-treated patients were surgically staged and known not to have lymph node metastases. Had patients with clinically unsuspected lymph node metastases been included in the radiation series, the resulting rates would undoubtedly have been higher.

A second line of evidence suggesting that the metastatic rates

TABLE 46-1. *Rates of metastasis of early-stage prostate cancer after 10 years*

Grade of lesion of diagnosis	Untreated (%)		After radiotherapy (%)	
	PORT	Pooled analysis	^{198}Au	^{125}I
Grade 1	2.7	19	29	30
Grade 2	13	42	50	51
Grade 3	41	57	66	70

were underestimated by the PORT team is provided by a recent pooled analysis of the literature on patients undergoing watchful waiting.[10] The 10-year progression rates in eight series averaged 19% for grade 1, 42% for grade 2, and 57% for grade 3 lesions. These rates are significantly closer to those derived from the interstitial radiation therapy data than to those used by the PORT team.

The third line of evidence that the metastatic rates used by the prostate PORT are inaccurate may be derived by reference to the number of deaths from prostate cancer known to have occurred during the last 20 to 25 years. This method is valid because death from prostate cancer must be preceded by the development of metastatic disease. If the PORT metastatic rates were accurate, the annual incidence of prostate cancer during the past 20 years would have had to exceed 250,000 cases per year to account for deaths already ascribed to prostate cancer during that time interval (J Beck, MD, personal communication). However, only about 200,000 cases of prostate cancer were diagnosed in the United States in 1994.

Because separate lines of evidence indicate that metastatic disease develops at a substantially higher rate in patients undergoing either no treatment or inadequate local treatment and because the metastatic rates used in the model do not explain the historic death rate of prostate cancer in this country, it appears certain that the rates of metastasis employed by the PORT team significantly underestimate the actual occurrence of metastatic disease. This may have resulted from the authors' heavy reliance on the Swedish studies of watchful waiting. These studies may not be appropriate to assess the natural history of prostate cancer because many of the men undergoing watchful waiting were elderly (mean age, 72 years in Johansson's series[11]) and had small-volume, well-differentiated prostate cancers treated by transurethral endoscopic resection of the prostate. Moreover, Johansson's study may be biased because the patients with the best prognosis were entered first in the trial. Only later were patients with higher, clinical stage B disease included in the watchful waiting program. Because survival curves are driven most by the patients entered first into any trial, entering the best-risk patients first may have had the effect of overestimating the benefits of watchful waiting. By comparison, most series of men undergoing radical prostatectomy have inadvertently entered the worst-risk patients first (i.e., those with relatively large-volume tumors diagnosed in the pre-PSA era). Because these patients are under follow-up for a longer period of time compared with those entered later, this procedure artifactually lowers the rate of disease control by surgery, as shown by comparison with a contemporary surgical series treating predominantly smaller, PSA-detected cancers. Since the Swedish study added the best patients first, the results of watchful waiting are probably overemphasized.

In addition, the Swedish studies may be misleading because of a bias introduced by the Swedish strategy of deliberately not screening for prostate cancer. In an environment in which there is no screening for prostate cancer, patients diagnosed with localized disease may tend to have tumors that grow slowly, because rapidly growing, fatal tumors (those that spend a relatively brief period of time in a localized stage) are less likely to be detected until they have metastasized. This may explain why Sweden has one of the highest cause-specific death rates from prostate cancer in the world while at the same time Swedish investigators report prolonged survival times for patients with untreated prostate cancer. This phenomenon also may explain why the majority of men with newly diagnosed prostate cancer in Johansson's regionally defined study area of Sweden did not have even clinically localized disease. A logical explanation is that the aggressive tumors are spreading beyond the prostate quickly and that only the very slow-growing, indolent tumors are detected before they escape the gland. Analysis of only the latter group of patients would be expected to yield misleading and overly optimistic estimates of the natural history of prostate cancer.

Application of either the brachytherapy or the pooled-analysis metastatic rates to the PORT model substantially changes the estimated benefit of radical prostatectomy compared with watchful waiting. Revision of this parameter only (leaving unchanged the assumptions of quality adjustment and complication rates from radical prostatectomy) yields a substantial increase in the benefit of radical prostatectomy across all tumor grades.

Disease-Control Capability of Radical Prostatectomy

The PORT model assumed that all men with pathologic extracapsular prostate cancer invariably progress to metastatic disease if treated with radical prostatectomy. Overall, 28% of men with grade 2 cancers and 65% of grade 3 cancers were projected to be treatment failures. Microscopic capsular penetration is the most common adverse pathologic finding in the approximately 30% of men with screening-detected prostate cancer who have pathologically advanced disease (Table 46-2). However, it appears that far fewer than half of such patients manifest disease failure after radical prostatectomy. This is evident from data by Partin and colleagues[12] and from Washington University (Catalona, WJ, personal communication, August, 1995), in which only 22% of patients observed for 5 years after radical prostatectomy for microscopic capsular penetration had a detectable level of serum PSA. Moreover, the clinical failure rate of these patients was less than 10%. Therefore, correction of the PORT model in this regard may further increase the estimated benefit of radical prostatectomy over that achieved by watchful waiting.

Complications and Morbidity of Radical Prostatectomy

The PORT model estimated that 1.1% of men undergoing radical prostatectomy die as a consequence of surgery. The op-

Table 46-2. *Estimated distribution of prostate cancers found by PSA-based screening*

Pathologic stage	Percentage
Small-volume, low-grade, organ-confined	10
Significant intracapsular volume or grade, organ-confined	60
Capsular penetration only	20
Other advanced histology (positive margins, lymph node or seminal vesicle involvement)	10

PSA, prostate-specific antigen.

TABLE 46-3. *Complications of radical prostatectomy for localized prostate cancer*

Complication	PORT (%)	Washington University (%)
Death	1.1	0.2
Major early complications	5.5	2.9
Stricture	22	4
Impotency	31	37
Incontinence	24	6

erative mortality at four major centers reported at the 1994 national meeting of the American Urological Association was 0.1%, and at the Washington University School of Medicine it has been reported to be 0.2%.[13,14] Table 46-3 compares the rates for major early complications and for late development of bladder neck stricture, impotency, or incontinence used in the PORT model with those found in contemporary experience at Washington University. Application of the Washington University mortality and complication rates to the PORT model would further enhance the indicated benefit of radical prostatectomy over watchful waiting.

Quality Adjustments

The quality adjustments used by the PORT decision analysis were derived from a consensus of clinical opinion and not from actual patient experience. Patients with metastatic cancer (an irreversible condition) were assigned a quality of life equal to or greater than that assigned to men with incontinence or a bowel injury, conditions that are surgically correctable. Moreover, the development of impotency (a reversible, nonlife-threatening condition) was estimated to be almost as debilitating as the development of metastatic cancer (a nonreversible, usually fatal condition). Finally, the model considered that, once a patient developed any of these complications, the quality of the remainder of his life was reduced. This is not appropriate for any health state except metastatic disease, because most complications are correctable by secondary surgical or medical intervention. Appropriate consideration of these issues would substantially improve the quality-adjusted benefit of radical prostatectomy over watchful waiting.

Utility Estimates

The Prostate PORT decision analysis did not consider any potential benefits of surgery beyond prevention of metastatic disease. Prevention (or delay) of the onset of local symptoms such as bladder outlet obstruction and alleviation of a patient's anxiety about having an inexorably growing cancer are two other benefits of surgery not incorporated into the model. For the PORT model to be considered valid, these issues must be addressed.

Application of the PORT Decision Analysis

In summary, the Prostate PORT model is an interesting starting point for further discussion about the optimal management of men with clinically localized prostate cancer. The practical usefulness of this model is in doubt, not only because of the deficiencies cited, but also because the model applies only to groups of men undergoing surgery or watchful waiting, and because the outcomes are reported as averages. Obviously, some patients undergoing surgery benefit immensely because they are cured of a lethal tumor, whereas the 1 man in 1000 who dies of surgery loses a great deal. The optimal management of an individual patient with clinically localized prostate cancer must rest on a detailed, individualized discussion of the problem and must not be based solely on impersonal knowledge derived from statistical analysis of large databases.[15]

CHOICE AND PERFORMANCE OF PROSTATE CANCER SCREENING TOOLS

The optimal means of screening for prostate cancer is of great interest to the urologic community. DRE, TRUS, and serum PSA testing have been evaluated individually and in combination as means of achieving early detection of prostate cancer. Although no uniformly agreed approach has been established, most authorities currently believe that the DRE and serum PSA testing should be performed initially, with TRUS and TRUS-guided biopsy as a secondary procedure in patients found to have an elevated serum PSA concentration or a suspicious DRE result, or both. Serial evaluations with serum PSA and DRE may be performed every 6 to 12 months.

Screening with DRE alone historically has been associated with very low detection rates (1% to 2.5%).[16] About 60% of the tumors detected by DRE-based screening are clinically advanced and not curable at the time of diagnosis, even if repeated DRE screening is performed on an annual basis.[17] Because DRE has a relatively low detection rate for potentially curable (i.e., pathologically organ-confined) prostate cancer, a rather low specificity, and a high rate of false-positive results (up to 80%), and because of the marked patient dissatisfaction associated with this examination, repeated DRE alone is not an appropriate means of screening for prostate cancer.

TRUS-based screening has, in general, been associated with higher cancer detection rates than DRE-based screening. In the best studies, detection rates approaching 5% have been achieved.[18] These relatively high rates, however, typically occur at the expense of biopsy of a high proportion of men undergoing screening. The rate of biopsy has been reported to approach 30% of the population screened by TRUS, a statistic that belies the rather subjective and nonspecific nature of TRUS interpretation. Because of the subjectivity of interpretation, the fact that a considerable proportion of tumors are ultrasonographically isoechoic with respect to normal tissues of the prostate, the expense, and the patient discomfort and dissatisfaction associated with this procedure, TRUS alone is not an inappropriate initial diagnostic tool for widespread prostate cancer screening.

PSA has many advantages as a screening tool compared with either the DRE or TRUS. PSA testing is relatively inexpensive and is an objective and quantitative test that is often, from the patient's point of view, preferable to either DRE or TRUS. In addition, serum PSA testing does not require a specially skilled examiner. Therefore, less professional time may be required in PSA-based screening programs compared with those based on

TRUS or DRE. These features, coupled with the known clinical superiority of PSA over DRE and TRUS in detection of prostate cancer among patients undergoing urologic evaluation for symptomatic disease,[19] have made serum PSA the primary screening tool for prostate cancer.

RESULTS OF PSA-BASED SCREENING PROGRAMS

Results With PSA Determination Alone

For approximately 2 years, beginning in the summer of 1989, slightly more than 10,000 men were enrolled in a PSA-based screening program at Washington University in St. Louis. Men older than 50 years of age who had no history of prostate surgery or prostate cancer volunteered to be evaluated. During this study, men whose serum PSA levels were less than 4 ng/mL were asked to return every 6 months for a repeat PSA determination. Men whose serum PSA levels exceeded 4 ng/mL returned for a repeat determination within a few weeks. If the second measurement was also higher than 4 ng/mL, DRE and TRUS were performed. Suspicious results on either the DRE or the TRUS scan led to biopsy with TRUS guidance.[20]

The initial results of this study have been published.[20,21] About one third of the volunteers were between 50 and 60, one half between 60 and 70, and the remainder older than 70 years of age. Overall, approximately 10% of volunteers were found to have an initial serum PSA concentration above 4 ng/mL. The probability of an elevated serum PSA concentration correlated with advanced age, but, for a given PSA level, the probability of cancer was similar for men of all ages, confirming that serum PSA determinations are a much more powerful predictor of the presence of prostate cancer than patient age.

About one third of men with an elevated serum PSA concentration were found to have prostate cancer on the basis of the initial evaluation, resulting in an overall 3% rate of cancer detection. This detection rate was achieved by biopsy of about 9% of the population. Some of the men with elevated serum PSA levels did not undergo biopsy because both their DRE and TRUS results were judged to be normal. The probability of prostate cancer varied directly with the serum PSA concentration. About one quarter of the men with an initial PSA level between 4 and 10 ng/mL were found to have prostate cancer, whereas almost 60% of those whose PSA level was higher than 10 ng/mL had prostate cancer. Overall, the DRE result was normal in 40% of the men who were found to have prostate cancer.

Addition of Digital Rectal Examination to PSA-Based Screening

A second program was undertaken to evaluate application of both DRE and serum PSA determination for initial screening.[22,23] If either test result was abnormal, patients underwent TRUS-guided biopsy of the prostate. Approximately 10% to 15% of patients screened in this manner had an elevated serum PSA level, almost 15% had a suspicious DRE result, and many men had abnormalities on both tests. Overall, about 20% of patients were referred for biopsy. About 50% of the men who had both an elevated PSA concentration and an abnormal DRE were found to have prostate cancer on TRUS-guided biopsy. Of those whose serum PSA was higher than 4 ng/mL but whose DRE was normal, only 25% were found to have prostate cancer. On the other hand, if the DRE result was suspicious but the PSA was within the normal range, prostate cancer was present only 10% of the time. Overall, about 20% of cancers detected in the screening program would not have been detected if PSA-based screening alone had been performed. Conversely, DRE-based screening alone would have missed about 45% of the cancers. This comparative study demonstrates that the DRE and serum PSA may be viewed as complementary diagnostic tests for prostate cancer but that serum PSA seems to detect more cancers than DRE overall.

TABLE 46-4. *Comparison of prostate cancer screening methods*

Item	Initial test: PSA alone	Initial test: PSA and DRE
Detection rate on initial evaluation	3%	4%–6%
Biopsy rate	9%	20%
Patients undergoing biopsy per cancer detected	3	4–5

DRE, digital rectal examination; *PSA*, prostate-specific antigen.

The combination of serum PSA and DRE screening results in a higher overall cancer detection rate than does use of either modality alone. Combined screening produces a detection rate of 4% to 6% (Table 46-4). This result is achieved at the expense of biopsy of about 20% of the population. In other words, 4 or 5 men must undergo biopsy to find a single case of prostate cancer. This compares unfavorably to screening with PSA alone, in which only about 3 patients must undergo biopsy to find one case of prostate cancer. The addition of the DRE to PSA-based screening also results in more biopsies per case of pathologically organ-confined prostate cancer than does PSA screening alone. This occurs because cancers that are palpable are apt to have spread beyond the prostate, whereas impalpable cancers that produce minimal serum PSA elevations are usually pathologically organ confined.

Stage of Cancers Detected on Initial PSA-Based Screening

Of all the cancers detected on initial evaluation in PSA-based screening programs, 97% to 99% are clinically localized to the prostate gland. Clinical staging included the findings on DRE, serum enzymatic prostatic acid phosphatase testing, radionuclide bone scan, and, in some cases, pelvic imaging with either computed tomography or magnetic resonance imaging. Pathologic staging (i.e., bilateral pelvic lymph node dissection and radical retropubic prostatectomy) indicates that men undergoing screening who have a PSA level of between 4 and 10 ng/mL have pathologically organ-confined disease about 70% of the time. On the other hand, only slightly more than 40% of men

TABLE 46-5. *Probability of detecting pathologically organ-confined prostate cancer by PSA-based screening*

Results of screening (ng/mL)	Percentage of cancers that are pathologically organ confined
INITIAL PSA TESTING	
4.0–10	65–70
>10	40–50
SERIAL PSA TESTING	
<4	80
4.0–10	70–75
>10	60–65

with cancer and a PSA level higher than 10 ng/mL are found to have pathologically organ-confined disease (Table 45-5).

Clinical Significance of Tumors Detected by PSA-Based Screening

Although there is no unequivocal means of determining the true biologic significance of an individual prostate cancer, the Gleason score and the tumor volume are among the most important predictors of overall biologic aggressiveness. More than 90% of the cancers detected through initial PSA screening either present bilaterally throughout the prostate, indicating a relatively high tumor volume, or are moderately or poorly differentiated (i.e., Gleason score ≥5), or both. Additional evidence of the medical importance of most tumors detected by PSA-based screening may be derived the fact that the 3% detection rate represents only one tenth of the cancers expected to be present in this population, based on the reported 30% autopsy prevalence of prostate cancer. It seems most likely that only the larger cancers are being detected with the ultrasound sampling techniques being employed. A third reason to believe that most of the tumors detected in this manner are clinically significant may be derived from detailed analysis of final tumor grade and stage in men who were initially found to have the most minute amounts of cancer at the time of detection. Among men with impalpable, well-differentiated prostate cancer that involved less than half of one biopsy core who undergo radical prostatectomy, 90% are found to have significantly higher-grade or higher-stage cancer on inspection of the entire prostate. Detailed analysis of 24 such men in our screening studies suggests that if the final pathologic stage and grade were known, only two or three patients (i.e., 8% to 12%) would be considered to have focal or incidental prostate cancer. Taken together, these arguments suggest that the large majority of cancers detected by PSA-based screening are apt to be biologically and clinically important.

Results of Serial PSA-Based Screening

Serial determination of serum PSA is an integral part of screening for prostate cancer with PSA testing. Men whose serum PSA concentration is less than 4 ng/mL initially but subsequently rises above 4 ng/mL are found to have prostate cancer about 40% of the time. Significantly, more than three quarters of the cancers detected among this group of patients are pathologically organ confined. Likewise, patients whose initial serum PSA level is greater than 4 ng/mL but whose initial biopsy is negative for cancer are found to have prostate cancer about one third of the time if a second, third, or fourth prostatic biopsy is performed, and almost 75% of the cancers detected on a subsequent biopsy are pathologically organ confined. Taken together, these results suggest that serial PSA screening may be associated with the highest probability of detecting pathologically organ-confined prostate cancer (see Table 46-5).

Potential Role of PSA Velocity and PSA Density in Serial PSA Screening

The ideal method of follow-up for patients with persistent serum PSA elevation and an initially negative prostatic biopsy has not been firmly established. In the PSA-based screening program, repeat biopsies of the prostate have been recommended every 6 months for patients with persistently elevated PSA values. Such serial reevaluation theoretically diagnoses 100% of the clinically detectable cases of prostate cancer occurring among this group of men (Table 46-6). This approach, however, exacts a fairly significant cost to the patient in terms of discomfort, morbidity, and expense. Identification of other tools that can guide the selection of only certain men for repeated biopsy would be beneficial. The PSA velocity (rate of change in PSA, or PSAV) and the PSA density (serum PSA concentration divided by prostate volume, or PSAD) have been investigated for their use in this setting.

PSAV may be a useful means of determining whether a patient has prostate cancer. A long-term, retrospective study[24] found that the serum PSA levels of men ultimately found to have prostate cancer usually rose at a faster rate than those of men with benign prostatic hyperplasia (BPH) or normal prostates. Patients with cancer typically had a PSAV exceeding 0.75 ng/mL per year. PSAV (also referred to as PSA slope) appears to be useful if more than 2 years of follow-up is available. For men monitored less than 2 years, the relatively high biologic and assay variation in PSA measurement precludes accurate measurement of PSAV. PSAV is also more meaningful in men whose initial serum PSA concentrations are normal and in men younger than 70 years of age. In the current screening study (Catalona WJ, personal communication, August, 1995), a PSAV of 0.8 ng/mL or more per year, sustained for more than 24 months, doubles the chance that cancer is present. Much longer follow-up is needed to clarify the role of PSAV in the serial evaluation of men in screening programs.

PSAD could improve the clinician's ability to differentiate, among patients with elevated PSA concentrations, those who have BPH from those who have prostate cancer.[25] The rationale

TABLE 46-6. *Probability of cancer detection on serial prostatic biopsy*

Serum PSA value (ng/mL)	First biopsy	Second biopsy	Third biopsy	Fourth biopsy
4–10	0.26	0.25	0.14	0.10
>10	0.57	0.47	0.16	0.10

TABLE 46-7. *Projected outcome of screening-detected prostate cancer treated by radical prostatectomy*

Pathologic stage detected by PSA screening	Percentage	Percentage free of biochemical or clinical disease at 5–10 years	Overall percentage of population free of disease at 5–10 years
Small-volume, low-grade, organ-confined	10	95	10
Significant-volume, low-grade, organ-confined	60	90	54
Capsular penetration only	20	70	14
Other advanced lesions	10	0	0
Total	100		78

for using PSAD is that consideration of the size of the prostate factors out of the total elevation in serum PSA that portion that is caused by BPH. In the Washington University PSA screening program (Andriole GL, personal communication, August, 1995), an initial PSAD greater than 0.15 has been associated with a 50% rate of cancer detection on serial biopsy, whereas fewer than 10% of men with a PSAD lower than 0.1 have been found to have prostate cancer, even if repeated biopsies were taken. These results suggest that PSAD is a potentially useful means of predicting which patients with elevated serum PSA and an initially negative biopsy of the prostate should undergo serial biopsy of the prostate gland.

Comparative evaluation of PSAV and PSAD in our screening studies suggests that they are comparable in predicting the presence of cancer.[26] It is anticipated that as the study matures PSAV will surpass PSAD as a predictive tool. Both measures miss some cancers, and the cancers missed are those most likely to be organ confined.

In the future, measurement of the free and bound fractions of PSA may help distinguish between patients with BPH and those with prostate cancer. Prostate cancer is associated with a lower percentage of free PSA.[27,28]

ABILITY OF RADICAL PROSTATECTOMY TO ALTER THE NATURAL COURSE OF SCREENING-DETECTED PROSTATE CANCER

Prostate-specific antigen–based screening and the profound increase in proportion of cancers detected at an early stage that it produces would not be beneficial unless it improved the results of therapy. Emerging experience suggests that radical prostatectomy offers a high probability of cure for those patients who have pathologically organ-confined disease. Moreover, those who have only early findings of capsular invasion by tumor also have a high probability of lifelong freedom from prostatic cancer after this treatment. Long-term studies (Partin et al[29]; WJ Catalona, personal communication) show that 85% to 95% of patients with pathologically organ-confined prostate cancer are free of PSA relapse (i.e., have undetectable serum PSA concentrations) at 5 to 10 years after radical prostatectomy, as are about 70% of men with only focal capsular penetration. In the era before serum PSA testing and widespread implementation of early detection programs, fewer than 50% of patients undergoing radical prostatectomy were found to have pathologically organ-confined prostate cancer, and only 5% to 10% had evidence of only minor degrees of capsular penetration. The current combination of early detection programs with anatomic radical prostatectomy may be expected to produce an overall 70% to 80% freedom from PSA relapse 10 years after surgery (Table 46-7). This is almost double the rate in older series of radical prostatectomy.

SUMMARY

The evolving experience with early detection and aggressive treatment programs has demonstrated that use of PSA and DRE increases not only the number of cancers detected but the proportion detected in an early pathologic stage. In general, 90% to 95% of tumors discovered in early detection programs are clinically localized, and 60% to 85% of these cancers are pathologically organ confined. In addition, only 5% to 15% of pathologically staged tumors are considered clinically unimportant (i.e., incidental, autopsy-type tumors) if judged by tumor volume and tumor grade criteria. These findings, coupled with the high cure rate resulting from radical prostatectomy for pathologically organ-confined lesions, suggest that institution of early detection programs significantly reduces prostate cancer-specific mortality and morbidity. The human and economic price of reducing prostate cancer deaths by this approach appears to be acceptable: both diagnostic- and treatment-induced morbidity have been significantly reduced, and the cost to diagnose and treat each case of prostate cancer is less than the per-case cost associated with breast or colon cancer screening. At a minimum, this early experience strongly supports the rationale for randomized prospective screening trials[30] and should defuse the concerns of some[31] that such trials are unethical.

REFERENCES

1. Parker LS, Tong T, Balden S, Wingo PA. Cancer Statistics, 1996 CA Cancer J Clin 1996;46:5.
2. Wilson J, Jungner G. Principles and practice of screening for disease. Public Health Papers 34. Geneva, World Health Organization, 1968.
3. Prorok PC, Connor RJ, Baker SG. Statistical considerations in cancer screening programs. Urol Clin North Am 1990;17:699.
4. Fleming C, Wasson JH, Albertsen PC, Barry MJ, Wennberg JE. A decision analysis of alternative treatment strategies for clinically localized prostate cancer. JAMA 1993;269:2650.
5. Krahn MD, Mahoney JE, Eckman MH, Trachtenberg J, Pauker SG, Detsky AL. Screening for prostate cancer. JAMA 1994;272:773.
6. Sonnenberg FA, Beck JR. Markov models in medical decision making: a practical guide. Med Decis Making 1993;13:322.
7. Wasson JH, Cushman CC, Bruskewitz RC, Littenberg BJ, Mulley AG, Wennberg JE. A structured literature review of treatment for localized prostate cancer. Arch Fam Med 1993;2:487.
8. Fuks Z, Leibel SA, Wallner KE, et al. The effect of local control on metastatic dissemination in carcinoma of the prostate: long term results

in patients treated with ^{125}I implantation. Int J Radiat Oncol Biol Phys 1991;21:537.
9. Lerner SR, Seale-Hawkins C, Carlton CE, Scardino PT. The risk of dying of prostate cancer in patients with clinically localized disease. J Urol 1991;146:1040.
10. Chodak GW, Thisted RA, Gerber GS, et al. Results of conservative management of clinically localized prostate cancer. N Engl J Med 1994; 330:242.
11. Johansson JE, Adami HO, Andersson SO, et al. A high 10 year survival rate in patients with early untreated prostate cancer. JAMA 1992;267: 2191.
12. Partin AW, Pound CR, Clemens JQ, Epstein JI, Walsh PC. Serum PSA after anatomic radical prostatectomy. Urol Clin North Am 1993;20: 713.
13. Andriole GL, Smith DS, Rao G, Goodnough L, Catalona WJ. Early complications of contemporary anatomic radical retropubic prostatectomy. J Urol. 1994;152:1858.
14. Catalona WJ, Basler JW. Return of erections and urinary continence following nerve-sparing radical retropubic prostatectomy. J Urol 1993; 150:905.
15. Tanenbaum SJ. Sounding board: what physicians know. N Engl J Med 1993;329:1268.
16. Optenberg SA, Thompson IA. Economics of screening for carcinoma of the prostate. Urol Clin North Am 1990;17:719.
17. Gerber GS, Thompson IM, Thisted R, Chodak GW. Disease-specific survival following routine prostate cancer screening by digital rectal examination. JAMA 1993;269:61.
18. Mettlin C, Lee F, Drago J, et al. The American Cancer Society National Prostate Cancer Detection Project. Cancer 1991;67:2949.
19. Cooner WH, Moseley BR, Rutherford CL, et al. Clinical application of transrectal ultrasonography for prostate specific antigen: the search for prostate cancer. J Urol 1988;139:758.
20. Catalona WJ, Smith DS, Ratliff TL, et al. Measurement of prostate specific antigen in serum as a screening test for prostate cancer. N Engl J Med 1991;324:1156.
21. Catalona WJ, Smith DS, Ratliff TL, Basler JW. Detection of organ-confined prostate cancer is increased through prostate specific antigen based screening. JAMA 1993;270:948.
22. Richie JP, Catalona WJ, Ahmann FR, et al. Effect of patient age on early detection of prostate cancer with serum prostate specific antigen and digital rectal examination. Urology 1993;42:365.
23. Catalona WJ, Richie JP, Ahmann FR, et al. Comparison of digital rectal examination and serum prostate specific antigen in the early detection of prostate cancer: results of a multicenter clinical trial of 6,630 men. J Urol 1994;151:1283.
24. Carter HB, Pierson JD, Medder EJ, et al. Longitudinal evaluation of prostatic specific antigen levels in men with and without prostate disease. JAMA 1992;267:2215.
25. Benson MC, Whang IS, Pantuk A, et al. Prostate specific antigen density: a means of distinguishing benign prostatic hypertrophy in prostate cancer. J Urol 1992;147:815.
26. McMurtry J, Keetch DW, Smith DS, Andriole GL, Catalona WJ. PSA density vs. PSA slope as predictors of prostate cancer in patients with initially negative prostatic biopsies. J Urol 1994;151:401A.
27. Stenman UH, Leinonen J, Alfthan H, Rannikko S, Tuhkanen K, Alfthan O. A complex between prostate-specific antigen and alpha 1-antichymotrypsin is the major form of prostate-specific antigen in serum of patients with prostatic cancer: assay of the complex improves clinical sensitivity for cancer. Cancer Res 1991;51:222.
28. Christensson A, Bjork T, Nilsson O, et al. Serum prostate-specific antigen complexed to alpha 1-antichymotrypsin as an indicator of prostate cancer. J Urol 1993;150:100.
29. Partin AW, Pound CR, Clemens Q, Epstein J, Walsh PC. Serum PSA after anatomic radical prostatectomy. Urol Clin North Am 1993;20: 713.
30. Kramer BS, Gohagan J, Prorok PC, Smart C. A National Cancer Institute sponsored screening trial for prostatic, lung, colorectal and ovarian cancers. Cancer 1993;71:589.
31. Adami HO, Baron JA, Rothman KJ. Ethics of a prostate cancer screening trial. Lancet 1994;343:958.

Principles and Practice of Genitourinary Oncology, edited by Derek Raghavan, Howard I. Scher, Steven A. Leibel, and Paul H. Lange. Lippincott-Raven Publishers, Philadelphia, © 1997.

CHAPTER 47

The Case for Conservative Therapy for Localized Prostate Cancer

Jan Adolfsson, Mark Austenfeld, and Ian Thompson

EXPERIENCE WITH SURVEILLANCE FOR LOCALIZED PROSTATE CANCER

The clinical course of prostate cancer is unpredictable. Before the era of endocrine therapy, the fate of patients with prostate cancer was illustrative of the natural course of the disease, and the prognosis at that time was almost uniformly poor.[1,2] This result was in part caused by the lack of effective therapy for metastatic disease but also by the advanced stage of disease at diagnosis in many patients. In more modern series, surveillance (also referred to as deferred treatment, observation, watchful waiting, or conservative treatment) has been employed for patients with clinically low-stage prostate cancer. With surveillance, no initial treatment is given and therapy is reserved for disease progression or development of symptoms. Surveillance customarily employs androgen deprivation, but in some series more aggressive local therapy has been used. This treatment policy is included among standard therapies in some parts of the world, especially in the Scandinavian countries. The rationale behind surveillance for patients with clinically localized prostate cancer is the combination of a usually protracted course of the disease and a high competing mortality risk among an older male population at diagnosis.

Incidental Prostate Cancer

In general, the prognosis for patients with nonpalpable prostate cancer that is diagnosed at the time of surgery for presumed benign prostatic hyperplasia is thought to be good if a policy of surveillance is implemented. More contemporary evidence does suggest that, with sufficient follow-up, a low but significant progression rate can be noted and that this risk is related to high-grade and high-volume disease.

Incidental prostate cancer can be segregated into low-volume (focal, T1a) and high-volume (diffuse, T1b) disease. This categorization is based on the volume of tumor in the resected specimen and varies with different staging systems. Because of differences in methods of sampling resected chips, categorization within these staging systems may be somewhat unreliable.[3]

With long-term follow-up, survival rates of 30% to 85% have been reported at 10 years for patients with incidentally detected disease. Progression-free survival rates range from 33% to 82%, and disease-specific survival rates as high as 93% for low-volume and 77% for high-volume disease have been reported. Table 47-1 illustrates the results in seven contemporary series. Several series provide only the rates of progression-free or overall survival.

For patients with incidental cancer who were studied for up to 25 years, rates of tumor progression ranging from 9% to 26% and disease-specific mortality rates of 4% to 9% have been reported.[4–11] The outcomes of the three largest of these series are similar.[5,9,10] Lowe and Listrom reported on 232 patients with low- or high-volume disease who were observed 1 to 26 years.[9] Overall, progression occurred in 60 patients (26%), and 15 (6%) died from prostate cancer. Cantrell and coworkers reported on 117 patients with low- or high-volume disease who were observed 2 to 15 years.[5] Fourteen patients (12%) had cancer progression, and 5 (4%) died from prostate cancer. Epstein and coworkers expanded the group of patients with low-volume disease in the previous study and reported on a total of 94 patients.[6] Progression occurred in 8 (9%), and 6 (6%) died from prostate cancer. However, among the 50 patients who showed no cancer progression before 8 years, the subsequent progression rate was 16% and the prostate cancer mortality rate was 12%. Finally, Zhang and coworkers reported on 132 patients with low-volume disease who had a mean follow-up period of 8 years.[10] Thirteen patients (10%) progressed, and none died from prostate cancer. Fifty-two of the patients in this study underwent a second transurethral resection: of the 38 patients without tumor, 8% progressed, and of the 12 with tumor, 25% progressed.

In general, for patients with incidental prostate cancer, greater risks of progression and death from prostate cancer are related to high-grade[5,7,9,11–13] and high-volume disease.[5,7–9,12–14] Content of DNA (DNA ploidy) was found to be prognostic in one study and nuclear roundness in another.[13,14]

TABLE 47-1. *Survival rates with conservative treatment of prostate cancer*

Investigators	Patients	Initial stage	Overall survival rate (%)			Progression-free survival rate (%)			Disease-specific survival rate (%)	
			5 y	10 y	15 y	5 y	10 y	15 y	5 y	10 y
INCIDENTAL CANCER										
Heaney et al, 1977[12]	33	Incidental	80	54	50	—	—	—	—	—
Blute et al, 1986[4]	23	A	100	85	—	—	—	—	—	—
Moskowitz et al, 1987[47]	40	T0b	91	65	—	—	—	—	—	—
Goodman et al, 1988[7]	69	A	50	30	—	—	—	—	—	—
Lowe and Listrom, 1988[9]	236	A	—	—	—	84	68	48	—	—
Waaler et al, 1990[11]	13	T0f	—	—	—	100	—	—	100	—
	53	T0d	—	—	—	80	—	—	93	—
Johansson et al, 1992[15]	72	T0l	72	39	—	89	82	—	95	93
	34	T0d	71	47	—	61	33	—	93	77
CLINICALLY ORGAN-CONFINED CANCER										
Moskowitz et al, 1988[47]	44	T1-T2	61	34	—	—	—	—	—	—
George, 1988[30]	105	Clinically localized	—	—	—	—	—	—	80*	—
Graverson et al, 1990[31]	50	VACURG I-II	70	55	32	—	—	—	—	—
Whitmore et al, 1991[23]	29	B1	92	90	67	55	30	26	—	—
	37	B2	88	65	33	70	37	0	—	—
	9	B3	84	65	63	73	60	0	—	—
Johansson et al, 1992[15]	117	T1-T2	63	40	—	56	43	—	93	85
	58	T0d-T2	78	58	—	60	50	—	94†	87†
Adolfsson et al, 1992[32]	122	T1-T2	51	—	—	—	—	—	99	84
Adolfsson et al, 1991[16],‡	61	T1-T2	—	85	—	—	—	—	98†	92†
Egawa et al, 1993[33]	52	A1-B	—	—	—	—	—	—	—	75
Stenzl and Studer, 1993[34]	34	T0-T2	67	34	—	—	—	—	89	87
Waaler et al, 1990[11]	28	T1-T2	—	—	—	—	—	—	70	—
CLINICALLY NOT ORGAN-CONFINED										
Adolfsson, 1993[17]	50	T3	—	37§	—	—	—	—	70§	—

* 90% in Figure 47-4.
† Patients less than 70 years of age.
‡ Subgroup of Adolfsson et al, 1992[32].
§ 9 years of follow-up.

Palpable, Clinically Localized Prostate Cancer

A growing international experience indicates that a surveillance strategy with treatment at the time of disease progression for patients with clinically localized palpable prostate cancer results in a significant rate of local progression, a moderate rate of distant progression, and a low rate of fatal disease during the first 10 years of follow-up after diagnosis. This experience is based on several studies from various parts of the world (see Table 47-1). The 10-year overall survival rate has been reported to range from 34% to 55%, and the 10-year disease-specific survival rate from 75% to 85%, for patients with disease clinically confined to the gland. One study reported a progression-free survival rate of 43% after 10 years of follow-up. The difference between overall and disease-specific survival rates indicates that many of the patients who die during 10 years of surveillance do so from causes not related to prostate cancer. In two series, patients younger than 70 years of age at diagnosis were analyzed separately; the disease-specific survival rate after 10 years was found to be 88% in one study and 92% in the other.[15,16] In one Scandinavian series, patients with clinically localized but palpably not confined prostate cancer were managed with surveillance.[17] The overall survival rate after 9 years was 37%, and the disease-specific survival rate was 70%. In this series, a higher proportion of patients died from prostate cancer than in the series of patients with tumors clinically confined to the prostate gland.

Combined Analyses of Surveillance Series

During 1993, two separate literature reviews with combined analyses of surveillance series for locally confined prostate cancer were published.[18,19] In one of the studies, the combined disease-specific survival rate after 10 years was calculated to be 84%.[18] The two studies used different methods to calculate rates of distant progression and of prostate cancer mortality. In the review of Wasson and colleagues,[19] the median annual rate of metastasis was 0.017%, with a 95% confidence interval (95% CI) of 0.011% to 0.043%; the annual mortality rate from prostate cancer in this study was 0.009% (95% CI = 0.006%–0.012%). In the report of Adolfsson, Steineck, and Whitmore,[18] the weighted mean number of patients at risk for development of metastasis was 0.025 (95% CI = 0.02%–0.031%), and the annual rate of prostate cancer mortality was 0.017% (95% CI = 0.013%–0.021%).

Recently, an international pooled analysis of original patient data from six different series employing surveillance for patients with clinically localized prostate cancer has been published.[20] Individual patient data were analyzed on 828 patients. For patients with well- or moderately differentiated tumors, the disease-specific survival rate after 10 years was 87%; for patients with poorly differentiated tumors, it was only 34%. In the same analysis, the metastasis-free survival after 10 years was 81% for patients with well-differentiated tumors, 58% for those with moderately differentiated tumors, and 26% for patients with poorly differentiated tumors.

Confounds in Series of Surveillance

Tumor Grade

Published surveillance series have been widely criticized because of their relatively high numbers of patients with well-differentiated tumors. In comparison with series of patients treated with radical prostatectomy or external beam radiation therapy, surveillance series have fewer patients with poorly differentiated disease, biasing to more favorable outcomes with surveillance. Mitigating against this bias is the fact that grading in surveillance series is uniformly based on prostate biopsy only (either core or fine-needle sampling), and if these grades were compared with grades established by radical prostatectomy, it is likely that the biopsy grade would be lower.[21,22]

Selection Bias

The question of selection bias is difficult to address for any management series because few authors give information on this issue. At one extreme in surveillance series is the Memorial Sloan-Kettering report, in which 75 patients were selected from more than 4000 during a specified period of time.[23] At the other extreme is the series of Johansson and associates,[15] in which the population at risk was well defined and the population studied comprised all those men with prostate cancer diagnosed during the period of study.

Age

Age constitutes a special problem in the assessment of surveillance for localized prostate cancer. In Adolfsson's review, there was a marked difference in mean age for patients undergoing the various treatments.[18] Patients in this review who underwent radical prostatectomy were approximately 10 years younger than patients monitored with surveillance. This difference may represent the selection of younger and usually fitter patients for surgical treatment rather than overinclusion of elderly patients on a program of surveillance. If age proves to be a prognostic factor (e.g., if prostate cancer follows a more aggressive course in younger men), the difference in mean age represents a major confound causing an unbalanced distribution of prognostic factors when comparing outcomes of radical surgery or irradiation and surveillance.

A second major bias can be injected by differences in age. Elderly men have shorter observation times because of higher competing mortality rates than younger men. Because prostate cancer usually affects the mortality hazard curve several years after diagnosis, older men with short observation times are exposed to shorter intervals of the hazard rate curve, whereas younger men with longer observation times are exposed to a longer and possibly more significant period of risk. Assuming that the hazard rate for prostate cancer mortality is not constant, this difference alone will make the rates for different age groups unequal. Only comparison of patients of similar age can eliminate this confound.

Duration of Follow-Up

The majority of outcome data available for surveillance in patients with clinically localized prostate cancer is valid for up to 10 years of follow-up. The relatively low metastasis-free survival rate after 10 years for patients with moderately differentiated tumors found in the pooled patient analysis may indicate an increase in tumor-related mortality in this group beyond 10 years of observation.[20] Supporting this concept is a Swedish series of surveillance for patients with localized prostate cancer that demonstrated an increase in prostate cancer mortality after 10 years of follow-up.[24] However, such an increase was not found in long-term survival data from Johansson and associates nor in an update of the Memorial Sloan-Kettering experience.[15]

Summary of Surveillance Experience

With up to 10 years of observation, patients with locally confined carcinoma of the prostate monitored on a program of surveillance seem to have a high rate of disease-specific survival. Patients with poorly differentiated tumors or tumors clinically localized but not confined to the prostate have a poorer prognosis, indicating that surveillance may not be appropriate for them. At this time, the outcome of surveillance for periods beyond 10 years of follow-up is unknown.

ASSISTING PATIENTS TO APPROPRIATELY SELECT SURVEILLANCE MANAGEMENT

Before making a decision regarding treatment of prostate malignancy, two competing outcomes should be considered: benefits and harms. In general, the benefits of treatment are the avoidance of harms associated with the disease: death from cancer or morbidity from disease progression. These treatment benefits are often achievable for localized prostate malignancy, with moderate variability among treatment options. Accompanying the chance of benefit with any treatment is a set of risks (complications) and side effects that together comprise the harms of treatment.

The degree of harm varies with the method of treatment delivery (e.g., technical differences among surgeons) and depends on the condition of the patient. Older patients are usually at greater risk of complications from intervention than younger, healthier men.[25] It is necessary to estimate chances of harm before treatment is selected. Variability in delivery of treatment is difficult to assess from available data, particularly as it applies to an individual patient. Information regarding the overall status

TABLE 47-2. *Prostate cancer case variables*

PATIENT CHARACTERISTICS

Physical status—Age, family history, comorbidity
Psychological status—Anxiety, fear, attitude, reliability

TUMOR CHARACTERISTICS

Stage—Volume, location, extension, serum level of prostate-specific antigen
Grade—Gleason pattern, DNA ploidy
Growth rate—Acceleration of serum prostate-specific antigen level

MEDICAL ACCESS

Physicians—Urologists, medical oncologists, radiation oncologists
Facilities—Hospital, radiotherapy

of the patient who is considering treatment is more accessible and more useful when estimating potential treatment harms.

Benefits from treatment for localized malignancy often depend on the character of the tumor. The degree of benefit varies according to the condition of the patient. For example, 20-year cure rates have greater value to a 50-year-old man than to an 80-year-old man. An attempt to quantitate relative benefits of treatment is also needed before therapy is selected. Variables to consider include patient characteristics, tumor status, and access to medical care (Table 47-2).

Patient Characteristics

Most localized prostate cancers are either well- or moderately differentiated,[20,22,26,27] and progression of disease is often slow and protracted.[15,28,29] The risk of morbidity or death from malignancy is low for the first 10 years after diagnosis.[15,16,20,23,25,30–34] Men with a relatively short natural life expectancy (<10 years) will therefore have little risk of cancer-related death or morbidity from cancer progression. These risks increase substantially after 10 years, and caution must be exercised for men expected to live longer.[24] In 1989, a 74-year-old man in the United States had an average of 9.9 years life remaining[35] (Table 47-3). Age alone, however, is not an accurate predictor of life expectancy or treatment outcome,[36] and information regarding family longevity and coexisting illness often influences these estimates. Exceptionally good health and

TABLE 47-3. *Expected years of life for men in the United States, 1989*

Age	Years
50	26.4
60	18.6
70	12.1
74	9.9
80	7.1
85	5.3

National Center for Health Statistics. Vital statistics of the United States, 1989. Vol II, Mortality, part A. US Public Health Service, DHHS Pub. No. (PHS) 93-1101. Washington DC, US Government Printing Office, 1993.

family history may reduce a patient's physiologic age by several years. Conversely, significant heart, lung, or vascular disease may add several years to the patient's physiologic age.

A general psychologic assessment is often useful before considering surveillance for localized disease. Not all men are emotionally prepared to allow a malignancy to slowly progress if treatment is available. The physician can usually get a sense of this comfort level or any anxiety by observing a patient's attitude or orientation regarding treatment during the interview.

For various reasons, some patients choose to avoid interactions with physicians. Surveillance still requires periodic monitoring of a patient's condition. For some individuals, a brief interval of opportunity for treatment (''doing something'') for a newly diagnosed malignancy is all that is psychologically tolerable. Ongoing surveillance for these men may be difficult to maintain.

Tumor Characteristics

Tumor Stage

Although surveillance for higher-stage tumors may at times be appropriate, reference here is made only to clinically confined (clinical stage T1 and T2) cancer of the prostate. Clinically confined cancers have a wide range of tumor volumes, and knowledge of tumor volume useful to predict rates of disease progression.[29,37] A variety of methods can be used to determine tumor volume. Although digital rectal examination (DRE) and transrectal ultrasonography of the prostate are useful if the tumors are palpable or sonolucent, accurate measurement with these techniques is not certain. The number or percentage of chips showing cancer after transrectal ultrasonography can be used to help estimate tumor volume for stage T1a or T1b lesions, as can the number and percent of each biopsy core having cancer for T1c tumors.[38,39] The total number or percentage of positive chips indirectly estimates the diffuseness or volume of diseased tissue in incidentally discovered malignancy.[40,41] Regardless of the method used, T1a malignancy usually progresses slowly and seldom becomes lethal within 10 years.[41]

Estimation of tumor size or location by physical examination is often inaccurate. This may account for observations that the progression rates of clinical T2a and T2b tumors are often similar.[23] More accurate estimates of tumor extent may be gleaned from the location and extent of malignancy found on the ultrasound-guided biopsy specimens.[39] Stamey and colleagues have carefully evaluated the information obtained from measurement of tumor length within the biopsy core.[29] Low prostatic volume was usually found if the tumor measured 3 mm or less in length.[42] If the biopsy was positive bilaterally, significantly higher tumor volumes were found at prostatectomy.[43]

Nonpalpable cancers (T1c lesions) suspected because of elevated levels of prostate-specific antigen (PSA) often represent significant malignancy. Despite the inability to palpate a nodule, these cancers most often involve the peripheral zone and morphologically are similar to their palpable counterparts.[44,45] Again, information from the biopsy core specimens is useful to estimate tumor volume and location.[29,39]

PSA values correlate with tumor extent,[28] and subsequent rises in serial serum PSA levels provide useful information to estimate the rate of tumor growth.[28] Increasing tumor volume usually occurs concomitantly with development of higher tumor grade, extension beyond the confines of the prostate, and metastatic potential.[29]

Tumor Grade

Although large-volume tumors progress more quickly than small-volume tumors, it is probably the higher grade of cancer associated with increased volume that is responsible for the accelerated growth rate. Although low-volume, high-grade tumors are uncommon, they do occur and represent a substantial threat to survival.[46] To date, tumor grade stands out as the single most useful predictor of metastatic progression and cancer mortality.[7,9,15,46,47]

The international pooled analysis by Chodak and colleagues[20] showed that men with high-grade localized tumors (grade 3, Gleason score 8 or higher) managed by surveillance stand a 74% chance of metastatic progression and a 66% chance of cancer-related death after 10 years. Those men with grade 1 or grade 2 malignancy experience only a 13% chance of cancer death, and their chance of metastatic progression is 19% (grade 1) to 42% (grade 2).

DNA Ploidy

In recent years, DNA ploidy analysis has been evaluated as a tool to predict biologic prostate cancer behavior.[26,27,48] In a retrospective analysis of prostate tumors in radical prostatectomy specimens, Montgomery and colleagues[27] found aneuploid tumors in 4%. All patients with aneuploid tumors had recurrent disease by 9.4 years of follow-up. Adolfsson and associates[26] prospectively analyzed DNA ploidy as it correlates to tumor progression in men placed on surveillance with grade 1 or grade 2 malignancy. Almost equal numbers of diploid and nondiploid tumors were found. Those men with nondiploid tumors progressed more quickly and more often than those whose tumors were considered diploid. Recently, Greene and colleagues found that even very small tumors can display nondiploid histograms.[48]

Medical Access

Ideally, access to physicians or medical facilities should not influence decisions regarding choice of medical management. However, there are still many men in the United States who, for various reasons, have limited access to medical care. There is a high likelihood that these men may be lost to follow-up because of lack of available health care or failure to seek health care. In remote areas, follow-up care may be limited by lack of physicians or facilities. In some situations, the treatment options (surgery or radiation) may be delivered only rarely or with less modern techniques, and the risks or harms caused by treatment variability may be relatively higher.

Ideally, cost of treatment should not limit access to medical care. There are, however, many men who are limited in their treatment choices by lack of insurance or by the restrictions of managed care contracts. These limitations may also need to be considered when deciding between treatment choices.

In summary, the patient's condition, including attitude, fear, and anxiety, should be assessed along with his tumor status and access to medical care before treatment choices are made. The ideal candidate for management of localized prostate cancer by surveillance is usually considered to be a man with well- or moderately differentiated tumor of relatively low volume. His life expectancy should be less than 10 years, as estimated by chronologic age and general health status. He should be comfortable with the proposal of living with the presence of prostate malignancy and the almost certain prospect that progression (although usually slow) will occur. A physician who is knowledgeable concerning prostate malignancy behavior should be available to perform follow-up visits within a facility that is easily accessible to the patient.

HOW TO IMPLEMENT SURVEILLANCE FOR PROSTATE CANCER

Two assumptions are fundamental to the policy of surveillance for the patient with carcinoma of the prostate. The first assumption is that the risk of disease progression is low. From the patient's standpoint, disease progression should be considered to consist of either the development of symptoms of prostate cancer or the need for treatment of the disease. The second assumption of surveillance is that one can successfully intervene to prevent disease progression. Intervention during surveillance is usually targeted either for cure of the disease or for palliation (or delay of progression). The two key words in this second assumption *successfully* and *prevent*. Although the first assumption is often met in patients with localized prostate cancer, the second is frequently a problem because of difficulties with implementation.

It is usually assumed that surveillance as a plan of management is employed after the diagnosis of localized disease, but a surveillance plan can be implemented at any time during the course of diagnosis or progression of the disease (Fig. 47-1). Examples include a decision not to perform a prostate biopsy in an octogenarian with congestive heart failure, a decision not

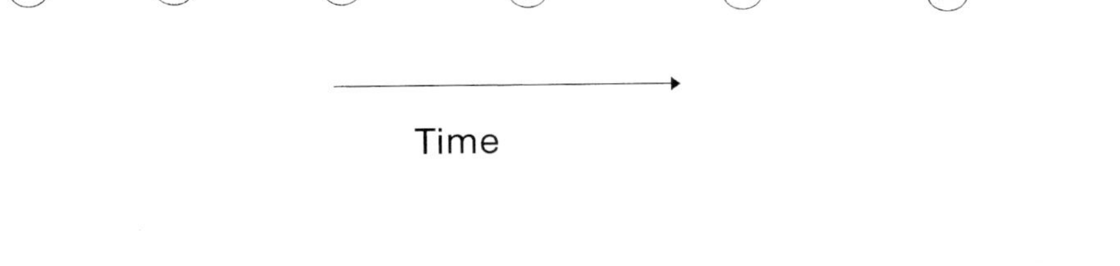

FIG. 47-1. Schema of surveillance. Although surveillance is usually thought to begin after prostate cancer diagnosis, this management plan can be initiated at any step.

to stage a cancer in a 74-year-old man with Gleason 2-2 tumor in one of eight prostate biopsies, and a decision to monitor a 74-year-old man who has a gradually rising PSA level 8 years after radical prostatectomy. In each of these examples, surveillance is being implemented in accordance with the two assumptions of therapy.

Strategies of Surveillance

When offering an eligible patient with prostate cancer surveillance as a method of treatment or follow-up, the physician must explain how this plan will be implemented. Two philosophic approaches can be used to guide surveillance. In the first approach, scheduled follow-up examinations are obtained, and if the results of any examination exceed a specific threshold (e.g., a 50% increase in PSA level), a change is considered, to include possible implementation of treatment for cure. In the second approach, no close follow-up is required, based on the recognition that the patient has a low risk of disease progression compared with other disease processes (comorbidities) and that most patients, with sufficient follow-up, will exceed some test threshold (e.g., abnormal DRE, increased PSA). These two surveillance philosophies differ radically in scheduled follow-up, but both have merit. Before embarking on a plan of surveillance with a given patient, the strategy to be used must be decided.

Follow-up Instruments for Surveillance

It is intuitively obvious that regular interaction between physician and patient is essential for follow-up of the patient on surveillance for prostate cancer. The development of obstructive voiding symptoms, weight loss, new unremitting pain, hematuria, or neurologic symptoms point to disease progression and should prompt evaluation. However, most of these symptoms or signs are associated with the development of regionally advanced or metastatic disease. This type of follow-up would therefore be most applicable to the second form of surveillance strategy. The first strategy, in which evidence of disease progression is sought to allow early intervention for cure or for delay of progression, requires more sensitive instruments. Two such instruments are available and are discussed separately here.

Digital Rectal Examination

If a prostate tumor is palpable (e.g., stage T2a), detection of an increase in size of the nodule would be one trigger for consideration of intervention for cure. The development of a palpable nodule in a T1c tumor should offer a similar opportunity. Unfortunately, the experience with DRE for prostate cancer suggests that palpable tumors are often locally advanced and are associated with high risk of recurrence. In an early screening series in which DRE was employed, 88% of tumors detected were locally confined, but 66% were assigned a higher stage after radical prostatectomy.[49] A more recent study found that 31% of DRE-detected tumors had extraprostatic spread at the time diagnosis.[50] The impact of the presence of T3 disease has been demonstrated by Paulson and colleagues, who noted that the 10-year disease-free survival rate dropped from 88% to 40% in those men with positive margins at radical prostatectomy.[51] These data suggest that DRE can be an insensitive method of follow-up for patients who are being monitored on a program of compulsive follow-up examinations designed to detect disease progression while cure is still possible.

Prostate-Specific Antigen

PSA level is an attractive determination to use as a trigger for intervention in a patient on a surveillance program. Because an exact numeric value is obtained, various thresholds for intervention can be used: an absolute value, percent change, doubling time, or some calculation of a second order rate of change. Each of these is discussed here in relation to detection of disease progression while the tumor is still confined to the prostate.

Most patients diagnosed with prostate cancer have an abnormal serum PSA value (>4.0 ng/mL) value at diagnosis.[50] For this reason, a meaningful increase in PSA level is a reasonable trigger to prompt intervention. Brawer and colleagues found that no patient whose serum PSA concentration exceeded 10 ng/mL had organ-confined disease.[52] In an analysis of 416 patients in whom pathologic stage was compared with preoperative PSA level, a rapid increase in risk of T3 disease was found to occur with PSA values of between 4 and 10 ng/mL.[53] Figure 47-2 demonstrates the relation between PSA and pathologic stage. It can be seen that the risk of extraprostatic disease increases significantly with relatively small increases in PSA level.

A number of authors have suggested that the rate of increase in PSA (PSA velocity, or PSAV) can predict the presence of carcinoma of the prostate. Brawer and his coworkers empirically chose a 20% annual increase as a threshold in their screening series, and Carter and colleagues, reviewing a group of patients with prostate cancer from the Baltimore Longitudinal Study of Aging (BLSA), found that an increase of 0.75 ng/mL per year was characteristic of patients with prostate cancer.[54,55] In both series, the number of patients evaluated was quite small (14 and 18, respectively), and the precision of these recommended values is therefore of concern. In addition, close inspection of the increases in PSA level in the BLSA patients shows that the rate of change follows what appears to be a second-

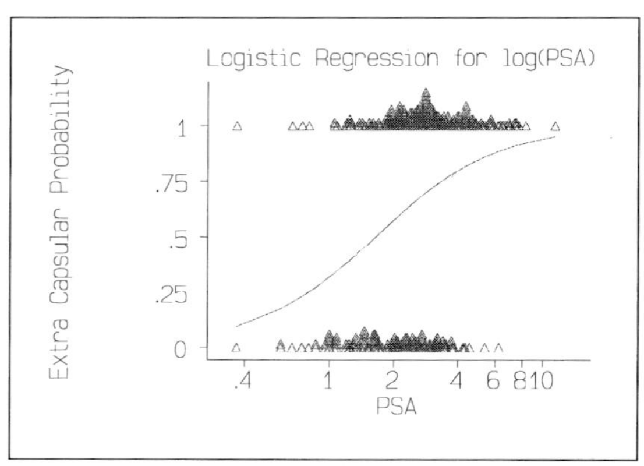

FIG. 47-2. Comparison of preoperative prostate-specific antigen (PSA) level and risk of extracapsular disease.

order curve (i.e., the rate of increase depends on the number of years of follow-up[2]).

The composite findings of these series using PSA or DRE suggest that most patients placed on a program of surveillance already have a substantial risk of extraprostatic disease at diagnosis. If it is desired to detect progressive disease before the development of extraprostatic disease, neither PSA nor DRE may be a sufficiently sensitive instrument for this purpose.

Implications of Effectiveness of Follow-up Instruments on Surveillance Philosophy

The discussion above, noting the poor performance of both DRE and PSA for follow-up during surveillance, suggests that if an aggressive follow-up philosophy is desired, there is a strong possibility of one of two errors. Because of the poor sensitivity of these instruments, disease progression beyond the confines of the prostate can occur before it is recognized. Conversely, if an overly sensitive threshold is chosen (e.g., a 20% increase in PSA), many patients may be overtreated. This is best illustrated in the series of patients who were observed without treatment by Whitmore and associates.[23] In this series, virtually every patient experienced disease progression with sufficient follow-up and would therefore have been treated in an aggressive surveillance regimen. However, only a small fraction of these patients developed metastatic disease or died of their disease during follow-up. The fraction of patients who would have benefited from an aggressive or highly sensitive plan of surveillance—that is, those whose progression would have been detected before development of extraprostatic disease and who would have experienced morbidity or mortality without such detection—may be quite small.

Other Issues

Disease Dedifferentiation

As has been stated, the ideal candidate for a surveillance strategy is the patient with well-differentiated, diploid disease. The determination of this status is usually made at the time of diagnosis. However, this feature can change with time, as reported by Adolfsson and Tribukait.[56] In their series of 84 patients who had multiple fine-needle aspirations while on a program of surveillance and had a median follow-up time of 47 months, an increase in ploidy was noted in 17 patients and an increase in cytologic differentiation was noted in 18. The troubling implication of this finding is that a patient with well-differentiated, diploid disease who embarks on a course of surveillance may be at high risk of disease dedifferentiation, and may thereby acquire a higher risk of disease progression.

Decision Styles and Management of Uncertainty

Conservative treatment for localized prostate cancer is not acceptable to all patients. Different styles of decision-making, how the issues are presented to the patient, and the age of the patient can all have an impact on whether the patient will find a surveillance strategy acceptable.[57,58,59] The decision to choose surveillance may in large part be based on risk aversion: avoidance of the immediate adverse consequences of treatment in exchange for acceptance of the risk of disease progression and symptoms which may occur at some time in the future. In many such decisions, the risk, albeit low, of immediate complications from treatment can lead to a choice of surveillance.[60] However, little is known of the psychological impact of the uncertainty associated with disease progression over long periods of time in patients who opt for no initial treatment. Individual patients may find one strategy more acceptable than another, and some, because of changes in decision-making styles or with further reconsideration of choices, may change their management decision over time.

CONCLUSIONS: IMPLEMENTATION OF SURVEILLANCE

For many patients with newly diagnosed prostate cancer, surveillance can be an excellent management choice. Optimal patients are those who have shorter life expectancy, who have lower-grade and lower-stage tumors, and whose decision-making style and anxiety level will allow them to accept this type of treatment. Before embarking on a strategy of surveillance, both physician and patient must agree on what follow-up tests will be performed, their frequency, and the treatment implications of test results. At all stages of this process, it is imperative that the physician educate the patient as much as possible concerning the nuances of the disease and its treatment. Through this process, the best treatment strategy for the individual patient can be chosen.

REFERENCES

1. Bumpus HC. Carcinoma of the prostate: a clinical study of 1000 cases. Surg Gynec Obstet 1926;43:150.
2. Nesbit RM, Plumb RT. Prostatic carcinoma: a follow-up on 795 patients treated prior to the endocrine era and a comparison of survival rates between these and patients treated by endocrine therapy. Surgery 1946; 20:263.
3. Paulson DF. Stage A prostatic adenocarcinoma. World J Urol 1989;7: 34.
4. Blute ML, Zincke H, Farrow GM. Long-term follow-up of young patients with stage A adenocarcinoma of the prostate. J Urol 1986;136: 840.
5. Cantrell BB, DeClerk DP, Egglestone JC, Boitnott JK, Walsh PC. Pathological factors that influence prognosis in stage A prostatic cancer: the influence of extent versus grade. J Urol 1981;125:516.
6. Epstein JL, Paull G, Eggleston JC, Walsh PC. Prognosis of untreated stage A1 prostatic carcinoma: a study of 94 cases with extended follow-up. J Urol 1986;136:837.
7. Goodman CM, Busuttil A, Chisholm GD. Age, and size and grade of tumour predict prognosis in incidentally diagnosed carcinoma of the prostate. Br J Urol 1988;62:576.
8. Haapiainen R. Latent (pTo) prostatic carcinoma: a retrospective study of frequency and natural history. Ann Chir Gynaecol 1986;75:172.
9. Lowe BA, Listrom MB. Incidental carcinoma of the prostate: an analysis of the predictors of progression. J Urol 1988;140:1340.
10. Zhang G, Wasserman NF, Sidi AA, Reinberg Y, Reddy PK. Long-term follow-up results after expectant management of stage A1 prostatic cancer. J Urol 1991;146:990.
11. Waaler G, Ludvigsen TC, Stenwig AE. Prognosis of incidental prostatic cancer in Aust-Agder County, Norway. Eur Urol 1990;18:179.
12. Heaney JA, Chang HC, Daly JJ, Prout GR. Prognosis of clinically

undiagnosed prostatic carcinoma and the influence of endocrine therapy. J Urol 1977;118:283.
13. Mohler JL, Partin AW, Epstein JL, et al. Prediction of prognosis in untreated stage A2 prostatic carcinoma. Cancer 1992;69:511.
14. McIntire TL, Murphy WM, Coons JS, et al. The prognostic value of DNA ploidy combined with histologic substaging for incidental carcinoma of the prostate gland. Am J Clin Pathol 1988;89:370.
15. Johansson JE, Adami HO, Andersson SO, Berstrom R, Holmberg L, Krussemo UB. High 10-year survival rate in patients with early untreated prostatic cancer. JAMA 1992;267:2191.
16. Adolfsson J, Carstensen J. Natural course of clinically localized prostate adenocarcinoma in men less than 70 years old. J Urol 1991;146:96.
17. Adolfsson J. Deferred treatment of low grade stage T3 prostate cancer without distant metastases. J Urol 1993;149:326.
18. Adolfsson J, Steineck G, Whitmore WF. Recent results of management of palpable clinically localized prostate cancer. Cancer 1993;72:310.
19. Wasson JH, Cushman CC, Bruskewitz RC, et al. A structured literature review of treatment for localized prostate cancer. Arch Fam Med 1993;2:487.
20. Chodak G, Thiested R, Gerber G, et al. Outcome following conservative management of patients with clinically localized prostate cancer. N Engl J Med 1994;330:242.
21. Catalona WJ, Stein AJ, Fair WR. Grading errors in prostatic needle biopsies: relation to the accuracy of tumor grade in predicting pelvic lymph node metastases. J Urol 1982;127:919.
22. Narayan P, Jajodia P, Stein R, Tanagho EA. A comparison of fine needle aspiration and core biopsy in diagnosis and preoperative grading of prostate cancer. J Urol 19889;141:560.
23. Whitmore WF, Warner JA, Thompson IM. Expectant management of localized prostate cancer. Cancer 1991;67:1091.
24. Aus G, Hogosson J, Norlen L. Risk of dying of prostate cancer in different stages, grades and age at diagnosis. J Urol 1994;151:278A. Abstract.
25. Fleming C, Wasson JH, Albertsen PC, Barry MJ, Wennberg JE. A decision analysis of alternative treatment strategies for clinically localized prostate cancer. JAMA 1993;269:2650.
26. Adolfsson J, Ronstrom L, Hedlund PO, Lowhagen T, Carstensen J, Tribukait B. The prognostic value of modal deoxyribonucleic acid in low grade, low stage untreated prostate cancer. J Urol 1990;14:1404.
27. Montgomery BT, Nativ O, Blute ML, et al. Stage B prostate adenocarcinoma: flow cytometric nuclear DNA ploidy analysis. Arch Surg 1990;125:327.
28. Schmid HP, McNeal JE, Stamey TA. Observations on the doubling time of prostate cancer: the use of serial prostate-specific antigen in patients with untreated disease as a measure of increasing cancer volume. Cancer 1993;71:2031.
29. Stamey TA, Freiha FS, McNeal JE, Redwine EA, Whittemore AS, Schmid HP. Localized prostate cancer: relationship of tumor volume to clinical significance for treatment of prostate cancer. Cancer 1993;71:933.
30. George NJR. Natural history of localized prostatic cancer managed by conservative therapy alone. Lancet 1988;5:494.
31. Graverson PH, Nielsson KT, Gasser TC, Corle DK, Madsen PO. Radical prostatectomy versus expectant treatment in stages I and II prostatic cancer: a fifteen-year follow-up. Urology 1990;36:493.
32. Adolfsson J, Castensen J, Lowhagen T. Deferred treatment in clinically localized prostatic carcinoma. Br J Urol 1992;69:183.
33. Egawa S, Go M, Kuwao S, Shoji K, Uchida T, Koshiba K. Long-term impact of conservative management of localized prostate cancer. Urology 1993;42:520.
34. Stenzl A, Studer UE. Outcome of patients with untreated cancer of the prostate. Eur Urol 1993;24:1.
35. National Center for Health Statistics. Vital statistics of the United States: 1989. Vol II, Mortality, part A. US Public Health Service, DHHS Pub. No. (PHS) 93-1101. Washington, DC: US Government Printing Office, 1993.
36. Corral DA, Bahnson RR. Survival of men with clinically localized prostate cancer detected in the eighth decade of life. J Urol 1994;151:1326.
37. Schmid HP, McNeal JE, Stamey TA. Clinical observations on the doubling time of prostate cancer. Eur Urol 1993;23:60.
38. Jewett HJ. The present status of radical prostatectomy for stages A and B prostatic cancer. Urol Clin North Am 1975;2:105.
39. Terris MK, McNeal JE, Stamey TA. Estimation of prostate cancer volume by transrectal ultrasound imaging. J Urol 1992;147:855.
40. Correa RJ Jr, Anderson RG, Gibbons RP, et al. Latent carcinoma of the prostate: Why the controversy? J Urol 1974;111:644.
41. Austenfeld M. Treatment of stage A1 prostate cancer: the case for observation. Semin Urol 1993;11:58.
42. Terris MK, McNeal JE, Stamey TA. Detection of clinically significant prostate cancer by transrectal ultrasound-guided systematic biopsies. J Urol 1992;148:829.
43. Daniels GF Jr, McNeal JE, Stamey TA. Predictive value of contralateral biopsies in unilaterally palpable prostate cancer. J Urol 1992;147:870.
44. Stormont TJ, Farrow GM, Myers RP, et al. Clinical stage B0 or T1c prostate cancer: nonpalpable disease identified by elevated serum prostate specific antigen concentration. Urology 1993;41:3.
45. Epstein JI, Carmichael MJ, Partin AW, Walsh PC. Small high grade adenocarcinoma of the prostate in radical prostatectomy specimens performed for nonpalpable disease: pathogenetic and clinical implications. J Urol 1994;151:1587.
46. Partin AW, Lee BR, Carmichael M, Walsh PC, Epstein JI. Radical prostatectomy for high grade disease: a reevaluation 1994. J Urol 1994;151:1583.
47. Moskowitz B, Nitecki S, Richter, Levin D. Cancer of the prostate: is there a need for aggressive treatment? Urol Int 1987;42:49.
48. Greene DR, Rogers E, Wessels EV, et al. Some small prostate cancers are nondiploid by nuclear image analysis: correlation of deoxyribonucleic acid ploidy status and pathological features. J Urol 1994;151:1301.
49. Thompson IM, Ernst JJ, Gangai MP, Spence CR. Adenocarcinoma of the prostate: results of routine urological screening. J Urol 1984;132:690.
50. Catalona WJ, Richie JP, Ahmann FR, et al. Comparison of digital rectal examination and serum prostatic specific antigen in the early detection of prostate cancer: results of a multicenter clinical trial of 6,630 men. J Urol 1994;151:1283.
51. Paulson DF, Moul JW, Walther PJ. Radical prostatectomy for clinical stage T1-2N0M0 prostatic adenocarcinoma: long-term results. J Urol 1990;144:1180.
52. Brawer MK, Chetner MP, Beatie J, Buchner DM, Vessella RL, Lange PH. Screening for prostatic carcinoma with prostate specific antigen. J Urol 1992;147:841.
53. Thompson IM, Zeidman EJ, Crawford ED, et al. In the era of prostate specific antigen, is prostate acid phosphatase necessary for staging prostate cancer? A Southwest Oncology Group Study. J Urol 1993;149:303A. Abstract.
54. Brawer MK, Beatie J, Wener MH, Vessella RL, Preston SD, Lange PH. Screening for prostatic carcinoma with prostate specific antigen: results of the second year. J Urol 1993;150:106.
55. Carter HB, Pearson J, Mouthier EJ, et al. Longitudinal evaluation of prostate-specific antigen levels in men with and without prostate disease. JAMA 1992;267:2215.
56. Adolfsson J, Tribukait B. Evaluation of tumor progression by repeated fine needle biopsies in prostate adenocarcinoma: Modal deoxyribonucleic acid value and cytological differentiation. J Urol 1990;144:1408.
57. Tversky A, Kahneman D. The framing of decisions and the psychology of choice. Science 1981;211:453.
58. Bergman L, Dekker G, VanLeeuwen FE, Huisman SJ, VanDam FSAM, VanDongen JA. The effect of age on treatment choice and survival in elderly breast cancer patients. Cancer 1991;67:2227.
59. Pierce PF. Deciding on breast cancer treatment: a description of decision behavior. Nurs Res 1993;42:22.
60. O'Meara JJ, McNutt RA, Evans AT, Moore SW, Downs SM. A decision analysis of streptokinase plus heparin as compared with heparin alone for deep-vein thrombosis. N Engl J Med 1994;330:1864.

Principles and Practice of Genitourinary Oncology, edited by Derek Raghavan, Howard I. Scher, Steven A. Leibel, and Paul H. Lange. Lippincott-Raven Publishers, Philadelphia, © 1997.

CHAPTER 48

Staging of Prostate Cancer

David A. Levy and Martin I. Resnick

As medical technology and diagnostic techniques continue to advance and provide increased longevity, a greater segment of the adult male population will be diagnosed with prostate cancer. In 1992, the American Cancer Society predicted that 133,000 newly diagnosed cases of prostate cancer would be recorded in the United States. By 1993, the number grew to 165,000, and prostate cancer became the most prevalent malignancy in American men.[1] The current prediction is that 317,100 new cases will be diagnosed and 41,400 men will succumb to the disease in 1996.[2] Furthermore, by the end of the century a 37% increase in annual mortality is anticipated among individuals diagnosed with prostate cancer.[3] Although the prevalence of the disease remains unchanged, the incidence is increasing at an astronomical rate, which may be attributable to the expanded use of serum prostate-specific antigen (PSA) testing coupled with an increased number of prostate biopsies being performed nationally. In 1954, autopsy studies indicated that 30% of 50-year-old men and 50% of 70-year-old men had pathologic evidence of prostate cancer.[4] It is doubtful that these statistics have changed over the decades; however, diligence in diagnosing individuals with the disease has clearly increased.

Despite more than 40 years of research effort and therapeutic intervention, medical advances have had little or no impact on the mortality of prostate cancer. More sensitive diagnostic and staging modalities are essential to improve cancer survival rates and minimize the morbidity associated with patient evaluation.

During the last two decades, the approach to evaluating men with prostate cancer has changed. Digital rectal examination (DRE) was the mainstay of detection and noninvasive staging, but this approach has been modified by the introduction of routine PSA determinations. Similarly, imaging modalities such as transrectal ultrasonography (TRUS) and magnetic resonance (MR) imaging have been thoroughly evaluated as potential means of detecting and staging asymptomatic disease. Laparoscopic lymph node dissection and radionuclide bone scanning play an integral part of the staging of many patients with the pathologic diagnosis of carcinoma of the prostate. Preliminary work with radioimmunoconjugates may prove to have merit as a noninvasive means of staging cancer in these patients.

The approach to the patient suspected of having a prostatic malignancy is based on a vast number of investigational studies. Anatomic studies of the prostate were conducted as early as 1912[5] in an effort to gain insight into the predilection for tumor involvement in particular regions of the gland. Uniform agreement on the glandular architecture remains debatable; however, there is considerable acceptance of the zonal anatomy as proposed by McNeal.[6,7] As described by McNeal,[8,9] the peripheral zone, which comprises approximately 75% of the normal gland, and the transition zone, the site of origin of benign prostatic hyperplasia, account for approximately 70% and 20%, respectively, of malignancies diagnosed within the prostate. The central zone comprises approximately 25% of the normal prostate and is the site of origin of approximately 10% of prostatic carcinomas.[10]

STAGING CLASSIFICATIONS

One of the earliest staging classification systems for carcinoma of the prostate was introduced by Whitmore in 1956.[11] This system, based on DRE and radiographic studies, was widely accepted and categorized the disease as follows:

Stage A: the presence of subclinical disease
Stage B: organ-confined disease without evidence of metastatic spread
Stage C: locally extensive disease beyond the prostate but without evidence of metastasis
Stage D: metastatic disease.

This system was the most commonly used staging system in the United States until its modification by Jewitt in 1975.[12] Jewitt subclassified stage A disease based on whether the disease was focal (A1) or diffuse (A2) as well as the histologic differentiation of the tumor. Stage B disease was subclassified as B1, implying focal unilateral involvement of the gland, and B2 or diffuse disease, involving both of the posterior lobes without capsular involvement. Stage C disease was subclassified into tumors having minimal extracapsular involvement (C1) or more extensive extracapsular tumor producing bladder outlet or ureteral obstruction (C2). Stage D disease indicated metastatic disease.[12]

A tumor, node, metastasis (TNM) system, adapted by the American Joint Committee for Cancer Staging and End Results Reporting, was introduced by Wallace and colleagues[13] in 1975.

This staging scheme was developed in an attempt to further subclassify prostate cancers based on quantitation of tumor burden from needle core biopsy specimens, lymph node involvement, palpable size of the lesions in the gland, and pathologic findings of capsular involvement.

In an effort to devise a uniform clinical staging system for patients diagnosed with prostate cancer, a modified TNM staging system was formulated by Whitmore and colleagues, acting as the Organ Systems Coordinating Center of the National Cancer Institute, in 1988.[14] This system has proved to be most versatile of the available schemata and can be used with tumors detected by means of TRUS, serum PSA levels, or DRE. (Table 48-1)

This modified TNM staging system incorporates the designations of the previously developed systems and defines stage TA disease as histologically confirmed but digitally undetectable. Substaging is based on the pathologic findings of the transurethral endoscopic resection specimen. There is some debate regarding what constitutes high- and low-grade disease, which can make differentiating A1 from A2 disease somewhat confusing. Combined Gleason scores of 5 or lower,[15] 6 or lower[16,17] and 7 or lower[18] have been used by different investigators to define low-grade (stage A1) disease. There is substantial data to suggest that a combined Gleason score of 6 or lower may be the appropriate endpoint for classifying a tumor as stage A1.[16,17]

Stage TAX disease indicates digitally unrecognizable disease and is further subclassified based on TRUS findings and serum PSA. The TAX stage in particular demonstrates the versatility of the modified TNM staging classification system. This system allows for flexibility and adaptability to developments in the use of PSA levels, ultrasonography, and possibly MR imaging and radioimmunoconjugates in evaluating patients with carcinoma of the prostate.

TABLE 48-1. *Organ systems coordinating center classification for clinical staging of prostate cancer*

PRIMARY TUMOR (T)	
TX	Anatomic relations indefinable (e.g., prior total prostatectomy)
TA	Digitally unrecognizable cancer (confirmed histologically and substaged if traditional TUR cancer)
TA1	≤5% of total surgical specimen and of low to medium grade
TA2	>5% of specimen, any grade, or ≤5% of specimen with any high grade
TAX	TA, but not A1 or A2
TAX-TRUS	Detected by ultrasonography, confirmed by biopsy
TAX-PSA	Detected by PSA, confirmed by biopsy
TAX-Asym	Detected by DRE as a normal feeling but asymmetric prostate
TB	Digitally palpated organ-confined cancer
TB1	≤½ of one lobe, regardless of location
TB2	>½ of one lobe but not >1 lobe
TB3	>1 lobe or bilaterally palpable cancer
TBX	Palpable, organ-confined cancer not otherwise characterized
TBX-asym	Abnormally firm (non-nodular)
TBX-sym	Abnormally firm (non-nodular)
TBC*	Palpable cancer extending beyond prostate capsule
TC1	Extension beyond margin unilaterally (may include seminal vesicle)
TC2	Extension bilaterally (may include seminal vesicle)
TC3	Extension into bladder, rectum, levator muscles, or pelvic side walls
LYMPH NODE STATUS (N)	
N0 (C and/or H)	No regional lymph node metastases, clinically (C) and/or histologically (H)
N1 (H)	Microscopic regional lymph node metastasis proved histologically
N2 (C and/or H)	Gross regional lymph node metastases
N3 (C and/or H)	Extraregional lymph node metastases
NX	Minimal requirements have not been met
DISTANT METASTASES (M)†	
M0	No evidence of metastases
M1	Elevated acid phosphatase only (3 consecutive elevations)
M2 (V and/or B)	Visceral (V) and/or bone (B) metastases
MX	Minimal requirements not met

DRE, digital rectal examination; PSA, prostate-specific antigen; TRUS, transrectal ultrasonography; TUR, transurethral resection.

* TBC, in addition to the TC categories, requires TB specification of the extent of the intracapsular cancer.

† Excludes lymph nodes.

From Whitmore WF Jr, Catalona WJ, Grayhack JT, et al. Organ systems program staging classification for prostate cancer. In: Coffey DS, Resnick MI, Dorr FA, Karr JP, eds. A multidisciplinary analysis of controversies in the management of prostate cancer. New York: Plenum Press, 1988:295.

Stage TB, clinically palpable organ-confined cancer is substaged as TB1, TB2, or TB3 based on the degree of glandular involvement as interpreted on DRE. The TBX classification is defined as palpable organ-confined disease not otherwise characterized. The TC1 designation implies tumor extension beyond the prostate capsule unilaterally, which may involve the seminal vesicle. TC2 indicates tumor extension beyond the capsule bilaterally, and TC3 indicates tumor extension into the bladder, rectum, levator ani muscles, or pelvic side walls.

Lymph node status is categorized as N0, which implies no regional lymph node metastases either clinically (C) or histologically (H). N1(H) is defined as histologically proven regional micrometastases, N2(C), N2(H), or N2(CH) depicts gross regional nodal disease, and N3(C) or N3(H) describes extraregional lymph node metastases. The NX designation is used when minimal requirements for staging have not been met.

Distant metastases are categorized based on serum prostatic acid phosphatase elevations as well as the detection of visceral or bony lesions. M0 denotes no evidence of distant metastases, and M1 designates only elevation of serum enzymatic acid phosphatase levels on three consecutive determinations, irrespective of the radioimmunoassay prostatic acid phosphatase determinations. M2 disease describes the individual with evidence of visceral (V) disease, bony (B) involvement, or both, and the MX classification is used when minimal requirements for staging have not been met.

In 1992, the Union Internationale Contre le Cancre–American Joint Committee on Cancer (UICC-AJCC) proposed a unifying TNM system for staging localized prostate cancer.[19,20] These criteria are depicted in Table 48-2. The utility of this particular system was evaluated by Zagars and colleagues.[21] In this study, 427 patients with clinically localized prostate cancer were followed for a mean of 32 months after definitive radiotherapy and had pretreatment and posttreatment PSA determinations; then the prognostic power of the UICC-AJCC system was compared to that of the Whitmore-Jewitt system. The actuarial incidence of relapse or rising serum PSA at 5 years was reported as follows:

Stage A2: 29%
Stage B: 41%
Stage C: 62%
T1a: 0%
T1b: 37%
T1c: 23%
T2a: 39%
T2b: 38%
T2c: 42%
T3a: 53%
T3c: 68%
T4b: >75%.

Overall, T1a, T1c, T1b/T2, T3, and T4 were significantly superior prognostically to the Whitmore-Jewitt system. This critical analysis proved conclusively that the UICC-AJCC system allows for the designation of a greater number of meaningful tumor categories which are prognostically superior to the Whitmore-Jewitt system. The UICC-AJCC system is the most applicable staging system for patients with carcinoma of the prostate and has become widely used since its inception.

TABLE 48-2. *AJCC definition of the primary tumor*

T1	Clinically inapparent tumor not palpable or visible by imaging
T1a	Tumor incidental histologic finding in 5% or less of tissue resected
T1b	Tumor incidental histologic finding in more than 5% of tissue resected
T1c	Tumor identified by needle biopsy (e.g., because of elevated PSA)
T2	Tumor confined within the prostate
T2a	Tumor involves one half of a lobe or less
T2b	Tumor involves more than one half of a lobe, but not both lobes
T2c	Tumor involves both lobes
T3	Tumor extends through the prostatic capsule
T3a	Unilateral extracapsular extension
T3b	Bilateral extracapsular extension
T3c	Tumor invades the seminal vesicles
T4	Tumor is fixed or invades adjacent structures other than the seminal vesicles
T4a	Tumor invades any of bladder neck, external sphincter, or rectum
T4b	Tumor invades levator muscles and/or is fixed to the pelvic wall

AJCC, American Joint Committee on Cancer; PSA, prostate-specific antigen.

Bearhs OH, Hanson DR, Hutter RVP, Kennedy BJ. Manual for staging of cancer. 4th ed. Philadelphia: JB Lippincott 1992: 181.

DIGITAL RECTAL EXAMINATION

Traditionally, DRE and digitally guided transrectal or transperineal biopsies were the mainstays of prostate cancer detection and diagnosis. This seemed reasonable considering the early anatomic studies that were carried out in an effort to gain insight into the predilection for tumor involvement in particular regions of the gland. However, even with a high index of suspicion of glandular abnormalities, detection rates rates using only DRE rarely exceed 1.7%.[22,23] Although DRE has been used in the detection of carcinoma of the prostate, it is not accurate in staging the disease.

The accuracy of clinical staging based on DRE alone approximates 50% in men with palpable lesions.[23] Furthermore, more than 70% of patients diagnosed by this modality prove to have more advanced disease on pathologic examination.[24] Finally, studies have demonstrated a false-negative rate as high as 36% for lesions believed to be suspicious based on the DRE.[25] Because of the high false-positive and false-negative rates, DRE in and of itself is inadequate for early detection or accurate staging of prostate cancer. Subsequently, serum PSA testing and various imaging modalities have been applied in attempts to detect both palpable and nonpalpable lesions within the glandular stroma and thereby enhance the rate of detection and accuracy of staging of prostatic carcinoma.

ULTRASONOGRAPHY

An additional discussion of the use and value of ultrasonography is contained in Chapter 45. Ultrasonography was first adapted for use by the medical community in 1942, when Dussik[26] placed transducers on patients' craniums in an attempt to localize brain tumors. Advances in ultrasonography continued over the next two decades,[27–29] and in 1963, A-mode ultrasonography was used to obtain the first ultrasound-generated images of the prostate.[30] It was not until 1967, however, that the first clinically useful TRUS-generated images of the prostate were obtained by Wantanabe and Katoh.[31] In 1968, using a 3.5-MHz transducer on a transrectal radial probe covered with a water-filled balloon, Watanabe and colleagues[32] demonstrated significant improvement in TRUS-generated images of the prostate. With the use of B-mode ultrasonography by Wantanabe in 1968 and the development of gray-scale presentation by Boyce and colleagues in 1976,[33] image quality improved significantly, and the diagnostic potential of ultrasonography was realized. Continued technological improvements in gray-scale imaging, the development of high-frequency (7-MHz) transducers, and the introduction of real-time ultrasonographic imaging in the early 1980s further expanded the diagnostic applications of ultrasonography. Transabdominal, transperineal, and transurethral techniques were evaluated in attempts to improve visualization of the prostate gland, but the majority of the investigators concluded that the most reliable and reproducible prostate images resulted from transrectal imaging techniques.[34–36]

Image Characteristics

The normal adult prostate as viewed on TRUS appears as a symmetrical, triangular, relatively homogeneous structure that is well delineated by its surrounding capsule. The capsule or margin is usually highly echogenic. The echogenicity of the peripheral zone is described as isoechoic and functions as the standard pattern against which other areas and zones are compared.[37,38] The central zone of the gland can at times produce a higher echogenic pattern than the peripheral zone, a phenomenon attributed to the presence of larger, more reflective glands and corpora amylacea in this region of the prostate.[39] In the majority of clinical situations, the central zone produces an isoechoic signal.[37,40] The transition zone of the gland prior to the development of benign hyperplasia is hypoechoic.[37]

Attempts to delineate a characteristic appearance of adenocarcinoma of the prostate based on gray-scale, TRUS-generated images has been unrewarding. Studies have indicated that prostate cancers may have variable echogenic patterns. Most early studies reported that carcinoma of the prostate appeared as a hyperechoic focus.[33,41–44] In 1985, Lee and colleagues[45] reported that the presence of a hypoechoic area in the peripheral zone of the prostate was a reliable criterion for the diagnosis of adenocarcinoma (Fig. 48-1). Subsequently, investigators have reported the association of adenocarcinoma with hyperechoic, hypoechoic, and isoechoic ultrasound-generated images. Rifkin and colleagues[46] reported on 130 men with pathologically proven adenocarcinoma of the prostate who underwent TRUS. The findings revealed that 69% of these men had purely hyperechoic cancers when compared to normal prostate and 27% had sonographically mixed tumors that ranged from predominantly hypoechoic to predominantly hyperechoic. These investigators concluded that there are no specific transrectal endosonographic characteristics that enable differentiation of carcinoma from benign processes within the gland. Similarly, Dahnert and colleagues[47] reviewed the ultrasonographic findings in 52 men who subsequently underwent radical prostatectomy for histologically proven adenocarcinoma of the prostate. In their series, 54% of the specimens manifested echopenic lesions, 22% of the lesions were hypoechoic, and 24% of the lesions were isoechoic. In a more recent study conducted by Shinohara and colleagues,[48] the inconsistent appearance of prostatic carcinoma on TRUS was confirmed; 60% of the lesions appeared as hypoechoic, 39% as isoechoic, and 1% as hyperechoic. Overall, the available data indicate that TRUS alone is unreliable in diagnosing adenocarcinoma of the prostate.

Initial studies revealed that ultrasonography has a definite role in staging locally advanced prostate cancer prior to definitive therapy. In 1980, Resnick and colleagues[49] reported on

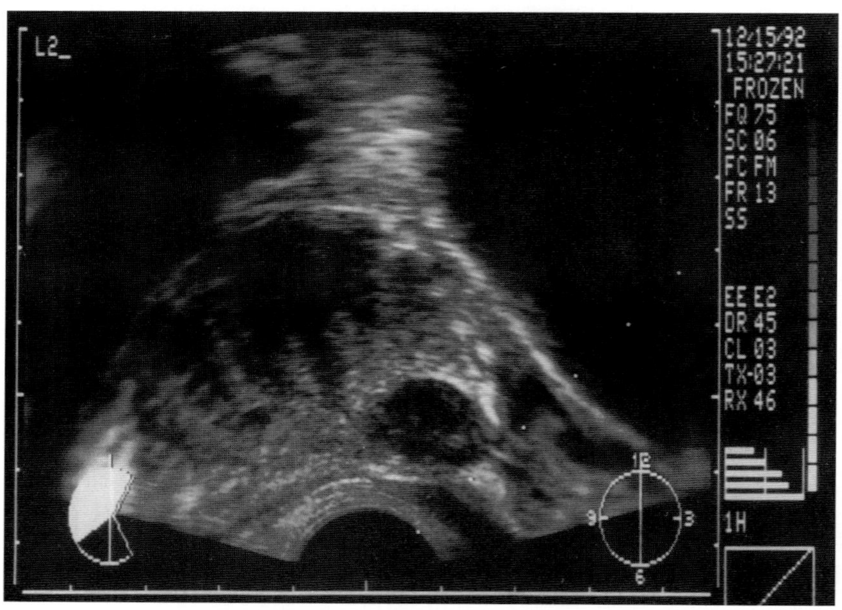

FIG. 48-1. Transverse transrectal ultrasonographic image of a prostate gland reveals a large, hypoechoic lesion located near the apex of the gland. The lesion was biopsy-confirmed cancer.

23 patients in whom the preoperative ultrasonographic staging coincided with the pathologic staging. Pontes and colleagues[50] reported on 31 patients with clinically localized prostate cancer who underwent preoperative TRUS and found an 89% sensitivity and 50% specificity for ultrasonographic prediction of capsular involvement and 100% sensitivity and 85% specificity for predicting seminal vesicle involvement. Errors occurred primarily because of the presence of microscopic invasive disease that was not detectable by ultrasonographic imaging. Fujino and Scardino[51] used ultrasonography to evaluate 50 patients with clinically localized prostate cancer. Ultrasonographic evaluation of 18 patients with previously untreated and clinically localized disease revealed that 8 (44%) actually had capsular involvement, which was confirmed by operative findings. Later studies were not as encouraging. Andriole and colleagues[52] evaluated 64 patients with clinically localized disease prior to radical prostatectomy; in this series, 43 of 48 patients (90%) with histologically localized disease were correctly staged by ultrasonography, whereas the remaining 5 patients were overstaged. Additionally, of 16 patients with locally advanced disease, 10 (62%) were understaged by preoperative ultrasonography, whereas 6 (38%) were correctly staged. The predictive value of a positive sonogram for extracapsular disease and seminal vesicle involvement in this study group was 55% and 100%, respectively. In a large, multicenter study, the accuracy of ultrasonography in staging prostate cancer was found to be 58% (126 of 219 patients), with a specificity of 46% ± 5% and a sensitivity of 68%.[53]

Ultrasonography is useful as an adjunctive means of evaluating a specific subgroup of patients with prostate cancer and may be useful in the assessment of seminal vesicle involvement. In a study of 73 patients undergoing radical prostatectomy, preoperative TRUS-guided biopsy was used to assess seminal vesicle involvement.[54] Terris and colleagues[54] reported that 20 (13.8%) of 145 preoperatively sampled seminal vesicles had pathologic evidence of tumor invasion. Overall, 21 seminal vesicles were thought to be suspicious for invasion based on the ultrasonographic images alone, whereas 124 were seminal vesicles were interpreted as benign. Pathologically, 13 (61.9%) of 21 suspicious seminal vesicles proved to have evidence of invasion, versus 7 (5.7%) of 124 in the benign group. The investigators concluded that preoperative TRUS-guided biopsy of the seminal vesicles may be useful in a select group of patients with carcinoma of the prostate.

One of the limitations of ultrasonography is the lack of sensitivity in differentiating between benign and malignant lesions within the gland with a high degree of certainty. Additionally, it is impossible to identify the extension of microscopic foci of tumor into the anatomic capsule or beyond. Although ultrasonography can be useful in staging patients with histologically proven carcinoma of the prostate, it is associated with considerable staging errors.

By combining DRE, TRUS, and serum PSA determinations, there are data to suggest that, based on tumor volume, it is possible to predict which tumors are surgically resectable, beyond cure, or have a low tendency to cause future morbidity, as discussed below.

PROSTATE-SPECIFIC ANTIGEN

PSA is a glycoprotein produced exclusively by prostatic epithelial cells, and it functions to hydrolyze the coagulum of the ejaculate.[55,56] This organ-specific protein was first discovered in seminal fluid by Hara and colleagues in 1971.[57] In 1979, Wang and colleagues[58] demonstrated the specificity of this protein for the prostate, as well as its differences from prostatic acid phosphatase. In 1980, Papsidero and colleagues[59] described the isolation of PSA from human serum and confirmed that the isolated form in the serum was identical to the antigen found in prostatic tissue. Subsequent studies of PSA led to the determination of accurate serum half-lives reported as 2.2 ± 0.8 days by Stamey and colleagues,[60] and 3.2 ± 0.1 days by Oesterling and colleagues.[61] Through further research, it was determined that as a result of the organ-specific properties of this protein, it had significant application in the monitoring of patients during and after therapy for prostate cancer. Subsequently, attempts to further define a possible role for PSA in the preoperative staging of patients with clinically localized adenocarcinoma of the prostate have been made. A more detailed account of PSA is contained in Chapter 41.

In 1987, Stamey and colleagues[60] illustrated that mean serum PSA levels consistently rise with increasing clinical disease stage. Abnormal PSA levels were reported in 122 (96%) of 127 patients studied, including 7 of 12 patients with stage A disease and all of the 115 patients with stage B through D disease. The strongest correlation of PSA level with tumor burden was demonstrated by plotting cancer volume versus serum PSA level in a log-log graph. Ercole and colleagues[62] studied 357 men with benign prostatic hypertrophy and 209 men with various stages of prostate cancer. These investigators designated a serum PSA level of 10 ng/mL or greater as evaluated by the Tandem assay as a substantial elevation, and their data indicate that of 74 men undergoing radical prostatectomy, when the serum PSA was substantially elevated, 59% (26 of 44 patients) had evidence of extracapsular disease, whereas 6.7% (2 of 30 patients) with organ-confined disease had similarly high preoperative serum PSA levels.

The shortcomings of PSA level as an accurate staging modality began to become apparent. Lange and colleagues[63] critically reported that the positive and negative predictive values (78% and 61%, respectively) for PSA to predict extracapsular disease were not sufficient to make this test useful as a sole means of noninvasively staging patients with carcinoma of the prostate. A study by Hudson and associates[64] demonstrated a significant overlap in serum PSA levels in men with various stages of disease. Of patients with clinical stage A or B disease, 62% (64 of 103 patients) had preoperative PSA values greater than 4 ng/mL versus 72% (31 of 43 patients) with clinical C or D lesions, and of 146 men evaluated in their series, 44% had PSA levels greater than 10 ng/mL, including 36% (37 of 103 patients) with clinical A or B disease. When compared with pathologic staging, these investigators found that preoperative PSA levels were inaccurate in predicting capsular penetration. There was a significant overlap of serum PSA levels among their study population regardless of clinical stage. These data indicate that serum PSA level alone is not a sensitive nor accurate indicator of clinical disease stage. There are no significant data to suggest that PSA level alone is a reliable indicator of extracapsular disease, particularly at serum levels close to the normal range, nor can serum PSA levels reliably predict that disease is confined to the gland.

It has been well established that elevated serum PSA levels can occur in the presence of benign or malignant prostatic tissue.

In the presence of cancer, Villers and associates[65] demonstrated that serum PSA levels increase at a rate proportional to the volume of intracapsular tumor; more specifically, at an average of 3.5 ng/mL per gram of intracapsular tumor, regardless of extracapsular spread. These researchers also examined serum PSA levels by polyclonal assay in relation to volume of disease, capsular penetration, and lymph node involvement.[65] In a study of 301 patients, the investigators were able to demonstrate that a serum PSA level lower than 10 ng/mL was associated with a 0% incidence of lymph node involvement, a less than 1% incidence of tumor volume greater than 12 mL, a 5% incidence of seminal vesicle involvement, and an 11% incidence of invasion into periprostatic fat. When compared to serum PSA level higher than 50 ng/mL, there was a 45% incidence of lymph node involvement, a 64% incidence of tumor volume greater than 12 mL, a 73% incidence of seminal vesicle invasion, and a 55% incidence of periprostatic fat invasion. Colberg and associates[66] reported that of 99 men with prostate cancer and a serum PSA level as determined by monoclonal assay greater than 10 ng/mL who underwent radical prostatectomy, the disease was organ confined in only 45% of the patients versus a 75% incidence of organ confinement in prostatectomy specimens of 145 patients with PSA levels ranging from 4.1 to 9.9 ng/mL.

These studies serve to illustrate that although predictions of extent of disease can be made with relative confidence when the PSA level is markedly elevated (i.e., 50 ng/mL or higher) there is considerable overlap of pathologic stage of disease at levels closer to the accepted values for normal. Furthermore, there is evidence to suggest that with increasing histologic grade, tumor cells may lose the ability to produce PSA; therefore, serum PSA levels in these patients may be lower than expected for their relative tumor burden.[67] Partin and colleagues[67] observed an inverse correlation between serum PSA levels and Gleason scores when adjusted for tumor volume and attributed this to decreased PSA production in areas of higher and more advanced tumor grade. This is in accordance with immunohistochemical studies of PSA production in relation to histologic tumor differentiation.[68,69] Overall, serum PSA determinations can suggest a relative state of tumor burden, but in and of itself it is neither specific nor predictive of extent of disease.

There are data to suggest that tumor volume is reliable predictor of extracapsular tumor growth. In a study of 176 radical prostatectomy specimens, capsular penetration was found in only 7% of tumors less than 4 mL in volume but in 86% of those tumors greater than 12 mL in volume.[17] Similarly, Villers and colleagues[65] reported seminal vesicle invasion in 6% of tumors less than 4 mL in volume versus 82% for lesions greater than 12 mL in volume. Stamey and McNeal[70] have demonstrated that cancer volumes of 4 mL or less are generally associated with a good prognosis, whereas tumors with volumes of 12 mL or greater are surgically incurable. Cancer volume is clearly a strong indicator of clinical stage and disease outcome, but unfortunately, there is no means by which the volume of tumor within the gland can be accurately assessed prior to initiation of therapy.

Gleason score also has been evaluated as a single predictor of disease progression. Epstein and colleagues[71] followed 185 individuals with clinical B disease for 5 years after radical prostatectomy and reported a significantly higher risk of disease progression in lesions with a Gleason score of 6.9 or higher versus tumors with a Gleason score of 5.8 or less. In this study, only 13% of tumors with a Gleason score lower than 7 showed evidence of disease progression, compared with 59% when the Gleason score was greater than 7.

The presence of bilateral disease in transrectal needle biopsy specimens of the prostate has also been shown to be a clinically significant prognostic indicator of relative disease status. In a study of 57 patients with clinical B1 lesions who underwent radical prostatectomy, Daniels and colleagues[72] reported that the presence of bilateral disease was associated with a 72% incidence of capsular penetration into periprostatic fat versus 28% for those with unilateral disease in preoperative needle biopsy specimens.

The measurement of serum PSA levels has a definite role, along with DRE and TRUS, in the evaluation of patients at risk for prostate cancer. Detection rates of prostatic carcinoma have increased dramatically with the combined use of these three modalities. PSA, like DRE and TRUS, has significant shortcomings; because of the lack of sensitivity of PSA as a reliable indicator of disease status and the inconsistency of stage of disease at lower serum PSA levels, the role of PSA in screening, staging, and early detection of prostate cancer remains debatable.[73,74] Reports have addressed staging probabilities based on PSA, Gleason score and the presence or absence of bilateral disease that can be applied to individuals with prostate cancer.[75,76] These data indicate that the best preoperative predictors of disease status for a given individual may be a combination of the Gleason score and the presence or absence of bilateral disease based on preoperative biopsy findings.

MAGNETIC RESONANCE IMAGING

In the 1980s, MR imaging became recognized as an accurate diagnostic modality for assessing urologic disorders.[77] Based on the inherent magnetic properties of different tissues, this imaging modality uses strong magnetic fields, radiowaves, and computers to generate anatomic images with significantly more contrast and detail than conventional radiography. Additionally, no ionizing radiation is involved in this type of imaging study; therefore, it is safer than conventional imaging techniques.

MR imaging is based on the magnetic properties of ions, which are naturally found in body tissues. All nuclei with an odd number of protons generate a small magnetic field with a particular vector that is randomly oriented in the absence of a strong magnetic field. The predominant ion manipulated in MR imaging is the hydrogen ion. When a strong magnetic field is applied, the nuclei of the hydrogen ions align themselves either parallel or antiparallel to the applied field. When the nuclei are in alignment, a radiofrequency coil or antenna applies a pulse of energy, thus generating a higher potential energy state for the nuclei. On termination of the applied pulse (i.e., during magnetic relaxation), the previously excited nuclei decay to their baseline energy levels and in doing so emit a radiofrequency that can be received by the coil. The signal is then interpreted by a computer and an image is produced. High-resolution imaging can be achieved with the use of local surface coils, which help to minimize associated background noise interference.[77,78] Tissue contrast in MR imaging depends on tissue proton density, T1, T2, and flow; T1 and T2 refer to the time constants describing the return of the excited ions to their baseline energy states after excitation by a radiofrequency pulse. The MR pulse can be manipulated to provide for maximal tissue contrast based on proton density, T1 and T2 times, and pulse duration.[77] With the use of body surface coils, the degree of contrast achievable is limited by the distance between the coil and the tissue to be imaged. With the development of endorectal surface coils, this distance has been dramatically reduced; consequently, imaging capabilities have improved significantly.[79]

The anatomy of the male pelvis as depicted by MR imaging using body surface coils has been described previously[80,81]; it was not until 1987 that a detailed report of the zonal anatomy of the normal prostate as depicted by MR imaging was available.[82] Hricak and colleagues[82] imaged 55 male subjects with the T2 technique, and anatomic differentiation of the peripheral, central, and transition zones and periprostatic tissue was demonstrated. The differentiation among the peripheral, central, and transition zones varied with patient age. In 31 of 32 men aged 25 to 35 years, the central zone was of low signal intensity and was well visualized, but in men older than 40 years of age, it could be visualized in only 8 of 23 patients. Transition and central zones proved to have similar imaging characteristics in older individuals and could be differentiated from each other only on the basis of their respective locations within the gland. This study illustrated both the potential application and limitations of body-surface MR imaging in the prostate.

A number of studies have been carried out in an attempt to differentiate between benign prostatic enlargement and carcinoma with body surface coils.[83–85] Studies have indicated that MR imaging cannot reliably differentiate benign from malignant processes confined to the gland nor stage carcinoma when present.[85,86] In a study of 28 patients with carcinoma of the prostate, Kahn and colleagues[85] reported that tumor was identified by MR imaging in 20 (70%) patients, and tumor volume was underestimated in 12 patients. Although the accuracy of MR imaging in predicting extraglandular tumor was 82%, the sensitivity was only 37.5%; furthermore, MR imaging identified only 10 of 19 patients with histologically proven benign hyperplasia. Similarly, in a report by Carter and colleagues,[87] the sensitivity of MR imaging in the detection of nonpalpable tumors within the prostate was only 58%, whereas the specificity was 48%; however, MR was 85% sensitive for anterior, nonpalpable lesions. In another series of 81 patients with a proven diagnosis of prostate cancer, body surface coil MR imaging failed to visualize the capsule in 17 of 37 (46%) patients.[88] Further attempts to evaluate with body surface coils patients who have carcinoma of the prostate have produced unreliable results.[89]

Quint and colleagues[89] attempted to determine tumor volume in 26 patients with prostate cancer. Only 20 of 31 lesions (65%) delineated on MR imaging corresponded to pathologically localized lesions. Additionally, tumor volume was underestimated in 11 of 20 patients and overestimated in 9 of 20. Furthermore, only 2 of 20 size estimates based on MR imaging were within 10% of the actual tumor volumes. Finally, body surface coil imaging was compared to TRUS and DRE in a large multicenter study involving 230 men with pathologically proven carcinoma. The accuracy of body coil MR imaging in staging the cancer was 69% versus 58% for TRUS, and the sensitivities were 77% for MR and 66% for TRUS.[53] The conclusion from these data is that MR imaging with a body surface coil does not provide accurate assessment of prostate cancer volume, nor can it differentiate carcinoma from benign hyperplasia. MR imaging is not recommended for staging patients with proven carcinoma, because the information obtained is not sufficiently reliable to affect clinical decision-making.

Body surface coil imaging of the prostate gland shows significantly more anatomic detail than does TRUS. Because of the variable tissue characteristics of carcinoma, MR imaging is not sufficiently sensitive to differentiate or diagnose carcinoma from benign hyperplasia. Overall, body surface coils did not provide enough resolution to accurately diagnose prostatic malignancies confined to the gland, and capsule visualization was at times poor. The advent of the endorectal surface coil provided for superior visualization of the anatomic capsule and periprostatic tissue, suggesting that endorectal MR imaging may have a significant role in the staging of localized disease.

The endorectal surface coils produced the anatomic detail necessary for the evaluation of patients with prostatic carcinoma. The images achieved with the T1-weighted technique using the endorectal surface coil depict the prostate as a homogeneous structure of medium signal intensity without zonal differentiation. T2-weighted images provide an accurate depiction of zonal glandular anatomy with a higher degree of tissue contrast compared with the surface coil technique. The peripheral zone appears as an area of high signal intensity, as do the seminal vesicles. The periprostatic venous plexus has a signal of lower intensity. The capsule has a signal intensity that is lower than that of the rest of the gland, and it is sharply delineated in the normal prostate.[90]

Endorectal surface coils can provide high-resolution images of the prostate[79,91] and have been used in attempts to stage prostate cancer. In a study of 22 patients with prostate cancer, MR imaging with an endorectal surface coil revealed an 82% accuracy rate in differentiating between stage B and stage C disease.[92] Only one tumor was overstaged and three were understaged, two of which had microscopic invasion of the capsule, seminal vesicle, or both. This study yielded an overall 16% increase in staging accuracy over that achievable with body-surface coil imaging. The sensitivity for detection of capsular invasion was 67%, a substantial improvement over the 44% sensitivity with body-surface coil images.[88]

MR imaging has been applied to the detection of pelvic lymph node metastases in patients with prostate cancer. The identification of suspicious lymph nodes is based primarily on the size of the particular node in question, with nodes larger than 1 cm considered to be enlarged.[93] MR imaging alone cannot differentiate between an inflammatory node and a pathologic node based solely on image characteristics; therefore, MR imaging lacks the necessary specificity to justify its use in the detection of pelvic lymph node metastases in patients with prostatic carcinoma.

Although the majority of MR studies conducted on the prostate have been carried out with body-surface coils, there is a potential role for MR with endorectal surface coils in the staging of patients with previously diagnosed carcinoma of the prostate. Some centers are using this technology to confirm bony metastases on a routine basis. MR imaging is not sufficiently sensitive or specific to be used as a routine diagnostic test; its cost also precludes this application. Additionally, there are insufficient data indicating the improved accuracy of MR imaging over TRUS in the staging of locally advanced prostate cancer. Additional studies using endorectal surface coils may provide the necessary information that will better define the role of MR imaging in the patient with prostate cancer.

COMPUTED TOMOGRAPHY

Computed tomography (CT) is a popular modality useful for imaging many different parts of the anatomy. The images generated by CT are the result of computer-assisted image generation techniques based on relative tissue density as measured by the attenuation of a radiation field applied to a limited area of the body by a circular scanner array. The density of tissues on CT scans are assigned Hounsfield units: water has a value of zero, air and fat have negative values, and dense body tissue has a positive value.

CT scanning has been applied to the assessment of genitourinary disorders and is particularly helpful in imaging the kidneys, adrenal glands, and urinary bladder. Additionally, accurate determination of prostatic volume is easily achieved with CT.[94,95] Before technological advances in ultrasonography, CT scanning seemed to have relative merit in the evaluation of patients with prostatic cancer. However, CT imaging lacks the sensitivity necessary to discern the internal architecture of the prostate gland,[94] and because of the relative homogeneity of prostatic tissue as well as the variable characteristics of carcinoma, CT scanning cannot differentiate between carcinoma and benign hyperplasia. Furthermore, the results of CT imaging in evaluating involvement of the anatomic capsule of the prostate or the seminal vesicles has been disappointing.[96,97]

CT imaging in the patient with carcinoma of the prostate has therefore been directed at improving the accuracy of preoperative noninvasive staging techniques. The usefulness of CT scanning in detection of extraprostatic disease has been evaluated in several studies.[98–101] The addition of CT scanning to more conventional techniques of assessing extracapsular disease (e.g., DRE) resulted in a sporadic improvement in accuracy of diagnosis ranging from 15% to 59%.[102,103] Comparing CT and TRUS, Salo and colleagues[103] demonstrated that ultrasonography is more accurate in detecting extracapsular invasion, with a sensitivity of approximately 86%, a specificity of 94%, and an accuracy of 90%, versus a sensitivity of 25% for CT scanning in the detection of capsular perforation. In the presence of palpably bulky disease, CT has sufficient resolution to demonstrate extracapsular disease and has been employed by some clinicians to differentiate between stage B2 and C disease.

Hricak and colleagues[104] studied 46 patients with palpable disease. The accuracy of clinical examination in this study was 61% and 39% of the patients were understaged, whereas CT provided 65% accuracy and 19% understaging. As in other studies, the inaccuracy of CT scanning was the result of its inability to delineate bladder base and seminal vesicle involvement. Furthermore, as with MR imaging, CT cannot differentiate a suspicious lymph node (>1 cm) from an abnormal lymph node (>1.5 cm) in regard to a benign inflammatory condition or a pathologic condition. The accuracy of CT scanning in the detection of lymph node involvement has therefore been low.[105]

Considering the cost, sensitivity, and specificity of CT scanning, there is little role for its routine use in assessing the patient with carcinoma of the prostate. CT lacks the resolution necessary to detect capsular penetration and seminal vesicle involvement to make it an effective adjunct in staging locally advanced disease. Even in conjunction with DRE and serum PSA determinations, CT scanning is suboptimal; TRUS provides better imaging at a considerably lower cost, avoids radiation exposure, and has a higher accuracy in the evaluation of this select group of patients. However, CT may have a role in the assessment of patients with a high likelihood of nodal involvement (e.g., stage C disease, Gleason score >7).

BONE SCINTIGRAPHY

In the patient with prostatic carcinoma, the skeleton is the most common site of metastases in those with advanced disease.[106] Plain radiographs of the skeletal system are not sufficiently sensitive to detect early tumor involvement of bone. To be detected by plain radiographs, a change in bony density of approximately 50% is usually needed.[107] The bony lesions that are detected are most often osteoblastic, but osteoclastic lesions may be present as well. A negative plain-film skeletal survey does not necessarily mean that a patient is free of bony involvement. As reported by Paulson in 1979,[108] 23% of patients found to have negative skeletal plain-film surveys have evidence of bony involvement on scintigraphy. Additionally, 16% of patients clinically staged as having stage A, B, or C disease are upstaged to stage D disease after radionuclide bone scan.[108] Bone scintigraphy is currently the most sensitive means of determining bony involvement by metastatic prostate cancer, but false-negative results can occur and have a reported incidence of approximately 8%.[109]

Radioisotopes used in bone scintigraphy are gradually taken up by metabolically active bone after intravenous injection. The exact mechanism of uptake has not been fully elucidated. The kidneys excrete any unadsorbed radionuclide. Technetium-99m phosphates and phosphonates are commonly used agents; both of these agents also provide some assessment of renal function during the bone scan.[110]

The relative indications for bone scintigraphy are symptoms of bone pain, elevated serum alkaline phosphatase levels in the absence of known hepatic disease, and markedly elevated serum PSA levels. In an early report of the results of bone scan findings in patients with adenocarcinoma of the prostate, as many as 43% of those with abnormal bone scans were asymptomatic (i.e., free of pain); furthermore, 23% had a normal serum alkaline phosphatase level, and prostatic acid phosphatase was normal in almost 40%.[111]

Serum PSA determinations have been used in an effort to better select those patients most likely to be at risk for bony involvement. The first large series correlating serum PSA levels and the incidence of a positive bone scan in newly diagnosed prostate cancer patients was reported by Chybowski and colleagues in 1991.[112] These investigators reported a negative predictive value of 99.7% for bone scans performed on 521 randomly selected and previously untreated patients who had serum PSA levels of less than 20 ng/mL as ascertained by Tandem assay. Clearly, these data suggest that a staging radionuclide bone scan is not warranted in patients who have a serum PSA level less than 20 ng/mL and are free of bone pain. The PSA criteria for bone scans was again substantiated in a report by Oesterling and colleagues[113] in which only 3 of 561 previously untreated prostate cancer patients with a serum PSA of

10 μg/mL or lower as determined by Tandem assay who underwent bone scintigraphy had a positive result. Furthermore, 0 of 467 men whose PSA level was 8 μg/mL or lower had a positive bone scan result. The associated false-negative results for a positive bone scan in patients with a serum PSA level of 8 μg/mL or lower was 0%, whereas that for patients with a serum PSA level of 10 μg/mL was 0.5%.[113]

Although bone scintigraphy is the most sensitive means by which bony involvement with prostate cancer can be detected, data suggest that it should be reserved for those individuals with symptoms of bone pain, serum PSA levels greater than 10 ng/mL, or both prior to intervention.

RADIOIMMUNOIMAGING

Radioimmunoimaging originated in the 1950s when Pressman and Korngold successfully isolated an antibody to a mouse murine tumor.[114,115] They were then able to iodinate the antibody, inject it into another mouse carrying the appropriate antigen, and subsequently demonstrate antigen targeting. Over the past 40 years, the field of immunology has virtually exploded with new developments; today, monoclonal antibodies as well as radioimmunoconjugates are employed in the diagnosis of colorectal, ovarian, breast, lung, and prostatic carcinoma.[116–121]

Site-specific immunoconjugates such as CYT-356 have been studied in prostate cancer. Lopes and colleagues[121] looked at in vivo imaging of human prostate cancer xenografts implanted into nude mice. CYT-356 labeled with indium-111 injected into the nude mice rapidly localized to and adequately imaged the human prostate adenocarcinoma xenografts. The localization to the xenografts was antigen specific, and no immunoconjugate localization to normal tissues was detected; thus, the labeled immunoconjugate accurately and specifically delineated the presence of human prostate cancer cells in the mice.

Human trials with the same immunoconjugate were carried out in 1991 by Wynant and colleagues.[122] In this study, 40 patients with known distant metastases received a single intravenous injection of the radiolabeled immunoconjugate. Bony metastases were detected in 21 of 38 patients (55%), including 12 of 14 patients (86%) receiving concomitant hormonal therapy. Furthermore, antibody imaging detected occult lesions in the bony pelvis and lumbar spine that were confirmed with follow-up imaging tests. No adverse effects from the test agent were reported. Additional studies have been conducted and demonstrate that even in the presence of hormone-refractory prostate cancer, intense staining patterns are present.[123]

The results of these studies suggest that there is potential for specific and sensitive prostate cancer imaging using site-specific immunoconjugates in a relatively noninvasive manner that poses little risk to the individual being studied. This type of imaging may have a role in the future detection, diagnosis, and staging of occult prostate cancer and certainly warrants further investigation.

CONCLUSIONS

As medical care continues to advance and the population ages, the incidence of adenocarcinoma of the prostate is expected to continue to rise. Early diagnostic and therapeutic modalities will continue to evolve in an effort to impact on the natural history of this disease process. TRUS will probably continue to have an important role in the diagnosis of prostate cancer, particularly when used in association with biopsy.

Future developments in radioimmunoscintigraphy will likely change the diagnostic approaches to prostate cancer. This technique seems to be both sensitive and specific and is associated with little morbidity. Radioimmunoimaging and immunotherapy are in an evolutionary stage; however, the prospects of gene manipulation and immunoimaging are encouraging and may alter the therapeutic approach to the patient with prostate cancer.

PELVIC LYMPHADENECTOMY

Pelvic lymphadenectomy for prostate cancer is primarily a staging procedure rather than a therapeutic one. In most cases, it is the last staging test performed prior to definitive therapy and is the best method for determining the status of the pelvic lymph nodes. Many experts believe that prostatectomy or radiotherapy are not warranted as definitive treatment if the lymph nodes are involved with cancer. The rationale and indications for the use of pelvic lymphadenectomy are described in detail elsewhere in the text.

The operation, conducted either laparoscopically or by open surgery, is performed before definitive treatment, but the exact timing of the surgery depends on the therapy planned and, to some extent, on physician preference. If a radical prostatectomy by the retropubic approach is contemplated, the lymphadenectomy is performed through the same incision and the prostatectomy done while the patient is under the same anesthesia if the lymph nodes are determined to be uninvolved grossly or by frozen section examination. If a radical perineal prostatectomy is planned, the lymphadenectomy requires a separate suprapubic procedure and can be performed during the same anesthesia or at a later time. The latter approach is preferred by some surgeons because there is a false-negative rate associated with frozen section versus permanent pathologic examination.

There has always been controversy regarding whether pelvic lymphadenectomy should be done, especially if the intended treatment is radiotherapy or perineal prostatectomy. With radiotherapy, lymphadenectomy delays therapy and increases complications somewhat. With perineal prostatectomy, a separate suprapubic procedure is required. As detailed elsewhere in the text, in the PSA era, the number of patients with lymph node involvement has decreased dramatically and the ability to preoperatively predict the probability of positive lymph nodes has increased. This capacity in turn has altered the decision-making process regarding whether and how radiotherapy or surgery will be done.

Technique

Pelvic lymphadenectomy involves the removal of the obturator and hypogastric lymph nodes; the lymphatics overlying the external iliac artery are usually preserved (Fig. 48-2). In the open pelvic lymphadenectomy, an infraumbilical midline incision extending to the pubis is made, the fascia of the anterior abdominal wall is incised, and the rectus abdominis is separated. The transversalis fascia is incised, and the space of Retzius is

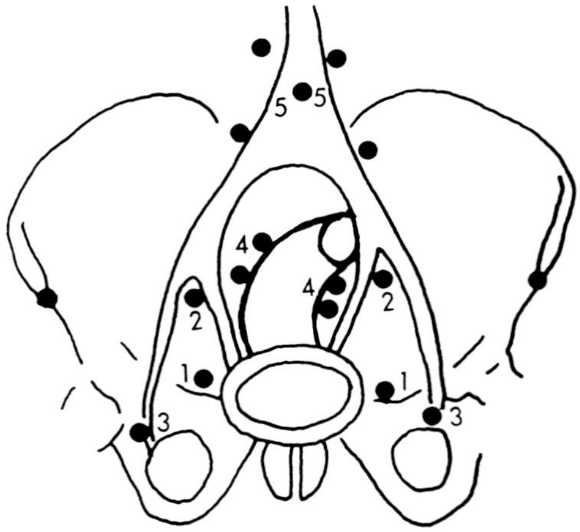

FIG. 48-2. The major lymphatics of the pelvis. Numbers 1 to 3 mark the limits of the lymph node dissection in prostate cancer: 1, obturator nodes; 2, hypogastric nodes; 3, node of Cloquet; 4, presacral; 5, common iliac/preaortic. (From Beahrs OH, Henson DE, Hutter RVP, Myers MH, eds, for the American Joint Committee on Cancer. Manual for staging of cancer. 3rd ed. Philadelphia: JB Lippincott, 1988:182.)

developed bluntly. Laterally, the peritoneum is mobilized from the external iliac vessels, thus exposing the deep circumflex iliac vessels caudally and the bifurcation of the common iliac vessels cranially.

The adventitia overlying the anterior aspect of the external iliac vein on the side ipsilateral to the pathologic finding in the prostate is incised, and the dissection is carried distally along the vein to the level of the femoral canal, at which point the node of Cloquet is removed. The obturator lymph nodes are dissected from the level of the obturator hiatus to the origin of the obturator artery. All lymphatic tissue is removed to the level of the bifurcation of the common iliac artery, at which point the lymphatics feeding to the lymph nodes in the angle of the internal and external iliac vessels are ligated and divided, allowing removal of the packet. The procedure is performed bilaterally.

A laparoscopic lymph node dissection is less invasive and permits sampling of tissue from similar locations. Through a stab incision just below the umbilicus, a Veress needle is introduced into the peritoneal cavity, and CO_2 insufflation is commenced to achieve a pneumoperitoneum. The Veres needle is removed, and the stab incision is enlarged to admit a 10-mm trocar through which peritoneoscopy is performed. Under direct visualization, 5-mm trocars are placed in the left and right lower abdomen and an 11-mm trocar is placed 3 cm above the pubic symphysis.

The left and right median umbilical ligaments are identified, as are the deep inguinal rings and the pulsation of the external iliac arteries. Through a transverse peritoneotomy, the iliac vessels are bluntly dissected, and the medial wall of the external iliac vein is carefully reflected laterally, thus exposing the obturator fossae. The dissection extends from the level of the deep circumflex iliac vessels and pubic bone to the juncture of the obliterated umbilical vessel with the hypogastric artery. The obturator nerve is identified, and all lymphatic tissue within the obturator fossae is removed.

The limits of the dissection are the obturator nerve inferiorly,

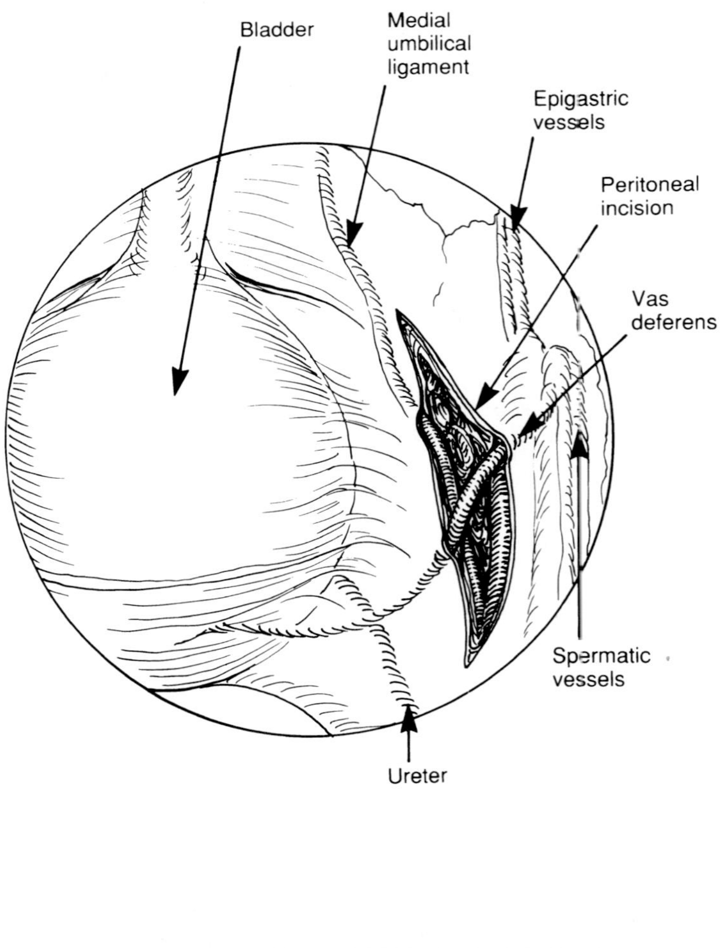

FIG. 48-3. Regional anatomy of the pelvic fossa and the important landmarks in laparoscopic lymph node dissection. (From Winfield HN. Urologic laparoscopic surgery. Atlas Urol Clin North Am 1993;1:33.)

the pelvic bone anteriorly, the external iliac vein laterally, the obliterated umbilical ligament medially, the origin of the hypogastric artery cranially, and the obturator foramen caudally (Fig. 48-3). Identical maneuvers are repeated on the opposite side. This technique results in an adequate lymphadenectomy that has proven to be an accurate means of surgically staging the patient who is at risk for metastatic prostate cancer.

REFERENCES

1. Boring CC, Squires TS, Tong T. Cancer statistics, 1993. CA Cancer J Clin 1993;43:7.
2. Parker SL, Tong T, Bolden S, Wingo PA. Cancer Statistics 1996. CA Cancer J Clin 1996;65:5.
3. Carter HB, Coffey DS. The prostate: an increasing medical problem. Prostate, 1990;16:39.
4. Frankes LM. Latent carcinoma of the prostate. J Pathol Biol 1954; 68:603.
5. Lowsley OS. The development of the human prostate gland with reference to the development of other structures at the neck of the urinary bladder. Am J Anat 1912;13:299.
6. McNeal JE. The prostate and prostatic urethra: a morphological synthesis. J Urol 1972;107:1008.
7. McNeal JE. Origin and evolution of benign prostatic enlargement. Invest Urol 1978;15:340.
8. McNeal JE. Normal histology of the prostate. Am J Surg Pathol 1988; 12:619.
9. McNeal JE. The prostate gland: morphology and pathobiology. Monographs Urol 1983;4:1.
10. McNeal JE. Regional morphology and pathology of the prostate. Am J Clin Pathol 1968;49:347.
11. Whitmore WF Jr. Hormone therapy in prostatic cancer. Am J Med 1956;21:697.
12. Jewitt HJ. The present status of radical prostatectomy for stages A and B prostatic cancer. Urol Clin North Am 1975;2:105.
13. Wallace DM, Chisholm GD, Hendry WF. TNM classification system for urologic tumors (UICC), 1974. Br J Urol 1975;47:1.
14. Whitmore WF Jr, Catalona WJ, Grayhack JT, et al. Organ systems program staging classification for prostate cancer. In: Coffey DS, Resnick MI, Dorr FA, Karr JP, eds. A multidisciplinary analysis of controversies in the management of prostate cancer. New York: Plenum Press, 1988:295.
15. Cantrell BB, DeKlerk DP, Eggleston JC, Boitnott JK, Walsh PC. Pathologic factors that influence prognosis in stage A prostatic cancer: the influence of extent versus grade. J Urol 1981;125:516.
16. McNeal JE, Bostwick DG, Klindrachuk RA, Redwine EA, Freiha FS, Stamey TA. Patterns of progression in prostate cancer. Lancet 1986; 1:60.
17. McNeal JE, Villers AA, Redwine EA, Freiha FS, Stamey TA. Capsular penetration in prostate cancer: significance for natural history and treatment. Am J Surg Pathol 1990;14:240.
18. Epstein JI, Paul G, Eggleston JC, Walsh PC. Prognosis of untreated stage A1 prostatic carcinoma: a study of 94 cases with extended follow-up. J Urol 1986;136:837.
19. Schroder FH, Hermanek P, Denis L, Fair WR, Gospodarowicz MK, Pavone-Macaluso M. The TNM classification of prostate cancer. Prostate Suppl 1992;4:129.
20. Beahrs OH, Henson DR, Hutter RVP, Kennedy BJ. Manual for staging of cancer. 4th ed. Philadelphia: JB Lippincott, 1992:181.
21. Zagars GK, Geara FB, Pollack A, von Eschenbach AC. The T classification of clinically localized prostate cancer. Cancer 1994;73:1904.
22. Chodak GW, Keller P, Schoenberg HW. Assessment of screening for prostate cancer using digital rectal examination. J Urol 1989;141: 1136.
23. Scardino PT. Early detection of prostate cancer. Urol Clin North Am 1989;16:635.
24. The Veterans Administration Co-Operative Urologic Research Group. Treatment and survival of patients with cancer of the prostate. Surg Gynecol Obstet 1967;124:1011.
25. Wantanabe H, Igari D, Tanahashi Y, Harada K, Saitoh M. Transrectal ultrasonography of the prostate. J Urol 1975;114:734.
26. Dussik KT. Uber die Moglichkeit hochfrequente mechanische Schwingungen als diagnostisches Hilfsmittel zu verwenden. Z Ges Neurol Psych 1942;174:153.
27. Martin JF. History of ultrasound. In: Resnick MI, Saunders RC, eds. Ultrasound in urology. Baltimore: William & Wilkins, 1984:1.
28. Wild JJ, Neal D. Use of high frequency ultrasonic waves for detecting changes of texture in living tissues. Lancet 1951;260:655.
29. Wild JJ, Reid JM. Application of echo-ranging techniques to the determination of structure of biological tissues. Science 1952;115:226.
30. Takahashi H, Ouchi T. The ultrasonic diagnosis in the field of biology. In: Japanese medicine and ultrasonics: the first report. 1963:7.
31. Wantanabe H, Katoh H. Diagnostic application of the ultrasonography for the prostate. J Urol 1968;59:279.
32. Wantanabe H, Kato H, Tanaka, Kato T, Terasawa Y. Diagnostic application of ultrasonotomography to the prostate. Japn J Urol 1968;59: 273.
33. Boyce WH, McKinney WM, Resnick MI, Willard J. Ultrasonography as an aid in the diagnosis and management of surgical diseases of the pelvis: special emphasis on the genitourinary system. Ann Surg 1976; 184:477.
34. Henneberry M, Carter MF, Neiman HL. Estimation of prostatic size by suprapubic ultrasonography. J Urol 1979;121:615.
35. Holm HH, Northeved A. A transurethral ultrasonic scanner. J Urol 1974;111:238.
36. Peeling WB, Griffiths GJ. Imaging of the prostate by ultrasound. J Urol 1984;132:217.
37. Cooner WH. Anatomy of the prostate as seen by ultrasound. AUA Update Series 1990;9:42.
38. Lee F. Transrectal ultrasound: diagnosis and staging of prostatic carcinoma. Urology Suppl 1989;33:5.
39. Denis JL, Braeckman J. Normal sonographic anatomy of the prostate. In: Resnick MI, ed. Prostatic ultrasonography. Philadelphia: BC Decker, 1990:41.
40. Kaye KW. Ultrasonographic anatomy of normal prostate gland: reconstruction by computer graphics. Urology 1990;35:12.
41. Peeling WB, Griffiths GJ, Evans KT, Roberts EE. Diagnosis and staging of prostate cancer by transrectal ultrasonography: a preliminary study. Br J Urol 1979;51:565.
42. Rifkin MD, Kurtz AB, Choi HY, Goldberg BB. Endoscopic ultrasonic evaluation of the prostate using a transrectal probe: prospective evaluation and acoustic characterization. Radiology 1983;149:265.
43. Resnick MI, Willard JW, Boyce WH. Ultrasonic evaluation of the prostatic nodule. J Urol 1978;120:86.
44. Abu-Yousef MM, Narayana AS. Prostatic carcinoma: detection and staging using suprapubic US. Radiology 1985;156:175.
45. Lee F, Gray JM, McLeary RD, et al. Transrectal ultrasound in the diagnosis of prostate cancer: location, echogenicity, histopathology and staging. Prostate 1985;7:117.
46. Rifkin MD, Frieland GW, Shortliffe L. Prostatic evaluation by transrectal endosonography: detection of carcinoma. Radiology 1986; 158:85.
47. Dahnert W, Hamper UM, Eggleston JC, Walsh PC, Sanders RC. Prostatic evaluation by transrectal sonography with histopathologic correlation: the echopenic appearance of early carcinoma. Radiology 1986; 158:97.
48. Shinohara K, Wheeler TM, Scardino PT. The appearance of prostate cancer on transrectal ultrasonography: correlation of imaging and pathological examinations. J Urol 1989;142:76.
49. Resnick MI, Willard JW, Boyce WH. Transrectal ultrasonography in the evaluation of the patient with prostatic carcinoma. J Urol 1980; 124:482.
50. Pontes JE, Eisenkraft S, Wantanabe H, Ohe H, Murphy GP. Preoperative evaluation of localized prostatic carcinoma by transrectal ultrasonography. J Urol 1985;134:289.
51. Fujino A, Scardino PT. Transrectal ultrasonography for prostatic cancer: its value in staging and monitoring the response to radiotherapy and chemotherapy. J Urol 1984;133:806.
52. Andriole GL, Coplen DE, Mikkelsen DJ, Catalona WJ. Sonographic and pathologic staging of patients with clinically localized prostate cancer. J Urol 1989;142:1259.
53. Rifkin M, Zerhouni E, Gatsonis C, et al. Comparison of magnetic resonance imaging and ultrasonography in staging early prostate cancer. N Engl J Med 1989;323:621.
54. Terris MK, McNeal JE, Freiha FS, Stamey TA. Efficacy of transrectal

ultrasound-guided seminal vesicle biopsies in the detection of seminal vesicle invasion by prostate cancer. J Urol 1993;149:1035.
55. Lee C, Keefer M, Zhao ZW, et al. Demonstration of the role of prostate-specific antigen in semen liquefaction by two-dimensional electrophoresis. J Androl 1989;10:432.
56. Lilja H, Lourell CB. The predominant protein in human seminal coagulate. Scand J Clin Lab Invest 1985;45:635.
57. Hara M, Inorre T, Fukuyama T. Some physio-chemical characteristics of gamma-seminoprotein, an antigenic compound specific for human seminal plasma. Japn J Legal Med 1971;25:322.
58. Wang MC, Valenzuela LA, Murphy GP, Chu TM. Purification of a human prostate specific antigen. Invest Urol 1979;17:159.
59. Papsidero LD, Wang MC, Valenzuela LA, Murphy GP, Chu TM. A prostate antigen in sera of prostatic cancer patients. Cancer Res 1980; 40:2428.
60. Stamey TA, Yang N, Hay AR, McNeal JE, Freiha FS, Redwine E. Prostate-specific antigen as a serum marker for adenocarcinoma of the prostate. N Engl J Med 1987;317:909.
61. Oesterling JE, Chan DW, Epstein JI, et al. Prostate specific antigen in the preoperative and postoperative evaluation of localized prostate cancer treated with radical prostatectomy. J Urol 1988;139:766.
62. Ercole CJ, Lange PH, Mathisen M, Chiou RK, Reddy PK, Vesella RP. Prostate specific antigen and prostatic acid phosphatase in the monitoring and staging of patients with prostate cancer. J Urol 1987; 138:1181.
63. Lange PH, Ercole CJ, Lightner DJ, Fraley EE, Vessella R. The value of serum prostate specific antigen determinations before and after radical prostatectomy. J Urol 1989;141:873.
64. Hudson A, Bahnson RR, Catalona WJ. Clinical use of prostate specific antigen in patients with prostate cancer. J Urol 1989;142:1011.
65. Villers AA, McNeal JE, Redwine EA, Freiha FS, Stamey TA. Pathogenesis and biological significance of seminal vesicle invasion in prostatic adenocarcinoma. J Urol 1990;143:1183.
66. Colberg JW, Smith DS, Catalona WJ. Prevalence and pathological extent of prostate cancer in men with prostate specific antigen levels of 2.9 to 4.0 ng/ml. J Urol 1993;149:507.
67. Partin AW, Carter HB, Chan DW, et al. Prostate specific antigen in the staging of localized prostate cancer: influence of tumor differentiation, tumor volume and benign hyperplasia. J Urol 1990;143:747.
68. Svanholm H. Evaluation of commercial immunoperoxidase kits for prostatic specific antigen and prostatic acid phosphatase. Acta Pathol Microbiol Immunol Scand A 1986;94:7.
69. Ellis DW, Leffers S, Davies JS, Ng ABP. Multiple immunoperoxidase markers in benign hyperplasia and adenocarcinoma of the prostate. Am J Clin Pathol 1984;81:279.
70. Stamey TA, McNeal JE. Adenocarcinoma of the prostate. In: Walsh PC, Retik AB, Stamey TA, Vaughan ED Jr, eds. Campbell's urology, 6th ed. Philadelphia: WB Saunders, 1992:1159.
71. Epstein JI, Carmichael M, Partin AW, Walsh PC. Is tumor volume an independent predictor of progression following radical prostatectomy? A multivariate analysis of 185 clinical stage B adenocarcinomas of the prostate with 5 years of followup. J Urol 1993;149:1478.
72. Daniels GF, McNeal JE, Stamey TA. Predictive value of contralateral biopsies in unilaterally palpable prostate cancer. J Urol 1992;147:870.
73. Catalona WJ, Ratliff TL, Yuan JJ. Serum prostate specific antigen as a first-line screening test for prostate cancer. [Abstract 499] J Urol 1990;143:313A.
74. Cooner WH, Mosley BR, Rutherford CL Jr, et al. Prostate cancer detection in a clinical urological practice by ultrasonography, digital rectal examination and prostate specific antigen. J Urol 1990;143: 1146.
75. Partin AW, Yoo J, Carter JB, et al. The use of prostate specific antigen, clinical staging and Gleason score to predict pathological stage in men with localized prostate cancer. J Urol 1993;150:110.
76. Epstein JI, Walsh PC, Carmichael M, Brendler CB. Pathological and clinical findings to predict tumor extent of non-palpable (stage T1C) prostate cancer. JAMA 1994;271:368.
77. Kressel H. Magnetic resonance imaging. In: Pollack HM, ed. Clinical urography. Philadelphia: WB Saunders, 1990:433.
78. Martin JF, Hajek P, Baker L. Inflatable surface coil for MR imaging of the prostate. Radiology 1988;167:268.
79. Schnall MD, Lenkinski RE, Pollack HM, Imai Y, Kressel HY. Prostate: MR imaging with an endorectal surface coil. Radiology 1989; 172:570.
80. Hricak H, Williams RD, Spring DB. Anatomy and pathology of the male pelvis by magnetic resonance imaging. AJR 1983;141:1101.
81. Buonocore E, Hesemann C, Pavlicek W. Clinical and in vitro magnetic resonance imaging of prostatic carcinoma. AJR 1984;143:1267.
82. Hricak H, Dooms DC, McNeal JE, et al. MR imaging of the prostate gland: normal anatomy. AJR 1987;148:51.
83. Ling D, Lee JKT, Heiken JP, Balfe DM, Glazer HS, McClennan BL. Prostatic carcinoma and benign prostatic hyperplasia: inability of MR imaging to distinguish between the two diseases. Radiology 1986; 158:103.
84. Carrol CL, Sommer FG, McNeal JE, Stamey TA. The abnormal prostate: MR imaging at 1.5 T with histopathologic correlation. Radiology 1987;165:521.
85. Kahn T, Burrig K, Schmitz-Drager B, Lewis JS, Furst G, Modder U. Prostatic carcinoma and benign prostatic hyperplasia: MR imaging with histopathologic correlation. Radiology 1989;173:847.
86. Bryan JP, Butler HE, Nelson AD, et al. Magnetic resonance imaging of the prostate. AJR 1986;146:543.
87. Carter HB, Bren RF, Tempany CM, et al. Nonpalpable prostate cancer: detection with MR imaging. Radiology 1991;178:523.
88. Bezzi M, Kressel HY, Allen KS, et al. Prostatic carcinoma: staging with MR imaging at 1.5 T1. Radiology 1988;169:339.
89. Quint LE, Van Erp JS, Bland PH, et al. Carcinoma of the prostate: MR images obtained with body coils do not accurately reflect tumor volume. AJR 1991;156:511.
90. Newhouse JH. Clinical use of urinary tract magnetic resonance imaging. Radiol Clin North Am 1991;29:455.
91. Schnall MD, Lenkinski RE, Pollack HM, Imai Y, Kressel HY. MR imaging with an endorectal surface coil. Radiol 1989;172(2):570.
92. Schnall MD, Imai Y, Tomaszewski J, Pollack HM, Lenkinski RE, Kressel HY. Prostate cancer: local staging with endorectal surface coil MR imaging. Radiology 1991;178:797.
93. Hricak H, Thoeni RF. Neoplasms of the prostate gland. In: Pollack HM, ed. Clinical urography, vol 2. Philadelphia: WB Saunders, 1990: 1381.
94. Van Engleshoven JMA, Kreel L. Computed tomography of the prostate. J Comput Assist Tomogr 1979;3:45.
95. Ohlsen H, Ekman P, Ringertz H. Assessment of prostatic size with computed tomography. Acta Radiol (Diagn) 1982;23:219.
96. Resnick MI. Noninvasive techniques in evaluating patients with carcinoma of the prostate. Urology 1981;17(Suppl 3):25.
97. Denis L, Appel L, Broos J, Declerq G. Evaluation of prostatic cancer by transrectal ultrasonography and CT scan. Acta Urol Belg 1980; 48:71.
98. Peterson RW. Computed tomographic evaluation of malignancies of the bladder and prostate. Comput Tomogr 1977;1:283.
99. Brizel HE, Livingston PAL, Grayson EV. Radiotherapeutic applications of pelvic computed tomography. J Comput Assist Tomogr 1979; 3:453.
100. Price JM, Davidson AJ. Computed tomography in the evaluation of the suspected carcinomatous prostate. Urol Radiol 1979;1:39.
101. Giri PGS, Walsh JW, Hazra TA, Texter JH, Koontz WW. Role of computed tomography in the evaluation and management of carcinoma of the prostate. J Radiol Oncol Biol Phys 1982;8:283.
102. Emory TH, Reinke DB, Hill AL, Lange PH. Use of CT to reduce understaging in prostatic cancer. AJR 1983;141:351.
103. Salo JO, Kivisaari L, Rannikko S, Lehtonen T. Computerized tomography and transrectal ultrasound in the assessment of local extension of prostatic cancer before radical prostatectomy. J Urol 1987;137: 435.
104. Hricak H, Dooms GC, Jeffrey RB, et al. Prostatic carcinoma: staging by clinical assessment, CT, and MR imaging. Radiology 1987;162: 331.
105. Sawczuk IS, deVere, White R, Gold RP, Olson CA. Sensitivity of computed tomography in evaluation of pelvic lymph node metastases from carcinoma of bladder and prostate. Urology 1983;21:81.
106. Whitmore WJ Jr. Natural history and staging of prostatic carcinoma. Urol Clin North Am 1984;11:209.
107. Lentle BC, McGowan DG, Dierich H. Technetium-99m polyphosphate bone scanning in carcinoma of the prostate. Br J Urol 1974;46: 543.
108. Paulson DF. The impact of current staging procedures in assessing disease extent of prostatic adenocarcinoma. J Urol 1979;121:300.
109. Ball JD, Maynard CD. Nuclear imaging in urology. Urol Clin North Am 1979;6:321.

110. Fine EJ, Blaufox MD. Urologic applications of radionuclides. In: Pollack HM, ed. Clinical urography, vol 2. Philadelphia: WB Saunders, 1990:518.
111. Schaffer DL, Pendegrass HP. Comparison of enzyme, clinical, radiographic, and radionuclide methods of detecting bone metastases from carcinoma of the prostate. Radiology 1976;121:431.
112. Chybowski FM, Larson Keller JJ, Bergstralh EJ, Oesterling JE. Predicting radionuclide bone scan findings in patients with newly diagnosed, untreated prostate cancer: prostate specific antigen is superior to all other parameters. J Urol 1991;145:313.
113. Oesterling JE, Martin SK, Bergstralh EJ, Lowe FC. The use of prostate-specific antigen in staging patients with newly diagnosed prostate cancer. JAMA 1993;269:57.
114. Pressman D, Korngold L. The in vivo localization of anti-Wagner osteogenic sarcoma antibodies. Cancer 1953;6:619.
115. Korngold L, Pressman D. The localization of antilymphosarcoma antibodies in the Murphy lymphosarcoma of the rat. Cancer Res 1954; 14:96.
116. Maguire RT, Schmelter RF, Pascucci VL, Conklin JJ. Immunoscintigraphy of colorectal adenocarcinoma: results with site-specifically radiolabeled B72.3 (^{111}In-Cyt-103). Antibodies, Immunoconjugates, and Radiopharmaceuticals 1989;2:257.
117. Nabi HA, Doerr RJ. Radiolabeled monoclonal antibody imaging (immunoscintigraphy) of colorectal cancers: current status and future perspectives. Am J Surg 1992;163:448.
118. Neal CE, Swan TL, Baker MR, Ellis RL, Katterhagen JG. Immunoscintigraphy of colorectal carcinoma utilizing ^{111}In. 1991;16:251.
119. Gallup DG. Multicenter clinical trial of ^{111}In-CYT-103 in patients with ovarian cancer. In: Maguire RT, Van Nostrand D, eds. Diagnosis of colorectal and ovarian carcinoma: application of immunoscintigraphic technology. New York: Marcel Dekker, 1992:111.
120. Keenan AM. Radiolabeled monoclonal antibodies: current status and future outlook. In: Freeman LM, Weissman HS, eds. Nuclear medicine annual. New York: Raven, 1988:171.
121. Lopes AD, Davis WL, Rosenstraus MJ, Uveges AJ, Gilman SC. Immunohistochemical and pharmacokinetic characterization of the site-specific immunoconjugate CYT-356 derived from antiprostate monoclonal antibody 7E11-C5. Cancer Res 1990;50:6423.
122. Wynant GE, Murphy GP, Horoszewicz JS, et al. Immunoscintigraphy of prostate cancer: preliminary results with ^{111}In-labeled monoclonal antibody 7E11-C5.3 (CYT-356). Prostate 1991;18:229.
123. Abel-Nabi H, Wright GL, Gulfo JV, et al. Monoclonal antibodies and radioimmunoconjugates in the diagnosis and treatment of prostate cancer. Semin Urol 1992;10:45.

Principles and Practice of Genitourinary Oncology, edited by Derek Raghavan, Howard I. Scher, Steven A. Leibel, and Paul H. Lange. Lippincott-Raven Publishers, Philadelphia, © 1997.

CHAPTER 49

Management of Stage A Prostate Cancer

Christopher Evans and Perinchery Narayan

Stage A prostate cancers are tumors incidentally identified in pathologic specimens after treatment for presumed benign prostatic hyperplasia (BPH). These cancers are further subdivided into stage A1 and A2 lesions based on tumor volume and grade, and in the TNM classification are called T1a and T1b, respectively. A new category of nonpalpable tumors, identified by increased levels of serum prostate-specific antigen (PSA), are classified as T1c tumors, and are discussed separately in Chapter 51. In this chapter, the term stage A refers only to A1 (T1a) and A2 (T1b) tumors.

The diagnosis and treatment of stage A prostatic cancer has been confounded by the inability to differentiate cancer from benign disease preoperatively, problems of variable natural history inherent in all prostatic cancers, and the difficulty of predicting residual disease and potential for progression based on examination of resected tissue. This chapter provides an overview of the definition, histopathologic features, natural history, and management strategies for stage A prostate cancer. In addition, the roles of grade and volume, repeat transurethral resection of the prostate (TURP), PSA and PSA-derived tests, transrectal ultrasonography (TRUS) and biopsy, DNA ploidy, and other markers in prognosis and follow-up of stage A prostate cancer are discussed.

DEFINITION

Stages T1a and T1b prostate cancer comprise nonpalpable cancers that are found incidentally during prostatectomy or TURP for presumed benign disease. The overall incidence of prostate adenocarcinoma in such procedures is 6% to 10%, but the incidence may be higher in older patients (up to 18% in men aged 60 to 69 years, and 37% in men aged 70 to 80 years).[1–8] In a Swedish population-based study, Johansson and colleagues used bone scans, chest radiographs, and intravenous pyelograms to stage clinically 654 new cases of prostate cancer. They identified 17% of these patients as having stage T1a or T1b disease.[9] The limitations in using only clinical and radiographic examinations to classify this stage of patient is apparent. Since the early appreciation of heterogeneity among stage A prostate cancers by Jewett,[10] several subclassifications of stage T1 prostate cancer have been proposed. Most subdivide stage T1 prostate cancer into stage T1a, or low-volume cancer, and stage T1b, or high-volume cancer.

Volume of stage T1a cancer has been variously defined as less than three foci, less than five foci, fewer than three chips involved, fewer than five chips involved, volume less than 2 cc, or tumor present in less than 5% of resected tissue.[11–16] Apart from volume, a significant factor in the division of stage T1 cancer into T1a and T1b subgroups is histologic grade. There is a spectrum of biologic behavior among stage T1 cancers that varies with the degree of cell differentiation. For practical purposes, patients with Gleason scores of 8 to 10 are classified as stage T1b even with volumes under 5% on TURP. Cantrell and associates have suggested that differences in prognosis between these cancers and stage T1 cancers with Gleason scores between 4 and 7 may be indistinct, and therefore they classify all these cancers as stage T1a.[11] However, even with Gleason scores of 4 to 7, patients with a large volume of cancer (>5%) have a different prognosis than those with a volume of less than 5%, as noted by Lowe and Listrom.[17] Based on the probability of progression, it appears more prudent to restrict the term T1a to cancers with volumes of less than 5% of total resected tissue and a grade of 4 or less by Gleason score (see Management Strategies).

The classification of stage T1 cancer initially came about as a result of diagnostic technique rather than on the basis of traditional staging techniques of grade and volume. Paulson and Robertson have suggested that the term stage A be discontinued in favor of ''organ-confined'' disease. They suggest that both stage A and stage B cancers be included in this category, because there is no evidence that there is any difference in prognosis between patients with stage A and B cancers if volume and grade are considered.[18]

HISTOPATHOLOGY

The diagnosis of stage T1a versus T1b prostate cancer depends in part on adequate tissue sampling. Epstein and associates initially submitted 12 g of TURP chips (10 cassettes) and reported a 91% detection of all stage T1a tumors.[19] Murphy and associates examined 6 g of tissue after TURP and missed only 10% of tumors.[20] They recommended that at least 10 g of TURP specimen be examined and, if any focus of cancer is found, that all chips be studied. Based on probability analysis, most pathologists agree that all chips must be examined if a single chip contains cancer.[21] Pathologic examination by step-sectioning techniques, as reported by Denton and associates,[6] increased the incidence of stage T1 cancer to 21% from the 6% identified by standard sectioning techniques. These techniques are probably also responsible for the increasing incidence of residual cancer being reported in radical prostatectomy specimens of stage T1 lesions, from 7% to 29% in earlier series[13,15,22] to 95% in more recent studies.[23]

Although stage T1a and T1b tumors are nonpalpable and are diagnosed by surgical techniques that excise the transition zone, these cancers are not confined to the transition zone. Greene and associates evaluated 42 post-TURP stage A radical prostatectomy specimens and found that 81% contained tumors in the transition zone and 93% in the peripheral zone.[24] TURP, however, had sampled tumors from both zones in only 8% of patients, transition zone cancer alone in 77%, and peripheral zone tumors alone in 31%. In related work, the total volume of cancer in stage A1 disease was found to be 1.55 cc, with 72% originating in the transition zone; this compared with a volume of 5.83 cc, with only 57% of transition zone origin, in stage A2 disease.[25] The transition zone tumors that are most frequently sampled by TURP are usually well differentiated,[26] in scattered foci,[27] and located anteromedially.[28] This tumor distribution differs from our unpublished pathologic data from stage T1c tumors, which reveal cancer in the transition zone in 6% of specimens, in the peripheral zone in 35%, and in both zones in 59%. Histopathologically, tumor extent in stage A2 cancer is extensive and often extracapsular. Christensen and associates, in a pathology review of 26 patients with stage A2 prostatic cancer who underwent radical prostatectomy, noted residual cancer in 100% of patients, with capsular penetration in 26%.[29]

Based on morphometric studies, McNeal and associates have divided stage A cancers into two groups: one group arise predominantly in the transition zone, are usually focal, and have small volumes, and the other group arise in the peripheral zone, invade the transition zone secondarily, and are larger in volume.[28,30] A significant number of focal transition zone cancers are located in the anterior portion of the transition zone distal to the verumontanum.[28,31] This has implications both in the search for residual disease after initial TURP and for obtaining adequate margins during radical prostatectomy.

Studies to determine precursor lesions for stage A cancer have not yielded conclusive findings. In one study undertaken to determine whether severe dysplasia was a precursor to stage A prostate cancer, Epstein and associates compared TURP specimens with radical prostatectomy specimens.[32] They found severe dysplasia in only 15% of TURP specimens and no correlation between dysplasia and stage A prostate cancer.

NATURAL HISTORY AND PROBABILITY OF PROGRESSION

Rich[33] and Moore[34] first drew the attention of urologists and pathologists to the existence of stage A cancers at autopsies in 1935. The prognostic significance of these tumors was subsequently recognized by Bauer and associates in 1960.[4] In 1972, Hanash and associates studied the progression of stage A prostate cancer in a group of untreated patients.[35] In patients with low-grade lesions, the 15-year life expectancy was normal, whereas in those with high-grade tumors, a normal 10-year but diminished 15-year life expectancy was noted.

The natural history of stage A disease is summarized in Table 49-1.[11,16,17,35–40] Cantrell and associates in 1981 reported on a group of 48 patients managed expectantly and found that 1 (2%) of 48 men with stage A1 tumors had clinically significant progression over 4 years, compared with 11 (33%) of 34 men with stage A2 cancers.[11] Subsequently, Epstein and associates' evaluation of 94 men with stage A1 disease monitored for a longer period showed a 16% progression rate at 8 years, suggesting that among men at risk, even stage A1 cancers carry a significant risk of progression.[38] Epstein's study suggested that risk of progression was independent of Gleason scores (in the 4 to 7 range) and of relative differences in volume among stage A1 cancers. Because 26 of the 94 patients died of unrelated causes, and an additional 18 patients who showed no evidence of progression were excluded from the study, Paulson and Robertson reanalyzed Epstein's data. This reanalysis suggested that the risk of death or progression was closer to 12% than 16%, as originally suggested.[18] Several other long-term follow-up studies of stage A1 patients treated expectantly have revealed progression rates of 5% to 16%.[37–39]

A correlation between grade, volume, and tumor progression was found in a study by Lowe and Listrom.[17] In an evaluation of 232 patients with stage A1 tumors, they reported an overall

TABLE 49-1. *Natural history of untreated stage A cancer*

Investigators	Stage	Patients	Mean age (y)	5-year progression rate (%)	5-year survival rate (%)	10-year survival rate (%)
Hanash et al, 1972[35]	A1, A2	50	—	14	86	52
Khalifa and Jarman, 1976[36]	A1, A2	43	68.9	44	56	31
Cantrell et al, 1981[11]	A2	14	69	32	68	—
Beynon et al, 1983[37]	A1, A2	27	73	33	67	—
Epstein et al, 1986[38]	A1	50	65	4; 16 (8 y)	96	84
Blute et al, 1986[16]	A1, A2	23	60	15; 32 (11 y)	85	68
Blute et al, 1986[16]	A1	15	62	15; 35 (11 y)	85	65
Lowe and Listrom, 1988[17]	A1, A2	33	62	45	55	—
Thompson and Zeidman, 1989[39]	A1	60	68	5 (7.5 y)	95	—
Roy et al, 1990[40]	A1	23	66.8	16 (8 y)	94	79
Mean			22.3	78.7		

TABLE 49-2. *Probability of progression based on Gleason score of volume of cancer*

Gleason score	Volume on transurethral resection (%)	Probability at 5 years*	Probability at 10 years*
2 or 3	<1	0.03–0.05	0.06–0.1
	1–5	0.08–0.12	0.15–0.22
4	<1	0.06–0.09	0.11–0.17
	1–5	0.14–0.21	0.25–0.36
	<5	0.31–0.44	0.51–0.67
5 or 6	1–5	0.24–0.35	0.41–0.56
	5	0.49–0.65	0.72–0.86
7–9	1–5	0.39–0.54	0.61–0.77
	>5	0.70–0.85	0.90–0.97

* Range represents the probability of progression from 65–75.

Modified with permission from Lowe AA, Listrom MB. Incidental carcinoma of the prostate: an analysis of the predictors of progression. J Urol 1988;140:1340.

progression rate of 9% at 9 years. They also analyzed the prognosis of subsets of stage A patients based on histologic grade and found that risk of progression increases in a linear fashion with grade, volume, and age (Table 49-2). A review of Table 49-2 suggests that a probability of progression of 31% to 44% exists at 5 years with a tumor volume of greater than 5%, even with a Gleason score of 4. A 24% to 35% risk of progression exists with Gleason scores 5 or 6 and volume of less than 5%. These findings were further supported by a study of 132 patients by Zhang and associates, who noted a 10% progression rate at a mean of 7 years of follow-up in stage A1 patients with Gleason scores of 4 or less.[41] These data indicate that the management approach to the subset of patients with Gleason grades between 4 and 6, tumor volume between 1% and 5%, and life expectancies of 10 years or more should take into account the significant likelihood of disease progression.

The presence of lymph node metastasis in patients with stage A disease is consistent with the natural history. Donohue and associates, reporting on 23 patients after pelvic lymphadenectomy, noted that 0 of 5 stage A1 patients had metastatic nodal spread, but 4 (22%) of 18 stage A2 patients had positive nodes. All of the primary tumors in patients with positive nodes were of high grade.[42] Golimbu and associates had similar results and found 0 of 4 patients with stage A1 disease and 6 (37.5%) of 16 patients with A2 disease to have nodal metastases.[14] A comparison with stage B1 lesions of similar grade revealed positive lymph nodes only in 17.6% of cases, despite the fact that patients with B1 disease had a higher incidence of capsular invasion (29%, versus 6% for patients with stage A2 disease).[14] Whitmore, in summarizing the natural history for stage A prostate cancers, reported the 10-year mortality rate to be less than 5% in patients with A1 lesions and more than 25% in those with A2 lesions.[43]

ROLE OF STAGING TRANSURETHRAL RESECTION OF THE PROSTATE

The differentiation between stage A1 and A2 tumors is based on the premise that adequate tissue sampling has occurred. However, not all TURP procedures adequately sample the anterior portion of the prostate or, perhaps, the areas close to the capsule in the lateral and posterior lobes. In an attempt to identify patients with residual cancers who may have been missed on initial TURP, repeat TURP has been advocated by some surgeons.

McMillen and Wettlaufer performed staging TURP on 27 patients with stage A1 disease.[44] Sixty-three percent of patients had no residual tumor in the specimen, 11% had a single focus detected, and 26% with residual tumor were restaged as having stage A2 disease. Carroll and associates reported similar results, with 10 (24%) of 42 patients whose disease was restaged to A2 after repeat TURP.[45] However, most investigators have found that, although residual cancer is detected on repeat TURP in a substantial fraction of patients with stage A1 disease, the actual incidence of upstaging to stage A2 is less than 10%. Drago and associates combined Carroll's data with four other series to study a total of 229 patients with stage A1 lesions.[12,13,22,46,47] Data from repeat TURP in this combined series yielded cancer in a mean of 24% of patients. However, the volume and grade of residual cancer detected on repeat TURP resulted in upstaging of only 7% to stage A2 disease.

Part of the reason for lack of restaging in these series may be inadequate tissue sampling of the anterior transition zone, distal to the verumontanum, where stage A1 cancers predominate. Most urologists do not resect this area for fear of producing incontinence.[28,30] Also, repeat TURP in stage A cancers is unlikely to identify residual disease present in the peripheral zone, apex, or areas adjacent to the capsule.[48] These areas are better sampled by TRUS-guided or systematic biopsies.

Even among patients whose tumors are upstaged to stage A2 by repeat TURP, only a few ultimately receive definitive therapy, because of age and coexisting medical illnesses. This was illustrated in the study by Zhang and associates, who reported on the outcome of 52 patients with stage A1 disease who were expectantly managed and had repeat TURP to detect residual disease.[41] Fourteen cancers demonstrated residual foci of tumor, of which three (25%) went on to progress locally. Only 8% of the 38 patients who had no residual disease on staging TURP had local progression. Although this makes a case for repeat TURP to detect residual disease, in actual practice only 2 patients (3.8%) received therapy based on the additional information. Repeat TURP for stage A disease was therefore not justified based on management strategy, because it did not significantly alter therapy. The authors did not advocate repeat TURP for stage A patients.

Epstein and associates have also argued that, even though residual tumor may be identified on repeat TURP, patients with residual tumor do not necessarily have a poorer prognosis.[38] In support of this argument, they cited their extended follow-up of 94 patients, in whom the classification of stage A1 disease based on the initial TURP was adequate to provide data that resulted in an overall progression rate of 16% at 8 years (or 12% as analyzed by Paulson). Lowe and Barry compared three modalities for predicting progression of stage A tumors: repeat TURP, progression probability tables (see Table 49-2), and the A1/A2 substaging system.[49] Among 96 patients studied, the probability tables correctly predicted disease progression in 92% of cases. Fifty-two of these patients underwent staging TURP, and disease-free survival was predicted accurately in 93%. These two modalities did not differ significantly, but both were superior to the 85% of patients predicted to be free of disease by the A1/A2 staging system. The combination of staging TURP and probability tables did not further improve predictive ability, and the authors concluded that the tables could be used alone to predict cancer progression.

Larsen and associates addressed the question whether data obtained from an initial TURP could predict the pathologic extent of stage A1 tumors.[50] They compared residual and total tumor volume and Gleason grade in 64 radical prostatectomy specimens from stage A1 tumors with those from stage A2 and B specimens. The TURP specimen tumor volume, percent, and grade did not statistically correlate with the residual tumor volume found in the radical prostatectomy specimens. Substantial tumor—defined as the presence of 1 cc or more of cancer, capsular penetration, or Gleason score greater than 8—was identified in 20% of stage A1 radical prostatectomy specimens. Six percent of patients had no residual tumor, and 74% had minimal tumor in this study. These results support the concept that a population of stage A1 patients harbor substantial residual tumor, which puts them at risk for significant disease progression over the next 6 to 10 years.

In summary, we conclude that, based on available data, repeat TURP results in reclassification of a small percentage of patients to stage A2. Only rarely does the additional information result in alteration of therapy. Furthermore, use of the progression probability tables introduced by Lowe and Listrom[17] may accurately identify those patients who will survive free of disease.

ROLE OF TRANSRECTAL ULTRASONOGRAPHY

TRUS has gained widespread application in the detection, staging, and follow-up of stage A prostate cancer (see Chaps. 46 and 49 for more details). Data about prostatic volume, tumor volume, and tumor location can be obtained with TRUS. TRUS is particularly useful in evaluating the peripheral zone, prostatic apex, and extracapsular extension, and it provides data not available by repeat TURP.

Sheth and colleagues compared TRUS results with pathologic analyses of TURP specimens in 29 patients with stage A prostate cancer.[51] Thirty hypoechoic peripheral lesions were identified, which correlated with 11 pathologic cancers. Nine tumors were not recognized during preoperative TRUS testing, eight of which were predominantly located in the transition zone. For this group of stage A patients, the sensitivity of TRUS was 55%, and the specificity was 37%.

Shinohara and associates evaluated the echogenic pattern of tumors as a function of the clinical stage.[52] One of 8 stage A1 lesions and 8 of 17 stage A2 lesions were hypoechoic and diagnostic of cancer, for a detection accuracy of 36%. The percentage of isoechoic patterns decreased from 87% in stage A1 to 53% in stage A2 tumors, to less than 30% in higher-stage carcinomas. The authors noted that most stage A1 tumors in their series were of small volume, in an anterior location, and isoechoic on TRUS.

Based on current technology and resolution capabilities, TRUS is most likely to be helpful in detecting residual disease in the peripheral zone and cancers in the transition zone that have a volume greater than 0.2 cc (diameter of 5 to 7 mm). In this regard, Terris and associates reported on the use of TRUS with guided biopsies to detect residual cancer in stage A patients after TURP or simple prostatectomy.[31] In one group, standard preoperative TRUS with biopsy identified residual cancer in 24% of patients, who then underwent radical prostatectomy. In a second group of patients, six TRUS-guided systematic biopsies were used to detect residual cancer, which was found in 28% of cases. This positive yield was increased to 47% in a third group of 47 patients, in whom four additional biopsies were performed in the anterior transition zone distal to the verumontanum.

Egawa and colleagues evaluated the ability of TRUS to identify residual tumor after TURP.[53] Eleven patients with stage A1 prostate cancer and 27 with stage A2 cancer, all of whom had had resection at least 3 weeks earlier, underwent TRUS before radical prostatectomy, and the sonograms were compared with the maps of the pathologic specimens. Hypoechoic areas were identified in 10 prostates by sonography, of which 8 were found to have cancer on the pathology specimen. Twenty-five additional hypoechoic lesions were noted retrospectively, and 15 of these contained cancer. In total, 47% of transition zone hypoechoic areas were malignant, compared with 88% of peripheral zone hypoechoic lesions. A breakdown by substage revealed residual cancer supported by sonography in 18% of patients with stage A1 and 22% of patients with stage A2 disease. Because stage A cancers are located anteriorly, the combination of TRUS and systematic biopsies of the anterior transition zone may yield a higher detection rate of residual cancer in stage A disease.

In patients with an initial diagnosis of stage A1 disease, TRUS with guided biopsies diagnoses an additional 18% to 28% of transition zone and peripheral zone cancers not detected by TURP or digital rectal examination (DRE). Systematic biopsies of the anterior transition zone further increase this detection rate to 47%. The question for stage A cancers, however, is whether the additional detection of residual cancer in the transition or peripheral zone implies a different prognosis for these patients who are classified as stage A1 by initial TURP. An argument could be made that the prognosis should be based on the progression probability tables,[17] which were derived from data generated before use of TRUS and systematic biopsies. This would not subject patients to the additional expense or morbidity caused by TRUS, systematic biopsies, or a second TURP. It therefore remains to be determined whether the additional data generated by TRUS and systematic biopsies provide information that translates into a survival advantage for patients when used to alter current management strategies.

ROLE OF SYSTEMATIC BIOPSIES

Before the introduction of PSA and TRUS with guided biopsies, it was suggested that patients with palpably benign disease should undergo a four-quadrant fine-needle aspiration of the prostate before prostatectomy.[54] Cytologic diagnosis correctly identified cancer in 3 of 4 patients with pathologic stage A2 tumors but did not detect cancer in any of 14 patients found to have pathologic stage A1 tumors by TURP. The failure to sample the transition zone of the prostate by fine-needle aspiration, and thereby to diagnose stage A1 tumors, can be appreciated. Coplen and colleagues performed systematic TRUS-guided biopsies in 73 men with the clinical diagnosis of BPH.[55] Seven patients (10%) were found to have prostate cancer, and of the remaining 67 men, 40 proceeded to TURP. In this group, 2 patients (5%) had prostate cancer. In this small population of men, PSA did not appear effective, because 6 of 9 patients with prostate cancer had normal PSA levels, and only 3 of 30 men with an elevated PSA value were eventually found to have cancer. The use of PSA and PSA density, discussed in the next section, may help to identify better those patients who should undergo TRUS with biopsies before prostatectomy for presumed benign disease.

The role of systematic biopsies in detecting residual cancer in stage A disease has not been evaluated extensively. In the study by Terris and associates,[31] the use of six systematic biopsies detected residual cancer in 3 of 16 patients with stage A1 and 4 of 9 with stage A2 disease, for a total yield of 28%. This was not very different from a previous group of 39 patients they had studied with TRUS-guided biopsies, in whom residual cancer was detected in 25%. These data suggest that systematic biopsies are probably just as accurate as TRUS with guided biopsies in detecting residual disease in patients with stage A disease. The information obtained from anterior transition zone biopsies may be the only additional feature of TRUS-guided biopsies that is not available from systematic biopsies. However, the relevance of both systematic biopsies and anterior transition zone biopsies in stage A1 disease detected after initial TURP is still evolving.

ROLE OF PROSTATE-SPECIFIC ANTIGEN

PSA is discussed in greater detail in Chapter 42. Briefly, PSA is a 33-kd serine protease which is normally present in the seminal vesicle coagulum.[56,57] PSA is secreted by normal, BPH, and malignant prostatic cells. Several studies have shown that PSA alone and in conjunction with DRE can improve detection rates of organ-confined cancers.[58–61] However, the value of PSA in defining tumor volume is still under investigation.

With regard to the use of PSA in evaluating the patient with symptoms of prostatism, the 1994 clinical practice guideline entitled *Benign Prostatic Hyperplasia: Diagnosis and Treatment,* published by the U.S. Department of Health and Human Services,[62] states the following:

> Measurement of PSA is optional in the initial evaluation. Testing for PSA increases the detection rate for prostate cancer over DRE alone and tends to detect cancer at an earlier stage. However, the PSA test does not discriminate well between patients with symptomatic BPH and those with prostate cancer, particularly if the cancers are pathologically localized and curable. There is significant overlap in PSA values between BPH and cancer patients. Also, there is a lack of consensus regarding the evaluation of minimally elevated PSAs. The test may trigger additional evaluation, including ultrasound and biopsy of the prostate. In addition, there is no evidence yet whether PSA testing does or does not lead to a decrease in morbidity and mortality from prostate cancer.

Table 49-3 shows the summary chart from the clinical practice guidelines comparing PSA levels for BPH and organ-confined prostate cancer from three studies.[63–65] Some authors believe that a PSA determination should be obtained in patients with obstructive symptoms and a family history of prostate cancer.[66] Despite the guidelines, it is likely that many urologists are incorporating the PSA test in their workup to evaluate the possibility of a stage T1c tumor.

A study by Monda and associates appeared shortly after the publication of the guidelines.[67] It evaluated the ability of PSA to distinguish between stage A1 prostate cancer and BPH and whether the use of PSA has affected the reported prevalence of stage A cancer. The authors retrospectively compared 499 patients who underwent TURP in the pre-PSA era (1986) with 467 patients who had a PSA test performed before TURP (1989 to 1990). The prevalence of stage T1a tumors was actually higher in patients who had PSA testing (7.3%) than in the earlier group (3.6%). This difference was not attributable to the volume resected nor to changes in methods of pathologic evaluation. PSA levels in patients with stage T1a tumors did not differ statistically from patients with BPH. The median PSA value for men with stage T1b tumors was significantly higher than for men with BPH (5.9 versus 3.4, $P = 0.01$). However, the percentage of patients with an elevated PSA concentration was greater in the stage T1b group compared with BPH patients only if the PSA level was greater than 10 ng/mL. Three percent of men having a PSA performed before TURP were found to have stage T1b cancers, compared with 5% of men who never had a preoperative PSA determination ($P = 0.11$). Therefore, the increased median PSA level in patients with stage T1b tumors, compared with BPH patients, did not translate into a significantly decreased prevalence of men found to have stage T1b tumors at the time of TURP.

TABLE 49-3. *Comparative PSA values for benign prostatic hyperplasia (BPH) and organ-confined prostate cancer*

	Percentage and number of patients with PSA in specified range (ng/mL)					
	0.0–4.0		4.1–10.0		≥10.1	
Investigators	BPH	Prostate cancer	BPH	Prostate cancer	BPH	Prostate cancer
Partin et al, 1990[63]	47% (34/72)	45% (83/185)	46% (32/72)	44% (82/185)	7% (5/72)	11% (20/185)
Lange et al, 1989[64]	79% (282/357)	45% (14/31)	18% (64/357)	32% (10/32)	3% (11/357)	23% (7/31)
Hudson et al, 1989[65]	79% (133/168)	38% (39/103)	19% (32/168)	26% (27/103)	2% (3/168)	36% (37/103)
Total	75% (449/597)	43% (136/319)	22% (129/597)	37% (119/319)	3% (19/597)	20% (64/319)
P value	$P < 0.001$		$P < 0.001$		$P < 0.001$	

The role of PSA in predicting residual disease after TURP was studied by Carter and associates.[68] They found that in a group of 67 patients with stage A disease who underwent radical prostatectomy, all stage A1 patients who had a PSA concentration of 1 ng/mL or less had residual tumor smaller than 0.5 cc, and all stage A patients with a PSA level higher than 10 ng/mL had a tumor volume greater than 0.5 cc. Overall, 51% of patients had values of PSA between 1 to 10 ng/mL, and serum PSA was not useful to predict tumor volumes in this group. These findings were partially confirmed by Voges and associates[23] in a study of radical prostatectomies for stage A prostate cancer. Seven of eight patients with a PSA value lower than 1 ng/mL had tumor volume smaller than 0.4 cc, and 19 of 20 patients with a PSA level higher than 2.5 ng/mL had tumor volume greater than 0.9 cc.

A statistically significant association between PSA, prostate gland volume, and age was also shown in a study of 408 patients by Babaian and associates.[69] They found a linear relation between the logarithm of the PSA level and patient age and between the PSA level and prostate volume. Multiple regression analyses revealed that mean PSA values increased by 26% per decade, and 32% for a 10-cc increase in prostate gland volume. Based on this data, they recommended systematic biopsies in those patients who had a PSA level between 4 and 10 mg/mL and a prostate volume of less than 25 cc as estimated by TRUS planimetry. Fewer than 2% of such patients had a PSA level greater than 4 ng/mL with no evidence of cancer. These studies were done in patients who had not undergone TURP. It remains to be seen whether determination of PSA values in relation to prostate volume after TURP can provide sufficient information regarding the prognostic value for patients with stage A disease.

A universal cutoff value of 4.0 ng/mL (by Tandem-R PSA assay) for a normal serum PSA concentration is not appropriate for all age groups of men. Oesterling reported the PSA concentration by decade of age for men 40 to 79 years old who had no evidence of prostate cancer (Table 49-4).[70] No men between 40 and 49 years of age had a PSA level higher than 4.0 ng/mL, and only 2% of men between the ages of 50 and 59 had a value greater than 4.0 ng/mL. Age-specific PSA reference ranges must be kept in mind when patients of different ages are evaluated.

In attempts to improve the accuracy of PSA as a screening tool, several other applications have been developed, including the calculation of PSA density (PSAD) and PSA velocity (PSAV) and the measurement of a complex formed between PSA and α_1-antichymotrypsin, known as PSA-ACT. Benson and associates studied the relation between PSA and prostate volume[71] and developed the PSAD quotient to help identify whether an elevated PSA level was caused by BPH or by a combination of BPH and cancer. PSAD is calculated by dividing the PSA level by the prostate volume. The prostate volume is obtained by the prolated ellipsoid formula, which is the product of the greatest three diameters on TRUS multiplied by 0.52. In Benson's study, the mean PSAD was 0.581 for prostate cancer and 0.044 for BPH ($P < 0.002$).

The PSAD value that best discriminates between cancer and BPH has not been clearly determined, but it probably is in the range 0.1 to 0.15. Shinohara and associates point out that a lower cutoff level increases the sensitivity for cancer detection.[72] They compared PSA to PSAD for predicting the presence of cancer on TRUS-guided biopsies in patients with nonpalpable prostate cancer. Both parameters were associated with the biopsy result ($P = 0.0034$ for PSA; $P = 0.0001$ for PSAD), but receiver-operator characteristic curves (sensitivity versus specificity) along a range of cutoff values revealed PSAD to be a superior predictor of the biopsy result ($P = 0.0013$). In a subset of 44 patients with normal DRE, normal TRUS studies, and PSA values in the 4 to 10 ng/mL range, cancer was demonstrated in 9 patients by biopsy. A PSAD cutoff of 0.1 would caused 86% of these patients to undergo biopsy and would have detected cancer in all 9. A cutoff of 0.15, on the other hand, would have resulted in biopsy for only 57% and would have missed detecting cancer in 2 (23%) of the 9 patients. Bazinet and associates also found PSAD to be useful for better selection of patients for TRUS and biopsy.[73] Their best PSAD cutoff value varied according to the PSA level and whether the DRE and TRUS results were positive or negative. As Cooner points out, however, patients must undergo TRUS in order to calculate the PSAD, and prostatic shapes are highly variable, with prostatic volume determinations very dependent on the skills of the operator.[74] Further experience with this technique will clarify its role as an adjunct in the diagnosis of nonpalpable, stage A tumors.

The rate of change of PSA determined serially over time (PSAV) may also be helpful to distinguish between patients with normal prostate, BPH, and prostate cancer. Carter and associates used serial frozen sera from the Baltimore Longitudinal Study of Aging to investigate this theory.[75,76] In a small group of patients, they found that the PSAV was greater in men with prostate cancer than in those with BPH, and greater in men with either disease than in men without BPH or cancer. BPH patients had a linear rise in PSA, whereas prostate cancer patients demonstrated an exponential increase in PSA. The change from a linear to an exponential rise occurred 7 to 9 years before the actual diagnosis of prostate cancer. In this study, a PSAV of 0.75 ng/mL per year or more correctly identified 72% of patients with cancer. This cutoff value also included 10% of BPH subjects as false-positives, for a sensitivity of 90%. Catalona and associates prospectively studied 224 men older than 50 years of age for 12 to 36 months who had a PSA level of 2.8 ng/mL or higher and a normal prostate examination. Patients then underwent prostate biopsy and were divided according to Carter's PSAV cutoff value of 0.75 ng/mL per year. Prostate cancer was found in 13 (23%) of 57 men with a mean PSAV value lower than the cutoff value and in 28 (23%) of 122 with a PSAV higher than the cutoff.[58] A larger, more extensive study

TABLE 49-4. *Serum prostate-specific antigen (ng/mL) and patient age*

Age range (y)	Median value	Interquartile range*	Reference range†
40–49	0.7	0.5–1.1	0–2.5
50–59	1.0	0.6–1.4	0–3.5
60–69	1.4	0.8–3.0	0–4.5
70–79	2.0	0.9–3.2	0–6.5

* The 25th to 75th percentile.
† Upper limit defined by the 95th percentile

Data from Oesterling JE, Cooner WH, Jacobsen SJ, Guess HA, Lieber MM. Influence of patient age on the serum prostate antigen concentration. Urol Clin North Am 1993;4:671.

is needed to verify whether PSAV accurately distinguishes between patients with cancer, those with BPH, and those with no prostatic disease, or between different tumor stages and stage A disease before prostatectomy.

Circulating forms of PSA in serum (unbound in its 30-kd form or complexed to other proteins) have recently been studied. Stenman and associates evaluated the forms of PSA in serum of patients with prostate cancer or BPH and found that a significant part of PSA immunoreactivity consisted of complexes larger than the monomeric form.[77] Specifically, a major proportion of the PSA was in the form of PSA-ACT, especially with increasing PSA concentrations. PSA was also complexed to α_1-protease inhibitor and, to a lesser extent, to α_2-macroglobulin and inter-alpha-trypsin inhibitor. PSA-ACT was more prevalent in patients with prostate cancer than in patients with BPH in the same total serum PSA range ($P < 0.001$). Two other studies have verified the formation of a PSA-ACT complex and elevation of this form in patients with prostate cancer.[78,79] Whether detection of PSA in a complexed form can lead to improved discrimination between prostate cancer and BPH remains to be determined.

ROLE OF DNA PLOIDY AND OTHER MARKERS

Nuclear DNA content is a laboratory determination that has been explored for its ability to predict prostate cancer progression. Evaluation of tumor cell DNA has shown that nuclear aberrations reflect malignancy and tumor cell behavior. Aneuploid prostatic tumors have a poorer prognosis and poorer response to hormonal therapy than do normal prostate cells.[80–82] In an analysis of archival material from patients with stage A prostate cancer, McIntire and associates used analysis of DNA ploidy to better predict disease progression.[83] Among 11 patients with stage A1 lesions, 1 had aneuploidy and subsequently died of metastatic disease; there was no disease progression in the remaining 10 nonaneuploid cases. In a group of 22 patients with stage A2 lesions, 6 (67%) of 9 with aneuploidy experienced disease progression, as did 2 (15%) of 13 with nonaneuploid tumors. The data suggest that flow cytometric determination of DNA ploidy may provide unique information that that can be used along with standard histologic analyses to predict disease progression. The heterogeneity of benign hyperplastic tissue, however, occasionally causes variation in the histograms that interferes with data interpretation. Recent data derived from static image analyses by Feulgen staining techniques and from fluorescence analyses suggest that these techniques may be better suited to the study of prostatic tissue than is flow cytometry.[84] Refinements in these techniques may eventually make DNA ploidy an important component in the prognostic evaluation of stage A prostate cancer.

The detection of genetic alterations in prostate cancer is being pursued by many investigators for potential diagnostic and therapeutic use. Changes in expression of tumor suppressor genes such as *P53* and the retinoblastoma gene; oncogenes such as *MYC*, *PDGFB* (formerly known as sis), *ERBB2*, and *RAS*; and cytokines such as transforming growth factor-beta$_1$ in prostate cancer have been reported.[85–91] Only van Veldhuizen and associates have specifically studied a genetic alteration in stage A prostate cancer.[92] Using a monoclonal antibody to *P53* and immunohistochemistry, they evaluated 36 tumor microfoci from 24 patients for abnormal *P53* expression, finding increased staining in 58% of the specimens. Although clinical application of genetic changes in prostate cancer is still investigational, it is likely to be of increasing importance in the near future.

MANAGEMENT

The major issue in stage A prostate cancer is quantification of risk of progression. Several techniques, such as TRUS, systematic biopsy, and PSA determination, can contribute additional information to the knowledge of grade and volume obtained on initial TURP. Additional techniques, such as DNA ploidy, genetic and proliferative markers, and further refinements in PSA measurements, may be helpful in the future. We outline here a cost-effective management strategy for stage A cancers based on current knowledge of natural history and prognosis (Fig. 49-1).

Patients with stage A prostate cancer are divided into three groups after initial TURP: those with low, intermediate, and high risk of progression. Patients with cancer volumes of less than 5% (after examination of a minimum of 12 g of TURP tissue, or of all chips if cancer is detected in any) and Gleason scores equal to 4 or less are classified as having low risk. Depending on age, medical health, and life expectancy, therapy for low-risk patients may consist of surveillance, irradiation, or surgery.

Patients with Gleason scores of 4 and volumes greater than 5% and those with Gleason scores of 5 or 6 and volumes less than 5% are said to have intermediate risk of progression. Patients in this group who are younger than 70 years of age and have a life expectancy of 10 years or more should be encouraged to have definitive therapy with surgery or radiotherapy. It is reasonable to subject the rest of this group to active surveillance.

Patients with Gleason scores of 5 to 6 and a volume of greater than 5% and those with Gleason scores of 7 or higher with any volume of disease should be classified as having high risk of progression. All patients in this group should undergo immediate therapy. The type of therapy varies and should be tempered by the age and medical fitness of the patient.

RESULTS OF THERAPY

Surveillance

Based on the known natural history of stage A cancer, it is reasonable for low-risk patients with stage A disease to opt for surveillance as therapy. Surveillance is probably adequate for patients who are older than 70 years of age and for younger patients whose other medical conditions give them a life expectancy of less than 10 years. The rationale for surveillance is based on the projection that fewer than 25% of these cancers will progress within 10 years and the fact that the presence or development of comorbid conditions over time is likely to cause death in a significant number of these patients before prostate cancer mortality would occur.

Several studies have evaluated the use of observation in the management of patients with organ-confined prostate cancer.[9,93–101] Chodak and others a pooled analysis of data from six of these investigations, comprising 828 patients.[102] Five-

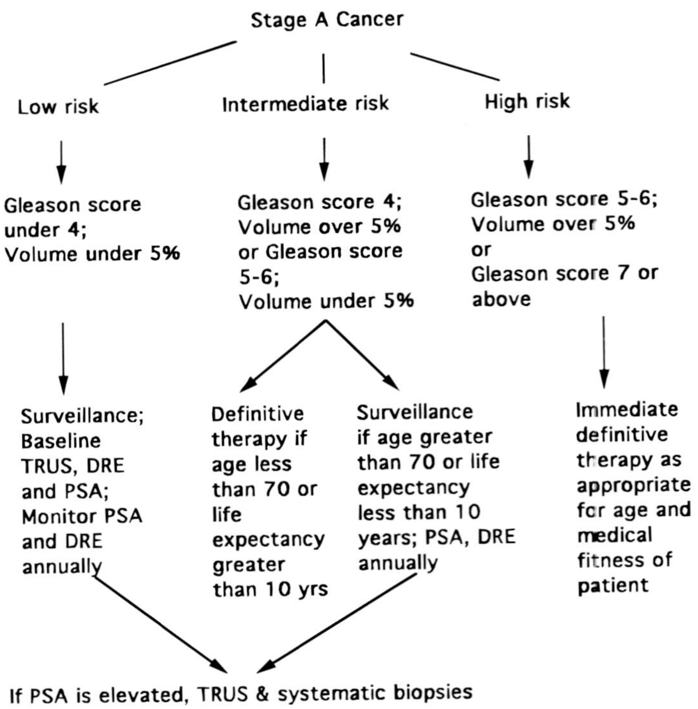

FIG. 49-1. Algorithm for therapy of stage A (T1a) cancer. DRE, digital rectal examination; PSA, prostate-specific antigen; TRUS, transrectal ultrasonography.

and 10-year disease-specific survival and metastasis-free survival rates were high in patients with low-grade tumors and focal disease, supporting the choice of conservative management in this group. Although the 10-year disease-free survival rate for patients with Gleason scores of 5 to 7 was 94%, the metastasis-free survival rate in this group was only 78%. The authors recommended observation for these patients also. However, these data underestimate the progression rate at 10 years as predicted by Lowe and Listrom.[17] Only 2 of 155 patients with focal disease had tumors with a Gleason sum greater than 8, not allowing for reasonable analysis of this group.

In the extended follow-up studies of stage A1 patients by Epstein and associates,[38] 26 (28%) of 94 men died from causes other than prostate cancer less than 4 years after diagnosis. Among 8 (16%) of 50 remaining patients whose cancer progressed, 6 (12%) died of cancer. Until randomized trials of surveillance versus definitive therapy are available, decisions on advocating surveillance for patients must be based on evaluation of incomplete data, individual patient preference, and philosophic approach.

Active surveillance of stage A patients involves periodic monitoring of serum PSA levels and annual DRE. Although there is no precise delineation of the levels of PSA elevation that can be said to be significant for prostate cancer versus BPH, a level of 0.3 ng/mL per gram of BPH has been calculated to be the serum PSA equivalent for BPH tissue.[103] A rapid rise of PSA without commensurate increase in transition zone volume should trigger a search for malignancy. Currently reported techniques of PSAD measurement do not distinguish transition zone volume from peripheral zone volume. At our center, we have devised a technique of measuring PSAD that is based on transition zone, peripheral zone, and tumor volume as detected by TRUS and Gleason grade of tumor.[104,105] As mentioned, both PSAD and PSAV may eventually prove to be valuable adjuncts in monitoring of these patients. Additional experience with the use of these methods to detect progression during surveillance is necessary before any of them can be fully advocated.

There are several assumptions that are made when placing patients on surveillance protocols. It is assumed that available follow-up studies such as PSA, TRUS, and DRE are adequate to detect progression. It must also be assumed that patients will be available for follow-up and that the optimum follow-up intervals are known. Furthermore, in patients who experience progression of disease it is presumed that the follow-up regimens will be adequate to detect progression before it is too late, that treatments given at that time will be tolerable and adequate, and that the remainder of the patient's life will be of reasonable quality.

In patients who are interested in pursuing therapy, detection of a rapid rise in PSA or an abnormal DRE result would warrant a TRUS and systematic biopsies of the prostate to identify the cause for the increased PSA level. The amount of increase in PSA within a year that should warrant TRUS is not yet clear. It is known that patients with PSA levels of less than 1 ng/mL have residual disease volumes of less than 0.5 cc and that those with PSA levels higher than 2.5 ng/mL have residual tumor volumes greater than 0.9 mL. The tumor doubling time of stage A tumors is calculated to be longer than 3 years. Therefore, it may be possible, based on the initial PSA values, to determine for a particular patient an inappropriate rise in PSA level, one that would be indicative of rapid versus slow progression. Again, the concept of PSAV may have significant application in these patients. Further management in these cases would depend on the detection of malignancy by biopsy. If no recurrence or residual disease is detected on biopsy, then annual PSA, TRUS, and biopsy testing may yield more definite information.

TABLE 49-5. *Radical prostatectomy in stage A prostate cancer*

Investigators	Patients	Stage	Mean age (y)	5-year disease-free survival rate (%)	10-year disease-free survival rate (%)
Partin et al, 1993[109]	161	Tla-Tlc	—	94	65
Middleton et al, 1986[107]	34	A2	—	94	65
Paulson et al, 1988[106]	105	A1, A2	64	85	81
Lowe and Listrom, 1988[17]	17	A	62	93	93
Zincke et al, 1991[108]	148	A1, A2	—	93	—
Mean			62	92	83

Radical Prostatectomy

In patients with intermediate- and high-risk stage A cancer, there is a high likelihood of disease progression. Radical prostatectomy should be considered the option of choice for patients in this category who seek definitive treatment, because surgery is the treatment most likely to produce the best long-term benefits.

Paulson and associates reported on a series of 76 stage A patients treated by radical prostatectomy.[106] Eleven (61%) of 18 were upstaged to stage A2 or C on examination of the radical prostatectomy specimen. There were no postoperative complications. Although there was disease recurrence or progression in 10 patients, the overall disease-free survival rate was 85% at 5 years and 75% at 10 years. Middleton and associates, in a series of 66 patients with stage A2 cancer who underwent radical prostatectomy, reported an 87% rate of disease-free survival at 5 years and 82% at 10 years.[107]

Another study of 148 patients with clinical stage A disease who underwent prostatectomy was reported by Zincke and colleagues.[108] Twenty-five percent of stage A1 and 9% of stage A2 patients were found to have no disease on examination of prostatectomy specimens, indicating that TURP had removed all detectable tumors. However, 12% of stage A1 patients were found to have stage C (extracapsular) disease. The overall survival rate was 92.5% at 5 years and 73.2% at 10 years after operation. Only 1 (3%) of 32 patients with stage A1 disease had clinical progression at 4 years, and the number of patients showing a progression by PSA determination was identical. Rates of clinical progression were higher among stage A2 patients (8 of 116, or 14%), and if an increase in PSA level was used to detect recurrence, the number further grew to 37 (32%). Postoperative complications in the form of incontinence were observed in 9% of patients, and 1 patient (0.7%) died in the postoperative period. A summary of the results of radical prostatectomy for stage A cancer is presented in Table 49-5.[17,106–109]

On the basis of these results, and in view of the slow progression rate after diagnosis of stage A cancers, radical prostatectomy is a good management approach in younger patients (<70 years) with a long life expectancy and in patients with intermediate- and high-risk disease. The incidence of postsurgical complications such as incontinence is influenced by the extent of prior TURP, the patient's preoperative sphincteric functional status, and the quality of bladder neck reconstruction and degree of sphincteric preservation during radical prostatectomy. In this regard, preoperative urodynamic studies are helpful. We often do not recommend surgery in patients in whom any degree of incontinence persists after initial TURP, especially if preoperative urodynamic studies reveal lower than normal urethral closure pressures (which are usually >60 cm of water in healthy patients).

Radiotherapy

Radiotherapy for stage A cancers has included both interstitial and external beam irradiation. A summary of results is presented in Table 49-6.[110–115] Zagars and associates previously reported a 90% survival rate in 32 patients treated with external beam radiation.[116] Complications occurred in 23% of these patients. Bagshaw and associates reviewed results of external beam irradiation in patients with stage A1 and A2 lesions and found little difference in stage-specific survival after 5 and 10 years (92% and 78%, respectively).[112] However, survival rates

TABLE 49-6. *Radiotherapy in stage A prostate cancer*

Investigators	Treatment period	Patients	Stage	5-year disease-free survival rate (%)	10-year disease-free survival rate (%)
Perez et al, 1986[113]	1967–1980	41	A2	80	69
Hanks et al, 1987[114]	1973–1975	60	A1, A2	84	77
Rounsaville et al, 1987[110]	1968–1981	49	A1, A2	85	71
Rosen et al, 1984[111]	1968–1978	25	A1, A2	82	65
Bagshaw et al, 1990[112]	1956–1985	85	A1, A2	87	77
Zagars et al, 1993[115]	1966–1988	101	A2	92	72
Mean				83	68

declined more rapidly with time in stage A2 patients than in stage A1 patients after 10 years. Overall, posttreatment survival rates have been good, with combined survival rates ranging from 80% to 92% at 5 years and from 45% to 77% at 10 years.

Results with interstitial radiotherapy have also been good. Morton and associates reported an 88% disease-free survival rate, and Kuban and associates found a disease-free survival rate of 100% at 5 years and 90% at 10 years.[117,118] Radiotherapy appears to yield results similar to those of surgery in stage A patients for up to 10 years, although 15-year data are not available in all studies. Irradiation is certainly a viable alternative in patients who are experiencing complications from initial TURP and to avoid the complications of incontinence in some patients.

Hormonal Therapy

Hormonal therapy is recommended as an option for patients with stage A cancers if age or medical fitness precludes other therapies. Patients with a high risk of progression for their age who do not desire or cannot tolerate surgery or irradiation may consider hormonal ablation. Whether this treatment improves survival, however, has not been demonstrated for this clinical scenario. Those patients on surveillance whose tumors progress but who desire less aggressive therapy should be considered for hormonal therapy.

CONCLUSION

The management of stages T1a and T1b prostate cancer necessitates an understanding of their definition and natural history. Tumor grade and volume, residual disease, patient age, and risk of cancer progression must be carefully assessed before a particular therapy is recommended. Within these limitations, safe, effective, and appropriate therapy can be offered to patients with stage A prostate cancer.

REFERENCES

1. Whitmore WF Jr. Hormone therapy in prostate cancer. Am J Med 1956;21:697.
2. Stillwell TJ, Malek RS, Engen DE, Farrow GM. Incidental adenocarcinoma after open prostatic adenectomy. J Urol 1989;141:76.
3. Bergman RT, Turner R, Barnes RW, Hadley HL. Comparative analysis of one thousand consecutive cases of transurethral prostatic resection. J Urol 1955;74:535.
4. Bauer WC, McGavran MH, Carlin MR. Unsuspected carcinoma of the prostate in suprapubic prostatectomy specimens. Cancer 1960;13:370.
5. Smith GG, Woodruff LM. The development of cancer of the prostate after subtotal prostatectomy. J Urol 1950;63:1077.
6. Denton SE, Choy SH, Volk WL. Occult prostatic carcinoma diagnosed by the step section technique of the surgical specimen. J Urol 1965;93:296.
7. Sheldon CA, Williams RD, Fraley EE. Incidental carcinoma of the prostate: review of the literature and critical reappraisal of classification. J Urol 1980;124:626.
8. Scott R, Mutchnik DL, Laskowski TZ, Schmalhorst WR. Carcinoma of the prostate in elderly men: incidence, growth characteristics and clinical significance. J Urol 1969;101:602.
9. Johansson JE, Adami HO, Andersson SO, Bergstroem R, Krusemo UB, Kraaz W. Natural history of localized prostatic cancer: a population-based study in 223 untreated patients. Lancet 1989;1:799.
10. Jewett HJ. The present status of radical prostatectomy for stages A and B prostatic cancer. Urol Clin North Am 1975;2:105.
11. Cantrell BB, DeKlerk DP, Eggleston JC, Boitnott JK, Walsh PC. Pathological factors that influence prognosis in stage A prostatic cancer: the influence of extent versus grade. J Urol 1981;125:516.
12. Boxer RJ. Adenocarcinoma of the prostate gland. Urol Surv 1977;27:75.
13. Parfitt HE Jr, Smith JA Jr, Gliedman JB, Middleton RG. Accuracy of staging in A1 carcinoma of the prostate. Cancer 1983;51:2346.
14. Golimbu M, Schinella R, Morales P, Kurusu S. Difference in pathological characteristics and prognosis of clinical A2 prostatic cancer from A1 and B disease. J Urol 1978;119:618.
15. Bridges CH, Belville WD, Insalaco SJ, Buck AS. Stage A prostatic carcinoma and repeat transurethral resection: a reappraisal 5 years later. J Urol 1983;129:307.
16. Blute ML, Zincke H, Farrow GM. Long-term followup of young patients with stage A adenocarcinoma of the prostate. J Urol 1986;136:840.
17. Lowe AA, Listrom MB. Incidental carcinoma of the prostate: an analysis of the predictors of progression. J Urol 1988;140:1340.
18. Paulson DF, Robertson CN. The relevance of stage A malignancy in prostatic cancer. Acta Oncol 1991;30:227.
19. Epstein JI, Oesterling JE, Walsh PC. The volume and anatomical location of residual tumor in radical prostatectomy specimens removed for stage A1 prostate cancer. J Urol 1988;139:975.
20. Murphy GP, Natarajan N, Pontes JE, et al. The national survey of prostate cancer in the United States by the American College of Surgeons. J Urol 1982;127:928.
21. Moore GH, Lawshe B, Murphy J. Diagnosis of adenocarcinoma in transurethral resectates of the prostate gland. Am J Surg Pathol 1986;10:165.
22. Sonda LP, Grossman HB, MacGregor RJ, Gikas PW. Incidental adenocarcinoma of the prostate: the role of repeat transurethral resection in staging. Prostate 1984;5:141.
23. Voges GE, McNeal JE, Redwine EA, Freiha FS, Stamey TA. The predictive significance of substaging stage A prostate cancer (A1 versus A2) for volume and grade of total cancer in prostate. J Urol 1992;147:858.
24. Greene DR, Wheeler TM, Egawa S, Dunn JK, Scardino PT. A comparison of the morphological features of cancer arising in the transition zone and in the peripheral zone of the prostate. J Urol 1991;146:1069.
25. Greene DR, Wheeler TM, Egawa S, Weaver RP, Scardino PT. Relationship between clinical stage and histological zone of origin in early prostate cancer: morphometric analysis. Br J Urol 1991;68:499.
26. Lee F, Gray JM, McLeary RD, et al. Transrectal ultrasound in the diagnosis of prostate cancer: location, echogenicity, histopathology, and staging. Prostate 1985;7:114.
27. Neerhut GJ, Wheeler TM, Dunn JK, et al. Residual tumor after TUR: pathologic features of stage A prostate cancer in the transurethral and radical prostatectomy specimens. J Urol 1988;139:315A.
28. McNeal JE, Price HM, Redwine EA, Freiha FS, Stamey TA. Stage A versus stage B adenocarcinoma of the prostate: morphological comparison and biological significance. J Urol 1988;139:61.
29. Christensen WN, Partin AW, Walsh PC, Epstein JI. Pathologic findings in clinical stage A2 prostate cancer: relation of tumor volume, grade and location to pathological stage. Cancer 1990;65:1021.
30. McNeal JE, Redwine EA, Freiha FS, Stamey TA. Zonal distribution of prostatic adenocarcinoma: correlation with histologic pattern and direction of spread. Am J Surg Pathol 1988;12:897.
31. Terris MK, McNeal JE, Stamey TA. Transrectal ultrasound imaging and ultrasound guided prostate biopsies in the detection of residual carcinoma in clinical stage A carcinoma of the prostate. J Urol 1992;147:864.
32. Epstein JI, Cho KR, Quinn BD. Relationship of severe dysplasia to stage A (incidental) adenocarcinoma of the prostate. Cancer 1990;65:2321.
33. Rich AR. On the frequency of occurrence of occult carcinoma of the prostate. J Urol 1935;33:215.
34. Moore RA. The morphology of small prostatic carcinoma. J Urol 1935;33:224.
35. Hanash KA, Utz D, Cook EN, Taylor WF, Titus JL. Carcinoma of the prostate: a 15 year follow-up. J Urol 1972;107:450.

36. Khalifa NM, Jarman WD. A study of 48 cases of incidental carcinoma of the prostate followed 10 years or longer. J Urol 1976;116:329.
37. Beyon LL, Bussutil A, Newsam JE, Chisholm GD. Incidental carcinoma of the prostate: selection for deferred treatment. Br J Urol 1983; 55:733.
38. Epstein JI, Paull G, Eggleston JC, Walsh PC. Prognosis of untreated stage A-1 prostate carcinoma: a study of 94 cases with extended follow-up. J Urol 1986;136:837.
39. Thompson IM, Zeidman EJ. Extended follow-up of stage A1 carcinoma of prostate. Urology 1989;33:455.
40. Roy CR, Horne D, Raife M, Pienkos E. Incidental carcinoma of prostate: long-term follow-up. Urology 1990;36:210.
41. Zhang G, Wasserman NF, Sidi AA, Reinberg Y, Reddy PK. Long-term results after expectant management of stage A1 prostatic cancer. J Urol 1991;146:99.
42. Donohue RE, Pfister RR, Wergel JW, Stonington OG. Pelvic lymph adenectomy in stage A prostatic cancer. Urology 1977;9:273.
43. Whitmore WF Jr. Natural history of low-state prostatic cancer and the impact of early detection. Urol Clin North Am 1990;17:689.
44. McMillen SM, Wettlaufer JN. The role of repeat transurethral biopsy in stage A carcinoma of the prostate. J Urol 1976;116:759.
45. Carroll PR, Leitner TC, Yen TS, Watson RA, Williams RD. Incidental carcinoma of the prostate: significance of staging transurethral resection. Urology 1985;133:811.
46. Drago JR, Badalament RA. Prostatic carcinoma: an overview. In: Crawford ED, Das S, eds. Current genitourinary cancer surgery. Philadelphia: Lea & Febiger, 1990:148.
47. Kopper B, Dhom G, Schwaiger R, Ziegler M. Staging of incidental carcinoma of the prostate by diagnostic secondary transurethral resection. J Urol 1984;131:241A. Abstract 550.
48. Zhang G, Wasserman NF, Kapoor DA, Smiley DG, Reddy PK. Early detection of local progressive disease from stage A1 prostate cancer (CAP) by transrectal ultrasonography (TRUS). J Urol 1991;145:215A. Abstract 9.
49. Lowe BA, Barry JM. The predictive accuracy of staging transurethral resection of the prostate in the management of stage A cancer of the prostate: a comparative evaluation. J Urol 1990;143:1142.
50. Larsen MP, Carter HB, Epstein JI. Can stage A1 tumor extent be predicted by transurethral resection tumor volume, percent or grade? A study of 64 stage A1 radical prostatectomies with comparison to prostates removed for stages A2 and B disease. J Urol 1991;146:1059.
51. Sheth S, Hamper UM, Walsh PC, Holtz PM, Epstein JI. Stage A adenocarcinoma of the prostate: transrectal US and sonographic-pathologic correlation. Radiology 1991;179:35.
52. Shinohara K, Wheeler TM, Scardino PT. The appearance of prostate cancer on transrectal ultrasonography: correlation of imaging and pathological examinations. J Urol 1989;142:76.
53. Egawa S, Greene DR, Flanagan WF, Wheeler TM, Scardino PT. Transrectal ultrasonography in stage A prostate cancer: detection of residual tumor after transurethral resection of the prostate. J Urol 1991;146:366.
54. Agatstein EH, Hernandez FJ, Layfield LJ, Smith RB, deKernion JB. Use of fine needle aspiration for detection of stage A prostatic carcinoma before transurethral resection of the prostate: a clinical trial. J Urol 1987;138:551.
55. Coplen DE, Andriole GL, Yuan JJ, Catalona WJ. The ability of systematic transrectal ultrasound guided biopsy to detect prostate cancer in men with the clinical diagnosis of benign prostatic hyperplasia. J Urol 1991;146:75.
56. Lilja H. A kallikrein-like serine protease in prostatic fluid cleaves the predominant seminal vesicle protein. J Clin Invest 1985;76:1899.
57. Wang MC, Valenzuela LA, Murphy GP, Chu TM. Purification of a human prostate specific antigen. Invest Urol 1979;17:159.
58. Catalona WJ, Smith DS, Ratliff TC, et al. Measurement of prostate specific antigen in serum as a screening test for prostate cancer. N Engl J Med 1991;324:1156.
59. Brawer MK, Chetner MP, Beatie J, Buchner DM, Vessella RL, Lange PH. Screening for prostatic carcinoma with prostate specific antigen. J Urol 1992;147:841.
60. Labrie F, Dupont A, Suburu R, et al. Serum prostate specific antigen as pre-screening test for prostate cancer. J Urol 1992;147:846.
61. Catalona WJ, Smith DS, Ratliff TL, Basler JW. Detection of organ-confined prostate cancer is increased through prostate-specific antigen-based screening. JAMA 1993;270:948.
62. McConnell JD, Barry MJ, Bruskewitz RC. Benign prostatic hyperplasia: diagnosis and treatment. Agency for Health Care Policy and Research Clinical Practice Guideline 1994;8:1.
63. Partin AW, Carter HB, Chan DW, et al. Prostate specific antigen in the staging of localized prostate cancer: influence of tumor differentiation, tumor volume and benign hyperplasia. J Urol 1990;143:747.
64. Lange PH, Ercole CJ, Lightner DJ, Fraley EE, Vessella R. The value of serum prostate specific antigen determinations before and after radical prostatectomy. J Urol 1989;141:873.
65. Hudson MA, Bahnson RR, Catalona WJ. Clinical use of prostate specific antigen in patients with prostate cancer. J Urol 1989;142:1011.
66. Bostwick DG, Cooner WH, Denis L, Jones GW, Scardino PT, Murphy GP. The association of benign prostatic hyperplasia and cancer of the prostate. Cancer 1992;70:291.
67. Monda JM, Barry MJ, Oesterling JE. Prostate specific antigen cannot distinguish stage T1a (A1) prostate cancer from benign prostatic hyperplasia. J Urol 1994;151:1291.
68. Carter HB, Partin AW, Epstein JI, Chan DW, Walsh PC. The relationship of prostate specific antigen levels and residual tumor volume in stage A prostate cancer. J Urol 1990;144:1167.
69. Babaian RJ, Camps JL, Frangos DN, et al. Monoclonal prostate specific antigen in untreated prostate cancer. Cancer 1991;67:2200.
70. Oesterling JE, Cooner WH, Jacobsen SJ, Guess HA, Lieber MM. Influence of patient age on the serum prostate specific antigen concentration. Urol Clin North Am 1993;4:671.
71. Benson MC, Wong IS, Pantuck A, et al. Prostate specific antigen density: a means of distinguishing benign prostatic hypertrophy and prostate cancer. J Urol 1992;147:815.
72. Shinohara K, Wolf JS, Narayan P, Carroll PR. Comparison of prostate specific antigen with prostate specific antigen density for 3 clinical applications. J Urol 1994;152:120.
73. Bazinet M, Meshref AW, Trudel C, et al. Prospective evaluation of prostate-specific antigen density and systematic biopsies for early detection of prostatic carcinoma. Urology 1994;43:44.
74. Cooner WH. Prostate cancer. J Urol 1994;151:103. Editorial.
75. Carter HB, Pearson JD, Metter J, et al. Longitudinal elevation of prostate-specific antigen levels in men with and without prostate disease. JAMA 1992;267:2215.
76. Carter HB, Pearson JD. PSA velocity for the diagnosis of early prostate cancer: a new concept. Urol Clin North Am 1993;20:665.
77. Stenman UH, Leinonen J, Alfthan H, Rannikko S, Tuhkanen K, Alfthan O. A complex between prostate-specific antigen and alpha 1 antichymotrypsin is the major form of prostate-specific antigen in serum of patients with prostatic cancer: assay of the complex improves clinical sensitivity for cancer. Cancer Res 1991;51:222.
78. Lilja J, Cockett AT, Abrahamsson PA. Prostate specific antigen predominantly forms a complex with alpha 1 antichymotrypsin in blood: implications for procedures to measure prostate specific antigen in serum. Cancer 1992;70:230.
79. Christensson A, Bjork T, Nilsson O, et al. Serum prostate specific antigen complexed to alpha 1 antichymotrypsin as an indicator of prostate cancer. J Urol 1993;150:100.
80. Zetterberg A, Esposti PL. Prognostic significance of nuclear DNA levels in prostatic carcinoma. Scand J Urol Nephrol 1980;55:53.
81. Friedlander ML, Hedley DW, Taylor IW. Clinical and biological significance of aneuploidy in human tumours. J Clin Pathol 1984;37: 961.
82. Stephenson RA, James BC, Gay H, Fair WR, Whitmore WF Jr, Melamed MR. Flow cytometry of prostate cancer: relationship of DNA content to survival. Cancer Res 1987;47:2504.
83. McIntire TL, Murphy WM, Coon JS, et al. The prognostic value of DNA ploidy combined with histologic substaging for incidental carcinoma of the prostate gland. Am J Clin Pathol 1988;89:370.
84. Koss LG, Bogdan C, Herz F, Wersto RP. Flow cytometric measurements of DNA and other cell components in human tumors: a critical appraisal. Hum Pathol 1989;20:528.
85. Peehl DM. Oncogenes in prostate cancer: an update. Cancer 1993; 71(Suppl 3):1159.
86. Bookstein R, Allred DC. Recessive oncogenes. Cancer 1993;71:1179.
87. Collins VP, Kunimi K, Bergerheim U, Ekman P. Molecular genetics and human prostatic carcinoma. Acta Oncol 1991;30:181.
88. Isaacs WB, Carter BS. Genetic changes associated with prostate cancer in humans. Cancer Surv 1991;11:15.
89. Kuhn EJ, Kurnot RA, Sesterhenn IA, Chang EH, Moul JW. Expres-

sion of the c-erbB-2 (HER-2/neu) oncoprotein in human prostatic carcinoma. J Urol 1993;150:1427.
90. Mellon K, Thompson S, Charlton RG. P53, c-erbB-2 and the epidermal growth factor receptor in the benign and malignant prostate. J Urol 1992;147:496.
91. Thompson TC, Truong LD, Timme TL, et al. Transforming growth factor beta 1 as a biomarker for prostate cancer. J Cell Biochem 1992; 16H:54.
92. Van Veldhuizen PJ, Sadasivan R, Cherian R, Dwyer T, Stephens RL. P53 expression in incidental prostatic cancer. Am J Med Sci 1993; 305:275.
93. Moskovitz B, Nitecki A, Richter LD. Cancer of the prostate: is there a need for aggressive treatment? Urol Int 1987;42:49.
94. Handley R, Carr TW, Travis D, Powell PH, Hall RR. Deferred treatment for prostate cancer. Br J Urol 1988;62:249.
95. Jones GW. Prospective, conservative management of localized prostate cancer. Cancer 1992;70:307.
96. Orestano F. Problems of the wait-and-see policy in incidental carcinoma of the prostate. In: Altwein JE, Faul P, Schneider W. eds. Incidental carcinoma of the prostate. New York: Springer-Verlag, 1991: 163.
97. Thompson IM. Observation alone in the management of localized prostate cancer: the natural history of untreated disease. Urology 1994; 43(Suppl 2):41.
98. Goodman CM, Busuttil A, Chisholm GD. Age, and size and grade of tumour predict prognosis in incidentally diagnosed carcinoma of the prostate. Br J Urol 1988;62:576.
99. George NJ. Natural history of localised prostatic cancer managed by conservative therapy alone. Lancet 1988;1:494.
100. Whitmore WF Jr, Warner JA, Thompson IM Jr. Expectant management of localized prostatic cancer. Cancer 1991;67:1091.
101. Adolfsson J, Carstensen J, Lowhagen T. Deferred treatment in clinically localised prostatic carcinoma. Br J Urol 1992;69:183.
102. Chodak GW, Thisted RA, Gerber GS, et al. Results of conservative management of clinically localized prostate cancer. N Engl J Med 1994;330:242.
103. Stamey TA, Kabalin JN, McNeal JE, et al. Prostate specific antigen in the diagnosis and treatment of adenocarcinoma of the prostate. II. Radical prostatectomy treated patients. J Urol 1989;141:1076.
104. Wolf JS Jr, Shinohara K, Carroll P, Narayan P. Improved prostate cancer staging: transrectal ultrasonography plus prostate specific antigen formula. J Urol 1992;147:292A. Abstract 318.
105. Wolf JS Jr, Shinohara K, Carroll P, Narayan P. Prostate cancer staging: accuracy of transrectal ultrasound enhanced by prostate specific antigen. Br J Urol 1992;70:534.
106. Paulson DF, Robertson JE, Daubert LM. Radical prostatectomy in stage A adenocarcinoma: long-term results. J Urol 1988;140:535.
107. Middleton RG, Smith JA Jr, Melzer RB, Hamilton PE. Patient survival and local recurrence rate following radical prostatectomy for prostatic carcinoma. J Urol 1986;136:422.
108. Zincke H, Blute ML, Fallen MJ, Farrow GM. Radical prostatectomy for stage A adenocarcinoma of the prostate: staging errors and their implications for treatment recommendations and disease outcome. J Urol 1991;146:1053.
109. Partin AW, Pound CR, Clemens JQ, Epstein JI, Walsh PC. Serum PSA after anatomic radical prostatectomy: the Johns Hopkins experience after 10 years. Urol Clin North Am 1993;20:713.
110. Rounsaville MC, Green JP, Vaeth JM, Purdon RP, Heltzel MM. Prostatic carcinoma: limited field irradiation. Int J Radiat Oncol Biol Phys 1987;13:1013.
111. Rosen EM, Cassady JR, Connolly J, Chaffey JT. Radiotherapy for localized prostate carcinoma. Int J Radiat Oncol Biol Phys 1984;10: 2201.
112. Bagshaw MA, Cox RS, Ramback JE. Radiation therapy for localized prostate cancer: justification by long-term follow-up. Urol Clin North Am 1990;17:787.
113. Perez AA, Pilepich MV, Zivnuska F. Tumor control in definitive irradiation of localized carcinoma of the prostate. Int J Radiat Oncol Biol Phys 1986;12:523.
114. Hanks GE. A ten year follow-up of 682 patients treated for prostate cancer with radiation therapy in the United States. Int J Radiat Oncol Biol Phys 1987;13:499.
115. Zagars GK, von Eschenbach AC, Ayala AG. Prognostic factors in prostate cancer: analysis of 874 patients treated with radiation therapy. Cancer 1993;72:1709.
116. Zagars GK, von Eschenbach AC, Johnson DE, Oswald MJ. The role of radiation therapy in stages A and B adenocarcinoma of the prostate. Int J Radiat Oncol Biol Phys 1988;14:701.
117. Morton JD, Peschel RE. Iodine-125 implants versus external beam therapy for stages A2, B, and C prostate cancer. Int J Radiat Oncol Biol Phys 1988;14:1153.
118. Kuban DA, El-Mahdi AM, Schellhammer PF. I-125 interstitial implantation for prostate cancer: what have we learned 10 years later? Cancer 1989;63:2415.

Principles and Practice of Genitourinary Oncology, edited by Derek Raghavan, Howard I. Scher, Steven A. Leibel, and Paul H. Lange. Lippincott-Raven Publishers, Philadelphia, © 1997.

CHAPTER 50

Management of Stage B (T1c-T2) Prostate Cancer

50.1 Surgical Management of Localized Prostate Cancer

Alan W. Partin and Patrick C. Walsh

DEFINITION AND DIAGNOSIS OF STAGE T1C-T2 PROSTATE CANCER

The term *localized adenocarcinoma of the prostate* refers to prostate cancer that is clinically confined within the prostatic capsule with no evidence of metastatic disease. Stage T1c and T2 prostate cancers are detected by prostatic biopsy prompted either by an elevated level of serum prostate-specific antigen (PSA) alone (stage T1c) or by a suspicious digital rectal examination (DRE) regardless of serum PSA level (stage T2).[1] Stage T1c disease represents nonpalpable disease detected in a man with an elevated serum PSA level who has undergone systematic sextant biopsies of the prostate. Stage T2 disease can be further subdivided into three biologically meaningful substages based on local tumor burden: stage T2a represents palpable disease occupying less than one half of a lobe of the prostate; stage T2b represents palpable disease occupying more than one half of a lobe but not more than one lobe of the prostate; and stage T2c represents palpable disease occupying more than one lobe of the prostate, either as one contiguous area of induration or as two distinct nodules on separate lobes. These staging subclassifications are based on the TNM Classification of Prostate Cancer[2] and assume clinically node-negative (N0) and clinically organ-confined (M0) nonmetastatic prostate cancer.

Men with stage T1c or T2 prostate cancer are often diagnosed during routine physical examination or as part of a routine workup of prostatism and do not present with symptoms that can be associated with prostate cancer. Present algorithms for the early detection of prostate cancer recommend an annual DRE and serum PSA determination for all men older than 50 years of age; for African Americans and men with a family history of prostate cancer, this testing should begin at age 40. All men with suspicious prostatic lesions detected by DRE (stage T2) and all men with serum PSA levels greater than 4.0 ng/mL (stage T1c) should be referred to a urologist for consideration of prostatic biopsy. This biopsy not only confirms the diagnosis of prostatic adenocarcinoma but provides additional information regarding the histologic grade of the tumor.

After a diagnosis of prostate cancer has been confirmed pathologically, evaluation of the patient for evidence of regional metastases to the pelvic lymph nodes or systemic metastases to bone must be made. Metastatic deposits to the regional pelvic lymph nodes are often microscopic. The resolution of present radiologic staging techniques—lymphangiography, computed tomography (CT), and magnetic resonance imaging (MRI)—is not accurate enough to determine lymph node status, and these modalities are not recommended for preoperative evaluation of men with clinically localized stage T1c and T2 prostate cancer. Although the clinical utility and cost-effectiveness of radionuclide bone scans for preoperative staging of men with clinical stage T1c and T2 prostate cancer has been questioned,[3] we strongly feel that this study should be performed and serves three main purposes: (1) to evaluate for metastatic disease to bone, (2) as a baseline study with which to compare future postoperative bone scans, and (3) to screen for obstruction of the upper urinary tract.

NATURAL HISTORY OF UNTREATED PROSTATE CANCER

Cure of prostatic cancer by any means requires excision or ablation of all viable cancer cells. Clinical stage T1c and T2 prostate cancer is often pathologically confined to the gland at the time of diagnosis, and men with these lesions are ideal candidates for radical surgical cure.[4] Although the optimal management of men with clinical stage T1c and T2 prostate cancer has remained a controversial topic, there exist no studies that demonstrate that any treatment other than radical prostatectomy produces better control of the primary tumor. Recognizing the protracted clinical course of prostatic cancer in many patients, it is reasonable to ask whether any form of therapeutic intervention modifies the course of the disease. At the present time, there are no long-term results comparing active therapy to no treatment. However, insight into the natural history of the disease can be inferred from two sources: results of deferred treatment and longitudinal studies of serum PSA.

Results of Deferred Therapy

There have been several attempts to evaluate the natural history of prostate cancer based on cohorts of patients who were observed initially until progression and then treated actively. One of the most recent and widely quoted studies is that of Johansson and colleagues.[5] They collected 223 patients with stage T1 and T2 prostate cancer for expectant therapy with delayed treatment; from 1977 through 1979, only patients with well-differentiated tumors were included; from 1979 through the end of the recruitment period, patients with younger than 75 years of age who had moderately or poorly differentiated tumors were randomly allocated to receive local radiation or no treatment. (No data were given on the patients treated with radiation therapy). The researchers further stratified these patients to provide "a sub-group who met current indications for radical prostatectomy, namely those who were younger than 70 years of age and had an occult but diffusely spread T1 or palpable T2 highly or moderately differentiated tumor." The results are summarized in the first columns of Table 50.1-1.

TABLE 50.1-1. *Comparison of patient characteristics and results in three series of men with prostate cancer**

Category	Johansson (all patients)	Johansson (patients <70 y)	Johns Hopkins (all patients)	Johns Hopkins (LN-negative patients)	Memorial (LN-negative patients)
Dates of study	3/77 to 2/84	3/77 to 2/84	6/75 to 12/87	6/75 to 12/87	1970 to 1985
Patients	223	58	561	501	679
Mean follow-up time in months (range)	123 (81–165)	Not given	75 (12–192)	74 (12–192)	97
Mean age	72	Not given	59	59	61
Stage					
T1	106 (47%)	Not given (all T1 or T2)	80 (14%)	75 (15%)	—
T2	117 (53%)		481 (86%)	476 (85%)	T2 590 (87%)
T3	—		—	—	T3 87 (13%)
Grade†					
Low (I)	148 (66%)	58 (100%)†	60 (11%)	57 (12%)	249 (37%)
Moderate (II)	66 (30%)		367 (70%)	343 (72%)	362 (53%)
High (III)	9 (4%)		103 (19%)	74 (16%)	41 (6%)
Patients with local progression					
T1	14		1	1	—
T2	36		23	20	44%
Total	50 (22%)	21 (36%)	24 (4%)	21 (4%)	
Patients with distant progression					
T1	12		5	3	—
T2	14		60	30	34%
Total	26 (12%)	7 (12%)	65 (12%)	33 (6.6%)	
Deaths from prostate cancer					
T1	9		1	1	—
T2	10		25	12	—
Total	19 (9%)	5 (9%)	26 (5%)	13 (3%)	
Actuarial 5-year PF, percent (95% CI)§	68 (61–75)	60 (47–73)	93 (89–94)	94 (91–96)	68
Actuarial 10-year PF, percent (95% CI)‖	53 (44–62)	50 (36–63)	69 (59–76)	79 (70–86)	44

CI, confidence intervals; *LN-negative,* no evidence of lymph node metastasis; *NS,* not significant; PF, likelihood of progression-free survival (i.e., free of local or distant recurrence).[12]

* Patients in the Johansson series[5] deferred therapy; patients in the Johns Hopkins series received staging pelvic lymphadenectomy followed, if negative, by radical prostatectomy; patients in the Memorial series[8] received interstitial radiotherapy with iodine-125.

† In the Johns Hopkins series, grading was based on Gleason score: low = Gleason score 2 to 4; moderate = Gleason score 5 to 6; high = Gleason score 7 to 10.

‡ Grade I/II.

§ Statistical comparisons of 5-year PF: Johns Hopkins (all patients) versus Johansson (all patients), $P < 0.001$; Johns Hopkins (all patients) versus Johansson (patients < 70 y), $P < 0.001$; Johns Hopkins (all patients) versus Johns Hopkins (LN-negative patients), NS.

‖ Statistical comparisons of 10-year PF: Johns Hopkins (all patients) versus Johansson (all patients), $P < 0.05$; Johns Hopkins (all patients) versus Johansson (patients < 70 y), $P < 0.05$; Johns Hopkins (all patients) versus Johns Hopkins (LN-negative patients), $P < 0.05$.

For comparison, we have included a series of 561 patients at The Johns Hopkins Hospital who were thought to be candidates for radical prostatectomy during the era 1975 to 1987.[12] Data are shown for all 561 patients who presented for radical prostatectomy and for the 501 patients who underwent surgery and had no evidence of lymph node metastases at staging pelvic lymphadenectomy (61 men were excluded from radical prostatectomy because of the finding of lymph node metastasis). From this comparison table, it is clear that the patients monitored by Johansson and colleagues were not comparable to those who underwent radical prostatectomy at The Johns Hopkins Hospital. They were older (average age of 72 years), one third had stage T1a disease (which is not a standard indication for radical prostatectomy in older men in the United States), and 66% had grade I tumors. Cytology was used for diagnosis in 50% of the cases, but most urologists in the United States would not perform a radical prostatectomy on the basis of a grade I cytology result without further confirmation of the presence of cancer. Another institution from Scandinavia has recently abandoned cytologic diagnosis in favor of core biopsy, because in their early experience with radical prostatectomy two patients were mistakenly operated on because of false-positive cytologic results. It is possible, then, that the series of Johansson and coworkers included a number of patients who did not have cancer. Furthermore, only 4% of the patients in that series had high-grade disease, compared with 19% in the Johns Hopkins series, which is more typical for patients with localized prostate cancer in the United States. The group of patients selected by Johansson and associates cannot be considered typical of men in the United States who are subjected to radical prostatectomy or radiation for the treatment of localized disease.

Johansson and colleagues also designated their study subjects as a group of "untreated" patients. This is misleading. By 10 years, about 50% of the patients had developed progression, and 84% of these men had undergone orchiectomy or treatment with estrogens. The progression rates and death rates from prostate cancer were probably even higher than those presented. One patient who "demonstrated no evidence of disease progression before death" was found at autopsy to have died of prostate cancer. Thus, it does not appear that the authors provided a critical analysis of progression or cause of death. Overall, 13% of the men in the study died of prostate cancer within 10 years. These results are not too dissimilar from those of Whitmore and associates results with expectant management, again of a very highly selected group of patients.[7] In that series, 27% of the patients who were observed 10 years or longer died of cancer and the disease progressed in 82%. As discussed later in this chapter, we believe that death rates at 10 years do not measure the efficacy of radical prostatectomy but rather reflect the number of men who presented with incurable disease and were needlessly subjected to treatment. Cancer-specific death rates at 15 and 20 years are more informative; comparative information on the short term must rely on quantitative end points such as elevation of serum PSA or evidence of metastasis on bone scan.

The study of Johansson and associates represents a well-selected group of patients, some of whom may not have had cancer and most of whom would not have been subjected to radical prostatectomy in the United States. Nevertheless, 47% of those patients had progression within 10 years. This progression rate is significantly higher than that found in the Johns Hopkins series, which contained patients with higher-grade and higher-stage tumors ($P < 0.05$). Johansson and colleagues have claimed that further follow-up would not increase the cancer-specific death rate. That may be true in a series in which the average age of the patients is 72, but it is not true in the series at Johns Hopkins, in which the average age was 59.

Also on Table 50.1-1, we have included data from the Memorial Sloan-Kettering Institute series of patients who received interstitial radiotherapy with iodine-125.[8] After 10 years, the disease of 56% of patients had progressed. Even in the most favorable subset of patients, the results were not good: at 10 years, metastases had developed in 20% of the node-negative stage T2 patients and in 30% of the patients with grade I disease. The authors stated, "These data suggest that the existence and regrowth of local residual disease in localized prostate cancer promotes an enhanced spread of metastatic disease, and that early and complete eradication of the primary tumor is required if long-term cure is to be achieved." This may be the most representative group of "untreated" patients yet reported for comparison with patients undergoing radical prostatectomy.

In patients who received inadequate interstitial radiotherapy with iodine-125, long-term follow-up has shown that local persistence of cancer is associated with progression to metastatic disease and death. This is consistent with the modern understanding of tumor biology and heterogeneity, in which progression beyond the organ is associated with dedifferentiation of the tumor and the proliferation of hormone-resistant cells that render the tumor incurable.

Chodak and colleagues[9] summarized the results of six nonrandomized studies totaling more than 800 men who were treated conservatively with observation and delayed hormonal therapy for clinically localized prostate cancer. Actuarial survival statistics demonstrated that grade was the most significant variable in predicting survival. Eighty-one percent of patients with grade I, 58% of those with grade II, and only 26% of those with grade III tumors demonstrating metastasis-free survival at 10 years. These studies and the summary presented by Chodak and colleagues[9] have been criticized severely for selection bias. The study by Whitmore and associates[7] consisted of 65 handpicked men who were selected for conservative management during a 40-year period. Johansson and colleagues[5] excluded 83 of 306 patients for their handpicked series. Moskowitz and colleagues[10] excluded 38% of the men in their study, and Jones[11] reported on only 233 of 312 men who underwent observation for clinically localized prostate cancer. As further evidence of selection bias in Chodak and colleague's meta-analysis, almost 60% of the men overall had grade I tumors, compared with only 11% in a large, single-institution study of almost 1000 men treated with radical prostatectomy for clinically localized disease.[12]

Almost 80% of patients with clinically localized prostate cancer in nonhandpicked series, present with grade II disease, and of this group, almost 80% have either clinical stage T1c or T2 disease.[12] Within the analysis of Chodak and associates, 42% of the men with grade II disease who were followed conservatively developed metastatic disease at 10 years, and 70% at 15 years. These progression statistics, although skewed by favorable selection bias within the individual studies, demonstrate the best data to date documenting the natural history of untreated clinical stage T1c and T2 prostate cancer. We believe that this high failure rate for conservative therapy justifies radical prostatectomy as the treatment of choice for men with clinically localized prostate cancer who are otherwise healthy and have a life expectancy or 10 to 15 years or longer.

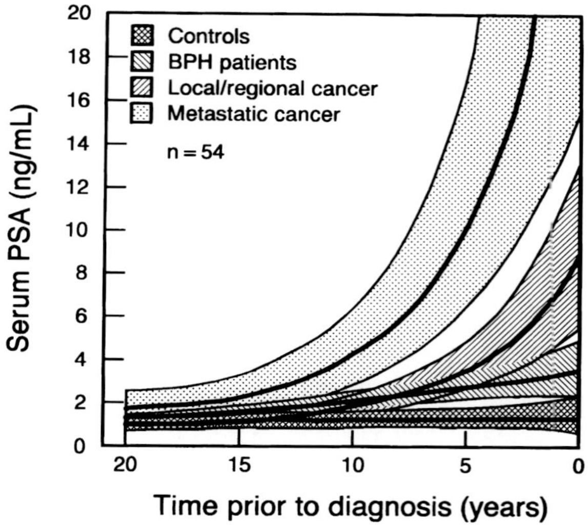

FIG. 50.1-1. Average prostate-specific antigen (PSA) velocity curves with 95% confidence intervals as a function of years before the diagnosis of the various prostatic disease states: controls, benign prostatic hyperplasia (BPH), local or regional cancer, and metastatic cancer. (Modified from Carter HB, Pearson JD. PSA velocity for the diagnosis of early prostate cancer: a new concept. Urol Clin North Am 1993;20:665, with permission.)

Longitudinal Studies of Serum Prostate-Specific Antigen

Insight into the natural history of untreated prostate cancer can also be obtained from longitudinal studies of serum PSA. Carter and colleagues evaluated serum PSA in men with normal prostates, benign prostatic hyperplasia, local or regional prostate cancer, or metastatic prostate cancer.[13,14] These patients were selected from the Baltimore Longitudinal Study of Aging, which is an ongoing, prospective aging study of the National Institute of Aging, Bethesda, Maryland. Carter and associates[13] evaluated the changes in serum PSA in these men during an average of 17 years before diagnosis. Fifteen years before diagnosis, men with metastatic prostate cancer had serum PSA levels significantly greater than those of men in any of the other three groups. In addition, the yearly rate of change of PSA (PSA velocity) in these patients was also significantly greater (Fig. 50.1-1); at an average of 9 years before the diagnosis of metastatic disease, PSA levels were increasing exponentially.[13] These data suggest that men with metastatic disease already have advanced disease 10 years before diagnosis and that death rates within the first decade after the diagnosis of prostate cancer do not measure the efficacy of any form of treatment. Rather, they reflect the number of patients with advanced disease at diagnosis who were subjected needlessly to treatment.

SELECTION OF CANDIDATES FOR RADICAL PROSTATECTOMY

The goal of radical prostatectomy should be the cure of prostatic cancer in patients who will live long enough to benefit from cure. First and foremost, the patient should be young and healthy enough to have a 10- to 20-year life expectancy. Studies of conservative therapy in men with localized prostatic cancer have demonstrated that 50% to 75% develop progression and 13% to 20% die of their disease during the first 10 years after diagnosis.[9] Although many patients require hormonal therapy or radiation therapy for palliation, radical prostatectomy is not necessary for men with a life expectancy shorter than one decade. In addition, in men older than 70 years of age, the disease is often pathologically more advanced than anticipated,[15] and postoperative impotence and incontinence are more common.

For patients who are young and healthy, the next important question is whether the disease has been detected at a time when cure is possible. In recent years, more men have been diagnosed at an earlier, curable stage. In the patient care evaluation studies of the American College of Surgeons, 43% of all staged patients with prostate cancer in 1974 were at stage T3 or T4, compared with only 33% in 1990.[16] With the use of serum PSA for early diagnosis of prostate cancer, it can be anticipated that more cancers will be detected at an earlier clinical stage.[17]

The ideal candidates for radical prostatectomy are patients with T1c or T2 disease. The combination of DRE, Gleason score, and PSA level is very useful in determining which patients are likely to have organ-confined disease and to benefit most from radical prostatectomy.[18] Because the expression of PSA is inversely related to the Gleason score (i.e., tumors that are more poorly differentiated produce less PSA per gram of tissue)[19] and because larger tumors are more likely to contain poorly differentiated disease, the Gleason score, clinical stage, and serum PSA level must be known to predict pathologic stage (Tables 50.1-2 and 50.1-3). For example, for a patient with stage T2b disease and a PSA concentration lower than 4 ng/mL, the likelihood of having organ-confined cancer is 67% if the tumor Gleason score is 5 but 31% if it is 8. For a patient with stage T2b disease but a PSA level of 4 to 10 ng/mL, the likelihood of having organ-confined cancer is 56% if the Gleason score is 5 and 22% if it is 8. Regardless of Gleason score, patients with T2b disease who present with PSA levels higher than 20 ng/mL have a likelihood of organ-confined disease of 1% to 11%.[18]

Patients with clinical stage T3 disease are not ideal candidates for radical prostatectomy. However, in a small number of patients with low-grade disease who have minimal extension beyond the prostate, cure is possible. Younger men who fall into this category may be considered candidates for radical prostatectomy.

The clinician must integrate these estimates of pathologic stage with the age of the patient. If the odds for organ-confined disease are not good and the patient is older, we encourage the patient to pursue palliation with external beam radiotherapy or hormonal therapy. In younger patients, however, it seems reasonable to offer radical prostatectomy even if the chances of organ-confined cancer are not great. With modern surgical techniques, the morbidity of radical prostatectomy is similar to that of external beam radiotherapy, and many young patients desire the chance to be cured.

There is increasing evidence that prostate cancers detected by PSA determination (i.e., stage T1c tumors) are most often significant cancers.[17,20,21] If an insignificant cancer is defined as a tumor volume of less than 0.2 cc, 89% of cancers detected by determination of a PSA level greater than 4.0 ng/mL would

TABLE 50.1-2. *Multivariate logistic regression analysis for prediction of pathologic stage by level of prostate-specific antigen (PSA), Gleason score, and TNM: clinical stage:* percentage likelihood of having organ-confined disease

Gleason score	PSA 0.0–4.0 ng/mL							PSA 4.1–10.0 ng/mL						
	T1a	T1b	T1c	T2a	T2b	T2c	T3a	T1a	T1b	T1c	T2a	T2b	T2c	T3a
2–4	100	85	92	88	76	82	—	100	78	82	83	67	71	—
5	100	78	81	81	67	73	—	100	70	71	73	56	64	43
6	100	68	69	72	54	60	42	100	53	59	62	44	48	33
7	—	54	55	61	41	46	—	100	39	43	51	32	37	26
8–10	—	—	—	48	31	—	—	—	32	31	39	22	25	12

Gleason score	PSA 10.1–20.0 ng/mL							PSA >20.0 ng/mL						
	T1a	T1b	T1c	T2a	T2b	T2c	T3a	T1a	T1b	T1c	T2a	T2b	T2c	T3a
2–4	100	—	—	61	52	—	—	—	—	33	20	7	—	—
5	100	49	55	58	43	37	26	—	—	24	32	—	3	—
6	—	36	41	44	28	37	19	—	—	22	14	1	4	5
7	—	24	24	36	19	24	14	—	—	7	18	4	5	3
8–10	—	11	—	29	14	15	9	—	—	3	3	—	2	2

be considered significant.[20] Based on these observations, Epstein and associates[20] have made recommendations to help clinicians determine the significance of a given PSA-detected prostate cancer (Table 50.1-4). It may be reasonable to observe some men with serial PSA measurements, DRE, and repeated biopsy if they fall into the favorable category, especially if they are older.

SURGICAL TECHNIQUE: AN ANATOMIC APPROACH

During the past 15 years, we have developed an anatomic approach to radical prostatectomy. This technique has been inappropriately termed a *nerve-sparing* technique. Nerve-sparing is only one of the important steps in the operative procedure. This technique emphasizes the principle of direct intraoperative visualization and identification of the extent of disease with wide excision of the neurovascular bundles if necessary.

Delineation of the anatomy of the dorsal vein complex enables this procedure to be performed in a bloodless field,[22] identification of the anatomy of the pelvic plexus makes it possible to preserve sexual function in most men,[23] and improved understanding of the anatomy of the striated urethral sphincter has reduced the frequency of postoperative incontinence. This procedure was developed based on sound anatomic and pathologic principles[24]: (1) the autonomic branches to the corpora cavernosa are located outside the capsule of the prostate and Denonvilliers' fascia; and (2) delineation of the anatomy of the cavernous nerves and their relation to the capsular vessels and prostatic fascia make it possible to obtain a wider margin of resection than is possible by blunt dissection[25] Previously during radical perineal prostatectomy or standard radical retropubic prostatectomy, the neurovascular bundles were not routinely resected.[26] Rather, they were divided and left in place during the procedure because their existence and significance was not appreciated. With reduced blood loss and improved understanding of the striated sphincter, it is also possible to perform a

TABLE 50.1-3. *Multivariate logistic regression analysis for prediction of pathologic stage by level of prostate-specific antigen (PSA), Gleason score, and TNM clinical stage: Percentage likelihood of having lymph nodes involved*

Gleason score	PSA 0.0–4.0 ng/mL							PSA 4.1–10.0 ng/mL						
	T1a	T1b	T1c	T2a	T2b	T2c	T3a	T1a	T1b	T1c	T2a	T2b	T2c	T3a
2–4	0	2	<1	1	2	4	—	0	2	1	1	2	5	—
5	0	4	1	2	4	8	—	0	4	1	2	5	10	8
6	0	8	2	3	9	17	15	0	9	2	4	11	19	16
7	—	15	2	7	18	31	—	0	18	3	8	20	34	28
8–10	—	—	—	13	32	—	—	—	30	5	15	35	53	30

Gleason score	PSA 10.1–20.0 ng/mL							PSA >20.0 ng/mL						
	T1a	T1b	T1c	T2a	T2b	T2c	T3a	T1a	T1b	T1c	T2a	T2b	T2c	T3a
2–4	0	—	—	1	3	—	—	—	—	6	2	7	—	—
5	0	5	3	2	6	13	11	—	—	9	3	—	29	—
6	—	11	4	5	13	22	20	—	—	8	9	18	53	31
7	—	21	7	9	24	39	35	—	—	24	11	44	62	55
8–10	—	41	—	17	40	59	54	—	—	41	35	76	73	65

TABLE 50.1-4. *Pathologic categorization of clinical stage T1c (nonpalpable, PSA-detected) prostate cancers*

INSIGNIFICANT CANCER

<3 cores involved with cancer *and*
No Gleason pattern 4 or 5 *and*
No single core with >50% involvement *and*
PSA density <0.1

Men with insignificant cancers can be observed with watchful waiting with serial DRE and PSA measurements and yearly biopsies, especially in older men.

SIGNIFICANT CANCER

≥3 cores involved with cancer *or*
Any Gleason pattern 4 or 5 *or*
Any single core with >50% involvement *or*
PSA density >0.1

Men with significant cancers should be offered definitive therapy according to age, life expectancy, and medical comorbidity.

DRE, digital rectal examination; *PSA*, prostate-specific antigen.

Modified from Epstein JI, Walsh PC, Carmichael M, Brendler CB. Pathologic and clinical findings to predict tumor extent of non-palpable (stage T1c) prostate cancer. JAMA 1994;271:368.

more precise dissection, to avoid injury to the pelvic floor musculature, and to achieve an accurate sutured vesicourethral anastomosis with coaptation of the mucosal surfaces, all of which have reduced the frequency of postoperative incontinence.[26]

RESULTS OF TREATMENT

A number of radical prostatectomy series have reported on the follow-up of men after surgery with respect to PSA level and pathologic stage of disease. Table 50.1-5 summarizes the demographic characteristics and outcomes of patients in these large series.

In the Johns Hopkins experience[12] of almost 1000 men who underwent radical prostatectomy, 11.2% were found to have an isolated elevation of serum PSA (>0.2 ng/mL, Hybritech, Tandem-R) as the only evidence of residual disease. The actuarial 5- and 10-year PSA progression-free likelihoods were 87% and 77%, respectively (Fig. 50.1-2). No patient who developed either local recurrence or distant metastases had an undetectable serum PSA level at the time of progression. At 10 years, actuarial data demonstrate that only 4% of men treated with radical prostatectomy for clinically localized disease had local recurrence, and 8% had distant metastases.

Two large radical prostatectomy series have confirmed our results (see Table 50.1-5). The Washington University series demonstrated actuarial PSA progression-free rates of 78% and 65% at 5 and 10 years, respectively, after radical prostatectomy in a cohort of almost 1000 men.[28] The Baylor group demonstrated PSA progression-free rates of 76% and 73% at 5 and 10 years, respectively, after radical prostatectomy in more than 500 men.[29] In three other large radical prostatectomy series, the long-term results were not as favorable. Researchers at the University of California at Los Angeles demonstrated PSA progression-free rates of 69% and 47% at 5 and 10 years, respectively, in a group of more than 600 men.[30] The Mayo Clinic series of more than 3000 men treated with radical prostatectomy demonstrated a 52% PSA progression-free rate at 10 years after surgery.[31] The Duke University series of 800 patients after radical perineal prostatectomy demonstrated 10-year actuarial progression-free survival rates (by PSA detection) of 70% if the disease was organ confined and 40% if the surgical margins were positive.[32] The differences in the results present by these large radical prostatectomy series may be explained by differences in surgical technique (retropubic versus perineal) and in patient selection.

At Johns Hopkins, the actuarial likelihood of an elevated

TABLE 50.1-5. *Comparison of patient characteristics and results in several radical prostatectomy series*

Institution	Investigators	Operation	Patients	Mean age (y)	Months follow-up (mean, range)	Percent T1 (%)	Percent T2 (%)	5-year PSA progression-free likelihood	10-year PSA progression-free likelihood
Johns Hopkins	Partin et al, 1993[12]	Retropubic	894	59 ± 6	53 (12–120)	17	83	87	77
Washington University	Catalona and Smith, 1994[28]	Retropubic	925	63 ± 7	28 (0–123)	21	79	78	65
Baylor University	Ohori et al, 1994[29]	Retropubic	500	63	36 (1–110)	22	78†	76	73
UCLA	Trapasso et al, 1994[30]	Retropubic	601	65	34* (12–237)	27	73	69	47
Duke University	Paulson et al, 1994[32]	Perineal	895	65	Not given	Not given	Not given	OC—85 SC—50 MP—40	OC—70 SC—40 MP—38
The Mayo Clinic	Zincke et al, 1994[31]	Retropubic	3,170	65 ± 4	60	7	93	70	52

PSA, prostate-specific antigen; *MP*, margin-positive; *OC*, organ-confined; *SC*, specimen-confined.
* Median.
† 4% Stage T3.

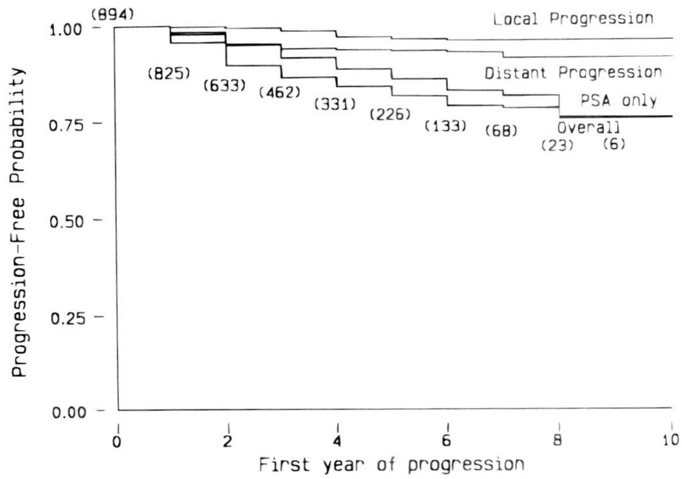

FIG. 50.1-2. Kaplan-Meier actuarial progression-free likelihood for overall progression, prostate-specific antigen (PSA) detectability only, local progression, and distant progression. Numbers in parentheses represent number of men in analysis at time interval. (Partin AW, Pound CR, Clemens JQ, Epstein JI, Walsh PC. Prostate-specific antigen after anatomic radical prostatectomy: the Johns Hopkins experience after ten years. Urol Clin North Am 1993; 20:713, with permission.)

serum PSA increased with increasing pathologic stage; the 10-year likelihood of freedom from PSA relapse was 85% for men with organ-confined disease, 82% with focal capsular penetration, 54% with established capsular penetration and Gleason score 2 to 6, 42% with established capsular penetration and Gleason score 7 to 10, and 43% with seminal vesicle involvement. No patient with evidence of lymph node metastasis had an undetectable serum PSA level at 10 years. Among the patients who had an isolated elevation of serum PSA level and subsequently underwent delayed radiotherapy to the prostatic bed, the PSA level fell to the undetectable range and remained there for at least 2 years in only 10%.

These data indicate that radical prostatectomy cures most men with organ-confined disease or with well- to moderately well-differentiated tumors that have penetrated the prostatic capsule to the extent at which it is possible to obtain a clear surgical margin. In men with capsular penetration and high-grade tumor or involvement of the seminal vesicles, cure is less likely. Cure is rarely, if ever, achieved in the presence of lymph nodal involvement.

SURGICAL COMPLICATIONS

The surgical complications of radical prostatectomy include bleeding, rectal injury, pulmonary embolus, and death from surgery.

Bleeding associated with radical retropubic prostatectomy has been greatly reduced by use of the anatomic studies of Reiner and Walsh,[22] and it is now possible to control bleeding, thereby reducing significant blood loss and improving exposure.[33] With the addition of autologous blood donations and the use of intraoperative clamps on the hypogastric arteries, transfusion of banked blood is necessary in only 2% of cases.[33]

Rectal injury is a rare complication, occurring in approximately 1% of cases.[34] If recognized intraoperatively, it can be repaired primarily without the need for a colostomy. In 1300 consecutive patients, there were 10 rectal injuries, and all were repaired primarily with no wound infections, pelvic abscesses, or rectourethral fistulae.[34]

Pulmonary embolus is the most significant postoperative complication that occurs after radical prostatectomy because of its associated mortality. Among 1300 consecutive patients undergoing radical prostatectomy at The Johns Hopkins Hospital, thromboembolic events occurred in 1.5%, and 2 patients (0.15%) died.[35]

QUALITY OF LIFE: CONTINENCE AND POTENCY

One of the most feared and disabling complications of radical prostatectomy is total urinary incontinence. The anatomic approach to radical prostatectomy has minimized urinary incontinence through several mechanisms: (1) precise anatomic dissection at the apex of the prostate in a bloodless surgical field; (2) preservation of the pelvic plexus and nerve branches that provide autonomic innervation to the striated urethral sphincter and smooth muscle complex; and (3) improved understanding of the striated urethral sphincter, which minimizes damage during ligation of the dorsal vein complex and division of its posterior components and enables an accurate reapproximation of the striated sphincter to the reconstructed bladder neck.[36]

After anatomic radical prostatectomy in the first 593 consecutive patients treated with radical prostatectomy in the Johns Hopkins series, complete urinary control was achieved in 92% and stress incontinence was present in 8%; 6% wore one or no pads per day, and stress incontinence was sufficient to require placement of an artificial sphincter in only 2 men (0.3%). No patient was totally incontinent.[4] Eighty-six percent of patients older than 70 years of age were completely dry. Although this decrease in continence rate did not reach statistical significance because of the small number of men older than age 70 (4%) in our series, we believe that this phenomenon is real. Continence was achieved in 94% of patients in whom both neurovascular bundles were preserved, in 92% of those with preservation of only one neurovascular bundle, and in 81% of those with excision of both neurovascular bundles; these differences did not reach statistical significance. There was no correlation between postoperative potency and urinary continence: 94% of potent patients and 90% of impotent patients were dry. These data suggest that anatomic factors other than preservation of autonomic innervation are primarily responsible for the improved urinary control associated with this approach to radical prostatectomy. Similar results have been reported from a number of other institutions.[37–39]

It is clear that the distal urethral sphincter mechanism is capable of maintaining passive urinary control in most but not all men. For the 8% of men in whom it is not sufficient, attempts at reconstruction of the bladder neck to provide an additional continence mechanism should be considered. Furthermore, because most of these patients have very mild problems, postoperative injection of collagen or autologous fat into the submucosa adjacent to the bladder neck may be all that is necessary to resolve this problem in the future.

Before the development of an anatomic approach to radical prostatectomy, almost all patients were rendered impotent by the operation. Because these patients had intact penile sensation and could achieve orgasm, injury to the pudendal nerve was not the reason for impotence. Rather, impotence arose from damage to the autonomic innervation to the corpora cavernosa. Before 1982, the exact anatomic location of the autonomic branches from the pelvic plexus to the corpora cavernosa was unknown. In that year, Walsh and Donker described the anatomy of the pelvic plexus and branches that innervate the corpora cavernosa and recommended minor modifications in the surgical procedure that could preserve potency.[23] It subsequently became clear that these nerves had typically been not excised with the specimen but merely cut and left in place. With further experience, we were able to demonstrate that it was possible to obtain a wider margin of excision than was previously possible by widely excising the nerves on one side without compromising sexual function in the majority of patients.[26]

We evaluated the recovery of sexual function in 600 consecutive patients aged 34 to 72 years who underwent an anatomic approach to radical prostatectomy between 1982 and 1988.[40] Of the 503 patients who were potent preoperatively and were monitored for a minimum of 18 months, 68% were potent postoperatively. Three factors were identified that correlated with the return of sexual function: age, clinical and pathologic stage of tumor, and surgical technique (preservation or excision of the neurovascular bundle) (Table 50.1-6). Sexual function was preserved in 91% of men younger than 50 years of age, in 75% of men aged 50 to 60 years, in 58% of men aged 60 to 70 years, and in 25% of men 70 years of age or older. Among men younger than 50 years of age, potency was similar in those who had both neurovascular bundles preserved and in those who had one neurovascular bundle widely excised. With advancing age (>50 years), sexual function was better in patients in whom both neurovascular bundles were preserved ($P < 0.05$). After adjustment for age, the relative risk of postoperative impotence was twofold greater if there was capsular penetration or seminal vesicle invasion ($P < 0.05$). For example, among patients aged 60 to 69 years with organ-confined cancer and preservation of both neurovascular bundles, 71% were potent; with preservation of both neurovascular bundles but involvement of the seminal vesicles, potency fell to 44%; and with wide excision of one neurovascular bundle and seminal vesicle invasion, potency fell to 17%.

TABLE 50.1-6. *Influence of age and preservation of the neurovascular bundles on retention of postoperative sexual function (percentage of patients retaining potency)*

		By status of neurovascular bundles	
Age (y)	Overall	Both intact	One excised
<50	91	90	91
50–60	75	82	58
60–70	58	69	47
>70	25	22	—

Data from Quinlan et al.: Sexual function following radical prostatectomy: Influence of preservation of neurovascular bundles. J Urol 1991;145:998.

Patients who have the best recovery of sexual function are those who are young (<50 years) and have organ-confined disease; these are also the patients who receive the most benefit from surgery. Successful preservation of sexual function after radical prostatectomy has been reported from a number of other institutions.[6,37,38,41–43] These data indicate that the return of sexual function in men older than 50 years of age is quantitatively related to preservation of autonomic innervation, along with other factors (e.g., vascular). In those men in whom it is necessary to excise the neurovascular bundle on one side, consideration in the future should be given to approaches that may restore autonomic function through nerve regeneration (e.g., partial excision of the bundle, cavernous nerve grafts).

COMPARISON WITH RADIOTHERAPY

Radiotherapy became popular as a treatment for localized prostate cancer when the morbidity associated with radical prostatectomy was greater than it is now. Enthusiasm for radiotherapy has declined in recent years because of decreased morbidity and because of uncertainty about the ability of irradiation to sterilize the lesion in younger men with localized disease.

Although overall survival rates appear to be equivalent in patients treated with radiotherapy and those treated with radical prostatectomy,[44] these rates are almost meaningless, for several reasons. First, almost all studies to date have been nonrandomized and have reported retrospective data from different institutions. Such data are not comparable, primarily because of differences in staging methodology. Overall, clinical stage has been determined primarily by DRE with variable ancillary diagnostic testing. The DRE is extremely subjective and comparisons of results from large, retrospective trials in which staging was done by many different physicians, including both urologists and radiotherapists, are unreliable. Urologists often understage borderline stage C lesions because "surgery is not done on stage C disease." Similarly, radiotherapists may overstage B lesions to solidify their recommendation of radiotherapy over surgery. On the other hand, radiotherapists are often referred patients who are not thought to be candidates for surgery because of the unfavorable grade or stage of their tumor. Overall survival rates are also of limited value if the follow-up is short, because most deaths occur from noncancer-related events.

Only one prospective trial has been reported in which patients with clinical stage T1b and T2 disease were randomly assigned to receive treatment with either radical prostatectomy or external beam radiotherapy.[45] Treatment failure was used as the end point for this study and was defined as either elevation of serum prostatic acid phosphatase on two consecutive follow-up examinations or the appearance of metastatic disease or parenchymal disease. The identification of cancer in the prostate on follow-up biopsy after irradiation did not signify treatment failure for purposes of evaluating relative treatment efficacy in this study. Using these criteria, 40% of men treated with external beam radiotherapy had failed treatment at 5 years, compared with only 10% of men undergoing radical prostatectomy. This study has been criticized because of flaws in design, execution, and reporting.[46] However, it is the only randomized study that has directly compared surgery with radiotherapy.

Because it is difficult to obtain meaningful data for comparison in the short term, interest has recently focused on two, more objective short-term end points in patients who have been treated with radiotherapy: evidence of recurrence on needle biopsy and elevation in serum PSA levels. Kabalin and associates[47] reported that multiple needle biopsies were positive in 16 of 17 patients with normal-feeling prostates 2 to 9 years after treatment with external beam radiotherapy. It is important to observe these patients prospectively to determine whether these positive biopsies predict subsequent clinical failure. Schellhammer and associates[48] reported that fewer than 10% of patients have undetectable serum PSA levels at 10 years after radiotherapy for localized prostate cancer. Therefore, in young men in whom durable long-term tumor-free survival is desired, radiotherapy in unlikely to be successful. On the other hand, the clinical progression-free survival rate at 10 years after irradiation was 65% for stage T1b, 40% for stage T2a, 35% for stages T2b or T2c, and 25% for stage T3 tumors. In older patients, if palliation of the local lesion is the major goal of treatment, radiotherapy may be suitable.

CONCLUSIONS

During the past decade, there have been a number of advances in the diagnosis and treatment of localized prostate cancer. Today, men are likely to be diagnosed at a younger age with earlier, curable disease. Men are also living longer; a man 65 to 70 years old has a 50% chance of living for another 15 years. In this review, we have emphasized that radical prostatectomy should be reserved for those patients who can be cured and who will probably live long enough to benefit from cure. These are also the patients who will have the best quality of life postoperatively.

Much of the progress in the technique of radical prostatectomy has been based on anatomic studies, by which the procedure has undergone a continuous evolution. Almost certainly, there will be further advances in anatomy and physiology that will improve the outcome of patients. At present, it is possible to cure most men with organ-confined cancer and many men with specimen-confined tumors. With the ability to perform wide excision of tumors, clinical rates of local recurrence are low, and most patients who fail treatment do so because of distant metastases. To improve the ability of radical prostatectomy to cure prostate cancer, diagnoses will have to be made at an earlier stage, before the cancer has escaped the prostate, or improved techniques for adjuvant chemotherapy or immunotherapy will have to be developed. Although the morbidity of radical prostatectomy is acceptable, simplified approaches to the management of stress incontinence must be formulated for the small minority of patients who develop this significant complication. Furthermore, with improved understanding of the physiology of penile erection, it may be possible to preserve or simply restore sexual function in almost every patient. With these developments, radical prostatectomy should maintain its well-deserved role in the cure of prostate cancer.

ACKNOWLEDGMENT

This work was supported by SPORE grant P50-CA58236-01 from the National Cancer Institute.

REFERENCES

1. Cooner WH, Mosely BR, Rutherford CL, et al. Prostate cancer detection in a clinical urological practice by ultrasonography, digital rectal examination and prostate specific antigen. J Urol 1990;143:1146.
2. Schroder FH, Hermanek P, Denis L, Fair WR, Gospodarowicz MK, Pavone-Macaluso M. The TNM classification of prostate cancer. Prostate Suppl 1992;4:129.
3. Bleustein DL, Bostwick DG, Bergstralh EJ, Oesterling JE. Eliminating the need for bilateral pelvic lymphadenectomy in select patients with prostate cancer. J Urol 1994;151:1315.
4. Morton RA, Steiner MS, Walsh PC. Cancer control following anatomical radical prostatectomy: an interim report. J Urol 1991;145:1197.
5. Johansson JE, Adami HO, Andersson SO, Bergstrom R, Holmberg L, Krusemo UB. High 10-year survival rate in patients with early, untreated prostatic cancer. JAMA 1992;267:2191.
6. Drago JR, Badalament RA, Nesbitt JA. Radical prostatectomy 1972–1987 single institutional experience: comparison of standard radical prostatectomy and nerve-sparing technique. Urology 1990;35:377.
7. Whitmore WF Jr, Warner JA, Thompson IM Jr. Expectant management of localized prostatic cancer. Cancer 1991;67:1091.
8. Fuks Z, Whitmore WF Jr, Liebel S, Nori D, Hilaris B. Local control is associated with decreased distant failure in early stage carcinoma of the prostate. Int J Radiat Oncol Biol Phys 1991;21:537.
9. Chodak GW, Thisted RA, Gerber GS, et al. Results of conservative management of clinically localized prostate cancer. N Engl J Med 1994;330:242.
10. Moskowitz B, Nitecki S, Richter LD. Cancer of the prostate: is there a need for aggressive treatment? Urol Int 1987;42:49.
11. Jones GW. Prospective, conservative management of localized prostate cancer. Cancer 1992;70(Suppl):307.
12. Partin AW, Pound CR, Clemens JQ, Epstein JI, Walsh PC. Prostate-specific antigen after anatomic radical prostatectomy: the Johns Hopkins experience after ten years. Urol Clin North Am 1993;20:713.
13. Carter HB, Pearson JD, Metter J, et al. Longitudinal evaluation of prostate-specific antigen levels in men with and without prostate disease. JAMA 1992;267:2215.
14. Carter HB, Morrell CH, Pearson JD, et al. Estimation of prostatic growth using serial prostate-specific antigen measurements in men with and without prostate disease. Cancer Res 1992;52:3323.
15. Alexander RB, Maguire MG, Epstein JI, Walsh PC. Pathological stage is higher in older men with clinical stage B1 adenocarcinoma of the prostate. J Urol 1990;141:880.
16. Mettlin C, Jones GW, Murphy GP. Trends in prostate cancer care in the United States, 1974–1990: observations from the patient care evaluation studies of the American College of Surgeons Commission on Cancer. CA Cancer J Clin 1993;43:83.
17. Catalona WJ, Smith DS, Ratliff TL, Basler JW. Detection of organ-confined prostate cancer is increased through prostate-specific antigen based screening. JAMA 1993;270:948.
18. Partin AW, Yoo JK, Carter HB, et al. The use of prostate-specific antigen, clinical stage and Gleason score to predict pathological stage in men with localized prostate cancer. J Urol 1993;150:110.
19. Partin AW, Carter HB, Chan DW, et al. Prostate-specific antigen in the staging of localized prostate cancer: influence of tumor differentiation, tumor volume and benign hyperplasia. J Urol 1990;143:747.
20. Epstein JI, Walsh PC, Carmichael M, Brendler CB. Pathologic and clinical findings to predict tumor extent of non-palpable (stage T1c) prostate cancer. JAMA 1994;271:368.

21. Stormont TJ, Farrow GM, Myers ML, et al. Clinical stage B0 or T1c prostate cancer: nonpalpable disease identified by elevated serum prostate-specific antigen concentration. Urology 1993;41:3.
22. Reiner WG, Walsh PC. An anatomical approach to the surgical management of the dorsal vein and Santorini's plexus during radical retropubic surgery. J Urol 1979;121:198.
23. Walsh PC, Donker PJ. Impotence following radical prostatectomy: insight into etiology and prevention. J Urol 1982;128:492.
24. Walsh PC, Lepor H, Eggleston JC. Radical prostatectomy with preservation of sexual function: anatomical and pathological considerations. Prostate 1983;4:473.
25. Walsh PC, Epstein JI, Lowe FC. Potency following radical prostatectomy with wide unilateral excision of the neurovascular bundle. J Urol 1983;138:823.
26. Walsh PC. Radical prostatectomy, preservation of sexual function, cancer control: the controversy. Urol Clin North Am 1987;14:663.
27. Steiner MS, Morton RA, Walsh PC. Impact of anatomical radical prostatectomy on urinary continence. J Urol 1991;145:512.
28. Catalona WJ, Smith DJ. Five-year tumor recurrence rates after anatomic radical retropubic prostatectomy for prostate cancer. J Urol 1994; 152:1837.
29. Ohori M, Goad JR, Wheeler TM, Eastmen JA, Thompson TC. Scardino PT. Can radical prostatectomy alter the progression of poorly differentiated prostate cancer? J Urol 1994;154:1818.
30. Trapasso JG, DeKernion JB, Smith RB, Dorey F. The incidence and significance of detectable levels of serum PSA after radical prostatectomy. J Urol 1994;152:1821.
31. Zincke H, Oesterling JE, Blute ML, Bergstralh EJ, Myers RP, Barett DM. Long-term (15 years) results after radical prostatectomy for clinically localized (stage T2c or lower) prostate cancer. J Urol 1994;152: 1850.
32. Paulson DF. Impact of radical prostatectomy in the management of clinically localized disease. J Urol 1994;152:1826.
33. Walsh PC. Radical retropubic prostatectomy. In: Walsh PC, Retik AB, Stamey TA, Vaughan ED Jr, eds. Campbell's urology, 6th ed. Philadelphia: WB Saunders, 1992:2865.
34. Borland N, Walsh PC. The management of rectal injury during radical retropubic prostatectomy. J Urol 1992;147:905.
35. Cisek LJ, Walsh PC. Thromboembolic complications following radical retropubic prostatectomy: influence of external pneumatic compression devices. Urology 1993;42:406.
36. Walsh PC, Quinlan DM, Morton RA, Steiner MS. Radical retropubic prostatectomy: improved anastomosis and urinary continence. Urol Clin North Am 1990;17:679.
37. Catalona WJ, Bigg SW. Nerve-sparing radical prostatectomy: evaluation of results after 250 patients. J Urol 1990;143:538.
38. Fowler JE Jr, Clayton M, Sharifi R, Mouli K, Ojeda L, Ray PS. Early experience with Walsh technique of radical retropubic prostatectomy. Urology 1987;29:242.
39. O'Donnell PD, Finan BF. Continence following nerve-sparing radical prostatectomy. J Urol 1989;142:1227.
40. Quinlan, Stutzman RE, Peters CA, Walsh PC, et al. Sexual function following radical prostatectomy: influence of preservation of neurovascular bundles. J Urol 1991;145:998.
41. Catalona WJ, Dresner ST. Nerve-sparing radical prostatectomy: extraprostatic tumor extension and preservation of erectile function. J Urol 1985;1149:1149.
42. Leandri P, Rossignol G, Gautier J-R, Ramon J. Radical retropubic prostatectomy: morbidity and quality of life. Experience with 620 consecutive cases. J Urol 1992;147:883.
43. Surya BV, Provet J, Dalbagni G, Johanson K-E, Brown J. Experience with potency preservation during radical prostatectomy. Urology 1988; 32:498.
44. Hanks GE. External beam radiation treatment for prostate cancer: still the gold standard. Oncology 1992;6:79.
45. Paulson DF, Lin GH, Hinshaw W, Stephan S. The Uro-Oncology Research Group: radical surgery versus radiotherapy for adenocarcinoma of the prostate. J Urol 1982;128:502.
46. Hanks GE. More on the Uro-Oncology Research Group report of radical surgery vs radiotherapy for adenocarcinoma of the prostate. Int J Radiat Oncol Biol Phys 1988;14:1053.
47. Kabalin JN, Hodge KK, McNeal JE, Freiha FS, Stamey TA. Identification of residual cancer in the prostate following radiation therapy: role of transrectal ultrasound guided biopsy and prostate specific antigen. J Urol 1989;142:326.
48. Schellhammer PF, El-Mahdi AM, Wright GL, Kolm P, Ragle R. Prostate-specific antigen to determine progression-free survival after radiation therapy for localized carcinoma of the prostate. Urology 1993;42: 13.

50.2 Radical Perineal Prostatectomy

David F. Paulson

Radical perineal prostatectomy is one of the two commonly accepted methodologies for surgical extirpation of the prostate. The operative procedure, once thought to be the ideal method for control of prostatic carcinoma, fell into disuse in the late 1960s and early 1970s, in part because of the belief that radical surgery was not a reasonable method for control of prostatic malignancy that was apparently organ confined and in part because of an increasing tendency of surgical training programs to provide only retropubic experience. Recently, it has become more acceptable to consider perineal prostatectomy as an equivalent method for surgical control of prostatic malignancy.

The perineum has long been recognized as the gateway to the prostate. In the late 1800s, surgeons began to describe perineal procedures for the management of both benign and malignant prostatic disease.[1] Gradually, over the next several decades, the perineal prostatectomy changed from a crude blunt dissection to a precise surgical exercise conducted under direct vision with hemostatic control, identification of local anatomic structures, and reconstruction of the urinary tract. Today, two surgical avenues for radical removal of the prostate exist: the radical perineal prostatectomy and the radical retropubic prostatectomy. These approaches seem to be equivalent in terms of cancer control.[2–4] Perineal prostatoseminal vesiculectomy has the advantage of providing a relatively avascular field, excellent exposure for reconstruction of the urethrovesical junction, and dependent postoperative drainage. Many surgeons have come to recognize that the elderly patient tolerates well the perineal approach, whereas retropubic prostatectomy is associated with delayed mobility, prolonged ileus, and restricted postoperative pulmonary function. The principal disadvantage of perineal prostatectomy is that it does not afford simultaneous exposure of the pelvic lymphatic drainage and determination of the presence or absence of lymph node extension. Two incisions therefore are necessary if the patient undergoing radical perineal prostatectomy is to have a preprostatectomy staging lymphadenectomy. Furthermore, although potency-preserving surgery can be accomplished by the perineal route, preservation of the periprostatic neurovascular plexus may be more difficult through the perineum than by the retropubic approach.

PATIENT SELECTION

Because surgical treatment of prostatic malignancy is considered appropriate only for patients with disease clinically confined to the prostate, preoperative staging maneuvers should be designed to ensure that that is the case. Patients are subjected to preoperative isotopic bone scanning to ensure that metastatic disease does not exist and also to provide a baseline against which future studies may be compared. Further, patients must have a serum acid phosphatase determination by colorimetric or enzymatic assay, with results within the normal range. Experience has indicated that patients whose serum acid phosphatase is abnormally elevated have an 85% probability of clinical failure at a distant site within 4 years after operative intervention. Finally, all reasonable efforts must be made to determine that the patient has no metastatic lymph node extension. This can be accomplished by staging pelvic lymphadenectomy through a lower abdominal incision or by laparoscopic surgery during an anesthesia before that needed for the perineal prostatectomy. Alternatively, this surgical staging can be accomplished under the same anesthesia.[5,6] However, studies have demonstrated that the probability of lymph node extension is so low in patients with nonpalpable disease whose prebiopsy serum concentration of prostate-specific antigen (PSA) is less than 20 ng/mL and whose Gleason sum is less than 7 that preoperative lymphadenectomy may be discarded and the patient may undergo radical perineal prostatectomy without physical assessment of the regional lymph nodes.[7–10]

PREOPERATIVE PREPARATION

The patient undergoes an osmotic mechanical bowel preparation the day before surgery, and nonabsorbable oral antibiotics are given the evening before surgery. On the morning of surgery, a neomycin enema is given 2 to 3 hours before the scheduled operative procedure. Broad-spectrum antibiotics are given parenterally as needed.

CONTRAINDICATIONS

Patients who have significant competing conditions that are expected to cause death within 10 years are not considered to be candidates for radical prostatectomy. Patients who have had an open transcapsular or transvesical prostatectomy are not thought to be candidates for perineal prostatectomy because of fixation of the prostatic capsule or bladder within the pelvis that may prevent an adequate urethrovesical anastomosis from being established. Patients who are massively obese may not be able to tolerate the exaggerated lithotomy position because the intraabdominal contents may drive the diaphragm into the chest and prevent adequate respiration, even at increased ventilatory pressures. Previous pelvic irradiation, other pelvic surgery, and abdominoperineal resection are not contraindications to surgery except in those instances in which the previous therapy has compromised the bladder neck.

OPERATIVE PROCEDURE

Positioning of the Patient

The procedure may be accomplished on a standard operating table using any form of leg support that is available (Fig. 50.2-1). My preference is to use candy-cane stirrups, wrapping the feet to ensure that the straps do not place excessive pressure on bony prominences. There is no need to wrap the legs, nor is there any need to place the legs in alternating pressure stockings. The patient is positioned far from the head of the table, the small of the back being brought to the edge of the table, with the buttocks extending approximately 8 to 12 inches over the end of the table. There is no necessity to use shoulder braces to stabilize the patient by producing counter pressure on the upper body and shoulders. With the patient properly positioned, the weight of the patient is borne across the upper back, and sandbags or folded towels placed beneath the sacrum and the small of the back maintain the elevation of the pelvis. The legs and feet are rotated toward the head and, if the patient has been properly positioned, the perineum is parallel to the floor. The ischial tuberosities can be palpated and should lie in a line parallel or just posterior to the anus (Fig. 50.2-2).

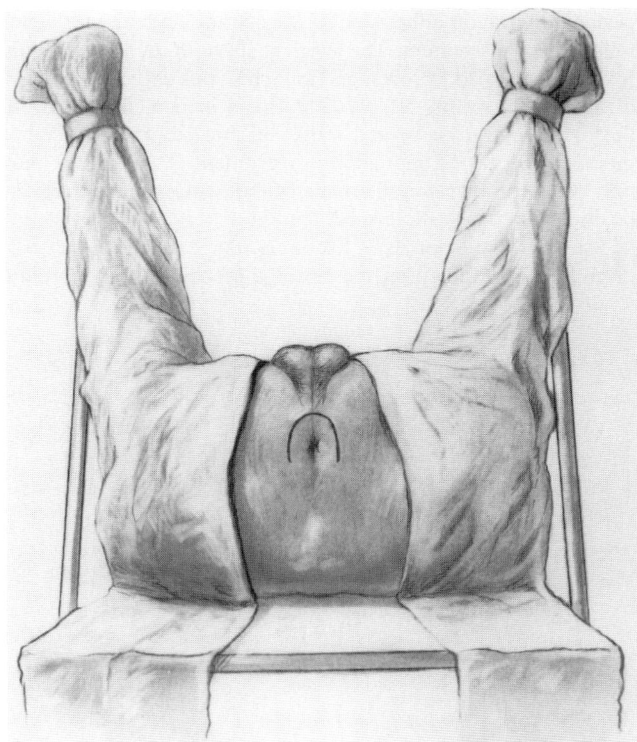

FIG. 50.2-1. In the exaggerated lithotomy position, the weight of the patient is borne across the upper back, and positioning is maintained by towels or pillows placed beneath the sacrum or small of the back.

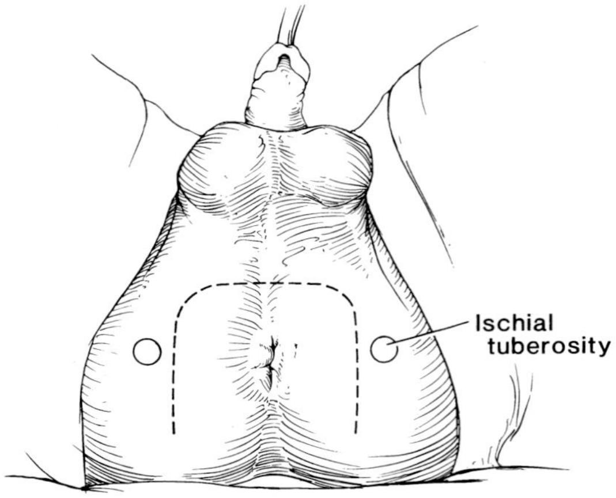

FIG. 50.2-2. The incision is a generous inverted U and is carried posteriorly to the anus.

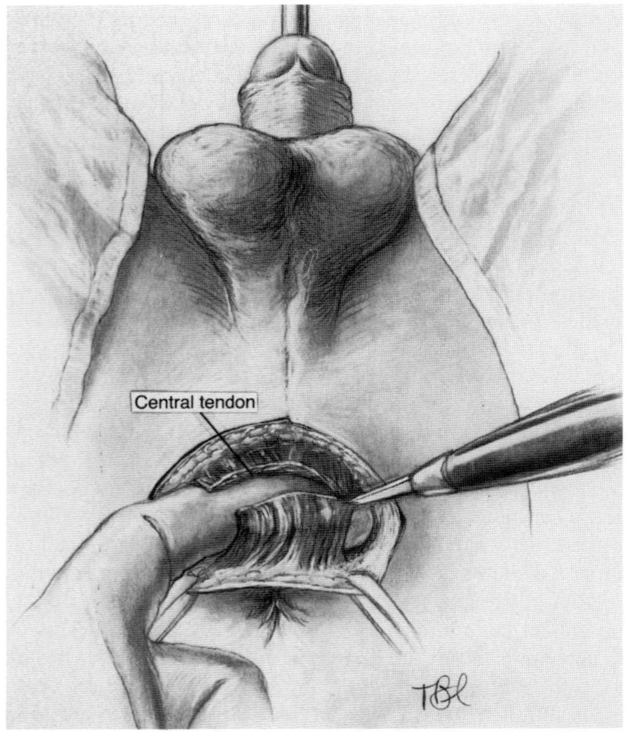

FIG. 50.2-4. The central tendon is isolated by placing a finger anterior to the rectum and is then divided at the skin margin.

Exposure of the Prostate

The Lowsley prostatic retractor is placed in the urethra and the bladder, and the blades are opened. In some cases, the Lowsley instrument is not necessary and may be replaced by a curved sound. The skin incision is made 1.5 cm anterior to the anal verge and extended posterolaterally on either side of the anus medial to the ischial tuberosities (see Fig. 50.2-2). The incision is continued behind the anus on either side. The ischial-rectal space now is opened by creating a defect in the superficial perineal fascia, on either side of the central tendon, with a cutting cautery instrument. The surgical space in the ischial-rectal fossa is developed by placing a finger into this defect perpendicular to the floor (Fig. 50.2-3). The finger is then curved toward the operating surgeon, and the overlying fibrofatty tissue is incised with the cutting cautery instrument. The surgeon then may place a finger on either side of the rectum and identify its position relative to the central tendon.

The central tendon is a fibromuscular band of tissue that originates posteriorly on the tip of the coccyx, flows around the rectum, and inserts on the perineal body. This fibromuscular tissue must be divided so that the anus and rectum can be displaced posteriorly. The surgeon passes a finger anterior to the rectum and beneath the central tendon and then divides the central tendon in its entirety with cautery, the line of incision being made as close as possible to the skin margin (Fig. 50.2-4). The surgeon may wish to mark the muscular extension of the central tendon with surgical clips or with a black silk suture so that it can be identified during final reconstruction of the perineum.

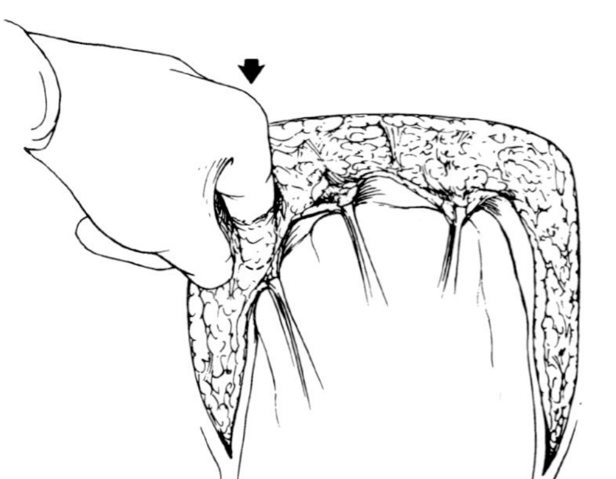

FIG. 50.2-3. The anus is excluded from the field by the use of drapes and Allis clamps. The fibrofatty tissue to either side of the midline is incised with cautery to permit access to the ischial rectal fossa.

After division of the central tendon, the anus drops posteriorly and, with upper traction on the perineal body, the rectourethralis can be identified, as can the glistening surface of the anterior rectal fascia (Fig. 50.2-5). By holding the Metzenbaum scissors in such a way that the curve of the scissors approximates the curve of the rectum and gently spreading the scissors on either side of the midline, the surgeon can, with blunt dissection, expose the anterior surface of the rectum and mobilize it on either side of the rectourethralis, to and beyond the level of the prostatic apex.

The next maneuver is designed to place the rectourethralis on tension. To accomplish this, an examining finger is inserted in the rectum and used to place downward pressure on the rectum while an assistant elevates the perineal body in the opposite direction. A finger may now be placed on either side of the rectourethralis to further open this space by blunt dissection. The rectourethralis is then incised, in the midline only, with the Metzenbaum scissors. The divided tissue is white and largely avascular. The series of cuts are made to the level of the prostate, at which point the rectum will be displaced posteriorly and the

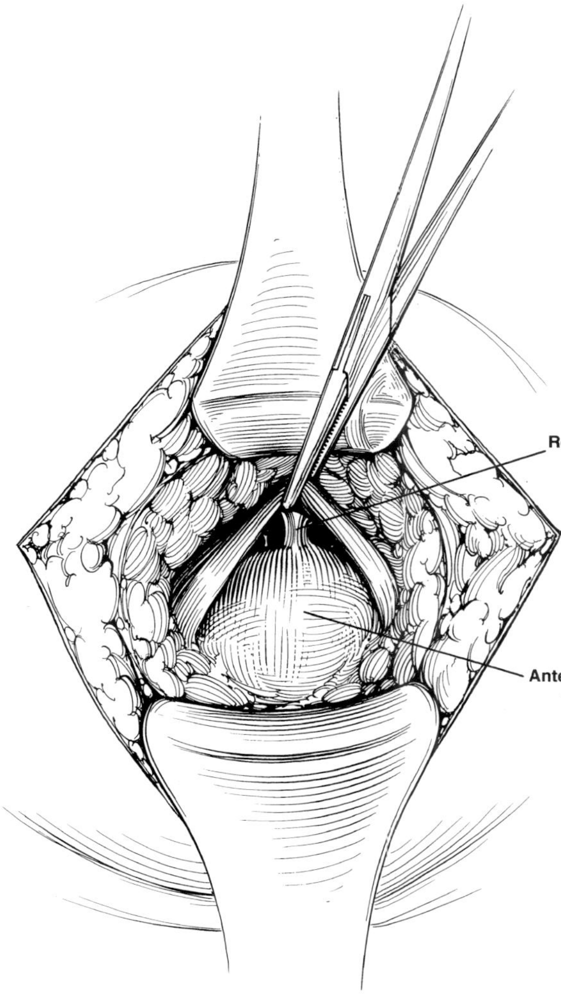

FIG. 50.2-5. The muscular fibers overlying the anterior rectal fascia are elevated and, with the anterior rectal fascia as a guide, a plane is established on either side of the rectourethralis to the base of the prostate.

prostate visualized anteriorly. The tissue that appears to either side of the midline is that portion of the levator sling that supports the prostate and the pelvis. Although this tissue may be divided, it is preferable to leave it intact so that the muscular sling can be brought together in the midline to support the urethrovesical anastomosis at the completion of the operative procedure.

The next maneuver is designed to fully expose the prostate laterally and posteriorly. This can easily be accomplished with the use of a bronchial or Kitner dissector. The surgeon places the instrument medial to the levator sling and lateral to the margin of the prostate, and, applying inward and downward pressure, separates the prostate and the neurovascular fascia from the levator sling to the level of the reflection of the endopelvic fascia onto the bladder. This is largely an avascular plane. After this area has been developed on both the right and left sides of the prostate, exposure is maintained by the use of baby Deaver retractors. Fixed retractors may be used, but it is my preference to use handheld retractors to facilitate exposure.

Attention is now turned to development of a plane between the rectum posteriorly and the prostate anteriorly. At this point in the procedure, the posterior aspect of the prostate is covered with musculature that is seemingly continuous with the anterior rectal surface. By downward pressure on the rectum, the margin between rectum and prostate can be identified, and these fibers can be divided with Metzenbaum or Strully scissors. After these muscular fibers have been divided, digital dissection establishes a plane between the prostate and seminal vesicles anteriorly and the rectal surface posteriorly.

Note that the Lowsley retractor has not been used at any time except to stabilize the prostate while it is being liberated from the levator sling on either side or while it is being elevated to permit identification of the plane between the rectum and the prostate posteriorly. Anterior or downward pressure on the handle of the Lowsley retractor would cause the prostate to move into the operative field and decrease markedly the amount of exposure between the bony pelvis and the prostatic surface. The movement is similar to pulling a cork from the inside of a wine bottle into the neck of the bottle and then attempting to dissect between the cork and the bottle neck.

Exposure of the Prostatic Apex, Urethra, and Neurovascular Fascia

After the prostate has been exposed laterally and posteriorly, it is time to expose the apex of the prostate, identify the urethra, determine whether the neurovascular fascia will be sacrificed unilaterally or bilaterally, and then divide the urethra from the apex of the prostate. To accomplish this, the surgeon should palpate the prostate laterally to determine whether there is palpable disease on the side of the negative biopsy. If there is any suggestion of disease on the side of the negative biopsy, it is my belief that the neurovascular fascia should be sacrificed on that side; in addition, the neurovascular fascia should always be sacrificed on the side of the positive biopsy.

With the prostate exposed and still covered posteriorly with fibromuscular tissue, the surgeon may palpate the Lowsley retractor in the urethra at the apex of the prostate. The fibers overlying the apex of the prostate and the urethra are incised, in the midline only, with scissors, and, by blunt dissection with a bronchial or Kitner dissector, the prostatic apex is displaced posteriorly and the urethra exposed in the midline. The dissector may then be pushed on either side of the urethra, medial to the neurovascular tissues that flow off the prostate and parallel to the urethra, to separate them from the urethra. After this plane has been established, if it is the intent of the surgeon to sacrifice the neurovascular fascia at the apex, the tissue is divided. If it is the intent of the surgeon to preserve the tissue, the neurovascular fascia is dissected with sharp dissection off the prostatic substance from the apex to the base of the prostate (Fig. 50.2-6). In either instance, the surgeon may, with digital dissection to the right and left of the urethra, separate prostatic substance from beneath the dorsal venous complex and liberate prostatic substance from the detrusor musculature. It may be necessary to excise some of the investing fascia on either side in order to further expose the apex of the prostate. After the apex of the prostate and the urethra have been fully mobilized, a right-angle clamp is placed around the urethra, the Lowsley retractor is removed, and the urethra is divided at the apex, the patient-side margin being tagged with 2-0 suture to permit its easy identification during reconstruction.

After division of the urethra, a Young prostatic tractor (or a straight Lowsley retractor) is passed through the urethra and into the bladder, and the blades are extended. The extended blades permit the surgeon to identify the bladder wall and also allow the surgeon to manipulate the operative specimen. Allis clamps or a tenaculum can be placed on the apex of the prostate to draw the prostate into the operative field and to permit identification of the plane between the prostate and the detrusor fibers. By blunt dissection, the surgeon develops the plane between the prostate and the detrusor to the right and the left of the bladder neck. The surgeon then sharply divides the bladder neck between the 10- and 2-o'clock positions, using curved Metzenbaum scissors, a large curved clamp passed through the prostatic urethra from apex to bladder neck, and a Foley catheter of any size grasped and brought out through the apex of the prostate, the Foley catheter being held as a loop and used for manipulation of the specimen.

With traction on the Foley catheter and the tenaculum, the prostate is further mobilized on either side of the bladder neck and cut away from the bladder laterally. There is no need to use surgical clips at this level; any bleeding points that are

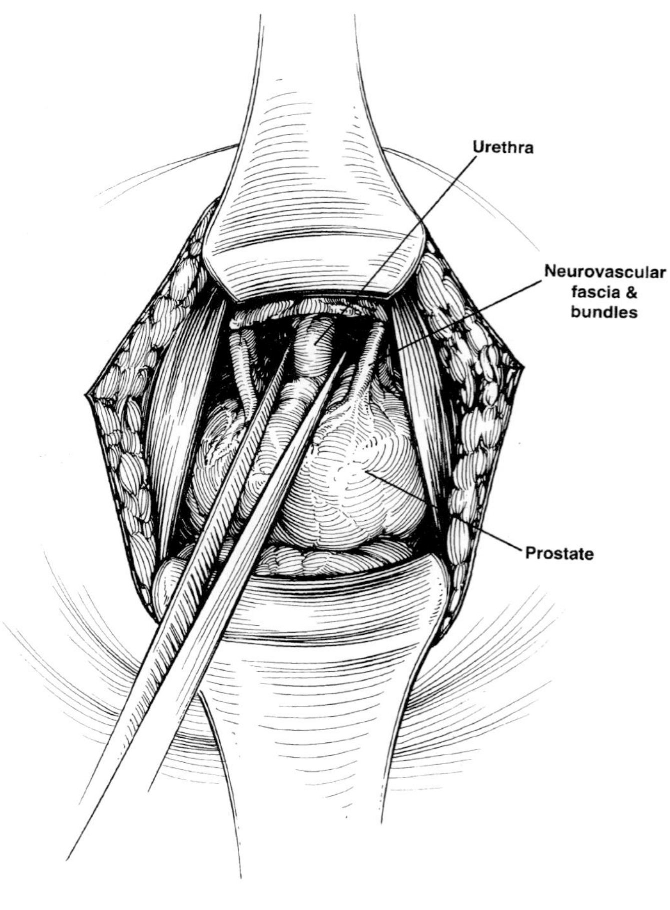

FIG. 50.2-6. The urethra may be exposed in the midline at the apex of the prostate; the neurovascular fascia may separate from the urethra. The fascial layer, which is adherent to prostatic substance, may be preserved or sacrificed in accordance with the extent of disease.

encountered can be successfully controlled after division with electrocautery. After the prostate is maximally mobilized but still adherent to the posterior bladder neck, the curved Metzenbaum scissors are passed behind the bladder neck and the posterior bladder neck is sharply divided. This now allows the bladder to retract into the pelvis.

With traction on the prostate to bring it further into the operative field, the surgeon then incises with scissors the fibromuscular tissue overlying the vasa deferens and seminal vesicles in the midline. This is an avascular structure, and these tissues may be divided with impunity. After the vasa deferens have been identified in the midline, the surgeon can begin to mobilize the lateral vascular pedicles to the prostate. This is accomplished by passing a right-angle clamp lateral to the seminal vesicles but medial to the vascular pedicle to the prostate (Fig. 50.2-7). After this space has been identified, the vascular pedicles may be controlled with surgical clips or they can be sharply divided and controlled by electrocoagulation. If desired, using the seminal vesicles as an anatomic marker, the seminal vesicles can be entirely encircled at the base of the prostate and the investing tissue sharply divided to fully mobilize the prostate. If, for technical reasons, the surgeon should decide not to so mobilize the prostatic specimen, the specimen may be elevated anteriorly by direct upward traction on the tenaculum, and the fibrous tissue (Denonvilliers' fascia) overlying the seminal vesicles and vasa deferens in the midline can be incised transversely. After this has been accomplished, a plane can be established, with the use of either a tonsillar clamp or a right-angle clamp, between the seminal vesicles medially and fibrovascular tissue posterolaterally, this tissue being controlled either with surgical clips before division or by electrocautery after division. After the fibrovascular tissue and vascular pedicles have been controlled on both the right and left sides, the specimen is held in place only by the seminal vesicles and vasa deferens.

The specimen is then displaced posteriorly, and each vas deferens is isolated in the midline, controlled with surgical clips, and divided. The specimen then can be elevated into the operative field and, with alternating sharp and blunt dissection, the seminal vesicles exposed, either in their entirety or for a distance of 2 to 3 cm. In those instances in which the surgeon elects not to remove the seminal vesicles in their entirety, they can be controlled at a distance of 2 to 3 cm from the prostate itself with surgical clips before division and removal of the specimen.

Control of Surgical Margins

The posterior bladder neck is grasped at the 6-o'clock position and bladder neck margins are taken, going from the 6- through the 8- to 12-o'clock positions and from the 6- through the 4- to 12-o'clock positions. A traction suture is placed at the 6-o'clock position, and tension is maintained on the posterior bladder neck by the weight of a Kelly clamp on this traction suture.

Attention is then turned to covering the raw detrusor fibers anteriorly with bladder mucosa. This is accomplished by using 4-0 absorbable suture and bringing the bladder mucosa up onto the raw surface of the detrusor from the 9- through the 12- to

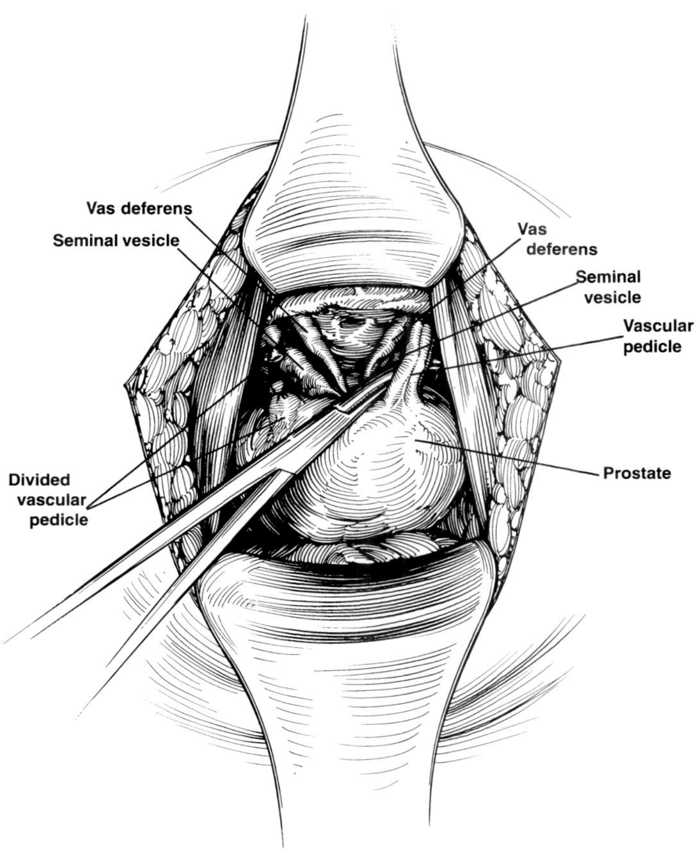

FIG. 50.2-7. The seminal vesicles bilaterally are the landmarks that the surgeon uses to identify the plane for control of the vascular pedicles of the prostate. A right-angle clamp may be passed lateral to the seminal vesicles and medial to the vascular pedicle. This tissue is divided sharply, and vascular control established either mechanically or with electrocautery.

3-o'clock positions. That portion of the detrusor that extends from the 3- through the 6- to 9-o'clock positions need not be covered with mucosa, because this is the portion that will later be enclosed within the "racket handle."

After the anterior bladder neck has been covered with vesical mucosa, 0-strength absorbable sutures are placed outside-inside, inside-outside, approximately 0.5 cm from the 12-o'clock midline position. These will later be brought through the perineal body and tied beneath the skin to support the direct urethrovesical anastomosis.

Urethrovesical Reconstruction

The surgeon now passes an 18F Foley catheter through the urethra. The previously placed 2-0 suture is used to identify the urethra as it penetrates the transverse perineal diaphragm, and 2-0 absorbable sutures are placed in the urethra at the 2-, 4-, 8-, and 10-o'clock positions. The two sutures placed at the 4- and 8-o'clock positons are driven into the mucosa-covered bladder neck approximately 0.5 cm from the 12-o'clock midline position, so as to produce a mucosa-to-mucosa approximation. The Foley catheter is placed into the bladder, and the balloon is inflated (Fig. 50.2-8). The bladder neck is closed from the 6- to the 12-o'clock position with interrupted 0-strength absorbable sutures, the closure being made tight around the 18F Foley catheter. At this point, the two urethral sutures which had been placed at the 10- and 2-o'clock positons are brought into the reconstructed bladder neck, approximately 0.5 cm to either side of the racket handle closure.

The four 2-0 absorbable sutures are then snugly tied. After the direct urethrovesical anastomosis has been secured, the four 2-0 absorbable sutures previously placed in the bladder neck anteriorly and the last two used in the racket handle posteriorly are brought through the transverse perineal body on the right and left side of the urethra, using a no. 8 surgeon's needle, and the sutures are tied securely beneath the skin.

The fibers previously identified as being a portion of the levator sling are brought together in the midline with interrupted 2-0 absorbable sutures to support the prostate, and the wound is drained with a Penrose drain. The central tendon is reconstructed with the use of interrupted absorbable 2-0 sutures, and the skin margins are then closed with vertical mattress sutures of 2-0 absorbable suture material.

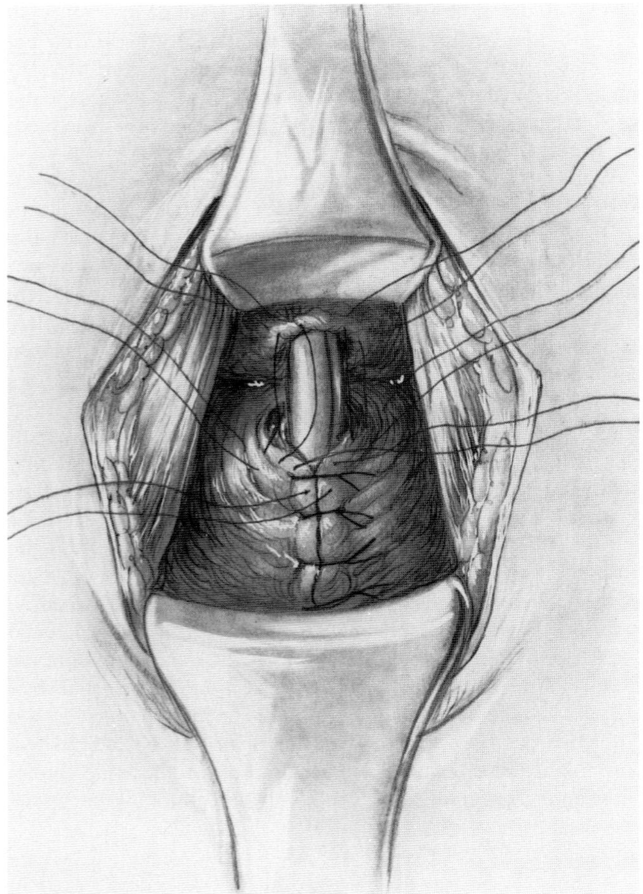

FIG. 50.2-8. The anastomosis between the urethra and bladder neck, closed initially from 6 to 12 o'clock with interrupted 1-0 absorbable sutures, is accomplished by four-quadrant 2-0 absorbable sutures. The direct anastomosis is supported by Dees' modification of the VEST suture technique, in which 1-0 absorbable sutures, at each quadrant of the vesical neck closure, are brought through the perineal body and secured anterior to anterior, posterior to posterior.

POSTOPERATIVE CARE

The patient is mobilized within 6 to 8 hours after surgery. Oral intake is initiated within 8 hours after surgery. The patient is given oral antibiotics plus a stool softener. Discharge is routinely achieved on the morning of the third or fourth postoperative day. The catheter is left in place for 18 days and is then removed by either the operating surgeon or the referring surgeon.

RESULTS

Cancer-specific survival is a function of the extent of disease in the histopathologic specimen and can be subdivided according to whether the malignancy is organ-confined, specimen-confined, or margin-positive (Figs. 50.2-9, 50.2-10, and 50.2-11).[11,12]

The time to continence for perineal prostatectomy is shown in Figure 50.2-12. Fifty percent of the patients surveyed in this review were continent the moment the catheter was removed.[2] Potency rates achieved with this procedure are presented in Table 50.2-1.[13–15]

The most remarkable difference between radical perineal and radical retropubic prostatectomy is in blood loss, as noted in Table 50.2-2. The relative costs also render a significant advantage to radical perineal prostatectomy (Table 50.2-3). Patients are discharged on the fourth or fifth postoperative day, and catheters are routinely removed 2 weeks after discharge. The rare patient with perineal urine leakage is maintained on catheter drainage until the leakage ceases, the catheter being removed after 5 days of dryness. Patients are observed and PSA determinations are obtained at 6-month intervals during the first 5 years and at yearly intervals thereafter.

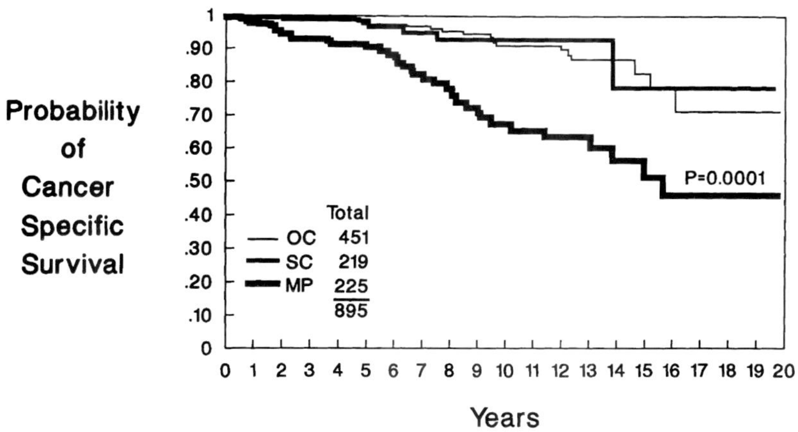

FIG. 50.2-9. Kaplan-Meier projection of cancer-specific survival for patients with organ-confined, specimen-confined, and margin-positive disease.

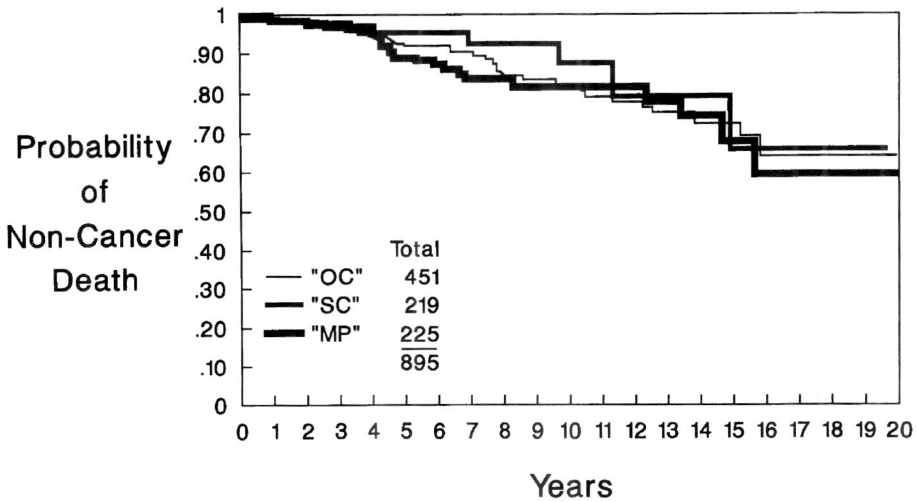

FIG. 50.2-10. Kaplan-Meier projection of noncancer deaths for patients with organ-confined, specimen-confined, and margin-positive disease.

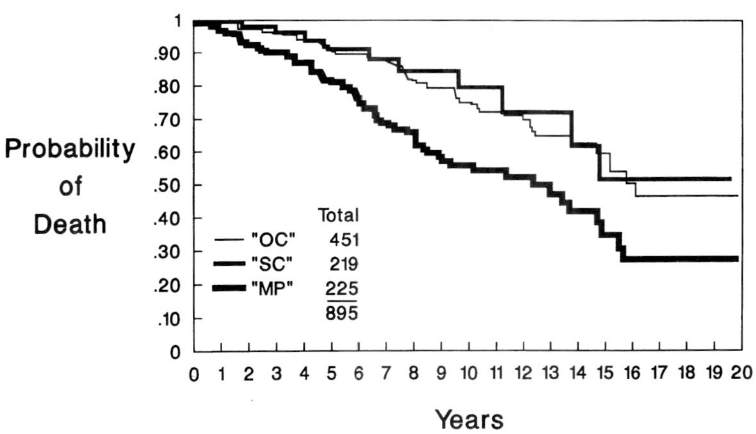

FIG. 50.2-11. Kaplan-Meier projection of overall deaths for patients with organ-confined, specimen-confined, and margin-positive disease.

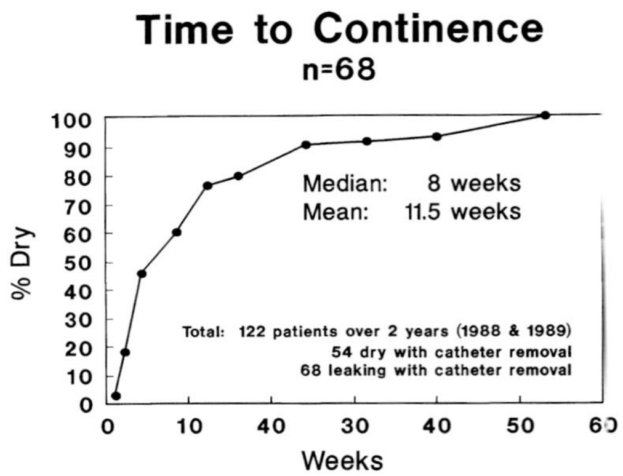

FIG. 50.2-12. Time to continence for 121 patients who underwent operation before the mucosal-to-mucosal anastomosis technique became available.

TABLE 50.2-1. *Potency among 122 consecutive patients undergoing radical perineal prostatectomy*

	Patients	Percentage
Potent before surgery	73 of 122	60
Thought to be candidates for potency preservation	22 of 74	30
Potent within 1 year after surgery	17 of 22	77

TABLE 50.2-2. *Mean operative parameters among 122 patients undergoing radical perineal prostatectomy and 51 patients undergoing radical retropubic prostatectomy*

Item	Perineal (n = 122)	Retropubic (n = 51)	*P* value
Age (y)	66.2	66.9	0.74
Preoperative HCT (%)	43.0	42.0	0.85
EBL (mL)	565	2000	<0.001
Transfusions (no. units)	0	3	<0.001
Operative time (min)	203	225	0 001
Anesthesia time (min)	268	290	0.192

EBL, estimated blood loss; HCT, hematocrit.

TABLE 50.2-3. *Relative costs of radical perineal prostatectomy (RPP) compared with radical retropubic prostatectomy (RRP)*

	RRP #1	RRP #2	RRP #3	RPP
Bed care	$3,241	$2,902	$3,932	$2,542
Operating room costs	2,503	2,556	2,832	1,813
Anesthesia	785	750	840	628
Recovery room	441	326	358	334
Transfusions	520	505	402	71
Average total cost	$11,418	$10,609	$12,565	$8,824
Average length of stay (d)	7.5	6.6	8.9	6.0

REFERENCES

1. Young HH. The early diagnosis and radical cure of carcinoma of the prostate: being a study of 40 cases and presentations of a radical operation which was carried out in 4 cases. Bull Johns Hopkins Hosp 1905;16:315.
2. Paulson DF, Frazier HA. Radical prostatectomy. In: Krane RJ, Siroky MB, Fitzpatrick JM, eds. Clinical urology. Philadelphia: JB Lippincott, 1994:1020.
3. Anscher MS, Prosnitz LR. Postoperative radiotherapy for patients with carcinoma of the prostate undergoing radical prostatectomy with positive surgical margins, seminal vesicle involvement and/or penetration through the capsule. J Urol 1987;138:1407.
4. Paulson DF, Moul JW, Walther PJ, Robertson JE. Postoperative radiotherapy of the prostate for patients undergoing radical prostatectomy with positive margins, seminal vesicle involvement and/or penetration through the capsule. J Urol 1990;143:1178.
5. Kramer SA, Cline WA, Farnham R, et al. Prognosis of patients with stage D1 prostatic adenocarcinoma. J Urol 1981;125:817.
6. Paulson DF. The prognostic role of lymphadenectomy in adenocarcinoma of the prostate. Urol Clin North Am 1980;7:615.
7. Paulson DF, Lin GH, Hinshaw W, Uro-Oncology Research Group. Radical surgery vs. radiotherapy for stage A2 and stage B (T1-2N0M0) adenocarcinoma of the prostate. J Urol 1982;128:502.
8. Paulson DF. Localized prostatic carcinoma: the case for radical surgery. In: Fitzpatrick J, Krane R, eds. The prostate. New York: Churchill Livingstone, 1989:327.
9. Whitesel JA, Donohue RE, Mani JH, et al. Acid phosphatase: its influence on the management of carcinoma of the prostate. J Urol 1984;131:70.
10. Paulson DF, Moul JW, Walther PJ. Radical prostatectomy for clinical stage T1-2N0M0 prostatic adenocarcinoma: long term results. J Urol 1990;144:1180.
11. Kaplan EL, Meier P. Nonparametric estimation from incomplete observations. J Am Stat Assoc 1958;53:457.
12. Cox DR. Regression models and life tables. J Roy Stat Soc B 1972;34:187.
13. Catalona WJ, Dresner SM. Nerve-sparing radical prostatectomy: extraprostatic tumor extension and preservation of erectile function. J Urol 1985;134:1149.
14. Eggleston JC, Walsh PC. Radical prostatectomy with preservation of sexual function: pathological findings in the first 100 cases. J Urol 1985;134:1146.
15. Walsh PC, Lepor H, Eggleston JC. Radical prostatectomy with preservation of sexual function: anatomical and pathological considerations. Prostate 1983;4:473.

Principles and Practice of Genitourinary Oncology, edited by Derek Raghavan, Howard I. Scher, Steven A. Leibel, and Paul H. Lange. Lippincott-Raven Publishers, Philadelphia, © 1997.

CHAPTER 51

Radiotherapy for Stage B (T1c, T2) Prostate Cancer

51.1 Contemporary Approaches Using External Beam Radiotherapy

Steven A. Leibel, Michael J. Zelefsky, Gerald J. Kutcher, and Zvi Fuks

Screening of men older than 50 years of age for abnormally elevated prostate-specific antigen (PSA) has resulted in an increase in the proportion of prostate cancer patients diagnosed with localized, early stage disease.[1] A National Cancer Institute Consensus Development Panel on the Management of Clinically Localized Prostate Cancer has concluded that both radical prostatectomy and radiotherapy are effective treatments, but there was no consensus regarding which is the most optimal mode of local therapy.[2] Because no conclusive information can be derived from randomized trials,[3] it is often difficult for patients and physicians to choose between these two modalities.

External beam irradiation was first used as a curative modality for localized prostate cancer in the 1950s, when the highly penetrating megavoltage beams from cobalt-60 (^{60}Co) teletherapy units[4–6] and linear accelerators[7] became available. Applied using the then newly developed methods of dosimetry and treatment planning, megavoltage radiotherapy permitted for the first time the delivery of tumoricidal doses to prostate tumors without excessive damage to the skin and the normal tissues surrounding the prostate.[8] Radiotherapy techniques for prostatic cancer have since advanced to improve precision and to further increase the dose. However, the basic therapeutic objectives have remained unchanged: attempt to permanently control organ-confined or locally advanced disease while producing minimal toxicity in the adjacent normal tissues.

This chapter examines contemporary external radiotherapy approaches in the treatment of localized stage T1 and T2 (A2 and B) carcinoma of the prostate. Experience accrued with conventional techniques indicates that external beam radiotherapy is reasonably effective in locally controlling T1 and T2 prostate tumors.[9,10] However, because biopsy for histologic confirmation of primary tumor control or failure has not been routinely performed, the true incidence of local control may be lower than the 65% to 88% commonly reported.[9–12] Furthermore, when posttreatment rise in serum PSA is used as a therapeutic endpoint, treatment failures after both radiotherapy and radical prostatectomy appear to be more common than previously recognized.[13–20]

Failure of radiotherapy to control organ-confined prostate cancer in most instances results from the persistence of prostatic tumor clonogens with inherent resistance to the radiation doses used. To avoid underdosage relative to the prescribed schedule or even a complete miss of part of the tumor-containing prostate, conventional radiotherapy techniques uniformly encompass significant portions of the bladder and rectum as safety margins included in the volume receiving the highest radiation doses. Consequently, attempts to increase the tumor dose are frequently restricted by the high sensitivity of the rectum and bladder to the effects of radiation. The recently introduced techniques of three-dimensional conformal radiotherapy (3D-CRT) provide a way to overcome these limitations on dose escalation. The three-dimensional approach uses sophisticated, computer-aided systems to plan and deliver prescribed radiation doses with high precision, accurately conforming the desired dose distribution to the entire three-dimensional anatomic configuration of the prostate while maximally excluding the surrounding normal tissues.[21,22] This approach has resulted in an improved ability to focus photon radiation beams on the entire prostate with reduced risk of underdosing parts of the tumor.[23] Concomitantly, the effective exclusion of normal tissues from the volume receiving high radiation doses has permitted tumor dose escalation to levels beyond those feasible with conventional two-dimensional radiotherapy with a decreased risk of normal tissue complications.[22] Clinical studies are underway to evaluate whether this strategy to increase the tumor dose will lead to improved local tumor control.[21,22] Photon-beam 3D-CRT techniques are routinely used at the Memorial Sloan-Kettering Cancer Center (MSKCC) to treat localized prostate cancer; preliminary results of this therapeutic approach in stages T1c and T2 tumors are summarized later in this chapter.

CONVENTIONAL TECHNIQUES OF EXTERNAL BEAM RADIOTHERAPY

When megavoltage radiotherapy techniques for the treatment of prostate cancer were introduced in the 1960s, computed tomography (CT) reconstruction of the prostatic anatomy was not available. The treatment field size and shape were estimated from the digital rectal examination and from plain radiographic simulator techniques using Foley catheter balloons placed adjacent to the bladder outlet and intravesical and intrarectal radiographic contrast media.[24] Because these localization techniques were in most instances suboptimal for accurate localization of the prostate and the seminal vesicles, treatment plans did not attempt to conform the irradiation fields to the target volume shape, and standard 6- × 6-cm to 8- × 8-cm rotational arc fields were most commonly used.[7,24] Although this approach may have provided adequate coverage for some small T1c and T2a tumors,[25] more bulky prostatic cancers were apparently underdosed in many patients, especially when the seminal vesicles were considered at risk.[23,26,27] Beginning in approximately 1970, treatment volumes were expanded to include the proximal echelons of the lymph node drainage of the prostate.[28]

Today, conventional treatment techniques are based on CT-assisted planning and include wide margins to avoid tumor tissue underdosage. Although elective irradiation of the pelvic lymph nodes has not been conclusively proven to be of benefit,[29,30] whole pelvic irradiation is frequently used for part of the treatment course when the anticipated risk of nodal involvement is 15% or higher (stage T2c and stages T2a and T2b with Gleason score ≥ 7).[30] When the whole pelvis is treated, a four-field technique designed to include the prostate, seminal vesicles, and the regional lymph nodes is usually employed.[30] The cross sections of the beams are shaped with customized cerrobend alloy blocks to shield the posterior wall of the rectum, the anal canal and sphincter, the small bowel, and the nonadjacent portions of the urethra and bladder.[28] The dose to this field is limited to 45 to 50 Gy in daily fractions of 1.8 to 2 Gy because of the limited tolerance of some pelvic organs to higher radiation doses. This dose level is, however, insufficient to control the intraprostatic tumor, and a boost to the primary target, designed to include the prostate and seminal vesicles with a 1- to 2-cm safety margin of normal tissue, is subsequently added. Target boosts of 20 to 25 Gy in daily dose fractions of 1.8 to 2 Gy are usually delivered with bilateral 120-degree arcs[8,23] or with four-field parallel opposed anterior, posterior, and lateral beam arrangements.[30] The boost technique raises the total dose to the prostate to 65 to 70 Gy. In T1 and small T2 lesions with a Gleason score of 6 or less, treatment is frequently confined to the prostate target volume only, omitting the distal two thirds of the seminal vesicles and the pelvic lymph node–bearing areas because of the low likelihood of spread to these regions.[28,30–32]

Patient Tolerance

Treatment with conventional external beam irradiation is relatively well tolerated, although approximately 60% of patients develop mild acute urinary symptoms (e.g., frequency, nocturia, urgency, dysuria) or mild rectal morbidity (e.g., discomfort, tenesmus, diarrhea) that require medication for relief.[33] Symptoms typically appear during the third week of treatment and resolve within days to weeks after its completion. Persistence of symptoms for longer than 3 months after completion of therapy or late complications developing 3 or more months after the completion of the course of treatment are significantly less common; serious complications that require hospitalization or surgical intervention occur in only 4.3% of patients.[34]

Shipley and colleagues[35] summarized the incidence of late sequelae in 331 stage T1-T2 patients treated at the Massachusetts General Hospital, at the MD Anderson Hospital, and in the Radiation Therapy Oncology Group (RTOG) trial 77-06. Tumor doses ranged between 63 and 74 Gy, and the median follow-up interval was 6.1 years. No patient developed a complication requiring major surgical intervention or prolonged hospitalization, and there were no fatal complications. Most late intestinal or rectal injuries (e.g., chronic diarrhea, proctitis, rectal and anal stricture, rectal bleeding) or urinary injuries (e.g., cystitis, hematuria, urethral or bladder neck stricture, incontinence) were not debilitating and usually resolved over time. Radiation injuries that altered the patient's performance status or those that necessitated minor surgical procedures were diarrhea (3.6%, 0% persisting); rectal bleeding (5.4%, 0.9% persisting) hematuria (5.1%, 0.9% persisting); bladder neck or urethral stricture (5.4%, 1.2% persisting); and urinary incontinence (0.4%). Urethral and bladder neck strictures and incontinence occurred primarily in patients who had undergone transurethral resections of the prostate before radiotherapy. Nearly all reported sequelae occurred within the first 3 to 4 years after treatment and only a few developed more than 5 years after treatment. The risk of late complications increases when radiation doses exceed 70 Gy.[34,36,37] The risk of rectal complications has also been correlated with the volume of anterior rectal wall receiving high doses.[38]

Sexual function was preserved in 73% to 82% of patients who were followed from 1 year to 15 months after irradiation.[39,40] However, erectile potency appears to diminish with advancing time after treatment; 33% to 61% of patients maintain their potency at 5 years or longer after irradiation.[35]

Long-Term Results

Table 51.1-1 summarizes published long-term results with conventional external beam irradiation. The 10-year disease-free survival rates range between 53% and 60% in stage T1b (stage A2) and between 27% and 85% in stage T2 (stage B) patients.[9,10,28,41,42] The corresponding 15-year survival rates are 39% to 50% and 15% to 50%, respectively.[28,41] Fifteen-year cause-specific survival rates range from 62% to 77%, and the 20-year rates vary from 55% to 73%.[43] Local recurrences determined clinically at 10 to 15 years after treatment vary from 12% to 35%.[9,10,41,42,44] Although comparisons between published radiotherapy and radical prostatectomy series may not be valid, the long-term therapeutic results of irradiated T1b and T2a patients are generally similar to those reported with radical prostatectomy.[10,39,45–51] Using a hazard function over successive 5-year intervals, Coleman and colleagues[52] demonstrated that despite differences in patient selection and the absence of

TABLE 51.1-1. *Results of external beam irradiation in stage T1b and T2 (A2 and B) carcinoma of the prostate*

			Survival rate (%)			Relapse-free survival rate (%)			Local relapse-free survival rate (%)		
Investigators	Stage	Patients	5 y	10 y	15 y	5 y	10 y	15 y	5 y	10 y	15 y
Bagshaw* et al, 1993[28]	T1	335	80	60	40	76	60	50	90	85	80
and Kaplan et al, 1992[44]	T2	242	80	55	30	66	40	35	80	70	65
Hanks et al, 1994[41]	T1 (A)	60	84	54	41	76	53	39	96	96	83
	T2 (B)	312	74	43	22	56	27	15	83	71	65
Perez et al, 1993[9]	T1b	48	85	70		78	60		90	80	
	T2	252	82	65		76	56		85	76	
Zagars et al, 1988[42]	T2	82	93	70		90	85		97	88	

* Stanford staging system.

surgical staging for most radiotherapy patients, stage for stage the rates of relapse were similar in the surgical and radiotherapy series. With the exception of very small tumors, there was a continuous risk of relapse throughout the follow-up period, suggesting that for larger tumors, the probability of cure is limited by the presence of extraprostatic disease.

There is limited data available on the long-term outcome of lymphadenectomy-staged patients treated by conventional external beam irradiation.[10,51,53] The 10-year cause-specific mortality in 104 pathologically staged patients with stage T1b and T2 node-negative disease, treated in the RTOG 77-06 trial, was only 14%. In this group of patients, 87% were clinically free of local recurrences, 79% were free of distant metastases, and 67% were free of any failure. The survival in this group of patients was nearly identical to the expected survival in a life table–generated age-matched control population throughout the 10 years of observation (63% observed versus 59% expected at 10 years).[10] These rates are similar to those reported in two radical prostatectomy series for clinical stage T1 and T2 node-negative disease followed for 10 years.[47,48,54]

Although most published data on primary tumor control have been based on digital rectal examination, additional increments in local failure of 21% to 27% were reported when biopsy specimens of the prostate were routinely obtained at 18 months or longer after external irradiation in stage T1b and T2 tumors.[55,56] In addition to stage and grade, the rates of positive biopsy specimens vary with factors related to the selection of patients for the procedure, whether the patient had elevated or rising serum PSA at the time of biopsy, and with the biopsy technique used.[55–59] Because the number of patients biopsied often do not correspond to the true denominators for the populations of patients treated at reporting institutions,[59] the true incidence of positive biopsy specimens in patients with normal digital rectal examinations after treatment remains uncertain.[60] Despite these reservations, it should be emphasized that a finding of a positive postirradiation biopsy specimen in a patient with a normal digital rectal examination is generally associated with an increased risk of a subsequent clinical local failure.[12,44,55] These data underscore the need for radiotherapy techniques to further improve local tumor control in prostatic carcinoma.

Serum PSA measurements also provide a sensitive and objective endpoint for monitoring the outcome of definitive therapy. Relapse after external beam irradiation[13,14,16,22,61,62] or radical prostatectomy[17–20] can be predicted when the serum PSA level is found to persistently rise after the completion of treatment, thus representing a harbinger for subsequent anatomic recurrence. Zietman and colleagues[14] compared the clinical relapse-free survival with PSA relapse-free survival in 85 patients with stage T1 and T2 tumors treated with external beam irradiation. PSA failure was defined as an increase of greater than 10% within the first 2 years after irradiation, or a PSA level of more than 1 ng/mL after a minimum follow-up of 2 years. Clinical relapse-free survival at 4 years was 71%, whereas the corresponding PSA relapse-free survival was only 41%. Freedom from PSA relapse was directly related to the pretreatment PSA value. For patients with an initial PSA level of 15 ng/mL or lower, the 4-year PSA relapse-free survival was 65%, whereas only 7% of patients with an initial PSA of more than 15 ng/mL were free of PSA relapse at 4 years, a rate similar to that observed in patients with T3 and T4 tumors with the same initial values of PSA. The shape of the survival curves in the latter patient groups suggest that pelvic nodal involvement, micrometastatic tumor dissemination, or both may have been present in the reported patients at the time of initial treatment; therefore, cure by the local therapy applied may be unlikely in such patients. Nonetheless, the true significance of PSA relapse using the strict criteria as offered by Zietman and colleagues[14] remains unknown, and correlation with subsequent local and distant failure is still required to resolve this issue.

Several other studies have reported PSA failure rates of as high as 65% to 80% in stage T1 and T2 patients at intervals of up to 10 years after external beam irradiation.[15,16] Although information on patient selection factors, pretreatment PSA levels, and patterns of anatomic failure were not presented in these reports, legitimate concerns have been raised regarding the ability of traditionally planned external beam irradiation given at conventional dose levels to completely eradicate the local tumor in the majority of treated patients.

THREE-DIMENSIONAL CONFORMAL RADIOTHERAPY

Several reasons for the failure of conventional techniques to locally eradicate prostatic tumors have been identified. Traditional approaches to tumor localization and treatment planning appear to have been insufficiently accurate to assure that the total prostatic target volume was properly encompassed by the prescribed dose.[63] This may have resulted from the use of inadequate imaging techniques for target volume definition, insuffi-

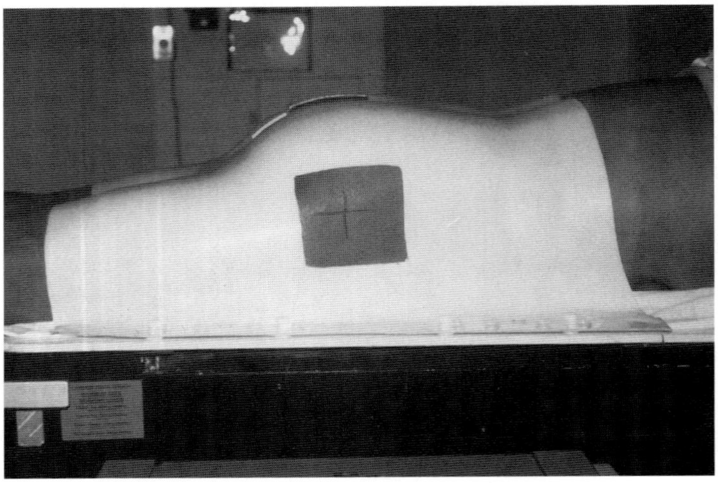

FIG. 51.1-1. Patient positioned within an individually fabricated thermoplastic immobilization device (Aquaplast, Wycoff, NJ). The cast is attached to a board on the treatment couch beneath the patient. (From Leibel SA, Heimann R, Kutcher GJ, et al. Three-dimensional conformal radiation therapy in locally advanced carcinoma of the prostate: preliminary results of a phase I dose-escalation study. Int J Radiat Oncol Biol Phys 1994;28:55.)

cient accuracy of the dose calculation methods available at the time, and from the restricted dose levels feasible with conventional approaches. The proximity of the prostate to the bladder and the rectum has limited the applicable prostate doses to less than 70 Gy when conventional radiotherapeutic techniques were used.[34,36,64]

As described previously, one of the main attributes of three-dimensional planning is the ability to effectively exclude the surrounding normal tissues. This process has been facilitated by new CT- and magnetic resonance imaging–based methods that provide complete anatomic and dose information for the entire tissue volume to be irradiated.[21,65] Because three-dimensional dose computations are highly labor intensive, requiring large numbers of dose computation points, the implementation of this approach is critically dependent on the availability of sophisticated computation algorithms and fast computer hardware. Such systems are also required for rapid displays of dose distributions to facilitate iterative techniques of planning and plan evaluation.[21] The recent introduction of fast computer workstations for treatment planning and of computer-aided treatment delivery systems (e.g., multileaf collimation and online real-time electronic portal imaging) have made it possible to implement external beam photon 3D-CRT in the routine management of prostate cancer in several institutions in the United States and Europe.[22,23,30,66–68]

Treatment Planning and Treatment Delivery Techniques

Several three-dimensional treatment simulation and planning techniques are now available for prostate cancer patients. In this chapter, the MSKCC system[20,65,69,70] is used as a model. Patients are treated while in the prone position within individually fabricated thermoplastic immobilization casts (Fig. 51.1-1). Simulation is performed using conventional simulators for patient localization and CT to derive anatomic data and define the treatment target volume. To decrease prostate and seminal vesicle positional variability as a result of organ motion, the simulation and each treatment session are performed after the patient empties his bladder. Careful attention should be given to the state of bladder filling to reduce the risk of tumor underdosage as a result of daily variations in prostate location and geometry.[71]

The target volume extends from 1 cm caudal to the apex of the prostate to 1 cm cephalad to the superior tips of the seminal vesicles. The targeted volume encompasses the prostate with a 1-cm margin, except posteriorly at the interface with the rectum, where a 0.6-cm margin is used. Three-dimensional reconstruction of the target volume and the surrounding normal tissues is performed and displayed using the beam's-eye-view technique.[21] A combination of six coplanar fields (two lateral opposed fields and two pairs of oblique fields) shaped by computer-driven multileaf collimators (MLCs) are used to deliver the treatment (Fig. 51.1-2).[22]

Dose distributions are calculated using a pencil-beam convolution algorithm with pixel-by-pixel inhomogeneity corrections.[72] The dose is prescribed to the maximum isodose surface distribution that completely encompasses the target volume. Dose inhomogeneity within the target volume varies from 4% to 7%. Dose-volume histograms[21] are used to ensure that no more than 30% of the rectal wall, 50% of the bladder wall, and 65% of the adjacent small bowel receives the prescription dose to decrease the risk of toxicity.[73] When radiation cannot be administered without exceeding these limits, a 3-month course of neoadjuvant androgen-deprivation therapy is given to decrease the target volume. Significant reductions in normal tissue volumes carried to the prescription dose have been observed in nearly 90% of patients treated with the neoadjuvant hormonal-deprivation approach.[73] No significant late rectal, bladder, or bowel complications have been observed with these strict treatment planning policies.[22]

The application of three-dimensional treatment plans generally involve large numbers of fields administered daily. The fast and accurate delivery of 3D-CRT plans has been facilitated by the recent introduction of automated computer-controlled MLCs capable of rapid delivery of large numbers of arbitrarily shaped fields. To ensure that treatment is delivered as planned, automated online electronic portal imaging has also become available. These systems enable fluoroscopy-like real-time imaging of the actual treatment fields. In the future, portal imaging may also improve the accuracy of three-dimensional treatment delivery by facilitating online automated corrections of patient

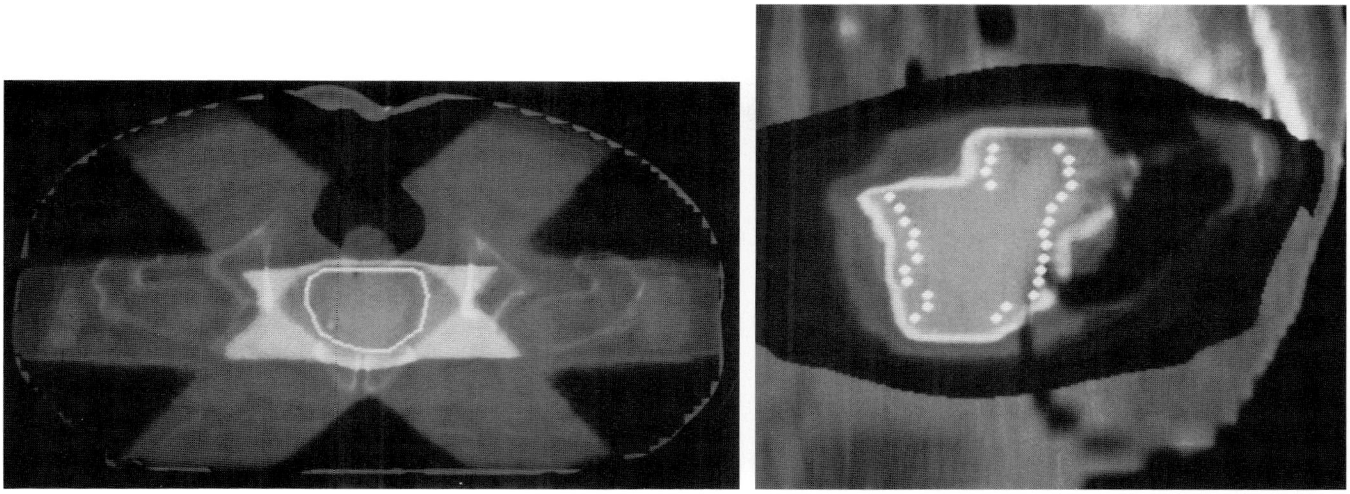

A B

FIG. 51.1-2. Midplane **(A)** axial and **(B)** sagittal dose-distribution displays of a six-field coplanar prostate treatment plan with 15-mV x-rays, consisting of one pair of lateral and two pairs of oblique fields. In this color-wash display, each band of the color spectrum corresponds to a dose range. The prescription dose is normalized to 100%. The red region represents the prescription isodose distribution (100---101%), while yellow corresponds to approximately 70---80%, green to 45---70%, and blue to 45% or less of the prescription dose. The planning target volume contour is outlined in yellow. (See Color Figure 51.1-2.)

setup errors during the treatment session through computer-driven feedback mechanisms.

Dose Escalation

As discussed previously, implementation of the 3D-CRT approach permits significant increases in tumor dose, which apparently is required to overcome the relative radiation resistance of prostatic tumor clonogens. A phase I dose-escalation study in prostate cancer patients receiving 3D-CRT is currently underway at MSKCC to establish the maximal tolerable doses that can be delivered with the three-dimensional approach. The target volume excludes the regional pelvic lymph nodes because studies failed to provide evidence for benefit in irradiating the lymph node–bearing areas.[29]

The dose-escalation study includes 432 patients in all disease stages treated between October 1988 and February 1994. Initially, the 3D-CRT dose levels used were 64.8 to 70.2 Gy given in daily increments of 1.8 Gy as classically used with conventional two-dimensional techniques.[74] When baselines for acute tolerance and late complications were established at these dose levels, the dose-escalation program was begun in patients with stages T2c and T3 tumors.[22,74] When 40 patients were treated with 75.6 Gy and no late toxicity was observed after a minimum follow-up of 1 year, this dose became available to patients with lower-stage disease. When the dose for T2c and T3 patients was escalated to 81 Gy, a restriction was imposed in the treatment plan design to limit the dose to 30% or less of the rectal volume to no more than 75.6 Gy. To meet this requirement, the final 9 Gy were delivered in five daily treatment fractions using a specially designed six- or eight-field coplanar beam arrangement with the rectum completely blocked in each field. A total of 46 patients were accrued into the 81-Gy dose level program and were been followed for a median of 18 months. No severe late complications have been observed in the 81 Gy patient group; therefore, escalation to 86.4 Gy was activated, and patients with T1c and T2 tumors became eligible to receive 81 Gy. Patients enrolled in the phase I dose-escalation study signed an informed consent form indicating that they were aware of the investigational nature of this clinical trial.

The results presented in this review entail 298 patients with T1c and T2 disease treated between October 1988 and February 1994. The characteristics of these patients are shown in Table 51.1-2. A total of 54 patients (15%) received androgen-deprivation therapy, either before referral for irradiation or as a planned neoadjuvant approach to meet the restrictions on normal tissue volumes carried to the prescription dose.[73] In each case, hormonal therapy was discontinued either before the beginning or after the completion of radiotherapy. The tumor target dose was 64.8 to 66.6 Gy in 60 patients, 70.2 Gy in 158 patients, 75.6 Gy in 59 patients, and 81 Gy in 21 patients. Late complications and disease status were determined at time of analysis in August 1994, and the median follow-up time was 14 months.

3D-CRT therapy at these dose levels was well tolerated. Acute gastrointestinal (GI) symptoms, when present, consisted of rectal discomfort, tenesmus, rectal bleeding (usually hemorrhoidal in origin) and minimal to mild diarrhea, and acute genitourinary (GU) symptoms included urinary frequency, nocturia, urgency, and dysuria. The majority of the patients (52%) had no acute toxicity or had mild (grade 1) symptoms that did not require therapeutic intervention. Only 15% of patients required medication for relief of GI symptoms and 39% for relief of acute GU symptoms, but for either type of toxicity, only one patient required interruption of treatment. The overall incidence of acute toxicity requiring medical intervention in this group of conformally treated patients compares favorably to the 60% observed in patients treated with conventional radiotherapeutic techniques in doses of 66 to 68.4 Gy.[33]

TABLE 51.1-2. *Characteristics of 298 stage T1c and T2 prostate cancer patients treated using three-dimensional conformal radiotherapy*

AGE (y)	
Median	69
Range	51–82
FOLLOW-UP (mon)	
Median	14
Range	6–63
CLINICAL STAGE	
T1c	67 (23%)
T2a	56 (19%)
T2b	84 (28%)
T2c	91 (30%)
GLEASON SCORE	
≤6	194 (65%)
≥7	104 (35%)
PRETREATMENT SERUM PROSTATE-SPECIFIC ANTIGEN LEVEL	
≤20	231 (78%)
>20	67 (22%)
TUMOR DOSE (Gy)	
64.8–66.6	60 (20%)
70.2	158 (54%)
75.6	59 (19%)
81	21 (7%)

Late complications were of minimal severity (grade 1 or 2), with none of the patients exhibiting severe grade 3 or 4 toxicities (Table 51.1-3). Although no intermediate or severe toxicities (grade 3 or higher) have been encountered in the patients receiving 75.6 Gy or 81 Gy, the length of follow-up in many of these patients is still too short to permit conclusions regarding morbidity at these dose levels.

Although this study was primarily designed to evaluate the toxicity associated with dose escalation, information on the initial response to treatment is also available. Posttherapeutic reduction of serum PSA levels to 4 ng/mL has been classically considered evidence for successful treatment because this value represents the upper limit of the normal range in the general male population. However, Willet and colleagues[75] demonstrated that the median PSA level after incidental irradiation of normal prostate glands was 0.65 ng/mL and that 70% of men receiving pelvic radiotherapy for rectal and other pelvic nonprostatic tumors had PSA values of 1 ng/mL or lower. Furthermore, long-term follow-up studies in irradiated prostate cancer patients indicate that those with persistent PSA values of 1 ng/mL or lower are less likely to develop prostatic relapses than those with levels of more than 1 but less than or equal to 4 ng/mL.[14,75–78] Hence, continuously maintained PSA levels of 1 ng/mL or more at 3 or more years after treatment has been accepted as a reliable endpoint for early evaluation of the efficacy of experimental radiotherapy protocols in prostate cancer.[78]

TABLE 51.1-3. *Incidence of late complications by grade* in 298 stage T1c and T2 prostate cancer patients treated using three-dimensional conformal radiotherapy to doses of 64.8 to 81 Gy*

	Complication	
Grade	Rectal	Urinary
None	255/298 (86%)	262/298 (88%)
Grade 1	33/298 (11%)	28/298 (9%)
Grade 2	10/298 (3%)	8/298 (3%)
Grade 3	0	0
Grade 4	0	0

* Radiation Therapy Oncology Group morbidity grading scheme.[36]

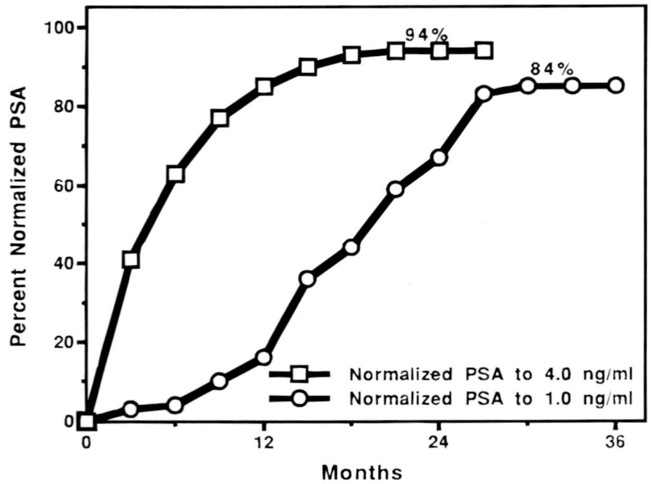

FIG. 51.1-3. Kaplan-Meier comparison of the cumulative times to posttreatment serum prostate-specific antigen (PSA) normalization to ≤4 ng/mL and to ≤1 ng/mL in 244 stage T1c and T2 patients who did not receive neoadjuvant hormonal therapy. The median time of PSA normalization to ≤4 ng/mL was 4.3 months, compared with 19.3 months for normalization to ≤1 ng/mL.

Testing these criteria of PSA response, Figure 51.1-3 shows a marked difference in the rate at which postirradiation PSA normalization to 4 ng/mL or lower and to 1 ng/mL or lower is achieved in patients who did not receive neoadjuvant androgen-deprivation therapy. The median times of PSA normalization to 4 ng/mL or lower and to 1 ng/mL or lower were 4.3 months and 19.3 months, respectively, whereas the 27-month actuarial PSA normalization rates to 4 ng/mL or lower and to 1 ng/mL or lower were 94% and 84%, respectively.

Table 51.1-4 shows that 29 patients (10%) had rising serum PSA levels, whether or not the PSA decreased to a nadir of 1 ng/mL or lower, at the time of their last follow-up visit, but only 7 (2%) developed clinically detectable anatomic relapses. The majority of anatomic relapses (5 of 7; 1% of the total number of patients) occurred at extraprostatic distant sites; only two patients (0.7%) had local recurrences in the prostate. All anatomic relapses occurred in patients with stage T2b or T2c tumors. One patient with stage T1c and 7 with T2a disease had a rising PSA level without evidence of anatomic relapse at the time of analysis. The 3-year actuarial overall survival was 94%, whereas the PSA relapse-free survival (from a PSA of ≤1 ng/

TABLE 51.1-4. *Clinical status at last follow-up in 298 stage T1c and T2c prostate cancer patients treated using three-dimensional conformal radiotherapy to doses of 64.8 to 81 Gy*

	Rising serum PSA level		Site of recurrence			
Stage	>4 ng/mL	>1 ng/mL	Local only	Distant only	Local and distant	Total
T1c	0	1	0	0	0	67
T2a	3	7	0	0	0	56
T2b	6	9	0	2	0	84
T2c	10	12	2	2	1	91
Total	19 (6%)	29 (10%)	2 (0.7%)	4 (1%)	1 (0.3%)	298

PSA, prostate-specific antigen.

mL) was 78%. The 3-year actuarial probability of survival without PSA relapse was 92% for stage T1c patients, 80% for T2a patients, 77% for T2b patients, and 67% for T2c patients (Fig. 51.1-4).

In addition to serving as a posttreatment outcome evaluation endpoint, the level of pretreatment PSA serves as a powerful predictor of the outcome after treatment.[13,14,61,62,76,79,80] The combination of pretreatment PSA and other pretreatment variables has been used in several studies to identify groups at high risk for relapse after treatment with surgery and radiotherapy.[13,22,62,80,81] A Cox proportional hazards regression analysis of the MSKCC series treated with 3D-CRT revealed that PSA (≤20 ng/mL versus >20 ng/mL), stage (≤T2c versus T3), and Gleason score (≤6 versus ≥7) were each significant, independent variables that affected the risk of subsequent PSA relapse.[22] However, when this multivariate analysis was restricted to T1c and T2 patients, pretreatment PSA level (≤20 ng/mL versus >20 ng/mL) turned out to be the only covariate that affected PSA relapse. The 3-year PSA relapse-free survival rate for T1c and T2 patients with a pretreatment PSA of 20 ng/mL or lower was 92%, compared to 38% for those with a PSA higher than 20 ng/mL ($P < .0001$).

Based on these findings, the rate of PSA normalization to 1 ng/mL or lower was examined in patients who had a pretreatment PSA of 20 ng/mL or lower. Figure 51.1-5 shows that the rate of PSA normalization was significantly greater in patients who presented with a PSA of 20 ng/mL or lower compared with those with a pretreatment PSA higher than 20 ng/mL ($P = .001$). Furthermore, Figure 51.1-6 shows a treatment dose effect on the rate of PSA normalization. Patients with pretreatment PSA values of 20 ng/mL or lower who received 70.2 Gy exhibited a significantly higher rate of PSA normalization to 1 ng/mL or lower than those who received 64.8 to 66.6 Gy ($P < .01$). Although a dose-response relation has not been observed thus far for patients treated with doses between 70.2 and 75.6 Gy, the follow-up of many of these patients is too short to draw even preliminary conclusions.

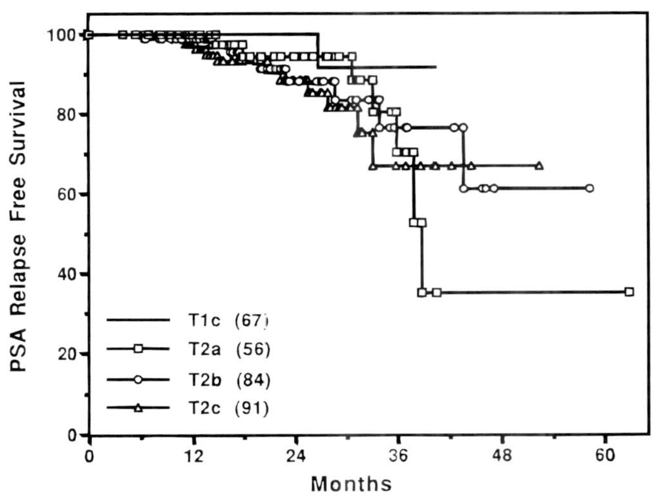

FIG. 51.1-4. Kaplan-Meier time-adjusted serum prostate-specific antigen relapse-free survival by stage in 298 T1c and T2 patients treated with three-dimensional conformal radiotherapy.

CONCLUSIONS AND FUTURE DIRECTIONS

The preliminary data available indicate a promising potential for 3D-CRT in the management of localized carcinoma of the prostate. The feasibility of safely escalating the radiation dose

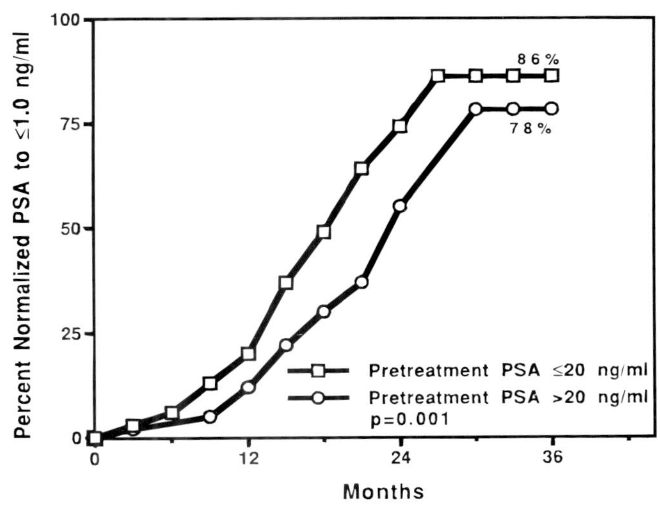

FIG. 51.1-5. Kaplan-Meier comparison of the cumulative time to posttreatment serum prostate-specific antigen (PSA) normalization to ≤1 ng/mL by pretreatment PSA in 244 stage T1c and T2 patients who did not receive neoadjuvant hormonal therapy. The rate of PSA normalization for patients with pretreatment PSA levels of ≤20 ng/mL was significantly higher than for those with pretreatment levels of >20 ng/mL ($P = .001$).

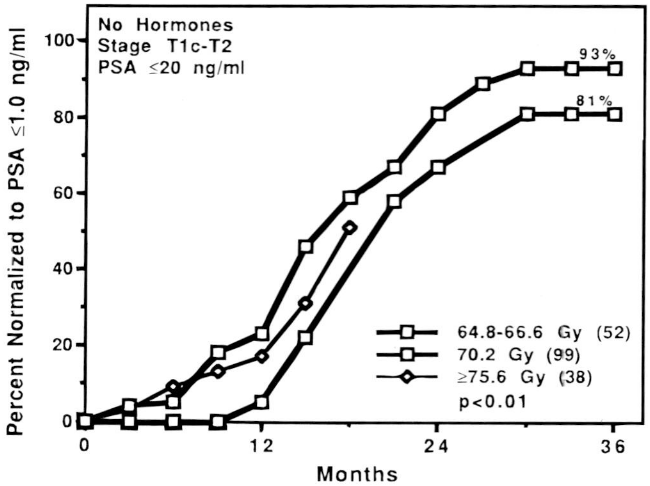

FIG. 51.1-6. Kaplan-Meier comparison of the cumulative time to posttreatment serum prostate-specific antigen (PSA) normalization to ≤1 ng/mL by dose in 189 stage T1c and T2 patients who had pretreatment PSA levels of ≤20 ng/mL and who did not receive neoadjuvant hormonal therapy. The rate of PSA normalization for patients who received 70.2 Gy was significantly higher than for those who received 64.8 to 66.6 Gy ($P < .01$).

to unprecedented levels has already been demonstrated. Furthermore, despite the use of higher doses, the incidence of both acute and late radiation morbidity has been reduced with 3D-CRT techniques. The current incidence of 0.7% (two grade 3 and one grade 4) for acute and late GI and GU toxicity in the entire group of 432 (stage T1-T3) 3D-CRT–treated patients is similar to the 0.6% incidence reported by Epstein and colleagues[82] for 108 patients treated with 3D-CRT techniques carried to 64 to 72 Gy. These rates compare favorably with the acute and late grade 3 GI and GU complication rate of 3.8% and the grade 4 rate of 2.5% reported in patients treated using standard radiotherapy techniques.[82] No severe late complications have been observed in patients receiving 75.6 Gy or 81 Gy. However, the follow-up of many of these patients is too short to permit definitive conclusions regarding the long-term safety of the higher dose levels as delivered by the MSKCC technique.

The preliminary therapeutic results of stage T1c and T2 patients treated with 3D-CRT also are encouraging. Patients who relapsed anatomically had T2b and T2c tumors, and the majority of these developed distant metastatic disease. The early PSA outcome data compare favorably with surgical series; short-term rates of freedom from PSA failure have ranged from 79% to 95% in patients with organ-confined disease and from 19% to 36% in those with more locally advanced tumors.[17–19]

Although several reports have demonstrated a relation between local control determined clinically with dose of 70 Gy or more delivered by conventional techniques in stage T3 tumors,[71,83] similar studies in T2 tumors have shown an advantage for doses of more than 60 Gy but not for more than 70 Gy.[71] The preliminary data from MSKCC suggest an improvement in the rate of PSA normalization to 1 ng/mL when the dose is increased from between 64.8 and 66.6 Gy to 70.2 Gy. The follow-up in many of the higher-dose patients is still too short to evaluate whether higher doses will be associated with higher initial rates of PSA normalization. With longer follow-up it will be important to determine whether maintenance of PSA at a level of 1 ng/mL or lower is dose dependent and an indicator for improved permanent local control.

Recent studies on the impact of local tumor control on subsequent metastatic dissemination suggest that clinical trials designed to test whether survival will be enhanced by improvements in local therapy should be restricted to node-negative patients only.[29] Based on the relation between the pretreatment PSA and subsequent chemical (PSA) outcome in stage T1c and T2 patients, it appears to be possible to distinguish clinically patients with a small probability of extraprostatic involvement (PSA ≤ 20 mg/mL) from those with a high likelihood of having either pelvic lymph node metastases or micrometastatic dissemination to remote sites (PSA > 20 ng/mL). Patients in the latter group should be considered for staging lymphadenectomy to select only node-negative patients as eligible for high-dose 3D-CRT. Combined with polymerase chain reaction detection methods of PSA-synthesizing cells in the peripheral circulation,[84] it may become possible to identify patients in whom combined modality therapy programs would be more appropriate.

As technical improvements are made in treatment planning and delivery and as methods are introduced to correct for treatment setup and organ motion–related uncertainties,[85] 3D-CRT is likely to improve on its current capacity for accuracy and safety in delivering high-dose radiotherapy for early stage prostate cancer. However, beyond technical progress, the ultimate success of this modality depends on the ability to improve local control and to affect disease-specific survival. If the current trend for improved results persists, it is expected that 3D-CRT will become the standard method of radiotherapy treatment of localized prostate cancer.

REFERENCES

1. Catalona WJ, Smith DS, Ratliff TL, et al. Measurement of prostate-specific antigen in serum as a screening test for prostate cancer. N Engl J Med 1991;324:1156.
2. Consensus Conference. The management of clinically localized prostate cancer. JAMA 1987;258:2727.
3. Zietman AL, Shipley WU. Randomized trials in loco-regionally confined prostate cancer: past, present and future. Semin Radiat Oncol 1993;3:210.
4. Budhraja SN, Anderson JC. An assessment of the value of radiotherapy in the management of carcinoma of the prostate. Br J Urol 1964;36:535.
5. George FW, Carlton CE Jr, Dykhuizen RF, Dillon JR. Cobalt-60 telecuritherapy in the definitive treatment of carcinoma of the prostate: a preliminary report. J Urol 1965;93:102.
6. Del Regato J. Radiotherapy in the conservative treatment of operable and locally inoperable carcinoma of the prostate. Radiology 1967;88:761.
7. Bagshaw MA, Kaplan HS, Sagerman RH. Linear accelerator supervoltage therapy. VII. Carcinoma of the prostate. Radiology 1965;85:121.
8. Ray GR, Cassady JR, Bagshaw MA. Definitive radiation therapy of carcinoma of the prostate: a report of 15 years experience. Radiology 1973;106:407.
9. Perez CA, Hanks GE, Leibel SA, Zietman AL, Fuks Z, Lee WR. Localized carcinoma of the prostate (stages T1B, T1C, T2, and T3). Review of management with external beam radiation therapy. Cancer 1993;72:3156.
10. Hanks GE, Asbell S, Krall JM, et al. Outcome for lymph node dissection negative T1-b, T2 (A-2,B) prostate cancer treated with external

beam radiation therapy in RTOG 77-06. Int J Radiat Oncol Biol Phys 1991;21:1099.

11. Kabalin JN, Hodge KK, McNeal JE, Freiha FS, Stamey TA. Identification of residual cancer in the prostate following radiation therapy: role of transrectal ultrasound guided biopsy and prostate specific antigen. J Urol 1989;142:326.
12. Kuban DA, El-Mahdi AM. Local control after radiation for prostatic carcinoma: significance and assessment. Semin Radiat Oncol 1993;3:221.
13. Zagars GK, von Eschenbach AC. Prostatic-specific antigen: an important marker for prostate cancer treated by external beam radiotherapy. Cancer 1993;72:538.
14. Zietman AL, Coen JJ, Shipley WU, Willett CG, Efird JT. Radical radiation therapy in the management of prostatic adenocarcinoma: the initial prostate specific antigen value as a predictor of treatment outcome. J Urol 1994;151:640.
15. Stamey TA, Ferrari MK, Schmid H-P. The value of serial prostate specific antigen determinations 5 years after radiotherapy: steeply increasing values characterize 80% of patients. J Urol 1993;150:856.
16. Schellhammer PF, El-Mahdi ASM, Wright GL Jr, Kolm P, Ragle P. Prostate-specific antigen to determine progress free survival after radiation therapy for localized carcinoma of the prostate. Urology 1993;42:13.
17. Stein A, deKernion JB, Smith RB, Dorey F, Patel H. Prostate specific antigen levels after radical prostatectomy in patients with organ confined and locally extensive prostatic cancer. J Urol 1992;147:942.
18. Frazier HA, Robertson JE, Humphrey PA, Paulson DF. Is prostate specific antigen of clinical importance in evaluating outcome after radical prostatectomy. J Urol 1993;149:516.
19. Osterling JE, Chan DW, Epstein JI, et al. Prostate specific antigen in the preoperative and postoperative evaluation of localized prostatic cancer treated with radical prostatectomy. J Urol 1988;139:766.
20. Zincke H, Blute ML, Fallen MJ, Farrow GM. Radical prostatectomy for stage A adenocarcinoma of the prostate: staging errors and their implications for treatment recommendations and disease outcome. J Urol 1991;146:1053.
21. Leibel SA, Kutcher GJ, Mohan R, et al. Three-dimensional conformal radiation therapy at the Memorial Sloan-Kettering Cancer Center. Semin Radiat Oncol 1992;2:274.
22. Leibel SA, Zelefsky MJ, Kutcher GJ, Burman CM, Kelson S, Fuks Z. Three-dimensional conformal radiation therapy in localized carcinoma of the prostate: interim report of a phase I dose-escalation study. J Urol 1994;152:1792.
23. Sandler HM, McShan DL, Lichter AS. Potential improvement in the results of irradiation for prostate carcinoma using improved dose distribution. Int J Radiat Oncol Biol Phys 1991;22:361.
24. Bagshaw MA. Definitive megavoltage radiation therapy in carcinoma of the prostate. In: Fletcher GH, ed. Textbook of radiotherapy. Philadelphia: Lea & Febiger, 1973:752.
25. Bagshaw MA. External radiation therapy of carcinoma of the prostate. Cancer 1980;45:1912.
26. Asbell SO, Schlager BA, Baker AS. Revision of treatment planning for carcinoma of the prostate. Int J Radiat Oncol Biol Phys 1980;6:861.
27. Pilepich MV, Prasad S, Perez CA. Computed tomography in definitive radiotherapy of prostatic carcinoma. Part 2. Definition of target volume. Int J Radiat Oncol Biol Phys 1982;8:235.
28. Bagshaw MA, Kaplan ID, Cox RC. Radiation therapy for localized disease. Cancer 1993;71:939.
29. Leibel SA, Fuks Z, Zelefsky MJ, Whitmore WF Jr. The effects of local and regional treatments on the metastatic outcome in prostatic carcinoma with pelvic lymph node involvement. Int J Radiat Oncol Biol Phys 1994;28:7.
30. Epstein BE, Hanks GE. Radiation therapy techniques and dose selection in the treatment of prostate cancer. Semin Radiat Oncol 1993;3:179.
31. Marks LB, Ancher MS. Radiotherapy for prostate cancer: should the seminal vesicles be considered target? Int J Radiat Oncol Biol Phys 1992;24:435.
32. Epstein JI, Carmichael M, Walsh PC. Adenocarcinoma of the prostate invading the seminal vesicle: definition and relation of tumor volume, grade and margins of resection to prognosis. J Urol 1993;149:1040.
33. Soffen EM, Hanks GE, Hunt MA, Epstein BE. Conformal static field radiation therapy treatment of early prostate cancer versus non-conformal techniques: a reduction in acute morbidity. Int J Radiat Oncol Biol Phys 1992;24:485.
34. Hanks GE. External-beam radiation therapy for clinically localized prostate cancer: patterns of care studies in the United States. Natl Cancer Inst Monogr 1988;7:75.
35. Shipley WU, Zietman AL, Hanks GE, et al. Treatment related sequelae following external beam radiation for prostate cancer: a review with an update in patients with stages T1 and T2 tumor. J Urol 1994;152:1799.
36. Lawton CA, Won M, Pilepich MV, et al. Long-term treatment sequelae following external beam irradiation for adenocarcinoma of the prostate: analysis of RTOG studies 7506 and 7706. Int J Radiat Oncol Biol Phys 1991;21:935.
37. Smit WGJM, Helle PA, van Putte WLJ, Wijnmaalen AJ, Seldenrath JJ, van der Werf-Messing BHP. Late radiation damage in prostate cancer patients treated by high dose external radiotherapy in relation to rectal dose. Int J Radiat Oncol Biol Phys 1990;18:23.
38. Benk VA, Adams JA, Shipley WU, et al. Late rectal bleeding following combined x-ray and proton high dose irradiation for stages T3-T4 prostate cancer. Int J Radiat Oncol Biol Phys 1993;26:551.
39. Bagshaw MA, Cox RS, Ray GR. Status of radiation treatment of prostate cancer at Stanford University. Natl Cancer Inst Monogr 1988;7:47.
40. Banker FL. The preservation of potency after external beam irradiation for prostate cancer. Int J Radiat Oncol Biol Phys 1991;15:219.
41. Hanks GE, Krall JM, Hanlon AL, Asbell SO, Pilepich MV, Owen JB. Patterns of care and RTOG studies in prostate cancer: long-term survival, hazard rate observations, and possibilities of cure. Int J Radiat Oncol Biol Phys 1994;28:39.
42. Zagars GK, von Eschenback AC, Johnson DE, Oswald MJ. The role of radiation therapy in stages A2 and B adenocarcinoma of the prostate. Int J Radiat Oncol Biol Phys 1988;14:701.
43. Bagshaw MA, Cox RS, Hancock SL. Control of prostate cancer with radiotherapy: long-term results. J Urol 1994;152:1781.
44. Kaplan ID, Prestidge BR, Bagshaw MA, Cox RS. The importance of local control in the treatment of prostatic cancer. J Urol 1992;147:917.
45. Jewett HJ, Walsh PC. Radical perineal prostatectomy for clinical stage T2 carcinoma of the prostate. J Urol 1982;127:704.
46. Gibbons RP, Correa RJ, Brannen GE. Total prostatectomy for localized prostatic cancer. J Urol 1982;131:73.
47. Middleton RG, Smith JA Jr, Melzer RB, Hamilton PE. Patient survival and local recurrence rate following radical prostatectomy for prostatic carcinoma. J Urol 1986;136:422.
48. Paulson DF, Moul JW, Walther PJ. Radical prostatectomy for clinical stage T1-T2NOMO prostatic adenocarcinoma: long-term results. J Urol 1990;144:1180.
49. Hanks GE. External beam radiation treatment for prostate cancer: still the gold standard. Oncology 1992;6:79.
50. Blute ML, Nativ O, Zincke H, Fallow GM, Therneau T, Lieber MM. Pattern of failure after radical retropubic prostatectomy for clinically and pathologically localized adenocarcinoma of the prostate: influence of tumor deoxyribonucleic acid ploidy. J Urol 1989;142:1262.
51. Kaplan ID, Cox PS, Bagshaw MS. Radiotherapy for prostatic cancer: patient selection and the impact of local control. Urology 1994;43:634.
52. Coleman CN, Beard CJ, Kantoff PW, Gelman R. Rate of relapse following treatment for localized prostate cancer: a critical analysis of retrospective reports. Int J Radiat Oncol Biol Phys 1994;28:303.
53. Lee RJ, Sause WT. Surgically staged patients with prostatic carcinoma treated with definitive radiotherapy: fifteen-year results. Urology 1994;43:640.
54. Corn BW, Hanks GE. Therapeutic options for clinically localized carcinoma of the prostate. Semin Radiat Oncol 1993;3:187.
55. Kuban DA, El-Mahdi AM, Schellhammer P. The significance of post-irradiation prostate biopsy with long-term follow-up. Int J Radiat Oncol Biol Phys 1992;24:409.
56. Crook J, Robertson S, Collin G, Zaleski V, Esche B. Clinical relevance of trans-rectal ultrasound, biopsy, and serum prostate-specific antigen following external radiotherapy for carcinoma of the prostate. Int J Radiat Oncol Biol Phys 1993;27:31.
57. Dugan TC, Shipley WU, Young RH, et al. Biopsy after external beam radiation therapy for adenocarcinoma of the prostate: correlation with original histological grade and current prostate specific antigen levels. J Urol 1991;146:1313.
58. Scardino PT, Wheeler TM. Local control of prostate cancer with radio-

therapy: frequency and prognostic significance of positive results of post-irradiation biopsy. Natl Cancer Inst Monogr 1988;7:95.
59. Hanks GE. Post treatment biopsies of the prostate: a stalking horse for improving local control. Int J Radiat Oncol Biol Phys 1992;24:572.
60. Zietman AL, Shipley WU, Willett GC. Residual disease after radical surgery or radiation therapy for prostate cancer: clinical significance and therapeutic implications. Cancer 1993;71:859.
61. Kaplan ID, Cox RS, Bagshaw MA. Prostate specific antigen after external beam for prostatic cancer: followup. J Urol 1993;149:519.
62. Pisansky TM, Cha SS, Earle JD, et al. Prostate-specific antigen as a pretherapy prognostic factor in patients treated with radiation therapy for clinically localized prostate cancer. J Clin Oncol 1993;11:2158.
63. Ten Haken RK, Perez-Tamayo C, Tesser RJ, McShan DL, Frass BA, Lichter A. Boost treatment of the prostate using shaped fixed fields. Int J Radiat Oncol Biol Phys 1989;6:193.
64. Hanks GE, Martz KL, Diamond JJ. The effect of dose on local control of prostate cancer. Int J Radiat Oncol Biol Phys 1988;15:1299.
65. Fuks Z, Leibel SA, Kutcher GJ, Mohan R, Ling CC. Three dimensional conformal treatment: a new frontier in radiation therapy. In: DeVita VT Jr, Hellman S, Rosenberg SA, eds. Important advances in oncology. Philadelphia: JB Lippincott, 1991:151.
66. Vijaykumar S, Awan A, Karrison T, et al. Acute toxicity during external-beam radiotherapy for localized prostate cancer: comparison of different techniques. Int J Radiat Oncol Biol Phys 1993;25:359.
67. Bijhold J, Lebesque JV, Hart AAM, Vijlbrief RE. Maximizing setup accuracy using portal images as applied to a conformal boost technique for prostatic cancer. Radiother Oncol 1992;24:261.
68. Roach M III, Pickett B, Rosenthal SA, et al. Defining treatment margins for six field conformal irradiation of localized prostate cancer. Int J Radiat Oncol Biol Phys 1994;28:267.
69. Mohan R, Barest G, Brewster LJ, et al. A comprehensive three-dimensional radiation treatment planning system. Int J Radiat Cncol Biol Phys 1988;15:481.
70. Leibel SA, Zekefsky MJ, Kutcher GJ, et al. The biological basis and clinical application of three-dimensional conformal external beam radiation therapy in carcinoma of the prostate. Semin Oncol 1994;21:580.
71. Melian E, Kutcher G, Leibel S, et al. Quantification and implications for three-dimensional conformal radiation therapy. (Abstract) Int J Radiat Oncol Biol Phys 1993;27(Suppl 1):137.
72. Mohan R, Chui CS. Use of Fourier transforms in calculating dose distributions for irregularly shaped fields for three dimensional treatment planning. Med Phys 1987;14:70.
73. Zelefsky MJ, Leibel SA, Burman CM, et al. Neoadjuvant hormonal therapy improves the therapeutic ratio in patients with bulky prostatic cancer treated with three-dimensional conformal radiation therapy. Int J Radiat Oncol Biol Phys 1994;29:755.
74. Leibel SA, Heimann R, Kutcher GJ, et al. Three-dimensional conformal radiation therapy in locally advanced carcinoma of the prostate: preliminary results of a phase I dose-escalation study. Int J Radiat Oncol Biol Phys 1994;28:55.
75. Willett CG, Zietman AL, Shipley WU, Coen JJ. The effect of pelvic radiation therapy on serum levels of prostate specific antigen. J Urol 1994;151:1579.
76. Ritter MA, Messing EM, Shanahan TG, Potts S, Chappell RJ, Kinsella TJ. Prostate-specific antigen as a predictor of radiotherapy response and patterns of failure in localized prostate cancer. J Clin Oncol 1992;10:1208.
77. Zagars GK. Prostate-specific antigen as a prognostic factor for prostate cancer treated with external beam radiotherapy. Int J Radiat Oncol Biol Phys 1992;23:47.
78. Zelefsky MJ, Leibel SA, Wallner KE, Whitmore WF Jr, Fuks Z. The significance of normal serum PSA in the follow-up after definitive radiation therapy for prostatic cancer. J Clin Oncol 1995;13:459.
79. Russell KJ, Dunatov C, Hafermann MD, et al. Prostate specific antigen in the management of patients with localized adenocarcinoma of the prostate treated with primary radiation therapy. J Urol 1991;146:1046.
80. Partin AW, Pound CR, Clemens JQ, Epstein JI, Walsh PC. Serum PSA after anatomic radical prostatectomy: the Johns Hopkins experience after 10 years. Urol Clin North Am 1993;20:713.
81. Partin AW, Yoo J, Carter HB, et al. The use of prostate specific antigen, clinical stage and Gleason score to predict pathological stage in men with localized prostate cancer. J Urol 1993;150:110.
82. Epstein B, Peter R, Martin E, Hunt M, Hanks G. Low complication rate with conformal radiotherapy for cancer of the prostate. (Abstract) Radiother Oncol 1992;24(Suppl):S100.
83. Perez CA, Pilepich MV, Zivnuska F. Tumor control in definitive irradiation of localized carcinoma of the prostate. Int J Radiat Oncol Biol Phys 1986;12:523.
84. Katz AE, Olsson CA, Raffo AJ, et al. Molecular staging of prostate cancer with the use of an enhanced reverse transcripase-PCR assay. Urology 1994;43:765.
85. Mageras GS, Melian E, Fuks Z, Leibel SA, Mohan R, Kutcher GJ. Incorporation of organ motion uncertainties into 3D prostate treatment plans. Int J Radiat Oncol Biol Phys (Abstract) 1994;30(Suppl 1):175.

51.2 Prostate Brachytherapy

Kent Wallner

Interest in prostate brachytherapy has fluctuated since the early 1900s. Barringer,[1] as head of urology at what is now the Memorial Sloan-Kettering Cancer Center (MSKCC), reported in 1917 on transperineal insertion of radium needles to treat prostate cancer. In the 1970s, retropubic iodine-125 (^{125}I) implants were popularized by Whitmore and colleagues,[2] also at MSKCC. Interest in brachytherapy waned in the 1980s because the suprapubic procedure was technically difficult to perform and poor local control rates were reported in some series.[3]

In the early 1980s, Holm and colleagues[4] introduced the use of transrectal ultrasonography (TRUS), allowing visualization of the needle location within the prostate. With TRUS or computed tomographic (CT) images, implants could be computer planned so that the the radiation dose would reliably conform to the shape of the prostate. Interest in brachytherapy was boosted further by the fact that transperineal procedures could be done on an outpatient basis.

PERMANENT OR TEMPORARY IMPLANTS

Prostatic brachytherapy can be done with permanent source placement or by temporary insertion of iridium-192 (^{192}Ir) inside hollow, flexible catheters. Current interest in prostate brachytherapy mainly involves the use of permanent sources. The primary advantage of permanent implants is that the procedure can be done on an outpatient basis, whereas temporary implants require overnight hospitalization. There is some interest in the use of high-dose-rate, remote after-loading ^{192}Ir for temporary implants, but no published results are available.

^{125}I is the most commonly used isotope for permanent implants. The minimum target dose of 140 to 160 Gy was arrived at empirically by Whitmore and colleagues.[2] Because of its low average energy (30 keV), ^{125}I requires minimal shielding and protection requirements. Its long half-life of 60 days allows its storage for several weeks prior to use.

One disadvantage of ^{125}I may be its low dose rate. The peripheral dose rate to the prostate with an ^{125}I implant of 160 Gy is approximately 8 cGy/hour, which is low compared to usual brachytherapy dose rates. A temporary ^{192}Ir implant, for instance, has a peripheral dose rate of approximately 40 cGy/hour. The low dose rate of ^{125}I has been cited as a reason for inferior local control rates in high-grade tumors[5,6]; however, the poor results for high-grade tumors are more likely the result of their more aggressive tumor biology. Nevertheless, because of the theoretical argument that ^{125}I dose rate is too low, the use of palladium-103 (^{103}Pd) has been introduced.

Similar to ^{125}I, ^{103}Pd is a low-energy isotope (21 keV) with minimal shielding requirements. ^{103}Pd has a half-life of only 17 days; therefore, the initial peripheral dose rate is approximately 20 cGy/hour (120-Gy total dose)—three times greater than that with a typical ^{125}I implant. Although there are theoretical arguments for and against use of ^{103}Pd, its benefit over ^{125}I is debatable. The advantage of ^{103}Pd's higher dose rate may be offset by the reduction in total dose delivered; the total dose with a ^{103}Pd implant is adjusted down from 160 Gy to 120 Gy because of the higher dose rate.[7] Use of ^{103}Pd is usually limited to moderately or poorly differentiated tumors, which presumably would be better treated with more rapid dose delivery. The disadvantages of ^{103}Pd are its greater cost and shorter shelf life. The total cost of ^{103}Pd sources for a full-dose implant is approximately 3000 U.S. dollars versus 1000 dollars for ^{125}I sources. Because of ^{103}Pd's shorter half-life, it can be stored for only 3 to 5 days before losing too much activity to be used. Considering the growing interest in prostate brachytherapy, it would be worthwhile to test the benefits of ^{103}Pd versus ^{125}I in a rigorous clinical trial.

TREATMENT PLANNING

One advantage of ultrasonography- and CT-planned prostate implants is that the prostate dimensions can be used to determine the proper amount and distribution of sources to adequately irradiate the prostate. The prostatic dimensions are taken from preimplant TRUS or CT images, usually at 5-mm intervals. The prostatic margins are digitized into a computer to reconstruct the prostate in three dimensions. Using the transverse images, a seed pattern and isodose distribution are calculated for each cross section. A preliminary isodose pattern is compared with the planning images, and alterations in seed placement can be made to adjust the coverage to the prostate, urethra, or rectum.

Planning images can be based on either ultrasonographic or CT images[8,9]; each has advantages and disadvantages. The advantage of ultrasonography over CT is its sharper delineation of the prostatic margin. The benefit of CT scanning over ultrasonography may be that CT produces less distortion of the prostatic contour. The degree of distortion with ultrasonography has not been quantified but is probably substantial, and it varies depending on probe position and the amount of water around the transducer. Remarkably good 5-year results have been reported with both methods. Obtaining superior results with transperineal implantation probably depends more on operator skill and appreciation of brachytherapy principles than the technology used.

TABLE 51.2-1. *General brachytherapy dose guidelines*

Isotope	Minimum prostatic dose (Gy)	External dose (Gy)
IMPLANT ALONE		
^{125}I	140–160	
^{103}Pd	110–120	
IMPLANT PLUS EXTERNAL IRRADIATION		
^{125}I	100–120	45–50
^{103}Pd	90–95	45–50
^{192}Ir	30–40	40–50

The dose is prescribed at the periphery of the prostate. It is intended as the minimum dose to the prostate. Because of the cumulative contribution from multiple sources, the dose to the center of the prostate is usually higher. High central doses may lead to urethral damage. However, the urethral dose can be reduced if sources are preferentially placed at the prostate periphery. In practice, it is difficult to keep the urethral dose below 250 Gy while delivering 150 Gy to the prostatic margins with ^{125}I. When using ^{103}Pd, it is possible to keep the urethral doses relatively lower because of this agent's more rapid falloff. This potential advantage of ^{103}Pd must be weighed against the increased possibility of cold spots within the target volume.

Brachytherapy doses for permanent or temporary implants were derived empirically based on experience at various institutions (Table 51.2-1). These doses are commonly adjusted to accommodate variations in treatment planning practices or experience at particular institutions.

PROCEDURE

The preparatory procedure varies somewhat among institutions. On the day prior to implantation, a diet to clear the lower colon is followed. Patients are limited to clear liquids for 24 hours prior to the procedure, and drink eight ounces of magnesium citrate the night before. Alternatively, an enema can be administered the morning of the procedure. The purpose of the preparatory diet is to facilitate use of TRUS and to minimize the likelihood of rectal contamination if the rectal wall is pierced during the procedure. Prophylactic antibiotics are routinely prescribed but probably are not necessary.[10]

To perform the implant, the patient is placed in the lithotomy position and given spinal or general anesthesia. A Foley catheter is placed to help identify the base of the prostate. A needle guide template is mounted against the perineum, and three or four needles are inserted (Fig. 51.2-1). The template has needle holes at 0.5 cm intervals. The first needles are chosen anteriorly, on each side of the urethra. They are inserted simultaneously to minimize lateral movement of the prostate. Subsequently, one or two posterior needles are placed. The position of the

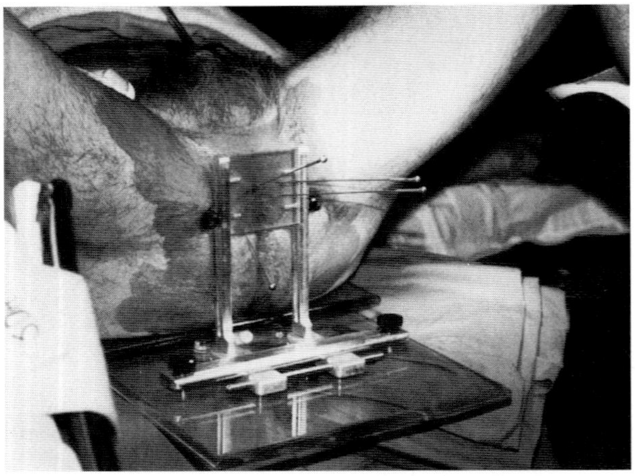

FIG. 51.2-1. View of template-guided transperineal prostate brachytherapy as performed at the Memorial Sloan-Kettering Cancer Center. The template is mounted against the perineum, and fluoroscopy, transrectal ultrasonography, or both are used to verify proper needle placement before radioactive sources are inserted.

needles is checked using TRUS, fluoroscopy, or both to determine their correct position relative to the preplan. If the placement does not match that intended, the needles are removed and the template is repositioned. Part of the positioning difficulty is the result of the unavoidable variance in patient positioning compared to that on the day the planning scans were made. Another source of difficulty is the mobility of the prostate when it is pierced with needles. Prostate motion during needle insertion is unavoidable and must be monitored throughout the procedure. Use of elaborate anchoring devices is probably not worthwhile. During actual insertion of sources, needle depth is gauged from the most proximal TRUS image or the Foley balloon as visualized fluoroscopically.

Sources can be placed with a Mick applicator or with spacer material in a preloaded configuration. There is no objective evidence as to which method is best. Fluoroscopy should be used to monitor seed placement during the procedure, because sources can migrate within the needle tracks.[11] Fluoroscopy is highly recommended, because it is impossible to reliably identify individual source placement using TRUS because of interference from other sources and needles already in place.

QUALITY ASSURANCE

TRUS, fluoroscopy, and computerization has dramatically improved the ability to perform precise implants. The encouraging results at some institutions reflect technically optimal technique. To obtain similarly good results, an effort must be made to assure good-quality implants. Assurance of implant quality requires some quantification of the dose to the prostate to verify that proper source placement was achieved based on postimplant x-ray films. Unfortunately, dosimetric evaluation of prostatic implants remains imprecise.

Total activity implanted and matched peripheral dose (MPD) have been the standard criteria for evaluating implant quality. Total activity is a very crude indication of quality because it gives no information regarding the relation of dose to the prostatic margins.

The MPD is calculated as the dose at which the isodose contour volume equals the volume of an ellipsoid having the same dimensions as those measured clinically for the target volume. The MPD is calculated from stereo-shift films. It is drawn in relation to the sources and does not necessarily correspond to the actual prostatic volume (Fig. 51.2-2). The MPD is an approximation of the dose to an approximation of the prostate volume. Reliance on such imprecise parameters as total activity or the MPD to evaluate implant quality leaves much to be desired. For patients implanted with ^{125}I at MSKCC, no relation has been noted between the MPD and urethral or rectal morbidity (Fig. 51.2-3).

Postimplant CT scans can be used to evaluate implant quality much more precisely than is possible using MPD. With CT images, the relation between the prostatic margin and the radiation dose lines can be determined. Accordingly, postimplant CT scans can be used to calculate the minimum prostatic dose, urethral dose, and rectal doses (Figs. 51.2-4 and 51.2-5). Wallner and colleagues[12] have shown that CT-based dosimetry can predict which patients are at higher risk of radiation-induced morbidity. Specifically, urethral doses greater than 400 Gy and rectal doses greater than 100 Gy are associated with a higher risk of postimplant complications. These researchers have also

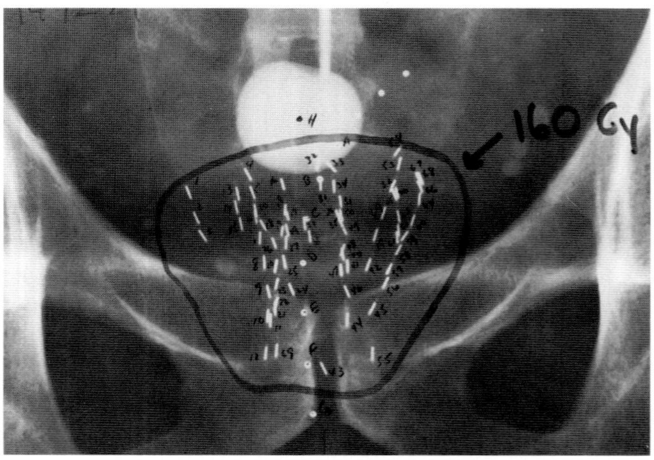

FIG. 51.2-2. Postimplant radiographs showing the 160-Gy isodose line.

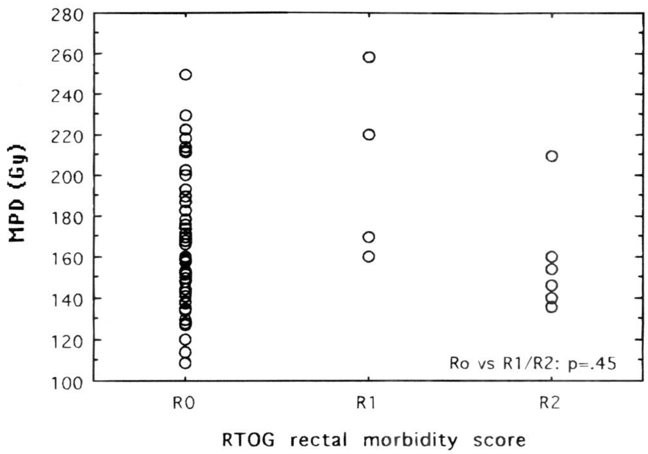

FIG. 51.2-3. Radiation Therapy Oncology Group (RTOG) rectal morbidity versus matched peripheral dose (MPD). The MPD had no correlation with rectal or urinary morbidity (P = .45). R1, painless bleeding; R2, rectal ulceration.

shown that CT-based dosimetry is a much more clinically meaningful way to determine radiation doses than are previously used parameters such as the total activity implanted, radioactivity per source, or MPD.[12]

Optimal assessment of implant quality should include CT-based dosimetry. Unfortunately, the cost of obtaining and analyzing postimplant CT scans could discourage their use, possibly jeopardizing implant quality control.

PATIENT SELECTION

Prostate brachytherapy can be used as the sole modality for patient selection, or it can be used in combination with external beam radiation therapy (EBRT). Selection of brachytherapy alone versus brachytherapy plus EBRT is based on the likelihood of extracapsular extension. Because of rapid dose falloff, brachytherapy alone can adequately treat only intracapsular disease and minimal transcapsular extension.

In general, brachytherapy alone is used for tumors clinical staged as T1 to T2a. Small stage T2b lesions that are well or moderately differentiated can be treated using implants alone, but the risk of extracapsular extension rises to 50% or more in higher-grade stage T2b tumors.[13] Brachytherapy alone should be discouraged for poorly differentiated tumors and in patients with prostate-specific antigen (PSA) levels greater than 20 ng/mL.

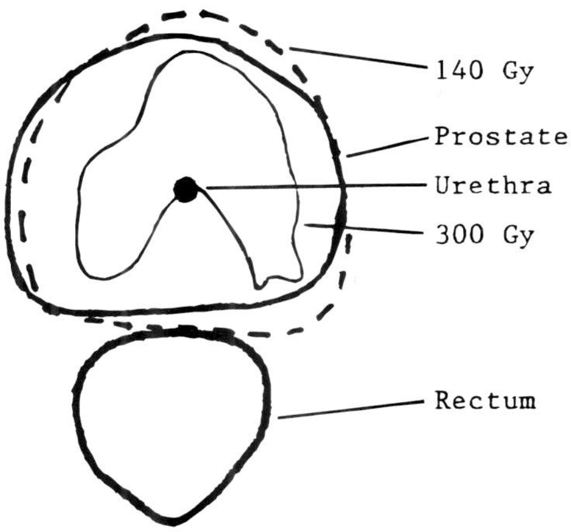

FIG. 51.2-5. Cross-sectional isodoses corresponding to the computed tomographic image in Figure 51.2-4. Coverage of the prostatic margin by the intended 140-Gy line is satisfactory. The central urethral dose is 300 Gy.

Patients who meet these guidelines for treatment with brachytherapy alone have a low likelihood of extraprostatic disease and probably do not need to undergo lymph node dissection or seminal vesicle biopsy. If higher-risk patients are selected for implantation, preimplant biopsy of pelvic lymph nodes and seminal vesicles should be performed.

For patients with a high risk of extraprostatic disease extension, implantation is combined with moderate-dose EBRT to allow wider coverage of the periprostatic tissues and seminal vesicles. Use of combined implant plus EBRT for high-stage tumors has produced results that compare favorably with EBRT alone.[14]

Patients with a prior history of transurethral resection of the prostate (TURP) should be approached cautiously. Some inves-

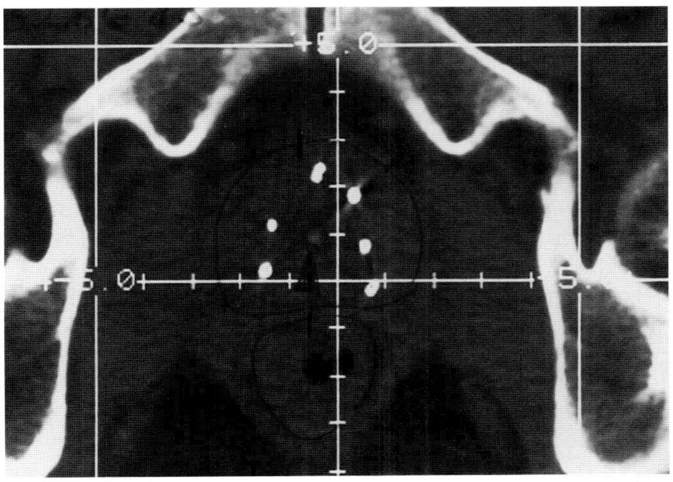

FIG. 51.2-4. On postimplant computed tomographic scan, radioactive sources are visible throughout the prostate. A catheter (*arrowhead*) is used to calculate the urethral dose.

tigators have reported higher rates of incontinence in such patients.[15] However, there has been no meticulous report regarding the effect of the degree of tissue resection or degree of post-TURP incontinence on the postimplant outcome. Patients who had a minimal tissue resection at the time of their TURP may be at less risk of postimplant incontinence. Additionally, it is likely that if an effort is made to keep the urethral dose low, the risk of incontinence will be lessened. More detailed reports regarding this topic are needed by those performing prostate brachytherapy.

HORMONAL MANIPULATION

Pretreatment hormonal manipulation is frequently used to shrink large prostates before implantation. The primary rationale behind this procedure is to facilitate coverage of the prostatic periphery, which may be blocked by the intervening inferior pubic rami.[16] The available TRUS needle templates do not allow for custom angling of the transperineal needles to allow coverage of the periphery of larger prostates. Preimplant hormonal shrinking of the prostate may also decrease the likelihood of postimplant morbidity.

There is little objective data to support or refute the concept of preimplant hormonal shrinking. At MSKCC, this procedure has not been used for men with larger prostates. I have found that men with larger prostates are more likely to develop postimplant urinary retention. The likelihood of long-term morbidity is greater in men with larger prostate volumes (Fig. 51.2-6). However, there was considerable overlap in prostate size between men who had Radiation Therapy Oncology Group (RTOG) grade 2 or higher urinary morbidity. The potential benefits of hormonal manipulation should be weighed against the possible side effects.

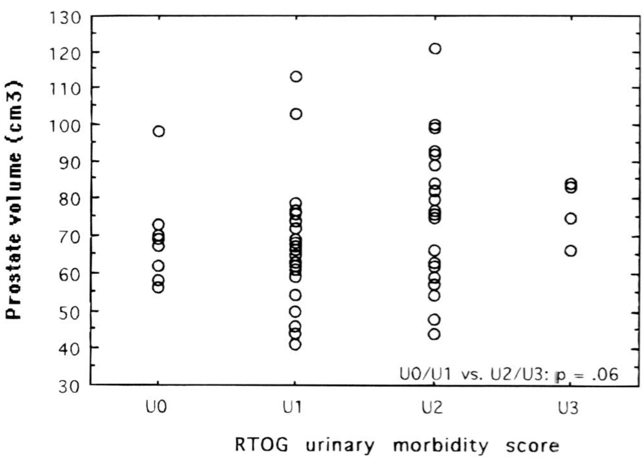

FIG. 51.2-6. Prostatic volume versus Radiation Therapy Oncology Group (RTOG) urinary morbidity at 1 year after radioactive source implantation. On average, patients with an RTOG morbidity of 2 or more had larger prostate volumes prior to implantation. Grade 2 urinary morbidity is the need for terazocin HCl (Hytrin). Patients did not receive preimplant hormonal therapy. U0, no morbidity; U1, RTOG grade 1 morbidity; U2, RTOG grade 2 morbidity; U3, RTOG grade 3 morbidity.

RESULTS

Temporary Implants

Long-term results with temporary ^{192}Ir implants have been reported by Syed and colleagues[14] at Long Beach Memorial Hospital. Patients with stage T1 to T3 lesions were treated with a combination of ^{192}Ir implants of 30 to 35 Gy plus 40 Gy of EBRT. High local control rates were achieved. The percent of positive biopsy specimens for well-differentiated or moderately differentiated T1 to T2 lesions is 15%, which is low compared with that for EBRT series. Unfortunately, fewer than one half of the patients were biopsied; therefore, there may have been a substantial selection bias.

Most impressive about the results of Syed and colleagues[14] is the leveling off of the survival curves after 5 years; this is generally not seen after prostatectomy or EBRT. This leveling off of the curves indicates cure of a large proportion of patients. Unfortunately, enthusiasm over these results must be tempered by the fact that the investigators did include rising PSA as a criterion for treatment failure. If tumor eradication was verified with PSA data, the efficacy of the technique would be more certain. No investigator has included PSA status in the follow-up of patients treated with ^{192}Ir implantation.

Permanent Implants

Results for permanent implants should be differentiated between those done using the retropubic method versus those done with newer, transperineal techniques. Investigators familiar with both methods generally agree that the transperineal technique is technically vastly superior. Because of monumental technical improvements, results with previously used retropubic techniques are irrelevant in determining the efficacy of newer techniques.

Several groups have accumulated 5-year data for transperineal implantation patients. Most notably, Blasko and colleagues[15] at Northwest Tumor Institute (NWTI) in Seattle, have analyzed disease-free survival after ^{125}I alone for 197 patients with clinical stage T1 or T2 prostatic carcinoma. Median follow-up was 3 years. Pretreatment serum PSA was elevated (>4.0 ng/mL) in 138 patients (70%). One hundred and fifty tumors were well differentiated (Gleason score of 2 to 4), 87 were moderately differentiated (Gleason score of 5 to 6) and 5 were indeterminate. Patients with a Gleason score of 7 or higher were excluded. The actuarial rate of chemical failure as determined by rising PSA or clinical failure at 5 years following implantation was only 7%. Fifteen patients were followed for 5 years or more. Although their failure rate was far lower than any published results for EBRT[17–19], enthusiasm for their results must be tempered somewhat by the fact that their series is heavily weighted with patients with low-grade tumors or a normal PSA prior to treatment. Patients with high-grade tumors were treated with a combination of EBRT and low-dose brachytherapy.

Actuarial 5-year results following transperineal implantation have also been collected by Wallner and colleagues[8] at MSKCC. Eighty-eight patients with clinical stage T1 or T2 prostatic carcinoma underwent ^{125}I prostate implantation from

1988 to 1994. The pretreatment characteristics were not as favorable as those in patients reported by Blasko and colleagues[15] and were more consistent with those reported in most EBRT or surgical series. Eighty-one patients (92%) had an elevated PSA before implantation (>4.0 ng/mL) and 67% had moderately differentiated tumors (Gleason score of 5 to 7). A rising PSA was defined as two consecutive increasing values, whether or not the value rose above the normal range. In this less selected group of patients, the actuarial freedom from failure at 5 years following implantation was 80%, with a median follow-up of 2 years. At last follow-up, 57% of patients had a PSA level of less than 1 ng/mL, and the PSA levels of some other patients was still decreasing. Similar to the results of Blasko and colleagues,[15] these results are comparable to or better than the results reported with prostatectomy in major surgical centers.

To appreciate just how promising the results from NWTI[15] and MSKCC[8] are, these results can compared to the PSA-based freedom from failure reported for stage T1/T2 patients from the Johns Hopkins experience (Fig. 51.2-7).[20] In making such a comparison, the patients have been grouped by pretreatment PSA level, which is the most objective gauge of likelihood of extraprostatic disease. Use of the Gleason score to stratify patients between series is clouded by the fact that assignment of Gleason score can be subjectively affected by the pathologist involved. When comparing results for patients with pretreatment PSA levels of 11 to 20 ng/mL, it is evident that the outcomes are similar between prostatectomy patients and those treated with ^{125}I implantation. Similar results are seen when comparing the PSA-based freedom from failure results for other pretreatment PSA levels.[12] Longer follow-up is needed to determine whether the apparent advantage of ^{125}I implantation over prostatectomy seen in patients with high PSA levels will hold at 10 and 15 years posttherapy. At this point, implantation appears to be comparable to or better than prostatectomy. This is especially true when considering that the implant patients are being compared to the most carefully selected group of surgical patients ever reported, based on the fact that 42% had a normal pretreatment PSA levels. Most other surgical series report results that are far less promising than those from Johns Hopkins.[21,22]

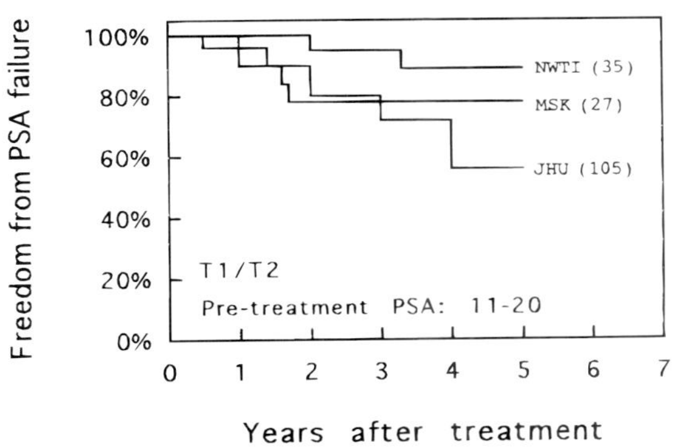

FIG. 51.2-7. Prostate serum antigen (PSA)–based freedom from failure for stage T1/T2 tumors and pretreatment PSA levels of 11–20 ng/mL, following I^{125} implantation at Memorial Sloan-Kettering Cancer Center (MSKCC) or Northwest Tumor Institute in Seattle (NWTI) versus radical prostatectomy at Johns Hopkins University (JHU). The number of patients in each series is shown in parentheses.

In contrast to the favorable results with transperineal implantation from MSKCC[8] and NWTI[15], Waehre and colleagues[23] at the Norwegian Radium Hospital reported poor results in patients treated with TRUS-guided transperineal ^{125}I implantation. Their findings can be traced to the low total activity of ^{125}I used. The average total radioactivity of ^{125}I used in the series by Wallner and colleagues[23] was 45 mCi. In marked contrast, Waehre and colleagues[23] used an average of 17 mCi. According to general dosimetry guidelines, 17 mCi would allow adequate irradiation of a prostate with an average dimension of 2.5 cm, which I believe to be smaller than a normal prostate gland. In addition to using a smaller amount of ^{125}I, no dosimetric evaluation of the implants was performed; the authors may not have been aware that their patients had been grossly underdosed. Without dosimetric evaluation of the implants, there can be no quality assurance. If brachytherapy is practiced without quality assurance, a poor outcome may result. These data are useful because they highlight the importance of good technique and a thorough working knowledge of brachytherapy.[24]

MORBIDITY

Detailed morbidity data following transperineal ^{125}I implantation has been reported by Kleinberg and colleagues[24] at MSKCC. Postoperative complications were rare. Of 150 patients receiving implants from 1988 to 1994, none have required a blood transfusion. Patients rarely required postoperative analgesics; when necessary, nonsteroidal antiinflammatory agents were sufficient. Most patients returned to work within 24 hours, although they were cautioned against heavy lifting for 1 week following implantation. Approximately 10% of patients required a Foley catheter for urinary retention, usually for less than 1 week.

Although serious postoperative complications are rare, some urinary symptoms caused by high-dose irradiation of the prostatic urethra are unavoidable. Symptoms of radiation-induced prostatitis appear approximately 2 to 3 weeks after implantation, peak at 4 to 6 weeks after implantation, and then gradually resolve. Marked urinary frequency and nocturia generally last for 3 to 12 months following implantation. Urinary symptoms following ^{125}I implantation tend to be more marked than those associated with conventional-dose EBRT.[24] It should be emphasized, however, that these side effects do not usually interfere substantially with a patient's lifestyle.

Postimplant urinary tract infections are uncommon, but should be ruled out if the clinical history is suggestive. Patients usually report substantial relief of radiation-induced prostatitis symptoms with selective α_1-blockers (e.g., terazocin HCl [Hytrin]).[25] Nonsteroidal antiinflammatory agents are also of some benefit, but not nearly so much as β-blockers. Phenazopyridine HCl (Pyridium) or catabolic steroids are rarely helpful. Vigorous exercise commonly alleviates symptoms temporarily.

The short-term morbidity reported by Kleinberg and colleagues[24] should be extrapolated with caution because there are some differences between their techniques and those used by others. There may be substantial differences in series in which brachytherapy is used only as a boost with EBRT and in series in which ^{103}Pd is used instead of ^{125}I. However, RTOG grades 1 or 2 morbidity have not been meticulously reported for ^{103}Pd or combined EBRT and brachytherapy.

Long-term morbidity following permanent ^{125}I implantation has been detailed by investigators at NWTI and MSKCC. The most common long-term complications are rectal ulceration and urethral necrosis. In the first 3 years of experience, 11% of patients implanted at MSKCC developed rectal ulcerations within 24 months of implantation.[8] These rectal ulcers nearly always healed spontaneously. However, patients with a prior history of pelvic irradiation or TURP are at greater risk of developing a prostatic-rectal fistula. The likelihood of rectal ulceration at MSKCC decreased to 2% from 1991 to 1994. The decreasing incidence of rectal complications is a reflection of increased experience and better application of dosimetric quality assurance guidelines.[12]

Blasko and colleagues[9] reported a 4% incidence of superficial urethral necrosis, which was associated with severe dysuria and sometimes with urinary incontinence. The risk of urethral necrosis was largely limited to patients with a prior history of TURP. The likelihood of urethral necrosis can probably be decreased if an effort is made to keep sources at least 1 cm from the urethra. Wallner and colleagues[8] reported a 9% incidence of urethral obstruction, requiring TURP within 2 years after implantation. However, they implanted many patients with large prostates, who would be expected to be at increased risk of postimplant obstructive symptoms.

Urinary incontinence in the absence of prior or subsequent TURP is unusual. At MSKCC, in patients who have not undergone TURP, there have been no instances of permanent incontinence.[8] At NWTI, none of 184 patients without TURP experienced incontinence. In contrast, of 90 patients with prior or subsequent TURP, there was a 17% likelihood of incontinence.[9]

More substantial morbidity has been reported following treatment with a combination of brachytherapy and EBRT. However, complications could usually be attributed to gross radiation overdose. Iverson and colleagues[26] reported rectal ulceration, colostomy, or severe radiation cystitis in 14 of 33 patients treated with 47-Gy whole-pelvic irradiation delivering 220 cGy/day followed by a full-dose (160-Gy) ^{125}I implant. Their unacceptable rate of complications reflects the high daily doses of whole-pelvic irradiation followed by a full-dose implant. If a combination of EBRT and implantation are used, the dose of each must be decreased by approximately 40%. The safety of high-quality brachytherapy plus reduced-dose EBRT is well documented by Syed and colleagues.[14]

Acute and long-term morbidity following brachytherapy is somewhat greater than that following conventional-dose EBRT. It is important to point out that the incidence of complications has decreased with experience in nearly all series reported, and that the complication rates summarized previously should be taken as somewhat worse than would be expected today. The phenomenal PSA-based tumor control rates at 5 years probably justify a slightly higher risk of complications as compared with conventional-dose EBRT.

PRESERVATION OF SEXUAL POTENCY

Impotency is the most common complication of curative treatment of prostate cancer. Much reference is made to the alleged potency-sparing effect of brachytherapy versus other forms of treatment. Unfortunately, there is remarkably little meticulous data regarding the effect of prostatectomy, EBRT, or brachytherapy on potency. Potency diminishes over time in these patients, such that stating a percent of patients still potent must include a reference to the time at which potency is measured. Little regard has been given to the effect of time when the effect of treatment on potency has been reported.

Wallner and colleagues[8] have reported the most detailed data regarding potency preservation after ^{125}I brachytherapy. Potency is defined as the ability to attain and maintain an erection sufficient for intercourse. In patients treated with ^{125}I, 90% maintained potency at 1 year after treatment. With longer follow-up, however, more patients lost potency. The actuarial potency rate at 5 years following ^{125}I implantation was 65%. This increased loss of potency with time probably represents a combination of natural loss with aging and long-term radiation-induced normal tissue changes, including microvascular and neurologic compromise. Younger patients clearly had less potency loss. Of 12 patients younger than 60 years of age at the time of implantation, none became impotent during a follow-up of as long as 5 years.

Potency after combined brachytherapy plus EBRT has never been meticulously reported. However, it may be lower than that reported after implantation alone.

The only series showing the long-term effect of EBRT on potency is from Stanford.[27] Potency was preserved in 54% of patients at 5 years after treatment, which is comparable to potency status after ^{125}I implantation at MSKCC (Fig. 51.2-8).[8] However Bagshaw and colleagues'[27] results should be viewed with caution, because they are based on an anonymous mail survey of a small percentage of patients treated and there is no mention of how potency was defined or the patients' ages at the time of treatment.

Long-term potency rates after nerve-sparing radical prostatectomy have not been reported. Large series of patients from Johns Hopkins Medical Center[20] and Washington University[13] have reported potency rates only at 1 or 2 years after surgery. With such short follow-up, maintenance of potency is achieved in approximately 60% of patients, with better results in younger patients. No surgical series has included actuarial calculations, which would almost certainly decrease the calculated potency rates substantially. The true incidence of impotency following nerve-sparing prostatectomy may be much higher, as suggested in a recent survey of Medicare patients.[28]

Potency preservation with ^{125}I brachytherapy probably compares favorably with that following EBRT or nerve-sparing prostatectomy. Unfortunately, it is impossible to make a definitive statement in this regard because of the lack of long-term data for all modalities. It would be a great service to patients if more investigators would publish their data regarding long-term potency preservation. The lack of published long-term data despite the large number of patients being treated at academic institutions raises suspicions that the potency-sparing effects of prostatectomy or EBRT may not be as good as what is generally believed.

CONCLUSIONS

There has been a resurgent interest in prostate brachytherapy spurred by improved technology that allows the performance of high-quality implants on an outpatient basis. PSA-based disease control rates from at least two institutions are comparable to

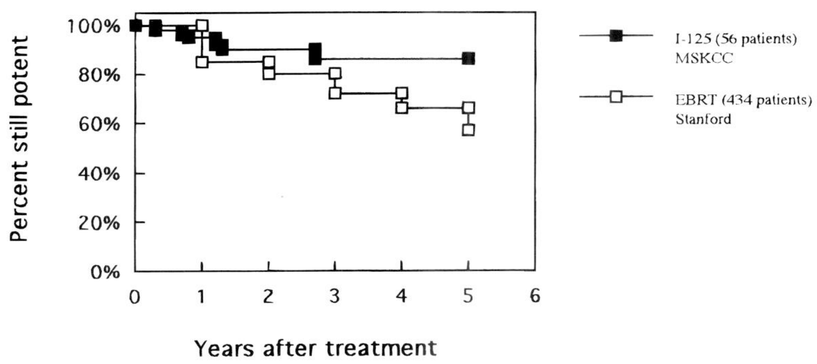

FIG. 51.2-8. Maintenance of potency after I^{125} brachytherapy at Memorial Sloan-Kettering Cancer Center (MSKCC) versus external beam radiotherapy (EBRT) at Stanford.

or better than those following prostatectomy at the most prestigious surgical centers. It is likely that brachytherapy will play a larger role in treatment of prostate cancer in the future. The role of brachytherapy for advanced-stage (T3) lesions is less clear, because limited PSA-based follow-up data has been reported.

REFERENCES

1. Barringer BS. Radium in the treatment of carcinoma of the bladder and prostate. JAMA 1917;68:1227.
2. Whitmore WF, Hilaris B, Grabstald H. Retropubic implantation of iodine 125 in the treatment of prostatic cancer. J Urol 1972;108:918.
3. Fuks Z, Leibel SA, Wallner KE, et al. The effect of local control on metastatic dissemination in carcinoma of the prostate: long term results in patients treated with 125-I implantation. Int J Radiat Oncol Biol Phys 1991;21:337.
4. Holm HH, Juul N, Pederson JR, Hansen H, Stroyer I. Transperineal 125-iodine seed implantation in prostatic cancer guided by transrectal ultrasonography. J Urol 1983;130:283.
5. Schellhammer PF, Ladaga LE, El-Mahdi A. Histological characteristics of prostatic biopsies after I-125 implantation. J Urol 1980;123:700.
6. Ling CC. Permanent implants using Au-198, Pd-103 and I-125: radiobiological considerations based on the linear quadratic model. Int J Radiat Oncol Biol Phys 1992;23:81.
7. Orton CG, Webber BM. Time-dose factor (TDF) analysis of dose rate effects in permanent implant dosimetry. Int J Radiat Oncol Biol Phys 1977;2:55.
8. Wallner KE, Roy J, Zelefsky M, Fuks Z, Harrison L. Short-term freedom from disease progression after I-125 prostate implantation. Int J Radiat Oncol Biol Phys 1994;30:405.
9. Blasko JC, Grimm PD, Ragde H. Brachytherapy and organ preservation in the management of carcinoma of the prostate. Semin Radiat Oncol 1993;3:240.
10. Packer MG, Russo P, Fair WR. Prophylactic antibiotics and Foley catheter use in transperineal needle biopsy of the prostate. J Urol 1984; 131:687.
11. Kaye KW, Olson DJ, Lightner DJ. Improved technique for prostate seed implantation: combined ultrasound and fluoroscopic guidance. J Endourol 1992;6:61.
12. Wallner KE, Roy J, Zelefsky M, Fuks Z, Harrison L. Dosimetry guidelines to minimize urethral and rectal morbidity following transperineal I-125 prostate brachytherapy. Int J Radiat Oncol Biol Phys 1995;32: 465.
13. Catalona WJ, Bigg SW. Nerve-sparing radical prostatectomy: evaluation of results after 250 patients. J Urol 1990;143:538.
14. Syed AM, Puthawala A, Austin P, Cherlow J. Temporary iridium-192 implant in the management of carcinoma of the prostate. Cancer 1992; 69:2515.
15. Blasko JC, Ragde H, Grimm PD. Transperineal ultrasound-guided implantation of the prostate: morbidity and complications. Scand J Urol Nephrol 1991;137(Suppl):113.
16. Wallner KE, Chiu-Tsao S, Roy J, et al. An improved method for transperineal prostate implants. J Urol 1991;146:90.
17. Kaplan ID, Co RS, Bagshaw MA. Prostate specific antigen after external beam radiotherapy for prostatic cancer: follow-up. J Urol 1993; 149:519.
18. Zeitman AL, Coen JJ, Shipley WU, Willett CG, Efird JT. Radical radiation therapy in the management of prostatic adenocarcinoma: the initial prostate specific antigen value as a predictor of treatment outcome. J Urol 1994;151:640.
19. Zagars GK, von Eschenbach AC. Prostate-specific antigen: an important marker for prostate cancer treated by external beam radiation therapy. Cancer 1993;72:538.
20. Partin AW, Pound CR, Clemens JQ, Epstein JI, Walsh PC. Serum PSA after anatomic radical prostatectomy: the Johns Hopkins experience after 10 years. Urol Clin North Am 1993;20:713.
21. Zeitman AL, Edelstein RA, Coen JJ, Babayan RK, Krane RJ. Radical prostatectomy for adenocarcinoma of the prostate: the influence of preoperative and pathologic findings on biochemical disease-free outcome. Urology 1994;43:828.
22. Stein A, deKernion JB, Smith RB, Dorey F, Patel H. Prostate specific antigen levels after radical prostatectomy in patients with organ confined and locally extensive prostate cancer. J Urol 1992;147:942.
23. Waehre H, Amellem O, Stenwig AE, et al. Deoxyribonucleic acid cytometry and histological findings before and after 125-iodine implantation of primary prostate cancer. J Urol 1992;148:838.
24. Kleinberg L, Wallner K, Roy J, et al. Treatment-related symptoms during the first year following transperineal I-125 prostate implantation. Int J Radiat Oncol Biol Phys 1994.
25. Kane MM, Fields DW, Vaughn ED. Medical management of benign prostatic hyperplasia. Urology 1990;36:5.
26. Iverson P, Nielsen L, Bak M, et al. Ultrasonically guided 125iodine seed implantation with external radiation in management of localized prostatic carcinoma. Urology 1989;34:181.
27. Bagshaw MA, Cox RS, Ray GR. Status of radiation of prostate cancer at Stanford University. NCI Monogr 1988;7:47.
28. Fowler FJ, Roman A, Barry MJ, Wasson J, Lu-Yao G, Wennberg JE. Patient-reported complications and follow-up treatment after radical prostatectomy. Urology 1993;42:622.

Principles and Practice of Genitourinary Oncology, edited by Derek Raghavan, Howard I. Scher, Steven A. Leibel, and Paul H. Lange. Lippincott-Raven Publishers, Philadelphia, © 1997.

CHAPTER 52

Management of Stage C (T3) Prostate Cancer

52.1 Nonradiation Therapy

Mark Frydenberg and Joseph E. Oesterling

Stage C (T3) prostate cancer includes all lesions that extend beyond the confines of the prostatic capsule and by definition excludes those patients with evidence of nodal or visceral metastasis on imaging studies. Many authors have subdivided stage C cancer in order to emphasize adverse pathologic features that could lead to a poorer prognosis. Initially, this stage was subdivided into C1 and C2 disease on the basis of seminal vesicle invasion,[1] but others have described three subdivisions. Stage C1 comprises those patients with invasion through the prostatic capsule with no tumor at the surgical margin and without seminal vesicle involvement. Stage C2 disease describes patients with tumor at the surgical margin but without seminal vesicle involvement, and stage C3 describes patients with invasion of the seminal vesicles with or without tumor at the surgical margin.[2] Despite the obvious prognostic implications, few studies stratify their results according to these stage C subdivisions.

In 1986, the results of a survey by The American College of Surgeons were published and demonstrated that 12% to 15% of all newly diagnosed cancers were clinical stage C. These cancers were treated by radiotherapy, with or without adjuvant antiandrogen therapy, in 39% of patients; hormonal therapy alone in 26%; transurethral resection of prostate (TURP) in 21%; and radical prostatectomy, with or without adjuvant antiandrogen or radiotherapy, in 14%.[3] Since the late 1980s there has been a wave of enthusiasm for the use of radical prostatectomy for the treatment of localized prostate cancer. This has occurred as a result of a marked diminution in the morbidity and mortality of the procedure in addition to the belief that the cancer may be cured if all the disease is eradicated. A survey conducted today may demonstrate different patterns of care in the management of prostate cancer, including locally extensive disease.

PROGNOSTIC FACTORS IN STAGE C PROSTATE CANCER

Some 40% to 50% of all patients undergoing radical prostatectomy for clinically localized disease have pathologic stage C cancer.[4–7] In the past, stage C cancer was not thought to be surgically curable because of the adverse prognostic implications once the tumor had breached the prostatic capsule. However, not all forms of extracapsular spread signify an equally poor prognosis. The lack of a well-defined prostate capsule and the limited periprostatic soft tissue make defining extracapsular cancer spread less certain in prostate cancer than in other tumors.

Extended survival in patients with limited extraprostatic disease treated by radical prostatectomy has been reported in the literature. De Kernion and Mukamel reported a disease-free survival rate of 81% at 8 years,[1] and Middleton and associates reported a rate of 87% at 5 years[8] in patients with capsular perforation only. Epstein and associates,[9] excluding patients with nodal or seminal vesicle involvement, found that 82% of patients with focal capsular penetration and 65% of those with established capsular penetration demonstrated no evidence of disease recurrence at 5 years, including no rise in serum prostate-specific antigen (PSA). It was also thought by the group at Johns Hopkins Hospital that the surgical margins may be artifactually positive as a consequence of the easily disruptable periprostatic soft tissues, and therefore the status of the margins may lose some prognostic significance. They demonstrated that progression of disease in patients with focal capsular penetration was correlated with an increase in grade of tumor (Gleason score of 7 or higher) but not margin positivity. Other studies have demonstrated that the 5-year risk of cancer progression is only 30% to 40% in patients with focally positive margins,[10] and studies from the Mayo Clinic did not identify margin positivity as an independent adverse prognostic variable on a multivariate analysis.[7] The Mayo Clinic study identified increasing tumor grade and, to a lesser extent, tumor volume as the most important adverse prognostic variables, but seminal vesicle involvement was not as important. There is almost universal agreement that the presence of high-grade (Gleason score of 7 or higher) disease is the best predictor of progression, including local recurrence.[11] Epstein and associates identified a 59% progression rate at 5 years if the Gleason score was 7 or more, but only 13% if it was less than 7.[11] Cheng and associates identified a 40% progression rate with high-grade (grade 3 or higher) tumors and a 20% rate with low-grade (less than grade 3) tumors at 5 years.[7] Schroeder and Belt found that grade 1, clinical stage C lesions treated with radical prostatectomy had a local recurrence rate of 0%, whereas grade 3 lesions had a local recurrence rate of 19%.[12]

In contrast to the results obtained from the Mayo Clinic, most series demonstrate seminal vesicle invasion to be a major adverse prognostic factor. Long-term follow-up of radical prostatectomy patients at the University of California at Los Angeles (UCLA) has demonstrated that seminal vesicle involvement by tumor significantly affects clinical progression and PSA-free survival despite the absence of nodal involvement.[13] Epstein and associates have described an 85% progression at 5 years in patients with seminal vesicle involvement,[11] and Fowler and Mills reported a 55% progression at 4 years.[14] However, Villers and colleagues at Stanford University[15] have demonstrated that tumor bulk and grade are more significant determinants of subsequent prostate cancer death than seminal vesicle invasion.

Others also support the importance of tumor volume and its independent correlation with extracapsular disease and positive margins.[16,17] However, transrectal ultrasonography does not allow accurate estimation of cancer volume, and only indirect evidence of tumor volume can be obtained by the number of positive biopsies[16] and the proportion of each biopsy core replaced by tumor.[18] Epstein and associates did not identify tumor volume as an independent adverse prognostic variable on a multivariate analysis when examining patients with stage B disease.[11]

Recently, nuclear DNA ploidy has been identified as a significant prognostic indicator for progression and disease-specific death, but it did not contribute significantly in addition to tumor grade or volume in a multivariate analysis.[19]

In summary, many variables influence outcome in surgically treated stage C prostate cancer, and, because many of them are interrelated, it is critical to test potential prognostic predictors by multivariate analysis. Tumor volume is difficult to assess accurately before surgery. Capsular penetration and margin positivity may not be as important prognostically as previously believed, and they are certainly are less significant than seminal vesicle invasion and histologic grade. Therefore, tumors of low and intermediate grades without seminal vesicle involvement have an acceptably low incidence of failure and are suitable for aggressive treatment by radical prostatectomy in selected patients.

ROLE OF CONSERVATIVE TREATMENT IN STAGE C PROSTATE CANCER

Is cure necessary in all cases of stage C prostate cancer? Adolfsson, from the Karolinska Institute in Sweden, has looked at a group of 50 patients with clinical stage C disease managed by surveillance initially and with delayed treatment of progression.[20] With a median follow-up of 6.5 years, 58% of patients required hormone therapy and 12% required radiotherapy. Metastases developed in 30% of patients, 22% died of prostate cancer, and 34% died from other causes, giving a cancer-specific survival rate of 70% at 9 years. This series was highly selected in that the median age of the patients was 71 years, and the tumors were described as small and were well to moderately differentiated in 96% of the patients. This study would have tended to select asymptomatic disease of low biologic activity in an elderly population with many competing causes of death, and therefore the cancer-specific survival may not reflect the overall experience with stage C disease managed conservatively. Stenzl and Studer examined a group of 24 patients with T3 or T4 disease managed conservatively, 14 with grade 2 disease and 10 with grade 3 disease.[21] Disease-specific survival was only 51% at 5 years and 0% at 10 years, with 47% of the patients dying of prostate cancer. This study demonstrates that patients with higher grades of disease have a significant risk of dying from their prostate cancer within a short interval, and therefore a more aggressive approach to treatment in younger patients with a 10-year life expectancy may be justified.

A conservative approach does not always mean a nonoperative approach, because there is a clear morbidity associated with leaving the prostate in situ. In the two studies just mentioned, TURP was required in 22%[20] and 57%[21] of patients, respectively. Tomlinson and associates described a group of patients with stage C prostate cancer, some of whom were treated by radical prostatectomy and others by conservative measures, including TURP with or without hormonal therapy.[22] Bladder neck obstruction occurred in 75% of patients managed conservatively, versus 4.3% of those undergoing radical surgery; ureteral obstruction occurred in 40% versus 4.3%; incontinence occurred in 30% versus 4.3%; urinary tract infection occurred in 80% versus 26%; and hematuria occurred in 45% versus 8.7%. Patients undergoing TURP required, on average, 23.4 readmission days to manage disease-related morbidity, whereas those treated by radical prostatectomy required only 1.6 days. The evidence demonstrates that radical prostatectomy affords excellent palliation from disabling symptoms and emphasizes the importance of achieving excellent local control in prostate cancer therapy.

RADICAL PROSTATECTOMY

The results of stage C prostate cancer treated by radical prostatectomy are summarized in Tables 52.1-1 and 52.1-2.

Monotherapy

Radical prostatectomy has infrequently been used alone in the treatment of stage C prostate cancer. Van den Ouden and associates prospectively performed radical prostatectomy in 100 patients with locally extensive prostate cancer as monotherapy.[23] Of these patients, 39 had lymph node metastasis and 2 had T4 disease and did not undergo radical prostatectomy. A further 9 patients with lymph nodal involvement did undergo surgery, all but 1 of whom subsequently progressed clinically or biochemically. Among the remaining 50 patients, there was an 18% overstaging error; these patients were found to have stage T2 disease at surgery, and none of them showed evidence of disease progression. Eighty-two percent of the 50 patients remained T3, and of these, 31% of the 82% showed no evidence of disease progression either clinically or biochemically. Therefore, with a median follow-up of almost 4 years, 38% of patients with negative lymph nodes show no evidence of disease progression (including PSA measurements). In this series, patients with high-grade tumors formed a subgroup with a particularly high risk of progression, and after this group was eliminated, there was no significant difference in time to progression be-

TABLE 52.1-1. *Disease-free survival rates for patients with stage C prostate cancer treated by radical prostatectomy*

Investigators	Survival rate (%) 5 y	8 y	10 y	15 y
Cheng et al, 1993[7]	78	—	56	48
Zincke et al, 1984[25]	71	—	52	48
Scott and Boyd, 1969[35]	61	—	51	29
Middleton et al, 1986[8]*	87	—	—	—
de Kernion and Mukamel, 1987[1]	—	81	—	—
Epstein et al, 1993[9]*	82†	—	—	—
	65‡	—	—	—
Flocks et al, 1975[27]	—	—	—	27.5
Morgan et al, 1993[24]§	51	—	—	—
Van den Ouden et al, 1994[23]§	38	—	—	—

* Patients with C1 disease.
† Patients with focal extracapsular extension.
‡ Patients with extensive extracapsular extension.
§ Patients with clinical stage C disease.

tween stage T3 and T0 to T2 tumors. In this series, seminal vesicle involvement and margin positivity did not have a significant independent effect on progression. Survival was not analyzed in this study because of the short follow-up.

Morgan and associates analyzed the results of 232 patients with clinical stage C disease treated with radical prostatectomy.[24] Forty-two percent had nodal involvement, and 22% had pathologic organ-confined disease. The 5-year disease-free survival rate was 51%, and once again advanced histologic grade and the presence of more than two involved lymph nodes was significantly associated with prostate cancer death on a multivariate analysis.

Surgery With Adjuvant Therapy

Local recurrence rates after radical prostatectomy vary. They can be as high as 30% to 75% without adjuvant treatment but are significantly lower if some type of adjuvant treatment (antiandrogen or radiotherapy) is used.[25,26] Schroeder and Belt[12] found a local recurrence rate of 14%, and Tomlinson and associates found a rate of 8.7% for patients who received adjuvant antiandrogen treatment.[22] Zincke and associates[25] found a local recurrence rate of 7.6% in patients receiving adjuvant hormonal treatment or radiotherapy. Flocks and colleagues[27] and Rosenberg and associates[28] observed local recurrence rates of 4.5% and 8%, respectively, after radical prostatectomy and simultaneous instillation of colloidal radioactive gold (^{198}Au). Despite this improvement in local control, there is little evidence to suggest a survival benefit with early adjuvant treatment. An analysis from the Mayo Clinic demonstrated significantly reduced rates of local, systemic and overall progression with early adjuvant treatment but no improvement in cause-specific or crude survival figures.[7] In that series, the cause-specific survival rate was 96%, 81%, and 66%, and overall nonprogression survival was 78%, 56%, and 48%, at 5, 10, and 15 years respectively. Orchiectomy and irradiation appeared to demonstrate similar efficacy in controlling local recurrences. The 5-year local recurrence-free survival rate was greater than 95% for both treatments, compared with 84% for patients who did not receive any adjuvant treatment.[7]

The rationale for any adjuvant treatment is that residual cancer cells may be the source of local or distant disease if left untreated. Anscher and Prosnitz[29] demonstrated that adjuvant radiotherapy decreased local recurrence from 27% to 10.5% in patients with seminal vesicle involvement, from 25% to 4.5% in patients with capsular penetration, and from 47% to 6% in patients with involved surgical margins. However, once again, there was no advantage in disease-free survival rates and only a trend to an improvement in the rates of death from prostate cancer.

Freeman and associates, at the University of Southern California,[30] have demonstrated a local recurrence rate of only 13% and a disease-specific survival rate of 78% after 10 years in patients treated with adjuvant radiotherapy after radical prostatectomy. The treatment was well tolerated, with no increased incidence of incontinence or strictures in patients undergoing radical prostatectomy alone, and no serious lasting effects on the rectal or bladder mucosa. Although the authors concluded that these survival rates were an improvement over historical controls, a nonrandomized concurrent series of patients with margin-positive disease who were treated with or without adjuvant radiotherapy at the same institution could not demonstrate a survival benefit.[31]

The timing of radiotherapy is similarly controversial. Zietman and associates[32] have addressed the issue of whether treatment should be given adjuvantly (for those with high risk of progression), at the time of failure as indicated by serum PSA, or when a clinical palpable recurrence is discovered. Their conclusion was that a larger tumor burden is associated with each of these steps and makes control of disease less likely. This certainly applied for patients with palpable recurrent disease, because salvage irradiation involved higher doses of external beam radiation than adjuvant treatment, carried a higher risk of morbidity, and had a lower probability of cure (<40% were disease-free 2 years after radiotherapy). McCarthy and associates[33] reported that 67% of patients who received adjuvant radiotherapy were without evidence of clinical or biochemical recurrence. Furthermore, 68% of patients who had an initially undetectable postoperative serum PSA level that began to rise during follow-up, and who then received treatment with irradiation, were disease free. These preliminary results (median fol-

TABLE 52.1-2. *Cause-specific survival rates for patients with stage C prostate cancer treated by radical prostatectomy*

Investigators	Survival rate (%) 5 y	10 y	15 y
Cheng et al, 1993[7]	96	81	66
Zincke et al, 1984[25]	94	81	66
Scott and Boyd, 1969[35]	—	79	68
Grups et al, 1990[45]*	—	71	—

* Patients to whom no immediate adjuvant treatment was given.

low-up, 2 to 3 years) indicate that no harm is incurred if radiotherapy is delayed until an elevated serum PSA concentration is detected. Those treated for a persistently elevated PSA levels postoperatively had a response rate of only 53%, and, after 3 years, only 33% were still free of disease, indicating failure of radiotherapy in those with more established residual disease.

Until results of prospective, randomized trials are available, patients in a high-risk category for progression (e.g., high grade, extensive margin positivity, involved seminal vesicle) may be considered for adjuvant radiotherapy. For those at lower risk, however, radiation may not alter the outcome of the disease, is expensive, is inconvenient to the patient, and may have some inherent morbidity.

Neoadjuvant Therapy and Surgery

In several surgical series, neoadjuvant therapy was used to down-stage the clinical stage C lesion. Gill and associates[34] used a 75-Gy dose of external beam radiation as neoadjuvant treatment before radical prostatectomy. Although there was clinical downstaging in 9 of 11 patients, 6 still had viable cancer on biopsy before surgery, and metastases developed in 2 of these patients.

Although neoadjuvant radiotherapy has not been widely adopted, preoperative antiandrogen therapy has increased in popularity recently. The rationale for its use is that if all the hormone-sensitive cells could be eliminated, then the remaining hormone-unresponsive cancer may be eradicated surgically. In the mid-1960s, Scott and Boyd[35] combined hormone therapy with radical surgery and observed a 15-year disease-free survival rate of 29% and a cause-specific survival rate of 68%. Hellstrom and associates[36] conducted a histopathologic study of androgen-deprived localized prostate cancers treated by radical prostatectomy. Patients in this study were given triptorelin (a luteinizing hormone–releasing hormone agonist) for 3 months, along with cyproterone acetate for 3 weeks to counter the flare effect. Residual cancer was found in all glands, with the predominant histologic changes being atrophy of glandular epithelium, nuclear pyknosis, intracytoplasmic vacuolation, squamous metaplasia in glands and ducts, and a relative increase in the ratio of stromal to epithelial tissue. In a separate report, this group revealed clinical downstaging in 27 of 40 cases, a 40% decrease in prostatic volume, and a decreased incidence of positive margins (58% versus 31%) compared with patients treated without neoadjuvant therapy.[37] The authors point out, however, that an easier dissection, as a result of decreased size and vascularity of the gland, may have contributed to the lower incidence of involved margins.

Schulman and associates have recently found an advantage in the ability of neoadjuvant hormone manipulation to downstage large stage B2/C lesions. Pathologic downstaging occurred in 18% of the treated group, compared with 5% of the control group, and positive margins were found in 25% and 40%, respectively.[38] Fair and associates examined a subgroup of patients with stage C prostate cancer treated with diethylstilbestrol, 3 mg/d for 8 to 32 weeks, before radical prostatectomy.[39] The final pathologic stage was B2 in 26%, which may not be significantly different than the 18% to 22% overstaging error identified when radical prostatectomy was used as monotherapy.[23] However, 10% of all cases were T0, and seminal vesicle involvement could not be confirmed pathologically in 2 patients with biopsy-proven seminal vesicle involvement preoperatively. The Memorial Sloan-Kettering group concluded that neoadjuvant treatment may have little effect on altering the potential for metastatic spread and no impact on survival, but it was worth investigating because there was little or no risk to the patient.

Oesterling and associates[40] examined a group of 21 patients with clinical stage B2 or C disease and paired them with a group matched for grade, PSA level, and tumor stage who did not receive any preoperative hormone therapy. They demonstrated a 98.5% median decrease in PSA level, a marked reduction in prostatic volume, but no significant differences in pathologic stage or in seminal vesicle or lymph node involvement. Paradoxically, capsular penetration and margin positivity were higher in those patients treated preoperatively with hormones. Kennedy and associates identified downstaging in only 2 of 7 patients,[41] and a study at UCLA demonstrated that only 25% of patients with stage C disease experienced downstaging.[42] Some data suggest improved operability after neoadjuvant therapy,[43] but other authors have not found any benefit.[42]

The current status of neoadjuvant hormonal therapy therefore remains unclear. The results of prospective, randomized trials should provide much-needed information. Currently, it seems that preoperative hormonal manipulation decreases prostatic volume and PSA level, may downstage a small percentage of patients, and, at least in some reports, has led to a decreased rate of positive margins. Whether these results translate into improved local control or disease-specific survival is speculative and requires longer follow-up.

One study has examined combined preoperative hormonal deprivation and chemotherapy to target both androgen-sensitive and hormone-insensitive cells.[44] This was achieved by combining total androgen blockade, with cisplatin (cDDP) or 5-fluorouracil, with mitomycin and calcium folinate. The authors reported clinical downstaging in 47.5%, but 38.8% were actually pathologically downstaged. They did note that if whole-mount sectioning was used, it may have allowed the identification of more pathologic stage C tumors, which would have lowered this percentage. A 20.4% incidence of nodal involvement was demonstrated, which differs from the 40% to 50% quoted for most other surgical series.[23,24] This approach, like that of neoadjuvant hormone therapy alone, deserves further consideration.

Safety of Radical Retropubic Prostatectomy in Stage C Disease

A study from Germany compared the complication rates according to clinical stage and found no significant difference between stage B and C tumors. They reported bowel injury in 5.2% of patients with stage B disease versus 3.6% in those with stage C tumors; ureteral injury occurred in 1.3% versus 0%; cardiovascular complications in 5.2% versus 5.4%; lymphocele in 12.2% versus 12.6%; incontinence in 4.5% versus 4.5%; and bladder neck contracture in 5.2% versus 4.5%.[45] These observations have been confirmed by others.[23] Radical prostatectomy is therefore an acceptable treatment alternative for stage C prostate cancer in selected patients with a life expectance longer than 10 years. It can be performed without increased morbidity and with acceptable survival rates and recurrence rates, especially if combined with adjuvant treatment in high-risk groups, and it provides effective palliation for obstructive symptoms.

ANDROGEN DEPRIVATION THERAPY

Despite its extensive use, there have been few clinical trials examining the role of endocrine manipulation alone in stage C disease. A study by the European Organization for Research on Treatment of Cancer Urological Group[46] demonstrated a 34% progression to D2 disease and a 22% death rate with only 2 years of follow-up. Another study showed that 28% of men with stage C disease who underwent immediate orchiectomy had progression to D2 disease within 2 years.[47] In 1973, the Veterans Administration Cooperative Urological Research Group reported on a large series of patients with stage C disease treated by hormonal therapy and found only a 20% survival rate after 10 years.[48] Because of its limited efficacy when used alone, hormonal therapy will probably continue to be used as an adjunct to other primary treatments.

TRANSURETHRAL RESECTION OF THE PROSTATE

Although TURP is one of the most common treatments for stage C prostate cancer, there has been little description in the literature of its long-term effects. A study by Gee and Cole[49] showed a 5-year overall survival rate of 66% and a 10-year survival rate of 20% after treatment of the initial lesion with TURP and orchiectomy. Of these patients, 11% needed to undergo repeat procedures for recurrent obstructive symptoms. Although on initial inspection the survival rate does not compare well with that for radical prostatectomy or radiotherapy, most of these lesions were of high grade, and 72% of the patients were 70 years of age or older. Of the 54 patients analyzed, 29 died of intercurrent disease, making the cause-specific survival rate about 75% at 10 years. This conservative treatment regimen may be a justifiable approach in patients older than 70 years of age at the time of diagnosis and in whom the life expectancy is not anticipated to exceed 10 years.

The question of whether TURP can cause tumor dissemination has been addressed by Jonasson and colleagues.[50] In their study, malignant cells were isolated from vena caval blood in 6 (67%) of 9 patients with adenocarcinoma of the prostate during TURP or prostatic massage. No cells were found in any of the patients undergoing a prostatic needle biopsy. Hanks[51] showed that patients with intermediate or poorly differentiated stage C cancer who underwent TURP as a method of diagnosis had a poor prognosis in terms of development of distant metastases and death. No adverse effects occurred in well-differentiated tumors. However, other studies have not confirmed this association and have demonstrated that, if grade and tumor volume are considered, TURP does not result in a poorer prognosis.[52–54]

EXPERIMENTAL THERAPIES

With the advancement of new technologies, other minimally invasive techniques are beginning to be implemented in prostate cancer patients. McKiel and associates recently described the use of cryosurgery in localized prostate cancer, including stage T3 cancer. Despite a negative biopsy rate of 90%, PSA levels were undetectable in only 33% at 3 months after treatment.[55] Cohen and associates reported that 27 of 29 patients with stage C disease treated with cryotherapy had negative biopsies at 3 months, with a fall of PSA level to a mean of 0.2 ng/mL.[56] This technology and that of focused ultrasound ablation are in the early phases of clinical trials, and the results will undoubtedly be of interest in the future.

CONCLUSION

As with most other stages of prostate cancer, meaningful and definitive conclusions are difficult to ascertain because of the lack of controlled, prospective, randomized studies comparing various treatments. Traditionally, stage C tumors have been considered lesions unsuitable for surgical removal. However, evidence suggests that radical prostatectomy may play a very definite role in this stage of disease. It can identify a subgroup of patients upstaged to clinical D1 disease who may benefit from adjuvant hormonal therapy, but it may also identify a smaller group downstaged to organ-confined disease who indeed may be cured by the procedure. It is associated with excellent overall and disease-specific survival rates, presumably because capsular penetration and margin positivity have been shown to be less ominous prognostic signs than were previously believed. Local recurrence rates have been low after radical prostatectomy, especially if it is combined with adjuvant treatment in patients with a high risk of progression. Surgery can be performed safely and may significantly palliate local symptoms. Serum PSA levels can also be used in follow-up to detect recurrent disease with a high degree of sensitivity; this may allow for earlier institution of adjuvant therapy if the tumor burden is still small.

The eventual decision as to how to manage patients with stage C prostate cancer depends on the age, general health, and 10-year life expectancy of the patient as well as the urologist's philosophy regarding the benefit of radical prostatectomy in reducing symptoms from the local tumor burden. Tumors with extensive extracapsular extension, high grade, and involved seminal vesicles or lymph nodes may well fail surgical therapy with curative intent, and irradiation as monotherapy is even less likely to be effective in this setting, given the reported high incidence of positive posttreatment biopsies and rising PSA levels. There are no definitive answers as to the best form or combinations of therapy, but we believe that radical prostatectomy may be the procedure of choice for some stage C prostate cancers in younger patients with life expectancies of longer than 10 years.

It seems appropriate to identify those patients with stage C prostate cancer who have evidence of seminal vesicle involvement. Most studies demonstrate that this feature is an independent adverse prognostic factor, associated with up to a 68% chance of progression over 5 years.[57] In patients who have palpable T2 disease but whose nomograms suggest T3 disease (PSA > 10 ng/mL), and in those with clinical T3 disease, routine transrectal ultrasonography-guided biopsies of the seminal vesicles bilaterally may be helpful. Biopsies in this setting identify involved seminal vesicles in 15% to 30% of cases, with a positive predictive value of 97% to 100%, a negative predictive value of 81% to 87.5%, and no adverse consequences for the subsequent surgical dissection.[58,59] A positive seminal vesicle biopsy may be sufficient evidence in itself to dissuade most urologists from attempting a surgical cure. However, for those wishing to proceed, a positive seminal vesicle biopsy in conjunction with a high-grade tumor (Gleason score above 7) on the preoperative biopsies makes the incidence of lymph node involvement 35% to 75%, sufficiently high for consideration of a laparoscopic lymph node dissection. Vallancien and associates have demonstrated only a 7% incidence of involved lymph nodes in the presence of negative seminal vesicle biopsies, so a laparoscopic lymph node dissection in those circumstances may not be necessary. Before radical prostatectomy, a cystoscopy should be performed to exclude trigonal involvement with tumor (T4), which occurs in approximately 2% of cases.[23] Although cystoprostatectomy and neobladder reconstruction may be considered in a young, healthy patient with T4 disease, there are no data to support its use. Because such locally extensive disease seems likely to fail treatment with distant metastases, these patients should probably not be considered for surgery other than in a trial setting.

After the decision has been made to perform a radical prostatectomy, preoperative neoadjuvant hormonal deprivation may be considered. This therapy poses little risk to the patient. Although lower positive margin rates have been reported with this treatment, this result may not translate into a significant survival advantage. Similarly, postoperative adjuvant treatment has not led to an improvement in cause-specific survival and is probably best reserved for those patients who are likely to develop a symptomatic local recurrence. A reasonable policy would be one of careful surveillance of the patient postoperatively, both clinically and biochemically, particularly noting the doubling time of any PSA elevations. In patients with extensive residual disease, a slow PSA rise should precede clinical recurrence by 1 to 3 years and allow for implementation of adjuvant radiotherapy before a palpable recurrence occurs, at which time irradiation would be less likely to eradicate the disease or normalize the PSA. A PSA level that has a doubling time of less than 1 year probably represents micrometastatic disease, and therefore hormonal therapy may be the preferred form of adjuvant treatment in that setting.[60]

The results of prospective, randomized trials examining the efficacy of neoadjuvant and adjuvant therapy in conjunction with surgery for stage C prostate cancer will be invaluable for future development of therapeutic approaches. New staging assays that could detect micrometastatic disease (e.g., PSA–reverse transcriptese–polymerase chain reaction assays, genetic markers) would help to identify and exclude patients who would not benefit from surgery. Continuing research into the fields of molecular biology and genetic therapy may provide new and exciting adjuvant treatments that can be used in conjunction with radical prostatectomy to treat patients with high-grade, stage C prostate cancer, a group who today continue to have a particularly unfavorable prognosis.

REFERENCES

1. de Kernion JB, Mukamel E. The management of stage C prostate cancer. Prog Clin Biol Res 1987;243B:403.
2. Gibbons RP, Cole BS, Richardson RG, et al. Adjuvant radiotherapy following radical prostatectomy: results and complications. J Urol 1986;135:65.
of disease 3. Schmidt JD, Mettin CJ, Natarian N, et al. Trends in the pattern of care for prostate cancer, 1974–1983: results of surveys by the American College of Surgeons. J Urol 1986;136:416.
4. Paulson DF, Stone AR, Walther PJ, Tucker JA, Cox EB. Radical prostatectomy: anatomical predictors of success or failure. J Urol 1986;136:1041.
5. McNeal JE, Villiers AA, Redwine EA, Freiha FS, Stamey TA. Capsular penetration in prostate cancer: significance for natural history and treatment. Am J Surg Pathol 1990;14:240.
6. Epstein JI. Evaluation of radical prostatectomy capsular margins of resection: the significance of margins designated as negative, closely approaching and positive. Am J Surg Pathol 1990;14:626.
7. Cheng WS, Frydenberg M, Bergstralh EJ, Larson-Keller JJ, Zincke H. Radical prostatectomy for pathologic stage C prostate cancer: influence of pathologic variables and adjuvant treatment on disease outcome. Urology 1993;42:283.
8. Middleton RG, Smith JA Jr, Melzer RB, Hamilton PE. Patient survival and local recurrence rate following radical prostatectomy for prostate carcinoma. J Urol 1986;136:422.
9. Epstein JI, Carmichael MJ, Pizov G, Walsh PC. Influence of capsular penetration on progression following radical prostatectomy: a study of 196 cases with long term follow up. J Urol 1993;150:135.
10. Ayala AG, Ro JY, Babaian R, Troncoso P, Grignon DJ. The prostatic capsule, does it exist? Its importance in the staging and treatment of prostatic carcinoma. Am J Surg Pathol 1989;13:21.
11. Epstein JI, Carmichael M, Partin AW, Walsh PC. Is tumor volume an independent predictor of progression following radical prostatectomy? A multivariate analysis of 185 clinical stage B adenocarcinoma of the prostate with 5 years of follow up. J Urol 1993;149:1478.
12. Schroeder FH, Belt E. Carcinoma of the prostate: a study of 213 patients with stage C tumors treated by total perineal prostatectomy. J Urol 1975;114:257.
13. Stein A, de Kernion JB, Smith RB, Dorey F, Patel H. Prostate specific antigen levels after radical prostatectomy in patients with organ confined and locally extensive prostate cancer. J Urol 1992;147:942.
14. Fowler JE Jr, Mills SE. Operable prostatic carcinoma: correlations among clinical stage, pathological stage, Gleason histological score and early disease free survival. J Urol 1985;133:49.
15. Villers AA, McNeal JE, Redwine EA, Freiha FS, Stamey TA. Pathogenesis and biological significance of seminal vesicle invasion in prostatic adenocarcinoma. J Urol 1990;143:1183.
16. Ackerman DA, Barry JM, Wicklund RA, Olson N, Lowe BA. Analysis of risk factors associated with prostate cancer extension to the surgical margin and pelvic node metastasis at radical prostatectomy. J Urol 1993;150:1845.
17. Voges GE, McNeal JE, Redwine EA, Freiha FS, Stamey TA. Morphological analysis of surgical margins with positive findings in prostatectomy for adenocarcinoma of the prostate. Cancer 1992;69:520.
18. Hodge KK, McNeal JE, Terris MK, Stamey TA. Random systematic versus directed ultrasound guided transrectal core biopsies of the prostate. J Urol 1989;142:71.
19. Hawkins CA, Bergstralh EJ, Zincke H. Influence of DNA ploidy on progression and survival in patients with stage pT3 prostate cancer following radical prostatectomy. J Urol 1994;151:255A. Abstract.
20. Adolfsson J. Deferred treatment of low grade stage T3 prostate cancer without distant metastases. J Urol 1993;149:326.
21. Stenzl A, Studer UE. Outcome of patients with untreated cancer of prostate. Eur Urol 1993;24:1.
22. Tomlinson RL, Currie DP, Boyce WH. Radical prostatectomy: palliation for stage C carcinoma of the prostate. J Urol 1977;117:85.
23. van den Ouden D, Davidson PJT, Hop W, Schroeder FH. Radical prostatectomy as monotherapy for locally advanced (stage T3) prostate cancer. J Urol 1994;151:646.
24. Morgan WR, Bergstralh EJ, Zincke H. Long term evaluation of radical prostatectomy as treatment for clinical stage C (T3) prostate cancer. Urology 1993;41:121.
25. Zincke H, Utz DE, Benson RC Jr, Patterson DE. Bilateral pelvic lymphadenectomy and radical prostatectomy for stage C adenocarcinoma of prostate. Urology 1984;24:532.
26. Schellhammer PF, El-Mahdi AM, Kuban DA. Local failure and related complications after definitive treatment of clinical stage C carcinoma of the prostate by irradiation or surgery. Semin Urol 1980;8:232.

27. Flocks RH, O'Donoghue EPN, Milleman LA, Culp DA. Management of stage C prostatic carcinoma. Urol Clin North Am 1975;2:163.
28. Rosenberg SJ, Loening SA, Hawtrey CE, Narayana AS, Culp DA. Radical prostatectomy with adjuvant radioactive gold for prostatic cancer: a preliminary report. J Urol 1985;133:225.
29. Anscher MS, Prosnitz LR. Postoperative radiotherapy for patients with carcinoma of the prostate undergoing radical prostatectomy with positive surgical margins, seminal vesicle involvement and/or penetration through the capsule. J Urol 1987;138:1407.
30. Freeman JA, Lieskovsky G, Cook DW, et al. Radical retropubic prostatectomy and post-operative adjuvant radiation for pathological stage C (Pc N0) prostate cancer from 1976 to 1989: intermediate findings. J Urol 1993;149:1029.
31. Paulson DP, Moul JW, Robertson JE, Walther DJ. Postoperative radiotherapy of the prostate for patients undergoing radical prostatectomy with positive margins, seminal vesicle involvement and/or penetration through the capsule. J Urol 1990;143:1178.
32. Zietman AL, Coen JJ, Shipley WU, Althausen AF. Adjuvant irradiation after radical prostatectomy for adenocarcinoma of the prostate: analysis of freedom from PSA failure. Urology 1993;42:292.
33. McCarthy JF, Catalona WE, Hudson MA. Effect of radiation therapy on detectable serum prostate specific antigen levels following radical prostatectomy: early versus delayed treatment. J Urol 1994;151:1575.
34. Gill WB, Marks JE, Straus FH, Sylora HO, Diamond HM. Radical retropubic prostatectomy and retroperitoneal lymphadenectomy following radiotherapy conversion of stage C to stage B carcinoma of the prostate. J Urol 1974;111:656.
35. Scott WW, Boyd HL. Hormone control and surgery: conversion into resectable lesion. JAMA 1969;2210:1078.
36. Hellstrom M, Haagman M, Branstedt S, et al. Histopathological changes in androgen deprived localized prostate cancer. Eur Urol 1993; 24:461.
37. Haagman M, Hellstrom M, Aus G, et al. Neoadjuvant GnRH agonist treatment (triptorelin and cyproterone acetate for flare protection) and total prostatectomy. Eur Urol 1993;24:456.
38. Schulman CC, Oosterhof GON, van Cangh PJ, de Bruyne FMJ, Witjes WPJ. Multicentre study of neoadjuvant combined androgen deprivation therapy in T2-T3, N0, M0 prostatic carcinoma. J Urol 1994;151:435A. Abstract.
39. Fair WR, Aprikan A, Sogani P, Reuter V, Whitmore WF Jr. The role of neoadjuvant hormonal manipulation in localized prostatic cancer. Cancer 1993;71:1031.
40. Oesterling JE, Andrews PE, Suman VJ, Zincke H, Myers RP. Preoperative androgen deprivation therapy: artificial lowering of serum prostate antigen without downstaging the tumor. J Urol 1993;149:779.
41. Kennedy TJ, Sonneland AM, Marlett MM, Troup RH. Luteinizing hormone releasing hormone downstaging of clinical stage C prostate cancer. J Urol 1992;147:891.
42. MacFarlane MT, Abi-Aad A, Stein A, Danella J, Belldegrun A, de Kernion JB. Neoadjuvant hormonal deprivation in patients with locally advanced prostate cancer. J Urol 1993;150:132.
43. Schulman CC, Sassine AM. Neoadjuvant hormonal deprivation before radical prostatectomy. Eur Urol 1993;24:450.
44. Kollermann MW, Sprenk P, Muhlfait V, Kahla H, Kollermann J. Downstaging of stage C prostatic carcinoma by inductive chemohormonal therapy? Eur Urol 1993;24:337.
45. Grups JW, Theiss M, Frohmuller HGW. Complications of radical prostatectomy: stage B versus stage C carcinoma of the prostate. Eur Urol 1990;18(Suppl):37. Abstract.
46. Pavone-Macaluso M, de Voogt HJ, Viggiano G, et al. Comparison of diethylstilbestrol, cyproterone acetate and medroxyprogesterone acetate in the treatment of advanced prostatic cancer: final analysis of a randomized phase III trial of European Organization for Research on Treatment of Cancer Urological Group. J Urol 1986;136:624.
47. Francini M, Veronesi A, Dal Bo V, et al. Radiotherapy versus orchiectomy in locally advanced prostate carcinoma: a randomized study. Eur Urol 1990;18(Suppl):130. Abstract.
48. Blackard CE, Byar DP, Jordan WP. Orchiectomy for advanced prostatic carcinoma. Urology 1973;1:553.
49. Gee WF, Cole JR. Symptomatic stage C carcinoma of prostate: traditional therapy. Urology 1980;15:335.
50. Jonasson O, Long L, Roberts S, McGrew E, McDonald JH. Cancer cells in the circulating blood during operative management of genitourinary tumors. J Urol 1961;85:1.
51. Hanks GE: External beam radiation therapy for clinically localized prostate cancer: patterns of care studies in the United States. Monogr Natl Cancer Inst 1988;7:75.
52. Zagars GK, von Eschenbach AC, Johnson DE, Oswald MJ. Stage C adenocarcinoma of the prostate: an analysis of 551 patients treated with external beam radiation. Cancer 1987;60:1489.
53. Babaian RJ, Archer JS. Dissemination of disease following transurethral resection for locally advanced prostate cancer. Urology 1988;31: 30.
54. Nativ O, Bergstralh EJ, Boyle ET Jr, Zincke H. Transurethral resection versus needle biopsy prior to radical prostatectomy for stage C prostate cancer: influence on progression and survival. Urology 1991;37:22.
55. McKiel CF Jr, Levine SR, Levine LA. PSA and post-treatment biopsy: results after cryosurgery for stages T1-T3 prostate cancer. J Urol 1994; 151:436A. Abstract.
56. Cohen JK, Miller RJ, Onik G. Cryosurgical ablation of the prostate in patients with clinical stage A, B and C adenocarcinoma of the prostate: outcome of PSA and biopsy at 3, 12 and 24 months. J Urol 1994;151: 375A. Abstract.
57. Catalona WJ, Smith DS. Five year tumor recurrence rates after anatomical radical retropubic prostatectomy for prostate cancer. J Urol 1994; 152:1387.
58. Vallancien G, Bochereau G, Wetzel O, Bretheau D, Drapotnich D, Bouganon J. Influence of pre-operative positive seminal vesicle biopsy on the staging of prostate cancer. J Urol 1994;152:1152.
59. Terris MK, McNeal JE, Freiha FS, Stamey TA. Efficacy of transrectal ultrasound guided seminal vesical biopsies in the detection of seminal vesicle invasion by prostate cancer. J Urol 1993;149:1035.
60. Trapasso JG, de Kernion JB, Smith RB, Dorey F. The incidence and significance of detectable levels of serum prostatic specific antigen after radical prostatectomy. J Urol 1994;152:1821.

52.2 Radiotherapy

Benjamin W. Corn and Gerald E. Hanks

This chapter concerns prostate tumors that are no longer confined to the gland but have extended locally beyond the prostatic capsule, invaded the seminal vesicles, or metastasized to regional lymph nodes. According to the American Cancer Society, such tumors are now diagnosed annually in more than 70,000 American men.[1] The local disease component was previously designated stage C in the classic Whitmore system[2] but is currently categorized as T3 in the 1992 revision of the American Joint Committee on Cancer staging system[3] that has been accepted by most international urologic oncology groups. The regional component of disease was previously denoted D1 by the American Urologic Association but is presently staged as N1-N3 depending on the size and number of lymph nodes involved (Table 52.2-1). This chapter separately analyzes the role of radiotherapy in the management of patients with T3 and node-positive disease. Issues related to surgical and endocri-

TABLE 52.2-1. *Comparison of three staging systems for prostate cancer*

AUA stage	AJCC stage (1988)	AJCC stage (1992)
A No palpable lesion A1 Focal A2 Diffuse B Confined to prostate B1 Small discrete nodule B2 Large or multiple nodules or areas C Localized to periprostatic area C1 No involvement of seminal vesicles, <70g C2 Involvement of seminal vesicles, >70g D Metastatic disease D1 Pelvic lymph nodes metastates or urethral obstruction causing hydronephrosis D2 Bone or distant lymph node or organ or soft tissue metastases	T0 No evidence of primary tumor T1a Three or fewer microscopic foci of carcinoma T1b More than 3 microscopic foci of carcinoma T2 Tumor present clinically or grossly, limited to the gland T2a Tumor 1.5 cm or less in greatest dimension with normal tissue on at least 3 slides T2b Tumor more than 1.5 cm in greatest dimension or in more than one lobe T3 Tumor invades the prostatic apex, or into or beyond the prostatic capsule, bladder neck, or seminal vesicle but is not fixed T4 Tumor is fixed or invades the adjacent structures other than those listed in T3 N1 Metastasis in a single lymph node, 2 cm or less in greatest dimension N2 Metastases in a single lymph node, more than 2 cm but not more than 5 cm in greatest dimension, or multiple lymph nodes, none more than 5 cm in greatest dimension N3 Metastasis in a lymph node more than 5 cm in greatest dimension M1 Distant metastasis	TX Primary tumor cannot be assessed T0 No evidence of primary tumor T1 Clinically inapparent tumor not palpable or visible by imaging T1a Tumor incidental histologic finding in 5% or less of tissue resected T1b Tumor incidental histologic finding in more than 5% of tissue resected T1c Tumor identified by needle biopsy (eg, because of elevated PSA) T2 Tumor confined within the prostate T2a Tumor involves half of a lobe or less T2b Tumor involves more than half of a lobe, but not both lobes T2c Tumor involves both lobes T3 Tumor extends through the prostatic capsule T3a Unilateral extracapsular extension T3b Bilateral extracapsular extension T3c Tumor invades the seminal vesicle(s) T4 Tumor is fixed or invades adjacent structures other than the seminal vesicles T4a Tumor invades any of: bladder neck, external sphincter, or rectum T4b Tumor invades levator muscles and/or is fixed to the pelvic wall NX Regional lymph nodes cannot be assessed N0 No regional lymph node metastasis N1 Metastasis in a single lymph node, 2 cm or less in greatest dimension N2 Metastasis in a single lymph node, more than 2 cm but not more than 5 cm in greatest dimension; or multiple lymph node metastases, none more than 5 cm in greatest dimension N3 Metastasis in a lymph node more than 5 cm in greatest dimension MX Presence of distant metastasis cannot be assessed M0 No distant metastasis M1 Distant metastasis M1a Nonregional lymph node(s) M1b Bone(s) M1c Other site(s)

AUA, American Urologic Association; *AJCC,* American Joint Committee on Cancer; *PSA,* prostate-specific antigen.

nologic management of these presentations have been addressed in Chapter 52.1.

RELIABILITY OF STAGING

Errors in Clinical Evaluation

The problem of pathologic upstaging of organ-confined disease has been well documented. Hanks summarized the literature[4] and concluded that 6% to 11% of clinical stage A patients and 19% to 66% of stage B patients have stage C disease. Frazier and colleagues recently analyzed 226 patients who underwent radical prostatectomy for presumed organ-confined disease at Duke University[5] on the basis of serum concentrations of prostate-specific antigen (PSA). They reported treatment failure in 66% of patients with positive margins, 39% of those with specimen-confined disease but only 10% of those with pathologically confirmed organ-confined disease.

The inaccuracies associated with the staging of clinical stage C (i.e., T3) disease are less clear, because few patients with involvement of the prostatic capsule or seminal vesicles are taken to the operating room for prostatectomy. In a series of 232 patients with clinical stage C disease who underwent prostatectomy at the Mayo Clinic, Morgan and associates[6] found that 22% had pathologic stage B disease. On the other hand, 42% had pathologic nodal involvement and were thus upstaged to D1 disease. It is not known whether these errors in clinical staging are typical of all patients presenting with stage T3 disease or whether these data are merely characteristic of the selected group with T3 tumors who can undergo prostatectomy.

Substaging of Stage T3 Prostate Cancer

Currently, T3 cancers are divided into three substages; those with unilateral extracapsular extension (T3a), those with bilateral extracapsular extension (T3b), and those with invasion of the seminal vesicle (T3c). Data from prostatectomy series imply that pathologic stage T3 disease represents a heterogeneous entity in which involvement of the seminal vesicles connotes a worse prognosis than involvement of the prostatic capsule. The meaning of clinical T3 substaging is less apparent.

Schellhammer[7] reported the experience from the Eastern Virginia Medical School. Among 26 patients with pathologic stage C disease, seminal vesicle involvement was associated with a 66% rate of distant failure and a 44% rate of local failure; 17 patients with capsular involvement only had no local failures and only 23% distant recurrence. In a report that included 28 patients with pathologic stage C tumors who underwent radical prostatectomy at the University of Utah, Middleton and colleagues[8] observed that 12 of 14 patients with capsular involvement alone were free of disease after 5 years of clinical follow-up (4 other patients were lost to follow-up), in contrast to only 5 of 10 patients with seminal vesicle involvement. Furthermore, in a report of 196 patients with capsular (but not seminal vesicle) involvement from Johns Hopkins, Epstein and associates[9] noted 82% progression-free survival at 5 years among patients with focal capsular penetration but only 65% among those with extensive capsular penetration ($P = 0.06$), suggesting that it is possible to elucidate differences among substages of pathologic stage T3 disease.

Scant *clinical* data are available to assess the validity of the current staging system. Zagars and associates[10] used the database from the M.D. Anderson Cancer Center in an attempt to discriminate between the respective substages. Only 4 patients had stage T3b disease, so patients with stages T3a and T3b were aggregated for purposes of analysis. Although patients with T3 disease had actuarial disease-free survivorship that was intermediate between those with T2 and T3 disease, no distinction could be made between the substages within stage T3. At the Fox Chase Cancer Center (FCCC), 111 patients irradiated for T3 disease were available for analysis.[11] At 3 years, the actuarial freedom from biochemical relapse of these patients was 41%. No significant differences were evident after separate analyses were run for T3a and T3b patients. Rather, multivariate analysis disclosed that the only significant predictor of treatment outcome was baseline PSA level (≤20 versus >20 ng/mL; $P < 0.0002$). It therefore appears that biochemical distinctions are superior to digital rectal examination which cannot reliably separate those patients with seminal vesicle involvement from those who have only the capsule involved by tumor.

STAGE T3: STANDARD MANAGEMENT

Clinical Criteria

The traditional standard of management for T3 adenocarcinoma of the prostate has been external beam radiotherapy. Several institutions have published long-term outcome data for this stage of disease (Table 52.2-2). At Stanford University, Bagshaw and associates[12] noted a 10-year survival rate of 35% and a 15-year survival rate of 18% among patients with T3 disease. Within that same group, the freedom from recurrence at 10 and 15 years was 28% and 23%, respectively. At the M.D. Anderson Cancer Center,[13] the 10- and 15-year survival rates for patients with stage C disease were 57% and 27%, respectively, and the disease-free survival rates were 45% and 40%. Ten-year data have also been published from Perez and associates[14] at Washington University in St. Louis, where the survival rate among 328 patients with stage C disease was 35%, and the rate of survival with no evidence of disease was 32%.

Hanks and colleagues generated survival curves and hazard rates from two large national databases: the Radiation Therapy Oncology Group (RTOG) and the Patterns of Care Study (PCS).[15] In contrast to the above results, which are subject to the biases associated with retrospective reports from single institutions, the RTOG and PCS experiences are representative of national averages in the United States. The hazard rates express the risk of death at a point in time. Comparison of the observed hazard rate for death from the RTOG and PCS patients with the expected hazard rate for a similar age population without cancer provides a rigorous assessment of cure. For stage C disease, an increased hazard rate is observed for up to 10 years, but the 15-year PCS hazard rate demonstrates a return to expected levels (Fig 52.2-1). This is reflected in the survival plots, in which observed survival and expected survival traces become parallel at 12 to 15 years. Although patients with stage C disease have an earlier and greater excess mortality than those with stage B disease (data not shown), the excess mortality is no

TABLE 52.2-2. *Long-term outcome of stage T3 prostate cancer treated by external irradiation: Clinical criteria*

Institution	Patients	10-y survival rate (%)	10-y FFR rate (%)	15-y survival rate (%)	15-y FFR rate (%)
Stanford[12]	348	35	28	18	23
MDACC[13]	551	57	45	27	40
Washington University[14]	328	35	32	NA	NA
RTOG[15]	503	38	NA	NA	NA
PCS[15]	296	32	65	23	NA

FFR, freedom from relapse; *NA,* data not available; *MDACC,* M.D. Anderson Cancer Center; *RTOG,* Radiation Therapy Oncology Group; *PCS,* Patterns of Care Study.

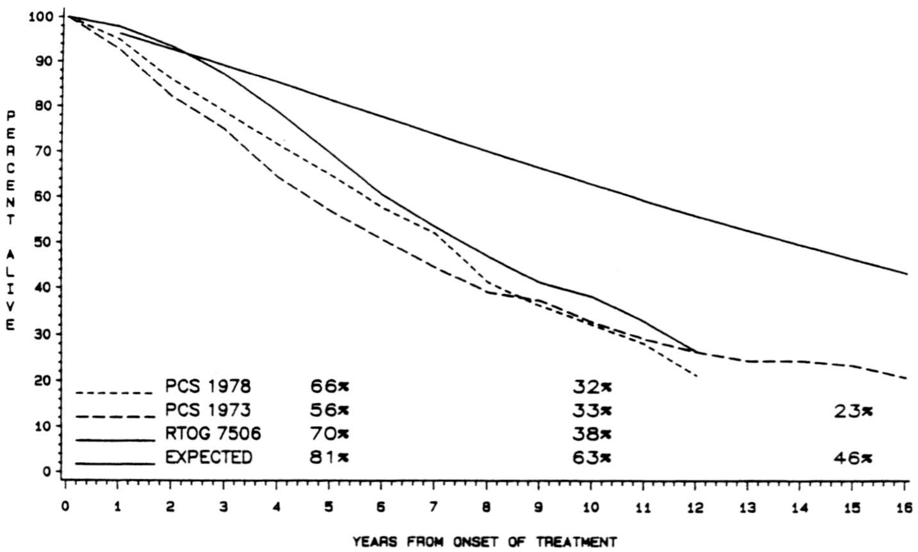

A

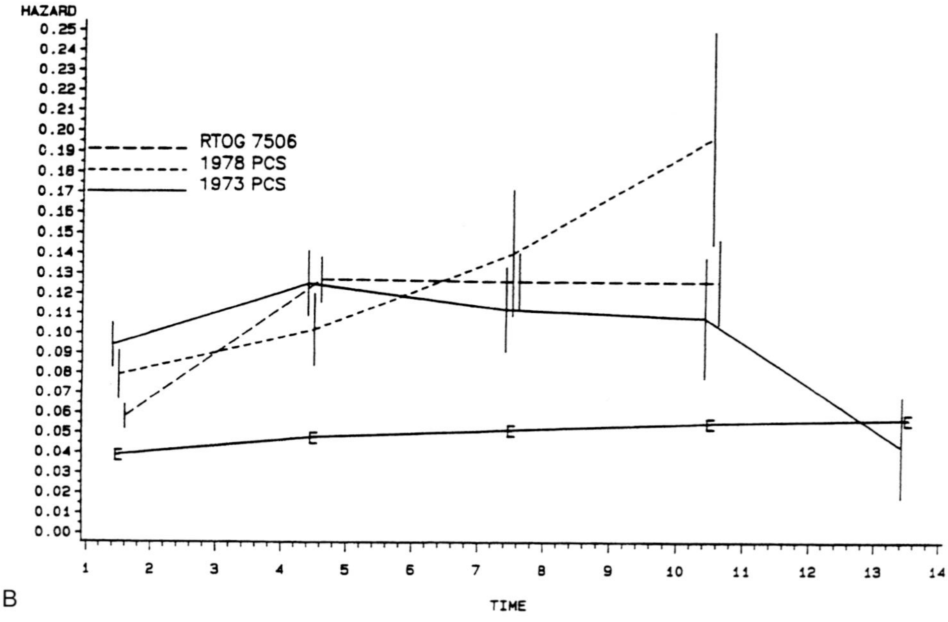

B

FIG. 52.2-1. (**A**) Long-term survival rates for T3,4 NX M0 prostate cancer treated with radiation in Patterns of Care Study (PCS) national surveys (1973 and 1978) and in Radiation Therapy Oncology Group (RTOG) 7506 compared with expected the survival rate. (**B**) Hazard rates for T3,4 NX M0 prostate cancer treated with radiation in PCS national surveys (1973 and 1978) and in RTOG 7506. The bar represents one standard deviation from the expected hazard rate, indicated by E. (Hanks GE, Krall JM, Hanlon AL, Asbell SO, Pilepich MV, Owen JB. Patterns of Care and RTOG studies in prostate cancer: long-term survival, hazard rate observations, and possibilities of cure. Int J Radiat Oncol Biol Phys 1993;28:39, with permission).

longer detectable by 15 years. Hanks and colleagues have speculated that this phenomenon may represent later intervention in the overall course of the disease for patients who are not going to be cured by the treatment, so that the excess mortality is fully expressed by 15 years. It is encouraging that even patients with large-volume disease (e.g., stage C [T3]) can be cured at 15 years according to the relatively strict criteria of the RTOG and PCS data, and that, of the 23% of patients who survived, three quarters remained free of any evidence of disease.

Fifteen-year observations represent unique demonstrations of the efficacy of external beam irradiation. Analogous data are not available for other cancer modalities such as surgery or hormonal manipulation. The patients in these reports were not staged with modern diagnostic tools; in particular, no patient had baseline PSA testing, none was monitored with interval PSA measurements. In addition, 40% to 60% of patients with stages T3/T4 disease would be expected to have positive lymph node involvement,[16] and such metastases (even if subclinical) would govern the natural history of the disease. Although there is some debate concerning the precise level of cure between institutions, the curative impact of irradiation is beyond question.

PSA-Based Outcome Data

Table 52.2-3 is a composite of the available data from institutions that have reported PSA-based results. Various outcome parameters have been used by the respective investigators. In general, it appears that 10% to 20% of T3 patients treated with definitive irradiation alone have no evidence of biochemical relapse at 3 to 4 years after treatment. It is essential to update these experiences as the data mature. Moreover, innovative strategies such as particle beams and combinations of radiotherapy with hormones (see later discussion) need to be evaluated by biochemical criteria. Only a commitment to rigorous PSA-based follow-up will allow valid comparison among therapeutic alternatives.

STAGE T3: INNOVATIVE STRATEGIES

Prophylactic Nodal Irradiation

Although theoretically appealing, the value of prophylactic nodal irradiation has never been established. Despite the completion of two prospective, randomized trials (one by the RTOG[41] and another by Stanford University[53]), the indications for prophylactic nodal irradiation remain controversial. Hanks[42] has drawn attention to the error in judgment of the RTOG in permitting both lymphangiography and computed tomography (CT) for determination of nodal status. As a result, this large study showed only that these imaging modalities cannot separate patients into different prognostic groups. The RTOG trial should not be construed as a negative study, but rather as one that could not probe the end point being tested because of poor study design. In contrast, the Stanford trial was well designed but the number of patients accrued was too small to demonstrate a significant benefit of prophylactic nodal irradiation. Our policy at FCCC continues to include elective irradiation of pelvic nodes for patients with stage T3 disease because of the considerable risk of nodal involvement.

Conformal Irradiation

Conformal irradiation is the delivery of radiation with beams that conform to the exact contour of the target volume (i.e., the prostatic bed plus other areas deemed to be at risk for recurrence with appropriate margins). The essential components of conformal treatment strategies include reproducible rigid immobilization, computer-driven three-dimensional treatment planning (e.g., CT-based planning), and radiation portal apertures that are configured to reflect the shape of the target. The department of radiation oncology at the FCCC published in 1992[17] the first description of this methodology, which included use of alpha cradle body casts (Smithers Medical Products, Akron, Ohio) extending from the thorax to the midthigh, urethrography and CT scanning performed in the treatment position, and beam's-eye view conformal portal apertures. This approach resulted in a 14% reduction of dose to the bladder and rectum, which translated into significant reductions of acute symptoms during treatment. For example, only 31% of the conformal group, compared with 60% of the conventionally treated group, required medications or treatment interruptions to combat acute reactions such as diarrhea, tenesmus, dysuria, and hematuria.[18]

In separate analyses using two different end points (PSA normalization at 1 year and biochemical freedom from relapse), investigators from FCCC have shown that conformal techniques are independently associated with significantly more tumor control than conventional irradiation strategies.[19,20] In each of these multivariate analyses, dose escalation did not emerge as an independent factor contributing to tumor control. This suggests that an inherent benefit of conformal techniques is the more accurate and precise deposition of the prescribed radiation dose within

TABLE 52.2-3. *Outcome of definitive radiotherapy in patients with T3 disease: PSA-based criteria*

Institution	No. of patients	Result
MGH[65]	76 (T3-T4)	26% 4-y freedom from biochemical relapse
FCCC[11]	111	20% 4-y freedom from biochemical relapse
Stanford[63]	36	15% 4-y freedom from biochemical relapse
University of Wisconsin[64]	10	20% free of biochemical failure (25-mo median follow-up)
Mayo Clinic[66]	44	9% relapse-free at 3 y
MDACC[67]	393	49% rising PSA at 5 y

FCCC, Fox Chase Cancer Center; *MGH,* Massachusetts General Hospital; *MDACC,* M.D. Anderson Cancer Center; *PSA,* prostate-specific antigen.

the target volume rather than the use of higher total doses of radiation.

Morbidity of Conventional and Conformal Irradiation

Several large databases have been used to determine the incidence of major complications after external beam irradiation. In the PCS, Hanks and colleagues[21] observed that 4.3% of 1633 patients receiving a median prostatic dose of 66 Gy had morbidity requiring hospitalization or surgical intervention. Lawton and associates[22] reviewed the RTOG experience of 1020 patients and found grades 3 to 5 toxicity (7.7% genitourinary; 3.3% gastrointestinal; 1.6% other) in 12.6% of men who received a median pelvic dose of 54 Gy and a median prostatic dose of 70 Gy. Perez and colleagues[50] reanalyzed the experience of 738 patients treated at Washington University and determined that technical factors such as treatment volume and dose have the greatest influence on severe late morbidities; for this reason, they encouraged the adoption of sophisticated conformal irradiation tactics.

Schultheiss and associates[23] have recently updated the FCCC conformal experience and found that only central axis dose is significantly related to the incidence of late gastrointestinal and genitourinary sequelae. In that series, the actuarial 5-year RTOG grades 3 to 5 toxicity levels were 13.8%, 7.9%, 4.2%, and 2.9% for central axis dose levels of 74 to 76.99, 71 to 73.99, 68 to 70.00, and 65 to 67.99 Gy, respectively. At the FCCC, our current conformal irradiation program does not include dose escalation above 70 Gy because higher doses have only been associated with increased severe late effects without an accompanying increase in freedom from biochemical relapse.

Neoadjuvant Hormonal Manipulation Plus Radiotherapy

Neoadjuvant hormonal manipulation before definitive radiotherapy has emerged as an integral concept in the treatment of locally advanced prostate cancer. The mechanism underlying the potential efficacy of this approach has been debated. Antecedent hormonal treatment may represent an effective form of "chemical tumor debulking."[24] Some hormones (e.g., estrogen) can inhibit intracellular metabolism of testosterone, on which prostate epithelial cells are dependent, and may exert a directly cytotoxic effect on tumor cells.[25] Although some have speculated that hormones may have an antagonistic effect when coupled with irradiation by shifting tumor cells to a theoretically quiescent phase of the cell cycle, recent evidence supports the concept that both radiation and hormonal manipulation may have their effects mediated through a common pathway of programmed cell death, or apoptosis.[26]

Several lines of clinical evidence are now emerging that support the integration of androgen blockade with irradiation. In a prospective trial (86-10),[27] the RTOG randomly assigned 457 patients with stage C tumors or "bulky" stage B tumors (i.e., stage B tumors with cross-sectional diameter of 24 cm^2 or higher) to a course of definitive radiotherapy (44 to 46 Gy of pelvic irradiation followed by a boost of 20 to 25 Gy to the prostate) with or without neoadjuvant total androgen deprivation (goserelin plus flutamide). The experimental arm in this study exhibited advantages at the 3-year end points of clinical local control (84% versus 71%; $P = 0.003$), disease-free survival (61% versus 43%; $P = 0.001$), and freedom from biochemical failure, defined as PSA levels lower than 4 ng/mL 1 year or more after therapy (46% versus 26%; $P = 0.0001$). No statistically significant differences were observed in distant failure (25% versus 30%; $P = .097$). Data are now maturing from a recently completed RTOG study (92-02) that treated all such patients with neoadjuvant androgen deprivation followed by irradiation but randomly assigned them to receive either maintenance hormones or no further treatment (GE Hanks, personal communication, October, 1994).

Zagars and colleagues[28] reported the results of a prospective, randomized trial from the M.D. Anderson Cancer Center in which 78 patients with stage C prostate cancer received either irradiation alone or irradiation and adjuvant diethylstilbestrol (DES). The radiotherapy consisted of 50 Gy to the pelvis followed by 20 Gy through reduced fields. The DES (daily dose of 5 mg at beginning of the study with protocol modification to 2 mg/d at the end of the study) was given immediately after the completion of radiotherapy and was continued indefinitely. Follow-up included determinations of acid phosphatase, but the study preceded the PSA era. Disease-free survival rates in the estrogen-treated group were significantly higher than in the group receiving only radiotherapy at 5, 10, and 15 years (71% versus 49%, 63% versus 43%, and 63% versus 35%, respectively; $P = 0.008$). Because of increased intercurrent disease mortality among those receiving estrogen therapy, there was no improvement in overall survival in the experimental arm.

Hyperfractionation

Forman and associates[29] at Wayne State University have used twice-daily administrations of radiotherapy to treat patients with T3/T4 prostate cancer. In a series of 25 men treated to total doses of 7800 cGy, 36% were alive without evidence of disease (PSA $\leq$4 ng/mL) at 1 year, and no increase in acute morbidities was encountered, compared with historical controls treated at one fraction per day. It is unclear whether the theoretic basis of hyperfractionation[68] dovetails with the biology of prostate cancer or whether it would be more prudent to offer hyperfractionated irradiation only to those patients with more aggressive tumors (e.g., low PSA doubling times).[30] Moreover, the researchers at Wayne State University may not have used a sufficiently rigorous end point for biochemical disease-free survival.

Protons

Shipley and colleagues[31] randomly assigned 202 patients with stage T3-T4 disease who were initially treated with 50.4 Gy of pelvic irradiation to receive either a 25.2 cobalt-Gy-equivalent (CGE) proton boost or a 16.8 CGE photon boost. At 7 years, there were no statistically significant differences between the study arms in overall survival, freedom from biochemical relapse, or freedom from local relapse. Among the subgroup with poorly differentiated tumors, however, there was a significant local control benefit associated with the use of protons instead of photons (85% versus 37%; $P = 0.001$). Regarding treatment-related morbidity, grade 1 and 2 rectal bleeding (32% versus 12%; $P = 0.002$) and urethral stricture (19% versus 8%; $P = 0.07$) were more common among those who received proton boosts. Reported outcome data did not include PSA-based criteria.

Neutrons

The RTOG[32] carried out a trial (no. 7704) that randomly assigned 91 patients with stage C or D1 disease to receive photon irradiation alone (50 Gy to the pelvis followed by a 20-Gy boost to the prostate) or a mixture of photon and neutron beams (identical prescription, with "photon equivalent doses" arrived at by summing the photon dose and the neutron dose and multiplying by the institutional *relative biologic equivalent* [RBE]).[3] After 8 years, the actuarial survival rate for the mixed beam cohort was 63%, compared with 13% for the patients receiving photons alone ($P = 0.01$). The "determinental" survival rates, adjusted by exclusion of the intercurrent deaths, were 82% and 54%, respectively ($P = 0.02$). Freedom from locally recurrent disease was 77% for the patients receiving mixed beam therapy and 31% for patients receiving photons alone ($P = 0.01$). Reported outcome data did not include PSA-based criteria.

In a subsequent study carried out by the Neutron Therapy Collaborative Working Group Trial, 182 patients with T3-T4 tumors or with positive pelvic lymph node involvement by prostate cancer were randomly assigned to receive either pure photon beam irradiation (5040 cGy to the pelvis, followed by a 2000-cGy boost) or neutron beam irradiation (13.6 nGy to the pelvis, with a 6.8-nGy boost). Although the neutron-treated study arm showed a clinical local control advantage (82% versus 60%), no increases in rates of overall survival or disease-free survival were found. Moreover, a significant increase in severe morbidity was observed in the neutron arm. Grade 4 morbidity occurred in 10 of 87 patients in the neutron-treated group, including 6 colostomies, but in only 1 of 85 patients in the photon-treated group.[33]

Although neutron and proton beams may hold some promise, from a practical perspective such forms of radiotherapy are not accessible to most oncologists. Conformal photon-based treatments, however, are easily transferable to community-based radiation oncology centers.[34]

Brachytherapy

The use of radioactive implants is considered here only briefly. To date, no prospective, randomized trial has compared treatment of similarly stratified patients with brachytherapy versus external beam irradiation or radical prostatectomy. Three institutions, however, have retrospectively compared the results in patients treated by either interstitial or external techniques within the same time period. Although selection factors would probably favor the patients with implantable disease, at each of these centers significantly more local failure was observed among stage C patients treated with implants compared with those receiving external therapy (67% versus 17%[35]; 44% versus 26%[36]; and 29% versus 17%[37] at the three institutions). A potentially more promising role for brachytherapy may come from its use in tandem with external beam treatment. In small series employing specially designed templates (as opposed to freehand implants), Syed and colleagues[38] reported 83% clinical control among 36 stage C patients treated with 35 Gy of interstitial irradiation followed by 40 Gy external beam irradiation, and Brindle and associates[39] described 89% actuarial 5-year disease-free survival among 51 patients with stage C or bulky stage B tumors treated with a similar dose combination. Because there are no published long-term or PSA-based results for the new brachytherapy technologies (CT- or ultrasound-guided template systems that theoretically allow better control of source localization), these approaches are not considered further.

LYMPH NODE METASTASES

Incidence

The risk of lymph node metastasis among prostate cancer patients is now being reassessed. In the past, approximately 25% of patients with clinical stage T1/T2 disease and at least 40% of patients with T3/T4 disease were found to have positive lymph node involvement.[16] A recent report of 521 consecutive patients who underwent surgical staging at Washington University School of Medicine between 1983 and 1991[40] revealed significantly lower rates of nodal disease (3.3% for A2, 5.3% for B1, and 9.7% for B2 cancers). These findings have been attributed to expanded efforts to detect prostate cancer at earlier stages. It is unclear whether institutions without commitments to such screening programs will confirm these results. Moreover, it is uncertain whether a lower frequency of nodal metastasis will be observed for stage T3 patients, because most prostatectomy series do not include these patients. Historical series suggest that patients with T3 disease are likely to have a 40% to 60% chance of harboring lymph node metastases.

The lone series that attempted to determine the benefit of prophylactic nodal irradiation[41] was flawed[42] by inconsistent lymph node assessment (e.g., CT, lymphangiography, lymphadenectomy). Ideally, patients with stage T3 disease should have their lymph nodes evaluated pathologically, because a large subset of these patients have nodal involvement. Prospective trials can then be designed to tailor the radiation portals of such patients to encompass the appropriate treatment volume (e.g., prostate, pelvis, paraaortic nodes).

Favorable Subsets

Surgical series that address node-positive disease have been detailed in Chapter 52.1. These surgical data are referred to here only for the sake of defining potentially curable subsets of patients with node-positive disease. It appears that "limited nodal involvement" confers a more favorable prognosis and presents the best opportunity for cure (Table 52.2-4). The definition of "limited nodal involvement" has varied between series. Prout and associates[43] found that the 5-year survival rate with no evidence of disease was 82% among those with only solitary nodal involvement but only 23% among those with multiple positive nodes. Similarly, Smith and colleagues[44] observed an advantage for patients with only a single positive node (44% versus 27% survival with no evidence of disease at 5 years). Steinberg and associates[45] distinguished between microscopic nodal involvement (80% 5-year survival rate) and

TABLE 52.2-4. *Influence of extent of nodal involvement on outcome*

Investigators	Patients	Degree of nodal involvement	Outcome at 5 y
Prout et al, 1980[43]	11	Solitary node	82% NED
	21	Multiple nodes	23% NED
Smith et al, 1984[44]	18	Solitary node	44% NED
	22	Multiple nodes	27% NED
Steinberg et al, 1990[45]	66	Microscopic	80% survival
	54	Microscopic	40% survival
Barzell et al, 1977[46]	18	Small volume (<3 cc)	70% free of metastases
	82	Large volume (>3 cc)	10% free of metastases

NED, no evidence of disease.

macroscopic nodal involvement (40% 5-year survival rate). Finally, Barzell and colleagues[46] found that patients with small-volume (<3 cc) nodal involvement had superior freedom from distant relapse when compared with those with large-volume (>3 cc) disease (70% versus 10% at 5 years).

Therapeutic Nodal Irradiation

Several investigators have reported small series of patients treated with therapeutic (as opposed to prophylactic) nodal irradiation (Table 52.2-5). Most of the published experiences suffer from small patient numbers, short follow-up, and clinical rather than PSA-based outcome criteria. At the Medical College of Wisconsin, Lawton and colleagues[47] treated 56 patients with stage D1 disease with external irradiation. Among the entire group, actuarial survival was 76% at 5 years and 33% at 10 years. The majority of patients in the series (59%) did not have pathologic documentation of nodal involvement but only radiographic evidence of adenopathy, and it is impossible to determine whether the favorable outcome reflected patients with only minimal nodal disease. Although the authors attributed the impressive results to meticulous workup, the staging of their patients did not exceed the standards of process established in a recent PCS newsletter.[48]

Whittington and associates[49] treated 41 patients with pathologically proven nodal metastases from prostate cancer with radiotherapy (55 Gy of pelvic irradiation to those with residual nodes measuring more than 1 cm, followed by prostatic boosts of 65 to 71 Gy) and concurrent hormonal manipulation. The hormonal treatment was either surgical (orchiectomy) or nonsurgical (leuprolide plus flutamide, leuprolide alone, or DES). Only 5 patients experienced relapse or biochemical failure. The remainder maintained normal PSA levels during a median follow-up period of 39 months. In comparison, 5 patients were offered concurrent irradiation and hormones at that institution but declined; all 5 of those patients relapsed within 18 months of radiotherapy.

Modig and colleagues[51] reported the preliminary results of a phase III trial carried out at the University of Umea in Sweden in which 91 patients with node-positive disease were randomly assigned to radiotherapy alone or radiotherapy with orchiectomy. After a median follow-up period of 4.5 years, the clinical recurrence rate (mostly in the form of bone metastases) was 72% among those treated by irradiation alone, compared with 20% among those who received irradiation and orchiectomy. Although the trial was prospectively randomized, the small number of patients enrolled in the study compromise the interpretation of the results.

Paulson and colleagues[52] described the results from a phase III trial that randomly assigned patients with stage D1 disease to either extended field radiotherapy (pelvis and paraaortic portals) or delayed hormonal manipulation (orchiectomy or DES). The study revealed an advantage to the radiotherapy group at

TABLE 52.2-5. *Node positive prostate cancer: Impact of therapeutic nodal irradiation*

Investigators	Determination of nodal status	Patients	Treatment	Disease-free survival rate (%) 5 y	10 y
Lawton et al, 1992[47]	Radiologic/pathologic	56	EB	60	33
Whittington et al, 1994[49]	Pathologic	41	EB + AD	88*	—
Modig et al, 1993[51]	Pathologic	19	EB + AD	72	—
		19	EB	20	—
Paulson et al, 1982[52]	Pathologic	41	EB	40	—
Bagshaw, 1984[53]	Pathologic	61	EB	45	20
Hanks et al, 1991[62]	Pathologic	86	EB	32	15
Lange et al, 1988[55]	Pathologic	36	RP + EB	69	—
Batata et al, 1980[57]	Pathologic	28	^{125}I + EB	21	—
Gervasi et al, 1989[59]	Pathologic	152	^{198}Au + EB	75	43

AD, androgen deprivation; ^{198}*Au,* gold implant; *EP,* external beam irradiation; ^{125}*I,* iodine implant; *RP,* radical prostatectomy.

* Nonactuarial calculations with median follow-up of 35 months.

34 months (70% versus 50% survival; $P = 0.056$); however, there were no outcome differences between the two arms at 5 years. The median time to first failure was also significantly prolonged in the radiotherapy group (23.9 versus 12.2 months; $P = 0.02$).

Bagshaw[53] reported a 10-year survival rate of 20% for 61 patients with positive lymph node involvement who received extended field irradiation after lymphadenectomy. Approximately 20% of these patients had positive paraaortic nodes in this report from Stanford University. It is conceivable that this finite long-term survivorship would have been improved if the analysis had been restricted to patients with positive pelvic nodes and if the lymph nodes had been treated in continuous rather than interrupted fashion (which was done to minimize acute morbidity while the prostatic bed was boosted).

Two institutions have employed pelvic irradiation after radical prostatectomy among patients found to have involved pelvic lymph nodes. Bahnson and associates[54] reported a 41% 5-year recurrence-free survival rate with a 50-month median time to failure among 6 patients who received 50 Gy of adjuvant pelvic irradiation after surgery. Lange and associates[55] prescribed 45 Gy to the pelvis and 60 Gy to the prostatic bed for 36 patients with stage D1 disease after surgery. The actuarial 5-year survival rate was 69% but the 95% confidence intervals were relatively wide (±18%), and recurrences were still being detected after 5 years.

Interstitial irradiation has also been used to combat stage D1 disease. The experience from the Memorial Sloan-Kettering Cancer Center involved bilateral pelvic lymphadenectomy followed by insertion of ^{125}I sources into the prostate to deliver a dose of 16,000 cGy over a 1-year period. In a recent update of the 345 patients so treated, Leibel and colleagues[56] found that by 10 years, fewer than one third had survived and more than 80% had failed with distant metastases.

Two centers interstitially irradiated the prostate itself with supplemental external irradiation to the nodes. In 1980, Batata and associates[57] added external beam radiotherapy (either to the pelvis or to the pelvis and paraaortic chimney) after pelvic lymphadenectomy and ^{125}I implantation. Twenty-eight patients treated with this approach derived no survival or local control advantage compared with other patients treated at the Memorial Sloan-Kettering Cancer Center with lymphadenectomy and brachytherapy alone. A similar concept was piloted by Gervasi and colleagues[58] at Baylor University, where the isotope used was radioactive gold (^{198}Au). Among 152 patients treated with this combined approach, the 5-, 10-, and 15-year disease-free survival rates were 75%, 43%, and 21%, respectively. It is difficult to understand how the Baylor experience for locoregionally advanced disease can appear superior to other strategies for treatment of node-positive prostatic cancer when the same methods yielded such poor results for early-stage disease.[4]

FUTURE DIRECTIONS

The revised clinical staging of prostate cancer has taken a few steps forward[2] but is still fraught with limitations. To be meaningful, a staging system must be capable of establishing prognostically useful breakpoints so that patients can be appropriately stratified for clinical trials. Further, a meaningful staging system can serve as a template for comparison of statistics reported by different institutions and evaluation of new therapeutic options. Traditionally, the staging of prostate cancer has been predicated on the anatomic extent of disease. Although such divisions have served uro-oncologists well in the past, data emerging from multiple departments of urology and radiation oncology[20,63,64,66] have shown that the anatomic divisions are overwhelmed in importance by histopathologic features (e.g., Gleason scoring system) and biochemical parameters (e.g., PSA data). The time has come to move toward a biochemical staging system, such as a PSA-based system, that incorporates anatomic, histopathologic, and even molecular[59] subdivisions. Such a system would describe the biologic potential of a given tumor and thereby surpass the current classification, which is still fundamentally based on the palpation of nodules during digital rectal examination.

CURRENT POLICIES AT FOX CHASE CANCER CENTER

We have been encouraged by the results achieved from the combination of irradiation and systemic therapy for locally ad-

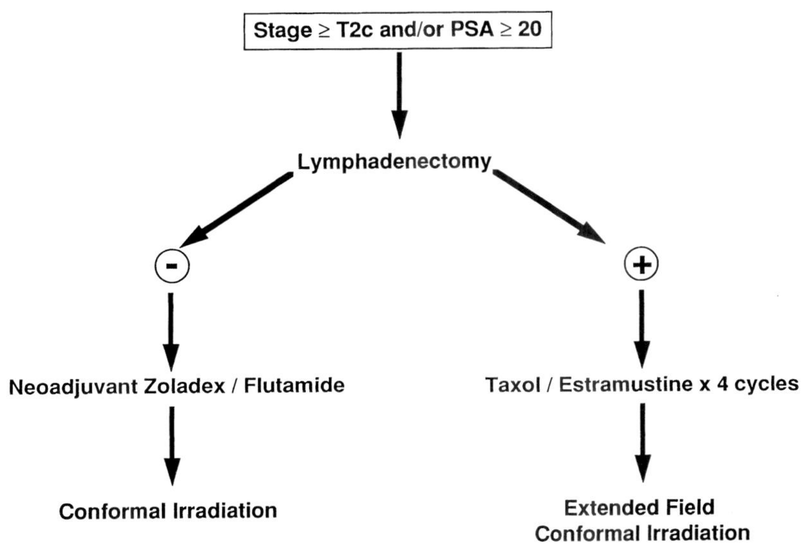

FIG. 52.2-2. Ongoing phase II protocol for patients with locally advanced prostate cancer (T3, N +) at Fox Chase Cancer Center.

vanced disease and believe that monotherapy is no longer the standard of management for patients with T3 disease and lymph node involvement. Although baseline PSA levels now appear to be the most potent independent predictor of outcome, nodal metastases are also important prognisticators. Patients with ''limited'' nodal disease represent a potentially curable subset that should be approached aggressively. Therefore, our prostate cancer patients with advanced stage disease (T2b or higher) or high baseline PSA levels (>20 ng/mL) are offered participation in a phase II protocol (Fig. 52.2-2) in which lymph nodes are assessed pathologically before treatment recommendations are formulated. Patients with negative nodal involvement are treated with neoadjuvant total androgen blockade (e.g., Lupron and flutamide), followed by conformal irradiation (68-Gy total dose in 2-Gy fractions). Those with positive lymph nodal involvement receive induction therapy with Taxol and estramustine (an active regimen for hormone-refractory prostate cancer[60,61]) followed by conformal extended field irradiation (paraaortic and pelvic nodes treated to 45 Gy; prostatic bed boosted to 68 Gy).

Locally advanced tumors challenge the clinical investigator to construct more aggressive strategies to transcend the poor results that are now considered state of the art. Because more than 70,000 American men are diagnosed annually with locoregionally advanced prostate cancer, it is important to prevail on physicians to enroll their patients in systematic prospective protocols in order to provide scientific solutions to this considerable oncologic problem.

REFERENCES

1. Cancer facts and figures—1994. Atlanta: American Cancer Society, 1994.
2. Montie JE. Staging system for prostate cancer. Semin Urol 1993;11:10.
3. Beahrs OH, Henson DE, Hutter RVP, Kennedy VJ, eds. Manual for staging of cancer, 4th ed. Philadelphia: JB Lippincott, 1992:185.
4. Hanks GE. The prostate. In: Moss WT, Cox JC, eds. Radiation oncology, 6th ed. St Louis: CV Mosby, 1989:487.
5. Frazier JA, Robertson JE, Humphrey PA, Paulson DJ. Is prostate specific antigen of clinical importance in evaluating outcome after radical prostatectomy. J Urol 1993;149:516.
6. Morgan WR, Bergstralh EJ, Zincke H. Long-term evaluation of radical prostatectomy as treatment for clinical stage C (T3) prostate cancer. Urology 1993;41:113.
7. Schellhammer PF. Radical prostatectomy. Patterns of local failure and survival in 67 patients. Urology 1988;3:191.
8. Middleton RG, Smith JA Jr, Melzer RB, Hamilton PE. Patient survival and local recurrence rate following radical prostatectomy for prostate carcinoma. J Urol 1986;136:422.
9. Epstein JI, Carmichael MJ, Pizov G, Walsh PC. Influence of capsular penetration on progression following radical prostatectomy: a study of 196 cases with long-term follow-up. J Urol 1993;150:135.
10. Zagars GK, Geara FB, Pollack A, von Eschenback AC. The T classification of clinically localized prostate cancer. Cancer 1994;73:1904.
11. Corn BW, Hanks GE, Schultheiss TE. Does the current subclassification of stage T3 adenocarcinoma of the prostate have clinical relevance? Urology 1995;45:484.
12. Bagshaw MA, Cox RS, Ray GR. Status of radiation treatment of prostate cancer at Stanford University. Monogr Natl Cancer Inst 1988;7:47.
13. Zagars Gk, von Eschenbach AC, Johnson DE, Oswald MJ. Stage C adenocarcinoma of the prostate: an analysis of 551 patients treated with external beam radiation. Cancer 1987;60:1489.
14. Perez CA, Pilepich MV, Garcia D, Simpson JR, Zivnuska F, Hederman MA. Definitive radiation therapy in carcinoma of the prostate localized to the pelvis: experience at the Mallinckrodt Institute of Radiology. Monogr Natl Cancer Inst 1988;7:85.
15. Hanks GE, Krall JM, Hanlon AL, Asbell SO, Pilepich MV, Owen JB. Patterns of care and RTOG studies in prostate cancer: long-term survival, hazard rate observations, and possibilities of cure. Int J Radiat Oncol Biol Phys 1993;28:39.
16. Hanks GE. External beam radiation treatment for prostate cancer: still the gold standard. Oncology 1992;6:79.
17. Soffen EM, Hanks GE, Hwang CC, Chu JCH. Conformal static field therapy for low volume low grade prostate cancer with rigid immobilization. Int J Radiat Oncol Biol Phys 1991;20:141.
18. Soffen EM, Hanks GE, Hunt MA, Epstein BE. Conformal static field radiation therapy treatment of early prostate cancer versus non-conformal techniques: a reduction in acute morbidity. Int J Radiat Oncol Biol Phys 1992;24:485.
19. Corn BW, Hanks GE, Schultheiss TE, Hunt MA, Lee WR, Coia L. Conformal treatment of prostate cancer: superior PSA response compared to standard treatment. Int J Radiat Oncol Biol Phys 1994. In press.
20. Lee WR, Hanks GE, Schultheiss TE, Corn BW, Hunt MA. Localized prostate cancer treated by external beam radiotherapy alone: serum PSA drive outcome analysis. J Clin Oncol 1994;13:464.
21. Hanks GE. The prostate. In: Cox J, ed. Radiation oncology. St Louis: CV Mosby. In press.
22. Lawton CA, Won M, Pilepich MV, et al. Long-term treatment sequelae following external beam irradiation for adenocarcinoma of the prostate: analysis of RTOG studies 7506 and 7706. Int J Radiat Oncol Biol Phys 1991;21:935.
23. Schultheiss TE, Hanks GE, Hunt MA, Corn BW, Lee WR. Incidence of and factors related to late complications in conformal and conventional radiation treatment of cancer of the prostate. Int J Radiat Oncol Biol Phy 1994;30:155.
24. Porter AT, Venner PM. The role of cytoreduction prior to definitive radiotherapy in locally advanced prostate cancer: the Canadian perspective. Prog Clin Biol Res 1990;8:231.
25. Corn BW, Hanks GE. Therapeutic options for clinically localized carcinoma of the prostate. Semin Radiat Oncol 1993;3:187.
26. Colombel M, Olsson CA, Ng PY, Buttyan R. Hormone-related apoptosis results from reentry of differentiated prostate cells onto a defective cell cycle. Cancer Res 1994;54:4313.
27. Pilepich MV, Caplan R, Al-Sarral M, et al. Phase III trial of hormonal cytoreduction in conjunction with definitive radiotherapy in locally advanced prostate carcinoma: the emerging role of PSA in the assessment of outcome. Int J Radiat Oncol Biol Phys 1993;27:246.
28. Zagars GK, Johnson DE, von Eschenbach AC, Hussey DH. Adjuvant estrogen following radiation therapy for stage C adenocarcinoma of the prostate: long-term results of a prospective randomized study. Int J Radiat Oncol Biol Phys 1988;14:1085.
29. Forman JD, Littrup P, Grignon D, Porter AT. Hyperfractionated conformal radiotherapy for locally advanced prostate cancer: results of a phase II dose escalation study. J Urol 1994;151:375. Abstract.
30. Hanks GE, D'Amico A, Epstein BE, Schultheiss TE. Prostatic-specific antigen doubling times in patients with prostate cancer: a potentially useful reflection of tumor doubling time. Int J Radiat Oncol Biol Phys 1993;27:125.
31. Shipley WU, Munzenrider JE, McManus PL, et al. Results of a randomized trial of total radiation dose for stage T3-T4 prostate cancer boosting with photons (to 67.2 CGE) or with conformal protons (to 75.6 CGE). ASTRO Abstract, 1994.
32. Russell KJ, Laramore GE, Krall JM, Thomas FJ, Maor MH, Hendrickson FR. Eight years experience with neutron radiotherapy in the treatment of stages C and D prostate cancer: updated results of the RTOG 7704 randomized clinical trial. Prostate 1987;11:183.
33. Perez CA, Hanks GE, Leibel SA, Zietman AL, Fuks Z, Lee WR. Localized carcinoma of the prostate (stages T1b, T2 and T3). Cancer 1993;72:3156.
34. Berk L, Epstein B, Hanks G. Conformal prostate treatment planning without multiplanar computer planning. Int J Radiat Oncol Biol Phys 1992;24:280.
35. Koprowski CD, Berkenstock KG, Borofski Am, et al. External beam irradiation versus 125-iodine implant in the definitive treatment of prostate carcinoma. Int J Radiat Oncol Biol Phys 1991;21:955.
36. Kuban DA, El-Mahdi AM, Schellhammer PF. I-125 interstitial implan-

tation for prostate cancer. What have we learned 10 years later? Cancer 1989;63:2415.

37. Morton JD, Peschel RE. Iodine-125 implants versus external beam therapy for stages A2, B and C prostate cancer. Int J Radiat Oncol Biol Phys 1988;14:1153.
38. Syed AM, Puthawala A, Austin P. Temporary iridium-192 implant in the management of carcinoma of the prostate. Cancer 1992;69:2515.
39. Brindle JS, Martinez A, Schray M. Pelvic lymphadenectomy and transperineal interstitial implantation of Ir-192 combined with external beam radiotherapy for bulky stage C prostatic carcinoma. Int J Radiat Oncol Biol Phys 1989;17:1063.
40. Petros JA, Catalona WJ. Lower incidence of unsuspected lymph node metastases in 521 consecutive patients with clinically localized prostate cancer. J Urol 1992;147:1574.
41. Pilepich MV, Krall JM, Johnson RJ, et al. Extended field (periaortic) irradiation in carcinoma of the prostate: analysis of RTOG 75–06. Int J Radiat Oncol Biol Phys 1986;12:345.
42. Hanks GE, Krall JM, Pilepich MV, et al. Comparison of pathologic and clinical evaluation of lymph nodes in prostate cancer: implications of RTOG data for patient management and trial design and stratification. Int J Radiat Oncol Biol Phys 1992;23:293.
43. Prout GR, Heaney JA, Griffin PP, Daly JJ, Shipley WU. Nodal involvement as a prognostic indicator in patients with prostatic carcinoma. J Urol 1980;124:226.
44. Smith JA, Haynes TH, Middleton RG. Impact of external irradiation on local symptoms and survival free of disease in patients with pelvic lymph node metastasis from adenocarcinoma of the prostate. J Urol 1984;131:705.
45. Steinberg GD, Epstein JI, Piantadosi S, Walsh PC. Management of stage D1 adenocarcinoma of the prostate: the Johns Hopkins experience 1974 to 1987. J Urol 1990;144:1425.
46. Barzell W, Bean MA, Hilaris BS, Whitmore WF. Prostatic adenocarcinoma: relationship of grade and local extent to the pattern of metastases. J Urol 1977;118:278.
47. Lawton CA, Cox JD, Glisch C, Murray KJ, Byhardt RW, Wilson JF: Is long-term survival possible with external beam irradiation for stage D1 adenocarcinoma of the prostate? Cancer 1992;69:2761.
48. Hanks GE. Carcinoma of the prostate. Patterns of Care Study Newsletter No. 4. American College of Radiology, 1990–1991.
49. Whittington R, Malkowicz B, Broderick G, Barnes M, Wein AJ. Combined hormone-radiation therapy for lymph node positive adenocarcinoma of the prostate. J Urol 1994:151.
50. Perez CA, Lee HK, Georgiou A, Logsdon MD, Lai PP, Lockett MA. Technical and tumor-related factors affecting outcome of definitive irradiation for localized carcinoma of the prostate. Int J Radiat Oncol Biol Phys 1993;26:581.
51. Modig H, Tomic R, Granfors I, Nyberg G. Prospective randomized trial in localized prostatic cancer: radiotherapy versus radiotherapy and orchiectomy. ASTRO Abstract, 1993;1323.
52. Paulson DF, Cline WA, Koefoot RB Jr, Hinshaw W, Stephani S, Uro-Oncology Research Group. Extended field radiation therapy versus delayed hormonal therapy in node positive prostatic adenocarcinoma. J Urol 1982;127:935.
53. Bagshaw MA. Radiotherapeutic treatment of prostatic carcinoma with pelvic node involvement. Urol Clin North Am 1984;11:297.
54. Bahnson RR, Garnett JE, Grayhack JT. Adjuvant radiation therapy in stages C and D1 prostatic adenocarcinoma: preliminary results. Urology 1986;27:403.
55. Lange PH, Reddy PK, Medini E, Levitt S, Fraley EE. Radiation therapy as adjuvant therapy after radical prostatectomy. Monogr Natl Cancer Inst 1988;7:141.
56. Leibel SA, Fuks Z, Zelefsky MJ, Whitmore WF. The effects of local and regional treatment on the metastatic outcome in prostatic carcinoma with pelvic lymph node involvement. Int J Radiat Oncol Biol Phys 1993;28:7.
57. Batata MA, Hilaris BB, Chu FCH, et al. Radiation therapy in adenocarcinoma of the prostate with pelvic lymph node involvement on lymphadenectomy. Int J Radiat Oncol Biol Phys 1980;6:149.
58. Gervasi LA, Mata J, Easley JD, et al. Prognostic significance of lymph nodal metastases in prostate cancer. J Urol 1989;142:332.
59. Katz AE, Olsson CA, Raffo AJ, et al. Molecular staging of prostate cancer with the use of an enhanced reverse transcriptase-PCR assay. Urology 1994;43:765.
60. Hudes GR, Greenberg R, Krigel RL, et al. Phase II study of estramustine and vinblastine, two microtubule inhibitors, in hormone-refractory prostate cancer. J Clin Oncol 1992;10:1754.
61. Hudes G, Obasaju C, McAleer C, et al. Phase I pharmacologic study of 96-hour infusional Taxol combined with estramustine. Proc ASCO 13:168, 1994. Meeting abstract.
62. Hanks GE, Asbell S, Krall JM, et al. Outcome of lymph node dissection negative T-ab, T-2 (A-2,B) prostate cancer treated with external beam radiation therapy in RTOG 77-06. Int J Radiat Oncol Biol Phys 1991; 21:1099.
63. Kaplan ID, Cox RS, Bagshaw MA. Prostate specific antigen after external beam radiotherapy for prostatic cancer: follow-up. J Urol 1993; 149:519.
64. Ritter MA, Messing EM, Shanahan TG, et al. Prostate-specific antigen as a predictor of radiotherapy response and patterns of failure in localized prostate cancer. J Clin Oncol 1992;10:1208.
65. Zeitman AL, Coen JJ, Shipley WU, Willett CG, Efird JT. Radical radiation therapy in the management of prostatic adenocarcinoma: the initial prostate specific antigen value as a predictor of treatment outcome. J Urol 1994;151:640.
66. Pisansky TM, Cha SS, Earle JD, et al. Prostate-specific antigen as a pretherapy prognostic factor in patients treated with radiation therapy for clinically localized prostate cancer. J Clin Oncol 1993;11:2158.
67. Zagars GK, Geara FB, Pollack A, von Eschenbach AC. The T classification of clinically localized prostate cancer. Cancer 1994;73:1904.
68. Peters LJ, Ang KK, Thames HD. Altered fractionation schedules. In: Perez CA, Brady LW, ed. Principles and practice of radiation oncology, 2nd ed. Philadelphia: JB Lippincott, 1992:97.

Principles and Practice of Genitourinary Oncology, edited by Derek Raghavan, Howard I. Scher, Steven A. Leibel, and Paul H. Lange. Lippincott-Raven Publishers, Philadelphia, © 1997.

CHAPTER 53

Stage D1 Prostate Cancer

Michael J. Rentzepis and Ralph deVere White

The least controversial point about D1 prostate cancer is its definition. Patients with stage D1 prostate cancer have various local tumor volumes (T0-3), histologic proof of tumor within the pelvic lymph nodes (N1-2), and no evidence of distant metastases. There is almost universal agreement that the number of patients with stage D1 disease is falling. A paper from Sgrignoli and colleagues[1] reported that the overall incidence of node-positive disease in patients undergoing radical prostatectomy is 7.5%. When patients with a Gleason score of 7 or lower were evaluated, this figure dropped to 5.5%. Only a few years ago there was an expected node-positive rate of up to 40% for high-local-volume, high-Gleason-score patients. What change in one decade has occurred to produce such a low rate of node-positive patients? Additionally, almost everyone agrees that there is a group of patients with node-positive prostate cancer who live for a long time. What is not agreed upon is whether any of the different treatment strategies leads to this prolongation of survival or to what degree it is tumor dependent.

The treatment of stage D1 prostate cancer remains controversial. There are no randomized, prospective studies available that can guide therapeutic decisions. Without this information, how can treatment be assigned for an individual patient? Regrettably, treatment decisions must be based on the inadequate knowledge of the natural history of the disease, tumor biology, and quality-of-life issues, together with the patient's comorbidities. Little is known about these variables; thus, treatment decisions are often made on an emotional basis by the doctor and patient.

The incidence of prostate cancer is approximately 200,000 cases per year.[2] Metastatic disease is present in as many as 30% of patients at the time of diagnosis, and about 5% to 7% have stage D1 disease.[3,4] This chapter reviews the natural history, detection, and treatment modalities of D1 prostate cancer. It also addresses the clinical usefulness of available molecular markers, including DNA ploidy analysis and polymerase chain reaction (PCR) technology.

STAGING AND NATURAL HISTORY

A decade ago, the incidence of pelvic lymph node metastasis was reported to be between 20% and 24%,[5–7] with the rate increasing as the tumor volume and grade increase. Since then, the rate has fallen to less than 10%. It is doubtful that the biology of the disease has changed; therefore this change must reflect prostate-specific antigen (PSA) screening and the early detection of cancers. Because patients with node-negative disease clearly do better than patients with node-positive disease, if patients with tumors of equal volume and grade have a lower incidence of node-positive disease than they did 10 years ago, this suggests that screening is beneficial. Detecting the presence of cancers in pelvic lymph nodes by noninvasive methods has proven to be totally unsatisfactory. The use of imaging technologies, particularly computed tomography (CT), has limited value. CT sensitivity ranges from 50% to 75%, and CT specificity ranges from 80% to 100%.[8–10] Magnetic resonance (MR) imaging is equally unsatisfactory. There are those who feel that if two tests are individually useless, putting them together may be more beneficial. With a 5% to 7% incidence of cancer-positive nodes and the low sensitivity and specificity of CT and MR, it is doubtful that there is added benefit in combining the two modalities, particularly in the climate of capitated health care. Other chapter address the use of laparoscopic lymph node dissection.

Attempts have been made to integrate PSA level and Gleason grading to predict those patients who are at greater risk for having positive lymph nodes. Harris and colleagues[12] constructed a table they used to predict the positive lymph node rate (Table 53-1). Using this table, 70% of the 484 patients had a less than 2.8% risk of having positive nodes. The practicality of this approach allows the surgeon to select patients who could proceed to radical prostatectomy by whatever approach he or she wishes to use without undergoing a staging lymphadenectomy. However, when the surgeon recognizes that even in patients with high-grade tumor the rate of positive lymph nodes is low, the value of these calculations lessens. If these calculations are used to predict which patients have positive lymph nodes, it can be assumed that a treatment strategy has been determined for treating patients with positive nodes and that this strategy is different than that for patients without positive nodes. However, this rationale could lead to treatment for no patients, in that treating node-positive patients may be fruitless and intervening in the course of node-negative patients may be unnecessary. The current problem is not in identifying patients with positive lymph nodes, but

TABLE 53-1. *Serum prostate-specific antigen level to predict positive lymph node rate*

PSA GS	<4 ng/mL	<5 ng/mL	<6 ng/mL	<7 ng/mL	8–10 ng/mL
<10	0	0.37	0.30	1.1	10
<15	0.7	1.1	1.2	2.5	10
<20	1.4	2.6	2.7	3.8	10
<20	18	21	16	18	30

GS; Gleason score; *PSA*; prostate-specific antigen

From Harris MJ; Bishoff JT; Reyes A, et al. Preoperative PSA and prostate biopsy Gleason's grade predictive of benign pelvic lymph nodes in men with prostate cancer, (Abstract 451) San Francisco: AUA, 1994:340A.

rather in devising a rational treatment approach for those with lymph node disease.

Although pelvic lymph node dissection (PLND) is not considered therapeutic, it may provide prognostic information. Approximately 70% of men with positive lymph nodes only can expect to live 5 years, but most series report a significant increase in mortality at the 10-year interval.[13–20] Several groups have examined the significance of tumor bulk and PLND specimens.[5,21,22] Smith and Middleton[14] reviewed 73 cases of PLND without prostatectomy. Five-year mortality was 28% for patients with a single positive node: 37% in the microscopically positive group, and 52% in the grossly positive group. Of those with a single positive node, 44% were disease-free at 5 years, in contrast to 15% in the grossly positive node group. As expected, these results become even worse over time. Golimbu and colleagues[22] demonstrated a 20% disease-free survival at 10 years; among patients with more than one positive node, none was alive and disease-free at 18 years. A contrasting viewpoint was provided by Gervasi and colleagues[5] in a study that showed little difference in 10-year survival among groups stratified by tumor volume. Patients with only one node, two nodes, or more than 2 nodes had an 80%, 84%, and 88% incidence, respectively, of distant metastatic disease at 10 years. All of these patients were treated with PLND, radioactive gold-198 (^{198}Au) to the prostate, and external beam irradiation to the pelvis.

An advance in the staging of prostate cancer has been the use of reverse transcriptase polymerase chain reaction (RT-PCR). Using this method, one PSA-expressing cell diluted in 100,000 lymphocytes can be detected.[23] Although RT-PCR can be used to stage tumors by looking for PSA-secreting cells in the blood or the bone marrow, how will this information guide therapy? If physicians are unable to decide how to treat patients with positive lymph nodes, it seems a far stretch to devise a way to treat patients based on RNA PCR of circulating cells, the presence of which may well be meaningless. This approach has not provided clinically useful information in other tumors.[24]

A report from Johns Hopkins[1] about stage D1 disease seems to indicate that the biology of the tumors being treated may be changing. In this report, a number of patients have relatively short follow-up times and, to some degree, the outcome is based on Kaplan-Meier tables. That notwithstanding, the group shows no prognostic significance based on the number of positive nodes or whether the positive nodes are unilateral or bilateral. The only prognostic factor was the Gleason grade of the biopsy specimen on which the diagnosis was made. If the Gleason grade was lower than 8, the likelihood of distant metastases was only 18% and 41% at 5 and 10 years, respectively, whereas 85% of men with a Gleason score of 8 to 10 had distant metastases by 5 years. Thus far, in the 114 patients in this group, only 2 have died of prostate cancer. All of these patients underwent radical prostatectomy.

Prostate cancer in the lymph nodes must be considered a systemic disease with varying rates of progression. The question to be answered is whether, in the setting of node-positive disease, the initiation of any immediate therapy (i.e., radical prostatectomy, radiotherapy, or hormonal therapy) improves patient outcome or is an added expense that causes a decrease in quality of life without any anticancer benefit.

ADJUVANT THERAPY

The situation at a clinical level is difficult. A patient presents to the urologist, is informed that he has no evidence of metastatic disease, and is therefore concentrating on the fact that with the local therapy of his choice, a good outcome is predicted. Having reviewed the options, he decides that he is going to live 10 to 15 years and therefore chooses a radical prostatectomy. He undergoes the operation, and positive lymph nodes are encountered. It is difficult at this point to stop the operation and tell the patient that neither surgery nor radiotherapy will help, and that he may live a long time but there is really nothing for the physician to do. It is for this reason that patients have tended to opt for treatment.

In earlier papers, the rate of progression for stage D1 prostate cancer was 50% at 5 years. Attempts have been made to stratify the patients based on tumor volume, PSA, and Gleason score. Of these, Gleason score and DNA ploidy are the best indicators of tumor activity. Patients with poorly differentiated tumors, however, behaved as if they had generalized micrometastatic disease; a Johns Hopkins report[1] underscores this point. Therefore, systemic therapy with hormones, instead of local or regional therapy, appears to be the most logical treatment for patients with stage D1 disease. Additionally, molecular staging by RT-PCR, peripheral blood, or similar studies of bone marrow biopsy specimens appears to indicate that these patients seems to be reasonable candidates for hormonal therapy, because the surgeon would be looking for reasons not to operate. However, appropriate clinical interpretation of the results of these studies will evolve over time. At this point, we would consider carrying out RNA PCR for PSA in bone marrow rather than in peripheral blood. Another approach would be to do immunohistochemistry of bone marrow aspirates or biopsy specimens.

Should these patients receive early adjuvant hormonal therapy? Based on the results of the European Organization for the Research and Treatment of Cancer (EORTC)[25] and intergroup studies,[26] patients with minimal metastatic disease fare best with maximum androgen ablation; therefore, if the physician is going to use hormonal therapy in patients with stage D1 disease, logically, he or she should use maximum androgen ablation. If these patients have long-term survival, and many do, should the physician subject them to the expense of maximum androgen ablation for that length of time? How does this affect their quality of life?

Van Aubel and colleagues[27] considered the effects of early hormonal intervention and reported that in 30 patients (21 of whom had high-grade disease) early orchiectomy resulted in 46% treatment failure at 45 months. In terms of when metastatic disease was discovered, these results appear to compare favorably with patients treated on a delayed basis. However, in a Johns Hopkins report[1] in which early hormonal therapy was not used, only 18% of patients had distant metastases at 33 months postoperatively. If the Johns Hopkins paper[1] is used as a control for the study of Van Aubel and colleagues,[27] it appears that early orchiectomy is associated with a worse outcome than delayed treatment. In comparing the various studies, the occurrence of metastasis is not the issue; the issue is that early hormonal treatment does not appear to prolong patient survival. In 1987, Zincke and colleagues[28] reported on 39 patients treated using PLND and early hormonal manipulation without removal of the prostate. The 5-year nonprogression rate was 56%.

Kramalowsky[29] reviewed 68 cases of patients with stage D1 disease who did not undergo radical prostatectomy. Thirty patients underwent hormonal therapy (22 by orchiectomy and 8 by exogenous antiandrogen treatment), 27 had delayed therapy (24 by orchiectomy and 3 by exogenous hormonal therapy), and 11 received no androgen deprivation. Minimum follow-up was 5 years. The median interval to development of bony metastases was 100 months in the immediate-treatment group versus 43 months in the delayed-treatment group. The median interval to death was 90 months in the delayed-treatment group versus 150 months in the immediate-treatment group, a difference that is not statistically significant. Therefore, early hormonal intervention may lead to an increased interval to progression; however, it may have no impact on the length of survival.

The situation is more complicated when looking at a recent paper from van den Ouden and colleagues,[30] in which patients diagnosed with prostate cancer, albeit unstaged, underwent either active surveillance or early orchiectomy. In this study, the actual survival was better in those patients who underwent active surveillance, suggesting that the early orchiectomy caused the hormone-sensitive cells to go into programmed cell death, or apoptosis, whereas the non–hormone-sensitive cells gained a growth advantage that led to earlier demise.

Other monotherapies have fared no better than early hormonal manipulation. Several authors have examined the use of radical prostatectomy alone in treating stage D1 disease.[31–34] One of the earliest studies was performed by McCullough and Leadbetter.[31] Only 4 of 17 patients remained tumor-free in follow-up ranging from 2 months to 10 years. In 1981, Kramer and colleagues[32] reported on 11 patients with median time to failure of 18.3 months and intermediate survival of 39.4 months. At the Mayo Clinic, Utz[33] reported a 5-year nonprogression rate of 18.5% in 52 patients. At Johns Hopkins,[18] only 3% of 64 patients treated with radical prostatectomy alone required another procedure to control local symptoms, in contrast to 23% and 24% of men requiring additional palliative surgery in the observation and radiotherapy groups, respectively; implying that radical prostatectomy was superior in controlling local symptoms. However, when the observation group is compared to the radical prostatectomy group, the radical prostatectomy group had 103 procedures to control local symptoms, whereas in the observation group, only 23 procedures were carried out. These results seem to favor the observation group over the radical prostatectomy group.

When reviewing papers from the Mayo Clinic,[35] Johns Hopkins,[1] and University of California at Los Angeles,[3] it is apparent that there is a group of patients with stage D1 disease who appear to have prolonged survival after radical prostatectomy. Everyone seems to agree that positive nodes in the setting of a high Gleason grade is a poor prognostic sign. Some researchers feel that volume of tumor is important and some feel that the size and number of nodes is important in patient outcome. However, none of these studies was able to show definitively that patient outcome was not dependent on the tumor biology, and radical prostatectomy may well confer absolutely no survival benefit.

Radiotherapy also has not been shown to offer an advantage in prolonged survival, regardless of its delivery via external beam or seed implants. The time to progression in radiotherapy studies ranges from 11 to 18 months.[36–39] The positive biopsy rate in the Stanford series[40] in patients with stage D1 disease is twice as high as that for patients who do not have positive nodes. Even irradiation therapists have not been extremely vociferous in proposing that these patients undergo radiotherapy. Studies rating the overall effectiveness of radiotherapy in treating prostate cancer, as judged by negative biopsy specimens, DNA ploidy, or Gleason score, indicate that it seems to be relatively ineffective in patients with node-positive disease.

Chemotherapy, either alone[41] or in combination with radiotherapy,[42] has not provided any significant increase in survival, and it adds to the expense and morbidity of treating stage D1 prostate cancer.

COMBINED THERAPY

The use of radical prostatectomy and subsequent hormonal therapy is based on the premise of local control and removal of future sources of metastatic disease followed by systemic therapy to treat presumed micrometastasis. This theory was put forth by Scott[43] in 1964, and refined by Scott and Boyd[43] in 1969, who performed orchiectomies on patients known to have gross capsular spread at the time of radical prostatectomy. Fifty-two percent disease-free survival at 10 years was considered an improvement over historical controls using hormones alone. In 1983, Zincke and Utz[45] reported on 100 patients at the Mayo Clinic who had undergone radical prostatectomy and PLND with a median follow-up of 5 years. Eighty percent of patients who did not receive adjuvant hormonal therapy progressed, compared with 10% of the 23 patients who underwent radical prostatectomy, PLND, and orchiectomy. Three criticisms of these results have emerged.

1. The study was uncontrolled and retrospective.
2. There were only 23 patients in the combined therapy group.
3. Eleven patients were treated with diethylstilbestrol instead

of orchiectomy, and all of these patients progressed within 5 years. It is possible that this subset of patients may not have been compliant with their medication, but it is interesting that the entire group appeared to fail.

From these results, it is difficult to conclude whether the favorable results are from the combined therapy or from the early use of hormone intervention.

The Mayo Clinic has, over the years, published data with increasing numbers of patients and different authors analyzing different subgroups. Taking all of these studies together, one is left with the impression that outcome is dependent on DNA ploidy and that it is impossible to show that surgery or early hormonal intervention in any way increased patient survival. In 1985, deKernion and colleagues[46] reported the outcome of 59 patients treated over a 10-year period using a variety of combination therapies. The 5-year survival across the board was 73%. For the radical prostatectomy subgroup, it was 85%; for the radical prostatectomy and hormonal therapy group, it was 100%; and in the radiotherapy and hormonal therapy group, it was 57%. In the breakdown by grade of disease, the well differentiated group fared better with an 85% 5-year survival versus 51% for the poorly differentiated group. It was noted that a patient selection bias could account for the improved statistics for the surgery group, because only 2 of 10 patients undergoing radical prostatectomy and hormonal therapy had five positive lymph nodes, compared with 12 of the 17 patients who underwent radiotherapy combined with hormonal therapy. The degree of nodal disease, however, does not correlate with survival, and it is the inherent tumor biology that may emerge as the principal determinant of patient outcome. The use of nuclear DNA ploidy analysis may offer a significant contribution toward the understanding of response to treatment and prediction of outcome.

NUCLEAR DNA PLOIDY ANALYSIS

Because prostate cancer appears to have a significant range of response to various therapies, efforts have been made to stratify a particular tumor's malignant potential in a variety of ways. Gleason grade and tumor stage have been identified as important variables, but they do not provide sufficiently precise information to formulate a plan for an individual patient. Although it can be said that most low-grade lesions have a more benign course than do tumors of poor differentiation, many tumors are within the intermediate or moderately differentiated group. In addition, some low-grade tumors go on to invade, whereas high-grade tumors remain localized.[47,48] Many studies have suggested that analysis of DNA ploidy may provide better prognostic information and better aid in choosing the direction of therapy.

DNA flow cytometry (FCM) has been shown to provide clinically relevant information in the management of patients with ovarian, breast, colorectal, and lung carcinoma; osteosarcoma; transitional cell carcinoma of the bladder; and prostate carcinoma.[49–58] FCM has been shown to be additive to pathologic grade and clinical stage, and the DNA histograms obtained predicted response to therapy and length of survival. Tribukait[59] reviewed the implications of DNA tetraploid and aneuploid tumors with regard to urologic malignancy and noted a poorer prognosis than for those tumors with a normal or diploid pattern.

Approximately 70% to 80% of localized prostate cancers are diploid. For the primary tumor, however, there is a DNA ploidy shift first seen as the tumor becomes locally invasive.[60–62] Disease progression is greater for the nondiploid tumors; at least one half of these tumors show progression. In contrast, approximately 15% of diploid cases can be expected to progress within 5 years, independent of stage from A2 to D1.[60–66]

DNA ploidy and progression of disease were first examined by the group at the Memorial Sloan-Kettering Cancer Center.[66] A total of 82 patients were reviewed, of which 49 had aneuploid tumors and 33 had diploid tumors. No difference existed between the two groups with regard to the number of positive nodes or tumor grade. Median survival time of the aneuploid and diploid groups was 5 and 8.8 years, respectively. Median disease-free survival was 4 and 2.1 years in the diploid and aneuploid groups, respectively; these data approached statistical significance.

The Mayo Clinic published a review of its use of DNA ploidy analysis in 1988.[62] The DNA ploidy pattern was found to have a profound association with prognosis. With a median follow-up of 7.5 years, 91 patients who had undergone radical prostatectomy and PLND were examined. Forty-two percent of specimens had diploid histograms, 45% were tetraploid, and 13% were aneuploid. High-grade tumors significantly correlated with DNA aneuploidy, whereas there was no statistical significance between diploid and tetraploid tumors and tumor grade. Seventy-five percent of patients with nondiploid patterns had disease progression, compared with 15% of patients with diploid patterns. Forty-three percent and 55% of patients with tetraploid and aneuploid tumors, respectively, died of prostate cancer 10 years after surgical treatment, whereas none of the patients with diploid tumors died of prostate cancer.

Using DNA ploidy analysis, the results at the Mayo Clinic can be more effectively explained.[67,68] Retrospective reviews show that patients with stage D1 disease and DNA-diploid cancers who received early hormonal therapy did not progress and had 100% survival at 10 years. Diploid tumors that did not receive immediate hormonal therapy had only a 43% nonprogression rate at 10 years. The late introduction of hormonal therapy gave a survival rate that was not significantly different from those patients who underwent immediate therapy. For patients with nondiploid tumors, the outcome was generally poor despite early or delayed hormonal intervention. When considering all of the drawbacks of immediate hormonal therapy (e.g., expense, loss of libido, other metabolic changes), its use must be seriously questioned.

DNA ploidy is now acknowledged by some urologists to be the single most important variable predicting disease progression or cause-specific survival in prostate cancer.[69] Within each Gleason score and pathologic stage, nondiploid tumors have approximately a threefold greater chance of disease progression and of causing cancer death than do diploid tumors. Babiarz and colleagues[70] reported on DNA ploidy comparison between primary tumors and metastatic lesions in stage D1 disease. Sixty-five percent and 35% of primary tumors were diploid and aneuploid, respectively, but for metastases, 30% were diploid and 70% were nondiploid. Of the 22 diploid carcinomas, 13 had aneuploid metastases. Seventy-seven percent of tumors in this group progressed to distant metastases in an average of 30 months. This study highlighted the importance of knowing the DNA ploidy for both the primary tumor and the metastatic lesion. In an update of 370 patients treated over 23 years with a median follow-up of 5 years, Zincke and colleagues[71] noted the following ploidy distribution: 138 (37%) diploid, 168 (45%) tetraploid, and 64 (17%) aneuploid. Early hormonal therapy was used in 80% of all ploidy classes, and it significantly improved nonprogression rates in all three classes (D > T > A). Diploid tumors treated using early hormonal therapy had a nonprogression rate of 95% and a survival rate of 98%. Two thirds of the diploid tumors progressed without early hormonal therapy. Nondiploid tumors, regardless of therapy, had no improvement in survival. It seems that DNA ploidy significantly affects the natural course of the disease and that hormonal therapy slows the progression of the disease but will not, for either DNA ploidy class, reduce cancer-associated mortality.

The argument about DNA ploidy has always been whether it is an independent variable. What has not been shown that if tumors are evaluated on the basis of DNA ploidy, information would be gained that is independent of that obtained by dividing the patients into those with Gleason scores of 8 to 10 and those with Gleason scores of 7 or less. There is little certainty about which patients with stage D1 diseases are benefitting from radical prostatectomy. It appears reasonable to perform DNA ploidy on the initial biopsy specimen and, if the tumor is aneuploid and positive nodes are found, the physician should not proceed with surgery. Although this approach appears logical, a report at Johns Hopkins[1] indicates that even in those with high-grade lesions, fewer than 10% of patients have positive nodes; therefore, how does the pathologist choose which biopsy specimens should undergo DNA ploidy analysis? If the physician has a high suspicion that a patient may have positive lymph nodes (i.e., high Gleason score, high PSA, high local tumor volume, but negative CT scan), then it is worth getting a DNA ploidy analysis before surgery. In such a patient, it is probably worth sending frozen sections for pathologic examination and discontinuing surgery at that point if the patient is node-positive. By extrapolation, it is evident that the number of patients that are going to require this approach is small, and therefore the number of patients for whom the treatment of stage D1 disease will change as a result is equally small. In choosing which specimens to submit for DNA ploidy analysis, the surgeon may ask himself or herself if the decision of whether or not to operate in the patient who is highly suspicious for positive lymph nodes might be affected by molecular staging of the bone marrow rather than the DNA ploidy of his local tumor.

TREATMENT GUIDELINES

At times, we hope that if we keep reviewing the information available lightning, clearly indicated treatment guidelines will become apparent for patients with stage D1 prostate cancer. Regrettably, this is not the case; often, the more articles the physician reviews, the more conflicting information is gathered, because in many series, the number of patients is relatively small. In some cases, even though there may be many reports in the literature, often the same patients, with additional data, are being used repetitively, and as a result, the overall weight of the information may not be as great as it appears. No randomized studies on the treatment of stage D1 prostate cancer are available, limiting the ability to predict how an individual patient's tumor is going to react to various treatment methods. The single best prognostic parameter available, and the one that is the easiest to obtain, is the grade of the tumor.

High-grade tumors that are node-positive are very unlikely to benefit from therapeutic intervention. The problem is what to do with lower-grade lesions that are node-positive. The physician can take the view that stage D1 disease is systemic and that delayed hormonal therapy is as effective as any other treatment modality and is less expensive and produces less morbidity than undergoing combinations based on radical prostatectomy. Conversely, the physician can take the view that 40,000 people die of prostate cancer each year, stage D1 disease is a significant risk, and radical prostatectomy can be performed with low morbidity and may eliminate any future local problems. In this view, the patient is given the benefit of the doubt in the hope that the surgeon is actually removing a significant tumor that, if left, would have gone on to cause local problems or be a source of future metastasis. Little proof exists that this is the case. In fact, even though local control is good following radical prostatectomy, the number of patients who die of metastatic prostate cancer with uncontrollable local symptoms is extremely small. Local control does not appear to be a strong argument for carrying out radical prostatectomy in patients with stage D1 disease.

If the physician chooses to use hormone therapy, maximum androgen ablation is the only choice. EORTC[25] and intergroup[26] studies show that patients with minimal metastatic disease have a longer survival if treated with maximum androgen ablation. When treating a patient early in the course of disease with maximum androgen ablation, why does the addition of flutamide appear to provide prolonged survival? If monotherapy is used and flutamide is added when the patient fails monotherapy, there appears to be no tumor response. Our hypothesis is that if monotherapy is used, the cells that are maximally androgen dependent go into apoptosis. Cells then emerge at G0, and a certain number of these adapt to a lower hormonal milieu. Once these cells have adapted, interfering with that milieu through flutamide is ineffective. Conversely, if flutamide is given before these cells have a chance to adapt, they also go into apoptosis. These results seem to indicate that greater tumor debulking takes place with maximum androgen ablation than with monotherapy. This line of reasoning may be used to support the use of intermittent hormone deprivation rather than continuous treatment.

Better biologic markers are needed on which to base the choice of treatment. In the node-positive patient with a high Gleason score or aneuploidy, radical prostatectomy appears to offer little survival advantage. With regard to other tumor characteristics, none of the currently available molecular probes really allow determination of outcome in an individual patient.

CONCLUSIONS

The only thing about stage D1 prostate cancer that is clear is its definition. The incidence of stage D1 disease has dropped dramatically over the past several years, and it is difficult to believe that this is the result of changing tumor biology. It must be concluded that this decline in incidence is one of the benefits of screening. Because there is only a 7% node-positive rate, it is not reasonable to submit everyone to DNA ploidy studies, molecular staging, or even frozen sections at the time of surgery.

In a managed health care system, routine CT and MR scans are not cost effective for staging. Regrettably, no definitive basis exists for choosing one form of treatment over any other. It is clear from the literature that there is a group of patients with node-positive disease who appear to do well with radical prostatectomy, but there is no way of knowing whether these patients would have done just as well without any immediate intervention. A study that is randomized between radical prostatectomy and no radical prostatectomy is needed; however, such a study, at least in the United States, will never be done. Thus, physicians are left with inadequate molecular and clinical information on which to base clinical decisions. Until this situation changes, the only thing that seems clear is that patients with high-grade, aneuploid, stage D1 disease will not do well, and if they can be identified preoperatively, they should not undergo surgery. Short of this, the physician must continue to tell patients that some people with stage D1 prostate cancer do well without treatment and then, with the patient, make what is more an emotional rather than a biologic decision regarding how to proceed.

REFERENCES

1. Sgrignoli AR, Walsh PC, Steinberg GD, et al. Prognostic factors in men with stage D1 prostate cancer: identification of patients less likely to have prolonged survival after radical prostatectomy. J Urol 1994; 152:1077.
2. Boring CC, Squires TS, Tong T, et al. Cancer statistics, 1994. CA Cancer J Clin 1994;44:7.
3. Danella JF, deKernion JB, Smith RB, et al. The contemporary incidence of lymph node metastases in prostate cancer: implications for laparoscopic lymph node dissection. J Urol 1993;149:1488.
4. Petros JA, Catalona WJ. Lower incidence of unsuspected lymph node metastases in 521 consecutive patients with clinically localized prostate cancer. J Urol 1992;147:1574.
5. Gervasi LA, Mata J, Easley JD, et al. Prognostic significance of lymph node metastasis in prostate cancer. J Urol 1989;142:332.
6. Donohue RE, Mani JH, Whitesel JA, et al. Pelvic lymph node dissection: guide to patient management in clinically locally confined adenocarcinoma of prostate. Urology 1982;20:559.
7. Fowler JE Jr, Whitmore WH Jr. The incidence and extent of pelvic lymph node metastases in apparently localized prostate cancer. Cancer 1981;47:2941.
8. Giri PG, Walsh JW, Hazra TA, et al. Role of computed tomography in the evaluation and management of carcinoma of the prostate. Int J Radiat Oncol Biol Phys 1982;8:283.
9. Golimbu M, Morales P, Al-Askari S, et al. CAT scanning in staging of prostatic cancer. Urology 1981;18:305.
10. Morgan CL, Calkins RF, Cavalcanti EJ. Computed tomography in the evaluation, staging, and therapy of carcinoma of the bladder and prostate. Radiology 1981;140:751.
11. Partin AW, Yoo H, Carter HB, et al. The use of prostate specific antigen, clinical stage and Gleason score to predict pathological stage in men with localized prostate cancer. J Urol 1993;150:110.
12. Harris MJ, Bishoff JT, Reyes A, et al. Preoperative PSA and prostate biopsy Gleason's grade predictive of benign pelvic lymph nodes in men with prostate cancer. (Abstract 451) San Francisco: AUA, 1994: 340.
13. Barzell W, Bean MA, Hilaris BS. Prostatic adenocarcinoma: relationship of grade and local extent to pattern of metastasis. J Urol 1977; 118:278.
14. Smith JA Jr, Middleton RG. Implications of volume of nodal metastases in patients with adenocarcinoma of the prostate. J Urol 1985;133:617.
15. Zincke H, Fleming TR, Furlow WL, et al. Radical retropubic prostatectomy and pelvic lymphadenectomy for high stage cancer of the prostate. Cancer 1981;47:1901.
16. Golimbu M, Prover J, Al-Askari S, et al. Radical prostatectomy for stage D1 prostate cancer. Urology 1987;30:427.
17. Ansher MS, Prosnitz LR. Prognostic significance of extent of nodal involvement in stage D1 prostate cancer treated with radiotherapy. Urology 1992;39:39.
18. Steinberg GD, Epstein JI, Piantadosi S, et al. Management of stage D1 adenocarcinoma of the prostate: the Johns Hopkins experience, 1974 to 1987. J Urol 1990;144:1425.
19. Grossman HB, Batata M, Hilaris B, et al. I-125 implantation for carcinoma of the prostate: further follow-up of first 100 cases. Urology 1982;20:591.
20. deKernion JB, Huang MH, Kaufman JJ, et al. Results of treatment of patients with stage D1 prostatic carcinoma. Urology 1985;26:446.
21. Smith JA Jr, Middleton RG. Implications of volume of nodal metastases in patients with adenocarcinoma of the prostate. J Urol 1985;133:617.
22. Golimbu M, Provet J, Al-Askari S, et al. Radical prostatectomy for stage D1 prostate cancer. Urology 1987;30:427.
23. Katz AE, Olsson CA, Raffo AJ, et al. Molecular staging of prostate cancer with the use of an enhanced reverse transcriptase-PCR assay. Urology 1994;43:765.
24. Osborne MP, Rosen PP. Detection and management of bone marrow micrometastases in breast cancer. Oncology 1994;8:25.
25. Denis LJ, Carneiro De Mura JL, Bono A, et al. Goserelin acetate and flutamide versus bilateral orchiectomy: a phase III EORTC trial (30853). Urology 1993;42:119.
26. Crawford ED, Eisenberger MA, Mcleod DG, et al. A controlled trial of leuprolide with and without flutamide in prostatic carcinoma. New Engl J Med 1989;321:419.
27. Van Aubel OGJM, Hoekstra WJ, Schroeder FH. Early orchiectomy for patients with stage D1 prostatic carcinoma. J Urol 1985;134:292.
28. Zincke H, Utz DC, Thule PM, et al. Treatment options for patients with D1 (T0-3, N1-2, MO) adenocarcinoma of prostate. Urology 1987; 30:307.
29. Kramalowosky EV. The value of testosterone deprivation in stage D1 carcinoma of the prostate. J Urol 1988;139:1242.
30. van den Ouden D, Tribukait B, Blom JHM, et al. Deoxyribonucleic acid ploidy of core biopsies and metastatic lymph nodes of prostate cancer patients: impact on time to progression. J Urol 1993;150:400.
31. McCullough DL, Leadbetter WF. Radical pelvic surgery for locally extensive carcinoma of the prostate. J Urol 1972;108:939.
32. Kramer SA, Cline WA Jr, Farnham R, et al. Prognosis of patients with stage D1 prostatic adenocarcinoma. J Urol 1981;125:817.
33. Utz DC. Radical excision of adenocarcinoma of prostate with pelvic lymph node involvement: surgical gesture or curative procedure? Urology 1984;24(Suppl):4.
34. Catalona WJ, Miller DR, Kavoussi LR. Intermediate-term survival results in clinically understaged cancer patients following radical prostatectomy. J Urol 1988;140:540.
35. Zincke H, Bergstralh E, Larsson-Keller J, et al. Stage D1 prostate cancer treated by radical prostatectomy and adjuvant hormonal treatment. Cancer 1992;70:311.
36. Paulson DF, Lin GH, Hinshaw W, et al. Radical surgery versus radiotherapy for adenocarcinoma of the prostate. J Urol 1982;128:502.
37. Bagshaw MA. Radiotherapeutic treatment of prostatic carcinoma with pelvic lymph node involvement. Urol Clin North Am 1984;11:297.
38. Bagshaw MA. Potential for radiotherapy alone in prostate cancer. Cancer 1985;55:2079.
39. Bagshaw MA. Radiation therapy for cancer of the prostate. In: Skinner DG, Lieskovsky G, eds. Management of genitourinary cancer. Philadelphia: WB Saunders, 1988:425.
40. Frieha FS, Bagshaw MA. Carcinoma of the prostate: results of post-irradiation biopsy. Prostate 1984;5:19.
41. Eisenberger MA, Abrams JS. Chemotherapy for prostatic carcinoma. Semin Urol 1988;6:303.
42. deVere White R, Babayan RK, Krikorian J, et al. Adjuvant chemotherapy for stage D1 adenocarcinoma of the prostate. Urology 1983;21: 270.
43. Scott WW. An evaluation of endocrine therapy plus radical perineal prostatectomy in the treatment of advanced carcinoma of the prostate. J Urol 1964;91:97.
44. Scott WW, Boyd HL. Combined hormone control therapy and radical prostatectomy in the treatment of selected cases of advanced carcinoma of the prostate: a retrospective study based upon 25 years of experience. J Urol 1969;101:86.
45. Zincke H, Utz DC. Radical surgery for D1 prostate cancer. Semin Urol 1983;1:253.

46. deKernion JB, Huang MY, Kaufman JJ, et al. Result of treatment of patients with stage D1 prostatic carcinoma. Urology 1985;26:446.
47. Oesterling JE, Brendler CB, Epstein JJ, et al. Correlation of clinical stage, serum prostatic acid phosphatase and preoperative Gleason grade with clinically localized adenocarcinoma of the prostate. J Urol 1987; 138:92.
48. Fan K, Peng CF. Predicting the probability of bone metastases through histological grading of prostate carcinoma: a retrospective correlative analysis of 81 autopsy cases with antemortem transurethral resection specimen. J Urol 1983;130:708.
49. Berman H, Kluin PM, Hermans J, et al. Prognostic significance of DNA ploidy in a series of 690 primary breast cancer patients. Int J Cancer 1990;45:34.
50. Kallioniemi OP, Punnanen R, Mattila J, et al. Prognostic significance of DNA index, multiploidy and S-phase fraction in ovarian cancer. Cancer 1988;61:335.
51. Kokal W, Gardine RL, Sheibani K, et al. Tumor DNA content in resectable, primary colorectal carcinoma. Ann Surg 1989;209:188.
52. Tirindelli-Danesi D, Teodori L, Mauro F, et al. Prognostic significance of flow cytometry in lung cancer: a 5 year study. Cancer 1987;60:844.
53. Look AT, Douglass EC, Meyer WH. Clinical importance of near-diploid stem lines in patients with osteosarcoma of an extremity. N Engl J Med 1988;318:1567.
54. deVere White RW, Deitch AD, West B, et al. The predictive value of flow cytometric information in the clinical management of stage 0 (Ta) bladder cancer. J Urol 1988;139:279.
55. Shaaban AA, Tribukait B, El-Bedeiwy AFA, et al. Prediction of lymph node metastases in bladder carcinoma with deoxyribonucleic acid flow cytometry. J Urol 1990;144:884.
56. Fradet Y, Tardiff M, Borget L, et al. Clinical cancer progression in urinary bladder tumors evaluated by multiparameter flow cytometry with monoclonal antibodies. Cancer Res 1990;50:432.
57. Fordham MVP, Burdge AH, Matthews J, et al. Prostatic carcinoma cell DNA content measured by flow cytometry and its relationship to clinical outcome. Br J Surg 1986;73:400.
58. Tribukait B. Rapid flow cytometry of prostatic fine needle aspiration biopsies. In: Karr JP, Coffey DS, Gardner W Jr, eds. Prognostic cytometry and cytopathlogy of prostate cancer. New York: Elsevier, 1988: 236.
59. Tribukait B. Flow cytometry in assessing the clinical aggressiveness of genitourinary neoplasms. World J Urol 1987;5:108.
60. deVere White RW, Deitch AD, Tesluk H, et al. Prognosis in disseminated prostate cancer as related to tumor ploidy and differentiation. World J Urol 1990;8:47.
61. Lee SE, Currin SM, Paulson DF, et al. Flow cytometric determination of ploidy in prostatic adenocarcinoma: a comparison with seminal vesicle involvement and histopathological grading as a predictor of clinical recurrence. J Urol 1988;140:769.
62. Winkler HZ, Rainwater LM, Myers RP, et al. Stage D1 prostatic adenocarcinoma: significance of nuclear DNA ploidy patterns studied by flow cytometry. Mayo Clin Proc 1988;63:103.
63. McIntire TL, Murphy WM, Coon JS, et al. The prognostic value of DNA ploidy combined with histologic substaging for incidental carcinoma of the prostate gland. Am J Clin Pathol 1988;89:370.
64. Montgomery BT, Nativ O, Blute ML, et al. Stage B prostate adenocarcinoma: flow cytometric nuclear DNA ploidy analysis. Arch Surg 1990; 125:327.
65. Nativ O, Winkler HZ, Ras Y, et al. Stage C prostate adenocarcinoma: flow cytometric nuclear DNA ploidy analysis. Mayo Clin Proc 1989; 64:911.
66. Stephenson RA, James BC, Gay H, et al. Flow cytometry of prostate cancer: relationship of DNA content to survival. Cancer Res 1987;47: 2564.
67. Zincke H. Extended experience with surgical treatment of stage D1 adenocarcinoma of prostate: significant influences of immediate adjuvant hormonal treatment (orchiectomy) on outcome. Urology 1989; 33(Suppl):27.
68. Zincke H. Combined surgery and immediate adjuvant hormonal treatment for stage D1 adenocarcinoma of the prostate: Mayo Clinic experience. Semin Urol 1990;8:175.
69. Lieber MM, Murtaugh PA, et al. DNA ploidy is prognostically more important than Gleason score or pathological stage: analysis of 494 patients who underwent radical prostatectomy for localized prostate carcinoma, 1967–1981. J Urol 1991;145:251A.
70. Babiarz JB, Peters-Gee JM, Crissman JD, et al. DNA quantitation in prostatic adenocarcinoma: a comparison between primary tumor and lymph node metastasis. J Urol 1991;145:215A.
71. Zincke H, Bergstrahl EJ, et al. Long term follow-up and comprehensive review of experience with radical prostatectomy (RP) for stage D1 prostate cancer. J Urol 1991;145:315A.

Principles and Practice of Genitourinary Oncology, edited by Derek Raghavan, Howard I. Scher, Steven A. Leibel, and Paul H. Lange. Lippincott-Raven Publishers, Philadelphia, © 1997.

CHAPTER 54

Neoadjuvant Hormonal Therapy in Prostate Cancer

Yu Wang and William R. Fair

Prostate cancer is the most common malignancy and the second leading cause of cancer mortality in North American men. In 1996, an estimated 317,000 new cases of prostate cancer will be diagnosed, with 43,000 men predicted to die from the disease.[1] The treatment of prostatic cancer using radical prostatectomy is effective if the disease is confined to the prostate. In a highly selected group of men (mean age, 59 years) with localized prostatic cancer, the overall 15-year survival rate after radical prostatectomy was equivalent to the expected survival rate of men in the same age group without prostatic cancer.[2]

Despite significant improvement in the staging of prostate cancer with serum acid phosphatase and prostate-specific antigen (PSA) levels, bone scans, computed tomography, magnetic resonance imaging, and transrectal ultrasonography (TRUS), pathologic understaging of apparently clinically localized carcinoma of the prostate remains a major clinical problem. Table 54-1 lists a compilation of 5 contemporary series involving more than 2000 patients with clinical T1 or T2 prostatic cancer treated with radical prostatectomy. Of these patients, only 927 (46%) had tumor confined to the prostate on pathologic examination.[3–7] Thus, 54% of tumors thought to be clinically localized (i.e., T1 or T2) are found to be beyond the prostate at pathologic examination following radical prostatectomy.

The impact of disease beyond the prostate has been shown to be associated with an earlier biochemical relapse after radical prostatectomy. Stein and colleagues[5] reported PSA relapse rates at a median follow-up of 34 months of 15% in patients with pathologic organ-confined involvement; 29% in those with extracapsular involvement, margin-positive involvement, or both; and 39% in those with seminal vesicle involvement. The combined clinical and biochemical (i.e., increased PSA level as the only manifestation of disease) failure rate at a median of 4 years following radical prostatectomy was 6% for patients with cancer confined to the prostate (n = 337), 26% for patients with extraprostatic extension but specimen confined disease (n = 122), and 79% for patients in whom the tumor involved the specimen margins, seminal vesicles, or regional lymph nodes (n = 127).[8] Frazier and colleagues[9] compared clinical failure and biochemical failure at various times for different pathologic stages after radical prostatectomy. With a median follow-up of 23 months, the PSA failure rates were 10% in patients with organ-confined disease, 39% in those with specimen-confined disease, and 66% in those with margin-positive disease. These investigators noted that the rate of biochemical failure at 2 years was similar to the clinical failure rate at 10 years after radical prostatectomy as measured by physical examination or imaging study in another group of patients reported from the same institution.[4,9] These data provide compelling evidence that tumor beyond the prostate at radical prostatectomy is associated with an earlier PSA relapse and that an early biochemical failure translates into clinical evidence of disease progression, although the biochemical failure may antedate clinical failure by as long as 8 years.

The challenge in the treatment of prostate cancer is to improve the rate of organ-confined disease at the time of radical prostatectomy, and hence possibly increase the long-term relapse-free and disease-specific survivals. Clearly, detection at an earlier stage of disease would help increase survival, but with the modalities available, it is unlikely that most prostate cancers will be detected at a time when the disease is totally confined to the prostate. Even in large series of patients having radical prostatectomy for stage T1c disease, only approximately 50% are pathologically organ confined.[10] Another approach to improve the rate of organ-confined disease is the use of combined modality therapy in an attempt to decrease the volume of tumor before surgery, such as neoadjuvant androgen deprivation therapy (ADT) followed by radical prostatectomy. This chapter reviews the use of neoadjuvant hormonal therapy in the settings of locally advanced and clinically localized prostate cancer. In addition, the pathologic features within the tumor after ADT are described.

RATIONALE FOR NEOADJUVANT THERAPY

Previous investigation in an animal model of prostatic cancer suggests that prostatic cancer is composed of a heterogenous mixture of "hormone-sensitive" and "hormone-insensitive"

Table 54-1. *Understaging of clinical T1/T2 tumors*

Investigators	Number of patients	Organ confined Number	Organ confined Percent
Catalona and Bigg, 1990[3]	250	142	57
Paulson et al, 1990[4]	441	242	55
Stein et al, 1992[5]	230	115	50
Rosen et al, 1992[6]	144	72	50
Partin et al, 1993[7]	955	356	37
Total	2020	927	46

cells.[11] The rationale for the use of neoadjuvant ADT is to eliminate the androgen-dependent tumor cells in the hope that these are responsible for the locally extensive tumor and that sufficient tumor regression may make it possible to remove any residual androgen-independent cells by surgical extirpation. The effect of ADT on hormone-sensitive malignant cells has been demonstrated in the androgen-dependent mouse Shionogi's mammary tumor model.[12] In that experiment, castration of the animals markedly depleted the relative stem cell population in the transplanted tumors. As a result, the propensity of malignant cells to form new tumors at the time of maximal castration effect (7 days) was significantly attenuated compared with that of tumor cells not treated with ADT or recurrent tumor cells after prolonged ADT. Therefore, it seems reasonable to conclude that in the setting of combined modality therapy, the ideal time to initiate additional treatment to augment hormonal manipulation would be when the ratio of stem cells to total cells is lowest (i.e., at the time of maximal ADT effect).

NEOADJUVANT ANDROGEN DEPRIVATION THERAPY IN LOCALLY ADVANCED PROSTATE CANCER

A number of studies have evaluated the possibility of downstaging locally advanced prostatic cancer by using neoadjuvant ADT before radical prostatectomy. None of these studies were randomized, and most were uncontrolled. Kennedy and colleagues[13] prospectively investigated the use of neoadjuvant luteinizing hormone–releasing hormone (LHRH) analogs for 2 to 5 months in seven patients with stage T3 prostatic cancer in an attempt to downstage the disease. They found that although substantial decreases in serum PSA level and prostatic volume occurred, only 2 patients (28%) experienced pathologic organ-confined disease after radical prostatectomy. In a similar uncontrolled study, Oesterling and colleagues[14] retrospectively evaluated 21 patients with stages T2c (n = 4) and T3 (n = 17) prostate cancer who received ADT prior to radical prostatectomy. Despite a dramatic decline in PSA levels (>98% reduction), only 1 patient (5%) had pathologic organ-confined disease. Similarly, Macfarlene and colleagues[15] demonstrated significant clinical shrinking of locally advanced prostatic cancer with reduction in prostatic volume and serum PSA levels after neoadjuvant ADT but not significant pathologic downstaging of the disease: 4 of 8 (50%) T2c and 3 of 12 (25%) T3 patients had pathologic organ-confined disease. Soloway and colleagues[16] reported pathologic extracapsular disease with or without positive margin in 23 of 37 (62%) T2b/T3 patients after neoadjuvant ADT and radical prostatectomy.

In a pilot study at Memorial Sloan-Kettering Cancer Center (MSKCC),[17] 55 patients with stages T2c (n = 18), T3 (n = 27), and D0 (persistently elevated serum acid phosphatase levels with no evidence of metastatic disease; n = 10) prostatic cancers were given diethylstilbestrol (DES), 3 mg/day for a minimum of 8 weeks (range, 8–32 weeks) before radical prostatectomy. A marked reduction in serum PSA levels occurred in all patients; 98% of patients had PSA levels reduced to the normal range of 0 to 4 ng/mL as measured by Hybritech assay, and 49% of patents had no measurable serum PSA level after 3 months of DES therapy. However, only 18 of the 55 patients (33%) had pathologic organ-confined disease.

A few studies have suggested that neoadjuvant ADT facilitates the dissection of the prostate during subsequent radical prostatectomy, with significant reduction in blood loss and operative time.[18,19] Other studies, however, did not demonstrate any difference in the ease or difficulty of surgery or in the amount of blood loss after preoperative hormonal ablation therapy. Our experience agrees with those who believe there is no appreciable decrease in surgical difficulty or blood loss following neoadjuvant ADT.[15,17]

A summary of the preceding clinical studies suggest that although neoadjuvant ADT results in a greater than 98% reduction in serum PSA levels and a 35% to 40% reduction of prostatic volume, most patients continue to exhibit disease beyond the prostate on final pathologic examinations. A clinical therapeutic response based on digital rectal examination (DRE), TRUS and serum PSA levels after hormonal therapy does not adequately predict final pathologic stage. Therefore, neoadjuvant ADT in the setting of locally advanced prostate cancer will not make a locally extensive lesion into a small tumor that could be predictably removed with negative surgical margins and organ-confined disease only.

NEOADJUVANT ANDROGEN DEPRIVATION THERAPY IN CLINICALLY LOCALIZED PROSTATE CANCER

Clinical understaging of localized prostate cancer had led some investigators to evaluate the combined use of neoadjuvant ADT and radical prostatectomy in patients with clinically localized stage T1 to T2 prostate cancer. Sassine and Schulman[19] retrospectively reviewed the records of 40 patients treated with a neoadjuvant LHRH agonist and an antiandrogen prior to radical prostatectomy. Of the 25 patients with clinical T2 disease, 15 (60%) had pathologic organ-confined disease. When the patients were stratified according to posttreatment PSA levels, 86% of patients with posttreatment PSA levels of less than 0.25 ng/mL had tumor confined to the gland. In another study, Monfette and colleagues[18] prospectively studied the use of temporary combination therapy with Tryptex (an LHRH agonist) and flutamide in 34 patients for 3 months prior to radical prostatectomy. Of these patients, 28 (83%) had clinical B1 or B2 disease. Overall, 10 of 34 (29%) patients had P0 disease (i.e., no cancer found in final specimen). Solomon and colleagues[20] studied the positive margin rates in 156 patients treated with an LHRH agonist and antiandrogen followed by radical prostatectomy (neoadjuvant group) and 119 patients treated with radical prostatectomy alone (control group). Of these patients, 140 in the neoadjuvant group and 118 in the control group had clinical T2 disease. The positive margin rates were significantly lower in the combination therapy group compared with those in the surgery alone group (11.5% versus 35.3%, respectively). None of these studies reported postsurgical PSA results as a marker of disease-free status.

Intrigued by the observation of marked regression with almost complete tumor disappearance in a small subset of patients with locally advanced disease, we embarked upon a prospective, nonrandomized, phase II study with concurrent controls to determine whether neoadjuvant ADT would increase the organ-confined disease rate in clinically localized prostate cancer. The patients in the study group were treated with a combination of an LHRH agonist (Zoladex) and an antiandrogen (flutamide) for 12 weeks before radical prostatectomy. Seventy-five patients (mean age, 62 years; range, 45–71 years) were entered in the study; six patients withdrew during the course of preoperative treatment, and 69 patients completed the protocol. During the same period, 72 men (mean age, 62 years; range, 45–72 years) served as concurrent controls. These patients were offered the protocol but declined participation, primarily because of geographic distance from MSKCC that would make coming back for the required monthly visits difficult or because of their desire for prompt surgery. Thus, the decision to participate in the protocol was based on patient selection, not physician selection. Comparison between the control and study groups did not show any significant differences with regard to age, grade of biopsy specimen, or initial serum PSA and prostatic acid phosphatase levels.

Clinical staging was according to the TMN classification.[21] Of the 69 patients in the study group who subsequently proceeded to radical prostatectomy and pathologic examinations, 10% had T1 lesions, 71% had T2 lesions, 13% had T2/T3 lesions, and 4% had T3 lesions. It was not possible to determine on the basis of two examiners whether those in the third group were T2 or T3 lesions. In the concurrent control group, the distribution of clinical stages were as follows: 23% had T1 lesions, 74% had T2 lesions, and 3% had T2/T3 lesions.

The mean serum PSA and acid phosphatase levels in the study group were 16 ng/mL and 0.5 U/L (normal, 0 to 0.6 U/L) respectively. After 1 month of treatment, the mean PSA level decreased to 2.1 ng/mL; at 2 months, the mean had fallen to 0.31 ng/mL; and at the time of surgery, the mean PSA level was 0.2 ng/mL. TRUS determination of prostatic volumes were performed before entry in the protocol and again after 8 weeks of hormonal therapy. The mean prostatic volume dropped from a prestudy value of 29.1 cm^3 to 17.8 cm^3 after 2 months of therapy, reflecting a decrease of 38% in mean prostatic volume.

Table 54-2 shows the comparison of the pathologic stages after radical prostatectomy between the study and control groups. Of the 69 patients who received neoadjuvant hormonal therapy, 3 (4%) had no tumor (P0) in the specimen, despite sectioning at 3-mm intervals; 48 (70%) had organ-confined (P2) disease; 13 (19%) had extracapsular disease, margin-positive (P3-P4) disease, or both; and 5 (7%) had nodal-positive (N +) disease. Of the 72 patients in the control group, 35 (48%) had P2 disease, 30 (42%) had P3-P4 disease, and 7 (10%) had N + disease. Therefore, 74% of those receiving neoadjuvant ADT had either no disease or disease confined to the prostate, compared with 48% of those treated with radical prostatectomy alone ($P < .05$). In addition, the margin-positive rate was only 10% in the neoadjuvant group, compared with 33% in the control group. More compelling evidence can be obtained by comparing the results of pathologic staging in patients thought to have clinical stage T2 disease before entering into the study. In 49 patients with clinical T2 disease who received neoadjuvant therapy, 77% had organ-confined disease, compared with only 45% in 53 concurrent controls. The margin-positive rate was 8% in the study group versus 34% in the control group (Table 54-3).

Table 54-2. *Distribution of pathologic stages of T1-T2 patients in the neoadjuvant phase II Memorial Sloan-Kettering Cancer Center trial (P = .003)*

	LHRH/flutamide plus surgery (n = 69)	Surgery only (n = 72)
P0	3 (4%)	0 (0%)
P2	48 (70%)	35 (48%)
P3-P4	13 (19%)	30 (42%)
Nodal-positive	5 (7%)	7 (10%)
Margin-positive	7 (10%)	24 (33%)

LHRH, leuteinizing hormone–releasing hormone.

Postprostatectomy PSA levels were measured in 66 patients in the neoadjuvant group and 70 patients in the concurrent control group. Median follow-up was 22 months. The PSA relapse rates (PSA levels > 0.2 ng/mL) in the neoadjuvant group was 11% for patients with pathologic organ-confined (P2) disease; 25% for those with extracapsular disease, margin-positive (P3-P4) disease, or both; and 67% for those with nodal-positive (N +) disease. In the control group, the PSA relapse rate was 9%, 17%, and 40% for P2, P3-P4 and N + diseases, respectively. The equivalent PSA relapse rates in patients with P2 disease in both the neoadjuvant and control groups implies that the final pathologic organ-confined status is an important determinant in predicting PSA relapse, regardless of how the organ-confined state was achieved. Whether the P2 patients in the neoadjuvant group will have a lower biochemical and clinical relapse rate on longer follow-up compared with P3-P4 patients in the control group remains to be seen.

The results of our phase II study were similar to those reported in a randomized study from Canada. Labrie and colleagues[22] compared the results of neoadjuvant ADT in 77 pa-

Table 54-3. *Distribution of pathologic stages of T2 patients in the neoadjuvant phase II Memorial Sloan-Kettering Cancer Center trial*

	LHRH/flutamide plus surgery (n = 49)	Surgery only (n = 53)
P0	3 (6%)	0 (0%)
P2	35 (71%)	24 (45%)
P3-P4	7 (14%)	24 (45%)
Nodal-positive	4 (8%)	5 (10%)
Margin-positive	4 (8%)	18 (34%)

LHRH, leuteinizing hormone–releasing hormone.

tients who received combination LHRH plus flutamide and radical prostatectomy (study group) to those of 65 patients who underwent radical prostatectomy alone (control group). The positive margin rate was 13% in the study group, compared with 38.5% in the control group. Clinical understaging (i.e., P stage > T stage) occurred in 19.5% of patients in the combined therapy group versus 61.5% of patients in the surgery-only group. At MSKCC, a single-institution prospective randomized clinical trial is underway comparing 3 months of neoadjuvant Zoladex and flutamide followed by radical prostatectomy to radical prostatectomy alone in patients with clinically localized prostate cancer. To be eligible for the study, all patients must have clinical T1-T2 adenocarcinomas of the prostate, good performance status and no prior hormonal therapy or radiotherapy. The end points of the study include clinical responses (e.g., changes in serum PSA levels and DRE and TRUS examinations), pathologic responses (e.g., final pathologic stage), and differences in the surgical procedure (e.g., amount of blood loss, operative time, complications) between the study and control groups. The statistical considerations in the randomized study are such that if approximately 54% of control patients are expected to have pathologic P3-P4 disease, and neoadjuvant ADT can reduce this figure by one half (i.e., to 27%), then a total population of 136 patients is required to have an 80% chance of detecting this difference at the 5% significance level. This sample size of 68 treated patients will allow the estimation of the response rate to hormonal therapy with a precision of more than 12% (95% confidence interval). At this time, 32 patients have been enrolled in the neoadjuvant arm and 33 patients have been enrolled in the control arm. Interim analysis of the results in patients who have completed the protocol showed that the pathologic organ-confined rate was 74% (20 of 27 patients) in the neoadjuvant group versus 50% (13 of 26 patients) in the control group. The margin-positive rate in the study group was 19%, compared with 40% in the control group.

PATHOLOGIC CHANGES ASSOCIATED WITH ANDROGEN DEPRIVATION THERAPY

Pathologic changes associated with ADT for prostate cancer have been described in several reports. Murphy and colleagues[23] reported a marked decrease in both the diameter and distribution density of neoplastic glands after hormonal therapy, as measured by morphometric analysis. Tetu and colleagues[24] reviewed the histopathology of 23 radical prostatectomies from patients pretreated with 3 to 6 months of an LHRH agonist and an antiandrogen. After combination therapy, the neoplastic glands showed marked atrophy with prominent basal cell layers, basal cell hyperplasia, and epithelial cell vacuolization. Hellstrom and colleagues[25] reported similar histologic changes, including nuclear pyknosis, which may be suggestive of programed cell death following androgen ablation.

The pathobiologic effects of neoadjuvant total androgen ablation therapy in clinically localized prostate cancer were described in 27 radical prostatectomy specimens from the nonrandomized phase II study at MSKCC.[26] The effects of ADT on serum PSA levels were intriguing. Although the PSA level dropped to no measurable amount in most patients, there was little correlation between serum PSA level and the PSA staining of the tumor on immunohistochemistry. In most men with an undetectable serum PSA level, PSA continued to be expressed abundantly as seen using immunohistochemistry in the residual cancer cells of radical prostatectomy specimens. Therapy-induced morphologic changes in residual carcinoma as seen using light microscopy consisted mainly of a loss of luminal architecture, prominent cytoplasmic vacuolization, nuclear condensation, and a decrease in the number of visible nucleoli. Electron microscopy demonstrated focal areas of necrosis, nuclear chromatin clumping, and cellular membrane disruption in the residual neoplastic cells, which may be morphologically suggestive of apoptosis. Therefore, the effects of neoadjuvant ADT on prostate cancer can be characterized by distinct pathologic features within residual tumor cells of the surgical specimens. The regression of carcinoma following preoperative ADT suggests that hormonal therapy can have a profound effect on a subset of prostatic carcinoma cells.

CONCLUSIONS

Radical prostatectomy gives excellent results in organ-confined carcinoma of the prostate, but available data indicate that most patients who have surgery for clinically localized prostatic cancer are found to have disease that is pathologically beyond the organ. Combination therapy with neoadjuvant ADT followed by radical prostatectomy in locally advanced (stage T3) lesions does not appear to be efficacious in downstaging most tumors into pathologically organ-confined disease. However, neoadjuvant ADT appears to have a marked impact on some clinically localized lesions compared with untreated controls, and complete tumor absence (P0) has been noted in a few patients. The effects of ADT on prostate cancer can be characterized by distinct pathologic changes, which may be associated with apoptosis of the hormone-sensitive cells within the tumor. Despite the improved pathologic staging of some patients after neoadjuvant ADT, survival benefits of combination therapy are not proven and await the results of longer follow-up postsurgery. However, the favorable impact of neoadjuvant ADT in clinically localized prostate cancer warrants further investigation with prospective randomized clinical trials.

REFERENCES

1. Parker, SL, Tong T, Bolden S, Wingo PA. Cancer statistics, 1996. CA Cancer J Clin 1996;65:5.
2. Gibbons RP, Correa RJ, Brannen GE, Mason JT. Total prostatectomy for localized prostatic cancer. J Urol 1984; 131:73.
3. Catalona WJ, Bigg SW. Nerve-sparing radical prostatectomy: Evaluation of results after 250 patients. J Urol 1990; 143:538.
4. Paulson DF, Moul JW, Walther PJ. Radical prostatectomy for clinical stage T1-2N0M0 prostatic adenocarcinoma: Long-term results. J Urol 1990; 144:1180.
5. Stein A, DeKernion JB, Smith RB, Dorey F, Patel H. Prostate specific antigen levels after radical prostatectomy in patients with organ confined and locally extensive prostate cancer. J Urol 1992; 147:942.
6. Rosen MA, Goldstone L, Lapin S, Wheeler T, Scardino PT. Frequency and location of extracapsular extension and positive surgical margins in radical prostatectomy specimens. J Urol 1992; 148:331.
7. Partin AW, Pound CR, Clemens JQ, Epstein JI, Walsh PC. Serum PSA after anatomic radical prostatectomy. The Johns Hopkins experience after 10 years. Urol Clin North America 1993; 20(4):713.
8. Morton RA, Steiner MS, Walsh PC. J Urol 1991; 145:1197.
9. Frazier HA, Robertson JE, Humphrey PA, Paulson DF. Is prostate

specific antigen of clinical importance in evaluating outcome after radical prostatectomy? J Urol 1993; 149:516.
10. Epstein JI, Walsh PC, Carmichael M, Brendler CB. Pathologic and clinical findings to predict tumor extent of nonpalpable (stage T1c) prostate cancer. JAMA 1994; 271:368.
11. Isaacs JT, Coffey DS. Adaptation versus selection as the mechanism responsible for the relapse of prostate cancer to androgen ablation therapy as studied in the Dunning R-3327-H adenocarcinoma. Cancer Res 1981; 41:5070.
12. Bruchovsky N, Rennie PS, Coldman AJ, Goldenberg SL, To M, Lawson D. Effects of androgen withdrawal on the stem cell composition of the Shionogi carcinoma. Cancer Res 1990; 50:2275.
13. Kennedy TJ, Sonneland AM, Marlett MM, Troup RH. Luteinizing hormone-releasing hormone downstaging of clinical stage C prostate cancer. J Urol 1992; 147:891.
14. Oesterling JE, Andrews PE, Suman VJ, Zincke H, Myers RP. Preoperative androgen deprivation therapy: Artificial lowering of serum prostate specific antigen without downstaging the tumor. J Urol 1993; 149:779.
15. Macfarlene MT, Abi-aad A, Stein A, Danella J, Belldegrun A, DeKernion JB. Neoadjuvant hormonal deprivation in patients with locally advanced prostate cancer. J Urol 1993; 150:132.
16. Soloway MS, Hachiya T, Civantos F, Murphy WM, Gomez CC, Ruiz HE. Androgen deprivation prior to radical prostatectomy for T2b and T3 prostate cancer. Urology 1994; 43(2):52.
17. Fair WR, Aprikian A, Sogani P, Reuter V, Whitmore WF. The role of neoadjuvant hormonal manipulation in localized prostatic cancer. Cancer 1993; 71:1031.
18. Monfette G, Dupont A, Labrie F. Temporary combination therapy with flutamide and tryptex as adjuvant to radical prostatectomy for the treatment of early stage prostate cancer. In: Labrie F, ed. Early stage prostate cancer: Diagnosis and choice of therapy. New York: Elsevier Science Publishers B.V., 1989:41.
19. Sassine AM, Schulman CC. Neoadjuvant hormonal deprivation before radical prostatectomy. Eur Urol 1993; 24(2):46.
20. Solomon MH, McHugh TA, Dorr RP, Lee F, Siders DB. Hormone ablation therapy as neoadjuvant treatment to radical prostatectomy. Clin Invest Med 1993; 16(6):532.
21. Schroder FH, Hermanek P, Denis L, Fair WR, Gospodarowicz MK, Pavone-Macaluso M. The TMN classification of prostate cancer. Prostate 1992; 4:129.
22. Labrie F, Dupont A, Cusan L, et al. Downstaging of localized prostate cancer by neo-adjuvant therapy with flutamide and lupron: The first controlled and randomized trial. Clin Invest Med 1993; 16(6):499.
23. Murphy WM, Soloway MS, Barrows GH. Pathologic change associated with androgen deprivation therapy for prostate cancer. Cancer 1991; 68:821.
24. Tetu B, Srigley JR, Boivin J, et al. Effect of combination endocrine therapy (LHRH agonist and flutamide) on normal prostate and prostatic adenocarcinoma: a histopathologic and immunohistochemical study. Am J Surg Pathol 1991; 15:111.
25. Hellstrom M, Haggman M, Brandstedt S, et al. Histopathological changes in androgen-deprived localized prostatic cancer: a study in total prostatectomy specimens. Eur Urol 1993; 24:461.
26. Armas OA, Aprikian AG, Melamed J, et al. Clinical and pathobiological effects of neoadjuvant total androgen ablation therapy on clinically localized prostatic adenocarcinoma. Am J Surg Pathol 1994; 18(10): 979.

Principles and Practice of Genitourinary Oncology, edited by Derek Raghavan, Howard I. Scher, Steven A. Leibel, and Paul H. Lange. Lippincott-Raven Publishers, Philadelphia, © 1997.

CHAPTER 55

Treatment of Local Failure of Prostate Cancer After Radiotherapy and Surgery

Marcelo Zerati and J. Edson Pontes

The concept of local failure following curative treatment for prostate cancer has changed significantly within the past few years. In the past, local failure following either radical prostatectomy or radiotherapy was based largely on the physical findings of either a nodule in the area of radical prostatectomy or on the findings of progression of local disease based on digital rectal examination in the case of radiotherapy. Local recurrences detected by these methods were usually late events, with a resulting poor outcome in response to any form of therapy. With the advent of prostatic-specific antigen (PSA) testing, new concepts have been developed regarding the value of early intervention based on the development of an abnormal PSA marker.

In this chapter, we discuss our viewpoints regarding local failure following radiotherapy and radical prostatectomy, with an emphasis on an aggressive treatment approach targeted toward the elimination of locally recurrent disease.

LOCAL FAILURE FOLLOWING RADIOTHERAPY

Radiotherapy is an effective means of treating localized prostate cancer; however, it has been known for many years that between 20% to 30% of patients continue to have positive biopsy specimens following radiotherapy.[1] The finding of a positive biopsy specimen in a previously irradiated patient is associated with an increased incidence of distant metastases and decreased survival compared with patients exhibiting negative biopsy specimens.[2,3] With the advent of PSA testing to evaluate patients after radiotherapy, it has been observed that approximately 80% of patients show progressive decrease of PSA in the first year following radiotherapy but that approximately one half of these patients showing an initial decrease will have progressively elevated PSA levels on subsequent follow-up.[4] The use of a progressively elevated PSA level in three consecutive measurements at 3-months intervals after initial stabilization following completion of radiotherapy is, in our opinion, an indication for biopsy. A positive biopsy in a patient with clinically localized disease with a life expectancy of 10 years is an indication for considering surgery as a treatment option. A complete metastatic workup is necessary, as well as a thorough endoscopic evaluation, including urodynamics, to assess the feasibility of bladder preservation.

Salvage Surgery After Radiotherapy

The concept of surgery after radiotherapy for prostate cancer is not new; several series have been reported.[5–14] In 1974, Estrada and Scardino[5] reported a patient who failed radiotherapy and was subsequently treated with perineal prostatectomy. Gill and colleagues[6] used radiotherapy to downstage the disease from T3 to T2 and then performed a radical prostatectomy. Four of 11 patients initially treated with this protocol were submitted to salvage prostatectomy; three patients were without evidence of progression at 1 to 2 years of follow-up.[6] Spaulding and Whitmore[7] reported on 35 patients treated with cystoprostatectomy or complete pelvic exenteration following radiotherapy failure for prostate cancer. Follow-up revealed that 35% were alive at 5 years postsurgery, and 22% (8 of 37) had no evidence of disease. Of these eight patients without evidence of disease at 5 years, only one failed later. Follow-up of the remaining patients ranged between 9 and 20 years.[7]

More recently, Neerhut and colleagues[8] reported on 16 patients who underwent salvage surgery after 1 to 10 years of definitive radiotherapy. The specimens were analyzed through whole-mount step sections, and in nine patients the tumor was resected completely (i.e., negative surgical margins) despite extracapsular extension in five patients and seminal vesical invasion in four patients.[8] Six patients had positive surgical margins, and one patient had negative margins but positive pelvic lymph nodes.[8] After a minimum follow-up of 20 months,[3–32] no patient had clinical recurrence, but two patients showed bony metastases.[8] Rainwater and Zincke[9] reported on 30 patients, 27 of whom underwent radical prostatectomy and 3 of whom underwent cystoprostatectomy. The course of irradiation varied among the patients from full dose in 17 patients to doses varying from 4000 to 7000 cGy in the remainder. Comparison between preoperative and pathologic staging revealed overstaging in 10% and understaging in 40% (12 patients), with eight patients having positive lymph nodes. When analyzing tumor grade and stage, adjuvant hormonal treatment, and DNA ploidy pattern for their impact on progression and survival, only DNA ploidy showed a positive correlation.[9] In 1991, Link and Freiha[10] reported on a series of 14 patients whose interval between radiotherapy and biopsy-proved recurrence was 61 months. Nine patients had capsular penetration, seven had positive seminal vesicles, and six had positive surgical margins. Three patients who had been treated with iodine-125 (^{125}I) implants required additional external beam irradiation because of elevated PSA levels without evidence of metastatic disease. Two patients developed symptomatic bone metastases and underwent bilateral orchiectomy. At the time of their report, six patients were alive without evidence of disease 1 to 54 months postoperatively (mean, 9 months).[10] Four patients had documented bony metastasis at 6 months postoperatively, and an additional four patients had detectable PSA levels but negative or equivocal bone scans.[10] Zincke[11] reported on his series of 62 patients who underwent surgery after failure of radiotherapy. Thirty-two patients underwent salvage prostatectomy, 23 underwent cystoprostatectomy, and 7 underwent total pelvic exenteration. There was a 5-year progression-free survival rate of 82% and a 5-year cause-specific survival rate of 90% for the patients undergoing salvage prostatectomy. Analysis of grade, DNA ploidy pattern, progression, death rates, and timing of hormonal treatment revealed that patients with poor prognosis (e.g., high grade tumors, aneuploidy, and no postoperative hormonal treatment) tended to have more aggressive surgery, exenterative procedures, or cystoprostatectomy. These patients also showed a higher rate of progression and higher death rates when compared with patients who had a good prognosis.[11] There was a statistically significant difference in favor of patients undergoing salvage prostatectomy rather than pelvic exenteration procedures, and Zincke stated that pelvic exenteration procedures seem to be of questionable benefit because of rapid disease progression.[11]

In another study, Ahlering and colleagues[12] reported on 34 patients with local failure after radiotherapy. Twenty-four patients underwent cystoprostatectomy and 11 patients underwent salvage prostatectomy.[12] Twenty-seven patients also received hormonal deprivation. The seven patients that did not receive hormones had moderately differentiated disease. On follow-up, 22 patients were alive without evidence of disease at a mean follow-up of 114 months (range, 64 to 153 months), 2 were alive with elevated PSA levels, 3 were alive with radiographically evident disease, and 7 died of disease with a mean follow-up of 96 months (range, 43 to 154 months).[12]

Our experience consists of 63 patients, 51 to 73 years of age, who underwent surgery after radiotherapy failure between 1982 and 1993.[13] This series can be divided in two groups. Group 1 includes 38 patients operated on at the Roswell Park Memorial Institute and at the Cleveland Clinic Foundation between 1982 and 1990, and group 2 includes 25 patients operated on from 1990 to 1993 at Wayne State University.[13]

In group 1, the diagnosis was based mostly on biopsy for clinical failure, with a follow-up prior to biopsy of 18 months to 2 years. Among these patients, 34 had received external beam radiotherapy, and 4 had been treated with brachytherapy with ^{125}I implants. Salvage prostatectomy was performed in 30 patients, and cystoprostatectomy was done in 8 patients. When comparing clinical versus pathologic stage, significant understaging became evident. Only 10 of 38 patients had disease confined to the prostate or capsular invasion only. The remainder of the patients had either seminal vesicle involvement (22 patients) or pelvic lymph node metastases (6 patients).[13] Thirty-three patients were followed for 5 to 11 years; 11 were alive without evidence of disease, 6 were alive with metastases, 13 died of prostate cancer, and 3 died as a result a second malignancy without prostate cancer.[13]

Among the 25 patients of group 2, most of the cases were diagnosed because of elevation in serum PSA levels. Twenty-two of these patients were treated with external beam radiotherapy, and three patients received brachytherapy. Seventeen salvage prostatectomies and eight cystoprostatectomies, two with continent urinary diversion, were performed.[13] Thirteen of 25 patients (50%) had disease confined to the prostate without capsular involvement or evidence of seminal vesicle or lymph node invasion. Eight of these patients had negative surgical margins and five had positive margins. Although the follow-up period in this group of patients is too short for evaluation of survival, with a minimal follow-up of 18 months, 12 of 25 patients had undetectable PSA levels in the absence of hormonal therapy.[13]

Preoperative Evaluation and Surgical Options

Potential candidates for surgery should undergo medical evaluation of any associated clinical conditions (e.g., diabetes, cardiac disease) that would impact on their life expectancy. Every attempt is made to rule out metastatic disease by performing bone and CT scans of the pelvis and abdomen. In our experience before the wide use of PSA testing, pathologic understaging occurred in about 73% of patients; more recently, this rate has decreased to approximately 50%.[13] Other contemporary series show similar rates of understaging in patients with clinical stage T2b disease.[11] During the decision-making process, patients must undergo complete endoscopic evaluation not only to try to assess extent of the disease but also to evaluate the functional status of the bladder. It is our opinion that small, contracted bladders should be removed even in the presence of a small tumor burden, because this is a frequent reason for urinary incontinence and decreased quality of life. The surgeon also must be prepared to change his or her surgical strategy during the operative procedure. Because a high percentage of understaging is to be expected, patients must be aware of the possibility of the need for more extensive surgery. Zincke[11] noted that occasionally surgery had to be modified because a different, higher-stage disease was found at operation, such as involvement of the bladder neck not detected during preoperative clinical studies, including cystoscopy. However Zincke[11] also mentioned that salvage pelvic exenterative procedures seem to be of questionable benefit because of rapid disease progression in these patients, who usually have high-stage, high-grade, nondiploid disease.[11]

Surgical Technique for Salvage Prostatectomy

The technique that we use for salvage prostatectomy has been published.[14] We believe that a combined retrograde and antegrade approach is important because of inherent difficulties associated with the procedure. The patient is placed in supine position with a flat sandbag under the sacrum. A standard modified pelvic lymphadenectomy is performed, if it has not been done previously. At the time of the prostatectomy, the patient is placed in hyperextended, slight reverse Trendelenburg position, which rotates the pelvis outward, facilitating visualization. The endopelvic fascia is opened bilaterally. The puboprostatic ligaments are transected at the pubis. The dorsal vein of the penis complex is controlled using a 00 polyglycol suture and a small needle. The urethra is then transected with placement of four sutures that will be used later for the final anastomosis. The prostate is then dissected from the rectum using sharp and blunt dissection. After the dissection is completed to the base of the prostate, or any time when the dissection is deemed difficult, an antegrade approach is chosen. The bladder neck is transected between the Foley balloon and the base of the prostate. After complete transection of the bladder neck, the ampullae of the vas deferens are identified bilaterally and ligated. The seminal vesicles are dissected and the specimen removed. The bladder neck is then approximated to the urethral stump with the sutures previously placed in the urethra.

Some patients must undergo salvage cystectomy; the technique for radical salvage cystectomy is described elsewhere.[15] In recent years, a significant proportion of our patients have undergone continent urinary diversion to the urethra; and our diversion of choice has been published.[16]

Complications

Several series have addressed the issue of complications during and after salvage surgery for prostate cancer. Although some reports state that radical salvage prostatectomies are technically uncomplicated,[10,17] the general feeling is that the procedure seems to be more technically demanding[8] in previously irradiated patients than in nonirradiated patients.[13] However, salvage prostatectomy is feasible, with an acceptable level of morbidity and mortality.[9,10,12,13,17] Intraoperatively significant fibrosis with obliteration of the surgical planes sometimes complicates the dissection of the prostate from the rectum[10,12]; as a result, the incidence of rectal injury varies from as low as 0% to as high as 19%.[7,10,12,17] When rectal injury occurs, it should be managed by primary closure in two planes. Sometimes a fistula may develop, necessitating a colostomy.[8] Intraoperative blood loss was not higher than that in patients undergoing standard radical prostatectomy, with a mean loss of 900 to 1000 mL.[8,10] Postoperative complications include impotence, incontinence, and bladder neck contracture.

Because little or no effort is made during surgery to preserve the neurovascular bundles, a very high incidence of impotence is expected. One series reports an incidence of impotence of 100%,[10] and another small series reports only 1 out of 5 patients have preserved sexual function 4 weeks after the procedure.[17] Urinary incontinence is also expected to be higher in previously irradiated patients than in nonirradiated patients. An incontinence rate of 27% has been reported at 6 months and at 1 year of follow-up.[8,11] Our series showed an incidence of 23% for complete incontinence and 17% for stress incontinence in the group operated on before 1990, and an incidence of 14% for complete incontinence and 12% for stress incontinence in patients operated on between 1990 and 1993.[13] When comparing incontinence with the type of previous radiotherapy, Ahlering and colleagues[12] showed that of the five patients with complete incontinence, only one had received external beam radiotherapy, whereas four had received brachytherapy. Total incontinence can be managed with the insertion of an artificial urinary sphincter.[8,10,12]

Bladder neck contracture and urethral strictures occurred in 19% to 25% of patients and can be managed by dilatation or visual direct urethrotomy.[8,11] The mortality rate after this procedure has been reported to be between 0%[8–10,12] and 3.2%.[13]

LOCAL FAILURE FOLLOWING RADICAL PROSTATECTOMY

Prostate cancer arises in the peripheral zone of the prostate in about 70% to 80% of cases.[18] With the advent of serial whole-mount sections from radical prostatectomy specimens, it has become evident that a large number of specimens thought to be organ confined have extraprostatic extension on pathologic examination.[19] The percentage of positive margins depends to a large extent on the initial stage of the disease and on the thoroughness of pathologic evaluation.

When analyzing prognostic factors in localized prostate cancer, we found that of 317 patients who underwent radical prostatectomy, 30% of those with T2a and 64% of those with T2b cancers had positive surgical margins.[20] Among the 152 patients with positive surgical margins, 84 (55.2%) had seminal vesicle involvement.[20] We reviewed 500 radical prostatectomies performed at Wayne State University from June 1990 to July 1993. This experience is similar to that of our previous series in that 37% of the T2a and 64% of the T2b cancers had positive surgical margins (Table 55-1).

The correlation between positive surgical margins and progression has been well established.[21] In a study by Epstein and colleagues,[21] patients were divided into three groups: those with negative margins (59%), those with focally positive margins (37%), and those with extensive positive margins (4%). The difference in progression between patients with negative margins and those with either focally or extensive positive margins was highly significant ($P < .0001$), regardless of the status of the seminal vesicles and lymph nodes.[21]

The risk of progression can also be estimated based on the correlation between surgical margins and Gleason score.[22] Progression in tumors with established penetration is adversely influenced by both the presence of positive margins and high Gleason score and can be stratified into three groups: negative

TABLE 55-1. *Relation between clinical stage and positive margins**

Stage	No. of patients	Positive margins	Negative margins
T1A	2	0	2
T1B	27	7	20
T1C	25	10	15
T2A	278	102 (37%)	176 (63%)
T2B	162	103 (64%)	59 (36%)
T3	6	5	1

* Five hundred patients treated at Wayne State University from June 1990 to July 1993.

TABLE 55-2. *Local recurrence following postop elective radiotherapy after radical prostatectomy*

Investigators	No. of patients	Positive margins, reactive seminal vesicles	Local recurrence (%)
Anscher and Prosnitz, 1987[25]	159	36 (postop elective radiotherapy)	6
		59 (no radiotherapy)	20
Hudson and Catalona, 1990[29]	21	7	28 (↑PSA)
Petrovich et al, 1991[30]	160	50	3 (clinical)
Freeman et al, 1993[31]	95	37	6 (clinical)
Link, et al, 1991[32]*	25	6	Unclear
Pontes and Forman, 1994, unpublished observations	34	15	27 (↑ PSA)

PSA; prostate-specific antigen.
* Delayed increase in serum PSA level favors long response.

margins and low grade; a combination of either positive margin or high grade, of which only one must be present; and positive margins and high grade.[21]

The mechanism of seminal vesicle involvement is closely related to capsular involvement and perforation of the capsule with migration of the cancer cells into the fatty tissues around the seminal vesicles.[19] The involvement of the seminal vesicles is prognostically associated with the development of metastases. In the original series of Jewett and colleagues,[23] no patient with seminal vesicle involvement survived 15 years without evidence of metastases. There is also a close association between seminal vesicle involvement and disease progression, because the majority of patients with lymph node metastases have seminal vesicle involvement.[24]

In identifying patients with local failure following radical prostatectomy, it is imperative to separate those patients at risk of developing distant metastases (i.e., those with seminal vesicle and lymph node involvement) from those with positive margins only (no seminal vesicle or lymph node involvement), who are at risk primarily of developing local recurrence. The latter group constitutes the ideal patients to be treated using local means of control.

Attempts at using radiotherapy as adjuvant treatment for patients failing radical prostatectomy have been made. Because in the past treatment was given for clinical local recurrence, the results of treatments were not as good as when given to patients diagnosed by early biopsy specimens following an elevated PSA level.

Because in the past treatment was given to patients not only with positive margins but often to those with seminal vesicle and lymph node involvement, the results of radiotherapy following radical prostatectomy has been controversial. Several series have addressed the effectiveness of local control and survival (Tables 55-2 and 55-3).

The effectiveness of adjuvant radiotherapy is reflected in the decrease of local recurrence, survival, or both. In all of the previously published series, there was a tendency to include patients who are at risk of developing distant metastases (see Table 55-2). Among 494 patients compiled from the literature, only 218 were ideal candidates for adjuvant radiotherapy (see Table 55-2). Among these patients, Anscher and Prosnitz[25] had the only comparative study of patients who did or did not receive postoperative radiotherapy. In their study, there was a clear advantage with postoperative radiotherapy; only 6% of patients receiving radiotherapy developed local recurrences, compared with 20% of those not treated with radiotherapy. Our results in patients with positive surgical margins and no seminal vesicle involvement are similar to those published by Hudson and Catalona[29] as they relate to elevated PSA levels as an indication of failure of radiotherapy (see Table 55-2).

Anscher and Prosnitz[25] reviewed 319 radical prostatectomies at Duke University and found 159 (50%) with positive surgical margins. Among these 159 patients, the actuarial survival of the 46 who received radiotherapy was 98% at 10 years, compared with 62% survival in the 113 patients who did not receive radiotherapy (P = .02; see Table 55-3)

Paulson and colleagues[26] reviewed the same 159 patients to analyze whether the benefits of radiotherapy actually existed. After analyzing local failure, death as a result of cancer, and death as a result of any cause, they concluded that postoperative adjuvant radiotherapy conferred no survival advantage.[26]

Meier and colleagues[27] analyzed 58 patients with positive margins after surgery at the University of California and Los Angeles. Nineteen patients received adjuvant radiotherapy and 39 patients did not. The actuarial survival and metastasis-free survival were similar for both groups; only when the patients with positive lymph nodes were excluded from the analysis did

TABLE 55-3. *Survival after postoperative radiotherapy following radical prostatectomy*

	No. of patients	Survival: Postoperative radiotherapy	Survival: No radiotherapy
Anscher and Prosnitz, 1987[25]	159	46 (10 y); 90%	113; 62% (P = .02)
Paulson et al, 1990[26]	159	No survival advantage	
Meier et al, 1992[27]	58	19	39
		No survival advantage	
Stein et al, 1992[28]	115	24 (5 y); 75%	91; 43% (P = .04)

the addition of radiotherapy result in improved recurrence-free survival (91% versus 46% at 10 years; $P = .04$).[27]

In another series of 115 patients with positive surgical margins, 24 patients received adjuvant radiotherapy.[28] At 5-year follow-up, considering PSA level as evidence of recurrence, the disease-free survival was 75% for the radiotherapy group and 43% for the surgery alone group ($P = .04$).[28]

At our institution, we base our decision regarding the need for adjuvant radiotherapy on a detailed pathologic report, available in every patient undergoing radical prostatectomy.

Patients who have a pathologically positive surgical margin with negative seminal vesicles and pelvic lymph nodes are potential candidates for postoperative radiotherapy. The decision of when to start radiotherapy is based on the postoperative PSA level. Patients with extensive positive margins whose postoperative PSA level never decreased to undetectable levels undergo radiotherapy as soon as continence returns following removal of the Foley catheter. Patients whose PSA level becomes undetectable, especially those with focal positive margins only, are followed at 3-month intervals and will receive radiotherapy if the PSA level becomes detectable. With this approach, we have selected a subgroup of patients in whom local control is still feasible despite the presence of positive margins. The impact of this approach and its associated survival is unknown, but excluding the patients who may have micrometastases, control of local disease may be important in halting progression to metastatic cancer. We believe that an aggressive approach to control local disease is important in the overall treatment of patients with localized prostate cancer, because it may impact on the prevention of metastasis as a result of progressive growth of local recurrence.

REFERENCES

1. Kurth KH, Altwein JE, Skoluda D, et al. Follow-up of irradiated prostatic carcinoma by aspiration biopsy. J Urol 1977;117:615.
2. Freiha FS, Bagshaw MA. Carcinoma of the prostate: results of postirradiation biopsy. Prostate 1984;5:19.
3. Scardino PT, Frankel JEF, Wheeler TM, et al. The prognostic significance of post-irradiation biopsy results in patients with prostatic cancer. J Urol 1986;135:510.
4. Stamey TA, Kabalin JN, Ferrari M. Prostate specific antigen in the diagnosis and treatment of adenocarcinoma of the prostate. III. Radiation treated patients. J Urol 1989;141:1084.
5. Estrada PC, Scardino PL. Total perineal prostatectomy after cobalt 60 therapy: report of a case. J Urol 1971;106:100.
6. Gill WB, Marks JE, Straus FH, Sylora HO, Diamond HM. Radical retropubic prostatectomy and retroperitoneal lymphadenectomy following radiotherapy conversion of stage C to stage B carcinoma of the prostate. J Urol 1974;111:656.
7. Spaulding JT, Whitmore WF Jr. Extended total excision of prostate adenocarcinoma. J Urol 1978;120:188.
8. Neerhut GJ, Wheeler T, Cantini M, Scardino PT. Salvage radical prostatectomy for radiorecurrent adenocarcinoma of the prostate. J Urol 1988;140:544.
9. Rainwater LM, Zincke H. Radical prostatectomy after radiation therapy for cancer of the prostate: feasibility and prognosis. J Urol 1988;140:1455.
10. Link P, Freiha FS. Radical prostatectomy after definitive radiation therapy for prostate cancer. Urol 1991;37:189.
11. Zincke H. Radical prostatectomy and exenterative procedures for local failure after radiotherapy with curative intent: comparison of outcomes. J Urol 1992;147:894.
12. Ahlering TE, Lieskovsky G, Skinner DG. Salvage surgery plus androgen deprivation for radioresistant prostatic adenocarcinoma. J Urol 1992;147:900.
13. Pontes JE. Salvage prostatectomy in recurrent carcinoma after radiotherapy. In: McGuire EJ, Catalona WJ, eds. Advances in urology, vol 8. St Louis: CV Mosby (in press).
14. Pontes JE, Montie JE. Surgical techniques for salvage prostatectomy. In: Schellhammer P, ed. Atlas of Urological Clinics of North America. Philadelphia: WB Saunders (in press).
15. Montie JE. Technique for radical cystectomy. Semin Urol 1983;1:42.
16. Montie JE, Pontes JE, Parulkar BG, Selby T. W stapled ileal neobladder formed entirely with absorbable staples. J Urol 1994;151:1188.
17. Thompson IM, Rounder JB, Spence CR, Rodriguez FR. Salvage radical prostatectomy for adenocarcinoma of the prostate. Cancer 1988;61:1464.
18. McNeal JE, Villers AA, Redwine EA, Freiha FS, Stanley TA. Capsular penetration in prostate cancer: significance for natural history and treatment. Am J Surg Pathol 1990;14:240.
19. Ohori M, Scardino PT, Lapin SL, Seale-Hawkins C, Link J, Wheeler TM. The mechanisms and prognostic significance of seminal vesicle involvement by prostate cancer. Am J Surg Pathol 1993;17:1252.
20. Pontes JE, Levin HS, Montie JE, Sakr W, Crissman J. Prognostic factors in localized prostate cancer. J Urol 1992;147:464a.
21. Epstein JI, Pizov G, Walsh PC. Correlation of pathologic findings with progression following radical prostatectomy. Cancer 1993;71:3582.
22. Epstein JI, Carmichael M, Pizov G, et al. Influence of capsular penetration on progression following radical prostatectomy: a study of 196 cases with long-term follow up. J Urol 1993;150:135.
23. Jewett JC, Eggleston JC, Yawn DH. Radical prostatectomy in the management of carcinoma of the prostate: probable cause of some therapeutic failures. J Urol 1972;107:1034.
24. Pontes JE, Wajsman Z, Huben RP, Wolf RM, Englander LS. Prognostic factors in localized prostatic carcinoma. J Urol 1985;134:1137.
25. Anscher MS, Prosnitz LR. Postoperative radiotherapy for patients with carcinoma of the prostate undergoing radical prostatectomy with positive surgical margins, seminal vesicle involvement and/or penetration through the capsule. J Urol 1987;138:1407.
26. Paulson DF, Moul JW, Robertson JE, Walther PJ. Postoperative radiotherapy of the prostate for patients undergoing radical prostatectomy with positive margins, seminal vesical involvement and/or penetration through the capsule. J Urol 1990;143:1178.
27. Meier R, Mark R, St Royal L, Tran L, Colburn G, Parker R. Postoperative radiation therapy after radical prostatectomy for prostate carcinoma. Cancer 1992;70:1960.
28. Stein A, deKernion JB, Dorey F, Smith RB. Adjuvant radiotherapy in patients post-radical prostatectomy with tumor extending through capsule or positive seminal vesicles. Urology 1992;39:59.
29. Hudson MA, Catalona WJ. Effect of adjuvant radiation therapy on prostate specific antigen following radical prostatectomy. J Urol 1990;143:1174.
30. Petrovich Z, Lieskovsky G, Langholz B, Luxton G, Jozsef G, Skinner DG. Radiotherapy following radical prostatectomy in patients with adenocarcinoma of the prostate. Int J Radiat Oncol Biol Phys 1991;21:949.
31. Freeman JA, Lieskovsky G, Cook DW, et al. Radical retropubic prostatectomy and postoperative adjuvant radiation for pathological stage C (PCNO) prostate cancer from 1976 to 1989: intermediate findings. J Urol 1993;149:1029.
32. Link P, Freiha FS, Stamey TA. Adjuvant radiation therapy in patients with detectable prostate specific antigen following radical prostatectomy. J Urol 1991;145:532.

Principles and Practice of Genitourinary Oncology, edited by Derek Raghavan, Howard I. Scher, Steven A. Leibel, and Paul H. Lange. Lippincott-Raven Publishers, Philadelphia, © 1997.

CHAPTER 56

Overview of Options for Localized Prostate Cancer

Paul F. Schellhammer, Deborah A. Kuban, and Anas M. El-Mahdi

Radical prostatectomy and external beam irradiation, the two major active intervention options directed toward treatment of localized prostate cancer, have been employed with widely varying levels of frequency and enthusiasm. Depending on the geographic locale, the decade of diagnosis, and the subspecialty interest of the treating physician, one or the other of these treatments has been specifically promoted.[1–3] The surgeons of North America recommend radical prostatectomy, radiation therapists recommend external beam irradiation, and physicians in Great Britain and Sweden favor expectant therapy. A wide variation in attitudes toward treatment exists in relatively homogeneous regions. Jonsson and colleagues[4] surveyed the Nordic countries and confirmed this (Fig. 56-1). In the United States, a Caucasian male residing in Seattle has a 6.4% likelihood of undergoing radical prostatectomy by age 75 years compared with a likelihood of 1.3% in Connecticut.[5] Outcome analysis of both radical prostatectomy and irradiation have uncovered areas of concern. Each modality has too often failed the prerequisite of successful local tumor therapy: namely, the complete ablation of local disease.

In the case of external beam radiotherapy, evidence supporting incomplete tumor ablation has come from several posttreatment biopsy studies, which find histopathology consistent with cancer even when digital rectal examination (DRE) demonstrates a favorable tumor response.[6–9] Although the viability of the tumor found on biopsy after irradiation has been questioned, the higher incidence of subsequent clinical and distant local failure among patients with positive biopsy specimen results has been well documented.[6–8] Biochemical evidence of early treatment failure is possible by measuring serum prostate-specific antigen (PSA) levels, which can identify patients at high risk of clinical failure by virtue of a postirradiation PSA nadir range higher than 1 to 2 ng/mL. Examination of biopsy material from the prostate in this cohort allows identification of histologic cancer in a large proportion of patients.[10–11] The presence of tumor at the specimen resection margin after radical prostatectomy raises concern regarding incomplete surgical removal. Even in centers where there has been a large volume of experience in performing radical prostatectomy, the incidence of positive margins for clinically organ-confined stage T1-2 (A/B) disease ranges from 20% to 50%.[12–16] Epstein[17] questioned equating a positive margin with residual tumor. He examined additional tissue that was identified as being adjacent to the positive prostate margin after prostatectomy. Of those with unequivocal margin-positive specimens, 40% had no tumor in the adjacent tissue. Of those with equivocal margin-positive specimens, 88% had no evidence of tumor in adjacent tissue, and all margin-negative specimens were accompanied by tumor-negative adjacent tissue specimens. Furthermore, in assessing the incidence of positive margins among series, it is important to recognize that the criteria employed to identify positive margins vary among pathologists.[17] However, although a positive margin finding may not be synonymous with residual tumor and may vary as a result of examiner subjectivity, patients with positive margins have a higher incidence of subsequent clinical and biochemical (i.e., PSA) failure than do patients with margin-negative specimens. This relation has been confirmed in several series.[18–21] When a detectable PSA level is included in the definition of failure, the probability of failing with margin-positive disease approaches 50% at 5 years.

Careful dissection at the apex, appropriate decisions regarding the use of bilateral or unilateral nerve-sparing or non–nerve-sparing technique, the establishment of a plane of dissection immediately anterior to the longitudinal rectal fibers to include Denonvilliers' fascia with the specimen, and wide resection of the lateral pedicles are all maneuvers that contribute to reducing the incidence of margin-positive specimens.[22] By careful attention to employing these factors, Stamey[22] reports a reduction in the incidence of margin-positive specimens to 18%. Although modern surgical techniques cannot be directly compared with those employed in past decades, the autopsy finding of unsuspected microscopic residual cancer at the vesicourethral anastomosis in 50% of patients who had radical perineal prostatectomy supports the contention that surgery is associated with a consistent incidence of failure to ablate all cancer.[23]

Logical strategies to improve the outcome of local therapy with surgery or irradiation include two avenues: more accurate staging to reduce the possibility of treating nonlocalized disease

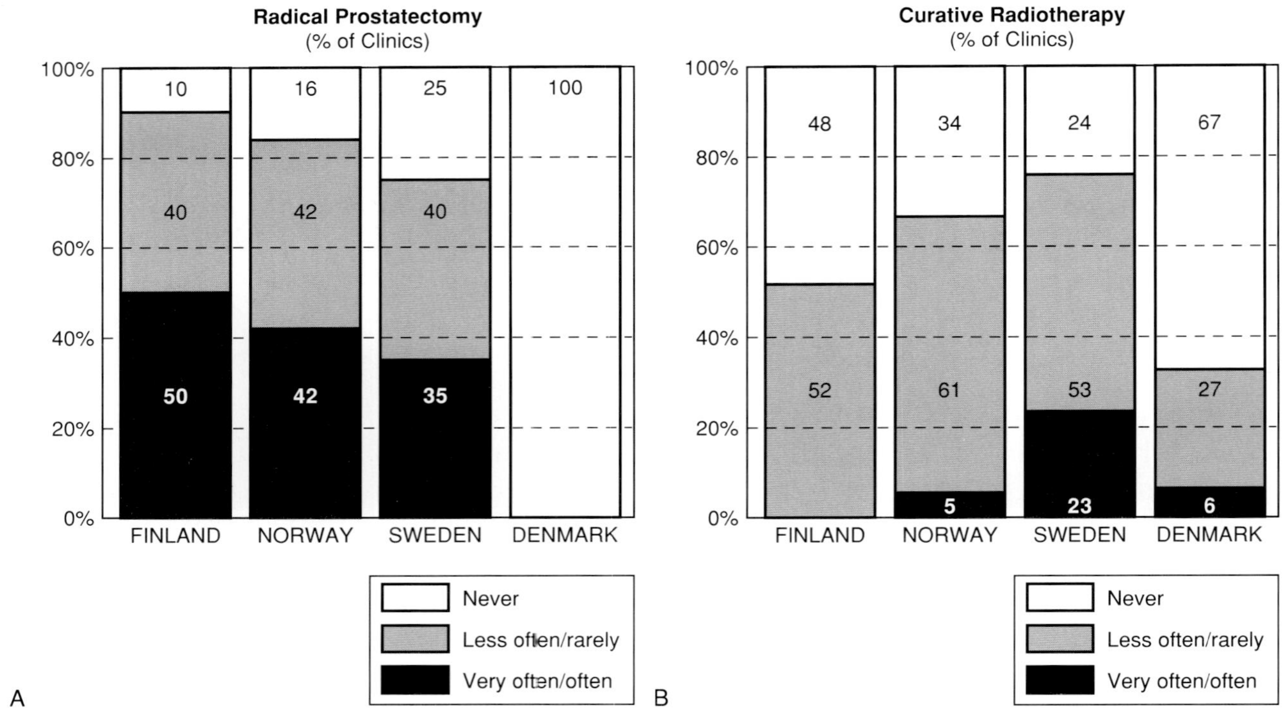

FIG. 56-1. Use of radical prostatectomy (**A**) and curative radiotherapy (**B**) in Scandinavia. Data are results of a survey in which representatives from surgical and urologic clinics were asked in a questionnaire how often they used a particular therapy in the treatment of clinically localized prostate cancer. Possible answers were "never," "rarely," "less often," "often," and "very often."[42]

and intensified initial therapy to increase the likelihood of complete ablation of local disease. The detection of low-volume metastases will always be difficult, but the introduction of radioimmunoisotope scans,[24] markers predictive of metastasis,[25] and other means of more accurate staging will identify a greater proportion of patients with minimal metastases who are incurable with local therapy. Intensification of initial therapy will include protocols testing the value of neoadjuvant androgen deprivation before radiotherapy and surgery, postirradiation adjuvant androgen deprivation, and postsurgical adjuvant irradiation. A host of new technologies, such as conformal therapy, hyperfractionated schedules for irradiation, heavy particle therapy, mixed photon–heavy particle therapy, and adjuvant hyperthermia protocols, are under investigation. New technologies have also revived old treatments. Ultrasonographically monitored interstitial brachytherapy using better isotopes,[26] remote high-dose afterloading with iridium-192, and ultrasonographically monitored cryoablation delivered via small, transperineally placed cryoprobes[27] are examples.

PROSPECTIVE RANDOMIZED TRIALS COMPARING TREATMENT OPTIONS

Comparative efficacy, morbidity, and quality-of-life assessment through analysis of prospective randomized trials for therapeutic options for localized prostate cancer are urgently needed. Despite the high prevalence and incidence of prostate cancer and the numerous controversies and questions surrounding the issue of treatment, few prospective randomized trials have been implemented. The only prospective randomized trial comparing radiotherapy with radical prostatectomy reported statistically superior progression-free survival in the surgical arm.[28] However, the trial arms contained approximately 50 patients each, and there were a number of concerns regarding the randomization process. A Southwest Oncology Group trial with a much larger cohort of patients (>500 patients per arm) was planned, but it closed because of failure to accrue patients, thereby demonstrating the great difficulty in the United States in randomizing patients to surgical versus nonsurgical options. The Prostate Intervention versus Observation Trial (PIVOT) initiative to randomize patients with localized prostate cancer to surgery or expectant therapy will face the same, and probably more formidable, obstacles regarding accrual. Scandinavian trials comparing expectant therapy to radical prostatectomy or radiotherapy are in progress. The Medical Research Council (MRC) in Great Britain is conducting a trial that will randomize 1800 patients to expectant or active treatment, consisting of radiotherapy or surgery according to the patient's choice after randomization. The results of these trials will require careful evaluation.

A prospective randomized trial initiated by the Veteran's Association Research Group in 1967 compared radical prostatectomy and placebo to placebo.[29] At 15 years' follow-up, there was no difference in survival between the two arms; however, only 94 of the 150 patients entered in the trial could be evaluated, and information concerning time to progression, subsequent interventions, and cause of death were unavailable. By the authors' admission, the trial was subject to too many uncertainties to provide meaningful conclusions. Furthermore, they noted that small series with uncertain results lead to more confusion than clarification.[29]

A prospective randomized trial was conducted by the MRC to test the benefits of radiotherapy, orchiectomy, and the combination of radiotherapy and orchiectomy in the treatment of patients with clinical stage B and C prostate cancer.[30] Approximately 100 patients were randomized into each arm between 1980 and 1985. After a follow-up period of 5 years, the incidence of metastasis was statically lower in the arms receiving orchiectomy alone and orchiectomy plus radiotherapy, demonstrating that androgen deprivation delayed the appearance of metastases. This benefit is expected when adding systemic therapy to local therapy and had been previously demonstrated in a smaller trial from the MD Anderson Cancer Center, which randomized patients with stage C disease to radiotherapy alone or radiotherapy plus diethylstilbestrol.[31] The MD Anderson trial also concluded that the combination of radiotherapy and estrogen therapy demonstrated better local control. This was also the finding of a large phase III study, Radiation Therapy Oncology Group (RTOG) trial 8610, which was preliminarily reported at the American Society of Clinical Oncology Meeting in 1993.[32] The RTOG 8610 trial randomized clinical stage B2 and C tumors to either radiotherapy alone or complete androgen blockade before and during radiotherapy. Approximately 220 patients entered each arm. At a median follow-up interval of 28 months, a statistically significant decrease in local failure, distant metastasis, and biochemical (i.e., PSA) failure was noted in the combined therapy arm. Determination of whether cancer mortality will be lower in the combined arm than in the monotherapy irradiation arm will only be available after a much longer follow-up period. The MD Anderson trial did not demonstrate a survival advantage with adjuvant hormone therapy. This could be explained by small sample size, by the confounding element of an excess of non–cancer-related morbidity secondary to estrogen, or by the fact that adjuvant androgen deprivation only serves to delay disease recurrence without decreasing cancer mortality.

The serum marker PSA has revolutionized assessment of the efficacy of a particular treatment modality in ablating cancer. The inordinately long time interval of 15 years required for clinical justification of success has probably been compressed to 5-year follow-up and is certainly less than 10 years. Regardless of the definitive treatment option studied, PSA monitoring has identified persistent tumor in patients who otherwise are judged as having obtained a clinical cure.[33–34] However, the time to interval clinical failure in a patient with a rising posttherapy PSA level may be sufficiently long to render the biochemical information of no pragmatic relevance, especially in the elderly. Nevertheless, the incidence of true cure—ablation of all cancer—is eroded with PSA monitoring, and the only reasonable conclusion is that, with time, persistent cancer will become a clinical problem in the majority of patients.

HISTORICAL SERIES

Because of the dearth of prospective randomized trials, the only avenue available for comparison of outcome among treatment modalities is through the analysis of retrospective reviews from a variety of reporting centers. An exhaustive analysis of the available literature was conducted by Adolfsson and colleagues[35] with the intent to compare the outcomes associated with radical prostatectomy, external beam irradiation, and expectant therapy. The study found that radical prostatectomy was associated with the highest 10-year disease-specific survival and the lowest incidence of progression to metastases, radiotherapy was associated with the lowest 10-year disease-specific survival and the highest incidence of progression to metastases, and the outcome of expectant therapy was between the two. The authors proposed that selection criteria were the primary determinants of end results and that treatment outcomes were therefore determined by the powerful effects of pretreatment selection of subjects.

Age, stage, grade and co-morbidity are well-recognized factors that introduce selection bias. Other selection factors are less well recognized. Two important examples of parameters that effect outcome but have not been routinely considered are the pretreatment PSA level and the race distribution of a treated cohort. Although a specific PSA level cannot identify with certainty the pathologic stage of a specific tumor, higher PSA levels are more frequently associated with advanced pathologic stage.[36] In a series reported by Zietman and colleagues,[37] a preirradiation PSA lower than 15 ng/mL was associated with a statistically higher progression-free status than a preirradiation PSA higher than 15 ng/mL within the same clinical stage category. In a large surgical series of clinical stage T1-2 (A/B) prostate cancer, the 5-year biochemical recurrence-free survival was determined by an undetectable PSA level; it was 92% when the pretreatment PSA was lower than 4 ng/mL but decreased incrementally with higher pretreatment PSA levels to a low of 45% when PSA was higher than 20 ng/mL.[38] Table 56-1 compares the distribution of pretreatment PSA levels for stage T1-2 (A/B) cancer from the surgical series from Johns Hopkins[38] and our surgical and irradiation series from Eastern Virginia Medical School. Analysis of our irradiation series showed that progressively elevated pretreatment PSA levels had an adverse impact on long-term outcome. It is evident that pretreatment PSA distribution will affect the outcome in compared series, even if they are matched by the traditional parameters of stage and grade. Another pretreatment prognostic factor that has been neglected is the race of the patient. In our irradiation series, an equal percentage of Caucasians and African Americans presented with clinical stage C disease.[39] However, grade analysis in patients with clinical stage C disease showed a higher incidence of poorly differentiated histology among African Americans. Therefore, as might be expected, the overall survival, cancer-specific survival, and freedom from progression of disease were statistically inferior for African-American men with stage C disease (Fig. 56-2). Although racial distribution differences between series may alter outcome, racial composition of treatment series has rarely been considered. These two examples of pretreatment PSA and race bias and the potential for other unknown factors that will alter outcome point to the necessity for prospective randomized trials in which such factors are balanced between treatment arms.

The advocates of surgery also differ in their approach to prostatectomy; some emphasize the benefits of the perineal approach, whereas others favor the retropubic technique. The two procedures have never been and probably never will be directly compared by prospective studies. A comparison study within

TABLE 56-1. *Incidence of PSA subsets within stage T1-2 (A-B) carcinoma of the prostate by treatment modality and location*

	No. of patients	Incidence by PSA level* (%)			
		≤4	>4–10	>10–20	>20
Johns Hopkins (surgery)	672	42	36	16	6
EVMS (surgery)	170	16	47	30	12
EVMS (radiation)	210	13	31	21	35

EVMS, Eastern Virginia Medical School; PSA, prostate-specific antigen.
* The distribution of PSA between rows 1 and 2 and between rows 2 and 3 are significantly different ($P < .0001$) by the Kruskal-Wallis test.
Data from reference 38.

a single institution reported similar incidences of positive margins and complications but a statistically significant lower amount of blood loss with the perineal approach. These urologists concluded that radical perineal and radical retropubic prostatectomy were equivalent cancer operations.[40] The major advantages of the perineal approach are decreased blood loss, decreased wound morbidity, shorter hospital stay and recovery, and more direct access to the area of urethrovesical anastomosis. The advantages of the retropubic route are a wider field of vision for resection, with the potential to decrease the positive margin rate. To paraphrase Stamey,[22] the limited access of the perineal exposure forces the surgeon to stay immediately adjacent to the prostate, whereas the retropubic exposure allows the prostate to be approached from the side walls of the pelvis. With the perineal approach, the limited view of the seminal vesicles deep within the operative field makes it necessary to enter Denonvilliers' fascia at the base of the prostate to reach the walls of the ampullae and seminal vesicles, potentially creating positive surgical margins in the 19% of cases with invasion of Denonvilliers' fascia. The reason the radical perineal prostatectomy results in less blood loss than radical retropubic prostatectomy is that the dorsal vein complex is pushed anteriorly by establishing a plane of dissection below the anterior fibromuscular stroma, which is fused imperceptibly with the fibrous tissue of the dorsal vein complex. Because this is not a natural plane of dissection, it is easy to penetrate the anterior fibromuscular tissue, expose underlying cancer, and produce a positive margin.[22] In his assessment of the positive apex margin data reported by Stamey,[22] Walther concluded "Although not specifically intending to do so, these authors [Stamey and colleagues] make a strong case for the value of radical perineal prostatectomy in achieving better cancer control at this critical site."[41] Arguments favoring one surgical approach over another will continue. The decision regarding the appropriate surgical approach will be based on the surgeon's training and familiarity with anatomy as well as his or her convictions regarding the relative merits of each approach in completely removing all cancer. The issue is probably best resolved by each surgeon performing the operation which he or she does best, but carefully monitoring the operative outcomes and studying the pathologic specimens with an interested pathologist.

EXPECTANT MANAGEMENT AS AN ALTERNATIVE TO ACTIVE TREATMENT

The purpose of early detection of prostate cancer by PSA testing is to identify disease of lesser volume and earlier stage in younger men so that local therapy can be applied more successfully (i.e., when the cancer is still organ confined). This movement evokes an elementary law of physics: namely, that a strong action is accompanied by an equal but opposite reaction. The reaction has promoted an increased interest in expectant therapy—also termed surveillance, watchful waiting, deferred therapy, or symptom-directed therapy—partly as a result

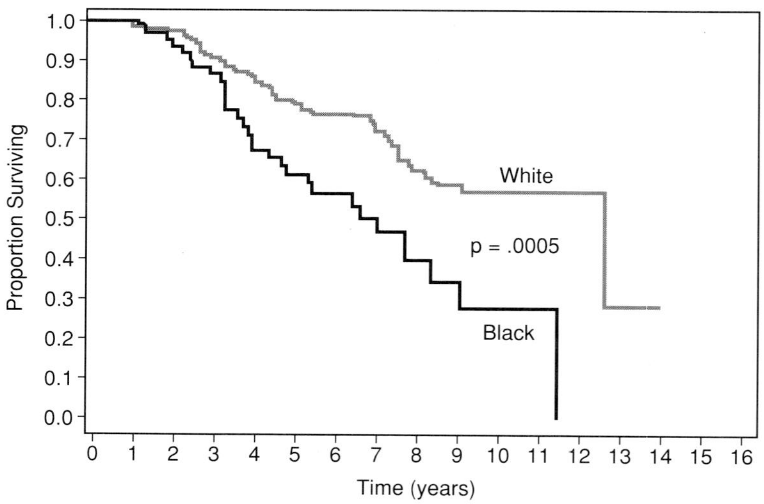

FIG. 56-2. Cancer-specific survival rates by race in patients with clinical stage C carcinoma treated by radiotherapy.

of dissatisfaction with treatment results and partly as a result of heightened interest in assessment of quality-of-life issues. Physicians have always been concerned about the quality of life of their patients, but they have not attempted to measure or to quantify this parameter in a uniform fashion. Furthermore, they have been more inclined to evaluate their perception of quality of a patient's outcome rather than the patient's personal view of quality of life. The instruments of assessment are new, unfamiliar, and difficult to standardize and analyze, but urologists need to become familiar with the concept of quality of life and the terms and instruments with which it is described and assessed. The quality-of-life parameters effected by invasive or active treatment of prostate cancer have served to direct more attention to expectant therapy, which at initial implementation is the option that interferes least with quality of life.

It is appropriate to look at enrollment criteria for expectant therapy protocols and recognize that they represent the efforts of physicians to identify patients who are more likely to die of a co-morbid disease than the prostate cancer. The most publicized of the expectant therapy protocols is that published by Johansson.[42] For the first 2 years of the study, only grade I patients, a cohort at low risk for prostate cancer death, were selected for expectant management, but not all grade I patients in the population-based sample were selected for expectant management; 199 patients had grade I histology, but only 166 were included in the expectant therapy protocol. The rest were excluded because they were not considered appropriate expectant therapy candidates; therefore, the outcome of grade I patients in this study should not be construed to predict the outcome expected for all patients with grade I cancer.

A meta-analysis compiles the results of six expectant therapy trials and provides important information.[43] The data permit calculation of time to metastases and time to death for grade I, II, and III cancer. For grade I patients identified as appropriate for expectant management, the metastatic rate (19%) at 10 years is very low. The pace of grade I disease is slow; however, the progression of grade II disease, which includes the majority of patients with prostate cancer, is faster, even among those patients selected for expectant management. Forty-two percent of patients with grade II disease develop metastases by 10 years, and 70% do so by 15 years. The median time to progression is 13 years. Because this study also reported that 50% of patients who progressed would subsequently die of prostate cancer within 3 years, it can be calculated that 25% of the entire grade II expectant therapy population will die by 16 (13 + 3) years (Fig. 56-3*A*).

This is information is useful when advising a 50-year-old patient with prostate cancer to undergo active therapy. His 26.3-year life expectancy as a Caucasian man (22.8 years for African-American men)[44] is significantly threatened by prostate cancer death. Conversely, for a 75-year-old patient, reasonable assurance can be given that his average life expectancy of 11.8 years as a Caucasian man (10.9 years for African-American men) probably will not be compromised by his prostate cancer. The meta-analysis reveals the situation to be dramatically different for a patient with grade III disease, in which the median time to progression is 5 years and 25% of the patients will be dead by 8 years (see Fig. 56-3*B*). Patients with grade III disease are not a favorable cohort from which to select individuals likely to die a from causes other than prostate cancer and therefore are not suitable for expectant management. The pace of progression of grade III prostate cancer is too rapid.

The results of this meta-analysis reflect the bias of the individual series, which was to select by disease stage, disease grade, patient age, and co-morbidity those individuals more likely to expire from causes other than prostate cancer. This selection in no way detracts from the value of expectant management as a therapeutic option. Selection is the exercise of the best judgment of the practiced clinician for his or her patient's welfare, and the favorable results reflect this. However, the results do not apply to the balance of patients who were excluded from this series and considered for other active-therapy options. Therefore, the results of any expectant series cannot mistakenly be thought to forecast outcome for the prostate cancer population in general. This same admonition applies to any series, whether it deals with expectant therapy, surgical therapy, radiotherapy, or hormonal therapy.

When a physician judges a patient to be at higher risk for death from cancer than for death from co-morbid disease, he or she will probably intervene and select an active-therapy option. If cancer mortality is reduced by treatment, one of two conclusions is reasonable: the treatment was successful in its objective or the initial patient selection was inappropriate (i.e., the patients were not actually at high risk for prostate cancer death). The only avenue to determine the correct conclusion is the prospective randomized trial. Until this information becomes available, patients must be advised and counseled regarding their treatment choices based on the outcomes of retrospective analysis. The Prostate Outcomes Research Team (PORT) has used decision modeling analysis to compare the active options of external beam irradiation and surgery to the expectant protocols using outcome and quality of life as endpoints.[45] The results favored active treatment only under specific circumstances. Using the most optimistic assumptions regarding treatment efficacy among men 60 to 65 years of age with moderately or poorly differentiated tumors, a benefit with radical prostatectomy and irradiation over watchful waiting was noted. Men with well-differentiated tumors did not benefit from active treatment because the rate of progression of disease was too slow to permit benefit to occur within the patient's life expectancy. For men 70 years of age or older, invasive therapy did not provide an advantage to watchful waiting, and when quality-of-life issues were considered, it actually proved disadvantageous or harmful.

The Markov model, which has been used to generate these assessments, requires precise figures for rate of metastasis after treatment of local disease. This figure, which is the linchpin in driving the outcome analysis, is not precisely known. The PORT team based their calculations on selected series which included 498 patients (381 stage A, 117 stage B) treated by expectant therapy and 299 patients (240 stage A, 59 stage B) treated by surgery.

The question regarding whether these small sample populations are representative of the whole population is a legitimate concern. Small changes in the rate of metastasis will generate different results. For example, using a rate of metastasis derived from the meta-analysis study rates, which differed from those used by the PORT analyses, Scardino and colleagues[46] reported a greater advantage with surgical therapy than that reported by the PORT study. Moreover, progression rates calculated from the series studied by PORT span wide confidence intervals. For example, the annual metastatic rate for stage A was calculated to range from .01 to .043 and for stage B was from .03 to .07; the annual cancer death rate for stage A was 0 to .009 and for

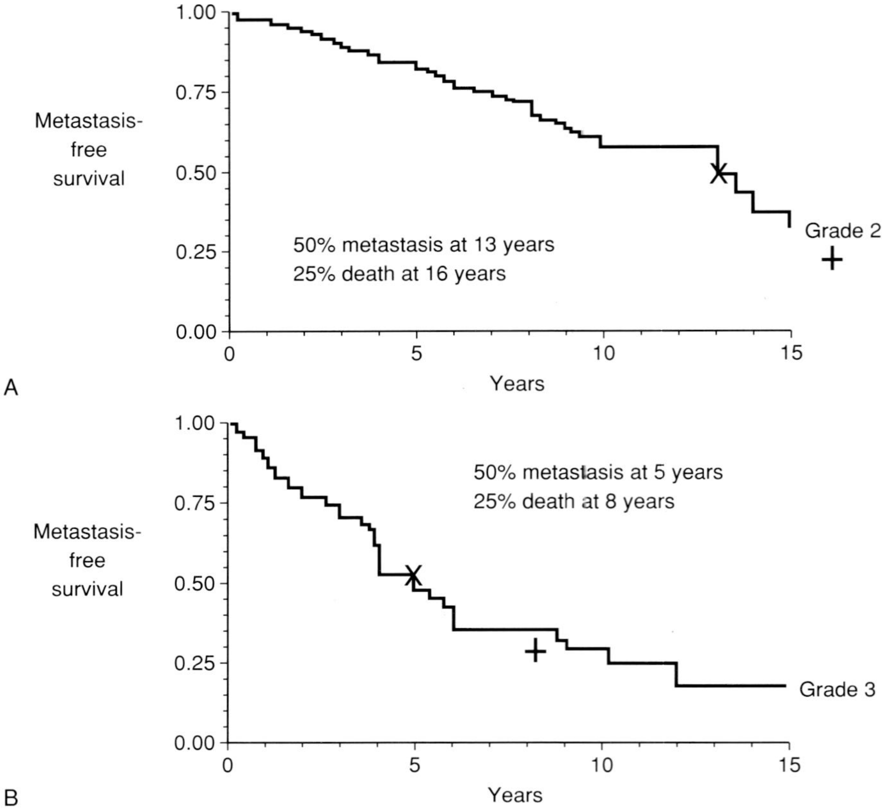

FIG. 56-3. (**A**) Metastasis-free survival rates for untreated patients with localized grade 2 prostate cancer according to tumor grade. (**B**) Metastasis-free survival rates for untreated patients with localized grade 3 prostate cancer according to tumor grade (From Chodak GW, Thisted RA, Gerber GS, et al. Results of conservative management of clinically localized prostate cancer. N Engl J Med 1994; 330:242.)

stage B was .007 to .027.[47] Small changes in these rates within these ranges would alter the measured endpoint. Before generalizing the variable results of these relatively small series to the overall population with prostate cancer, more data is necessary. Furthermore, the utility values placed on treatment morbidity are somewhat arbitrary and need to be refined.

TREATMENT SELECTION

How are treatment options selected and what are the relative proportions of each treatment in urologic practice? The American College of Surgeons' data reveal that in the decade from 1974 to 1983, 72.9% of stage A and 28.1% of stage B patients were treated by transurethral resection only (expectant therapy); 4.4% and 13.6% of those with stage A and B disease, respectively, were treated by radical prostatectomy; and 12.2% and 35.8% of those with stage A and B disease, respectively, were treated by irradiation.[48] Selection by age of patient is not available from this data. A 1990 update from the American College of Surgeons described changing trends from the 1984 statistics.[49] Overall, the use of radical prostatectomy had increased from 8.9% to 21.4%; expectant therapy had decreased from 36.1% to 28.9%, and use of irradiation was stable at 22.6%. Specific analysis by stage, grade, and age were not reported. We reviewed our experience at Eastern Virginia Medical School between 1988 and 1993 with attention to the assignment of therapy options by age. Our patient population is generally representative of a community experience rather than a referral practice. For example, of the newly diagnosed patients who presented during this 6-year interval, 80% had their biopsy in our department, identifying us as the primary urologists. The patients were divided into those aged younger than 70 years or those 70 years of age and older. When analyzed by year of diagnosis, there has been a progressive rise in the use of radical prostatectomy for T1-2 (A/B) disease and a progressive decrease in the use of irradiation in men younger than 70 years of age. Expectant therapy in this age group has been stable at 10% to 15%. For men 70 years or older, the incidence of radiotherapy and expectant therapy is consistent at 40% to 50% each, and the incidence of surgery is less than 10% (Fig. 56-4).

Expectant management should be considered more frequently as age increases. Whether the age cutoff point employed is 70, 72, or 75 years depends on physiologic age and the patient's attitude toward active versus deferred treatment. However, with advancing age, expectant therapy becomes more appropriate, and surgical therapy becomes less desirable. In a study of radical prostatectomy reimbursed under Medicare, preoperative mortality rose from less than 1% for males less than 75 years of age to more than 4.6% for those older than 80 years.[2] There are some who would consider this decision as reflecting good clinical judgment (discussed previously); however, others may deem it as discriminatory. An article in *Cancer* in 1991 entitled "Patterns of Care Related to Age of Men with Prostate Cancer"[50] examined the assignment of therapies for patients with prostate cancer by patient age. Older patients were more frequently assigned to observation or androgen deprivation, whereas younger patients were more frequently directed to surgery or radiotherapy. The media seized on this apparent

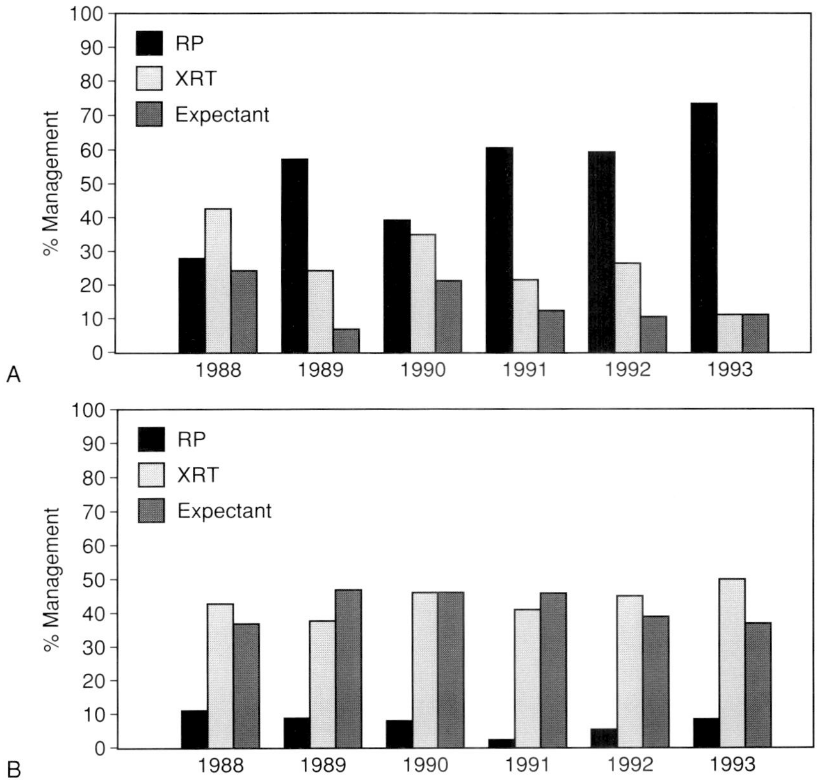

FIG. 56-4. Treatment selection for clinical stage T1/T2 (A/B) carcinoma of the prostate for men less than 70 years old (**A**) and aged 70 years or older (**B**) by year at Eastern Virginia Medical School. RP, radical prostatectomy; XRT, radiotherapy.

discrimination and published the following provocative headline "Study in Prostate Cancer Reinforces Theory of Medical Bias Against the Elderly." Lost in the reporting were the risks associated with active therapy. Although these risks have been reported from single centers of excellence by the treating physicians, there is a lack of broad-based assessment of treatment morbidity and impact on quality of life from the patients perspective.

TREATMENT MORBIDITY

Fowler and colleagues[51] conducted a patient survey to estimate the probability of complications and follow-up treatment as perceived by the patient. Five percent of Medicare patients who underwent radical prostatectomy between 1988 to 1990 were included. Respondents reported their current status with respect to continence and sexual function. Also tabulated were postsurgical treatments for persistent cancer or to correct surgical complications.

From the sample as a whole, 63% of men reported current problems with urinary wetness. Thirty-one percent responded that they wear pads, adult diapers, or a clamp to deal with leakage. Complete lack of control, evidenced by a permanent indwelling urinary catheter, was reported by 2%; 6% reported that they had had another surgical intervention in an attempt to correct incontinence or improve continence.

Prior to the radical prostatectomy, 91% of the patients claim to have had some erectile function. Following surgery, only 11% said they had erections firm enough for intercourse during the month prior to the survey.

Twenty percent of patients have had at least one dilation or other surgical procedure for stricture; 11% had more than one procedure. The more time that had elapsed since surgery, the higher the risk of treatment failure as reflected by the increasing incidence of additional cancer treatments. Within 2 years postsurgery, 16% required treatment; at 3 and 4 years postsurgery, these figures were 22% and 28%, respectively (Table 56-2).

Using essentially the same survey instrument, the University of Wisconsin obtained data from patients who had been treated with radical prostatectomy[52,53] and irradiation: 93 surgical patients were polled and 86 (92%) responded; 119 irradiation patients were polled and 106 (91%) responded. For the surgical group, mean posttreatment follow-up was 22.5 months and mean age at treatment was 64 years; for the irradiation group, mean posttreatment follow-up was 31 months and mean age at treatment was 71 years. This study reported a morbidity rate higher than might have been predicted (see Table 56-2); however despite these complications, 74% were satisfied with surgery, and 88% said they would have surgery again. Only 8% rated their medical care or outcome as poor. For the irradiated patients, 82% were satisfied with therapy, 92% would have irradiation again, and only 5% rated their care or outcome as poor.

As noted in these surveys, local cancer recurrence is a legitimate cause of morbidity stemming from treatment failure. We retrospectively analyzed treatment failure morbidity related to surgery and irradiation. The most immediate and significant consequence of local failure is the high association with subsequent distant failure. In our Eastern Virginia Medical School experience with external beam irradiation, there was a statisti-

TABLE 56-2. *Incidence and type of treatment morbidity by type of therapy*

Type of morbidity	University of Wisconsin patients (%) Radiotherapy (n = 106)	Radical prostatectomy (n = 87)	Radical prostatectomy (n = 757)
No current urinary dripping	61	26	37
Dripping at least some urine daily	28	59	47
Dripping more than a few drops of urine daily	13	30	23
Using pad	10	47	31
Dripping urine when coughing	21	48	43
Dripping urine with full bladder	38	59	44
Surgery to correct incontinence	2	3	6
Recalled being able to have erection before treatment	78	84	91
No partial or full erection since treatment	50	53	61
No erection in past month	19	15	17
Erection in the past month but not firm enough for intercourse	19	16	11
Erection firm enough for intercourse	13	16	11
Treatment for impotence	11	17	15
Urethral strictures	6	20	20
More than one treatment for urethral strictures	3	12	11

cally higher incidence of distant failure within each stage and grade when patients with local failure were compared with patients with local disease c control.[54] In addition to the association with subsequent metastases, local failure can produce significant local morbidity. This was especially the case in attempts to treat those with clinical stage C disease, in whom, despite androgen deprivation at failure, there was a significant morbidity after radical prostatectomy and irradiation.[55] Efforts to improve local control are obviously important, but local persistent or recurrent disease is not the paramount obstacle in dealing with failure of prostate cancer treatment. In analyzing our data to determine what if any additional benefit could be achieved by assuming that ideal irradiation would provide local control in 100% of patients, an overall survival advantage of approximately 10% to 15% was calculated.[56] The group of patients who fail at distant sites with or without clinical local failure present the greater problem. The development of effective therapy for systemic disease must proceed in tandem with efforts to improve local control.

CONCLUSIONS

Urologists have used their best judgment and intuition to construct general and individualized treatment pathways for patients with prostate cancer. As in so many other areas of medicine, treatment recommendations have evolved through the formative opinions of mentors and the accumulation of personal experience as well as within the constraints of the economic, cultural, and social climate of practice. However, these pathways of clinical judgment are under challenge by observations of wide practice variation and practitioner uncertainty.[56] The urologic community is witnessing the implementation of a number of clinical trials to test the validity and benefit of practice concepts previously deemed intuitively sound. Documentation beyond expert testimony or consensus statement are being sought before recommending a particular intervention. The Prostate, Lung, Colon and Ovary (PLCO) screening trial was designed to determine whether prostate cancer mortality is reduced with annual PSA and DRE screening.[57] Although screening for breast cancer by mammography has demonstrated the capacity to reduce breast cancer mortality in many trials, this information cannot be automatically transferred to prostate cancer. The PLCO trial will compare mortality between men randomized to the screened arm versus men randomized to a routine care, nonscreened, control arm.

The PIVOT protocol[58] will test the specific advantage of the time-honored procedure of radical prostatectomy against expectant or deferred therapy with androgen deprivation at the time of symptomatic or metastatic progression. As new technology and treatments are instituted (e.g., cryosurgery; conformal, heavy particle, and interstitial radiotherapy; high-intensity focused ultrasonography; neoadjuvant and adjuvant combinations), trials assessing comparative efficacy, cost, and morbidity will be necessary.

The PIVOT study should logically have preceded the PLCO study, because the utility of screening for early detection of cancer rests on the presumption of effective therapy for the cancer detected. If effective therapy is not available, then early detection is useless. However, the time necessary to complete these trials sequentially is long; therefore, they are being conducted simultaneously. Even so, time is a critical issue. The results of these trials will not be available for more than 15 years, and there is no guarantee that these trials will be completed or that their findings will be conclusive. In the interim, approximately 200,000 new cases of and approximately 40,000 deaths from cancer of the prostate will occur yearly. The clinical urologist will continue to face the dilemma of what treatment course is advisable. He or she can best do this by offering responsible direction toward expectant management to men with low-volume, low-grade tumors who have an anticipated life expectancy of less than 10 years and whose co-morbidity is likely to determine longevity. There is risk in this recommendation, and this risk, as with the risk of active intervention, must be made an appropriately shared risk through patient education and participation in the decision. The challenge is to identify tumor markers that characterize the biologic activity of prostate cancer so that decisions regarding active treatment versus surveillance for younger men can be made with a greater degree of certainty than is currently possible.

REFERENCES

1. Moore M, O'Sullivan B, Tannock I. How expert physicians would wish to be treated if they developed genitourinary malignancies. J Clin Oncol 1991;6:1736.
2. Lu-Yao GL, McLerran D, Wasson J, Wennberg JE, Patient Outcomes Research Team. An assessment of radical prostatectomy: time trends, geographic variation, and outcomes. JAMA 1993;269:2633.
3. Mettlin C, Murphy GP, Menck H. Trends in treatment of localized prostate cancer by radical prostatectomy: observations from the commission on cancer national cancer database, 1985–1990. Urology 1994; 43(4):488.
4. Jonsson PM, Danneskiold-Samsøe B, Heggestad T, Iversen P, Leisti S. Management of early prostatic cancer in the Nordic countries: variations in clinical policies and physicians' attitudes toward radical treatment options. A Nordic Evaluation of Medical Technology (NEMT) survey. Int J Technol Assess 1995;11:66.
5. Lu-Yao GL, Greenberg ER. Changes in prostate cancer incidence and treatment in USA. Lancet 1994;343:251.
6. Scardino PT, Wheeler TM. Local control of prostate cancer with radiotherapy: frequency and prognostic significance of positive results of postirradiation prostate biopsy. NCI Monogr 1988;7:95.
7. Schellhammer PF, El-Mahdi AM, Higgins EM, Schultheiss TE, Ladaga LE, Babb TJ. Prostate biopsy after definitive treatment by interstitial iodine implant or external beam radiation therapy. J Urol 1987;137: 897.
8. Miller EB, Ladaga LE, Schellhammer PF, et al. Reevaluation of prostate biopsy after definitive radiation therapy. Urology 1993;41(4):311.
9. Freiha FS, Bagshaw MA. Carcinoma of the prostate: results of postirradiation biopsy. Prostate 1984;5:19.
10. Dugan T, Shipley W, Young R, et al. Biopsy after external beam radiation therapy for adenocarcinoma of the prostate: correlation with original histological grade and current prostate specific antigen levels. J Urol 1991;146:1313.
11. Goad JR, Chang S, Ohori M, et al. PSA after definitive radiotherapy for clinically localized prostate cancer. Urol Clin North Am 1993;20(4): 727.
12. Stamey TA, Villers AA, McNeal JE, et al. Positive surgical margins at radical prostatectomy: importance of the apical dissection. J Urol 1990;143:1166.
13. Rosen MA, Goldstone L, Lapin S, et al. Frequency and location of extracapsular extension and positive surgical margins in radical prostatectomy specimens. J Urol 1992;148:331.
14. Wahle S, Reznicek M, Fallon B, Platz C, Williams R. Incidence of surgical margin involvement in various forms of prostatectomy. Urology 1990;36:23.
15. Ackerman DA, Barry JM, Wicklund RA, et al. Analysis of risk factors associated with prostate cancer extension to the surgical margin and pelvic node metastasis at radical prostatectomy. J Urol 1993;150:1845.
16. Catalona WJ, Bigg SW. Nerve-sparing radical prostatectomy: evaluation of results after 250 patients. J Urol 1990;143:538.
17. Epstein JI. Evaluation of radical prostatectomy capsular margins of resection: the significance of margins designated as negative, closely approaching, and positive. Am J Surg Pathol 1990;14:626.
18. Morton RA, Steiner MS, Walsh PC. Cancer control following anatomical radical prostatectomy: an interim report. J Urol 1991;145:1197.
19. Frazier HA, Robertson JE, Humphrey PA, Paulson DF. Is prostate specific antigen of clinical importance in evaluating outcome after radical prostatectomy. J Urol 1993;149:516.
20. Paulson DF, Moul JW, Walther PJ. Radical prostatectomy for clinical stage T1-2N0M0 prostatic adenocarcinoma: long-term results. J Urol 1990;144:1180.
21. Epstein JI, Carmichael MJ, Partin AW, et al. Is tumor volume an independent predictor of progression following radical prostatectomy? A multivariate analysis of 185 clinical stage B adenocarcinomas of the prostate with 5 years of follow-up. J Urol 1993;149:1478.
22. Stamey TA. Techniques for avoiding positive surgical margins during radical prostatectomy. Atlas Clin North Am 1994;2(2):37.
23. Oesterling JE, Epstein JI, Walsh PC. Long-term autopsy findings following radical prostatectomy. Urology 1982;29:584.
24. Abdel-Nabi H, Wright GK, Gulfo JV, et al. Monoclonal antibodies and radioimmuno-conjugates in the diagnosis and treatment of prostate cancer. Semin Urol 1992;10(1):45.
25. Veltri RW, Epstein JI, Partin AW, et al. Multivariate statistical modeling of biomarkers as predictors of recurrence following radical prostatectomy. Am Urol Assoc Abstr 1994;452;340A.
26. Blasko JC, Ragde H, Grimm PD. Transperineal ultrasound guided implantation of the prostate: morbidity and complications. Scand J Urol Nephrol 1991;137(Suppl):113.
27. Onik GM, Cohen JK, Reyes GD, et al. Transrectal ultrasound-guided percutaneous radical cryosurgical ablation of the prostate. Cancer 1993; 72:1291.
28. Paulson DF, Lin GH, Hinshaw W, et al. Radical surgery versus radiotherapy for adenocarcinoma of the prostate. J Urol 1982;128:502.
29. Madsen PO, Graverson PH, Gasser TC, et al. Treatment of localized prostate cancer: radical prostatectomy versus placebo: a 15-year follow-up. Scand J Urol Nephrol 1988;110(Suppl):95.
30. Fellows GJ, Clark PB, Beynon LL, et al. Treatment of advanced localised prostatic cancer by orchiectomy, radiotherapy, or combined treatment. Br J Urol 1992;70:304.
31. Zagars GK, Johnson DE, von Eschenbach AC, et al. Adjuvant estrogen following radiation therapy for stage C adenocarcinoma of the prostate: long-term results of a prospective randomized study. Int J Radiat Oncol Biol Phys 1988;14:1085.
32. Pilepich MV, Krall J, Al-Sarraf M, et al. A phase III trial of androgen suppression before and during radiation therapy (RT) for locally advanced prostatic carcinoma: preliminary report of RTOG protocol 8610. [Abstract 703] Proc Am Soc Clin Oncol 1993;12:229.
33. Stein A, deKernion JB, Smith RB, et al. Prostate-specific antigen levels after radical prostatectomy in patients with organ-confined and locally extensive prostate cancer. J Urol 1992;147:942.
34. Schellhammer PF, El-Mahdi A, Wright GL, et al. Prostate specific antigen to determine progression-free survival after radiation therapy for localized carcinoma of the prostate. Urology 1993;42(1):13.
35. Adolfsson J, Steineck G, Whitmore WF Jr. Recent results of management of palpable clinically localized prostate cancer. Cancer 1993; 72(2):310.
36. Oesterling JE, Chan DW, Epstein JI, et al. Prostate-specific antigen in the preoperative and postoperative evaluation of localized prostatic cancer treated with radical prostatectomy. J Urol 1988;139:766.
37. Zietman AL, Coen JJ, Shipley WU, Willett CG, Efird JT. Radical radiation therapy in the management of prostatic adenocarcinoma: the initial prostate specific antigen value as a predictor of treatment outcome. J Urol 1994;151:640.
38. Partin AW, Pound CR, Clemens JQ, Epstein JI, Walsh PC. Serum PSA after anatomic radical prostatectomy: the Johns Hopkins experience after 10 years. Urol Clin North Am 1993;20:713.
39. Kim JA, Kuban DA, El-Mahdi AM, Schellhammer PF. Race as a prognostic indicator in definitively irradiated prostatic carcinoma. [Abstract] Radiology Suppl 1993;189(P):184.
40. Frazier HA, Robertson JE, Paulson DF. Radical prostatectomy: the pros and cons of the perineal versus retropubic approach. J Urol 1992; 147:888.
41. Walther PJ. Radical perineal vs. retropubic prostatectomy: a review of optimal application and technical considerations in the utilization of these exposures. Eur Urol 1993;24(Suppl 2):34.
42. Johansson JE, Adami HO, Andersson SO, Bergström R, Holmberg L, Krusemo UB. High 10-year survival rate in patients with early, untreated prostatic cancer. JAMA 1992;267:2191.
43. Chodak GW, Thisted RA, Gerber GS, et al. Results of conservative management of clinically localized prostate cancer. N Engl J Med 1994; 330:242.
44. Life table: statistical abstract of the United States, 1991: the national date book. Washington DC: US Department of Commerce Economics and Statistics Administration, Bureau of the Census 1991:73.
45. Fleming C, Wasson JH, Albertsen PC, Barry MJ, Wennberg JE. A decision analysis of alternative treatment strategies for clinically localized prostate cancer: Prostate Patient Outcomes Research Team. JAMA 1993;269:2650.

46. Scardino PT, Beck JR, Miles BJ. Letter to the editor. N Engl J Med 1994;330:1831.
47. Wasson JH, Cushman CC, Bruskewitz RC, et al. A structured literature review of treatment for localized prostate cancer. Arch Fam Med 1993; 2:487.
48. Schmidt JD, Mettlin CJ, Natarajan N, et al. Trends in patterns of care for prostatic cancer, 1974–1983: results of surveys by the American College of Surgeons. J Urol 1986;136:416.
49. Mettlin C, Jones GW, Murphy GP. Trends in prostate cancer care in the united states, 1974–1990: observations from the Patient Care Evaluation Studies of the American College of Surgeons Commission on Cancer. CA Cancer J Clin 1993:43:83.
50. Bennett CL, Greenfield S, Aronow H, Ganz P, Vogelzang NJ, Elashoff RM. Patterns of care related to age of men with prostate cancer. Cancer 1991;67:2633.
51. Fowler FJ Jr, Barry MJ, Lu-Yao G, Roman A, Wasson J, Wennberg JE. Patient-reported complications and follow-up treatment after radical prostatectomy: the national Medicare experience: 1988–1990 [Updated June 1993] Urology 1993;42:622.
52. Jonler M, Messing EM, Rhodes PR, Bruskewitz RC. Sequelae of radical prostatectomy. Brit J Urol 1994;74:352.
53. Jonler M, Ritter MA, Brinkmann R, Messing EM, Rhodes PR, Bruskewitz RC. Sequelae of definitive radiation therapy for prostate cancer localized to the pelvis. Urology 1994;44:876.
54. Kuban DA, El-Mahdi AM, Schellhammer PF. The potential benefit of improved local tumor control in prostate carcinoma. Presented at the 76th Annual Meeting of the American Radium Society, April 22-26, 1994, Southampton, Bermuda.
55. Schellhammer PF, Whitmore RB III, Kuban DA, et al. Morbidity and mortality of local failure after definitive therapy for prostate cancer. J Urol 1989;141:570.
56. Eddy DM. The challenge. JAMA 1990;263:287.
57. Gohagan JK, Early Detection Branch, Early Detection and Community Oncology Program, DCPC, NCI, NIH. A 16-year randomized screening trial for prostate, lung, colon, and ovarian cancer (PLCO).
58. Wilt TJ, VA-CSP-407 NCI T94-01310 PIVOT. Phase III randomized study of prostatectomy vs expectant observation with palliative therapy for stage I/II prostate cancer (PIVOT).

Principles and Practice of Genitourinary Oncology, edited by Derek Raghavan, Howard I. Scher, Steven A. Leibel, and Paul H. Lange. Lippincott-Raven Publishers, Philadelphia, © 1997.

CHAPTER 57

Hormonal Manipulation for Metastatic Prostate Cancer

57.1 Androgen Withdrawal Therapy: New Perspectives in the Treatment of Prostate Cancer

S. Larry Goldenberg and Nicholas Bruchovsky

The ablation of testicular function for the palliative treatment of prostate cancer was first attempted in the 1930s with radioorchiectomy.[1] This proved less effective than surgical orchiectomy, which was introduced about a decade later by Huggins and Hodges[2] and became the gold standard of treatment. No other treatment exists that equals or surpasses androgen ablation in checking the growth of prostate cancer and reducing its volume in 60% to 80% of patients. However, for reasons that remain unknown, the cell death process induced by androgen ablation fails to eliminate the entire malignant cell population. The result is inevitable progression to a state of androgen-independent tumor growth.

The past decade has seen a proliferation of therapeutic alternatives. Drugs affecting the hypothalamic production of luteinizing hormone–releasing hormone (i.e., LHRH analogs) and drugs blocking the peripheral effects of androgens (i.e., steroidal and nonsteroidal antiandrogens) have been used alone or in various combinations to achieve medical castration. Many questions remain regarding their differing efficacies, toxicities, and costs and whether or not a new gold standard of therapy has been attained. This chapter discusses the issues of tumor regulation, androgen independence, and complete and incomplete androgen-deprivation strategies. It also reviews new strategies of hormonal therapy in early stages of disease and intermittent androgen suppression.

ESSENTIAL MECHANISMS OF ANDROGEN-MEDIATED TUMOR REGULATION

In normal conditions, three essential levels of androgen-mediated regulation determine the size of the prostate and can be activated to check malignant growth (Fig. 57.1-1)[3]: positive effects on initiation of DNA synthesis and cell proliferation; negative or inhibitory effects that limit the number of cells in the prostate; and apoptosis (i.e., autophagic lysis), a form of controlled cell death that occurs in the prostate when androgens are withdrawn and results in the active elimination of cells from the epithelial compartment of the gland.

Androgen dependence is the clinical manifestation of apoptosis after androgen withdrawal in both normal and malignant tissues.[4] In the early stages of prostate cancer, only the second, or negative, type of regulation is missing.[4] Because the other two mechanisms are still functional, androgen ablation has the double effect of triggering apoptosis and inhibiting DNA synthesis and cell proliferation. Even in malignancy, the ability to undergo apoptosis is acquired as a feature of differentiation under the influence of androgens; thus, in the absence of androgens, it is impossible for dividing cells to differentiate and become preapoptotic again.[4,5] This explains why recurrent tumor growth is characterized by androgen independence.

LIMITATIONS OF ANDROGEN WITHDRAWAL THERAPY

An increased rate of progression to androgen independence is a serious limitation of conventional androgen ablation.[6] It has been appreciated for some time that progression to androgen independence is initiated by androgen withdrawal.[6] Foulds[7] and Noble[8] have both demonstrated that because the tumor cell is responsive to its environment, efforts to kill the cell by withdrawing androgens from their cellular milieu results immediately or after a delay in the induction of progressive autonomy. Restoring the environment to its normal state of hormonal balance may offer a pathway for the repair of cellular mechanisms and reverse aberrant metabolic pathways. Treatment goals should change from an attempt to kill every cancer cell by

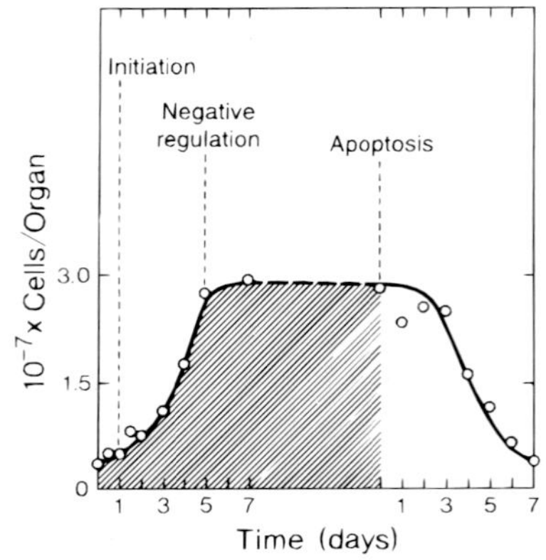

FIG. 57.1-1. Androgenic regulation of the prostate occurs in three steps: initiation of DNA synthesis and cell proliferation by androgens; negative feedback regulation; apoptosis (i.e., autophagic lysis).

potent androgen ablation approaches to an attempt to regain biologic control of the tumor cells' growth and response to subsequent androgen ablation.[9]

In the absence of androgens, it seems that androgen-dependent cells generate proteins that limit the amount of cell death in the population of malignant cells. New growth factors that substitute for androgens in stimulating the growth of tumor cells may also be produced. Androgen withdrawal based on the use of LHRH agonists and antiandrogens may be slightly more effective than surgical orchiectomy in bringing about the death of tumor cells, but ultimately, the cell death pathway is circumvented by survival mechanisms and new growth factors.

PROGNOSTIC INDICATORS DURING ANDROGEN WITHDRAWAL THERAPY

A summary of prognostic indicators during androgen withdrawal therapy in patients with advanced prostate cancer is provided in Table 57.1-1.

Serum Prostate-Specific Antigen Level Response to Therapy

Serial prostate-specific antigen (PSA) determinations appear to be a reliable marker for disease response and progression, with minimal random fluctuations between measurements in patients with metastatic tumor.[10–12] We have observed that at least 32 weeks of treatment are necessary to bring the serum PSA level into the normal range in about 70% of men with advanced prostate cancer.[13] In the remaining 30% of patients, serum PSA levels will decrease temporarily and then increase; if a plateau is reached, it will be short-lived or stabilize outside of the normal range. This is usually a sign of early progression to androgen independence and is associated with a poor prognosis. In a series by Bruchovsky and colleagues,[13] if the serum PSA level remains above 4 ng/mL between 24 and 32 weeks of treatment, the median survival time is only 18 months. Conversely, if the serum PSA level is below 4 ng/mL between 24 and 32 weeks of therapy, the median survival time is much greater (40 months). It has been observed that the rate of normalization is faster between 0 and 10 weeks than in the succeeding interval between 10 and 32 weeks of initial treatment.[13] From this point onward, the serum PSA level remains abnormal in about 30% of patients (as described previously), with little chance of treatment producing a normal result beyond 32 weeks.

Nature and Burden of Metastatic Disease

Potent androgen withdrawal therapy is highly effective in inducing the regression of the primary prostatic tumor and soft tissue metastases. However, even the strongest forms of androgen withdrawal therapy cannot cure metastatic prostate cancer because of an inherent inability to eliminate the more lethal, skeletal component of the disease. In a series of 51 patients treated with cyproterone acetate plus low-dose diethylstilbestrol (DES), 41 of 49 patients (84%) with evaluable local and metastatic soft tissue disease responded with a reduction in tumor volume.[14] In contrast, significant improvement occurred in only 13 (27%) of the 48 initially abnormal bone scans. This difference clearly demonstrates the relative resistance of skeletal metastases to potent androgen withdrawal therapy, as has also been noted by other investigators.[15]

Matzkin and colleagues[16] documented that patients with fewer than six metastatic deposits as seen on bone scan had a significantly better 2-year survival than those with more extensive disease. Both the National Cancer Institute (NCI) Intergroup study[17] and the European Organization for the Research and Treatment of Cancer (EORTC) 30853 trial[18] showed that the number and location of bone metastases have a strong effect on treatment outcome. The good-prognosis group (i.e., those

Table 57-1. *Summary of prognostic indicators in advanced prostate cancer*

Prognostic indicator	Risk category: Good	Risk category: Poor
Prostate-specific antigen level at 24 and 32 weeks of therapy	Normal	Elevated
Number of bone metastases	≤5	>5
Tumor grade	Well to moderately well differentiated	Poorly-differentiated
Tumor ploidy	Diploid	Aneuploid
Pretreatment hemoglobin	≥85 g/L	<85 g/L
Pretreatment testosterone	≥300 ng/dL	<300 ng/dL
Alkaline phosphatase	<1.25 × ULN	>1.25 × ULN

ULN, upper limit of normal.

with 5 or fewer metastases confined to the axial skeleton) and patients with good performance status tended to derive the most benefit from treatment.

Other Prognostic Factors

The grade and ploidy of the primary tumor are important predictors of cancer behavior.[19] A low pretreatment serum testosterone level (<300 ng/dL),[16] the presence of anemia (hemoglobin <85 g/L), and an elevated alkaline phosphatase (>1.25 times the upper limit of normal) are all considered important negative prognostic indicators.[15,20]

"ONE-TIME" CONTINUOUS CASTRATION

The synthesis of testosterone by the Leydig's cells of the testis is stimulated by pituitary luteinizing hormone (LH) and accounts for 90% or more of the dihydrotestosterone formed in the prostate. The remaining sources of testosterone are weak adrenal androgens and dietary sources. Serum testosterone, by acting as a negative feedback signal to the hypothalamus, regulates the secretion of LHRH and thus also of LH. As summarized in Figure 57.1-2, methods of medical and surgical castration eliminate 90% of testosterone from the blood, antiandrogens prevent the translocation of the cytoplasmic form of androgen receptor into the nucleus, and 5α-reductase inhibitors prevent the conversion of testosterone to dihydrotestosterone.

Initiation of Therapy

We believe that it is intuitively evident that treatment should commence at the time of diagnosis of locally advanced or metastatic disease. The NCI Intergroup[17] and EORTC 30853[18] studies have clearly demonstrated that in patients with low-volume disease and good performance status, there is a longer time to disease progression and increased overall survival. A clinical trial of oral estrogen therapy in men with locally extensive cancer has shown that the chances of developing metastases within 5 years can be decreased from 50% to 20% by therapy.[21] Experimental data from studies on animal models of prostate cancer indicate that androgen withdrawal therapy is more effective when started early in the treatment of a tumor.[22–24]

Patients with good prognostic characteristics at the time of diagnosis respond well for a prolonged period of time. Patients with poor prognostic factors, and especially those with failure of PSA normalization at 32 weeks, die within 18 months. Decisions about therapy must also take into consideration the implications of impotence, the impact of drug effects on quality of life, and the fact that no form of treatment can guarantee prevention of androgen-independent progression.

Surgical Castration

"One-time" surgical castration is associated with minimal morbidity and mortality, is cost-effective, and has guaranteed patient compliance. With 60% to 80% response rates, it has always been the standard against which all other forms of male hormone withdrawal are measured. The main advantage of bilateral orchiectomy in managing advanced symptomatic disease is the rapid lowering of serum testosterone. Lin and colleagues[25] found that the castration time for surgical orchiectomy ranged from 3 to 12 hours (mean, 8.6 hours). The corresponding time for oral estrogen castration was from 21 to 60 days (mean, 38.3 days). The major disadvantages of surgical castration are that it is irreversible, causes hot flushes in 40% of patients, and arguably causes significant psychological trauma.[26,27]

Medical (Nonsurgical) Castration

Estrogen Therapy

The first form of so-called medical castration involved the daily administration of oral estrogen, which acts at the hypotha-

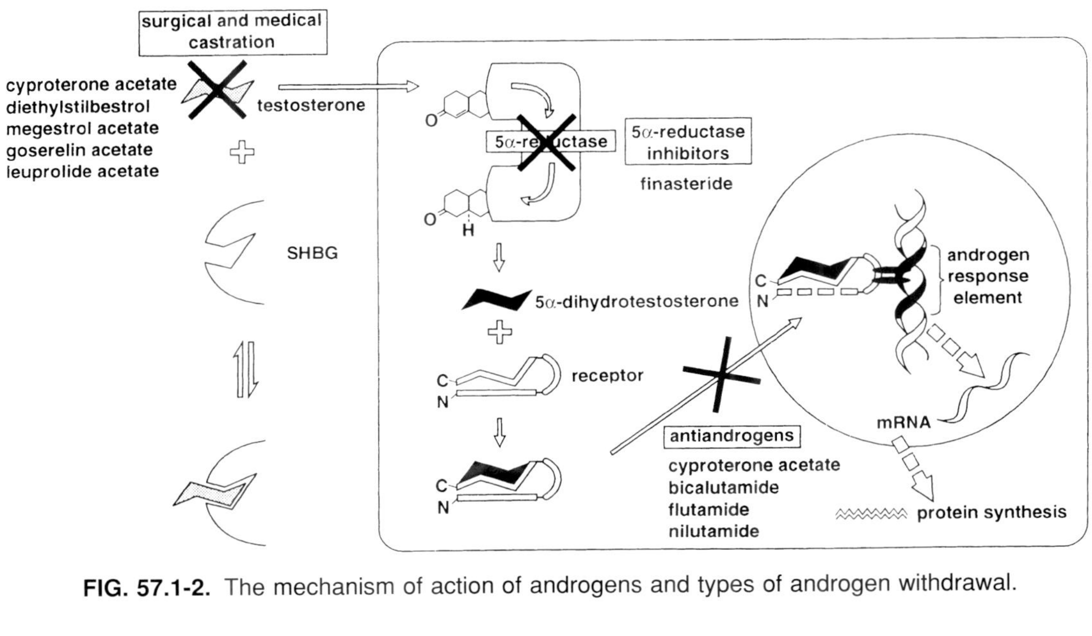

FIG. 57.1-2. The mechanism of action of androgens and types of androgen withdrawal.

lamic level to shut off the production of LHRH. A cascade of effects ultimately reduces the synthesis of testosterone by the testes. The results of estrogen therapy are discussed in detail in Chapter 57.2.

Although estrogen therapy is effective and relatively cheap, it does have significant side effects. Besides decreasing libido and depressing sexual function, it causes gynecomastia. This complication can be prevented by a single dose of radiation to the breast area. Estrogen can also lead to fluid retention, with the possibility of weight gain, edema, congestive heart failure, deep vein thrombosis, pulmonary embolus, myocardial infarction, and stroke.[21,28,29] For these reasons and because of the development of safer alternative drugs, estrogen has lost much of its popularity as therapy for the management of prostate cancer.

Luteinizing Hormone–Releasing Hormone Analogs

The development of LHRH analogs[30] such as leuprolide acetate and goserelin acetate has made nonsurgical castration the preferred option for many patients. Available in depot forms, these drugs are easily administered and produce castration levels of serum testosterone. Therapy consists of leuprolide acetate (7.5 mg) or goserelin acetate (3.6 mg) repeated every 4 weeks. Leuprolide acetate is formulated as microspheres for intramuscular injection, and goserelin acetate is formulated as a cylindrical plug for subcutaneous injection.

LHRH agonists are synthetic analogs of natural gonadotropin-releasing factor, and because of minor changes in amino acid composition, they possess greater potency than the parent hormone. After administration, a paradoxic effect is observed, consisting of an initial stimulation of pituitary release of LH and follicle-stimulating hormone (FSH) followed after 1 to 2 weeks by a gradual inhibition of these hormones.[29] In synchrony with the LH and FSH levels, the concentration of serum testosterone first rises and then falls to castration levels. This transient elevation of serum testosterone may initially stimulate tumor growth (i.e., flare reaction), and about 10% of patients experience exacerbation of pain.[29,31–33] After the initial rise, which lasts 2 to 3 days, serum testosterone levels decrease into the castration range over 10 to 14 days. To avoid the possibility of flare reaction complications, antiandrogens are sometimes administered, either temporarily or on a continuous basis, prior to or concurrently with an LHRH agonist. LHRH analogs cause frequent hot flushes (63%),[33] loss of libido and potency, and are readily reversible; there is a delay of at least 12 weeks after the last injection before serum testosterone returns to normal.[29,34] LHRH analogs have been shown to be equivalent to estrogen therapy[29] and orchiectomy[33] but are contraindicated as monotherapy in patients with impending spinal cord compression or advanced urinary tract obstruction because of the risk of disease flare reaction.

Steroidal Antiandrogens

There are two principal steroidal antiandrogens: cyproterone acetate and megestrol acetate. Clinical and animal studies have found cyproterone acetate to be more efficacious than megestrol acetate.[35] These agents, because of their progestational activity, override normal negative feedback inhibition. The result is antigonadotropic suppression of LHRH, LH, and consequently, androgen production by the testes. Serum testosterone decreases slowly to a plateau concentration that is usually about 30% of normal. It has been observed that cyproterone acetate therapy alone is unable to completely suppress gonadotropin release and androgen production; its effect apparently weakens after 6 to 9 months of therapy.[36,37] However, the predominant activity of cyproterone acetate is competitive inhibition of androgens at the target cell level.[38] Following administration of cyproterone acetate, the concentrations of dihydrotestosterone and nuclear androgen receptor are reduced. The strong antiandrogenic action in the prostate inhibits the effects of the noncastration level of serum testosterone.

Taking advantage of the synergism between progestational and estrogenic compounds,[35,39] Goldenberg and colleagues[14] studied the effects of a low dose of DES (0.1 mg/day orally) combined with cyproterone acetate (200 mg/day orally) in 51 patients with stage D2 prostate cancer. The rapid decrease of serum testosterone into the castration range (often within 1 week and in all patients by 2 months; mean, 25 days) could not be ascribed to DES alone, because at a dose of 0.1 mg daily, DES has no effect on serum testosterone.[40] Furthermore, the weakening of the antigonadotropic effect of cyproterone acetate expected after 6 to 9 months of treatment was not evident with the coadministration of DES.

An overall objective response rate of 98% was observed. The actuarial median time to progression was 17 months and the median survival time, 24 months. True surviving fractions at 12, 24, 36, and 60 months were 84, 51, 34 and 15 percent, respectively.[14] It was concluded that cyproterone acetate plus low-dose DES could be used as a potent form of androgen withdrawal therapy to bring about regression of the primary tumor and soft tissue metastases with a high degree of reliability.

Therapy with either progestational agent features reversibility of effects, as well as the side effects of loss of libido and potency, some nipple tenderness and breast swelling, loss of energy, occasional shortness of breath, rare occurrences of depression, and deep vein thrombosis. The frequency of hot flushes with cyproterone acetate or megestrol acetate* is low.

Nonsteroidal Antiandrogens

The nonsteroidal or pure antiandrogens act only at the cellular level, without any gonadotropic or progestational effects. The interruption of the normal negative feedback mechanism results in compensatory release of LH and elevated serum testosterone. The normal or slightly raised testosterone level permits the preservation of libido and potency in 70% to 80% of patients[41,42] but causes concern over whether peripheral blockade provides sufficient androgen withdrawal.[43] For this reason, nonsteroidal antiandrogens are generally used in combination with bilateral orchiectomy or LHRH analogs to obtain total androgen blockade. The three drugs in this class are flutamide (750 mg daily), nilutamide (300 mg daily) and bicalutamide (Casodex; 50 mg daily), all of which are structurally related.

The use of flutamide as monotherapy for prostate cancer has been described in several small, inconclusive, nonrandomized

* Megestrol acetate may also have some androgenic funtion and its use may result in a tumor flare in 10% of cases.

clinical trials.[41,42,44] The most frequent side effects are gynecomastia as a result of unopposed estrogen, diarrhea, and nausea. Hepatocellular toxicity may occur and, although usually reversible, has caused death in some cases.[45] The flutamide withdrawal syndrome should be considered in patients progressing while on total androgen blockade with a pure antiandrogen.[46]

Nilutamide has toxicities that include visual disturbances (light-dark adaptation), mild nausea, alcohol intolerance, and rarely, the serious condition of acute interstitial pneumonitis.[47,48]

The newest of this class of antiandrogen is bicalutamide, which is still under investigation. The major advantage of this drug is once-per-day dosing and less toxicity, which nevertheless includes breast tenderness, gynecomastia, and diarrhea.[49,50]

TOTAL ANDROGEN BLOCKADE

Numerous clinical trials have explored the possibility that combined androgen blockade offers an advantage over standard therapy. This issue is addressed in Chapter 57.2. Both the NCI Intergroup[17] and EORTC 30853[18] studies demonstrated improved time to progression and overall survival, particularly in patients with minimal disease burden, but this has not been a consistent trend in other clinical trials. It remains unclear whether differences between trials reflect random variations or reproducible results that ultimately emerge with the inclusion of larger numbers of patients. A detailed meta-analysis of 22 international studies involving 5710 patients with advanced prostate cancer has been reported.[51,52] This study showed that 26.2% of 2720 patients in the combined androgen blockade group and 22.8% of 2705 patients in the partial deprivation group were projected to be alive at 5 years after initiation of therapy. In this analysis, those in the combined androgen blockade group were judged to have a 7% reduced risk of death. However, the standard deviation was 4%; therefore, the gap between the two groups was not statistically significant. A final conclusion of this meta-analysis awaits further follow-up in some of the included trials. The validity of such an overview analysis has been discussed by Blumenstein.[53]

Although the results remain inconclusive, it does appear that androgen withdrawal based on the combined use of LHRH agonists and antiandrogens may be slightly more effective than surgical orchiectomy in bringing about the death of tumor cells in a subset of patients with minimal skeletal or soft tissue metastases.

REVERSIBLE ANDROGEN WITHDRAWAL

Reversible androgen withdrawal therapy usually takes the form of nonsurgical castration combined with an antiandrogen. The criteria for an ideal combination include rapid suppression of androgen, rapid reversibility, absence of flare reaction, absence of hot flushes, low toxicity, dose-response effect, and ease of administration. The most commonly used agents are LHRH agonists combined with a nonsteroidal antiandrogen. This combination features rapid onset of action; reduced or no risk of clinical flare reaction; high incidence of hot flushes; frequent antiandrogen-related nausea, vomiting, and diarrhea; occasional hepatotoxicity; loss of libido and potency; reversibility; and reduced compliance because of gastrointestinal symptoms.

We prefer to utilize lead-in therapy[13] with cyproterone acetate (100 mg/day) and DES (0.1 mg/day) administered for 4 weeks; this reduces the serum testosterone level into the castration range within 3 to 7 days in most patients and eliminates the possibility of a flare reaction. The LHRH agonist is started and DES is stopped after 4 weeks of lead-in therapy, but cyproterone acetate is continued to prevent hot flushes. Serum testosterone level recovers to the normal range 8 to 16 weeks after termination of therapy. This regimen features rapid onset of action, no risk of flare reaction, very low incidence of hot flushes, few if any side effects other than loss of libido and potency, dose-response effect, predictable reversibility, and excellent compliance.

Strategies

Cytoreduction (Combined Modality Therapy)

A better understanding of the biology of prostate cancer has highlighted the fact that the risk of systemic spread is already appreciable at the time of initial diagnosis. Under such conditions, the results of radical therapy will be less than optimal, although it may still be indicated for control of local or regional disease. Preoperative treatment for 3 to 8 months with a reversible androgen withdrawal agent affords the possibility of downstaging the primary tumor and eradicating micrometastases. Theoretically, this approach should result in improved survival and is the subject of several ongoing trials (see Chap. 54). We studied the concept of prolonging the course of neoadjuvant therapy until the PSA level reaches its nadir or becomes undetectable.[54] This occurred in 85% of patients by 8 months. Of individuals treated for at least 6 months, 91% had disease that was pathologically confined to the gland, and the majority of tumors were focal or of small volume.

Adjuvant Therapy

The role of hormone withdrawal therapy in patients with pathologic stage C disease following radical prostatectomy has not been studied. The advantage of this form of therapy is that both local and subclinical metastatic disease may be responsive. In animal studies, Henry and Isaacs[22] demonstrated that the probability of cure decreased as the size of the primary tumor increased if there was a delay in starting adjuvant chemotherapy. Similarly, Isaacs[23] demonstrated that androgen ablation therapy is optimally effective when used as early as possible. In clinical trials, Zincke and colleagues[55] combined the use of surgery and immediate androgen ablation in 43 patients with pathologic stage C prostate cancer. These patients did as well as a historical group who had pathologic stage B prostate cancer. These observations are consistent with the results of Benson and colleagues,[56] who projected a 76% 10-year survival in 40 patients treated using radical prostatectomy and immediate orchiectomy.

Bruchovsky and colleagues[24] have demonstrated that androgen withdrawal produces a 2 logarithm cell kill in the androgen-dependent Shionogi's mouse mammary carcinoma model. This implies that a tumor should be treated when fewer than 100 stem cells are present in each metastatic lesion. If it is assumed that failure rates following local therapy are the result of metastatic disease present at the time of initial treatment, then immediate hormone withdrawal may lead to killing of sufficient stem cells in small metastatic foci to cure early disseminated disease. The optimal duration of adjuvant hormonal therapy has not been established. Regression of soft tissue tumor commonly occurs within 3 to 6 months of initiation of therapy, suggesting that 6 to 12 months of treatment may be sufficient to achieve sustained tumor control. This would be consistent with the observations of Spirnak and Resnick[57] who noted that patients treated with orchiectomy for metastatic disease experienced regression of prostatic tumor within 6 months.

Intermittent Androgen Suppression

In attempting to avert or delay progression to the androgen-independent state, it has been hypothesized that if malignant cells that survive androgen withdrawal are forced into a normal pathway of differentiation by androgen replacement,[58] then apoptotic potential might be restored, thus setting the stage for another response to androgen withdrawal (Fig. 57.1-3). The results of experiments on animal tumor models suggest that intermittent androgen suppression delays progression to androgen independence but does not prevent it. In both experimental (Fig. 57.1-4) and clinical carcinomas (Fig. 57.1-5), apoptosis can be induced multiple times using successive cycles of androgen withdrawal and replacement.

The potential for a full recovery from the side effects of therapy makes it possible to alternate a patient between periods of treatment and no treatment. Only those patients whose serum PSA level has reached a stable or decreasing value in a normal range between 24 and 32 weeks of therapy should be considered eligible for intermittent androgen suppression with interruption of the therapy at 36 weeks. When the patient is off treatment, the function of the testes and the concentration of serum testosterone slowly return to normal over a period of 8 to 14 weeks. Quality of life is improved with recovery of sexual function and a normal sense of well being. In response to this incremental androgenic stimulus, atrophic cells are recruited into a normal pathway of differentiation in which the risk of progression is low. With the associated movement through the division cycle, the cells once again become preapoptotic, making it possible to repeat therapy.

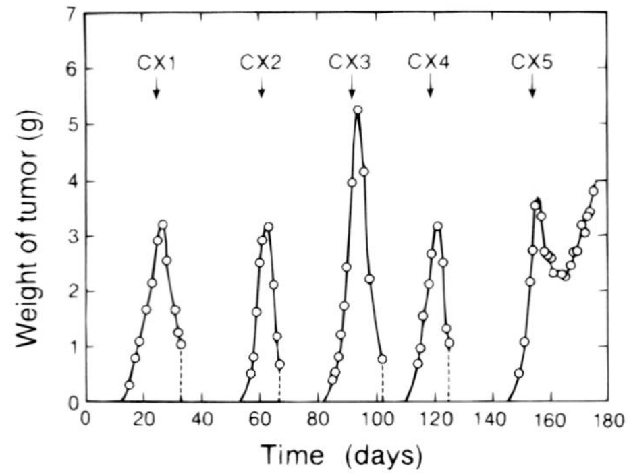

FIG. 57.1-4. Effects of intermittent androgen suppression on Shionogi's carcinoma. About 5 – 10^6 Shionogi's carcinoma cells were injected into a male DDS-strain mouse. When the tumor reached a weight of 3 g, the host animal was castrated (CX1–CX5). After the tumor had regressed to a weight of 1 g, it was implanted into a noncastrated male mouse. This cycle of transplantation and castration was repeated five times. (From Akakura K, Bruchovsky N, Goldenberg SL, Rennie PS, Buckley AR, Sullivan LD. Effects of intermittent androgen suppression on androgen-dependent tumours: apoptosis and serum prostate specific antigen. Cancer 1993; 71:2782.)

Whether intermittent androgen suppression and its effects on tumor progression alter survival in a beneficial or adverse way is unknown, although the possibility of an improved outcome has been considered by Klotz and colleagues.[59] The experience of Goldenberg and colleagues[60] confirms that treatment of patients by intermittent androgen suppression is clinically tenable. Observations were made on a group of 47 patients (clinical

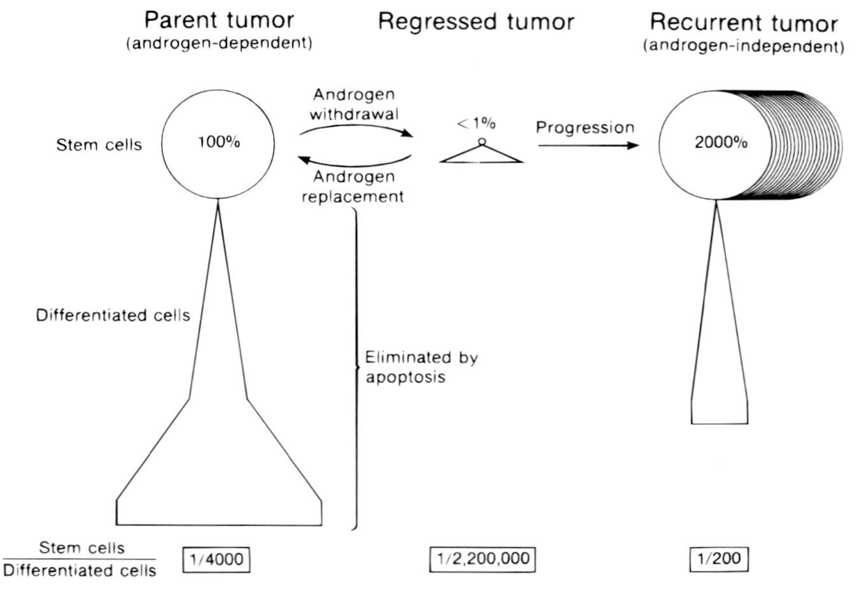

FIG. 57.1-3. Model of stem cell composition of the androgen-dependent Shionogi's carcinoma. The ratio of stem cells to differentiated cells changes after androgen withdrawal. Androgen replacement stimulates the differentiation of stem cells in the regressed tumor, and apoptotic potential is recovered. (From Akakura K, Bruchovsky N, Goldenberg SL, Rennie PS, Buckley AR, Sullivan LD. Effects of intermittent androgen suppression on androgen-dependent tumours: apoptosis and serum prostate specific antigen. Cancer 1993;71:2782.)

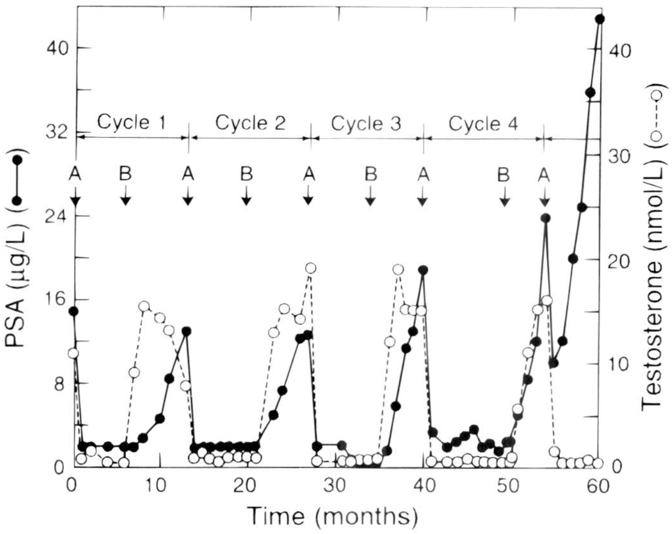

FIG. 57.1-5. Effects of intermittent androgen suppression on prostate cancer in a 57-year-old man with a single lumbar metastasis and local progression of previously irradiated, stage C, moderately differentiated carcinoma. Androgen suppression started at time A and was interrupted at time B, yielding treatment intervals of 6, 7, 7, and 9 months and no-treatment intervals of 7, 7, 6, and 5 months, respectively. ○, serum testosterone; ●, serum prostrate serum antigen (PSA). (Adapted from Akakura K, Bruchovsky N, Goldenberg SL, Rennie PS, Buckley AR, Sullivan LD. Effects of intermittent androgen suppression on androgen-dependent tumours: apoptosis and serum prostate specific antigen. Cancer 1993;71:2782.)

stages: 14 patients with D2 disease, 10 with D1, 19 with C, 2 with B2 and 2 with A2) with a mean follow-up time of 125 weeks. Treatment with combined androgen blockade was continued for at least 6 months until a serum PSA nadir was observed. Medication was then withheld until the serum PSA level increased to a mean value between 10 and 20 ng/mL. This cycle of treatment and no treatment was repeated until the regulation of serum PSA became androgen independent. With each of the first two treatment cycles, the overall mean percentage time off therapy was between 41% and 45%. Serum testosterone returned to the normal range within an average of 8 weeks of discontinuing treatment. The off-treatment period in both cycles was associated with an improvement in the patient's sense of well being and the recovery of libido and potency in men who reported normal or near-normal sexual function before the start of therapy. In 7 patients with stage D2 disease, the cancer progressed to an androgen-independent state. The mean and median times to progression were similar to the expected results with continuous androgen ablation. More information will become available from planned clinical trials of intermittent androgen suppression.

TREATMENT OF EMERGENCY CONDITIONS

Urinary retention is a common presentation of patients with prostate cancer. Rapid relief of urethral obstruction can be obtained with catheterization and subsequent transurethral resection. Procedures that result in a rapid decline of serum testosterone can also be used to bring about regression of the obstructing lesion, particularly in the high-risk surgical patient or the individual with extensive local disease.[61] Orchiectomy and the use of cyproterone acetate or ketoconazole are recommended for this purpose.

When a patient presents with signs of impending spinal cord compression or hydronephrosis, it is reasonable to add an agent such as cyproterone acetate to conventional management. The use of an LHRH agonist is not advised, because an acute elevation in the concentration of serum testosterone may stimulate tumor growth and exacerbate the condition.

Coagulation disorders complicating prostatic cancer have been well-recognized entities for some time but remain rare. The disseminated intravascular coagulation syndrome that occurs is most likely the result of a slow, continuous release of thromboplastic material from tumor cells, with fibrinolysis occurring secondarily. In addition to appropriate replacement of blood, platelets, and clotting factors, prompt treatment of the cancer is required to correct the underlying pathophysiologic defect. This has been carried out successfully with high-dose intravenous DES diphosphate (Honvol)[62] or ketoconazole.[63]

TREATMENT OF HOT FLUSHES

The normal neuroendocrine mechanism for control of thermoregulation is centered within the hypothalamus.[31] When orchiectomy or LHRH agonist therapy leads to a peripheral androgen deficit, inhibitory factors, presumably opioid peptides, which are normally stimulated in the presence of sex steroids, are no longer released from the hypothalamus. This results in increased central adrenergic activity, with release of norepinephrine and inappropriate stimulation of thermoregulatory centers; body heat is lost through peripheral vasodilation and manifests as hot flushes.

This effect can be blocked by the administration of central antiadrenergic medication (clonidine)[64] or steroids with central inhibitory action such as exogenous testosterone (which is clearly contraindicated in prostate cancer), estrogens[65] (which are relatively contraindicated because of side effects) or progestogens.[66] Low-dose megestrol acetate[67] or cyproterone acetate in a dose of 100 mg/day orally has been successful in significantly suppressing hot flushes with a minimum of side effects.[13,68,69] Repression of hot flushes cannot be achieved with pure nonsteroidal antiandrogens (e.g., flutamide), which lack a central antigonadotrophic effect.

CONCLUSIONS

The history of androgens is old and prodigious, yet the hormonal nature of androgens was not discovered until the early

20th century. Fifty years ago, prostate cancer was proven to be responsive to orchiectomy and estrogen therapy, and various types of androgen withdrawal therapies have become increasingly accepted as conventional treatment. Reversible treatments based on the use of LHRH analogs and antiandrogens offer flexibility and have a number of applications in the therapy of patients with different stages of prostate cancer. Of considerable interest is the use of neoadjuvant and adjuvant endocrine manipulations. Intermittent androgen suppression offers the potential for long-term control of prostate cancer while maximizing quality of life. In the near future, it is likely that the indications for the use of antiandrogens will expand, as will the number of antiandrogenic agents.

REFERENCES

1. Sharifi R, Kiefer J. History of endocrine manipulation in the treatment of carcinoma of the prostate: who was first? J Endocrinol Invest 1987; 10(Suppl 2):91.
2. Huggins C, Hodges CV. Studies on prostate cancer. I. Effect of castration, estrogen, and androgen injection on serum phosphatases in metastatic carcinoma of the prostate. Cancer Res 1941;1:293.
3. Bruchovsky N. Androgens and antiandrogens. In: Holland JF, Frei III E, Bast RC, Kufe DW, Morton DL, and Weichselbaum RR, eds. Cancer medicine, 3rd ed. Philadelphia: Lea & Febiger, 1993:884.
4. Bruchovsky N, Brown EM, Coppin CM, et al. The endocrinology and treatment of prostate tumour progression. In: Coffey DS, Bruchovsky N, Gardner WA Jr, Resnick MI, Karr JP, eds. Current concepts and approaches to the study of prostate cancer: progress in clinical and biological research. New York: Alan R Liss, 1987:348.
5. Akakura K, Bruchovsky N, Goldenberg SL, Rennie PS, Buckley AR, Sullivan LD. Effects of intermittent androgen suppression on androgen-dependent tumours: apoptosis and serum prostate specific antigen. Cancer 1993;71:2782.
6. Gleave M, Hsieh J-T, Wu H-C, von Eschenbach AC, Chung LWK. Serum prostate specific antigen levels in mice bearing human prostate LNCaP tumors are determined by tumor volume and endocrine and growth factors. Cancer Res 1992;52:1598.
7. Foulds L. Neoplastic development, vol. 1. New York: Academic Press, 1969:69.
8. Noble RL. Hormonal control of growth and progression in tumors of Nb rats and a theory of action. Cancer Res 1977;37:82.
9. Schipper H, Goh CR, Lim Wang T. Rethinking cancer: should we control rather than kill? Part 2. Cancer J Oncol 1993;3:220.
10. Maatman TJ. The role of prostate specific antigen as a tumor marker in men with advanced adenocarcinoma of the prostate. J Urol 1989; 141:1378.
11. Stamey TA, Kabalin JN, Ferrari T, Yang N. Prostate specific antigen in the diagnosis and treatment of adenocarcinoma of the prostate IV: antiandrogen-treated patients. J Urol 1989;141:1088.
12. Matzkin H, Eber P, Todd B, van der Zwaag R, Soloway MS. Prognostic significance of changes in prostate-specific markers after endocrine treatment of stage D2 prostatic cancer. Cancer 1992;70:2302.
13. Bruchovsky N, Goldenberg SL, Akakura K, Rennie PS. LHRH agonists in prostate cancer: elimination of flare reaction by pretreatment with cyproterone acetate and low-dose diethylstilbestrol. Cancer 1993;72: 1685.
14. Goldenberg SL, Bruchovsky N, Rennie PS, Coppin CM. The combination of cyproterone acetate and low dose diethylstilbestrol in the treatment of advanced prostatic carcinoma. J Urol 1988;140:1460.
15. Fossa SD, Heilo A, Lindegaard M, Skinningrud A, Ous S. Clinical significance of routine follow-up examinations in patients with metastatic cancer of the prostate under hormone treatment. Eur Urol 1983; 9:262.
16. Matzkin H, Perito PE, Soloway MS. Prognostic factors in metastatic prostate cancer. Cancer 1993;72:3788.
17. Crawford ED, Eisenberger MA, McLeod DG, et al. A controlled trial of leuprolide with and without flutamide in prostatic carcinoma. N Engl J Med 1989;321:419
18. Denis LJ, Whelan P, Carneiro De Moura JL, et al. Goserelin acetate and flutamide versus bilateral orchiectomy. Urology 1993;42:119.
19. Soloway MS. The importance of prognostic factors in advanced prostate cancer. Cancer 1990;66:1017.
20. Mulders PFA, Dijkman GA, Fernandez del Moral P, Theeuwes AGM, Debruyne FML, Members of the Dutch Southeastern Urological Cooperative Group. Analysis of prognostic factors in disseminated prostatic cancer. Cancer 1990;65:2758.
21. Byar DP, Corle DK. Hormone therapy for prostate cancer: results of the Veterans Administration Cooperative Urological Research Group studies. NCI Monogr 1988;7:165.
22. Henry JM, Isaacs JT. Relationship between tumor size and the curability of metastatic prostatic cancer by surgery alone or in combination with adjuvant chemotherapy. J Urol 1988;139:1119.
23. Isaacs JT. The timing of androgen ablation therapy and/or chemotherapy in the treatment of prostatic cancer. Prostate 1984;5:1.
24. Bruchovsky N, Rennie PS, Coldman AJ, Goldenberg SL, To M, Lawson D. The effects of androgen withdrawal on the stem cell composition of the Shionogi carcinoma. Cancer Res 1990;50:2275.
25. Lin BJT, Kuang-Kuo C, Ming-Tsun C, Chang LS. The time for serum testosterone to reach castrate level after bilateral orchiectomy or oral estrogen in the management of metastatic prostate cancer. Urology 1994;43:834.
26. Cassileth BR, Soloway MS, Vogelzang NJ, et al. Patients' choice of treatment in stage D prostate cancer. Urology 1989;33:57.
27. Chadwick DJ, Gillatt DA, Gingell JC. Medical or surgical orchidectomy: the patients' choice. Br Med J 1991;302:572.
28. Veterans Administrative Cooperative Urological Research Group. The effect of treatment on survival of patients with cancer of the prostate. Surg Gynecol Obstet 1967;124:1011.
29. The Leuprolide Study Group. Leuprolide versus diethylstilbestrol for metastatic prostate cancer. N Engl J Med 1984;311:1281.
30. Coy DH, Schally AV. Gonadotropin releasing hormone analogues. Ann Clin Res 1978;10:139.
31. Neumann F, El Etreby MF, Habenicht UF, Radlmaier A, Bormacher K. Pharmacological basis of androgen deprivation by various antiandrogens and their combination with LHRH agonists. In: Klosterhalfen H, ed. Endocrine management of prostatic cancer. Berlin: de Gruyter, 1988:57.
32. Schroeder FH, Lock T, Chada DR, et al. Metastatic cancer of the prostate managed with buserelin versus buserelin plus cyproterone acetate. J Urol 1987;137:912.
33. Kaisary AV, Tyrrell CJ, Peeling WB, Griffiths K. Comparison of LHRH analogue (Zoladex) with orchiectomy in patients with metastatic prostate cancer. Br J Urol 1991;67:502.
34. Soloway MS, Chodak G, Vogelzang NJ, et al. Zoladex versus orchiectomy in the treatment of advanced prostate cancer: a randomized trial. Urology 1991;37:46.
35. Rennie PS, Bruchovsky N, Goldenberg SL, et al. Relative effectiveness of alternative androgen withdrawal therapies in initiating regression of rat prostate. J Urol 1988;139:1337.
36. Tunn UW, Graff J, Senge TH. Treatment of inoperable prostatic cancer with cyproterone acetate. In: Schroeder FH, ed. Androgens and antiandrogens. The Netherlands: Weesp, Schering Nederland BV, 1983:149.
37. Goldenberg SL, Bruchovsky NB. Use of cyproterone acetate in prostate cancer. Urol Clin North Am 1991;18:111
38. Neumann F, Humpel N, Senge TH, Schenck B, Tunn U. Cyproterone acetate: biochemical and biological basis for treatment of prostatic cancer. In: Jacobi GH, Hohenfellner R, eds. Prostate cancer. Baltimore: Williams & Wilkins, 1982:269.
39. Salhanick HA, Hisaw FL, Zarrow MX. The action of estrogen and progesterone on the gonadotropin content of the pituitary of the monkey. J Clin Endocrinol Metabol 1952;12:310.
40. Kent JR, Bischoff AJ, Arduino LJ, et al. Estrogen dosage and suppression of testosterone levels in patients with prostatic carcinoma. J Urol 1973;109:858.
41. Prout GR Jr, Keating MA, Griffin PP, Schiff SF. Long-term experience with flutamide in patients with prostatic carcinoma. Urology 1989; 34(Suppl):37.
42. Sogani PC, Vagaiwala MR, Whitmore WF Jr. Experience with flutamide in patients with advanced prostate cancer without prior endocrine therapy. Cancer 1984;54:744.
43. Schroeder FH. Pure antiandrogens as monotherapy in prospective studies of prostatic carcinoma. In: EORTC Genitourinary Group mono-

graph 8: treatment of prostatic cancer—facts and controversies. New York: Wiley-Liss, 1990:93.
44. Airhart RA, Barnet T, Sullivan J, et al. Flutamide therapy of carcinoma of the prostate. South Med J 1978;71:798.
45. Wysowski DK, Freiman JP, Tourtelot JB, Horton ML. Fatal and nonfatal hepatotoxicity associated with flutamide. Ann Intern Med 1993; 118:860.
46. Scher HI, Kelly WK. Flutamide withdrawal syndrome: its impact on clinical trials in hormone-refractory prostate cancer. J Clin Oncol 1993; 11:1566.
47. Decensi AU, Boccardo F, Guarneri D, et al. Monotherapy with nilutamide, a pure nonsteroidal antiandrogen, in untreated patients with metastatic carcinoma of the prostate. J Urol 1991;146:377.
48. DuPlessis DJ. Castration plus nilutamide vs castration plus placebo in advanced prostate cancer. Urology 1991;37(Suppl):20.
49. Denis L. A new nonsteroidal antiandrogen. In: Murphy GP, Khoury S, eds. Therapeutic progress in urologic cancer. New York: Alan R Liss, 1989:95.
50. Waymont B, Blackledge G, Tyrrell CJ, Robinson MRG, Williams JL. Efficacy and safety of the non-steroidal antiandrogen Casodex in early clinical trials for advanced prostate cancer. Br J Cancer 1990;62:499.
51. Denis L, Murphy GP. Overview of phase III trials on combined androgen treatment in patients with metastatic prostate cancer. Cancer 1993; 72(Suppl 12):3888.
52. Prostate Cancer Trialists' Collaborative Group. Maximum androgen blockade in advanced prostate cancer: an overview of 22 randomized trials with 3283 deaths in 5710 patients. Lancet 1995;346:265.
53. Blumenstein BA. Some statistical considerations for the interpretation of trials of combined androgen therapy. Cancer 1993;72(Suppl 12): 3834.
54. Gleave M, Goldenberg SL, Bruchovsky N, Jones EC. Long-term neoadjuvant hormonal therapy prior to radical prostatectomy in localized prostate cancer. (Abstract) J Urol 1994;151(5):435.
55. Zincke H, Utz DC, Thule PM, Taylor WF. Treatment options for patients with stage D1 (T0-3, N1-2, Mo) adenocarcinoma of prostate. Urology 1987;30:307.
56. Benson MC, Hoke G, Veenema RJ, Olsson CA. Radical retropubic prostatectomy and bilateral orchiectomy: editorial comment. J Urol 1986;135:1205.
57. Spirnak JP, Resnick ML. Transrectal ultrasonography. Urology 1984; 23:461.
58. Akakura K, Bruchovsky N, Goldenberg SL, Rennie PS, Buckley AR, Sullivan LD. Effects of intermittent androgen suppression on androgen-dependent tumours: apoptosis and serum prostate specific antigen. Cancer 1993;71:2782.
59. Klotz LH, Kerr HW, Morse MJ, Whitmore WF Jr. Intermittent endocrine therapy for advanced prostate cancer. Cancer 1986;58:2546.
60. Goldenberg SL, Bruchovsky N, Gleave ME, Sullivan LD, Akakura K. Intermittent androgen suppression in the treatment of prostate cancer: a preliminary report. Urology 1995;45:839.
61. Fleischmann JD, Catalona WJ. Endocrine therapy for bladder outlet obstruction from carcinoma of the prostate. J Urol 1985;134:498.
62. Goldenberg SL, Fenster HN, Perler Z, McLoughlin MG. Disseminated intravascular coagulation in carcinoma of prostate. Urology 1983;22: 130.
63. Lowe FC, Somers WJ. The use of ketoconazole in the emergency management of disseminated intravascular coagulation due to metastatic prostatic cancer. J Urol 1987;137(5):1000.
64. Parra RO, Gregory JG. Treatment of post-orchiectomy hot flashes with transdermal administration of clonidine. J Urol 1990;143:753.
65. Steinfeld AD, Rheinhardt C. Male climacteric after orchiectomy in a patient with prostatic cancer. Urology 1980;16:620.
66. Charig CR, Rundle JS. Flushing: long-term side effect of orchiectomy in treatment of prostatic carcinoma. Urology 1989;33:175.
67. Loprinzi LL, Michalak JC, Quella SK, et al. Megestrol acetate for the prevention of hot flashes. N Engl J Med 1994;331:347.
68. Eaton AC, McGuire N. Cyproterone acetate in the treatment of post-orchiectomy hot flushes: double-blind cross-over trial. Lancet 1983;2: 1336.
69. Moon TD. Cyproterone acetate for treatment of hot flashes after orchiectomy. (Letter) J Urol 1985;134:155.

57.2 Androgen Deprivation Strategies for Metastatic Prostate Cancer

Maha H. Hussain and E. David Crawford

Since the original observations of Huggins and Hodges,[1] a great deal of information has been accumulated regarding androgenic physiology[2,3] and molecular actions,[4] the development of bioassays to measure androgenic activity, the cloning of the androgen receptor complementary DNA with the sequencing of the receptor protein,[5,6] the expansion of the armamentarium for the hormonal therapy of prostate cancer, and evolution in therapeutic philosophy away from the intent to palliate symptoms toward early intervention in the management of patients with asymptomatic metastatic disease with the hope of improving survival. Nevertheless, issues relating to the optimal androgen deprivation therapy, the role of adrenal androgens, cost, and quality of life versus survival improvement are not settled and remain controversial.

This chapter reviews the basic rational and outcome of various therapeutic strategies and explores potential future directions in the systemic treatment of advanced, hormone-naive prostate cancer.

PHYSIOLOGY OF ANDROGEN DEPRIVATION

The hormonal dependence of prostatic cancer was documented in the early 1940s by Huggins and Hodges.[1] Although the regulatory role of androgens in the normal prostate gland and in prostate cancer is complex, it is clear that testosterone and its metabolites play the major role.[2,3,7,8] Luteinizing hormone–releasing hormone (LHRH) is released from the hypothalamus in a pulsatile manner, stimulating the anterior pituitary to release luteinizing hormone (LH), which stimulates testosterone production by the Leydig's cells. More than 90% of circulating testosterone is produced by the testes. After medical or surgical castration, circulating levels of androgens are still noted, and dihydrotestosterone (DHT) remains detectable in prostatic tissue.[9] Such observations signified the potential role of adrenal androgens, which account for 5% to 10% of the total circulating pool of androgens, in prostate cancer growth and progression.[10,11] This concept is not universally supported, and adrenal androgens alone do not support physiologic development of the prostate.[12] These weak androgens are produced by the adrenal cortex under the control of adrenocorticotropic hormone and are converted to testosterone by the enzyme 17β-hydroxysteroid dehydrogenase within the prostate. Upon entering the prostate, testosterone is converted to DHT by 5α-reductase in an irreversible enzymatic process.[3] The relative potency of testosterone and DHT is dependent on the target tissue[13,14]; although they both bind to the same androgen receptor protein, DHT has a much higher affinity for the receptor based on increased efficiency in stability of binding, increased thermostability, and more effective upregulation of the receptor.[15] In the prostate nucleus, the DHT receptor complex binds to specific DNA sites modulating gene transcription of specific androgen-dependent genes.[16]

STRATEGIES FOR ANDROGEN DEPRIVATION

Androgen deprivation can be accomplished using a variety of methods.

A. Monotherapy
   1. Bilateral orchiectomy
   2. Nonsurgical castration
      a. Suppression or interruption of hypothalamic-pituitary-testicular axis (e.g., estrogens, LHRH analogs)
      b. Inhibition of DHT action by interfering with receptor-steroid binding or nuclear translocation (e.g., steroidal and nonsteroidal antiandrogens)
      c. Adrenal suppression (e.g., ketoconazole, aminoglutethimide)
B. A combination of primary gonadal suppression plus antiandrogens

OUTCOME OF MONOTHERAPY TRIALS

Therapy of advanced prostate cancer revolves around the primary suppression of gonadal function. This was previously accomplished by surgical of medical castration by oral estrogen. The rapid onset of symptomatic relief, immediate and massive reduction in circulating testosterone, and minimal adverse effects made bilateral orchiectomy the gold standard in prostate cancer therapy. Testosterone levels remain in the castrate range indefinitely,[17,18] and no compensatory adrenal androgen secretion occurs.[19] diethylstilbestrol (DES) has demonstrated an effectiveness equivalent to that of orchiectomy in lowering plasma levels of testosterone to castrate levels. The Veterans Administration Cooperative Urological Research Group (VACURG) conducted a series of studies starting with the evaluation of 5 mg of DES relative to orchiectomy.[20] It was concluded that 5-mg DES therapy is complicated by an increased risk of cardiovascular deaths. No overall survival differences between the hormonal therapy arm and the placebo arm were detected; this was attributed to the increased number of cardiovascular deaths in the DES arm. DES did appear to be more effective than orchiectomy in preventing cancer deaths.[21] A second trial compared placebo, 0.2 mg, 1 mg, and 5 mg of DES.[22] This study confirmed the high risk for cardiovascular complications with the 5-mg DES dose, necessitating the early termination of the study, and concluded that 1-mg DES therapy had the same beneficial effects on delaying cancer progression when compared to the 5-mg dose. A modest effect on survival was observed with 1-mg DES beginning at diagnosis as compared with placebo. Subsequently, 1-mg DES was found to be somewhat more effective in delaying progression, but no survival improvement was detected when compared with premarin, provera, and provera plus 1 mg of DES.[22] In its final analysis, European Organization for the Research and Treatment of Cancer trial 30805 (EORTC 30805)[23] confirmed the equivalence of 1-mg DES therapy to orchiectomy.

The isolation, structural characterization, and synthesis of LHRH ushered in a new era in androgen deprivation.[24,25] By substituting D-leucine for glycine at position 6, agonists with higher potency and longer half-life have been synthesized.[26–28] In the United States, two LHRH analogs are available in the clinic: leuprolide and goserelin. The use of these agents was significantly enhanced by the availability of the depot formulation.[29–31] Both agents have been investigated in phase II trials[32–35] and randomized phase III trials.[31,36] Most notable of these is the Leuprolide Study Group[36] report on a randomized study comparing leuprolide to DES. No differences were detected between leuprolide and DES in the overall response rates (86% versus 85%, respectively) or 1-year survival (87% versus 78%, respectively).[36] Patients receiving DES experienced more frequent painful gynecomastia, nausea and vomiting, edema, and thromboembolism than did those receiving leuprolide. Goserelin was compared to orchiectomy and DES in two multicenter randomized trials in the United Kingdom.[31] In these studies, goserelin was comparable to orchiectomy or DES in response rate, time to progression, and survival. Of significance is the observation that in addition to a faster response to depot goserelin, 15% of patients receiving DES required cessation of therapy during the first 3 months of therapy because of side effects. This led to the conclusion that goserelin was superior to DES in terms of achieving an earlier response and having a better side effect profile. Another LHRH agonist, buserelin, was found to be comparable to orchiectomy in response, relapse rate, and survival.[37]

The outcomes of monotherapy studies indicate a subjective and objective improvement in 60% to 85% of patients, a median progression-free survival of 12 to 18 months, and a median survival of 24 to 30 months.[32,36,38] Collective data from randomized trials strongly indicate that LHRH agonists are equivalent in efficacy to the gold standard therapy and superior in terms of physical and psychological side effects. Moreover, when given the choice, patients choose an LHRH agonist over bilateral orchiectomy.[30] This issue brings to light the importance of patients' perceptions of therapy and quality of life, which has become one of the studied end points of clinical trials in this disease.

COMBINED ANDROGEN DEPRIVATION

Despite a gratifying initial response to primary androgen deprivation, virtually all patients progress in a predictable and irreversible manner to androgen independence. The possibility that a tumor clone or clones may be or will adapt to become sensitive to lower levels of androgens, necessitating the elimination of all sources of androgens including the small amount produced by adrenal glands, provides the basis for combined androgen deprivation (CAD). This concept is not new; what is relatively new is the implementation of this form of therapy at the time of initial diagnosis of D2 disease, as opposed to when progression has occurred following monotherapy. The latter approach is seldom successful.[39,40] Advocates of CAD cite observations suggesting that adrenal androgens contribute 16% to 20% of total DHT in the prostate[41] and the persistence of relatively high intracellular DHT levels despite castrate-range serum testosterone levels.[42–44] This was shown by Geller and colleagues[42,43] in a study in which untreated cancer patients had approximately 5 ng of DHT per gram of prostatic tissue, compared with approximately 2 ng per gram of prostatic tissue in orchiectomized or DES treated patients. It has been proposed that the persistence of measurable tissue DHT results from the continued conversion of adrenal androgen precursors to testosterone and subsequently to DHT in the prostatic cells.[45] Therefore, the addition of antiandrogens that prevent androgens from expressing their activity at the target site should enhance the efficacy of primary androgen deprivation. Additional support for CAD stems from the desire to block the effects of the transient elevation in serum testosterone and potential flare reaction associated with LHRH agonist monotherapy. Because antiandrogens neutralize the action of androgens at the target cell level[46,47] the addition of a pure antiandrogen to an LHRH agonist would be desirable. Rennie and colleagues[48] reported that the effectiveness of an antiandrogen is a function of its ability to reduce the amount of functionally active androgen receptor in the nucleus of the target cell. Although this could be accomplished to varying degrees by different methods of androgen deprivation,[49] it is thought that the nuclear depletion of the androgen receptor is more complete using therapies that combine primary gonadal suppression with a steroidal or nonsteroidal antiandrogen.[49] However, a major criticism of this assumption is the lack of supporting direct experimental evidence.[49,50]

Experimentally, in the androgen-sensitive Shionogi's mammary carcinoma, androgen resistance was induced in the absence of androgens, but androgen sensitivity was maintained in the absence of androgens when flutamide was added.[51] Investigating the effect of flutamide treatment in the presence or absence of concomitant LHRH agonist on secondary sex organ weight indicated that CAD therapy had an additive effect in reducing prostatic and seminal vesicle weight higher than that observed with each drug alone[44]; however, the results with CAD were comparable to those seen after surgical castration. The activity of ornithine decarboxylase (ODC), a specific marker of androgenic activity in the rat prostate, was measured after flutamide or LHRH agonist monotherapy and with combination therapy.[51] Although daily monotherapy had no significant effect on ODC activity, combination treatment resulted in a marked drop in ODC activity, indicating the need for more complete blockade of androgens before significant inhibition of ODC activity can be detected.

Outcome of Combined Androgen Deprivation Trials

In 1982, Labrie and colleagues[52] reported that 8 of 9 metastatic prostate cancer patients responded to combined androgen therapy. Although the number of patients studied was small, these results seem to support the hypothesized potential role for adrenal androgens in prostate cancer progression. Their observation was followed by flurry of clinical trials attempting to confirm these findings. Table 57.2-1 summarizes the characteristics and outcomes of some of the randomized studies. One of the largest of the confirmatory trials with a high statistical power was the National Cancer Institute Intergroup Trial 0036 (INT-0036) reported by Crawford and colleagues.[53] Leuprolide plus placebo was compared with leuprolide plus flutamide. A 19% increase in the median time to progression, 26% increase in the median overall survival (35 months versus 29 months), and 26% increase in the response rate in favor of the CAD arm was reported.[53] A striking benefit was noted in progression-free and overall survival of patients labeled as having a good prognosis (defined as having minimal disease as evidenced by absence of metastases in ribs, long bones, skull, or soft tissue other than lymph nodes, and Eastern Cooperative Oncology Group performance status 0 to 2) in favor of CAD arm (48 versus 19 months and 61 versus 42 months, respectively). Unpublished survival analysis excluding the good-prognosis patients indicated that CAD still holds a survival advantage. Although the initial report of the EORTC 30853 study of orchiectomy versus Zoladex plus flutamide, published after 2 years of follow-up, was negative,[54] an updated analysis concluded that CAD was superior in both subjective and objective median time to progression. The difference in objective median time to progression was 48 weeks, with a 7-month prolongation in survival.[55] Like the INT-0036 investigation,[53] this study demonstrated that the benefit of the CAD was most evident in patients with minimal disease. Although several large, well-designed studies confirm the superiority of CAD (see Table 57.2-1), there still is controversy regarding the validity of this approach. The conflicting opinions stem to some degree from the misinterpretation of a number of reportedly negative trials that had insufficient statistical power, as discussed by Blumenstein,[56] and a too-small sample size to clearly detect a moderate decrease in mortality.[57] This is complicated by the fact that many of the "negative" reports were early analyses of ongoing clinical trials.[56] The experience with EORTC 30853 emphasizes the need to await mature data and avoid early reporting.

Attempting to overcome difficulties caused by small sample sizes and enhance statistical power, a systematic overview (i.e., meta-analysis) of all CAD trials is underway.[58] It remains to be seen whether this analysis will resolve the controversy. It is our belief that meta-analyses cannot replace well-designed randomized trials. A detailed discussion of the statistical principles of the meta-analysis has been provided by Blumenstein.[58]

In addition to controversies stemming from the interpretation of the outcome of the clinical trials, a variety of other issues have been raised regarding CAD. For example, critics of this approach point out that adrenal androgens have yet to be implicated in the recurrent growth of prostate cancer[12,49,59]; therefore, the elimination of flare reaction by an antiandrogen is the strongest justification for this approach and the reason to which the superiority of CAD can be attributed.[49] If this was the case, a survival advantage in favor of CAD would not be expected in studies using bilateral orchiectomy as a control arm, as demonstrated by the EORTC 30853[55] and the Anandron International Study Group trials.[60] Furthermore, the statistically significant higher response rates observed in these trials together with

Table 57-2. *Summary of selected randomized trials investigating combined androgen deprivation*

Investigator	Treatment arms	RC No. of evaluable D2 patients	RR Time to progression (weeks)	Median survival (months)	Comments
Robinson, 1993[53]	Orch vs Orch plus CPA vs DES	328	ND	ND	Increase DES Cardiovascular toxicity
Klijn et al, 1993[82]	Orch vs Buserelin plus CPA for 2 wk vs buserelin plus continuous CPA	347	ND	ND	
Tyrell et al, 1993[84]	Gos vs Gos plus Flut	301	ND	26.9 vs 29 (ND)	Flut dose, 250 mg bid
Iverson et al, 1993[83]	Orch vs Gos plus Flut	262	16.8 vs 16.5	27.6 vs. 22.7 (ND)	9% Had local disease May or may not have had nodal disease only
Keuppens et al, 1990[54]	Orch vs Gos plus Flut	327	48-weeks advantage for CAD (P = .00)	7 month advantage for CAD (P = .05)	Survival advantage increased to 15 mo for death by cancer (P = .02)
Jacknegt et al, 1993 [60]	Orch vs Orch plus Nilu	457	14.7 vs 20.8 (P = .004)	29.8 vs 37.1 (P = .04)	
Crawford et al, 1989[53]	Leup plus placebo vs Leup plus Flut	603	14 vs 17	29 vs 35 (P = .035)	
Hucher et al, 1993[85]	Orch plus placebo vs Orch plus Nilu	1056	Odds of progression reduced in CAD (P = .05)	Odds of death reduced (NS)	Higher response rate for CAD (P < .001); Meta-analysis

BUS, buserdin; CAD, combined androgen deprivation; CPA, cyproterone acetate; DES, diethylstilbestrol; Flut, flutamide; Gos, goserelin; Leup, leuprolide; ND, no difference; Nilu, nilutamide; NS, not significant; Orch, bilateral orchiectomy.

the INT-0036[53] response data suggest that a higher initial tumor kill is the more likely explanation. Nevertheless, confirmatory and definitive answers will be provided by the current INT-0105, a double-blinded evaluation of orchiectomy plus placebo versus orchiectomy plus flutamide. The accrual goal of this study was 1248 eligible patients; this number was computed based on the effect size actually observed for INT-0036.[53] INT-0105 completed accrual in 1994 with 1387 patients; more registrations were allowed to maximize the amount of data collected on specific subgroups, particularly good-prognosis and African American patients. It is anticipated that outcome of INT-0105 will be reported within 2 years from its closure.[58]

Another issue that is being discussed nationally, in general and in terms of prostate cancer, because of the changing climate of health care and economics, is the issue of cost-effectiveness of CAD. Primarily, the "marginal" survival benefit to the majority of patients led to concerns in this regard. However, there is a paucity of data, and cost-effectiveness studies in this disease are in their infancy. In a recent report, Bennett and colleagues[61] developed a decision analysis model of the natural history of prostate cancer to study a hypothetical cohort of 70-year-old men with bony metastases and good performance status to compare orchiectomy versus orchiectomy plus flutamide or LHRH agonist versus LHRH agonist plus flutamide. CAD disease-specific relative efficacy in reducing progression was based on published randomized studies. This model demonstrated that CAD has an incremental cost-effectiveness similar to or less than that of other accepted treatments such as dialysis.[61] Considering the striking survival benefit of good-prognosis prostate cancer patients with CAD, the shift toward more stage D2 patients with smaller tumor burdens as a result of the widespread use and sensitivity of prostate-specific antigen (PSA) as a screening tool, it is logical to conclude that the cost-effectiveness of CAD can only improve.

FUTURE DIRECTIONS

Whether the addition of an antiandrogen to primary gonadal suppression exerts its effects through inhibiting the binding of DHT to the androgen receptor in addition to decreasing the concentration of DHT in the prostate gland or through some other mechanism, the fact remains that such an approach is proven in a randomized controlled fashion to be statistically superior. Although translating statistical superiority to clinically relevant superiority when such benefit is relatively marginal for the majority of patients is a difficult task that is complicated by lack of data on cost-effectiveness and unmeasurable impact on quality of life, it is important to emphasize that by any standard considering treatment of metastatic solid tumors, outcome for D2 prostate cancer receiving CAD is favorable. A survival advantage of 6 months or greater associated with treatment of metastatic solid tumors would be considered a significant achievement.

Despite the favorable patient response to CAD, progression to hormone refractory status is almost always the rule, with a median survival of 40 weeks. Two primary hypotheses have been offered to explain this progression: the adaptation model and the clonal selection model.[62–64] The common denominator between the two theories is androgen deprivation. Noble[65] and others[64] have suggested that progression to autonomy is a function of the withdrawal of the hormone that is necessary for the tumor growth and not the result of the regression process. This observation is supported by the accumulating experimental data suggesting that androgen withdrawal triggers a complex process with changes occurring at stem cell and molecular levels. It has been suggested, using androgen-dependent experimental models, that clinical progression is the result of a massive expansion in the androgen-independent components of the stem cell compartment.[66] These changes appear to be a reflection of changes occurring at a molecular level aiming at self-preservation; therefore, progression at a cellular-molecular level seems to occur despite a clinically evident response. Experimentally, during the active cell death process (i.e., apoptosis) following androgen deprivation, a variety of novel RNAs and proteins are induced, the expression of several constitutive gene products is markedly enhanced, and a number of androgen-repressed genes are also induced.[66–68] Of these genes, testosterone-repressed prostate message-2 (*TRPM2*) is receiving a great deal of attention.[69,70] It was originally cloned from regressing rat ventral prostate tissue after castration or treatment with an antiandrogen. Clusterin, the *TRPM2* gene product, is a potent inhibitor of complement-induced cytolysis and as such acts as a stabilizer of cell membranes. A variety of genes have been implicated in the prevention of the apoptotic process, some of which appear to have increased expression following androgen deprivation. *BCL2* and *P53* are two examples. *BCL2* is normally expressed in the androgen-independent, nonapoptotic basal cell of prostatic glandular epithelium.[71,72] It is unique in that it has been shown to extend the viability of cells by overriding the normal mechanisms of programed cell death.[73] Experimentally, enhanced *BCL2* expression results from androgen deprivation and is associated with the conversion of androgen-dependent prostate cancer to androgen-independent prostate cancer.[73] Recent data suggest that *P53* is induced after androgen withdrawal[74] and that *P53* plays a role in blocking the apoptotic pathway.[75,76] Enhanced *MYC* expression in the rat prostate gland was observed postcastration.[77] *MYC* is involved in the regulation of mitosis and apoptosis. In the presence of critical growth stimuli, *MYC* acts as a classic protooncogene stimulating mitosis.[78] The simultaneous overexpression of *BCL2* abrogates the capacity of increased *MYC* expression to induce apoptosis.[78] Collectively, the emerging experimental data, although not complete, suggests the need for a change in strategy in attacking metastatic prostate cancer. If the outcome of therapy and impact on survival is to be improved, a variety of issues must be addressed in the design of future clinical trials:

Discover mechanisms of progression to androgen independence.
Explore mechanisms to delay progression to androgen independence.
Devise innovative therapies that will induce active cell death and eradication of the stem cells.

Appropriate patient selection and stratification are critical factors. Implicit in this approach is maximizing benefit from hormone therapy for those who are likely to profit from it, bearing in mind enhancing quality of life and targeting poor-prognosis patients early for more aggressive therapy incorporating chemotherapeutic agents to eradicate stem cells, particularly the androgen-independent ones.

Mechanisms to delay progression to androgen independence are being explored. These studies are based on observations, described previously, that progression is associated with the activation of previously androgen-repressed genes, some of which may code for autocrine or paracrine growth factors that substitute for androgens in maintaining the viability of the tumorigenic stem cells.[79] Therefore, replacing androgens before the initiation of progression should cause the surviving stem cells to give rise to an androgen-dependent tumor amenable to retreatment by androgen withdrawal. This provides the rational for intermittent androgen deprivation. In experimental models, this approach resulted in threefold prolongation of the duration of androgen dependence,[79] and although clinical data are limited, studies done using variable methods of intermittent androgen deprivation suggest that this intriguing concept should be further investigated.[79–81] In addition to delaying progression and potentially improving survival, this approach is attractive because it is associated with improved quality of life and potentially reduced cost of therapy. These data provide the rational for a phase III study coordinated by the Southwest Oncology Group evaluating intermittent androgen deprivation compared with continuous androgen deprivation in metastatic prostate cancer patients, with survival and quality of life as the primary end points.

CONCLUSION

In our view, CAD is the best available therapy for metastatic prostate cancer and as such should be considered the standard treatment. Although debate about this issue may continue, it is time that researchers move ahead with innovative treatment strategies that incorporate the vast and rapidly accumulating experimental data. Although developing novel therapeutic strategies for metastatic prostate cancer should be the focus of research efforts, the real target is earlier stages of prostate cancer, in which the adjuvant applications of such therapies are more likely to have a greater impact on survival.

Note Added in Proof

This is a thorough review of aspects of the published literature on combined androgenic blockade. However, it is important to note that Drs. Hussain and Crawford have been selective in their choice of studies for citation and in their critical assessment of some of the negative trials. A contrary view, opposed to the routine use of combined androgenic blockade, is presented in reference 52 of section 1 of this chapter. (D.R.)

REFERENCES

1. Huggins C, Hodges CV. Studies on prostatic cancer. I. The effect of castration, of estrogen and of androgen injection on serum phosphatases in metastatic carcinoma of the prostate. Cancer Res 1941;1:293.
2. Anderson KM, Liao S. Selective retention of dihydrotestosterone by prostatic nuclei. Nature 1968;219:277.
3. Bruchovsky N, Wilson JD. The conversion of testosterone to 5-alpha-androstan 17-beta-oL-3-one by rat prostate in vivo and in vitro. J Biol Chem 1968;243:2012.
4. Bruchovsky N, Wilson JD. The intranuclear binding of testosterone and 5-alpha androstan-17 beta-oL-3-one by rat prostate. J Biol Chem 1968;243:5953.
5. Chang C, Kokontis J, Liao S. Molecular cloning of human and rat complementary DNA encoding androgen receptors. Science 1988;240:324.
6. Lubahn DB, Joseph DR, Sullivan PM, Willard HF, French FS, Wilson EM. Cloning of human androgen receptor complementary DNA and localization to the X chromosome. Science 1988;240:327.
7. Geller J, Albert JD, Endocrine therapy: predictors of response to prostatic cancer. Semin Urol 1983;1(4):291.
8. Bruchovsky N. Comparison of the melabotites formed in the rat prostate following in vitro administration of seven natural androgens. Endocrinology 1971;89:1212.
9. Geller J, Albert JD, Nachstheim DA, Losa D. Comparison of prostatic cancer tissue DHT levels at time of relapse following orchiectomy or estrogen therapy. J Urol 1984;132:693.
10. Barrett-Connor E, Garland C, McPhillips JB, Khaw KT, Wingard DL. A prospective, population-based study of androstenedione, estrogen, and prostatic cancer. Cancer Res 1990;50:169.
11. Labrie, Trudel C, Li S, Martel C, Couet J, Labrie F. Combination of an antiandrogen and 5 alpha-reductase inhibitor: a further step towards total androgen blockade? Endocrinology 1991;129:566.
12. Osterling JE, Epstein JI, Walch PC. The inability of adrenal androgens to stimulate the adult human prostate: an autopsy evaluation of men with hypogonadotropic hypergonadism and panhypopituitarism. J Urol 1986;136:1030.
13. Conovatchel WJ, Imperato-McGinley J. Pathogenesis and the role of medical management. Geriatr Nephrol Urol 1992;2:1.
14. Wilson JD. Syndromes of androgen resistance. Biol Reprod 1992;46:168.
15. Grino PB, Griffin JE, Wilson JD. Testosterone at high concentration interacts with the human androgen receptor similarly to dihydrotestosterone. Endocrinology 1990;126:1165.
16. Coffey DS, Peinta KJ. New concepts in studying the control of normal and cancer growth of the prostate. Prog Clin Biol Res 1987;239:1.
17. Robinson MRG, Thomas BS. Effects of hormonal therapy on plasma testosterone levels in prostatic carcinoma. Br Med J 1971;4:391.
18. Young HH, Kent JR. Plasma testosterone levels in patients with prostatic carcinoma before and after treatment. J Urol 1968;99:788.
19. Walsh PC, Siiteri PK. Suppression of plasma androgens by spironolactone in castrated men with carcinoma of the prostate. J Urol 1975;114:254.
20. Veterans Administration Cooperative Urological Research Group. Treatment and survival of patients with cancer of the prostate. Surg Gynecol Obstet 1967;124:1011.
21. Blackard CE, Byard DP, Jordan WP Jr. Orchiectomy for advanced prostatic carcinoma: a re-evaluation. Urology 1973;1:553.
22. Byar DP, Corle DK. Hormone therapy for prostate cancer: results of the Veterans Administration Cooperative Urological Research Group Studies. NCI Monogr 1988;7:165.
23. Robinson MRG. A further analysis of European Organization for Research and Treatment of Cancer Protocol 30805: orchidectomy versus orchidectomy plus cyproterone acetate versus low-dose diethylstilbestrol. Cancer 1993;72(Suppl 12):3855.
24. Schally AV, Arimura A, Baba Y, et al. Isolation and properties of the FSH and LH-releasing hormone. Biochem Biophys Res Commun 1971;43:393.
25. Baba Y, Matsuo M, Schally AV. Structure of the porcine LH and FSH releasing hormone. II. Confirmation of the proposed structure by conventional sequential analyses. Biochem Biophys Res Commun 1971;44:459.
26. Monahan MW, Amos MS, Anderson HA, et al. Synthetic analogs of the hypothalamic luteinizing hormone releasing factor with increased agonist or antiagonist properties. Biochemistry 1973;12:4616.
27. Coy DH, Vilchez-Martinez JA, Coy EJ, Schally AV. Analogs of luteinizing hormone-releasing hormone with increased biological activity produced by D-amino acid substitutions in position 6. J Med Chem 1976;19:423.
28. Fujino M, Lobayashi S, Obayashi M, Shinagawa S, Fukuda T. Structure-activity relationships in the C-terminal part of luteinizing hormone releasing hormone (LH-RH). Biochem Biophys Res Commun 1972;49:863.
29. Sharifi R, Soloway M, The Leuprolide Study Group. Clinical study of leuprolide depo formulation in the treatment of advanced prostate cancer. J Urol 1990;143:68.
30. Cassileth BR, Soloway MS, Vogelzang NJ, et al. Patients choice of treatment in stage D prostate cancer. Urology 1989;33(Suppl 5):57.
31. Peeling WB. Phase III studies to compare goserelin (Zoladex) with orchiectomy and with diethylstilbestrol in the treatment of prostatic carcinoma. Urology 1989;33(Suppl 5):45.
32. Eisenberger MA, O'Dwyer PJ, Friedman MA. Gonadotropin-hormone-releasing hormone analogues: a new therapeutic approach for prostatic carcinoma. J Clin Oncol 1986;4:414.
33. Smith JA Jr, Glode LM, Wettlaufer JN, et al. Clinical effects of gonadotropin-releasing hormone analogue in metastatic carcinoma of the prostate. Urology 1985;25:106.
34. Trachtenberg J. The treatment of metastatic prostatic cancer with a potent luteinizing hormone-releasing hormone analogue. J Urol 1983;129:1140.
35. Waxman JH, Wass JA, Hendry WF, et al. Treatment with gonadotropin releasing hormone analogue in advanced prostatic cancer. Br Med J 1983;286:1309.
36. The Leuprolide Study Group. Leuprolide versus diethylstilbestrol for metastatic prostate cancer. N Engl J Med 1984;311:1281.
37. Koutsilieris M, Faure N, Tolis G, Laroche B, Robert G, Ackman CFD. Objective response and disease outcome in 59 patients with stage D2 prostatic cancer treated with either buserelin or orchiectomy. Urology 1986;27:221.
38. Byar DP. The Veterans Administration Cooperative Urological Research Group studies of cancer of the prostate. Cancer 1973;32:1126.
39. Eichenberger T, Trachtenberg J. Effects of high dose ketoconazole in patients with androgen-independent prostatic cancer. Am J Clin Oncol 1988;11(Suppl 2):S104.
40. Grayhack JT. Adrenalectomy and hypophysectomy for carcinoma of the prostate. JAMA 1969;210:1075.
41. Harper ME, Pike A, Peeling WB, Griffiths K. Steroids of adrenal origin metabolized by human prostatic tissue both in vivo and in vitro. J Endocrinol 1974;60:117.
42. Geller J, Albert J, Loza D, Geller S, Stoeltzing W, Dela Vega D. DHI concentration in human prostate cancer tissue. J Clin Endocrinol Metabol 1978;46:440.
43. Geller J, Albert JD, Nachstheim DA, Losa D. Comparison of prostatic cancer tissue DHT levels at the time of relapse following orchiectomy or estrogen therapy. J Urol 1984;132:693.
44. Fransworth WE, Brown JR. Androgen of the human prostate. Endocr Res Commun 1976;3:105.
45. Labrie F. Mechanism of action and pure antiandrogenic properties of flutamide. Cancer 1993;72:3816.
46. Neri RO, Peets EA. Biological aspects of antiandrogens. J Steroid Biochem 1975;6:815.
47. Simard J, Luthy IA, Gray J, Belanger A, Labrie F. Characteristics of interaction of the antiandrogen flutamide with the androgen receptor in various target tissues. Mol Cell Endocrinol 1986;44:261.
48. Rennie PS, Bruchovsky N, Goldenberg SL, Lawson D, Fletcher T, Foekens JA. Relative effectiveness of alternative androgen withdrawal therapies in initiating regression of rat prostate. J Urol 1988;139:1337.
49. Bruchovsky N. Androgens and antiandrogens. In: Holland J, Frei E III, Bast R Jr, et al, eds. Cancer medicine, 3rd ed, vol. 1. Philadelphia: Lea & Febiger, 1991:884.
50. Bruchovsky N, Brown EM, Coppin CM, et al. The endocrinology and treatment of prostate tumor progression. In: Coffey DS, Bruchovsky N, Gardner WE Jr, Resnick MI, Karr JP, eds. Current concepts and approaches to the study of prostate cancer: progress in clinical and biological research. New York: Alan R Liss, 1987:348.
51. Luthy I, Labrie F. Development of androgen resistance in mouse mam-

mary tumor cells can be prevented by the antiandrogen flutamide. Prostate 1987;10:89.
52. Labrie F, Dupont A, Belanger A, et al. New hormonal therapy in prostatic carcinoma: combined treatment with an LHRH agonist and an antiandrogen. Clin Invest Med 1982;5:267.
53. Crawford ED, Eisenberger MA, McLeod DG, et al. A controlled trial of leuprolide with and without flutamide in prostatic carcinoma. N Engl J Med 1989;321:419.
54. Keuppens F, Denis L, Smith PH, et al. Zoladex R and flutamide versus bilateral orchiectomy: a randomized phase III trial EORTC 30853 study. Cancer 1990;66(5):1045.
55. Keuppens F, Whelan P, Carneiro de Moura JL, et al. Orchidectomy versus goserelin plus flutamide in patients with metastatic prostate cancer (EORTC 30853). Cancer 1993;72:3863.
56. Blumenstein BA. Some statistical considerations for the interpretation of trials of combined androgen therapy. Cancer 1993;72:3834.
57. Denis L, Murphy GP. Overview of phase III trials on combined androgen treatment in patients with metastatic prostate cancer. Cancer 1993; 72:3888.
58. Blumenstein BA. Overview analysis issues using combined androgen overview analysis as an example. Urol Oncol 1995;1:95.
59. Schulze H, Osterling JE, Isaacs JT, Coffey DS. Hormonal therapy of prostate cancer: limitations in the total androgen ablation concept. In: Coffey DS, Resnick MI, Dorr FA, Karr JP, eds. A multidisciplinary analysis of controversies in the management of prostate cancer. New York: Plenum Press, 1986:215.
60. Jacknegt RA, for the Anandron International Study Group. Total androgen blockade with the use of orchiectomy and nilutomide (anandron) or placebo as treatment of metastatic prostate cancer. Cancer 1993;72: 3874.
61. Bennett CL, McLeod DG, Hillner BE. Estimating the cost-effectiveness of total androgen blockade for stage D2 prostate cancer. (Abstract) Proc Am Soc Clin Oncol 1994;13:724.
62. Isaacs JT, Kyprianou N. Development of androgen independent tumor cells and their implications for the treatment of prostatic cancer. Urol Res 1987;15:133.
63. Coffey DS, Isaacs JT. Prostate tumor biology and cell kintics-theory. Urology 1981;27(Suppl 3):40.
64. Isaacs JT. The timing of androgen ablation therapy and/or chemotherapy in the treatment of prostatic cancer. Prostate 1984;5:1.
65. Noble RL. Hormonal control of growth and progression in tumors of Nb rats and a theory of action. Cancer Res 1977;37:82.
66. Bruchovsky N, Rennie PS, Coldman AJ, Goldenberg SL, To M, Lawson D. Effects of androgen withdrawal on the stem cell composition of the Shionogi carcinoma. Cancer Res 1990;50:2275.
67. Furuya Y, Sato N, Akakura K, et al. Paracrine growth stimulation of androgen responsive Shionogi carcinoma 115 by its autonomous subline (Chiba subline 2). Cancer Res 1990;50:4979.
68. Rennie PS, Bruchovsky N, Coldman AJ. Loss of androgen dependence is associated with an increase in tumorigenic stem cells and resistance to cell-death genes. J Steroid Biochem Mol Biol 1990;37:843.
69. Tenniswood MP, Guenette RS, Lakins J, Mooibroek M, Wong P, Welsh J. Active cell death in hormone-dependent tissues. Cancer Metast Rev 1992;11:197.
70. Bandyk MG, Sawczuk IS, Olsson CA, Katz AE, Buttyan R. Characterization of the products of a gene expressed during andorgen-programmed cell death and their potential use as a maker of urogenital injury. J Urol 1990;143:407.
71. Hockenberg DM, Zutter M, Hickey W, Nahm M, Korsmeyer SJ. bcl-2 protein is topographically restricted in tissues characterized by apoptotic cell death. Proc Natl Acad Sci U S A 1991;88:6961.
72. Kyprianou N, English HF, Isaacs JT. Programmed cell death during regression of PC-82 human prostate cancer following androgen ablation. Cancer Res 1990;50:3748.
73. McDonnell TJ, Troncoso P, Brisbay S, et al. Expression of protooncogene bcl-2 in the prostate and its association with emergence of androgen-independent prostate cancer. Cancer Res 1992;52:6940.
74. Colombel M, Olsson CA, Ng P, Buttyan R. Hormone-regulated apoptosis results from reentry of differentiated prostate cells onto a defective cell cycle. Cancer Res 1992;52:4313.
75. Lane DP. A death in the life of P53. Nature 1993;362:786.
76. Debbas M, White E. Wild-type P53 mediates apoptosis by E1A which is inhibited by E1B. Genes Develop 1993;7:546.
77. Buttyan R, Zakeri Z, Lockshin R, Wolgemuth D. Cascade induction of c-fos, c-myc, and heat shock 7ok transcripts during regression of rat ventral prostate gland. Mol Endocrinol 1988;2:650.
78. Kerr JFR, Winterford CM, Harmon BV. Apoptosis: its significance in cancer and cancer therapy. Cancer 1994;73:2013.
79. Akakura K, Bruchovsky N, Goldenberg SL, Rennie PS, Buckley AR, Sullivan LD. Effects of intermittent androgen suppression or androgen-dependent tumors. Cancer 1993;71:2782.
80. Klotz LH, Herr HW, Morse MJ, Whitmore WF Jr. Intermittent endocrine therapy for advanced prostate cancer. Cancer 1986;58:2546.
81. Vahlensieck W, Wegner G, Lehmann HD, Franzen G, Steffens L, Wahlby S. Comparison between continuous and intermittent administration of estracyt in the treatment of carcinoma of the prostate. Urol Res 1985; 13:209.
82. Klijn JGM, de Voogt HJ, Studer UE, Schroder FH, Sylvester R, De Pauw M. Short term versus long term addition of cyproterone acetate to buserelin therapy in comparison with orchidectomy in the treatment of metastatic prostate cancer. Cancer 1993;72:3858.
83. Iversen P, Rasmussen F, Klarskov P, Christensen IJ. Long term results of Danish Prostatic Cancer Group Trial 86. Goserilin acetate plus flutamide versus orchiectomy in advanced prostate cancer. Cancer 1993; 72:3851.
84. Tyrrell CJ, Altwein JE, Klippel F, et al. Multicenter randomized trial comparing Zoladex with Zoladex plus flutamide in the treatment of advanced prostate cancer. Survival update. Cancer 1993;72:3878.
85. Hucher M, de Gery A, Bertagna C. Anandron (nilutamide) combined with orchiectomy in stage D prostate cancer patients: overview of seven randomized placebo controlled studies. Cancer 1993;72:3886.

Principles and Practice of Genitourinary Oncology, edited by Derek Raghavan, Howard I. Scher, Steven A. Leibel, and Paul H. Lange. Lippincott-Raven Publishers, Philadelphia, © 1997.

CHAPTER 58

Management of Androgen-Independent Prostatic Cancer

Howard I. Scher and Christopher J. Logothetis

The cornerstone of treatment for advanced prostate cancer involves the manipulation of the hypothalamic-gonadal-pituitary axis to negate the stimulatory actions of androgens on the malignant prostate. This is generally effected by medical or surgical castration with or without agents that inhibit adrenal androgen synthesis. As discussed in Chapter 57, although significant palliation is observed in the majority of cases, the effects are not durable, and signs of treatment failure become manifest in a median of 12 to 18 months. Several lines of laboratory and clinical evidence explain the acquisition of the androgen-independent phenotype. The relative dependence on androgens for prostate cancer cell survival and growth has been hypothesized as an important distinguishing feature predicting androgen-independent growth. The range of dependence on androgens for successful growth may distinguish prostate cancers into recognizable categories: androgen-dependent, androgen-sensitive, and androgen-independent. Androgen-dependent cancer cells require androgens for continued growth and survival.[1] Androgen-sensitive cancer cells show a decrease in growth rate but are not lethally injured when androgens are withdrawn. Androgen-independent cells grow and proliferate without androgens and are the primary cell population responsible for the mortality of the disease. Improving survival will require a better understanding of and inhibition of androgen-independent progression as well as more effective treatment of the androgen-independent cell population.

PATTERNS OF PROGRESSION

Relapsed prostate cancers encompass a spectrum of diseases that differ in clinical presentation and prognosis. For example, a clinically undetectable tumor that presents with small, incremental increases in prostate-specific antigen (PSA) may never become clinically manifest or contribute to the death of the patient. In contrast, a patient with diffuse bony metastases who is progressing is likely to die of the disease. The approach to each of these clinical situations is different. Before the general availability of PSA determinations, the most common clinical presentation of relapsing disease was symptoms related to tumor growth, such as pain in an osseous site, or a change in urination from local tumor regrowth. Less commonly, soft tissue disease, such as an enlarging lymph node or visceral lesion, is documented. In one series of patients who presented with soft tissue and osseous disease, 25% of bone lesions improved after hormone therapy opposed to 82% of soft tissue lesions, whereas progression was four times more frequent in bone than in soft tissue.[2] Plain radiographs typically show an osteoblastic pattern, one of the hallmarks of prostate cancers that have spread to the skeleton, with a distribution that parallels sites of hematopoiesis in the marrow. The propensity for prostate cancers to spread and proliferate in bone is not a chance event[3] and can present management problems as a result of the difficulties of assessing response in bone and because an improvement in clinical symptoms does not necessary mean that tumor cell kill has been achieved.

The addition of PSA testing to routine clinical practice has changed the management of prostate cancer in all stages. It has resulted in a decrease in the proportion of patients who present with advanced metastatic disease.[4] It has also led to a stage migration wherein more patients receive hormonal therapy for asymptomatic elevations in PSA after radical surgery or external beam irradiation, or low-volume regional nodal disease documented at laparotomy as the only sign of spread. The same meticulous monitoring of PSA levels after androgen ablation has also produced an increase in the proportion of patients who demonstrate sequential elevations in PSA as the first and only manifestation of androgen independence. Management of these patients, who are not only asymptomatic but typically have no evidence of disease by conventional imaging studies, is controversial. Some physicians defer treatment until a predetermined level of PSA is reached, whereas others wait until symptoms develop. In the absence of curative treatment, the relative toxicity of a proposed intervention also impacts on the decision of when to institute therapy.

For patients who present with distant metastases or who are symptomatic at the time androgen ablation is initiated, documentation of a rise in PSA level indicates a predictable adverse outcome. In one series of patients treated with either orchiectomy alone or a gonadotropin-releasing hormone analog plus flutamide, sequential elevations in PSA level antedated progression on a radionuclide bone scan by a median of 6 months and clinical symptoms by a median of 10 months.[5] This justifies the consideration of a change in treatment when PSA levels rise prior to the development of clinical symptoms.

There is a distinct pattern of relapse that occurs in 10% to 15% of cases in which rapid progression is documented locally or in a visceral site after a period of apparent stability. Frequently, serum PSA levels are disproportionately low relative to total tumor burden, and the striking bone tropism associated with typical prostatic adenocarcinomas is absent. Bone lesions, when present, are osteolytic as opposed to osteoblastic. In these cases, a repeat biopsy frequently shows cells with neuroendocrine features interspersed throughout the tumor.

The clinical heterogeneity of relapsing prostate cancers has significant therapeutic implications. As such, a uniform treatment recommendation for all patients with relapsing disease cannot be made. Treating patients with a wide range of clinical behavior with similar therapy risks misinterpreting the results of treatments that may have a unique effect on a subset of these cancers. Each patient must be evaluated individually and the clinical background of the relapse considered. This involves an evaluation of tumor factors such as the extent, sites, and proliferative capacity, and host factors such as estimated life expectancy of the patient in the context of medical comorbidities. It must also be recognized that much of the literature on which treatment recommendations are currently based was generated prior to the availability of PSA determinations. Posttherapy PSA changes permit a more accurate assessment of disease activity in relapsed patients, and provide a useful surrogate endpoint to evaluate new agents. As more patients are treated who have received less prior treatment, have a good performance status, and have adequate bone marrow reserve, it will become apparent that prostate cancers are not as resistant to treatment as previously believed. This section focuses on the evolution of a treatment approach designed to clarify the clinical status of a patient so that therapy can be optimized for individuals and new strategies investigated.

BIOLOGY OF PROGRESSION

A series of genetic changes are required to develop a malignancy. These generally involve two classes of genes: oncogenes, which lead to an increase in cell number, and tumor suppressor genes, which inhibit this process.[6] In normal adult tissues, the stimulatory and inhibitory influences are balanced so that there is no net accumulation of cells. Although the tissues are self-renewing, growth rates and death rates are equivalent.

Investigators have shown stage-dependent differences in the expression of specific oncogenes and tumor suppressor genes in prostate cancer from different stages. For example, overexpression of *HRAS* appears to be more common in metastatic prostate cancers than in those that are clinically localized.[7] In the normal prostate, tumor suppressor genes such as the retinoblastoma (*RB1*) and *P53* genes are constitutively expressed. In the malignant phenotype, the function of a tumor suppressor gene may be abrogated. Mutations in *P53* were initially thought to occur rarely in prostatic carcinomas because less than 5% of primary hormone-naive tumors stain positive for this tumor suppressor gene. However, when pathologic specimens from metastatic hormone-independent tumors are evaluated, about 50% of samples are positive for *P53*.[8–10] The biologic behavior of these tumors is likely to be different.

Specific chromosomal regions associated with metastatic ability have also been identified. These include the long arm of chromosome 16 (16q22.1), where the E-cadherin gene is located.[11] E-cadherin is a Ca^{2+}-dependent cell-surface glycoprotein found on epithelial cells that functions as a Ca^{2+}-dependent epithelial cell-cell adhesion molecule. Loss of expression enhances invasiveness and motility of epithelial cells. Similarly, C-CAM, another cellular adhesion molecule, appears to be lost very early in malignancy. All carcinomas and a portion of the prostatic intraepithelial neoplasias lose C-CAM. Prostatic intraepithelial neoplasia is considered a premalignant lesion of prostatic carcinoma and the central suppressive event that, when deregulated, permits the growth of the malignancy. Studies suggest that transfection of C-CAM back into the tumor cells results in suppression of the tumor.

Evolution to Hormone Independence

Medical or surgical castration results in the apoptotic regression of a portion of the tumor; the surviving cells may lie dormant or undergo the same sequence of expansion, metastatic seeding, and proliferation despite castrate levels of androgen. In these cases, alternative signaling pathways are activated to permit androgen-independent growth. It has been shown that progression to androgen independence coincides with the enhanced expression of the *BCL2* oncogene.[12] This oncogene is unique in that its expression inhibits the rate of death of cancer cells without affecting their rate of cell proliferation. Blocking the programed cell death normally induced by androgen ablation allows these cells to become androgen independent.[12] Strategies to increase death rates of cancer cells by, for example, increasing intracellular calcium are under investigation.[13]

Growth Factor and Growth Factor Receptor Interactions

A number of polypeptide growth factors have been shown to contribute to prostate cancer cell growth. These factors include the transmembrane receptor tyrosine kinases such as epidermal growth factor receptor (EGFR) and its natural ligand transforming growth factor-α (TGFA), the insulin-like growth factors (IGFs), and members of the fibroblast growth factor families.[14,15] IGFs are potent mitogens for human prostate cancer cells[16–20] and osteoblasts[21] via interaction with IGF receptors. Elevated levels of serum IGF binding proteins have been reported in patients with metastatic human prostate cancer.[22] Additionally, as prostate cancers progress from androgen-dependent to androgen-independent states, they begin to synthesize and secrete PSA in the absence of androgen.[23–25] A factor representing a PSA-stimulating autocrine factor (PSAF) has been identified that may correlate with an androgen-refractory state.[25] PSA itself may be a direct mitogen for prostate cancer growth through selective proteolysis. The release of IGF from the IGF binding protein is an example of such activation by PSA.[26] The predilection of prostate epithelial cells for bone and the proliferation in the bone microenvironment is also the result of a bidirectional interaction whereby bone cells produce growth-promoting substances and prostate cancer cells produce soluble mediators that promote osteoblast proliferation.[27–31]

Neuroendocrine Differentiation

Neuroendocrine cells are intimately associated with the prostate and can be identified by immunostaining of the normal and malignant gland. Cohen and coworkers[32] first demonstrated that neuron-specific enolase (NSE) and chromogranin staining increased in patients with more advanced tumors and predicted an adverse outcome. Abrahamsson and coworkers[33] also observed that there was an increased density of neuroendocrine cells associated with tumor progression. A number of neuropeptides have been identified in prostatic tissues and their effects on proliferation evaluated experimentally. Bombesin, which is produced by prostatic epithelial cells, binds to receptors on the same cells to function in an autocrine fashion.[34,35] Elevated serum levels of bombesin and NSE have been identified in patients with androgen-independent disease. The effect of bombesin is similar to that observed in small cell lung cancers. Serotonin, a potent epithelial cell mitogen, is produced in prostatic stroma and is believed to act via a paracrine interaction by binding to the 5-H1A serotonin receptor isoform on prostatic epithelial cells. Blockade of the receptor decreases proliferation and invasion in vitro and tumor growth in vivo.[36]

It is likely that there is some redundancy in the signaling processes that contribute to androgen-independent growth. It is also likely that different pathways may be more active in one patient's tumor relative to another patient's tumor. Additional studies that directly characterize tumors from patients in different stages, in different sites, and before and after androgen ablative therapy are needed. For these studies, it is also important to classify correctly the associated clinical status from which the specimens were derived. The clinical observation that a tumor is proliferating in the absence of androgen does not necessarily mean that the tumor is resistant to all forms of hormonal manipulations. These same considerations are important when evaluating the results of reported clinical trials.

INTERPRETING CLINICAL TRIALS IN RELAPSED DISEASE

No therapeutic intervention has been demonstrated to improve survival in a randomized controlled clinical trial for patients with relapsed disease.[37,38] Although several trials are ongoing, current treatment recommendations are for the most part based on the results of single-arm phase II trials. Numerous single agents and combinations of agents have been tried.[39] Even in cases that do respond to treatment, the duration of response is usually short, and treatment-related toxicities can be significant. On the surface, it appears that chemotherapy should not be used. A review of the reported trials provides some insight into the reasons outcomes have been so poor. Patient, tumor, and methodologic issues must be considered in formulating a treatment approach.

Patient Factors

In many studies, the patient population enrolled is not clearly defined with respect to prior therapy and extent of disease. This is particularly true for hormonal therapies, in which patients who have received one or and those who have received as many as five different hormone manipulations are included in the same trial.[40–42] Many chemotherapeutic drugs have a steep dose-rate dose-response relation. The ability to deliver adequate doses of an agent may be limited by the percent of bone marrow that is compromised by tumor or that has been previously exposed to radiotherapy. Intercurrent medical problems can also limit drug delivery.[37,38] When a patient progresses after androgen ablation, castrate levels of testosterone are assumed; however, documentation of castrate levels in clinical trials is not routine.

Tumor Factors

A proportion of patients who progress on one hormone treatment may respond to a second hormone. Operationally, these patients are androgen independent but not hormone independent. Agents that have shown efficacy include inhibitors of adrenal synthesis such as ketoconazole,[43–46] corticosteroids,[40,47–49] and aminoglutethimide[50–54]; antiandrogens such as flutamide[55]; and hormonal agents such as estrogens,[56,57] estramustine phosphate[37,58,59] and progestational agents.[60,61] More recently, responses have been observed with the withdrawal of antiandrogens such as flutamide[62–64] and casodex[65,66] in patients with castrate levels of testosterone. This biologic phenomenon is of great interest and may indicate that select patients whose tumors exhibit androgen-independent growth may benefit from further hormonal manipulations. In general, however, these secondary responses are short-lived and may benefit only a small proportion of patients. These observations further emphasize the importance of distinguishing androgen independence from hormonal independence.

Unfortunately, in many trials the rates and adequacy of hormonal manipulations are not adequately explored, which can have a profound influence on the results reported. This clarification is important when considering interventions for patients who are asymptomatic yet show progression of disease manifest by a rise in PSA levels, because it is likely that hormonal interventions may be significantly less toxic than some chemotherapeutic options. We have proposed that certain basic information be required to place a patient on a clinical trial. Inclusion of this information in the clinical protocol will allow the completion of a trial in a uniform population. All patients with cancers that exhibit androgen-independent growth must have castrate levels of serum testosterone as well as objective clinical or biochemical evidence of progression. Those who are being treated with a combined androgen blockade regimen including an antiandrogen should have the antiandrogen withdrawn and be observed until progression is again documented or for a minimum of 6 weeks before initiating any new therapies.

Failure to employ uniform and objective criteria of androgen-independent growth may account for some of the differences in reported results of therapy. It may also explain the frequency of secondary hormonal responses following failure of primary therapy for androgen-independent prostate cancer progression. In particular, it may have contributed to the differences in reported outcomes with the combination of suramin and hydrocortisone.[42]

TABLE 58-1. *Selected results with conventional chemotherapeutic agents in hormone-refractory prostatic cancer using different endpoints*

Agent	References	No. of patients	Response rate (%)	95% Confidence interval
Adriamycin weekly	81	12	33[a]	7–60
	81	25	84[b]	70–98
	71	32	12[a]	1–32
Adriamycin + ketoconazole	96	38	55[d]	38–71
	96	12	58[a]	
Vinblastine	176	39	21[c,d]	8–33
Estramustine	104		21	9–34
Estramustine plus vinblastine	177	24	54[f]	34–74
Estramustine plus vinblastine	109	37	46[f]	30–62
Estramustine plus vinblastine	95	23	52[f]	31–73
Estramustine plus vinblastine	95, 177, 178	19	42[a]	20–61
Estramustine plus oral etoposide	93	42	52[b]	36–68
	93	18	50[a]	26–74
Taxol	110	22	5	1–23
Mitomycin	179	31	29[a]	13–45
FAM (5-fluorouracil, adriamycin, mitomycin)	67	78	41[d]	30–52
Mitoxantrone	36	38	50[e]	34–66
Mitoxantrone (infusion)	82	13	16[f]	0–35
Mitoxantrone + prednisone	83	25	36[g]	18–57
	83	13	52[b]	25–82
	83	25	20[f]	7–41

[a] Measurable disease only.
[b] National Prostatic Cancer Project response criteria (includes stable disease).
[c] Administered by continuous infusion.
[d] M. D. Anderson criteria (180).
[e] Subjective improvement.
[f] >50% decline in PSA.
[g] Palliative response based on present pain intensity (PPI) and analgesic score.

Trial Methodology: Outcomes Based on Measurable, Osseous, and PSA-Only Disease

The endpoints and patient populations used for phase II trials in relapsed prostate cancer are as follows:

Endpoints
- Objective regression in measurable disease
- Decline in serum PSA level
- Quality of life
  - Functional indices
  - Pain relief, change in analgesic, or both
- Time to progression
- Time to need for change in therapy
- Survival

Patient population
- PSA only
- Osseous only
- Measurable disease
- Initial therapy in poor-prognosis patients

Discerning tumor response in bone, the most common site of spread of prostatic cancers, is difficult. This has led some investigators to restrict clinical trial entry to patients with measurable disease. Using this approach at Memorial Sloan-Kettering Cancer Center (MSKCC), 10 single-agent trials were completed, with partial responses in 0% to 24% of cases[70–75] and an overall median survival of 6.3 months.[76] The limited efficacy of these agents may reflect several factors: that the agent is inactive, that an adequate trial was not conducted because of the advanced nature of the disease in the population treated, or because measurable disease does not reflect true prostate cancer. As an illustration of the latter factor, in several of our measurable disease trials, lymph node metastases were shown to regress at the same time that osseous lesions progressed. Although this may relate to the inherent insensitivity of bone lesions, it also suggests that outcomes based on measurable disease regression alone may not translate to patients with osseous spread.

Standardized phase II response criteria based on measurable disease regression cannot be applied for osseous lesions.[77] Recognizing this, many groups have developed independently criteria for response which are for the most part not comparable. The inclusion of subjective criteria in many of the trials is similarly problematic, because these outcomes are difficult to reproduce on a large scale. It therefore is not surprising that a wide range of response proportions have been reported for a given chemotherapeutic agent. The influence of criteria on outcome is shown by the results using mitoxantrone, in which a response proportion of 16% was observed using posttherapy PSA changes as the outcome measure[78] and a response proportion of 50% was observed when subjective criteria were used as the outcome measure.[79] Weekly administration of Adriamycin produced regression in measurable disease in 33% (4 of 12) of cases in one series. In contrast, using a set of criteria that included ''stable disease'' as a response category,[80] an 84% response proportion was reported for the same patient population.[81] A similar range in outcomes based on different response criteria have been observed for mitoxantrone.[36,82,83] Table 58-1 summarizes a series of trials with several traditional chemotherapeutic agents.

Other investigators have used randomized design based on "time to progression" as the outcome measure.[84,85] In these trials, care must be taken to insure that an adequate number of patients are enrolled, that the criteria for progression are well defined and reproducible, and that patients are reevaluated at fixed time intervals with the same testing procedures. Additionally, these trials probably should not be undertaken unless there is sufficient evidence of antitumor activity in a patient population in whom response can be assessed. Perhaps the greatest difficulty with early trials is that the criteria for progression used did not consider changes in PSA.

Posttherapy PSA Decline as a Clinical Trial Endpoint

Changes in PSA levels correlate with the activity of prostate cancers in all stages. PSA testing provides the opportunity to screen more agents rapidly and reproducibly.[86] Additionally, although the absolute levels of PSA are lower in androgen-independent tumors, more than 90% of patients with relapsing disease have elevated PSA levels.[87] A justification for using posttherapy PSA levels as a clinical trial endpoint is provided by the clinical observation that for patients with metastatic disease, elevations in PSA precede radiographic and clinical signs of progression by a matter of months.[88] Similarly, patients with persistently elevated PSA levels after androgen ablation have such poor outcomes that a change in treatment is justified. The null hypothesis under study in these trials is that agents that do not produce a defined degree of decline in PSA on multiple determinations for a defined duration are inactive and do not warrant further investigation.

It is recognized that PSA levels can change as a function of hormonal status[89] or by the chemotherapy itself, independent of an effect on cell kill. For example, we observed midcycle declines in PSA after administration of trimetrexate,[75] while suramin has been shown to inhibit PSA release in vitro.[90] Retinoic acid can result in an increase in PSA levels, whereas dimethylformamide inhibits PSA mRNA expression.[91] Immunohistochemical evaluations of prostatic tumors for PSA show that not all cells are positive.[92] These data show that PSA levels may fluctuate independent of cell kill, and that decreases in PSA may simply reflect an effect on PSA-positive cells, with the non–PSA-positive cells surviving and continuing to proliferate.

Many groups have reported results based on posttherapy PSA declines; however, there is no uniform definition for PSA response. For example, some investigators report a range of percentage declines,[56,93] others a mean decrease,[94] and others fixed percentages ranging from 40%[55] to 50%[70,95,96] to 80%[41] as the endpoint. The criteria in use at MSKCC are as follows:

Complete response: normalization of serum PSA level for three successive evaluations, 2 or more weeks apart
Partial response: decline of PSA value by ≥80% (without normalization) for three successive evaluations
Stabilization: patients who do not meet the criteria for partial response or progression for at least 90 days
Progression: three consecutive increases in PSA[19] to >50% above baseline

Standardization of reporting is essential. More important is that no criteria have been validated through correlations with changes in measurable disease or in relation to survival in phase III trials using a survival endpoint. An outline of the approach to screen new agents based on PSA change is shown in Figure 58-1. Prior to entry on trial, we require three successive elevations in PSA despite castrate levels of testosterone. Baseline values should exceed 40 ng/dL (>20 ng/mL if the prostate has been removed) prior to entry. For response, we require three biweekly determinations a minimum of 2 or more weeks apart. For progression, we require a more than 50% rise from baseline on two successive occasions. These criteria were based on a trial in patients with measurable disease in which all patients who showed elevations developed symptoms in a relatively short period of time.[75] Agents that show antitumor activity can then be tested in patients with measurable disease. If antitumor activity is confirmed in the first validation of the outcome (step II), the agent or agents can then be tested in a large-scale phase III trial using survival as the endpoint (steps III and IV).

To assess what degree of decline in PSA level correlates with survival in patients with hormone-refractory disease treated with systemic therapies, we performed a multivariable analysis of patients treated with relapsed disease for prognostic factors for survival. Of 20 factors considered, whether or not a patient showed a 50% or greater decline in PSA posttherapy was most significant. The median survival of patients showing a 50% decline from baseline in PSA (23 cases) versus those who did not show a 50% decline (91 cases) was 20.76 versus 8.11 months (logrank test, $P = .0002$). For an 80% decline (8 cases) the median survival has not been reached, compared with 8.57 months for the 106 patients who did not meet this criterion (logrank test, $P = .02$).[97] This model was subsequently validated on an independent data set of 91 patients treated in Norway.[98] The prognostic significance of a more than 50% decline in PSA from baseline has been confirmed by other groups.[93,96,99] It is unknown whether a 50% decline is as stringent as an 80% decline. It is possible, however, that the less stringent criterion may be equally valid, because it will capture patients whose PSA levels do not decline or increase after treatment. It is likely that many of these patients were formerly considered stable.

Survival

Agents with activity in phase II investigations can be tested for an impact on survival by comparing the experimental treatment with a standard therapy or best supportive care. Sample size considerations and the comparative morbidity of the experimental treatments must also be considered when designing such trials. The National Prostatic Cancer Project was one of the first groups to conduct randomized comparisons using single agents versus best supportive care.[100] They reported an increase in the *mean* survival time for cyclophosphamide versus standard therapy; however, no improvement in *median* survival was shown on a reanalysis. A 70% to 80% improvement in median survival would have been required for the experimental group relative to the control for statistical significance to be reached.[37] Low-dose prednisone has been used as the control arm in several such studies based on the palliative effects observed in a phase II trial.[49]

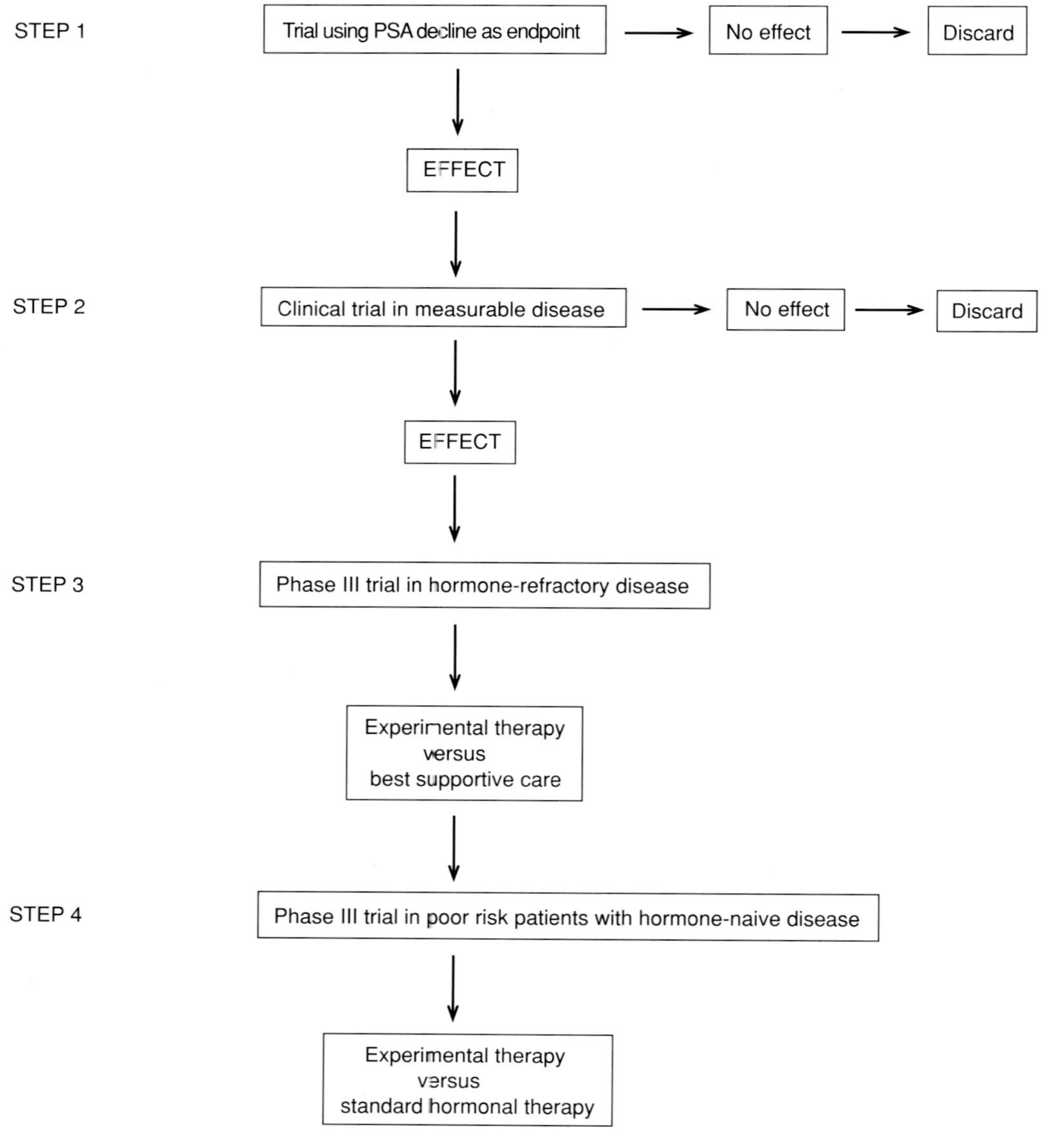

APPROACH TO THE PATIENT

In our clinics, a patient who presents for treatment of relapsed disease is first characterized on the basis of whether he is in fact castrate. In some cases of patients receiving gonadotropin-releasing hormone analogs, incomplete suppression of testosterone may occur. A patient showing progression on a pure antiandrogen may respond to a hormonal manipulation that lowers testosterone levels.[101] For patients treated with combined androgen blockade with a gonadotropin-releasing hormone analog or orchiectomy plus an antiandrogen, a trial of antiandrogen withdrawal is evaluated as the initial therapeutic maneuver. This rationale is based on the results of three independent trials showing that the selective discontinuation of flutamide in patients who have progressed on combined androgen blockade can result in biochemical, clinical, and radiographic improvement.[62–64] In two of the reports describing flutamide-withdrawal responses, objective clinical benefit was documented in patients who had progressed on multiple hormone therapies and chemotherapy,[62,64] a clear indication that their treating physicians had considered them to be hormone refractory.

It is also important to maintain androgen ablative therapies in patients who have not undergone surgical castration, because a proportion of cells in a relapsing tumor remain sensitive to testosterone. In one study in which androgens were given in an attempt to make cells more susceptible to chemotherapy[102] or radioisotopes, life-threatening complications or disease flares were seen in some patients. Similarly, megesterol acetate can cause clinically significant exacerbation of the disease.[60]

Results With Traditional Chemotherapeutic Agents

Until the criteria for response have been standardized and validated in the PSA era, it is best to report outcomes based on PSA declines; measurable disease regression and other modalities should be evaluated separately. Many agents are currently undergoing reevaluation. The results demonstrate that some of the traditional agents indeed have activity and suggest that agents that are administered on a chronic basis appear most active. The data also show that prostate cancers are not as resistant to therapy as previously believed.

Two trials evaluating a doxorubicin-based combination are illustrative. The first study combined weekly doxorubicin (15 mg/m^2) and 5-fluorouracil (250 mg/m^2/day) administered by continuous infusion. Objective responses (>50% reduction in PSA or >50% regimen in measurable disease) were observed in 61% (11 of 18; 95% confidence interval, 39% to 84%) of patients.[103] The second study, from MD Anderson, which combined ketoconazole (1200 mg daily) and Adriamycin (20 mg/m^2 weekly by 24-hour infusion), resulted in an overall response proportion using MD Anderson criteria of 55% (21 of 38; 95% confidence interval, 38% to 71%), including a more than 50% reduction in PSA on three consecutive occasions in 55% and measurable disease regression in 7 of 12 (58%; 95% confidence interval, 28% to 85%) cases.[96] Toxicities included grade 3 or 4 stomatitis and acral erythema in 29% and anal and urethral mucositis in 13% of patients. Myelosuppression was significant, and 63% of patients developed clinical signs of adrenal insufficiency. Nevertheless, if activity is confirmed with additional testing, phase III trials using these combinations appear to be justified.

Targeted Approaches

Several translational approaches have been investigated with promising preliminary results. Phase III investigations have likewise been initiated.

Microtubules Inhibition

Estramustine phosphate inhibits microtubule assembly. It has a different mechanism than the vinca alkaloids vinblastine and vincristine, which exert their antimitotic effects by binding to tubulin. As single agents, estramustine (14 mg/kg/day) produced a greater than 50% decline in PSA in 21% (95% confidence interval, 9% to 34%) of cases,[104] whereas vinblastine administered by continuous infusion produced tumor regression in 21% of cases.[105] Based on in vitro studies showing synergy with the vinca alkaloids,[106,107] a two-drug regimen was developed. At MSKCC, estramustine (10 mg/kg/day orally) combined with vinblastine (4 mg/m^2 weekly for 6 weeks) produced a more than 50% decline in PSA in 13 of 24 (54%; 95% confidence interval, 34% to 74%) and measurable disease regression in 2 of 5 cases. Myelosuppression was minimal.[77] Using these same endpoints, but a slightly different dose schedule, Amato[108] observed PSA declines in 11 of 22 and measurable disease regression in 3 of 7 cases, and Hudes and colleagues[109] observed PSA declines in 17 of 37 (46%; 95% confidence interval, 35% to 62%) and measurable disease response in 3 of 7 cases, respectively. Combining the results, 43% (35 of 82; 95% confidence interval, 32% to 53%) of patients showed PSA regressions, and 42% (8 of 19; 95% confidence limits, 20% to 64%) showed measurable disease response. Two phase III trials comparing the combination to vinblastine are ongoing. Taxol, an agent that also acts on tubulin and is active against a number of tumors, showed minimal activity in a phase II trial in patients with measurable hormone-refractory tumors. Overall, only 1 of 22 patients (5%; 95% confidence interval, 0% to 13%) responded using PSA or measurable disease as response criteria.[110] When combined with estramustine, responses were observed in a number of cases.[110a]

Nuclear Matrix

The nuclear matrix, an RNA-protein network in the nucleus, is altered by transformation to the malignant state.[111] It functions to control chromatin organization and nuclear shape, which are important for the regulation of both DNA replication and gene expression. A unique set of nuclear matrix proteins have been described in prostate cancer cells.[112] In vitro, estramustine alone and etoposide alone have modest effects on prostate cancer cell growth. In combination, synergy is observed through an effect on the nuclear matrix.[112a] Based on these results, a phase II trial of estramustine (15 mg/kg daily) and oral etoposide (100 mg daily for 21 days) was investigated. Using posttherapy PSA changes as response criteria, 52% showed a more than 50% decline, and 9 of 18 (50%; 95% confidence interval, 26% to 74%) patients with measurable disease showed a complete (3 cases) or partial response (6 cases).[112b] These results are noteworthy based on the limited activity observed with etoposide as a single agent in this disease.[113–115]

Growth Factor Inhibitors

Suramin is a polyanionic compound with a variety of biologic effects that include the inhibition of binding of growth factors to their receptors. Other effects include inhibition of glycosaminoglycan degradation, membrane associated ion pumps, protein kinase C, glycolysis, and cell motility.[116] Based on the observation that suramin blocked a number of the polypeptide growth factors believed to contribute to prostate cancer cell growth and proliferation,[117,118] the results of in vitro and in vivo studies using prostate cancer cell lines,[117,119] and the effects of suramin on adrenal steroidogenesis,[120] clinical trials were initiated against human prostate cancers.

Reported results from several centers are summarized in Table 58-2. Thirty-five percent (35 of 111; 95% confidence interval, 20% to 42%) of patients with measurable disease showed a greater than 50% reduction in size, and 44% (71 of 166; 95% confidence interval, 34% to 54%) showed a greater than 50% decline in PSA. Toxicities include polyradiculopathy, myelopathy, renal insufficiency, coagulopathy, and vortex keratopathy. A therapeutic window was suggested on the basis of phase I investigations, which led to complex dosing schema with computer-based modeling and plasma concentration monitoring.[121] The durability of the responses seen led to the investigation of simplified schedules, several of which are under study.[122–124] The most frequent mode of administration involves repeated short infusions that maintain plasma concentrations over a period of several weeks.[99] More recently, it has been shown that computer modelling is not required, and that maintaining plasma concentrations in a defined range may not

TABLE 58-2. *Reported results with suramin and hydrocortisone*

			Measurable Disease		PSA (>50% decrease)	
Center	Reference	Schedule	No. of patients	PR	No. of patients	PR
National Cancer Institute	41	Infusion*	14	7 (50%)	32	15 (47%)
University of Arizona	180	Infusion*	15	7 (42%)	15	7 (42%)
MSKCC-MDAH-Mayo Clinic	†	Infusion*	36	3 (9%)	36	8 (22%)
Walter-Reed	‡	Infusion*		NR	20	10 (50%)
Brussels	181	Infusion‖		NR	9	4 (44%)
Gustave Roussy	¶	Infusion‖		NR	5	3 (60%)
South Africa	182	Infusion*	25	5 (20%)		NR
University of Maryland	183	Interm#	18	7 (40%)	67	40 (60%)
MSKCC	184	Cohort A**	7	1 (14%)	19	4 (21%)
		Cohort B††	6	1 (20%)	6	1 (17%)
		Cohort C‡‡	4	0 (20%)	28	4 (23%)
University of Chicago	185	Day 1, 2, 8, 9[7]‖‖		N.R.	12	9 (75%)
Total			125	29 (26%)	211	79 (37%)

MDAH, MD Anderson Cancer Center; MSKCC, Memorial Sloan-Kettering Cancer Center; NR, no response; PR, partial responding.
* Loading dose followed by infusion of 350 mg/m^2/day to a target of 280–300 μg/mL.
† Christian M, unpublished study, 1991.
‖ Loading dose followed by infusion of 400 or 500 mg/m^2/day to target of 300 μg/mL.
¶ Armand JP, Droz JP, personal communication, 1990.
\# Intermittent bolus infusions maintaining concentrations in range of 200–300 μg/mL until dose-limiting toxicities are observed.
** Loading dose, continuous infusion for 1 week, intermittent bolus administrations to maintain concentrations in range of 200–300, 175–275, or 150–250 μg/mL.
†† Adaptive control without computer simulation maintaining plasma concentrations in the range of 150–250 μg/mL.
‡‡ Empiric schedule without adaptive control.
‖‖ Empiric schedule giving 1730 mg/m^2 in month 1 and 865 mg/m^2 in months 2 and 3.
‡Dawson N, personal communication, 1990.

be necessary for therapeutic efficacy. A potentially confounding factor of the clinical trials is that all patients receive hydrocortisone replacement therapy as part of treatment.[125] A randomized trial of suramin and hydrocortisone versus hydrocortisone alone has been initiated.

Anaplastic Small Cell Tumors

The clinical presentation of this variant of androgen-independent prostatic cancer has been previously described. This tumor presents in its pure form with a dominant small cell component responsible for its clinical manifestation in one third of the cases, whereas in two thirds of cases it is an acquired phenomenon. It is viewed as a histologic continuum and progression from the adenocarcinoma component. In most cases, a mixture of cells with neuroendocrine features stain positively for neuropeptides such as serotonin, bombesin, somatostatin, calcitonin, or PTH-related protein.[126] Prior to initiating trials, the predictive value of neuroendocrine elements in identifying this unique subset of patients must be confirmed, and the expression of these elements must be controlled in prospective clinical trials focused on adenocarcinoma in these elements alone.

Recognition of this entity is important because these tumors are sensitive to regimens used to treated small cell tumors of the bronchus, such as etoposide and cisplatin (EP) or cyclophosphamide and Adriamycin and vincristine (CAV), treatments that are generally not recommended for conventional adenocarcinomas.[127–129] Other strategies under investigation include the inhibition of serotonin-mediated progression by specific inhibitors of bombesin and inhibition of organ-specific progression. In many cases, elevated serum levels of bombesin, NSE, or chromogranin can be documented. Direct correlations with survival, however, have not been performed. The role of castration in the outcome of patients with small cell carcinoma has not been validated. Similarly, the role of neuroendocrine elements and the influence of selection of therapy in otherwise typical adenocarcinoma of the prostate has not yet been established.

OSSEOUS METASTASES

In phase II chemotherapy trials for relapsing patients, we have observed that soft tissue sites are more responsive than osseous lesions. Even among responding patients, 80% of progressions occur in bone. These results suggest that the microenvironment of the skeleton is uniquely permissive for prostate cancer cell proliferation and survival. Growth factors that have been implicated in this process include IGF, which can be isolated from bone osteoblasts[130]; transferrin[131]; and basic fibroblast growth factor.[132] A review of these growth factors is provided elsewhere.[3] Each of these factors can selectively stimulate prostate cancer cells in vitro.

To investigate these interactions further, investigators coinnoculated LNCaP cells with fibroblasts from bone, prostate, lung and kidney into athymic male nude mice.[24,25] PSA levels were shown to correlate with tumor volume. By maintaining these cell lines in castrated hosts, a number of sublines were developed. One of these sublines, C4-2, acquired androgen independence as shown by its ability to proliferate and to metastasize to bone in a castrate environment. This cell line was also shown to secrete PSA autonomously.[24,25] This was shown to be the result of PSAF, which may serve as a marker for androgen-independent progression. A similar factor has been found in bone marrow samples from patients with osseous lesions that proliferate without androgens. Our preliminary analysis showed that 22 of 43 patient samples were positive.

To selectively attack prostate cancer cells in the skeleton, a number of bone-seeking radioisotopes have been investigated. These agents were traditionally used for imaging. By using short-range emitters, normal marrow can be spared and all areas of the skeleton treated simultaneously. As discussed in more detail elsewhere in this text, one agent, strontium-89 (^{89}Sr) was approved for use in 1994 based on the results of randomized comparisons.[133] This agent was shown to have a tumor-to-marrow ratio of 10 : 1, and more than 50% of an injected dose is taken up in the bone matrix.[134] Although the results of individual trials vary, palliation has been reported in up to 75% of cases treated with a 4-mCi dose. Few data, however, are available regarding the effect of the compound on PSA levels.

Two diphosphonates, 186-ReHEDP rhenium-186 (Tin) hydroxy ethylidene diphosphonate and Sm-153-EDTMP samarium-153 phosphonic acid 1,2-ethyanediyl bis nitrilobis (methylene) tetrakis-monohydrate are also in trial.[78,135] The radioactive moieties of these compounds emit gamma energies that can be imaged and short-range beta energies that are therapeutic. Localization to bone is provided by the diphosphonate moiety. Re-186-HEDP was originally developed at the University of Cincinnati and has shown significant palliation for patients with painful lesions.[136,137] In a phase II trial at MSKCC, palliation was observed; however, the effect on PSA was less consistent.[138] A dose response, however, was suggested, because the proportion of patients demonstrating PSA declines increased with higher levels of administration. Similar results have been observed using 153-Sm-EDTMP. At doses of 1 to 3 mCi/kg, pain relied was observed in 17 of 19 patients (87%), and PSA declines were noted in 7 (35%) cases.[139]

The cumulative results reported with ^{89}Sr, 186-Re-HEDP and 153-Sm-153 show differences between the proportion of patients who are palliated relative to the proportion who show permanent declines in PSA level. This may represent a placebo effect, a local effect on mediators of bone pain or osteoclasts, or a limited effect on the tumor cells at the site of isotope deposition with no effect on the central portion of the lesion. In our experience, unless there is some degree of tumor cell kill achieved, pain palliation is not durable.[140,141] It is also possible that these agents exert their effect by inhibiting the release of local mediators such as prostaglandins or growth factors, or through a direct toxic effect on bone cells. Several strategies are under study to increase the efficacy of these agents. These include administration of higher activities, combining them with agents that inhibit the repair of sublethal radiation damage, and combining them with chemotherapy programs that have independent activity against a tumor.

TRANSLATIONAL APPROACHES BASED ON TUMOR BIOLOGY

The evolution of treatment approaches emphasizes the importance of direct characterization of the cancers of individual patients. At MSKCC, patients with relapsed disease undergo a repeat biopsy of the refractory tumor to determine the presence or absence of a neuroendocrine component, in which case aggressive chemotherapy may be recommended, and for the selection of specific treatments that target the cell surface. Preliminary results have shown that primary and hormone-refractory metastatic lesions are different with respect to the expression of EGFR[142] and prostate-specific membrane antigen (PSMA).[143,144] Clinical trials with agents directed to these cell-surface targets are ongoing.

Angiogenesis Inhibition

Growth of a tumor mass beyond a certain size requires new blood vessel formation.[145] Pathologic studies show that the microvessel density of latent prostate cancers is lower than that of clinically manifest tumors. Mean microvessel counts are higher in primary tumors that have metastasized than in those that have not.[146] Several agents that inhibit angiogenesis are undergoing study, including interferon, pentosan polysulfate,[147] and TNP-470, a semisynthetic analog of Fumagillin.[148] Inhibiting angiogenesis may reduce the rate of metastatic progression as well as reduce the ability of a tumor that has metastasized to grow larger than a certain size. Although these agents may have modest effects alone, they may be particularly useful in combination studies.

Differentiation

Trials designed to convert a prostate cancer to a less malignant form are also under study. Such an approach has been successfully applied using all-trans retinoic acid in acute promyelocytic leukemia.[149] Agents that act via the steroid hormone receptor superfamily have been mentioned previously. Other compounds under study include phenylacetate, which in addition to being cytostatic in cell culture, converts cells to a nonmalignant phenotype.[150] Synergy with suramin, a putative growth factor inhibitor that has undergone extensive testing in hormone-refractory disease,[123] has also been observed. Other strategies under study are focused on inhibiting signal transduction pathways with agents such as genistein, a component of soy now available as a dietary supplement[151]; tiazofurin, which inhibits inosine monophosphate dehydrogenase and down regulates *MYC* and *RAS*[152]; and lovostatin, an inhibitor HMGCoA reductase involved in the synthesis of RAS.[153]

Retinoids

Retinoic acid binds to nuclear receptors, which are transcriptional factors that may regulate particular differentiation programs. The receptors are members of the nuclear steroid receptor superfamily and have both DNA and ligand binding properties. All-trans retinoic acid was evaluated in the clinic on the basis of the direct cytotoxicity observed in vitro,[119] differentiation effects,[154] inhibitory effects on tumor development in animal models, and effects on TGFα expression in germ cell tumor cell lines.[155] Fong and colleagues[154] showed that retinoic acid inhibits EGF- and TGFα-induced proliferation of LNCaP cells by 30% and 60%, respectively. A possible role in chemoprevention was shown in a separate study. Fenretinide [*N*-(4-hydroxyphenyl)retinamide] was shown in Lobund-Wistar rats to decrease the incidence of primary tumors from 88% to 21% and metastatic tumors from 61% to 16% that spontaneously develop after treatment with *N*-methyl-nitosourea and testosterone propionate.[156] These agents are currently under study. Along similar lines, Miller and colleagues[157] described the presence of biologically active 1α,25-dihydroxyvitamin D_3 receptors on LNCaP cells.

Cell-Surface Targets

Antibodies to Growth Factor Receptors

Our initial studies focused on EGFR based on the observation that human prostate tumor–derived cell lines synthesize TGFα in culture,[97,158–161] that prostatic tumor cells express EGFR in vitro and in vivo,[162,163] that TGFA or EGF added to cultured cells is mitogenic,[97,158,164] and that monoclonal antibodies to EGFR[165] inhibit human prostate cancer cell growth.[158,166] ERBB2 (formerly known as Her2/neu) is highly expressed in prostate tissues.[167–169] Monoclonal antibody 4D5 against ERBB2 inhibits the growth of cells with high levels of the receptor.[170] EGF, ERBB2 ligand, and other growth factors exert their effects by binding to and stimulating a transmembrane tyrosine kinase receptor.

The observation that the staining pattern for EGFR and its ligand TGFA changes as prostate cancers metastasize and develop androgen independence suggests that EGFR could be a therapeutic target. A clinical trial evaluating DAB_{389}EGF in patients whose tumors express high levels of EGFR is ongoing. This molecule is a fusion toxin produced by expressing a fusion gene in bacteria and consists of sequences of EGF and the toxic portion of the diphtheria toxin molecule. Inside a cell, the toxin is released. Similarly, trials evaluating antibodies to ERBB2 are also ongoing.

TAG-72

TAG-72 is a panadenocarcinoma antigen that is expressed on prostate cancer cells. In 35 adenocarcinomas of the prostate, TAG-72 expression was seen in 100% of well differentiated, 82% of moderately differentiated, and 58% of poorly differentiated tumors.[171] In a second study, five of six prostate cancer tissue samples stained positive for both monoclonal antibodies B72.3 and CC-49 in a study comparing the two.[172] Clinical trials using 131-I-CC49, a second-generation antibody to TAG-72, are ongoing at the University of Alabama and MSKCC.

Prostate-Specific Membrane Antigen

7El1.C5 is a mouse monoclonal antibody raised against a membrane antigen on the LNCaP human-derived prostate cancer cell line. The antigen, PSMA, is restricted to prostatic tissue and skeletal and cardiac muscle cytoplasm using immunohistologic techniques.[173] The gene has been cloned and relative tissue specificity confirmed.[143] Preliminary studies show staining of both primary and metastatic tumors, with a suggestion that a higher percentage of cells stain in androgen-independent metastatic (90%) than in primary (50%) lesions.[174] An immunoconjugate of the antibody labeled with indium-111 was successful in imaging prostate cancers in humans.[175] More recently, the beta-emitter yttrium-90 has been attached to the antibody CYT-356 (^{90}Y-CYT-356) and is in trial.

CONCLUSIONS

Androgen-independent prostate cancer is a heterogeneous disease that continues to be a therapeutic challenge. A variety of treatment options are available that can provide objective tumor regression and palliate the symptoms of the disease. Increased understanding of the biology of the disease has led to the rapid translation of promising strategies from research trials to the clinic. These include strategies that inhibit blood vessel formation and thereby render tumors less malignant. Additionally, as contemporary trials define the patients populations more clearly, and the outcomes are reported in a more consistent and reproducible fashion, treatment selection will be refined and outcomes will improve. This is particularly important for the small cell variant of the disease.

REFERENCES

1. Isaacs JT, Lundmo PI, Berges R, Martikainen P, Kyprianou N, English HF. Androgen regulation of programmed cell death of normal and malignant prostatic cells. J Androl 1992;13:457.
2. Goldenberg SL, Bruchovsky N, Rennie PS, Coppin CM. The combination of cyproterone acetate and low dose diethylstilbestrol in the treatment of advanced prostatic carcinoma. J Urol 1988;138:1460.
3. Scher HI, Chung LWK. Bone metastases: improving the therapeutic index. Semin Oncol 1994;21:630.
4. Murphy GP. Report on the American Urologic Association/American Cancer Society scientific seminar on the detection and treatment of early-stage prostate cancer. CA Cancer J Clin 1994;44:91.
5. Newling DWW. Orchiectomy versus zoladex and flutamide in the treatment of newly diagnosed metastatic prostate cancer. Cancer 1993; 72:3793.
6. Isaacs WB, Carter BS. Genetic changes associated with prostate cancer in humans. Cancer Surv 1993;11:15.
7. Sumiya H, Masai M, Akimoto S, Yatani R, Shimazaki J. Histochemical examination of expression of ras p21 protein and R 1881-binding protein in human prostatic cancers. Eur J Cancer 1990;26:786.
8. Effert PJ, Neubauer A, Walther PJ, Liu ET. Alterations of the P53 gene are associated with the progression of a human prostate carcinoma. J Urol 1992;147:789.
9. Navone NM, Troncoso P, Pisters L, Conti CJ. High frequency of p53 mutation in bone marrow metastases of human prostate carcinoma. J Natl Cancer Inst 1993;85:1657.
10. Bookstein R, MacGrogan D, Hilsenbck SG, Sharkey F, Allfred DC. p53 is mutated in a subset of advanced-stage prostate cancers. Cancer Res 1993;53:3369.
11. Umbas R, Schalken JA, Aalders TW, et al. Expression of the cellular adhesion molecular E-cadherin is reduced or absent in high-grade prostate cancer. Cancer Res 1992;52:5104.
12. McDonnell TJ, Troncoso P, Brisbay SM, et al. Expression of the protooncogene bcl-2 in the prostate and its association with emergence of androgen-independent prostate cancer. Cancer Res 1992;52:6940.

13. Furuya Y, Isaacs JT. Proliferation independent programmed cell death as a therapeutic target for pros cancer. Cancer Bull 1994;46:173.
14. Steiner MS. Role of peptide growth factors in the prostate: a review. Urology 1993;42:99.
15. Tanaka A, Miyamoto K, Minamino N, et al. Cloning and characterization of an androgen-induced growth factor essential for the androgen-dependent growth of mouse mammary carcinoma cells. Proc Natl Acad Sci 1992;89:8928.
16. Polychronakos C, Janthyly U, Lehous J, Koutsilieris M. Mitogenic effects of insulin and insulin-like growth factors on PA-III rat prostate adenocarcinoma cells: characterization of the receptors involved. Prostate 1991;19:313.
17. Kaicer EK, Blat C, Harel L. IGF-1 and IGF-binding proteins: stimulatory and inhibitory factors secreted by human prostatic adenocarcinoma cells. Growth Factors 1991;4:231.
18. Iwamura M, Sluss PM, Casamento JB, Cockett ATK. Insulin-like growth factor 1: action and receptor characterization in human prostate cancer cell lines. Prostate 199322:243.
19. Pietrzkowski Z, Mulholland G, Gomella L, Jameson BA, Wernicke D, Baserga R. Inhibition of growth of prostatic cancer cell lines by peptide analogues of insulin-like growth factor 1. Cancer Res 1993; 53:1102.
20. Cohen P, Peehl DM, Lamson G, Rosenfeld RG. Insulin-like growth factors (IGFs), IGF receptors, and IGF-binding proteins in primary cultures of prostate epithelial cells. J Clin Endocrinol Metab 1991; 73:401.
21. Polychronakos C, Janthly U, Lehoux JG, Koutsilieris M. Mitogenic effects of insulin and insulin-like growth factors on PA-III rat prostate adenocarcinoma cells: characterization of the receptors involved. Prostate 1991;19:313.
22. Kanety H, Madjar Y, Dagan Y, et al. Serum insulin-like growth factor-binding protein-2 (IGFBP-2) is increased and IGFBP-3 is decreased in patients with prostate cancer: correlation with serum prostate-specific antigen. J Clin Endocrinol Metab 1993;77:229.
23. Gleave ME, Hsieh JT, Wu HC, von Eschenbach AC, Chung LW. Serum prostate specific antigen levels in mice bearing human prostate LNCaP tumors are determined by tumor volume and endocrine and growth factors. Cancer Res 1992;52:1598.
24. Wu HC, Hsieh JT, Gleave ME, Brown NM, Pathak S, Chung LWK. Derivation of androgen-independent human LNCaP prostatic cancer cell sublines: role of bone stromal cells. Int J Cancer 1994 (in press).
25. Hsieh JT, Wu HC, Gleave ME, von Eschenbach AC, Chung LWK. Autocrine regulation of prostate specific antigen expression in a human prostatic cancer (LNCaP) subline. Cancer Res 1993;53:2852.
26. Cohen P, Peehl DM, Rosenfeld RG. The IGF axis in the prostate. (Abstract) 1992 International Symposium on Biology of Prostate Growth 16, Washington, DC 1992.
27. Story MT, Livingston B, Baeten L, et al. Cultured human prostate-derived fibroblasts produce a factor that stimulates their growth with properties indistinguishable from basic fibroblast growth factor. Prostate 1989;15:355.
28. Story MT, Sasse J, Jacobs SC, Lawson RK. Prostatic growth factor: purification and structural relationship to basic fibroblast growth factor. Biochemistry 1987;26:3843.
29. Koutsilieris M, Rabbani SA, Goltzman D. Effects of human prostatic mitogens on rat bone cells and fibroblasts. J Endocrinol 1987;115: 447.
30. Jacobs SC, Pinka D, Lawson RK. Prostatic osteoblast factor. Invest Urol 1979;17:195.
31. Koutsilieris M. Osteoblastic metastasis in advanced prostate cancer. Anticancer Res 1993;13:443.
32. Cohen RJ, Glezerson G, Haffejee Z. Prostate-specific antigen and prostate-specific acid phosphatase in neuroendocrine cells of prostate cancer. Arch Pathol Lab Med 1992;116:65.
33. Abrahamsson PA, Falkmer S, Falt K, Grimelius L. The course of neuroendocrine differentiation in prostatic carcinomas: an immunohistochemical study testing chromogranin A as an "endocrine marker." Pathol Res Pract 1989;185:373.
34. Shimoda J. Effects of bombesin and its antibody on growth of human prostatic carcinoma cell lines. Nippon Hinyokika Gakkai Zasshi 1992; 83:1459.
35. Milovanovic SR, Radulovic S, Groot K, Schally AV. Inhibition of growth of PC-82 human prostate cancer line xenografts in nude mice by bombesin antagonist RC-3095 or combination of agonist [D-Trp6]-luteinizing hormone-releasing hormone and somatostatin analog RC-160. Prostate 1992;20:269.
36. Hoosein NM, Logothetis CJ, Chung LWK. Differential effects of peptide hormones bombesin, vasoactive intestinal polypeptide, and somatostatin analog RC-160 on the invasive capacities of human prostatic carcinoma cell lines. (Abstract) J Urol 1992;147:333A.
37. Halpern J, Catane R. Oral estramustine phosphate (Estracyt): a broad phase II study. J Med 1984;15:35.
38. Cordon-Cardo C, Bander NH, Fradet Y, et al. J Histochem Cytochem 1984;32:1035.
39. Eisenberger MA. Chemotherapy for prostate carcinoma. Natl Cancer Inst Monogr 1988:151.
40. Harland SJ, Duchesne GM. Suramin and prostate cancer: the role of hydrocortisone. Eur J Cancer 1992;28A:1295.
41. Myers C, Cooper M, Stein C, et al. Suramin: a novel growth factor antagonist with activity in hormone-refractory metastatic prostate cancer. J Clin Oncol 1992;10:881.
42. Kelly WK, Scher H, Bajorin D, et al. The contribution of hydrocortisone to the observed response proportion of suramin. (Abstract) Proc Am Soc Clin Oncol 1994;13:231.
43. Muscato JJ, Ahmann TA, Johnson KM, Wilding W, Monaghan G, Schlossman DM. Optimal dosing of ketoconazole and hydrocortisone leads to long response in hormone refractory prostate cancer. Proc Am Soc Clin Oncol 1994;13:701.
44. Trachtenberg J, Pont A. Ketoconazole therapy for advanced prostate cancer. Lancet 1984;2:433.
45. Jubelirer SJ, Hogan T. High dose ketoconazole for the treatment of hormone refractory metastatic prostate carcinoma: 16 cases and review of the literature. J Urol 1989;142:89.
46. Williams G, Kerle DJ, Ware H, et al. Objective responses to ketoconazole therapy in patients with relapsed progressive prostatic cancer. Br J Urol 1986;58:45.
47. Miller GM, Hinman F. Cortisone treatment in advanced carcinoma of prostate. J Urol 1954;72:485.
48. Robinson MR, Shearer RJ, Fergusson JD. Adrenal suppression in the treatment of carcinoma of the prostate. Br J Urol 1974;46:555.
49. Tannock I, Gospodarowicz M, Meakin W, Panzarella T, Stewart L, Rider W. Treatment of metastatic prostatic cancer with low-dose prednisone: evaluation of pain and quality of life as pragmatic indices of response. J Clin Oncol 1989;7:590.
50. Geller J, Albert JD. Adrenal androgen blockade in relapsed prostate cancer. Eur J Cancer Clin Oncol 1985;21:1127.
51. Drago JR, Santen RJ, Lipton A, et al. Clinical effect of aminoglutethimide, medical adrenalectomy, in treatment of 43 patients with advanced prostatic carcinoma. Cancer 1984;53:1447.
52. Worgul TJ, Santen RJ, Samojlik E, et al. Clinical and biochemical effect of aminoglutethimide in the treatment of advanced prostatic carcinoma. J Urol 1983;129:51.
53. Rostom AY, Folkes A, Lord C, Notley RG, Schweitzer FA, White WF. Aminoglutethimide therapy for advanced carcinoma of the prostate. Br J Urol 1982;54:552.
54. Robinson MR. Aminoglutethimide: medical adrenalectomy in the management of carcinoma of the prostate. A review after 6 years. Br J Urol 1980;52:328.
55. Fossa SD, Hosbach G, Paus E. Flutamide in hormone-resistant prostatic cancer. J Urol 1990;144:1411.
56. Ferro MA, Gillatt D, Symes MO, Smith PJB. High-dose intravenous estrogen therapy in advanced prostatic carcinoma: use of prostate-specific antigen to monitor response. Urology 1989;34:134.
57. Droz JP, Kattan J, Bonnay M, Chraibi Y, Bekradda M, Culine S. High-dose continuous-infusion fosfestrol in hormone-resistant prostate cancer. Cancer 1992;71:1123.
58. Boccardo F, Decensi A, Guarneri D, Martorana G, Giberti C, Giuliani L. Estramustine phosphate (estracyt) following androgens in men with refractory stage D2 prostate cancer. Cancer Chemother Pharmacol 1988;22:172.
59. Soloway MS, Beckley S, Brady MF, et al. A comparison of estramustine phosphate versus cis-platinum alone versus estramustine phosphate plus cis-platinum in patients with advanced hormone refractory prostate cancer who had had extensive irradiation to the pelvis or lumbosacral area. J Urol 1983;129:56.
60. Sasagawa I, Satomi S. Effect of high-dose medroxyprogesterone acetate on plasma hormone levels and pain relief in patients with advanced prostatic cancer. Br J Cancer 1990;65:278.

61. Johansson JE, Lingardh G. High-dose medroxyprogesterone in the treatment of advanced therapy-resistant prostatic carcinoma. Eur Urol 1985;11:9.
62. Scher HI, Kelly WK. The flutamide withdrawal syndrome: its impact on clinical trials in hormone-refractory prostatic cancer. J Clin Oncol 1993;11:1566.
63. Dupont A, Gomez J, Cusan L, Koutsilieris M, Labrie F. Response to flutamide withdrawal in advanced prostate cancer in progression under combination therapy. J Urol 1993;150:908.
64. Sartor O, Cooper M, Weinberger M, et al. Surprising activity of flutamide withdrawal, when combined with aminoglutethimide, in treatment of "hormone-refractory" prostate cancer. J Natl Cancer Inst 1994;86:222.
65. Small EJ, Carroll PR. Prostate-specific antigen decline after casodex withdrawal: evidence for an antiandrogen withdrawal syndrome. Urology 1994;43:408.
66. Nieh PT. Withdrawal phenomenon with the antiandrogen casodex. J Urol 1995;153:1070.
67. Logothetis CJ, Samuels ML, von Eschenbach AC, et al. Doxorubicin, mitomycin-C, and 5-fluorouracil (DMF) in the treatment of metastatic hormonal refractory adenocarcinoma of the prostate, with a note on the staging of metastatic prostate cancer. J Clin Oncol 1983;6:368.
68. Shain SA, Lin AL, Koger JD, Karaganis AG. Rat prostate cancer cells contain functional receptors for transforming growth factor-beta. Endocrinology 1990;126:818.
69. Knudson G, Grinis G, Lopez Majano V, et al. Bone scan as a stratification variable in advanced prostate cancer. Cancer 1991;68:316.
70. Seidman AD, Scher HI, Petrylak D, Dershaw D, Curley T. Estramustine and vinblastine: use of prostate specific antigen as a clinical trial endpoint in hormone-refractory prostatic cancer. J Urol 1992;147:931.
71. Tong WP, Scher HI, Petrylak DP, Smart-Curley T, Dnistrian A, Vasquez J. A rapid assay of suramin in plasma. J Liq Chromat 1991;13:2269.
72. Scher HI, Yagoda A, Ahmed T, Watson RC. Methylglyoxal-bis(guanylhydrazone) in hormone-resistant adenocarcinoma of the prostate. J Clin Oncol 1985;3:224.
73. Scher H, Yagoda A, Watson RC, Serber M, Whitmore W. Phase II trial of doxorubicin in bidimensionally measurable prostatic adenocarcinoma. J Urol 1984;131:1099.
74. Scher HI, Yagoda A. Bone metastases: pathogenesis, treatment, and rationale for use of resorption inhibitors. Am J Med 1987;82:6.
75. Scher HI, Curley T, Geller N, et al. Trimetrexate in prostatic cancer: preliminary observations on the use of prostate-specific antigen and acid phosphatase as a marker in measurable hormone-refractory disease. J Clin Oncol 1990;8:1830.
76. Eisenberger MA, Simon R, O'Dwyer PJ, Wittes RE, Friedman MA. A reevaluation of nonhormonal cytotoxic chemotherapy in the treatment of prostatic carcinoma. J Clin Oncol 1985;3:827.
77. Scher HI, Yagoda A. Clinical trials in prostatic cancer: methodology and controversies. In: Bruce AW, Trachtenberg J, eds. Adenocarcinoma of the prostate. New York: Springer-Verlag, 1987:197.
78. Raghavan D, Pearson BS, Coorey GJ, et al. Management of hormone-resistant prostate cancer: experience at Royal Prince Alfred Hospital. In: Johnson DE, Logothetis CJ, vonEschenbach AC, eds. Systemic therapy for genitourinary cancers. Chicago: Year Book Medical, 1989:245.
79. Kantoff PW, Bryant P, Block C, Rieker P, George MJ. Fourteen day constant infusion of mitoxantrone HCL for hormone refractory carcinoma of the prostate (HRCaP): a pilot dose finding study. Proc Am Soc Clin Oncol 1991;10:175.
80. Slack NH, Mittelman A, Brady MF, Murphy GP. The importance of the stable category for chemotherapy treated patients with advanced and relapsing prostate cancer. Cancer 1980;46:2393.
81. Kolbeck S, Watson L, Ozkara H, Croft B, Gillenwater J. Magnetic resonance imaging in the evaluation of metastasis to bone from prostate caner. (Abstract) J Urol 1992;147:419A.
82. Maygarden SJ, Strom S, Ware JL. Localization of epidermal growth factor receptor by immunohistochemical methods in human prostatic carcinoma, prostatic intraepithelial neoplasia, and benign hyperplasia. Arch Pathol Lab Med 1992;116:269.
83. Moore MJ, Osoba D, Murphy D, et al. Use of palliative end points to evaluate the effects of mitoxantrone and low-dose prednisone in patients with hormonally resistant prostate cancer. J Clin Oncol 1994;12:689.
84. Newling DW, Fossa S, Tunn U, Kurth KH, De Pauw M, Sylvester R. Comparison of the effects of high dose estramustine phosphate and mitomycin C on the time to progression and length of survival of patients with progressive, advanced endocrine-independent prostatic cancer: an interim analysis of EORTC-GU Group Study No. 30865. J Steroid Biochem Mol Biol 1990;37:971.
85. Newling DW, Fossa SD, Tunn UW, Kurth KH, De Pauw M, Sylvester R. Mitomycin C versus estramustine in the treatment of hormone resistant metastatic prostate cancer: the final analysis of the European Organization for Research and Treatment of Cancer: Genitourinary Group prospective randomized phase III study (30865). J Urol 1993;150:1840.
86. Scher HI. Prostatic cancer: where do we go from here? Curr Opin Oncol 1991;3:568.
87. Leo ME, Bilhartz DL, Bergstralh EJ, Oesterling JE. Prostate specific antigen in hormonally treated stage D2 prostate cancer: is it always an accurate indicator of disease status? J Urol 1991;145:802.
88. Newling DW, Dennis L, Vermeylen K. Orchiectomy versus goserelin and flutamide in the treatment of newly diagnosed metastatic prostate cancer. Cancer Suppl 1993;72:3793.
89. Montgomery BT, Young CY, Bilhartz DL, et al. Hormonal regulation of prostate-specific antigen (PSA) glycoprotein in the human prostatic adenocarcinoma cell line LNCaP. Prostate 1992;21:63.
90. Bussemakers MJ, van de Ven WJ, Debruyne FM, Schalken JA. Identification of high mobility group protein I(Y) as potential progression marker for prostate cancer by differential hybridization analysis. Cancer Res 1991;51:606.
91. Peehl DM, Wong ST, Stamey TA. Vitamin A regulates proliferation and differentiation of human prostatic epithelial cells. Prostate 1993;23:69.
92. Gallee MP, Visser de Jong E, van der Korput JA, et al. Variation of prostate-specific antigen expression in different tumour growth patterns present in prostatectomy specimens. Urol Res 1990;18:181.
93. Pienta KJ, Redman B, Hussain M, et al. Phase II evaluation of oral estramustine and oral etoposide in hormone-refractory adenocarcinoma of the prostate. J Clin Oncol 1994;12:2005.
94. Gerber GS, Chodak GW. Prostate specific antigen for assessing response to ketoconazole and prednisone in patients with hormone refractory metastatic prostate cancer. J Urol 1990;144:1177.
95. Amato RJ, Logothetis CJ, Dexeus FH, Sella A, Kilbourn RG, Fitz K. Preliminary results of a phase II trial of estramustine (EMCYT) and vinblastine (VLB) for patients with progressive hormone refractory prostate carcinoma (HRPC). (Abstract) Proc Am Assoc Cancer Res 1991;32:86.
96. Sella A, Kilbourn R, Amato R, et al. Phase II study of ketoconazole combined with weekly doxorubicin in patients with androgen-independent prostate cancer. J Clin Oncol 1994;12:683.
97. Wilding G, Valverius E, Knabbe C, Gelmann EP. Role of transforming growth factor alpha inhuman prostate cancer cell growth. Prostate 1989;15:1.
98. Kelly WK, Scher HI, Mazumdar M, Vlamis V, Schwartz M, Fossa SD. Prostate specific antigen as a measure of disease outcome in hormone-refractory prostatic cancer. J Clin Oncol 1993;11:607.
99. Eisenberger MA, Reyno LM, Jodrell DI, et al. Suramin, an active drug for prostate cancer: interim observations in a phase I trial. J Natl Cancer Inst 1993;85:611.
100. Murphy GP, Gibbons RP, Johnson DE, et al. A comparison of estrmustine phosphate and streptozotocin in patients with prostatic carcinoma who had extensive irradiation. J Urol 1977;118:288.
101. Kasimis B, Howard L, Bamberger M, et al. Sequential therapy with the antiandrogen Casodex (C) (ICI 176334), and castration (CST) in patients (PTS) with stage D2 prostate cancer (PC): the results of CST. Proc Am Soc Clin Oncol 1993;12:252.
102. Manni A, Bartholomew M, Caplan R, et al. Androgen priming and chemotherapy in advanced prostate cancer: evaluation of determinants of clinical outcome. J Clin Oncol 1988;6:1456.
103. Koch P, Bayer G, McGovern J, Saphner T. Continuous infusion 5-fluorouracil (5FU) and weekly doxorubicin for hormone resistant prostate cancer. Proc Am Soc Clin Oncol 1992;11:207.
104. Yagoda A, Smith JA, Soloway MS, et al. Phase II study of estramustine phosphate in advanced hormone refractory prostatic cancer with increasing prostate specific antigen levels. (Abstract) J Urol 1991;145:384A.
105. Dexeus F, Logothetis CJ, Samuels ML, et al. Continuous infusion of

vinblastine for advanced hormone-refractory prostate cancer. Cancer Treat Rep 1985;69:885.

106. Nilsson S, Nordgren H, Karlberg L, et al. Expression of estramustine-binding protein (EMBP) and the proliferation-associated antigen Ki-67 in prostatic carcinomas. Scand J Urol Nephrol Suppl 1988;110: 31.
107. Heim W, Ahlgren J, Lokich J, Rosenthal CJ. Long term continuous infusion (CI) of 5-fluorouracil (5-FU) in the treatment of metastatic prostate cancer: a phase II Mid-Atlantic Oncology Group (MAOP) study. Proc Am Soc Clin Oncol 1991;10:179.
108. Amato RJ, Ellerhorst J, Bui C, Logothetis CJ. Estramustine and vinblastine for patients with progressive androgen-independent adenocarcinoma of the prostate. Urol Oncol 1995;1:168.
109. Hudes GR, Greenberg R, Krigel RL, et al. Phase II study of estramustine and vinblastine, two microtubule inhibitors, in hormone-refractory prostate cancer. J Clin Oncol 1992;10:1754.
110. Roth B, Yeap B, Wilding G, Kasimis B, McLeod D, Loehrer P. Taxol (NSC 125973) in advanced, hormone-refractory prostate cancer: an ECOG phase II trial. Proc Am Soc Clin Oncol 1992;11:196.
110a. Hudes GR, Natan FE, Khater C, et al. Paclitaxel plus estramustine in metastatic hormone-refractory prostate cancer. Sem Oncol 1995;22: 41.
111. Partin AW, Getzenberg RH, Carmichael MJ, et al. Nuclear matrix protein patterns in human benign prostatic hyperplasia and prostate cancer. Cancer Res 1993;53:744.
112. Pienta KJ, Lehr JE. A common set of nuclear matrix proteins in prostate cancer cells. Prostate 1993;23:69.
112a. Pienta KJ. Estramustine and etoposide act synergistically at the level of the nuclear matrix to inhibit prostate cancer growth in vitro and in vivo. (Abstract) Society for Basic Urologic Research 1992;6.
112b. Pienta KJ, Redman B, Hussain M, et al. Phase II evaluation of oral etoposide and oral estramustine in hormone-refractory adenocarcinoma of the prostate. J Clin Oncol 1994;12:2005.
113. Scher HI, Sternberg C, Heston WD, et al. Etoposide in prostatic cancer: experimental studies and phase II trial in patients with bidimensionally measurable disease. Cancer Chemother Pharmacol 1986;18:24.
114. Trump DL, Loprinzi CL. Phase II trial of etoposide in advanced prostate cancer. Cancer Treat Rep 1984;68:1195.
115. Walther PJ, Williams SD, Troner M, et al. Phase II study of etoposide for carcinoma of the prostate. Cancer Treat Rep 1986;60:771.
116. Baxter LT, Jain RK. Transport of fluid and macromolecules in tumors. II. Role of heterogeneous perfusion and lymphatics. Microvasc Res 1990;40:246.
117. La Rocca RV, Danesi R, Cooper MR, et al. Effect of suramin on human prostate cancer cells in vitro. J Urol 1991;145:393.
118. Myers CE, Stein C, LaRocca R, Cooper M, Cassidy J, McAtee N. Suramin: an antagonist of heparin-binding tumor growth factors with activity against a broad spectrum of human tumors. (Abstract) Proc Am Soc Clin Oncol 1989;8:66.
119. Peehl DM, Wong ST, Stamey TA. Cytostatic effects of suramin on prostate cancer cells cultured from primary tumors. J Urol 1991;145: 624.
120. Stein CA, Saville W, Yarchoan R, Broder S, Gelmann EP. Suramin and function of the adrenal cortex. Ann Intern Med 1986;104:286.
121. Stein CA, La Rocca RV, Thomas R, McAtee N, Myers CE. Suramin: an anticancer drug with a unique mechanism of action. J Clin Oncol 1989;7:499.
122. Eisenberger MA, Reyno LM, Jodrell DI, et al. Suramin, an active drug for prostate cancer: interim observations in a phase I trial. J Natl Cancer Inst 1993;85:611.
123. Scher HI, Kelly WK. Suramin: defining the role in the clinic: principles and practice of oncology. PPO Updates 1993;9:1.
124. Kobayashi D, Vokes EE, Janisch L, et al. A phase I cohort study of suramin (SUR) in patients with advanced cancer (CA). Proc Am Soc Clin Oncol 1993;12:161.
125. Veldscholte J, Voorhorst-Ogink MM, Bolt-de Vries J, van Rooij HCJ, Trapman J, Mulder E. Unusual specificity of the androgen receptor in the human prostate tumor cell lines LNCaP: high affinity for progestagenic and estrogen steroids. Biochim Biophys Acta 1990;1052:187.
126. Iwamura M, di Sant'Agnese PA, Wu G, Cockett ATK, Abrahamsson P, Deftos LJ. Parathyroid hormone-related protein is expressed by prostatic neuroendocrine cells. Urol 1994;43:667.
127. Amato RJ, Logothetis CJ, Hallinan R, Ro JY, Sella A, Dexeus FH. Chemotherapy for small cell carcinoma of prostatic origin. J Urol 1992;147:935.
128. Scher HI, Cordon-Cardo C. Current and future therapeutic strategies in metastatic hormonal resistant prostate cancer: therapy based on phenotype. Probl Urol 1993;7:226.
129. Logothetis CJ, Hoosein NM, Hsieh J-T. The clinical and biologic study of androgen independent prostate cancer (AI PCa). Semin Oncol 1994;21:620.
130. Nicholson GL, Winkelhake JL. Organ specificity of blood-borne tumour metastasis determined by cell adhesion. Nature 1975;255:230.
131. Wu He W, Fischer LM, Sun S, et al. Molecular cloning of the androgen receptors from divergent species with polymerase chain reaction technique: complete cDNA sequence of the mouse androgen receptor and isolation of androgen receptor cDNA probes from dog, guinea pig, and clawed frog. Biochem Biophys Res Commun 1990;171:697.
132. Maxon HR, Thomas SR, Hertzberg VS, et al. Relation between effective radiation dose and outcome of radioiodine therapy for thyroid cancer. N Engl J Med 1983;309:937.
133. Carroll PR, Sugimura K, Cohen MB, Hricak H. Detection and staging of prostate carcinoma after transurethral resection or open enucleation of the prostate: accuracy of magnetic resonance imaging. J Urol 1992; 147:402.
134. Blake GM, Zivanovic MA, McEwan AJ, Ackery DM. Sr-89 therapy: strontium kinetics in disseminated carcinoma of the prostate. Eur J Nucl Med 1986;12:447.
135. Claringbold PG, Turner JH. A phase II study of the treatment of painful multifocal skeletal metastases with single and repeated dose samarium-153-ethylenediaminetetramethylene phosphonate (Sm-153-EDTMP). Proc Am Soc Clin Oncol 1991;10:108.
136. Maxon HR,III, Schroder LE, Thomas SR, et al. Re-186(Sn) HEDP for treatment of painful osseous metastases: initial clinical experience in 20 patients with hormone-resistant prostate cancer. Radiology 1990; 176:155.
137. Isaacs JT, Coffey DS. Adaptation versus selection as the mechanism responsible for the relapse of prostatic cancer to androgen ablation as studied in the Dunning R-3327 H adenocarcinoma. Cancer Res 1981;41:5070.
138. Curley T, Scher H, Thaler H, et al. Phase II trial of 186-rhenium hydroxyethylidene diphosphonate (^{186}Re-HEDP) as treatment of painful bone metastases from prostatic cancer (PC). (Abstract) Proc Am Soc Clin Oncol 1992.
139. Sutkowski D, Sensibar J, Kozlowski J, Lee C. Effect of TGF-B on proliferation of PC3 cells in culture. (Abstract) J Urol 1992;147:415A.
140. Scher HI, Curley T, Geller N, et al. Gallium nitrate in prostatic cancer: evaluation of antitumor activity and effects on bone turnover. Cancer Treat Rep 1987;71:887.
141. Sullivan W, Guthrie T, Gaddis T, Swartz D. Gallium nitrate (GN) and doxorubicin (DOX) therapy of hormone refractory prostate cancer (HRPC): effects on parameters of pain, performance status (PS) and prostate specific antigen (PSA). Proc Am Soc Clin Oncol 1993;12: 150.
142. Kaisary AV. Current clinical studies with a new nonsteroidal antiandrogen, Casodex. Prostate Suppl 1994;5:34.
143. Israeli RS, Powell CT, Fair WR, Heston WDW. Molecular cloning of a complementary DNA encoding a prostate-specific membrane antigen. Cancer Res 1993;53:227.
144. Axelrod HR, Gilman SC, D'Aleo DJ, et al. Preclinical results and human immunohistochemical studies with 90-Y-CYT-356: a new prostate cancer therapeutic agent. (Abstract) J Urol 1992;147:361.
145. Folkman J, Watson K, Ingber D, Hanahan D. Induction of angiogenesis during the transition from hyperplasia to neoplasia. Nature 1992; 339:58.
146. Weidner N, Carrol PR, Flax J, Blumenfeld W, Folkman J. Tumor angiogenesis correlates with metastasis in invasive prostate carcinoma. Am J Pathol 1993;143:401.
147. Nguyen N, Pienta KJ. Pentosan inhibits angiogenesis in vitro and this appears to correlate with the inhibition of prostate tumor-associated angiogenesis in vivo. Proc Am Assoc Cancer Res 1993;34.
148. Zukiwski A, Gutterman J, Bui C, et al. Phase I trial of the angiogenesis inhibitor TNP-470 in patients with androgen independent prostate cancer. Proc Am Soc Clin Oncol 1994;13:795.
149. Warrell RP, Frankel SR, Miller WH. Differentiation therapy of acute promyelocytic leukemia with tretinoin (all-trans-retinoic acid). N Engl J Med 1991;324:1385.
150. Samid D, Shack S, Myers CE. Selective growth arrest and phenotypic reversion of prostate caner cells in vitro by nontoxic pharmacological concentrations of phenylacetate. J Clin Invest 1993;91:2288.

151. Bergan R, Kyle E, Neckers L. Genistein: a protein-tyrosine kinase inhibitor inhibits the growth of prostate C cells. Breast and prostate cancer symposium II Y 502, 1994.
152. Borden E, Lotan R, Levens D, Young C, Waxman S. Differentiation therapy of cancer: laboratory and clinical investigations. Cancer Res 1993;53:4109.
153. Pienta K, Meyer L. Treatment and prevention of prostate cancer. Proc Am Assoc Cancer Res 1994;35:678.
154. Kelly WK, Scher HI, Muindi J, et al. Phase II trial of all-trans retinoic acid in patients with adenocarcinoma of the prostate. Proc Amer Assoc Cancer Res 1993;34:203.
155. Miller WH, Warrell RP, Frankel S, et al. Novel retinoic acid receptor-gamma transcripts in acute promyelocytic leukemia responsive to all-trans retinoic acid. J Natl Cancer Inst 1990;82:1932.
156. Pollard M, Luckert PH, Sporn MB. Prevention of primary prostate cancer in Lobund-Wistar rats by N-(4-hydroxyphenyl)retinamide. Cancer Res 1991;51:3610.
157. Werthman P, Khanna OP, Gonick P, et al. Carcinoma of prostate in men aged fifty and under: therapeutic options. Urology 1992;39:48.
158. Hofer DR, Sherwood ER, Bromberg WD, Mendelsohn J, Lee C, Kozlowski JM. Autonomous growth of androgen-independent human prostatic carcinoma cells: role of transforming growth factor α. Cancer Res 1991;51:2780.
159. Logothetis CJ, von Eschenbach AC, Samuels ML, Trindade A, Johnson DE. Doxorubicin, mitomycin, and 5-FU (DMF) in the treatment of hormone-resistant stage D prostate cancer: a preliminary report. Cancer Treat Rep 1982;66:57.
160. Rochlitz CF, Damon LE, Russi MB, Geddes A, Cadman EC. Cytotoxicity of ketoconazole in malignant cell lines. Cancer Chemother Pharmacol 1988;21:319.
161. Connolly JM, Rose DP. Secretion of epidermal growth factor and related polypeptides by the DU 145 human prostate cancer cell line. Prostate 1989;15:177.
162. Tillotson JK, Rose DP. Density-dependent regulation of epidermal growth factor receptor expression in DU 145 human prostate cancer cells. Prostate 1991;19:53.
163. Traish AM, Wotiz HH. Prostatic epidermal growth factor receptors and their regulation by androgens. Endocrinology 1987;121:1461.
164. MacDonald A, Habib FK. Divergent responses to epidermal growth factor in hormone sensitive and insensitive human prostate cancer cell lines. Br J Cancer 1992;65:177.
165. Kawamoto T, Sato JD, Le A, Polikoff J, Sato GH, Mendelsohn J. Growth stimulation of A431 cells by epidermal growth factor: identification of high affinity receptors for epidermal growth factor by an anti-receptor monoclonal antibody. Proc Natl Acad Sci U S A 1983; 80:1337.
166. Fong CJ, Sherwood ER, Mendelsohn J, Lee C, Kozlowski JM. Epidermal growth factor receptor monoclonal antibody inhibits constitutive receptor phosphorylation, reduces autonomous growth, and sensitizes androgen-independent prostatic carcinoma cells to tumor necrosis factor alpha. Cancer Res 1992;52:5887.
167. Myers RB, Srivasta S, Oselschlager dK. Expression of p160ereb-3 and p185erbB-2 in prostatic intraepithelial neoplasia and prostatic adenocarcinoma. (Abstract) J Natl Cancer Inst 1994;86:1140.
168. Bostwick DG. c-erbB-2 oncogene expression in prostatic intrapeithelial neoplasia: mounting evidence for a precursor role. J Natl Cancer Inst 1994;86:1108.
169. Zhau HYE, Siles RA, Chung LWK. The c-erb B/2 oncogene in human prostate cancer growth and progression. In: Khan SA, Stancel GM, eds. Protooncogenes and growth factors in steroid hormone induced growth and differentiation. New York: CRC Press, 1994:207.
170. Hudziak RM, Lewis GD, Fendly BM, Shepard HM, Ullrich A. p185HER2 monoclonal antibody has antiproliferative effects in vitro and sensitizes human breast tumor cells to tumor necrosis factor. Mol Cell Biology 1989;9:1165.
171. Mazur MT, Shultz JJ. Evaluation of Immunoreactivity to monoclonal antibody B72.3. Am J Clin Pathol (Abstract) 1990;93:466.
172. Molinolo A, Simpson JF, Thor A, Schlom J. Enhanced tumor binding using immunohistochemical analyses by second generation anti-tumor-associated glycoprotein 72 monoclonal antibodies versus monoclonal antibody B72.3 in human tissue. (Abstract) Cancer Res 1990;50:1291.
173. McNeal JE, Villers AA, Redwine EA, Freiha FS, Stamey TA. Histologic differentiation, cancer volume, and pelvic lymph node metastasis in adenocarcinoma of the prostate. Cancer 1990;66:1225.
174. Huggins C, Hodges CV. Studies on prostatic cancer, effect of castration, of estrogen and of androgen injection on serum phosphatases in metastatic carcinoma of the prostate. Cancer Res 1941;1:293.
175. Babaian RJ, Sayer J, Podoloff DA, Steelhammer LC, Bhadkamkar VA, Gulfo JV. Radioimmunoscintigraphy of pelvic lymph nodes with 111-indium-labeled monoclonal antibody CYT-356. J Urol 1994;152: 1952.
176. Kaplan EL, Meier P. Nonparametric estimation from incomplete observations. J Am Statist Assoc 1958;53:457.
177. Seidman AD, Scher HI, Petrylak D, Dershaw DD, Curley T. Estramustine and vinblastine: use of prostate specific antigen as a clinical trial end point for hormone refractory prostatic cancer. J Urol 1992;147: 931.
179. Westermark B, Heldin CH. Platelet-derived growth factor as a mediator of normal and neoplastic cell proliferation. Med Oncol Tumor Pharmacother 1986;3:177.
180. Ahmann FR, Schwartz J, Dorr R, Salmon S. Suramin in hormone resistant metastatic prostate cancer: significant anticancer activity but unanticipated toxicity. (Abstract) Proc Am Soc Clin Oncol 1991;10: 178.
181. Sato Y, Rifkin DB. Autocrine activities of basic fibroblast growth factor: regulation of endothelial cell movement, plasminogen activator synthesis, and DNA synthesis. J Cell Biol 1988;107:1199.
182. Rapoport BL, Ansell S, Coccia-Portugal MA, et al. Phase II clinical study of suramin in combination with mitomycin-C in patients with hormone refractory prostate cancer. Proc Am Soc Clin Oncol 1991; 10:177.
183. Eisenberger MA, Sinibaldi V, Reyno LM, et al. Phase I clinical evaluation of a pharmacologically guided regimen of suramin in patients with hormone-refractory prostate cancer. J Clin Oncol 1995;13:2174.
184. Kelly WK, Scher HI, Mazumdar M, et al. Suramin and hydrocortisone: determining drug efficacy in andragen-independent prostate cancer. J Clin Oncol 1995;13:2214.
185. Kobayashi K, Vokes EE, Vogelzang NJ, et al. Phase I study of suramin given by intermittent infusion without adaptive control in patients with advanced cancer. J Clin Oncol 1995;13:2196.

Principles and Practice of Genitourinary Oncology, edited by Derek Raghavan, Howard I. Scher, Steven A. Leibel, and Paul H. Lange. Lippincott-Raven Publishers, Philadelphia, © 1997.

CHAPTER 59

Management of Pain Associated With Prostate Cancer

Nathan I. Cherny and Kathleen M. Foley

Patients with prostate cancer are heterogeneous in their experience of pain. Pain is an uncommon presenting symptom in prostate cancer. In one survey, only 68 of 614 new cases presented with pain.[1] In contrast, pain is a common and important clinical problem among patients with advanced prostate cancer. One survey of patients receiving outpatient treatment for their genitourinary cancers found that 84% had tumor-related pain and that their pain was inadequately relieved in two thirds of these cases.[2] In a study of patients admitted for hospice care, 52% of patients with a diagnosis of prostate cancer had severe pain at presentation.[3]

Unrelieved pain interferes with physical functioning and social interaction and is strongly associated with heightened psychological distress.[4] Relief of pain is a compelling therapeutic goal for physicians who care for these patients. Despite the widespread acceptance of a highly effective therapeutic strategy for the management of cancer pain, surveys suggest that 40% to 50% of patients in routine practice settings fall to achieve adequate pain relief.[2,5] Clinicians are frequently ill equipped to treat pain; patients who complain of severe pain may not be believed,[6] assessment is often inadequate,[5] and knowledge of pain management approaches is often rudimentary.[5,7]

CANCER PAIN SYNDROMES

Cancer pain syndromes are defined by the association of particular pain characteristics and physical signs with specific complications of the underlying disease or its treatment. Cancer-related pain syndromes may be acute or chronic and are usually associated with distinct etiologies, pathophysiologies, and prognostic and therapeutic implications.

Temporal Classification

Cancer-related acute pain syndromes are most commonly the result of diagnostic or therapeutic interventions. Although some tumor-related pains have an acute onset (e.g., pain from a pathologic fracture), most persist unless effective treatment for the underlying lesion is provided. In contrast, chronic tumor-related pain is usually insidious in onset, often increases progressively with tumor growth, and may regress with tumor shrinkage in response to anticancer therapy. Although overt pain behaviors and sympathetic hyperactivity are often absent, cancer-related pain may be associated with affective disturbances (e.g., anxiety, depression) and vegetative symptoms (e.g., asthenia, anorexia, sleep disturbance).[8]

Transitory exacerbations of severe pain over a baseline of moderate pain or less are described as "breakthrough pains."[9] Breakthrough pains are common in both acute and chronic pain states. These exacerbations may be precipitated by volitional actions of the patient (e.g., movement, micturition, cough, defecation; i.e., incident pains) or nonvolitional events (e.g., bowel distention). Spontaneous fluctuations in pain intensity can also occur without an identifiable precipitant.

Most chronic cancer-related pains are caused directly by the tumor. Bone pain and compression of neural structures are the two most common causes.[10–12] The chronic cancer pain syndromes encountered in patients with prostate cancer are presented in Table 59-1.

Common Pain Syndromes in Prostate Cancer

Bone Pain

Bone metastases are the most common cause of chronic pain in cancer patients[13] and are overwhelmingly the most common site of metastases from prostate cancer. Although bone pain is usually associated with direct tumor invasion of bony structures, more than 20% of patients with bony metastases are pain-free,[14] and patients with multiple bony metastases typically report pain in only a few sites.[14] The factors that convert a painless lesion to a painful one are unknown. Bone metastases generate pain by several mechanisms, including endosteal or periosteal nociceptor activation by mechanical distortion or release of chemical mediators and tumor growth into adjacent soft tissues and

TABLE 59-1. *Chronic cancer pain syndromes in prostate cancer*

TUMOR-RELATED PAIN SYNDROMES
Bone pain
Multifocal or generalized bone pain
Multiple bony metastases
Marrow expansion
Vertebral syndromes
Atlantoaxial destruction and odontoid fractures
C7-T1 syndrome
T12-L1 syndrome
Sacral syndrome
Back pain and epidural compression
Pain syndromes of the bony pelvis and hip
Headache and facial pain
Base of skull metastases
Painful cranial neuralgias
Tumor involvement of the peripheral nervous system
Malignant lumbosacral plexopathy
Tumor-related mononeuropathy
Pain syndromes of the viscera and miscellaneous tumor-related syndromes
Malignant perineal pain
Ureteric obstruction
Bladder pain
CHRONIC PAIN SYNDROMES ASSOCIATED WITH CANCER THERAPY
Postchemotherapy pain syndromes
Avascular necrosis of femoral or humeral head
Chronic pain associated with hormonal therapy
Gynecomastia with hormonal therapy for prostate cancer
Chronic Postsurgical pain syndromes
Postsurgical pelvic floor myalgia
Chronic Postradiotherapy pain syndromes
Plexopathies
Chronic radiation myelopathy
Chronic radiation enteritis and proctitis
Burning perineum syndrome
Osteoradionecrosis

Adapted from Cherny NI, Portenoy RK. Cancer pain: principles of assessment and syndromes. In: Wall PD, Melzack R, eds. Textbook of pain, 3rd ed. Edinburgh: Churchill Livingstone, 1994:787.

nerves.[13] Bony metastases can be associated with specific clinical syndromes (Table 59-2). The vertebrae are the most common sites of bony metastases,[15] and vertebral metastases from prostate cancer metastasize most commonly to the lumbosacral spine.[15]

Back Pain and Epidural Spinal Cord Compression

Tumors of the prostate account for 10% to 20% of patients who develop epidural compression of the spinal cord or cauda equina.[16] Most incidences of epidural compression are caused by posterior extension of a vertebral body metastasis into the epidural space. Less commonly, epidural compression is caused by tumor extension from the posterior arch of the vertebra or infiltration of a paravertebral tumor through the intervertebral foramen. Because the most salient determinant of treatment efficacy is the degree of neurologic impairment at the time therapy is initiated,[17] early identification of any such impairment is essential. Treatment generally involves the administration of corticosteroids and radiotherapy.[18,19] Surgical decompression is considered in some patients with radioresistant tumors, in those who have previously received maximal radiotherapy to the involved field, and in those with spinal instability.[16,20]

Lumbosacral Plexopathy

Prostate cancer is among the primary tumors most frequently associated with malignant lumbosacral plexopathy.[21,22] Neoplastic infiltration or compression of the lumbosacral plexus may be associated with pain in the lower abdomen, inguinal region, buttock, or leg.[22] Such infiltration or compression must be distinguished from less common causes of pain such as radiation-induced plexopathy and other conditions that may mimic lumbosacral plexopathy. Epidural or leptomeningeal metastases can potentially resemble lumbosacral plexopathy and should be considered in the diagnostic evaluation. Lumbosacral plexopathy is rare in patients with prostate cancer.

Pain is the first symptom reported by most patients with malignant lumbosacral plexopathy; numbness, paresthesias, or weakness follow weeks to months later. Coccygeal plexopathy, with prominent sphincter dysfunction and perineal sensory loss, can occur with low pelvic tumors such as those arising from the bladder or prostate. Cross-sectional imaging with either computed tomography (CT) or magnetic resonance imaging, is the usual diagnostic procedure to evaluate lumbosacral plexopathy. When using CT scanning techniques, images should include bone and soft tissue windows.

Malignant Perineal Pain

Tumors of the distal genitourinary system are among those most commonly responsible for perineal pain.[23] Severe perineal pain following antineoplastic therapy may precede evidence of detectable disease and should be viewed as a potential harbinger of progressive or recurrent cancer.[23] This phenomenon is often caused by microscopic perineural invasion by recurrent disease. The pain, which is typically described as constant and aching, is often aggravated by sitting or standing, and may be associated with tenesmus or bladder spasms.[23] Tumor invasion of the musculature of the deep pelvis can also result in a constant perineal ache that is exacerbated with upright posture. Digital examination of the pelvic floor may reveal local tenderness or palpable tumor.

CANCER PAIN ASSESSMENT

Cancer pain assessment has two major objectives: the accurate characterization of the pain, including the pain syndrome and inferred pathophysiology, and the evaluation of the impact of the pain and the role it plays in the overall suffering of the patient. The pain-related history must elucidate the relevant pain characteristics as well as the responses of the patient to previous disease-modifying and analgesic therapies. The use of a validated pain assessment tool such as a 100-mm visual analog scale for pain intensity,[24] or an instrument such as the Memorial

TABLE 59-2. *Specific pain syndromes associated with bony metastases*

Syndrome	Clinical features
VERTEBRAL	
Atlantoaxial destruction Odontoid fractures	Nuchal or occipital pain radiating over the posterior aspect of the skull to the vertex. Exacerbated by flexion of the neck. Pathologic fracture may result in secondary subluxation with ensuing compression of the spinal cord at the cervicomedullary junction.
C7-T1 syndrome	Pain referred to the interscapular region. May be missed if radiographic evaluation is mistakenly targeted to the painful area caudal to the site of damage. May be obscured by overlying bone and mediastinal shadows. Bone scintigraphy may assist in targeting additional diagnostic imaging procedures, particularly CT or MR.
T12-L1 syndrome	T12 or L1 vertebral lesions can refer pain to the ipsilateral iliac crest or the sacroiliac joint. Imaging procedures directed at pelvic bones will therefore miss the source of the pain.
Sacral syndrome	Severe focal pain radiating to buttocks, perineum, or posterior thighs may accompany destruction of the sacrum. Often exacerbated by sitting or lying and relieved by standing or walking. Lateral spread to involve muscles that rotate the hip (e.g., the pyriformis muscle) may produce a malignant "pyriformis syndrome" characterized by buttock or posterior leg pain that is exacerbated by internal rotation of the hip.
PELVIC	
hip joint syndrome	Localized hip pain that is aggravated by weight bearing and movement of the hip. The pain may radiate to the knee or medial thigh, and occasionally this is the only site of pain. The weight-bearing function of these structures contributes to the propensity of incident pain with ambulation. CT and MR techniques are most sensitive and demonstrate the extent of adjacent soft tissue involvement.
BASE OF SKULL	
Orbital	Progressive ipsilateral retroorbital and supraorbital pain.
Parasellar	Unilateral supraorbital and frontal headache with or without diplopia opthalmoparesis, papilledema, hemianopsia, or quadrantinopsia.
Middle cranial Fossa	Facial numbness or paresthesias in the distribution of the second or third divisions of the trigeminal nerve referred to the cheek or jaw.
Jugular foramen	Hoarseness or dysphagia, pain referred to the ipsilateral ear or mastoid, and occasionally glossopharyngeal neuralgia, with or without syncope.
Occipital condyle	Unilateral occipital pain worsened with neck flexion, with or without stiffness of the neck.
Clivus	Vertex headache, often exacerbated by neck flexion. Lower cranial nerve (VL–XII) dysfunction may become bilateral.
Sphenoid sinus	Bifrontal headache radiating to the temporal region and intermittent retroorbital pain.

CT, Computed tomography; MR, magnetic resonance.

Pain Assessment Card[25] or the Brief Pain Inventory[26] can provide a format for communication between the patient and health care professionals and can also be used to monitor the adequacy of therapy.

The consequences of pain, such as impairment in activities of daily living; psychological, familial, and professional dysfunction; disturbed sleep, appetite, and vitality; and financial concerns, must also be assessed. A physical examination, including a neurologic evaluation, is a necessary part of the initial pain assessment. The need for a thorough neurologic assessment is justified by the high prevalence of painful neurologic conditions in this population.[27,28] Careful review of previous laboratory and imaging studies can provide important information about the cause of the pain and the extent of the underlying disease. Investigations are often required to clarify the pain diagnosis, the extent of disease, and the patients physiological status.[27] Pain should be managed during the diagnostic evaluation, because adequate relief will improve compliance and reduce the level of distress associate with procedures. No patient should be inadequately evaluated because of poorly controlled pain.

The evaluation should enable the clinician to appreciate the precise nature of the pain syndrome, its impact, and concurrent symptoms and problems that further undermine quality of life. The findings of this evaluation should be reviewed with the patient and appropriate others so that problems can be prioritized to reflect their importance to the patient and goals of therapy can be discussed. The formulation of the goals of care provides an essential context for therapeutic intent and, consequently, therapeutic decision-making.[29] When patients equally prioritize optimal comfort and function, the therapeutic intent is to achieve an adequate degree of relief without compromising cognitive and physical function. When comfort is the overriding goal of care, it may be appropriate to continue effective therapies even if they impair function.

MANAGEMENT OF CHRONIC CANCER PAIN

Most cancer patients can attain satisfactory relief of pain through an approach that incorporates primary treatments, oral or parenteral analgesic therapy, and at times, other noninvasive techniques (e.g., psychological or rehabilitative interventions). Patients who fall to attain adequate relief despite these approaches may require the more invasive anesthetic or neurosurgical approaches (Fig. 59-1).

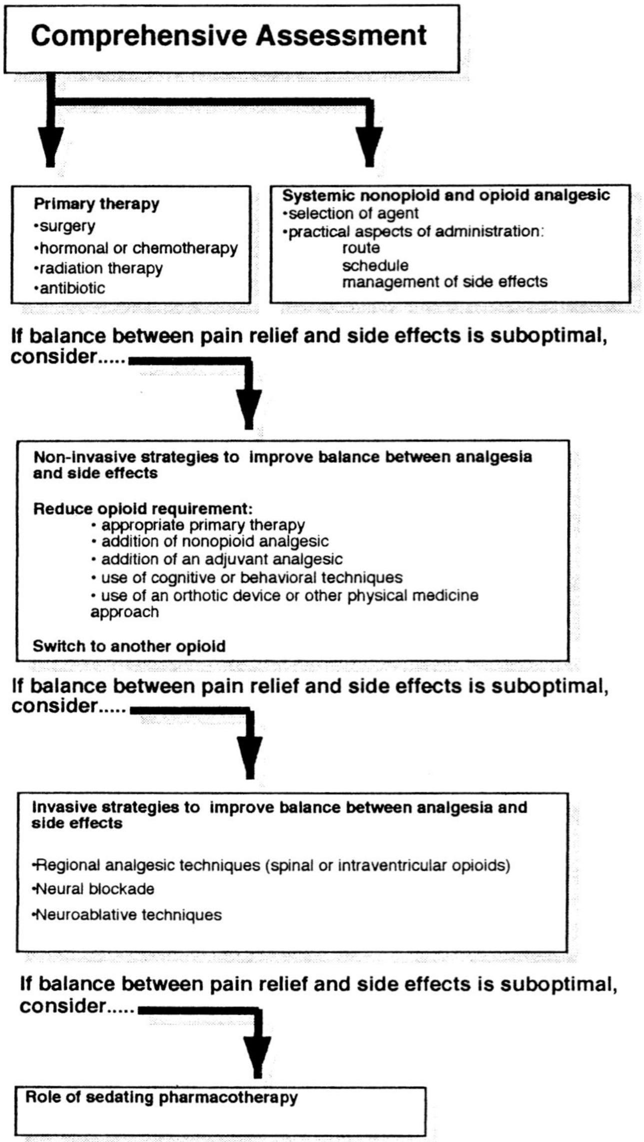

FIG. 59-1. Strategy for the management of cancer pain. (Adapted from Cherny NI, Portenoy RK. Cancer pain management: current strategy. Cancer Suppl 1993;72(11):3393.)

Role of Primary Therapy

The assessment process may reveal a cause for the pain that is amenable to primary therapy. Pain that is produced by tumor infiltration may respond to antineoplastic treatment with hormonal therapy, radiotherapy, surgery, or chemotherapy, and pain caused by infection may be relieved with antibiotic therapy or drainage procedures. Specific analgesic treatments are usually required as an adjunct to the primary therapy.

Hormonal Therapy

Hormonal therapy is the first line of approach in the management of pain caused by metastatic prostate cancer. Among previously untreated patients, pain relief can be anticipated in 60% to 75% of patients whether they are treated with orchidectomy, diethylstilbestrol, androgen antagonists, or luteinizing hormone–releasing factor (LHRF) agonist therapy. Initiation of LHRF hormonal therapy for prostate cancer produces a transient symptom flare in 5% to 25% of patients.[30,31] The flare is presumably caused by an initial stimulation of luteinizing hormone release before suppression is achieved.[30] The syndrome typically presents as an exacerbation of bone pain or urinary retention; spinal cord compression and sudden death have also been reported.[31] Symptom flare is usually observed within the first week of therapy and lasts for 1 to 3 weeks in the absence of androgen antagonist therapy. Coadministration of an androgen antagonist during the initiation of LHRF agonist therapy can prevent this phenomenon.[32–34]

Chronic gynecomastia and breast tenderness are common complications of antiandrogen therapies for prostate cancer.[30] The incidence of this syndrome varies among drugs; it is frequently associated with diethylstilbestrol,[35] is less common with flutamide and cyproterone,[36–38] and is uncommon with LHRF agonist therapy.[30] Gynecomastia in the elderly must be distinguished from primary breast cancer or a secondary cancer in the breast.[29]

Radiotherapy

External beam radiotherapy has a pivotal role in the treatment of cancer pain caused by bone metastases[39,40] and epidural neoplasm.[39] Although there is a paucity of data regarding the efficacy of radiotherapy in the management of pelvic plexopathic pain, clinical experience suggests that palliative radiotherapy for malignant lumbosacral plexopathy often yields partial relief of short duration.[41] Data specific to lumbosacral plexopathy caused by prostate cancer are lacking, but the overall response rate to radiotherapy for locoregional recurrence is in excess of 50%.[42]

For patients with a solitary site of bone pain, local radiotherapy is effective in more than 80% of patients.[43] Dose fractionation should be influenced by the anticipated duration of survival of the patient and the site of the lesion; large, single-fraction treatment (4 to 8 Gy), which has a shorter duration of analgesic effect, is suitable for patients with a short life expectancy.[44]

For patients with multiple sites of bone pain, radiotherapeutic options include multifocal radiotherapy, hemibody radiotherapy (HBR) and systemic radiopharmaceuticals. HBR or sequential upper and lower HBR can relieve pain in 50% to 85% of patients.[42] The onset of pain relief is more rapid with a single dose of 6 to 8 Gy within 48 hours than with fractionated therapy.[45] The median time to pain relapse was approximately 2 to 6 months for patients who received a single dose and 6 to 11 months for those who were treated with a fractionated schedule.[45] Significant transient acute radiation toxicity, predominantly gastrointestinal toxicity and bone marrow suppression, occurs in the majority of patients, and radiation pneumonitis and alopecia can occur with upper-body therapy.

Radiopharmaceuticals are systemically administered radionuclides that are sequestered focally at sites of bone metastases. The radionuclides are administered alone or can be linked to a bisphosphonate compound. Strontium-89 (^{89}Sr) is a beta-particle–emitting calcium analog that has been approved by the

FDA for the treatment of bone pain caused by hormone-refractory metastatic prostate cancer. It has a half-life of 50 days and is sequestered in metastases at a level that is 2 to 25 times that harbored in normal bone.[46] In phase II studies of patients with prostate cancer, 60% to 95% of patients reported pain relief,[47–50] which was complete in 10% to 25%.[47–50] A flare response, characterized by transient worsening of pain 1 to 2 days after administration, occurs in 15% to 20% of patients.[51] This flare usually resolves after 3 to 5 days, and most affected patients subsequently develop a good analgesic response.[51] Treatment with ^{89}Sr can compromise marrow reserve; leukocyte and platelet counts generally fall by 20% to 35%.[52] A platelet count higher than 60,000/mm^3 is recommended.[51] In responding patients, pain relief usually develops within 6 weeks and is sustained for a median duration of 6 months.[48] ^{89}Sr can be administered alone or in combination with nonmyelotoxic chemotherapy[53] or external beam radiotherapy,[54] and it can be administered to patients who have previously been treated with HBR.[55] The usual dose is 40 to 60 mCi/kg (2.5 to 5 MCi total), and the therapy can be repeated at 3-month intervals.[51] In a Canadian multicenter trial involving 126 patients with endocrine-resistant advanced prostate cancer receiving external beam radiotherapy, treatment with a single injected dose of 400-MBq ^{89}Sr significantly improved overall pain control, delayed the requirement for further external beam radiotherapy, and was associated with an enhanced quality of life compared with placebo-treated controls.[54]

Systemically administered phosphorus-32 (^{32}P) orthophosphate has been used to relieve pain from osteoblastic metastases for more than 50 years.[56] In a review of 28 studies involving 494 patients with prostate cancer, Silberstein and colleagues[56] found that 77% achieved pain relief, which was complete in one fifth of responders. After a brief flare of pain, analgesia generally developed within 14 days, and the median duration of response was 5 months. The extent of the hematologic toxicity is not well described and has been variably characterized as tolerable[56] and severe.[57] Other radiopharmaceuticals with similar activity that are under investigation include samarium-153-ethylenediaminetetramethylene phosphonic acid[58–62] and rhenium-186-hydroxyethylidene diphosphonate.[63,64]

Although direct comparative data of HBR and radiopharmaceutical therapies are lacking, retrospective surveys using matched patient populations indicate that response rates and duration are similar in the two modalities and that radiopharmaceutical therapy is better tolerated by patients.[65,66] Data comparing the various radiopharmaceuticals is lacking.

Chemotherapy

The therapeutic index of chemotherapy in the management of cancer pain is related to the balance between its antineoplastic efficacy and cost factors of toxicity and outpatient opportunity. In a phase II trial of estramustine phosphate and vinblastine in hormone-refractory prostate cancer, a major reduction in pain was observed in 12 of 28 patients with assessable pain. Analgesic response was closely related to decreases in serum prostate-specific antigen (PSA) level, with 93.7% specificity, 50% sensitivity, and positive predictive value of 85.7%.[67]

Surgery

Surgery may have a role in the relief of symptoms caused by specific problems such as obstruction of a hollow viscus, unstable bony structures, and compression of neural tissues.[68] In all cases, the potential benefits must be weighed against the risks of surgery, the anticipated length of hospitalization and convalescence, and the predicted duration of benefit.[68]

Antibiotics

Antibiotics may be analgesic when the source of the pain involves infection, as illustrated by the treatment of chronic sinus infection, pelvic abscess, pyonephrosis, and osteitis pubis.[69,70] Occasionally, infection may be occult and confirmed only by the symptomatic relief provided by empiric treatment with these drugs.[71]

The Analgesic Ladder Approach to Systemic Pharmacotherapy

The World Health Organization's "Three Step Analgesic Ladder" (Fig. 59-2) provides a useful approach to drug selection for cancer pain[72,73]:

Step I: patients with mild to moderate cancer-related pain should be treated with a non-opioid analgesic, which should be combined with an adjuvant analgesic if a specific indication for one exists.

Step II: patients who are relatively nontolerant and present with moderate to severe pain or who fail to achieve adequate relief after a trial of a non-opioid analgesic should be treated with a so-called "weak" opioid (e.g., codeine, oxycodone, propoxyphene); this drug is typically combined with a non-opioid and may be coadministered with an adjuvant analgesic.

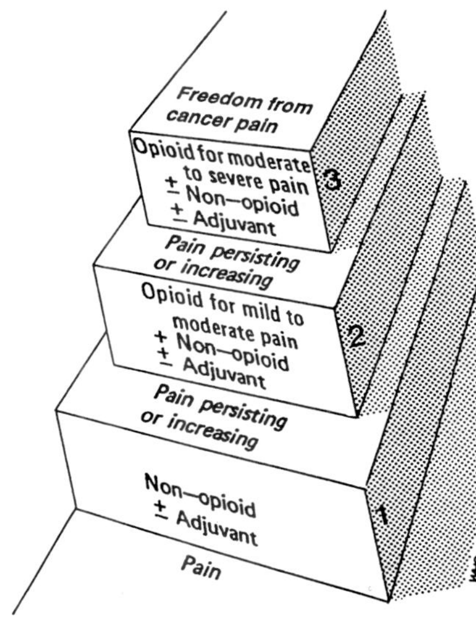

FIG. 59-2. The three-step "analgesic ladder" proposed by an expert committee of the Cancer Unit of the World Health Organization.

Step III: patients who present with severe pain or fail to achieve adequate relief following appropriate administration of drugs on the second step of the analgesic ladder should receive a so-called ''strong'' opioid, which may also be combined with a non-opioid analgesic or another adjuvant drug.

Some patients whose pain is refractory to this approach benefit from a combination of invasive anesthetic or neurosurgical treatments. Such patients should have access to specialists in pain management or palliative medicine, who can provide additional expertise in addressing these complex problems.

Systemic Analgesic Pharmacotherapy

Non-opioid Analgesics

The non-opioid analgesics (Table 59-3) are useful alone for mild to moderate pain described in step I of the analgesic ladder and provide additive analgesia when combined with opioid drugs in the treatment of more severe pain. Unlike opioid analgesics, non-opioid analgesics have a ceiling effect for analgesia, and they do not produce tolerance or physical dependence. Safe administration of non-opioid analgesics requires familiarity with their potential adverse effects. Aspirin and other nonsteroidal antiinflammatory drugs (NSAIDs) have a broad spectrum of potential toxicity, and caution is required in the administration of these agents to patients at increased risk, including the elderly; those with blood clotting disorders, ulcer diathesis, or impaired renal function; and those receiving concurrent corticosteroid therapy.[74] The nonacetylated salicylates, such as choline magnesium trisalicylate and salsalate, have less of an effect on platelet aggregation and no effect on bleeding time at usual clinical doses; these drugs are preferred in patients who have a bleeding diathesis and a strong indication for an antiinflammatory drug. Acetaminophen has fewer adverse effects than do NSAIDs, and although acetaminophen-induced hepatic toxicity is a rare occurrence, patients with chronic alcoholism and liver disease can develop severe hepatotoxicity, even when the drug is taken in usual therapeutic doses.

Opioid Analgesics

Selecting an Appropriate Drug

All patients with pain of moderate or greater severity should receive a trial of opioid therapy, irrespective of the pathophysiologic mechanism underlying the pain.[75] The pure agonist opioids (Table 59-4) have no clinically relevant ceiling effect with regard to analgesia and are the most commonly used drugs in cancer pain management. Patients with moderate pain are usually treated with a conventional opioid (e.g., codeine, dihydrocodeine, hydrocodone, oxycodone, propoxyphene).[72,73] These drugs can be prescribed as a single agent, but they are more commonly available as combination products containing

TABLE 59-3. *Commonly prescribed non-opioid analgesics*

Chemical class	Generic name	Half-life (h)	Starting dose (mg)	Maximum recommended dose (mg/day)	Comments
NONACIDIC					
p-Aminophenol derivatives	Acetaminophen	3–4	750 q4h	3000	
ACIDIC					
Salicylates	Aspirin	3–12	650 q4–6h	5000	
	Diflunisal	8–12	500 q12h	1500	Less GI toxicity than aspirin
	Choline Magnesium Trisalicylate	8–12	1000 q12h	4000	No effect on platelet function at usual doses
	Salsalate	8–12	1000 q12h	4000	No effect on platelet function at usual doses
Proprionic acids	Ibuprofen	3–4	400 q6h	4200	Available over the counter
	Naproxen	1–3	250 q12h	1000	
	Tenoprofen	2–3	200 q6h	3200	
Acetic acids	Indomethacin	4–5	25 q12h	200	Available in sustained-release and rectal preparations
	Sulindac	14	150 q12h	400	
	Diclofenac	2	25 q8h	200	
	Ketorolac	4–7	30 q6h	240	Available in oral or parenteral preparations
Oxicams	Piroxicam	45	20 q24h	40	
Fenamates	Mefenamic acid	2	250 q6h	1000	
Pyranocarboxylic acids	Etodolac	7	1000 q24h	2000	

GI, gastrointestinal.
Adapted from Cherny NI, Portenoy RK. Cancer pain management: current strategy. Cancer Suppl 1993;72(11):3393.

TABLE 59-4. *Opioid agonist drugs*

Drug	Dose (mg) equianalgesic to 10 mg IM morphine: IM	PO	Half-life (h)	Duration of action (h)	Comments
FOR MODERATE PAIN					
Codeine	130	200	2–3	2–4	Usually combined with a nonopioid; available over the counter
Oxycodone*	15	30	2–3	2–4	Used for step 2 of the analgesic ladder formulated in combination with a nonopioid
Propoxyphene	100	50	2–3	2–4	Usually combined with nonopioid; norpropoxyphene accumulation in patients with renal impairment may cause seizures
FOR SEVERE PAIN					
Morphine	10	30 (repeated dose) 60 (single dose)	2–3	3–4	M6G accumulation in renal failure may predispose to additional toxicity; wide range of formulations; on WHO essential drug list
Oxycodone	15	30	2–3	2–4	Formulated as single agent; can be used for severe pain
Hydromorphone	1.5	7.5	2–3	2–4	
Methadone	10	20	15–190	4–8	Plasma accumulation may lead to delayed toxicity; dosing should be initiated on an as needed basis
Meperidine	75	300	2–3	2–4	Not recommended for cancer pain
Oxymorphone	1	10 (PR)	2–3	4–4	No oral formulation available; less histamine release than other opioids
Levorphanol	2	4	12–15	4–8	Plasma accumulation may lead to delayed toxicity
Fentanyl transdermal system	**	**		48–72	Patches available to deliver 25, 50, 75 and 100 μg/h

M6G, morphine–6–sulfate; WHO, World Health Organization
* When combined with a nonopioid.
** Transdermal fentanyl 100 μg/h = parenteral morphine sulfate 2–4 mg/h.
Adapted from Cherny NI, Portenoy RK. Cancer pain management: current Strategy. Cancer Suppl 1993;72(11):3393.

acetaminophen. The doses of these combination products can be increased until the maximum dose of the non-opioid coanalgesic is attained (e.g., 3000 mg of acetaminophen); beyond this dose, the opioid contained in the combination product could be increased as a single agent, or the patient could be switched to an opioid conventionally used in step III of the analgesic ladder.

Patients who present with severe pain are usually treated with an opioid customarily used in step III. For the patient without major organ failure who is opioid naive, any of the available agonist opioids can be selected. Short–half-life opioid agonists (e.g., morphine, hydromorphone, fentanyl, oxycodone, oxymorphone) are generally favored because they are easier to titrate than the long–half-life drugs, which require a longer period to approach steady-state plasma concentrations. Among the short–half-life opioids, the range of available formulations often influences specific drug selection. For ambulatory patients who are able to tolerate oral opioids, morphine sulfate is usually preferred because it is easy to titrate in its immediate-release form and is also available as a controlled-release preparation that allows a 8- to 12-hour dosing interval. The long–half-life drugs (e.g., methadone, levorphanol) are not used as first-line opioids because they can be difficult to titrate, particularly if delayed toxicity develops as plasma concentrations gradually rise following an increase in dose increments.

It is always important to review the patient's response to previous trials of opioid therapy. If the current opioid is well tolerated, it is usually continued unless difficulties in dose titration occur or the required dose cannot be administered conveniently. If dose-limiting side effects develop, a trial of an alternative opioid should be considered. In a series of 100 consecutive patients referred to the pain service at Memorial Sloan-Kettering, 44 patients required a switch in their opioid therapy, and 20 patients required more than one change. Among the patients who survived to be discharged, there was an increase in the proportion of patients with no adverse effects (18% to 41%) and a diminished requirement for coanalgesics and therapies to manage adverse effects (86% to 54%).[76] The existence of different degrees of incomplete cross-tolerance to various receptor-mediated opioid effects (e.g., analgesia, side effects) may explain the utility of these sequential trials.[77–79] To safely implement the technique of sequential opioid trials, the clinician must be familiar with at least three opioid drugs used in the management of severe pain and have the ability to calculate appropriate starting doses using equianalgesic dosing data.

Meperidine is not recommended in the management of cancer pain. Meperidine is *N*-demethylated to normeperidine, which is an active metabolite that is twice as potent as a convulsant and one half as potent as an analgesic than its parent compound.

Accumulation of normeperidine after repetitive meperidine administration can result in central nervous system excitability characterized by subtle mood effects, tremors, multifocal myoclonus, and occasionally, seizures.[80] Patients with renal impairment may accumulate the active metabolites of meperidine (normeperidine) and morphine (morphine-6-glucuronide); caution is required in the administration of these drugs in these patients.

Selecting an Appropriate Route

Opioids should be administered by the least invasive and most convenient route that can provide adequate analgesia. The oral route is usually the most appropriate. For patients who have impaired swallowing or gastrointestinal obstruction, alternative noninvasive routes, including the transdermal, rectal and sublingual routes, are feasible. A transdermal formulation of fentanyl that delivers 25, 50, 75, or 100 μg per hour is available. The dosing interval for each system is usually 72 hours, but there is wide interindividual pharmacokinetic variability,[81] and some patients require a dosing interval of 48 hours. Rescue doses for breakthrough pain can be provided by an alternative short-acting opioid or the oral transmucosal formulation of fentanyl.[82,83] Rectal suppositories containing morphine, hydromorphone, and oxymorphone are available, and controlled-release morphine tablets can also be administered rectally.[84] The potency of opioids administered rectally approximates that of oral dosing.[85] Sublingual administration of an injectable formulation can be a useful approach in some patients who transiently lose the ability to receive oral dosing.

Parenteral routes of administration should be considered for patients who have impaired swallowing or gastrointestinal obstruction, those who require the rapid onset of analgesia, and those who are highly tolerant and require doses that cannot otherwise be conveniently administered. Repeated parenteral bolus injections, which can be delivered by the intravenous (IV), intramuscular (IM) or subcutaneous (SC) routes, may be appropriate in some situations but are often complicated by toxicity at peak concentration or pain breakthrough at trough levels. Although repetitive IM injections are commonly prescribed, they are painful, offer no pharmacokinetic advantage, and their use is not recommended. Repeated bolus doses, if required, can be administered without frequent skin punctures through the use of an indwelling IV or SC infusion device. To deliver repeated SC injections, a 27-gauge infusion device (i.e., "butterfly") can be left under the skin for as long as 1 week.[86]

Continuous infusions avoid the problems associated with the bolus effect and may be administered IV or SC.[86] Ambulatory infusion devices vary in complexity, cost, and ability to provide patient-controlled rescue doses as an adjunct to a continuous basal infusion (discussed later). Morphine, hydromorphone, oxymorphone, and fentanyl can be administered by these routes. Methadone is relatively irritating and is not recommended for SC infusion.[87] Studies suggest that dosing with SC administration can proceed in a manner identical to that with continuous IV infusion.[88,89] To maintain the comfort of an infusion site, the SC infusion rate should not exceed 5 mL/hour. Patients who require high doses may benefit from the use of concentrated solutions, which in selected cases can be compounded specifically for continuous SC infusion. Continuous IV infusion may be the most appropriate way of delivering an opioid when there is a need for infusion of a large volume of solution or when using methadone. If continuous IV infusion must be continued on a long-term basis, establishment of a permanent central venous port is recommended.

Switching drug-delivery routes requires careful attention to relative potency (see Table 59-4). It is generally prudent to perform the switch in a gradual, stepwise manner over a 2- to 3-day period.

Selecting a Dosing Schedule

Patients with continuous or frequently recurring pain generally require scheduled around-the-clock dosing. All such patients should also be offered a rescue dose, which is a supplemental dose given on an as-needed basis to treat pain that breaks through the regular schedule. The integration of scheduled dosing with rescue doses provides a method for safe and rational stepwise dose escalation and is applicable to all routes of opioid administration (Table 59-5). The rescue drug is usually identical to that administered on a continuous basis. The frequency with which it is available to the patient depends on the drug's time to peak effect for the drug and the route of administration; oral rescue doses are offered up to every 1 to 2 hours, and parenteral rescue doses are offered up to every 15 to 30 minutes. The size of the rescue dose should be equivalent to approximately 5% to 15% of the 24-hour baseline dose.

Controlled-release formulations can lessen the inconvenience associated with around-the-clock drug administration.[90] Controlled-release oral morphine sulfate and transdermal fentanyl are widely used, and controlled-release formulations of oxycodone and hydromorphone are under development. Controlled-release preparations of morphine sulfate typically achieve peak plasma levels 3 to 5 hours after administration and have a duration of effect of 8 to 12 hours. Controlled-release and immediate-release formulations of oral morphine are dose equivalent; a switch from one to the other is done on a milligram-to-milligram basis when the effective around-the-clock dose is identified. These formulations should not be used to rapidly titrate the dose in patients with severe pain.

Patient-controlled analgesia (PCA) is a technique of parenteral drug administration in which the patient controls a pump that delivers bolus doses of an analgesic according to parameters set by the physician. Use of a PCA device allows the patient to carefully titrate the opioid dose to his or her individual analgesic needs. Long-term PCA in cancer patients is accomplished via the SC or IV route using a ambulatory infusion device. The more technologically advanced of these devices have programmable variables, including infusion rate, rescue dose, and lock-out interval.[86] The option for bolus dosing is generally administered in conjunction with a continuous opioid infusion.

Dose Selection and Titration

Patients in severe pain who are opioid naive should generally begin with one of the opioids conventionally used for severe pain at a dose equivalent to 5 to 10 mg IM morphine every 3 to 4 hours. If a switch from one opioid drug to another is re-

TABLE 59-5. *Examples of stepwise dose escalation of morphine sulfate administered as an oral immediate-release preparation and an oral controlled-release preparation and continuous infusion*

	Oral controlled release with immediate-release rescue dosing		Intravenous infusion with intravenous rescue doses	
Step*	Around the clock dose (mg)	Rescue dose as needed q1h (mg)	Rescue dose (mg/hr)	As needed q15–30 min (mg)
1	30 q12h	7.5	3	2
2	30 q8h	15	5	2.5
3	60 q12h	15	7	3.5
4	100 q12h	30	10	5
5	100 q8h	30	15	7.5
6	200 q12h	45	20	10
7	200 q8h	60	30	15

*Indications for progression from one step to the next: more than 2 rescue doses in any 4-hour interval or more than 6 rescue doses in 24 hours.

Adapted from Cherny NI, Portenoy RK. Pharmacotherapy of cancer pain. In: Arbit E, ed. Management of cancer-related pain. Mount Kisko: Futura, 1993:65.

quired, the equianalgesic dose table (see Table 71-4) is used as a guide to determining the starting dose. For patients with good pain control but unacceptable side effects, the starting dose of the new drug should be reduced to 50% to 75% of the equianalgesic dose. However, if pain control is poor, the starting dose of the new drug should be 75% to 100% of the equianalgesic dose. After any change from one opioid to another, patients must be monitored to assess the adequacy of analgesia and to detect the development of side effects. Subsequent dose adjustments are usually necessary.

Inadequately relieved pain should be addressed through a stepwise escalation of the opioid dose until adequate analgesia is reported or unmanageable side effects supervene. A dose increment of 30% to 50% is safe and sufficiently large to observe a meaningful change in effects. In most cases, gradual dose escalation allows identification of a favorable balance between analgesia and side effects that remains stable for a prolonged period.[3] In a retrospective study of 100 patients with advanced cancer, the average daily opioid requirement was equivalent to 400 to 600 mg of IM morphine, but approximately 10% of patients required more than 2000 mg, and one patient required more than 30,000 mg per 24 hours.[91] The absolute dose is immaterial as long as the balance between analgesia and side effects remains favorable. Patients who develop dose-limiting side effects during dose titration require another analgesic approach or a technique to reduce opioid toxicity (discussed later). The rate of dose titration is determined by the severity of the pain; patients with very severe pain should be managed by repeated parenteral dosing every 15 to 30 minutes until pain is partially relieved. The hourly maintenance dosing after parenteral loading with a short–half-life opioid can be estimated by dividing the total loading dose by twice the elimination half-life of the drug.[92] For example, the starting maintenance dose for a patient who required an IV loading dose of 60 mg of morphine sulfate, which has a half-life of approximately 3 hours, would be 10 mg/hour. Patients with less severe pain can undergo more gradual dose escalation.

Adverse Effects of Opioids and Their Management

An understanding of the strategies used to prevent or manage common opioid toxicities is needed to optimize the balance between analgesia and side effects. The most common adverse effects are constipation, nausea and vomiting, and somnolence or cognitive impairment. Other important dose-limiting adverse effects include dysphoria, myoclonus, and respiratory depression.

The likelihood of opioid-induced constipation is so great that laxative medications should be prescribed prophylactically to most patients, particularly those who are elderly or have coexisting gastrointestinal pathology. A combination of a softening agent (e.g., docusate) and a cathartic (e.g., senna, bisacodyl, phenolphthalein) is frequently used.

The incidence of opioid-induced nausea has been estimated to be 10% to 40%.[93] Tolerance to these effects often develops rapidly, and routine prophylactic administration of an antiemetic is not usually indicated except in patients with a history of severe opioid-induced nausea. Three putative mechanisms may produce nausea and vomiting: a direct effect on the chemoreceptor trigger zone, enhanced vestibular sensitivity, and delayed gastric emptying. If nausea is associated with early satiety, bloating, or postprandial vomiting, all of which are features of delayed gastric emptying, metoclopramide is the most reasonable initial treatment. Patients with vertigo, or prominent movement-induced nausea, may benefit from the use of an antivertiginous drug such as scopolamine or meclizine. If signs of neither gastroparesis nor vestibular dysfunction are prominent, treatment is usually begun with a neuroleptic such as prochlorperazine or metoclopramide. If these drugs are ineffective at relatively high doses, other options include a trial of an alternative opioid or treatment with an antihistamine (e.g., diphenhydramine, hydroxyzine), neuroleptic (e.g., haloperidol, chlorpromazine, droperidol), benzodiazepine (e.g., lorazepam), steroid (e.g., dexamethasone), or serotonin antagonist (e.g., ondansetron).

The initiation of opioid therapy or significant dose escalation is often associated with somnolence or cognitive impairment that usually persists for days to weeks.[94] Although tolerance often develops, some patients continue to have intolerable effects, particularly if other contributing factors exist. The following stepwise management strategy is useful:

1. Eliminate nonessential central nervous system depressant medications and evaluate the patient for concurrent causes,

including sepsis, metabolic derangement, or intracerebral or leptomeningeal metastases.
2. If analgesia is satisfactory, reduce the opioid dose by 25%.
3. If analgesia is unsatisfactory, switch to a different opioid drug.
4. If analgesia is satisfactory and lethargy persists, consider the addition of a psychostimulant such as methylphenidate (starting dose, 510 mg twice daily), dextroamphetamine (starting dose, 5 to 10 mg twice daily), or pemoline (starting dose, 18.75 to 35.5 mg twice daily).
5. If hallucinations or delirium persist despite dose reduction, consider a trial of haloperidol (starting dose, 0.5 mg three times daily).
6. If these problems continue to persist, consider the addition of a non-opioid or adjuvant analgesic (which may allow reduction in opioid dose), a switch to a different opioid drug, or an anesthetic or neurolytic technique.

Myoclonus is a common dose-related adverse effect of opioids, which, like somnolence and cognitive impairment, is often determined by multiple factors other than the opioid. If the myoclonus is symptomatic and distressing, it can be treated empirically with clonazepam.[95]

Among cancer patients whose opioid dose is carefully titrated, respiratory depression is a rare occurrence. Although tolerance may develop rapidly to this effect,[96] the observation that some patients on stable opioid therapy develop sedation or respiratory depression after anesthetic or neurodestructive procedures suggests that other pain-related factors may also play a role in the ability to tolerate high-dose opioid therapy.[96] Reduction of the opioid dose is usually necessary after anesthetic or neurolytic techniques. Clinically significant respiratory depression is always accompanied by other signs of central nervous system depression, including somnolence and mental clouding. Respiratory distress associated with tachypnea and anxiety is never a primary opioid event, and alternative explanations (e.g., pneumonia, pulmonary embolism) should be sought. Because of the risk of systemic withdrawal and the return of pain, naloxone should only be administered for symptomatic respiratory depression. If the patient is arousable and the peak plasma levels of the opioid have already been reached, naloxone should not be administered; the opioid dose should be withheld and the patient monitored and kept awake until improvement is noted. If the patient is becoming progressively obtunded, is unarousable, or has severe respiratory depression, naloxone should be administered using small bolus injections of dilute solution (0.4 mg in 10 mL saline) that are titrated against respiratory rate.[97,98] Because naloxone has a short half-life, patients receiving slow-release morphine, transdermal fentanyl, or methadone may require repeated doses or a naloxone infusion to prevent recurrence of respiratory depression.

Physical and Psychological Dependence

Opioids should never be withheld in the management of patients with chronic cancer pain because of fear of physical and psychological dependence (i.e., addiction). Physical dependence is not a clinical problem if patients are warned to avoid abrupt discontinuation of the drug, a tapering schedule is used if treatment cessation is indicated, and opioid antagonist drugs, including agonist-antagonist analgesics, are avoided.

Psychological dependence, or addiction, refers to a psychological and behavioral syndrome characterized by a continued craving for an opioid drug to achieve a psychic effect (i.e., psychological dependence) and associated aberrant drug-related behaviors (e.g., compulsive use, continued use despite harm to self or others). Addiction should be suspected if patients demonstrate compulsive use, loss of control over drug use, and continuing use despite harm. The term addiction should never be used when physical dependence is meant. The medical use of opioids is rarely associated with the development of addiction.[99–101] In the largest prospective study, only 4 cases of iatrogenic addiction could be identified among 11,882 patients with no prior history of addiction who received at least one opioid preparation in the hospital setting.[102] Extensive clinical experience in the use of opioids for patients with chronic cancer pain affirms that that the risk of addiction in this population is extremely low.[72,73]

Patients who continue to experience unrelieved pain and express concern about opioid availability and the need for dose escalation are often accused of drug-seeking behaviors. Pain relief, usually produced by dose escalation, eliminates these requests. This syndrome has been termed "pseudo-addiction."[103] Misunderstanding of these phenomena may lead the clinician to inappropriately stigmatize the patient with the label of "addict," which may compromise care and erode the doctor-patient relationship. In the setting of unrelieved pain, the request for increases in drug dose requires careful assessment, renewed efforts to manage pain, and avoidance of stigmatizing labels.

Noninvasive Interventions for Patients Unable to Attain an Acceptable Balance Between Relief and Side Effects of Systemic Opioids

Even with optimal management of adverse effects, some patients do not attain an acceptable balance between pain relief and the side effects of an opioid. Several noninvasive interventions can improve this balance by reducing the opioid requirement. These include the concurrent use of an appropriate primary therapy; alternative pharmacologic approaches including non-opioid analgesics, adjuvant analgesics, or switch to another opioid; and the use of psychological or rehabilitative techniques

Adjuvant Analgesics

Adjuvant analgesics are drugs that have a primary indication other than pain but have analgesic effects in some painful conditions. These drugs play an important role in improving the analgesic outcome in some patients who cannot otherwise attain an acceptable balance between pain relief and opioid side effects. Adjuvant analgesics can be broadly divided into general-purpose analgesics and those with specific utility for either neuropathic or bone pain.

Corticosteroids

Corticosteroids are the most widely used general-purpose adjuvant analgesics.[104] These drugs may ameliorate pain and produce beneficial effects on appetite, nausea, mood, and malaise.[105,106] In a study of low-dose prednisone (7.5 to 10 mg daily) in the management of patients with hormone-refractory prostate cancer complicated by symptomatic bone metastases, 14 of 38 patients had improved pain relief at 1 month, and 7 patients (19%) maintained this improvement for 3 to 30 months (median, 4 months). Reduction in pain was associated with improvement in other dimensions of quality of life and in the scale for overall well-being. Pain relief was generally associated with a decrease in serum concentration of adrenal androgens.[106] The painful conditions that commonly respond to corticosteroids include raised intracranial pressure, acute spinal cord compression, superior vena cava syndrome, metastatic bone pain, neuropathic pain caused by infiltration or compression by tumor, symptomatic lymphedema, and hepatic capsular distention.[104] Patients with advanced cancer who experience pain and other symptoms that may respond to steroids are usually given a small dose (e.g., dexamethasone, 1 to 2 mg twice daily). An acute episode of severe pain related to a neuropathic lesion (e.g. plexopathy, epidural spinal cord compression) or bony metastasis that cannot be promptly reduced with opioids may respond dramatically to a short course of relatively high doses of a corticosteroid (e.g., dexamethasone, 100 mg IV, followed initially by 96 mg/day in divided doses). In all cases, once pain reduction is achieved, the dose should be gradually lowered to the minimum level needed to sustain relief.

Adjuvant Drugs for Bone Pain

The management of bone pain frequently requires the integration of opioid therapy with multiple ancillary approaches. Although a meta-analysis of NSAID therapy in cancer pain that reviewed data from 1615 patients in 21 trials found no specific efficacy in bone pain and analgesic effects equivalent only to weak opioids,[107] some patients appear to benefit greatly from the addition NSAIDs.

Bisphosphonate drugs inhibit osteoclast activity and are used in the management of hypercalcemia. In patients with prostate cancer, pamidronate[108–112] and clodronate[113–116] have also been demonstrated to relieve bone pain. Sodium etidronate demonstrated no beneficial effects.[117] Parenteral administration of pamidronate every 2 weeks is generally well tolerated, and the risk of symptomatic hypocalcemia is low. An appropriate starting dose is 60 mg administered by slow infusion over 2 to 4 hours. Although the data in support of calcitonin[118] and gallium nitrate[119,120] in the management of bone pain is limited, these agents should be considered in difficult cases and are worthy of further evaluation. Although clinically significant, the magnitude of pain relief observed with these approaches is not dramatic, and most patients continue to require other analgesic approaches.

Adjuvant Drugs for Neuropathic Pain

Neuropathic pains such as those observed in patients with lumbosacral plexopathy can be difficult to treat, and the use of adjuvant drugs can contribute substantially the successful management of these problems. For the purpose of drug selection, it is useful to distinguish, based on the patient's history and physical examination, between continuous and lancinating neuropathic pain (Table 59-6).[121] Furthermore, because of the great interpatient and intrapatient variability in the response to adjuvant drugs in this setting, including those within the same class, sequential trials of adjuvant analgesics are frequently required.

TABLE 59-6. *Adjuvant analgesics for neuropathic pain based on clinical characteristics*

Continuous pain	Lancinating pain
Antidepressants	Anticonvulsant drugs
Amitriptyline	Carbamazepine
Doxepin	Oxcarbazepine
Imipramine	Phenytoin
Desipramine	Clonazepam
Nortriptyline	Valproate
Trazodone	Baclofen
Maprotiline	Oral local anesthetics
Oral local anesthetics	
Mexiletine	
Clonidine	

Adapted from Cherny NI, Portenoy RK. Cancer pain management: current strategy. Cancer Suppl 1993;72(11):3393.

Other Noninvasive Techniques

Psychological Therapies

Although all cancer patients benefit from psychological assessment and support, some will benefit from specific psychological interventions used in the management of pain. Cognitive-behavioral interventions can help reduce the perception of distress caused by the pain through the development of coping skills and the modification of thoughts, feelings, and behaviors,[122] and relaxation techniques can reduce muscular tension and emotional arousal and enhance pain tolerance.[123]

Physiatric Techniques

Physiatric techniques can be used to enhance analgesia and optimize function in the patient with chronic cancer pain. Therapeutic modalities such as electrical stimulation (including transcutaneous electrical nerve stimulation), heat, or cryotherapy can be useful adjuncts to standard analgesic therapy. Treatment of lymphedema with the use of wraps, pressure stockings, or pneumatic pump devices can both improve function and relieve pain and heaviness.[124] Orthotic devices can immobilize and support painful or weakened structures, and assistive devices can enhance comfort for patients with pain precipitated by weight bearing or ambulation.

Invasive Interventions for Patients Unable to Attain an Acceptable Balance Between Relief and Side Effects of Systemic Pharmacotherapy

Patients who are unable to achieve a satisfactory balance between analgesia and side effects with systemic analgesic therapies may be candidates for the use of invasive anesthetic and neurosurgical techniques. These approaches may reduce the requirement for systemically administered opioids. Techniques such as intraspinal opioid and local anesthetic administration can achieve this end without compromising neurological integrity. The use of neurodestructive procedures should be based on an evaluation of the likelihood and duration of analgesic benefit, the immediate and long-term risks, the likely duration of survival of the patient, and the anticipated length of hospitalization.

Epidural and Intrathecal Opioids

The delivery of low opioid doses near the sites of action in the spinal cord may decrease supraspinally mediated adverse effects. In the absence of randomized trials comparing the various intraspinal techniques with other analgesic approaches, the indications for the selection of a spinal route remain empirical. Compared with neuroablative therapies, spinal opioids have the advantage of preserving sensation, strength, and sympathetic function. Reserving these techniques for patients with persistent dose-limiting toxicity from systemic opioid therapy, Hogan and colleagues[125] reported that only 16 of 1205 cancer patients with pain required use of these routes. Contraindications include bleeding diathesis, profound leukopenia, and sepsis. A temporary trial of spinal opioid therapy should be performed to assess the potential benefits of this approach before implantation of a permanent catheter. The addition of a low concentration of a local anesthetic (e.g., 0.125% to 0.25% bupivacaine) to an epidural opioid has been demonstrated to increase analgesic effect without increasing toxicity. The potential morbidity for these procedures indicates the need for a well-trained clinician and long-term monitoring.

Neurodestructive Procedures

For patients with unilateral pelvic or lower limb pain, cordotomy or rhizotomy can be considered. Cordotomy involves interruption of the anterolateral spinothalamic tract to produce contralateral loss of pain and temperature sensibility.[126,127] The percutaneous technique is generally preferred[126]; open cordotomy is usually reserved for patients who are unable to lie in the supine position or are not cooperative enough to undergo a percutaneous procedure.[126] Significant pain relief is achieved in more than 90% of patients during the period immediately following cordotomy.[126–128] The neurologic complications of cordotomy, which include paresis, ataxia, and bladder dysfunction, are usually transient but are protracted and disabling in approximately 5% of cases.[128] The most serious potential complication is respiratory dysfunction, which may result from phrenic nerve paralysis or sleep-induced apnea in patients who undergo bilateral high cordotomy.[129] The potential for this complication relatively contraindicates bilateral high cervical cordotomies or unilateral cervical cordotomy ipsilateral to the site of the only functioning lung.

Rhizotomy involves the selective destruction of the dorsal nerve roots either surgically or by the instillation of a neurolytic solution into the epidural or intrathecal space.[127,130] Satisfactory analgesia is achieved in about 50% of patients who undergo epidural or intrathecal neurolysis.[131] In contrast to cordotomy, rhizotomy is useful for patients with bilateral pain. Complications of lumbosacral neurolysis include paresis (5% to 20%), sphincter dysfunction (5% to 60%), impairment of touch and proprioception, and dysesthesias. Although neurologic deficits are usually transient, the risk of increased disability as a result of weakness, sphincter incompetence, and loss of positional sense suggests that these techniques be reserved for patients with limited function and preexistent urinary diversion. Patient counseling regarding the risks involved in these techniques is essential.

Severe pain limited to the perineum may be treated by neurolysis of the S_4 nerve root via the ipsilateral posterior sacral foramen, a procedure that carries a minimal risk of motor or sphincter impairment.[132] Intercostal and paravertebral neurolysis are alternatives to rhizotomy for patients with chest wall pain. Visceral pain arising from pelvic structures can be treated with blockade of the superior hypogastric nerve plexus, which is located immediately anterior to the sacral promontory.[133]

Pituitary ablation by chemical or surgical hypophysectomy can be considered for patients with multifocal pain syndromes that are refractory to opioid therapy and are unsuitable for any regional neuroablative procedure.[134] Pain relief has been observed from pain associated with both hormone-dependent and hormone-independent tumors.[134]

Therapy for Patients With Refractory Pain: The Role of Sedation

For some patients with advanced disease, adequate relief of physical pain may be achieved only at the cost of profound sedation.[135] The incidence of this situation is controversial and has been variably estimated at 5% to 52% of patients with far-advanced cancer.[136] Increasing attention has been focused on the use of sedation to manage intractable pain and suffering in patients who fall to benefit from optimal therapy.[136] The patient with advanced cancer and uncontrolled symptoms may choose transitory use of sedating therapy while continuing trials of analgesic approaches. Alternatively, a strategy can be designed to provide adequate sedation until death.

The ethical basis of the latter approach is predicated on informed consent and an acknowledgment of the "principle of double effect," which distinguishes between the compelling primary therapeutic intent (i.e., to relieve suffering) and unavoidable untoward consequences (i.e., the potential for accelerating death).[137] This approach recognizes the right of dying patients to adequate relief of pain and the right of all patients to choose among appropriate therapeutic options.[136] No patient should have to ask to be killed because of persistently unrelieved pain; conversely, no patient should be sedated without appropriate informed consent of the patient or proxy. The process of informed decision-making requires candid discussion that clarifies the prevailing clinical predicament and presents the alternative analgesic options, including sedation.

REFERENCES

1. Chisholm GD, Rana A, Howard GCW. Management options for painful carcinoma of the prostate. Semin Oncol 1993;20(Suppl 2):34.

2. Cleeland CS, Gonin R, Hatfield A, et al. Pain and its treatment in outpatients with metastatic cancer. N Engl J Med 1994;330(9):592.
3. Brescla FJ, Portenoy RK, Ryan M, Krasnoff L, Gray G. Pain, opioid use, and survival in hospitalized patients with advanced cancer. J CIin Oncol 1992;10(1):149.
4. Helm HM, Oel TP. Comparison of prostate cancer patients with and without pain. Pain 1993;53(2):159.
5. Von Roenn JH, Cleeland CS, Gonin R, Hatfield A, Pandya KJ. Physician's attitudes and practice in cancer pain management: a survey from the Eastern Cooperative Oncology Group. Ann Intern Med 1993; 119(2):121.
6. Grossman SA, Sheidler VR, Swedeen K, Mucenski J, Piantadosi S. Correlation of patient and caregiver ratings of cancer pain. J Pain Symptom Manage 1991;6(2):53.
7. Weissman DE, Gutmann M, Dahl JL. Physician cancer pain education: a report from the Wisconsin Cancer Pain Initiative. J Pain Symptom Manage 1991;6(7):445.
8. McCaffery M, Thorpe DM. Differences in perception of pain and the development of adversarial relationships among health care providers. In: Hill CS, Fields WS, ed. Advances in pain research and therapy, vol 11. Drug treatment of cancer pain in a drug oriented society. New York: Raven Press, 1989:19
9. Portenoy RK, Hagen NA. Breakthrough pain: definition, prevalence and characteristics. Pain 1990;41(3):273.
10. Banning A, Sjogren P, Henriksen H. Pain causes in 200 patients referred to a multidisciplinary cancer pain clinic. Pain 1991;45(1):45.
11. Daut RL, Cleeland CS. The prevalence and severity of pain in cancer. Cancer 1982;50:1913.
12. Twycross RG, Fairfield S. Pain in far-advanced cancer. Pain 1982; 14:303.
13. Nielsen OS, Munro AJ, Tannock IF. Bone metastases: pathophysiology and management policy. J Clin Oncol 1991;9(3):509.
14. Palmer E, Henrikson B, McKusick K, Strauss HW, Hochberg F. Pain as an indicator of bone metastasis. Acta Radiol 1988;29(4):445.
15. Cumming J, Hacking N, Fairhurst J, Ackery D, Jenkins JD. Distribution of bony metastases in prostatic carcinoma. Br J Urol 1990;66(4): 411.
16. Grant R, Papadopoulos SM, Greenberg HS. Metastatic epidural spinal cord compression. Neurol Clin 1991;9(4):825.
17. Turner S, Marosszeky B, Timms I, Boyages J. Malignant spinal cord compression: a prospective evaluation. Int J Radiat Oncol Biol Phys 1993;26(1):141.
18. Zelefsky MJ, Scher HI, Krol G, Portenoy RK, Leibel SA, Fuks ZY. Spinal epidural tumor in patients with prostate cancer: clinical and radiographic predictors of response to radiation therapy. Cancer 1992; 70(9):2319.
19. Flynn DF, Shipley WU. Management of spinal cord compression secondary to metastatic prostatic carcinoma. Urol CIin North Am 1991; 18(1):145.
20. Bridwell KH. Treatment of metastatic prostate cancer of the spine. Urol Clin North Am 1991;18(1):153.
21. Jaeckle KA. Nerve plexus metastases. Neurol Clin 1991;9(4):857.
22. Jaeckle KA, Young DF, Foley KM. The natural history of lumbosacral plexopathy in cancer. Neurology 1985;35:8.
23. Stillman M. Perineal pain: diagnosis and management, with particular attention to perineal pain of cancer. In: Foley KM, Bonica JJ, Ventafrida V, ed. Advances in pain research and therapy, vol 16. Second International Congress on Cancer Pain. New York: Raven Press, 1990: 359.
24. Agency for Health Care Policy and Research: Acute Pain Management Panel. Management of cancer pain: clinical practice guideline number 9. Washiñgton: US Department of Health and Human Services, 1994.
25. Fishman B, Pasternak S, Wallenstein SL, Houde RW, Holland JC, Foley KM. The Memorial Pain Assessment Card: a valid instrument for the evaluation of cancer pain. Cancer 1987;60:1151.
26. Daut RL, Cleeland CS, Flanery RC. Development of the Wisconsin Brief Pain Questionnaire to assess pain In cancer and other diseases. Pain 1983;17(2):197.
27. Gonzales GR, Elliot KJ, Portenoy RK, Foley KM. The impact of a comprehensive evaluation in the management of cancer pain. Pain 1991;47:141.
28. Clouston P, De Angelis L, Posner JB. The spectrum of neurologic disease in patients with systemic cancer. Ann Neurol 1992;31:268.
29. Cherny NI, Portenoy RK. Cancer pain: principles of assessment and syndromes. In: Wall PD, Melzack R, ed. Textbook of pain, 3rd ed. Edinburgh: Churchill Livingstone, 1994:787.
30. Chrisp P, Sorkin EM. Leuprorelin: a review of its pharmacology and therapeutic use in prostatic disorders. Drugs Aging 1991;1(6):487.
31. Thompson IM, Zeldman EJ, Rodriguez FR. Sudden death due to disease flare with luteinizing hormone-releasing hormone agonist therapy for carcinoma of the prostate. J Urology 1990;144(6):1479.
32. Labrie F, Dupont A, Belanger A, Lachance R. Flutamide eliminates the risk of disease flare in prostatic cancer patients treated with a luteinizing hormone-releasing hormone agonist. J Urol 1987;138(4): 804.
33. Lungimayr G. 'Zoladex' versus 'Zoladex' plus flutamide in the treatment of advanced prostate cancer: first interim analysis of an international trial. International Prostate Cancer Study Group. Prog Clin Biol Res 1989;303(1):145.
34. Crawford ED, Nabors W. Hormone therapy of advanced prostate cancer: where we stand today. Oncology 1991;5(1):21.
35. Eberlein TJ. Gynecomastia. In: Harris JR, Hellman S, Henderson IC, Kinne D, eds. Breast diseases. Philadelphia: JB Lippincott, 1991:46.
36. Delaere KP, Van Thillo E. Flutamide monotherapy as primary treatment in advanced prostatic carcinoma. Semin Oncol 1991;5(1):13.
37. Neumann F, Kalmus J. Cyproterone acetate in the treatment of sexual disorders: pharmacological base and clinical experience. Exper Clin Endocrinol 1991;98(2):71.
38. Goldenberg SL, Bruchovsky N. Use of cyproterone acetate in prostate cancer. Urol Clin North Am 1991;18(1):111.
39. Bates T. A review of local radiotherapy in the treatment of bone metastases and cord compression. Int J Radiat Oncol Biol Phys 1992; 23(1):217.
40. Bates T, Yarnold JR, Blitzer P, Nelson OS, Rubin P, Maher J. Bone metastasis consensus statement. Int J Radiat Oncol Biol Phys 1992; 23(1):215.
41. Bosch A. Radiotherapy. Clin Oncol 1984;3(1):47.
42. Perez CA, Cosmatos D, Garcia DM, Eisbruch A, Poulter CA. Irradiation in relapsing carcinoma of the prostate. Cancer 1993;71:1110.
43. Tong D, Gillick L, Hendrickson FR. The palliation of symptomatic osseous metastases: final results of the study by the Radiation Therapy Oncology Group. Cancer 1982;50:893.
44. Ashby M. The role of radiotherapy in the management of cancer-related pain. In: Arbit E, ed. Management of cancer-related pain. Mount Kisko: Futura, 1993:121.
45. Zelefsky MJ, Scher HI, Forman JD, Linares LA, Curley T, Fuks Z. Palliative hemiskeletal irradiation for widespread metastatic carcinoma of the prostate. Int J Radiat Oncol Biol Phys 1989;17:1281.
46. Breen SL, Powe JE, Porter AT. Dose estimation in strontium-89 radiotherapy of metastatic prostatic carcinoma. J Nucl Med 1992;33(7): 1316.
47. Robinson RG, Spicer JA, Preston DF, Wegst AV, Martin NL. Treatment of metastatic bone pain with strontium-89. Int J Radiat Appl Instrum B 1987;14(3):219.
48. Laing AH, Ackery DM, Bayly RJ, et al. Strontium-89 chloride for pain palliation in prostatic skeletal malignancy. Br J Radiol 1991; 64(765):816.
49. Lewington VJ, McEwan AJ, Ackery DM, et al. A prospective, randomised double-blind crossover study to examine the efficacy of strontium-89 in pain palliation in patients with advanced prostate cancer metastatic to bone. Eur J Cancer 1991;27(8):954.
50. Haesner M, Buchall K, Pink V, Lips H. The efficacy of therapy using 89Sr-strontium chloride in 200 patients with bone metastases of a prostatic cancer. Nuklearmedizin 1992;31(2):48.
51. Robinson RG. Strontium 89: precursor targeted therapy for relief of blastic metastatic disease. Cancer Suppl 1993;72(11):3433.
52. Fossa SD, Paus E, Lochoff M, Backe SM, Aas M. Strontium-89 in bone metastases from hormone resistant prostate cancer: palliation effect and biochemical changes. Br J Cancer 1992;66(1):177.
53. Mertens WC, Porter AT, Reid RH, Powe JE. Strontium-89 and low-dose infusion cisplatin for patients with hormone refractory prostate carcinoma metastatic to bone: a preliminary report. J Nucl Med 1992; 33(8):1437.
54. Porter AT, McEwan AJ. Strontium-89 as an adjuvant to external beam radiation improves pain relief and delays disease progression in advanced prostate cancer: results of a randomized controlled trial. Semin Oncol 1993;20:38.
55. McEwan AJB, Porter AT, Venner PM, Amyotte G. An evaluation of

the safety and efficacy of strontium-89 in pain palliation in patients who have previously received wide field radiotherapy. Antibody Immunoconj Radiopharm 1990;3:91.
56. Silberstein EB, Elgazzar AH, Kapilivsky A. Phosphorus-32 radiopharmaceuticals for the treatment of painful osseous metastases. Semin Nucl Med 1992;22(1):17.
57. Porter AT, Davis LP. Systemic radionuclide therapy of bone metastases with strontium-89. Oncology 1994;8(2):93.
58. Holmes RA. (153Sm)EDTMP: a potential therapy for bone cancer pain. Semin Nucl Med 1992;22(1):41.
59. Sandeman TF, Budd RS, Martin JJ. Samarium-153-labelled EDTMP for bone metastases from cancer of the prostate. Clin Oncol (R Coll Radiol) 1992;4(3):160.
60. Turner JH, Claringbold BG, Heatherington EL, Sorby P, Martindal AA. A phase 1 study of samarium-153 ethylenedl-amenetetramethylene phosphonate therapy for disseminated skeletal metastases. J Clin Oncol 1989;7:1926.
61. Turner JH, Claringbold PG. A phase II study of treatment of painful multifocal skeletal metastases with single and repeated dose samarium-153 ethylenediaminetetramethylene phosphonate. Eur J Cancer 1991;27(9):1084.
62. Collins C, Eary JF, Donaldson G, et al. Samarium-153-EDTMP in bone metastases of hormone refractory prostate carcinoma: a phase I/II trial. J Nucl Med 1993;34(11):1839.
63. Maxon H, Thomas SR, Hertzberg VS, et al. Rhenium-186 hydroxyethylidene diphosphonate for the treatment of painful osseous metastases. Semin Nucl Med 1992;22(1):33.
64. Maxon H, Schroder LE, Hertzberg VS, et al. Rhenium-186(Sn)HEDP for treatment of painful osseous metastases: results of a double-blind crossover comparison with placebo. J Nucl Med 1991;32(10):1877.
65. Dearnaley DP, Bayly RJ. A'Hern RP, Gadd J, Zivanovic MM, Lewington VJ. Palliation of bone metastases in prostate cancer. Hemibody irradiation or strontium-89? Clin Oncol (R Coll Radiol) 1992;4(2): 101.
66. Aziz H, Chol K, Sohn C, Yaes R, Rotman M. Comparison of 32P therapy and sequential hemibody irradiation (HBI) for bony metastases as methods of whole body irradiation. Am J Clin Oncol 1986; 9(3):264.
67. Hudes GR. Greenberg R. Krigel RL, et al. Phase II study of estramustine and vinblastine, two microtubule inhibitors, in hormone-refractory prostate cancer. J Clin Oncol 1992;10(11):1754.
68. Boraas M. Palliative surgery. Semin Oncol 1985;12(4):368.
69. Burney RE, Faulkner DJ. Recurrent abdominal abscess caused by retained colorectum after proctocolectomy. Surgery 1988;104(3):580.
70. Butch RJ, Wittenberg J, Mueller PR, Simeone JF, Meyer JE, Ferrucci JJ. Presacral masses after abdominoperineal resection for colorectal carcinoma: the need for needle biopsy. Am J Roentgenol 1985;144(2): 309.
71. Coyle N, Portenoy RK. Infection as a cause of rapidly increasing pain in cancer patients. J Pain Symptom Manage 1991;6:266.
72. World Health Organization. Cancer pain relief and palliative care. Geneva: World Health Organization, 1990.
73. World Health Organization. Cancer pain relief. Geneva: World Health Organization, 1986.
74. Brooks PM, Wood AJJ. Nonsteroidal antiinflammatory drugs-differences and similarities. N Engl J Med 1991;324:1716.
75. Portenoy RK, Foley KM, Inturrisi CE. The nature of opioid responsiveness and its implications for neuropathic pain: new hypotheses derived from studies of opioid infusions. Pain 1990;43(3):273.
76. Cherny NI, Chang V, Frager G, et al. Opioid pharmacotherapy in the management of cancer pain: a survey of strategies used by pain physicians for the selection of analgesic drugs and routes of administration. 1995;76:1283.
77. Galer BS, Coyle N, Pasternak GW, Portenoy RK. Individual variability in the response to different opioids: report of five cases. Pain 1992; 49(1):87.
78. Crews JC, Sweeney NJ, Denson DD. Clinical efficacy of methadone in patients refractory to other mu-opioid receptor agonist analgesics for management of terminal cancer pain: case presentations and discussion of incomplete cross-tolerance among opioid agonist analgesics. Cancer 1993;72(7):2266.
79. MacDonald N, Der L, Allan S, Champion P. Opioid hyperexcitability: the application of alternate opioid therapy. Pain 1993;53(3):353.
80. Elsendrath SJ, Goldman B, Douglas J, Dimatteo L, Van DC. Meperidine-lnduced delirium. Am J Psychiatr 1987;144(8):1062.
81. Portenoy PK, Southam M, Gupta SK, et al. Transdermal fentanyl for cancer pain repeated dose pharmacokinetics. Anesthesiology 1993; 78:36.
82. Fine PG, Marcus M, DeBoer AJ, Van der Oord B. An open label study of oral transmucosal fentanyl citrate (OTFC) for the treatment of breakthrough cancer pain. Pain 1991;45:149.
83. Stanley TH, Hague B, Mock DL, et al. Oral transmucosal fentanyl citrate (lollipop) premedications in human volunteers. Anesth Analg 1989;69:21.
84. Wilkinson TJ, Robinson BA, Begg EJ, Duffull SB, Ravenscroft PJ, Schneider JJ. Pharmacokinetics and efficacy of rectal versus oral sustained-release morphine in cancer patients. Cancer Chemother Pharmacol 1992;31(3):251.
85. Hanning CD. The rectal absorption of opioids. In: Benedetti C, Chapman CR, Giron G, eds. Advances in pain research and therapy, vol 14. Opioid analgesia. New York: Raven Press, 1990:259.
86. Coyle N, Cherny NI, Portenoy RK. Subcutaneous opioid infusions in the home. Oncology 1994;8(4):21.
87. Bruera E, Fainsinger R, Moore M, Thibault R, Spoldi E, Ventafridda V. Local toxicity with subcutaneous methadone: experience of two centers. Pain 1991;45:141.
88. Waldmann CS, Eason JR, Rambohu IE, Hanson GC. Serum morphine levels: a comparison between continuous subcutaneous infusions and intravenous infusions in postoperative patients. Anesthesia 1984; 39(8):768.
89. Moulin DE, Kreeft JH, Murray PN, Bouquillon AI. Comparison of continuous subcutaneous and intravenous hydromorphone infusions for management of cancer pain. Lancet 1991;337:465.
90. Arkinstall WW, Goughnour BR, White JA, Stewart JH. Control of severe pain with sustained-release morphine tablets v. oral morphine solution. Can Med Assoc J 1989;140(6):653.
91. Coyle N, Adelhardt J, Foley KM, Portenoy RK. Character of terminal illness in the advanced cancer patient: pain and other symptoms during last four weeks of life. J Pain Symptom Manage 1990;5:83.
92. Edwards WT, Breed RJ. Treatment of postoperative pain in the post anesthesia care unit. Anesthesiol Clin North Am 1990;8:235.
93. Campora E, Merlini L, Pace M, et al. The incidence of narcotic induced emesis. J Pain Symptom Manage 1991;6(7):428.
94. Bruera E, Macmillan K, Hanson J, MacDonald RN. The cognitive effects of the administration of narcotic analgesics in patients with cancer pain. Pain 1989;39(1):13.
95. Eisele JH, Grigsby EJ, Dea G. Clonazepam treatment of myoclonic contractions associated with high dose opioids: a case report. Pain 1992;49(2):231.
96. Foley KM. Clinical tolerance to opioids. In: Basbaum AI, Bessom JM, eds. Towards a new pharmacotherapy of pain, dahlem konfrenzen. Chichester: John Wiley & Sons, 1991:181.
97. Goldfrank L, Weisman RS, Errick JK, Lo MW. A dosing nomogram for continuous infusion of intravenous naloxone. Ann Emerg Med 1986;15(5):91.
98. Bradberry JC, Reabel MA. Continuous Infusion of naloxone in the treatment of narcotic overdose. Drug Intelligence and Clinical Pharmacy 1981;15:85.
99. Schuster CR. Does treatment of cancer pain with narcotics produce junkies? In: Hill CS, Fields WS, eds. Advances in pain research and therapy, vol 11. Drug treatment of cancer pain in a drug oriented society. New York: Raven Press, 1989:1.
100. Chapman CR, Hill HF. Prolonged morphine self-administration and addiction liability. Cancer 1989;63:1636.
101. Foley KM. Controversies in cancer pain: medical perspective. Cancer 1989;63:2257.
102. Porter J, Jick H. Addiction rare in patients treated with narcotics. (Letter) N Engl J Med 1980;302:123.
103. Weissman DE, Haddox JD. Opioid pseudoaddiction—an iatrogenic syndrome. Pain 1989;36:363.
104. Ettinger AB, Portenoy RK. The use of corticosteroids in the treatment of symptoms associated with cancer. J Pain Symptom Manage 1988; 3:99.
105. Della Cuna GR, Pellegrini A, Piazzi M. Effect of methylprednisolone sodium succinate on quality of life in preterminal cancer patients: a placebo-control multicenter study. Eur J Cancer Clin Oncol 1989;29: 1817.

106. Tannock I, Gospodarowlcz M, Meakin W, Panzarella T, Stewart L, Rider W. Treatment of metastatic prostatic cancer with low-dose prednisone: evaluation of pain and quality of life as pragmatic indices of response. J Clin Oncol 1989;7:590.
107. Berkey CS, Eisenberg E, Carr DB, Chalmers TC, Mosteller F. Nonsteroidal anti-inflammatory drugs (NSAIDs) for cancer pain: meta-analysis: 7th World Congress on Pain. (Abstract 5) Seattle: IASP Publications, 1993.
108. Thiebaud D, Leyvraz S, von Fliedner V, et al. Treatment of bone metastases from breast cancer and myeloma with pamidronate. Eur J Cancer 1991;27(1):37.
109. Morton AR, Cantrill JA, Pillai GV, McMahon A, Anderson DC, Howell A. Sclerosis of lyric bony metastases after aminohydroxyprpylidene bisphosphonate (APD) in patients with breast cancer. Br J Med 1988;297:772.
110. van Holten Verzantvoort ATM, Zwinderman AH, Aaronson NK, et al. The effect of supportive pamidronate treatment on aspects of quality of life of patients with advanced breast cancer. Eur J Cancer 1991;27(5): 544.
111. Clemens MR, Fessele K, Helm ME. Multiple myeloma: effect of daily dichloromethylene bisphosphonate on skeletal complications. Ann Hematol 1993;66(3):141.
112. van Holten-Verzantvoort AT, Kroon HM, Bijvoet OL, et al. Palliative pamidronate treatment in patients with bone metastases from breast cancer. J CIin Oncol 1993;11(3):491.
113. Adami S, Mian M. Clodronate therapy of metastatic bone disease in patients with prostatic carcinoma. Cancer Res 1989;116:67.
114. Elomaa I, Kyimala T, Tammela T, et al. Effect of oral clodronate on bone pain: a controlled study in patients with metastatic prostatic cancer. Int Urol Nephrol 1992;24(2):159.
115. Vorreuther R, Klotz T, Engelking R. Clodronate in the palliative therapy of bone-metastasized prostatic carcinoma. Urologe A 1992;31(2): 63.
116. Ernst DS, MacDonald RN, Paterson AHG, Jensen J, Brasher P, Bruera E. A double blind, crossover trial of I.V. clodronate in metastatic bone pain. J Pain Symptom Manage 1992;7:4.
117. Smith JA. Palliation of painful bone metastases from prostate cancer using sodium etidronate: results of a randomized, prospective, double-blind, placebo-controlled study. J Urol 1989;141:85.
118. Roth A, Kolaric K. Analgesic activity of calcitonin in patients with painful osteolytic metastases of breast cancer. Oncology 1986;43:283.
119. Warrell RP, Lovett D, Dilmanian FA, Schnieder R, Heelan RT. Low-dose gallium nitrate for prevention of osteolysis in myeloma: results of a pilot randomized study. J Clin Oncol 1993;11(12):2443.
120. Scher HI, Curley T, Geller N, et al. Gallium nitrate in prostatic cancer: evaluation of antitumor activity and effects on bone turnover. Cancer Treat Rep 1987;71(10):887.
121. Cherny NI, Portenoy RK. Cancer pain management: current strategy. Cancer Suppl 1993;72(11):3393.
122. Fishman B. The treatment of suffering in patients with cancer pain: cognitive behavioral approaches. In: Foley KM, Bonica JJ, Ventafridda V, eds. Advances in pain research and therapy, vol 16. Second International congress on cancer pain. New York: Raven Press, 1990: 301.
123. Linton SL, Melin L. Applied relaxation in the management of cancer pain. Behav Psychother 1983;11:337.
124. Brennan MJ, Management of lymphedema: review of pathophysiology and treatment. J Pain Symptom Manage 1992;7:110.
125. Hogan Q, Haddox JD, Abram S, Weissman D, Taylor ML, Janjan N. Epidural opiates and local anesthetics for the management of cancer pain. Pain 1991;46(3):271.
126. Arbit E. Neurosurgical management of cancer pain. In: Foley KM, Bonica JJ, Ventafrida V, ed. Advances in pain research and therapy, vol 16. Second international congress on cancer pain. New York: Raven Press, 1990:289.
127. Ischia S, Luzzani A, Ischia A, Magon F, Toscano D. Subarachnoid neurolytic block (L5-S1) and unilateral percutaneous cervical cordotomy in the treatment of pain secondary to pelvic malignant disease. Pain 1984;20(2):139.
128. Tasker RR, Tsuda T, Howrylyshn P. Percutaneous cordotomy—the lateral high cervical technique. In: Schmidek HH, Sweet WH, eds. Operative neurosurgical technique indications: methods and results. New York: Grune & Stratton, 1988:1191.
129. Polatty RC, Cooper KR. Respiratory failure after percutaneous cordotomy. South Med J 1986;79:367.
130. Hellendoorn SM, Overweg van Kints J. Perineal pain: a case report. Eur J Surg Oncol 1988;14(2):197.
131. Cousins MJ, Dwyer B, Gibb D. Chronic pain and neurolytic blockade. In: Cousins MJ, Bridenbaugh PO, eds. Neural blockade in clinical anesthesia and management of pain, 2nd ed. Philadelphia: JB Lippincott, 1988:1053.
132. Robertson DH. Transsacral neurolytic nerve block: an alternative approach to intractable perineal pain. Br J Anaesth 1983;55(9):873.
133. Plancarte R, Amescua C, Patt RB, Aldrete JA. Superior hypogastric plexus block for pelvic cancer pain. Anesthesiology 1990;73(2):236.
134. Levin AB, Ramirez LL. Treatment of cancer pain with hypophysectomy: surgical and chemical. In: Benedetti C, Chapman CR, Moricca G, eds. Advances in pain research and therapy, vol 7. Recent advances in the management of pain. New York: Raven Press, 1984:631.
135. Ventafridda V, Ripamonti C, De Conno F, Tamburini M, Cassileth BR. Symptom prevalence and control during cancer patients' last days of life. J Palliat Care 1990;6(3):7.
136. Cherny NI, Portenoy RK. Sedation in the treatment of refractory symptoms: guidelines for evaluation and treatment. J Palliat Care 1994;10(2) (in press).
137. Latimer EJ. Ethical decision-making in the care of the dying and its applications to clinical practice. J Pain Symptom Manage 1991;6:329.

PART IV

Testis Cancer

Principles and Practice of Genitourinary Oncology, edited by Derek Raghavan, Howard I. Scher, Steven A. Leibel, and Paul H. Lange. Lippincott-Raven Publishers, Philadelphia, © 1997.

CHAPTER 60

Testicular Germ Cell Tumors

Molecular Biology and Genetics

J. Wolter Oosterhuis, Bauke de Jong, Ethan Dmitrovsky, and Leendert H. J. Looijenga

GERM CELL TUMORS AND TERATOMAS

Testicular germ cell tumors belong to the group of germ cell tumors and teratomas, a heterogeneous group of neoplasms that occur in the gonads and in specific extragonadal localizations. Origin, pathobiology, clinical behavior, and treatment response of male germ cell tumors may differ depending on the site of the tumors, their histology, and the age of the patient.[1–3]

The gonadal and some of the extragonadal germ cell tumors are derived from germ cells. Some other extragonadal tumors may not be derived from germ cells and have been termed teratomas.[4–6] This chapter discusses the molecular biology and genetics of testicular germ cell tumors.

Testicular Germ Cell Tumors

Germ cell tumors of the adult testis are divided into two entities according to the World Health Organization (WHO) classification: seminomas and nonseminomatous germ cell tumors (nonseminomas).[7] Seminomas are composed of cells that are considered the neoplastic counterparts of primitive germ cells (gonocytes). Nonseminomas have embryonal carcinoma cells as their stem cells, which may differentiate into extraembryonic tissues (trophoblast and yolk sac), embryonic (somatic) tissues, or both in a caricature of embryonic development. Most nonseminomas have a mixture of these components. Embryonal carcinoma is the most common pure variant of nonseminoma. Semimona and nonseminomatous elements may occur simultaneously and may be geographically separate or mixed. Such tumors belong to the nonseminomas according to the WHO classification. The British classification recognizes these neoplasms as a separate entity known as combined tumor.[8] The classification of germ cell tumors as seminoma or nonseminoma is clinically important because the therapy for these tumors can differ. Seminomas and nonseminomas of the adult testis have a common precursor: carcinoma in situ (CIS), a neoplastic growth of cells that, like seminoma cells, resemble primitive germ cells.[9] CIS spreads along the basement membrane of seminiferous tubules within the space normally occupied by spermatogonia.[10] When testicular parenchyma is left adjacent to seminoma or nonseminoma, it frequently contains seminiferous tubules with CIS.[11]

Germ cell tumors of the infantile testis are a separate entity from those of the adult testis. Seminoma does not occur, and the nonseminomas are either pure yolk sac tumors or pure teratomas. CIS, as it presents in the adult testis, is not found in the seminiferous tubules adjacent to an infantile yolk sac tumor or teratoma.[12]

Spermatocytic seminoma typically occurs in elderly men. It is distinct from seminoma in its morphology and pathogenesis and does not have CIS as a precursor lesion.[13–15]

Advances in the genetics and molecular biology of testicular germ cell tumors are reviewed in the following sections. Ploidy, chromosomal abormalities, tumor suppressor genes and oncogenes, genomic imprinting, and methylation are reviewed. We propose a pathogenetic model of testicular germ cell tumors of adults that takes these new data into account, and the clinical relevance of the genetic and molecular findings are discussed.

PLOIDY

Germ cell tumors of the adult testis are virtually always aneuploid, with a rather broad range around a triploid DNA content. The median DNA index (i.e., ratio of the DNA content of tumor to normal cells) of seminomas is hypertriploid, significantly higher than the DNA index of nonseminomas, which is in the hypotriploid range.[16,17] This significant difference in ploidy is also found in the seminoma and nonseminoma components of combined tumors.[16] The different histologic components of nonseminomas usually have the same ploidy.[16]

The distribution of the ploidy values can be explained by assuming that early in tumor evolution the tumor cells doubled their DNA content and subsequently lost DNA by a net loss of chromosomes.[18] Measurements by image analysis of the DNA content of CIS before development of an invasive germ cell tumor have in some cases demonstrated near-tetraploid cells, which supports the concept of early polyploidization.[19] CIS adjacent to seminoma and nonseminoma is hypertriploid with the same range as seminoma,[17,20] suggesting that much of the karyotype evolution in germ cell tumors of adults takes place in the preinvasive stage.

Polyploidization of tumor cells in the course of tumor progression is not uncommon.[18] The finding that about 10% to 15% of testicular germ cell tumors and CIS have hypertetraploid DNA contents suggests that these tumors have undergone a second round of polyploidization during tumor progression.[20] The fact that virtually all testicular germ cell tumors of adults and CIS are polyploid could mean that the primitive germ cells from which these tumors originate are particularly prone to polyploidization. Conceivably, polyploidization itself could be the first oncogenetic event endowing the polyploid cell with growth advantage over its normal counterparts.[4]

Although cell fusion cannot be ruled out, endoreduplication is the most likely mechanism of polyploidization.[21] It has been suggested that defective bridge formation plays a role in the neoplastic process of the primitive germ cells[22] and might explain their propensity for polyploidyzation. It has been proposed that the polyploid character of seminomas and nonseminomas of the adult testis indicates that they arise from germ cells in the testis blocked in the first meiotic division.[23] The phenotype of CIS cells strongly argues against this hypothesis. Microscopically, immunohistochemically, and ultrastructurally, CIS cells resemble primitive germ cells well before the stage of spermatogonia. For example, the membranous staining for placental-like alkaline phosphatase, which is characteristic of seminoma and CIS cells, is not found in normal spermatogenesis or in spermatocytic seminoma but is found in germ cells in the embryo[24] and in the testes of infants.[12]

Infantile testicular germ cell tumors are usually diploid.[16] When polyploid, the DNA content is more in the tetraploid range. In this respect they resemble the malignant germ cell tumors of the anterior mediastinum.[25] The ploidy of spermatocytic seminoma is also different from that of testicular germ cell tumors of the adult testis.[13,26,27] They are often diploid, and when aneuploid, they are very rarely peritriploid. These ploidy findings suggest that these tumors are pathogenetically different from adult testicular germ cell tumors.

CLASSIC AND INTERPHASE CYTOGENETICS

The discovery of isochromosome 12p [i(12p)] in testicular germ cell tumors of adults by Atkin and Baker in 1982[28] has greatly stimulated interest in the cytogenetics of germ cell tumors. Germ cell tumors are among the solid tumors of which the highest numbers of karyotypes have been published.[29]

The interpretation of the aberrant chromosome was initially questioned, but its identity as i(12p) has been well established by chromosome painting.[30] Additional molecular analysis showed uniparentalness of the p-arms of i(12p).[31,32] These molecular findings oppose the view that differences in the size of the centromeric regions of i(12p) and normal chromosome 12 are explained as the result of nonsister chromatid exchange.[33,34] Isochromosome 12p may be derived from the paternal or the maternal chromsome 12, but within one tumor, it is reported to derive from a single parent.[31,32]

Geurts van Kessel and colleagues[35] made the observation that in tumors with i(12p), the heterozygosity of 12q, the long arm of chromosome 12 is retained, arguing that in testicular germ cell tumors of adults, polyploidization preceeds the formation of i(12p).

In large series it has been shown that i(12p) is present in roughly 80% of examined germ cell tumors, including seminomas, nonseminomas, and residual mature teratoma after chemotherapy.[36,37] Tumors lacking i(12p) often had other chromosomal abnormalities involving 12p.[38,39] Chromosome painting has revealed that all examined testicular germ cell tumors of adults without i(12p) have other abnormalities involving 12p, resulting in overrepresentation of 12p material (Fig. 60-1).[40] Like the invasive tumors, CIS may have i(12p).[41] The consistent finding of overrepresentation of 12p in testicular germ cell tumor of adults and its precursor, CIS,[42] suggests that it plays an important role in the biology of these tumors. The gene or genes that are overrepresented on 12p and that directly contribute to the development of germ cell tumors need to be defined.

Isochromosome 12p was not present in two cases of infantile yolk sac tumor[43] nor in the first karyotyped spermatocytic seminoma; however, it has been demonstrated in dysgerminomas and nonseminomas of the ovary, germ cell tumors of the anterior mediastinum,[44,45] and one germ cell tumor of the midline of the brain.[46] Isochromosome 12p is also identified in acute leukemia, which can occur subsequent to the diagnosis of a mediastinal germ cell tumor.[47] All tumors, whether located in the gonads, the anterior mediastinum, or the midline of the brain, that may have i(12p) share the same histologic spectrum, including seminoma, dysgerminoma, and germinoma; similar tumors are

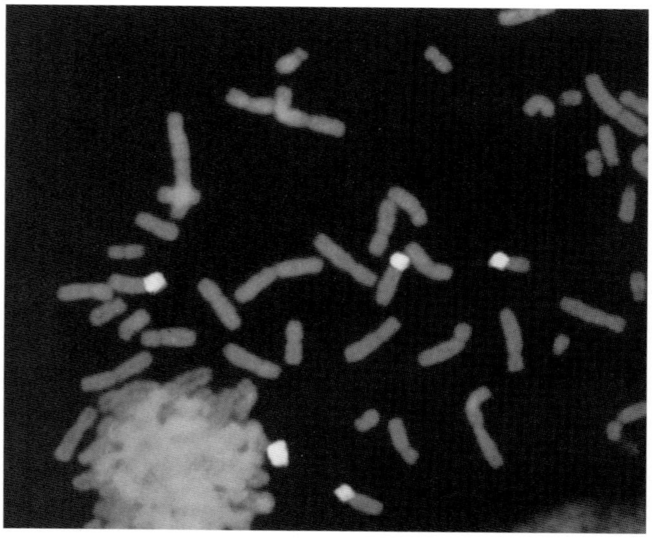

FIG. 60-1. Metaphase of which chromosome 12p is "painted," showing the short arms of the normal chromosomes 12, the isochromosome 12p [i(12p)], and 12p material in marker chromosomes. The centromeres of chromosome 12p and i(12p) are visualized with a specific probe.

found in the testis, the ovary, and in extragonadal sites, respectively. These tumors are also prone to polyploidization. Taken together, these findings suggest that the gonadal and extragonadal germ cell tumors of the adult testicular type originate from similar primitive germ cells.[45]

In a large series of untreated primary testicular germ cell tumors consisting of 26 seminomas, 60 nonseminomas, and 32 residual mature teratomas, consistent structural chromosomal abnormalities other than i(12p) were not found.[48] Other investigators report the clustering of 12q deletions.[49] Some structural rearrangements have been correlated with histologic subtype,[37,50] for example, rearrangements of 1p32-36 and 7q11.2 with teratoma and rearrangement of 1p22 with yolk sac tumor.

The comparison of the karyotypes of different components within one tumor specimen has been possible in selected cases. CIS and its invasive counterparts were compared,[41] as were different components of mixed nonseminomas[51,52] and the seminoma and nonseminoma components of combined tumors.[53–55] These selective analyses revealed that the compared components often had common chromosomal abnormalities, suggesting a clonal origin for these histopathologically dissimilar tumors. De Graaff and colleagues[52] have reported a similar karyotype in the mature teratoma and in the choriocarcinoma component of a single nonseminoma. Because teratomas and choriocarcinomas often have different clinical courses, it may be that cytogenetic abnormalities alone do not account for the different biologic properties of these distinct germ cell tumor subtypes.

Numerical analysis has shown that seminomas have modal chromosome numbers in the hypertriploid range and that nonseminomas and residual mature teratomas have modal chromosome numbers in the hypotriploid range, which is in agreement with the analysis of DNA content. De Jong and colleagues[36] have found a nonrandom pattern of overrepresentation and underrepresentation of chromosomes that is to a large degree similar in seminomas and nonseminomas. Chromosomes 7, 8, 12, and X are overrepresented, and chromosomes 11, 13, 18, and Y are underrepresented. The speculation is that the overrepresented chromosomes harbor oncogenes and the underrepresented chromosomes harbor tumor suppressor genes. In addition, these researchers found that some chromosomes, particularly 15 and 22, are present in higher numbers in seminomas than in nonseminomas.[36] The different chromosomal constitution of seminomas and nonseminomas may relate to the different developmental potential of the two tumor types. The excess copies of chromosome X are visible as X chromatin in nonseminomas but not in seminomas.[56]

In situ hybridization with centromere-specific probes has allowed numerical analysis of chromosomes in interphase nuclei.[42,57–59] Using this approach, a higher than normal number of copies of chromosome 1 has been demonstrated in the nuclei of CIS cells in seminiferous tubules and in semen. A CIS cell with one or two copies of chromosome 1 will go undetected with this method.[42]

Using probe pα12H8 specific for the centromeric region of chromosome 12[60] and commercially available probes for the centromeric regions of chromosomes 1 and 15, the numbers of centromeric regions of these chromosomes in seminoma, nonseminoma, and adjacent CIS were compared.[42] The karyotypic data indicate that seminoma contains a higher number of copies of chromosome 15 than does nonseminoma. This result was confirmed by in situ hybridization. Surprisingly, it was demonstrated that this numerical difference is not restricted to the invasive components but is also present in the adjacent CIS. This finding highlights a novel difference between CIS adjacent to seminoma and nonseminoma, despite a similar phenotype. In situ hybridization showed in general that the number of copies of a particular chromosome is similar in CIS and the adjacent invasive component, suggesting that both the noninvasive and invasive component within the same testis underwent a similar karyotypic evolution.[42]

Combined tumors do not reflect the pattern seen in pure seminoma and nonseminoma regarding the copy number of chromosome 15.[61] Some combined tumors have a low copy number, such as nonseminoma in the CIS, the seminoma, and the nonseminoma components. Other tumors have a high copy number in these components, similar to seminoma. Some combined tumors have a pattern similar to pure seminoma and nonseminoma, with a high copy number in the seminoma component and its adjacent CIS and a low copy number in the nonseminoma component and its adjacent CIS. These results indicate that there is more to determine the subsequent histopathology of a CIS lesion than the chromosome 15 copy number. In situ hybridization data reveal that, in keeping with the results of karyotyping, the seminoma and nonseminoma components within combined tumors most often have a monoclonal origin. The nonseminoma component may be derived directly from CIS or possibly from the invasive seminoma component. A minority of the combined tumors seem to be biclonal, with the seminoma and nonseminoma component each derived from its own CIS.

TUMOR SUPRESSOR GENES AND PROTOONCOGENES

In principle two types of genes are involved in malignant transformation: the protooncogenes and the tumor suppressor genes.[62] Both classes of genes are important in the regulation of normal proliferation and differentiation. The protooncogenes can be activated, due to point mutations, small insertions, deletions or translocations, to become oncogenes which act in a dominant manner. In contrast, the tumor suppressor genes generally act in a recessive manner. Involvement of tumor suppressor genes usually requires loss of function. Familial cancer syndromes are caused by mutated tumor suppressor genes which are transmitted through the germ line.[63,64] Transmission of oncogenes through the germ line has not been reported.

Tumor Suppressor Genes

Indicative for the loss of tumor suppressor gene activity in the development of cancer is the presence of consistent genetic deletions. These may be detectable by cytogenetics when relatively large chromosomal regions are involved, otherwise they may be identified by screening for loss of heterozygosity.[65]

Cytogenetic analysis suggests that tumor suppressor genes, localized on chromosomes 1 and 11, may be involved in testicular germ cell tumors.[66] In addition, specific underrepresentation of chromosomes (e.g., 11, 13, 18) may indicate the presence of tumor suppressor genes on these chromosomes. Chromosomes 1, 2, 3, 5, 6, 7, 11, 12, 13, 15, 16, 19 and 22 have, to varying degrees, been screened for loss of heterozygosity.[35,67–73] The results vary among the studies, even when the same probes were used in the same histologic subtypes. Loss of heterozygosity is rarely found in more than 30%, which is the expected figure assuming random loss of parts of chromosomes from a near-triploid cell. Some investigators have highlighted a role for loss of tumor suppressor activity localized on the long arm of chromosome 12.[70] Others have not confirmed the molecular finding of frequent deletions on 12q.[35,67,68,72] Whether or not a tumor suppressor gene located on 12q plays an important role in germ cell tumorigenesis awaits elucidation in further studies.

None of the chromosomal regions containing a putative tumor suppressor gene is consistently involved in testicular germ cell tumors except the short arm of chromosome 11, bands p13 and p15.5.[69] However, there is no indication that the tumor suppressor gene *WT1*, which maps to 11p13,[74] is inactivated in testicular germ cell tumors.[73]

Expression of the retinoblastoma (*RB1*) gene, analyzed by Western and Northern blotting, is found only in the teratoma component of testicular germ cell tumors, without gross genomic alterations.[75] Immunohistochemistry shows *P53* expression in testicular germ cell tumors of all histologic types, including CIS, with more intense staining in embryonal carcinoma than in seminoma.[76] No mutations in the coding regions of *P53* were found in a series of 22 testicular germ cell tumors and in the germ line of 17 members of families with an increased risk for the development of this cancer.[77] In contrast, mutations affecting exons 5, 7, or 8 were reported in 4 of 17 primary seminomas of Chinese patients.[78]

The familial occurrence of testicular germ cell tumors in first-degree relatives and identical twins suggests that mutations predisposing for testicular germ cell tumors may be carried in the germ line.[79] Such mutations, which may affect tumor suppressor genes, have not been identified by high resolution banding[80] nor by linkage analysis. A higher susceptibility for testicular germ cell tumors may be associated with rare alleles of *HRAS*, which have an increased incidence in individuals with bilateral tumors and in those who present at a young age (<20 years).[81] An increased level of constitutional chromosome instability might be a predisposing factor.[82,83]

In one elegant study, linkage analysis was carried out in strain 129 inbred mice, which have an inherited susceptibility to spontaneous testicular germ cell tumors. A candidate linkage to the *Ter* locus on mouse chromosome 18 was found. The human homolog of this locus is located on chromosome 5q. The primary effects of the *Ter* allele are codominantly inherited. *Ter* is neither necessary nor sufficient for tumorigenesis, but it dramatically increases tumor susceptibility.[84] This kind of inheritance would be difficult to analyze in the human population.

Protooncogenes

Overrepresentation of chromosomes 7, 8, 12, and X in testicular germ cell tumors may indicate the involvement of oncogenes located on these chromosomes. Of particular interest in testicular germ cell tumors is the short arm of chromosome 12. The consistent overrepresentation of 12p material in testicular germ cell tumors indicates its importance in their pathogenesis. The *KRAS* gene, located on 12p, has been studied as a candidate gene in comparison with other *RAS* genes. A low incidence of *KRAS* codon 12 mutations (<15%) has been found in all available studies on human primary testicular germ cell tumors.[85–89] In contrast, conflicting data have been reported for *NRAS*. One study showed mutations at codon 12 or 61 in 13 of 20 seminomas and in 2 of 3 nonseminomas.[86] Another study, which comprised only seminomas, revealed *NRAS* codon 61 mutations in 4 of 14 tumors.[85] A low incidence of mutations and no mutations were found in *NRAS* 12 and 61, respectively, in three studies comprising 68 seminomas and 91 nonseminomas.[87–89] A consistent finding is the absence of mutations in *NRAS* 13; *HRAS* 12, 13, and 61; and *KRAS* 13 and 61 in testicular germ cell tumors and derived cell lines.[85–92] *PTHRP*, a gene mapped to 12p, was expressed in all seminomas and choriocarcinoma components but not in embryonal carcinoma and teratoma.[93]

Some candidate oncogenes and tumor suppressor genes have been studied in testicular germ cell tumors on the DNA, RNA, or protein level. The MYC oncogene product is present at higher levels in seminoma than in different components of nonseminoma.[94] Enhanced *NMYC* expression correlated with a diminished *RB1* expression in one seminoma.[95] Expression of *NMYC* without gene amplification was also detected in primary seminoma and embryonal carcinoma, whereas no expression was found in primary teratoma components. This study also showed that *LMYC* is not expressed by testicular germ cell tumors.[96]

In testicular germ cell tumors, a gene dosage increase for *PDGFA* was found, without enhanced expression.[97] This study showed no consistent alterations in *NRAS, MYC, KIT, MYB, ABL, HRAS, P53,* or *ERBB2* on either the DNA or the RNA level. In addition, expression of *HSTF1* was found in testicular germ cell tumors without obvious differences in gene copy number, whereas *INT2* was not expressed.[93,98] A differential expression of *HSTF1* has also been reported in a embryonal carcinoma cell line and in primary testicular germ cell tumors.[99] These results are partly supported by studies of 70[100] and 24[93] testicular germ cell tumors that revealed *HSTF1* expression in the majority of nonseminomas and in a minority of seminomas. In contrast to this pattern of *HSTF1* expression in germ cell tumors, all examined tumors expressed transforming growth factor-α (*TGFA*).[101] One study[100] showed expression of *KIT* in 80% of seminomas and 7% of nonseminomas. Using three nonseminoma cell lines (NT2D1, 2102EP and 240A) and primary testicular germ cell tumors (10 seminomas, 12 nonseminomas, 2 combined tumors), another study reported expression of stem cell factor (*SCF*) and *KIT*.[70] Three percent of seminomas and 50% of nonseminomas show *SCF* expression, whereas 30% of seminomas and no nonseminomas express *KIT*. CIS also expresses the KIT protein.[102]

Testicular germ cell tumors rarely contain *P53* mutations.[103] This could account for the relatively stable genome,[104] explaining why homogeneously staining regions and double minutes are not documented in large numbers of karyotyped primary tumors.[48] Karyotypic evolution in testicular germ cell tumors is characterized by tetraploidization and a steady net loss of chromosomes, resulting in a predictable pattern of overrepresentation and underrepresentation, of which overrepresentation of 12p is the most conspicuous. The involvement of those oncogenes and tumor suppressor genes examined thus far do not highlight a consistent deregulation that could point to a frequent initiation event in germ cell tumorigenesis.

DIFFERENTIATION POTENTIAL OF GERM CELL TUMORS

An inverse relation between differentiation and malignancy can be seen in germ cell tumors. Some cultured germ cell tumor cell lines mature when treated with differentiation-inducing agents, including retinoic acid and hexamethylene bisacetamide (HMBA).[105] These differentiated cells have reduced proliferative and tumorigenic potentials compared with undifferentiated cells. Inhibition of the malignant phenotype can also occur when teratocarcinomas are fused to a normal blastocyst, giving rise to chimeric mice that are developmentally normal.[106]

Differentiation induction as a clinical treatment for germ cell tumors is conceptually appealing, and preclinical studies provide support for this view. For example, mice bearing syngeneic teratocarcinomas have prolonged survival when fed retinoic acid compared with untreated control mice.[107] Antitumor responses are also reported for murine teratocarcinomas following intratumor injection of a differentiation-inducing agent.[108] It is also known that treatment of the multipotent human embryonal carcinoma cell line NTERA-2 clone D1 (NT2/D1)[109] in culture with all-trans retinoic acid induces cellular maturation and a marked reduction in the tumorigenic potential of differentiated versus undifferentiated teratocarcinoma cells.[110] These responses are mediated through a specific retinoic acid receptor, RARG.[111]

Several male germ cell tumor cell lines exist; these provide useful tools for exploring mechanisms involved in human teratocarcinoma differentiation. Although cell lines that are derived from nonseminomatous tumors of diverse histopathologic subtypes have been described,[109,112–114] no cell line has yet been established from a seminomatous tumor. The unique in vitro growth requirements for seminomas are not known.[115,116] Germ cell tumor lines that are sensitive[109] and resistant[111] to retinoic acid have been isolated. Cisplatin-resistant germ cell tumor lines have also been derived.[117] Whether mechanisms responsible for sensitivity to chemotherapeutic agents and differentiation-inducing agents are linked is not known.[118,119]

Clinical germ cell tumors may retain the capacity to differentiate. This is reflected in the frequent identification of mature teratoma[120,121] containing differentiated cellular components within patient-derived tumors. Mature teratomas can be the predominant cellular elements remaining after successful treatment of malignant germ cell tumors with combination chemotherapy. Although teratomas have a small but identifiable risk of malignant degeneration,[122] teratomas, unlike the highly proliferative embryonal carcinomas from which they arise, have a reduced clinical growth potential.

These in vitro and in vivo potentials for maturation of germ cell tumors make them attractive clinical models for differentiation-based therapy.[123] Perhaps retinoic acid will enhance the differentiation potential already evident in these tumors. Preclinical studies in other cell systems indicate that in vitro retinoid sensitivity can predict clinical response to treatment, as seen in acute promyelocytic leukemias, which are sensitive to the cytodifferentiation actions of all-trans retinoic acid both in vitro[124] and in vivo.[125–127]

A clinical trial testing the activity of 13-*cis*-retinoic acid in the treatment of chemotherapy-refractory germ cell cancers was conducted at Memorial Hospital.[128] No complete responses were seen, but some patients had stable disease for several months, an uncommon finding in this clinical setting. One patient had extensive teratoma at autopsy, suggesting that this retinoid may have exhibited clinical antitumor actions through maturation of this germ cell cancer. Whether other retinoids will have greater clinical antitumor activity than 13-*cis*-retinoic acid in relapsed germ cell cancer patients is under study at Memorial Hospital.

GENOMIC IMPRINTING AND METHYLATION

The spectrum of different embryonal and extraembryonal tissues present in testicular germ cell tumors suggests that mechanisms involved in regulation of early embryonic development are involved in their pathogenesis. During the 1980s it was discovered that genomic imprinting, a non-Mendelian form of inheritance, plays an important role in early embryonic development. Pronuclear transfer experiments in mice showed that the developmental potential of a manipulated diploid zygote was determined by the parental origin of the two haploid sets of chromosomes.[129] Uniparental embryos always die early in pregnancy, they rarely survive beyond day ten. Androgenotes, zygotes with an exclusively paternal genome, show a poor development of somatic tissues, but the extraembryonic tissues, in particular the trophoblast, develop relatively well. In contrast, the gynogenotes, zygotes with a completely maternally derived genome, have a relatively normal development of somatic tissues and a very poor growth of the trophoblast.[130] Apparently for normal embryonic development certain chromosomal regions must be acquired through the father and some through the mother.[130,131] This difference in functionality between homologous chromosomal regions based on parental origin is defined as genomic imprinting.[129] Sometime during the development of the primordial germ cell to the mature gamete, the genomic constitution of both paternally and maternally imprinted chromosomes, present in the normal zygote, has to be changed into either a completely maternal pattern during oogenesis, or into a completely paternal pattern during spermatogenesis.[132] It is somewhere along this route, that testicular germ cell tumors are initiated.

Several murine genes have a uniparental pattern of expression during normal development. The *H19* and *Igf2*-receptor genes are only expressed from the maternal allele,[133,134] while *Igf2* and *Snrpn* are expressed from the paternal allele.[135–137] The yolk sac shows allele specific expression of the *Ins1* and *Ins2* genes.[138] Murine complete androgenotes express both *H19* and *Igf2*, while gynogenotes lack expression of these genes.[139] The human homologs of *H19*, *Igf2* and *Snrpn* have the same imprinting as in the mouse,[140–143] while only a minority of individuals show imprinting of the *IGF2* receptor with exclusive expression of the maternal allele.[144–146] *H19* and *IGF2* are localized on the short arm of chromosome 11, band 15.5, approximately 200 kb apart.[147] Both genes are important in early development.[135,148,149] A tumor suppressor activity of *H19* RNA was recently suggested.[150]

Disturbance of the monoallelic pattern of expression, referred to as relaxation of imprinting or loss of imprinting, has been reported in human renal Wilms' tumors and in one rhabdoid tumor.[151,152] Biallelic expression of the *IGF2* gene was found in the majority of cases, and in a minority for *H19*. In addition, loss of imprinting has been reported in approximately 40% of lung cancers.[153] In contrast, retention of uniparental expression of *IGF2* is reported in hepatoblastoma.[154]

The mechanisms involved in the specific expression of either the maternal or paternal allele of imprinted genes are not yet elucidated. That DNA methylation plays a role is illustrated by mice deficient in DNA methyltransferase activity.[155] These mutants, which die in utero around day 11 post coitum, express both parental alleles of *H19*, but the genes for *Igf2* and *Igf2* receptor are not expressed.[156,157] This pattern is in agreement with the different methylation status of these genes during normal development.[158–161] *H19* is expressed from the demethylated allele, while the opposite is found for *Igf2* and its receptor. Apparently methylation is required for monoallelic expression of the imprinted genes, but it may have opposite effects.

The suspicion that genomic imprinting might play a role in the pathogenesis of testicular germ cell tumors is based on the assumption that the dermoid cyst of the ovary is the human counterpart of the mouse gynogenote, which favors somatic differentiation. Indeed the dermoid cyst of the ovary which is exclusively composed of somatic tissues is the result of parthenogenetic activation of a meiotic ovum, of which the chromosomes most likely have completed erasement and contain new female imprinting.[130,162] On the other hand the complete mole is the human counterpart of the mouse androgenote which favors trophoblast development. The complete mole consists only of trophoblastic tissue and results from the fertilization of an empty ovum by two sperm. It has, therefore, an exclusively male imprint.[130,162]

Testicular germ cell tumors appear to be derived from primitive germ cells. It is not known when precisely in the development of the primordial germ cell to a mature sperm erasement takes place and the new uniparental pattern of imprinting is established. It is conceivable that testicular germ cell tumors are derived from primitive germ cells in different stages of these processes, and that their developmental potential is more or less determined by the imprinting status of these cells.

We hypothesize that the pluripotent character of nonseminoma requires a biparental imprinting. The finding by Lothe[69] and us [72] that the maternal copy of 11p and of chromosome 22 are preferentially retained in testicular germ cell tumors suggests nonequivalence of the paternal and the maternal copy of chromosomes 11 and 22, compatible with a biparental imprinting pattern. Further support for this assumption comes from our results with the probes DN34 and PW71,[73] which indicate retention of both the paternal and maternal methylation pattern of chromosomal region 15q12. These findings suggest that the primitive germ cell from which a nonseminoma is derived still has its original somatic imprint, and is not yet erased: a preerased precursor cell.

Seminomas on the other hand, when probed with DN34 and PW71, may show a methylation pattern as nonseminoma, however the majority show a demethylated pattern, which is compatible with a paternal imprint. The fact that this pattern was even found on a maternally derived chromosome 15 suggests that the genome had been erased, and had acquired a fresh paternal imprinting. These results suggest that most seminomas are malignant counterparts of cells which are in or even past the process of erasement and renewed imprinting. This imprinting status could be inherent to the cell of origin or acquired during the tumor evolution.

The biallelic expression of the *H19* and *IGF2* genes in both seminoma and nonseminoma[163] is not explained by the imprinting status of the presumed precursor cell. It may be due to a different regulation of imprinted genes in primordial germ cells and somatic cells. Since a qualitative RT-PCR technique was used, there is no indication of the relative level of expression of the paternal and maternal allele. Therefore, leakiness of the imprinted allele cannot be excluded. Another possible explanation would be loss of imprinting as a result of tumor progression, as demonstrated in most Wilms' tumors for *IGF2*.[151]

The on average hypertriploid DNA content of CIS and seminoma and the hypotriploid DNA content of nonseminoma, with highly consistent overrepresentation and underrepresentation of certain parts of chromosomes makes for a more complex situation. Paternally and maternally imprinted genes may reside on different chromosomes. Disturbed ratios between parts of these chromosomes may result in mimicking of a paternal or a maternal pattern of genomic imprinting, and thereby favor either trophoblastic or somatic differentiation.

PATHOGENETIC MODEL: A WORKING HYPOTHESIS

In keeping with current concepts in tumor biology,[164] we hypothesize that a primitive germ cell, initiated prior to erasement, when it still has a biparental imprinting, may be activated, or reprogrammed, to pluripotency. If the initiated cell is further down the road of maturation towards spermatogenesis, and therefore has undergone erasement and perhaps already new paternal imprinting, reprogramming to a pluripotent cell is less likely. Thus the neoplastic cell will retain the phenotype of a primitive germ cell, perhaps resulting in seminoma.

It is challenging to try to combine this hypothesis on the role of genomic imprinting with current models of the pathogenesis of testicular germ cell tumors (Fig. 60-2). An early, perhaps the initiating, event is polyploidization of a primitive germ cell and not necessarily a mutation.[84] The tetraploid cell is more prone to mitotic errors. Due to this genetic instability, it may nonrandomly loose or gain chromosomes during progression. The net effect is reduction of the DNA content. The polyploid cells have survival and growth advantage over their normal counterparts which may be further enhanced by an increasing number of copies of 12p.

These events, polyploidization, nonrandom loss or to a lesser extent gain of chromosomes and overrepresentation of 12p are apparently very similar for initiated preerased early primitive germ cells and the initiated erased late primitive germ cells. This is not surprising since both cell types grow as CIS in the seminiferous tubules, in the niche of spermatogonia, with tightly controlled growth conditions. The different developmental potential of the precursor cells may only become apparent at the invasive stage. It is also only after invasion that the difference in ploidy between seminoma and nonseminoma starts to develop. Between early invasion and clinical presentation nonseminoma might lose additional chromosomes compared to the in situ stage, while seminoma does not. This may be directly related to the change in phenotype in nonseminoma after invasion. Certain parts of chromosomes with genes coding for factors which are necessary for growth as phenotypically seminoma cells in the seminiferous tubule may not be adjusted to sustain

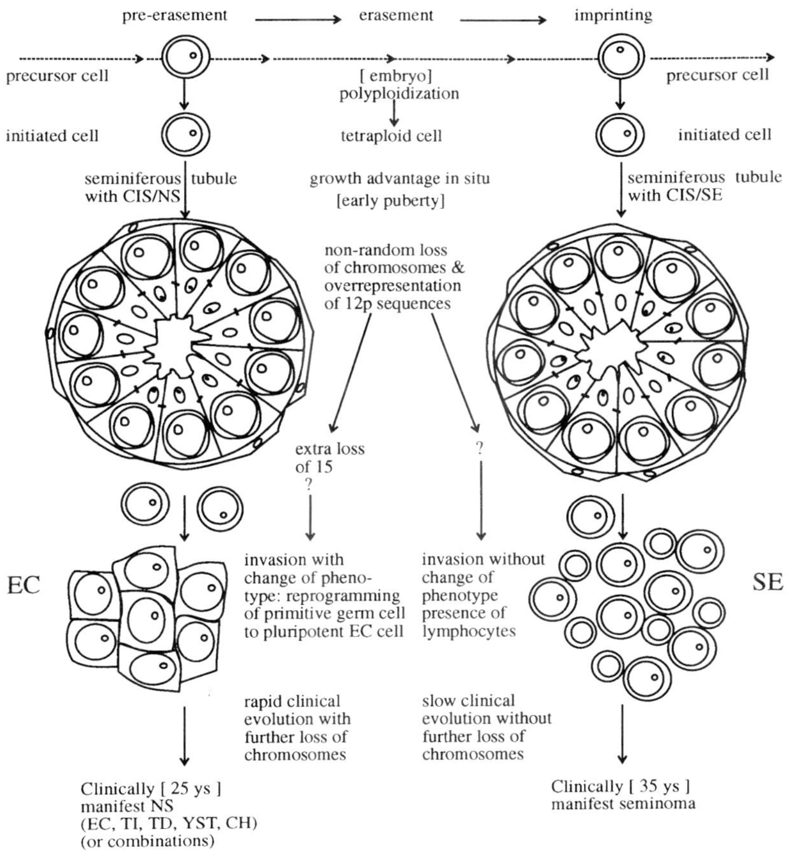

FIG. 60-2. Model of the pathogenesis of germ cell tumors of the adult testis. CH, choriocarcinoma; CIS, carcinoma in situ; ES, embryonal carcinoma; NS, nonseminoma; SE, seminoma; TD, teratoma differentiated; TI, teratoma immature; YST, yolk sac tumor.

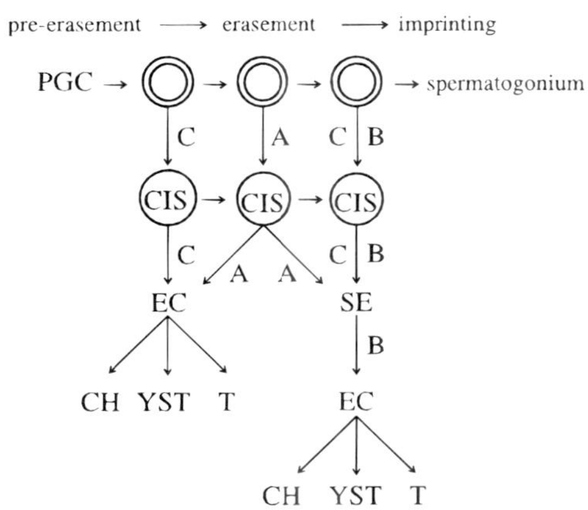

FIG. 60-3. Three different mechanisms are used to explain the origin of combined tumors. Mechanism A assumes a bipotent primitive germ cell as precursor. In mechanism B, the nonseminoma component is derived from a seminoma component. In mechanism C, the seminoma and nonseminoma components each have their own independent carcinoma in situ. When mechanisms A and B apply, the seminoma and nonseminoma component are monoclonal. When mechanism C applies, the combined tumor is of biclonal origin. CH, choriocarcinoma; EC, embryonal carcinoma; PGC, primordial germ cell; SE, seminoma; T, teratoma; YST, yolk sac tumor.

the growth of a nonseminomatous tumor. This might not be the case for seminoma. The differences which do occur between CIS of nonseminoma as compared to CIS of seminoma, e.g. the extra loss of copies of chromosomes 15, may relate to characteristics of the early preerased primitive germ cell. Alternatively, the initiation of both seminoma and nonseminoma may affect a primitive germ cell at the same stage of maturation, while during progression of seminoma in the in situ or invasive stage, further differentiation along the spermatogenic lineage takes place. This model is in principle similar to the one described, except that changes during tumor progression determine the developmental potential of the tumor cells, rather than the inherent characteristics of the initiated primitive germ cell.

In this model combined tumors might originate from primitive germ cells which are between the development of the precursor cell of nonseminoma versus seminoma (mechanism A, Fig. 60-3). This figure illustrates two more scenarios for the development of combined tumors: development of the nonseminoma component from an invasive seminoma component (mechanism B, see Fig. 60-3); development of the nonseminoma and seminoma component each from its own CIS (mechanism C, see Fig. 60-3).

CLINICAL RELEVANCE

Research into the genetics and molecular biology of testicular germ cell tumors has significantly increased our understanding of their pathogenesis. Although the clinical relevance of these studies is still evolving some clinical correlations and applications have emerged.

Hyperpentaploidy is associated with progression in patients who present in clinical stage I.[165] Hypertetraploid tumor stem lines and multiple aneuploid stem lines are more often found in men who present with metastatic disease. These patients may also have a higher chance of relapse. The combination of hypertetraploidy and multiple aneuploid stem lines is particularly unfavorable.[166] Earlier studies had failed to show a correlation between ploidy and clinical behavior.[16,167] A high percentage of tumor cells in S-phase is also prognostically unfavorable.[168] Studies which prospectively compare the prognostic value of ploidy and percentage of S-phase cells with known prognostic factors in a multivariate analysis of a large patient material are lacking.

Since testicular germ cell tumors of adults are virtually always peritriploid,[16] this characteristic can be diagnostically helpful, in particular in the differential diagnosis between a metastasis of a testicular germ cell tumor and a primary extragonadal germ cell tumor which may be diploid.[25] One has to be cautious, however, because firstly, extragonadal germ cell tumors can be aneuploid, and secondly, absence of an aneuploid stem line can be due to technical errors.

The i(12p) is so specific for the adult testicular type of germ cell tumors that it can be used as a diagnostic tool. Bosl and colleagues[169] have shown that subsets of poorly differentiated cancers of the midline of the body contain the i(12p) and are undifferentiated germ cell tumors which respond relatively favorably to the chemotherapy regimens of germ cell tumors. The i(12p) may be demonstrated by karyotyping or by in situ hybridization with a probe for the centromere of chromosome 12.[169] The signal of i(12p) is different from the signal of the normal chromosome 12. With Southern analysis the excess copies of 12p can be demonstrated and is consistent with the diagnosis of a germ cell tumor.[169] The prognostic significance of structural chromosomal abnormalities, including the copy number of 12p, remains to be established. The number of copies of i(12p) does not relate to stage of disease,[169,170] nor is it predictive for outcome[169,170] although this was suggested in earlier reports.[44,68,171]

To date there are no molecular markers which allow detection of minimal disease in testicular germ cell tumors at the time of clinical presentation or after treatment. One of the challenges of the molecular study of testicular germ cell tumors is to find specific markers which allow the noninvasive detection of CIS, when it is curable without sacrificing the testis.[4]

The majority of patients with male germ cell cancer can be cured even when disseminated disease is present. However, subsets of advanced-staged patients are either refractory to initial treatment or relapse after treatment with cisplatin-based chemotherapy. Despite major advances in the treatment of germ cell cancer there exist poor-risk patients at the time of presentation. At Memorial Hospital a mathematical model has been developed to discriminate between good-risk and poor-risk patients.[172] Although other definitions of poor risk are proposed[173–175] most investigators agree that some germ cell cancer patients have a reduced cure rate based on clinical or biologic features at presentation.

The molecular biologic and genetic studies summarized in this chapter can prove useful as diagnostic tools that might discriminate between poor-risk or good-risk germ cell tumors. These studies may help predict those patients at higher risk for relapse of germ cell tumors. These basic laboratory investigations of germ cell tumors could lead to an improved understanding of the mechanisms involved in the cytodifferentiation, transformation, and chemotherapeutic sensitivity or resistance of these tumors. Basic studies have practical clinical applications incorporating biologic findings into the design of germ cell tumor clinical trials that would lead to clinical improvements in the management especially of poor-risk patients. This could yield an improved diagnostic and classification system based on the unique biologic and genetic features of germ cell cancers.

REFERENCES

1. Mostofi FK, Sobin LH. Histological typing of testis tumours. Geneva: World Health Organization, 1977.
2. Gonzalez-Crussi F. Extragonadal teratomas. Washington, DC: Armed Forces Institute of Pathology, 1982.
3. Jacobsen GK, Talerman A. Atlas of germ cell tumours. Copenhagen: Munksgaard, 1989.
4. Oosterhuis JW, Looijenga LHJ. The biology of human germ cell tumours: retrospective speculations and new prospectives. Eur Urol 1993;23:245.
5. Walt H, Oosterhuis JW, Stevens LC. Experimental testicular germ cell tumorigenesis in mouse strains with and without spontaneous tumours differs from development of germ cell tumours of the adult human testis. Int J Androl 1993;16:267.
6. Hoffner L, Deka R, Chakravarti A, Surti U. Cytogenetics and origins of pediatric germ cell tumors. Cancer Genet Cytogenet 1994;74:54.
7. Ulbright TM. Germ cell neoplasms of the testis. Am J Surg Pathol 1993;17:1075.
8. Pugh RCB. Combined tumours. In: Pugh RCB, ed. Pathology of the testis. Oxford: Blackwell, 1976:245.
9. Skakkebaek NE, Berthelsen JG, Giwercman A, Müller J. Carcinoma-in-situ of the testis: possible origin from gonocytes and precursor of all types of germ cell tumours except spermatocytoma. Int J Androl 1987;10:19.
10. Holstein AF. Cellular components of early testicular cancer. Eur Urol 1993;23:9.
11. Jacobsen GK, Henriksen OB, Van der Masse H. Carcinoma in situ of testicular tissue adjacent to malignant germ-cell tumors: a study of 105 cases. Cancer 1981;47:2660.
12. Jørgensen N, Giwercman A, Müller J, Skakkebæk NE. Immunohistochemical markers of carcinoma in situ of the testis also expressed in normal infantile germ cells. Histopathology 1993;22:373.
13. Dekker I, Rozeboom T, Delemarre J, Dam A, Oosterhuis JW. Placental-like alkaline phosphatase and DNA flow cytometry in spermatocytic seminoma. Cancer 1992;69:993.
14. Burke AP, Mostofi FK. Spermatocytic seminoma: a clinicopathologic study of 79 cases. J Urol Pathol 1993;1:21.
15. Cummings OW, Ulbright TM, Eble JN, Roth LM. Spermatocytic seminoma: an immunohistochemical study. Hum Pathol 1994;25:54.
16. Oosterhuis JW, Castedo SMMJ, De Jong B, et al. Ploidy of primary germ cell tumors of the testis: pathogenetic and clinical relevance. Lab Invest 1989;60:14.
17. El-Naggar AK, Ro JY, McLemore D, Ayala AG, Batsakis JG. DNA ploidy in testicular germ cell neoplasms: histogenetic and clinical implications. Am J Surg Pathol 1992;16:611.
18. Shackney SE, Smith CA, Miller BW, et al. Model for the genetic evolution of human solid tumors. Cancer Res 1989;49:3344.
19. Müller J, Skakkebæk NE. Microspectrophotometric DNA measurements of carcinoma-in-situ germ cells in the testis. Int J Androl Suppl 1981;4:211.
20. De Graaff WE, Oosterhuis JW, De Jong B, et al. Ploidy of testicular carcinoma in situ. Lab Invest 1992;66:166.
21. Vorechovsky I, Mazanec K. Cytogenetic investigation of gonadal carcinomas in situ in syndromes of abnormal sexual differentiation. In: Oosterhuis JW, Walt H, Damjanov I, eds. Pathobiology of human germ cell neoplasia. Berlin: Springer-Verlag, 1991:45.

22. Gondos B. Ultrastructure of developing and malignant germ cells. Eur Urol 1993;23:68.
23. Chaganti RSK, Rodriguez E, Mathew S. Origin of adult male mediastinal germ-cell tumours. Lancet 1994;343:1130.
24. Koide O, Iwai S, Baba K, Iri H. Identification of testicular atypical germ cells by an immunohistochemical technique for placental alkaline phosphatase. Cancer 1987;60:1325.
25. Oosterhuis JW, Rammeloo RHU, Cornelisse CJ, Jong de B, Dam A, Sleijfer DT. Ploidy of malignant mediastinal germ-cell tumors. Hum Pathol 1990;21:729.
26. Takahashi H. Cytometric analysis of testicular seminoma and spermatocytic seminoma. Acta Pathol Japon 1993;43:121.
27. Looijenga LHJ, Olie RA, Van der Gaag I, et al. Seminomas of the canine testis; counterpart of spermatocytic seminoma of men? Lab Invest 1994;74:490.
28. Atkin NB, Baker MC. Specific chromosome change, i(12p), in testicular tumours? Lancet 1982;8311:1349.
29. Mitelman F. Catalog of chromosome aberrations in cancer, 4th ed. New York: Wiley-Liss, 1991.
30. Suijkerbuijk RF, van de Veen AY, van Echten J, et al. Demonstration of the genuine iso-12p character of the standard marker chromosome of testicular germ cell tumors and identification of further chromosome 12 aberrations by competitive in situ hybridization. Am J Hum Genet 1991;48:269.
31. Peltomäki P, Lothe RA, Børresen AL, Fosså SD, Brøgger A, de la Chapelle A. Chromosome 12 in human testicular cancer: dosage changes and their parental origin. Cancer Genet Cytogenet 1992;64:21.
32. Sinke RJ, Suijkerbuijk RF, De Jong B, Oosterhuis JW, Geurts van Kessel A. Uniparental origin of i(12p) in human germ cell tumors. Genes Chromosom Cancer 1993;6:161.
33. Mukherjee AB, Murty VVVS, Rodriquez E, Reuter VE, Bosl GJ, Chaganti RSK. Detection and analysis of origin of i(12p), a diagnostic marker of human male germ cell tumors by fluorescent in situ hybridization. Genes Chromosom Cancer 1991;3:300.
34. Rodriquez E, Mathew S, Mukherjee AB, Reuter VE, Bosl GJ, Chaganti RSK. Analysis of chromosome 12 aneuploidy in interphase cells from male germ cell tumors by fluorescence in situ hybridization. Genes Chromosom Cancer 1992;5:21.
35. Geurts van Kessel A, Van Drunen E, De Jong B, Oosterhuis JW, Langeveld A, Mulder MP. Chromosome 12q heterozygosity is retained in i(12p)-positive testicular germ cell tumor cells. Cancer Genet Cytogenet 1989;40:129.
36. De Jong B, Oosterhuis JW, Castedo SMMJ, Vos A, Te Meerman GJ. Pathogenesis of adult testicular germ cell tumors: a cytogenetic model. Cancer Genet Cytogenet 1990;48:143.
37. Rodriquez E, Mathew S, Reuter V, Ilson DH, Bosl GJ, Chaganti RSK. Cytogenetic analysis of 124 prospectively ascertained male germ cell tumors. Cancer Res 1993;52:2285.
38. Castedo SMMJ, De Jong B, Oosterhuis JW, et al. "i(12p) negative" testicular germ cell tumors. A different group? Cancer Genet Cytogenet 1988;35:171.
39. Rodriquez E, Houldsworth J, Reuter VE, et al. Molecular cytogenetic analysis of i(12p)-negative human male germ cell tumors. Genes Chromosom Cancer 1993;8:230.
40. Suijkerbuijk RF, Sinke RJ, Meloni AM, et al. Overrepresentation of chromosome 12p sequences and karyotypic evolution in i(12p)-negative testicular germ-cell tumors revealed by fluorescence in situ hybridization. Cancer Genet Cytogenet 1993;70:85.
41. Vos A, Oosterhuis JW, De Jong B, Buist J, Schraffordt Koops H. Cytogenetics of carcinoma in situ of the testis. Cancer Genet Cytogenet 1990;46:75.
42. Looijenga LHJ, Gillis AJM, Van Putten WLJ, Oosterhuis JW. In situ numeric analysis of centromeric regions of chromosomes 1, 12, and 15 of seminomas, nonseminomatous germ cell tumors, and carcinoma in situ of human testis. Lab Invest 1993;68:211.
43. Oosterhuis JW, Castedo SMMJ, De Jong B, et al. Karyotyping and DNA flow cytometry of an orchidoblastoma. Cancer Genet Cytogenet 1988;36:7.
44. Bosl GJ, Dmitrovsky E, Reuter VE, et al. Isochromosome of chromosome 12: clinically useful marker for male germ cell tumors. J Natl Cancer Inst 1989;81:1874.
45. Oosterhuis JW, Castedo SMMJ, De Jong B. Cytogenetics, ploidy and differentiation of human testicular, ovarian and extragonadal germ cell tumours. Cancer Surv 1990;9:321.
46. De Bruin TWA, Slater RM, Defferrari R, et al. Isochromosome 12p-positive pineal germ cell tumor. Cancer Res 1994;54:1542.
47. Chaganti RSK, Ladanyi M, Samaniego F, et al. Leukemic differentiation of a mediastinal germ cell tumor. Genes Chromosom Cancer 1989;1:83–87.
48. Van Echten J, Oosterhuis JW, Looijenga LHJ, et al. No recurrent structural abnormalities in germ cell tumors of the adult testis apart from i(12p). Genes Chromosom Cancer 1995;14:133–144.
49. Samaniego F, Rodriguez E, Houldsworth J, et al. Cytogenetic and molecular analysis of human male germ cell tumors: chromosome 12 abnormalities and gene amplification. Genes Chromosom Cancer 1990;1:289.
50. Castedo SMMJ, De Jong B, Oosterhuis JW, et al. Chromosomal changes in human primary testicular nonseminomatous germ cell tumors. Cancer Res 1989;49:5696.
51. De Graaff WE, De Jong B, Oosterhuis JW, et al. Cytogenetic analysis of the mature and immature teratoma components of a metastatic testicular nonseminomatous germ cell tumor. Cancer Genet Cytogenet 1991;57:59.
52. De Graaff WE, Oosterhuis JW, De Jong B, et al. Cytogenetic analysis of the mature teratoma and the choriocarcinoma component of a testicular mixed nonseminomatous germ cell tumor. Cancer Genet Cytogenet 1992;61:67.
53. Berger CS, Pennington RD, Dobbs RM, Haddad FS, Sandberg AA. Cytogenetic aspects of germ cell tumors of the testis. Cancer Genet Cytogenet 1987;28:43.
54. Haddad FS, Sorini PM, Somsin AA, et al. Familial double testicular tumors: identical chromosome changes in seminoma and embryonal carcinoma of the same testis. J Urol 1988;139:748.
55. Castedo SMMJ, De Jong B, Oosterhuis JW, Seruca R, Buist J, Schraffordt Koops H. Cytogenetic study of a combined germ cell tumor of the testis. Cancer Genet Cytogenet 1988;35:159.
56. Atkin NB, Baker MC. X-chromatin, sex chromosomes, and ploidy in 37 germ cell tumors of the testis. Cancer Genet Cytogenet 1992;59:54.
57. Emmerich P, Jauch A, Hofmann M-C, Walt H. Interphase cytogenetics in paraffin embedded sections from human testicular germ cell tumor xenografts and in corresponding cultured cells. Lab Invest 1989;61:235.
58. Walt H, Emmerich P, Cremer T, Hofmann M-C, Bannwart F. Supernumerary chromosome 1 in interphase nuclei of atypical germ cells in paraffin-embedded human seminiferous tubules. Lab Invest 1989;61:527.
59. Giwercman A, Hopman AHN, Ramaekers FCS, Skakkebæk NE. Carcinoma in situ of the testis: detection of malignant germ cells in seminal fluid by means of in situ hybridization. Am J Pathol 1990;136:497.
60. Looijenga LHJ, Smit VTHBM, Wessels JW, et al. Localization and polymorphism of a chromosome 12-specific α satellite DNA sequence. Cytogenet Cell Genet 1990;53:216.
61. Gillis AJM, Looijenga LHJ, De Jong B, Oosterhuis JW. Clonality of combined testicular germ cell tumors of adults. Lab Invest 1994;71:874.
62. Bishop JM. Molecular themes in oncogenesis. Cell 1991;64:235.
63. Cavenee WK, Hansen MF, Nordenskjold M, et al. Genetic origin of mutations predisposing to retinoblastoma. Science 1985;228:501.
64. Malkin D, Li FP, Strong LC, et al. Germ line p53 mutations in a familial syndrome of breast cancer, sarcomas, and other neoplasms. Science 1990;250:1233.
65. Knudson AG. Antioncogenes and human cancer. Proc Natl Acad Sci U S A 1993;90:10914.
66. Parrington JM, West LF, Povey S. Loss of heterozygosity in hypotriploid cell cultures from testicular tumours. Hum Genet 1987;77:269.
67. Radice P, Pierotti MA, Lacerenza S, et al. Loss of heterozygosity in human germinal tumors. Cytogenet Cell Genet 1989;52:72.
68. Peltomäki P, Halme A, de la Chapelle A. Human testicular cancer: changes in autosomal dosage. Cancer Genet Cytogenet 1990;48:1.
69. Lothe RA, Hastie N, Heimdal K, Fosså SD, Stenwig AE, Børresen AL. Frequent loss of 11p13 and 11p15 loci in male germ cell tumours. Genes Chromosom Cancer 1993;7:96.
70. Murty VVVS, Houldsworth J, Baldwin S, et al. Allelic deletions in the long arm of chromosome 12 identify sites of candidate tumor

suppressor genes in male germ cell tumors. Proc Natl Acad Sci U S A 1992;89:11006.
71. Looijenga LHJ, Abraham M, Gillis AJM, Saunders GF, Oosterhuis JW. Testicular germ cell tumors of adults show deletions of chromosomal bands 11p13 and 11p15.5, but no abnormalities within the zinc-finger regions and exons 2 and 6 of the Wilms' tumor 1 gene. Genes Chromosom Cancer 1994;9:153.
72. Looijenga LHJ, Gillis AJM, Hoekstra JW, Sinke RJ, Geurts van Kessel A, Oosterhuis JW. Involvement and parental origin of chromosomes 12 and 22 in testicular germ cell tumors of adults. (submitted).
73. Looijenga LHJ, Gillis AJM, Oosterhuis JW. Chromosome 15 allelic imbalances and parental methylation status in germ cell tumors of the adult testis. (submitted).
74. Gessler M, Poustka A, Cavenee W, Nene RL, Orkin SH, Bruns GA. Homozygous deletion in Wilms tumours of a zinc-finger gene identified by chromosome jumping. Nature 1990;343:774.
75. Strohmeyer T, Reissmann P, Cordon-Cardo C, Hartmann M, Ackermann R, Slamon D. Correlation between retinoblastoma gene expression and differentiation in human testicular tumors. Proc Natl Acad Sci U S A 1991;88:6662.
76. Bartkova J, Bartek J, Lukas J, et al. P53 protein alterations in human testicular cancer including pre-invasive intratubular germ-cell neoplasia. Int J Cancer 1991;49:196.
77. Peng HQ, Hogg D, Malkin D, et al. Mutations of the p53 gene do not occur in testis cancer. Cancer Res 1993;53:3574.
78. Wei YD, Jiafu Z, Xi QS, et al. P53 gene mutations in Chinese human testicular seminoma. J Urol 1993;150:884.
79. Waterhouse JAH. Epidemiology of testicular tumors. J R Soc Med 1985;78:3.
80. Lothe RA, Heimdal K, Lier ME, Fosså SD, Møller P, Brøgger A. High resolution chromosome banding in search of germ line mutations applied on testicular cancer patients. Cancer Genet Cytogenet 1992; 59:62.
81. Ryberg D, Heimdal K, Fosså SD, Børresen AL, Haugen A. Rare Ha-ras1 alleles and predisposition to testicular cancer. Int J Cancer 1993; 53:938.
82. Gundy S, Baki M, Bodrogi I, Czeizel A. Persistance of chromosomal abberations in blood lymphocytes of testicular cancer patients. Oncology 1990;47:410.
83. van den Berg-de Ruiter E, de Jong B, Mulder NH, te Meerman GJ, Koops HS, Sleijfer DT. Chromosomal damage in peripheral blood lymphocytes of patients treated for testicular cancer. Hum Genet 1990; 84:191.
84. Asada Y, Varnum DS, Frankel WN, Nadeau JH. A mutation in the Ter gene causing increased susceptibility to testicular teratomas maps to mouse chromosome 18. Nature Genet 1994;6:363.
85. Mulder MP, Keijzer W, Verkerk A, et al. Activated ras genes in human seminoma: evidence for tumor heterogeneity. Oncogene 1989;4:1345.
86. Ganguly S, Murty VV, Samaniego F, Reuter VE, Bosl GJ, Chaganti RS. Detection of preferential NRAS mutations in human male germ cell tumors by the polymerase chain reaction. Genes Chromosom Cancer 1990;1:228.
87. Moul JW, Theune SM, Chang EH. Detection of ras mutations in archival testicular germ cell tumors by polymerase chain reaction and oligonucleotide hybridization. Genes Chromosom Cancer 1992;5:109.
88. Ridanpää M, Lothe RA, Önfelt A, Fosså SD, Børresen AL, Husgafvel-Pursiainen K. K-ras oncogene codon 12 point mutations in testicular cancer. Environ Health Perspect 1993;101:185.
89. Olie RA, Looijenga LHJ, Boerrigter L, et al. N- and KRAS mutations in human testicular germ cell tumors: incidence and possible biological implications. Genes Chromosom Cancer 1995;12:110–116.
90. Wang L, Vass W, Gao C, Chang KSS. Amplification and enhanced expression of the c-Ki-ras2 in human embryonal carcinomas. Cancer Res 1987;47:4192.
91. Dmitrovsky E, Murty VVVS, Moy D, et al. Isochromosome 12p in non-seminoma cell lines: karyologic amplification of c-ki-ras_2 without point-mutational activation. Oncogene 1990;5:543.
92. Tesch H, Fürbass R, Casper J, et al. Cellular oncogenes in human teratocarcinoma cell lines. Int J Androl 1990;13:377.
93. Shimogaki H, Kitazawa S, Maeda S, Kamidono S. Variable expression of hst-1, int-1, and parathyroid hormone-related protein in different histological types of human testicular germ cell tumors. Cancer 1993; 6:81.
94. Sikora K, Evan G, Stewart J, Watson JV. Detection of the c-myc oncogene product in testicular cancer. Br J Cancer 1985;52:171.
95. Saksela K, Mäkelä TP, Alitalo K. Oncogene expression in small-cell lung cancer cell lines and a testicular germ-cell tumor: activation of the N-myc gene and decreased RB mRNA. Int J Cancer 1989;44:182.
96. Misaki H, Shuin T, Yao M, Kubota Y, Hosaka M. Expression of myc family oncogenes in primary human testicular cancer. Nippon Hin Gakk Zasshi 1989;80:1509.
97. Peltomäki P, Alfthan O, de la Chapelle A. Oncogenes in human testicular cancer: DNA and RNA studies. Br J Cancer 1991;63:851.
98. Yoshida T, Tsutsumi M, Sakamoto H, et al. Expression of the HST1 oncogene in human germ cell tumors. Biochem Biophys Res Commun 1988;155:1324.
99. Schofield PN. Developmental tumours. Br Med Bull 1991;47:227.
100. Strohmeyer T, Peter S, Hartmann M, et al. Expression of the hst-1 and c-kit protooncogenes in human testicular germ cell tumors. Cancer Res 1991;51:1811.
101. Miller WH Jr, Maerz WS, Kurie J, et al. All-trans-retinoic acid and hexamethylene bisacetamide (HMBA) regulate TGF-α and Hst-1/kFGF expression in differentiation sensitive but not in resistant human teratocarcinoma. Differentiation 1994;55:145.
102. Rajpert-De Meyts E, Skakkebæk NE. Expression of the c-kit protein product in carcinoma-in-situ and invasive testicular germ cell tumours. Int J Androl 1994;17:85.
103. Boyle P, Zaridze DG. Risk factors for prostate and testicular cancer. Eur J Cancer 1993;29A:1048.
104. Harris CC. P53: at the crossroads of molecular carcinogenesis and risk assessment. Science 1993;262:1980.
105. Baselga J, Dmitrovsky E. Human teratocarcinomas and retinoic acid-mediated tumor differentiation. In: Hong WK, Lotan R, eds. Retinoids in oncology. New York: Marcel Dekker, 1993:285.
106. Illmensee K, Mintz B. Totipotency and normal differentiation of single teratocarcinoma cells cloned by injection into blastocysts. Proc Natl Acad Sci U S A 1976;73:549.
107. Strickland S, Sawey MJ. Studies on the effect of retinoids on the differentiation of teratocarcinoma stem cells in vitro and in vivo. Develop Biol 1980;78:76.
108. Speers WC. Conversion of malignant murine embryonal carcinomas to benign teratomas by chemical induction of differentiation in vivo. Cancer Res 1982;42:1843.
109. Andrews PW. Retinoic acid induces neuronal differentiation of a cloned human embryonal carcinoma cell line in vitro. Develop Biol 1984;103:285.
110. Dmitrovsky E, Moy D, Miller WH Jr, Li A, Masui H. Retinoic acid causes a decline in TGF-α expression, cloning efficiency, and tumorigenicity in a human embryonal carcinoma cell line. Oncogene Res 1990;5:233.
111. Moasser MM, DeBlasio A, Dmitrovsky E. Response and resistance to retinoic acid are mediated through the retinoic receptor τ in human teratocarcinomas. Oncogene 1994;9:833.
112. Vogelzang NJ, Bronson D, Savino D, et al. A human embryonal-yolk sac carcinoma model system in athymic mice. Cancer 1985;55:2584.
113. Pera MF, Blasco MJ, Mills J. Cultured stem-cells from human embryonal carcinoma, and its comparison with two types of yolk-sac carcinoma. Int J Cancer 1987;40:334.
114. Andrews PW, Oosterhuis JW, Damjanov I. Cell lines from human germ cell tumors. In: Robertson, EJ ed. Teratocarcinomas and embryonic stem cells. Oxford: IRL Press, 1987:227.
115. Berends JC, Schutte SE, Van Dissel-Emiliani FMF, De Rooij DG, Looijenga LHJ, Oosterhuis JW. Significant improvement of the survival of seminoma cells in vitro by use of a rat sertoli cell feeder layer and serum-free medium. J Natl Cancer Inst 1991;83:1400.
116. Olie RA, Looijenga LHJ, Dekker MC, et al. Heterogeneity in the in vitro survival and proliferation of human seminoma cells. Br J Cancer 1995;71:13.
117. Timmer-Bosscha H, Timmer A, Meijer C, et al. Cis-diamminedichloroplatinum(II) resistance in vitro and in vivo in human embryonal carcinoma cells. Cancer Res 1993;53:5707.
118. Guchelaar HJ, Timmer-Bosscha H, Dam-Meiring A, et al. Enhancement of cisplatin- and etoposide cytotoxity after all-trans retinoic acid induced cellular differentiation of a murine embryonal carcinoma cell line. Int J Cancer 1993;55:442.
119. Timmer-Bosscha H, De Vries EGE, Oosterhuis JW, Mulder NH. Differential effects of all-trans-retinoic acid, docosahexaenoic acid, and

hexadecylphosphocholine on cisplatin-induced cytotoxicity and apoptosis in a cisplatin sensitive- and resistant human embryonal carcinoma cell line (submitted).
120. Hong WK, Wittes RE, Hadju ST, Cvitkovic E, Whitmore WF, Golbey RB. The evolution of mature teratoma from malignant testicular tumors. Cancer 1977;40:2987.
121. Oosterhuis JW, Suurmeyer AJH, Sleyfer DT, Schraffordt Koops H, Oldhoff J, Fleuren GJ. Effects of multiple-drug chemotherapy (cis-diammine-dichloroplatinum, bleomycin, and vinblastine) on the maturation of retroperitoneal lymph node metastases of nonseminomatous germ cell tumors of the testis. Cancer 1983;51:408.
122. Ahmed T, Bosl GJ, Hajdu SI. Teratoma with malignant transformation in germ cell tumors in man. Cancer 1985;56:860.
123. Wouda S, Timmer B, Mulder NH, Dam A, Koudstaal J, Oosterhuis JW. Retinoic acid and cisdiaminodichloroplatinum in the treatment of murine teratocarcinomas in vivo in a nullipotent model. J Immunother 1993;13:261.
124. Chomienne C, Ballerini P, Balitrand N, et al. All-trans retinoid acid in acute promyelocytic leukemias. II. In vitro studies: structure-function relationship. Blood 1990;76:1710.
125. Huang ME, Ye YC, Chen SR, et al. Use of all-trans retinoic acid in the treatment of acute promyeolocytic leukemia. Blood 1988;72:567.
126. Castaigne S, Chomienne C, Daniel MT, et al. All-trans retinoic acid as a differentiation therapy for acute promyelocytic leukemia. I. Clinical results. Blood 1990;76:1704.
127. Warrell RP, Frankel SR, Miller WH, et al. Differentiation therapy of acute promyelocytic leukemia with tretinoin (all-trans retinoic acid) N Engl J Med 1991;324:1385.
128. Gold EJ, Bosl GJ, Itri LM. Phase II trial of 13-cis-retinoic acid in patients with advanced nonseminomatous germ cell tumors. Cancer Treat Rep 1984;68:1287.
129. Solter D. Differential imprinting and expression of maternal and paternal genomes. Ann Rev Genet 1988;22:127.
130. de Groot N, Hochberg A. Gene imprinting during placental and embryonic development. Mol Reprod Devel 1993;36:390.
131. Cattanach BM, Beechy CV. Autosomal and X-chromosomal imprinting. Development 1990;(Suppl 63–72).
132. Rossant J. Immortal germ cells? The derivation of permanent pluripotent stem cell lines directly from mouse germ cells in vitro promises to provide a new source of stem cells for genetic manipulation of mammals. Curr Biol 1993;3:47.
133. Bartolomei MS, Zemel S, Tilghman SM. Parental imprinting of the mouse H19 gene. Nature 1991;351:153.
134. Barlow DP, Stöger R, Herrmenn BG, Saito K, Schweifer N. The mouse insulin-like growth factor type-2 receptor is imprinted and closely linked to the true locus. Nature 1991;349:84.
135. DeChiara TM, Robertson EJ, Efstratiadis A. Parental imprinting of the mouse insuline-like growth factor II gene. Cell 1991;64:849.
136. Rappolee DA, Sturm KS, Behrendtsen O, Schultz GA, Pedersen RA, Werb Z. Insulin-like growth factor II acts through an endogenous growth pathway regulated by imprinting in early mouse embryos. Genes Develop 1992;6:939.
137. Leff SE, Brannan CI, Reed ML, et al. Maternal imprinting of the mouse Snrpn gene and conserved linkage homology with the human Prader-Willi syndrome region. Nature Genet 1993;2:259.
138. Giddings SJ, King CD, Harman KW, Flood JF, Carnaghi LR. Allele specific inactivation of insulin 1 and 2, in the mouse yolk sac indicates imprinting. Nature Genet 1994;6:310.
139. Mutter GL, Stewart CL, Chaponot ML, Pomponio RJ. Oppositely imprinted genes H19 and insulin-like growth factor 2 are coexpressed in human androgenetic trophoblast. Am J Hum Genet 1993;53:1096.
140. Zhang Y, Tycko B. Monoallelic expression of the human H19 gene. Nature Genet 1992;1:40.
141. Giannoukakis N, Deal C, Paquette J, Goodyer CG, Polychronakos C. Parental genomic imprinting of the human IGF2 gene. Nature Genet 1993;4:98.
142. Ohlsson R, Nystroem A, Pfeifer-Ohlsson S, et al. IGF2 is parentally imprinted during human embryogenesis and in the Beckwith-Wiedemann syndrome. Nature Genet 1993;4:94.
143. Glenn CC, Porter KA, Jong MTC, Nicholls RD, Driscoll DJ. Functional imprinting and epigenetic modification of the human SNRPN gene. Hum Mol Genet 1993;2:2001.
144. Kalscheuer VM, Mariman EC, Schepens MT, Rehder H, Ropers HH. The insulin-like growth factor type-2 receptor gene is imprinted in the mouse but not in humans. Nature Genet 1993;5:74.
145. Ogawa O, McNoe LA, Eccles MR, Morison IM, Reeve AE. Human insulin-like growth factor type I and type II receptors are not imprinted. Hum Molec Genet 1993;2:2163.
146. Xu Y, Goodyer CG, Deal C, Polychronakos C. Functional polymorphism in the parental imprinting of the human IGF2R gene. Biochem Biophys Res Comm 1993;197:747.
147. Glaser T, Housman D, Lewis WH, Gerhard D, James C. A fine structure deletion map of human chromosome 11p: analysis of the J1 series hybrids. Somat Cell Molec Genet 1989;15:477.
148. Brunkow ME, Tighman SM. Ectopic expression of the H19 gene in mice causes prenatal lethality. Genes Dev 1991;5:1092.
149. Poirier F, Chan CTJ, Timmons PM, Robertson EJ, Evans MJ, Rigby PWJ. The murine H19 gene is activated during embryonic stem cell differentiation in vitro and at the time of implantation in the developing embryo. Development 1991;113:1105.
150. Hao Y, Crenshaw T, Moulton T, Newcomb E, Tycko B. Tumour-suppressor activity of H19 RNA. Nature 1993;365:764.
151. Ogawa O, Eccles MR, Szeto J, et al. Relaxation of insulin-like growth factor II gene imprinting implicated in Wilms' tumour. Nature 1993; 362:749.
152. Wang HC, Fedoroff S. Banding in human chromosomes treated with trypsin. Nature 1972;235:52.
153. Suzuki H, Ueda R, Takahashi T. Altered imprinting in lung cancer. Nature Genet 1994;6:332.
154. Davies SM. Maintenance of genomic imprinting at the IGF2 locus in hepatoblastoma. Cancer Res 1993;53:4781.
155. Li E, Bestor TH, Jaenisch R. Targeted mutation of the DNA methyltransferase gene results in embryonic lethality. Cell 1992;69:915.
156. Li E, Beard C, Jaenisch R. Role of DNA methylation in genomic imprinting. Nature 1993;366:362.
157. Surani MA. Silence of genes. Nature 1993;366:302.
158. Sasaki H, Jones PA, Chaillet JR, et al. Parental imprinting: potentially active chromatin of the repressed maternal allele of the mouse insulin-like growth factor II (Igf2) gene. Genes Dev 1992;6:1843.
159. Bartolomei MS, Webber AL, Brunkow ME, Tilghman SM. Epigenetic mechanisms underlying the imprinting of the mouse H19 gene. Genes Dev 1993;7:1663.
160. Ferguson-Smith AC, Sasaki H, Cattanach BM, Surani MA. Parental-origin-specific epigenetic modification of the mouse H19 gene. Nature 1993;362:751.
161. Stöger R, Kubicka P, Liu CG, et al. Maternal-specific methylation of the imprinted mouse igf2r locus identifies the expressed locus as carrying the imprinting signal. Cell 1993;73:61.
162. Tycko B. Genomic imprinting: mechanism and role in human pathology. Am J Pathol 1994;144:431.
163. Van Gurp RJLM, Oosterhuis JW, Kalscheuer V, Mariman ECM, Looijenga LHJ. Biallelic expression of the H19 and IGF_2 genes in human testicular germ cell tumors. J Natl Cancer Inst 1994;86:1070.
164. Sell S, Pierce GB. Maturation arrest of stem cell differentiation is a common pathway for the cellular origin of teratocarcinomas and epithelial cancers. Lab Invest 1994;70:6.
165. Allhoff E, Wittekind C, Liedke S, Tanke H, Jonas U. The modular image analysis computer for assessment of prognosis in testicular tumors. Verh Dtsch Ges Pathol 1990;74:196.
166. De Graaff WE, Sleijfer DTh, De Jong B, Dam A, Schraffordt Koops H, Oosterhuis JW. Significance of aneuploid stemlines in testicular nonseminomatous germ cell tumors. Cancer 1993;72:1300.
167. Fosså SD, Nesland JM, Waehre H, Amellem O, Pettersen EO. DNA ploidy in the primary tumor from patients with nonseminomatous testicular germ cell tumors clinical stage I. Cancer 1991;67:1874.
168. Sledge GW Jr, Eble JN, Roth BJ, Wuhrman BP, Fineberg N, Einhorn LH. Relation of proliferative activity to survival in patients with advanced germ cell cancer. Cancer Res 1988;48:3864.
169. Bosl GJ, Ilson DH, Rodriguez E, Motzer RJ, Reuter VE, Chaganti RSK. Clinical relevance of the i(12p) marker chromosome in germ cell tumors. J Natl Cancer Inst 1994;86:349.
170. De Graaff WE, Van Echten-Arends J, Oosterhuis JW, et al. Cytogenetic abnormalities and clinical stage in testicular nonseminomatous germ cell tumors. Cancer Genet Cytogenet 1993;70:12.
171. Delozier-Blanchet CD, Walt H, Engel E, Vuagnat P. Cytogenetic studies of human testicular germ cell tumours. Int J Androl 1987;10:69.
172. Bosl GJ, Geller NL, Cirrinione C, et al. Multivariate analysis of prog-

nostic variables in patients with metastatic testicular cancer. Cancer Res 1983;43:3403.
173. Birch R, Willaims S, Cone A, et al. Prognostic factors for favourable outcome in disseminated germ cell tumors. J Clin Oncol 1986;4: 400.
174. Logothetis CJ, Samuels ML, Selig D, et al. Improved survival with cyclic chemotherapy for nonseminomatous germ cell tumors of the testis. J Clin Oncol 1985;3:326.
175. Ozols RF, Ihde DC, Linehan WM, Jacob J, Ostchega Y, Young RC. A randomized trial of standard chemotherapy versus a high-dose chemotherapy regimen in the treatment of poor prognosis nonseminomatous germ-cell tumors. J Clin Oncol 1988;6:1031.

Principles and Practice of Genitourinary Oncology, edited by Derek Raghavan, Howard I. Scher, Steven A. Leibel, and Paul H. Lange. Lippincott-Raven Publishers, Philadelphia, © 1997.

CHAPTER 61

Epidemiology of Testicular Cancer

A. J. Swerdlow

Testicular cancer is not common, accounting for 1% to 2% of all cancers in men in most white populations and affecting about 1 in 250 men in the United States by 65 years of age, with a lower risk in most nonwhite people.[1] At young-adult ages, however, testicular cancer is the most common cancer in white men in many countries, constituting 28% of all cancers other than nonmelanoma skin cancer at 20 to 34 years of age in men in the United States (SEER registries areas) in 1983 to 1987. Because incidence at young ages is increasing in white populations across the world, the epidemiology of testicular cancer and the search for its etiology are of considerable importance. This chapter outlines the descriptive epidemiology of testicular cancer and the extent to which etiologic clues can be gained from the epidemiology. Analytic epidemiologic studies attempting to find specific causes of the malignancy are also discussed.

DESCRIPTIVE EPIDEMIOLOGY

Time Trends

Incidence

Incidence rates of testicular cancer have increased steadily in white populations around the world for as far back as data are available, doubling about every 30 years. In Connecticut and Denmark, with the longest-running population-based cancer registries in the world, there are increases in incidence since their earliest data, for 1935 and 1943, respectively.[2–4] The recorded rate of increase in recent years varies somewhat among white populations and is particularly high in Eastern Europe.[5] When rates are analyzed by birth cohort (i.e., generation), increasing rates are found at young-adult ages for more recent compared with less recent cohorts.[2,3] It seems likely that most or all of the increase is real and not an artifact of improvements in registration or diagnostic changes: a large increase has been seen in areas with good cancer registration over periods when registration completeness was high; it has occurred at ages for which clinical investigation of potential cases was likely to be reasonably complete and diagnostic accuracy high; nearly all cases were histologically confirmed[3,6]; and changed histologic criteria do not explain the increase.[7] The increase appears to have affected seminoma and nonseminoma germ cell tumors similarly[2,4,8] but has not affected non–germ cell tumors. When examined by age, there has been a great increase in incidence in young adults, but rates in children and in older men have not increased.

In nonwhite populations, the trends are less clear. In US blacks, there is evidence that rates have not increased[9,10]; in Singapore Chinese, there has been an increase from 0.5 per 100,000 (age standardized to the World Standard Population) in 1950 to 1961[11] to 0.9 per 100,000 in 1983 to 1987[1]; and in New Zealand Maoris, rates have increased from 3.4 per 100,000 in 1962 to 1966[12] to 6 per 100,000 in 1983 to 1987[1]; and in Japan, both incidence[5] and mortality[13] rates have increased substantially. Trends in most other low-risk populations are difficult to assess because of the small numbers of tumors occurring and because there was no long-running, good-quality cancer registration.

In Denmark, men born in the early 1940s (i.e., during World War II), and to a lesser extent the late 1930s, have had a lower risk of testicular cancer at each age throughout life than that expected from the overall trends in incidence rates by birth cohort.[4] A similar dip in rates for those 15 to 64 years of age has been shown in Norway for those born during World War II and in British Colombia for those born in the late 1930s and early 1940s.[5]

Mortality

Mortality rates from testicular cancer also increased until the 1970s but since then have declined greatly as a result of advances in treatment. Where data are available, increasing rates at young ages until the 1970s can be seen for more than half a century—since 1910 in Australia,[14] 1911 in England and Wales,[15] and 1914 in the United States[16]—but at older ages (>60 years), rates have decreased or have not risen consistently.

Since the early 1970s, mortality has greatly decreased with the introduction of effective chemotherapy for teratomas. In Denmark, relative 10-year survival is now over 80% for teratomas and over 90% for seminomas.[17] As a result, mortality data are no longer useful as a proxy for incidence when assessing time trends or geography of testicular cancer. The date at which

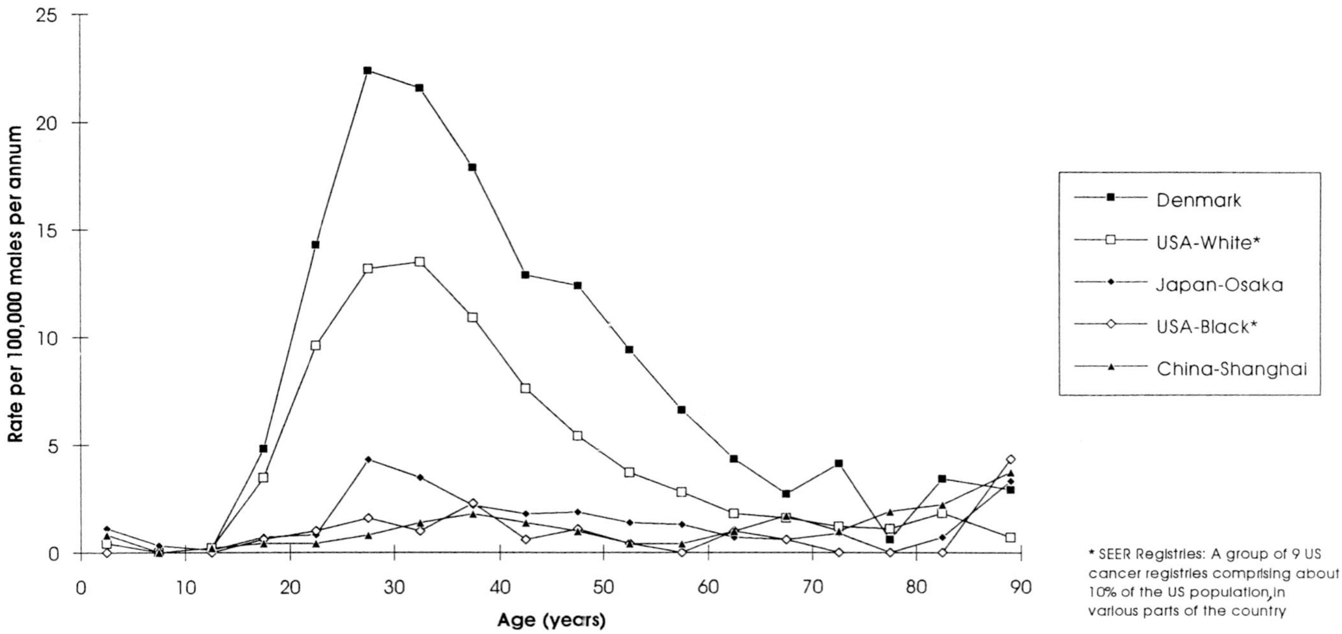

FIG. 61-1. Age-specific incidence of testicular cancer in males in various populations between 1983 and 1987. (Data from Parkin DM, Muir CS, Whelan SL, Gao Y-T, Ferlay J, Powell J, eds. Cancer incidence in five continents, vol 6, no 120. Lyon: International Agency for Research on Cancer, 1992.)

the downturn in rates started varied somewhat among countries; it occurred in the 1980s in several East European countries, presumably because of the later introduction of modern chemotherapy compared with the Western world.

Age

The age distribution of testicular cancer in white men (Fig. 61-1) is highly characteristic of the tumor: there is a small peak at about 2 years of age, then low rates until 15 years of age, after which rates climb rapidly to a peak in young adults, followed by a second decline and then a slow rise or plateau after the age of about 65 years. The childhood testicular cancers are mainly of the germ cell histology, as is the young adult peak (teratoma with a peak at about 25 to 29 years of age and seminoma with a peak at about 35 to 39 years of age), whereas the malignancies occurring after age 65 years are mainly non–germ cell, principally lymphomas. The shape of the age curve in US blacks, shown by Brown and colleagues[2] and also in Figure 61-1, but based on smaller numbers and therefore more unstable, shows the same general features as that in whites, with peaks in young children, young adults, and the elderly, but only in children are the rates similar to those in whites.

Ethnic Group

The incidence of testicular cancer is generally much lower in nonwhite than in white men. This is likely to reflect ethnic rather than environmental or behavioral differences because it applies also to comparisons among ethnic groups living in the same area—for instance, blacks, Japanese, Chinese, and whites in areas of the United States that have cancer registration. A notable exception to this is Polynesians; there are high rates of testicular cancer in Maoris and native Hawaiians. There are also fairly high rates in native Alaskans and American Indians. Italian migrants to high-risk countries appear to retain low risks.[18] Rates in Chinese and Japanese ethnic men in the United States, although well below those in whites, are higher than those in China and Japan.[1,19]

Geography

The highest recorded incidence rates of testicular cancer internationally are in Denmark (8.4 per 100,000 per year) and Switzerland (6.2 to 8.8 per 100,000 per year in different areas).[1] There are sizable variations across the remainder of Europe, with risks generally lower in Iberia and Eastern Europe than elsewhere. US, Canadian, New Zealand, and Australian rates for white men, as in much of Europe, are around 3 to 6 per 100,000 per year.[1] Rates in Asia, Africa, and South America are generally much lower than those in white, non-Hispanic populations. In the United States, the highest rates are in the west[2]; in England and Wales, the risk in young adults tends to be greatest in the south and southeast[20]; and in Scandinavia, the variation in rates is mainly among countries rather than by region within countries,[21] with a more than 4-fold difference between the highest risk, in Denmark, and the lowest, in Finland.[1]

Socioeconomic Group

In whites in several countries, testicular cancer incidence has been shown to be greater in higher than in low socioeconomic groups, although recent Danish data do not show such a trend.[22]

Urban Versus Rural Residents

On average, there is a slightly greater risk of testicular cancer in whites in urban than in rural populations.[23] In Denmark, where long-term data have been analyzed separately by degree of urbanization, a large increase in rates occurs with each increasing urbanization stratum.[3]

Marital Status

Findings on the relation of testicular cancer risk to marital status are inconsistent.

Month of Birth

No consistent evidence of a temporal cycle in month of birth and testicular cancer cases has been found.[24]

Laterality

Testicular cancer is slightly more common in the right than in the left testis. About 55% of unilateral cancers occur on the right side; cryptorchidism also is more common on the right. There is a tendency for the percent of right-sided testicular cancers to decrease with increasing age.[6,25,26] Only about 0.2% of testicular cancers are bilateral at first presentation.[27]

Descriptive Epidemiology as an Indicator of Etiology

The distinctive features of the descriptive epidemiology of testicular cancer suggest the types of factors that are likely to be the main causes of this malignancy and define which etiologic theories are plausible. For instance, the large increase in risk in young adults over time and the large variation in risk between genetically similar populations suggest a major contribution of behavioral or environmental factors in the etiology of testicular cancer, and hence great scope for prevention if these factors can be identified. The key factors must have increased steadily in white populations over several decades, except perhaps in certain countries during the World War II. The rising incidence and associations with high socioeconomic status and relatively rich countries suggest that the factors relate to modern lifestyles or exposures. The age distribution, which is very different from the exponential rise with age seen for most cancers, suggests that unlike these malignancies, testicular cancer is not the result of cumulative exposure to a carcinogen over life, but rather to an age-dependent factor or age-specific (e.g., prenatal) susceptibility.

The etiologic studies described in the following sections have tried to go beyond these generalities to find specific causal factors. Except for studies based on small numbers of children,[28–30] all of these studies were restricted to germ cell malignancies in young men or have effectively been studies of this group because they included relatively few cancers that occur at older ages or are of the non–germ cell variety. When seminoma and nonseminoma histologies were analyzed separately, they did not give consistent evidence of qualitative differences in etiology; when quantitative differences were found consistently, they are described.

UNDESCENDED TESTIS

The only specific factor known to be associated with a substantial proportion of cases of testicular cancer is maldescended testis, a history of which is present in about 10% of white men with this malignancy. There is little information on testicular cancer in relation to cryptorchidism in nonwhite men, but one study suggests that cryptorchidism may be present in a much greater proportion than 10% of cases in blacks,[31] although ethnic differences in the proportion with orchidopexy complicate interpretation.

The relative risk of testicular cancer in white men with undescended testis has been investigated in numerous case-control studies[9,28,32–44] and in two cohort studies following 506[45] and 224[46] cryptorchid boys. Although results in individual studies have varied considerably, it seems likely that the relative risk of testicular malignancy in a man with cryptorchidism compared with that in a man with bilateral descent is around or slightly greater than five. Thus, a white boy with undescended testis in the United States has about a 2% chance of developing testicular cancer by the age of 65 years. It should be noted that the increase in risk is essentially for men who have undescended testis beyond infancy. The risk in the majority of patients with undescended testis present at birth whose testis has descended spontaneously in infancy, usually before 3 months of age, is unknown. If these men have a risk similar to those whose maldescent continues beyond infancy, then the proportion of cases of testicular cancer associated with cryptorchidism at birth might be considerably higher (~20% or more).

The risk of testicular cancer in a unilaterally cryptorchid boy is mainly on the undescended side, with a risk about five times that on the descended side.[40] This implies that the relative risk on the descended side compared with risk in a descended testis of a boy without cryptorchidism is about 1 to 1.5. This is also the conclusion drawn, although with wide confidence intervals, from studies presenting direct analyses of risk in descended testes opposite maldescended testes, in which relative risks of 1.1,[38] 1.4,[44] and 1.6[42] have been found.

The risk of testicular cancer appears to be much higher in persons with abdominal than in inguinal maldescent, although quantification of abdominal risk is not well delineated because of the comparative rarity of this malformation. Risk is also greater in men with bilateral maldescent than in those with unilateral maldescent, and available evidence suggests that the difference in risk between these groups is more than twofold (i.e., that each testis is at higher risk than in a unilaterally cryptorchid man). Bilateral cryptorchidism is some times associated with abdominal maldescent, however, and it has not yet been established whether the abdominal position or the bilaterality is the underlying association with high risk.

There is evidence that raised risk in the undescended testis is particularly for seminoma; in several series, the proportion of seminomas associated with maldescent is greater than the proportion of nonseminomas,[47] although in case-control studies, the relative risk for seminoma is only slightly greater[39,40,42] or is not different than that for nonseminoma.[33,43] In several studies, the proportion of seminomas was lower if orchidopexy had been performed than if the maldescent was uncorrected.[26,40,48]

It is clinically and theoretically important to know whether orchidopexy, or at least orchidopexy at a sufficiently young age, can prevent testicular cancer. There is evidence that orchidopexy before puberty can prevent to some extent the degenerative changes of cryptorchidism.[42] The evidence to date on age at orchidopexy in relation to testicular cancer risk is encouraging but not conclusive. Two US studies and one in the United Kingdom have found a lower risk of testicular cancer in males with earlier correction,[38,42,44] with the youngest age-at-correction category 5 to 7 years or younger than 10 years, depending on the study, whereas another UK study found no association with age at orchidopexy.[49] These studies have included few subjects with orchidopexy at younger than 5 years of age, the effect of which remains essentially unevaluated. This is important because degenerative histologic changes in the cryptorchid testis begin by 2 years of age[50]; therefore, early correction may be critical to successful prophylaxis. Damage to the germinative epithelium is also seen in the contralateral descended testis, although it occurs less often and later,[50] suggesting that correction of position may not be a total solution. Cancer in situ of the testis has been found in 2% to 3% of men with a history of maldescent.[51]

In the largest study to date,[44] although not in two smaller studies,[38,42] the risk in uncorrected maldescent was slightly lower than that after orchidopexy. In other studies[26,52] the proportion of malignancies ipsilateral to maldescent was greater after orchidopexy than in uncorrected maldescent, also implying that complications of orchidopexy (e.g., trauma, damage to the blood supply) may *increase* the risk of testicular cancer. Further investigation of this, preferably using recorded operation data, is needed.

Risk of testicular cancer in a descended testis opposite a maldescended testis and the effect of orchidopexy on risk are important in relation to the possible mechanism of the association of testicular cancer with cryptorchidism. One possibility is that the effects of maldescent on the testis (e.g., raised testicular temperature and, if inguinal, increased risk of trauma) are carcinogenic. Alternatively, maldescent and testicular cancer may both be the results of the same prenatal etiologic process, or both mechanisms might apply. If maldescent causes testicular cancer, risk would be expected to be reduced by sufficiently early orchidopexy, provided the operation itself does not cause damage leading to malignancy, and risk in a descended testis opposite a maldescended testes would be expected to not be raised. If maldescent and testicular cancer have systemic etiologic factors in common, orchidopexy would be expected to ineffective in preventing malignancy and risk would be expected to be raised in a descended testis opposite a maldescended testis because both testes are exposed to the same systemic prenatal environment. As discussed previously, there is insufficient evidence to answer fully any of these questions, although it is clear that the risk in the testis opposite maldescent is much less than that in the maldescended testis, implying that most of the risk in a maldescended testis is either a consequence of the maldescent or a reflection of local factors prenatally affecting one testis more than the other.

If testicular cancer and cryptorchidism do share etiologic factors, time trends in cryptorchidism rates would be likely predictors of future trends in testicular cancer. This would imply, disconcertingly, that testicular cancer incidence is likely to continue to rise for several decades to come. In the United Kingdom, there is good evidence that incidence of cryptorchidism has almost doubled from the 1950s to the 1980s,[53] and in the United States, the frequency of cryptorchidism appears to have increased since the early 1940s.[9] Another implication is that investigation of prenatal etiologic factors for cryptorchidism, which is much easier than similar studies for adult testicular malignancy because the disease manifests much sooner after birth, may be illuminating in the search for the causes of testicular cancer; this has spurred several investigations of the etiology of undescended testis.

INGUINAL HERNIA

Inguinal hernia has been found to be a risk factor for testicular cancer in several case-control studies,[9,28,32,33,35–40,44] with risk generally greater for hernia diagnosed in childhood than for adult-diagnosed hernia. Inguinal hernia is often associated with cryptorchidism, but in two large studies[32,44] the risk associated with childhood hernia was significant even in individuals who were not cryptorchid. There has not been a consistent relation found between side of hernia and side of malignancy.[40]

OTHER GENITOURINARY ABNORMALITIES

There has been limited evidence for an association of testicular cancer with several other genitourinary abnormalities, including hydrocele,[9,37,40] varicocele,[54] renal infections, implying possible renal abnormalities,[33] and in children, various other congenital genitourinary malformations.[28–30] The association of testicular cancer with cryptorchidism, hernia, and hydrocele suggests that abnormality of the overall process of testicular descent and subsequent closure of the processus vaginalis is related to the etiology of testicular cancer, or there may be an association with genitourinary congenital malformation generally. Additionally, there is evidence of increasing incidence of cryptorchidism and perhaps other male genitourinary abnormalities, and also of several risk factors in common among testicular cancer, cryptorchidism, and childhood inguinal hernia (e.g., low birth weight, twinning)[55] and families in which several of these factors appear to be familial (discussed later). Cryptorchidism is associated with raised risk of inguinal hernia and other genitourinary malformations.[56] All of this suggests that the etiology of these malformations and that of testicular cancer are intimately linked.

PRENATAL ETIOLOGIC FACTORS

The raised risk of testicular cancer in association with cryptorchidism, inguinal hernia, and probably other congenital genitourinary malformations suggests the possibility of a prenatal etiology of testicular cancer, and several other factors also point to this. The age distribution of the tumor is that which would be expected from a prenatally caused cancer with a 20- to 30-year induction period, and there is a model for such an etiology in the causation of vaginal adenocarcinoma in young women by in utero exposure to diethylstilbestrol (DES) taken by the mother, nearly always during the first trimester of pregnancy. The age distribution of these vaginal adenocarcinomas in young women is analogous to that for testicular cancer in young men, although with a peak at a slightly younger age. The apparently low risk in Danes and Norwegians born during World War II, if confirmed in other populations whose supply of food and other goods was severely disrupted during the War, would strongly imply an etiologic factor acting primarily before or soon after birth, because men born a few years before World War II do not appear to have been affected. Several case-control studies have attempted to investigate prenatal risk factors for testicular cancer, but almost all have had to rely on histories of the exposure variables, from 20 or 30 years earlier, from the subjects or their mothers, with considerable potential for misclassification and possibly bias.

Most studies,[33,36,41,57] but not all,[39,58] have found a raised relative risk for low birth weight, prematurity, or both (in one instance, the results were simply described as not significant[43]), and relative risks have varied from 1.0[39,58] to 12.5[57] for low birth weight, which was variously defined. Only two of the studies used birth certificate or obstetric case-note data rather than recall to ascertain birth weights, and these found differing results: no raised risk in one study[58] and a raised risk in the other.[59] There have also been reports of raised risk in relation to the following factors[9,28,33–36,39,41,43,55,56,57,60–62]:

- excessive maternal nausea in a first index pregnancy
- high maternal weight for height
- older maternal age in a first index pregnancy
- x-ray exposure, especially to the mother's abdomen, during the index pregnancy
- use of sedatives or alcohol in the index pregnancy
- unusual maternal bleeding or spotting in the index pregnancy
- threatened miscarriage
- maternal exposure to various infectious diseases in the index pregnancy
- delivery by Cesarean section
- first-born child
- small siblingship size of the child
- having male siblings
- right-handedness of the child (which might be of prenatal origin)
- child who is a twin

The latter factor, found in three case-control studies[28,36,55] but not a fourth,[57] has also emerged as a risk factor, although not significant, in a cohort study for dizygotic as opposed to monozygotic twins.[63] None of the previously listed factors has been found consistently and repeatedly, which may reflect the use of data based on recall with the exceptions noted previously: the differing designs of the studies, especially with respect to control selection; the small size of several of the studies; and the likely indirectness of the measures chosen in relation to the underlying etiologic variables.

Henderson and colleagues[64,65] have developed an etiologic hypothesis that may explain several of the previously described findings: that the underlying cause of both testicular cancer and cryptorchidism may be exposure in utero during the first trimester of pregnancy, when maternal estrogen levels are rising rapidly, to a raised level of free, unbound maternal estrogen. They hypothesize that estrogen may affect differentiating germ cells permanently, causing cryptorchidism and also, both in cryptorchid boys and others without overt genitourinary abnormality, adversely affecting germ cell development in ways that raise the risk of future malignancy. Dysgenetic cells would then remain dormant until, under the stimulus of rising pituitary gonadotrophin levels at puberty, they divide and become overtly malignant, die, or revert to normal.

Evidence on the prenatal estrogen theory is tantalizing but inconclusive. Analyses of testicular cancer risk in relation to maternal pharmacologic exposure to estrogens during pregnancy by hormonal treatments, pregnancy tests, and inadvertent use of oral contraceptives after conception were based on small numbers and, overall, have been inconclusive.[9,33,34,36,39,57] Therapeutic DES exposure occurred in too few cases to account for more than a small fraction of testicular cancers, especially outside the United States; oral contraceptive exposure after conception may be appreciable worldwide for more recent cohorts. Endogenous estrogens and estrogens originating from the diet could potentially be a far more important risk factor,[66] but the evidence thus far has been indirect. There is evidence that several of the prenatal factors described previously, although they have not been found consistently as risk factors for testicular cancer, may be associated with high free estrogen levels, either because of raised estrogen levels or decreased levels of sex hormone binding globulin.[33,36,55] Such evidence is available for maternal obesity, first-born status, dizygotic twin birth, maternal nausea, handedness of subject, and maternal age in a first pregnancy. For instance, free estradiol levels have been found to be raised in first pregnancies compared with second pregnancies,[67] and raised estradiol levels in the first trimester have been found in hyperemetic women.[68] The maternal estrogen hypothesis is strengthened by findings that estrogen administration can cause cryptorchidism and probably testicular cancer in mice,[36,69] that normal testicular descent in the third trimester of pregnancy is under hormonal control,[70] that maternal bioavailable estradiol levels are raised in the first trimester of pregnancy of cryptorchid boys,[71] and that cryptorchidism and hypoplastic testes in man can be caused by exogenous estrogens; however, evidence of the latter is inconsistent.[36,41,71]

Blacks have low rates of testicular cancer and cryptorchidism, but black women have been found to have higher, although not significantly so, free estradiol and significantly higher testosterone levels in early gestation of a first pregnancy than do white women.[72] Henderson and colleagues[72] suggest that maternal testosterone may counteract the effects of estrogens, explaining the low testicular cancer rates in blacks, and thus that the balance of testosterone and estrogen levels in the mother may be relevant to testicular cancer risk.

POSTNATAL HORMONAL FACTORS AND SEXUAL ACTIVITY

The age-incidence curve of testicular cancer in children and young adults approximately parallels testosterone and gonadotrophin levels, with a peak of testicular cancer in childhood, following high levels of these hormones in infancy, and a rising incidence of testicular cancer a few years after puberty, parallelling high levels of the hormones in young men.[73] The parallels are less clear at older ages. The age peaks of testicular cancer may reflect increased cell division or other changes that depend on high hormone levels. A raised risk in association with atrophy (discussed later) would agree with this hypothesis, because atrophy can lead by feedback to high gonadotrophin levels. Cryptorchidism is also associated with high gonadotrophin levels.[74]

Evidence to support these hypotheses is weak. Although hormonal abnormalities have been found at presentation in a high percentage of men with testicular cancer, it is not clear whether these abnormalities predate the tumor.[73] There have been case reports of testicular cancer in men receiving hormonal treatment for infertility or in those abusing androgens,[73] but case-control data on risk in relation to hormone intake are few and inconclusive,[39,73] as are results for indirect variables that may reflect or affect endogenous hormone levels.[73] Severe acne, which may reflect high testosterone levels, has been associated with *decreased* testicular cancer risk in two studies[36,75] but not a third.[39]

The young-adult peak of testicular cancer might also suggest a relation to sexual activity; however, the available evidence does not indicate any relation between testicular cancer risk and sexual activity,[35,73,76] specifically homosexuality.[44] No association has been found between testicular cancer and history of venereal disease.[35,40,75]

AGE AT PUBERTY

In a case-control study, Forman and colleagues[44] found a significant trend of raised risk for testicular cancer in relation to early age of puberty. One other study supports this finding,[39] whereas three other studies found no such relation.[36,43,73] Variables concerning puberty in males are likely to be recalled poorly by adult cases and controls, and although it is not immediately obvious why such recall should be biased between cases and controls, it is nevertheless possible that bias occurred. Because age at male puberty appears to be declining over time, a relation to testicular cancer risk would give a potential explanation for the secular increase in testicular cancer incidence. A relation between testicular cancer and age at puberty may imply that childhood nutrition was important to testicular cancer risk.

ACTIVE VERSUS SEDENTARY LIFESTYLES

Forman and colleagues[44] found a raised risk of testicular cancer in relation to lack of exercise in adulthood and, independently, in relation to a sedentary adult lifestyle. Hours of physical exercise at the age of university entrance was not related to testicular cancer risk in a cohort study.[61] Exercise may affect gonadotrophin levels.[44] Lack of exercise and sedentariness are factors that probably have been increasing over time and therefore may have contributed to the rising incidence of testicular cancer; however, these factors require additional study.

RISK OF CANCER IN A CONTRALATERAL TESTIS

Five to six percent of men with unilateral testicular cancer have cancer in situ in the opposite testis,[51] and prior testicular cancer is a major risk factor for development of malignancy contralaterally. In follow-up of 2850 testicular cancer patients in Denmark, the cumulative risk of contralateral malignancy was 5.2% by 25 years after the first primary, with a significantly greater risk after nonseminoma (8.4%) than after seminoma (3.6%) primary tumors.[27] The relative risk of testicular cancer compared with risk in the general population for a man with previous testicular malignancy was 24.8, 29.2 after nonseminoma and 21.7 after seminoma. The relative risk was constant by time after initial primary tumor, and there was a significantly lower risk after cisplatin therapy than after other treatments. Raised serum follicle-stimulating hormone level after treatment of the initial tumor may be a risk factor for a second, contralateral testicular cancer.[77]

MUMPS ORCHITIS AND OTHER VIRAL INFECTIONS

There is appreciable but inconclusive evidence that mumps orchitis is a rare cause of testicular cancer. There have been numerous case reports of testicular cancer after mumps orchitis.[78] In a cohort study of 132 men with mumps orchitis in Rochester, Minnesota, two subjects developed testicular cancer, both occurring in testes that were atrophic after the orchitis.[79] A raised risk in relation to a history of mumps orchitis was seen in three case-control studies,[40,75,76] and raised risk for orchitis of unspecified cause was seen in another.[37] Orchitis is an uncommon complication of mumps that occurs more frequently when mumps occurs at older ages. Mumps orchitis can cause permanent damage to the germinal epithelium.[80] Later infections with childhood viruses are often more severe; it therefore seems possible that late infections with other common childhood viruses with gonadotropic properties may be a cause of a larger proportion of testicular cancers, and may potentially explain the young-adult peak in incidence of the tumor, the rising incidence and association with high socioeconomic conditions, and the raised risk in certain, but not all, studies for first-born males[33,36,39,55,57,62] and men from small sibships.[33,35,55,60,61] Investigations of this association are few and are inconclusive. Serologic studies have sometimes shown elevated antibody titers, but not consistently, against cytomegalovirus (CMV), varicella, herpes simplex virus (HSV), and Epstein-Barr virus (EBV).[81–83] The increased antibody levels, when found, occurred after the incidence of the testicular cancer and may be the result of decreased immunologic control of latent viruses because of the presence of testicular cancer or its treatment. EBV DNA was not detected in testicular cancer cells in two of three studies,[83] CMV DNA was not detected in one study,[83] and HSV DNA was detected in some tumors in one study.[83] One case-control study has found a protective effect of a history of infectious mononucleosis,[39] implying that late infection with EBV is unlikely to be a cause of testicular malignancy.

INFERTILITY AND TESTICULAR ATROPHY

Current data suggest that infertility is a rare causal association of testicular cancer. Cancer in situ of the testis has been found in 0.4 to 1.1% of infertile men,[51] not clearly a greater prevalence than in the general population. The largest case-control study of testicular cancer to date[44] found low fertility or sterility was a borderline significant risk factor, present in only 13 out of 487 testicular cancer cases who had tried to conceive and were not bilaterally cryptorchid. Further patients might have had low fertility sufficient to conceive, and might not have sought clinical help. Other studies of testicular cancer risk in relation to previously diagnosed infertility have had mixed results,[43,73,75] but again indicate that at most this accounts for a low proportion of cases. Indirect assessment of infertility, by consideration of the proportion of patients who have fathered children before cancer incidence, has not shown raised risk.[33,35,36] Many patients with testicular cancer are severely oligospermic or azoospermic at presentation, but this may often be an effect of the tumor rather than an etiologic factor present before the cancer.[84] It has been claimed,[85] although disputed,[86,87] that sperm counts are declining over time in Western populations, and it has been hypothesized that both the falling counts and the rising rates of testicular cancer and cryptorchidism might be the result of rising levels of estrogen exposure in utero.[66]

Two case-control studies have found raised risk of testicular cancer in relation to prior testicular atrophy, even after exclusion of cryptorchid patients,[40,43] and in series without control data substantial proportions of testicular cancers have been reported in atrophic testes.[40] Cryptorchidism also leads to small testes that fail to achieve normal histologic development (e.g., tubular immaturity, arrest of spermatogenesis),[56] and mumps orchitis can lead to atrophy. Thus atrophy might be a common pathway for several different sources of raised risk of testicular cancer.

TEMPERATURE AND TRAUMA

One possible reason for the raised risk of malignancy in cryptorchid testes is the raised temperature of the testis in this position. Studies of risk in relation to wearing tight underpants, use of saunas and hot baths, and occupational heat exposure[34,39,43,54,75,76,88] have not been supportive of such an association. These types of exposures to heat are intermittent, however, and it remains possible that the continuous raised temperature associated with cryptorchidism and varicocele may be carcinogenic.

Patients with testicular cancer frequently report previous trauma, and the inguinal cryptorchid testis is at increased risk of trauma. There is considerable scope for recall bias regarding trauma, however, and additionally, presentation for trauma may result in the diagnosis of malignancies that are already present. Questions on previous trauma, and on occupational and recreational activities in which trauma might occur,[35,43,75,76,88] do not provide consistent evidence of etiology; however, the possibility remains that trauma sufficiently severe to cause atrophy might be etiologic for testicular cancer.

OCCUPATION

A large number of occupations have been associated with testicular cancer in specific populations, often as a cluster of a small number of cases noticed in a particular workforce. None of these occurrences has been found consistently enough to provide convincing evidence of an association except for that with professional and other high-social-class occupations, which could be the result of social class–related lifestyle variables rather than occupation per se, or may to some extent relate to the sedentary nature of their work (discussed previously). The age distribution of occupational exposures compared with that of testicular cancer suggests that such exposures cannot be among the main causes of the malignancy. Men with occupations that have been reported to be associated with raised risk include farmers, oil and natural gas extraction workers,[37] police officers exposed to hand-held radar,[89] metal workers,[90] filling station and printing industry workers,[35] podiatrists,[91] methyl bromide workers,[92] those with jobs involving heat exposure,[76] leather tanners exposed to dimethylformamide,[93] aircraft repairmen,[94] naval personnel equivalent to automobile mechanics,[95] those with occupational exposures to fertilizers, phenols, and fumes or smoke,[43] and Vietnam veterans.[96]

UNCOMMON GENETIC ABNORMALITIES

Based on case reports, it is clear that patients with *XY gonadal dysgenesis* are at greatly raised risk of gonadal malignancy,[97] although there has not been epidemiologic quantification of the risk. Based on clinical reports, risk is not as obviously raised in forms of gonadal dysgenesis without a Y chromosome, despite raised gonadotrophin levels[97]; epidemiologic quantification of risk is needed. Cancer in situ has been found in testes of 25% (4 of 12) of patients with *androgen-insensitivity syndrome* (i.e., testicular feminization)[51]; in those with complete androgen insensitivity, whose testes are usually intraabdominal, several cases of testicular cancer have been reported, and risk is probably increased[97] but has not been quantified. Based on six cases, raised risk of testicular cancer has been suggested in patients with *ichthyosis,* an uncommon genetic skin disease in which testicular abnormalities are often found.[98] Several cases of testicular cancer have been reported in patients with *Down's syndrome,*[40,99,100] but it is not clear whether there is a raised risk. Men with Down's syndrome often have testicular dysgenesis and atrophy, a raised incidence of cryptorchidism, and elevated plasma concentrations of gonadotrophins. Based on small numbers of cases, a possible association has been suggested between testicular cancer and *Marfan's syndrome.*[100] Risk of testicular cancer is not obviously raised in *Klinefelter's disease,*[97,100] but epidemiologic quantification of risk would be of considerable interest because these patients have seminiferous tubule dysgenesis and raised gonadotrophin levels.

GENETIC FACTORS

The large difference in risk of testicular cancer between whites and blacks, and to a lesser extent between whites and other nonwhite groups, even when both populations are living in the same geographic area and thus presumably share many exposures,* suggests an appreciable genetic component in the etiology of testicular cancer. There are more than 100 case reports of families in which one or more first-degree relatives of an index case have had testicular cancer[101]; in some instances, four brothers have been affected.[102,103] In several instances, the families have also included several individuals with

*Although for in utero exposures, only second-generation or later generations of immigrants (e.g., most blacks in the United States) can share the host-country exposure.

undescended testis, inguinal hernia, or other genitourinary abnormalities,[55,104,105] suggesting that the inherited predisposition may be, more widely, to genitourinary abnormality. In a cohort study,[61] testicular cancer risk was significantly raised for university-aged men reporting cancer in either parent. In case-control studies, Tollerud and colleagues[104] and Forman and colleagues[101] found a sixfold relative risk of testicular cancer in men who had a first-degree relative with this disease. Forman and colleagues[101] found a relative risk of 9.8 for individuals who had a brother with testicular cancer; these individuals were estimated to have a 2.2% chance of developing testicular cancer by the age of 50 years. There is evidence that familial cases may be younger and more often have bilateral testicular cancer than nonfamilial cases.[101] Several studies have suggested possible associations of testicular cancer with particular HLA haplotypes,[106,107] but others have found no association[101]; overall, there is no consistent evidence for an HLA-related risk.[101]

OTHER FACTORS

Allergy has been found to be a risk factor for testicular cancer in some studies[40,108] but not in others.[22,33,75] A history of pneumonia was a significant risk factor in a cohort study[61] and a nonsignificant risk factor in a case-control study.[40] Vasectomy does not appear to be associated with testicular cancer from consideration of the case-control literature overall[44,109]; this lack of association is also present in large cohort studies with confidence intervals that preclude appreciably raised risks.[110,111] No consistent relation between risk and height, weight, or body mass index of the subject has been found.[22,61,73,75,76] Testicular cancer risk does not appear to be associated with smoking.[33,35,61,75,76] Individual studies have found raised risk in relation to having a sibling with a birth defect[43] or a mother[39] or sister[55] with breast cancer, which might relate to maternal or familial hormone levels. Raised risk has been found for males with a first-degree relative with a history of meningitis[55] or epilepsy.[30,55] Decreased risk has been found in men whose mothers have had severe menopausal menorrhagia.[36] Previous nontesticular malignancy is a risk factor for testicular cancer.[26,112]

In international, population-based registration data, the incidence of testicular cancer correlates strongly with geographic differences in fat consumption.[113] Diet could affect hormone levels of mothers and sons and therefore may underlie several of the mechanisms of risk discussed previously (e.g., exposure to maternal estrogen levels, postnatal hormone levels especially at puberty, age at puberty). Data on diet in relation to testicular cancer have been very limited and inconclusive.[73]

CONCLUSIONS

Testicular cancer incidence continues to increase in white populations for reasons that remain unknown. Certain risk factors have been clearly demonstrated, notably undescended testes, inguinal hernia, previous primary cancer in the opposite testis, first-degree family members with testicular cancer, and XY gonadal dysgenesis, but even for these factors important issues remain to be investigated. Several other factors, such as mumps orchitis, seem likely to be risk factors also, but are less well established. It appears probable that key events leading to testicular cancer occur prenatally. The most attractive prenatal hypothesis, which potentially explains many features of the epidemiology of the malignancy, is that relating to prenatal estrogen exposure,[64,65] but this is not yet well established, and other alternative mechanisms remain possible.[56] It is likely there are also postnatal influences on etiology; gonadotrophin levels seem one likely influence, which may explain several findings in the literature; however, this association also is not yet well established. Future epidemiologic investigation of these issues promises to be fascinating, but not easy.

REFERENCES

1. Parkin DM, Muir CS, Whelan SL, Gao Y-T, Ferlay J, Powell J, eds. Cancer incidence in five continents, VI, no 120. Lyon: IARC Scientific Publications, 1992.
2. Brown LM, Pottern LM, Hoover RN, Devesa SS, Aselton P, Flannery JT. Testicular cancer in the United States: trends in incidence and mortality. Int J Epidemiol 1986;15:164.
3. Østerlind A. Diverging trends in incidence and mortality of testicular cancer in Denmark, 1943–1982. Br J Cancer 1986;53:501.
4. Møller H. Clues to aetiology of testicular germ cell tumours from descriptive epidemiology. Eur Urol 1993;23:8.
5. Coleman MP, Estève J, Damiecki P, Arsalan A, Renard H. Trends in cancer incidence and mortality, no 121. Lyon: IARC, 1993.
6. Spitz MR, Sider JG, Pollack ES, Lynch HK, Newell GR. Incidence and descriptive features of testicular cancer among United States whites, blacks, and Hispanics, 1973–1982. Cancer 1986;58:1785.
7. Stone JM, Sandeman TF, Ironside P, Cruickshank DG, Matthews JP. Time trends in accuracy of classification of testicular tumours, with clinical and epidemiological implications. Br J Cancer 1992;66:396.
8. Forman D, Møller H. Testicular cancer. Cancer Surv 1994;19/20:323.
9. Schottenfeld D, Warshauer ME, Sherlock S, Zauber AG, Leder M, Payne R. The epidemiology of testicular cancer in young adults. Am J Epidemiol 1980;112:232.
10. Van den Eeden SK, Weiss NS. Is testicular cancer incidence in blacks increasing? Am J Public Health 1989;79:1553.
11. Doll R, Payne P, Waterhouse J. Cancer incidence in five continents: a technical report. Geneva: UICC, 1968.
12. Doll R, Muir C, Waterhouse J. Cancer incidence in five continents, vol 2. Geneva: UICC, 1970.
13. Lee JAH, Hitosugi M, Petersen GR. Rise in mortality from tumors of the testis in Japan, 1947–70. J Natl Cancer Inst 1973;51:1485.
14. Holman D, Armstrong B. Cancer mortality trends in Australia 1910–1979. Perth: Cancer Council of Western Australia, 1982.
15. Davies JM. Testicular cancer in England and Wales: some epidemiological aspects. Lancet 1981;1:928.
16. Petersen GR, Lee JAH. Secular trends of malignant tumors of the testis in white men. J Natl Cancer Inst 1972;49:339.
17. Møller H, Friis S, Kjaer SK. Male genital organs. Acta Pathol Microbiol Immunol Scand 1993;(Suppl 33):122.
18. Geddes M, Parkin DM, Khlat M, Balzi D, Buiatti E, eds. Cancer in Italian migrant populations, no 123. Lyon: IARC, 1993.
19. Bernstein L, Ross RK. Cancer in Los Angeles county: a portrait of incidence and mortality 1972–1987. Los Angeles: University of Southern California, 1991.
20. Swerdlow A, dos Santos Silva I. Atlas of cancer incidence in England and Wales 1968–85. Oxford: Oxford University Press, 1993.
21. Jensen OM, Carstensen B, Glattre E, Malker B, Pukkala E, Tulinius H. Atlas of cancer incidence in the Nordic countries. Helsinki: Puna Musta, 1988.
22. Davies TW, Prener A, Engholm G. Body size and cancer of the testis. Acta Oncol 1990;29:287.
23. Doll R. Urban and rural factors in the aetiology of cancer. Int J Cancer 1991;47:803.
24. Kinlen LJ, Willows AN. Cancer of the testis and month of birth. Br J Cancer 1987;55:579.
25. Swerdlow AJ, Skeet RG. Occupational associations of testicular cancer in Southeast England. Br J Ind Med 1988;45:225.

26. Stone JM, Cruickshank DG, Sandeman TF, Matthews JP. Laterality, maldescent, trauma and other clinical factors in the epidemiology of testis cancer in Victoria, Australia. Br J Cancer 1991;64:132.
27. Østerlind A, Berthelsen JG, Abildgaard N, et al. Risk of bilateral testicular germ cell cancer in Denmark: 1960–1984. J Natl Cancer Inst 1991;83:1391.
28. Li FP, Fraumeni JF Jr. Testicular cancers in children: epidemiologic characteristics. J Natl Cancer Inst 1972;48:1575.
29. Sakashita S, Koyanagi T, Tsuji I, Arikado K, Matsuno T. Congenital anomalies in children with testicular germ cell tumor. J Urol 1980; 124:889.
30. Swerdlow AJ, Stiller CA, Kinnier Wilson LM. Prenatal factors in the aetiology of testicular cancer: an epidemiological study of childhood testicular cancer deaths in Great Britain, 1953–73. J Epidemiol Commun Health 1982;36:96.
31. Abratt RP, Reddi VB, Sarembock LA. Testicular cancer and cryptorchidism. Br J Urol 1992;70:656.
32. Morrison AS. Cryptorchidism, hernia, and cancer of the testis. J Natl Cancer Inst 1976;56:731.
33. Henderson BE, Benton B, Jing J, Yu MC, Pike MC. Risk factors for cancer of the testis in young men. Int J Cancer 1979;23:598.
34. Loughlin JE, Robboy SJ, Morrison AS. Risk factors for cancer of the testis. N Engl J Med 1980;303:112.
35. Coldman AJ, Elwood JM, Gallagher RP. Sports activities and risk of testicular cancer. Br J Cancer 1982;46:749.
36. Depue RH, Pike MC, Henderson BE. Estrogen exposure during gestation and risk of testicular cancer. J Natl Cancer Inst 1983;71:1151.
37. Mills PK, Newell GR, Johnson DE. Testicular cancer associated with employment in agriculture and oil and natural gas extraction. Lancet 1984;1:207.
38. Pottern LM, Brown LM, Hoover RN, et al. Testicular cancer risk among young men: role of cryptorchidism and inguinal hernia. J Natl Cancer Inst 1985;74:377.
39. Moss AR, Osmond D, Bacchetti P, Torti FM, Gurgin V. Hormonal risk factors in testicular cancer: a case-control study. Am J Epidemiol 1986;124:39.
40. Swerdlow AJ, Huttly SRA, Smith PG. Testicular cancer and antecedent diseases. Br J Cancer 1987;55:97.
41. Gershman ST, Stolley PD. A case-control study of testicular cancer using Connecticut tumour registry data. Int J Epidemiol 1988;17:738.
42. Strader CH, Weiss NS, Daling JR, Karagas MR, McKnight B. Cryptorchism, orchiopexy, and the risk of testicular cancer. Am J Epidemiol 1988;127:1013.
43. Haughey BP, Graham S, Brasure J, Zielezny M, Sufrin G, Burnett WS. The epidemiology of testicular cancer in upstate New York. Am J Epidemiol 1989;130:25.
44. Forman D, Pike MC, Davey G, et al. Aetiology of testicular cancer: association with congenital abnormalities, age at puberty, infertility, and exercise. Br Med J 1994;308:1393.
45. Giwercman A, Grindsted J, Hansen B, Jensen OM, Skakkebaek NE. Testicular cancer risk in boys with maldescended testis: a cohort study. J Urol 1987;138:1214.
46. Benson RC Jr, Beard CM, Kelalis PP, Kurland LT. Malignant potential of the cryptorchid testis. Mayo Clin Proc 1991:66:372.
47. Chilvers C, Pike MC. Cancer risk in the undescended testicle. Eur Urol Update Series 1992;1:74.
48. Halme A, Kellokumpu-Lehtinen P, Lehtonen T, Teppo L. Morphology of testicular germ cell tumours in treated and untreated cryptorchidism. Br J Urol 1989;64:78.
49. Pike MC, Chilvers C, Peckham MJ. Effect of age at orchidopexy on risk of testicular cancer. Lancet 1986;1:1246.
50. Mengel W, Hienz HA, Sippe WG II, Hecker WCh. Studies on cryptorchidism: a comparison of histological findings in the germinative epithelium before and after the second year of life. J Pediatr Surg 1974; 9:445.
51. Giwercman A, von der Maase H, Skakkebaek NE. Epidemiological and clinical aspects of carcinoma in situ of the testis. Eur Urol 1993; 23:104.
52. Depue RH, Pike MC, Henderson BE. Cryptorchidism and testicular cancer. J Natl Cancer Inst 1986;77:830.
53. John Radcliffe Hospital Cryptorchidism Study Group. Cryptorchidism: a prospective study of 7500 consecutive male births, 1984–8. Arch Dis Child 1992;67:892.
54. Karagas MR, Weiss NS, Strader CH, Daling JR. Elevated intrascrotal temperature and the incidence of testicular cancer in noncryptorchid men. Am J Epidemiol 1989;129:1104.
55. Swerdlow AJ, Huttly SRA, Smith PG. Prenatal and familial associations of testicular cancer. Br J Cancer 1987;55:571.
56. Fram RJ, Garnick MR, Retik A. The spectrum of genitourinary abnormalities in patients with cryptorchidism, with emphasis on testicular carcinoma. Cancer 1982;50:2243.
57. Brown LM, Pottern LM, Hoover RN. Prenatal and perinatal risk factors for testicular cancer. Cancer Res 1986;46:4812.
58. Malone KE, Daling JR. Birth weight and the risk of testicular cancer. J Natl Cancer Inst 1986:77;829.
59. Depue RH, Pike MC, Henderson BE. Birth weight and the risk of testicular cancer. J Natl Cancer Inst 1986;77:829.
60. Morrison AS. Some social and medical characteristics of army men with testicular cancer. Am J Epidemiol 1976;104:511.
61. Whittemore AS, Paffenbarger RS Jr, Anderson K, Lee JE. Early precursors of urogenital cancers in former college men. J Urol 1984;132: 1256.
62. Prener A, Hsieh C-C, Engholm G, Trichopoulos D, Jensen OM. Birth order and risk of testicular cancer. Cancer Cause Control 1992;3:265.
63. Braun MM, Caporaso NE, Brinton L, Page WF. Re: twin membership and breast cancer risk. Am J Epidemiol 1994;140:575.
64. Henderson BE, Ross RK, Pike MC, Casagrande JT. Endogenous hormones as a major factor in human cancer. Cancer Res 1982;42:3232.
65. Henderson BE, Ross RK, Pike MC, Depue RH. Epidemiology of testis cancer. In: Skinner DG, ed. Urologic cancer. New York: Grune & Stratton, 1983:237.
66. Sharpe RM, Skakkebaek NE. Are oestrogens involved in falling sperm counts and disorders of the male reproductive tract? Lancet 1993;341: 1392.
67. Bernstein L, Depue RH, Ross RK, Judd HL, Pike MC, Henderson BE. Higher maternal levels of free estradiol in first compared to second pregnancy: early gestational differences. J Natl Cancer Inst 1986;76: 1035.
68. Bernstein L, Depue R, Ross R, Henderson BE. Higher pregnancy levels of estradiol and sex-hormone binding globulin in hyperemetic women: a case-control study. Am J Epidemiol 1986;124:509.
69. Walker AH, Bernstein L, Warren DW, Warner NE, Zheng X, Henderson BE. The effect of in-utero ethinyl oestradiol exposure on the risk of cryptorchid testis and testicular teratoma in mice. Br J Cancer 1990; 62:599.
70. Hutson JM. A biphasic model for the hormonal control of testicular descent. Lancet 1985;2:419.
71. Bernstein L, Pike MC, Depue RH, Ross RK, Moore JW, Henderson BE. Maternal hormone levels in early gestation of cryptorchid males: a case-control study. Br J Cancer 1988;58:379.
72. Henderson BE, Bernstein L, Ross RK, Depue RH, Judd HL. The early in utero oestrogen and testosterone environment of blacks and whites: potential effects on male offspring. Br J Cancer 1988;57:216.
73. Swerdlow AJ, Huttly SRA, Smith PG. Testis cancer: post-natal hormonal factors, sexual behaviour and fertility. Int J Cancer 1989;43: 549.
74. Werder EA, Illig R, Torresani T, et al. Gonadal function in young adults after surgical treatment of cryptorchidism. Br Med J 1976;2: 1357.
75. Brown LM, Pottern LM, Hoover RN. Testicular cancer in young men: the search for causes of the epidemic increase in the United States. J Epidemiol Commun Health 1987;41:349.
76. Lin RS, Kessler II. Epidemiologic findings in testicular cancer. Am J Epidemiol 1979;110:357.
77. Wanderas EH, Fosså SD, Heilo A, Stenwig AE, Norman N. Serum follicle stimulating hormone—predictor of cancer in the remaining testis in patients with unilateral testicular cancer. Br J Urol 1990;66: 315.
78. Kaufman JJ, Bruce PT. Testicular atrophy following mumps: a cause of testis tumour? Br J Urol 1963;35:67.
79. Beard CM, Benson RC Jr, Kelalis PP, Elveback LR, Kurland LT. The incidence and outcome of mumps orchitis in Rochester, Minnesota, 1935 to 1974. Mayo Clin Proc 1977;52:3.
80. Adamopoulos DA, Lawrence DM, Vassilopoulos P, Contoyiannis PA, Swyer GIM. Pituitary-testicular interrelationships in mumps orchitis and other viral infections. Br Med J 1978;1:1177.
81. Mueller N, Hinkula J, Wahren B. Elevated antibody titers against

cytomegalovirus among patients with testicular cancer. Int J Cancer 1988;41:399.
82. Algood CB, Newell GR, Johnson DE. Viral etiology of testicular tumors. J Urol 1988;139:308.
83. Heinzer H, Dieckmann K-P, Huland E. Virus-related serology and in situ hybridization for the detection of virus DNA among patients with testicular cancer. Eur Urol 1993;24:271.
84. Schilsky RL. Infertility in patients with testicular cancer: testis, tumor, or treatment? J Natl Cancer Inst 1989;81:119.
85. Carlsen E, Giwercman A, Keiding N, Skakkebaek NE. Evidence for decreasing quality semen during past 50 years. Br Med J 1992;305: 609.
86. Tummon IS, Mortimer D. Decreasing quality of semen. Br Med J 1992;305:1228.
87. Bromwich P, Cohen J, Stewart I, Walker A. Decline in sperm counts: an artefact of changed reference range of "normal"? Br Med J 1994; 309:19.
88. Swerdlow AJ, Huttly SRA, Smith PG. Is the incidence of testis cancer related to trauma or temperature? Br J Urol 1988;61:518.
89. Davis RL, Mostofi FK. Cluster of testicular cancer in police officers exposed to hand-held radar. Am J Ind Med 1993;24:231.
90. Rhomberg W, Schmoll HJ. High incidence of metalworkers among patients with testicular cancer. In: Niebergs HE, ed. Prevention and detection of cancer, part 1, vol 2. New York: Marcel Dekker, 1978: 1737.
91. Rose LI, Weiss W, Gibley CW Jr, Borowski G, Levy RA. Carcinoma of the testis in podiatrists. Ann Intern Med 1983;99:636.
92. Wong O, Brocker W, Davis HV, Nagle GS. Mortality of workers potentially exposed to organic and inorganic brominated chemicals, DBCP, TRIS, PBB and DDT. Br J Ind Med 1984;41:15.
93. Levin SM, Baker DB, Landrigan PJ, et al. Testicular cancer in leather tanners exposed to dimethylformamide. Lancet 1987;2:1153.
94. Ducatman AM, Conwill DE, Crawl J. Germ cell tumors of the testicle among aircraft repairmen. J Urol 1986;136:834.
95. Garland FC, Gorham ED, Garland CF, Ducatman AM. Testicular cancer in US Navy personnel. Am J Epidemiol 1988;127:411.
96. Tarone RE, Hayes HM, Hoover RN, et al. Service in Vietnam and risk of testicular cancer. J Natl Cancer Inst 1991;83:1497.
97. Verp MS, Simpson JL. Abnormal sexual differentiation and neoplasia. Cancer Genet Cytogenet 1987;25:191.
98. Lykkesfeldt G, Bennett P, Lykkesfeldt AE, et al. Testis cancer: ichthyosis constitutes a significant risk factor. Cancer 1991;67:730.
99. Braun DL, Green MD, Rausen AR, et al. Down's syndrome and testicular cancer: a possible association. Am J Pediatr Hematol Oncol 1985; 7:208.
100. Dexeus FH, Logothetis CJ, Chong C, Sella A, Ogden S. Genetic abnormalities in men with germ cell tumors. J Urol 1988;140:80.
101. Forman D, Oliver RTD, Brett AR, et al. Familial testicular cancer: a report of the UK family register, estimation of risk and an HLA Class 1 sib-pair analysis. Br J Cancer 1992;65:255.
102. Gedde-Dahl T, Hannisdal E, Klepp OH, et al. Testicular neoplasms occurring in four brothers: a search for a genetic predisposition. Cancer 1985;55:2005.
103. Goss PE, Bulbul MA. Familial testicular cancer in five members of a cancer-prone kindred. Cancer 1990;66:2044.
104. Tollerud DJ, Blattner WA, Fraser MC, et al. Familial testicular cancer and urogenital developmental anomalies. Cancer 1985;55:1849.
105. Anderson KC, Li FP, Marchetto DJ. Dizygotic twinning, cryptorchism and seminoma in a sibship. Cancer 1984;53:374.
106. De Wolf WC, Lange PH, Einarson ME, Yunis EJ. HLA and testicular cancer. Nature 1979;277:216.
107. Pollack MS, Vugrin D, Hennessy W, Herr HW, Dupont B, Whitmore WF Jr. HLA antigens in patients with germ cell cancers of the testis. Cancer Res 1982;42:2470.
108. Vena JE, Bona JR, Byers TE, Middleton E Jr, Swanson MK, Graham S. Allergy-related diseases and cancer: an inverse association. Am J Epidemiol 1985;122:66.
109. Lynge E, Knudsen LB, Møller H. Vasectomy and testicular cancer: epidemiological evidence of association. Eur J Cancer 1993;29A: 1064.
110. Nienhuis H, Goldacre M, Seagroatt V, Gill L, Vessey M. Incidence of disease after vasectomy: a record linkage retrospective cohort study. Br Med J 1992;304:743.
111. Møller H, Knudsen LB, Lynge E. Risk of testicular cancer after vasectomy: cohort study of over 73000 men. Br Med J 1994;309:295.
112. Schoenberg BS. Multiple primary malignant neoplasms: the Connecticut experience, 1935–1964. Recent Results Cancer Res 1977;58:1.
113. Armstrong B, Doll R. Environmental factors and cancer incidence and mortality in different countries, with special reference to dietary practices. Int J Cancer 1975;15:617.

Principles and Practice of Genitourinary Oncology, edited by Derek Raghavan, Howard I. Scher, Steven A. Leibel, and Paul H. Lange. Lippincott-Raven Publishers, Philadelphia, © 1997.

CHAPTER 62

Pathology of Testicular Tumors

Ivan Damjanov

GERM CELL TUMORS AND TERATOMAS

Testicular tumors account for approximately 1% of all neoplasms in males. Although these tumors may originate from several intratesticular and paratesticular cells, and even cells that are not limited to testes (e.g., hematopoietic and mesenchymal connective tissue cells), the vast majority of tumors are of germ cell origin. For practical reasons, in most epidemiologic and statistical references, testicular neoplasms are equated with germ cell tumors, which comprise approximately 95% of all testicular tumors. Similarly, this chapter is devoted primarily to germ cell tumors.

In clinical practice, for prognostic and therapeutic purposes, the first step taken by the pathologist is to determine whether a tumor is derived from germ cells or from some other cell type (Fig. 62-1). Non–germ cell tumors, which account for 5% of all tumors, are easily classified into several categories, the most important of which are the sex cord cell tumors such as Sertoli cell, Leydig cell, granulosa cell, and primitive gonadal stromal tumors. The remaining non–germ cell tumors originate from nonspecific stromal cells (e.g. fibroblasts, angioblasts, nerve sheath cells, smooth or striated muscles), rete testis, or the mesothelium of tunica vaginalis. Metastatic tumors are rare in the testis, but they must be considered as well, especially in very young or very old patients.

CLASSIFICATION OF TESTICULAR GERM CELL TUMORS

Several classifications of testicular germ cell tumors are in use (Table 62-1). These classifications are derived from the studies of histogenesis or histopathology of testicular tumors.[1–3] However, because this approach has not produced generally acceptable schemes, most pathologists use some modification of the histogenetic or histopathologic classifications. These intricate details of complex pathologic classifications are often ignored by clinicians, because morphologic aspects of tumors bear very little clinical significance.

Germ cell tumors are classified for clinical purposes in two major groups: seminomas or nonseminomatous germ cell tumors (NSGCT). The differentiation of seminomas from NSGCT, which are also sometimes called nonseminomas, is relatively simple and can be made easily on microscopic examination of adequately sampled tumors.[4] Approximately 40% of germ cell tumors are seminomas, 35% are NSGCT, and 15% are mixed seminomas and NSGCT. Because the stem cells of the NSGCT component are more malignant than seminoma, mixed tumors are treated as NSGCT.

Three rare tumor types are separate from these two main groups of germ cell tumors: spermatocytic seminomas, yolk sac tumors (YSTs), and teratomas. Biologically, clinically, and probably histogenetically, these tumors are distinct from other germ cell tumors.[4]*

Applying the paraphrase of Oscar Wilde's aphorism about truth, it could be said that the testicular germ cell tumors are rarely pure, and their classification rarely simple. Nevertheless, subclassification of NSGCT into pure embryonal carcinomas (EC), teratocarcinomas, choriocarcinomas, and polyembryomas is of limited clinical value. Enumeration of various components and the use of morphologic terms advocated in the British classification is useful mostly for morphologic studies.[3] Although the prognostic value of such detailed morphologic analysis is questionable, it should not be discounted a priori until data from the various multivariate clinicopathologic therapeutic studies in progress are compiled.[5]

SEMINOMA

Seminoma is the most common testicular tumor.[6] On gross examination, the tumors are lobulated or irregularly nodular and compress the remaining testicular parenchyma. On cross section, the tumor appears firm and grayish white or yellow, with occasional foci of necrosis or hemorrhage. Histologically, the tumor is composed of relatively large, polygonal, clear cells arranged into broad sheets, strands, or groups, delimited in part by connective tissue septa (Fig. 62-2). The septa are infiltrated with lymphocytes, macrophages, plasma cells, and occasional multinucleated giant cells. Although the tumors usually appear sharply demarcated from the normal testicular parenchyma, mi-

* This view is controversial and many investigators believe that there is a histologic continuum between germ cell tumors, teratoma, and yolk sac tumors. (D.R.)

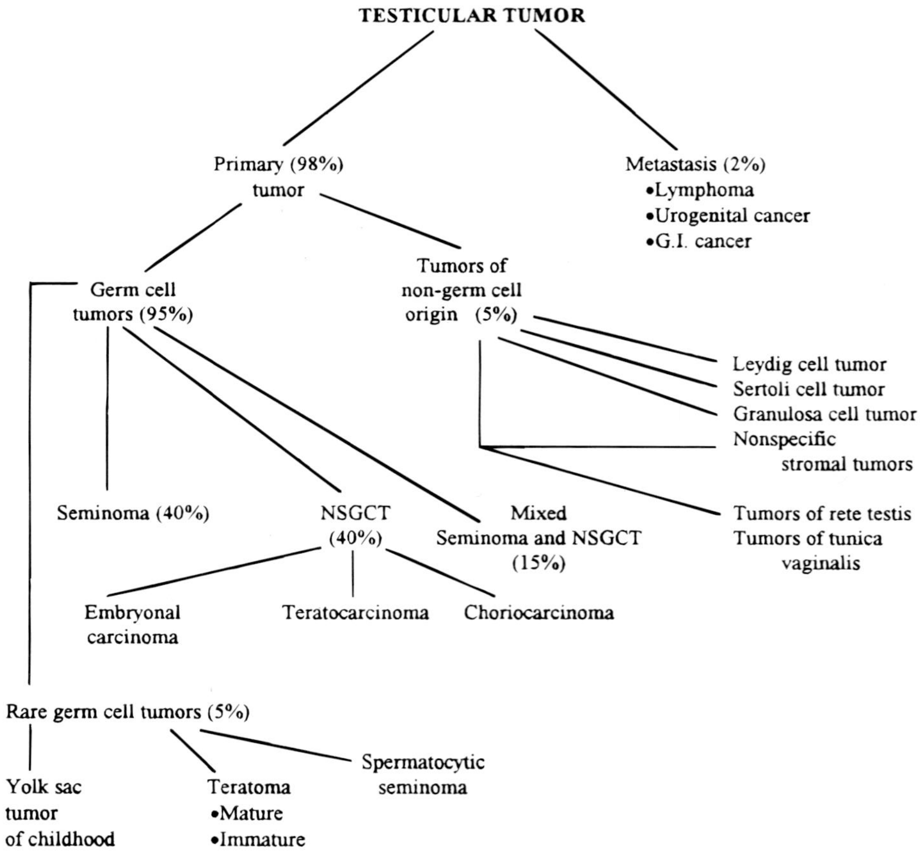

FIG. 62-1. Algorithm for histopathologic diagnosis of testicular tumors. G.I., gastrointestinal; NSGCT, nonseminomatous germ cell tumors.

croscopic extension of tumor cells between the seminiferous tubules is often present (Fig. 62-3). Intratubular growth of seminoma is a common finding, which should not be confused with carcinoma in situ (CIS). Pagetoid spread of seminoma cells may extend into the rete testis.[6] CIS is almost invariably present in the seminiferous tubules adjacent to the tumor.[7]

Several variants of seminoma have been described. Such subclassifications are of no practical clinical value. For example, the term *anaplastic seminoma* was previously used for tumors showing cytologic pleomorphism and high mitotic activity.[8] However, the survival of patients with these tumors is not different from those with classic seminoma[6,9]; therefore, the value of this concept has been challenged and abandoned. Morphologic variants such as cribriform and sclerosing seminoma (Fig. 62-4)[10] or tubular seminoma[11] do not deserve to be treated as distinct clinicopathologic forms. Nevertheless, it is important for the pathologist to be aware of these entities so as not to be confounded by them.

TABLE 62-1. *Comparison of classifications of germ cell tumors of the testis*

Dixon and Moore, 1953[1]	Mostofi and Sobin, 1977[2]	Pugh, 1976[3]
Group I Seminoma Spermatocytic seminoma	Seminoma Spermatocytic seminoma	Seminoma Spermatocytic seminoma
Group II Embryonal carcinoma	Embryonal carcinoma, adult-type	Malignant teratoma, undifferentiated
Group III Teratoma, pure	Teratoma Mature Immature	Teratoma, differentiated
Group IV Teratoma with carcinoma or sarcoma	Teratoma with malignant areas other than seminoma, embryonal carcinoma, or choriocarcinoma	Malignant teratoma, intermediate
Group V Teratoma with embryonal carcinoma or choriocarcinoma	Embryonal carcinoma and teratoma (teratocarcinoma)	Malignant teratoma, intermediate
Not listed	Infantile embryonal carcinoma	Yolk sac tumor; orchioblastoma
Not listed	Polyembryoma	Not listed

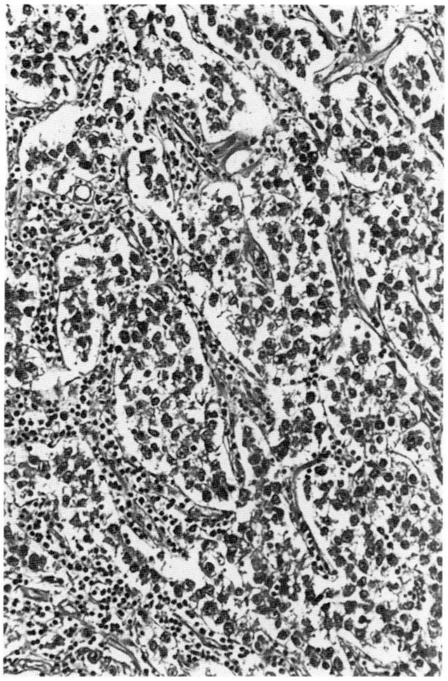

FIG. 62-2. This seminoma is composed of polygonal cells with clear cytoplasm. The connective tissue septa are infiltrated with lymphocytes. H&E stain; original magnification ×160.

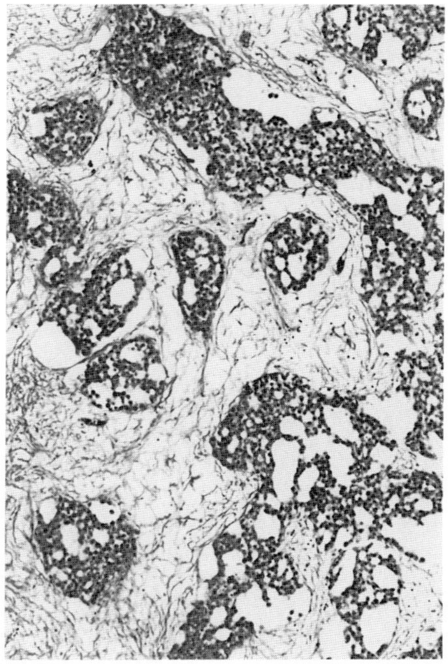

FIG. 62-4. This cribriform and sclerosing seminoma is composed of round cells that have clear cytoplasm but are smaller than typical seminoma cells. The tumor cells form groups that are encased in abundant stroma. There are no lymphoid infiltrates in the stroma. H&E stain; original magnification × 160.

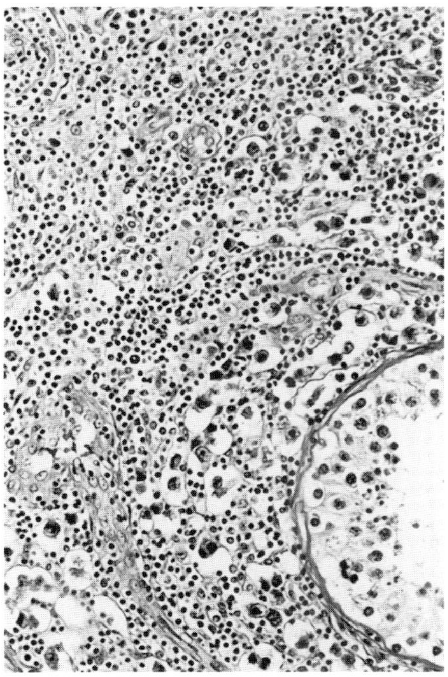

FIG. 62-3. Seminoma infiltrating the interstitium between the seminiferous tubules. H&E stain; original magnification ×240.

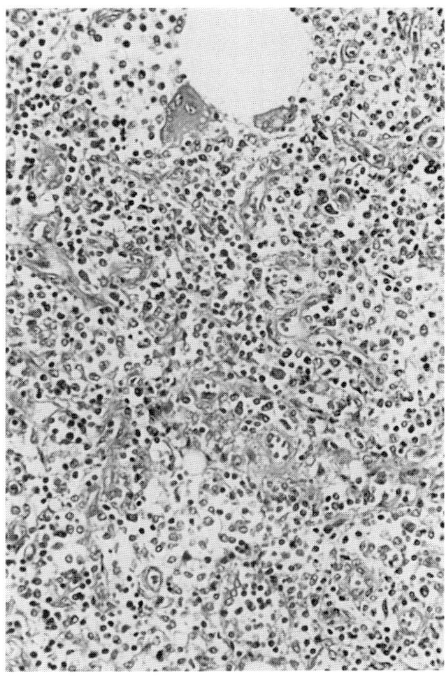

FIG. 62-5. Seminoma with trophoblastic cells, which are large, multinucleated cells that correspond to syncytiotrophoblastic cells. H&E stain; original magnification ×160.

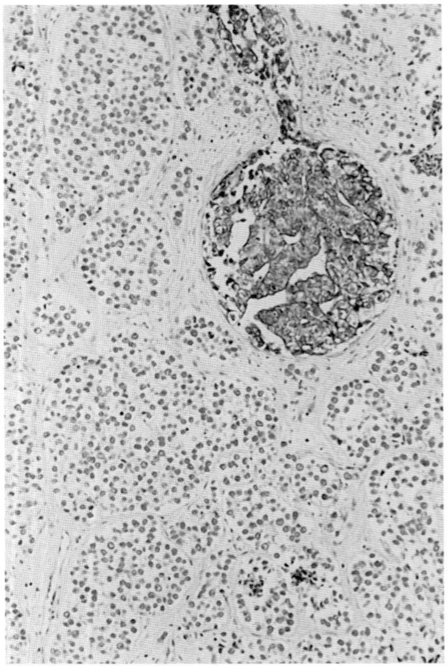

FIG. 62-6. This specimen of mixed seminoma and embryonal carcinoma, stained with antibodies to keratin, shows a positive focus of embryonal carcinoma, whereas the seminoma cells are nonreactive. Immunoperoxidase stain for keratin; original magnification ×160.

At least 15% of seminomas contain trophoblastic giant cells (Fig. 62-5),[12] which might be mistaken for choriocarcinomatous elements. These giant cells are positive for human chorionic gonadotropin (hCG), but the hCG level in serum is less often elevated.

Histochemical studies of seminomas are rarely indicated but may be helpful in complex cases, especially those that are overgrown by lymphocytes and resemble lymphoma. Seminoma cells are rich in glycogen, which is readily demonstrable by the periodic acid–Schiff (PAS) reaction. Immunohistochemically, seminoma cells react with antibodies to placental alkaline phosphatase (PLAP).[13,14] In paraffin sections, seminoma cells are mostly unreactive with antibodies to keratins, although in frozen sections, many tumors contain keratin-positive cells.[15] Apparently, either most seminomas contain very little keratin, or the immunoreactive epitopes of keratins are not readily detectable in paraffin-embedded tissue. This fact is most useful for distinguishing seminomas from EC cells. EC cells invariably contain keratin filaments, which are demonstrable immunohistochemically in routinely prepared tissue sections. The contrast between keratin-positive EC cells and keratin-negative seminoma cells is striking in mixed tumors (Fig. 62-6). Trophoblastic giant cells also react with antibodies to keratins. However, in contrast to EC cells, which usually express keratins 8 and 18, trophoblastic giant cells, like normal trophoblastic cells, express keratin 7.[16]

EMBRYONAL CARCINOMA

EC, originally defined more as a concept[1] than a morphologic entity, is nevertheless a distinct form of testicular neoplasia. For clinical purposes, EC is best considered as one of the NSGCT tumors, and it is of only academic interest to determine whether it is pure (single-cell type) or combined with other cell types.

From the point of developmental biology, EC is a tumor composed of cells that correspond to early embryonic cells.[4] These cells are undifferentiated but theoretically could differentiate into both embryonic cells forming the three germ layers (i.e., ectoderm, mesoderm, and endoderm) and extraembryonic derivatives (i.e., trophoblast, and yolk sac).[4] EC cells could also be developmentally nullipotent and unable to differentiate into any other cell type.

On gross examination, EC usually presents as a soft, irregular mass that is poorly demarcated from the testicular tissue surrounding it. On cross section, EC appears as brownish tan, partially hemorrhagic tissue with irregular areas of necrosis. Histologically, EC is composed of anaplastic cells that have irregularly shaped nuclei and indistinct cell borders (Fig. 62-7), which accounts for crowding of cells and apparent overlapping of their nuclei in histologic sections. EC cells may grow also in solid sheets or form papillary and glandular structures. Areas of necrosis, hemorrhage, and "smudging" are common.[6]

Pure EC is rare, and I agree with Ulbright[6] that this tumor does not account for more than 2% to 3% of all testicular neoplasms. In contrast to this view are the reports that EC represent 15% to 30% of all testicular tumors[17,18]; this only reflects the fact that EC cells cannot be reliably distinguished morphologically from yolk sac carcinoma cells and other embryonic cell types (Fig. 62-8). Theoretically, yolk sac components could be distinguished from EC cells by their immunoreactivity with antibodies to alphafetoprotein (AFP), but this prediction cannot always be proved in routinely prepared slides. Other more-differentiated embryonic or fetal cell types derived from EC cannot

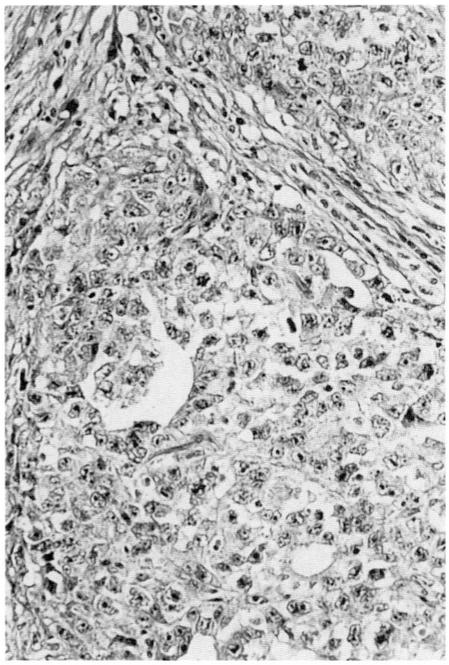

FIG. 62-7. This embryonal carcinoma is composed of anaplastic cells arranged in solid sheets. H&E stain; original magnification × 240.

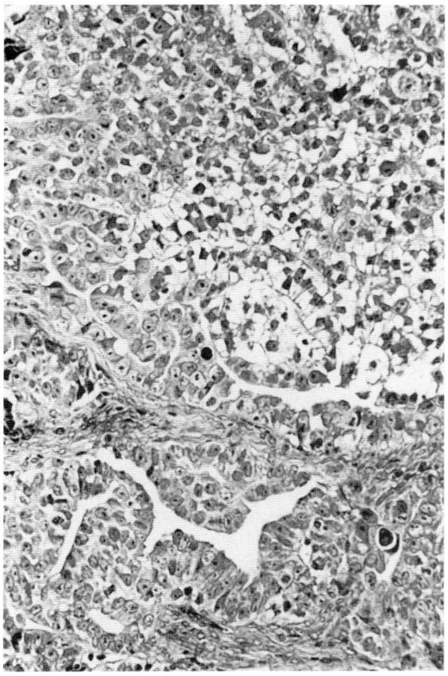

FIG. 62-8. Embryonal carcinoma cells appear compact, whereas yolk sac carcinoma cells have clear cytoplasm and have a papillary gland–like arrangement. H&E stain; original magnification ×240.

be recognized unequivocally by using routine microscopy or immunohistochemistry.

Immunohistochemistry is of limited value for the identification of EC cells. These tumor cells express keratins and are positive for alkaline phosphatase. The alkaline phosphatase of EC cells is of the intestinal type[19] rather than of the placental type as in seminomas. However, this distinction between seminoma and EC noted in cell lines in vitro has not been explored rigorously using clinical human tumor material. None of the commercially available antibodies are suitable for such studies. There are no reliable immunohistochemical means for distinguishing EC from yolk sac carcinoma cells and other embryonic cells. Antibody TRA-1-60, which is reactive with a surface glycoconjugate of EC cells (Fig. 62-9) and is released into the circulation of tumor-bearing patients,[20] is a useful marker, but it needs to be evaluated further because the epitope recognized by this monoclonal antibody is not limited to EC cells.

TERATOCARCINOMA

Teratocarcinoma is a term that has been received with skepticism by clinical pathologists and is thus used sporadically. The concept of teratocarcinomas has been developed by experimental pathologists who have shown that EC cells can differentiate into various somatic and extraembryonic cells.[4,21] According to this experimental tumor model in mice, teratocarcinomas are composed of EC cells, which are their undifferentiated stem cells and various differentiated descendants of these cells. EC cells correspond to embryonic cells from the cleavage stages of development (i.e., cells that could give rise to both the embryo and the embryonic membranes). Teratocarcinomas contain EC cells and various somatic and extraembryonic tissues. The finding of structures resembling early embryo, so called embryoid bodies (Fig. 62-10),[22] is yet another proof that ECs are equivalent to early embryonic cells.

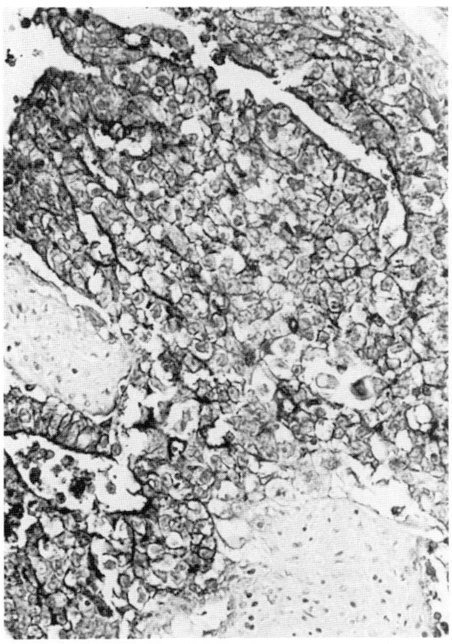

FIG. 62-9. This embryonal carcinoma, consisting of TRA-1-60–positive cells and TRA-1-60–negative cells which could not be further classified. Immunoperoxidase stain with antibody to TRA-1-60; original magnification × 240.

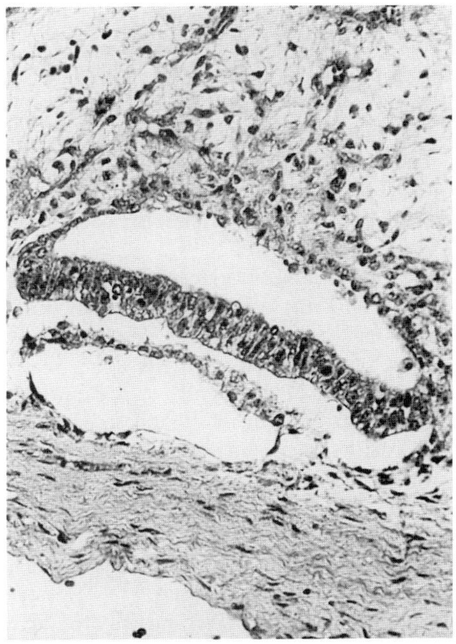

FIG. 62-10. This embryoid body from a teratocarcinoma consists of an embryonic plate composed of columnar cells and vesicles corresponding to early endoderm. H&E stain; original magnification ×240.

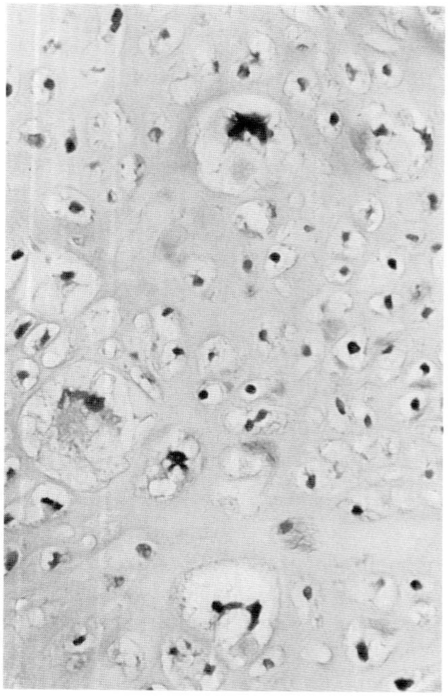

FIG. 62-11. Cartilage from a teratocarcinoma shows cellular atypia such as enlargement and irregularity of nuclei. Some lacunae contain more than one cell, as would be expected in normal tissue. H&E stain; original magnification ×240.

Pathologists opposed to the use of the term teratocarcinoma call such tumors malignant mixed germ cell tumors or simply NSGCT. It is also common to use one of these terms and then enumerate the various tissues found in the tumor. In practical terms, irrespective of the terminology, it is important to realize that the EC cells (i.e., the malignant stem cells of teratocarcinoma) have the same malignant potential as the EC cells in pure ECs of the testis. The differentiated derivatives of EC cells, whether in form of somatic tissues (e.g., squamous epithelium, neural tissue, bone) or extraembryonic tissues (e.g., yolk sac, trophoblast), have a limited propensity for growth and invasion. Such cells may show morphologic signs of malignancy (Fig. 62-11) but are, for practical purposes, benign.[6] Secondary malignant tumors derived from differentiated components of teratocarcinomas are rare.

The malignant stem cells of teratocarcinoma may metastasize to distant sites, producing tumors that have the same complex histologic appearance. However, the metastases may also be composed of EC cells or somatic cells exclusively. Somatic cell tumors that appear histologically as benign teratomas are presumably derived from stem cells that have completely differentiated into somatic tissues and in this process lost their malignancy. The stem cells in the primary metastasizing teratocarcinomas may also differentiate into somatic, nonproliferating cells, in which case both the primary and metastatic tumor histologically appear as benign teratomas. Many metastasizing teratomas of this type have been reported.[23,24] Metastatic tumors composed of "benign" tissues are commonly found in the lungs or lymph nodes of patients in whom the primary teratocarcinoma was resected and the disease was treated subsequently by chemotherapy.[25] It is thought that chemotherapy eradicates ECs, which are more sensitive to cytotoxic drugs than the somatic tissues, while leaving the resistant, well-differentiated somatic tissues intact.

Teratocarcinomas contain various tissues. From the clinical viewpoint, the most important of these are the yolk sac and trophoblastic cells, which account for the presence of AFP and hCG in the serum of two thirds of these patients.[26] Examination of other tissues in the teratocarcinoma has little clinical value. The morphologic findings that have prognostic significance in these NSGCTs were analyzed by multivariate logistic regression analysis by Moul and colleagues.[27] It was found that vascular invasion and percentage of EC have predictive value for staging tumors and are better indicators for formulating therapy. All other morphologic parameters were found to be less important.

Teratocarcinomas may contain seminoma cells. Such tumors are called *mixed gem cells tumors*, or NSGCT with seminoma. The presence of seminoma has no prognostic significance[27] in these tumors, which are clinically treated as NSGCT.

YOLK SAC TUMOR

YST, also known as yolk sac carcinoma or endodermal sinus tumor, occurs in two forms: as a pure YST of infancy or as a component of teratocarcinomas.[6] Histologically, this tumor is composed of cells resembling those in seen in the primary and secondary yolk sac in extraembryonic parts of the early human conceptus.

In teratocarcinomas, YST elements are found in about 50% of cases. YST cells and EC cells cannot always be distinguished from each other. The juxtaposition of EC and YST cells often results in a double-layered pattern composed of ribbons of typi-

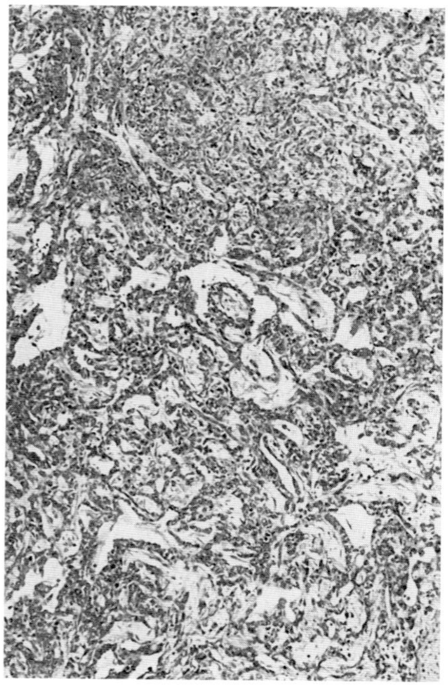

FIG. 62-12. Yolk sac tumor is composed of cuboidal and flattened epithelial cells arranged in a complex manner. H&E stain; original magnification ×160.

cal EC cells and flattened YST cells. The flattened cells strongly react with antibody to AFP.[6] Cuboidal YST cells often do not react with antibody to AFP and therefore cannot be always identified unequivocally as representing yolk sac components.

YSTs of infancy and childhood, which represent the most common testicular tumor in children under the age of 5 years,[28] have an extremely variegated histologic appearance (Fig. 62-12). A dozen histologic patterns are recognized.[29,30] These patterns, which have been reviewed in an article by Ulbright,[6] are endodermal sinus, reticular, papillary, glandular/alveolar, solid, myxomatous, sarcomatoid, macrocystic, polyvesicular vitelline, hepatoid, and parietal. Morphologic classification of tumors according to the prevailing histologic patterns has no clinical prognostic significance. Infants and children with YSTs have an excellent prognosis.

CHORIOCARCINOMA

Choriocarcinoma is an extremely rare tumor in the testis, accounting for less than 0.5% of all testicular neoplasms.[6] The tumor is composed of mononuclear cytotrophoblastic and multinucleated syncytiotrophoblastic cells (Fig. 62-13). On gross examination, these tumors appear as hemorrhagic nodules and are associated with distant metastases that are present at the time of diagnosis. Choriocarcinoma has an abysmal prognosis.

Choriocarcinomatous elements are found in approximately 10% of NSGCT tumors, accounting for the elevated level of hCG in these patients.[6,26] Tumors associated with elevated hCG levels in serum have a poor prognosis.

TERATOMA

Teratomas are tumors composed of benign somatic tissues. Testicular teratomas are rare as opposed to ovarian teratomas, which represent the most common germ cell tumor in females. Mature testicular teratomas are typically found in children.[28] These tumors are composed of mature somatic tissues such as skin, neural tissues, various glands, and pigmented retinal epithelium (see Fig. 62-13). Immature teratomas composed of less-differentiated somatic tissues are rare in the testis. Malignant transformation of benign teratomas has been reported but occurs rarely.[6]

It is important to note that the benign teratomas of postpubertal testes should not be grouped with the mature teratomas of prepubertal children. Postpubertal teratomas may be composed of the same mature somatic tissue yet be present with metastases. Such tumors are best considered as mature teratocarcinomas that have lost their malignant stem cells (EC cells) in the process of maturation. The mature metastases of these tumors probably represent derivatives of EC cells that have differentiated after settling in the lungs or lymph nodes.[24] It is hard to imagine that complex benign tissues could enter the blood stream and metastasize to distant sites. The factors that have influenced the maturation of EC cells in these tumors are poorly understood.

SPERMATOCYTIC SEMINOMA

Spermatocytic seminoma, initially described as a variant of seminoma, is a distinct tumor of uncertain histogenesis.[4,6] This tumor occurs in elderly patients, and in contrast to all other

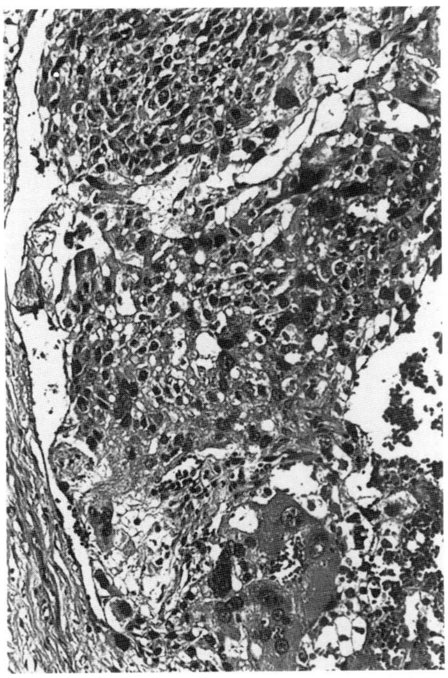

FIG. 62-13. Choriocarcinoma is composed of clear mononuclear cells, which correspond to cytotrophoblastic cells, and multinucleated syncytiotrophoblastic cells. H&E stain; original magnification ×240.

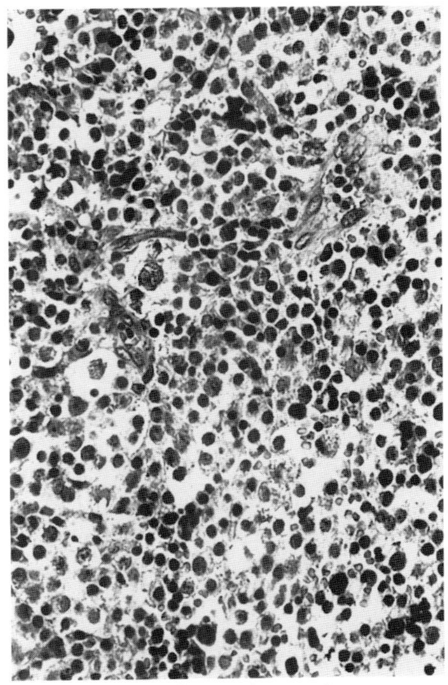

FIG. 62-14. Spermatocytic seminoma is composed of three cell types: small, dark, round cells; intermediate cells with vesicular nuclei; and large cells. H&E stain; original magnification ×240.

germ cell tumors, it does not occur in the ovary and does not arise in tissues outside of the testis.

On gross examination, spermatocytic seminoma is multinodular, and on cross section, it may be solid or multicystic. The cut surface often appears mucoid and shows areas suffused with blood. Histologically, the tumor is composed of a mixed population of small, medium, and large cells which may be multinucleated and could assume giant cell proportions (Fig. 62-14).[31] In contrast to the classic seminoma, spermatocytic seminoma does not contain septa infiltrated with lymphocytes, it is not associated with intratubular CIS, it is unreactive with antibodies to PLAP, and it does not stain with PAS because the cells do not contain glycogen.[32] Spermatocytic seminoma is never associated with NSGCT. Spermatocytic seminomas are benign tumors with a good prognosis. It has been reported that some of these tumors may be associated with sarcoma[33] and have a poor prognosis.

GONADAL STROMAL TUMORS

Gonadal stromal tumors account for 3% to 5% of all testicular tumors. These tumors are classified as Leydig cell tumors, Sertoli cell tumors, granulosa cell tumors, and undifferentiated stromal tumors.

Leydig Cell Tumors

Leydig cell tumors are composed of cells that have the morphologic features and some of the functions of normal Leydig cells.[34] On gross examination, Leydig cell tumors are usually small and firm and appear brown on cross section. Histologically, these tumors are composed of polygonal cells with round or slightly indented vesicular nuclei and well-developed granular or vacuolated cytoplasm (Fig. 62-15). Reinke's crystalloids, which are diagnostic of Leydig cells, are found in occasional cells in about 20% of tumors.

Leydig cell tumors may be benign or malignant. There are no reliable histologic signs of malignancy, and the prognosis depends on the clinical assessment of tumor spread.

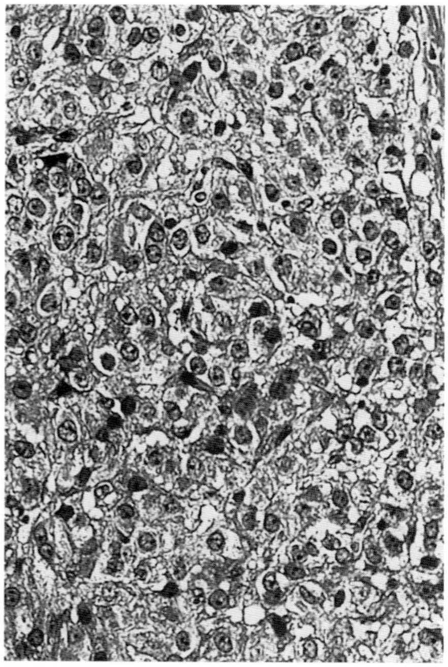

FIG. 62-15. Leydig cell tumor is composed of cells that have round nuclei and well-developed cytoplasm and are arranged into solid sheets. H&E stain; original magnification ×240.

Sertoli Cell Tumors

Sertoli cell tumors are rare neoplasms that can occur in any age group. Most Sertoli cell tumors are benign, but at least 10% are malignant.[35]

Histologically, Sertoli cell tumors may present in several forms. In the best-differentiated form, the tumors are composed of well-differentiated tubules, whereas in the least differentiated form, they are composed of elongated spindle cells arranged without any distinct pattern. Intermediate forms that recapitulate tubulogenesis to some extent are also found (Fig. 62-16). Large cell calcifying Sertoli cell tumor is a unique variant associated with endocrine disturbances. This tumor presents as a bilateral or multifocal lesion in about 50% of cases.[36]

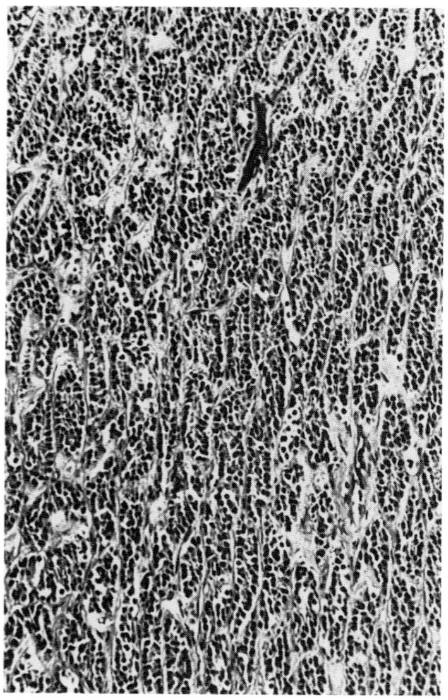

FIG. 62-16. Sertoli cell tumor is composed of cells arranged into sheets reminiscent of immature tubules. H&E stain; original magnification × 160.

Granulosa Cell Tumors

Granulosa cell tumors of the testis are rare tumors that resemble either the adult or the juvenile granulosa cell tumors of the ovary.[37] These tumors are benign.

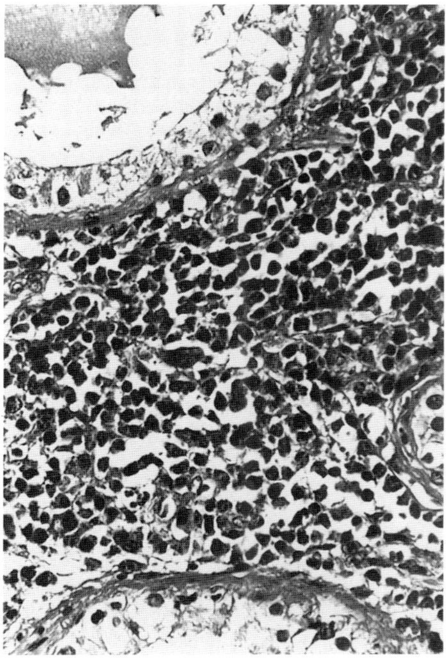

FIG. 62-17. In lymphoma, neoplastic lymphoid cells infiltrate the interstitial spaces of the testis. H&E stain; original magnification × 240.

OTHER TUMORS

Tumors of nonspecific testicular stroma are rare. These tumors resemble those in other locations and are classified accordingly as fibromas, lipomas, rhabdomyosarcomas, or neurofibrosarcomas, among others.

Metastases

Metastases to the testes are rare. The most common are metastases of lymphomas (Fig. 62-17).[38] Metastases of solid tumors are usually related to primary lesions in the urogenital tract or the gastrointestinal tract. These adenocarcinomas must be distinguished from primary adenocarcinomas of the rete testis[39] or remnants of the müllerian ducts.[40]

CLINICAL SIGNIFICANCE OF THE PATHOLOGY REPORT

Pathologic findings are essential for classifying testicular tumors and are important for determining the prognosis and choosing the therapy. The pathology report must include a detailed description of the gross and microscopic features of the tumor; the extent of the tumor invasion into the normal tissues, vessels, and lymphatics; and the presence of microscopic metastases in the lymph nodes or resected tissues from distant sites. Microscopic data are essential for staging tumors of the testis. The pathologic data should, however, not be considered without reference to the clinical and laboratory findings. With clinical and laboratory data, the pathology data are best used for multivariate analysis of the disease and planning various treatment modalities.

REFERENCES

1. Dixon FJ, Moore RA. Tumors of the male sex organs. In: Atlas of tumor pathology, sec 8, fasc. 31 and 32. Washington DC: Armed Forces Institute of Pathology, 1953.
2. Mostofi FK, Sobin LH. International histological classification of tumors of testes. Geneva: World Health Organization, 1977.
3. Pugh RCB, ed. Pathology of testis. Oxford: Blackwell, 1976.
4. Damjanov I. Pathobiology of human germ cell neoplasia. Recent Results Cancer Res 1991;123:1.
5. Sesterhenn IA, Weiss RB, Mostofi FK, et al. Prognosis and other clinical correlates of pathologic review in stage I and II testicular carcinoma: a report from the Testicular Cancer Intergroup Study. J Clin Oncol 1992;10:69.
6. Ulbright TM. Germ cell neoplasms of the testis. Am J Surg Pathol 1993;17:1075.
7. Jacobsen GK, Hendricksen OB, von der Maase H. Carcinoma in situ of testicular tissue adjacent to malignant germ-cell tumors: a study of 105 cases. Cancer 1981;47:2660.
8. Johnson DE, Gomez JJ, Ayala AG. Anaplastic seminoma. J Urol 1975; 114:80.
9. Boba VS, Mittal BB, Hoover SV, Kepka A. Classical and anaplastic seminoma: difference in survival. Radiology 1988;167:849.
10. Damjanov I, Niejadlik DC, Rabuffo JF, Donadio JA. Cribriform and sclerosing seminoma devoid of lymphoid infiltrates. Arch Pathol Lab Med 1980;104:527.
11. Young RH, Finlayson N, Scully RE. Tubular seminoma: report of a case. Arch Pathol Lab Med 1989;113:414.
12. Butcher DN, Gregory WM, Gunter PA, Masters JRW, Parkinson MC. The biological significance of hCG-containing cells in seminoma. Br J Cancer 1985;51:473.
13. Manivel JC, Jessurun J, Wick MR, Dehner LP. Placental alkaline phosphatase immunoreactivity in testicular germ-cell neoplasms. Am J Surg Pathol 1987;11:21.
14. Mostofi FK, Sesterhenn IA, Davis CJ Jr. Immunopathology of germ cell tumors of the testis. Semin Diagn Pathol 1987;4:320.
15. Fogel M. Lifschitz-Mercer B, Moll R, et al. Heterogeneity of intermediate filament expression in human testicular seminomas. Differentiation 1990;45:242.
16. Damjanov I, Osborn M. Miettinen M. Keratin 7 is a marker for a subset of trophoblastic cells in human germ cell tumors. Arch Pathol Lab Med 1990;114:81.
17. Nochomovitz LE, DeLa Torre FE, Rosai J. Pathology of germ cell tumors of the testis. Urol Clin Am 1977;4:359.
18. Vugrin D, Chen A, Feigl P, Laszlo J. Embryonal carcinoma of the testis. Cancer 1988;61:2348.
19. Benham FJ, Andrews PW, Knowles BB, Bronson DL, Harris H. Alkaline phosphatase isoenzymes as possible markers of differentiation in human testicular teratocarcinomas cell lines. Dev Biol 1981;88:279.
20. Marrink J, Andrews PW, van Brummen et al. TRA-1-60: a new serum marker in patients with germ cell tumors. Int J Cancer 1991;49:369.
21. Pierce GB Jr, Abell MR. Embryonal carcinoma of the testis. Pathol Annu 1970;5:27.
22. Marin-Padilla M. Origin, nature and significance of the "embryoids" of human teratomas. Virchows Arch 1965;340:105.
23. Kusuda L, Leidich RB, Das S. Mature teratoma of the testis metastasizing as mature teratoma. J Urol 1986;135:1020.
24. Moran CA, Travis WD, Carter D, Koss MN. Metastatic mature teratoma in lung following testicular embryonal carcinoma and teratocarcinoma. Arch Pathol Lab Med 1993;117:641.
25. Brodsby GL. Pathology of testicular germ cell tumors. Hematol Oncol Clin North Am 1991;5:1095.
26. Toner GC, Geller NL, Tan C, Nisselbaum J, Bosl GJ. Serum tumor marker half-life during chemotherapy allows early prediction of complete response and survival in nonseminomous germ cell tumors. Cancer Res 1990;50:5904.
27. Moul JW, McCarthy WF, Fernandez EB, Sesterhenn IA. Percentage of embryonal carcinoma and of vascular invasion predicts pathological

stage in clinical stage I nonseminomatous testicular cancer. Cancer Res 1994;54:362.
28. Kay R. Prepubertal testicular tumor registry. J Urol 1993:150:671.
29. Talerman A. Germ cell tumors. In: Talerman A, Roth LM, eds. Pathology of the testis and its adnexa. New York: Churchill Livingstone, 1986:29.
30. Ulbright TM, Roth LM, Brodhecker CA. Yolk sac differentiation in germ cell tumors: a morphologic study of 50 cases with emphasis on hepatic, enteric and parietal yolk sac features. Am J Surg Pathol 1986; 10:151.
31. Burke AP, Mostofi FK. Spermatocytic seminoma: a clinicopathologic study of 79 cases. J Urol Pathol 1993;1:21.
32. Cummings OW, Ulbright TM, Eble JN, Roth LM. Spermatocytic seminoma: an immunohistochemical study. Hum Pathol 1994;25:54.
33. True LD, Otis CN, Delprado W, Scully RE, Rosai J. Spermatocytic seminoma of testis with sarcomatous transformation: a report of five cases. Am J Surg Pathol 1988;12:75.
34. Kim I, Young RH, Scully RE. Leydig cell tumors of the testis: a clinicopathological analysis of 40 cases and review of the literature. Am J Surg Pathol 1985;9:177.
35. Nielsen K, Jacobsen GK. Malignant Sertoli cell tumor of the testis. An immunohistochemical study and a review of the literature. Acta Pathol Microbiol Immunol Scand 1988;96:755.
36. Tetu B, Ro JY, Ayala AG. Large cell calcifying Sertoli cell tumor of the testis: a clinocopathologic, immunohistochemical and ultrastructural study of two cases. Am J Clin Pathol 1991;96:717.
37. Jimenez-Quintero LP, Ro JY, Zavala-Pompa A, et al. Granulosa cell tumor of the adult testis: a clinicopathologic study of several cases and a review of the literature. Hun Pathol 1993;24:1120.
38. Ferry JA, Harris NL, Young RH, Coen J, Zietman A, Scully RE. Malignant lymphoma of the testis, epididymis, and spermatic cord: a clinicopathologic study of 69 cases with immunophenotypic analysis. Am J Surg Pathol 1994;18:376.
39. Orozco RE, Murphy WM. Carcinomas of the rete testis: case report and review of the literature. J Urol 1993;150:974.
40. DeNictolis M, Tommasoni S, Fabris G, Prat J. Intratesticular serous cystadenoma of borderline malignancy: a pathological, histochemical and DNA content study of a case with long-term follow-up. Virchows Arch A Pathol Anat Histopathol 1993:423:221.

Principles and Practice of Genitourinary Oncology, edited by Derek Raghavan, Howard I. Scher, Steven A. Leibel, and Paul H. Lange. Lippincott-Raven Publishers, Philadelphia, © 1997.

CHAPTER 63

Carcinoma in Situ of the Testis

Aleksander Giwercman and Niels E. Skakkebæk

Unlike most other solid tumors, cancer of the testis has its peak of incidence at a young age, between 20 and 40 years.[1] In fact, in the Western world, this is the most common malignant disease in men of this age. The treatment of patients with testicular cancer represents a special challenge because the youth of the survivors makes their quality of life such an important factor.[2] The discovery of the preinvasive stage of *carcinoma in situ* (CIS) as a precursor of testicular germ cell tumors,[3] however, has made possible the early diagnosis of testicular neoplasia. This discovery may in future reduce the need for aggressive therapy and may thereby limit the extent of serious side effects in patients who have achieved complete cure.[2] Additionally, studies of CIS of the testis not only have given new information relevant to clinical management of testicular neoplasia, but also have contributed to our understanding of the biology of cancer of the testis. In this chapter, histologic and immunohistochemical features of CIS are described in relation to the origin and diagnosis of this early neoplasia. Moreover, high-risk groups and the management of CIS, in view of the spontaneous course of this condition, are discussed.

MORPHOLOGIC ASPECTS OF CIS

CIS cells are usually located inside the seminiferous tubules at the site usually occupied by spermatogonia.[4] In routine histologic preparations, CIS cells show a close resemblance to seminoma cells. They are larger than spermatogonia, the nucleus is irregular in shape with coarse chromatin clumps, the nucleoli are distinct, and the intracytoplasmatic glycogen content is high.[4,5] At the ultrastructural marker level, however, CIS cells differ from the cells of seminomas,[5] and the DNA content of CIS, which is nearly tetraploid, seems to be higher than that of seminomas.[6,7]

In typical cases, in adults, CIS cells are located in one row along a thickened basement membrane with Sertoli cells as the only other cell type. In some cases, however, CIS cells may be found in tubules with ongoing spermatogenesis. Although CIS cells are usually found within the seminiferous tubules, they may invade the interstitial tissue, a finding that clearly demonstrates the malignant potential of these cells. Other evidence indicating the invasive ability of CIS cells is the occasional presence in the epithelium of the rete.[4]

CIS cells have also been seen in testes during the first months of life.[8,9] These cells are usually scant but are morphologically similar to the CIS cells found in adult testes. Furthermore, they resemble normal infantile germ cells, and they are scattered throughout the whole tubular diameter, not located along the basal membrane, as in adults.

CIS is usually associated with infiltration of mononuclear leukocytes in the interstitial tissue or even in the tubules.[9a] Such infiltration, the significance of which is not yet known, was found in approximately 70% of cases with CIS without invasive growth and in all cases of CIS accompanied by microinvasion or a tumor. In infantile testes with CIS, such leukocyte infiltration may also be found, although it is less frequent.

MARKERS OF CIS CELLS

CIS cells possess several ultrastructural, immunohistochemical, and chromosomal features by which they differ from spermatogonia and other germ cells of the normal spermatogenic epithelium. Studies of such markers have provided valuable information, which is important not only for diagnosis but also for studies on the pathogenesis and other biologic features of CIS.

Ultrastructural Markers

In semithin sections, large quantities of glycogen, a subplasmalemmal margin of microfilaments and cytoplasmic processes, have been found to be characteristic of CIS cells, by which they bear an extraordinary resemblance to gonocytes during the early embryonic period.[5,10–12] This resemblance has been confirmed by electron microscopic studies showing the so-called dense core vesicles, Nuage bodies, and lack of intercellular bridges, all features of early fetal germ cells.[13,14]

Immunohistochemical Markers

In nearly all cases of CIS, an immunohistochemical reaction with antibodies against placental-like alkaline phosphatase has been seen.[15–18] This marker is also usually seen in the cells of seminoma and to a varying degree in embryonal carcinomas. Alkaline phosphatase is also a well-known marker of fetal germ cells.[15,18,19] Immunohistochemically, alkaline phosphatase present in CIS is usually demonstrated by means of antibodies raised against placental alkaline phosphatase. Malignant germ cells contain a distinct type of this enzyme, the germ cell akaline phosphatase, which immunohistochemically cross-reacts with placental-like alkaline phosphatase, however.[18]

CIS cells have also been shown to possess antigens recognized by monoclonal antibodies M2A, 43-9F, and TRA-1-60, which react against different carbohydrate epitopes on the cell surface.[20–22] All three markers have also been found in fetal germ cells, with a peak of expression between the seventh and the 11th week of gestation, which means during the period of differentiation of the male gonad.[22a] M2A is also expressed by seminomas, but not by nonseminomas,[23] whereas 43-9F is a good marker of embryonal carcinoma (EC) and reacts only weakly or not at all with seminoma cells.[24] TRA-1-60 was originally raised against a human EC cell line,[25] and it reacts immunohistochemically with EC tissue but also to some degree with seminomas.[22]

High expression of the protooncogene *KIT* (formerly designated c-kit) has been found in CIS cells. *KIT* is known as a marker of early germ cells and seminomas.[26]

Chromosomal Markers

Densitometric studies performed on tissue samples have clearly demonstrated that CIS cells possess an aneuploid, near-tetraploid DNA content.[27] Studies on chromosomes of CIS germ cells have been hampered by lack of established CIS cell lines, however, and so have had only limited access to metaphase chromosomes. The limited information available has indicated that isochromosome 12p, which is a striking characteristic of seminomas as well as nonseminomas, may also be present in CIS cells.[28] By means of in situ hybridization, which allows studies of chromosomes in interphase nuclei, investigators have shown that numeric aberration of chromosome 12, a characteristic feature of germ cell tumors, is also seen in CIS cells.[29,30] The gene encoding for the so-called *stem cell factor,* a ligand for *KIT* protooncogene, is located on the long arm of chromosome 12. Whether *KIT* plays a role in the etiology and pathogenesis of testicular cancer is not yet known, however.

In situ hybridization has also provided other interesting information on the biology of CIS. These results are described in more detail elsewhere.[30]

POSSIBLE ORIGIN

As indicated earlier, CIS germ cells share several structural and immunologic characteristics with early embryonic germ cells. Consequently, investigators have proposed that CIS originates from a malignant transformation of fetal gonocytes.[31] Such transformation may take place during the first few weeks of fetal development, a period that seems to be critical for the development of the male gonad. The assumption of embryonal origin of CIS is also supported by epidemiologic data. Thus, boys born in Denmark during World War II had a significantly lower risk of testicular cancer than those born before and after this war.[32,33] This finding points to the importance of prenatal factors in the pathogenesis of testicular germ cell tumors and thereby also of CIS.

The worldwide increase in the incidence of testicular cancer seen during the past half-century has been accompanied by an apparent increase of other abnormalities of male genital organs. Thus, mean sperm density seems to have declined by 50% from 1940 to 1990.[34–36] Additionally, some data indicate a simultaneous rise in the frequency of testicular maldescent and hypospadias.[37–40] The connection among cryptorchidism, testicular neoplasia, and poor semen quality is well known. According to one hypothesis, all these abnormalities of male reproductive organs have a common fetal origin and are due to increased levels of maternal estrogens during early fetal development of the male gonad.[41] The experience with sons of mothers treated with diethylstilbestrol during early pregnancy[42] seems to support this hypothesis, which, however, remains to be proved.

SPONTANEOUS COURSE

In adults, in nearly 100% of cases, CIS cells are found in the tissue adjacent to testicular tumors, with spermatocytic seminoma as the only exception.[43,44] Thus, the consensus is that all testicular germ cell tumors in adults, except spermatocytic seminoma, have CIS as a precursor. Germ cell cancers found in the testes of adolescent boys seem to have a similar origin, whereas early infantile tumors may have a different etiology and pathogenesis. Moreover, extragonadal germ cell tumors, mainly those located mediastinally and intracranially, may not be related to CIS cells.[45]

Whereas clinicians and investigators generally accept that germ cell tumors, with the foregoing exceptions, are preceded by CIS, the spontaneous course of CIS is not completely known. Some parallels have been drawn between CIS in other sites, such as the uterine cervix, and CIS of the testis. Because the former only progresses to a cancer stage in approximately 50% of cases, investigators have been suggested that only half the men with CIS of the testis will develop a tumor. CIS germ cells seem to differ from CIS in other organs, however. Thus, although after 5 years of observation only 50% of men with CIS will develop a tumor, this figure increases if the time of observation is prolonged.[46,47] Unlike CIS of the cervix uteri, spontaneous regression of testicular CIS has not been reported. Because up to 40 years may elapse between the development of first and second testicular cancer,[48] however, CIS cells apparently have the potential to stay dormant for a long time before they progress into a tumor. Therefore, the likelihood is that untreated adult CIS will progress into a tumor.

Progression of CIS diagnosed at the age of 10 years to an adult CIS pattern and consequently to a seminoma has been reported.[8,47] Present knowledge does not allow to us draw any firm conclusions regarding the spontaneous course of CIS diagnosed in children, however.

Evidence indicates an early fetal origin of CIS cells.[31,49] What triggers the conversion from the CIS stage to a tumor and which factors are responsible for the development of these cells into seminoma and nonseminoma are unknown. The age distribution of testicular cancers, with a maximum peak between 20 and 40 years of age, may indicate that the sex steroids or gonadotropins, the secretions of which rapidly increase during puberty, are involved in the pathogenesis of testicular cancer.[49]

PREVALENCE IN DIFFERENT SUBGROUPS

Information on the prevalence of CIS in the *general male population* is limited. In a Danish autopsy study, no cases of CIS were found among 399 men aged 18 to 50 years, who died suddenly and unexpectedly; however, 3 of the men had previously had a testis removed: 2 because of cancer and 1 because of CIS. Thus, the overall freqency of malignant testicular disease was 0.8%.[50] The prevalence of CIS just after puberty, before CIS progresses to a tumor, is probably close to this figure because it can be assumed that the 2 men previously treated for testicular cancer would have been dignosed as having CIS if they had had a biopsy performed at a younger age. The lifetime risk of testicular cancer in Denmark is approximately 0.7%, and because this figure is close to the 0.8% frequency of malignancy, it supports the idea that most CIS progresses to a tumor stage.

Good epidemiologic data exist on the prevalence of CIS in the *contralateral testis of men with a unilateral testicular cancer*. In a Danish study, based on biopsies from 600 contralateral testes, CIS was found in 34, a figure corresponding to 5.7%.[47,51] Investigators have claimed that the high prevalence of contralateral CIS is a specific Danish phenomenon, because Denmark has one of the highest incidences of testicular cancer in the world. Additionally, based on some old studies, investigators suggested that only 2% to 3% of all men with testicular cancer have bilateral disease.[52] This suggestion indicates that either the prevalence of bilateral testicular neoplasia is higher in Denmark than in other countries or that only a proportion of CIS cases progesses into tumor stage. In these early studies on bilateral testicular cancer, however, no statistical correction was made for lethal outcome of the primary disease before a second tumor developed or for delay in the rise of the second cancer because of chemotherapy given for metastases from the first tumor. More recent epidemiologic studies have shown that the prevalence of bilateral testicular cancer, after correction for the foregoing factors, is in fact close to 5%.[53–55] Additionally, a study of more than 1000 contralateral biopsies has shown that 4.6% of German patients with testicular cancer harbour CIS in the contralateral testis.[54,56] No data are available from other countries.

Men with a *history of cryptorchidism* comprise a well-known risk group for testicular cancer. Based on studies from the 1940s, investigators have claimed that the relative risk of developing cancer in a maldescended testis is of a magnitude 40 to 50.[57,58] More recent studies, however, have confirmed that these men have an increased risk of testicular cancer, but the relative risk is of a magnitude 4 to 5.[59,60] A compilation of published data on testicular biopsies from maldescended testes has shown that a total of 17 cases of CIS were found in a total of 599 testes. Based on these data, the prevalence of CIS in maldescended testes was estimated to be 2% to 3%.[61]

Infertility is usually considered a risk factor for testicular cancer. Impairment of semen quality is often seen in men with testicular neoplasia. Male infertility is a common clinical designation covering different histopathologic conditions, however. Some of these conditions, such as obstructive azoospermia without an effect on spermatogenesis and the presence of Sertoli cells without germ cells in the testis, are not expected to increase the risk of testicular cancer. Thus, the available data, based on retrospective studies of testicular biopsies from men evaluated for infertility, do not answer the question whether infertile men have an increased risk of malignancy. These studies, based on heterogeneous groups of infertile men, showed frequencies of CIS varying from 0.4% in a British study, to 0.6% in a Swiss study, to 1% in a German trial, and finally to 1.1% in a Danish study.[4,62–64] Our present experience may indicate the need to focus on infertile men who have atrophic testes, low sperm counts, or a history of cryptorchidism,[65] but no such data are available.

Other individuals have rare clinical conditions associated with a high risk of testicular CIS. Thus, in one study, 40% of men with *assumed extragonadal germ cell tumor,* without any clinical sign of testicular tumor, were found to have CIS of the testis.[66] The gonadal neoplasia was only found in patients who had a retroperitoneal tumor, either isolated or with a mediastinal component, whereas no CIS was found in men with cancer limited to the mediastinum. *Intersex individuals,* both those with androgen insensitivity syndrome and those with gonadal dysgenesis, have a high risk of malignant gonadal disease.[9,67]

Information on the prevalence of CIS in different populations is important in planning screening programs for early testicular neoplasia and for counseling patients who belong to a high-risk group.

DIAGNOSIS

Patients with CIS, except intersex individuals, do not present with any characteristic clinical features. The testis harboring CIS is often atrophic and slightly tender, and the patient may have noted some shrinkage of the gonad. Otherwise, the CIS gives no warning of the threatening tumor, and even the classic germ cell tumor markers in serum are negative. Surgical testicular biopsy is the only reliable method for diagnosis of CIS.

Testicular Biopsy

Worldwide, thousands of biopsies have been performed as part of the examination of infertile men.[68] The biopsy can be performed, using local anesthesia, by the so-called "open-window technique," and a standard biopsy specimen is 3 mm in diameter. Complications are few and are usually insignificant, the most common being inflammation of the skin and minor hematoma.[68,69] A rise in the serum titer of antisperm antibodies has been seen in some men following the biopsy. This transitory immunologic reaction has no clinical implications, however.[70] No spread of malignant cells has been observed after biopsy from a testis harboring CIS, but biopsy should be avoided if a palpable tumor is present.

The sensitivity of biopsy in the diagnosis of CIS has been questioned. Experimental and clinical data indicate that testicular biopsy in adults is a sensitive tool in the diagnosis of CIS, because of the dispersed character of this neoplasia.[71,72] Despite the high number of biopsies performed worldwide, fewer than 10 cases of a negative biopsy followed by cancer development have been published.[73] Among more than 1500 of our high-

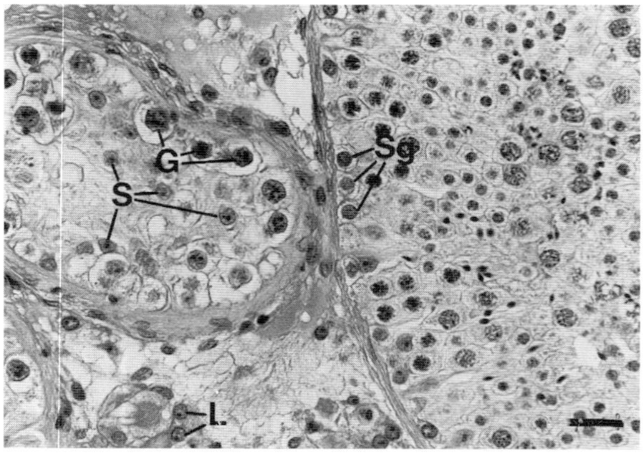

FIG. 63-1. Testicular biopsy of carcinoma in situ. Note a tubule with normal-appearing Sertoli cells (*S*) and carcinoma in situ germ cells (*G*) possessing several characteristics of malignancy. Beside the tubule with carcinoma in situ is another tubule with ongoing spermatogenesis including normal spermatogonia (*Sg*). In addition, the Leydig cells (*L*) appear normal. (Stieve's fixative; iron-hematoxylin and eosin staining; bar, 25 μm.)

risk patients who underwent a biopsy, only 1 developed a tumor during an observation period of up to 10 years.[74] Although we do not have any exact estimate of the sensitivity of a biopsy, available data indicate that this procedure is reliable, and if the biopsy is negative, the risk of subsequent cancer development, even in high-risk patients, is lower than in the general population. Because evidence indicates a fetal origin of CIS, cases of negative biopsy followed by a tumor should be explained by the occasional focal distribution of CIS, rather than by transformation of benign cells to CIS after the biopsy.

CIS changes may also be overlooked during routine histologic examination,[62] particularly if formalin is used as a fixative for tthe testicular biopsy specimen.[75] This fixative is unfit for preserving the histologic features of the testis and makes the diagnosis of CIS with routine hematoxylin and eosin staining impossible. We recommend Stieve's fixative or Bouin's fixative, which preserves the morphologic features of the testis as well as the known antigens of CIS cells.

Immunohistochemical staining with antibodies against placental-like alkaline phosphatase or some of the previously mentioned monoclonal antibodies may facilitate the diagnosis of CIS. This method is especially useful if the tissue has been fixed in formalin[16] (Figs. 63-1 through 63-4).

The foregoing considerations pertain to postpubertal biopsies. We do not have sufficient data on the sensitivity of a biopsy performed during infancy; however, the number of CIS cells before puberty is probably low and may be difficult to determine.[76]

Other Invasive Methods

Because surgical biopsy is not suitable as a general screening method, but rather is a tool to investigate high-risk groups, the demand exists for an alternative diagnostic procedure. Needle biopsy has been proposed as a possibility for obtaining tissue for assessment of testicular histologic features. The sensitivity of this method has not been proved, however, and our unpublished data, based on our limited experience, may indicate that a needle (Tru-Cut) biopsy is not sufficiently reliable in the diagnosis of CIS.

Investigators have reported that CIS cells may be aspirated by means of fine-needle technique and may be identified by means of immunocytochemistry or by flow cytometry because of their aneuploidy.[77,78] Data proving the sensitivity of this method are not yet available.

Noninvasive Methods

Although needle biopsy techniques may represent an improvement in screening for CIS, implementing screening programs would be more feasible if an easy and noninvasive method of detecting early testicular neoplasia were developed.

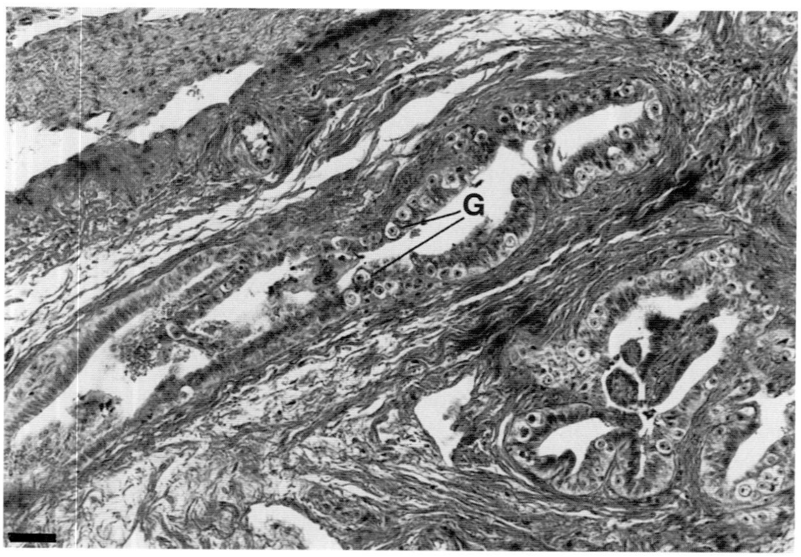

FIG. 63-2. Rete testis with invasive growth of CIS germ cells (*G*). (Histologic procedure as in Figure 63-1; bar, 50 μm.)

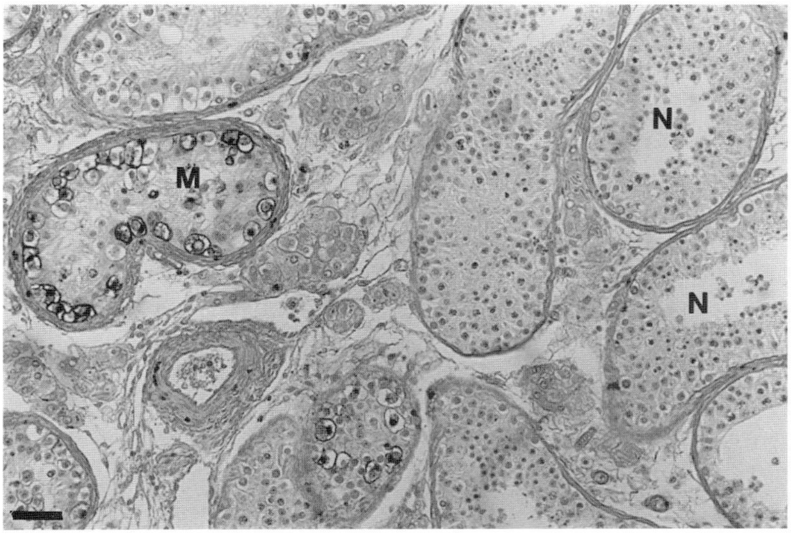

FIG. 63-3. Immunohistochemical staining with monoclonal antibody TRA-1-60. Note the positive staining in tubules with malignant CIS cells (*M*). The staining is mainly located at the surface of CIS cells. No staining occurs in tubules with normal spermatogenesis (*N*). (Stieve's fixative; immunoperoxidase streptavidin-biotin technique; counterstained with iron-hematoxylin; bar, 50 μm.)

Theoretically, to diagnose CIS by means of seminal analysis should be possible; the CIS cells are located inside the seminiferous tubules and are therefore expected to be exfoliated into semen, as are all types of normal germ cells.[79]

One of the major problems in the detection of CIS by semen analysis, however, is the identification of exfoliated cells, because the morphologic features of seminal cells other than sperm are poorly preserved. Therefore, recognition by using specific markers of CIS cells has been undertaken. By use of DNA flow cytometry[80] and in situ hybridization[81] for detection of aneuploidy and by means of immunocytochemical staining,[82] investigators have shown that CIS cells are exfoliated into seminal fluid. A need still exists for the development of a method sufficiently reliable to be used in large-scale screenings, however.[61]

Ultrasound may also be a useful tool in screening for CIS. Testes with CIS have an irregular echo pattern, which is, however, not specific for this early neoplasia. The method may possibly be used for identifying patients at particularly high risk of CIS, to whom a biopsy should be offered.[83–85] The results of the ultrasound scan depend on the equipment used and on the investigator. The pathophysiology of the irregular echo pattern of CIS testes has not yet been elucidated.

MANAGEMENT

Adults

As with other clinical aspects of CIS, most information on management pertains to adults. In such patients, management depends on whether the disease is *unilateral* or *bilateral*.

In men with unilateral CIS, such as infertile men or those with a history of cryptorchidism, orchidectomy is the treatment of choice. The patient can be assured that he is cured, although the standard staging procedure, including serum markers and

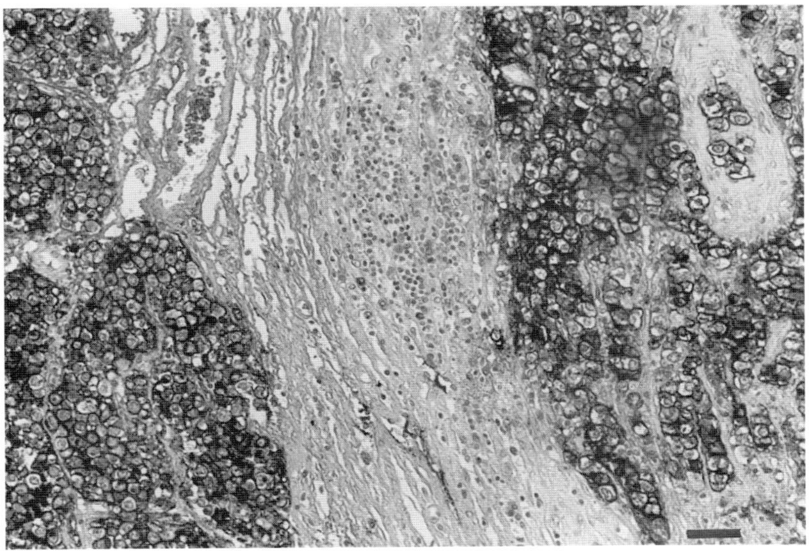

FIG. 63-4. Embryonal carcinoma reacting strongly with the monoclonal antibody TRA-1-60. (Immunoperoxidase technique as in Figure 63-3; bar, 50 μm.)

computed tomographic scanning, may be advisable. Early diagnosis is of great benefit to the patient by preventing the development of invasive cancer. Because CIS cells displace the cells of normal spermatogenesis, the testis harboring CIS ususally does not contribute to total sperm production.[86] The Leydig cell function of one testis is assumed to be sufficient to maintain normal testosterone levels. Androgen production should be assessed in these men to disclose possible signs of hypogonadism, however. Testicular cancer may occur as a bilateral disease, and patients with a history of unilateral cryptorchidism may have an increased risk of malignancy even in the normally descended testis. Therefore, a testis should not be removed because of CIS before a biopsy from the other gonad shows no evidence of CIS.

Patients with bilateral testicular neoplasia, typically those who had one testis removed because of cancer and who have CIS in the contralateral gonad, represent a therapeutic challenge. The high risk of tumor development in the remaining gonad[47] implicates the need for a second orchidectomy and, thus, the need for life-long androgen replacement therapy in these young individuals. Despite the possibility of giving testosterone to hypogonadal men, none of the existing methods of substitution has been ideal for these patients, who often experience changes in sexual function and other symptoms of hypogonadism.[52] In an attempt to avoid bilateral castration, localized irradiation was introduced in 1985 as treatment of CIS in the contralateral gonad.[87]

The goals of radiotherapy were to eradicate CIS cells to prevent cancer development and to preserve sufficient Leydig cell function. The first group of 20 patients, who received 10 doses of 2 Gy each of localized irradiation, has been followed for up to 9 years.[51] Follow-up biopsies performed 3 months and 2 years after the 20-Gy irradiation showed a uniform pattern of Sertoli cells, without germ cells. None of the 20 patients has developed a second tumor, and this observation, combined with the uniform lack of germ cells, indicates that all CIS cells were eradicated.[88] Thus, the first goal of radiotherapy has been achieved. Generally, no changes in libido or sexual function have been observed in this group. Significant increases in luteinizing hormone levels and decreases in human chorionic gonadotropin-stimulated testosterone concentration in serum have indicated some degree of Leydig cell involvement, however. The decline in basal testosterone has not reached the level of statistical significance, but because of the youth of these men, the development of clinically noticeable hypogonadism cannot be excluded.[88] Thus, lower doses of irradiation are being tested to find a treatment that eradicates CIS without affecting the Leydig cells. Our limited experience with giving 18 Gy or 16 Gy instead of 20 Gy indicates that these doses are sufficient to prevent cancer, whereas data on their effect on androgen production are not yet available.

The opponents of radiotherapy for CIS have claimed that such treatment may decrease the fertility of such men.[52]* The alternative for these patients is not life-long preservation of testicular function, however, because, untreated, CIS will progress to a tumor necessitating a second orchidectomy. For patients to maintain their own androgen production and not be dependent on full androgen replacement therapy is an advantage. Additionally, data indicate that men with CIS in the contralateral testis are infertile even before radiotherapy. Thus, in a group of 38 English men, none fathered a child during a period of 0.5 to 14 years between the diagnosis of first and second testicular cancer.[89] Furthermore, in a group of men harboring CIS in the contralateral gonad, a median sperm density of 0.3 million/mL was found, and only 1 of the 16 men had a sperm count in the range in which fertilization without the use of assisted reproduction techniques was considered probable.[86] Techniques such as *intracytoplasmatic sperm injection* allow fertilization using ejaculates with extremely low numbers of sperm, however. For this reason, all men with CIS who are candidates for radiotherapy need to have their semen examined, and the possibility of cryopreservation should be considered.

Consequently, in our opinion, radiotherapy must be offered to all men with contralateral CIS, if they are not treated with cytotoxic drugs for metastases from the primary tumor. The management of this group of patients who receive chemotherapy is still problematic, because no good data on the effect of chemotherapy on CIS exist. Disappearance of CIS from follow-up biopsies in men treated with chemotherapy has been reported,[90] but CIS cells may also reappear in the biopsy.[91] The best proof of resistance of CIS cells to cytotoxic drugs is that a second testicular tumor may arise even in men who receive chemotherapy after the diagnosis of the first gonadal cancer.[92] Thus, our clinical practice is not to offer radiotherapy first, but rather to observe patients with contralateral CIS who receive cytotoxic drugs. If CIS is present in one of the regular follow-up biopsies, testicular radiotherapy should be given. The need exists for data on the effect of cytotoxic drugs on CIS cells in relation to the dose and the type of drugs given, however.

Investigators have proposed that even patients without metastases should be given chemotherapy for contralateral CIS. In view of the many systemic side effects of chemotherapy and the unpredictable outcome with respect to contralateral cancer, we do not recommend such treatment.

Children

We cannot give general guidelines for the management of infantile CIS because our experience in the diagnosis and spontaneous course of CIS in this age group is so limited. The treatment of such patients should be a matter of individual preference. In many prepubertal patients, the diagnosis is made because of an intersex condition that requires careful consideration involving several medical specialists. These patients are known to have an extremely high risk of gonadal tumor, however, and removal of the gonad at a young age is often recommended.

The sensitivity of testicular biopsy performed before puberty may not be high. Thus, if no CIS is found in a prepubertal high-risk patient, the patient's course should be followed and the biopsy repeated after puberty.

CONCLUSIONS

The research on CIS of the testis has given us valuable information on the biology of testicular germ cell cancer. Increasing evidence indicates a fetal origin of germ cell neoplasia, and

*Editor's note: In addition, the late effects of low-dose radiotherapy to this tie in young men have not yet been defined.

further studies on CIS may provide us with information clarifying the etiology and pathogenesis of cancer of the testis.

In our clinical work, we should of course be happy about the excellent results in treatment of even advanced forms of testicular cancer. These young men pay a price for these benefits, however; their quality of life may be seriously affected, and the long-term consequences of aggressive chemotherapy are not yet known. Therefore, our goal should be to diagnose testicular neoplasia at the stage of CIS, before the need for adjuvant chemotherapy.

Testicular biopsy is the only method for reliable diagnosis of CIS at present. If a reliable noninvasive technique for early diagnosis becomes available, clinicians may consider whether screening for CIS should be offered to all young men.

In the meantime, testicular biopsy needs to be considered in some selected groups. The risk of malignant disease is so high in intersex individuals and in men with assumed extragonadal germ cell cancer that histologic examination of the gonads seems mandatory. Men with a history of cryptorchidism, a condition often seen in infertility clinics, should be informed about the magnitude of the cancer risk, and a biopsy may be recommended both as screening for CIS and as part of the infertility assessment. In men with unilateral testicular cancer, biopsy of the contralateral testis is recommended, especially at the time of primary orchidectomy. Because CIS can be cured by means of localized irradiation, the patient who has contralateral CIS can avoid bilateral castration if the diagnosis of neoplasia is made at this preinvasive stage.

ACKNOWLEDGMENT

The studies of our group were financially supported by grants from the Danish Cancer Society (Nos. 91-032 and 92-016).

REFERENCES

1. Prener A, Österlind A. Cancer in Denmark. Copenhagen, Danish Cancer Registry, 1985:44.
2. Hansen SW. Late-effects after treatment for germ-cell cancer with cisplatin, vinblastine, and bleomycin. Thesis. Copenhagen, Lægeforeningens Forlag, 1992:1.
3. Skakkebæk NE. Possible carcinoma-in-situ of the testis. Lancet 1972; 2:516.
4. Skakkebæk NE. Carcinoma in situ of the testis: frequency and relationship to invasive germ cell tumours in infertile men. Histopathology 1978;2:157.
5. Holstein AF, Schütte B, Becker H, Hartmann M. Morphology of normal and malignant germ cells. Int J Androl 1987;10:1.
6. Müller J, Skakkebæk NE. Microspectrophotometric DNA measurements of carcinoma-in-situ germ cells in the testis. Int J Androl 1981; (Suppl 4):211.
7. Oosterhuis JW, Castedo SMMJ, de Jong B, et al. Ploidy of primary germ cell tumors of the testis. Lab Invest 1989;60:14.
8. Müller J, Skakkebæk NE, Nielsen OH, Græm N. Cryptorchidism and testis cancer: atypical infantile germ cells followed by carcinoma in situ and invasive carcinoma in adulthood. Cancer 1984;54:629.
9. Müller J, Skakkebæk NE, Ritzén EM, Plöen L, Petersen KE. Carcinoma in situ of the testis in children with 45,X/46,XY gonadal dysgenesis. J Pediatr 1985;106:431.

9a. Jahnukainen IC, Jørgensen N, Pöllänen P, et al. Testicular mononuclear cell infiltrates in normal males and in patients with germ cell neoplasia. J Pathol (in press).

10. Holstein AF, Körner F. Light and electron microscopical analysis of cell types in human seminoma. Virchows Arch A Pathol Anat Histopathol 1974;363:97.
11. Gondos B. Ultrastructure of developing and malignant germ cells. Eur Urol 1993;23:68.
12. Gondos B, Berthelsen JG, Skakkebæk NE. Intratubular germ cell neoplasia (carcinoma in situ): a preinvasive lesion of the testis. Ann Clin Lab Sci 1983;13:185.
13. Nielsen H, Nielsen M, Skakkebæk NE. The fine structure of a possible carcinoma-in-situ in the seminiferous tubules in the testis of four infertile men. APMIS 1974;82:235.
14. Albrechtsen R, Nielsen MH, Skakkebæk NE, Wewer U. Carcinoma in situ of the testis: some ultrastructural characteristics of germ cells. APMIS 1982;90:301.
15. Hustin J, Collette J, Franchimont P. Immunohistochemical demonstration of placental alkaline phosphatase in various states of testicular development and in germ cell tumours. Int J Androl 1987;10:29.
16. Giwercman A, Cantell L, Marks A. Placental-like alkaline phosphatase as a marker of carcinoma-in-situ of the tesits: comparison with monoclonal antibodies M2A and 43-9F. APMIS 1991;99:586.
17. Manivel JC, Jessurun J, Wick MR, Dehner LP. Placental alkaline phosphatase immunoreactivity in testicular germ-cell neoplasms. Am J Surg Pathol 1987;11:21.
18. Hofmann MC, Millan JL. Developmental expression of alkaline phosphatase genes: reexpression in germ cell tumours and in vitro immortalized germ cells. Eur Urol 1993;23:38.
19. McKay DG, Hertig AT, Adams EC, Danziger S. Histochemical observations on the germ cells of human embryos. Anat Rec 1953;117:210.
20. Giwercman A, Marks A, Bailey D, Baumal R, Skakkebæk NE. A monoclonal antibody as a marker for carcinoma in situ germ cells of the human adult testis. APMIS 1988;96:667.
21. Giwercman A, Lindenberg S, Kimber SJ, Andersson T, Müller J, Skakkebæk NE. Monoclonal antibody 43-9F as a sensitive immunohistochemical marker of carcinoma in situ of human testis. Cancer 1990; 65:1135.
22. Giwercman A, Andrews PW, Jørgensen N, Müller J, Græm N, Skakkebæk NE. Immunohistochemical expression of embryonal marker TRA-1-60 in carcinoma in situ and germ cell tumors of the testis. Cancer 1993;72:1308.

22a. Jørgensen N, Rajpert-DeMeyts E, Green N, et al. Expression of immunohistochemical markers for testicular carcinoma *in situ* by normal human fetal germ cells. Lab Invest 1995;72:223.

23. Bailey D, Baumal R, Law J, et al. Production of monoclonal antibody specific for seminomas and dysgerminomas. Proc Natl Acad Sci USA 1986;83:5291.
24. Visfeldt J, Giwercman A, Skakkebæk NE. Monoclonal antibody 43-9F: an immunohistochemical marker of embryonal carcinoma of the testis. APMIS 1992;100:63.
25. Andrews PW, Banting G, Damjanov I, Arnaud D, Avner P. Three monoclonal antibodies defining distinct differentiation antigens associated with different high molecular weight polypeptides on the surface of human embryonal carcinoma cells. Hybridoma 1984;3:347.
26. Rajpert-De Meyts E, Skakkebæk NE. Expression of the c-kit protein product in carcinoma-in-situ and invasive testicular germ cell tumours. Int J Androl 1994;17:85.
27. Müller J, Skakkebæk NE, Lundsteen C. Aneuploidy as a marker for carcinoma-in-situ of the testis. APMIS 1981;89:67.
28. de Jong B, Oosterhuis JW, Castedo SMMJ, Vos A, te Meerman GJ. Pathogenesis of adult testicular germ cell tumors: a cytogenetic model. Cancer Genet Cytogenet 1990;48:143.
29. Vos AM, Oosterhuis JW, de Jong B, Buist J, Schraffordt Koops H. Cytogenetics of carcinoma in situ of the testis. Cancer Genet Cytogenet 1990;46:75.
30. Oosterhuis JW, Gillis AJM, van Putten WJL, de Jong B, Looijenga LHJ. Interphase cytogenetics of carcinoma in situ of the testis: numeric analysis of the chromosomes !, 12 and 15. Eur Urol 1993;23:16.
31. Skakkebæk NE, Berthelsen JG, Giwercman A, Müller J. Carcinoma-in-situ of the testis: possible origin from gonocytes and precursor of all types of germ cell tumours except spermatocytoma. Int J Androl 1987;10:19.
32. Møller H. Decreased testicular cancer risk in men born in wartime. J Natl Cancer Inst 1989;81:1668.
33. Møller H. Clues to the aetiology of testicular germ cell tumours from descriptive epidemiology. Eur Urol 1993;23:8.
34. Carlsen E, Giwercman A, Keiding N, Skakkebæk NE. Evidence for decreasing quality of semen during past 50 years. Br Med J 1992;305:609.
35. Auger J, Czyglik F, Kunstmann JM, Jouannet P. Significant decrease of semen characteristics of fertile men from Paris area during the last 20 years. Hum Reprod 1994;9(Suppl 4):72. Abstract.
36. Van Waeleghem K, De Clercq N, Vermeulen L, Schoonjans F, Comhaire F. Deterioration of sperm quality in young Belgian men during recent decades. Hum Reprod 1994;9(Suppl 40):73. Abstract.

37. Chilvers C, Pike MC, Forman D, Fogelman K, Wadsworth MEJ. Apparent doubling of frequency of undescended testis in England and Wales in 1962–81. Lancet 1984;2:330.
38. Jackson MB, John Radcliffe Hospital Cryptorchidism Research Group. The epidemiology of cryptorchidism. Horm Res 1988;30:153.
39. Källén B, Bertollini R, Castilla E, et al. A Joint International Study on the Epidemiology of Hypospadias. Acta Paediatr Scand 1986;(Suppl)324:5.
40. Anonymous. An increasing incidence of cryptorchidism and hypospadias? Lancet 1985;1:1311.
41. Sharpe RM, Skakkebæk NE. Are oestrogens involved in falling sperm counts and disorders of the male reproductive tract? Lancet 1993;341:1392.
42. Stillman RJ. In utero exposure to diethylstilbestrol: adverse effects on the reproductive tract and reproductive performance in male and female offspring. Am J Obstet Gynecol 1982;142:905.
43. Jacobsen GK, Henriksen OB, von der Maase H. Carcinoma in situ of testicular tissue adjacent to malignant germ-cell tumors: a study of 105 cases. Cancer 1981;47:2660.
44. Müller J, Skakkebæk NE, Parkinson MC. The spermatocytic seminoma: views on pathogenesis. Int J Androl 1987;10:147.
45. Oosterhuis JW, Looijenga LHJ. The biology of human germ cell tumours: retrospective speculations and new prospectives. Eur Urol 1993;23:245.
46. Skakkebæk NE, Berthelsen JG, Müller J. Carcinoma-in-situ of the undescended testis. Urol Clin North Am 1982;9:377.
47. von der Maase H, Rørth M, Walbom-Jørgensen S, et al. Carcinoma in situ of contralateral testis in patients with testicular germ cell cancer: study of 27 cases in 500 patients. Br Med J 1986;293:1398.
48. Philipsen JP, Gimbel HM. Cancer of the testis in an 80-year-old man with a former contralateral testicular cancer. Ugeskr Laeger 1994;156:2908.
49. Rajpert-De Meyts E, Skakkebæk NE. The possible role of sex hormones in the development of testicular cancer. Eur Urol 1993;23:54.
50. Giwercman A, Müller J, Skakkebæk NE. Prevalence of carcinoma-in-situ and other histopathological abnormalities in testes from 399 men who died suddenly and unexpectedly. J Urol 1991;145:77.
51. von der Maase H, Giwercman A, Müller J, Skakkebæk NE. Management of carcinoma-in-situ of the testis. Int J Androl 1987;10:209.
52. Grigor KM, Rørth M. Should the contralateral testis be biopsied? Round table discussion. Eur Urol 1993;23:129.
53. Õsterlind A, Berthelsen JG, Abildgaard N, et al. Risk of bilateral testicular germ cell cancer in Denmark: 1960–1984. J Natl Cancer Inst 1991;83:1391.
54. Dieckmann K-P, Loy V. Prevalence of bilateral testicular germ cell tumors and early detection by testicular intraepithelial neoplasia. Eur Urol 1993;23(Suppl 2):22.
55. Thompson J, Williams CJ, Whitehouse JMA, Mead GM. Bilateral testicular germ cell tumours: an increasing incidence and prevention by chemotherapy. Br J Urol 1988;62:374.
56. Loy V, Dieckmann K-P. Prevalence of contralateral testicular intraepithelial neoplasia (carcinoma in situ) in patients with testicular germ cell tumour. Eur Urol 1993;23:120.
57. Gilbert JB, Hamilton JB. Studies in malignant testis tumors. III. Incidence and nature of tumors in ectopic testes. Surg Gynecol Obstet 1940;71:731.
58. Campbell HE. Incidence of malignant growth of the undescended testicle. Arch Surg 1942;44:353.
59. Henderson BE, Benton B, Jing J, Yu MC, Pike MC. Risk factors for cancer of the testis in young men. Int J Cancer 1979;23:598.
60. Giwercman A, Grindsted J, Hansen B, Jensen OM, Skakkebæk NE. Testicular cancer risk in boys with maldescended testis: a cohort study. J Urol 1987;138:1214.
61. Giwercman A. Carcinoma-in-situ of the testis: screening and management. Scand J Urol Nephrol 1992;148(Suppl):1.
62. Pryor JP, Cameron KM, Chilton CP, et al. Carcinoma in situ in testicular biopsies from men presenting with infertility. Br J Urol 1983;55:780.
63. Nüesch-Bachmann IH, Hedinger C. Atypische Spermatogonienals Präkanzerose. Schweiz Med Wochenschr 1977;107:795.
64. Schütte B. Early testicular cancer in severe oligozoospermia. In: Holstein AF, Leidenberger F, Hölzer KH, Bettendorf G, eds. Carl Schirren Symposium: advances in andrology. Berlin, Diesbach Verlag, 1988:188.
65. Berthelsen JG, Skakkebæk NE, von der Maase H, Sørensen BL, Mogensen P. Screening for carcinoma in situ of the contralateral testis in patients with germinal testicular cancer. Br Med J 1982;285:1683.
66. Daugaard G, Rørth M, von der Maase H, Skakkebæk NE. Management of extragonadal germ-cell tumors and the significance of bilateral testicular biopsies. Ann Oncol 1992;3:283.
67. Müller J, Skakkebæk NE. Testicular carcinoma in situ in children with androgen insensitivity (testicular feminisation) syndrome. Br Med J 1984;288:1419.
68. Rowley MJ, Heller CG. The testicular biopsy: surgical procedure, fixation, and staining technics. Fertil Steril 1966;17:177.
69. Bruun E, Frimodt-Møller C, Giwercman A, Lenz S, Skakkebæk NE. Testicular biopsy as an outpatient procedure in screening for carcinoma-in-situ: complications and the patient's acceptance. Int J Androl 1987;10:199.
70. Hjort T, Linnet L, Skakkebæk NE. Testicular biopsy: indications and complications. Eur J Pediatr 1982;138:23.
71. Berthelsen JG, Skakkebæk NE. Distribution of carcinoma-in-situ in testes from infertile men. Int J Androl 1981;(Suppl 4):172.
72. Mumperow E, Lauke H, Holstein AF, Hartmann M. Further practical experiences in the recognition and management of carcinoma in situ of the testis. Urol Int 1992;48:162.
73. Dieckmann K-P, Kaup F, Loy V. False-negative biopsy for testicular intraepithelial neoplasia. J Cancer Res Clin Oncol 1993;119:1.
74. Giwercman A, Berthelsen JG, Müller J, von der Maase H, Skakkebæk NE. Screening for carcinoma-in-situ of the testis. Int J Androl 1987;10:173.
75. Schütte B. The importance of fixatives for detection of carcinoma-in-situ (CIS) in testicular tissue. Andrologia 1988;20:422.
76. Müller J. Abnormal infantile germ cells and development of carcinoma-in-situ in maldeveloped testes: a stereological and densitometric study. Int J Androl 1987;10:543.
77. Brackenbury ET, Hargreave TB, Howard GCW, McIntyre MA. Seminal fluid analysis and fine-needle aspiration cytology in the diagnosis of carcinoma in situ of the testis. Eur Urol 1993;23:123.
78. Nagler HM, Kaufman DG, O'Toole KM, Sawczuk IS. Carcinoma in situ of the testes: diagnosis by aspiration flow cytometry. J Urol 1990;143:359.
79. World Health Organization. WHO laboratory manual for the examination of human semen and sperm-cervical mucus interaction, 3rd Ed. Cambridge, Cambridge University Press, 1992.
80. Giwercman A, Clausen OPF, Skakkebæk NE. Carcinoma in situ of the testis: aneuploid cells in semen. Br Med J 1988;296:1762.
81. Giwercman A, Hopman AHN, Ramaekers FCS, Skakkebæk NE. Carcinoma in situ of the testis: detection of malignant germ cells in seminal fluid by means of in situ hybridization. Am J Pathol 1990;136:497.
82. Giwercman A, Marks A, Skakkebæk NE. Carcinoma-in-situ germ-cells exfoliated from seminiferous epithelium into seminal fluid. Lancet 1988;1:530.
83. Lenz S, Giwercman A, Skakkebæk NE, Bruun E, Frimodt-Møller C. Ultrasound in detection of early neoplasia of the testis. Int J Androl 1987;10:187.
84. Lenz S, Giwercman A, Elsborg A, Cohr K-H, Jelnes JE. Ultrasonic testicular texture and size in 444 men from the general population: correlation to semen quality. Eur Urol 1993;24:231.
85. Giwercman A, Lenz S, Skakkebæk NE. Carcinoma-in-situ in atrophic testis selected for biopsy by abnormal ultrasound pattern. Br J Urol 1993;72:118.
86. Giwercman A, von der Maase H, Rørth M, Skakkebæk NE. Semen quality in testicular tumour and CIS in the contralateral testis. Lancet 1993;341:384.
87. von der Maase H, Giwercman A, Skakkebæk NE. Radiation treatment of carcinoma-in-situ of testis. Lancet 1986;1:624.
88. Giwercman A, von der Masse H, Berthelsen JG, Rørth M, Bertelsen A, Skakkebæk NE. Localized irradiation of testes with carcinoma in situ: effects on Leydig cell function and eradication of malignant germ cells in 20 patients. J Clin Endocrinol Metab 1991;73:596.
89. Fordham MVP, Mason MD, Blackmore C, Hendry WF, Horwich A. Management of the contralateral testis in patients with testicular germ cell cancer. Br J Urol 1990;65:290.
90. von der Maase H, Berthelsen JG, Jacobsen GK, et al. Carcinoma-in-situ of testis eradicated by chemotherapy. Lancet 1985;1:98.
91. von der Maase H, Meinecke B, Skakkebæk NE. Residual carcinoma-in-situ of contralateral testis after chemotherapy. Lancet 1988;1:477.
92. Fosså SD, Aass N. Cisplatin-based chemotherapy does not eliminate the risk of a second testicular cancer. Br J Urol 1989;63:531.

Principles and Practice of Genitourinary Oncology, edited by Derek Raghavan, Howard I. Scher, Steven A. Leibel, and Paul H. Lange. Lippincott-Raven Publishers, Philadelphia, © 1997.

CHAPTER 64

Testicular Cancer

Presentation, Assessment and Prognosis

Alan Horwich and Dean Bajorin

PRESENTATION

The characteristic and usual presentation of a testicular germ cell tumor (GCT) is that of a painless, hard, swollen testis. However, 10% to 20% of patients complain of pain in the testis, and a larger number have had episodic pain in the past.[1,2] Pain may be secondary to hemorrhage within the testis, and in 15% to 20% of cases the symptom seems to date from an episode of trauma.[1,3] The presence of pain and local tenderness often leads to the erroneous diagnosis of epididymoorchitis; this can be a cause of significant delay in instituting appropriate treatment.[2]

Ninety to 95% of men with GCTs present with a testicular primary lesion, although in about 5% of these the primary lesion is occult within the testis[4] and is disclosed by testicular ultrasonography. GCTs may also arise at extragonadal sites, especially in the retroperitoneum, mediastinum, and pineal area.[5] Another cause of occult presentation is when the primary lesion appears to have regressed; this is suspected when histologic section of the testis reveals a scar in the patient with metastatic GCT.[6]

Other symptoms and signs of metastatic or extragonadal tumors depend on the site and volume of disease. Retroperitoneal lymphadenopathy can be a cause of severe backache that usually is unrelated to posture or recent physical exertion, and larger masses can cause ureteric obstruction, renal displacement, duodenal obstruction, or bleeding. Occasionally, there is posterior extension, which may invade bone or cause spinal cord compression. Lung metastases may cause cough or hemoptysis, but dyspnea is unusual unless the disease is very extensive. Gynecomastia and galactorrhea may occur and usually are associated with endocrine metabolism disorder secondary to a high serum concentration of human chorionic gonadotrophin (hCG).

The pattern at presentation is influenced by the histologic subtype of the tumor. Figure 64-1 shows that patients with nonseminomatous tumors present at an earlier age than those with seminomas; median ages are approximately 25 and 35 years, respectively. In patients with nonseminoma, the average length of history of symptoms is just under 3 months.[7] However, with primary testicular seminoma, the history of testicular abnormality may be 1 to 2 years in duration.

The stage distribution is also distinct, as shown in Figure 64-2, which is based on new patients at the Royal Marsden Hospital (RMH) between 1980 and 1993, staged by tumor marker analysis and computed tomography (CT) of the thorax, abdomen, and pelvis. For seminoma, approximately 70% of patients present at RMH stage I, 25% present with retroperitoneal metastases, and more widespread metastases are distinctly uncommon. However, for all nonseminomatous tumors, about 50% present at stage I, and in the context of metastatic disease, the vast majority of patients have retroperitoneal lymphadenopathy, lung metastases, or a combination of both. Widespread extranodal involvement is more typical of trophoblastic tumors than tumors of other histologic types.[8] For seminoma, extranodal metastases are rare; characteristic sites include lung, pleura, liver, and bone. In nonseminoma, extranodal metastases predominantly affect the lung. Liver, bone, and brain involvement are uncommon.

In patients with testicular nonseminoma, there is some evidence of a change in stage distribution in successive patient cohorts comparing those presenting between 1976 and 1982 with those presenting between 1982 and 1986. Table 64-1 shows patients from multicenter prognostic factor analyses relating to these two treatment periods,[9,10] and the data is presented in terms of the volume of metastatic disease. Between 1976 and 1982, 30% of patients presented with large-volume disease, whereas in the later time period, disease volume fell to 13%; this is probably the result of greater public awareness of testicular cancer.

Additionally, in testicular seminoma, there is evidence for a recent change in stage distribution, with both an increase in the proportion of patients presenting with stage I disease and a reduction in the mean maximum diameter of the primary tumor.[10]

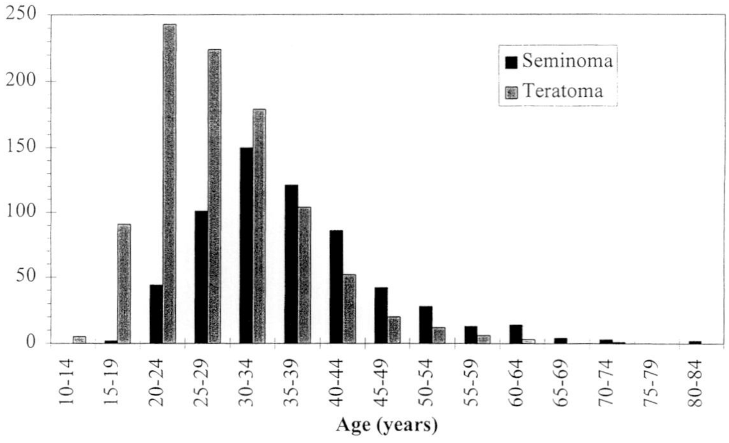

FIG. 64-1. Incidence of seminoma and all nonseminoma by age group. (Data from Royal Marsden NHS Trust, 1980–1988.)

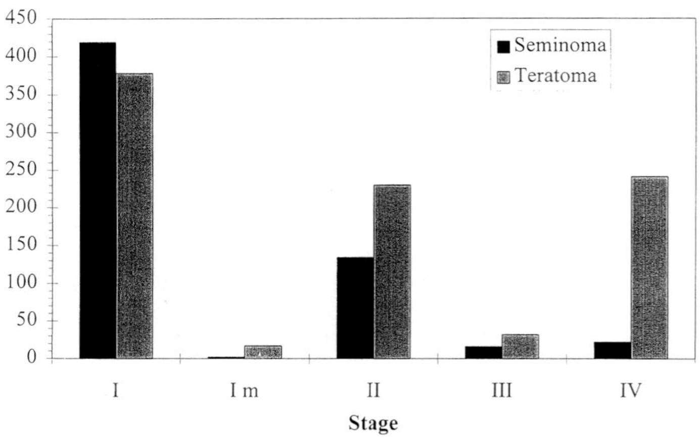

FIG. 64-2. Stage distribution of testicular germ cell tumors staged by computed tomographic scanning. (Data from Royal Marsden NHS Trust, 1980–1989.)

TABLE 64-1. *Medical Research Council prognostic factors analysis*

		Treatment period 1976–1982		Treatment period 1982–1986	
Category	Stage	No. of patients	3-yr survival (%)	No. of patients	3-yr survival (%)
Small volume	I M	18	83	78	95
	II III AB	106	87	253	92
	IV L1 L2 AB	70	75	200	90
Large volume	IIC IIIC	104	85	82	82
	IV L1 L2 C	43	77	37	89
Very large volume	IV L3 H+ Bo Br	117	54	145	60

A, abdominal nodes ≤2 cm; B, abdominal nodes 2–5 cm; Bo, bone; Br, brain; C, abdominal nodes ≥5 cm; H+, liver; L1, 3 or fewer lung metastases; L2, more than 3 lung metastases, all smaller than 2 cm in diameter; L3, more than 3 lung metastases with at least 1 larger than 2 cm in diameter; M, marker positive.

From MRC Working Party on Testicular Tumours, Peckham MJ. Prognostic factors in advanced nonseminomatous germ-cell testicular tumours: results of a multicentre study. Lancet 1985;1:8; and Mead GM, Stenning SP, Parkinson MC, et al. The second Medical Research Council Study of prognostic factors in nonseminomatous germ cell tumours. J Clin Oncol 1992;10(1):85.

DIAGNOSIS

The initial diagnosis is based on careful clinical examination of the testis. This should be performed first with the patient standing. A testis containing a tumor is usually heavier and lies lower than the normal testis, whereas an inflammatory condition or torsion of the testis tends to raise it. With the patient in the prone position, the testis can be held stably in one hand while using the thumb, index, and middle fingers of the other hand to palpate to assess its consistency and to localize any areas of induration. A small tumor is identifiable as a hard swelling within the body of the testis, but as the tumor becomes larger, the testis appears to be uniformly replaced by harder and heavier tissue. At this stage, there is a loss of the sensation of pain on gentle pressure.

In cases of doubt, testicular ultrasonography or assay of serum tumor markers may help to elucidate the diagnosis.[11,12] However, there is a false-negative rate with ultrasonography of the order of 5% to 12%,[13] and when doubt continues to exist, the testicle should be explored surgically. An alternative approach for a primary tumor or a metastasis is fine needle biopsy, although this may create the risk of track recurrence.

Clinically, the differential diagnosis includes epididymitis, torsion of the testis, tuberculosis, gumma, and granulomatous orchitis. Surgical exploration offers a definitive diagnosis and also provides a specimen for pathologic definition of the tumor subtype. Where there is a testicular lesion, the diagnosis is rarely difficult. However, for anaplastic extragonadal presentation, the histopathologic diagnosis may be supported by staining for tumor markers. Alphafetoprotein (AFP), hCG, or both are expressed in about 75% of nonseminomas, and staining for placental alkaline phosphotase can be helpful in identifying seminoma (see Chap. 65). When markers are not expressed, a strong clue to the diagnosis can be provided by cytogenetic analysis to identify the isochromosome 12p (see Chap. 60).[14]

Early diagnosis and appropriate referral are important to maximize the cure rate of these tumors. As discussed in the following section, prognosis relates to the extent of disease at presentation. Bosl and colleagues[15] have shown that the median delay for stage I tumors was 75 days, for stage II tumors was 101 days, and for stage III tumors was 134 days. Some of this delay in diagnosis is the result of ignorance of the disease among the general public and could be corrected by education programs in school. However, another component of the delay in diagnosis is medical misdiagnosis.[1,2] Erman[16] found that the correct diagnosis was established at the first consultation in only 43% of patients.

The prognostic importance of delayed diagnosis is suggested by the retrospective prognostic factor analyses performed by the Medical Research Council (MRC).[8,9] However, the RMH analyses (Table 64-2) showed an inverse relation between delay and survival[7]; this may be because rapidly progressing tumors led to a more urgent presentation.

Diagnosis should be followed by appropriate referral to a physician with particular experience in the management of GCT. A recent observational study based on 440 men with nonseminoma showed that the risk of dying more than doubled if the patient was not managed in a specialist testicular tumor unit.[17]

TABLE 64-2. *Distribution of patients with adverse prognostic factors in relation to length of delay in diagnosis*

	Delay in diagnosis (days)		
Prognostic factor	0–49	50–99	100 or more
STAGE			
I	45	42	39
II	17	15	27
III and IV	22	20	30
Total	84	77	96
MARKERS			
Low*	25	22	32
High	17	14	26
Total	42	36	58
TUMOR VOLUME			
Stage I marker negative	42	41	38
Small†	29	23	26
Large†	7	8	16
Very large†	6	5	16
Total	84	77	96

* Alphafetoprotein <500 IU 1^{-1} and human chorioric gonadotropin <IU 1^{-1}.

† As classified by Medical Research Council Working Party on Testicular Tumors, Peckham MJ. Prognostic factors in advanced non-seminomatous germ-cell testicular tumors: results of a multicentre study. Lancet 1985;1:8.

Data from Royal Marsden NHS Trust, 1980–1986.

From Chilvers CED, Saunders M, Bliss JM, Nicholls J, Horwich A. Influence of delay in diagnosis in prognosis in testicular teratoma. Br J Cancer 1989;59:126.

PATIENT INVESTIGATION

Investigation of the patient must include an evaluation of the patient's general medical fitness to tolerate treatment, an assessment of the extent of the tumor, and the information necessary to estimate prognosis.

History and Examination

The pattern of symptoms may indicate the extent of metastatic disease, and as previously discussed, backache may be a clue to the development of retroperitoneal lymphadenopathy or renal obstruction. Gynecomastia or galactorrhea, especially in the context of other evidence of widespread metastases, may be a sign of a trophoblastic tumor, alerting the clinician to the potential for rapid disease progression.[8] Other particular points to establish from the patient history include a past medical history of maldescent,[7] because this contributes to judgment of risk of a contralateral testicular tumor.[18] A history of previous inguinal surgery can alter the pattern of lymph node metastasis such that first-station nodes may be in the inguinal region rather than in the paraaortic region.[19] A full family history is important, since there is evidence for genetic predisposition.[20] Physical examination can provide a strong clue for the diagnosis of testicular tumor, as described previously. The physical examination should include careful palpation of the contralateral testis as well as the assessment of potential sites of metastases. Other measures of general medical health should always include cardiovascular assessment, complete blood count, and assessment of renal and liver function.

Disease Extent

Tumor marker analyses are particularly well developed for GCTs because of the sensitivity and specificity of assays for tumor product, hCG, and AFP.[19] Other markers, such as placental-like alkaline phosphatase[21] and serum lactate dehydrogenase (LDH),[22] can be useful in both diagnosis and assessment of prognosis. When serum markers are assessed following orchidectomy, a sequence of markers is more informative than a single assay because of the finite time for clearance of markers from the serum, even in patients without metastases. The maximum rate of decline in AFP concentration is a halving time of approximately 5 days (36 hours for hCG); thus, the finding of an elevated marker following orchidectomy may not indicate the presence of metastases. However, a sequence of markers showing a rise in serum concentration always indicates metastatic disease. There is a potential for using these markers for radioimmunoscintigraphy; however, this approach remains experimental.[23,24]

Staging of the Retroperitoneum

Left testicular tumors predominantly affect the left paraaortic nodes just beneath the renal vessels and, subsequently, the preaortic nodes. Right-sided tumors commonly metastasize to the interaorticocaval nodes, the precaval nodes, and the right paraaortic region in general; however, 20% of right-sided tumors involve contralateral nodes. Crossover is much more rare for left-sided tumors.[25,26] Pedal lymphography may miss involvement of the echelon node, which characteristically is located adjacent to the right renal hilum.[27,28]

Historically, retroperitoneal nodes were investigated by bipedal lymphography, because this modality could identify involvement of external iliac, common iliac, and paraaortic chains, with metastases appearing as a filling defect within the node. Bipedal lymphography is sensitive, but only in a limited range of abdominal structures; furthermore, the procedure is uncomfortable for patients and time-consuming. Even when facilities are available, bipedal lymphography has largely been superseded by CT of the abdomen and pelvis. Sensitivity and specificity of CT depend on the scanning protocol and the criteria for defining lymph node abnormality.[29,30] At a conventional level of 15-mm-diameter nodal size, the specificity of defining involvement was 98%, compared with 67% if the threshold for diagnosing metastasis was reduced to a node of 5-mm in diameter.[31] In practice, the site of enlarged nodes is taken into account, as is the degree of node enlargement, and in doubtful cases, the assessment can be supplemented either by bipedal lymphography or by a repeat of the CT scan 4 to 6 weeks later.

The abdominal CT scan can also reveal evidence of renal outflow obstruction or metastases in other organs such as the liver. The examination is well tolerated by patients and can reveal abnormalities in the echelon nodes and also in the upper retroperitoneal and retrocrural nodes. CT provides a better definition of lymph node size and therefore lymphography.

Retroperitoneal lymphadenopathy can also be detected by abdominal ultrasonography, especially in a thin patient with bulky disease[32,33] or liver disease.[34] Nevertheless, there is limit to the sensitivity of radiologic techniques to detect small-volume lymph node involvement. Evidence from surgical series or surveillance policies in stage I cancers suggest that false-negative results occur in 30% to 40% of patients with stage I nonseminoma[35,36] and in 15% to 20% of patients with stage I seminoma of the testis.[37–39]

Retroperitoneal Lymph Node Dissection

Retroperitoneal lymph node dissection (RPLND) is a sensitive method of detecting retroperitoneal lymph node involvement and is in widespread use in the United States and some European countries, although not in the United Kingdom. This technique is not only regarded as diagnostic but is also therapeutic, with a high chance of curing patients with limited nodal involvement.[35] This technique is mainly used in patients with nonseminomatous tumors, and traditionally, the approach used is a bilateral dissection of nodes around the inferior vena cava, aorta, and ipsilateral common iliac vessels.[40,41] The probability of detecting nodal metastases using this technique can be predicted by the presence of lymphatic or vascular invasion in the primary tumor.[42–44] RPLND has the advantage of highly accurate staging, which is a guide to prognosis and the need for adjuvant chemotherapy. The problems with RPLND are that if the nodal histology is positive, there remains a 30% to 50% relapse risk which requires either close surveillance or adjuvant chemotherapy, and if the node dissection is negative, there remains a 10% relapse risk in the thorax which requires surveillance. Additionally, the traditional bilateral dissection causes loss of ejaculation[45] as a result of dissection of autonomic nerves; however, nerve-sparing techniques have been developed.[46] These techniques require both skill and specific experience, and the use of RPLND in all patients is being questioned.[47–49]

Staging of the Thorax

A simple chest x-ray film is a very useful screen for lung or mediastinal metastases; however, these may be detected with greater sensitivity using a thoracic CT scan.[50,51]

Summary of Initial Assessment

The investigation of patients with testicular GCTs begins with confirmation of the diagnosis, usually following orchidectomy. Basic investigations include CT scan of the thorax and abdomen and assay of serum tumor markers; additionally, patients should have assessments of their general medical health, fertility, contralateral testis, and psychosocial adjustment. In selected patients, it is reasonable to perform baseline lung function and auditory function tests to monitor the effects of bleomycin and cisplatin, respectively. Central nervous system screening should be reserved for those with an hCG level higher than 10^5 U/L or those with multiple lung metastases; magnetic resonance (MR) is probably more sensitive than CT of the brain in this regard. When surgery of enlarged lymph nodes is contemplated, their relation to the renal vessels and inferior vena cava should be established by contrast radiography or MR.

HISTOLOGY OF TESTIS TUMORS

The vast majority of primary testis tumors arise from germinal cells and are either seminomatous or nonseminomatous tumors. There have been numerous attempts to classify the histology of testicular GCTs. The system used in the United States has evolved from the Dixon and Moore classification[52] with modification by the World Health Organization (WHO) classification systems reported by Mostofi and Sobin.[53] In contrast, pathologists in the United Kingdom use the British Testicular Tumor Panel classification system of Pugh.[54]

One major difference between the two classification systems is the use of the term *teratoma*. In the British system, the term teratoma includes all nonseminomatous germ cell tumor (NSGCT) components, which are then divided into subsets of differentiated, intermediated, and undifferentiated tumors. In the WHO system, the use of the term teratoma is restricted to a subset of tumors with low malignant potential, and embryonal carcinoma is the term representing the most undifferentiated form of teratoma. Despite these differences, correlations between the two systems are readily apparent (Table 64-3).

Fewer than 5% of testis tumors are nongerminal neoplasms and are grouped as tumors of the gonadal stroma. These tumors are more frequently seen in children and, as a group, behave in a more benign fashion. These include Sertoli cell tumors, Leydig cell tumors, and granulosa-theca cell tumors.[55]

SERUM TUMOR MARKERS OF PROGNOSTIC IMPORTANCE IN GERM CELL TUMORS

Human Chorionic Gonadotrophin

hCG, a glycoprotein normally secreted by the placenta during pregnancy, is composed of two subunits: the α-subunit, which is identical to that of pituitary glycoprotein hormones (luteinizing hormone [LH], follicle-stimulating hormone [FSH] and thyroid-stimulating hormone [TSH]), and the β-subunit, which has some homology with the α-subunit of LH, FSH, and TSH but is uniquely distinct in the terminal 29 amino acids.[56] hCG is produced by syncytiotrophoblastic cells, and elevated values can be found in patients with pure seminoma as well as in those with nonseminomatous histologies.[57] The presence of hCG does not imply the presence of choriocarcinoma, which is a histologic GCT variant with both syncytiotrophoblasts and cytotrophoblasts.

A variety of radioimmunoassays for the β-subunit are available to determine hCG levels in serum. Results of various types of assays for hCG may differ substantially; until recently, the ratio of milliinternational units (mIU) to nanograms (ng) was not standardized among the various kits, making direct interinstitutional comparisons impossible.[58] The adoption of the World Health Organization Third International Standard (code number 75/537), which has a mIU-ng ratio of 9.3 : 1, will establish uniformity for this assay; most radioimmunoassay vendors now conform to this standard.

As a result of earlier detection of disease and the phenomenon of stage migration, only 40% of patients with advanced disease present with elevated values of hCG compared with approximately 60% in earlier clinical trials, and the degree to which the hCG level is elevated has decreased over time.[59,60] Approximately 7% to 18% of patients with pure seminoma present or develop an elevated hCG level in the course of their disease.[61,62] False elevations of hCG have been reported in GCT patients as a result of treatment-induced hypogonadism, either from cross-reactivity of the antibody with LH in the assay for hCG or from the pituitary production of hCG.[63–65]

Alphafetoprotein

AFP, a glycoprotein with a molecular weight of approximately 70 kd, is produced in the liver, gastrointestinal tract,

TABLE 64-3. *Classification systems for germ cell tumors*

Dixon and Moore, 1952[52]	Mostofi and Sobin, 1977[53]	Pugh, 1976[54]
	TUMORS OF ONE HISTOLOGIC TYPE	
Seminoma	Seminoma	Seminoma
	Spermatocytic seminoma	Spermatocytic seminoma
	Seminoma with high mitotic index	
Embryonal carcinoma	Embryonal carcinoma	Malignant teratoma, undifferentiated
	Polyembryoma	
Teratoma, adult	Teratoma	Teratoma, differentiated
	Mature	
	Immature with malignant areas	
	Yolk sac tumor	Yolk sac tumor, child
		Malignant teratoma, undifferentiated, adult
	Choriocarcinoma	Malignant teratoma, trophoblastic
	TUMORS OF MORE THAN ONE HISTOLOGIC TYPE	
Teratoma with embryonal carcinoma (teratocarcinoma)	Embryonal carcinoma with teratoma (teratocarcinoma)	Malignant teratoma, intermediate
	Choriocarcinoma and any other types	Malignant teratoma, trophoblastic
	Other combinations	Combined tumor when seminoma present

and yolk sac of the fetus. The normal adult concentration of AFP is usually less than 15 ng/mL. AFP is detected using a radioimmunoassay, and values are reported predominantly in nanograms per milliliter (ng/mL) or kilounits per liter (kU/L).[66] The ratio of kU to ng is 1.2 : 1, which makes conversions simpler than those with hCG.

The production of AFP is restricted to endodermal sinus tumors and embryonal carcinoma. An elevated level of AFP in a patient with pure seminoma as determined by histology reflects undetected nonseminomatous components. As has been observed with hCG, there has been a decline in the degree of AFP elevation as a consequence of stage migration.[67] Elevated serum levels of AFP have also been observed in patients with other tumors and in those with benign conditions such as ataxia telangiectasia and hepatocellular injury with regeneration.[68]

Lactate Dehydrogenase

The serum level of LDH has independent significance in advanced GCT patients. LDH has a relatively constant rate of degradation among patients, and increases in the serum level are influenced primarily by tumor burden, growth rate, and cell proliferation and death. LDH is elevated in approximately 60% of NSGCT patients with advanced disease and 80% of patients with advanced seminoma. LDH is more frequently elevated than hCG or AFP in both metastatic NSGCT and seminoma.[62,69]

The serum level of LDH comprises multiple isoenzymes, and performance of the assays vary in pH, the temperature at which the reaction is conducted, and whether the reaction is measured by conversion of lactate to pyruvate or vice versa. Methodologic differences result in different distributions of normal values, but conversion among laboratories is possible by converting to multiples of the upper limit of normal.[70,71]

STAGING CLASSIFICATION OF TESTIS TUMORS

Multiple staging systems are currently in use for the clinical management of GCT patients. The staging systems differ in the number of stages (3 versus 4, respectively) and the classification of size and sites of metastases. Unfortunately, no single staging system is optimal, resulting in the use of multiple systems. A comparison of the clinical staging systems is shown in Table 64-4. Most clinicians in North America use the T,N,M staging of the American Joint Committee on Cancer (AJCC) and Union Internationale Contre le Cancre (UICC) for stage I and II disease, with separation of stage II into A, B, and C categories.[40,60,70] In Europe, use of the RMH staging system[9] predominates and is the standard for studies performed by the MRC and the European Organization for Research and Treatment of Cancer (EORTC).[4,9] All classification systems are similar for stage I and II disease. Major differences occur for more advanced disease. The RMH system uses four stages with stage IV disease representing extralymphatic disease, whereas the AJCC/UICC system classifies all patients with disease beyond the retroperitoneal lymph nodes as stage III. Deficiencies in all staging systems are present because size and sites of disease alone do not accurately reflect prognosis at all stages. In general, a combination of extent of disease and the values of serum tumor markers are more predictive of GCT patients' prognosis. These observations have resulted in the development of other classification systems for patient allocation to clinical trials in GCT patients with advanced disease, many of which do not include classic staging.

PROGNOSIS

Prognostic Factors in Clinical Stage I Disease

The primary tumor should be evaluated to carefully assess all tumor elements to ascertain the correct histologic diagnosis. The local extent of the tumor is assessed to determine if the tumor is restricted to the testes, including the rete testis (T1), invades beyond the tunica albuginea or into the epididymis (T2), invades into the spermatic cord (T3), or invades into the scrotum (T4), and whether or not there is evidence of vascular or lymphatic invasion (see Table 64-4).

Prognostic factors for the development of metastatic disease based on the clinical characteristics of the primary tumor have been studied extensively (Table 64-5). For patients with stage I nonseminomatous tumors, the presence of either lymphatic invasion, vascular invasion, or both has been associated with the highest risk of metastases.[72–75] Some studies[72] distinguished vascular invasion from lymphatic invasion; however, it is not possible to reliably distinguish lymphatic invasion from invasion of capillaries. Therefore, vascular and lymphatic invasion are considered as vascular invasion, enhancing its prognostic role.

Another important prognostic factor for the development of metastatic disease in patients with stage I NSGCT is the histology of the primary tumor.[72] The presence of malignant teratoma, undifferentiated (MTU), increases the potential for metastases, and the presence of yolk sac tumor (YST) in the primary tumor decreases the likelihood of progression. The former probably reflects a lower frequency of the most undifferentiated tumor (embryonal carcinoma) or the more benign behavior of tumors with greater differentiation.

The presence of an elevated AFP level prior to orchiectomy is also associated with a lower incidence of metastatic disease.[74] AFP is produced by YST, and 99% of tumors containing YST have evidence of AFP, either by immunohistochemistry or elevated serum levels.[75] The independent significance of AFP may in part reflect incomplete reporting of YST elements by pathologists.

Patients with clinical stage (CS) I seminoma who are observed rather than treated with radiotherapy have approximately a 15% incidence of relapse.[76] Despite evidence for multiple prognostic factors in stage I nonseminomatous tumors, unequivocal prognostic factors for relapse in CSI seminoma patients have not been identified. Prognostic factors for relapse were studied in 194 CSI patients treated with radiotherapy as initial management at the Princess Margaret Hospital from 1981 to 1991.[77] Three factors were associated with subsequent relapse on univariate analysis: anaplastic histology, invasion of the tunica, and invasion of the epididymis. However, other studies have failed to identify tumor size, histology (anaplastic seminoma), T stage or vascular invasion as prognostic factors for relapse in CSI patients treated with conventional therapy.[78,79] The prognostic value of vascular invasion in CSI seminoma patients in surveillance studies has also been studied.[37]

TABLE 64-4. *Staging systems in germ cell tumors*

	Boden-Gibbs		AJCC/UICC		RMH
I(A)	Tumor confined to testes	I	p Tany, NO, MO	I	Disease confined to testis
		pTX	Primary tumor cannot be assessed		
		pTO	No evidence of primary tumor (e.g., histologic scar in testis)	IM	Rising or persistently elevated postorchiectomy marker
		pTis	Intratubular tumor; preinvasive cancer		
		pT1	Tumor limited to the testis, including the rete testis		
		pT2	Tumor invades tunica albuginea or epididymis		
		pT3	Tumor invades the spermatic cord		
		pT4	Tumor invades the scrotum		
II(B)	Spread to RP nodes	II	RP Adennopathy	II	RP Adenopathy
		NX	Regional lymph nodes cannot be assessed		
		NO	No regional lymph node metastasis		
	A RP nodes <2 cm*	N1	Metastasis in a single lymph node ≤2 cm		A RP Adenopathy <2 cm
	B RP nodes 2–5 cm*	N2	Metastasis in a single lymph node 2–5 cm		B RP Adenopathy 2–5 cm or multiple lymph nodes, none >5 cm
	C RP nodes >5 cm*	N3	Metastasis in a lymph node >5 cm		C RP Adenopathy >5 cm
III(C)	Spread beyond RP nodes	III	Disease beyond RP nodes	III	Supradiaphragmatic lymphadenopathy
		M1	Distant metastasis		IIIO No abdominal disease
					ABC RP disease as per stage II
					IV IV Extralymphatic metastases
					L_1 ≤3 lung metastases
					L_2 >3 lung metastases, all <2 cm
					L_3 >3 lung metastases, any >2 cm
					H+, Liver involvement
					Bo+, Bone involvement
					Br+, Brain involvement

* Modifications used in clinical practice but not reported in original publication.
L, lung; RMH, Royal Marsden Hospital; RP, retroperitoneal; AJCC, American Joint Committee on Cancer.

The prognostic value of elevated levels of hCG prior to orchiectomy has been examined extensively. The incidence of elevated levels of hCG in seminoma varies from 5% to 40%, most likely reflecting the heterogeneity of patients and the variability of hCG assays. Studies have concluded a relation of elevated hCG level with both a poor prognosis and a lack of prognostic importance.[80,81] Given the generally excellent prognosis of patients with CSI disease, these data have not resulted in modification of therapy in patients with preorchiectomy elevations of hCG.

Prognostic Factors in Clinical Stage II Disease

The number and size of retroperitoneal lymph nodes found at RPLND for patients with nonseminomatous tumors have prognostic importance (Table 64-6).[82–87] Most studies show that the cutoff point for a low (≤35%) incidence of recurrent disease is fewer than 6 nodes involved with tumor with the largest smaller than 2 cm and no evidence of extranodal tumor extension. Patients with more extensive tumor involvement generally have a recurrence rate of 50% or greater.

The histology of the primary tumor and the presence or absence of vascular invasion in patients with stage II disease have been evaluated for potential prognostic value in addition to lymph node involvement. No consistent prognostic potential of these factors has been demonstrated.

The clinical extent of retroperitoneal lymph node involvement in patients with stage II seminoma is the most important factor in predicting outcome. Generally, the bulkier the tumor, the more likely relapse will occur despite radiotherapy. However, the definition of bulky disease is not uniform. All investigators agree that patients with tumors that have a transverse diameter of 10 cm or more are likely to relapse after radiotherapy. However, some investigators feel that 5 cm rather than 10 cm is the cutoff point above which relapse is likely. One report from the Princess Margaret Hospital demonstrates that approximately 40% of patients with masses between 5 and 10 cm relapse after primary radiotherapy.[77]

The prognostic value of hCG has also been examined in stage

TABLE 64-5. *Multivariate analyses for factors predictive of metastatic disease in patients with clinical stage I nonseminomatous germ cell tumor*

Investigators	Study end point	No. of patients	Factors significant on multivariate analysis (increased [I] or decreased [D] risk)
Swedish-Norwegian Testicular Cancer Group[44]	PSII at RPLND	187	Vascular invasion (I) Elevated preorchiectomy AFP (D) Embryonal Ca (I) YST (D)
	Relapse in PSI	190	Vascular invasion (I) Orchiectomy-RPLND interval (D) Teratoma elements (D)
	All relapses	258	Vascular invasion (I) Teratoma present (D) Orchiectomy-RPLND interval (D) Elevated preorchiectomy AFP (D)
Medical Research Council[72]	Relapse after orchiectomy	259	Vascular invasion (I) Lymphatic invasion (I) Presence of YST (D) Presence of MTU (I)
Royal Marsden Hospital[73] Testicular Tumor Unit	Relapse after orchiectomy	126	Lymphatic invasion (I) Histology, MTU vs MTI (I)
AFIP*[75]	PSII at orchiectomy	459	Vascular invasion (I) Histology, embryonal (I) vs teratoma or YST (D)

* Relations between prognostic variables were explored using a proportional hazard model.

AFIP, Armed Forces Institute of Pathology; AFP, alphafetoprotein; MTU, malignant teratoma undifferentiated; MTI, malignant tumor intermediate; PSI, pathologic stage I; PSII, pathologic stage II; RPLND, retroperitoneal lymph node dissection; YST, yolk sac tumor.

II disease. Most investigators have reported that hCG elevations in stage II disease do not confer a poor prognosis.[59,62]

Prognostic Factors in Clinically Advanced Disease

Prognostic factors for response and survival in GCT patients with advanced disease treated with cisplatin-based therapy have been studied extensively. Prognostic factors found to have significance for either response or survival are shown in Table 64-7. These studies demonstrate that the extent of disease and serum tumor markers are important prognostic factors; however, the use of these factors in the clinic varies substantially. The classification systems that have been developed using these factors have taken three distinct approaches: the extent of disease and serum tumor markers used as continuous variables; the sites and size of metastatic disease and serum tumor markers used as discrete variables; the size and extent of disease alone without the use of serum tumor markers.

The use of extent of disease plus serum tumor markers as continuous variables is exemplified by the Memorial Sloan-Kettering Cancer Center (MSKCC) Model.[88] Logistic regression was used to determine prognostic factors for complete responders. These were $\log_{10}$ (LDH + 1), $\log_{10}$ (hCG + 1), and the total number of metastases (TOTMET), defined as 0 (markers only), 1 site, and 2 or more sites of disease, exclusive of the size or number of metastases at any particular site. AFP level did not attain statistical significance as a prognostic factor and was not used in the model. The probability of a given patient (i) attaining a complete response was determined by the following equation:

$$P_i = \exp H_i/(1 + \exp H_i)$$

where $H_i = 8.514 - 1.973 \log (\text{LDH} + 1) - 0.530 \log (\text{hCG}$

TABLE 64-6. *Prognostic factors for relapse in patients with pathologic stage II nonseminoma using both number and size of lymph nodes*

Investigators	Criteria for low risk of relapse	Relapse vs high risk (%)
Vogelzang et al, 1983[82]	<2 cm, <6 nodes	33 vs 60
Vugrin et al, 1981[83]	<6 nodes, 2 cm, no extranodal extension	0 vs 35
Pizzocaro and Monfardini, 1984[99]	<3 cm, no extranodal extension	27 vs 73
Skinner,* 1969[85]	<6 nodes, <2 cm, no extranodal extension	18 vs 38
Richie and Kantoff, 1991[86]	<6 nodes, <2 cm, no extranodal extension	8 (good risk only)
Williams et al, 1987[98]	Microscopic	40
	<2 cm	53
	>2 cm	60
	Extranodal extension	20

* Includes patients treated with non–cisplatin-containing chemotherapy.

TABLE 64-7. *Factors that have prognostic significance in patients with advanced germ cell tumors*

Investigators	Histology	Primary site	Metastatic sites			LDH	HCG	AFP
			Size	Number	Location			
Williams et al, 1987[98]	No	NE	Yes	No	NE	Yes	Yes	No
Pizzocaro and Monfardini, 1984[99]	No	No	No	NE	No	NE	Yes	Yes
Medical Research Council Working Party in Testicular Tumors and Peckham, 1985[9]	No	No	Yes	NE	Yes	NE	Yes	Yes
Newlands et al, 1983[100]	No	No	Yes	NE	Yes	NE	No	Yes
Horwich et al, 1987[101]	No	No	Yes	Yes	Yes	NE	Yes	No
Stoter et al, 1987[102]	No	No	No	NE	No	NE	Yes	Yes
Droz et al, 1985[103]	No	No	No	NE	No	NE	Yes	NS
Logothetis et al, 1986[104]	No	No	Yes	Yes	Yes	No	Yes	Yes
Birch et al, 1986[106]	No	No	Yes	Yes	Yes	Yes	Yes	Yes
Krag Jacobsen et al, 1984[10]	Yes	Yes	Yes	No	Yes	No	Yes	Yes
Aass et al, 1991[105]	Yes	Yes	No	Yes	Yes	Yes	Yes	No
Bajorin et al, 1988[96]	Yes	Yes	No	No	Yes	Yes	Yes	Yes

AFP, alphafetoprotein; HCG, human chorionic gonadotropin; LDH, lactate dehydrogenase; NE, not evaluated.

+ 1) − 1.111 TOTMET. hCG was expressed in mass units (ng/mL). Good risk assignment was equated with values of P_i greater than or equal to 0.5, whereas patients with a P_i or less than 0.5 were considered poor risk. All patients with extragonadal NSGCT were considered poor risk. The predictive ability of this model has been confirmed in more than 500 patients allocated to MSKCC NSGCT trials since 1982. Complete response rates ranged from 40% to 51% in poor-risk trials and from 91% to 95% in good-risk trials.[89–92]

The MRC Working Party on Testicular Tumors performed two reviews of prognostic factors.[9,80] The first study involved 458 patients treated between 1976 and 1982 at six British centers and represents the combined use of specific sites of disease, tumor measurements, and serum tumor marker levels to predict prognosis.[80] Patients were staged according to the RMH staging classification.[93] AFP and hCG were identified pretreatment, but LDH was not evaluated. Factors associated with poor survival included paraaortic nodes larger than 5 cm; more than three lung metastases, one or more larger than 2 cm (i.e., bulky pulmonary metastases); liver or bone metastases; the number of sites of metastasis; age older than 30 years; AFP level higher than 500 kU/L; and hCG level higher than 1000 IU/L. On the basis of these factors, good, intermediate, and poor prognostic groups of GCT patients were identified (see Table 64-1). The worst prognosis was seen in patients with very large-volume tumors (defined as bulky pulmonary disease or involvement of liver, bone, or central nervous system) and high marker elevations, as defined previously. The criteria outlined in Table 64-1 are used to allocate patients to GCT trials conducted by both the MRC and the EORTC. The second trial analyzed 795 patients from 13 centers.[9] Independent factors for survival included the presence of bone, liver, or brain metastases; elevated AFP levels (>1000 kU/L) or hCG levels (>1000 IU/L); mediastinal mass larger than 5 cm; more than 20 lung metastases; increasing age; and absence of MTU (embryonal carcinoma) in the primary tumor.

The Indiana University (IU) classification system[106] uses tumor bulk alone without the use of serum tumor markers (Table 64-8). The IU staging system has been applied in good-risk patients in a prospective trial of three versus four cycles of BEP therapy; complete-response rates were 97% to 98%, and disease-free survival rates were 91% to 92%.[94] In a randomized trial of poor-risk patients, the response rates were 49% to 54%,

TABLE 64-8. *The Indiana University classification system*

MINIMAL DISEASE

1. Elevated human chorionic gonadotropin and/or alphafetoprotein only
2. Cervical nodes, with or without nonpalpable retroperitoneal nodes
3. Unresectable, but nonpalpable, retroperitoneal disease
4. Minimal pulmonary metastases (<5 per lung field, <2 cm) with or without nonpalpable abdominal disease

MODERATE DISEASE

5. Palpable (≥10 cm) abdominal mass as only disease
6. Moderate pulmonary metastases (5–10 pulmonary metastases per lung field, <3 cm); a mediastinal mass <50% of the intrathoracic diameter; or a solitary pulmonary metastasis >2 cm, with or without nonpalpable abdominal disease

ADVANCED DISEASE

7. Advanced pulmonary metastases: mediastinal mass >50% of the intrathoracic diameter; >10 pulmonary metastases per lung field; or multiple pulmonary metastases, >3 cm, with or without nonpalpable abdominal disease
8. Palpable abdominal mass plus pulmonary metastases
    8.1 Minimal pulmonary
    8.2 Moderate pulmonary
    8.3 Advanced pulmonary
9. Hepatic, osseous, or central nervous system metastases

From Birch R, Williams S, Cone A, et al. Prognostic factors for favorable outcome in disseminated germ cell tumors. J Clin Oncol 1986;4:400.

TABLE 64-9. *Proposed classification for good-, intermediate-, and poor-risk classifications by the International Germ Cell Tumor Collaborative Group*[97]

	CLASSIFICATION OF MARKER STATUS		
	LDH	HCG (ng/mL)*	AFP (ng/mL)
Good	$<1.5 \times N$	<1000	<1000
Intermediate	$1.5 \times N \leq LDH \leq 10 \times N$	1000–10,000	1000–10,000
Poor	$>10 \times N$	$>10,000$	$>10,000$

CLASSIFICATION STATUS

NONSEMINOMATOUS GERM CELL TUMOR

Good

Testis or RP primary, no evidence of nonpulmonary visceral metastases, good markers

Intermediate

Testis or RP primary, no evidence of nonpulmonary visceral metastases, intermediate markers

Poor

Testis or RP primary, with or without evidence of nonpulmonary visceral metastases, poor markers

Testis or RP primary, evidence of nonpulmonary visceral metastases, any markers

Mediastinal primary, with or without evidence of nonpulmonary visceral metastases, any markers

SEMINOMA

Good

Any primary, no evidence of nonpulmonary visceral metastases, any marker

Intermediate

Any primary, evidence of nonpulmonary visceral metastases, any marker

* For HCG, 1 ng/mL is approximately 5 mIU/mL.

AFP, alphafetoprotein; HCG, human chorionic gonadotropin; LDH, lactate dehydrogenase; RP, retroperitoneal.

From Mead GM. International consensus prognostic classification for metastatic germ cell tumors treated with platinum-based chemotherapy: final report of the International Germ Cell Cancer Collaborative Group (IGCCCG). Proc Am Soc Clin Oncol 1995;14:235.

and the 16-month disease-free survival rates were 42% to 48%.[95]

Comparisons of good- and poor-risk criteria allow a more comprehensive understanding of the differences in patient allocation to clinical trials exerted by the different approaches and their impact on trial results. A study of the criteria previously used by EORTC, IU, the National Cancer Institute, and MSKCC performed in 118 consecutive NSGCT patients treated using MSKCC protocols demonstrated that the use of different risk criteria resulted in marked differences in outcome.[96] The allocations of patients to either good- or poor-risk categories by all four sets of criteria were in agreement in only 56% of patients.

The use of diverse eligibility criteria for allocation to clinical trials and the implications of these criteria resulted in the formation of the International Germ Cell Cancer Collaborative Group. This group analyzed data from GCT trials in Europe, North America, and Australia to determine independent prognostic factors for use in one classification system. This study, with more than 3000 GCT patients, found that the pretreatment levels of LDH, hCG, and AFP; the site of the primary tumor (mediastinal versus testis or retroperitoneal); and the presence of nonpulmonary visceral metastases were independent factors for survival.[97] This study defined good-, intermediate- and poor-prognosis groups of patients based on their response to chemotherapy so that uniform eligibility criteria could be used for all clinical trials in patients with advanced GCTs (Table 64-9).

Summary of Prognostic Factors

The prognosis of patients with GCTs is dependent on stage of disease, extent of disease, histology, and the degree of elevated serum tumor markers. Despite the differences in histologic classification and staging, studies for prognostic factors in patients with disease confined to the testis and the retroperitoneum are remarkably consistent in their findings. In contrast, studies for prognostic factors and their use in patients with more advanced GCTs are quite disparate in both their findings and their use for allocation of patients to clinical trials. The latter differences have been reconciled with the adoption of one international classification system that can be used for all patients with GCTs.

REFERENCES

1. Stephen RA. The clinical presentation of testicular tumours. Br J Urol 1962;34:448.
2. Sandeman TF. Symptoms and early management of germinal tumours of the testis. Med J Aust 1979;2:281.
3. Thompson IM, Wear J, Almond C, Schewe EJ, Sala J. An analytical survey of one hundred and seventy eight testicular tumours. J Urol 1961;85:173.
4. Horwich A. Testicular germ cell tumours: an introductory overview. In: Horwich A, ed. Testicular cancer: clinical investigation and management. London: Chapman & Hall Medical, 1991:1.
5. Raghavan D. Malignant extragonadal germ cell tumours in adults. In: Horwich A, ed. Testicular cancer: clinical investigation and management. London: Chapman & Hall Medical, 1991:297.
6. Azzopardi JG, Mostofi FK, Theiss EA. Lesions of testes observed in certain patients with widespread choriocarcinoma and related tumors. Am J Pathol 1961;38:207.
7. Chilvers CED, Saunders M, Bliss JM, Nicholls J, Horwich A. Influence of delay in diagnosis on prognosis in testicular teratoma. Br J Cancer 1989;59:126.
8. Andreyev HJN, Dearnaley DP, Horwich A. Testicular non-seminoma with high serum human chorionic gonadotrophin: the trophoblastic teratoma syndrome. Diagn Oncol 1993;3:67.

9. Medical Research Council Working Party on Testicular Tumours, Peckham MJ. Prognostic factors in advanced non-seminomatous germ-cell testicular tumours: results of a multicentre study. Lancet 1985;1:8.
10. Krag Jacobsen G, Barlebo H, Olsen J, et al. Testicular germ-cell tumours in Denmark 1976-1980: pathology of 1058 consecutive cases. Acta Radiol 1984;23(4):239.
11. Tiptaft RC, Nicholls BM, Hately W, Blandy JP. The diagnosis of testicular swelling using water-path ultrasound. Br J Urol 1982;54: 759.
12. Vick CW, Bird KI, Rosenfield AT, Richter J, Taylor KJ. Ultrasound of the scrotal contents. Urol Radiol 1982;4:147.
13. Ozols RF, Idhoe D, Jacob J, et al. Randomized trial of PV BV [high dose (HD) cis-platinum (P), vinblastine (Ve), bleomycin (B), VP.16 (V)] versus PVeB in poor prognosis non-seminomatous testicular cancer (NSTC). Proc Am Soc Clin Oncol 1984;3:155.
14. Atkin NB, Baker MC. i(12): specific chromosomal marker in seminoma and malignant teratoma of the testis? Cancer Genet Cytogenet 1983;10:199.
15. Bosl GJ, Vogelzang NJ, Goldman A, et al. Impact of delay in diagnosis on clinical stage of testicular cancer. Lancet 1981;2:970.
16. Erman P. Delay in the diagnosis of testicular cancer. Lakartidningen 1980;77:4275.
17. Harding MJ, Paul J, Gillis CR, Kaye SB. Management of malignant teratoma: does referral to a specialist unit matter? Lancet 1993; 314(8851):999.
18. Berthelsen JG, Skakkebaek NE, Von der Maase H, Sorensen BL. Screening for carcinoma in situ of the contralateral testis in patients with germinal testicular cancer. Br Med J 1982;285:1683.
19. Mason MD. Tumour markers. In: Horwich A, ed. Testicular cancer: clinical investigation and management. London: Chapman & Hall Medical, 1991:33.
20. Forman D, Oliver RTD, Brett AR, et al. Familial testicular cancer: a report of the UK family register, estimation of risk and an HLA Class 1 sib-pair analysis. Br J Cancer 65(2):1992;65(2):255.
21. Horwich A, Tucker DF, Peckham MJ. Placental alkaline phosphatase as a tumour marker in seminoma using the H17E2 monoclonal antibody assay. Br J Cancer 1985;51:625.
22. Stoter G. Preliminary results of BEP (bleomycin, etoposide, cisplatin) versus EP in low volume metastatic (LVM) testicular non-seminomas: an EORTC study. Proc Am Soc Clin Oncol 1987;6:110.
23. Javadpour N, Kim EE, Deland FH, Salyer JR, Shah U, Goldenberg DM. The role of radioimmunodetection in the management of testicular cancer. JAMA 1981;246:45.
24. Begent RHJ. Radioimmunolocalisation of germ cell tumours. In: Jones WG, Ward M, Anderson CK, eds. Germ cell tumours II. Oxford: Pergamon Press, 1986.
25. Ray B, Steven I, Hajdu SI, Whitemore WF Jr. Distribution of retroperitoneal lymph node metastases in testicular germinal tumors. Cancer 1974;33:340.
26. Dixon AK, Ellis M, Sikora K. Computed tomography of testicular tumours: distribution of abdominal lymphadenopathy. Clin Radiol 1986;37:519.
27. Rouviere H. Anatomy of the human lymphatic system. Michigan: Edward Brothers, 1938:216.
28. Samuels ML, Lanzotti VJ, Holoye PY, Howe CD. Stage III testicular cancer: complete response by substage to velban plus continuous bleomycin infusion (VB-3). Proc Am Assoc Cancer Res 1977;18:146.
29. Lien HH, Fossa SD, Ous S. Lymphography in retroperitoneal metastases in non-seminoma testicular tumor patients with a normal CT scan. Acta Radiol 1983;24:319.
30. Tesoro-Tess JD, Pizzocaro G, Zanoni F, Musumeci R. Lymphangiography and computerized tomography in testicular carcinoma: how accurate in early state disease? J Urol 1986;133(6):967.
31. Lien HH, Stenwig AE, Ous S. Influence of different criteria for abnormal lymph node size on reliability of computed tomography in patients with nonseminomatous testicular tumor. Acta Radiol 1986;27:199.
32. Poskitt KJ, Cooperberg PL, Sullivan LD. Sonography and CT in staging nonseminomatous testicular tumors. Am J Roentgenol 1985;144: 939.
33. Robinson B, Kingston J, Nogueira Costa R, Malpas JS, Barrett A, McElwain TJ. Chemotherapy and irradiation in childhood Hodgkin's disease. Arch Dis Child 1984;59:1162.
34. Husband JE, Peckham MJ, MacDonald JS. The role of abdominal computed tomography in the management of testicular tumours. J Comput Assist Tomogr 1980;4:1.
35. Donohue JP, Thornhill JA, Foster RS, Rowland RG, Bihrle R. Primary retroperitoneal lymph node dissection in clinical stage A non-seminomatous germ cell testis cancer: review of the Indiana University experience 1965–1989. Br J Urol 1993;71(3):326.
36. Horwich A. Current issues in the management of clinical stage I testicular teratoma. Eur J Cancer 1993;29A(7):933.
37. Horwich A, Alsanjari N, A'Hern R, Nicholls J, Dearnaley DP, Fisher C. Surveillance following orchidectomy for stage I testicular seminoma. Br J Cancer 1992;65:775.
38. von der Maase H, Specht L, Jacobsen GK, et al. Surveillance following orchidectomy for stage I seminoma of the testis. Eur J Cancer 1993; 29A(14):1931.
39. Warde PR, Gospodarowicz MK, Goodman PJ, et al. Results of a policy of surveillance in stage I testicular seminoma. Int J Radiat Oncol Biol Phys 1993;27(1):11.
40. Whitmore WFJ. Surgical treatment of clinical stage I non-seminomatous germ cell tumors of the testis. Cancer Treat Rep 1982;66:5.
41. Tamburini M, Filiberti A, Barbieri A, et al. Psychological aspects of testis cancer therapy: a prospective study. J Urol 1989;142(6):1487.
42. Fosså S. Testicular cancer in young Norwegians. J Surg Oncol 1988; 39:43.
43. McKeen EA, Bodurtha J, Meadows AT, Douglass EC, Mulvhill JJ. Rhabdomyosarcoma complicating multiple neurofibromatosis. J Pediatr 1978;93:992.
44. Klepp O, Olsson AM, Henrikson H, et al. Predicting metastases in clinical stage I testicular teratoma: multivariate analysis of a large multicentric study (SWENOTECA). Abstract No. O787. Book of Abstracts, 5th European Conference on Clinical Oncology (ECCO), September 2–7, 1989.
45. Donohue JP, Rowland RG. Complications of retroperitoneal lymph node dissection. J Urol 1981;125:338.
46. Donohue JP, Thornhill JA. Retroperitoneal lymphadenectomy in staging and treatment the development of nerve-sparing techniques. In: Horwich A, ed. Testicular cancer: clinical investigation and management. London: Chapman & Hall Medical, 1991:175.
47. Sujka SK, Huben RP. Clinical stage I nonseminomatous germ cell tumors of testis: observation vs retroperitoneal lymph node dissection. Urology 1991;38(1):29.
48. Horwich A. Comments and critique: current issues in the management of clinical stage I testicular teratoma. Eur J Cancer 1993;29A(7):933.
49. Yarnold JR, Jelliffe AM, Vaughan Hudson G. Patterns of relapse following radiotherapy for Hodgkin's disease. Clin Radiol 1982;33: 137.
50. Husband JE, Grimer DP. Staging testicular tumours: the role of CT scanning. J Royal Soc Med 1985;58:429.
51. Lien HH, Lindskold L, Fossa SD, Aass N. Computed tomography and conventional radiography in intrathoracic metastases from nonseminomatous testicular tumor. Acta Radiol 1988;29(5):547.
52. Dixon FJ, Moore RA. Atlas of tumour pathology. Washington DC: Armed Forces Institute of Pathology, 1952:32.
53. Mostofi FK, Sobin LH. International histological classification of tumours of testes. Geneva: World Health Organization, 1977.
54. Pugh RCB. Testicular tumours. In: Pugh RCB, ed. Pathology of the testis. Oxford: Blackwell Scientific Publications, 1976:139.
55. Mostofi FK, Theiss EA, Ashley DJB. Tumors of specialized gonadal stroma in human male patients. Cancer 1959;12:944.
56. Vaitukaitis JL. Human chorionic gonadotrophin as a tumor marker. Ann Clin Lab Sci 1974;4:276.
57. Mostofi FK. Pathology of germ cell tumors of testis: a progress report. Cancer 1980;45:1735.
58. Nisselbaum JS. Argument in favor of using mass units to calibrate and report concentrations of human choriogonadotropin. Clin Chem 1986;32:1998.
59. Bosl GJ, Geller NL, Cirrincione C, et al. Serum tumour markers in patients with metastatic germ cell tumours of the testis: a ten year experience. Am J Med 1983;75:29.
60. Bosl GJ, Geller NL, Chan EYW. Stage migration and the increasing proportion of complete responders in patients with advanced germ cell tumors. Cancer Res 1988;48:3524.
61. Javadpour N, McIntire KR, Waldmann TA. Human chorionic gonadotrophin (HCG) and alpha-fetoprotein (AFP) in sera and tumor cells

of patients with testicular seminoma: a prospective study. Cancer 1978;42:2768.
62. Motzer RJ, Bosl GJ, Geller NL, et al. Advanced seminoma: the role of chemotherapy and adjunctive surgery. Ann Intern Med 1988;108: 513.
63. Catalona WJ, Vaitukaitis JL, Fair WR. Falsely positive specific human chorionic gonadotrophin assays in patients with testicular tumors: conversion to negative with testosterone administration. J Urol 1979;122: 126.
64. Odell WD, Griffin J. Pulsatile secretion of human chorionic gonadotrophin in normal adults. N Engl J Med 1987;317:1688.
65. Fowler JEJ, Platoff GE, Kubrock CA. Commercial radioimmunoassay for beta subunit of human chorionic gonadotrophin: falsely positive determinations due to elevated serum luteinizing hormone. Cancer 1982;49:136.
66. The Medical Research Council Working Party on Testicular Tumours. Prognostic factors in advanced non-seminomatous germ-cell testicular tumours: results of multicentre study. Lancet 1985;1:8.
67. Pizzocaro G, Zanoni F, Salvioni R, Milani A, Piug L. Difficulties of a surveillance study omitting retroperitoneal lymphadenectomy in clinical stage I non-seminomatous germ cell tumors of the testis. J Urol 1987;138(6):1393.
68. Staples J. Alphafetoprotein, cancer, and benign conditions. Lancet 1986;2:1277.
69. Bosl GJ, Gluckman R, Geller NL, et al. VAB-6: an effective chemotherapy regimen for patients with germ-cell tumors. Am J Clin Oncol 1986;4(10):1493.
70. Bosl GJ, Geller N, Bajorin D, et al. A randomized trial of Etoposide + Cisplatin versus VAB-6 (Vinblastine + Bleomycin + Cisplatin + Cyclophosphamide + Dactinomycin) in patients with good prognosis germ cell tumor. J Clin Oncol 1988;6(8):1231.
71. Bajorin DF, Mazumdar M, Motzer RJ, Vlamis V, Bosl GJ. Model comparisons predicting germ cell tumor (GCT) response to chemotherapy. (Abstract) Proc Am Soc Clin Oncol 1994;13(715):232.
72. Freedman LS, Parkinson MC, Jones WG, et al. Histopathology in the prediction of relapse of patients with stage I testicular teratoma treated by orchidectomy alone. Lancet 1987;2:294.
73. Hoskin P, Dilly S, Easton D, Horwich A, Hendry WF, Peckham MJ. Prognostic factors in stage I non seminomatous germ cell testicular tumours managed by orchiectomy and surveillance: implications for adjuvant chemotherapy. J Clin Oncol 1986;4:1031.
74. Klepp O, Olsson AM, Henrikson H, et al. Prognostic factors in clinical stage I nonseminomatous germ cell tumors of the testis: multivariate analysis of a prospective multicentre study (SWENOTECA). J Clin Oncol 1990;8:509.
75. Sesterhenn IA, Weiss RB, Mostofi FK. Prognosis and other clinical correlates of pathologic review in stage I and II testicular carcinoma: a report from the Testicular Cancer Intergroup Study. J Clin Oncol 1992;10:69.
76. Horwich A. Surveillance for stage I seminoma of the testis. In: Horwich A, ed. Testicular cancer: clinical investigation and management. London: Chapman & Hall Medical, 1991:109.
77. Gospodarowicz MK, Warde PR, Panzarella T. The Princess Margaret Hospital experience in the management of stage I and II seminoma: 1981 to 1991. In: Germ cell tumors III, vol. 1. Oxford: Pergamon Press, 1994:177.
78. Vaeth M, Schultz HP, Von der Maase H, et al. Prognostic factors in testicular germ cell tumours: experiences from 1058 consecutive cases. Acta Radiol Oncol 1984;32:271.
79. Zagars GK, Babaian RJ. Stage I testicular seminoma: rationale for post-orchiectomy radiation therapy. Int J Radiat Oncol Biol Phys 1987;13:155.
80. Butcher DN, Gregory WM, Gunter PA, Masters JRW, Parkinson MC. The biological and clinical significance of HCG-containing cells in seminoma. Br J Cancer 1985;51:473.
81. Peckham MJ, Hamilton CR, Horwich A, Hendry WF. Surveillance after orchidectomy for stage I seminoma of the testis. Br J Urol 1987; 59:343.
82. Vogelzang NJ, Fraley EE, Lange PH. Stage II non seminomatous testicular cancer: a 10 year experience. J Clin Oncol 1983;1:171.
83. Vugrin D, Whitmore W, Cvitkovic E. Adjuvant chemotherapy with VAB-3 of stage II-B testicular cancer. Cancer 1981;48:233.
84. Ozols RF, Ihde DC, Linehan WM. Management of high risk patients with advanced testis cancer: National Cancer Institute approach. Semin Oncol 1988;15:335.
85. Skinner D. Non seminomatous testis tumors: a plan of management based on 96 patients to improve survival in all stages by combined therapeutic modalities. J Urol 1969;115:65.
86. Richie JP, Kantoff PW. Is adjuvant chemotherapy necessary for patients with stage B1 testicular cancer? J Clin Oncol 1991;9(8):1393.
87. Williams SD, Stablein DM, Einhorn LH. Immediate adjuvant chemotherapy versus observation with treatment at relapse in pathological stage II testicular cancer. N Engl J Med 1987;317:1433.
88. Bosl GJ, Geller NL, Cirrincione C, et al. Multivariate analysis of prognostic variables in patients with metastatic testicular cancer. Cancer Res 1983;43:3403.
89. Bosl GJ, Geller NL, Vogelzang NJ, et al. Alternating cycles of etoposide plus cisplatin and VAB-6 in the treatment of poor-risk patients with germ cell tumors. J Clin Oncol 1987;5(3):436.
90. Motzer R, Cooper K, Geller NL. Carboplatin, etoposide, and bleomycin for patients with poor risk germ cell tumors. Cancer 1990;65: 2465.
91. Bajorin DF, Sarosdy MF, Pfister DG, et al. Randomized trial of etoposide and cisplatin versus etoposide and carboplatin in patients with good-risk germ cell tumours: a multiinstitutional study. J Clin Oncol 1993;11(4):598.
92. Bajorin DF, Sarosdy MF, Bosl GJ, Weisen S, Heller G. A randomized trial of etoposide + carboplatin (EC) vs etoposide + cisplatin (EP) in patients (PTS) with metastatic germ cell tumors (GCT). Proc Am Soc Clin Oncol 1991;10:168.
93. Peckham MJ. Investigations and staging: general aspects and staging classification. In: Peckham M, ed. The management of testicular tumours. London: Edward Arnold, 1971:89.
94. Einhorn LH, Williams SD, Loehrer PJ, et al. Evaluation of optimal duration of chemotherapy in favorable-prognosis disseminated germ cell tumors: a Southeastern Cancer Study Group Protocol. J Clin Oncol 1989;7(3):387.
95. Loehrer PJ, Einhorn LH, Elison P, et al. Phase II study of cisplatin (P) plus etoposide (VP-16) with either bleomycin (B) or ifosfamide (I) in advanced stage germ cell tumours (GCT): an intergroup trial. Proc Am Soc Clin Oncol 1993;12:261.
96. Bajorin D, Katz A, Chan E, Geller N, Vogelzang N, Bosl GJ. Comparison of criteria for assigning germ cell tumour patients to "good risk" studies and "poor risk" studies. J Clin Oncol 1988;6(5):786.
97. Mead GM. International consensus prognostic classification for metastatic germ cell tumors treated with platinum-based chemotherapy: final report of the International Germ Cell Cancer Collaborative Group (IGCCCG). Proc Am Soc Clin Oncol 1995;14:235.
98. Williams SD, Stablein DM, Einhorn LH, et al. Immediate adjuvant chemotherapy versus observation with treatment at relapse in pathological stage II testicular cancer. N Engl J Med 1987;317(23):1433.
99. Pizzocaro G, Monfardini S. No adjuvant chemotherapy in selected patients with pathologic stage II non seminomatous germ cell tumors of the testis. J Urol 1984;131:677.
100. Newlands ES, Begent RHJ, Rustin GJS, Parker D, Bagshawe KD. Further advances in the management of malignant teratomas of the testis and other sites. Lancet 1983;1:948.
101. Horwich A, Easton D, Husband J. Prognosis following chemotherapy for metastatic malignant teratoma. Br J Urol 1987;59:578.
102. Stoter G, Sylvester R, Sleijfer DT, et al. Multivariate analysis of prognostic factors in patients with disseminated nonseminomatous testicular cancer: results from a European Organization for Research on Treatment of Cancer multiinstitutional phase III study. Cancer Res 1987;47(10):2714.
103. Droz JP, Kramar A, Caillaud JM. A multivariate analysis of prognostic factors in advanced stages of non seminomatous germ cell tumors of the testis (NSGCTT). Prog Clin Biol Res 1985;203:269.
104. Logothetis CJ, Samuels ML, Selig DE, et al. Cyclic chemotherapy with cyclophosphamide, doxorubicin and cisplatin plus vinblastine and bleomycin in advanced germinal tumors: results with 100 patients. Am J Med 1986;81(2):219.
105. Aass N, Klepp O, Cavallin-Stahl E, et al. Prognostic factors in unselected patients with nonseminomatous metastatic testicular cancer: a multicenter experience. J Clin Oncol 1991;9(5):818.
106. Birch R, Williams S, Cone A, et al. Prognostic factors for favorable outcome in disseminated germ cell tumors. J Clin Oncol 1986;4:400.

Principles and Practice of Genitourinary Oncology, edited by Derek Raghavan, Howard I. Scher, Steven A. Leibel, and Paul H. Lange. Lippincott-Raven Publishers, Philadelphia, © 1997.

CHAPTER 65

Management of Stage I-II Seminoma

Mary K. Gospodarowicz and Padraig R. Warde

Testicular cancer is the commonest malignant disease in young men. Racial and geographic variations in the incidence of testis tumors are considerable, and the number of new cases is rising.[1–3] Approximately 50% of patients present with pure seminoma. The disease affects men aged 20 to 50 years, with a median age at presentation of 35 years. Cryptorchidism is a well-established risk factor, and certain HLA types such as BW41 have also been implicated.[4] At presentation, 75% of these patients have no disease outside the testis. Approximately 20% of patients present with metastatic spread to the retroperitoneal lymph nodes.

The following chapter reviews the management of patients with stage I and II seminoma with particular emphasis on unresolved questions and new treatment approaches.

DIAGNOSIS AND PATIENT ASSESSMENT

Presenting symptoms include painless swelling of the testis (70% to 80%), found either on self-examination or during a routine checkup, testicular pain (20% to 30%), or both (5% to 10%).[5] Less often, patients report hematospermia, shrinkage of the testis, hardening of the testis, or symptoms due to metastases, such as back or abdominal pain. Little formal screening or promotion of testicular self-examination exists. No clear association has been shown between a longer duration of symptoms and a higher stage of disease.[6,7]

The diagnosis is established by histologic examination of the tumor at orchiectomy, but it may also be established by needle biopsy.[8] Serum tumor markers should be obtained before or during orchiectomy, mainly to identify an apparent pure seminoma with an elevated alphafetoprotein (AFP), implying the presence of nonseminomatous elements. Typical or classic seminoma is the most common histologic type (70% to 85%). Anaplastic seminoma occurs in 10% to 30% of cases and is associated with more advanced stage and less favorable outcome.[9–11] Spermatocytic seminoma is rare, occurring mainly in elderly men, and metastases have been described in few cases, but they are much less common than in typical seminoma.[12–14] Occasionally, the tumor first appears in paratesticular tissues or with metastatic disease without an apparent primary tumor in the testis.[15,16]

All patients presenting with a testicular tumor should have a full history and physical examination. A history of cryptorchidism, orchidopexy, inguinal or scrotal surgery, and comorbid illnesses such as inflammatory bowel disease, previous abdominopelvic surgery, and infections should be noted. The initial laboratory investigations should include a complete blood count and renal function tests. AFP and β-human chorionic gonadotropin (β-hCG) should be measured again after orchiectomy, and levels should be interpreted in light of their known half-lives. A persistent elevation of β-hCG after orchiectomy indicates the presence of residual disease. Placental leukocyte alkaline phosphatase (PLAP) has proved to be a disappointing marker for seminoma, and its role should be regarded as investigational.[17,18]

Computed tomography (CT) of the abdomen and pelvis is performed to document the size, location, and transverse diameter of any abnormal retroperitoneal lymph nodes.[19] When lymph nodes larger than 10 mm in diameter are considered abnormal, the overall accuracy of CT scans to detect lymph node metastases has been reported to be approximately 70%.[20,21] CT is also useful in demonstrating the position of normal kidneys and in identifying renal abnormalities such as horseshoe or pelvic kidney for planning radiotherapy. Lymphography has been recommended for those with negative CT scans, but its value has also been questioned.[19] Lymphography has been advised in particular for patients considered for surveillance.[22] Although the concept that this imaging technique may improve on the accuracy of CT is appealing, experience in nonseminomatous germ cell testis tumors (NSGCTs) has been disappointing. Pizzocaro and associates, in a series of 114 patients with such tumors and a normal CT scan, found an abnormal lymphographic study in 6 patients, whereas retroperitoneal lymph node dissection (RPLND) revealed abnormal lymph nodes in 26 patients.[23] Magnetic resonance imaging (MRI) has little advantage over CT,[24] and earlier hopes that T1- and T2-weighted images would detect smaller disease have not been realized.[25] All patients should have a chest radiograph, but because skip metastases are uncommon in seminoma, thoracic CT is not required for patients with a normal CT scans of the abdomen and pelvis. CT of the thorax should be performed in the presence of abdominal disease, however.[26] A baseline ultrasound of the contralateral testicle should be obtained in all cases. Biopsy of the contralat-

TABLE 65-1. *Seminoma staging classification*

Stage	Criteria
Stage I	No clinical evidence of metastases beyond testicle
State II	Infradiaphragmatic lymph node metastases: A. Maximum diameter <2 cm B. Maximum diameter >2 ≤5 cm C. Maximum diameter >5 ≤10 cm D. Maximum diameter >10 cm
Stage III	Supradiaphragmatic nodal involvement (infradiaphragmatic nodes recorded as A, B, C, D as for stage II)
Stage IV	Parenchymal metastatic disease

Thomas G, Jones W, Van Oosterom A, Kawai T. Consensus statement on the investigation and management of testicular seminoma 1989. Prog Clin Biol Res 1990;357:285. Review.

eral testicle, either during orchiectomy or at the time of referral to a specialist center, should be considered, to allow early detection of carcinoma in situ (CIS) in the contralateral testis. If CIS is detected, it can be successfully treated with modest doses of radiotherapy to the testicle (see Chap. 63). Sperm banking should be offered if the patient is going to have radiotherapy or chemotherapy.

The current TNM staging classification systems of the International Union Against Cancer (Union Internationale Contre le Cancer; UICC) or of the American Joint Committee on Cancer (AJCC) for testicular tumors are not universally used.[27,28] Other staging classifications have been favored by some clinicians, and the designation of stage II and its substages differs among classifications. A modification of the Royal Marsden Hospital staging classification accepted at the 1989 Leeds Consensus Meeting is increasingly used worldwide and is used in this chapter (Table 65-1).[29]

TREATMENT

For over 50 years, patients with seminoma have usually been treated with orchiectomy and radiotherapy. This approach has been successful, with long-term survival obtained in 80% to 90% of patients. These results are as much a function of the pattern of presentation favoring localized disease as evidence of the exquisite radiosensitivity of seminoma. In the past decade, with improvements in diagnosis, staging, and treatment, the routine use of radiotherapy in seminoma has been questioned.

Initial management involves radical orchiectomy in all cases. An inguinal approach is recommended to allow high division of the spermatic cord. The scrotal approach does not appear to compromise the outcome, however, provided the scrotal cavity is not contaminated by tumor.* Possible approaches to the post-orchiectomy management of patients with stage I and II seminoma include radiotherapy, surveillance in stage I disease, RPLND, and chemotherapy. The success of surveillance in stage I NSGCTs and the establishment of curative chemotherapy for advanced disease have led to reexamination of the standard treatment policies for stage I seminoma. The low relapse rates after radiotherapy and the lack of apparent serious morbidity have dissuaded many clinicians from abandoning the traditional treatment approach, however.

*Editor's note: Scrotal violation should be avoided because of the widely held view that it is associated with altered patterns of spread and a worse prognosis.

Stage I Seminoma

Radiotherapy

Considerable experience in treating stage I seminoma with retroperitoneal radiation has been accumulated (Table 65-2).[30–51] With the use of moderate-dose radiation (25 to 35 Gy), in-field disease control has been observed in 92% to 98% of patients.

The lymphatic drainage of the testis is directly to the paraaortic lymph nodes. Minor differences are noted in the distribution of metastases from left or right testis tumors. The left testicular vein drains to the left renal vein, and the lymphatic drainage is primarily to the lymph nodes in the paraaortic area directly below left renal hilum. On the right side, the testicular vein drains directly to the inferior vena cava below the level of the renal vein, and, therefore, paracaval and interaortocaval nodes are the first to be involved in right-sided tumors. Pelvic and inguinal lymph node involvement is rare. Factors predisposing patients to inguinal lymph node involvement and inguinal relapse are well established and include a past history of scrotal or inguinal surgery, seminoma involving a cryptorchid testis, scrotal orchiectomy with incision of the tunica albuginea, and tumor invasion of the tunica vaginalis or lower third of the epididymis.[52,53] Disruption of lymphatic vessels in the spermatic cord during inguinal surgery has induced anastomoses between testicular lymphatic vessels and regional lymphatics destined for inguinal or pelvic lymph nodes. A connection with the contralateral inguinal lymph nodes may be established, but this situation is rare. A few patients with inguinal relapse may have no apparent predisposing factors.[52,54]

Standard postorchiectomy radiotherapy in stage I seminoma is directed to the paraaortic and ipsilateral pelvic lymph nodes. At the Princess Margaret Hospital in Toronto, parallel opposed anteroposterior fields are treated with 6- 18-MeV linear accelerator photons. The treatment volume includes the paraaortic and ipsilateral pelvic lymph nodes and is based on the information obtained from CT scans of the abdomen and pelvis to avoid excessive irradiation of renal parenchyma. This plan is called "hockey stick" in North America and "dog leg" in the United Kingdom and Europe.[55] Field-shaping blocks are used to protect the suprahilar renal parenchyma while covering the renal hilar lymph nodes, especially in left-sided presentations. The radiation fields extend from the T11 vertebral level to the inguinal ligament and are typically 9 to 10 cm wide. No attempt is made to treat the hypogastric or contralateral pelvic lymph nodes. The penis is moved out of the field. The contralateral testis is placed in a scrotal shield to protect fertility and hormonal function. Verification simulator and port films are routinely obtained. The dose of 25 Gy is prescribed at midplane and is delivered in 20 daily fractions. Inguinal lymph nodes are not routinely treated, but the radiation field is extended to cover the inguinal area in patients with risk factors for inguinal lymph

TABLE 65-2. *Results of retroperitoneal radiotherapy in Stage I seminoma*

Investigators	No. of patients	Survival rate (%)	Relapse rate (%)
Allhoff et al, 1991[30]	64	100	3.1
Brunt and Scoble, 1992[32]*	25	100	4
Bayens et al, 1992[31]	132	99	5
Duncan and Munro, 1987[34]	103	96	5
Dosmann and Zagars, 1993[33]	282	97†	3
Epstein et al, 1990[35]	42	100	2
Fossa et al, 1989[36]	365	99	4
Germa Lluch et al, 1993[37]	36	100	0.3
Giacchetti et al, 1993[38]	184	96	2
Gospodarowicz et al, 1994[39]	194	100	5
Hannum and Vugrin, 1990[40]	48	97	4
Kellokumpu and Halmer 1990[41]	129	95	6
Lai et al, 1994[42]	95	97	2
Lindeman and Tiver, 1991[43]	73	90	2
Read and Johnston, 1993[44]‡	94	98	1
Singhal et al, 1993[45]	56	96	7
Sommer et al, 1990 [46]	133	100	0
Stein et al, 1993[47]	64	94	9.3
Thomas, 1985[48]	150	99	1.3
Tongaonkar et al, 1993[49]	71	100	7.4
Willan and Megowan, 1985[50]	149	98	7
Yeoh et al, 1993[51]	69	96	1.4

* Paraaortic radiotherapy alone: 17 patients.
† Disease-free survival.
‡ Paraaortic radiotherapy alone: 94 patients.

node involvement. Scrotal irradiation is avoided, even in patients with scrotal violation.

An alternative field arrangement, used at the M. D. Anderson Cancer Center in Houston, involves parallel opposed portals to the paraaortic lymph nodes (T10-L5) and an anterior field only for the pelvic and inguinal lymph nodes.[56] The advantage of a hockey-stick field is that it avoids a junction that could form an overlap or gap, and the dose distribution is more homogeneous than with separate fields. The advantage of having separate abdominal and pelvic fields is the decreased weight of shielding used daily.

The low incidence of pelvic lymph node involvement in stage I seminoma has led to the suggestion to limit the radiation volume to the paraaortic lymph nodes alone. Occasional reports of patients thus treated have consistently shown excellent results, with no pelvic treatment failures.[32,44] Only a large body of experience, or a large prospective randomized trial, can determine the risks and benefits of such therapy, however. Nevertheless, some centers have changed their policy to treat the paraaortic lymph nodes alone. The Medical Research Council Testicular Study Group in the United Kingdom has conducted a prospective randomized trial of the traditional paraaortic and pelvic irradiation versus paraaortic irradiation alone, but the results of this trial have not yet been reported. To control the small risk of supradiaphragmatic recurrence, prophylactic mediastinal irradiation has been used in some centers, but has been both unnecessary and harmful (see the section of this chapter on stage II seminoma). Such therapy is not recommended in stage I seminoma.

The in-field control rate after retroperitoneal radiotherapy is close to 100%, and no in-field failures were seen in a cohort of 194 patients with stage I seminoma treated at the Princess Margaret Hospital between 1981 and 1991.[31,36,39,41,42,57–59] The minimum dose of radiation required to control occult retroperitoneal disease has not been defined. Published reports include radiation doses ranging from 2500 cGy[60] to 4000 cGy.[36] Isolated local treatment failures have been reported at 1500 cGy[61] and at 2100 cGy.[60] Read and Johnston described 91 patients who underwent treatment to the paraaortic area only with a radiation dose of 2000 cGy in 8 fractions, with alternate fields treated daily.[44] With a median follow-up of 34 months, no local treatment failures have been reported.

Approximately 5% of patients are expected to have a relapse outside the treatment volume (see Table 65-2). Relapse is most common in the first 18 months after diagnosis of primary seminoma, but it may occur later.[31] In the Princess Margaret Hospital experience, 10 of 11 relapses occurred at 6 to 18 months from first diagnosis, and 1 patient experienced a relapse at 72 months.[39] A small proportion of patients, usually with predisposing factors, have a relapse in the inguinal lymph nodes. The pattern of relapse has been well documented, with the majority of relapses occurring in supraclavicular lymph nodes, mediastinum, lung, or bone. Uncommon sites of isolated metastases, such as brain, bone, and tonsil have also been noted.[33,62–64]

The cause-specific survival rate in stage I seminoma approaches 100%.[31,36,41,42,57–59] The overall survival rate ranges between 92% and 99% at 5 to 10 years, however. Most deaths are due to intercurrent illness, but concern exists that premature deaths may be occurring from radiation-induced cancers. With such excellent treatment results, the prognostic factors for relapse are often not apparent. Up to 1 in 20 patients treated with postorchiectomy radiotherapy develops disease recurrence, however. Factors that predispose patients to distant relapse include anaplastic histologic features and locally extensive tumor with invasion of the tunica albuginea, epididymis, or spermatic cord, but the predictive of these factors value is low.[9,39] Recognition of factors strongly predictive for early disease dissemination beyond the retroperitoneal lymph nodes would help to identify those patients who possibly would better be treated with initial chemotherapy.

Surveillance

Although adjuvant retroperitoneal radiotherapy continues to be the standard management of stage I seminoma, interest been increasing over the past 10 years in surveillance, with treatment reserved for patients who have a relapse. The reasons for considering surveillance include the possibility of reducing overall treatment morbidity, the availability of CT to stage and to follow patients' courses more accurately, and the development of curative chemotherapy regimens.

Several prospective nonrandomized studies of surveillance have been conducted (Table 65-3).[30,37,65–69] The largest reported experience with surveillance is from the Danish Testicular Carcinoma Study Group.[68] With a median follow-up of 48 months, the crude relapse rate in 261 patients was 19%. The other studies with adequate follow-up (>36 months) have reported similar relapse rates.[39,66] The predominant site of relapse in all studies was in the paraaortic lymph nodes: 41 of 49 (82%) relapses in the Danish study and 24 of 27 (89%) in the Princess Margaret Hospital series.[68,69] The median time to relapse ranged from 12 to 18 months, but late relapses (>4 years) have also been reported. In the Princess Margaret Hospital series, late relapse occurred in 5 of 27 (19%) patients who experienced a relapse. Only 2 of the 727 patients in the surveillance series died of disease (see Table 65-3); an additional 2 died of the results of chemotherapy-induced neutropenia.[68]

Prognostic factors for relapse have been studied in the three large surveillance studies.[66,68,69] In the Danish study, with univariate analysis, tumor size, histologic subtype, necrosis, and invasion of the rete testis predicted relapse.[68] On multivariate analysis, tumor size was the only significant factor. The cumulative risk of relapse after 4 years was 6% in patients with tumors less than 3 cm in diameter, 18% in patients with tumors 3 to 6 cm, and 36% in patients with tumors 6 cm or larger. In the Princess Margaret Hospital series, age at diagnosis was the only factor predictive for relapse on univariate analysis.[69] The risk of progression at 5 years was 26% in patients 34 years old or younger, in contrast to a 10% risk in those older than 34 years of age. Age was not a significant factor in the Danish study, and it was not analyzed in the Royal Marsden Hospital study. The only significant factor in the Royal Marsden Hospital study was the presence of lymphatic or vascular invasion (9% versus 17% relapse rate). At relapse, most patients were treated with retroperitoneal radiotherapy. In the Danish, Princess Margaret Hospital, and Royal Marsden Hospital studies, the proportion of patients treated with radiotherapy at relapse was 76%, 74%, and 71%, respectively. The incidence of second relapse after radiotherapy was less than 20% in the Princess Margaret Hospital and Danish series. The likelihood of detecting tumor progression in the retroperitoneal lymph nodes when their size is less than 5 cm, and therefore suitable for radiotherapy, depends on the frequency of follow-up CT scans of the abdomen and pelvis. One of the concerns about surveillance is the potential for more patients to require chemotherapy, which involves a prolonged and more toxic course of treatment. In the Princess Margaret Hospital experience from 1981 to 1991, equal numbers of patients managed with surveillance (8 of 172) and adjuvant radiotherapy (8 of 194) received chemotherapy.[39] This concern is difficult to address, because, in some centers, chemotherapy was used electively at relapse.[37,70]

The most attractive feature of surveillance is the avoidance of unnecessary treatment in a majority of patients. Surveillance must not compromise survival, however, and knowing that only 4 disease-related deaths have occurred in the 727 patients under surveillance (see Table 65-3) is reassuring. Surveillance requires a commitment to close and prolonged follow-up from both patients and clinicians. It can produce considerable anxiety in some patients and should not be considered mandatory when other equally effective management options are clearly available. Another concern relates to patient compliance with follow-up because failure to detect relapse early may compromise the patient's safety. On a smaller scale, however, failure to keep follow-up appointments may also compromise the outcome for patients treated with radiotherapy. In the future, it should be possible to identify patients at low risk of relapse and to recommend surveillance to selected patients only.

Other Treatment Approaches

RPLND is a frequently forgotten treatment option in stage I seminoma. Even so, it is a reasonable approach for patients

TABLE 65-3. *Results of surveillance in Stage I seminoma*

Investigators	No. of patients	Follow-up median (mo)	Relapse (no. of pts)	Survival: carcinoma in situ (%)
Allhoff et al, 1991[30]	33	—	3	100
Charig et al, 1990[65]	15	31	5	100
Germa Lluch et al, 1993[37]	45	34	5	100
Horwich et al, 1992[66]	103	62	17	100
Oliver et al, 1994[70]	26	18	4	100
Ramakrishnan et al, 1992[67]	72	44	13	100
von der Masse et al, 1993[68]	261	48	49	98.9
Warde et al, 1993[69]	172	50	27	99
Total	727			

unwilling to comply with surveillance and unable to be treated with radiotherapy, such as patients with a second testicular tumor or previous retroperitoneal radiotherapy for other disease. RPLND may be also appropriate in patients with another concurrent or previous malignant disease, in whom histologic examination of lymph nodes would be relevant to management.

Chemotherapy with cisplatin and etoposide or carboplatin has been effective in the treatment of advanced seminoma (see Chap. 66). Oliver and colleagues suggested a short course of carboplatin alone for patients with stage I seminoma, and although preliminary results of this approach look promising, further experience is needed to assess this potentially simpler treatment option.[70] The toxicity of chemotherapy and the potential for late relapse in patients treated with adjuvant chemotherapy should not be overlooked, however.[71]

Stage II Seminoma

Stage II seminoma includes a wide spectrum of disease extent. Staging is based on the transverse diameter of the largest retroperitoneal lymph node mass (see Table 65-1). The definition of stage II seminoma and its substages has varied over time, and the literature must be interpreted with caution. The most common presentation is with stage IIA disease. The frequency of stage IIA disease depends on the staging investigations performed, and it is more commonly seen when stage allocation is based on lymphography alone. Presentations with stage IID disease are rare, and only retrospective studies are available to study patterns of treatment failure and treatment outcome in this group of patients. The traditional approach to the management of stage II seminoma is radiotherapy to the paraaortic and pelvic lymph nodes. With this approach, excellent local disease control can be expected, but the patient has an increasing risk of distant relapse with increasing bulk of retroperitoneal metastases.

Radiotherapy

The technique of radiotherapy in stage II seminoma is similar to that used in stage I disease. In patients with small (<2 cm) and solitary paraaortic lymph nodes, no alterations in the radiation dose or technique are required. In patients with more extensive metastases, the radiation field is extended to cover the common iliac lymph nodes bilaterally. The treatment volume also commonly includes the contralateral external iliac lymph nodes, but no evidence indicates that such practice is necessary except in patients with risk factors for contralateral pelvic relapse, such as seminoma in an undescended testis. A dose of 25 Gy is usually delivered to the entire treatment volume and is followed by a boost of 10 Gy to the involved lymph nodes. The planning process ideally includes a CT-based plan and distribution to ensure appropriate coverage of the disease, without excessive irradiation of the kidneys. If CT-based planning is not available, intravenous contrast is injected to localize both kidneys relative to the treatment volume. The question of including the inguinal lymph nodes or scrotum in the radiation volume is analogous to the problem in stage I seminoma, but bulky (>5 cm) paraaortic lymph nodes have been associated with an increased risk of inguinal lymph node involvement.[52]

Until the early 1980s, with the exception of some centers in the United Kingdom and Canada, most patients with stage II seminoma received elective mediastinal and supraclavicular irradiation.[72,73] The rationale for this policy was based on the recognition of the orderly spread of seminoma from the abdominal to the supraclavicular and mediastinal lymph nodes. Such treatment reduced the supradiaphragmatic treatment failure rate.[33] The last decade, however, this practice has been abandoned for the following reasons:

1. Supradiaphragmatic irradiation does not affect the risk of haematogenous metastases to the lung or bone.
2. Effective salvage chemotherapy is available for supradiaphragmatic relapse.
3. The use of elective supradiaphragmatic irradiation may compromise bone marrow reserve for salvage chemotherapy.
4. Mediastinal irradiation has been associated with an increased risk of premature cardiac death.

Supradiaphragmatic relapses may be limited to lymph node involvement in the left supraclavicular fossa. Dosmann and Zagars have suggested and have implemented the use of elective irradiation to the left supraclavicular lymph nodes in patients with stage IIA-IIC seminoma.[33] Such therapy would not affect bone marrow reserve or the heart and may indeed reduce the overall risk of relapse, but further information on the incidence and pattern of relapse is needed to assess the risks and benefits of this approach fully. All patients should have a follow-up CT scan of the abdomen to assess the completeness of response to abdominal irradiation. In stage IIA disease, complete regression of retroperitoneal adenopathy is commonly seen toward the end of the patient's course of radiotherapy, but in patients with bulky disease, a residual mass may be noted for 12 to 18 months after treatment. Follow-up CT scanning abdomen should be continued until complete response has been documented.

The ultimate local control rates with radiotherapy in stage II seminoma have not been well described. Most reports include patients diagnosed and treated without the benefit of CT evaluation of disease extent. Before the availability of CT, the extent of abdominal disease was poorly defined, and relapse was inadequately documented. Even with CT, the difficulties in estimating local control are compounded by the frequent persistence of a residual mass after treatment of bulky retroperitoneal disease.[43,74,75] In the Princess Margaret Hospital experience, only 2 of 72 patients with stage II seminoma who were treated with radiotherapy failed to achieve local control of the disease.[39] One patient, with a 5-cm paraaortic mass, was found to have a pure embryonal carcinoma at salvage RPLND, and the second patient, who had a 6-cm mass at diagnosis, refused chemotherapy, developed progressive abdominal disease after radiotherapy, and died after refusing further treatment. Data from other contemporary series of patients with stage II seminoma include only an occasional in-field recurrence.[31–33,35,41–43,59,76,77] The presence of nonseminomatous tumor in metastatic lymph nodes, or at relapse, in patients with pure seminoma has been documented in several series.[33,39,76] Failure to achieve complete tumor regression in the retroperitoneal lymph nodes in a patient with pure seminoma should alert the clinician to the possible presence of nonseminomatous tumor. If the residual mass is small and continues to regress, observation is recommended. On occasion, regression is minimal, and a persistent mass may be observed for several years. The management of such patients has been controversial, and few data exist on the risk of continuing observation rather than intervention. The need for RPLND in patients with a residual mass after chemotherapy of seminoma has been questioned, and the indications for surgery have been revised to include only a residual mass larger than 3 cm in diameter, rather than resecting smaller masses or diffuse fibrotic changes (see Chap. 66).[74,78] An elective resection of a persistent mass is useful to exclude the presence of teratoma and to obviate the need for continuous monitoring of the abdomen. Another factor in local treatment failure after irradiation is the possibility of a geographic or marginal miss. Efforts to spare renal parenchyma occasionally result in inadequate coverage of the renal hilar lymph nodes. This error may lead to recurrence of the disease at the margin of the treatment volume, and such situations require salvage RPLND or chemotherapy.

The majority of relapses occur outside the irradiated area. The main risk factor predictive of distant relapse is the initial extent of retroperitoneal lymph node disease. In the absence of supradiaphragmatic radiotherapy, the treatment failure rate for patients with stage IIA and IIB seminoma is 10% to 20%.[10] The treatment failure rate for patients with stage IIC seminoma has been reported to be between 20% and 50%, and the relapse rate for patients with stage IID seminoma is in excess of 50%. In 72 patients with stage II seminoma who were treated with retroperitoneal irradiation at the Princess Margaret Hospital, the size of retroperitoneal lymph nodes was the most important predictor of relapse and survival. Six of 56 patients with stage IIA and IIB disease had relapses, and 2 of these had a biopsy-proved embryonal carcinoma at relapse.[39] The 5-year actuarial relapse rate was 11% for patients with stage IIA-IIB disease and 56% for those with stage IIC-IID disease. The 5-year survival rate in stage IIA-IIB disease was 96%, and it was 75% in stage IIC-IID disease. In stage IIC, characterized by retroperitoneal lymph nodes 5 to 10 cm in diameter, 7 of 14 patients treated with radiotherapy had relapses, 6 in distant sites. The sites of relapse included supraclavicular lymph nodes, bone, mediastinum, and lung. Of the 4 patients with relapse in bone, 3 presented with spinal cord compression.

Chemotherapy

Chemotherapy has been used with success in the management of advanced stage II seminoma, with local control rates comparable to those obtained with radiotherapy, as long as the clinician bears in mind the difficulties in evaluating the presence of viable residual disease (see Chap. 66). The toxicity of chemotherapy should not be ignored, however (see Chap. 71). RPLND is an alternative strategy for stage IIA-IIB seminoma, especially in patients with limited retroperitoneal involvement and contraindications to the use of radiotherapy. The toxicity of RPLND compares favorably with that of chemotherapy in stage IIA-IIB disease.

Our experience supports the use of chemotherapy in all patients with stage IIC-IID disease, and, possibly, some patients with multiple lymph nodes 3 to 4 cm in diameter may also be better treated with chemotherapy.[39] Unfortunately, the total burden of infradiaphragmatic disease has not been analyzed as a possible prognostic factor for distant relapse, and our own data are not sufficient to answer this question.

Special Management Problems

Elevated β-Human Chorionic Gonadotropin

Gonadotropins can be secreted by most types of testicular tumors, including pure seminoma. Histologic studies have shown that hCG is secreted by syncytiotrophoblastic giant cells. In pure seminoma, the frequency of hCG production measured in peripheral blood is reported to be between 8% and 13%,[79–81] and in some reports it is even higher: 39% to 68%.[82,83] Mumperow and Hartmann reported a much higher incidence of hCG secretion by pure seminoma, by measuring β-hCG levels in blood from the testicular vein and the antecubital fossa.[84] They found elevated β-hCG levels in the cubital vein in 26% of patients and in the testicular vein in 80% of patients. Syncytiotrophoblastic cells were found in only 39% of patients with elevated serum β-hCG (cubital or testicular).

The main question regarding seminomas that secrete β-hCG is whether these tumors have a prognosis inferior to that of tumors that do not secrete hCG. The interpretation of the literature is confounded by the lack of attention to the decay of β-hCG levels after orchiectomy. Reports of seminoma treated in the 1960s and 1970s have claimed a worse prognosis.[57,85,86] These reports may have included tumors with components of NSGCTs, or they may have failed to consider an elevated β-hCG level in the context of known disease extent. More recent reports, taking disease extent into account, have failed to confirm a worse outcome in patients with tumors that secrete β-hCG.[81,87,88] Weissbach, in a large prospective study of seminoma, found that 31% of patients had tumors that secreted β-hCG.[89] Tumors that produced β-hCG were more likely to have metastases in retroperitoneal lymph nodes. Stage by stage, however, no difference was noted in their risk of later relapse. These results imply that the detection of β-hCG is an indicator of tumor burden (primary or metastatic) rather than a sign of tumor aggressiveness.

Few reports exist of pure seminoma with high postorchiectomy β-hCG levels, without evidence of metastases. If the level of β-hCG reflects tumor burden, and if imaging of the retroperitoneal lymph nodes does not reveal metastases, then the possibility of occult disease outside the retroperitoneum must be considered. In such patients, chemotherapy, rather than retroperitoneal radiotherapy, may be the preferred treatment approach, although these patients probably can be successfully treated with radiotherapy. Unfortunately, few modern data are available to resolve this issue.

Cryptorchidism

Pure seminoma accounts for a large proportion of testicular germ cell tumors occurring in cryptorchidism.[90] Nevertheless, presentation of seminoma in uncorrected cryptorchidism is rare.[90,91] Although previous reports suggested that seminoma presenting in an undescended testis is associated with an inferior outcome, more recent reports do not support this finding.[91] A painful groin mass and abdominal pain were the presenting symptoms in more than half the patients with tumors in an undescended testis. Gauwitz and Zagars, in a report of 26 patients with seminoma in undescended testis, found 9 patients with seminoma in an inguinal testis and 17 with tumor in a pelvic testis.[91] The size of the primary tumor was larger in pelvic than in inguinal seminoma. The incidence of metastatic involvement (62%) was also much higher than in seminoma presenting in a scrotal testis (25%). Patients with primary pelvic tumors had a higher incidence of nodal involvement (76%) than those with inguinal presentations (33%). In addition, 69% of patients with nodal metastases had pelvic lymph node involvement, in comparison with only 14% in patients with seminoma arising in a scrotal testis.[91] A small proportion of patients had peritoneal metastases, mostly those with pelvic seminoma, although 1 patient had an inguinal primary tumor. The postorchiectomy management of seminoma presenting in cryptorchidism depends on the location of the primary tumor and the extent of disease. Stage I and II disease, other than in patients with large nodal metastases (>5 cm), is treated with radiotherapy. For patients with stage I and II seminoma arising from an undescended testis, comparable survival can be achieved by giving similar doses of radiation and adjusting the size of the paraaortic and pelvic radiation fields to cover the known extent of disease.[91,92] In patients with pelvic lymph node involvement, irradiation of whole pelvis is recommended. The prognosis of patients with seminoma arising from an undescended testis depends more on the stage and extent of disease than on its origin.

Horseshoe Kidney or Pelvic Kidney

Horseshoe kidney occurs in approximately 1 in 400 of the general population.[93] An association also exists between renal fusion abnormalities and cryptorchidism, which, in turn, is associated with an increased incidence of testicular neoplasms. The association of horseshoe kidney and testicular tumors may occur more commonly, because it represents another abnormality in the development of the urogenital ridge.[94] Because of this anomaly, variation in the normal pathways of lymphatic spread may be expected. Two main problems are recognized in the management of seminoma associated with horseshoe kidney or pelvic kidney. One is related to the technical problem of delivery of radiotherapy. In some patients with horseshoe kidney, a large part of the renal parenchyma directly overlies the regional lymph nodes and is within the standard radiation volume. The delivery of a standard radiation dose would be associated with an unacceptable risk of radiation nephritis. The second problem is related to the possible abnormalities in lymphatic drainage of the testis and therefore the possibility of relapse when standard radiation fields are used. The unusual patterns of relapse observed in patients managed by surveillance confirm concerns regarding abnormal lymphatic pathways.[95] For these reasons, postorchiectomy surveillance in patients with stage I disease and chemotherapy in patients with stage II disease have usually been the treatments of choice. RPLND is another option for patients unwilling to follow the surveillance program, however. Reports in the literature suggest that RPLND is both safe and effective in selected patients.[96,97]

Renal Transplantation

Seminoma has been reported after renal transplantation.[98–100] Dieckmann and coworkers reported a case of stage I seminoma in a patient who had undergone renal transplantation and who was receiving cyclosporine. The patient was managed with routine postoperative radiotherapy and remained well 2 years after therapy.[101] Villalona-Calero and associates reported 2 patients with stage I disease, 1 managed with radiotherapy and the other with surveillance, with no recurrence at up to 2 years.[102] Stage I and II seminoma in patients who have undergone renal transplantation has usually been treated with postoperative radiotherapy. Concerns regarding potential damage to the transplanted kidney may dictate surveillance, however. Short-term follow-up of these patients does not suggest a higher risk of relapse, but available data are limited.

Patients Positive for Human Immunodeficiency Virus

Several reports have documented the presentation and course of testis tumors in patients positive for human immunodeficiency virus (HIV).[103–109] Moyle and associates found 3 patients with seminoma among 2205 known HIV-positive patients (136 per 100,000), which is 68 times the expected incidence.[106] Testis tumors in HIV-positive patients are most commonly NSGCTs.[105] Some reports suggested that the pattern of presentation in HIV-associated seminoma is similar to that of non-HIV–related seminoma, but reports also suggest an increased frequency of bilateral tumors.[107,108] Staging of testis tumors in HIV-positive patients may be difficult, especially in those with normal tumor markers and retroperitoneal adenopathy because the enlarged retroperitoneal lymph nodes may be benign. Most patients with stage I and II HIV-related seminoma and a good performance status have been treated with the usual radiotherapy, although surveillance has also been used in this population. Retroperitoneal radiotherapy has resulted in a prolonged decrease in the CD4 count.[110] The concern that wide-field irradiation and chemotherapy both worsen immunosuppression and may precipitate HIV-related infection has led to a recommendation for surveillance in stage I seminoma.[108] The risk of early tumor dissemination may be greater in HIV-positive than in HIV-negative patients, however. In patients without severe infections, chemotherapy may be well tolerated without risk of activation of HIV-related infections.[103] In some series, stage I patients managed with surveillance had tumor progression in the retroperitoneal lymph nodes and required treatment soon after diagnosis. Few data exist on the therapy, pattern of relapse, and survival of patients with HIV and seminoma, however. As in other malignant diseases in these patients, the prognosis is related more to the severity of acquired immunodeficiency syndrome (AIDS) and its complications. Further information regarding the tolerance and response of these patients to radiotherapy and chemotherapy will be helpful in determining the optimal treatment strategy.

Noncompliant Patients

Because the cure rate for patients with stage I and II seminoma approaches 100%, problems with patient compliance with treatment or follow-up recommendations may affect the outcome more than the choice of therapy. Every large cancer center has experience with a patient who refuses conventional therapy or who fails to attend follow-up appointments and eventually dies of disease. Little attention has been given to this problem, and it is important to examine factors contributing to lack of compliance. Patient education regarding the diagnosis, available treatment options, and outcome in testis tumors and the need for regular evaluation should be given high priority.

FOLLOW-UP MANAGEMENT

Patients with stage I or II seminoma have a low risk of disease recurrence. In most instances, recurrent disease is curable with further treatment, and, consequently, appropriate follow-up is essential. The follow-up schedule is similar for patients treated with radiotherapy or chemotherapy or for those in surveillance programs. Our policy is to assess patients with stage I and II seminoma treated with retroperitoneal radiotherapy at 3-month intervals in the first 2 years, 4-month intervals in the third year, 6-month intervals in years 4 to 6, and annually thereafter. Patients are seen with a chest radiograph, and the tumor marker estimation is continued only for the first 3 years. Patients with stage II seminoma have follow-up abdominal CT scans until the retroperitoneal disease has resolved. The schedule for surveillance is not much different, but it includes regular imaging of the abdomen and pelvis at 4-month intervals for the first 3 years, 6-month intervals in years 4 to 6, and annually thereafter. This schedule continues to evolve as more extensive data on the pattern of progression on surveillance become available. The follow-up of chemotherapeutically treated patients is similar to those managed with radiotherapy. The management of a persistent retroperitoneal mass is discussed earlier in this chapter. Whatever the choice, observation versus resection, ultimately, the frequency, duration, and interpretation of abdominal imaging become a problem. In most instances, resection of any discrete residual mass is appropriate.

Histologic confirmation of any relapse is strongly advocated. Although the majority of patients have a relapse with the same histologic features as the primary tumor, the occurrence of NSGCTs at relapse has been reported.[10,39,111] In addition, the use of etoposide and platinum-based agents alone may not be the optimal treatment for NSGCTs, especially if bulky disease is present. Another confounding factor in follow-up is the reported association of sarcoidosis and testis tumors. Sarcoidosis, usually manifested as hilar adenopathy or, less commonly, lung nodules, has been reported to distort the true extent of seminoma at presentation and lead to false diagnosis of relapse.[112–115] No evidence suggests that coexistent sarcoid affects the outcome of patients with seminoma.

Late relapse is an infrequent but well-recognized event in patients with seminoma. In a study of 512 patients with seminoma treated at the Norwegian Radium Hospital between 1972 and 1982, 6 patients had relapses more than 36 months after diagnosis.[116] In the Princess Margaret Hospital experience, 6 patients had relapses more than 4 years after diagnosis.[39] Patients with seminoma are at prolonged risk of relapse, and relapse has been reported as late as 19 years after orchiectomy. Both patients and physicians should be aware of relapse patterns, and measures to permit early diagnosis of relapse should be instituted. Patients should also be informed of the small but significant risk of tumor in the contralateral testis. Metachronous occurrence of a contralateral testis tumor can occur more than 20 years after the first tumor. To expect patients to comply with such a long follow-up for a remote risk of relapse is unreasonable. Long-term follow-up (>10 years) is not cost effective, and most late recurrences are noted by the patient himself, or patients present with symptoms.

MANAGEMENT OF RECURRENT DISEASE

The management of recurrent disease depends on previous therapy, extent of disease, and histologic features at relapse. Patients who develop disease progression while they are under surveillance, and those who have not had previous retroperitoneal radiotherapy, are managed similarly to new patients with seminoma. Depending on the extent of disease, they receive either radiotherapy alone—for those with retroperitoneal or inguinal relapse smaller than 5 cm in diameter, or chemotherapy—for those with metastases larger than 5 cm or distant disease. Patients who are not candidates for radiotherapy may be treated with RPLND. The management of recurrent disease after treatment depends on the previous therapy, extent of disease and histology at relapse. Patients who have relapses after radiotherapy are usually managed with chemotherapy. The exception is isolated inguinal relapse, which may be effectively treated with local irradiation or surgical excision. The choice of chemotherapy depends on the histologic features of recurrent disease. In patients with unknown histologic features at relapse, using chemotherapy appropriate for NSGCTs may be safer than relying on the two-drug combination of etoposide and cisplatin. Most recurrences are detected on follow-up visits. Occasionally, however, pain due to bone metastases may be attributed to benign causes and not investigated. Spinal cord compression may develop within weeks of the onset of symptoms. This devastating complication of relapse has been described before, but it has not been emphasized sufficiently in the literature.[56,117]

SECOND TESTICULAR TUMORS

Patients with testicular tumors are at increased risk of developing a tumor in the contralateral testis.[118,119] The relative risk, as compared with the general population, in 1909 patients with testicular cancer diagnosed in the Netherlands with a median follow-up of 7.7 years was 35.7.[120] This increased risk was confined to those patients treated with radiotherapy or with surgery alone. The cumulative risk of developing a second testicular tumor at 25 years of follow-up was reported to be as high as 5.2% by Osterlind and associates in 1991.[121] These investigators reported on the follow-up of 2850 patients with testicular tumors in Denmark diagnosed between 1960 and 1984 and found the risk of developing a second testicular primary tumor to be 9.4% in 224 patients treated with surgery alone, 4.7% in 1994 patients treated with radiotherapy, and 4.3% in 582 patients given chemotherapy. The risk was greater in patients with nonseminomatous tumors (8.4%) than in those with seminomas (3.6%). No second testicular tumors were observed in Manchester, where routine prophylactic radiotherapy was given to the contralateral testis.[122] Patients with second testis cancers and subsequent second orchiectomy have an unsatisfactory quality of life because of hormonal imbalance. Needle biopsy followed by radiotherapy or partial orchiectomy followed by radiotherapy has been proposed in an attempt to preserve hormonal function.[8]

At a minimum, patients with testicular cancer should be taught testicular self-examination and should have a baseline ultrasound study of the contralateral testis. Considerable controversy exists over the need for biopsy of the contralateral testis to detect CIS.[123] The overall incidence of CIS in the contralateral testis is approximately 5%, which is similar to the cumulative risk of developing a second testicular carcinoma. Risk factors for CIS have been identified, and the management of patients with CIS is discussed in Chapter 63. When a tumor in the contralateral testis is diagnosed, orchiectomy is usually performed. Postorchiectomy management depends on the extent of disease and treatments used for the first tumor. For patients with stage I disease previously treated with radiotherapy, surveillance or RPLND may be used. In patients with stage II disease, the choice of RPLND or chemotherapy depends on the extent of disease.

COMPLICATIONS

Early Complications

The radiation doses used in treatment of seminoma are lower than those used for other malignant diseases, and the short-term complications have been assumed to be minor. The morbidity caused by abdominal irradiation has not been well documented, however. A minor degree of nausea occurs in most patients, but fewer than 50% develop vomiting. Approximately 10% of patients develop severe nausea and vomiting requiring regular antiemetics and are unable to complete normal daily tasks. Antiemetic drugs control nausea in most patients, and the availability of ondansetron has improved symptom control in patients with severe nausea and vomiting. Diarrhea develops in a minority of patients. Significant depression of white blood cells and platelets is uncommon and rarely requires treatment interruption. In spite of outpatient therapy, many patients are unable to continue full employment or to study while receiving radiotherapy. Weakness and lassitude requiring additional rest develop in many patients. Reports in the literature describe isolated cases of bowel obstruction, although this complication only occurs with higher radiation doses.[46]

Late Complications

Late complications of radiotherapy for seminoma are uncommon. Only major complications are usually recorded, and the incidence of severe hepatic, renal, bladder, and bowel damage is reported to be less than 1%.[124] No risk of radiation myelitis exists with adjuvant postorchiectomy radiotherapy. Indeed, no severe complications are expected unless the patient has an underlying medical problem, or a technical error occurs. The only well-documented complication is an increased incidence of peptic ulceration in patients treated with a radiation dose of 30 to 45 Gy.[125] This complication was observed in a retrospective study; other reports did not make the same observation.

Reproductive Complications

Testicular germinal epithelium is exquisitely sensitive to ionizing radiation. Although the contralateral testis is not in the radiation field, scatter dose can be significant, and it may cause profound depression of spermatogenesis and may compromise future fertility. A radiation dose between 20 and 50 cGy may produce temporary aspermia, and doses greater than 50 cGy may preclude recovery of spermatogenesis. The use of scrotal shielding reduces the scattered radiation dose, but it cannot ensure protection of spermatogenesis in all patients. The use of sperm banking is recommended for patients who wish to optimize their chances for future fertility and who are to be treated with radiotherapy. In men who recover spermatogenesis after radiotherapy for seminoma, no evidence indicates an increased incidence of genetic abnormalities in their subsequent offspring.[126]

Psychological Problems

Most studies of the psychosocial well-being of patients after treatment for testicular cancer have analyzed patients without considering the different treatment modalities used. The majority of the studies show that most patients do not have any serious psychological sequelae of their diagnosis or treatment.[127–129] Indeed, some patients report an improved outlook on life compared with their premorbid state and also compared with control groups.[127,130] Some patients, however, do experience severe psychological symptoms, mainly in the areas of sexual activity, infertility, distress, and social upheaval.[131] Schover and associates reported that 19% of 84 patients who received radiotherapy for seminoma had low rates of subsequent sexual activity.[132] Fifteen per cent had erectile dysfunction, and 10% had difficulty reaching orgasm. Data on the psychological morbidity associated with surveillance programs are sparse, but the evidence suggests that these patients may have fewer sexual problems than those who undergo treatment.[130] These patients may have other significant problems with anxiety regarding relapse and social or work-related problems associated with the follow-up necessary in surveillance programs, however. Open discussions with clinicians, active participation in treatment decisions, and continuous support after therapy has been completed are helpful in alleviating anxiety regarding therapy, its effects, and outcome.

Cardiac Complications of Mediastinal Irradiation

Mediastinal irradiation has been associated with an increased incidence of coronary artery disease, valvular heart disease, and pericardial disease.[133,134] Until recently, however, serious cardiac complications were considered unlikely in patients who received mediastinal radiotherapy, because the radiation doses used in seminoma were low. Lederman and colleagues, in a cohort of 124 patients with seminoma, 57 of whom received mediastinal irradiation, found 4 patients with heart disease.[135] One had a fatal myocardial infarction, 1 an uncomplicated myocardial infarction, 1 constrictive pericarditis, and 1 valvular and ischemic heart disease requiring surgery. Two additional patients died suddenly, of possible cardiac causes, and all 6 events occurred in the group treated with mediastinal irradiation. In the Patterns of Care Study in the United States, Hanks and associates found an increased incidence of cardiac disease in patients treated with mediastinal radiotherapy, as compared with those treated with infradiaphragmatic radiotherapy alone.[136] The true incidence of cardiac disease associated with mediastinal radiotherapy is not known, and patients and physicians should be educated about the risk of radiation-related heart disease.

Second Malignant Tumors

A distinction must be made between second testis tumors, which reflect a common risk factor for this disease, and unrelated malignant diseases that may be treatment induced (see Chap. 71). Treatment-induced malignant diseases have been reported after both radiotherapy and chemotherapy of Hodgkin's disease, malignant lymphoma, and ovarian and other cancers.[137,138] Numerous isolated occurrences of second nontesticular tumor after treatment of seminoma with radiotherapy have been reported, although in such cases any association between radiotherapy and the second malignant tumor must be of speculative rather than proved causative relationship.[139–141] More convincing data come from long-term studies of large groups of patients with testis tumors who received radiotherapy. An increased risk of second cancers has been documented in the Netherlands and in Denmark,[120,142] and because this increased risk is expressed more than 10 to 15 years after radiotherapy, it may not be apparent in series with shorter follow-up.

CONCLUSIONS

The survival of patients with stage I and II seminoma is excellent, and the overall risk of relapse is low. Postorchiectomy radiotherapy to the retroperitoneal and ipsilateral pelvic lymph nodes with a dose of 25 Gy is considered a standard approach in stage I disease.[29] Nonetheless, higher radiation doses continue to be given in many centers, and this higher dosage contributes to the early and late morbidity of therapy. When postorchiectomy radiotherapy is prescribed, pelvic and inguinal lymph nodes should be treated in patients with known risk factors. If fertility is a concern, a surveillance policy may be the preferred management option, rather than treatment with less than adequate radiation fields. Scrotal relapse has not been reported in the last decade, and the use of scrotal irradiation is not necessary.[143] In patients considered for radiotherapy, without prior scrotal or inguinal surgery, the clinician should consider limiting the radiation volume to the paraaortic lymph nodes alone. Until further data on patterns of relapse are available, however, such patients should be monitored for pelvic recurrence. With regional nodal control virtually assured, no follow-up imaging of the retroperitoneum is required for patients treated with radiotherapy.

Surveillance is a viable alternative management option in stage I seminoma. The morbidity resulting from adjuvant radiotherapy is not immediately apparent because the early side effects of therapy are usually easily controlled with antiemetic and antidiarrheal medication. The social and economic costs to the patient and the health care system associated with the use of routine postoperative radiotherapy are considerable, however, and concern still exists regarding the potential induction of second cancers by radiation.[120,138,140] Although the policy of routine treatment with adjuvant radiotherapy has been deemed successful, whether this success is due to the efficacy of treatment or to the low incidence of metastases is unclear. The surveillance data indicate that only 15% to 20% of all stage I seminomas are at risk for relapse, and the relapse rate despite retroperitoneal radiotherapy is 4% to 5%. Therefore, only about 3 of 4 patients at risk are spared relapse by routine postorchiectomy abdominal radiotherapy. For the majority of patients with stage I disease, adjuvant treatment is unnecessary. The concerns expressed regarding surveillance in seminoma, as compared with NSGCTs, include the absence of a reliable tumor marker and the need for prolonged observation. Despite the value of markers in NSGCTs, however, the majority of these patients in surveillance programs have relapses with normal tumor markers in the retroperitoneal lymph nodes.[144] The only distinction between routine adjuvant radiotherapy and surveillance is the need for monitoring of the retroperitoneum. The surveillance experience suggests the risk of relapse after 5 years is uncommon. Newer data by Oliver and associates suggest that chemotherapy should be investigated as a novel management for stage I seminoma.[70] Clearly, further experience is required before this suggestion can be considered a viable treatment alternative.

Available data suggest that almost 100% of patients with stage I seminoma are cured whether radiotherapy or surveillance is chosen for postorchiectomy management. Physicians may view one management option as preferable, but individual patient preferences must be considered. These preferences may be based on the side effects associated with both approaches; for example, young patients in whom fertility is an issue may choose surveillance, whereas for others surveillance may be inconvenient and adjuvant treatment may be preferred.

The choice of therapy, assessment of response, and management of residual retroperitoneal mass in patients with stage II seminoma continue to be controversial.[77,145–147] In general, radiotherapy is recommended for patients with retroperitoneal lymph nodes less than 5 cm in diameter, and chemotherapy is used for those with masses 5 cm or more in diameter, although some centers continue to recommend radiotherapy for retroperitoneal disease smaller than 10 cm in diameter.[33,145] Occurrence of NSGCTs at relapse confirms the hypothesis for the common origin of all germ cell testis tumors and narrows the artificial distinction between the approach to the management of seminoma and that of nonseminomatous tumors.[111]

Overall survival in stage I and II seminoma is excellent, and relapse after therapy is uncommon. These results have been achieved with careful assessment of disease extent, risk factors, knowledge of relapse patterns, and diligence in treatment delivery. With effective salvage chemotherapy available for relapse, a less than rigorous approach to the initial management of patients with seminoma may evolve. A nonchalant approach to patients, poor application of accepted treatment methods, and disregard to follow-up may lead to deaths in patients with an otherwise curable tumor. Continuous vigilance and audit of treatment failures and late effects are required to optimize the survival and quality of life of patients with this disease.

REFERENCES

1. Gudlaugsson E, Magnusson B, Hallgrimsson J. Tumours in Iceland. 13. Malignant tumours of the testis: a histological classification, epide-

miological considerations and survival. Acta Pathol Microbiol Immunol Scand 1990;98:173.
2. Halme A, Kellokumpu-Lehtinen P, Lehtonen T. Trends in incidence and results of treatment of testicular germ cell tumours in Finland 1972–1983. Acta Oncol 1989;28:777.
3. Stone JM, Cruickshank DG, Sandeman TF, Matthews JP. Trebling of the incidence of testicular cancer in Victoria, Australia (1950–1985). Cancer 1991;68:211.
4. Dieckmann KP, von Keyserlingk H. HLA association of testicular seminoma. Klin Wochenschr 1988;66:337.
5. Kennedy B, Schmidt J, Winchester D, Peace B, Natarajan N, Mettlin C. National survey of patterns of care for testis cancer. Cancer 1987; 60:1921.
6. Moul JW, Paulson DF, Dodge RK, Walther PJ. Delay in diagnosis and survival in testicular cancer: impact of effective therapy and changes during 18 years. J Urol 1990;143:520.
7. Sandeman TF. Symptoms and early management of germinal tumors of the testis. Med J Aust 1979;2:281.
8. Bos SD, Ypma AF. Synchronous bilateral seminoma testis treated with unilateral orchiectomy and contralateral irradiation: a therapeutic option. Case report. Scand J Urol Nephrol 1993;27:559.
9. Bobba VS, Mittal BB, Hoover SV, Kepka A. Classical and anaplastic seminoma: difference in survival. Radiology 1988;167:849.
10. Evensen JF, Fossa SD, Kjellevold K, Lien HH. Testicular seminoma: histological findings and their prognostic significance for stage II disease. J Surg Oncol 1987;36:166.
11. Schultz HP, von der Maase H, Rorth M, et al. Testicular seminoma in Denmark 1976–1980: results of treatment. Acta Radiol (Oncol) 1984;23:263.
12. Matoska J, Ondrus D, Hornak M. Metastatic spermatocytic seminoma: a case report with light microscopic, ultrastructural, and immunohistochemical findings. Cancer 1988;62:1197.
13. Schoborg TW, Whittaker J, Lewis CW. Metastatic spermatocytic seminoma. J Urol 1980;124:739.
14. Talerman A. Spermatocytic seminoma: clinicopathological study of 22 cases. Cancer 1980;45:2169.
15. Dichmann O, Engel U, Jensen DB, Bilde T. Juxtatesticular seminoma. Br J Urol 1990;66:324.
16. Simpson AH, Calvert DG, Codling BW. The shrinking seminoma. J R Soc Med 1990;83:187.
17. Munro AJ, Nielsen OS, Duncan W, et al. An assessment of combined tumour markers in patients with seminoma: placental alkaline phosphatase (PLAP), lactate dehydrogenase (LD) and beta human chorionic gonadotrophin (beta hCG). Br J Cancer 1991;64:537.
18. Nielsen OS, Munro AJ, Duncan W, et al. Is placental alkaline phosphatase (PLAP) a useful marker for seminoma? Eur J Cancer 1990; 26:1049.
19. MacVicar D. Staging of testicular germ cell tumours. Clin Radiol 1993;47:147. Review.
20. Lien HH, Stenwig AE, Ous S, Fossa SD. Influence of different criteria for abnormal lymph node size on reliability of computed tomography in patients with non-seminomatous testicular tumor. Acta Radiol (Diagn) 1986;27:199.
21. Stomper PC, Fung CY, Socinski MA, Jockelson MS, Garnick MB, P RJ. Detection of retroperitoneal metastases in early-stage non-seminomatous testicular cancer: analysis of different CT criteria. AJR Am J Roentgenol 1987;149:1187.
22. Thomas GM. Stage I, II seminoma: then and now. Int J Radiat Oncol Biol Phys 1993;26:545. Editorial.
23. Pizzocaro G, Nicolai N, Salvioni R, et al. Comparison between clinical and pathological staging in low stage nonseminomatous germ cell testicular tumors. J Urol 1992;148:76.
24. Ellis JH, Bies JR, Kopecky KK, et al. Comparison of NMR and CT imaging in the evaluation of metastatic retroperitoneal lymphadenopathy from testicular carcinoma. J Comput Assist Tomogr 1984;8:709.
25. Hogeboom WR, Hoekstra HJ, Mooyaart EL, et al. The role of magnetic resonance imaging and computed tomography in the treatment evaluation of retroperitoneal lymph-node metastases of non-seminomatous testicular tumors. Eur J Radiol 1991;13:31.
26. See WA, Hoxie L. Chest staging in testis cancer patients: imaging modality selection based upon risk assessment as determined by abdominal computerized tomography scan results. J Urol 1993;150:874.
27. Beahrs OH, Henson DE, Hutter RV, Kennedy BJ. American Joint Committee on Cancer: manual for staging of cancer, 4th ed. Philadelphia, JB Lippincott, 1992.
28. Hermanek P, Sobin LH. UICC International Union Against Cancer: TNM classification of malignant tumors, 4th ed, 2nd rev. Berlin, Springer-Verlag, 1992.
29. Thomas G, Jones W, VanOosterom A, Kawai T. Consensus statement on the investigation and management of testicular seminoma 1989. Prog Clin Biol Res 1990;357:285. Review.
30. Allhoff EP, Liedke S, de Riese W, Stief C, Schneider B. Stage I seminoma of the testis: adjuvant radiotherapy or surveillance? Br J Urol 1991;68:190.
31. Bayens YC, Helle PA, Van PW, Mali SP. Orchidectomy followed by radiotherapy in 176 stage I and II testicular seminoma patients: benefits of a 10-year follow-up study. Radiother Oncol 1992;25:97.
32. Brunt AM, Scoble JE. Para-aortic nodal irradiation for early stage testicular seminoma. Clin Oncol 1992;4:165.
33. Dosmann MA, Zagars GK. Post-orchiectomy radiotherapy for stages I and II testicular seminoma [see comments]. Int J Radiat Oncol Biol Phys 1993;26:381.
34. Duncan W, Munro AJ. The management of testicular seminoma: Edinburgh 1970–1981. Br J Cancer 1987;55:443.
35. Epstein BE, Order SE, Zinreich ES. Staging, treatment, and results in testicular seminoma: a 12-year report. Cancer 1990;65:405.
36. Fossa SD, Aass N, Kaalhus O. Radiotherapy for testicular seminoma stage I: treatment results and long-term post-irradiation morbidity in 365 patients. Int J Radiat Oncol Biol Phys 1989;16:383.
37. Germa Lluch JR, Climent MA, Villavicencio H, et al. Treatment of stage I testicular tumours. Br J Urol 1993;71:473.
38. Giacchetti S, Raoul Y, Wibault P, Droz JP, Court B, Eschwege F. Treatment of stage I testis seminoma by radiotherapy: long-term results—a 30-year experience. Int J Radiat Oncol Biol Phys 1993;27: 3.
39. Gospodarowicz MK, Warde PR, Panzarella T, et al. The Princess Margaret Hospital experience in the management of stage I and II seminoma: 1981 to 1991. Adv Biosci 1994;91:177.
40. Hannun Y, Vugrin D. Long-term survival in patients treated for testicular seminoma. J Surg Oncol 1990;43:177.
41. Kellokumpu LP, Halme A. Results of treatment in irradiated testicular seminoma patients. Radiother Oncol 1990;18:1.
42. Lai PP, Bernstein MJ, Kim H, Perez CA, Wasserman TH, Kucik NA. Radiation therapy for stage I and IIA testicular seminoma (see comments). Int J Radiat Oncol Biol Phys 1994;28:373.
43. Lindeman GJ, Tiver KW. Management of testicular seminoma at Westmead Hospital from 1980 to 87. Aust N Z J Surg 1991;61:211.
44. Read G, Johnston RJ. Short duration radiotherapy in stage I seminoma of the testis: preliminary results of a prospective study. Clin Oncol 1993;5:364.
45. Singhal S, Dixit S, Vyas RK, Neema JP, Murthy RR, Baboo HA. Post-orchiectomy management in stage I testicular seminoma: elective irradiation or surveillance? Australas Radiol 1993;37:205.
46. Sommer K, Brockmann WP, Hubener KH. Treatment results and acute and late toxicity of radiation therapy for testicular seminoma. Cancer 1990;66:259. Review.
47. Stein ME, Kessel I, Luberant N, Kuten A. Testicular seminoma stage I: treatment results and long-term follow-up (1968–1988). J Surg Oncol 1993;53:175.
48. Thomas GM. Controversies in the management of testicular seminoma. Cancer 1985;55:2296.
49. Tongaonkar HB, Dalal AV, Kelkar DS, Kulkarni JN, Kamar MR. Stage I testicular tumours: the TATA Memorial Hospital experience. J Surg Oncol 1993;54:114.
50. Willan BD, McGowan DG. Seminoma of the testis: a 22-year experience with radiation therapy. Int J Radiat Oncol Biol Phys 1985;11: 1769.
51. Yeoh E, Razali M, O'Brien PC. Radiation therapy for early stage seminoma of the testis: analysis of survival and gastrointestinal toxicity in patients treated with modern megavoltage techniques over 10 years. Australas Radiol 1993;37:367.
52. Mason MD, Featherstone T, Olliff J, Horwich A. Inguinal and lilac lymph node involvement in germ cell tumours of the testis: implications for radiological investigation and for therapy. Clin Oncol 1991; 3:147.
53. Stein M, Steiner M, Suprun H, Robinson E. Inguinal lymph node metastases from testicular tumor. J Urol 1985;134:144.

54. Klein FA, Whitmore WJ, Sogani PC, Batata M, Fisher H, Herr HW. Inguinal lymph node metastases from germ cell testicular tumors. J Urol 1984;131:497.
55. Dobbs J, Barrett A, Ash D. Practical radiotherapy planning. 2nd ed. London, Edward Arnold, 1992:229.
56. Zagars GK. Management of stage I seminoma: radiotherapy. In: Horwich A, ed. Testicular cancer: investigation and management. London, Chapman and Hall Medical, 1991:83.
57. Babaian RJ, Zagars GK. Testicular seminoma: the M. D. Anderson experience. An analysis of pathological and patient characteristics, and treatment recommendations. J Urol 1988;139:311.
58. Hamilton C, Horwich A, Easton D, Peckham MJ. Radiotherapy for stage I seminoma testis: results of treatment and complications. Radiother Oncol 1986;6:115.
59. Zagars GK. Stage I testicular seminoma following orchidectomy: to treat or not to treat (comment). Eur J Cancer 1993;14:1923. Review.
60. Dosoretz DE, Shipley WU, Blitzer PH, et al. Megavoltage irradiation for pure testicular seminoma: results and patterns of failure. Cancer 1981;48:2184.
61. Lester SG, Morphis J2, Hornback NB. Testicular seminoma: analysis of treatment results and failures. Int J Radiat Oncol Biol Phys 1986; 12:353.
62. Abdeen N, Souhami L, Freeman C, Yassa M, Roman T. Radiation therapy of testicular seminoma: a 15-year survey. Am J Clin Oncol 1992;15:87.
63. Raina V, Singh SP, Kamble N, et al. Brain metastasis as the site of relapse in germ cell tumor of testis. Cancer 1993;72:2182.
64. Rathmell AJ, Mapstone NP, Jones WG. Testicular seminoma metastasizing to palatine tonsil. Clin Oncol 1993;5:185.
65. Charig MJ, Hindley AC, Lloyd K, Golding SJ. "Watch policy" in patients with suspected stage I testicular seminoma: CT as a sole staging and surveillance technique. Clin Radiol 1990;42 40.
66. Horwich A, Alsanjari N, A'Hern R, Nicholls J, Dearnaley DP, Fisher C. Surveillance following orchidectomy for stage I testicular seminoma. Br J Cancer 1992;65:775.
67. Ramakrishnan S, Champion AE, Dorreen MS, Fox M. Stage I seminoma of the testis: is post-orchidectomy surveillance a safe alternative to routine postoperative radiotherapy? Clin Oncol 1992;4:284.
68. von der Maase H, Specht L, Jacobsen GK, et al. Surveillance following orchidectomy for stage I seminoma of the testis (see comments). Eur J Cancer 1993;14:1931.
69. Warde PR, Gospodarowicz MK, Goodman PJ, et al. Results of a policy of surveillance in stage I testicular seminoma. Int J Radiat Oncol Biol Phys 1993;27:11.
70. Oliver RT, Edmonds PM, Ong JY, et al. Pilot studies of 2 and 1 course carboplatin as adjuvant for stage I seminoma: should it be tested in a randomized trial against radiotherapy? Int J Radiat Oncol Biol Phys 1994;29:3.
71. Boyer M, Raghavan D. Toxicity of treatment of germ cell tumors. Semin Oncol 1992;19:128.
72. Hanks GE, Herring DF, Kramer S. Patterns of care outcome studies: results of the national practice in seminoma of the testis. Int J Radiat Oncol Biol Phys 1981;7:1413.
73. Thomas GM, Rider WD, Dembo AJ, et al. Seminoma of the testis: results of treatment and patterns of failure after radiation therapy. Int J Radiat Oncol Biol Phys 1982;8:165.
74. Fossa SD, Borge L, Aass N, Johannessen NB, Stenwig AE, Kaalhus O. The treatment of advanced metastatic seminoma: experience in 55 cases. J Clin Oncol 1987;5:1071.
75. Gregory C, Peckham MJ. Results of radiotherapy for stage II testicular seminoma. Radiother Oncol 1986;6:285.
76. Evensen JF, Fossa SD, Kjellevold K, Lien HH. Testicular seminoma: analysis of treatment and failure for stage II disease. Radiother Oncol 1985;4:55.
77. Smalley SR, Earle JD, Evans RG, Richardson RL. Modern radiotherapy results with bulky stages II and III seminoma. J Urol 1990;144: 685.
78. Herr HW, Bosl G. Residual mass after chemotherapy for seminoma: changing concepts of management. J Urol 1987;137:1234.
79. Mann K, Siddle K. Evidence for free beta-subunit secretion in so-called human chorionic gonadotropin-positive seminoma. Cancer 1988;62:2378.
80. Mirimanoff RO, Shipley WU, Dosoretz DE, Meyer JE. Pure seminoma of the testis: the results of radiation therapy in patients with elevated human chorionic gonadotropin titers. J Urol 1985;134:1124.
81. Mirimanoff RO, Sinzig M, Kruger M, et al. Prognosis of human chorionic gonadotropin-producing seminoma treated by postoperative radiotherapy. Int J Radiat Oncol Biol Phys 1993;27:17.
82. Paus E, Fossa SD, Risberg T, Nustad K. The diagnostic value of human chorionic gonadotrophin in patients with testicular seminoma. Br J Urol 1987;59:572.
83. Swartz DA, Johnson DE, Hussey DH. Should an elevated human chorionic gonadotropin titer alter therapy for seminoma? J Urol 1984; 131:63.
84. Mumperow E, Hartmann M. Spermatic cord beta-human chorionic gonadotropin levels in seminoma and their clinical implications. J Urol 1992;147:1041.
85. Morgan DA, Caillaud JM, Bellet D, Eschwege F. Gonadotrophin-producing seminoma: a distinct category of germ cell neoplasm. Clin Radiol 1982;33:149.
86. Norgaard PB, Schultz HP, Arends J, et al. Tumour markers in testicular germ cell tumours: five-year experience from the DATECA Study 1976–1980. Acta Radiol (Oncol) 1984;23:287.
87. Dieckmann KP, Due W, Bauer HW. Seminoma testis with elevated serum beta-hCG: a category of germ-cell cancer between seminoma and nonseminoma. Int Urol Nephrol 1989;21:175. Review.
88. Mauch P, Weichselbaum R, Botnik K. The significance of positive chorionic gonadotrophins in apparently pure seminoma of the testis. Int J Radiat Oncol Biol Phys 1979;5:887.
89. Weissbach L, Bussar-Maatz R. HCG-positive seminoma. Eur Urol 1993;2:29.
90. Batata MA, Whitmore W Jr., Chu FC, et al. Cryptorchidism and testicular cancer. J Urol 1980;124:382.
91. Gauwitz MD, Zagars GK. Treatment of seminoma arising in cryptorchid testes. Int J Radiat Oncol Biol Phys 1992;24:153.
92. Sham JS, Choy D, Chan KW, Choi PH. Seminoma of normally-descended and cryptorchid testis. Eur J Surg Oncol 1990;16:33.
93. Bauer SB, Perimutter AD, Retik AB. Anomalies of the upper urinary tract. In: Walsh PC, Retik AB, Stamey TA, Vaughan ED Jr., eds. Campell's urology, 6th ed. Philadelphia, WB Saunders, 1992:1357.
94. Li FP, Fraumeni JF. Testicular cancers in children: epidemiologic characteristics. J Natl Cancer Inst 1972;48:1575.
95. Elyan SA, Reed DH, Ostrowski MJ, Williams MV, Dixon AK. Problems in the management of testicular seminoma associated with a horseshoe kidney. Clin Oncol 1990;2:163.
96. Key DW, Moyad R, Grossman HB. Seminoma associated with crossed fused renal ectopia. J Urol 1990;143:1015.
97. Sogani PC, Whitmore W Jr. Retroperitoneal lymphadenectomy for germ cell tumor of testis in association with horseshoe kidney. Urology 1981;18:446.
98. Fisher KS, Birtch AG. Seminoma in renal transplant patients: a patient report and review of the literature. Curr Surg 1990;47:181. Review.
99. Nellans RE, Raver J. Seminoma in a renal transplant recipient. J Urol 1986;113:871.
100. Viddeleer AC, Lycklama A, Nijeholt GAB, Beekhuis-Brussee JAM. A late manifestation of testicular seminoma in the bladder in a renal transplant recipient: a case report. J Urol 1992;148:401.
101. Dieckmann KP, Due W, Offermann G. Testicular seminoma in an immunosuppressed renal transplant recipient. Br J Urol 1989;63:549.
102. Villalona CM, Ducker T, Holasek M, Najarian I, Kennedy BJ. Management of testicular seminoma following organ transplantation. Med Pediatr Oncol 1992;20:338.
103. Damstrup L, Daugaard G, Getstoft J, Rorth M. Effects of antineoplastic treatment of HIV-positive patients with testicular cancer. Eur J Cancer Clin Oncol 1989;23:983.
104. Green ST, Nathwani D, Goldberg DJ, Paterson PJ, Kennedy DH. Urological manifestations of HIV-related disease: a case of AIDS-associated testicular seminoma, Kaposi's sarcoma and possible intracranial lymphoma. Br J Urol 1991;67:188. Review.
105. Logothetis CJ, Newell GR, Samuels ML. Testicular cancer in homosexual men with cellular immune deficiency report of 2 cases. J Urol 1985;133:484.
106. Moyle G, Hawkins DA, Gazzard BG. Seminoma and HIV infections. Int J STD AIDS 1991;2:293.
107. Roehrborn CG, Worrell JT, Wiley EL. Bilateral synchronous testis tumors of different histology in a patient with the acquired immunodeficiency syndrome related complex. J Urol 1990;144:353.

108. Wilkinson M, Carroll PR. Testicular carcinoma in patients positive and at risk for human immunodeficiency virus. J Urol 1990;144:1157.
109. Wilson WT, Frenkel E, Vuitch F, Sagalowsky AI. Testicular tumors in men with human immunodeficiency virus. J Urol 1992;147:1038.
110. De Ruysscher D, Waer M, Vandeputte M, Aerts R, Vantongelen K, van der Schueren E. Changes of lymphocyte subsets after local irradiation for early stage breast cancer and seminoma testis: long-term increase of activated (HLA-DR +) T cells and decrease of "naive" (CD4-CD45R) T lymphocytes. Eur J Cancer 1992;10:1729.
111. de Jong B, Oosterhuis JW, Castedo SM, Vos A, te Meerman GJ. Pathogenesis of adult testicular germ cell tumors: a cytogenetic model. Cancer Genet Cytogenet 1990;48:143.
112. Blacher EJ, Maynard JF. Seminoma and sarcoidosis: an unusual association. Urology 1983;26:288.
113. Fossa SD, Abeler V, Marton PF, Lien HH, Hoie J. Sarcoid reaction of hilar and paratracheal lymph nodes in patients treated for testicular cancer. Cancer 1985;56:2212.
114. Geller RA, Kuremsky DA, Copeland JS, Stept R. Sarcoidosis and testicular neoplasm: an unusual association. J Urol 1977;118:487.
115. Urbanski J, Alison RE, Jewett MAS, Gospodarowicz MK, Sturgeon JFG. Association of germ cell tumours of the testis and intrathoracic sarcoid-like lesions. Can Med Assoc J 1987;137:416.
116. Borge N, Fossa SD, Ous S, Stenwig AE, Lien HH. Late recurrence of testicular cancer. J Clin Oncol 1988;6:1248.
117. Thomas G. Management of metastatic seminoma: role of radiotherapy. In: Horwich A, ed. Testicular cancer: investigation and management. London, Chapman and Hall Medical, 1991:117.
118. Bokemeyer C, Schmoll HJ, Schoffski P, Harstrick A, Bading M, Poliwoda H. Bilateral testicular tumours: prevalence and clinical implications. Eur J Cancer 1993;6:874.
119. Ondrus D, Matoska J, Hornak M. Bilateral germ cell tumors of the testis. Neoplasma 1993;40:329.
120. van Leeuwen F, Stiggelbout AM, van den Belt-Dusebout AW, et al. Second cancer risk following testicular cancer: a follow-up study of 1,909 patients. J Clin Oncol 1993;11:415.
121. Osterlind A, Berthelsen JG, Abildgaard N, et al. Risk of bilateral testicular germ cell cancer in Denmark: 1960–1984. J Natl Cancer Inst 1991;83:1391.
122. Read G, Robertson AG, Blair V. Radiotherapy in seminoma of the testis. Clin Radiol 1983;34:469.
123. Grigor KM, Rorth M. Should the contralateral testis be biopsied? Round table discussion. Eur Urol 1993;23:129.
124. Coia LR, Hanks GE. Complications from large field intermediate dose infradiaphragmatic radiation: an analysis of the patterns of care outcome studies for Hodgkin's disease and seminoma. Int J Radiat Oncol Biol Phys 1988;15:29.
125. Hamilton CR, Horwich A, Bliss JM, Peckham MJ. Gastrointestinal morbidity of adjuvant radiotherapy in stage I malignant teratoma of the testis. Radiother Oncol 1987;10:85.
126. Senturia YD, Peckham CS, Peckham MJ. Children fathered by men treated for testicular cancer. Lancet 1985;2:766.
127. Cassileth B, Steinfeld A. Pyschological preparation of the patient and family. Cancer 1987;60:547.
128. Fossa SD, Aass N, Kaalhus O. Testicular cancer in young Norwegians. J Surg Oncol 1988;39:43. Review.
129. Kaasa S, Aass N, Mastekaasa A, Lund E, Fossa SD. Psychosocial well-being in testicular cancer patients. Eur J Cancer 1991;27:1091.
130. Tinkler SD, Howard GC, Kerr GR. Sexual morbidity following radiotherapy for germ cell tumours of the testis. Radiother Oncol 1992; 25:207.
131. Moynihan C. Psychosocial assessments and counselling of the patient with testicular cancer. In: Horwich A, ed. Testicular cancer: investigation and management. London, Chapman and Hall Medical, 1991: 353.
132. Schover LR, Gonzales M, von Eschenbach A. Sexual and marital relationships after radiotherapy for seminoma. Urology 1986;27:117.
133. Corn BW, Trock BJ, Goodman RL. Irradiation-related ischemic-heart disease. J Clin Oncol 1990;8:741.
134. Stewart JR, Fajardo LF. Radiation induced heart disease: an update. Prog Cardiovasc Dis 1984;28:173.
135. Lederman GS, Sheldon TA, Chaffey JT, Herman TS, Gelman RS, Coleman CN. Cardiac disease after mediastinal irradiation for seminoma. Cancer 1987;60:772.
136. Hanks GE, Peters T, Owen J. Seminoma of the testis: long-term beneficial and deleterious results of radiation. Int J Radiat Oncol Biol Phys 1992;24:913.
137. Jacobsen GK, Mellemgaard A, Engelholm SA, Moller H. Increased incidence of sarcoma in patients treated for testicular seminoma. Eur J Cancer 1993;5:664.
138. Kaldor JM, Day NE, Band P, et al. Second malignancies following testicular cancer, ovarian cancer and Hodgkin's disease: an international collaborative study among cancer registries. Int J Cancer 1987; 39:571.
139. Amichetti M, Boi S. Postirradiation sarcoma in a patient treated for testicular seminoma. Oncology 1993;50:264.
140. Coleman MP, Bell CM, Fraser P. Second primary malignancy after Hodgkin's disease, ovarian cancer and cancer of the testis: a population-based cohort study. Br J Cancer 1987;56:349.
141. O'Brien WM, Abbondanzo SL, Chun BK, Manz HJ, Maxted WC. Neurogenic fibrosarcoma following radiation therapy for seminoma. Urology 1989;33:420.
142. Moller H, Mellemgaard A, Jacobsen GK, Pedersen D, Storm HH. Incidence of second primary cancer following testicular cancer. Eur J Cancer 1993;5:672.
143. Kennedy L, Hendry WF, Peckham MJ. The significance of scrotal interference in stage I testicular cancer managed by orchiectomy and surveillance. Br J Urol 1986;58:705.
144. Sturgeon JF, Jewett MA, Alison RE, et al. Surveillance after orchidectomy for patients with clinical stage I nonseminomatous testis tumors. J Clin Oncol 1992;10:564.
145. Gospodarowicz MK, Thomas GT, Sturgeon JFG. The optimal treatment of patients with stage II seminoma with moderate size retroperitoneal metastases (5–10 cm). Curr Opin Urol 1991;1:76.
146. Mason BR, Kearsley JH. Radiotherapy for stage 2 testicular seminoma: the prognostic influence of tumor bulk. J Clin Oncol 1988;6: 1856.
147. Thomas G. Progress and controversies in the management of seminoma. Prog Clin Biol Res 1990;357:217. Review.

Principles and Practice of Genitourinary Oncology, edited by Derek Raghavan, Howard I. Scher, Steven A. Leibel, and Paul H. Lange. Lippincott-Raven Publishers, Philadelphia, © 1997.

CHAPTER 66

Management of Stage III-IV (C) Seminoma

Robert Dreicer and Mark A. Ritter

Patients presenting with pure seminoma represent approximately 40% of all testicular cancers per year. Because the majority of patients with seminoma present with stage I disease, the numbers of patients with advanced disease are limited, even at centers with wide experience. Radiotherapy as sole treatment for stage III and IV seminoma is mostly of historical interest only. Many patients receiving radiotherapy alone were treated in the era preceding computed tomography (CT) and serum tumor markers, and, therefore, their treatment planning did not benefit from the better imaging and biologic information currently available. The results for radiotherapy as primary treatment indicate a control of disease in only 30% to 40% of patients,[1–8] percentages clearly inferior to results with cisplatin-based chemotherapy.*

Historically, the role of cisplatin-based combination therapy in the management of advanced seminoma lagged behind its use in patients with nonseminoma. Given the exquisite radiosensitivity of seminomas, the bulk of early experience with chemotherapy was in radiotherapy failures. Over the past decade, increasing experience with primary chemotherapy of patients with advanced disease has led to an emerging consensus that patients presenting with bulky disease (≥5 cm) should receive cisplatin-based therapy as primary treatment. The impetus of the change was the recognition that cisplatin-based therapy yielded long-term disease-free survival in 85% of patients, and, more recently, with the introduction of serotonin antagonist antiemetics and recombinant colony-stimulating factors, three to four courses of cisplatin-based therapy are increasingly well tolerated.[9–11]

Despite the extraordinary effectiveness of cisplatin-based therapy in advanced seminoma, several management issues remain controversial, including the role of carboplatin-based regimens, the contribution of bleomycin, the surgical management of residual masses, and the role of adjuvant radiotherapy.

CHEMOTHERAPEUTIC SALVAGE OF RADIOTHERAPY FAILURES

Approximately 70% of patients who have a relapse after receiving primary radiotherapy for seminoma can obtain long-term disease-free survival after treatment with chemotherapy (Table 66-1). The most widely held theory for the disparity of response rates for patients pretreated with radiotherapy (70%), compared with those obtained in untreated patients (85%), is increased myelosuppression leading to a decrease in delivered dose intensity. In the Memorial Sloan-Kettering Cancer Center (MSKCC) series reported by Motzer and colleagues, a statistically significant difference in white blood cell nadir from similar cisplatin-based combination therapy was observed in patients pretreated with radiotherapy, when compared with patients treated primarily with chemotherapy.[12] In the series reported by Schuette and associates, 2 of 9 patients pretreated with radiotherapy required dose modifications and subsequently died of progressive disease.[13] Loehrer and colleagues, reporting the Southeastern Cancer Study Group experience, noted a statistically significant increase in thrombocytopenia in patients pretreated with radiotherapy.[14] Fosså and associates demonstrated a statistically significant reduction in vinblastine dose intensity secondary to myelosuppression in their radiotherapy-pretreated patients.[15] Other series with patients treated with comparable regimens suggest a trend toward increased myelosuppression and decreased dose intensity in patients pretreated with radiotherapy.[16,17] Some evidence in the literature suggests that a dose-response relationship exists between prior radiotherapy and the ability to salvage patients who receive more extensive fields (mediastinal plus abdominal) versus limited fields.[14,15] Other reports have suggested an increase in mortality secondary to cardiac events or second cancers in patients pretreated with radiotherapy, although data regarding these nonmyelosuppressive complications are limited.[18] All the referenced studies used cisplatin-based therapy before the availability of myeloid colony-stimulating factors; hence the impact on these agents cannot be assessed. Nonetheless, thrombocytopenia appears to represent a critical issue in the absence of an effective platelet-stimulating agent.

CHEMOTHERAPY AS INITIAL THERAPY OF ADVANCED SEMINOMA

In the early 1980s, investigators at Indiana University and at the MSKCC reported response rates of 63% to 89% to cisplatin-based combinations in patients with advanced seminoma.[19,20]

*Editor's note: Of course, the use of radiotherapy for stage III-IV seminoma predated the use of cytotoxic chemotherapy for these tumors, and hence effective salvage for treatment failures was not available.

TABLE 66-1. *Results of platinum-based salvage chemotherapy in patients with seminoma relapsing after primary radiotherapy*

Investigators	No. of patients	Salvage therapy	Complete response (%)	Disease-free survival (%)
Clemm et al, 1986[16]	7	VIP	5 (71)	5 (71)
Mencel et al, 1994[21]	18*	VAB-6, EP, EC, VAB-6 alternating with EP	13 (72)	13 (72)
Fosså et al, 1987[15]	15	PVB/BEP	13 (83)	4 (67)
Vugrin et al, 1981[20]	6	CDDP/CTX	5 (83)	4 (67)
Pizzocaro et al, 1986[55]	12	PVB/BEP	9 (75)	6 (50)
Schuette et al, 1985[13]	9	PVB/PVBA CDDP/IFX	7 (78)	7 (78)
Loehrer et al, 1987[14]	33	PVB/BEP PVBA	20 (61)	
Peckham et al, 1985[49]	13	PVB/BEP EP/CBDCA		10 (77)
Gietema et al, 1991[56]	8	PVB/BEP	4 (50)	7 (88)
Wilkinson et al, 1988[57]	25	PVB/BEP CTX/VP-16	7 (26)	14 (52)
Srougi et al, 1985[58]	3	VAB-6	3 (100)	3 (100)
Total	149	—	86 (63)	79 (70)

* Includes 4 patients who received combined chemotherapy and radiotherapy.

VIP, vinblastine, ifosfamide, and cisplatin; *VAB-6*, cisplatin, vinblastine, bleomycin, cyclophosphamide, and dactinomycin; *EP*, etoposide and cisplatin; *EC*, etoposide and carboplatin; *PVB*, cisplatin, vinblastine, and bleomycin; *BEP*, cisplatin, etoposide, and bleomycin; *CDDP*, *CTX*, cyclophosphamide; *PVBA*, PVB plus doxorubicin; *IFX*, ifosfamide; *CBDCA*, carboplatin.

Mature experiences from various centers have been reported over the past several years (Table 66-2). Mencel and colleagues reported the MSKCC experience in 142 patients with advanced seminoma.[21] All patients were treated with platinum-based combinations including cisplatin, vinblastine, bleomycin, cyclophosphamide, and dactinomycin (VAB-6), etoposide and cisplatin (EP), and VAB-6 alternating with EP or etoposide and carboplatin. Durable responses were obtained in 86% of patients, with a median follow-up of 43 months. The highest proportional durable response was achieved in patients receiving EP. Given these findings, in addition to the results of a randomized trial of VAB-6 versus EP demonstrating at least equal efficacy with less vascular toxicity and neurotoxicity, investigators at the MSKCC have adopted four cycles of EP as standard therapy for patients with advanced seminoma.[22]

In a series of 42 previously untreated patients with advanced

TABLE 66-2. *Results of cisplatin-based combination chemotherapy in untreated patients with seminoma*

Investigators	No. of patients	Salvage therapy*	Complete response (%)	Disease-free survival (%)
Clemm et al, 1986[16]	11	VIP	9 (82)	9 (82)
Mencel et al, 1994[21]	124†	VAB-6, EP, EC, VAB-6 alternating with EP		108 (87)
Fosså et al, 1987[15]	40	PVB/BEP	36 (90)	33 (83)
Pizzocaro et al, 1986[55]	19	PVB/BEP	18 (95)	17 (89)
Loehrer et al, 1987[14]	27	PVB ± A/BEP	21 (87)	
Peckham et al, 1985[49]	31	PVB/BEP EP/CBDCA		29 (93)
Gietema et al, 1991[56]	25	PVB/BEP	9 (36)	20 (80)
Wilkinson et al, 1988[57]	10	PVB/BEP CTX/VP-16	1 (10)	5 (50)
Friedman et al, 1985[17]	8	PVB	3 (38)	6 (75)
Srougi et al, 1985[58]	10	VAB-6	10 (100)	10 (100)
Total	305	—	107 (71)	237 (85)

* Includes some patients who received adjuvant radiotherapy.

† Includes 4 patients who received combined chemotherapy and radiotherapy.

VIP, vinblastine, ifosfamide, and cisplatin; VAB-6, cisplatin vinblastine, bleomycin, cyclophosphamide, and dactinomycin; EP, etoposide and cisplatin; EC, etoposide and carboplatin; PVB, cisplatin, vinblastine, and bleomycin; BEP, cisplatin, etoposide, and bleomycin; CBDCA, carboplatin; CTX, cyclophosphamide.

seminoma treated in Europe and Indiana University with cisplatin, vinblastine, and bleomycin (PVB), 35 (83%) achieved a complete response with chemotherapy alone. With a minimum follow-up of 2 years, 33 (79%) remained alive and disease-free.[23] Fosså and colleagues treated 39 patients with advanced seminoma with PVB or cisplatin, etoposide, and bleomycin (BEP) for four cycles. Thirty-six patients obtained a complete remission, and 3 had a partial remission. The majority of these patients had adjuvant radiotherapy, surgery, or both. With a minimum follow-up of 3 years, 33 patients (85%) remained alive and disease-free.[15]

The role of bleomycin in the management of patients with advanced seminoma remains controversial. Levi and associates performed a randomized trial of cisplatin and vinblastine (PV) versus PVB in 218 patients with good risk germ cell cancer.[24] Six percent of randomized patients had pure seminoma. Patients treated on the PVB arm of the study had significantly more toxicity, including leukopenia, anemia, thrombocytopenia, and renal and pulmonary complications. After a minimum of 4 years of follow-up, 7% of patients treated on the PV arm of the trial had relapses, in contrast with 5% of those in the PVB arm of the study. After salvage therapy, deaths from progressive malignant disease occurred in 15% of patients initially treated with PV, compared with 5% of those treated with PVB. These investigators note, however, that the increase in deaths in the PV arm of the trial was partially offset by the higher proportion of toxic deaths seen in the PVB arm of the study.

Both the Eastern Cooperative Oncology Group (ECOG) and the European Organization for the Research and Treatment of Cancer (EORTC) have performed randomized trials evaluating the role of bleomycin. In the ECOG trial, three cycles of BEP were compared with three cycles of EP in good risk patients. This study was closed early after an unacceptably high incidence of failure was observed in the EP arm. These investigators concluded that bleomycin was an essential component of this combination.[25] The EORTC study compared four cycles of EP with BEP in 180 good risk patients.[26] In an early analysis, rates of both complete remission and relapse were similar; however, a reanalysis of the data is in progress. Although the optimal chemotherapy regimen for the initial therapy of patients with advanced seminoma remains disputable, four cycles of either BEP or EP should be considered the current standard.

SALVAGE THERAPY FOR CHEMOTHERAPY FAILURES

Published experience regarding the role of salvage chemotherapy in patients with advanced disease in whom primary chemotherapy fails is limited. Historically, some patients who have had relapses outside the primary treatment fields have been retreated with radiotherapy and have been rendered long-term survivors.[8] As with nonseminomatous germ cell cancer, patients who have relapses after primary chemotherapy may be salvaged with alternative cisplatin-based therapy such as etoposide, ifosfamide, cisplatin (VIP) in patients in whom PVB has failed or vinblastine, ifosfamide, and cisplatin (VeIP) in patients whose relapses have occurred after treatment with BEP.[27,28] Levi and colleagues treated 51 patients who either failed to achieve a complete response or had a relapse after complete response to PVB with the combination of VP-16, dactinomycin, and methotrexate. In this multiinstitutional trial, therapy was well tolerated, and 15 patients (29%) were ultimately rendered disease-free, long-term survivors.[29] Ultimately, even in heavily pretreated or cisplatin-refractory patients, 15% to 44% of patients may be rendered long-term survivors with high-dose chemotherapy and autologous bone marrow or peripheral stem cell rescue.[30,31]

ROLE OF CARBOPLATIN-BASED THERAPY

Given the widely recognized sensitivity of seminoma to cisplatin-based combination therapy, clinical investigation has been directed at reducing the toxicity and expense associated with the management of these patients. Occasional reports have suggested modifications of standard cisplatin combinations such as that noted by Berkmen, who decreased the dose intensity of vinblastine and bleomycin in the PVB regimen with a reported a complete response rate of 97%.[32] The majority of these efforts have concentrated on evaluating the role of carboplatin as a single agent or in combination, however.

In 1989, Horwich and associates reported their early experience with carboplatin in 34 patients with advanced seminoma, 14 of whom had received prior radiotherapy.[33] Carboplatin, 400 mg/m^2, was administered as an intravenous infusion every 28 days for a total of four to six cycles. Thirty-two of 33 evaluable patients responded (97%), with 14 (42%) achieving a complete response. Therapy was well tolerated, with no neurotoxicity, ototoxicity, significant renal damage, or episodes of neutropenic sepsis. In a follow-up report involving 70 patients with a median follow-up of 3 years, the actuarial 3-year relapse-free survival rate was 77%, and the overall survival rate was 91%.[34] Sixteen patients had relapses, with 12 successfully salvaged with cisplatin-based combination therapy. Twenty of the 70 patients received postcarboplatin radiotherapy, and this subgroup had a significantly lower relapse rate than those patients treated with chemotherapy alone.

Bajorin and associates compared EP with etoposide and carboplatin (EC) in a large multicenter trial of patients with good risk germ cell tumors.[35] Two-hundred seventy patients were randomized to receive EP at 21-day intervals, versus EC given in 28 day cycles. Sixty-nine patients with seminoma were equally divided between the two treatment regimens. The overall complete response rates were equivalent for the EC and EP arms of the trial, at 88% and 90%, respectively; however, at a median follow-up of 22.4 months, those patients treated with EC had significantly inferior event-free and relapse-free survival rates. In patients with seminoma, the complete response rates were comparable, with 87% and 94% for the EP and EC arms of the study, respectively. Four (13%) of the EC-treated patients had relapes, however, versus none of the EP group.

A large randomized trial in Europe compared four cycles of BEP with four cycles of carboplatin, etoposide, and bleomycin (CEB) in patients with good risk nonseminomatous disease. Patients treated with CEB had a significant increase in the number of disease-related deaths as well as a significantly inferior failure free-survival, in comparison with patients treated with BEP.[36] Whether this result is directly applicable to patients with seminoma is unclear.

Because the overriding principle in the management of patients with good-risk disease must remain therapeutic efficacy, carboplatin-based therapy appears to have no standard role in the majority of patients with advanced seminoma, although it may have useful application in the patient with comorbid diseases that preclude the use of cisplatin.

MANAGEMENT OF THE RESIDUAL MASS

In contrast to the widely accepted management of residual masses in patients with nonseminomatous disease, the role of adjunctive surgery in patients with extensive seminomas represents a dilemma for the majority of oncologists who practice outside centers with clearly defined management strategies.

The rationale for surgical resection of residual masses in patients with nonseminomatous germ cell tumors is to identify and treat patients whose masses harbor residual carcinoma or teratoma, found in 20% and 40% of resections, respectively.[37] The surgical approach, retroperitoneal lymph node dissection (RPLND), is well defined, and, in experienced hands, is highly effective.[38,39] Several important differences complicate the management approach to the residual mass in patients with seminoma. Unlike in nonseminomatous germ cell cancer, the presence of teratoma in residual masses in patients with seminoma is uncommon.[40] Additionally, the well-described extensive fibrotic reaction in these tumors after chemotherapy makes complete resection difficult and leads to an increase in perioperative morbidity.[17,41]

Bulky seminomas often do not completely regress radiographically after chemotherapy,[42] but only a minority of such residual abnormalities contain tumor. An average of only about 10% of pretreatment sites of bulky disease contain histologic evidence of seminoma when these sites are surgically explored after completion of chemotherapy.[14,15,17,40,43–45]

Puc and colleagues reported their experience in 104 patients with advanced seminoma. A total of 55 patients had postchemotherapy surgical resections or biopsy, and 49 patients were carefully monitored. Only two of 74 (3%) patients with residual masses < 3 cm developed progressive disease compared with eight of 30 (27%) patients with residual masses ≥ 3 cm.[59] Herr and Bosl described two distinct presentations of residual radiographic abnormalities that may predict the likelihood of residual disease.[41] The most common is dense scar tissue surrounding the great vessels resulting from an ''implosion'' of tumor mass in response to systemic therapy leading to a CT pattern consistent with retroperitoneal fibrosis. Alternatively, some patients have a well-defined, discrete mass of 3 cm or larger. For these lesions, investigators at MSKCC advocate surgical extirpation, because they acknowledge that complete RPLND is rarely possible with the pattern of retroperitoneal fibrosis.[41] This approach, based on literature review, has been supported by other investigators.[46]

Investigators at Indiana University have taken a different approach to the management of the residual mass. In a series of 36 patients with advanced seminoma treated with cisplatin combination therapy, 21 had radiographic evidence of a residual mass. Nine of these 21 patients had masses larger than 3 cm in diameter. Only 3 of the 21 patients underwent RPLND, and all had evidence of necrotic fibrous tissue. With a median follow-up of 41 months, 19 of 21 patients (8 of 9 with masses >3 cm) had no evidence of radiographic or clinical progression.[47] Although they acknowledge the limitations of their data, Schultz and colleagues[47] suggest that close follow-up with routine tumor markers, chest radiographs, and CT scans every 3 months for 1 year and then every 6 months subsequently is appropriate, in lieu of surgical intervention or routine adjuvant radiotherapy. This more conservative approach is supported by other investigators.[16,48,49]

Fosså and colleagues evaluated the predictive value of pretreatment and posttreatment radiographic assessment of residual masses on patient outcome.[50] Forty-six patients with advanced seminoma with retroperitoneal, mediastinal, or pulmonary disease were evaluated. All patients were treated with a minimum of three cycles of cisplatin-combination chemotherapy and were radiographically assessed with CT scans. All patients underwent adjunctive radiotherapy, surgery, or both. In the 11 patients with retroperitoneal tumors treated surgically, 1 chemotherapy failure was found in 5 patients with residual masses larger than 10 cm^2, and 1 failure occurred in 6 patients with masses smaller than 10 cm^2. When all patients were considered, patients with masses larger than 10 cm^2 were at significantly higher risk of harboring residual viable tumor. Size was not a predictor for either residual tumor or relapse in patients with mediastinal or pulmonary metastases. Given the high relapse rate in nonirradiated areas in their series, Fosså and associates advocate the routine use of adjuvant radiotherapy to sites of initial disease.[15] These investigators acknowledge that, whereas radiotherapy appears to decrease local recurrence, it does not affect relapses outside the radiation field.[50] In contrast, Mencel and colleagues propose adjuvant radiotherapy only in patients with residual masses larger than 3 cm that have not been explored.[21]

Thus, results vary with respect to large residual masses and can support the following opposite conclusions: (1) that further evaluation and therapy is warranted; and (2) that observation with intervention only on progression is preferable. Several noninvasive techniques have the potential to characterize the residual mass in patients with advanced seminoma more clearly. Willan and associates[51] evaluated the role of gallium scans in patients with testicular seminomas. In their series of 77 patients who underwent pretherapy and posttherapy imaging, this technique was reported to have a sensitivity and specificity of 83% and 95%, respectively. Unfortunately, all these patients were evaluated in the pre-CT era, a likely factor in the sensitivity and specificity reported. Additionally, this study did not evaluate the role of gallium imaging as a means of assessing the residual mass.[51] Investigators at MSKCC and Indiana University conducted a prospective study to assess the ability of gallium scans to determine whether residual masses consist of viable tumor or necrotic tissue. In 27 evaluable patients they found 8 false positive scans at time of diagnosis and two of 19 follow-up studies were falsely negative. They concluded that gallium scans have minimal value in the management of these patients.[52] Another potentially interesting approach uses positron emission tomography (PET). In a preliminary report, investigators at Indiana University evaluated 15 patients with nonseminomatous germ cell cancer with PET-2-fluorodeoxyglucose imaging before planned adjuvant surgery.[52] Three patients were found to have residual tumor, and 12 had either necrotic fibrous tissue or teratoma. PET imaging was able to distinguish viable tumor from necrosis or teratoma. Although the inability to distinguish teratoma from fibrosis remains a significant problem in patients with nonseminoma, the potential to separate tumor from fibrosis suggests a promising role of this imaging modality in patients with seminoma. We hope that these studies will shed further light on the significance of persisting radiologic abnormalities.

In conclusion, the database from which to make definitive recommendations on the value of postchemotherapy radiation therapy in stage III and IV seminoma, as well as in chemotherapy-treated patients with bulky stage II tumors, is inadequate. Radiotherapy should not be considered in all patients with postchemotherapy masses, but the occurrence of local failures after chemotherapy, the low local failure rates observed in series using adjuvant radiation, and the finding, at least in some studies, of residual tumor in many large residual masses suggest that consolidative radiotherapy may have potential value in selected patients. Potential, location-dependent late effects of radiation, such as cardiac toxicity,[53] must be considered in any treatment decision.

REFERENCES

1. Duncan W, Munro AJ. The management of testicular seminoma: Edinburgh 1970–1981. Br J Cancer 1987;55:443.
2. Andrews CF, Micaily B, Brady LW. Testicular seminoma: results of a program of megavoltage irradiation. Am J Clin Oncol 1987;10:491.
3. Ball D, Barrett A, Pechkham MJ. The management of metastatic seminoma testis. Cancer 1982;50:2289.
4. Smalley SR, Earle JD, Evans RG, Richardson RL. Modern radiotherapy results with bulky stages II and III seminoma. J Urol 1990;144:685.
5. Lester SG, Morphis JG, Hornback NB. Testicular seminoma: analysis of treatment results and failures. Int J Radiat Oncol Biol Phys 1986; 12:353.
6. Doornbos JF, Hussey DH, Johnson DE. Radiotherapy for pure seminoma of the testis. Radiology 1975;116:401.
7. Thomas GM. Controversies in the management of testicular seminoma. Cancer 1985;55:2296.
8. Dosoretz DE, Shipley WU, Blitzer PH, et al. Megavoltage irradiation for pure testicular seminoma: results and patterns of failure. Cancer 1981;48:2184.
9. Marks LB, Anscher MS, Shipley WU. The role of radiation therapy in the treatment of testicular germ cell tumors. Hematol Oncol Clin North Am 1991;5:1143.
10. Lederman GS, Herman TS, Jochelson M, et al. Radiation therapy of seminoma: 17-year experience at the Joint Center for Radiation Therapy. Radiother Oncol 1989;14:203.
11. Thomas GM, Rider WD, Dembo AJ, et al. Seminoma of the testis: results of treatment and patterns of failure after radiation therapy. Int J Radiat Oncol Biol Phys 1982;8:165.
12. Motzer RJ, Bosl GJ, Geller NL, et al. Advanced seminoma: the role of chemotherapy and adjunctive surgery. Ann Intern Med 1988;108: 513.
13. Schuette J, Niederle N, Scheulen ME, Seeber S, Schmidt CG. Chemotherapy of metastatic seminoma. Br J Cancer 1985;51:467.
14. Loehrer PJ, Birch R, Williams SD, Greco FA, Einhorn LH. Chemotherapy of metastatic seminoma: the Southeastern Cancer Study Group experience. J Clin Oncol 1987;5:1212.
15. Fosså SD, Borge L, Aass N, Johannessen NB, Stenwig AE, Kaalhus O. The treatment of advanced metastatic seminoma: experience in 55 cases. J Clin Oncol 1987;5:1071.
16. Clemm C, Hartenstein R, Willich N, Boening L, Wilmanns W. Vinblastine-ifosfamide-cisplatin treatment of bulky seminoma. Cancer 1986; 58:2203.
17. Freidman EL, Garnick MB, Stomper PC, et al. Therapeutic guidelines and results in advanced seminoma. J Clin Oncol 1985;3:1325.
18. Pizzocaro G, Salvioni R, Piva L, Faustini M. Mortality following cisplatin combination chemotherapy for advanced testicular seminoma pretreated with radiotherapy. Proc Am Soc Clin Oncol 1987;6:418. Abstract.
19. Einhorn LH, Williams SD. Chemotherapy of disseminated seminoma. Cancer Clin Trials 1980;3:313.
20. Vugrin D, Whitmore WF, Batata M. Chemotherapy of disseminated seminoma with combination of cis-diamminedichloroplatinum (II) and cyclophosphamide. Cancer Clin Trials 1981;4:423.
21. Mencel PJ, Motzer RJ, Mazumdar M, et al. Advanced seminoma: treatment results, survival and prognostic factors in 142 patients. J Clin Oncol 1994;12:120.
22. Bosl GJ, Geller NL, Bajorin D, et al. A randomized trial of etoposide + cisplatin versus VAB-6 in patients with good prognosis germ cell tumors. J Clin Oncol 1988;6:1231.
23. van Ooosterom AT, Williams SD, Cortes-Funes H, et al. The treatment of advanced seminoma with combination chemotherapy. In: Jones WG, Ward AM, Anderson CK, eds. Germ cell tumour II. Oxford, Pergamon, 1986:229.
24. Levi JA, Raghavan D, Harvey V, et al. The importance of bleomycin in combination chemotherapy for good-prognosis germ cell carcinoma. J Clin Oncol 1993;11:1300.
25. Loehrer PJ, Elson P, Johnson DH, et al. A randomized trial of cisplatin plus etoposide with or without bleomycin in favorable prognosis disseminated germ cell tumors: an ECOG study. Proc Am Soc Clin Oncol 1991;10:540. Abstract.
26. Stoter G, Kaye S, Jones W, et al. Cisplatin and VP16 in good risk patients with disseminated non-seminomatous testicular cancer: a randomized EORTC GU Group Study. Proc Am Soc Clin Oncol 1987;6: 432. Abstract.
27. Loehrer PJ, Einhorn LH, Williams SD. VP-16 plus ifosfamide plus cisplatin as salvage therapy in refractory germ cell cancer. J Clin Oncol 1986;4:528.
28. Einhorn LH, Weathers T, Loehrer PJ, et al. Second line chemotherapy with vinblastine, ifosfamide and cisplatin after initial chemotherapy with cisplatin, VP-16 and bleomycin in disseminated germ cell tumors: long term followup. Proc Am Soc Clin Oncol 1992;11:599. Abstract.
29. Levi JA, Thomson D, Harvey V. Effective salvage chemotherapy with etoposide, dactinomycin, and methotrexate in refractory germ cell cancer. J Clin Oncol 1990;8:27.
30. Broun ER, Nichols CR, Kneebone P, et al. Long-term outcome of patients with relapsed and refractory germ cell tumors treated with high-dose chemotherapy and autologous bone marrow rescue. Ann Intern Med 1192;117:124.
31. Siegert W, Beyer J, Strohscheer I, et al. High-dose treatment with carboplatin, etoposide, and ifosfamide followed by autologous stem-cell transplantation in relapsed or refractory germ cell cancer: a phase I/II study. J Clin Oncol 1994;12:1223.
32. Berkmen F. Reduced dose PVB treatment of stage IIC-IV testicular seminoma. Eur J Surg Oncol 193;19:24.
33. Horwich A, Dearnaley DP, Duchesne GM, Williams M, Brada M, Peckham MJ. Simple nontoxic treatment of advanced metastatic seminoma with carboplatin. J Clin Oncol 1989;7:1150.
34. Horwich A, Dearnaley DP, A'Hern R, et al. The activity of single-agent carboplatin in advanced seminoma. Eur J Cancer 1992;28A:1307.
35. Bajorin DF, Sarosdy MF, Pfister DG, et al. Randomized trial of etoposide and cisplatin versus etoposide and carboplatin in patients with good-risk germ cell tumors: a multiinstitutional study. J Clin Oncol 1993;11:598.
36. Horwich A, Sleijfer D, Fosså S, et al. A trial of carboplatin-based combination chemotherapy in good prognosis metastatic testicular non seminoma. Proc Am Soc Clin Oncol 1994;13:709. Abstract.
37. Einhorn LH. Testicular cancer as a model for curable neoplasm: the Richard and Hinda Rosenthal Foundation award lecture. Cancer Res 1981;41:3275.
38. Donohue JP, Rowland RG. The role of surgery in advanced testicular cancer. Cancer 1984;54:2716.
39. Toner GC, Panicek DM, Heelan RT, et al. Adjunctive surgery after chemotherapy for nonseminomatous germ cell tumors: recommendations for patient selection. J Clin Oncol 1990;10:1683.
40. Motzer F, Bosl G, Heelan R. Residual mass: an indication for further therapy in patients with advanced seminoma following systemic chemotherapy. J Clin Oncol 1987;5:1064.
41. Herr HW, Bosl G. Residual mass after chemotherapy for seminoma: changing concepts of management. J Urol 1987;137:1234.
42. Stomper PC, Jochelson MS, Griedman EL, Garnick MB, Richie JP. CT evaluation of advanced seminoma treated with chemotherapy. AJR Am J Roentgenol 1986;146:745.

43. Schultz HP, von der Maase H, Rorth M. Testicular seminoma in Denmark 1976–1980: results of treatment. Acta Radiol Oncol 1984;23: 263.
44. Kamat MR, Kulkarni JN, Tongaonkar HB, Ravi R. Value of retroperitoneal lymph node dissection in advanced testicular seminoma. J Surg Oncol 1992;51:65.
45. Stanton GF, Bosl GJ, Whitmore WJ, et al. VAB-6 as initial treatment of patients with advanced seminoma. J Clin Oncol 1985;3:336.
46. Ellison MF, Mostofi FK, Flanigan RC. Treatment of the residual retroperitoneal mass after chemotherapy for advanced seminoma. J Urol 1988;140:618.
47. Schultz SM, Einhorn L, Conces DJ, et al. Management of postchemotherapy residual mass in patients with advanced seminoma: Indiana University experience. J Clin Oncol 1989;7:1497.
48. Wettlaufer JN. The management of advanced seminoma. Semin Urol 1984;2:257.
49. Peckham MJ, Horwich A, Hendry WF. Advanced seminoma: treatment with cis-platinum-based combination chemotherapy or carboplatin (JM 8). Br J Cancer 1985;52:7.
50. Fosså SD, Kullmann G, Lien HH, Stenwig AE, Ous S. Chemotherapy of advanced seminoma: clinical significance of radiological findings before and after treatment. Br J Urol 1989;64:530.
51. Willan BD, Penney H, Castor WR, et al. The usefulness of gallium-67 citrate scanning in testicular seminoma. Clin Nucl Med 1987;10: 831.
52. Warren GP, Einhorn LH. Gallium scans in the evaluation of residual masses after chemotherapy for seminoma. J Clin Oncol 1996;13:2784.
53. Stephens A, Donohue J, Hutchins G, Einhorn LH. Positron emission tomography evaluation of residual radiographic abnormalities in postchemotherapy germ cell tumors. Proc Am Soc Clin Oncol 1994;13: 721. Abstract.
54. Hanks GE, Peteres T, Owen J. Seminoma of the testis: long-term beneficial and deleterious results of radiation. Int J Radiat Oncol Biol Phys 1992;24:913.
55. Pizzocaro G, Salvioni R, Piva L, Zanoni F, Milani A, Faustini M. Cisplatin combination chemotherapy in advanced seminoma. Cancer 1986;58:1625.
56. Gietema JA, Willemse PHB, Mulder NH, Oldhoff J, de Vries EGE, Sleijfer DT. Alternating cycles of PVB and BEP in the treatment of patients with advanced seminoma. Eur J Cancer 1991;27:1376.
57. Wilkinson PM, Read G, Magee B. The treatment of advanced seminoma with chemotherapy and radiotherapy. Br J Cancer 1988;57:100.
58. Srougi M, Simon SD, De Góes GM. Vinblastine, actinomycin D, bleomycin, cyclophosphamide and cis-platinum for advanced germ cell testis tumors: Brazilian experience. J Urol 1985;134:65.
59. Puc HS, Heelan R, Mazumda M, et al. Management of residual mass in advanced seminoma: Results and Recommendations from the Memorial Sloan-Kettering Cancer Center. J Clin Oncol 1996;14:454.

Principles and Practice of Genitourinary Oncology, edited by Derek Raghavan, Howard I. Scher, Steven A. Leibel, and Paul H. Lange. Lippincott-Raven Publishers, Philadelphia, © 1997.

CHAPTER 67

Controversies in the Treatment of Early Stage Nonseminomatous Testicular Cancer

Michael A. S. Jewett, Paul H. Lange, and Derek Raghavan

In the past 20 years, progress in the management of testicular cancer has been dramatic, and the approach to management and the expectations of success have changed completely. Essential factors in this evolution include the improvement in our understanding of the biology of the disease,[1] with the identification of specific tumor markers and the definition of reliable prognostic determinants, the modification of the approaches to surgery, a reduced role for radiation, and the introduction of combination chemotherapy as curative treatment for patients with metastatic disease. These changes have had a particular impact on the treatment of early-stage disease, especially in the context of the increased precision of staging and prognostication and the "safety net" provided for most patients by chemotherapy in the event of failure of primary treatment.

PATHOBIOLOGY OF EARLY-STAGE TESTICULAR CANCER

The majority of testicular cancers are germ cell tumors, originating from primordial germ cells that arise in the genital ridges, which have the capacity to differentiate along two major lines: seminoma and nonseminoma germ cell tumors (NSGCTs).[1] The most common type of seminoma is the classic variant, which is composed of uniform, round, or polygonal cells with abundant cytoplasm and a centrally placed nucleolus, as discussed in Chapter 62. Less commonly, spermatocytic and anaplastic variants have been described, although the anaplastic variant sometimes represents a misdiagnosed NSGCT.[2] The histologic subtype of seminoma has no prognostic implication, although some series have suggested that anaplastic seminoma is associated with a higher relapse rate. In the older series, the anaplastic variant may have represented misdiagnosed embryonal carcinoma or yolk sac carcinoma. Several histologic variants are included in the group of NSGCTs, including embryonal carcinoma, mature and immature teratoma, endodermal sinus tumor, and choriocarcinoma[3]; frequently, NSGCT is composed of several of these elements and may consist of elements of undifferentiated cancer, trophoblastic tissue, and varying components of somatic differentiation.[1,3] Fewer than 5% of testicular cancers consist of lymphomas and other non–germ cell tumors,[4] and these are not covered in this chapter.

Testicular tumors usually follow an orderly pattern of spread, from the testis to the surrounding supportive tissues or up the spermatic cord, to regional and distant lymphatics, and sometimes to visceral sites by blood-borne metastasis. Much of the literature on the distribution of metastases antedates the availability of effective treatment of advanced disease and the awareness of the entity of testis cancer in the community; accordingly, a higher proportion of involvement of unusual sites, such as peritoneum, spleen, pancreas, adrenal glands, has been recorded[5] than applies to current clinical practice.

The predictable natural history of this disease is important in influencing the approach to the surgery of the retroperitoneum for the patient with established testicular cancer. Prognostic factors defined for stage I (A) testicular tumors should influence the considerations of management (see the discussion on staging later in this chapter).

Tumor Markers

Both seminomas and NSGCTs are characterized by the production of tumor markers, oncofetal proteins that are elaborated and released by the tumor cells. Although many such proteins have been documented in association with these germ cell tumors, two have found a particular role in patient management: alphafetoprotein (AFP) and human chorionic gonadotropin (hCG). Both proteins can be demonstrated in the blood of patients with testis cancer, or in germ cell tumor tissues immunohistochemically, using immunofluorescent or immunoperoxidase assays; however, certain fixatives (e.g., formalin) can reduce the staining of AFP.[6]

AFP, a single-chain polypeptide with a molecular weight of about 70,000, is produced by tissues with hepatic, gastrointestinal, and yolk sac differentiation. In the normal human fetus, AFP is a major serum protein that reaches peak levels at about the 12th week of gestation and then declines. Its function is not completely known, although it appears to act as an albumin-like protein in the fetus and may have an immunoregulatory function.[7] In the context of testicular tumors, it is specifically associated with yolk sac tumors (endodermal sinus tumors) and embryonal carcinoma. Occasionally, raised blood levels of AFP are associated with apparently pure seminoma; this phenomenon reflects an occult focus of NSGCT, hepatic abnormalities (such as hepatitis), or histologic misdiagnosis in which the solid variant of yolk sac carcinoma is mistaken for seminoma.[2] AFP is not absolutely specific to hepatic and germ cell tissues and may be found in association with other malignant tumors, predominantly those of the gastrointestinal tract. AFP characteristically has a half-time in the human circulation of 5 to 7 days, providing a useful characteristic for monitoring of residual disease after orchiectomy or of the persistence of viable tumor after lymph node dissection or chemotherapy.[6]

hCG, a glycoprotein hormone with a molecular weight of approximately 38,000, is produced by trophoblastic tissues, including the placenta, syncytiotrophoblastic giant cells, and choriocarcinomas (both gestational and germ cell tumors).[8] Occasionally, hCG is associated with other malignant tumors (e.g., lung cancer, ovarian cancer, bronchogenic cancer, pancreatic cancer, and non-Hodgkin's lymphoma) as an ectopic hormone, although this phenomenon may be explained by the presence of scattered syncytiotrophoblastic giant cells. hCG may be found in association with both seminomas and nonseminomatous germ cell tumors. The half-life of this complex protein is approximately 24 to 36 hours. Of importance, the molecula shares a common alpha chain with luteinizing hormone and follicle-stimulating hormone, and thus accurate and specific measurement of hCG can best be obtained from assays using antibodies raised against the beta subunit of the molecule. Patients with testicular cancer frequently have impaired gonadal function, with consequent elevation of circulating luteinizing hormone or follicle-stimulating hormone, and this elevation can cross-react with the less specific assays of hCG that do not measure the beta chain of the molecule.

Other tumor markers have been documented in association with germ cell tumors, including lactic acid dehydrogenase (LDH), the placental isoenzyme of alkaline phosphatase, ferritin, carcinoembryonic antigen, fibronectin, and human placental lactogen. Apart from LDH, however, none has found its way into routine clinical use, and none seems to confer any particular diagnostic or prognostic information. In the system of prognostic classification at the Memorial Sloan-Kettering Cancer Center, New York, LDH is included as an independent determinant of outcome for advanced disease (see Chap. 64).

Some controversy exists regarding the prognostic implications of AFP and hCG (see Chap. 64). In the past, investigators suggested that the absolute levels of AFP or hCG merely reflected tumor bulk and thus did not independently portend a worse prognosis.[9] More recently, studies have shown that raised levels of hCG, in particular, and of AFP in selected series are associated independently with a worse prognosis in patients with advanced disease. In a patient with clinical stage I (stage A) disease, however, whether high levels of these markers before orchiectomy are associated with a worse prognosis if the blood levels normalize according to normal half-life times after orchiectomy is unclear.

Both serum AFP and hCG should be measured in such a patient because either or both can be elevated when the tumor is "active." When both markers are used, they are indispensable for monitoring treatment. Serum LDH, although nonspecific, should also be measured initially and serially, especially in patients thought to have metastatic disease.

The monitoring of disease status by tumor markers is not perfect. Before initial therapy, the sensitivity is proportional to the stage of disease (approximately 40% in stage I (stage A), 50% to 70% in stage II (stage B), and 80% to 90% in stage III-IV (stage C). Active germ cell malignancy can be present despite negative markers. In some cases, the presence of a defined "tumor" mass, in association with negative markers, may suggest the presence of pure seminoma or differentiated or mature teratoma.

SURGERY FOR THE PRIMARY TUMOR

Inguinal orchiectomy is the treatment of choice of primary testicular cancer; this procedure allows both diagnosis and definitive treatment to be effected in one step. Certain principles should be followed, irrespective of the details of surgical approach. A confident diagnosis should be attempted before surgery; alternative diagnoses, such as testicular torsion and orchitis, should be excluded, if possible. To aid in this process, a careful history and examination, testicular ultrasonography, and (when possible) rapid assay of the AFP and hCG, may help. Testicular ultrasonography is accurate in distinguishing between testicular and paratesticular masses, but it is less useful in defining whether an intratesticular mass represents a benign or malignant process.

Important features in the patient's history that may suggest the presence of a testicular germ cell tumor include the onset, nature, and duration of the symptoms, family history, prior maldescent of the testicles, recent development of gynecomastia, history of infertility, and history of testicular cancer. On physical examination, enlargement of the testis, often with induration and a craggy quality, raises the suspicion of tumor; other classic features that increase the level of suspicion include the physical features of metastatic disease, such as an abdominal mass, supraclavicular adenopathy, or evidence of the dyspnea associated with lung metastases. Investigators have suggested that germ cell tumors may be associated with congenital genitourinary or musculoskeletal anomalies[1] and with multiple atypical nevi,[10] and the presence of such features should also increase the level of suspicion of an underlying testicular germ cell tumor, depending on the clinical context.

When orchiectomy is anticipated, the correct surgical approach requires inguinal exploration, with soft clamp control of the spermatic cord before manipulation, to avoid the potential for tumor cell dissemination. If not previously done, blood should be drawn for measurement of routine hematologic and biochemical indices and for estimation of serum tumor markers. Because differences among histologic patterns may be subtle, examination by a pathologist who specializes in tumors is important in achieving the correct diagnosis.[11] Accordingly, the specimen should be sent for extramural review, if such a specialist is not available on site, with an emphasis on accurate histologic definition and T staging of the primary tumor (in particular, including the definition of vascular and lymphatic involvement). In addition, immunohistochemical staining for the presence of AFP or hCG gives additional information about the nature of the tumor.

On occasion, if the diagnosis is truly in doubt, inguinal exploration, with short-term spermatic cord clamping, and careful examination, with or without a frozen section, may define the diagnosis. Rarely, bivalving the testis may be helpful, although the clinician can make no guarantee that the testis will function normally if bivalved and then sutured and returned to the scrotum without orchiectomy. In our view, returning the testis to the scrotum without taking some type of biopsy, even if the surgeon is confident that the patient has no clinical evidence of cancer, is a fundamental error.

In most cases, a transscrotal incision is contraindicated during exploration of a suspected testicular tumor, and a transscrotal needle aspiration should be avoided unless the unequivocal diagnosis is hydrocele without underlying cancer. The reason is that the transscrotal route exposes the patient to different lymphatic drainage routes. Before the era of effective chemotherapy, if a transscrotal incision were performed and a testicular tumor found, subsequent hemiscrotectomy and even an inguinal lymphadenectomy would have been recommended. Today, if a transscrotal incision is made and a testicular tumor found, then the incision should be converted to an inguinal one, the tumor and spermatic cord should be completely excised, and perhaps a wide excision of the scrotal incision should be completed if gross tumor spillage has occurred during the procedure. Subsequently, the surgeon should be alert for local inguinal recurrence, but otherwise, it is appropriate to follow the patient's course in the usual manner.

Technique of Orchiectomy

The incision for a radical orchiectomy is made parallel to the inguinal ligament as for an inguinal hernia repair. The external ring is identified and the external oblique fascia is sharply incised, taking care not to injure the ilioinguinal nerve lying beneath it. The spermatic cord is then bluntly dissected and is encircled first at the tubercle and then proximally deep into the internal inguinal ring.

The spermatic cord is then encircled and is "occluded" with a noncrushing clamp (a time-honored maneuver designed to prevent escape of tumor cells during subsequent testicular manipulation, and probably prudent, if not scientifically validated). The testicle is then pushed into the operative field by pressing the scrotum upward. The testicle is then freed from its scrotal attachments and is wrapped in a towel to prevent tumor spillage into the wound. At this point, if the diagnosis is certain, the spermatic cord is clamped as proximally as possible and is amputated, and the proximal end is ligated with a colored permanent suture, so if retroperitoneal lymph node dissection is required, it can be excised with the retroperitoneal spermatic cord. If the diagnosis is uncertain, the testicle can be "explored" and frozen section diagnosis made, taking special care to avoid tumor spillage. In general, if any doubt exists, the testicle should be removed because leaving a tumorous testicle in place should be avoided if at all possible.

STAGING THE TUMOR

Either before definitive surgery, during which the diagnosis of cancer is anticipated, or after the procedure, a formal staging process is mandatory, to define the extent of disease and thus to determine the nature of treatment required (see Chap. 4). In addition to the usual clinical assessment, including a careful history and physical examination, the following additional investigations are required:

1. Routine blood work, including complete blood count to determine whether the patient has an associated infection or bone marrow infiltration (rare, unless the tumor is a testicular lymphoma), and biochemical screen to determine the presence of renal tract dysfunction (e.g., obstruction of ureters from a lymph node mass) or biochemical evidence of hepatic involvement (uncommon in testis cancer) are necessary. We previously documented an unanticipated high frequency of hypercholesterolemia in treated patients with germ cell tumors,[12] and therefore we usually check pretreatment serum lipids as part of routine medical prophylactic care.
2. The circulating tumor markers, AFP and hCG, should also be measured; ideally, the first specimens should be obtained before surgical treatment of the primary tumor. As noted earlier, AFP and hCG have predictable serum half-life values, and prolongation of these half-life times usually denotes the presence of occult metastatic disease, which remains after orchiectomy and implies the need for further investigation and treatment.[6]
3. Chest radiographs (posteroanterior and lateral) are indicated to exclude large pulmonary metastases or evidence of mediastinal lymph node involvement; occasionally, pectus excavatum is associated with germ cell tumors of the testis, a finding that may be important if general anesthesia is planned.
4. Computed tomographic (CT) scans of the abdomen and pelvis are indicated to define the extent of lymph node enlargement; if the early use of systemic therapy is not anticipated, then a CT scan of the chest may give added information by indicating the presence of occult pulmonary deposits not visualized on plain chest radiographs (see Chap. 4). By contrast, a CT scan of the chest also yields an occasional false-positive result, especially in the context of a negative abdominal scan and normal chest radiograph[13]; thus, the clinical context must be considered carefully, and isolated radiologic abnormalities may require a fine needle biopsy if tumor markers are negative.
5. Magnetic resonance imaging (MRI) has become available for the assessment of metastatic involvement; however, whether this technology offers any benefit over CT scanning in the routine workup of a patient with testicular cancer is unclear (see Chap. 4).
6. CT or MRI scanning of the brain is not routinely necessary unless symptoms of intracranial metastasis are present or unless the predominant histologic type of the primary tumor is choriocarcinoma, which tends to metastasize to the brain. In patients with multiple pulmonary metastases, a CT or MRI scan of the brain is also prudent, although this clinical presentation is often associated with elements of choriocarcinoma anyway.

On completion of the staging protocol, a stage classification can be attributed to the tumor. Three common systems of classification are used in current clinical practice, each developed to

TABLE 67-1. *Stage classification of testicular cancer*

Description	Royal Marsden Hospital*	Conventional US system†	AJCC classification‡
Cancer limited to testis	I	A	I
Cancer in abdominal nodes	II	B	II
Involved mediastinal and supradiaphragmatic lymph nodes	III	C	III
Visceral metastases	IV	C	III

* Subclassifications A, B, and C, depending on volume of disease. Data from Peckham MJ, Barrett A, McElwain TJ, Hendry WF, Ragharan D. Non-seminoma germ cell tumours (malignant teratoma) of the testis: results of treatment and an analysis of prognostic factors. Br J Urol 1981;53:162.

† Data from Einhorn LH. Testicular cancer as a model for a curable neoplasm: the Richard and Hinda Rosenthal Foundation Award lecture. Cancer Res 1981;41:3274.

‡ American Joint Committee on Cancer. Staging Manual, 4th ed. Philadelphia, JB Lippincott, 1992.

allow prognostication and the allocation of appropriate treatment to the individual patient with a specific stage of disease (Table 67-1).[9,14,15]

In addition to the assessment of regional and distant metastases, the potential risk factors within the primary tumor itself (T staging) must be defined, and thus expert histologic review is mandatory because some of these histologic features are subtle.[11]

Although no consensus exists, most clinicians agree that the following factors are adverse prognostic determinants for primary testicular cancer: the presence of vascular or lymphatic invasion within the primary tumor; advanced T stage, with extension to the rete testis, epididymis, spermatic cord, or through the tunica albuginea; the presence of embryonal carcinoma; the absence of endodermal sinus tumor; and the persistence of raised circulating serum tumor markers after orchiectomy (Table 67-2).[16–29] What is more controversial is whether these factors function as independent prognostic determinants on multivariate analysis. Similarly, the prognostic significance of surgical scrotal interference or violation of the tunica albuginea during the diagnostic process is controversial. Less clearly defined are the prognostic implications of tumor size, side of the tumor, and duration of antecedent symptoms, although most reports have suggested that these prognostic factors are not significant.

A formal reassessment of the prognostic implications of these factors is in progress, under the auspices of the American Joint Committee on Cancer (AJCC) and the International Union Against Cancer (Union Internationale Contre le Cancer; UICC), and some modifications to the current system of TNM staging of these tumors will probably be made, to create a uniform international system of prognostic classification. Specifically, prognostic groups will be formulated, based on the location and amount of disease as determined by CT imaging, as well as on the presence or amplitude of AFP, hCG, and LDH levels. In addition, indices from the primary tumor, such as vascular invasion and the proportion of embryonal carcinoma, will be taken into consideration.

TABLE 67-2. *Prognostic factors for Stage I(A) NSGCT*

	Adverse prognostic factors					
Investigators	Vascular-lymphatic invasion	Advanced T stage	Embryonal carcinoma	Persistent markers	Size	Presurgery marker levels
Sandeman and Matthews, 1979[16]	+	+	+	?	?	?
Raghavan et al, 1982[17]	?	+	+	+	?	–
Raghavan et al, 1982[18]	?	+	–	?	–	?
Vaeth et al, 1984[19]	+	+	?	+	–	–?
Hoskin et al, 1986[20]	+	+	+	excluded	–	–
Freedman et al, 1987[21]	+	+	+	excluded	–	?
Dunphy et al, 1988[22]	+	?	+	excluded	–	?
Raghavan et al, 1988[23]	?	+	–	excluded	?	–
Thompson et al, 1988[24]	+	–?	+?	?	?	?
Klepp et al, 1990[25]	+	+	+	?	–	–
Pont et al, 1990[26]	+	–	?	?	?	?
Rorth et al, 1991[27]	+	?	+	excluded	?	?
Sesterhenn et al, 1992[28]	+	+	+	?	?	?
Sturgeon et al, 1992[29]	+	?	+	excluded	?	?

+ denotes prognostic implication in series; – denotes no prognostic implication in series; ? denotes factor not assessed/not documented (in many of these series, numbers were insufficient to allow definite conclusions regarding some uncommon prognostic factors).

TREATMENT AFTER ORCHIECTOMY: STAGE I (STAGE A) TUMORS

Seminoma

The type of tumor and the extent of disease determine the requirements for optimal treatment. In most instances, treatment is predicated on the use of adjuvant radiotherapy to the draining lymph nodes. The policy of active surveillance, in which patients undergo a meticulous program of scrutiny without additional adjuvant therapy after inguinal orchiectomy, has been assessed. These issues are covered in detail in Chapter 65.

Nonseminoma Germ Cell Tumors

In the case of stage I NSGCT, the current choice of treatment rests between retroperitoneal lymph node dissection (RPLND) or a policy of active surveillance. Because the demonstration that adjuvant radiotherapy has little role in the management of stage I NSGCT,[9] RPLND has been regarded as the standard of treatment in that it gives both diagnostic and prognostic information and provides definitive treatment for patients with micrometastatic nodal involvement.

Radical surgery for testicular cancer was first attempted during the last century, but not until the anatomic description of the lymphatic drainage of the testis[30] was the approach to retroperitoneal surgery rationalized. Similarly, RPLND was first carried out toward the end of the nineteenth century, but it was not standardized until the military experience of the American forces during World War II.[31] Improvements in anesthesia, with positive-pressure ventilation, allowed the development of thoracoabdominal exposure[32] and its application to RPLND for testicular cancer. Cooper, Leadbetter, and Chute championed this approach and were able to resect contralateral retroperitoneal tissue.[33] The transabdominal approach, first reported by Tavel, with mobilization of the posterior peritoneum by incising from the cecum to the ligament of Treitz to expose the renal pedicles as well as aorta and vena cava, is now more commonly used.[34] Mallis and Patton[35] extended the skin incision from xiphoid to pubis and mobilized colon onto the chest to enhance visualization of the retroperitoneum.

The early templates of surgical dissection, which required resection of all retroperitoneal lymph node tissue, were associated with incompetent ejaculation, with associated infertility, a high price for a young man to pay. The potential also existed for the other complications of major abdominal surgery, including the formation of adhesions, the occurrence of pulmonary emboli or wound infections, and occasional development of a lymphocele or lymphatic leakage.

Nerve-Sparing Retroperitoneal Surgery

In the past 20 years, information has led to the development of techniques for retroperitoneal lymphadenectomy that have allowed the preservation of ejaculatory function in most cases. This information has been derived from careful mapping of the pattern of retroperitoneal metastases and has allowed the development of template surgery,[36,37] as well as a better understanding of the anatomy and function of the sympathetic nerves controlling ejaculation.[38]

Certain techniques have been reported.[39] Donohue and associates[40–42] evolved a refined technique of template surgery, limiting the boundaries of surgery, with nerve sparing within the dissected zone. Richie,[43,44] using a thoracoabdominal approach, limits his complete bilateral dissection on the contralateral side to a level above the inferior mesenteric artery in the absence of gross disease, preserving antegrade ejaculation in 94% of cases.

Template surgery has not always worked, however, presumably because of variation in sympathetic anatomy, and it has not always been possible in stage II (stage B) disease, in which bilateral dissection is mandatory. Surgeons have come to realize that preservation of the appropriate nerves within the surgical boundaries can be achieved, and when these techniques are applied, the preservation rate increases to nearly 100% for stage I (A) disease and to more than 95% for stage II tumors.[41,42,45]

A review of the anatomy of the retroperitoneal sympathetic nerve tracts is important to understand surgical nerve-sparing techniques (Fig. 67-1). Seminal emission results from sympathetic stimulation of the seminal vesicles and vas deferens with deposition of semen into the posterior urethra. The sympathetic fibers arise from the sympathetic trunk as postganglionic nerves (specifically T12-L3). The paired sympathetic trunks run along the medial margin of the psoas, lateral to the lumbar vertebrae. The ganglia comprising the sympathetic chain in this area number usually 4 or 5 (range 2 to 6), and are rounded or fusiform, with a diameter of 1 to 10 mm. Variation of number with fusion of adjacent ganglia is common. The overlying aorta partly conceals the left trunk, with the right trunk partly covered anteriorly by the inferior vena cava. The lumbar sympathetic nerves arise from the ganglia opposite the first, second, and third lumbar vertebral bodies. These nerves course in a variable fashion anteromedially to form a network of fibers lying on the anterior surface of the aorta. In addition, the surgeon often sees small groups of ganglion cells. Condensation of these nerve fibers and ganglions occurs with the formation of several nerve plexuses: superior mesenteric, inferior mesenteric, and hypogastric. These plexuses vary in location, with their nomenclature approximating adjacent aortic branches (intermesenteric nerves, which have no constant pattern, connect the plexuses). The lowest (hypogastric) plexus can usually be found anterior to the bifurcation of the aorta and in the interiliac angle. From there, the right and left inferior hypogastric nerves run inferiorly to form the pelvic nerves that eventually supply sympathetic fibers to the bladder, prostate, urethra, periurethral glands, vas deferens, and seminal vesicles.

Technique

Before undertaking RPLND, the standard precautions, as for any major surgical procedure, are required, including preoperative assessment and attention to intercurrent medical disorders. Clear and careful explanation of the aims and details of the procedure are required, including a statement regarding the potential risks of incompetent ejaculatory function and other surgical complications that may occur despite the attempt at nerve sparing. If possible, the patient may be encouraged to bank sperm in case of postoperative ejaculatory dysfunction. The

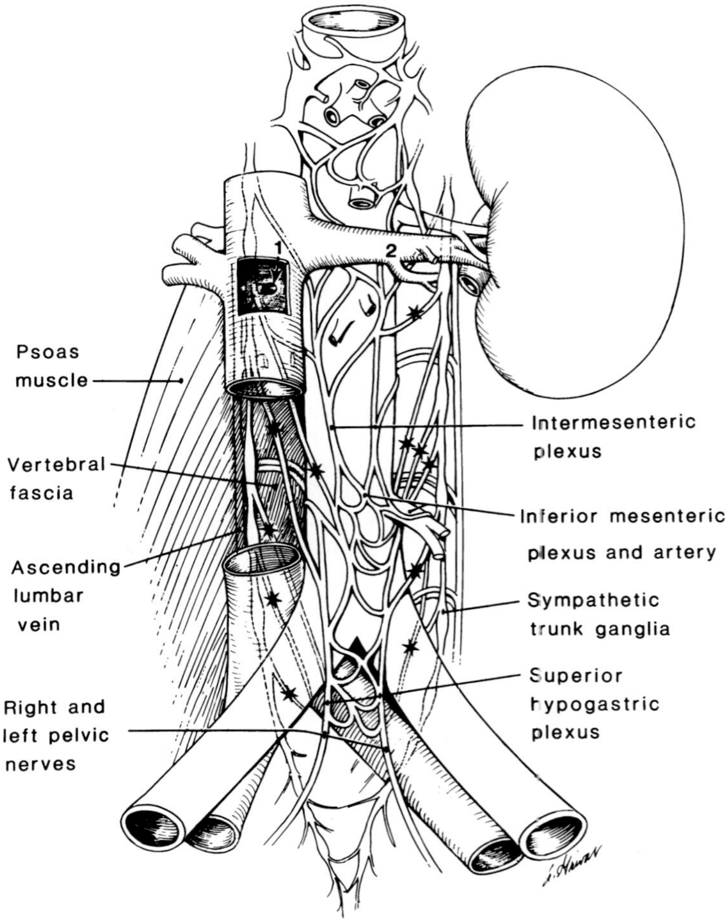

FIG. 67-1. Anatomy of the retroperitoneal nerve tracts. The asterisks represent lumbar splanchnic nerves.

patient is encouraged to cease smoking, or at least to stop for as long as possible before surgery. The patient is usually given a mechanical bowel preparation (e.g., 500 mL of 10% mannitol by mouth). To ensure adequate hydration, an intravenous infusion of normal saline is commenced the evening before the procedure.

The RPLND is usually performed through a midline abdominal incision, xiphoid to mid- to lower abdomen.[41,42,45] The laparotomy is then carefully performed to assess the extent of retroperitoneal disease and to exclude other pathologic processes. The small bowel and right colon are mobilized so they can be rotated out of the abdomen and placed onto the patient's chest. The hepatic flexure is taken down, followed by incision of the posterior peritoneum along the right colic gutter to the cecum. Care is taken to identify the right ureter during mobilization of the right colon, and the rest of the small bowel mesentery is incised cephalad to the ligament of Treitz. Lymphatics are coagulated or ligated when divided. The inferior mesenteric vein is routinely divided. Division of the vein allows rotation of the pancreas anteriorly to allow better access to the retroperitoneum. Using blunt and sharp dissection, the plane is developed between the bowel, including the pancreas and the anterior leaf of the perinephric fascia. These structures are then wrapped with moist packs, are placed into a bowel bag, and lifted out of the abdomen onto the patient's chest.

With the retroperitoneum fully exposed, the limits of dissection can be defined. For clinical stage I disease, in which no gross disease is visible intraoperatively, the surgeon can use limited boundaries of dissection, as discussed subsequently. For stage II disease, however, most surgeons perform a bilateral dissection and, when appropriate, preserve the appropriate sympathetic nerves within these boundaries. The boundaries for a bilateral dissection are the ureters laterally; the superior margin is the inferior border of the superior mesenteric artery extended bilaterally at a level 1 to 2 cm above the renal arteries; and the inferior border extends at least to the midpoint of the ipsilateral external iliac artery and to the bifurcation of the contralateral common iliac artery including the aortic bifurcation. Posteriorly, the anterior spinal ligament and the psoas muscles are cleared. Templates can be defined within these areas.

Dissection is begun by incising the retroperitoneal tissue in the midline, anterior to the inferior vena cava. The left side of the cava is exposed from the left renal vein to its origin at the left common iliac vein by peeling the adipose and lymphatic tissue medially, taking care to cauterize or ligate small vessels. The inferior vena cava is carefully rolled laterally with ligation, and division of the left lumbar veins is required. The right sympathetic chain lies posterior to the midline of the vena cava. The right lumbar veins can be followed posteriorly behind the vena cava as a guide to identify it. Although these lumbar veins normally run medial to the sympathetic chain, occasionally they can be lateral and may even branch around the sympathetic chain. From the fusiform ganglia, fine postganglionic nerve fibers can be seen coursing anteromedially and inferiorly to the right side of the aorta. These fibers are the lumbar splanchnic nerves and can be individually skeletonized from the underlying interaortocaval lymphatic tissue that is ultimately mobilized posteriorly from the anterior spinal ligament and is withdrawn inferiorly, leaving the web of sympathetic nerves.

Before proceeding further, the left ureter is visualized by creating a plane across the midline anterior to the retroperitoneal lymphatic tissue but behind the inferior mesenteric artery, mesocolic fat, and other soft tissues. This dissection may require division of the inferior mesenteric artery, but it should be several centimeters distal to its origin. The left ureter can be exposed to the perinephric tissue to visualize the left psoas muscle; the left paraaortic retroperitoneal adipose tissue containing the lymph nodes is thus left intact. This bulk of tissue is carefully reflected medially to expose the left sympathetic chain. The lumbar vessels on the left are also identified with this dissection as they course directly medially past the sympathetic chain. Again, as with right-sided vessels, they occasionally are lateral or bifurcate around the chain. These vessels can be sacrificed as needed. The lumbar splanchnic nerves are identified originating from the sympathetic ganglia coursing medially and anteriorly. Superiorly, a branch may be present anterior to the renal artery coming from a higher ganglion, but this structure may be difficult to preserve.

At this point, the surgeon has a sense of the individual patient's sympathetic anatomy, which is variable. The aorta can now be exposed in the midline by mobilizing the left renal vein and by splitting the soft tissue over it. Dissection is carried close to the aorta. The individual sympathetic nerve branches, having been identified on both right and left sides from preceding dissection, are seen on the anterior and lateral surfaces of the aorta. They are skeletonized, taking care to preserve those branches that form variable plexuses on the anterior aorta. This allows withdrawal of the interaortocaval lymphatic tissue and the left paraaortic tissue from between the anterior spinal ligament posteriorly and the nerves anteriorly. The plexus at and below the level of the level of the inferior mesenteric artery condenses to form the two hypogastric nerves that pass over the aorta and proceed inferiorly into the pelvis. Identification and preservation of these two nerves allow all lymphatic tissue over the aortic bifurcation and common iliac veins down to the sacral promontory to be removed without sacrificing ejaculation. Most surgeons limit the dissection inferiorly to a point approximately midway along the ipsilateral external iliac artery and to the bifurcation of the contralateral common iliac artery. The remnant of the spermatic cord is removed ipsilaterally from its insertion on the inferior vena cava (right) or renal vein (left) to the inguinal area to include the suture used to tie the spermatic cord during radical orchiectomy. As much of the vas deferens as can easily be removed is also taken.

Frequently, nodal metastases or tumor masses are immediately adjacent to nerves or even involve them. Preserving all postganglionic nerves is not necessary to ensure ejaculation. Therefore, the surgeon should not hesitate to sacrifice nerves unilaterally or even in a limited manner bilaterally to ensure complete removal of the cancer.

The retroperitoneum defined by the selected surgical margins should now be clear of all lymphatic and fatty tissue surrounding the great vessels, with the postganglionic sympathetic nerves remaining beside and on the aorta. The contents of the bowel bag are placed back into the patient's abdomen, and the large and small bowel peritoneal reflections are closed in their normal relationships using a running suture of 1 chromic gut. The abdominal incision is closed using a running 1 polyglycolic suture with interrupted figure-of-eight sutures. Drains are not used.

The management of the patient postoperatively is usually straightforward and uncomplicated. The aggressive replacement of isotonic fluids and colloid intraoperatively and immediately postoperatively is required because of third-space losses into the large, raw retroperitoneal space. Postoperatively, the patient often has a positive fluid balance of 4 to 6 L. Central venous pressure readings and hourly urine output give a reasonable estimation of intravascular volume. Nasogastric suction is continued until the postoperative ileus resolves, usually within 2 to 4 days. Routinely, the indwelling urethral catheter is removed on the first postoperative morning to decrease the risk of urethral stricture and infection. Diet is increased stepwise after the removal of the nasogastric tube. Chest physiotherapy and early mobilization of the patient help to minimize postoperative complications. The average patient is discharged from hospital on the sixth postoperative day.

Perioperative Complications

Intraoperative complications are unusual and are mainly confined to vascular damage of the renal or great vessels. Topical papaverine to reduce vessel spasm is used throughout the procedure. Vascular injury is rare unless a large mass of tumor is present. In removing a bulky mass from the aorta, care is taken to define the appropriate plane of dissection. Dissection in a subadvential plane on the aorta, thereby leaving a weakened vessel for potential aneurysmal dilatation, is easy. If an appropriate plane of dissection cannot be developed, it may be safer to resect part of the vessel wall with primary closure or placement of a synthetic graft. In addition, vein or Gortex patches have been used to close defects of the vena cava.

The meticulous obliteration of lymphatics by ligature or cautery decreases the incidence of lymphocele and ascites postoperatively. Occasionally, a lymphocele can become symptomatic because of a local mass effect, resulting in vague abdominal or flank discomfort. Rarely, obstruction of the small bowel or ureter can occur secondary to the lymphocele mass. Management usually is by percutaneous drainage (if the patient is symptomatic), using ultrasound or CT scans for guidance. Most lymphoceles resolve spontaneously, however.

Early postoperative complications of RPLND are similar to those of any major abdominal procedure. Aggressive chest physical therapy should be commenced immediately postoperatively in all patients to avoid the risk of atelectasis or pneumonia.

Experience with nerve-sparing surgery has established this as the technique of choice for patients undergoing RPLND in the absence of gross disease adjacent to the sympathetic nerve roots. The procedure used can be either thorough bilateral lymphadenectomy with nerve identification and sparing or by dissection of a template or zone that conforms to the likely sites of occult metastases. Because a left-sided tumor does not usually metastasize to the right side, removal of the lymph nodes in the left paraaortic region from the left renal vein inferiorly is usually sufficient. On the right side, the intraaortal caval nodes below the renal vein as well as the right lateral vena cava nodes should be removed. As previously mentioned, the lumbar sympathetic nerves within the boundaries can usually be spared. With these techniques, the rates of preservation of seminal emission and antegrade ejaculation exceed 90%. The nerves can be electrostimulated intraoperatively to aid in the identification of the dominant fibers.[47]

In some centers, laparoscopic lymph node dissection is being investigated,[48] with the intention of further reducing the morbidity of surgery; whether this procedure will produce the same *cure* rates will require the test of time because the ultimate local relapse rate has not yet been defined.

Active Surveillance

The policy of active surveillance was first implemented for patients with stage I NSGCT. The initial programs required careful staging as well as meticulous and frequent follow-up.[20,23] The initial protocols required monthly follow-up visits for the first 6 to 12 months after orchiectomy, with careful physical examination and the measurement of tumor markers, with alternating chest radiographs and CT scans of chest and abdomen or pelvis. Subsequently, the frequency of visits decreased over the ensuing 3 to 5 years. More recently, with an experience of more than 10 years, the frequency and intensity of follow-up visits have been reduced, without loss of safety, as discussed later.

Relapse rates in the range of 17% to 40% have been identified, with a cumulative relapse rate of approximately 30% in the experience of more than 500 such patients (Table 67-3).[20,23,24,27,29] The published literature requires careful and detailed evaluation; many series include few cases and short durations of follow-up. Series with relapse rates at the higher end of the spectrum may well represent inappropriate selection of cases or an absence of review of histologic features or staging investigations from outside centers (with consequent inappropriate inclusion into a surveillance program).[49] More than 50% of first relapses have occurred in the retroperitoneal lymph nodes (see Table 67-3),[20,23,29] and the majority have been associated with elevations of serum tumor marker levels. Less frequently, marker-only relapses (raised tumor marker levels without an obvious site of recurrence) or pulmonary metastases have been documented.[20,23,29]

Having identified the pattern of spread and relapse in an accumulated experience of more than 1000 cases undergoing active surveillance, the frequency of follow-up visits and of CT scans has been reduced; however, surveillance should not be done in an unsupervised or unstructured fashion. Investigators at several referral centers have now begun to see patients with more advanced-stage disease (with a concomitantly worse prognosis) at the time of first relapse who participated in active surveillance programs carried out by inexperienced clinicians or in centers without appropriate protocols to ensure patient compliance with the meticulous schedules of follow-up mandatory for optimal results.

Early studies of the treatment of stage I testicular cancer revealed a series of adverse prognostic factors, including advanced T stage[17,18] and vascular or lymphatic infiltration[16] From the studies of active surveillance, much additional information has been gleaned regarding the natural history of testicular cancer and its pattern of relapse. In addition, late relapses may occur (beyond 5 years), in particular associated with the histologic type of immature teratoma (teratocarcinoma), and thus annual surveillance should be maintained indefinitely. At particular risk of relapse are patients with vascular or lymphatic invasion[19,20,21,25,50] and those with advanced T stage.[21,23] Investigators have also suggested that histologic features of embryonal cancer are an adverse prognostic determinant,[20,21] and the presence of endodermal sinus tumor is a favorable prognostic factor,[21] although this has not always been maintained in multivariate analyses of these factors. Care should be taken in the interpretation of some series with small numbers in which the absence of prognostic impact may only have reflected the small numbers of observations. Even in the definitive work of Hoskin and associates,[20] the study of the significance of invasion of the spermatic cord was marred by the assessment of this feature in only a small proportion of the cases.

Investigational protocols using adjuvant chemotherapy have been developed to prevent recurrence in high-risk groups with primary tumors characterized by vascular invasion, unfavorable histologic features, or advanced T stage.[26,51] The intention of these studies is to reduce the relapse rate and to control occult metastases as early as possible with the use of smaller cumulative doses of chemotherapy. Although the early results suggest a marked reduction in relapse rates, longer follow-up will be required before such treatment can be defined as standard, particularly in view of the potential late complications of systemic chemotherapy.[52]

TREATMENT AFTER ORCHIECTOMY: SMALL-VOLUME LYMPH NODE METASTASES

Seminoma

On completion of a staging workup, evidence of small volume lymph node involvement (i.e., lymph nodes or lymph node

TABLE 67-3. *Patterns of relapse in surveillance of Stage I nonseminomatous germ cell tumors*

Investigators	No. of patients	Major sites* of relapse	Relapse rate (%)	"Cure" rate (%)	Median follow-up (mo)
Freedman et al, 1987[21]	259	R, L	32	98	30
Dunphy et al, 1988[22]	93	R, L	30	?	34
Raghavan et al, 1988[23]	46	R, L	28	95	40
Rorth et al, 1991[27]	77	R	30	100	64
Sturgeon et al, 1992[29]	105	R	35	99	60

R, retroperitoneal lymph nodes; *L*, lungs.

masses measuring less than 2 to 3 cm) is occasionally found. In the case of seminoma, such patients are usually treated by radiotherapy to the ipsilateral lymph nodes in the pelvis, with extension to the paraaortic chain (including the involved nodes) (see Chap. 65). Although the trend has been toward dose reduction, most clinicians use a standard dose of 30 to 35 Gy to ensure local tumor control.

Nonseminomatous Germ Cell Tumors

In the case of NSGCT, the optimal management of early-stage II (stage B or N1 to N2) disease is controversial. Clinicians generally agree that radiotherapy has no routine role. Some proponents of RPLND, however, advocate a standard surgical approach as offering both diagnosis and definitive treatment, and they cite surgical cure rates of up to 50%, particularly in patients with only microscopic evidence of lymph node involvement.[40–45] With this approach, chemotherapy can be used to salvage most relapsing patients.

The alternative approach is to offer first-line cytotoxic chemotherapy to such patients,[53] based on cure rates approaching 100% for patients with small-volume metastases limited to the retroperitoneal nodes; the attraction of this approach is that it limits the morbidity of surgery, but this advantage may be offset by the acute toxicity of chemotherapy and the potential for late complications.[52] No randomized trial has attempted to resolve this issue, and the decision is usually predicated on the biases of the clinician and the preferences of the patient.

One important randomized trial is relevant to the issue: 195 patients with *resected* pathologic stage II NSGCT were randomly allocated to receive two cycles of adjuvant chemotherapy or to undergo a program of observation with salvage chemotherapy at the time of relapse.[54] The group of patients included patients with N2 to N3 disease, however. Of the 98 patients who were observed, nearly 48 (49%) had relapses, but the majority were salvaged with chemotherapy, and 93 were alive and free of disease at the time of reporting. Conversely, of 97 patients allocated to adjuvant chemotherapy, 6 had relapses, although only 1 of these patients had actually received chemotherapy before the recurrence, and 94 of the 97 survived; the investigators concluded that no statistically significant difference in outcome existed.[54]

Another particularly controversial issue is the management of the patient with marker-only disease (i.e., without evidence of specific lymph node or other metastases, but with persistent elevation of serum marker levels after orchiectomy). RPLND identifies a proportion of patients with occult lymphatic involvement and achieves a cure in some of them[42–45]; however, up to 50% of patients undergoing surgery eventually require chemotherapy. Analogous to small-volume nodal metastases, the cure rates with cytotoxic chemotherapy are close to 100%, although the risk of additional late toxicity is significant, as compared with surgery alone. In patients with of marker-only disease, many centers use initial combination chemotherapy,[9,55,56] and they reserve surgery for the occasional patient in whom persistent lymph node enlargement is subsequently identified on a scan.[57]

With the potential for iatrogenic disorders associated with the treatment for testis cancer,[52] these patients must be surveyed for the range of potential problems outlined earlier, including the complications of surgery, radiotherapy, or chemotherapy and the late sequelae of the disease itself.

TESTIS CANCER AND FERTILITY

The association of testicular cancer and infertility is well documented, but it is not completely understood. Testicular cancer is known to occur in association with cryptorchidism and with certain congenital anomalies of the genitourinary tract[1]; cryptorchidism, in turn, is associated with gonadal hypofunction and subsequent infertility. Investigators have also suggested that maternal ingestion of estrogens during pregnancy may be a risk factor for the subsequent development of testicular cancer in male offspring, and this factor is also associated with developmental anomalies of the testes. At least 50% of patients with newly diagnosed testis cancer have subnormal semen quality.[58] Up to half of patients who have no treatment beyond orchiectomy recover fertility spontaneously. The reason for this reversible impairment is unknown, but it may relate to endocrine or psychological factors, and in some cases it may be due to the function of hCG in some tumors. Carcinoma in situ is usually associated with poor semen quality (see Chap. 63), and it is commonly first diagnosed in men undergoing testicular biopsy for the investigation of infertility.

In addition to the underlying risk of infertility in association with testicular cancer, most available therapies carry a risk of inducing infertility. The conventional techniques of RPLND may damage the sympathetic nerves that normally produce seminal emission by contraction of the seminal vesicles and closure of the bladder neck before ejaculation, with consequent loss of antegrade ejaculatory function.[38,45,59] As noted earlier, this problem can be restricted by limiting retroperitoneal dissection to the most likely sites of metastasis, such as the primary regional lymphatics, with preservation of contralateral sympathetic ganglion nerves.[39,42,43] This approach appears to be safe, although a theoretic risk of a higher local postsurgical relapse rate remains, and longer periods of assessment will be required before a final level of risk can be defined. Another option for the patient who is not prepared to undergo a restricted (template) lymphadenectomy, or for the patient in whom disrupted ejaculation occurs despite the procedure, is to use sympathomimetic drugs or electrically stimulated ejaculation.[45]

Radiotherapy may also cause sterility, depending on the doses and fields selected. Even with the low doses of abdominal irradiation used for prophylaxis after orchiectomy for stage I (stage A) seminoma (25 to 30 Gy), permanent aspermia may be induced, despite scrotal shielding; in this context, recovery after a period of acute suppression of spermatogenesis is more common.[52,60]

Combination chemotherapy can also impair fertility.[52] It usually produces aspermia during the first 12 months after initiation of treatment, although recovery often occurs, especially since the elimination of conventional alkylating agents from standard regimens. We estimate that more than half the patients who are fertile before chemotherapy will regain fertility beyond 6 to 12 months after completion of treatment. No substantial risk of fetal abnormality appears to exist among the offspring of males treated with standard chemotherapy regimens for germ cell tumors, although available data are inadequate for a definitive opinion.

CONCLUSIONS

The past 2 decades have seen a major revolution in the management of early-stage NSGCT, with the deletion of radiotherapy from most management programs and the development of treatment based on well-defined prognostic determinants in the primary tumor. Although RPLND remains the standard, active surveillance has been shown to be safe and effective, at least in expert hands, with apparent cure rates higher than 95%.

The emphasis is on the reduction of the toxicity of standard treatment. Modified templates of surgery are being applied, with the intention of reducing the chance of incompetent ejaculation and the morbidity of surgery. These approaches will require the validation of time to demonstrate that they are not associated with a higher prevalence of late in-field relapse.

Limited-dose adjuvant chemotherapy is being tested in patients with high-risk tumors, with the intention of achieving cure without the necessity of the full doses required for patients with established relapse (and thus reducing the potential for side effects, such as infertility and leukemia). We must exercise caution in this approach to the reduction of the overall toxicity of treatment, however. Two trials of modified, less toxic chemotherapy for advanced disease (in which carboplatin replaced cisplatin and bleomycin was deleted from the standard chemotherapy regimen, respectively) were associated with a *reduction* in the cure rate.

In any situation that may lead to the increased use of chemotherapy, such as in active surveillance, we should not forget the potential for leukemogenesis[52,61] and the other late complications of these drugs, in particular late cardiovascular complications.[52] Although investigators have commonly suggested that etoposide-based regimens for testis cancer are associated with leukemogenesis only with large cumulative doses,[61] we have reported a case of iatrogenic leukemia in a patient treated on relapse after active surveillance with only four cycles of cisplatin, etoposide, and bleomycin.[62] Similarly, few detailed studies of the prevalence of late complications of these chemotherapy regimens have been published.[52] Until more definitive information of this type is available, we should attempt to alter our approaches to the treatment of early-stage testicular cancer only in the context of carefully researched, well-structured clinical trials.

REFERENCES

1. Raghavan D, Neville AM. The biology of testicular tumours. In: Innes-Williams D, Chisholm G, eds. Scientific foundations of urology, 2nd ed. London, William Heinemann Medical Books, 1992:785.
2. Raghavan D, Sullivan AL, Peckham MJ, Neville AM. Elevated serum alphafetoprotein and seminoma: clinical evidence for a histologic continuum? Cancer 1982;50:982.
3. Mostofi FK, Price EB Jr. Tumors of the male genital system: atlas of tumor pathology, 2nd series, fascicle 8. Washington, DC, Armed Forces Institute of Pathology, 1979:1.
4. Hamilton CR, Horwich A. Rare tumours of the testis and paratesticular tissues. In: Williams CJ, Krikorian J, Green MR, Raghavan D, eds. Textbook of uncommon cancer. Chichester, NY, Wiley Liss, 1988: 225.
5. Johnson DE, Appelt G, Samuels ML, Luna M. Metastases from testicular carcinoma: study of 78 autopsied cases. Urology 1976;8:234.
6. Lange PH, Raghavan D. Clinical applications of tumor markers in testicular cancer. In: Donohue JP, ed. The management of testicular cancer. Baltimore, Williams & Wilkins, 1983:111.
7. Gitlin D, Boesman M. Serum alpha-fetoprotein, albumin and gamma-G-globulin in the human conceptus. J Clin Invest 1966;45:1826.
8. Vaitukaitis JL. Human chorionic gonadotrophin: a hormone secreted for many reasons. N Engl J Med 1979;301:324.
9. Peckham MJ, Barrett A, McElwain TJ, Hendry WF, Raghavan D. Nonseminoma germ cell tumours (malignant teratoma) of the testis: results of treatment and an analysis of prognostic factors. Br J Urol 1981;53: 162.
10. Raghavan D, Zalcberg J, Grygiel JJ, et al. Multiple atypical nevi: a cutaneous marker of germ cell tumors. J Clin Oncol 1994;12:2284.
11. Segelov E, Cox KM, Raghavan D, et al. The impact of histological review on clinical management of testicular cancer. Br J Urol 1993; 71:736.
12. Raghavan D, Cox K, Childs A, Grygiel J, Sullivan D. Hypercholesterolemia after chemotherapy for testis cancer. J Clin Oncol 1992;10:1386.
13. Fernandez FB, Colon E, McLeod DG, et al. Efficacy of radiographic chest imaging in patients with testicular cancer. Urology 1994;44:548.
14. Einhorn LH. Testicular cancer as a model for a curable neoplasm: the Richard and Hinda Rosenthal Foundation Award Lecture. Cancer Res 1981;41:3274.
15. American Joint Committee on Cancer (AJCC). Testis. In: AJCC, eds. Staging manual, 4th ed. Philadelphia, JB Lippincott, 1992:187.
16. Sandeman TF, Matthews JP. The staging of testicular tumors. Cancer 1979;43:2514.
17. Raghavan D, Peckham MJ, Heyderman E, et al. Prognostic factors in clinical stage I NSGCT of the testis. Br J Cancer 1982;45:167.
18. Raghavan D, Vogelzang NJ, Bosl GJ, et al. Tumor classification and size in germ-cell testicular cancer: influence on the occurrence of metastases. Cancer 1982;50:1591.
19. Vaeth M, Schultz HP, von der Maase H, et al. Prognostic factors in testicular germ cell tumours. Acta Radiol Oncol 1984;23:271.
20. Hoskin P, Dilly S, Easton D, et al. Prognostic factors in stage I nonseminomatous germ cell tumors managed by orchiectomy and surveillance: implications for adjuvant chemotherapy. J Clin Oncol 1986;4: 1031.
21. Freedman LS, Parkinson MC, Jones WG, et al. Histopathology in the prediction of relapse of patients with stage I testicular teratoma treated by orchiectomy alone. Lancet 1987;2:294.
22. Dunphy CH, Ayala AG, Swanson DA, Ro JY, Logothetis CJ. Clinical stage I nonseminomatous and mixed germ cell tumors of the testis: a clinicopathologic study of 93 patients on a surveillance protocol after orchiectomy alone. Cancer 1988;62:1202.
23. Raghavan D, Colls B, Levi J, et al. Surveillance for stage I non-seminomatous germ cell tumours of the testis: the optimal protocol has not yet been defined. Br J Urol 1988;61:522.
24. Thompson PI, Nixon J, Harvey VJ. Distant relapse in patients with stage I non-seminomatous germ cell tumor of the testis on active surveillance. J Clin Oncol 1988;6:1597.
25. Klepp O, Olsson AM, Henrikson H, et al. Prognostic factors in clinical stage I nonseminomatous germ cell tumors of the testis: multivariate analysis of a prospective multicenter study. J Clin Oncol 1990;8:509.
26. Pont J, Holtl W, Kosak D, et al. Risk-adapted treatment choice in stage I nonseminomatous testicular germ cell cancer by regarding vascular invasion in the primary tumor: a prospective trial. J Clin Oncol 1990; 8:16.
27. Rorth M, Jacobsen GK, von der Masse H, et al. Surveillance alone versus radiotherapy after orchidectomy for clinical stage I nonseminomatous testicular cancer. J Clin Oncol 1991;9:1543.
28. Sesterhenn IA, Weiss RB, Mostofi FK, et al. Prognosis and other clinical correlates of pathologic review in stage I and II testicular carcinoma: a report from the Testicular Cancer Intergroup Study. J Clin Oncol 1992;10:69.
29. Sturgeon JFG, Jewett MAS, Alison RE, et al. Surveillance after orchidectomy for patients with clinical stage I nonseminomatous testis tumor. J Clin Oncol 1992;10:564.
30. Most J. Ueber die lymphagefaesse des hoden. Arch Anat Entwicklungsgesch 1899:113, cited in: Staubitz WJ. Historical perspectives on node dissection. In: Donohue JP, ed. Testis tumors. Baltimore, Williams & Wilkins, 1983:159.
31. Lewis LG. Radical operation for tumors of the testis. JAMA 1948;137: 828.
32. Chute R, Soutter L, Kerr WS. The value of the thoracoabdominal incision in the removal of kidney tumors. N Engl J Med 1949;241:951.
33. Cooper JF, Leadbetter WF, Chute R. The thoracoabdominal approach

for retroperitoneal gland dissection: its application to testes tumors. Surg Gynecol Obstet 1950;90:486.
34. Van Buskirk KE, Young JG. The evolution of the bilateral antegrade retroperitoneal lymph node dissection in the treatment of testicular tumors. Mil Med 1968;10:575.
35. Mallis N, Patton JF. Transperitoneal bilateral lymphadenectomy in testis tumors. J Urol 1958;80:501.
36. Ray B, Hajdu SI, Whitmore WF Jr. Lymph node metastases in the retroperitoneum from nonseminomatous testis cancer. J Urol 1982;128: 315.
37. Donohue J, Zachary J, Maynard BL. Distribution of nodal metastases in nonseminomatous testis cancer. J Urol 1982;128:315.
38. Lange PH, Narayan P, Fraley EE. Fertility issues following therapy for testicular cancer. Semin Urol 1984;2:264.
39. Jewett MAS, Kong Y-SP, Goldberg SD, et al. Retroperitoneal lymphadenectomy for testis tumor with nerve sparing for ejaculation. J Urol 1988;139:1220.
40. Foster RS, Donohue JP. Nerve sparing retroperitoneal lymphadenectomy. Urol Clin N Am 1993;20:117.
41. Donohue JP, Thornhill JA, Foster RA, Rowland RG. Primary retroperitoneal lymph node dissection in clinical stage A nonseminomatous germ cell testis cancer. Br J Urol 1993;71:326.
42. Donohue JP, Thornhill JA, Foster RS, Rowland RG, Bihrle R. Retroperitoneal lymphadenectomy for clinical stage A testis cancer (1965-1989): modifications of technique and impact on ejaculation. J Urol 1993;149:237.
43. Richie JP. Modified retroperitoneal lymphadenectomy for patients with clinical stage I testicular cancer. In: Ratliff TL, Catalona W, eds. Urologic oncology. Boston, Kluwer Academic Publishers, 1989:35.
44. Richie JP. Clinical stage I testicular cancer: the role of modified retroperitoneal lymphadenectomy. J Urol 1990;144:1160.
45. Lange PH, Chang WY, Fraley EE. Fertility issues in the therapy of nonseminomatous testicular tumors. Urol Clin North Am 1987;14:731.
46. Jewett MAS. Nerve sparing retroperitoneal lymphadenectomy for carcinoma of the testis. Urol Clin North Am 1990;17:449.
47. Dieckmann K-P, Huland H, Gross AJ. A test for the identification of relevant sympathetic nerve fibers during nerve sparing retroperitoneal lymphadenectomy. J Urol 1992;148:1450.
48. Klotz L. Laparoscopic retroperitoneal lymphadenectomy for high-risk stage I nonseminomatous germ cell tumor: report of four cases. Urology 1994;43:752.
49. Sturgeon JFG, Herman JG, Jewett MAS, et al. A policy of surveillance alone after orchidectomy for clinical stage I non-seminomatous testis tumours. Proc Am Soc Clin Oncol 1983;2:142.
50. Moriyama N, Daly JJ, Keating MA, et al. Vascular invasion as a prognosticator of metastatic disease in non-seminomatous germ-cell tumors of the testis. Cancer 1985;56:2492.
51. Sandeman TF, Yang C. Results of adjuvant chemotherapy for low-stage nonseminomatous germ cell tumors of the testis with vascular invasion. Cancer 1988;62:1471.
52. Boyer M, Raghavan D. Toxicity of treatment of germ cell tumors. Semin Oncol 1992;19:128.
53. Horwich A, Norman A, Fisher C, et al. Primary chemotherapy for stage II nonseminomatous germ cell tumors of the testis. J Urol 1994;151: 72.
54. Williams SD, Stablein DM, Einhorn LH, et al. Immediate adjuvant chemotherapy versus observation with treatment at relapse in pathological stage II testicular cancer. N Engl J Med 1987;317:1433.
55. Levi JA, Thomson D, Sandeman T, et al. A prospective study of cisplatin-based combination chemotherapy in advanced germ cell malignancy: role of maintenance and long-term follow-up. J Clin Oncol 1988;6:1154.
56. Levi JA, Raghavan D, Harvey V, et al. The importance of bleomycin in combination chemotherapy for good prognosis germ cell carcinoma. J Clin Oncol 1993;11:1300.
57. Davis BE, Herr HW, Fair WR, Bosl GJ. The management of patients with nonseminomatous germ cell tumors of the testis with serologic disease only after orchiectomy. J Urol 1994;152:111.
58. Presti JC, Herr HW, Carroll PR. Fertility and testis cancer. Urol Clin North Am 1993;20:173.
59. Pizzocarro G. Retroperitoneal lymphadenectomy in clinical stage I nonseminomatous germinal testis cancer. Eur J Surg Oncol 1986;12:25.
60. Fossa SD, Aass N, Kaalhus O. Long-term morbidity after infradiaphragmatic radiotherapy in young men with testicular cancer. Cancer 1989;64:404.
61. Pedersen-Bjergaard J, Daugaard G, Hansen SW, et al. Increased risk of myelodysplasia and leukemia after etoposide, cisplatin and bleomycin for germ-cell tumours. Lancet 1991;338:359.
62. Segelov E, Raghavan D, Kronenberg H. Acute leukemia following chemotherapy including etoposide for testicular carcinoma. Aust N Z J Med 1993;23:718.

Principles and Practice of Genitourinary Oncology, edited by Derek Raghavan, Howard I. Scher, Steven A. Leibel, and Paul H. Lange. Lippincott-Raven Publishers, Philadelphia, © 1997.

CHAPTER 68

Management of Stage II and Good-Risk Stage III and IV Nonseminomatous Germ Cell Tumors

Gerrit Stoter, Patrick J. Loehrer Sr, and John Levi

The availability of cisplatin has made metastatic testicular cancer a curable disease in about 80% of cases.[1,2] Initially, cisplatin was added to the most active regimen of vinblastine and bleomycin (PVB), but vinblastine has been replaced by etoposide (BEP) because this combination is at least as effective as PVB and is less toxic.[3] Much effort has been invested in the delineation of prognostic factors and models with the aim of arriving at a reliable, uniform predictive model to discriminate patients with a good prognosis from those who have a less good (i.e., intermediate) or poor prognosis. To this end, major research groups from the United States, Canada, Europe, and Australia have formed the International Germ Cell Cancer Collaborative Group (IGCCCG) prognostic model.

STAGE II

The curative potential of cisplatin-based combination chemotherapy has redressed the role of surgery and radiotherapy in all stages of germ cell cancer. In the era before cisplatin, bilateral radical lymph node dissection, radiotherapy, or both were considered treatments of choice in stage I and stage II disease. After the introduction of cisplatin, the majority of European and Australian institutes changed their policies and turned to induction chemotherapy, even for patients with operable stage II disease, denoted by retroperitoneal lymph nodes smaller than 3 cm in diameter on computed tomographic (CT) scan.

Investigators from the Royal Marsden Hospital have reported a series of 122 stage II patients, 58 of whom had lymph node metastases smaller than 2 cm (IIA) and 64 of whom had lymph nodes with a diameter of 2 to 5 cm (IIB).[4] After a median observation period of 5.5 years following platinum induction chemotherapy, 97% of patients were free of disease. Debulking lymphadenectomy was done in patients with a residual post-chemotherapy mass. This procedure was required in 10 (17%) patients with stage IIA and in 25 (39%) patients with stage IIB disease. The resection specimen contained cancer in only one patient.

In the United States, the basic approach to resectable stage II disease is bilateral radical retroperitoneal lymph node dissection. Controversy exists as to the role of adjuvant chemotherapy following surgery.[5]

The U.S. Intergroup performed a study of bilateral retroperitoneal lymph node dissection with randomization for adjuvant chemotherapy with two cycles of cisplatin combination chemotherapy versus no further treatment.[6] Forty-eight (49%) of 98 patients on the observation arm relapsed; two died despite adequate chemotherapy, two died of non–disease-specific reasons, and one died after refusal of chemotherapy. Six (6%) of 97 patients on the adjuvant chemotherapy arm relapsed, five of these did so before the start of chemotherapy. One patient died despite salvage chemotherapy. Two patients died of non–disease-specific reasons. Because the survival in both arms was similar after a median follow-up of 4 years, the results of this study can be used to argue in favor of either treatment approach. However, these and other investigators stress the need for bilateral dissection,[7–12] with the attendant disadvantage of perioperative and long-term morbidity, including persistent anejaculation. This side effect can be largely avoided by modern nerve-sparing techniques, particularly in patients with small nodal metastases.[13–15]

There is worldwide consensus that unresectable stage II tumor—defined as retroperitoneal metastases larger than or equal to 3 cm in diameter—should be treated with induction chemotherapy, which must be followed by debulking surgery when there is residual tumor.[16–21]

Patients with minimal-volume stage II disease (i.e., markers only or nodal metastasis <3 cm in diameter) are candidates for retroperitoneal lymph node dissection or primary chemotherapy. Patients with advanced stage II disease should be treated with induction chemotherapy, and postchemotherapy lymphadenectomy should be reserved for patients with residual tumor mass.

DEFINITION OF GOOD-RISK TESTICULAR CANCER

Although the management of germ cell tumors has greatly improved, it is well recognized that patients with disseminated disease have diverse prognoses. Proper identification of prognostic subsets is critical, because patients with a poor prognosis should be considered for investigational therapy aimed at improving complete response and cure rates, whereas good-prognosis patients are candidates for clinical trials aiming at reduction of side effects while maintaining the high cure rate. Several staging systems have been devised as a means of differentiating good-prognosis from poor-prognosis patients.

In the United States, the staging systems most commonly used include the Indiana University staging system[1,2,22] and a system described by investigators at Memorial Sloan-Kettering Cancer Center (MSKCC).[23] Although the specific clinical parameters found to influence prognosis vary somewhat between these classifications, extent of disease (i.e., tumor bulk) is the common denominator.

The Indiana University staging system was developed using data derived from several prospective trials conducted by the Southeastern Cancer Study Group (SECSG) and is based on readily available clinical data (i.e., physical examination, CT scans, laboratory data).[1,2,22] This classification system separates metastatic patients into three clinically distinct groups: minimal, moderate, or advanced metastatic disease (Table 68-1). The Indiana University system allows patients to be divided into two prognostic groups: good prognosis, denoted as minimal or moderate disease, and poor prognosis, denoted as advanced disease. More than 90% of patients with minimal or moderate disease achieve long-term disease-free status with cisplatin combination chemotherapy. Conversely, patients with advanced disease suffer a much higher failure rate (approximately 50%).

TABLE 68-1. *Indiana University staging system*[22]

MINIMAL
Elevated marker or markers post–retroperitoneal lymphadenectomy
Cervical nodes
Unresectable nonpalpable retroperitoneal disease
<5 Pulmonary metastases per lung field and largest <2 cm
MODERATE
Palpable abdominal mass but no supradiaphragmatic disease
5–10 Metastases per lung field and largest <3 cm
OR
Solitary pulmonary mass >2 cm
ADVANCED
Primary mediastinal nonseminomatous germ-cell tumor
OR
>10 Metastases per lung field
OR
Multiple metastases >3 cm
Palpable abdominal mass with supradiaphragmatic disease
Liver, bone, or central nervous system metastases

TABLE 68-2. *Memorial Sloan-Kettering Cancer Center staging system*[23]

GOOD-RISK DISEASE
All seminomas
Testicular NSGCT with probability of CR >0.5 calculated by prob CR = $\exp^k (1 + \exp/h)$
where h = 8.514 − 1.973 log (LDH + 1) − 0.530 log (hCG + 1) − 1.111 TOTMET, and TOTMET = 0, 1, or 2, depending on whether there are 0, 1, or 2 or more sites of metastases
POOR-RISK DISEASE
All patients with NSGCT of extragonadal origin
Testicular NSGCT with probability of CR <0.5

CR, complete response; hCG, human chorionic gonadotrophin; LDH, lactate dehydrogenase; NSGCT, nonseminomatous germ cell tumor; TOTMET, total metastases.

Investigators at MSKCC also identified several clinical variables as important determinants for successful outcome following cisplatin therapy.[23] A mathematic formula was devised that incorporates the logarithm of the pretreatment values of serum lactate dehydrogenase (LDH) and human chorionic gonadotropin (hCG), along with the total number of metastatic sites (Table 68-2). The value derived from this equation has been found to correlate well with complete response rates. A value greater than 0.5 is associated with a high probability of achieving a favorable response, whereas a value of less than 0.5 is associated with a poor outcome. For example, among patients treated with cisplatin-based combination chemotherapy at MSKCC between 1982 and 1985, 95% (77 of 81) of those identified as good-prognosis patients achieved an initial complete response, compared with only 38% (14 of 37) of poor-prognosis patients.[24]

In Europe, the mostly used staging systems are derived from studies reported by the European Organization on Research and Treatment of Cancer (EORTC)[25] and the Medical Research Council (MRC) Working Party on Testicular Tumours.[26] In the latter report, three distinct prognostic groups were described, using such pretreatment factors as tumor volume and serum levels of alphafetoprotein (AFP) and hCG (Table 68-3).

Analyses from the Australasian Germ Cell Trial Group (AGCTG) involved initial evaluation of relevant prognostic factors in a study of 253 cisplatin-treated patients with advanced disease.[27] Multivariate analysis showed that total tumor diameter of all involved sites and serum hCG levels were independent prognostic factors. This model was confirmed and refined in a subsequent study of 220 patients.[28] When these two studies, which include 460 patients evaluable for prognostic variables, were evaluated together, AFP was added as an independent prognostic factor.

In an attempt to reach a consensus with regard to one uniform prognostic model, the first International Consensus Meeting involving all representative research groups worldwide was held in 1987. Published and forthcoming data[22–33] were discussed, and it was recognized that the models showed great similarities but could not be amalgamated because of the different parameters studied.[34] Hence, the IGCCCG was established, with the goal of collecting source data from patients who had been treated in the framework of platinum chemotherapy study protocols. At the first meeting of the IGCCCG in May 1994, the database contained information on more than 5000 patients.[35]

TABLE 68-3. *Medical Research Council staging system*

I. Lymphogram negative, no evidence of metastases
  IM. No evidence of metastases, but persistently elevated serum AFP and/or hCG levels
II. Paraaortic node metastases
  A Metastases <2 cm diameter
  B Metastases 2–5 cm diameter
  C Metastases >5 cm diameter
III. Supradiaphragmatic lymph node involvement
  O No abdominal disease
  A, B, C As in stage II
IV. Extralymphatic metastases (abdominal status A, B, C, as in stage II)
  Lung status
    L_1, ≤3 metastases
    L_2, multiple metastases, none >2 cm diameter
    L_3, multiple metastases, one >2 cm diameter
  Liver status
    H+, liver involvement
Small-volume disease: stages IM, IIAB, IIIAB, IVABL$_{1-2}$
Large-volume disease: stages IIC, IIIC, IVCL$_{1-2}$
Very-large-volume disease: L_3 pulmonary disease, H+, CNS disease, or bone metastases
Serum tumor markers: prechemotherapy AFP titres >500 kU/L and hCG titres >1000 IU/L

AFP, alphafetoprotein; CNS, central nervous system; hCG, human chorionic gonadotrophin.

At the second meeting of the IGCCCG in September 1994, a consensus was reached with regard to the definition of good prognosis patients:

- absence of a mediastinal nonseminomatous primary lesion
- no liver, bone, or brain metastases
- serum hCG <1000 ng/mL
- serum AFP <1000 ng/mL
- serum LDH <1.5 times upper limit of an institution's normal value

Patients with none, one, or more than one of these unfavorable variables are divided in three prognostic groups, with approximate cure rates of 90% in the good-prognosis category (no unfavorable factors), 60% in the intermediate-prognosis group (one unfavorable factor), and 20% to 40% in the poor-prognosis category (>1 unfavorable factor).[32,33,35]

With the establishment of these three prognostic categories, it became apparent that two thirds of patients with metastatic germ cell tumors have a good prognosis and a probability of cure of more than 90%.

OPTIMIZING TREATMENT IN GOOD-PROGNOSIS PATIENTS

Given the high cure rate of more than 90% in good-prognosis patients, it is clear that attempts to improve the cure rates of presently available chemotherapy regimens would be extremely difficult. Accordingly, investigators have turned their efforts to reducing toxicity of therapy in these patients. These efforts have included reduction in the number of treatment cycles and alteration of the composition of induction regimens. Because much of the toxicity associated with standard chemotherapy regimens is related to vinblastine or bleomycin, attention has focused on these agents. As mentioned previously, etoposide can be substituted for vinblastine in the PVB regimen without loss of effectiveness but with improvement in the toxicity profile.[3,36,37] Table 68-4 shows the different chemotherapy regimens referred to in this chapter.

Fewer Cycles

Using the Indiana classification system, the SECSG conducted a randomized prospective trial in 184 good-prognosis patients (i.e., minimal to moderate disease) in which patients were randomized to receive either three or four cycles of BEP.[38] Overall, 99% of minimal-disease and 95% of moderate-disease patients achieved an initial disease-free status. Among the 88 patients randomized to three cycles of BEP, 86 (98%) achieved disease-free status (minimal disease, 98%; moderate disease, 98%), compared with 93 of 96 (97%) randomized to receive four cycles of BEP (minimal disease, 100%; moderate disease, 93%). Relapse rates were virtually identical, with 6% and 5% on the respective treatment arms. With a minimum follow-up of 1 year, the overall disease-free survival was 92% in both treatment arms. On a per course basis, hematologic, gastrointestinal, renal, and neurologic toxicities were comparable. However, because of the shorter duration of 9 instead of 12 weeks of treatment, patients randomized to three cycles of BEP had less toxicity overall. Thus, the deletion of the fourth cycle of BEP substantially reduced the toxicity, cost, and inconvenience of this regimen without sacrificing therapeutic efficacy. These data have resulted in three cycles of BEP becoming the preferred regimen in the United States for good-prognosis metastatic germ cell tumors as defined by the Indiana University system.

Fewer Drugs

From 1982 to 1986, MSKCC investigators conducted a randomized comparison of their standard cisplatin-based induction chemotherapy VAB-6 and a two-drug regimen of etoposide plus cisplatin (EP; see Table 68-4) in 164 good-prognosis patients.[39] Good prognosis was defined by their previously described model and also included patients with testicular or extragonadal pure seminoma. Seventy-nine of 82 (96%) patients receiving VAB-6 and 76 of 82 (93%) patients receiving EP achieved disease-free status. Relapse from complete response was essentially identical (11% versus 12%, respectively). Thirty-one patients entered into this trial would have been classified as poor prognosis using the Indiana University staging system; 20 of these patients received VAB-6 and 11 received EP. Of the 20 patients receiving VAB-6, 19 (95%) achieved a complete response, whereas 9 (81%) of the 11 patients given EP also had a complete response. Relapse-free and overall survival were similar in the two treatment regimens. Patients treated with EP had less vomiting, mucositis, and magnesium wasting; higher leukocyte and platelet nadirs; and no pulmonary toxicity. These data led the investigators to consider four cycles of EP as the standard induction chemotherapy in good-prognosis germ cell cancer patients.

TABLE 68-4. *Treatment scheme*

Regimen	Drugs	Schedule
PVB	Cisplatin 20 mg/m^2 d 1–5 Vinblastine 0.3 mg/kg d 1, 2 Bleomycin 30 mg d 1, 8, 15	Repeat every 3 wk × 4; consider surgery after 4 cycles
VAB-6	Vinblastine 4 mg/m^2 d 1 Cyclophosphamide 600 mg/m^2 d 1 Dactinomycin 1 mg/m^2 d 1 Bleomycin 30 mg d 1 Bleomycin 20 mg d 1–3 Cisplatin 120 mg/m^2 d 4	Repeat every 4 wk × 3; no bleomycin in third cycle; consider surgery after 3 cycles
BEP	Cisplatin 20 mg/m^2 d 1–5 Bleomycin 30 mg d 1, 8, 15 Etoposide 100 mg/m^2 d 1–5 (U.S.) Etoposide 120 mg/m^2 d 1, 3, 5 (Europe)	
EP	Etoposide 100 mg/m^2 d 1 (U.S.) Etoposide 120 mg/m^2 d 1, 3, 5 (Europe) Cisplatin 20 mg/m^2 d 1–5	Repeat every 3 wk × 4; consider surgery after 4 cycles

Deletion of Bleomycin

In addition to the previously mentioned MSKCC study, which deleted a number of drugs in addition to bleomycin,[39,40] other study groups have reported their experience from randomized trials investigating the relative merits of bleomycin.

The EORTC conducted a trial comparing four cycles of cisplatin and etoposide, with or without bleomycin, in patients with good prognoses.[41,42] Good prognosis was defined as lung metastases smaller than 2 cm, serum AFP levels lower than 1000 IU/L, hCG levels lower than 10,000 IU/L, and lymph node metastases smaller than 5 cm in diameter. The etoposide schedule was based on the Royal Marsden regimen[36,37] comprising 120 mg/m^2 administered intravenously on days 1, 3 and 5, rather than the Indiana University scheme of 100 mg/m^2 on days 1 through 5.

In an interim analysis of 313 evaluable patients,[42] a complete response was reported in 154 of 160 patients (96%) treated with four cycles of BEP, compared with 140 of 153 patients (92%) treated with four cycles of EP (P = .13). Overall toxicity was much greater in the group receiving BEP: leukocytes were lower than 2,000/μL in 45% versus 25% patients, respectively; platelets were lower than 75,000/μL in 29% versus 18%; skin toxicity occurred in 34% versus 3%; and pulmonary toxicity occurred in 30% versus 0%. Relapse occurred in six patients on BEP (3.9%) and five on EP (3.6%) at a median follow-up of 3 years (P = .96). There were four deaths (2.2%) among patients treated with BEP, compared to seven deaths (3.9%) among patients receiving EP (P = .31). This study showed no significant differences in complete response rate, relapse rate, or overall survival.

The AGCTG has reported a randomized study of cisplatin and vinblastine, with or without bleomycin.[28] Good prognosis was defined as a total tumor diameter smaller than 10 cm in the absence of liver, bone, and brain metastases. Patients were treated with cisplatin 100 mg/m^2 on day 1 and vinblastine 6 mg/m^2 on days 1 and 2. This cycle was repeated every 3 weeks. After the achievement of maximum response, two more cycles were given. Forty percent of the patients received five or more cycles. Bleomycin was administered at a dose of 30 mg intramuscularly weekly for a maximum of 12 weeks.

Complete response to chemotherapy alone was achieved in 96 (87%) of 110 evaluable patients on PVB and in 88 (82%) of 108 evaluable patients on PV (P = .29). In addition, seven and eight patients, respectively, were rendered free of disease by surgery. The cause-specific death rate was significantly higher in the PV arm, in which 16 patients (15%) died of malignant disease, compared with 6 (5%) in the PVB arm (P = .02). The excess of tumor-related deaths in the PV arm was partly counterbalanced by a higher rate of toxic death in the PVB arm as a result of bleomycin-related lung toxicity (two patients) and neutropenic sepsis (four patients). In the PV arm, only one patient died of sepsis.

The Eastern Cooperative Oncology Group further elaborated on the results of their previous work, which showed no evidence that three cycles of BEP were inferior to 4 cycles.[38] They performed a randomized study of three cycles of cisplatin and etoposide (EP), with or without bleomycin (BEP).[43] Grade 3 or 4 hematologic toxicity was slightly greater with the bleomycin-containing regimen (57% versus 45%). Interestingly, there was no recorded pulmonary toxicity in either arm. Of the 86 patients randomized to BEP, 82 (95%) achieved disease-free status, compared with 78 of 86 (90%) patients treated with EP. However, the investigators noted a statistically significant increase in the number of unfavorable events—defined as relapse, persistent or progressive carcinoma, or death—among patients treated with EP. Of 86 patients receiving EP, only 60 (70%) remained continuously disease-free, whereas 74 of 86 (86%) patients treated with BEP remained disease-free (P = .03). Because of the untoward number of unfavorable events among patients receiving EP, the study was closed early.

These studies suggest that bleomycin may be deleted from cisplatin and etoposide combination regimens provided that four cycles of induction chemotherapy are given. It should be noted that the deletion of bleomycin may compromise the efficacy of treatment; the design of the trials mentioned did not allow the detection of a survival difference of less than 10%.

It is unclear whether the recommended dose of etoposide should be 100 mg/m^2 days 1 through 5 or 120 mg/m^2 days 1, 3, and 5. It should be noted in this respect that the EORTC study used ultragood-prognosis criteria comparable to the minimal-disease criteria of the Indiana University classification system.

Therefore, it is advisable to use the 100 mg/m^2 dose five times if four cycles of EP are to be given to minimal- and moderate-disease patients. It is evident that bleomycin cannot be deleted when three cycles of BEP are given.

Substituting Carboplatin for Cisplatin

Soon after the introduction of carboplatin, evidence began to appear that showed that its side effects were different from those of cisplatin[44] and that carboplatin might have a different therapeutic spectrum.[45] The dose-limiting side effects of cisplatin are renal and neurologic toxicity, whereas the predominant adverse effect of carboplatin is myelosuppression. Early observations on the activity of carboplatin suggested that there might be incomplete cross-resistance in ovarian cancer.[45] The activity of carboplatin as a single agent in the treatment of nonseminomatous germ cell tumor was demonstrated in a pilot study of 12 chemotherapy-naive patients.[46]

Calvert and colleagues[47] recommend that the optimal dose of carboplatin should be based on glomerular filtration rate (GFR) and the plasma concentration versus time curve (AUC). An AUC of 5 to 7 mg/mL × min is advised, from which the desired dose of carboplatin can be calculated by using the following formula[47,48]:

$$\text{Dose} = \text{AUC}\ (\text{GFR} + 25)$$

Other investigators have used fixed doses per square meter in their studies.[49–51]

The Royal Marsden Hospital experience with carboplatin, etoposide, and bleomycin (CEB) has been reported.[52,53] Eligibility included stages IM, IIA-IIC, IIIAB, IVO-IVC L_1, and IVO-IVB L_2 (see Table 68-3).

After a median follow-up of 40 months, nine patients (7%) had failed CEB. There was suggestive evidence that the failure rate was related to an AUC of less than 5 mg/minute/mL or a carboplatin dose of less than 400 mg/mL × min. The use of carboplatin resulted in considerable hematologic toxicity; 60 patients (56%) experienced WHO grade 3 to 4 leukopenia, and 39 patients (36%) developed grade 3 to 4 thrombopenia. Only 11 patients (9%) had impaired renal function.[53]

In a randomized trial conducted by investigators at MSKCC in conjunction with the Southwest Oncology Group cisplatin plus etoposide (EP) was compared to carboplatin plus etoposide (EC) in good-prognosis testis cancer patients as defined by the MSKCC model but also including patients with extragonadal stage IIC or stage III seminoma.[54] Two hundred and seventy patients were randomized to receive either four cycles of EP given every 3 weeks or four cycles of EC administered every 4 weeks. The carboplatin dose was 350 to 400 mg/m^2 on day 1 in the first 22 patients, but was subsequently increased to 500 mg/m^2 because of the lack of serious hematologic toxicity. Etoposide was administered at a dose of 100 mg/m^2 on days 1 through 5 in both arms.

Complete response was observed in 121 (90%) of 134 patients treated with EP and in 115 (88%) of 131 patients on EC (P = .32). Unfavorable events, defined as incomplete response or relapse, occurred in 17 (13%) patients treated with EP and in 32 (24%) patients treated with EC (P = .02). Disease-free survival after a median follow-up of 22 months was significantly worse in patients treated with EC (P = .005). In addition, hematologic toxicity with EC was considerably more severe than that with EP; 37% of patients on EC and 23% of patients on EP developed neutropenic fever (P = .016). This study showed that carboplatin cannot replace cisplatin when these drugs are given in combination with etoposide alone.

The MRC and the EORTC have completed a randomized trial of B_1EP versus CEB.[55] B_1EP denotes a regimen composed of bleomycin 30 mg on day 1; etoposide 120 mg/m^2 on days 1, 3, and 5; and cisplatin 20 mg/m^2 on days 1 through 5. The CEB regimen was identical with regard to dose and schedule of etoposide and bleomycin; the carboplatin dose was calculated as specified previously with a target AUC of 5 mg/mL × min. Carboplatin was given every 3 weeks, and dosages of less than 400 mg/m^2 were avoided.

A total of 598 patients were randomized. Good prognosis was defined as retroperitoneal lymph node metastases smaller than 10 cm in transverse diameter; fewer than 20 lung metastases; mediastinal or supraclavicular mass smaller than 5 cm in largest diameter; no bone, brain, or liver metastases; serum AFP level lower than 1000 IU/L, and serum hCG level below 10,000 IU/L. These prognostic factors were well balanced in the two treatment arms.

Unfavorable outcome, defined as incomplete response or progressive disease, was observed in 29 (9.6%) of 299 patients on B_1EP and in 56 (18.7%) of 299 patients on CEB (P = .002). Disease-free survival at 1 year was 90% on B_1EP, compared with 80% on CEB. The difference between the arms was most apparent in stage III and IV disease. CEB was associated with more bone marrow toxicity but less renal toxicity. This study shows that carboplatin cannot be substituted for cisplatin, even when the regimen contains bleomycin in addition to etoposide.

CONCLUSIONS AND PERSPECTIVES

The development of cisplatin-based combination chemotherapy has yielded a probability of cure of 90% or more in good-prognosis patients. Based on the consensus definition of good prognosis, this subset comprises about two thirds of patients.

In the past decade, large-scale randomized trials have been conducted with the goals of reducing toxicity and treatment burden in good-prognosis patients. The following are conclusions that can be drawn from these studies.

- BEP is the preferred induction regimen.
- Three cycles of BEP may be as effective as four cycles, but a small reduction in treatment efficacy cannot be excluded.
- Carboplatin cannot replace cisplatin.
- Bleomycin should not be routinely deleted from a combination regimen. Studies are needed to evaluate the possibilities for mitigation of total dose.
- It is unclear whether the administration of etoposide 120 mg/m^2 days 1, 3 and 5 is as effective as 100 mg/m^2 days 1 through 5.

These questions have led to the initiation of new trials in Europe and Australia.

The MRC and EORTC are preparing to perform a trial with a double-randomization design addressing the relative merit of three or four cycles of BEP, as well as the relative merit of a 3-day instead of a 5-day treatment cycle.

Three cycles of BEP with nine weekly administrations of bleomycin versus the same three cycles of BEP plus a fourth cycle of EP will be evaluated. Cycles will be given every 3 weeks. Cisplatin is given at a dose of 20 mg/m^2 days 1 through 5 and etoposide at 100 mg/m^2 days 1 through 5. The 5-day schedule of cisplatin and etoposide, as specified previously, versus the same total dose of drugs delivered over 3 days will be evaluated.

The objectives of the study are to compare the cure rates of the experimental treatment arms (three cycles of BEP, 3 days of BEP) by testing the hypothesis of therapeutic equivalence. Therefore, a disease-free survival difference of 5% or more at 2 years after initiation of therapy must be ruled out; this requires a total of 775 patients enrolled in the study. A quality-of-life assessment and a health-economics (i.e., cost-benefit) analysis will be prospectively carried out in this study.

The Australian and New Zealand Germ Cell Trials Group has initiated a study of good-prognosis patients, comparing two different regimens of BEP. The standard arm of the study comprises three cycles of BEP with 9 weekly administrations of bleomycin and etoposide 100 mg/m^2 days 1 through 5 versus four cycles of BEP in which 30 mg of bleomycin is given every 3 weeks and etoposide is administered at a dose of 120 mg/m^2 days 1, 3, and 5.[55]

In addition to comparisons of response, disease-free survival, and overall survival, assessments of toxicity, quality of life, and costs will be made. This study will therefore evaluate shortened duration of administration of cisplatin and a reduction in the total dose of bleomycin. It seems plausible that these studies will contribute to the maximum therapeutic refinement that can possibly be achieved in good-prognosis germ cell tumor patients.

REFERENCES

1. Einhorn LH. Testicular cancer: a model for a curable neoplasm. Cancer Res 1981;41:3275.
2. Einhorn LH. Treatment of testicular cancer: a new and improved model. J Clin Oncol 1990;8:1777.
3. Williams SD, Birch R, Einhorn LH, et al. Treatment of disseminated germ-cell tumors with cisplatin, bleomycin, and either vinblastine or etoposide. New Engl J Med 1987;316:1435.
4. Horwich A, Norman A, Fisher C, Hendry WF, Nicholis J, Dearnaley DP. Primary chemotherapy for stage II nonseminomatous germ cell tumours of the testis. J Urol 1994;151:72.
5. Motzer RJ, Bosl GJ. Role of adjuvant chemotherapy in patients with stage II nonseminomatous germ-cell tumors. Urol Clin North Am 1993;20:111.
6. Williams SD, Stablein DM, Einhorn LH, et al. Immediate adjuvant chemotherapy versus observation with treatment at relapse in pathological stage II testicular cancer. New Engl J Med 1987;317:1433.
7. Donohue JP, Zachary JM, Maynard BR. Distribution of nodal metastases in nonseminomatous testicular cancer. J Urol 1982;128:315.
8. Sesterhenn IA, Weiss RB, Kash Mostofi F, et al. Prognosis and other clinical correlates of pathologic review in stage I and II testicular carcinoma: a report from the Testicular Cancer Intergroup Study. J Clin Oncol 1992;10:69.
9. McLeod MG, Weiss RB, Stablein DM, et al, for the Testicular Cancer Intergroup Study. Staging relationship and outcome in early stage testicular cancer: a report from the Testicular Cancer Intergroup Study. J Urol 1991;145:1178.
10. Pizzocaro G, Nicolai N, Salvioni R, et al. Comparison between clinical and pathological staging in low stage nonseminomatous germ cell testicular tumors. J Urol 1992;148:76.
11. Socinski MA, Garnick MB, Stomper PC, Fung CF, Richie JP. Stage II nonseminomatous germ cell tumors of the testis: an analysis of treatment options in patients with low volume retroperitoneal disease. J Urol 1988;140.
12. Richie JP, Kantoff PW. Is adjuvant chemotherapy necessary for patients with stage B1 testicular cancer? J Clin Oncol 1991;9:1393.
13. Donohue JP, Foster RS, Geier G, et al. Preservation of ejaculation following nerve sparing retroperitoneal lymphadenectomy. J Urol 1988;138:206.
14. Jewett MAS, Kong Y-SP, Goldberg SD, et al. Retroperitoneal lymphadenectomy for testis tumor with nerve sparing for ejaculation. J Urol 1988;139:1220.
15. Donohue JP, Thornhill JA, Foster RS, Rowland RG, Bihrle R. Primary retroperitoneal lymph node dissection in clinical stage A non-seminomatous germ cell testis cancer. Review of the Indiana University experience 1965–1989. Br J Urol 1993;71:326.
16. Harding MJ, Brown IL, Macpherson SG, Turner MA, Kaye SB. Excision of residual masses after platinum based chemotherapy for non-seminomatous germ cell tumours. Eur J Cancer Clin Oncol 1990;23:1689.
17. Toner GC, Panicek DM, Heelan RT, et al. Adjunctive surgery after chemotherapy for nonseminomatous germ cell tumors: recommendations for patient selection. J Clin Oncol 1990;8:1683.
18. Bajorin DF, Herr H, Motzer RJ, Bosl GJ. Current perspectives on the role of adjunctive surgery in combined modality treatment for patients with germ cell tumors. Semin Oncol 1992;19:148.
19. Fosså SD, Qvist H, Stenwig AE, Lien HH, Ous S, Giercksky KE. Is postchemotherapy retroperitoneal surgery necessary in patients with nonseminomatous testicular cancer and minimal residual tumor masses? J Clin Oncol 1992;10:569.
20. Hendry WF, A'Hern RP, Hetherington JW, Peckham MJ, Dearnaley DP, Horwich A. Para-aortic lymphadenectomy after chemotherapy for metastatic non-seminomatous germ cell tumours: prognostive value and therapeutic benefit. Br J Cancer 1993;71:208.
21. Fox EP, Weathers TD, Williams SD, et al. Outcome analysis for patients with persistent nonteratomatous germ cell tumor in postchemotherapy retroperitoneal lymph node dissection. J Clin Oncol 1993;11:1294.
22. Birch R, Williams S, Cone A, et al. Prognostic factors for favorable outcome in disseminated germ cell tumors. J Clin Oncol 1986;4:400.
23. Bosl GJ, Geller NL, Cirrincione C, et al. Multivariate analysis of prognostic variables in patients with metastatic testicular cancer. Cancer Res 1983;43:3403.
24. Bajorin D, Katz A, Chan E, et al. Comparison of criteria for assigning germ cell tumor patients to "good-risk" and "poor-risk" studies. J Clin Oncol 1988;6:786.
25. Stoter G, Sylvester R, Sleijfer D, et al. Multivariate analysis of prognostic factors in patients with disseminated non seminomatous testicular cancer: results from a European Organization for Research on Treatment of Cancer multiinstitutional phase III study. Cancer Res 1987;47:2714.
26. Medical Research Council Working Party on Testicular Tumours. Prognostic factors in advanced non seminomatous germ-cell testicular tumours: results of a multicenter study. Lancet 1985;1:8.
27. Levi JA, Thomson D, Sandeman T, et al. A prospective study of ciplatin-based combination chemotherapy in advanced germ cell malignancy: role of maintenance and long-term follow-up. J Clin Oncol 1988;6:1154.
28. Levi JA, Raghavan D, Harvey V, et al. The importance of bleomycin in combination chemotherapy for good-prognosis germ cell carcinoma. J Clin Oncol 1993;11:1300.
29. Droz JP, Kramar A, Ghosn M, et al. Prognostic factors in advanced nonseminomatous testicular cancer: a multivariate logistic regression analysis. Cancer Res 1988;62:564.
30. Mead GM, Stenning SP, Parkinson MC, et al. The second Medical Research Council study of prognostic factors in nonseminomatous germ cell tumors. J Clin Oncol 1992;10:85.
31. Stoter G, Sleijfer DTh, Kaye SB, et al, for the EORTC GU-Group. Prognostic factors in metastatic nonseminomatous germ cell tumours: an interim analysis of the EORTC GU-Group experience. Eur Urol 1993;23:202.
32. Stoter G, Sylvester R, for the EORTC Genito-Urinary Tract Cancer Cooperative Group. Prognostic factors in disseminated non-seminomatous testicular cancer. Proc Am Soc Clin Oncol 1994;13:230
33. Bajorin DE, Mazumdar M, Motzer RJ, Vlamis V, Bosl GJ. Model

comparison predicting germ cell tumor (GCI) response to chemotherapy. Proc Am Soc Clin Oncol 1994; 13:232.
34. Stoter G, Bosl GJ, Droz JP, et al. Prognostic factors in metastatic germ cell tumors. In: Newling DWW, Jones WG, eds. EORTC Genitourinary Group monograph 7: prostate cancer and testicular cancer. New York: Wiley-Liss, 1990:313.
35. Mead GM, Stenning SP, on behalf of the IGCCCG. Prognostic factors for metastatic germ cell cancers treated with platinum-based chemotherapy: the International Germ Cell Cancer Collaborative Group (IGCCCG) project to standardise risk criteria. Proc Am Soc Clin Oncol 1994;13:251.
36. Peckham MJ, Barrett A, Liew KH, et al. The treatment of metastatic germ cell testicular tumors with bleomycin, etoposide and cisplatin (BEP). Br J Cancer 1983;47:613.
37. Dearnaley DP, Horwich A, A'Hern R, et al. Combination chemotherapy with bleomycin, etoposide and cisplatin (BEP) for metastatic testicular teratoma: long-term follow-up. Eur J Cancer 1991;27:684.
38. Einhorn LJ, Williams SD, Loehrer PJ, et al. Evaluation of optimal duration of chemotherapy in favorable prognosis disseminated germ cell tumors: a Southeastern Cancer Study Group protocol. J Clin Oncol 1989;7:387.
39. Bosl GJ, Geller NL, Bajorin D, et al. A randomized trial of etoposide + cisplatin versus vinblastine + bleomycin + cisplatin + cyclophosphamide + dactinomycin in patients with good prognosis germ cell tumors. J Clin Oncol 1988;6:1231.
40. Bajorin DF, Geller NL, Weisen SF, Bosl GJ. Two-drug therapy in patients with metastatic germ cell tumors. Cancer 1991;67:28.
41. Stoter G, Kaye S, Jones W, et al. Cisplatin and VP-16 ± bleomycin (BEP vs EP) in good risk patients with disseminated nonseminomatous testicular cancer: a randomized EORTC GU Group study. Proc Am Soc Clin Oncol 1987;6:110.
42. Stoter G, Kaye S, Jones W, et al. Cisplatin (P) and VP16 (E) ± Bleomycin (B), (BEP) vs. (EP) in good risk patients with disseminated nonseminomatous testicular cancer: a randomized EORTC GU Group study. Onkologie 1991;14S4:17.
43. Loehrer PJ, Elson P, Johnson DH, et al. A randomized trial of cisplatin plus etoposide with or without bleomycin in favorable-prognosis disseminated germ cell tumors: an ECOG study. (Abstract 540) Proc Am Soc Clin Oncol 1991;10:169.
44. Calvert AH, Harland SJ, Newell DR, et al. Early clinical studies with cis-diammine-1,1-cyclobutanedicarboxylate platinum II. Cancer Chemother Pharmacol 1982;9:140.
45. Evans BD, Raju KS, Calvert AH, Harland SJ, Wiltshaw E. JM8 (cisdiammine-1,1-cyclobutanedicarboxylate platinum II): a new platinum analogue active in the treatment of advanced ovarian carcinoma. Cancer Treat Rep 1983;67:997.
46. O'Reilly SM, Rustin GJS, Smith DB, Newlands ES. Single agent activity of carboplatin in patients with previously untreated non-seminomatous germ cell tumours. Ann Oncol 1992;3:163.
47. Calvert AH, Newell DR, Gumbrell LA, et al. Carboplatin dosage: prospective evaluation of a simple formula based on renal function. J Clin Oncol 1989;7:1748.
48. Calvert AH. Combining cisplatin and carboplatin complementary or contradictory? Ann Oncol 1991;2:89.
49. Motzer RJ, Bosl GJ, Tauer K, Golbey R. Phase II trial of carboplatin in patients with advanced germ cell tumours refractory to cisplatin. Cancer Treat Rep 1987;71:197.
50. Trump DL, Elson P, Brodovsky H, Vogl SE. Carboplatin in advanced, refractory germ cell neoplasms: a phase II Eastern Cooperative Oncology Group study. Cancer Treat Rep 1987;71:989.
51. Williams SD, Nichols CR, Jansen J. Use of carboplatin in the treatment of testicular cancer. Semin Oncol 1989;16:42.
52. Horwich A, Dearnaley DP, Nichols J, et al. Effectiveness of carboplatin, etoposide, and bleomycin combination chemotherapy in good-prognosis metastatic testicular non-seminomatous germ cell tumors. J Clin Oncol 1991;9:62.
53. Childs WJ, Nicholls EJ, Horwich A. The optimisation of carboplatin dose in carboplatin, etoposide and bleomycin combination chemotherapy for good prognosis metastatic nonseminomatous germ cell tumours of the testis. Ann Oncol 1992;3:291.
54. Bajorin DF, Sarosdy MF, Pfister DG, et al. Randomized trial of etoposide and cisplatin versus etoposide and carboplatin in patients with good-risk germ cell tumours: a multiinstitutional study. J Clin Oncol 1993;11:598.
55. Horwich A, Sleijfer D, Fosså S, et al. A trial of carboplatin-based combination chemotherapy in good prognosis metastatic testicular nonseminoma. Proc Am Soc Clin Oncol 1994;13:231.

Principles and Practice of Genitourinary Oncology, edited by Derek Raghavan, Howard I. Scher, Steven A. Leibel, and Paul H. Lange. Lippincott-Raven Publishers, Philadelphia, © 1997.

CHAPTER 69

Management of Poor-Risk Germ Cell Tumors

Craig R. Nichols, Hans J. Schmoll, Robert J. Motzer, and Jean-Pierre Droz

The history of the development of effective chemotherapy for disseminated germ cell tumors can be divided into three distinct eras: the pre-cisplatin era, in which a variety of single agents and vinblastine-bleomycin combinations were investigated; the early cisplatin era, in which cisplatin-based combination therapy was first developed and tested; and the modern era, in which clinical investigations with cisplatin combinations are adapted to the perceived risk of failure. In this modern era, trials in good-risk patients attempt to maintain equivalent high cure rates with diminished toxicity, and trials in poor-risk patients attempt to improve therapeutic outcome by the addition of new drugs or providing higher doses of existing drugs.

By the mid-1980s, well tolerated, effective, cisplatin-based combination chemotherapies were available; cisplatin, etoposide, and bleomycin (BEP) and vinblastine, Actinomycin D, cyclophosphamide, cisplatin, and bleomycin (VAB-6) were the most broadly applied chemotherapeutic agents for disseminated germ cell cancer.[1] Initial attempts at developing predictive prognostic models allowed for the development of clinical trials based on risk of failure with these standard combinations.[2,3] Trials in patients with good-risk features examined the value of bleomycin in the drug combinations, the number of courses required for cure, and the role of substituting the cisplatin analog carboplatin for cisplatin in the combination.[4–7] Trials in patients with poor-risk features attempted to determine the optimal cisplatin and etoposide dosage, examined the role of ifosfamide and other new drugs in addition to standard combination of cisplatin etoposide and bleomycin, and delineated the role of high-dose chemotherapy with autologous stem cell support. These investigations are reviewed in some detail in this chapter, and a discussion of prognostic features and future directions for clinical investigations of poor-risk germ cell tumors is provided.

PROGNOSTIC FACTORS

With the growing base of clinical experience in germ cell tumors, investigators have become increasingly able to identify patients with good-risk features, who are suitable for therapies of diminished intensity, and less fortunate patients presenting with poor-risk features, in whom more intense, higher-risk approaches are reasonable. Therapy for poor-risk disease is evolving, becoming more complex, intense, and associated with increased short-and long-term complications; therefore, the imperative to properly define the patient's risk category has assumed increased importance.

Prognostic Classifications

The most widely used prognostic classification is the Indiana University classification.[2] Patients deemed at poor risk have either advanced pulmonary or retroperitoneal disease or liver, brain, and bone metastases.[2] This classification has been validated in an independent patient population. Risk assessment using the Indiana University classification is a simple system based on anatomic extent of disease and tumor bulk. This system is easily applied to nearly every clinical setting and reproducibly identifies the bulk of patients with excellent prognoses (>90% long-term survival with modern cisplatin-based treatments) and patients in whom cure is less reliably obtained (~60% long-term survival). This system does not employ serum marker values, histologic subtype, or lactate dehydrogenase (LDH) into the classification of risk. The only recent change has been the addition of any primary mediastinal nonseminomatous germ cell tumor into the advanced disease (i.e., poor-risk) category. Attempts to refine this system may add some additional prognostic ability.

Within the Indiana University classification system, the group that consistently has the lowest disease-free survival is the group of patients with primary mediastinal nonseminoma. Between 1978 and 1993, 88 patients with mediastinal nonseminoma were identified. All patients received modern cisplatin-based chemotherapy, most in randomized clinical trials conducted under the direction of Indiana University. Forty-eight of 88 (55%) patients with mediastinal nonseminoma obtained disease-free status, either with chemotherapy alone (28% or 32%) or with subsequent surgery; 17 patients achieved the status of "no evidence of disease" by resection of teratoma and 3 by resection of cancer for a total of 23%. Of those obtaining disease-free status, 31 were continuously free of disease with a median follow up in excess of 30 months (range, 4 to 144 months). Relapse from disease-free status occurred in 17 of the 48 patients, with 8 patients developing recurrent germ cell tumor, 7 developing an associated hematologic neoplasm, and 2 developing sarcomatous recurrences. A total of 48 patients had persistent or recurrent nonseminomatous germ cell tumor after primary treatment. Three of these patients (6%) are long-term survivors. Thus, it appears that a substantial majority of patients with mediastinal nonseminoma fail to obtain durable complete remission, and salvage therapy is, for the most part, ineffective. Most investigators and prognostic models consider all such patients to be poor risk.

Prognostic Mathematical Models

Two mathematical models allow determination of the probability that a patient will attain complete response status when treated with standard therapy (Table 69-1). Both of these systems use serum tumor markers as continuous variables rather than as discrete variables with cutoff levels. This approach allows the absolute value of the marker level to enter the model and presumably adds to the performance of the model.

1. The Memorial Hospital model uses three factors: human chorionic gonadotropin (HCG) levels, LDH levels, and number of involved sites.[3] The alphafetoprotein (AFP) level failed to attain significant prognostic value in this model.
2. The Institut Gustave-Roussy model uses two factors: HCG levels and AFP levels.[8]

These models attempt to provide a spectrum of probability of complete response in a patient population, which allows meaningful study of stage migration.

Other Prognostic Studies

Other prognostic models, based on multivariate analyses, have been developed by the Medical Research Council (MRC) and the European Organization for the Research and Treatment of Cancer (EORTC). These systems use tumor markers as discrete values with cutoff levels rather than as absolute values.

The second MRC multivariate analysis defines a poor prognostic group as one that includes patients who have at least one of the following adverse prognostic factors[9]:

- presence of liver, bone, or brain metastases
- elevated serum tumor markers (AFP ≥ 1 ng/mL, HCG ≥ 10 IU/L)
- mediastinal mass larger than 5 cm in diameter
- presence of 20 or more lung metastases

The EORTC conducted a multivariate analysis of prognostic factors.[10] Patients with poor outcome had three or four of the following factors: 10 or more lung metastases, maximum diameter of retroperitoneal lymph nodes larger than 5 cm, presence of supraclavicular metastases, and serum HCG levels of 10,000 mIU/L or higher.

A consensus conference was convened to address the multiplicity of prognostic systems and attempt to develop a system that could serve as a unified approach to assigning risk to patients with disseminated germ cell tumors.[11] Many large institutions from throughout Europe and the United States pooled patient information in this effort. More than 6000 cases were analyzed, and several themes became apparent. Mediastinal nonseminomatous germ cell tumors were clearly associated with poor outcome. The presence of nonpulmonary visceral disease was a commonly accepted adverse feature. The issue

TABLE 69-1. *Prognostic models for germ cell tumors*

	Indiana University[30]	MSKCC[3]	IGR[8]	MRC[9]	EORTC[10]
Poor prognostic factors	Group 7: mediastinum/thorax > 50% > 10 lung metastases < 20 mm > 2 lung metastases > 3 cm Group 8: palpable abdominal mass + any metastases Group 9: liver, bone, brain	$Pi = \exp(hi)/[1 + \exp(hi)]$ $h = 8.514$ $- 1.976 \log(HCG + 1)$ $- 0.53 \log(HCG + 1)$ $+ 1.111\ TOTMET$	$h = 1.9$ $- 0.0033 \sqrt{AFP}$ $- 0.021 \sqrt{HCG}$ $+ 0.000033\ HCG$	Liver, bone, brain AFP ≥ 1000 ng/mL or HCG ≥ 10 IU/L Mediastinal mass > 5 cm ≥ 20 Lung metastases	Supraclavicular metastasis HCG ≥ 10 IU/L Retroperitoneal lymph nodes > 5 cm ≥ 10 Lung metastases
Poor prognostic group	Groups 7, 8, or 9	Pi < 0.50	Pi < 0.70	One factor	3 or 4 factors
Percent of patients		18	30	34	9
Percent complete response	60	40	60	68	60

AFP, alphafetoprotein; EORTC, European Organization for the Research and Treatment of Cancer; HCG, human chorionic gonadotropin; IGR, Institut Gustave Roussy; MRC, Medical Research Council; MSKCC, Memorial Sloan-Kettering Cancer Center.

of the prognostic impact of marker elevation was less clear, but it seemed possible to augment the prognostication based on anatomic distribution with the addition of the level of elevation of AFP, HCG and LDH levels. Publication of this internationally defined prognostic system is pending, but it is hoped that this system will, at the least, allow translation of study results using one prognostic system to a more general and widely accepted system.

Tumor Marker Decline as a Prognostic Factor

Investigators at Memorial Hospital emphasized the role of tumor marker decline after the first cycle of chemotherapy as a prognostic factor.[12] A prognostic model was performed in which the tumor marker half-life was calculated between the first two values measured after day 7 from start of chemotherapy. The cutoff values for HCG and AFP half-life were 3 days and 7 days, respectively.

This study included patients with both good risk and poor risk initial characteristics. Patients with normal half-life clearance of AFP and HCG had an 81% complete response rate, those with long half-life clearance had a 19% complete response rate. This factor was independent from other prognostic factors.[12] Additional studies failed to confirm this observation.[13,14,15,16]

Biologic Predictors of Outcome

The ability to assign risk on the basis of available clinical parameters has been maximized. Which system is the most accurate is debatable, but most commonly employed systems can assign prognosis correctly in the vast majority of patients. Efforts at an producing an internationally defined prognostic system may assist in supplementing local prognostic schemes and allow for accurate comparison of results among studies. However, the next level of prognostication will likely come from measurement of available and experimental biologic predictors of outcome. None of these biologic parameters have been investigated thoroughly enough to recommend widespread usage, but future prognostic systems will almost certainly incorporate one or more of these parameters.

Ploidy and proliferative index have been investigated as prognostic parameters in a variety of tumors, including germ cell tumors.[17,18] Within the advanced-disease category as defined by the Indiana University Staging system, Sledge and colleagues analyzed ploidy and proliferative index as predictors of outcome.[19] In this study, ploidy was not predicative of survival, but proliferative index appeared to be a strong predictor of outcome. In the group of patients with a proliferative index above the mean, survival was 37.7 $\pm$ 11 months, compared with a mean survival of 85.6 $\pm$ 7.6 months for patients below the mean. In a multivariate analysis, proliferative index remained the most significant variable in the model ($P < .001$) compared with log(HCG) ($P = .016$, histology ($P = .045$), treatment employed (P = not significant), or DNA index (P = not significant). Further attempts to validate these preliminary findings in the Eastern Cooperative Oncology Group study of cisplatin and etoposide with either bleomycin or ifosfamide in advanced germ cell tumors are ongoing.

Other groups are using similar approaches to assess the impact of cytogenetic findings and oncogene expression in determining outcome. The appearance of a nonrandom chromosomal abnormality in the majority of germ cell tumors has renewed hope that a new understanding of the molecular mechanisms of this disease may be attainable in the near future, with an attendant benefit for the therapy of patients with advanced disease. The identification of an isochromosome of the short arm of chromosome 12 [i(12p)] was initially reported by Atkin and Baker[20,21] and is present in as many as 90% of germ cell tumor specimens. The identification of i(12p) in numerous cell types, including seminoma, nonseminoma, and mature teratoma, as well as in testicular and extragonadal primary lesions and even in carcinoma in situ of the testis, strongly suggest that this chromosomal event plays a role in the process of transformation.[22–27]

Additionally, Bosl and colleagues[27] suggested that the number of copies of i(12p) present has prognostic importance. In their analysis, 4 of 11 patients (36%) with a normal karyotype or fewer than two additional copies of i(12p) had residual viable carcinoma after chemotherapy or failed induction therapy, compared with 6 of 6 patients with more than three copies of i(12p) ($P = .035$). Importantly, three of the latter six patients had been categorized as good risk by the Memorial Hospital prognostic model.[3] Further confirmation of these observations in large clinical trials in advanced disease are required; however, this cytogenetic abnormality may ultimately prove to be an independent prognostic factor.

Investigators have begun to analyze host-related factors as predictors of outcome. In no other malignancy is the identification of resistance to a single chemotherapeutic agent so closely related to poor outcome as cisplatin is in germ cell tumors. The ability to identify inherent (de novo) resistance to this agent at the time of diagnosis would allow the identification of patients destined to fail standard treatment and the early entry of these patients in clinical trials of novel therapeutic approaches. The analysis of potential mechanisms of cisplatin resistance can be broadly grouped into studies of platinum adduct formation, excision and repair capacity, and endogenous thiol content. Investigation of the role of cisplatin resistance in predicting poor outcome offers the possibility of identification of such patients early in the course of treatment.[28,29] It is hoped that such studies will lead to a biologically based prognostic system or a hybrid classification with clinical and biologic parameters that accurately explain the diversity of response seen in patients with germ cell tumors.

CLINICAL TRIALS IN POOR-RISK GERM CELL TUMORS

Randomized Trials

The one third of patients with disseminated testicular cancer who present with poor prognostic features remain a therapeutic challenge. The emphasis in the initial treatment of these poor-risk patients is on the exploration of cisplatin-intense regimens and the use of etoposide and other newer agents. The initial clue to the importance of including etoposide as a component of initial therapy came from the randomized comparison of BEP versus PVB.

Among 72 patients with advanced disease as classified by the Indiana University system, 37 were randomized to receive PVB and 35 to receive BEP.[30] There was a significant difference in disease-free survival; 63% of patients receiving BEP remained disease-free compared with only 38% of patients receiving PVB ($P = .06$).

Preclinical models and dose-intensity analysis of clinical trials suggest a steep dose-response relation for cisplatin. This relation has been exploited in the design of several clinical trials of intensive cisplatin therapy in patients with poor-prognosis germ cell cancer. Ozols and colleagues[31] at the National Cancer Institute in the United States reported the results of a randomized trial of aggressive, high-dose cisplatin therapy versus PVB in poor-risk testicular cancer patients. There was a 2 : 1 randomization of poor-risk patients to receive aggressive treatment with cisplatin 40 mg/m^2 days 1 to 5 with vinblastine bleomycin and etoposide in standard doses versus classic PVB with cisplatin given at 20 mg/m^2 days 1 to 5. Thirty-four patients were randomized to receive the aggressive treatment, whereas 18 were given PVB. Of patients receiving the aggressive arm, 88% obtained a complete response, compared with 67% of patients receiving PVB. The PVB arm had a high incidence of relapse, with 41% of patients having disease recurrence compared with 17% of the patients receiving PVB. Overall, 68% of the group randomized to the aggressive treatment arm remained disease-free, compared with only 33% of the patients receiving standard therapy. Unfortunately, accompanying this apparent improvement in outcome was substantial increase in toxicity. There was significantly more myelosuppression and hearing loss in the patients receiving the high-dose cisplatin therapy.

Whether the apparent superiority of the high-dose regimen in this trial was attributable to the high-dose cisplatin, the inclusion of etoposide, or to other factors was not clear. The Southeastern Cancer Study Group (SECSG) trial of PVB versus BEP showed a clear-cut advantage for the etoposide-containing arm.

Rigid testing of the impact of high-dose cisplatin therapy in disseminated germ cell cancer was accomplished in the successor trial of the SECSG in advanced germ cell cancer.[32] This trial enrolled only patients with advanced disease as defined by the Indiana University classification system. Patients were assigned at random to receive standard doses of etoposide and bleomycin and either standard-dose cisplatin (20 mg/m^2 daily for 5 days) or high-dose cisplatin (40 mg/m^2 daily for 5 days). Between 1984 and 1989, 159 patients with advanced disseminated germ cell cancer were enrolled in the study, of which 153 were evaluable for toxicity and response. Among 76 patients assigned to high-dose therapy, 52 (68%) became disease-free with chemotherapy alone or with chemotherapy and subsequent surgery. Among 77 patients on the standard-dose arm, 56 (73%) became disease-free with chemotherapy alone or with chemotherapy plus surgical resection of residual disease. Eleven patients relapsed from disease-free status, three of whom were receiving high doses and eight of whom were receiving standard doses. Overall, 74% of patients receiving the high-dose cisplatin were alive and 63% were continuously free of disease, compared to 74% alive and 61% continuously free of disease on the standard-dose arm. In addition, the high-dose arm was associated with significantly more ototoxicity, neurotoxicity, gastrointestinal toxicity, and myelosuppression. This large randomized trial found no therapeutic benefit to dose escalation of cisplatin beyond standard doses.[32]

In follow-up to the SECSG trial of cisplatin dose intensity, the Eastern Cooperative Oncology Group conducted a trial testing the substitution of ifosfamide for bleomycin.[33] From 1987 to 1992, 304 patients with advanced-stage disseminated germ cell cancer as defined by the Indiana University classification system were entered on this trial, which randomized patients to either four standard courses of BEP or to four courses of VIP with etoposide (75 mg/m^2 daily for 5 days), ifosfamide (1.2 g/m^2 daily for 5 days), and cisplatin (20 mg/m^2 daily for 5 days). In the preliminary analysis, 278 patients were fully evaluable for survival and toxicity. Of 128 patients randomized to VIP, 69 (54%) became disease-free, compared with 61 of 125 (49%) patients randomized to BEP (P = not significant). Sixty-two patients (48%) on VIP and 52 patients (42%) on BEP were continuously free of disease (P = not significant). Grade IV or greater toxicity, primarily hematologic, was significantly greater on the VIP arm ($P < .0001$). There were five therapy-related deaths on each arm. This preliminary analysis failed to demonstrate benefit for the experimental arm (i.e., VIP) relative to standard therapy with BEP as treatment for poor-risk germ cell tumor.

ONGOING STUDIES

Other ongoing trials in poor-risk patients incorporated high-dose cisplatin therapy with newer agents or bone marrow transplantation. Although preliminary results are encouraging, randomized comparisons of these new therapies to standard-dose cisplatin-based therapy are needed to evaluate the role of these innovative approaches.

Several groups are investigating the addition of other active agents to the traditional three-drug regimen or modest dose escalation with the addition of growth factors or stem cells. At Indiana University, a pilot trial of the five-drug regimen VIP/VB (standard dose VIP plus vinblastine 0.18 mg/kg day 1 and bleomycin 30 U weekly plus G-CSF).[34] Twenty patients were entered in this phase II trial. Toxicity was significant but manageable. There was only one therapy-related death, which occurred in a patient who died of bleomycin lung disease during postchemotherapy surgery. Twelve of the eighteen patients evaluable for response obtained complete remission, and two additional patients obtained a marker-negative partial remission with residual but minimal radiographic abnormalities at 4<ps> and 10<ps> months posttherapy. With a minimum follow-up of 3 months, 10 patients remained progression free.

The EORTC/MRC trial for poor-risk germ cell cancer compared bleomycin; oncovin and cisplatin; and etoposide, ifosfamide, and cisplatin (BOP/VIP) to standard therapy with BEP. The French trial for poor-risk disease compares BEP to the MD Anderson regimen of CISCA/VB. Accrual to both of these important trials has been completed and analysis is pending.

Investigators in Hannover and other institutions in Germany have attempted to intensify therapy for poor-risk patients by incorporating growth factors and peripheral blood progenitor cell support to give high-dose, repetitive chemotherapy cycles. In the most recent update of this phase I/II trial, patients with poor-risk disseminated germ cell tumors were given repetitive cycles of cisplatin 25 to 30 mg/m^2 on days 1 to 5, etoposide 100 to 250 mg/m^2 on days 1 to 5, and ifosfamide 2 g/m^2 on days 1 to 5 over 22 days for four cycles. At the highest dose levels, support with growth factors and peripheral blood progenitor cells were required. With these supportive care techniques, this high-dose therapy was tolerated with no dose-limiting myelosuppression, mucositis, renal toxicity, or neurotoxicity. Three of the 32 patients at the highest dose levels died related to therapy. Of the 23 patients who were evaluable for response, 20 (83%) obtained disease-free status, and 3 patients have relapsed. Accrual to this important exploratory trial is ongoing.

The experience at Charing Cross using alternating regimens has served as a basis for some studies in poor-prognosis germ cell cancer. POMB-ACE chemotherapy uses vincristine, methotrexate, bleomycin, and cisplatin alternating with etoposide, Actinomycin D, and cyclophosphamide. In the original report, 106 out of 193 fully evaluable patients had large-volume metastatic disease as defined by the Royal Marsden staging (abdominal disease >5 cm or lung metastases >2 cm).[35] Of these 106 patient, more than 80% had prolonged survival. In a smaller series of 60 patients with more advanced disease, overall survival was 70%.[36]

Investigators at MD Anderson incorporated some of the principles of alternating therapy and attempted to intensify therapy by shortening the interval between cycles of individually effective therapies.[37] In a small pilot trial, poor-risk patients received rapidly alternating cycles of BOP (7-day delay), CISCA (14 days), POMB (10 days), ACE (14 days). In 17 patients, remission was achieved after an average of 3.5 cycles. Of 11 patients evaluable for response, 8 achieved disease-free status (73%). Toxicity was substantial, with significant requirements for red blood cell and platelet transfusions, but there were no therapy-related deaths. Accrual of patients into this study is ongoing.

This series of phase II trials suggests that more intensive, nonmyeloablative chemotherapy can be given safely. Therapeutic results are not obviously better than those achieved with less intense, standard therapy. The impact of intensive chemotherapy approaches require randomized comparisons to standard treatment.

High-Dose Chemotherapy as Primary Treatment

A trial from the Institut Gustave-Roussey has been reported in which poor-risk patients were randomized to receive conventional therapy with cisplatin, vinblastine, etoposide, and bleomycin or similar therapy followed by a single high-dose cycle of cisplatin, etoposide, and cyclophosphamide.[38] Patients were randomized to receive either the double-dose cisplatin, vinblastine, bleomycin, and etoposide regimen described by Ozols and colleagues[31] or a modified regimen with etoposide 100 mg/m^2 on days 1 to 5, vinblastine 0.2 mg/kg on day 1, cisplatin 40 mg/m^2 on days 1 to 5, and bleomycin 20 U continuous infusion on days 1 to 5 followed by bolus injections on days 8, 15, and 22 of each cycle. Two such cycles were given, followed by high-dose consolidation with cisplatin 40 mg/m^2 on days 1 to 5, etoposide 350 mg/m^2 on days 1 to 5, and cyclophosphamide 1.6 g/m^2 on days 1 to 4, with autologous bone marrow support.

Between 1988 and 1991, 115 patients who were classified as poor risk by the Institut Gustave-Roussey prognostic model were enrolled in this study.[38] One patient was incorrectly determined to have poor-risk features and was ineligible. Fifty-seven patients were randomized to each arm. In the conventional arm, six patients failed to complete treatment because of progressive disease (4), refusal (2), or toxic death (1). In the high-dose arm, 16 patients did not complete treatment because of early death prior to transplant (6), refusal (3), toxic death (2), poor performance status (1), or human immunodeficiency virus infection (1). In a long follow-up, 40 of 57 (70%) patients were progression-free on the standard-therapy arm, compared with 33 of 57 (58%) patients on the high-dose arm.

This trial failed to demonstrate any advantage for the high-dose arm.[38] As with many emerging new treatments, however, the high-dose arm of this trial would be considered substandard by modern criteria; different prognostic factors have emerged as important predictors of outcome. Accordingly, a large scale trial is being conducted in poor-risk patients that will compare standard therapy (i.e., BEP) to brief conventional therapy followed by two cycles of high-dose carboplatin, etoposide, and cyclophosphamide. It is hoped that this trial will define the role of high-dose chemotherapy as the primary therapy in poor-risk disease. This trial concept is based on the preliminary experience of high-dose chemotherapy as primary treatment from Memorial Sloan-Kettering, in which patients with poor predicted complete response rates (<0.5) treated with VAB-6 and or those patients exhibiting marker decline consistent with a prolonged half-life (>7 days AFP, >3 days HCG).[39] Twenty-eight patients were entered into the study, and 22 patients proceeded to receive two cycles of high-dose carboplatin, etoposide, and cyclophosphamide plus ABMT. Overall, 12 of the 22 patients (55%) receiving high-dose therapy and 15 of 27 (56%) patients overall achieved disease-free status, two via resection of residual carcinoma. Eleven patients remained continuously free of disease with a median follow-up of 31 months.

STANDARD MANAGEMENT OF POOR-RISK GERM CELL TUMORS

In this rare subset of an uncommon illness for which significant therapeutic questions remain, all such patients should be referred for participation in clinical trials. Off protocol or in patients who are too ill to travel, standard management should include prompt initiation of combination chemotherapy with standard BEP for a planned four cycles of treatment. In some cases, serologic confirmation of suspected germ cell tumor is sufficient to initiate therapy for patients in extremis from massive tumor dissemination. Patients presenting with brain metastases should receive modern, curative-intent radiotherapy as well as chemotherapy.

Patients should receive chemotherapy on schedule with as few delays as possible. Concerns regarding myelosuppression at the scheduled time of the next cycle (day 22) are often overblown. Despite low white blood cell counts, almost all of these young, otherwise healthy patients have evidence of incipient hematologic recovery. Therapy should be initiated in these patients, and only if no recovery is seen over the course of the 5-day treatment is the last day of etoposide held.

Patients should have tumor markers obtained and compared to previous values with each cycle of therapy. If markers are not falling consistent with the half-life (HCG, 18 hours; AFP, 5 days), considerations of alternative salvage treatments should be made. In this situation, the possibility of occult disease at a sanctuary site (e.g., central nervous system, testis) must be considered and involvement of these areas ruled out before labeling the program as a failure.

Depending on the stage at diagnosis, 20% to 50% of patients who undergo induction chemotherapy for disseminated germ cell tumor have significant residual radiographic abnormalities. It is common practice for patients facing extensive postchemotherapy resection to discontinue bleomycin after the tenth dose and not receive the eleventh and twelfth week of bleomycin. In this subset of patients, postchemotherapy resection of residual disease is often performed to remove residual teratoma or viable cancer. Several points bear emphasis in this setting. Consideration of postchemotherapy should be made only if the serum AFP and HCG have normalized. Patients with persistently elevated serum markers should be considered for salvage chemotherapy rather than surgical debulking. Postchemotherapy resection of residual abnormalities is rarely urgent, and sufficient time should be taken to allow the patient to recover from the effects of induction chemotherapy. Typically, patients are taken to surgery 6 weeks after the last course of chemotherapy. Third, repeat imaging of the areas of abnormality should be performed before surgery. In some patients, continued involution of residual masses occurs after the completion of therapy and surgical resection is not necessary.

Patients with persistent retroperitoneal disease undergo resection using either a midline or thoracoabdominal approach. Resection of residual radiographic abnormalities after induction chemotherapy for disseminated nonseminomatous germ cell cancer has a surprisingly low rate of significant complications. The most common intraoperative complication is injury to the renal vessels, which can be repaired at the time of surgery in most cases. Significant postoperative complications include wound infections, ileus, prolonged atelectasis, and pneumonia. Development of lymphoceles can occur and may be mistaken for recurrent disease on abdominal computed tomography scans. Overall, significant morbidity is rare, and operative mortality is almost nonexistent; however, the majority of patients undergoing bilateral radical retroperitoneal lymphadenectomy are rendered infertile as a result of retrograde ejaculation. Developments in urologic surgery have allowed for preservation of the sympathetic fibers that control ejaculation while maintaining the therapeutic template of the cancer surgery. Depending on the extent of residual disease, many patients retain ejaculatory function after undergoing resection of residual disease after chemotherapy.

Patients with unilateral disease in the pulmonary parenchyma or mediastinum can achieve resection of this supradiaphragmatic disease through a thoracotomy incision. Patients with combined thoracic and abdominal disease frequently require a median sternotomy as well as a midline abdominal approach. Patients who have received bleomycin as part of induction chemotherapy require specialized management. These patients may have subtle restrictive pulmonary disease and diminished carbon monoxide diffusion capacity. Care should be taken during anesthesia to avoid overhydration and to use colloid rather than crystalloid fluid replacement. Most importantly, inspired O_2 concentration should not exceed 25% in the intraoperative period nor during postoperative recovery.

The histopathologic findings in postchemotherapy surgical specimens help define the need for further treatment. In early reports, about 40% of patients had teratoma, 40% had fibrous necrotic debris, and 20% had residual viable germ cell cancer. Analysis of more recent series suggests that the incidence of persistent cancer is decreasing. In a study of optimal duration of chemotherapy in minimal-extent disseminated germ cell cancer, 14 of 107 patients were found to have residual teratoma in the postchemotherapy specimen, and no patient was found to have viable carcinoma.[4] In the same study, 19 of 77 patients with moderate volume disease were found to have teratoma, whereas only 6 patients had residual cancer.[4] In a study of 153 advanced-disease patients, 30 had residual teratoma, and only 6 had persistent germ cell cancer.[32] This apparent decrease in the incidence of residual cancer has also been reported by others and is partly the result of better selection of patients for surgery and improvements in primary chemotherapy.

Patients with persistent cancer identified and totally removed at postchemotherapy surgery require special management. If the surgical margins are free of tumor, all sites of known disease are removed and the serum tumor markers remain normal; patients should receive two postoperative cycles of cisplatin-based therapy similar to induction therapy. Patients with unresectable disease, positive surgical margins, or elevated tumor markers should be considered for full salvage therapy using new agents and more prolonged courses of therapy. About two thirds of patients receiving additional postoperative cisplatin-based chemotherapy after total resection of residual viable cancer remain free of disease.[40]

NEW AGENTS

The development of new active compounds offers the best hope of significantly changing the prospect for cure in recurrent or resistant germ cell tumors and better therapy for patients presenting with poor-risk features. Several classes of drugs are being investigated, including the taxanes and the topoisomerase I inhibitors. Preliminary information suggests a possible role for paclitaxil in the treatment of germ cell tumors, and other phase II studies are underway.[41] In addition, the use of differentiating agents in the rare clinical setting of malignant non–germ cell elements developing in the background of germ cell tumor is being investigated.

CONCLUSIONS

Depending on what system of classification is used, only about one half of all patients with poor-risk disseminated germ cell tumors survive their illness. Standard therapy in this setting is four timely cycles of cisplatin, etoposide, and bleomycin as a combination regimen, with aggressive and complete resection of residual radiographic abnormalities when necessary. The foci of clinical investigations in this area are twofold. First is the exploration of more intensive scheduling or dosing with existing active agents. The randomized intergroup trial of BEP compared with abbreviated BEP plus high-dose carboplatin, etoposide, and cyclophosphamide will serve to validate or refute the role of high-dose chemotherapy in the management of patients with poor-risk germ cell cancer. Second, ongoing efforts to define new agents with activity in treating germ cell tumors are critical to developing alternative regimens. Perhaps most important will be enhanced biologic understanding of these unique malignancies, which will serve to discriminate between clinically identical but biologically diverse presentations as well as yield new targets for rationally designed therapeutics.

REFERENCES

1. Einhorn L. Treatment of testicular cancer: a new and improved model. J Clin Oncol 1990;8:1777.
2. Birch R, Wiliams S, Cone A, et al. Prognostic factors for favorable outcome in disseminated germ cell tumors. J Clin Oncol 1986;4(3): 400.
3. Bosl G, Geller N, Cirrincione C, et al. Multivariate analysis of prognostic variables in patients with metastatic testicular cancer. Cancer Res 1983;43:3403.
4. Einhorn LH, Williams SD, Loehrer PJ, et al. Evaluation of optimal duration of chemotherapy in favorable-prognosis disseminated germ cell tumors: a Southeastern Cancer Study Group protocol. J Clin Oncol 1989;7(3):387.
5. Loehrer PJ, Elson P, Johnson DH, Williams SD, Trump DL, Einhorn LH. A randomized trial of cisplatin plus etoposide with or without bleomycin in favorable prognosis disseminated germ cell tumors. Proc Am Soc Clin Oncol 1991;10:169.
6. Levi J, Raghavan D, Harvey V, et al. The importance of bleomycin in combination chemotherapy for good prognosis germ cell carcinoma. J Clin Oncol 1993;11:1300.
7. Bajorin D, Sarosdy M, Pfister D, et al. A randomized trial of etoposide cisplatin vs. etoposide and carboplatin in patients with good-risk germ cell tumors: a multiinstitutional study. J Clin Oncol 1993;11:598.
8. Droz J, Kramer A, Ghosn M, et al. Prognostic factors in advanced nonseminomatous testicular cancer: a multivariate logistic regression analysis. Cancer 1988;62:564.
9. Mead G, Stenning S, Parkinson M, et al. The second Medical Research Council study of prognostic factors in nonseminomatous germ cell tumors. J Clin Oncol 1992;10:85.
10. Stoter G, Sylvester R, Sleifer D, et al. Multivariate analysis of prognostic factors in patients with disseminated non seminomatous testicular cancer: results from a European Organization for Research on Treatment of Cancer multi-institutional phase III study. Cancer Res 1987; 47:2714.
11. Mead G, Stenning S. Prognostic factors for metastatic germ cell cancers treated with platinum-based chemotherapy: the International Germ Cell Cancer Collaborative Group (IGCCCG) project to standardise risk criteria. Proc Am Soc Clin Oncol 1994;13:251.
12. Toner G, Geller N, Tan C, et al. Serum tumor marker half-life during chemotherapy allows early prediction of complete response and survival in nonseminomatous germ cell tumors. Cancer Res 1990;50:5904.
13. Horwich A, Peckham M. Serum tumor marker regression rate following chemotherapy for malignant teratoma. Eur J Cancer Clin Oncol 1984; 20:1463.
14. Lange P, Vogelzang N, Goldman A, Kennedy B, Fraley E. Marker half-life analysis as a prognostic tool in testicular cancer. J Urol 1982; 128:708.
15. Thompson D, Haddow J. Serial monitoring of serum alpha-fetoprotein and chorionic gonadotropin in males with germ cell tumors. Cancer 1979;43:1820.
16. Stevens M, Horwich A. Prognostic significance of serum marker half-life in metastatic testicular teratoma. J Clin Oncol 1995 (in press).
17. Fossa S, Pettersen E, Thorud E, et al. DNA flow cytometry in human testicular cancer. Cancer Lett 1985;28:55.
18. Quirke P, Dyson J, Sutton J, et al. Assessment of germ cell tumors of the testis by flow cytometry and histopathology. In: Jones W, ed. Germ cell tumors II. Oxford: Pergammon Press, 1986:45.
19. Sledge G, Eble J, Roth B, Wuhrman B, Fineberg N, Einhorn L. Relation of proliferative activity to survival in patients with advanced germ cell cancer. Cancer Res 1988;48:3864.
20. Atkin N, Baker M. Specific chromosome change, i(12p) in testicular tumors? Lancet 1982;2:1349.
21. Atkin N, Baker M. i(12p): Specific chromosomal marker in seminoma and malignant teratoma of the testis? Cancer Genet Cytogenet 1983; 10:199.
22. Castedo S, de Jong B, Oosterhuis J, et al. Chromosomal changes in human primary non-seminomatous germ cell tumors. Cancer Res 1989; 49:5696.
23. Castedo S, de Jong B, Oosterhuis J, et al. Chromosomal changes in mature residual teratomas following chemotherapy. Cancer Res 1989; 49:672.
24. Castedo S, de Jong B, Oosterhuis J, et al. Cytogenetic analysis of ten human seminomas. Cancer Res 1989;49:439.
25. Vos A, Oosterhuis J, de Jong B, et al. Cytogenetics of carcinoma in situ of the testis. Cancer Genet Cytogenet 1990;46:75.
26. Samaniego F, Bosl G, Geller N, Penenberg D, Golbey R. Identification of prognostic variables in patients (PTS) with germ cell tumor (GCT) within the poor risk subgroup. Proc Am Soc Clin Oncol 1988;7:132.
27. Bosl G, Dmitrovsky E, Reuter V, et al. Isochromosome of chromosome 12: useful marker for male germ cell tumors. J Natl Cancer Inst 1989; 81:1874.
28. Reed E, Ozols R, Tarone R, et al. Platinum-DNA adducts in leukocyte DNA correlate with disease response in ovarian cancer patients receiving platinum-based chemotherapy. Proc Natl Acad Sci U S A 1987; 84:5024.
29. Reed E, Ozols R, Tarone R, et al. The measure of cisplatin-DNA adduct levels in testicular cancer patients. Carcinogenesis 1988;9:1909.
30. Williams S, Birch R, Einhorn L, Irwin L, Greco F, Loehrer P. Treatment of disseminated germ cell tumors with cisplatin, bleomycin, and either vinblastine or etoposide. New Engl J Med 1987;316:1435.
31. Ozols RF, Ihde DC, Linehan M, Jacob J, Ostchega Y, Young RC. A randomized trial of standard chemotherapy v a high-dose chemotherapy regimen in the treatment of poor prognosis nonseminomatous germ-cell tumors. J Clin Oncol 1988;6(6):1031.
32. Nichols C, Williams S, Loehrer P, et al. Randomized study of cisplatin dose intensity in advanced germ cell tumors: a Southeastern Cancer Study Group and Southwest Oncology Group protocol. J Clin Oncol 1991;9:1163.
33. Loehrer P, Einhorn L, Elson P, et al. Phase III study of cisplatin (p) plus etoposide (VP-16) with either bleomycin (B) or ifosfamide (I) in advanced stage germ cell tumors (GCT): an intergroup trial. Proc Am Soc Clin Oncol 1993 1993;12:261.
34. Blanke C, Loehrer P, Einhorn L, Nichols C. A phase II trial of VP-16 plus ifosfamide plus cisplatin plus vinblastine plus bleomycin (VIP/VB) with filgrastim for advanced stage testicular cancer. Proc Am Soc Clin Oncol 1994;13:234.
35. Newlands E, Rustin G, Begent R, et al. Further advances in the management of malignant teratomas of the testis and other sites. Lancet 1983; 1:948.
36. Cullen M, Harper P, Woodroffe C, et al. Chemotherapy for poor risk germ cell tumours: an independent evaluation of the POMB/ACE regime. Br J Urol 1988;62:454.
37. Amato R, Hutchinson L, Striegel A. Modulation of Dose Intensity (DI) by Reducing Chemotherapy (CHT) Intervals in Patients (pts) with High Volume Non-seminomatous Germ cell tumors (HV-GCT). Proc Am Soc Clin Oncol 1994;13:253.
38. Droz J, Pico J, Biron P, et al. No evidence of a benefit of early intensified chemotherapy (HDCT) with autologous bone marrow transplantation (ABMT) in first line treatment of poor risk non seminomatous germ cell tumors. Proc Am Soc Clin Oncol 1992;11:197.
39. Motzer R, Mazumdar M, Gulati S. Phase II trial of high dose carboplatin and etoposide with autologous bone marrow transplantation in first line therapy for patients with poor-risk germ cell tumors. J Natl Cancer Inst 1993;85:1828.
40. Fox E, Weathers T, Williams S, et al. Outcome analysis for patients with persistent germ cell carcinoma in post chemotherapy retroperitoneal lymph node dissections. J Clin Oncol 1993;11:1294.
41. Motzer R, Bajorin B, Schwartz L, et al. Phase II trial of paclitaxel shows antitumor activity in patients with previously treated germ cell tumors. J Clin Oncol 1994;12:2277.

Principles and Practice of Genitourinary Oncology, edited by Derek Raghavan, Howard I. Scher, Steven A. Leibel, and Paul H. Lange. Lippincott-Raven Publishers, Philadelphia, © 1997.

CHAPTER 70

Cytoreductive Surgery for Nonseminomatous Germ Cell Cancer

John P. Donohue, Richard S. Foster, Randall G. Rowland, and Richard Bihrle

Advanced testicular cancer is best treated with combination platinum-based chemotherapy as primary therapy. Those with more bulky tumors who obtain a partial remission should have residual tumor completely resected. This effectively restages the patient, provides therapeutic benefit to many, and determines the need for additional chemotherapy. If carcinoma is found in the resected specimen, ''salvage'' chemotherapy is required. If the resection is grossly complete, most in this group survive (Fig. 70-1).[1] The postoperative relapse potential is related to the site of the disease (i.e., mediastinal or retroperitoneal), histology (i.e., sarcomatous elements or none), and bulk of disease (i.e., massive, moderate, or small).[2–4]

Two groups of patients should be considered. The first group had partial remissions with primary therapy. The second group had complete remissions after primary chemotherapy but relapsed and then achieved partial remissions after salvage chemotherapy. Members of the first group who do not have complete resolution of findings on abdominal computed tomography (CT) scans or on abdominal ultrasound scans after chemotherapy are considered as candidates for radical retroperitoneal lymph node dissection (RPLND). If the residual mass is high in the abdomen and extends into the retrocrural area or apparently involves the diaphragm and has extended into the chest, a combined abdominal and thoracic approach is indicated.

Depending on the circumstances of the individual case, a thoracoabdominal incision or a median sternotomy in combination with the midline abdominal incision is used. When patients have residual unilateral chest disease in the parenchyma or the mediastinum, a thoracotomy incision alone is sufficient, assuming the abdominal findings have completely normalized after chemotherapy or were normal initially. If bilateral chest disease is present, particularly in the posterior mediastinum, separate thoracotomy incisions may be indicated. If the bilateral chest disease is in any other location, adequate exposure can be obtained through a median sternotomy. Any of these approaches can be used in combination with a midline abdominal incision if there is residual disease in the abdomen (Table 70-1).

If any patient in the first group, having undergone primary cytoreductive chemotherapy, has a persistently elevated serum marker, such as alphafetoprotein (AFP) or beta human chorionic gonadotropin (β-HCG), he is treated with salvage chemotherapy rather than surgical resection, based on the knowledge that active disease is present.

The indications for surgery for members of the second group of patients are the same as for the first: evidence of only a partial remission. If a patient had an elevated AFP or β-HCG level, he would be a candidate for further chemotherapy rather than surgical treatment. There are occasional exceptions to this rule: If the patient has exhausted all chemotherapeutic regimens that have any likelihood of success and has a limited focus of disease deemed resectable. Table 70-1 summarizes the indications for surgery.

The technical portions of the retroperitoneal node dissection have been previously described.[5–7] A full bilateral RPLND is indicated in most cases. Tissue analysis from full RPLND specimens confirms the diverse nature of histologic changes in the patients who have had widespread metastatic disease.[8] A simple biopsy or ''lumpectomy'' is a potentially dangerous practice, because it risks missing tumor elsewhere in the retroperitoneum. Figures 70-2 through 70-7 illustrate basic technical points in postchemotherapy dissections.

RESULTS OF CYTOREDUCTIVE SURGERY

Our experience at Indiana University with postchemotherapy dissections exceeds 800 cases. We have a 2-year follow-up of 557 patients, who are divided according to the histologic classification of their resected specimen (Table 70-2). Fully one third of our postchemotherapy RPLND experience consists of patients referred after prior surgical RPLND attempts elsewhere. We have studied 248 patients who failed locally after prior RPLND; 179 of these (72%) have no evidence of disease (NED), 52 have died of disease (21%), and 17 are living with disease (7%).

Patients with partial remissions after primary chemotherapy or patients who had relapsed after primary therapy and had partial responses to salvage chemotherapy were present in all groups. In the combined series, about two fifths had fibrotic-

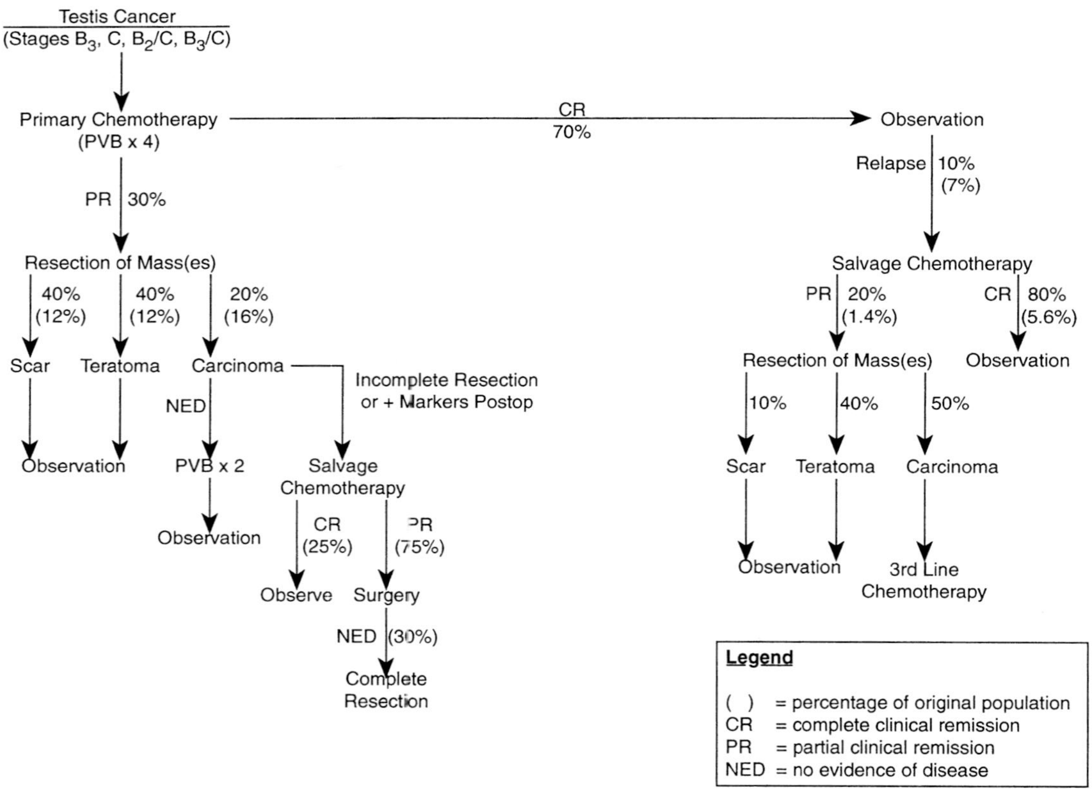

FIG. 70-1. Treatment scheme for disseminated testis cancer at Indiana University

cystic-necrotic tissue, two fifths had teratomas (mature or immature), and one fifth had carcinomas.[2] In general, the patients that have only necrotic or fibrocystic tissue at the time of exploration do extremely well postoperatively. Initially, the relapse rate was thought to be 10% for patients with teratomas. Loehrer and associates[4] reported relapses in 16 of 54 patients with surgically resected teratomas after a minimum follow-up of 18 months. Nine of these teratoma patients relapsed with carcinoma, and 7 relapsed with recurrent teratoma. In the group of 9 patients with recurrent carcinoma, 4 have been rendered disease free with subsequent treatment, 2 are alive with disease, and 3 are dead. In the group of 7 patients with recurrent terato-

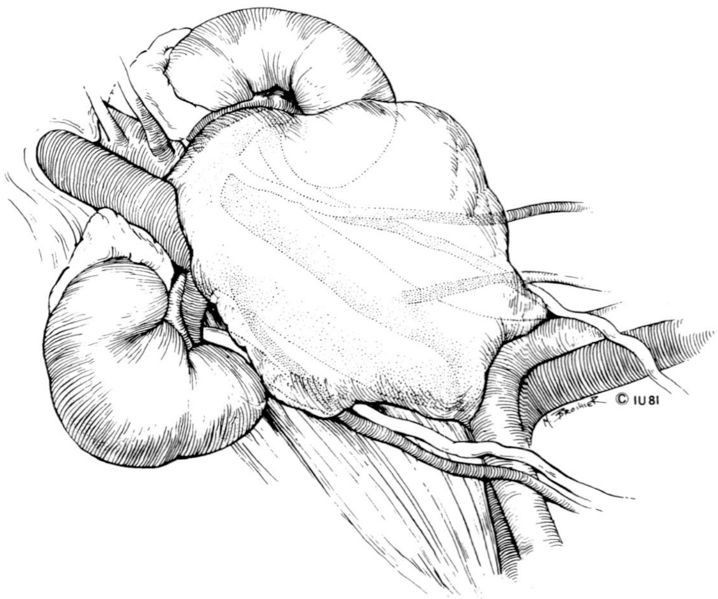

FIG. 70-2. Schematic representation of a tumor in the retroperitoneum after primary chemotherapy. Extensive tumor may still involve the great vessels or ureters. The bowel and mesenteric divisions are made to expose the tumor in its entirety. Using the split and roll technique, vascular control can be obtained and the tumor removed.

TABLE 70-1. *Histologic findings in surgery after chemotherapy*

Group	No. of patients	Fibrotic-cystic necrotic tissue (%)	Teratoma (%)	Carcinoma (%)
RPLND only 2.5	51*	16 (31.5)	16 (31.5)	19 (37)
Thoracotomy only 12, 13	48	14 (30)	17 (35)	17 (35)
RPLND + thoracotomy 13	24†	4 (17)	13 (54)	7 (29)
	123	34 (28)	46 (37)	43 (35)

* These patients represent partial remissions after primary chemotherapy and relapse after complete remission who went on to have partial remissions with salvage chemotherapy.

† In 17 patients, the pathology in the chest and retroperitoneum agreed, and in 7, they differed.

RPLND, retroperitoneal lymph node dissection.

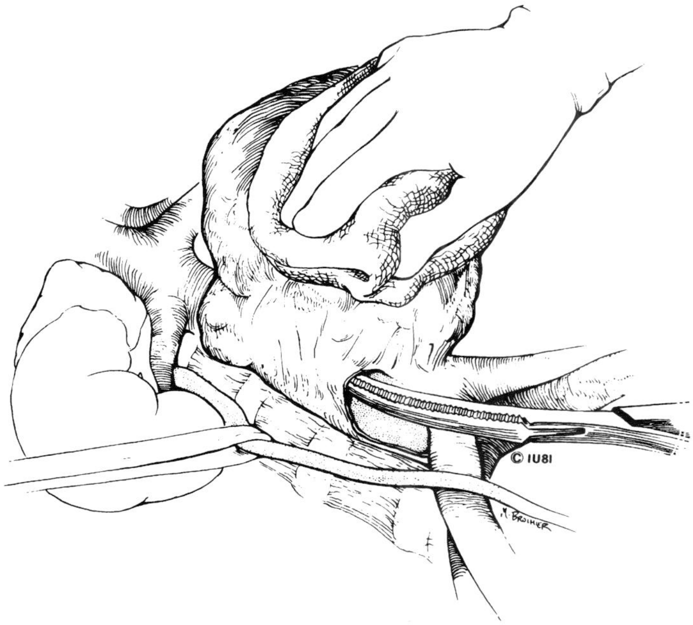

FIG. 70-3. The tumor can be dissected off the anterior vena cava, usually in the subadventitial plane below the fibrous capsule of the tumor. Rarely, the vena cava may be ablated or involved with tumor thrombus. In such cases, the vena cava can be resected or a thrombectomy done. The vena cava is a low-pressure system, and subadventitial dissection does not provide a later spontaneous rupture.

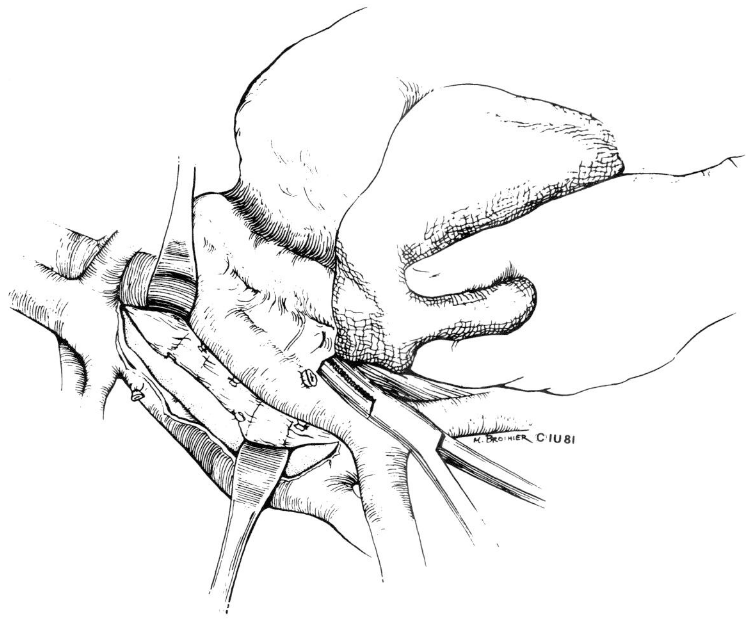

FIG. 70-4. Tumor is dissected free of the vena cava, after caval lumbars have been ligated and divided. Dissection from the aorta requires care in preserving as much adventitia as possible. Complete subadventitial dissection may weaken the aortic wall. In this high-pressure system, rupture can occur spontaneously or intraoperatively, and it is difficult to repair without some adventitial tissue. An approach that preserves adventitia on the aorta is shown.

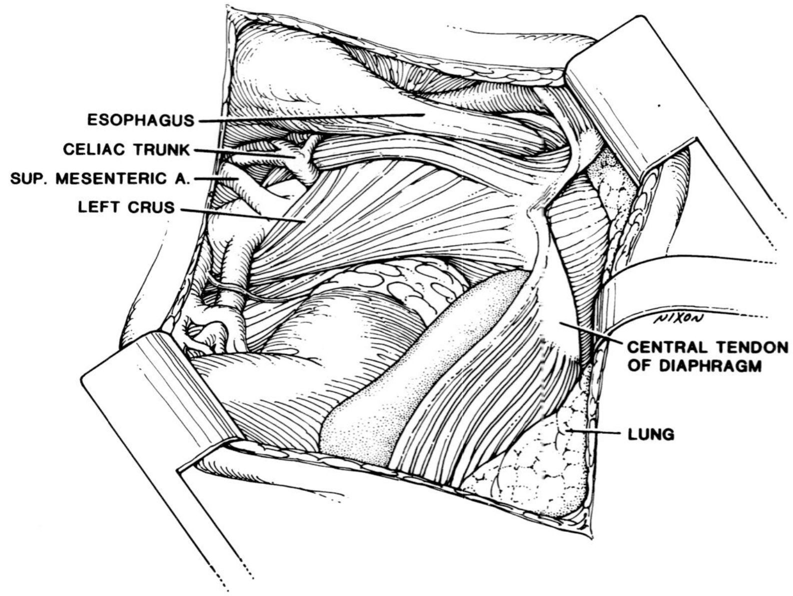

FIG. 70-5. The left lower chest, upper abdomen, and retroperitoneum are exposed with a thoracoabdominal incision through the 8th, 9th or 10th intercostal space. The incision extends across the rectus muscle and into the peritoneal cavity. This permits simultaneous access to the renal vessels and superior mesenteric and celiac arterial bases. The crus of the diaphragm is exposed; under it lies the tumor to be resected.

mas, 2 have died of inoperable progressive disease, and 5 are disease free, although 2 have required multiple surgical procedures. The fact that relapses tend to occur near sites of previous resection points to the necessity of complete dissection in these patients at the time of their cytoreductive surgery.

If a patient's diagnosis was originally made by means other than orchiectomy and there was an abnormal testis discovered by history, examination, or ultrasound, the testicle should be removed at the time of surgery because of the possibility of persistence of the primary tumor. The originally involved testis should also be removed, even if the patient had an apparently complete response to chemotherapy. In 42% of such patients, teratoma or carcinoma was found in the testicle that was removed after chemotherapy.[9] This suggests that there may be a blood-testis barrier in the testis that inhibits the effectiveness of chemotherapy in this organ.

Despite the increased risks for patients who have undergone primary or salvage chemotherapy before resection of residual disease, the complication and death rates are acceptable. We reported 49 patients who underwent surgery for advanced disease; 45 had received previous chemotherapy.[10] The total complication rate for this postchemotherapy group with advanced disease was 26%, and the death rate was 2%, compared with an overall complication rate of 12% and a death rate of 0.5% for patients who were operated on for lesser-stage disease (stage I or II). Similar findings were reported by Skinner's group.[11]

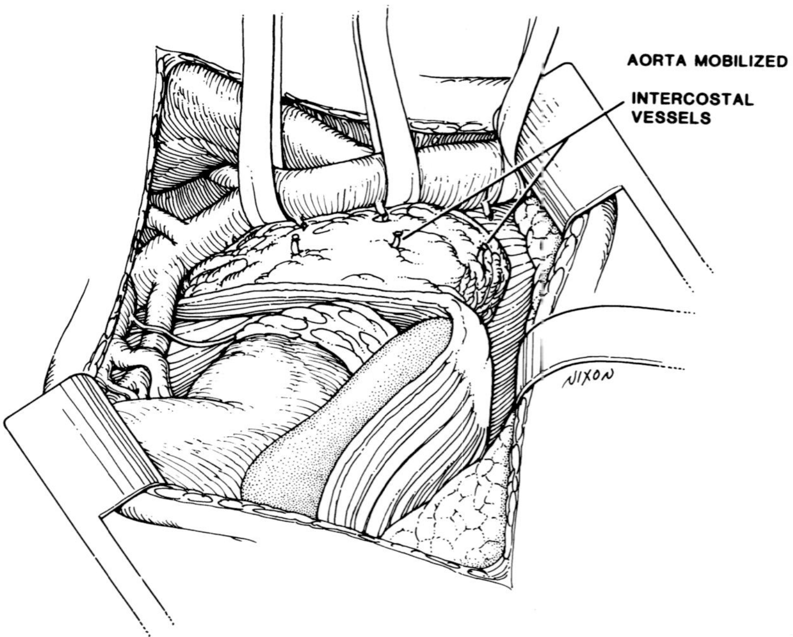

FIG. 70-6. The crus of the diaphragm is divided, exposing the underlying posterior mediastinal mass (i.e., retrocrural tumor), which extends above the renal artery. It may extend into the chest (i.e., posterior, inferior mediastinum) for a number of thoracic interspaces. The intercostal vessels are exposed, doubly ligated, and divided to assist in the mobilization of the aorta.

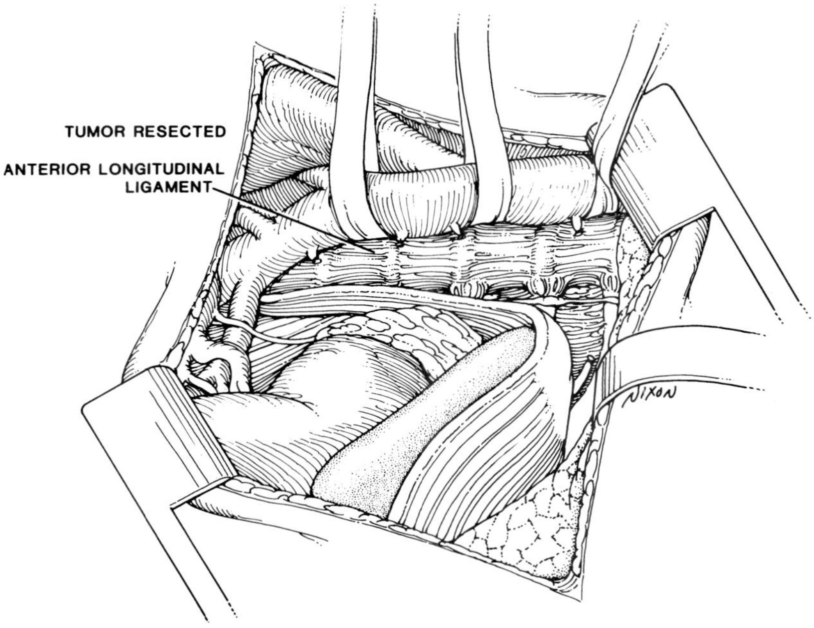

FIG. 70-7. After the aorta is mobilized, the tumor can be resected off the posterior body wall. The anterior spinous ligaments and posterior rib articulations are seen. The intercostal foramina can be secured with clips or suture ligatures and cautery, achieving control of proximal (i.e., aortic) and distal control of the intercostal vessels. The tumor is safely removed in this setting. The esophagus is on the right side and slightly anterior to the aorta; it is not seen with this exposure.

Fifty-two patients in their group were operated on for advanced disease. The complication rate was 23%, and the death rate was 4%.

Clinical experience with certain patterns of response to chemotherapy led us to recognize another group of patients who almost invariably have necrosis alone in the residual tumor: patients with pure seminoma in the primary testis tumor. Many have noticed that these patients had only necrosis in resected tumors after chemotherapy and, if observed without surgery, had stable partial remissions and no progression after treatment of bulky metastatic disease with platinum-based chemotherapy programs. A second group is likely to have necrosis only in resected tissue.[3] These patients had pure embryonal carcinoma in their primary tumors and had more than 90% reduction in tumor mass, as measured on sequential CT scans after treatment. The much cytoreduced, small lesions resected after chemotherapy were entirely necrotic in this subset of patients treated. A pure embryonal primary testis tumor and an impressive cytoreductive response to chemotherapy treatment ≥90% were required to achieve this histologic response of necrosis only. In retrospect, we may conclude that these patients were cured by their chemotherapy. In contrast, Toner and colleagues,[12] reporting the results from the Memorial Sloan-Kettering, Cancer Center, have not found uniform necrosis in such patients and contend that RPLND is still required.

Our findings somewhat parallel our earlier experience of patients with seminoma who were found to have necrosis with great regularity when their residual metastases were resected after chemotherapy. This led to a general consensus that they could be followed safely, especially if they had smaller lesions and some measurable response to earlier treatment. Others chose to use consolidation radiotherapy, particularly for bulky residual tumors. Relapses in these seminoma patients with partial remissions observed expectantly have been few. Unlike the seminoma patients, patients with pure embryonal cancer and advanced disease must have a dramatic radiographic response (>90%) to be likely to have necrosis only. Anything less runs the risk for some persistent tumor elements with growth potential.

One of the special challenges in postchemotherapy surgery is the patient with a bulky teratoma. This tumor must be well resected, operating in several stages if necessary (e.g., chest, supraclavicular, abdominal and pelvic), because it will not regress; most progress as "mature and immature teratomas", and some have malignant changes. Several factors are associated with increased relapse and survival risks. We found that the

TABLE 70-2. *Status after chemotherapy*

(1975–1990)	Total	NED* (%)	LWD	UNK	DOD	DOp	DOC
Fibrosis	150	139 (93)	2	0	8	1	0
Teratoma	273	244 (89)	11	0	12	3	3
NSGCT cancer	121	63 (52)	11	1	41	5	0
NGC cancer	13	5 (39)	1	4	3	0	0
Total	557	451 (81)	25	5	64	9	3

* Disease-free survival (NED) = 451/557 = 81%. Overall survival (NED plus LWD) = 476/557 = 85%.
NED, no evidence of disease; LWD, living with disease; UNK, unknown; DOD, dead of disease; DOp, died with 30 days post op; DOC, died of operative complications; NSGCT, nonseminomatous germ cell tumor; NGC, non-germ cell cancer.

univariate factors predictive for relapse included tumor burden, immature teratoma with non–germ cell elements, and site (e.g., mediastinum); only immature teratoma with non–germ cell elements and site predicted for survival.[4] Immature teratoma and mature teratoma had similar relapse-free intervals and overall survival intervals.

RESECTION OF EXTENSIVE BULKY TUMOR

Surgery for massive metastatic disease in testis cancer has become reasonable and appropriate in view of the great advances in chemotherapy for advanced disease. Most patients have their bulky disease reduced in volume and downgraded histologically to a more mature teratomatous or even necrotic form. Some tumors persist with malignant element as well. This critical information guides postoperative medical management. Those with persistent malignant tumors require further salvage chemotherapy. Those with only teratomas or necrosis in the specimen can be managed expectantly. Often these retroperitoneal tumors are massive. They must be resected completely, because local or regional recurrence is possible, particularly for the more extensive, bulky tumors.[4] This area represents one of the ultimate surgical challenges. Total tumor extirpation is required, with exceptional demands on vascular isolation and preservation. An aggressive ablative purpose must be combined with thoughtful and delicate dissection.

EN BLOC NEPHRECTOMY WITH RESECTION OF BULKY TUMOR

The renal hilum easily becomes involved with bulky metastatic nonseminomatous germ cell tumor (NSGCT) because the genital ridge originates just medial to the metanephrogenic blastema. In the course of its descent, the testis leaves its own venous and lymphatic drainage near its site of origin. The primary zone of metastatic spread is paraaortic, just below the renal vessels. When confronted with a difficult dissection involving the renal vessels, it may be the more practical choice to do a nephrectomy en bloc with the tumor resection. This is particularly true in secondary cases that have already failed a prior RPLND attempt elsewhere. Such cases represent almost 40% of our referrals; hence, the relatively large number of nephrectomies in our post chemotherapy RPLND series.

An en bloc nephrectomy can save time of dissection in the hilum, provide wider tumor clearance, provide better paraaortic and suprahilar crural exposure, and reduce tumor recurrence locally. Our data (Tables 70-3 and 70-4) indicate that the outcomes for this difficult subset of patients who require en bloc nephrectomy are at least as good or marginally better than the easier patients who do not require nephrectomy. This supports the principle of completeness and the value of appropriate radicality.

TABLE 70-3. *Postchemotherapy surgery for advanced testis cancer*

Nephrectomy: relapse	Fibrosis	Teratoma	Cancer
Unknown	0	2	3
No	25	28	21
Yes (cancer)	2	3	5
Yes (teratoma)	0	8	0
Yes (unknown)	0	1	1
Other	0	1	0
Total nephrectomies	27	43	30

TABLE 70-4. *Postchemotherapy surgery for advanced testis cancer*

Nephrectomy current status	Fibrosis	Teratoma	Cancer
NED	26	35	19
Living with disease	0	1	3
DOD	1	4	6
D. op. complic.	0	2	2
D. 2nd (other) causes	0	1	0
Unknown	0	0	0
Total nephrectomies	27	43	30

NED, no evidence of disease; DOD, dead of disease; *D. Op.,* dead of operative complications; *D. 2nd,* dead of other causes.

EXTENDED SUPRAHILAR AND POSTERIOR MEDIASTINAL DISSECTION

The requirements of retroperitoneal dissection sometimes extend to nodal disease that is paraaortic, retrocrurual, and posterior mediastinal; such is the extension of the lymphatic drainage from the abdomen into the chest. Precrural tissues below the diaphragm consists largely of splenic lymphatics, ganglia, and nerves from the superior mesenteric and celiac axis. Paraaortic tumor below the renal arteries usually spreads into the posterior mediastinum at the level of the renal arteries and through the aortic hiatus in the diaphragm. This situation is created by the right and left crus of the diaphragm, which inserts on the anterior spinous ligaments around the aorta. The diaphragmatic fibers decussate superior to the celiac axis, and the aortic hiatus is created in something of an inverted U shape. The lymphatics course lateral and posterior to the aorta as it passes the diaphragm. Positive nodes in this area are reliably demonstrated by upper abdominal and chest CT scans. We reserve dissection in this area only for patients who have demonstrated tumor after chemotherapy. It is inappropriate and unnecessary to dissect these retrocrural paraaortic nodes in cases of low-stage disease.

The technique of this dissection is based on the volume of disease. Patients with bulky nodal disease require a thoracoabdominal approach. The choice of a right or left approach depends on the distribution of nodes as viewed on the CT scan. The left thoracoabdominal approach through an 8th, 9th, or 10th interspace incision is usually adequate. For extremely large retrocrural or posterior mediastinal disease, we may resort to a thoracotomy several interspaces higher.

Figures 70-4 through 70-6 demonstrate the principles of dissection in this area, which are much the same as the principles of surgery in the abdomen. First, the parietal pleura must be incised with the overlying fibers of the diaphragm as they condense to form the crus. This exposes the lateral aspect of the aorta and the posterolateral nodal tissue, which can sometimes be fairly bulky. The parietal pleural incision is carried cephalad to the pulmonary hilum if necessary.

The "split and roll" technique is used to mobilize the aorta in the chest. We are mindful of the fact that the anterior spinal artery arises from the thoracic aorta cephalad to T8. Nonetheless, we have often divided the intercostals from this level through T12 bilaterally without any untoward effect on spinal cord function. The intercostal vessels must be prospectively identified and secured between ligatures and clips and then divided if the aorta is to be appropriately mobilized and elevated in the mediastinum. It is crucial to approach this posterolaterally. Only in this manner can the aorta be well visualized with its intercostal posterior branches. An anterior sternal splitting incision is a difficult and inappropriate approach to posterior mediastinal dissection, particularly in the inferior portion of the mediastinum. It is better to approach this with a lateral thoracotomy combined with a midline transperitoneal approach.

If each intercostal segment can be secured with clips and ligatures, the aorta can be elevated away from the posterior spinous ligament with Penrose drains, for example. This permits clearance of the posterior mediastinal nodal tissue with attendant preservation of the aorta, esophagus, and contralateral crus, which can be visualized as the nodes are stripped off the anterior spinous ligaments. Occasionally, posterior passage of the vessels through foramina T8 through T12 requires electrocautery or suture ligation for control.

If the dissection is extensive, we make no effort to reconstruct the pleura. We instead close the chest in the traditional manner, with insertion of a chest tube that usually remains in place for several days, depending on the amount of chest drainage.

Several principles apply in the management of these patients postoperatively. Our treatment options are based on the histopathology of the resected tissue. If there are still active malignant elements in the tumor, two courses of salvage chemotherapy are indicated. If only teratoma or necrosis and scar tissue are found, we recommend close follow-up, with interval CT scans of the chest at least semiannually and obtaining more frequent serum marker levels and chest films, usually on a 2-month schedule.

RESECTION OF THE GREAT VESSELS DURING EXTENSIVE RPLND SURGERY

Although it is infrequently necessary, extensive vascular repair or resection is sometimes required in the course of extended postchemotherapy testis tumor dissections. In most cases, the tumor can be dissected from the great vessels with the usual split and roll technique, but the tumor sometimes involves the wall of the great vessel or, in the case of the venous system, invades the vessel as a tumor thrombus.

We reviewed our vascular surgical experience after approximately 500 postchemotherapy RPLNDs.[13] We had to resect the infrarenal vena cava 45 times. In most of these cases, the vena cava was directly involved with tumor thrombus. In the early years, we resected several vena cavas with active tumor thrombus from extensive retroperitoneal tumor before chemotherapy. In later years, this problem was largely eliminated with prior chemotherapy for reducing extensive disease. Occasionally, we still find tumor thrombus in the vena cava in the form of necrotic tumor covered by fibronous thrombus or teratoma. On two occasions, despite salvage chemotherapy for relapsing, advanced disease, active tumor with malignant elements was found as intracaval tumor thrombus.[13]

This procedure should not be undertaken lightly, because there is significant morbidity with caval resection. The morbidity can include immediate venous congestion of the lower extremities and continued extravasation of lymphatic tissue into a third space (i.e., retroperitoneum). In analyzing our postoperative complications, we noticed a greater frequency of abdominal ascites in patients who had caval resection. Abdominal ascites is an added risk factor for any patient who has the vena cava resected.

The technique of caval resection is relatively simple. A vessel is mobilized by dividing the various lumbar tributaries and mobilizing it as completely as possible in the infrarenal area. Usually, there are several major lumbar vessels just below the level of the renal vessels, and these should be secured to obtain 360-degree clearance. Normally, we use the vascular staple clamp for this, but it can also be oversewn with any vascular suture material in a continuous suture while controlled in vascular clamps.

The distal extent of the caval resection should be as limited as possible. It is preferable to leave both iliac veins intact. This is not always possible, however, and on occasion, we have resected the venous structures below the hypogastric venous entry (i.e., external iliac level). This compounds the felony of lower extremity venous stasis and lymphedema, which gradually reverses. The major morbidity is the risk for transient abdominal ascites in these patients, presumably secondary to massive alternate lymphatic drainage along the body wall, with leakage into a large third space created by the dissection. The absence of venous connections for lymphatic drainage is probably the culprit in such cases.

AORTIC REPAIRS

In the same cohort of postchemotherapy RPLND patients, we have had to use interposition aortic or tube grafts or bifurcated aortoiliac grafts in 10 patients. One of these procedures was done on an emergent basis in a patient who ruptured his aorta while in the recovery room after an extended subadventitial dissection hours earlier. Fortunately, he was rescued and had a remarkably smooth postoperative course. The other four procedures were done in a planned manner because of evident aortic involvement with tumor seen during the RPLND procedure. In each of these remaining four cases, it was apparent that the aortic wall was so heavily involved and so damaged by the tumor dissection that it should be replaced. The decision can be made more easily if the dissection is clearly required in the subadventitial plane and the aortic wall is pale, "cheesy," and poorly controlled with suture ligature. In such patients, it is safer to resect the involved segment and replace it with an interposition Dacron tube graft. Five of the 9 patients did very well postoperatively, showing that the need for aortic resection does not preclude a good oncologic outcome. In rare circumstances, it may be necessary to achieve complete local excision and resultant cure.[14]

The technique is essentially the same as that used in aortic aneurysm repair. Care is taken to develop a safe cuff below the renal arteries, which is virtually always possible in testis tumor cases. In none of the 5 patients was a shunt necessary for aortic involvement in the suprarenal area. We commonly use a running 4-0 Prolene suture to anastomose the tube graft, which has been sized and preclotted. The distal limb of the dissection must also be prepared at the time of the interposition graft to minimize the distal ischemic time. A 360 degree, continuous 4-0 Prolene suture is suitable for the distal anastomosis. Care is taken to backflush the graft by removing the distal clamps first and then under low-pressure conditions reviewing the integrity of the graft and the connections. The cephalad clamp is then removed. Any additional hemostasis can be obtained at the suture line. Normally, this is unnecessary, and simple digital occlusion and time is all that is needed for hemostasis. Depending on the time required, heparinization is used and then reversed with protamine. Normally, we use 1 mg/kg of heparin and reverse it with about two thirds of the dose of protamine. In the event of a patch graft or a relatively brief clamping, no heparinization is required.

Based on these experiences, it is prudent to attempt the dissection in the extraadventitial plane whenever possible. This should obviate the need for grafting.

TECHNICAL CONSIDERATIONS AND SURGICAL PRINCIPLES

The technique of postchemotherapy RPLND employs basic vascular surgical principles. Figures 70-1 through 70-3 show the basic strategy of postchemotherapy RPLND for residual bulk disease, the split and roll technique. The tumor should be dissected completely off both great vessels, and tissues within the original retroperitoneal template of nodal drainage should be swept off the posterior body wall and foramina en bloc, if possible. A full bilateral RPLND is indicated in postchemotherapy dissections with few exceptions. Normally, the exposure is the same as described for low-stage disease. in most cases, the root of the small bowel mesentery is incised, the posterior attachments to the cecum and the mesocolon of the right side are divided, and bowel is mobilized up and away from the anterior aspect of Gerota's fascia and placed on the chest in a bowel bag. It is common to need additional exposure in such cases. We usually divide the inferior mesenteric vein between silk ligatures and then mobilize the left colonic mesentery. We also usually divide the inferior mesenteric artery to complete mobilization of the left colonic mesentery and retract this away from the tumor and the retroperitoneal nodes. Most of these patients have their lumbar postganglionic fibers dissected in the preaortic dissection in this area and are not able to ejaculate if they have had complete dissections in the lower periaortic zone. This contrasts with current nerve-sparing techniques for low-stage disease wherein ejaculation is preserved.

A basic strategy is to begin anterior to the great vessels in the iliac or left renal venous area. The longitudinal split is made over the great vessels, sometimes retracting tumor laterally as this is done. It is usually helpful to divide the lumbar vessels to better retract the great vessels off and away from the tumor. If all the lumbar vessels are divided and the vessels are elevated from the tumor, the tumor can be resected from the posterior body wall. The lumbar vessels are controlled at the foramina with clips or suture ligatures. Bovine cautery, using an extender if necessary, is usually helpful in these postchemotherapy dissections.

Suprahilar disease can take two forms. Direct extension from a massive infrahilar tumor may project into the suprahilar zone. In this case, it is usually precrural and can be rolled down and away from the great vessels. Occasionally, it needs to be removed en bloc, with one kidney or the other being inseparable from the renal hilum. Tables 70-4 indicates that en bloc nephrectomy in such difficult cases has favorable outcomes in terms of relapse and survival, equivalent to outcomes in standard lower-volume postchemotherapy RPLND cases. The maxim of ''when in doubt, take it out'' (i.e., do an en bloc nephrectomy with the specimen) seems to apply in difficult postchemotherapy reoperation cases.

The usual path of lymph flow into the chest from the retroperitoneum is periaortic and posterior. CT scans have taught us that most suprahilar positive nodal disease is in the retrocrural zone. As this becomes larger, it is more expedient to do a thoracoabdominal approach (Figs. 70-4 through 70-6). This reflects the essential nature of a posterior mediastinal fixed tumor. For early and low-volume involvement, this part of the dissection can still be done through the anterior approach, even if it requires splitting the crus for a few centimeters. This area can be repaired by direct suture reapproximation of the crura and the posterior ligamentous attachments of the spine. The cysterna chyli is found anywhere from L1 to T10 in the posterior periaortic retrocrural space together with the azygos and hemiazygos venous systems. This can usually be recognized as such. It must be handled with great care, and the suture should be ligated or clipped at its base to avoid leakage and subsequent ascites. About 1% of our advanced cases develop postoperative ascites, which can usually be managed conservatively with hyperalimentation and then oral feedings with a medium- and short-chain triglyceride diet. Surgical intervention with peritoneal venous shunting, for example, is a rarely needed alternative to conservative management.

SUMMARY

Management of retroperitoneal recurrent tumor remains a great challenge. Accurate radiographic and clinical restaging and careful consultation with the prior treating physicians can provide valuable insights into the history of each patient's disease. This helps with the choice of incision and exposure requirements. The surgeon must be prepared for all contingencies in the abdomen and chest, including vascular resections. Our experience suggests more than 80% of patients can be rendered free of disease (see Table 70-3).

REFERENCES

1. Einhorn LH, Donohue JP. *Cis*-Diammine-dichloroplatinum, vinblastine and bleomycin combination chemotherapy in disseminated testicular cancer. Ann Intern Med 1977;87:293.
2. Donohue JP, Rowland RG. The role of surgery in advanced testicular cancer. Cancer 1984;54:2716.
3. Donohue JP, Rowland RG, Kopecky K, et al. Correlation of computerized tomographic changes and histologic findings in 80 patients having radical retroperitoneal lymph node dissection after chemotherapy for testis cancer. J Urol 1987;137:1176.
4. Loehrer PJ, Williams SD, Clark SA, et al. Teratoma following chemo-

therapy for nonseminomatous germ cell tumor (NSGCT): a clinicopathologic correlation. J Urol 1986;135:1183.

5. Donohue JP, Einhorn LH, Williams SD. Cytoreductive surgery for metastatic testis cancer: considerations of timing and extent. J Urol 1980;123:876.
6. Donohue JP. Surgical management of testis cancer. In: Einhorn LH, ed. Testicular tumors: management and treatment. New York: Masson Publishing, 1980:29.
7. Donohue JP, Rowland RG, Bihrle R. Transabdominal retroperitoneal lymph node dissection. In: Diagnosis and management of genitourinary cancer. Philadelphia: WB Saunders, 1988:802.
8. Donohue JP, Roth LM, Zachary JM et al. Cytoreductive surgery for metastatic testis cancer: tissue analysis of retroperitoneal masses after chemotherapy. J Urol 1982;127:1111.
9. Griest A, Williams SD, Einhorn LH, Donohue JP, Rowland RG, Estes N. Pathologic findings at orchiectomy following chemotherapy for disseminated testicular cancer. Proc Am Soc Clin Oncol, 1983;2:139.
10. Donohue JP, Rowland RG. Complications of retroperitoneal lymph node dissection. J Urol 1981;125:338.
11. Skinner GD, Melamed A, Lieskovsky G. Complications of thoracoabdominal retroperitoneal lymph node dissection. J Urol 1982;127:1107.
12. Toner G, Manicek DM, Heelan RT, et al. Adjunctive surgery after chemotherapy for nonseminomatous germ cell tumors: recommendations for patient selections. J Clin Oncol 1990;1:8.
13. Donohue JP, Thornhill JA, Foster RS, et al: Resection of the inferior vena cava during RPLND for metastatic germ cell cancer: indications and results. J Urol 1991;146:346.
14. Donohue JP, Thornhill JA, Foster RS, Birhle R. Vascular considerations in postchemotherapy retroperitoneal lymph node dissection: part I, vena cava; part II, aorta. World J Urol 1994;12:182.

Principles and Practice of Genitourinary Oncology, edited by Derek Raghavan, Howard I. Scher, Steven A. Leibel, and Paul H. Lange. Lippincott-Raven Publishers, Philadelphia, © 1997.

CHAPTER 71

Side Effects of Treatment

Michael J. Boyer and Bruce J. Roth

The advances in the management of testicular cancer described in the preceding chapters have resulted in long-term survival for the majority of men who develop this disease. In parallel with these advances has been a growing awareness of the adverse effects of treatment. Although the acute toxicities of treatment for testicular cancer have been recognized for some time, the type and incidence of long-term or late side effects have only been systematically investigated recently. In particular, attention has been turned to those side effects that either are long-lasting, such as persistent hearing impairment after cisplatin-based chemotherapy, or first appear after the conclusion of treatment, such as second cancers or leukemia. What constitutes a "late" or "chronic" side effect of treatment is not clearly defined. The majority of studies have considered adverse effects that persist beyond 12 months or that first appear more than 12 months after the conclusion of treatment. This chapter reviews both the early and late side effects of chemotherapy for testicular cancer, as well as examining efforts made to reduce the toxicity of therapy. The side effects of radiotherapy are reviewed in Chapter 65.

TOXICITY OF CHEMOTHERAPY FOR GERM CELL TUMORS

The management of metastatic testicular cancer was revolutionized by the introduction of effective, cisplatin-based chemotherapy. Previously, metastatic testicular cancer was treated with minimally effective drug combinations that were associated with modest toxicity.[1,2] The incorporation, in the 1970s, of cisplatinum into combination regimens resulted not only in high cure rates, but also in novel patterns of acute and chronic toxicity. Because most patients with metastatic testicular cancer are now cured of their malignant disease, a major focus of recent clinical trials has been the reduction of toxicity.

The acute toxicity of treatment with combination chemotherapy regimens for metastatic testicular cancer has been well documented. The pattern of short-term side effects is a reflection of the toxicities of each of the drugs that comprise the combinations, and therefore, it varies based on the drugs and doses used. More recently, studies focusing on the long-term toxicities of chemotherapy have been completed and published. This section reviews both early and delayed side effects of chemotherapy.

Gastrointestinal Toxicity

The major short-term gastrointestinal toxic effects of chemotherapy for testicular cancer have been nausea and vomiting, diarrhea, paralytic ileus or constipation, and mucositis. Cisplatin and vinblastine, as used in the cisplatin, vinblastine, bleomycin (PVB) regimen,[3,4] have accounted for much of this toxicity, with a contribution also from methotrexate, actinomycin D, and ifosfamide in men receiving salvage therapy or treatment for poor-prognosis disease.[5] More recent developments, including the use of effective antiemetics such as ondansetron,[6,7] the replacement of vinblastine by etoposide,[8] and the use of the two-drug combination of etoposide and cisplatin (EP),[9] have reduced the degree of gastrointestinal toxicity in many patients. Thus, abdominal cramps, which occurred in 20% of patients treated with PVB, now occur in only 5% of men receiving bleomycin, etoposide, and cisplatin (BEP),[8] whereas the volume of emesis in patients treated with EP is reduced in comparison with that occurring with the older VAB-VI regimen.[9]

Nephrotoxicity

Cisplatin is a nephrotoxin, producing renal damage that may be associated with several patterns of histologic change. These patterns include acute focal necrosis of the distal convoluted tubules and collecting ducts, dilatation of convoluted tubules, and the formation of casts.[10] Less commonly, changes may occur in the proximal tubules. The alterations in renal function associated with these histologic abnormalities have been studied extensively.[11] In early-phase studies, before the routine use of forced diuresis, significant nephrotoxicity occurred in up to 36% of patients.[11] The incidence of renal complications of cisplatin has been reduced dramatically by modern schedules of administration, which incorporate forced diuresis,[8,12] and significant renal impairment occurs in fewer than 10% of patients.[12] Furthermore, the duration of administration of cisplatin (1-day versus 5-day schedules) has little influence on the frequency or severity of renal dysfunction.[9,13]

Although cisplatin is responsible for most of the nephrotoxicity observed during the treatment of testicular cancer, other drugs, may also contribute to this problem. In particular, methotrexate (as used in the POMBACE regimen for tumors with a poor prognosis),[14] may exacerbate the renal damage caused by cisplatin. Furthermore, the use of aminoglycoside antibiotics, for example, in the management of febrile neutropenia, may also contribute to renal impairment. Care should be taken when these agents and other nephrotoxins are administered to patients treated with cisplatin.

The acute nephrotoxicity that results from combination chemotherapy for germ cell tumors may lead to long-term changes in renal function. Various methods have been used to assess renal function after treatment with cisplatin-based chemotherapy, and results of these studies are summarized in Table 71-1. These studies have demonstrated consistently a decrease in renal function that persists more than 12 months after the conclusion of therapy; this finding suggests that some of the changes induced by cisplatin-based chemotherapy are irreversible. A few investigators have reported reversal of the changes induced by chemotherapy, but these findings have been observed in a small number of patients only.[15–17] In some studies, the severity of persistent renal impairment has correlated with the dose of cisplatin administered.[18–20] Because the dose of cisplatin administered to patients in many of these studies was the same, a dose-response relationship may have been difficult to demonstrate even if it did exist. The greatest deterioration in renal function was noted in patients treated with a combination of chemotherapy and abdominal radiotherapy.

In contrast to the changes described for glomerular function, persistent changes in renal tubular function occur less commonly. Although such changes, most commonly identified by magnesium wasting, have been reported after chemotherapy for testicular cancer,[21–23] tubular function appears to be normal in the majority of patients.

Despite the demonstration of long-term changes in renal function after the use of cisplatin-based chemotherapy for testicular cancer, overt renal failure has not been reported as a problem in series of patients with long-term follow-up.[19,21,24,25] The majority of patients who have been treated for this disease are still young, however, and whether clinically apparent renal disease will become evident remains to be seen as this population of men ages.

Vascular Toxicity

Small-vessel vascular toxicity after chemotherapy for testicular cancer is common and is manifest clinically as Raynaud's phenomenon. Although case reports of this side effect have implicated single-agent bleomycin therapy,[26] small-vessel vascular toxicity has most commonly been associated with the combination of vinblastine and bleomycin.[27–30] Vogelzang and associates reported a 21% incidence of digital ischemia with vinblastine and bleomycin alone and a 41% incidence if these agents were combined with cisplatin.[31] This symptom can persist long after the completion of treatment, and in the Indiana University series with a median follow-up of 8.5 years, 49% of patients reported some symptoms of digital cold hypersensitivity, although most patients graded this effect as mild. This finding is in keeping with most other series, which report persisting Raynaud's phenomenon in 23% to 45% of men.[21,24,31–38] Most attempts to treat this condition with vasodilators have been unsuccessful, although some investigators have successfully used calcium-channel blockers.[39] As etoposide has replaced vinblastine as part of combination chemotherapy, the incidence of Raynaud's phenomenon has not diminished,[8] al-

TABLE 71-1. *Long term follow-up of renal function after cisplatin based chemotherapy (many of the patients in these series also underwent retroperitoneal lymphadenectomy)*

Investigators	No. of patients	Follow-up (mo)	Median cisplatin dose	Measure of renal function	Result
Fjeldborg et al, 1986[132]	22	16–52	452 mg/m^2	a	12.5% fall in GFR
Daugaard et al, 1988[20]	30	?	1200 mg	a	30% fall in GFR
Hansen et al, 1988[16]	34	43–97	583 mg/m^2	a	8–15% fall in GFR
Hamilton et al, 1989[15]	22	8–59	400 mg/m^2	a	19% fall in GFR
Macleod et al, 1988[17]	17	6–60	720 mg	a	28% fall in GFR
Groth et al, 1986[133]	25	12	600 mg/m^2	b	29% fall in GFR
Stoter et al, 1989[33]	57	84–120	400 mg/m^2	c	Increase in creatinine clearance in 21%
Stuart et al, 1990[55]	24	7–63	350 mg/m^2	c	Elevated creatinine clearance in 12.5%
Moul et al, 1989[18]	114	1–24 y	?	c	Elevated creatinine clearance in 8%
Aass et al, 1990[19]	43	36–60	36 Gy	d	8% fall in ERPF
	57	36–60	743* mg	d	8% fall in ERPF
	15	36–60	1280* mg	d	35% fall in ERPF
	15	36–60	775 mg +40 Gy	d	20% fall in ERPF
Bissett et al, 1990[24]	74	13–125	400 mg/m^2	e	23% fall in creatinine clearance
Boyer et al, 1990[21]	30	48–126	400 mg/m^2	e	Below normal in 43%
Osanto et al, 1992[25]	36	18–112	483 mg/m^2	e	20% fall in creatinine clearance

* Some patients received maintenance chemotherapy with cisplatin.

a, ^{51}Cr-EDTA clearance; *b*, ^{99m}Tc-DTPA clearance; *c*, serum creatinine; *d*, ^{131}I hippuran clearance; *e*, creatinine clearance.

Boyer MJ, Raghavan D. Long-term morbidity of testicular cancer treatment. Prob Urol 1994;8:154.

TABLE 71-2. *Major vascular events after treatment with cisplatin-based chemotherapy (total number of patients excludes those who died of nonvascular causes)*

Author	No. of patients	No. of events	Time after chemotherapy	Ages (y)	Type of event	Other risk factors	Deaths
Bissett et al, 1990[24]	74	4	?	?	IHD, 2 with previous MI	Yes, in 4	—
Doll et al, 1986[45]	23	4	7 d–18 mo	21–27	2 MI, 2 CVA	Yes, in 1	—
Stoter et al, 1989[33]	59	3	16–62 mo	45–58	2 MI, 1 PVD	Yes, in 1	2
Samuels et al, 1987[46]	65	5	6 d–46 mo	23–58	3 MI, 1 CVA, 1 rectal infarct	Yes, in 1	5
Boyer et al, 1990[21]	30	1	58 mo	63	IHD	Yes	—
Roth et al, 1988[36]	229	6	36–69 mo	27–55	4 MI, 2 IHD	Yes, in 5	3
Gietema et al, 1992[38]	57	1	75 mo	39	MI	Yes*	—

IHD, ischemic heart disease; *MI,* myocardial infarction; *CVA,* cerebrovascular accident; *PVD,* peripheral vascular disease.

Boyer MJ, Raghavan D. Long-term morbidity of testicular cancer treatment. Prob Urol 1994;8:154.

though it has not been reported in the early follow-up of patients treated with cisplatin and etoposide alone.[9]

Although a recognized association exists between cisplatin-based chemotherapy for testicular cancer and small-vessel disease, that combination chemotherapy places the patient at risk for the development of major vascular events is less clear. Acute cardiac ischemia has been reported after the administration of vinblastine alone,[40] vinblastine and bleomycin,[41] vinblastine and cisplatin,[42] and the PVB combination,[21,24,33,43–46] as have cerebral ischemic events[45,46] (see Table 71-2). To implicate chemotherapy definitively as the cause of these events is difficult because comorbid factors may be involved, including tobacco use, mediastinal radiotherapy, and family history. Similarly, as patients are followed for increasing periods after treatment, the underlying frequency of cardiovascular disease in that age range will also increase. An interesting observation has been the increase in serum cholesterol levels after combination chemotherapy,[21,38,47] a change that may, in the long term, affect the cardiovascular risk of treated patients. Because of difficulty in analyzing the anecdotal reports listed, an analysis was undertaken of a large randomized trial in pathologic stage II nonseminomatous disease in which patients received postoperative adjuvant chemotherapy or were observed and treated with chemotherapy at the time of relapse.[48] With a median follow-up of over 5 years, no evidence was found of an increased risk of acute cardiovascular complications in the patients receiving chemotherapy. These findings are important given the increasing use of combination chemotherapy in earlier-stage disease.

Neurotoxicity

Neural toxicity after chemotherapy for germ cell tumors may take the form of a chronic, predominantly sensory peripheral neuropathy, autonomic neuropathy, or auditory damage. Although cisplatin may produce each of these problems, the use of combinations that contain other neurotoxic agents, such as the vinca alkaloids, makes the occurrence of problems, particularly neuropathies, more likely.[4,12,49,50] Consequently, these toxicities are becoming less common as the use of vinca alkaloids in the first-line management of testicular cancer has decreased.

Paresthesia, a common symptom during treatment, occurs in up to 80% of patients. After the conclusion of therapy, however, it disappears in the majority of patients, and the reported incidence of persisting paresthesia ranges from 7% to 51%.[18,21,24,32,36,38,51,52] By contrast, asymptomatic damage to the peripheral nerves has been detected by neurophysiologic testing in 50% to 76% of patients.[21,51] In patients treated more recently with regimens containing etoposide in place of vinblastine,[8] or carboplatin in place of cisplatin,[53] peripheral neuropathy is less common, although long-term follow-up data for these patients are lacking.

Although not the subject of intensive study, impairment of autonomic function has been recognized after cisplatin-based chemotherapy for testicular cancer.[34,54] Orthostatic hypotension may occur in the early posttreatment phase, but it rarely constitutes a long-term problem.[34] When autonomic function was studied specifically, abnormalities in parasympathetic function were detected in 2 of 26 men, with borderline abnormalities in a further 8 patients.[54] Sympathetic function was normal in all these men.

Impairment of auditory function is the most common persistent toxicity after cisplatin-containing chemotherapy for germ cell tumors. The basis for this damage is believed to be cisplatin-induced death of hair cells in the organ of Corti. The major clinical manifestation of this damage is tinnitus, which persists in 11% to 33% of men.[21,32,33] Clinically significant subjective hearing loss is less frequent, although difficulty in hearing against a noisy background is a common complaint. In contrast to the clinical manifestations, audiometric abnormalities are common. The typical audiometric change is bilateral sensorineural hearing loss, occurring at 4 to 8 kHz. This pattern has been detected in 28% to 75% of patients in large series.[21,24,25,55] Only a weak correlation between the dose of cisplatin administered and the severity of hearing loss has been demonstrated in men with testicular cancer, although such a relationship exists in patients receiving cisplatin for other malignant diseases.[56] Furthermore, the schedule of cisplatin administration may be important in determining the degree of auditory toxicity.[13] Single-day administration schedules are associated with higher peak plasma levels, and this may result in greater ototoxicity than a 5-day schedule.

Myelosuppression

Myelosuppression affecting all blood elements occurs after treatment with chemotherapy for testicular cancer. As with other acute toxicities, the pattern of changes reflects the choice of drug and the dose used. Thus, although cisplatin causes a mild, progressive anemia, carboplatin, vinblastine, and etoposide all cause neutropenia and thrombocytopenia. The commonly used combination chemotherapy regimens cause World Health Organization (WHO) grade 3 or 4 neutropenia in 40% to 50% of patients and grade 3 to 4 thrombocytopenia in 15%,[8,57] although the EP combination produces slightly less myelosuppression.[9] Despite this high incidence of bone marrow suppression, with modern management, including the use of granulocyte-colony-stimulating factor, toxic deaths from febrile neutropenia should occur only rarely. Persistent myelosuppression after the conclusion of therapy has not been a significant problem.

Pulmonary Toxicity

Pneumonitis, most commonly induced by the antitumor antibiotic bleomycin, is the principal respiratory side effect of chemotherapy for testicular cancer.[58,59] This disorder may be exacerbated by cigarette smoking or prior pulmonary irradiation. In a small proportion of patients, pneumonitis progresses to irreversible pulmonary fibrosis. In modern practice, deaths from bleomycin pulmonary toxicity are rare, but they may still occur. To minimize this event, monitoring of the diffusing capacity for carbon monoxide (DLCO) is usually performed; controversy remains, however, over whether other tests or even clinical signs are more appropriate indicators.[59,60]

The occurrence of pulmonary fibrosis after treatment with bleomycin is dose related, with a higher incidence with doses above 400 mg. Despite this finding, toxicity has been noted at lower doses.[58] Pulmonary symptoms are uncommon after the conclusion of chemotherapy for testicular cancer; such symptoms occur in fewer than 20% of patients, and persistent reductions in the level of DLCO beyond 12 months seem to be confined to smokers.[21,61,62]

Second Malignant Diseases

Pooled data from cancer registries suggest that survivors of testis cancer are at as much as a 30% increased risk of developing a second malignant disease, compared with the general population;[63] this risk may be related to the testicular cancer itself, or it may be related to therapy. The most common second cancer in these patients is a contralateral testicular tumor. This tumor is not considered to be a consequence of treatment, and chemotherapy administered for an initial primary lesion may actually have some protective effect on the development of a contralateral primary tumor.[64] Similarly, the appearance of hematologic malignant diseases in patients with primary mediastinal nonseminomatous germ cell tumors appears to be part of a larger syndrome, and it is not related to therapy.[65,66]

Most of the remainder of observed second cancers in these patients are probably attributable to therapy. Evidence is sufficient from the treatment of other malignant diseases that curative therapy for a first malignant tumor may be the initiating event for a second, unrelated tumor.[67–69] An increased risk of therapy-related second malignant diseases in patients with testicular cancer has been associated both with radiotherapy and combination chemotherapy.

The leukemogenic capabilities of chemotherapy, particularly with alkylating agents, have been demonstrated in solid tumors, and a summary of anecdotal reports of patients with germ cell tumor in the era before the availability of etoposide revealed that the majority of patients had prolonged exposure to alkylating agents, simultaneous radiotherapy, or nonseminomatous tumors of mediastinal origin, all confounding factors in the development of subsequent leukemia.[70] Reports of acute nonlymphocytic leukemia after therapy with standard doses of PVB have been anecdotal.[71] In a review of over 650 patients with testicular cancer at Indiana University who were treated with PVB, no cases of leukemia were reported.[65]

Increasing evidence suggests the leukemogenic potential of topoisomerase II inhibitors, specifically etoposide and teniposide. Etoposide-induced leukemia has been recognized in patients treated for childhood acute lymphoblastic leukemia,[72,73] as well as for both small and non–small cell lung cancer.[74–76] The following characteristics distinguish these leukemias from those caused by alkylating agents: a shorter interval from treatment to appearance of the disease, with a mean of 33 months for etoposide-induced leukemia versus 58 to 73 months for alkylating agents; a predominance of monocytic phenotypes; and specific cytogenetic abnormalities, most commonly balanced translocations involving 11q23 or 21q22.[77–79] These phenoptypic and genotypic characteristics have also been seen with other agents known to target topoisomerase II, including 4-epidoxorubicin.[80]

Etoposide has replaced vinblastine in combination chemotherapy for germ cell tumors because of decreased neurotoxicity and increased efficacy, paricularly in the group of patients with "poor-risk" disease.[8] As expected, case reports exist of patients with germ cell tumors who were treated with etoposide and who subsequently developed leukemia.[77,81] In retrospective reviews of large series of patients with germ cell tumors who were treated with etoposide, a small but fixed rate of leukemias was detected: in Denmark, 4 of 212 patients;[82] at Memorial Hospital, New York City, 2 of 340 patients;[83] and at Indiana University, 2 of 348 patients.[84] Although the specific risk factors in an individual patient are unclear, one study has suggested that the total dose of etoposide is not related to the subsequent development of leukemia, but that schedules with more frequent administration (weekly or twice weekly) are much more likely to result in this complication.[73] The implications of this observation for schedules that involve dosing daily for 5 days, or long-term oral administration (21 of each 28 days), are unclear. This rare complication of therapy (0.5% to 4%) is easily outweighed by the benefits of etoposide in advanced disease. These factors need to be considered when selecting chemotherapy in patients with low-volume disease, however, in whom an alternative form of therapy, such as observation or retroperitoneal lymph node dissection (RPLND), produces an equivalent cure rate.

PSYCHOSOCIAL SEQUELAE OF TESTICULAR CANCER AND ITS TREATMENT

Because most patients with testicular cancer are treated with curative therapy and can expect to survive without recurrence for another 40 to 60 years, evaluating the immediate and long-term psychosocial impact of such therapy on the patient and his family is appropriate. The literature on the posttreatment psychological and social adjustment of these patients is confusing, and in many cases it is contradictory. This confusion arises from several causes, including the following: the use of small, retrospective, anecodotal series versus propspective analysis; the use of unvalidated in-house questionnaires versus standardized measurement tools; significant variations in the time since completion of therapy; the inconsistent use of proper control groups; and the evaluation of patients treated with outmoded, toxic forms of therapy. In general, data have been generated in three specific areas: (1) general psychological dysfunction; (2) sexual dysfunction and psychological impact of decreased fertility; and (3) social functioning as it relates to employment and to spousal and other interpersonal relationships.

Psychological Dysfunction

Several studies have suggested that the psychological consequences of therapy for testicular cancer in the first 6 months include anxiety and depression in 6% to 20% of patients, and the type and severity of symptoms are related to the modality of treatment.[85,86] The consensus is that most patients who have completed therapy by at least a year have adjusted well to their situation.[85,87–90] A small proportion (10% to 30%), however, continues to suffer moderate to severe feelings of nervousness, anxiety, and depression,[85,87] although the rates vary significantly based on the instrument used. Patients who have sexual difficulties,[90,91] who are unemployed,[92] or who have financial problems[92] appear to be at a higher risk of developing significant psychological morbidity in the posttreatment period. In contrast, these same studies demonstrated no influence of age, marital status, time since diagnosis, infertility, or previous history of psychiatric disorder on the level of psychological distress. When compared with patients with other malignant diseases, specifically Hodgkin's disease, patients with testis cancer reported more focused symptoms, such as a decrease in sexual enjoyment and poor health habits.[93] In a similar comparison with cardiac patients, however, cured cancer patients (32% testicular cancer, 50% Hodgkin's disease) were found to have subjective well-being similar to age-matched neighborhood controls.[94] Most of the patients who have reported psychological distress after therapy have cited either sexual dysfunction or alterations in social relationships as the major areas of difficulty.

Sexual Dysfunction

Apart from the fertility issues related to both the disease and its therapy, which are discussed elsewhere in this chapter, investigators have found significantly disparate rates of sexual dysfunction in patients after therapy. Although several investigators note no impairment in sexual function,[85,92,95] others report more dysfunction in these patients than in either controls or the patient's pretherapy status,[90,91] with estimates that 10% to 50% of patients are affected. In married couples, the patient considers the problem more severe than his spouse does.[95] The modality of therapy chosen has a major impact on the level of dysfunction; patients who have undergone a classic bilateral RPLND with its attendant, almost universal incidence of retrograde ejaculation[96] report the highest rate of dysfunction. Increasing use of modified template or nerve-sparing procedures, and increasing use of surveillance in patients with clinical stage I nonseminomatous disease, should reduce the incidence of this complication, however.

Interpersonal Relationships

Divorce rates among treated patients appear to be no higher than in the general population.[90,92] The proportion of couples who report some strain in the relationship due to cancer varies, but when present, such strain is usually related to a perception of sexual dysfunction. These patients are able to maintain their current level of employment or to continue with plans for further education.[36,90,92] Finally, some patients have been reluctant to reveal their diagnosis to employers, for fear of discrimination in general or job loss in particular. This perception may be reinforced by the patient who is told by a physician that he is cured of his testicular cancer but is denied health or life insurance. Increasing attention needs to be given to such issues in long-term survivors of testicular cancer, and physicians providing follow-up care need to be willing to prompt discussions of these topics with patients and their families on an ongoing basis.

FERTILITY

Before discussing the effects of different modalities of therapy on the fertility of patients with testis cancer, the clinician must realize that a significant percentage of these patients have reduced fertility at diagnosis, before the institution of any therapy. Many studies have now demonstrated both endocrine and exocrine gonadal dysfunction, and 40% to 80% of these patients have oligospermia or azoospermia at diagnosis,[97–104] with apparently more severe oligospermia in patients with a history of cryptorchidism or those with pure seminoma histologically.[98] Although the exact origin of this hypofertile state is unclear, several potential hypotheses have emerged. One possibility is that this condition represents an autoimmune phenomenon because of the following: (1) antisperm antibodies can be identified in the sera of over 70% of patients before orchiectomy; (2) the titer of these antibodies decreases with therapy directed against the malignant disease; and (3) the incidence of antibody positivity increases with increasing stage of the tumor.[105] Other investigators have suggested a paracrine-endocrine model in which tumor-secreted human chorionic gonadotropin stimulates production of estradiol by normal testicular tissue, with resulting impairment of spermatogenesis.[106]

Each specific modality of treatment for testicular cancer (surgery, radiotherapy, and chemotherapy) can exacerbate the impaired fertility of the patient. The psychological impact of potential sterility in a young man with a normal life expectancy can be significant,[107] and it should be taken into consideration when choosing among equally curative treatment options. For years, the standard approach in patients with clinical stage A or low-volume clinical stage B nonseminomatous disease involved RPLND. Until the mid-1980s, full, bilateral RPLND was routinely performed, which compromised postganglionic sympathetic efferents, resulting in retrograde ejaculation and subsequent infertility in more than 90% of patients. Because of the predictable pattern of nodal involvement based on the location of the primary testicular primary,[108] attempts to limit the template of dissection were undertaken,[109] although as many as 25% to 30% of patients still suffered retrograde ejaculation as a result. The development of nerve-sparing RPLND, however, has preserved antegrade ejaculation in 99% of patients,[110,111] although such techniques may not be appropriate in patients undergoing postchemotherapy resection of residual disease. Moreover, increasing use of surveillance alone (in place of staging RPLND in patients with clinical stage A nonseminomatous disease) will further reduce the incidence of infertility attributable to surgical intervention.[112,113]

Other studies have analyzed the effects of nonsurgical intervention, specifically radiotherapy and combination chemotherapy. The administration of low-dose abdominal radiotherapy for early-stage seminoma impairs spermatogenesis, and this condition is most severe in patients with pretreatment oligospermia.[114] The effects of combination chemotherapy can be categorized as those that alter the endocrine function of the testis or those that impair spermatogenesis directly, reflecting chemotherapy-induced damage both to Leydig cells and to germinal epithelium.

The most frequent endocrine dysfunction after chemotherapy is an elevation of serum gonadotropins. Both luteinizing hormone and follicle-stimulating hormone are elevated for at least 2 years after completion of chemotherapy,[104,115–118] and treated patients have more significant rises in these two hormones after stimulation with gonadotropin-releasing hormone than untreated controls.[115] The elevation of follicle-stimulating hormone is less significant in younger patients,[115] as well as in patients who completed therapy at least 18 to 24 months previously.[115,117] The incidence of azoospermia appears to be higher in patients with more significant elevations of follicle-stimulating hormone,[104] presumably because of effects on the hormonal microenvironment in the testicle. The specific agents used in combination chemotherapy may also determine the degree of endocrine dysfunction, with etoposide-containing regimens having a greater effect on the level of follicle-stimulating hormone.[119] Testosterone and adrenal androgen levels are unaffected by chemotherapy,[116,118] although dihydrotestosterone levels are elevated acutely during treatment, presumably because of a cisplatin-induced increase in hepatic androgen 5-α-reductase activity.[116] The long-term persistence of abnormalities may be more closely related to a patient's age and pretherapeutic gonadal function than to the therapy itself.[118]

The short-term impairment of spermatogenesis by combination chemotherapy is profound, but unlike in Hodgkin's disease, many patients have a return to spermatogenesis within 1 to 3 years after completion of therapy. The reported incidence of persistent azoospermia more than 2 years after therapy has ranged from 0% to 40%,[97,104,120,121] and a history of radiotherapy, age older than 30 years, or therapy lasting longer than 6 months all appear to increase the likelihood of remaining azoospermic.[122] Similarly, the incidence of oligospermia or azoospermia may be increased in patients treated with etoposide-containing regimens.[123] Almost 50% of patients followed-up for 2 to 5 years after chemotherapy have total sperm counts return to their pretherapeutic levels[97,121] Children fathered by men who received short-course, intensive chemotherapy do not have an increased frequency of congenital malformations.[36,124]

REDUCING THE TOXICITY OF THERAPY FOR TESTICULAR CANCER

The improved prospects for the cure of patients with germ cell tumors of the testicle have resulted in attempts to reduce the toxicity of treatment. Several strategies have been used, including the introduction of the policy of active surveillance for men with stage I nonseminomatous germ cell tumors, a reduction in the intensity of treatment, and efforts to protect normal tissues.

Surveillance for Stage I Disease

The policy of active surveillance, in which patients with stage I nonseminomatous germ cell tumors are followed-up meticulously without undergoing radiotherapy or retroperitoneal lymphadenectomy, was introduced in an effort to avoid treatment that may be unnecessary in some patients. The details of this approach to treatment are beyond the scope of this chapter and are discussed elsewhere in this volume (Chaps. 65 and 67). Provided a well-structured follow-up schedule is maintained, surveillance appears to be safe and effective in reducing the number of patients exposed to potentially toxic therapy,[125] although some patients who may not otherwise have received chemotherapy do so. Little information is available, however, regarding the possible late hazards of frequent radiologic imaging in young males, and this issue will require further study.

Reduction of the Intensity of Treatment

In an effort to reduce toxicity, regimens for the treatment of testis cancer have been modified. These modifications have included a reduction in the number of cycles of chemotherapy administered,[126] the substitution of etoposide for vinblastine,[8] and the omission of bleomycin.[9,127] Although early results suggested that these approaches resulted in less acute toxicity, data from long-term follow-up of patients treated with these regimens suggest that the omission of bleomycin is associated with an increased risk of death from cancer.[127] Although efforts to devise less toxic regimens are appropriate, these newer regimens must produce the same high cure rate as the regimens they replace.

Protection of Normal Tissues

Several approaches to protect normal tissues against the toxic effects of chemotherapy are being evaluated. For example, Ozols and colleagues suggested that the administration of cisplatin with hypertonic saline protects against nephrotoxicity, although this study did not make clear whether the altered hydration schedule was the major contributor to this effect.[128] The use of hematopoietic growth factors, with a view to protection of the bone marrow against the effects of chemotherapy, has become common practice.[129] Whether the colony-stimulating factors will stimulate tumor growth or will reduce the efficacy of cytotoxic treatment remains the subject of intensive scrutiny, because the growth of epithelial tissues may be influenced by these agents.[130]

A fundamental principle in the attempts to reduce the adverse effects of treatment is that the reduction in toxicity must not be at the expense of the efficacy of therapy. Appropriate evaluation of new reduced-toxicity treatment programs must be carried out before their acceptance into general use. Thus, although the omission of bleomycin from regimens for patients with a good prognosis disease reduces pulmonary toxicity, such a strategy is associated with a higher rate of cancer-related deaths.[127,131] A failure to assess rigorously the impact of strategies designed to reduce toxicity on the effectiveness of anticancer therapy could result in unnecessary deaths, clearly an unacceptable situation in this highly curable cancer.*

REFERENCES

1. Li MC, Whitmore WF, Golbey R. Effects of combined drug therapy on metastatic cancer of the testis. JAMA 1960;174:1271.
2. MacKenzie AR. Chemotherapy of metastatic testis cancer: reslts on 154 patients. Cancer 1966;19:1369.
3. Einhorn LH. Testicular cancer as a model for a curable neoplasm: the Richard and Hinda Rosenthal Foundation Award Lecture. Cancer Res 1981;41:3274.
4. Peckham MJ, Barrett A, McElwain TJ, Hendry WF, Raghavan D. Non-seminoma germ cell tumours (malignant teratoma) of the testis: results of treatment and an analysis of prognostic factors. Br J Urol 1981;53:162.
5. Levine E, Raghavan D. Treatment of refractory testis cancer: salvage or savage chemotherapy? Eur J Cancer 1991;27:932.
6. Marty M, Pouillart P, Scholl S, et al. Comparison of the 5-hydroxytryptamine 3 (serotonin) antagonist ondansetron (GR 38032F) with high dose metoclopramide in the control of cisplatin-induced emesis. N Engl J Med 1990;322:816.
7. Einhorn LH, Nagy C, Werner K, Finn AL. Ondansetron: a new antiemetic for patients receiving cisplatin chemotherapy. J Clin Oncol 1990;8:731.
8. Williams SD, Birch R, Einhorn LH, Irwin L, Greco FA, Loehrer PJ. Treatment of disseminated germ-cell tumors with cisplatin, bleomycin, and either vinblastine or etoposide. N Engl J Med 1987;316:1435.
9. Bosl GJ, Geller NL, Bajorin D, et al. A randomized trial of etoposide + cisplatin versus vinblastine + bleomycin + cisplatin + cyclophosphamide + dactinomycin in patients with good-prognosis germ cell tumors. J Clin Oncol 1988;6:1231.
10. Gonzales-Vitale JC, Hayes DM, Cvitkovic E, Steinberg SS. The renal pathology in clinical trials of cis-platinum (II) diamminedichloride. Cancer 1977;39:1362.
11. Prestayko AW, D'Aoust JC, Issell BF. Cisplatin (cis-diamminedichloroplatinum II). Cancer Treat Rev 1979;6:17.
12. Levi JA, Thomson D, Sandeman T, et al. A prospective study of cisplatin-based combination chemotherapy in advanced germ cell malignancy: role of maintenance and long-term follow-up. J Clin Oncol 1988;6:1154.
13. Williams SD, Stablein DM, Einhorn LH, et al. Immediate adjuvant chemotherapy versus observation with treatment at relapse in pathological stage II testicular cancer. N Engl J Med 1987;317:1433.
14. Newlands ES, Bagshawe KD, Begent RHJ, Rustin GJS, Crawford SM, Holden L. Current optimum management of anaplastic germ cell tumours of the testis and other sites. Br J Urol 1996;58:307.
15. Hamilton CR, Bliss JM, Horwich A. The late effects of cis-platinum on renal function. Eur J Cancer Clin Oncol 1989;25:185.
16. Hansen SW, Groth S, Daugaard G, Rossing N, Rorth M. Long-term effects on renal function and blood pressure of treatment with cisplatin, vinblastine, and bleomycin in patients with germ cell cancer. J Clin Oncol 1988;6:1728.
17. MacLeod PM, Tyrell CJ, Keeling DH. The effect of cisplatin on renal function in patients with testicular turnouts. Clin Radiol 1988;39:190.
18. Moul JW, Robertson JE, George SL, Paulson DF, Walther PJ. Complications of therapy for testicular cancer. J Urol 1989;142:1491.
19. Aass N, Foss SD, Aas M, Lindegaard MW. Renal function related to different treatment modalities for malignant germ cell tumours. Br J Cancer 1990;62:842.
20. Daugaard G, Rossing N, Rorth M. Effects of cisplatin on different measures of glomerular function in the human kidney with special emphasis on high dose. Cancer Chemother Pharmacol 1988;21:163.
21. Boyer M, Raghavan D, Harris PJ, et al. Lack of late toxicity in patients treated with cisplatin containing chemotherapy for metastatic testicular cancer. J Clin Oncol 1990;8:21.
22. Schilsky RL, Barlock A, Ozols RF. Persistent hypomagnesemia following cisplatin chemotherapy for testicular cancer. Cancer Treat Rep 1982;66:1767.
23. Bosl GJ, Leitner SP, Atlas SA, Sealey JE, Preibisz JJ, Scheiner E. Increased plasma renin and aldosterone in patients treated with cisplatin-based chemotherapy for metastatic germ-cell tumors. J Clin Oncol 1986;4:1684.
24. Bissett D, Kunkeler L, Zwanenburg L, et al. Long-term sequelae of treatment for testicular germ cell tumours. Br J Cancer 1990;62:655.
25. Osanto S, Bukman A, Van Hoek F, Sterk PJ, De Laat JA, Hermans J. Long-term effects of chemotherapy in patients with testicular cancer. J Clin Oncol 1992;10:574.
26. Adoue D, Arlet P. Bleomycin and Raynaud's phenomenon. Ann Intern Med 1984;100:770.
27. Teutsch C, Lipton A, Harvey HA. Raynaud's phenomenon as a side effect of chemotherapy with vinblastine and bleomycin for testicular carcinoma. Cancer Treat Rep 1977;61:925.
28. Rothberg H. Raynaud's phenomenon after vinblastine-bleomycin chemotherapy. Cancer Treat Rep 1978;62:569.
29. Soble AR. Chronic bleomycin associated Raynaud's phenomenon. Cancer Treat Rep 1978;62:570.
30. Chernicoff DSP, Bukowski RM, Young JR. Raynaud's phenomenon after bleomycin treatment. Cancer Treat Rep 1978;62:570.
31. Vogelzang NJ, Bosl GJ, Johnson K, Kennedy BJ. Raynaud's phenomenon: a common toxicity after combination chemotherapy for testicular cancer. Ann Intern Med 1981;95:288.
32. Aass N, Kaasa S, Lund E, Kaalhus O, Skard Heier M, Foss SD. Long-term somatic side-effects and morbidity in testicular cancer patients. Br J Cancer 1990;61:151.
33. Stoter G, Koopman A, Vendrik CPJ, et al. Ten-year survival and late sequelae in testicular cancer patients treated with cisplatin, vinblastine, and bleomycin. J Clin Oncol 1989;7:1099.
34. Vogelzang NS. Vascular and other complications of chemotherapy for testicular cancer. World J Urol 1984;2:32.
35. Vogelzang NJ, Torkelson JL, Kennedy BJ. Hypomagnesemia, renal dysfunction, and Raynaud's phenomenon in patients treated with cisplatin, vinblastine, and bleomycin. Cancer 1985;56:2765.
36. Roth BJ, Greist A, Kubilis PS, Williams SD, Einhorn LH. Cisplatin-based combination chemotherapy for disseminated germ cell tumors: long-term follow-up. J Clin Oncol 1988;6:1239.
37. Hansen SW, Olsen N. Raynaud's phenomenon in patients treated with cisplatin, vinblastine and bleomycin for germ cell cancer: measurement of vasoconstriction response to cold. J Clin Oncol 1989;7:940.
38. Gietema JA, Sleijfer DT, Willemse PHB, et al. Long-term follow-up of cardiovascular risk factors in patients given chemotherapy for disseminated nonseminomatous testicular cancer. Ann Intern Med 1992;116:709.
39. Hantel A, Rowinsky E, Donehower R. Nifedipine and oncologic Raynaud's phenomenon. Ann Intern Med 1988;108:767.
40. Lejonc JL, Vernant JP, Macquin I, Castaigne A. Myocardial infarction following vinblastine treatment. Lancet 1980;2:692.
41. Vogelzang NJ, Frenning DH, Kennedy BJ. Coronary artery disease after treatment with bleomycin and vinblastine. Cancer Treat Rep 1980;53:1159.
42. Subar M, Muggia FM. Apparent myocardial ischemia associated with vinblastine administration. Cancer Treat Rep 1986;70:690.
43. Edwards GS, Lane M, Smith FE. Long-term treatment with cis-dichlorodiamineplatinum(II)-vinblastine-bleomycin: possible association with severe coronary artery disease. Cancer Treat Rep 1979;63:551.

*Editor's note: Although my colleagues and I agree that most second malignant diseases may be due to iatrogenic factors, the usual carcinogens (e.g., cigarette smoking) may play a role, as may unsuspected associations. For example, the statistical association of malignant melanoma among patients with germ cell tumors is probably a function of the high prevalence of multiple atypical nevi in this population group.[134] Patients should be followed in the long term for evidence of such unexpected associations.

44. Bodensteiner D. Fatal coronary artery fibrosis after treatment with bleomycin, vinblastine, and cis-platinum. South Med J 1981;74:898.
45. Doll DC, List AF, Greco FA, Hainsworth JD, Hande KR, Johnson DH. Acute vascular ischemic events after cisplatin-based combination chemotherapy for germ-cell tumors of the testis. Ann Intern Med 1986;105:48.
46. Samuels BL, Vogelzang NJ, Kennedy BJ. Severe vascular toxicity associated with vinblastine, bleomycin, and cisplatin chemotherapy. Cancer Chemother Pharmacol 1987;19:253.
47. Raghavan D, Cox K, Childs A, Grygiel J, Sullivan D. Hypercholesterolemia after chemotherapy for testis cancer. J Clin Oncol 1992;10: 1386.
48. Nichols CR, Roth BJ, Williams SD, et al. No evidence of acute cardiovascular complications of chemotherapy for testicular cancer: an analysis of the Testicular Cancer Intergroup study. J Clin Oncol 1992;10: 760.
49. Kaplan RS, Wiernik PH. Neurotoxicity of antineoplastic drugs. Semin Oncol 1982;9:103.
50. Thompson SW, Davis LE, Kornfeld M, Hilgers RD, Standefer JC. Cisplatin neuropathy: clinical, electrophysiologic, morphologic and toxicologic studies. Cancer 1984;54:1269.
51. Hansen SW, Helweg-Larsen S, Trojaborg W. Long-term neurotoxicity in patients treated with cisplatin, vinblastine, and bleomycin for metastatic germ cell cancer. J Clin Oncol 1989;7:1457.
52. Foss SD, Kreuser ED, Roth GJ, Raghavan D, and Members of the Consensus Group. Long-term side effects after treatment of testicular cancer. Prog Clin Biol Res 1990;357:321.
53. Hudes GR, Greenberg R, Krigel RL, et al. Phase II study of estramustine and vinblastine, two microtubule inhibitors, in hormone refractory prostate cancer. J Clin Oncol 1992;10:1754.
54. Hansen SW. Autonomic neuropathy after treatment with cisplatin, vinblastine, and bleomycin for germ cell cancer [see comments]. Br Med J 1990;300:511.
55. Stuart NSA, Woodroffe CM, Grundy R, Cullen MH. Long-term toxicity of chemotherapy for testicular cancer: the cost of cure. Br J Cancer 1990;61:479.
56. Vermorken JB, Kapteijn TS, Hart AAM, Pinedo HM. Ototoxicity of cisdiamminedichloroplatinum(II): influence of dose, schedule and mode of administration. Eur J Cancer 1983;19:53.
57. Dearnaley DP, Horwich A, A'Hern R, et al. Combination chemotherapy with bleomycin, etoposide and cisplatin (BEP) for metastatic testicular teratoma: long-term follow-up. Eur J Cancer 1991;27:684.
58. Ginsberg SJ, Comis RL. The pulmonary toxicity of antineoplastic agents. Semin Oncol 1982;9:34.
59. Comis RL. Detecting bleomycin pulmonary toxicity: a continued conundrum. J Clin Oncol 1990;8:765.
60. McKeage MJ, Evans BD, Atkinson C, Perez D, Forgeson GV, Dady PJ. Carbon monoxide diffusing capacity is a poor predictor of clinically significant bleomycin lung. J Clin Oncol 1990;8:779.
61. Senan S, Paul J, Thomson N, Kaye SB. Cigarette smoking is a risk factor for bleomycin-induced pulmonary toxicity. Eur J Cancer 1992; 28A:2084. Letter.
62. Lehne G, Johansen B, Fossa SD. Long-term follow-up of pulmonary function in patients cured from testicular cancer with combination chemotherapy including bleomycin. Br J Cancer 1993;68:555.
63. Kaldor JM, Day NE, Band P, et al. Second malignancies following testicular cancer, ovarian cancer and Hodgkin's disease: an international collaborative study among cancer registries. Int J Cancer 1987; 39:571.
64. van Leeuwen FE, Stiggelbout AM, van den Belt-Dusebout AW, et al. Second cancer risk following testicular cancer: a follow-up study of 1,909 patients. J Clin Oncol 1993;11:415.
65. Nichols CR, Hoffman R, Einhorn LH, Williams SD, Wheeler LA, Garnick MB. Hematologic malignancies associated with primary mediastinal germ-cell tumors. Ann Intern Med 1985;102:603.
66. Nichols CR, Roth BJ, Heerema N, Griep J, Tricot G. Hematologic neoplasia associated with primary mediastinal germ-cell tumors. N Engl J Med 1990;322:1425.
67. Kaldor JM, Day NE, Pettersson F, et al. Leukemia following chemotherapy for ovarian cancer. N Engl J Med 1990;322:1.
68. Pedersen-Bjergaard J, Larsen SO. Incidence of acute nonlymphocytic leukemia, preleukemia, and acute myeloproliferative syndrome up to 10 years after treatment of Hogkin's disease. N Engl J Med 1982; 307:965.
69. Greene MH, Boice JD, Greer BE, Blessing JA, Dembo AJ. Acute nonlymphocytic leukemia after therapy with alkylating agents for ovarian cancer. N Engl J Med 1982;307:1416.
70. Redman JR, Vugrin D, Arlin ZA, et al. Leukemia following treatment of germ cell tumors in men. J Clin Oncol 1984;2:1080.
71. Van Imhoff GW, Sleijfer DT, Breuning MH, Anders GJPA, Mulder NH, Halie MR. Acute nonlymphocytic leukemia 5 years after treatment with cisplatin, vinblastine, and bleomycin for disseminated testicular cancer. Cancer 1986;57:984.
72. Winick NJ, McKenna RW, Shuster JL, et al. Secondary acute myeloid leukemia in children with acute lymphoblastic leukemia treated with etoposide (see comments). J Clin Oncol 1993;11:209.
73. Pui CH, Ribeiro RC, Hancock ML, et al. Acute myeloid leukemia in children treated with epipodophyllotoxins for acute lymphoblastic leukemia. N Engl J Med 1991;325:1682.
74. Ratain MJ, Kaminer LS, Bitran JD, et al. Acute nonlymphocytic leukemia following etoposide and cisplatin combination chemotherapy for advanced non–small cell carcinoma of the lung. Blood 1987;70: 1412.
75. Johnson DH, Porter LL, List AF, Hande KR, Hainsworth JD, Greco FA. Acute nonlymphocytic leukemia after treatment of small cell luung cancer. Am J Med 1986;81:962.
76. Markman M, Pavy MD, Abeloff MD. Acute leukemia following intensive therapy for small-cell carcinoma of the lung. Cancer 1982;50: 672.
77. DeVore R, Whitlock J, Hainsworth JD, Johnson DH. Therapy-related acute nonlymphocytic leukemia with monocytic features and rearrangement of chromosome 11q. Ann Intern Med 1989;110:740.
78. Whitlock JA, Greer JP, Lukens JN. Epipodophyllotoxin-related leukemia. Cancer 1991;68:600.
79. Pedersen-Bjergaard J, Phillip P. Balanced translocations involving chromosome bands 11q23 and 21q22 are highly characteristic of myelodysplasia and leukemia following therapy with cytostatic agents targetting at DNA-topoisomeraase II. Blood 1991;78:1147.
80. Pedersen-Bjergaard J, Sigsgaard TC, Nielsen D, et al. Acute monocytic or myelomonocytic leukemia with balanced chromosome translocations to band 11q23 after therapy with 4-epi-doxorubicin and cisplatin or cyclophosphamide for breast cancer. J Clin Oncol 1992;10: 1444.
81. Oliver RTD, Ong JYH, Raja MA, Sperandio P, Gibbons B, Walker M. Secondary pre-leukaemia and etoposide. Lancet 1991;338:1269.
82. Pedersen-Bjergaard J, Hansen SW, Larsen SO, Daugaard G, Philip G, Rorth M. Increased risk of myelodysplasia and leukaemia after etoposide, cisplatin, and bleomycin for germ-cell tumours. Lancet 1991;338:359.
83. Bajorin DF, Motzer RJ, Rodriguez E, Murphy B, Bosl GJ. Acute nonlymphocytic leukemia in germ cell tumor patients treated with etoposide-containing chemotherapy. J Natl Cancer Inst 1993;85:60.
84. Nichols CR, Breeden ES, Loehrer PJ, Williams SD, Einhorn LH. Secondary leukemia associated with a conventional dose of etoposide: Review of serial germ cell protocols. J Natl Cancer Inst 1993;85:36.
85. Foss SD, Aass N, Kaalhus O. Testicular cancer in young Norwegians. J Surg Oncol 1988;39:43.
86. Malec JF, Romsaas MS, Trump DL. Psychological and personality disturbance among patients with testicular cancer. J Psycosoc Oncol 1985;3:55.
87. Kaasa S, Aass N, Mastekaasa A, Lund E, Fossa SD. Psychosocial well-being in testicular cancer patients. Eur J Cancer 1991;27:1091.
88. Gritz ER, Wellisch DK, Landserk JA. Psychosocial sequelae in long-term survivors of testicular cancer. J Psychosoc Oncol 1989;6:41.
89. Schover LR, von Eschenbach AC. Sexual and marital counselling with men treated for testicular cancer. J Sex Marital Ther 1984;10: 29.
90. Rieker PP, Fitzgerald EM, Kalish LA, et al. Psychosocial factors, curative therapies, and behavioural outcomes: a comparison of testis cancer survivors and a control group of healthy men. Cancer 1989; 64:2399.
91. Rieker PP, Edbril SD, Garnick MB. Curative testis cancer therapy: psychosocial sequelae. J Clin Oncol 1985;3:1117.
92. Moynihan C. Testicular cancer: the psychological problems of patients and their relatives. Cancer Surv 1987;6:477.
93. Bloom JR, Fobair P, Gritz E, et al. Psychosocial outcomes of cancer: a comparative analysis of Hodgkin's disease and testicular cancer. J Clin Oncol 1993;11:979.

94. Olweny CL, Juttner CA, Rofe P, et al. Long-term effects of cancer treatment and consequences of cure: cancer survivors enjoy quality of life similar to their neighbours. Eur J Cancer 1993;29A:826.
95. Gritz ER, Wellisch DK, Wang H, Siau J, Landsverk JA, Cosgrove MD. Long-term effects of testicular cancer on sexual functioning in married couples. Cancer 1989;64:1560.
96. Narayan P, Lange PH, Fraley EE. Ejaculation and fertility after extended retroperitoneal lymph node dissection for testicular cancer. J Urol 1982;127:685.
97. Hansen PV, Trykker HPE, Andersen J. Testicular function in patients with testicular cancer treated with orchiectomy alone or orchiectomy plus cisplatin based chemotherapy. J Natl Cancer Inst 1989;81:1246.
98. Hansen PV, Trykker HPE, Andersen J, Helkjaer PE. Germ cell function and hormonal status in patients with testicular cancer. Cancer 1989;64:956.
99. Hansen SW, Berthelsen JG, von der Maase H. Long-term fertility and Leydig cell function in patients treated for germ cell cancer with cisplatin, vinblastine, and bleomycin versus surveillance. J Clin Oncol 1990;8:1695.
100. Hendry WF, Stedronska J, Jones CR, Blackmore CA, Barrett A, Peckham MJ. Semen analysis in testicular cancer and Hodgkin's disease: pre- and post-treatment findings and implications for cryopreservation. Br J Urol 1983;55:769.
101. Jewett MAS, Thachil JAV, Harris JF. Exocrine function of testis with germinal testicular tumour. Br Med J 1983;286:1849.
102. Berthelsen JG, Skakkebaek NE. Gonadal function in men with testis cancer. Fertil Steril 1983;39:68.
103. Swerdlow AJ, Huttly SRA, Smith PG. Testis cancer: post-natal hormonal factors, sexual behaviour and fertility. Int J Cancer 1989;43:549.
104. Fossa SD, Ous S, Abyholm T, Norman N, Leob M. Post-treatment fertility in patients with testicular cancer. II. Influence of cisplatin based combination chemotherapy. Br J Urol 1985;57:210.
105. Guazzieri S, Lembo A, Ferro G, et al. Sperm antibodies and infertility in patients with testicular cancer. Urology 1985;26:139.
106. Morrish DW, Venner PM, Siy O, Barron G, Bhardwaj D, Outhet D. Mechanisms of endocrine dysfunction in patients with testicular cancer. J Natl Cancer Inst 1990;82:412.
107. Rieker PP, Fitzgerald EM, Kalish LA. Adaptive behavioural responses to potential infertility among survivors of testis cancer. J Clin Oncol 1990;8:347.
108. Donohue JP, Zachary J, Maynard B. Distribution of nodal metastases in non-seminomatous testis cancer. J Urol 1982;128:315.
109. Fossa SD, Klepp O, Ous S, et al. Unilateral retroperitoneal lymph node dissection in patients with non-seminomatous testicular tumor in clinical stage 1. Eur Urol 1984;10:17.
110. Donohue JP, Thornhill JA, Foster RS, Rowland RG, Bihrle R. Retroperitoneal lymphadenectomy for clinical stage A testis cancer (1965 to 1989): modifications of technique and impact on ejaculation. J Urol 1993;149:237.
111. Donohue JP, Foster RS, Rowland RG, Bihrle R, Jones J, Geier G. Nerve-sparing retroperitoneal lymphadenectomy with preservation of ejaculation. J Urol 1990;144:287.
112. Read G, Stenning SP, Cullen MH, et al. Medical Research Council prospective study of surveillance for stage I testicular teratoma. J Clin Oncol 1992;10:1762.
113. Peckham MJ, Barrett A, Horwich A, Hendry WF. Orchiectomy alone for stage 1 testicular non-seminoma: a progress report on the Royal Marsden Hospital study. Br J Urol 1983;55:754.
114. Fossa SD, Abyholm T, Normann N, Jefne V. Post-treatment fertility in patients with testicular cancer: influence of radiotherapy in seminoma patients. Br J Urol 1986;58:315.
115. Leitner SP, Bosl GJ, Bajournas D. Gonadal dysfunction in patients treated for metastatic germ-cell tumors. J Clin Oncol 1986;4:1500.
116. LeBlanc GA, Kantoff PW, Ng SF, Frei E, Waxman DJ. Hormonal perturbations in patients with testicular cancer treated with cisplatin. Cancer 1992;69:2306.
117. Nijman JM, Koops HS, Kremer J, Sleijfer DT. Gonadal function after surgery and chemotherapy in men with stage II and III nonseminomatous testicular tumors. J Clin Oncol 1987;5:651.
118. Aass N, Fossa SD, Theodorsen L, Norman N. Prediction of long-term gonadal toxicity after standard treatment for testicular cancer. Eur J Cancer 1991;27:1087.
119. Hartlapp JH, Brensing KA, Voss KH, Deitenbeck R, Mumperow E. Long-term impairment of the gonadal function after cisplatin-based chemotherapy in 140 patients with testicular cancer. Proc Am Soc Clin Oncol 1990;9:516.
120. Nijman JM, Schraffordt Koops H, Kremer J, Sleijfer DT. Gonadal function after surgery and chemotherapy in men with stage II and III nonseminomatous testicular tumors. J Clin Oncol 1987;5:651.
121. Drasga RE, Einhorn LH, Williams SD, Patel DN, Stevens EE. Fertility after chemotherapy for testicular cancer. J Clin Oncol 1983;1:179.
122. Rustin GJS, Pektasidis D, Newland ES. Fertility and second tumours after treatment of germ cell tumours. In: Jones WG, Ward AM, Anderson CK, eds. Germ cell tumours II. New York, Pergammon, 1986: 483.
123. Poirier S, Einhorn LH, Rubin L. Evaluation of reproductive capacity in germ-cell tumor patients following chemotherapy with cisplatin, VP-16 and bleomycin. Proc Am Soc Clin Oncol 1992;11:379. Abstract.
124. Senturia YD, Peckham CS. Children fathered by men treated with chemotherapy for testicular cancer. Eur J Cancer 1990;26:429.
125. Boyer M, Raghavan D. Active surveillance for stage I non-seminomatous germ cell testis tumors: practice and pitfalls. Prog Clin Biol Res 1990;350:309.
126. Einhorn LH, Williams SD, Loehrer PJ, et al. Evaluation of optimal duration of chemotherapy in favorable-prognosis disseminated germ cell tumors: a Southeastern Cancer Study Group protocol. J Clin Oncol 1989;7:387.
127. Levi JA, Raghavan D, Harvey V. The role of bleomycin in combination chemotherapy for good prognosis germ cell carcinoma. J Clin Oncol 1993;11:1300.
128. Ozols RF, Ihde DC, Linehan WM, Jacob J, Ostchega Y, Young RC. A randomized trial of standard chemotherapy v a high-dose chemotherapy regimen in the treatment of poor prognosis nonseminomatous germ-cell tumors. J Clin Oncol 1988;6:1031.
129. Morstyn G, Campbell L, Souza LM, et al. Effect of granulocyte colony stimulating factor on neutropenia induced by cytotoxic chemotherapy. Lancet 1988;1:667.
130. Bussolino F, Wang JM, Defilippi P, et al. Granulocyte- and granulocyte-macrophage-colony stimulating factors induce human endothelial cells to migrate and proliferate. Nature 1989;337:471.
131. Loehrer PJ, Elson P, Johnson DH, Williams AN, Trump DL, Einhorn LH. A randomized trial of cisplatin (P) plus etoposide (E) with or without bleomycin (B) in favourable prognosis disseminated germ cell tumors (GCT): an ECOG study. Proc Am Soc Clin Oncol 1991; 10:A540. Abstract.
132. Fjeldborg P, Sorensen J, Helkjaer PE. The long-term effect of cisplatin on renal function. Cancer 1986;58:2214.
133. Groth S, Nielsen H, Sorensen JB, Christensen AB, Pedersen AG, Rorth M. Acute and long-term nephrotoxicity of cis-platinum in man. Cancer Chemother Pharmacol 1986;17:191.
134. Raghavan D, Zalcberg JR, Grygiel JJ, et al: Multiple atypical nevi: a cutaneous marker of germ cell tumors. J Clin Oncol 1994;12:2284.

Principles and Practice of Genitourinary Oncology, edited by Derek Raghavan, Howard I. Scher, Steven A. Leibel, and Paul H. Lange. Lippincott-Raven Publishers, Philadelphia, © 1997.

CHAPTER 72

Extragonadal Germ Cell Tumors

Ramesh A. Shivdasani and Philip W. Kantoff

DEFINITION OF EXTRAGONADAL GERM CELL TUMORS AND THEIR RELATION TO PRIMARY GONADAL TUMORS

As the term is generally applied in clinical practice, an extragonadal germ cell tumor (EGGCT) is a germ cell neoplasm displaying one of the histologies associated with gonadal origin but found in a different location and in the absence of a detectable gonadal mass. Because the term encompasses mature teratomas, it is important to recognize that not all EGGCTs are frankly malignant at presentation. Additionally, because a subset of tumors with the histologic appearance of undifferentiated carcinoma possesses serum marker and clinical characteristics consistent with germ cell origin,[1,2] it is necessary to broaden the definition of EGGCT to include this important group of malignancies.

Whether the tumor arose de novo in an extragonadal site or spread there by metastasis from a primary gonadal mass is central to the consideration of EGGCTs. Most investigations report series of male patients with testes that are normal on palpation and occasionally include cases with normal sonographic examinations. Although high-resolution ultrasonography may increase the likelihood of detecting a testicular mass,[3] blind testicular biopsy is not practiced in the United States. In series in which histologic examination of the testes has been reported after biopsy, orchiectomy, or autopsy, the results are conflicting. Some investigators have found microscopic tumor foci in the testes of all patients with extragonadal presentation of a germ cell tumor[4]; others have done so in a minority of patients[5,6] or only in those patients with evidence of retroperitoneal disease.[7,8] Although it is possible that regression of testicular primary tumors, with or without residual scarring, may occur and the metastases be confused with EGGCT, two lines of evidence support the existence of EGGCT as a distinct entity. First, these tumors occur not only in sites that are common for metastasis of gonadal primaries, such as the mediastinum, but also as solitary lesions in sites where such metastases are distinctly unusual, such as the pineal gland. Even within the mediastinum, EGGCTs are found almost exclusively in an anterior superior distribution, whereas metastatic gonadal tumors do not display a regional preference. Secondly, pure yolk sac histology, which is very rare among primary gonadal tumors in adults, may be encountered in primary mediastinal masses. An association between EGGCTs and cryptorchidism has never been reported.

It is therefore appropriate to regard EGGCTs as a distinct group of neoplasms with characteristic biologic properties and treatment considerations (Table 72-1). At the same time, it is useful to narrow the definition of EGGCT to exclude germ cell tumors present in the lower abdomen or retroperitoneum, because these lesions are more likely to be associated with an occult or regressed gonadal primary tumor[7] and the clinical behavior in this group more closely parallels that observed with gonadal primary lesions.[9,10]

EGGCTs share a number of properties with their gonadal counterparts: occurrence in young adults, mostly men; midline location; association with elevated serum levels of alphafetoprotein (AFP) and the β-subunit of human chorionic gonadotropin (β-hCG); common detection of the isochromosome 12p karyotypic abnormality and other nonrandom chromosomal breaks; and sensitivity to cisplatin-based chemotherapy. However, they also differ in important respects, which justifies their consideration as a distinct disease entity. Specifically, patients with EGGCT often demonstrate greater tumor bulk and have a poorer prognosis than do patients with gonadal primary tumors. Whether this is the result of differences in biology or a longer preclinical period is controversial. In addition, patients with EGGCT are more likely to have clinical or karyotypic evidence of Klinefelter's syndrome, and they develop leukemia at a much higher frequency than do patients with gonadal primary tumors. In this chapter, the similarities and differences between gonadal germ cell tumors (GCTs) and EGGCTs are highlighted in each area of discussion.

CELL OF ORIGIN

The cell of origin in EGGCTs is a source of considerable controversy; however, the notion that both GCTs and EGGCTs arise from primordial germ cells seems likely and has dominated the literature. One alternative possibility, that EGGCTs develop from primitive rests of totipotential cells remaining from the earliest embryonic divisions,[11] has received neither experimental support nor wide acceptance.

TABLE 72-1. *Clinical and biologic features of extragonadal germ cell tumors*

SHARED WITH GONADAL GERM CELL TUMORS
Occurrence in young adults, mostly men
Midline locations
Metastasis to lung, liver, and bone
Seminomatous and nonseminomatous histologic subtypes
Elevated serum tumor markers (β-hCG, AFP)
i(12p) karyotypic abnormality
Sensitivity to cisplatin-based combination chemotherapy
DISTINCT FROM GONADAL GERM CELL TUMORS
Increased tumor bulk at presentation
Anterior superior mediastinal predominance
High frequency of patients with Klinefelter's syndrome
High frequency of development of hematologic malignancies

During human embryogenesis, the genital ridges, one on each side of the midline, are formed after the fifth week of gestation. Primordial germ cells arise from the primitive ectoderm in the fourth or fifth week of gestation in the most caudal part of the yolk sac, near the allantois. Primordial germ cells are difficult to distinguish morphologically from the surrounding cells, although they can be recognized by their high level of alkaline phosphatase activity. These cells subsequently migrate toward the gonadal ridges along a midline course that includes the mesentery and the coelomic epithelium of the gut.[12] Analysis of the phenotype of Steel and W mutations in mice indicates that proliferation and migration of the germ cells is controlled at least in part by the c-kit ligand (i.e., stem cell factor).[13,14] The demonstration of germ cell passage along a midline course, with concomitant mitosis,[12] has led to the speculation that a small fraction may be arrested in extragonadal sites during this journey and subsequently undergo malignant transformation. Although this represents the likely scenario, arrested passage of germ cells has never been documented. Additionally, although these primordial germ cells are considered to be totipotential cells, their normal differentiation within the gonadal environment is always along a gamete lineage; it is only with malignant transformation that they manifest the full spectrum of embryonic and extraembryonic differentiation. The histologic type of tumor that results depends on the degree of further differentiation: seminomas (germinomas) differentiate along a gametic (spermatocytic) lineage, embryonal carcinomas result from embryonic differentiation, and endodermal sinus (yolk sac) tumors or choriocarcinomas follow from extraembryonic differentiation.

Cytogenetic studies point to a premeiotic germ cell as the one that is transformed to generate GCTs.[15–17] More specifically, it has been suggested that the precursor cell in males is the meiotic midprophase (zygotene to diplotene) spermatocyte, which would normally complete gametogenesis rather than undergo further divisions.[18]

EPIDEMIOLOGY

GCTs account for fewer than 1% of all malignancies in men in the United States. The Surveillance, Epidemiology and End Results database indicates that the vast majority are testicular primaries; extragonadal neoplasms represent 1% to 5% of all GCTs, with an estimated 100 to 200 new diagnoses annually. GCTs account for approximately 3% of all malignancies in children and adolescents in the United States. Extragonadal tumors are more common than gonadal primary lesions in young children; the reverse is true in adolescents.

More than 90% of EGGCTs in adults occur in men; sacrococcygeal teratomas, which occur exclusively in infants and young children, are more common in girls than in boys.[19–21] There is a wider range of age at presentation with EGGCTs than is typical for gonadal tumors, and the median age of presentation in adults is 5 to 10 years older with EGGCTs than with gonadal tumors in most series.

Although the majority of ovarian tumors in adults are of epithelial origin, more than 60% of ovarian tumors in girls are derived from germ cells, and ovarian GCTs in children are more common than testicular cancer.[21] The extremely low incidence of EGGCTs in women has precluded their consideration independently; their discussion in the literature is either included with series of mostly male patients or limited to case reports. There is, however, no indication that the biologic properties of EGGCTs differ between men and women; therefore, the principles outlined in this chapter are broadly applicable.

HISTOPATHOLOGY

Like their counterparts of gonadal origin, EGGCTs occur in several characteristic histologic patterns that reflect stages of normal embryonic and fetal development. An understanding of the classification of these histologic types is best achieved by appreciating that GCTs arise from primordial germ cells, which are totipotential and can recapitulate embryonic and fetal developmental processes during their differentiation. Histologies corresponding to both embryonic and extraembryonic structures are represented within the spectrum. The following are the histologic subtypes of GCTs and EGGCTs:

A. Seminoma (germinoma/dysgerminoma)
B. Nonseminomatous germ cell tumors
   Endodermal sinus (yolk sac)
   Embryonal carcinoma
   Choriocarcinoma
   Mature and immature teratoma

Seminoma (Germinoma)

The terms germinoma (or dysgerminoma) and seminoma are synonymous and refer to a tumor in which the malignant cells undergo differentiation along a spermatocytic (gamete) lineage; both terms are in wide clinical use. The microscopic appearance of this tumor is characterized by a monotonous pattern of large round cells with central vesicular nuclei and, generally, a clear cytoplasm with well-defined cell borders. Lymphoid infiltrates of varying density may be present. The classification of a pure or classic seminoma is applied only when no other embryonic differentiation is present; alternately, the tumor is considered to harbor both seminomatous and nonseminomatous components. In the latter case, the clinical behavior of tumor typically reflects the most aggressive histologic component, although the tumor is regarded and treated as a mixed GCT. Serum tumor markers are not usually elevated in association with seminomas, which is consistent with their nonembryonic differentiation, although β-hCG may be elevated in a small fraction of cases, even when nonseminomatous elements are not appreciated microscopically. Elevation of serum AFP levels is incompatible with a diagnosis of pure seminoma.

In unselected series of GCTs or EGGCTs, seminoma is the most common histologic subtype, accounting for 25% to 50% of cases. The exquisite sensitivity of this subtype of germ cell neoplasms to radiotherapy and cisplatin-based combination chemotherapy has contributed significantly to its curability, which justifies its consideration in a category distinct from all other histologic subtypes.

Nonseminomatous Germ Cell Tumors

It has been a consistent finding in series of patients with EGGCT that yolk sac and choriocarcinoma histologies are more commonly represented in comparison with gonadal primary lesions.[10,22–25] Although one of the following histologies may be present exclusively, nonseminomatous GCTs are most often of mixed composition and may also harbor seminomatous elements.

Yolk Sac (Endodermal Sinus) Tumor

As the name suggests, and as demonstrated by morphogenetic[26] and ultrastructural[27] studies, yolk sac tumors represent malignant differentiation along the lineage of the embryonic yolk sac. They are characterized by the presence of primitive-looking cells that occur in reticular, tubulopapillary, or solid patterns and have perivascular structures called Schiller-Duval bodies. Serum levels of AFP are almost invariably elevated[28,29]; cellular AFP may be detected in tumor sections by immunohistochemistry,[30] in addition to α_1-antitrypsin and keratin.[29] Unfortunately, the distinction between elements of yolk sac and embryonal carcinoma appears to reflect institutional pathologist bias more than strictly defined histologic or immunocytochemical criteria.

Yolk sac tumors are the most common histologic subtype of GCTs in children. In adults, yolk sac histology seems to be more common in EGGCTs compared with gonadal primary lesions, and some authors have attributed the historically poorer prognosis associated with EGGCTs to this difference.

Embryonal Carcinoma

The classification and use of this category in the clinical literature is confusing, probably as a result of institutional biases in pathologic diagnosis. Some clinical series report the presence of embryonal elements in virtually all patients,[22] whereas others report it in almost none, with a high fraction of patients with yolk sac tumors.[31,32] This is because embryonal carcinoma does not have a characteristic histologic pattern, but rather resembles an anaplastic or poorly differentiated carcinoma with variable presence of papillary, tubular, or reticular features. The distinction of embryonal carcinoma from tumors comprised exclusively of yolk sac elements is based on cells of larger size, the presence of nucleoli, and negative immunoperoxidase staining for AFP. Takei and Pearl[33] have suggested that embryonal carcinomas are formed as a result of overgrowth and anaplasia of endodermal elements within yolk sac tumors, which may explain why both elements are commonly present together. In adults, the clinical behavior of embryonal and yolk sac carcinomas appears to be similar.

Choriocarcinoma

Two main cell types are identified adjacent to vascular sinusoids: cytotrophoblasts and syncytiotrophoblasts, corresponding to the cellular components of the placenta. Both elements are required for the histologic diagnosis of pure choriocarcinoma, which is rare; however, trophoblastic foci found within nonseminomatous GCTs qualify as choriocarcinomatous components. Cytotrophoblasts are polygonal cells with abundant clear cytoplasm, sharp outlines, and a central vesicular nucleus. Syncytiotrophoblasts are multinucleated large cells with eosinophilic cytoplasm. Extensive hemorrhage and necrosis within the tumor are characteristic of choriocarcinoma, and the vascular invasive properties of the placenta may favor the hemorrhage and hematogenous metastasis associated with this subtype. Circulating and cytoplasmic β-HCG are commonly detected, whereas levels of AFP usually are normal.

Teratoma

Mature teratoma is an entity in which mature or well-differentiated elements derived from one or more of the three germinal layers are present within the tumor. However, growth and metastasis can occur; therefore, mature teratoma warrants complete staging and surgical treatment. In immature teratomas, foci of poorly differentiated cells or mitotic figures coexist with the mature elements, and these tumors are associated with a variably higher incidence of malignant transformation. It is likely that all of the elements within a teratoma are clonally derived. Thus, the biologic behavior of these tumors merely mirrors the range of potential or frank malignant transformation within the daughters of that clone. The vagueness associated with the distinction between mature and immature teratomas can be minimized, and the management of patients with these tumors optimized, by careful examination of the histopathology and detailed consultation with an experienced pathologist.

It is important to note that in Great Britain, all nonseminomatous tumors are classified as malignant teratomas, with subcategories that correlate directly with each of the above described germinal malignancies.[34] This is not the terminology applied in this chapter.

GENETICS AND CHROMOSOMAL ABNORMALITIES

Except for rare anecdotes of GCTs diagnosed in siblings and twins, there is no evidence for familial inheritance in most cases. There is a clear association between EGGCT and Klinefelter's syndrome, which is discussed further later in this chapter. The diagnosis of EGGCT has been reported in patients with Down's syndrome[15] and Li-Fraumeni syndrome,[35] but the patient num-

TABLE 72-2. *Anatomic locations of extragonadal germ cell tumors (EGGCTs)*

COMMON
Mediastinum
Pineal and suprasellar regions
Sacrococcyx (infants and young children only)
CONTROVERSIAL
Retroperitoneum (metastatic vs true EGGCT?)
RARE (CASE REPORTS)
Vagina
Prostate
Liver and gastrointestinal tract
Orbit

bers have been too small to establish biologically or clinically meaningful relations between these diseases and GCTs.

The characteristic cytogenetic abnormality associated with both GCTs and EGGCTs is isochromosome 12p, or i(12p), in which the long arm of chromosome 12 is lost and the short arm is duplicated, with symmetry around the centromere.[17,18] i(12p) is detected with a frequency of approximately 70% in primary tumors and up to 100% in metastatic deposits and presumably results from aberrant chromatid exchanges in recombination-defective prophase gametocytes. Additional nonrandom chromosomal breaks are encountered with some frequency in 1p, 3p, 6q, 7q, 12q, and 15p.[18,36] The most common nonrandom abnormalities in germ cell–derived tumor cell lines are encountered in chromosome 1.[37] The genetic consequences of these chromosomal abnormalities are unknown, but the frequent increase in copy number of 12p suggests that this is an early event in the development of germ cell malignancies. Increased expression of genes located on this chromosome arm may favor or trigger neoplastic transformation; alternately, loss of 12q may result in relief of protection afforded by a tumor suppressor gene.

In experimental mice, deletion of the gene encoding α-inhibin, a member of the transforming growth factor-β family of growth factors, results in development of gonadal stromal tumors.[38] No corresponding genetic defect pertaining to GCTs has been described.

ANATOMIC LOCATIONS OF EXTRAGONADAL GERM CELL TUMORS

Although rare cases of EGGCT have been reported in the prostate,[20,39] orbit,[40] vagina,[20,41,42] stomach,[43] and liver[24,44], usually in children, three midline sites dominate the presentation of EGGCTs (Table 72-2). In decreasing order of frequency, these are the mediastinum, the pineal region, and the sacrococcyx. As discussed previously, GCTs in the retroperitoneum are best regarded as originating from a gonadal primary, even at the risk of neglecting a subset that may arise de novo. In addition, the syndrome of EGGCT presenting as a metastatic carcinoma of unknown primary lesion has received considerable attention in the literature and is discussed briefly later in this chapter.

Mediastinum

The mediastinum is the most common location for EGGCTs in adolescents and adults, and, after the sacrococcyx, is the second most common location in young children. GCTs account for 1% to 3% of all mediastinal malignancies. In larger series of patients with mediastinal GCTs, approximately 50% have mature teratoma; the remainder harbor frankly malignant histologies.[32,45] Malignant EGGCTs occur almost exclusively in an anterior superior distribution (Fig. 72-1) within or adjacent to the thymus, and 85% to 100% of cases have been reported in males.

Although a minority of patients may be diagnosed incidentally after detection of a mass on chest radiography, the majority are symptomatic at presentation.[46] Because symptoms may not occur until the tumors are quite large, patients with mediastinal GCTs tend to present at a more advanced stage than patients with gonadal tumors. The most common symptoms are nonspecific, relate to tracheobronchial compression or local pulmonary invasion, and include cough, dyspnea, and chest pain. Occasionally, symptoms related to obstruction of the superior vena cava may be present, and hemoptysis may accompany advanced tumors of nonseminomatous histology, particularly choriocarcinoma. Chest x-rays reveal an anterior mediastinal mass and, together with computed tomographic (CT) scans, are useful in evaluating the extent of disease. Serum tumor markers may be elevated depending on the histology and are useful both in diagnosis and in following the response to treatment. Gallium-67 (^{67}Ga) scanning may have similar utility, because the majority of seminomas and some nonseminomatous GCTs are gallium-avid.[47]

A tissue specimen is imperative, because the differential diagnosis includes highly curable neoplasms of germinal and lymphoid origin. This is true even in the presence of elevated serum tumor markers because mild elevations may be seen in non–germ cell malignancies, and identification of all germ cell components by histopathology is crucial in determining both prognosis and optimal therapy. Although surgery remains the primary treatment for mediastinal mature teratoma, it is not the optimal first-line treatment of other mediastinal GCTs in the era of cisplatin-based chemotherapy. The need for a complete histologic diagnosis makes open surgical biopsy preferable to a mediastinoscopic approach, so that an adequate tissue specimen can be obtained. The exceptions are cases in which thoracic surgery is contraindicated, initial mediastinoscopic findings are diagnostic, or best medical management dictates aggressive cisplatin-based combination chemotherapy as the appropriate initial treatment.

Mediastinal GCTs may be associated with both local invasion and distant metastases. Invasion of adjacent structures, including the pericardium, bronchi, great vessels, and anterior chest wall, have been reported. The most common sites of metastases are the lungs, liver, and skeletal system.

Central Nervous System

Metastases from primary gonadal tumors do not typically deposit in the central nervous system (CNS) without concomitant retroperitoneal or pulmonary deposits; thus, midline CNS tumors represent a distinct subset of EGGCTs, with histopathol-

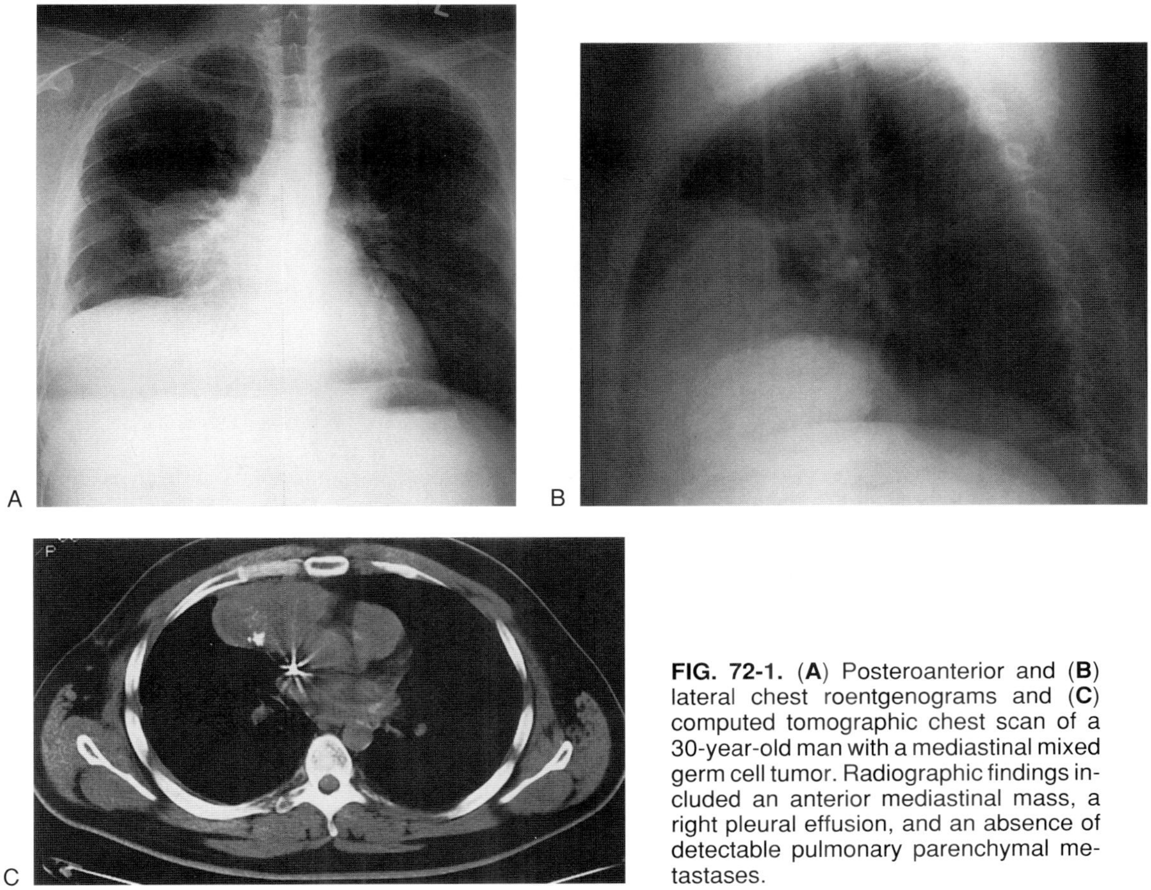

FIG. 72-1. (A) Posteroanterior and (B) lateral chest roentgenograms and (C) computed tomographic chest scan of a 30-year-old man with a mediastinal mixed germ cell tumor. Radiographic findings included an anterior mediastinal mass, a right pleural effusion, and an absence of detectable pulmonary parenchymal metastases.

ogy identical to that seen in other locations.[48,49] Within the CNS, these tumors tend to localize in the pineal gland, in the suprasellar region, and around the third ventricle (Fig. 72-2). These lesions constitute fewer than 1% of all intracranial neoplasms in adults in the United States, but comprise approximately 2.5% of intracranial neoplasms in Japanese adults[50] and 5% to 10% in U.S. children.[51] As many as two thirds of pineal tumors in children and one half of pineal tumors in adults are of germ cell origin.[52] In this location, germinoma (seminoma) is by far the most common histology, generally diagnosed in males in the second decade of life. Teratomas occur at one-fifth the frequency of germinomas, and other germ cell histologies are rare[52,53]; yolk sac and embryonal cell histology are almost never seen in pure form, and only rarely are they admixed

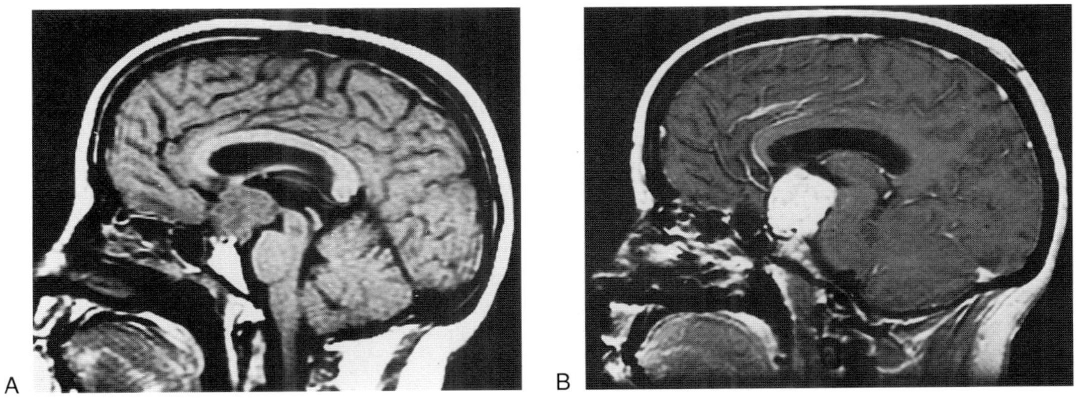

FIG. 72-2. Sagittal T1-weighted magnetic resonance images of the head (A) without and (B) with gadolinium enhancement from an 11-year-old girl with a suprasellar nonseminomatous germ cell tumor (*arrows*).

with other germ cell elements.[49,51] Although the differential diagnosis of a suprasellar mass is broad, the syndrome of "multiple midline tumors" (i.e., separate pineal and suprasellar masses) almost always represents germinoma. Suprasellar germinomas occur throughout the first three decades of life, with equal frequency in males and females. i(12p) has been reported in at least one case of nongerminomatous pineal GCT,[54] implying common pathogenetic mechanisms with other GCTs.

The clinical presentation of CNS GCTs usually involves headache and decreased visual acuity; it may include Parinaud's triad (i.e., paralysis of upward gaze, pupillary areflexia, and paralysis of convergence), hydrocephalus, diabetes insipidus, hypopituitarism, and precocious puberty.[55,56] Serum β-hCG levels are elevated in as many as 40% of patients, and AFP levels are increased in only a small minority; cerebrospinal fluid (CSF) levels of these markers may be increased if leptomeningeal seeding has occurred.[57] The size and location of suprasellar and pineal tumors is best defined by CT; germinomas have equal or slightly greater density than normal brain tissue, do not typically display calcification, and enhance uniformly with contrast, whereas teratomas may show evidence of tissues derived from all three germinal layers. In contrast, non-GCTs may be either isodense, as in pineocytoma or pineoblastoma, or have decreased density, as in astrocytoma, compared with surrounding tissue. The role of magnetic resonance imaging in diagnosis and staging continues to be investigated.

Initial reports of high mortality associated with biopsy of masses in the pineal region and the desire to avoid seeding of the subarachnoid space led to a period of presumptive treatment that has been superseded in the era of stereotactic CNS surgery.[58] CSF cytology and tumor markers also may help in yielding a diagnosis. In the event that biopsy cannot be performed and clinical or radiographic features and tumor markers do not provide a diagnosis, rapid response to a trial of 2000-cGy radiotherapy to the tumor bed yields a presumptive diagnosis of germinoma.[59,60]

Metastasis of primary CNS GCTs outside of the CNS is exceedingly rare.[61] Germinomas in particular may be locally invasive and spread through the cerebrospinal axis with an incidence of 10% to 15%.[52,62,63] An increase in incidence, to as much as 57%, in patients who have undergone surgical manipulation, including biopsy, has been noted by some[55] but disputed by others.[64] The clinical significance of positive CSF cytology is unclear, because some patients with this finding have prolonged disease-free survival even in the absence of spinal axis irradiation.[50] Abdominal metastases occurring via ventriculoperitoneal shunts have been reported for both germinomatous and nongerminomatous intracranial EGGCTs,[65,66] albeit rarely.

The 5-year survival of patients with CNS germinomas treated with radiotherapy using a dose of 5000 cGy to the tumor bed is between 65% and 90%.[52,56,67,68] The need for extended field or spinal axis irradiation is controversial in view of the relatively low incidence of spinal or intracranial recurrences; toxicities, including growth retardation, associated with spinal irradiation in children; and less than satisfactory results with salvage therapy. Although the trend to avoid irradiation of the entire neural axis has received support from retrospective clinical data,[52,67] the presence of extensive intracranial disease and multiple tumor foci probably serve as reasonable indications for extended field irradiation, whereas evidence for ventricular or meningeal seeding have been used to justify treatment of the spinal axis.

Compared with germinomas, results of external beam irradiation in the treatment of nongerminomatous intracranial GCTs have been uniformly poorer, even when combined with adjuvant chemotherapy. In the Royal Marsden experience, patients with teratoma had an 18% 5- or 10-year survival, even though most recurrences were confined to the primary site,[68] whereas survival beyond 1 year in patients with yolk sac or embryonal cell histology is extremely rare.[69,70] Conclusive recommendations are difficult, because only small numbers of patients have been studied. However, promising results following treatment of 10 patients with metastatic CNS GCTs and of a single patient with a primary intracranial GCT with the POMB/ACE regimen (cisplatin, vincristine, methotrexate, bleomycin, actinomycin D, cyclophosphamide, and etoposide) suggests that, as with nonseminomatous GCTs in other locations, an aggressive chemotherapy regimen may be the preferred method of treatment.[71] Rare instances of tumor regression and patient survival after treatment of recurrent intracranial GCTs with systemic cisplatin and etoposide further demonstrate effective delivery of cytotoxic agents to CNS disease sites.[72,73]

Sacrococcyx

Sacrococcygeal GCTs occur exclusively in children, in whom they represent the most common site for this group of neoplasms; 39% of all (i.e., gonadal and extragonadal) GCTs present in this location.[21] Sacrococcygeal teratomas are also the most common neoplasms in the newborn, and although they can become evident at any age, more than 50% are noted in the neonatal period.[74] The disease is three to five times more common in girls than in boys. The differential diagnosis includes meningomyelocele, hemangioma, and lipoma for predominantly external masses and chordoma, neuroblastoma, and anterior meningocele for presacral masses.

The Surgical Section of the American Academy of Pediatrics has divided sacrococcygeal teratomas into four types according to location.[74] Predominantly external buttock masses constitute type I tumors; types II and III have both external and internal components, with the former predominating in type II and the latter in type III; and exclusively presacral masses are classified as type IV tumors. About one half of sacrococcygeal teratomas have both external and internal (i.e., pelvic, abdominal, or both) components. Sacrococcygeal teratomas may be extremely vascular, and type I tumors, particularly, may manifest with hemorrhage. Tumors with a significant intrapelvic component frequently invade or obstruct surrounding structures, including the bladder and rectum. Other presenting symptoms include peripheral edema, abdominal distension, and leg weakness, which may indicate intraspinal extension. Rectal examination plays a critical role in the diagnosis of presacral masses.[21] Remarkably, most patients lack radiographic evidence of bony sacrococcygeal abnormalities,[75] and although cystic lesions with calcifications are more often benign than malignant, neither of these radiographic features is completely reliable.

Approximately one half of all sacrococcygeal GCTs are benign teratomas; one fourth harbor immature components without frank malignancy; and the remainder are frankly malignant. Yolk sac and embryonal carcinoma are the most frequently encountered malignant histologies.[76,77] Although tumor size did not correlate with malignant content in the largest survey,[74] fewer than 10% of tumors diagnosed before the age of 2 months, but up to 50% of those diagnosed at a later age, had a malignant component. Similarly, there is an increased risk of malignancy in recurrent disease, in primary tumors that have gone unrecognized for a long period, and in association with immature (undifferentiated) teratoma.[76] All these data suggest the occurrence of malignant transformation within teratomas and underscore the importance of surgical resection after diagnosis.

Surgical excision, including the coccyx, is the primary treatment modality for sacrococcygeal teratomas.[76,78] If malignant histologic components are detected, the prognosis is substantially worse, and adjuvant chemotherapy is indicated[77]; if the pathology reveals only mature teratoma, close follow-up rather than further treatment is necessary. The optimal management of immature teratoma remains under investigation, although conservative follow-up is the norm.

Metastatic Carcinoma of Unknown Primary Source

Patients with poorly differentiated or undifferentiated carcinoma of unknown primary site constitute a heterogeneous group with diverse clinical presentations. Within this group, the clinical characteristics of a significant minority, perhaps up to 30%, parallel those of patients with EGGCT.[1,2,79,80] In contrast, the proportion of patients who fit this description within the group that carries the light microscopic diagnosis of poorly differentiated adenocarcinoma, poorly differentiated neuroendocrine carcinoma, or poorly differentiated neoplasm, which implies the inability to distinguish between lymphoma, carcinoma, or sarcoma, among others, appears to be much smaller.[80–82] Clinical characteristics associated with metastatic, poorly differentiated, or undifferentiated carcinoma of unknown primary site are as follows[79]:

- age younger than 50 years
- predominantly male patients
- frequent primary involvement of midline structures (e.g., mediastinum, retroperitoneum), lungs, or lymph nodes
- elevated serum levels of AFP or β-hCG
- clinical evidence of rapid tumor growth
- sensitivity to cisplatin-based chemotherapy

These clinical features are consistent with histologically atypical forms of GCTs and justify the inclusion of this group of malignancies within the broader framework of EGGCTs.

Several points regarding this categorization are worth noting. The true origin of these neoplasms may remain obscure in the majority of patients, even after detailed immunohistochemistry and electron microscopy of biopsy specimens or autopsy[79]; therefore, the presumption of a germ cell malignancy is based on clinical rather than pathologic features. The consideration of a neoplasm as an unrecognized EGGCT is based on a constellation of features and not exclusively on serum levels of AFP, β-hCG, or both. Tumor markers may be elevated in only a minority of patients (<20% in the large Vanderbilt University series[79]) and, unless they are very high, are not diagnostic, because mild elevations can be present in the context of nongerminal malignancies.[83,84] Dramatic responses to therapy have been observed in patients who lack the clinical features listed previously, whereas other patients with clinically typical features are unresponsive to therapy.[85] Thus, EGGCTs account for only a fraction of cases of poorly differentiated carcinoma of unknown primary site.

The median age of patients with poorly differentiated carcinoma is about 40 years[80]; the majority are men; and the predominant sites of metastasis are the mediastinum, retroperitoneum, and peripheral lymph nodes. In contrast, patients with poorly differentiated adenocarcinoma tend to be older; many more are female; and the dominant sites of metastases are the lungs, liver, and bone. A pulmonary or gastrointestinal primary site may be identified at some point in a significant fraction of these patients. Both groups of patients have documented responses to cisplatin-based combination chemotherapy, although the response and cure rates are considerably higher in those with poorly differentiated carcinoma.

The biologic understanding of poorly differentiated or undifferentiated carcinomas of unknown primary site remains primitive, and the management of patients with this histologic diagnosis is incompletely defined. Although dramatic responses and long-term survival can occur with cisplatin-based treatment, clinical and pathologic features that predict responsiveness to therapy remain undefined.

ASSOCIATION WITH OTHER DISEASES

Hematologic Disorders

The association between EGGCTs and hematologic disorders represents one of the most intriguing and biologically unique aspects of these malignancies. Since the original recognition of this association in 1985,[86,87] more than 25 cases have been reported. All affected patients have been young men with primary mediastinal presentation of nonseminomatous GCTs; yolk sac differentiation has been noted in the majority.[88] In the largest series reported,[88] the median time from diagnosis of EGGCT to that of the hematologic disorder was 6 months; one third of the patients presented with both disorders simultaneously. Although acute lymphocytic leukemia and acute myeloid leukemias of other subtypes have been reported, acute megakaryoblastic leukemia is the most common pathologic diagnosis, and other disorders of the megakaryocyte lineage predominate, including idiopathic thrombocytopenia,[89,90] essential thrombocytosis, and myelodysplastic syndrome with abnormal megakaryocytes.[88] Rare cases associated with malignant histiocytosis[91] or systemic mastocytosis[32] have also been reported.

Hematologic neoplasms associated with EGGCT tend to be very aggressive, with patients either dying before treatment, not responding to antileukemic therapy, or achieving only brief remissions. Although patients with nonmalignant platelet disorders may display a chronic course,[88,89] the reported median survival of patients with leukemia is less than 1 month.[88]

Several lines of evidence indicate that the development of these rare hematologic disorders in patients with EGGCT is not coincidental, and EGGCT is not related to therapy. A number of patients have been diagnosed with both disorders either simultaneously or prior to treatment with cytotoxic agents; abnormalities involving chromosomes 5 and 7, frequently seen in treatment-related leukemias, have not been noted at a high frequency; and leukemias following treatment with cisplatin are exceedingly rare.

The most attractive explanation for the association between EGGCT and hematologic neoplasms is that a subpopulation of the clonally expanded totipotential germ cells within mediastinal GCTs undergo hematopoietic differentiation. Because primordial germ cells and hematopoietic precursors both arise within the yolk sac during development, the high frequency of yolk sac differentiation within mediastinal GCTs associated with hematologic disorders is consistent with this hypothesis. Histologic,[92] immunohistochemical,[93] and cytogenetic[93,94] demonstration of hematopoietic precursors or blast cells within resected mediastinal GCTs and the presence of the i(12p) karyotypic abnormality in a subset of the hematologic malignancies[88] lend further support to this theory.

Nonhematologic Malignancies

The presence within GCTs of teratoma elements with the capacity for somatic differentiation may favor the development of non–germ cell malignancies within the teratomatous components. Indeed, sarcomas of various histologies, particularly embryonal rhabdomyosarcoma, are the most common nongerminal malignancies detected in mediastinal GCTs.[95] These malignancies appear to develop within teratomatous components and are not related to treatment of the GCT. In one small series that did not achieve statistical significance, the development of sarcomas within EGGCTs was found to be three times more frequent than in testicular neoplasms, although this was rare in both cases.[96] The development of sarcomas in EGGCTs may reflect the more advanced stage of presentation of EGGCTs than testicular neoplasms in most cases; however, it should be emphasized that actual progression of immature teratoma into frank malignancy has never been demonstrated convincingly.

Sarcomas that resist initial cisplatin-based combination chemotherapy for GCTs may be resected surgically but respond poorly to further treatment with cisplatin[96] and are associated with a particularly poor prognosis.[97] Their treatment with other regimens has not been evaluated systematically.

Klinefelter's Syndrome

Klinefelter's syndrome is a male genetic disorder characterized by the 47,XXY karyotype, small and soft testes, sterility, eunuchoid habitus, gynecomastia, high circulating levels of follicle-stimulating hormone (FSH), and up to a 20-fold increased risk of developing carcinoma of the breast.[98,99] In addition, more than 30 cases of mediastinal GCTs and at least 10 cases of GCTs in other extragonadal locations have been reported in patients with Klinefelter's syndrome.[100–104] Although these patients may develop primary gonadal tumors, the frequency of extragonadal presentation appears to be considerably greater. In contrast to mediastinal GCTs that occur in the absence of Klinefelter's syndrome, nonseminomatous histologies with or without teratoma predominate (although pure seminoma has been reported), and the median age at presentation is about 10 years earlier.[103] Development of a GCT may be the first presentation of Klinefelter's syndrome in a subset of young patients in whom other clinical features of the disorder are absent or occult.[103,105] Consistent with this is the finding that the 47,XXY karyotype is noted incidentally with a frequency of 8% to 18% in small series of selected patients with EGGCTs.[103,106]

It remains unclear whether the development of GCTs in patients with Klinefelter's syndrome is a result of the primary genetic abnormality, of errors during embryonic development, or of the abnormal hormonal milieu. Survival and the response to treatment of EGGCTs in patients with Klinefelter's syndrome does not appear to be different from that in other groups of patients.

PROGNOSIS AND PROGNOSTIC FACTORS

The extent of disease prior to treatment is widely accepted as the most important prognostic factor in advanced GCTs.[107] Therefore, a number of schemes to quantitate the extent of disease have been developed which incorporate tumor size, levels of serum tumor markers, and sites and number of metastases.[108–110] The position of extragonadal tumors within these schemes has been controversial, largely because of the small numbers of patients in this category. Adding to the confusion, the outcome of patients with EGGCTs, even after the introduction of cisplatin-based combination chemotherapy, has been variable among different research groups. Some investigators have found consistently poorer outcomes for patients with nonseminomatous EGGCTs,[10,22,23,111,112] whereas others have found little or no difference between EGGCTs and testicular GCTs of similar stage treated with intensive cisplatin-based combination chemotherapy.[113,114]

These differences in published results probably relate to the small numbers of patients, to the lack of completely uniform or appropriately intensive treatment in some of the studies, and perhaps to the relative proportion of patients with retroperitoneal versus mediastinal tumors. In the Vanderbilt and Indiana University experience, application of the Indiana Classification of Extent of Disease[109] and multivariate analysis suggested that extragonadal primary sites per se do not adversely affect outcome.[113] This result led the authors to conclude that the poor prognosis historically associated with EGGCTs in comparison with gonadal primary lesions stems more from the the greater frequency of advanced disease at diagnosis than from intrinsic biologic differences between the two subsets of germ cell neoplasms. Although the dominant location of EGGCTs in the mediastinum lowers the likelihood of symptoms at early stages so that most patients present with advanced disease,[46,113] some investigators have noted that patients with mediastinal nonseminomatous GCTs fare poorly even with low disease bulk.[112] Thus, the relative contributions of disease burden and of biologic differences to the overall differences in outcome between patients with gonadal and extragonadal GCTs remains unknown. In contrast, the outcome in various series of patients with extragonadal seminoma appears to be the same as in patients with primary gonadal disease,[115] which indicates that there is no difference in intrinsic sensitivity to therapy based on location of the primary tumor for this histologic subtype of GCTs.

Prognostic factors other than stage of disease have been suggested in small and retrospective series; age of patients may have some impact on outcome,[32] and the greater frequency of yolk sac and choriocarcinoma histologies among patients with EGGCTs may contribute to the poorer prognosis historically associated with these malignancies. None of these results has, however, retained significance in multivariate analyses in larger series of patients that were treated uniformly.[31]

TREATMENT

Seminoma

Radiotherapy

Even before the advent of cisplatin therapy, the locoregional treatment of extragonadal seminomas was associated with high response rates and cures. In retrospective reviews of patients with mediastinal seminoma who were treated with a combination of surgical resection and postoperative irradiation, the long-term survival ranged from 50% in patients who were symptomatic at diagnosis[116] to 80% in asymptomatic patients.[117] In these early and uncontrolled studies, these results typically reflect radiation doses of 3000 to 3500 cGy, although long-term survival has been reported with as little as 1500 cGy of external beam irradiation. Remarkably, radiotherapy has resulted in long-term survival and probably cure, even when employed as the sole treatment modality, in patients with discrete and multiple distant metastases discovered over a period of years.

Although these results are retrospective and include selected patients, they demonstrate the remarkable radiosensitivity of seminomas and highlight the common biology between those in gonadal and extragonadal locations. However, because mediastinal seminomas are almost always associated with extensive local invasion or distant metastases at diagnosis,[116–118] relapse rates with radiotherapy approach 50%, and patients with adequate locoregional control often succumb to metastatic disease.[118] Additionally, retrospective subgroup analysis within several patient series indicates that initial radiotherapy may reduce the likelihood of future cure, either by reducing the response rate to chemotherapy or by compromising the ability to deliver curative doses without toxicity.[111,115,118,119] Therefore, cisplatin-based combination chemotherapy has largely replaced surgery and radiotherapy as the initial treatment modality in patients with mediastinal seminoma. This is in contrast to CNS germinomas, which only rarely spread outside the CNS and consequently are highly curable by irradiation alone, and in which the blood-brain barrier may impair drug delivery to the tumor site.

The long-term survival of patients with CNS seminoma treated with radiotherapy alone is on the order of 65% to 85%. Doses of 4500 to 5000 cGy to the region of the tumor routinely are delivered over 5 to 6 weeks; it is unclear whether lower doses would be equally effective. Because there is a 10% to 15% incidence of leptomeningeal metastasis, which may be increased following surgical manipulation and decreased with prophylactic spinal-axis irradiation of 3000 cGy, there has been debate about the need for routine craniospinal treatment.[50,60,67] In view of the relatively low incidence of leptomeningeal metastasis in the absence of surgery and the morbidity associated with craniospinal treatment in children, use of this modality is controversial and subject to the physician's preferences. Salvage treatment with systemic chemotherapy has not been studied systematically, but anecdotal reports of success indicate a possible role for this treatment in the event of disease recurrence.[62]

Chemotherapy

In the experience of several large centers and groups, cisplatin-based combination chemotherapy regimens developed for the treatment of nonseminomatous GCTs appear to have comparable efficacy in the treatment of gonadal and extragonadal seminomas. The Southeastern Cancer Study Group trial reported by Loehrer and colleagues[119] showed a complete response (CR) rate of 75% with the use of cisplatin, bleomycin, and etoposide (BEP) or cisplatin, bleomycin, and vinblastine with (PVB-A) or without (PVB) doxorubicin. Response rates up to 90% have been reported using either the five-drug VAB-6 regimen or cisplatin and etoposide at Memorial Hospital,[115] and various cisplatin-based regimens have been effective in smaller series of patients.[112,114,120] With variable lengths of follow-up, it appears that the survival rate closely parallels the CR rate.

Surgery

Surgical resection of residual masses after treatment of nonseminomatous GCT reveals teratoma or viable carcinoma in about 60% of patients and necrotic tumor in about 40%. In contrast, in analogous studies in patients with seminoma, necrosis with fibrous reaction is the predominant finding in both gonadal and extragonadal disease[25]; residual viable tumor may be detected in only about 10% of patients,[119] although the proportion may be as high as 40% when the mass is larger than 3 cm in diameter.[121] Consequently, the management of residual masses detected radiographically after chemotherapy of gonadal and extragonadal seminomas is controversial. Various authors agree that residual masses smaller than 3 cm in diameter should be followed carefully with serial imaging studies, with institution of salvage chemotherapy or radiotherapy in the event of relapse. Some investigators argue that residual masses larger than 3 cm should be treated with adjunctive irradiation or with surgical excision, even though the majority of such patients would be treated unnecessarily[115,121]; others have demonstrated that these patients can also be followed safely.[122] These recommendations have been made on the basis of results in relatively small numbers of patients, and the question remains open to debate. ^{67}Ga and positron emission tomography are under investigation as means for determining the need for treatment of residual masses.[47]

In CNS germinoma, the role of neurosurgery is limited to decompression and shunting in the event of increased intracranial pressure.[52,123] At the time of the diagnostic procedure, stereotactic biopsy rather than debulking surgery is indicated.

Nonseminomatous Germ Cell Tumors

Treatment Results

Economou and colleagues[124] reviewed the published experience in treatment of mediastinal nonseminomatous GCT before

1978 and noted a 3% survival rate beyond 16 months. Although durable remissions have occurred after treatment of metastatic nonseminomatous GCTs with a variety of cytotoxic agents, either singly or in combination, the best results and significant cure rates have been reported only after the incorporation of cisplatin (CDDP) into the treatment regimen.[107] However, virtually all initial reports on treatment of EGGCT, even with cisplatin-based combination chemotherapy, revealed disappointing results and form the basis for the notion that extragonadal primary tumors represent a particularly virulent subset of germ cell malignancies.

In a Southwest Oncology Group (SWOG) study of 19 men treated with cisplatin-based (50 to 75 mg/m^2 every 4 weeks) combination chemotherapy, Feun and colleagues[111] reported complete and overall response rates of 19% and 56%, respectively, with a median duration of 2 months; all responses occurred in patients with retroperitoneal disease. Sixteen of these patients had metastases at presentation, the median Karnofsky's performance score was 40%, and 11 patients had been treated previously. Although further dose escalation was not practical in this group, the CDDP dosing was probably suboptimal and, together with the previously described factors, may have contributed to the poor results.

Garnick and colleagues[22] reported one CR with chemotherapy alone and 9 CR with a combination of chemotherapy and surgery in 15 patients with EGGCTs. The relapse rate was 50%, and median duration of response was 40 months. Israel and colleagues[23] and Toner and colleagues[10] reported the CR rate to be approximately 40% with a combination of chemotherapy and surgery, with median survival of 18 months and only 5 long-term survivors of 29 patients. Logothetis and colleagues[112] reported a 40% disease-free survival among 30 previously untreated men; the duration of follow-up was not specified. In a review of 25 patients, Hainsworth and colleagues[113] reported a CR in 14 patients who received a combination of chemotherapy and surgery, with 89% survival (median, 30 months) among responders. Patients with yolk sac histology were excluded from this study; when analyzed separately, only 1 of 10 such patients achieved a durable CR with multimodality treatment.[125] In 1993, Childs and colleagues,[114] Delgado and colleagues,[120] and Dulmet and colleagues[32] reported 38% to 73% disease-free survival after chemotherapy and surgery in small numbers of selected, previously untreated men.

Each of the previously described studies was retrospective in nature and lacked uniformity both in treatment and in patient selection; most included patients with primary retroperitoneal disease. In 31 patients with mediastinal nonseminomatous GCT treated prospectively with cisplatin-based chemotherapy of uniform intensity, Nichols and colleagues[31] reported a 39% CR rate with chemotherapy alone, which increased to 58% with the addition of surgery; 83% of those patients rendered disease-free remained alive and free of disease with a median follow-up of 55 months. In an intergroup trial that included 43 patients with EGGCTs, response data for individual sites and survival data were not presented.[126] In the only other prospective (SWOG) trial with adequate maturity,[25] chemotherapy consisted of cycles of cisplatin, vinblastine, and bleomycin (PVB) alternating with cycles of cisplatin, etoposide, bleomycin, and doxorubicin (EBAP). Of 17 patients with mediastinal nonseminomatous GCTs, 14 achieved a CR after chemotherapy plus surgery, resulting in long-term survival between 60% and 70%.[25] Thus, response rates appear slightly better in prospective studies and the results approach but remain inferior to those achieved with testicular tumors. The results with chemotherapy are summarized in Table 72-3.

The relative rarity of nonseminomatous GCTs in the CNS has precluded systematic treatment or meaningful analysis of outcome, and long-term survival has been reported only infre-

TABLE 72-3. *Results of treatment of nonseminomatous extragonadal germ cell tumors*

Investigators	Patients*	Chemotherapy†	Surgery‡	Complete response (%)¶	Survival (%)‖
RETROSPECTIVE					
Feun et al, 1980[111]	12	Modified PVB	No	0	0
Hainsworth et al, 1982[13]#	19	PVB ± doxorubicin	Yes	68	60
Garnick et al, 1983[22]	9	PVB	Yes	44	11
Logothetis et al, 1985[112]	15	Various (CDDP)	Yes	NS	27
Toner et al, 1991[10]	32	Various (CDDP)	Yes	38	14
Childs et al, 1993[114]	11	Various (CDDP)	Yes	82	73
Dulmet et al, 1993[32]	14	PVB	Yes	57	36
Delgado et al, 1993[120]	18	Various (CDDP)	Yes	44	38
PROSPECTIVE					
Nichols et al, 1990[31]	31	PVB, BEP	Yes	58	48
Bukowski et al, [25]	17	PVP, EBAP	Yes	75	63

* In keeping with arguments made elsewhere in this chapter, analysis in this table, when possible, excludes patients with retroperitoneal disease. Note the small size of all studies.

† Only patients treated with cisplatin based regimens are included.

‡ In most cases surgery was directed at radiographically detected masses post chemotherapy.

¶ Complete response was achieved with chemotherapy plus surgery.

‖ When possible, disease-free survival is represented.

\# This study excluded patients with endodermal sinus histology and did not separate analysis by tumor site.

CDDP, cisplatin-based regimens; NS, not stated.

quently. In this disease, the previously mentioned success with the POMB/ACE regimen[71] indicates a role for aggressive first-line treatment with a combination chemotherapy including cisplatin and intrathecal and high-dose intravenous methotrexate.

Radiotherapy

Many of the previously described reports included patients who received external beam irradiation at some point in the course of the disease; in general, this did not impact significantly on response or survival. The notion that extragonadal nonseminomatous GCTs are relatively radioresistant has been confirmed in one retrospective series, which included patients treated with radiation doses greater than 4000 cGy and patients treated with a combination of radiotherapy and chemotherapy.[127]

Salvage Chemotherapy

Failure of primary treatment is common; results with salvage chemotherapy have been similarly disappointing. Motzer and colleagues[128] reported that none of 14 patients who had failed primary chemotherapy were cured with secondary treatment. Similarly, Saxman and colleagues[129] showed that only 5 of 73 (7%) patients with EGGCTs who had been treated with salvage chemotherapy, including 28 patients treated with autologous bone marrow transplantation (ABMT), were long-term disease-free survivors.

Surgery

Radical resection of residual masses is indicated where appropriate[130,131]; long-term survival has been reported even when thoracic surgery has necessitated prosthetic replacement of the superior vena cava.[32,132] Indeed, surgery is an integral component in the overall management of patients with nonseminomatous EGGCTs and contributes significantly to improved cure rates.[25,31] Despite the theoretical possibility of an occult gonadal primary tumor in patients with EGGCTs, the data do not support the notion of the gonads behaving as a sanctuary site in this disease. Consequently, orchiectomy or blind testicular biopsy is not indicated in successfully treated patients.

Treatment of Teratomas

The primary treatment of nonseminomatous GCTs of extragonadal origin associated with elevated serum tumor markers is cisplatin-based combination chemotherapy. This includes patients with biopsy evidence of pure teratoma, in whom the assumption is that the teratoma is admixed with other nonseminomatous elements. As with testicular GCTs, full resection of residual masses is indicated when serum tumor markers have normalized following completion of chemotherapy. If necrosis, fibrosis, or teratoma is found at this time, continued observation is appropriate, with the expectation of long-term survival. Conversely, if residual carcinomatous elements are detected, further therapy is indicated.

Surgery remains the primary treatment of patients with normal serum marker levels and histologic evidence of teratoma. Consideration of chemotherapy is based on the presence of carcinomatous elements revealed on pathologic evaluation of the resected specimen.

Treatment in Children

Because nonteratomatous GCTs respond to cisplatin-based combination chemotherapy in all age groups, it stands to reason that in general, the treatment of children with GCTs should be similar to that of adults. Indeed, excellent results with standard regimens such as PVB and BEP have been reported in the pediatric population.[133] Most reports of chemotherapy trials in children have, however, included either inconsistent treatments or regimens containing drugs with little proven additional benefit such as cyclophosphamide and actinomycin D.[134] Outside of a clinical trial, it is probably preferable to attempt to induce remission and minimize toxicity by use of a standard adult regimen such as BEP in the management of children with EGGCTs. This is particularly true because several studies have demonstrated the short- and long-term safety of cisplatin-based combination chemotherapy regimens.[133,135] Surgery and radiotherapy remain the cornerstones of management for teratomas and CNS germinomas, respectively.

Conclusions

Perhaps the most important concept to emerge from this discussion is that between 30% and 60% of unselected patients with EGGCTs are likely to enter remission with standard cisplatin-based combination chemotherapy, followed by surgery if necessary; the majority of these responders will likely enjoy long-term survival. This appears to be true even for patients with high disease burden at presentation and for those with histologies that traditionally have been considered unfavorable. The remaining patients respond to treatment either only for short durations or not at all and usually succumb to the disease. In both groups, as discussed previously, the prognosis of a small proportion of patients is further hampered by the development of hematologic malignancies that are resistant to treatment.

Together with the results summarized in Table 72-3, this discussion leads to the following conclusions. Patients with extragonadal nonseminomatous GCTs, as a group, fare worse than those with gonadal primary tumors or patients with seminomas in any location. This is a uniform observation, whether the poorer prognosis for those with extragonadal nonseminomatous GCTs stems from more advanced stage of presentation or from differences in biology. The primary treatment modality for patients with extragonadal nonseminomatous GCTs should be intensive cisplatin-based combination chemotherapy, which provides the greatest likelihood of inducing a complete remission and long-term survival. The most commonly used chemotherapy regimens are listed in Table 72-4. Surgery remains an important component of the management of these patients and may be required in addition to chemotherapy to achieve a disease-free state. The literature supports a policy of aggressive surgical intervention when residual masses are detected radiographically. The role of radiotherapy is less well-defined but

TABLE 72-4. *Combination chemotherapy regimens for treatment of extragonadal germ cell tumors*

BEP
Bleomycin 30 U IV bolus d 2, 9, and 16
Etoposide (VP-16) 100 mg/m² BSA IV daily for 5 d
Cisplatin 20 mg/m² BSA IV daily for 5 d
VIP
Etoposide (VP-16) 75 mg/m² BSA IV daily for 5 d
Ifosfamide 1200 mg/m² BSA IV daily for 5 d
Cisplatin 20 mg/m² BSA IV daily for 5 d

Both combinations are delivered over 21-day cycles. BSA, body surface area.

appears to be more limited; this modality is best reserved for palliative control of discrete masses. The surgical or clinical detection of viable cancer after induction chemotherapy portends a particularly ominous prognosis, perhaps worse than that of comparable patients with primary gonadal tumors; therefore, patients with this finding are reasonable candidates for investigational therapies. Unfortunately, results with salvage regimens, including ABMT, have been disappointing.

Future Directions

The optimal chemotherapy regimen for treatment of EGGCTs remains undefined. However, principles in the management of primary gonadal GCTs are likely to extend to EGGCTs as well. Whether VIP as initial therapy for poor-risk GCTs, including EGGCTs, is superior to BEP has been examined in a randomized prospective study; preliminarily, no apparent benefit was seen with VIP.[136] The role of dose-intensive chemotherapy with ABMT has also been explored in patients with relapsed and refractory GCTs, including extragonadal disease, with disappointing results.[137] Clinical trials in progress will help determine whether the outcome in these patients can be improved with the use of high-dose chemotherapy and ABMT as initial treatment.

REFERENCES

1. Fox RM, Woods RL, Tattersall MHN, McGovern VJ. Undifferentiated carcinoma in young men: the atypical teratoma syndrome. Lancet 1979;1:1316.
2. Richardson RL, Schoumacher RA, Fer MF, et al. The unrecognized extragonadal germ cell cancer syndrome. Ann Intern Med 1981;94:181.
3. Kirschling RJ, Kvols LK, Charboneau JW, Grantham JG, Zincke H. High-resolution ultrasonographic and pathologic abnormalities of germ cell tumors in patients with clinically normal testes. Mayo Clin Proc 1983;58:648.
4. Asif S, Uehling DT. Microscopic tumor foci in testes. J Urol 1968;99:776.
5. Azzopardi JG, Mostofi FK, Theiss EA. Lesions of testes observed in certain patients with widespread choriocarcinoma and related tumors. Am J Pathol 1965;38:207.
6. Cox JD. Primary malignant germinal neoplasms of the mediastinum. Cancer 1975;36:1162.
7. Luna MA, Valenzuela-Tamariz J. Germ-cell tumors of the mediastinum, postmortem findings. Am J Clin Pathol 1976;65:450.
8. Daugaard G, von der Maase H, Olsen J, Rorth M, Skakkebaek NE. Carcinoma-in-situ testis in patients with assumed extragonadal germ-cell tumors. Lancet 1987;2:528.
9. McAleer JJA, Nicholls J, Horwich A. Does extragonadal presentation impart a worse prognosis to abdominal germ-cell tumors? Eur J Cancer 1992;28A:825.
10. Toner GC, Geller NL, Lin SY, Bosl GJ. Extragonadal and poor risk nonseminomatous germ cell tumors. Cancer 1991;67:2049.
11. Schlumberger HG. Teratoma of the anterior mediastinum in the group of military age. Arch Pathol 1946;41:398.
12. Witschi E. Migration of the germ cells of human embryos from the yolk sac to the primitive gonadal folds. Contrib Embryol 1948;32:67.
13. Mintz B, Russell ES. Gene induced embryological modifications of primordial germ cells in the mouse. J Exp Zool 1957;134:207.
14. Russell ES. Hereditary anemias of the mouse; a review for geneticists. Adv Genet 1979;20:357.
15. Linder D, Hecht F, McCaw BK, Campbell JR. Origin of extragonadal teratomas and endodermal sinus tumors. Nature 1975;254:597.
16. Wang N, Perkins KL, Bronson DL, Fraley EE. Cytogenetic evidence for premeiotic transformation of human testicular cancers. Cancer Res 1981;41:2135.
17. Samaniego F, Rodriguez E, Houldsworth J, et al. Cytogenetic and molecular analysis of human male germ cell tumors: chromosome 12 abnormalities and gene amplification. Genes Chromosome Cancer 1990;4:239.
18. Chaganti RSK, Rodriguez E, Mathew S. Origin of adult male mediastinal germ-cell tumors. Lancet 1994;343:1130.
19. Mahour GH, Woolley MM, Trivedi AN, Landing BH. Sacrococcygeal teratoma: a 33 year experience. J Pediatr Surg 1975;10:183.
20. Mann JR, Pearson D, Barrett A, et al. Results of the United Kingdom Children's Cancer Study Group's malignant germ cell tumor studies. Cancer 1989;63:1657.
21. Ablin A, Isaacs AJ. Germ cell tumors. In: Pizzo PA, Poplack DG, eds. Principles and practice of pediatric oncology. Philadelphia: JB Lippincott, 1993:867.
22. Garnick MB, Canellos GP, Richie JP. Treatment and surgical staging of testicular and primary extragonadal germ cell cancer. JAMA 1983;250:1733.
23. Israel A, Bosl GJ, Golbey RB, Whitmore W Jr, Martini N. The results of chemotherapy for extragonadal germ-cell tumors in the cisplatin era: the Memorial Sloan-Kettering Cancer Center experience (1975 to 1982). J Clin Oncol 1985;3:1073.
24. Logothetis CJ. The case for relevant staging of germ cell tumors. Cancer 1990;65:709.
25. Bukowski RM, Wolf M, Kulander BG, et al. Alternating combination chemotherapy in patients with extragonadal germ cell tumors: a Southwest Oncology Group study. Cancer 1993;71:2631.
26. Teilum G, Albrechtsen R, Norgaard-Pedersen B. The histogenetic-embryologic basis for reappearance of AFP in endodermal sinus tumors (yolk sac tumors) and teratomas. Acta Pathol Microbiol Scand 1975;83:80.
27. Nogales-Fernandez F, Silverberg SG, Bloustein PA, Martinez-Hernandez A, Pierce GB. Yolk sac carcinoma (endodermal sinus tumor): ultrastructure and histogenesis of gonadal and extragonadal tumors in comparison with normal human yolk sac. Cancer 1977;39:1462.
28. Talerman A, Haije WG, Baggerman L. Serum alpha-fetoprotein (AFP) in patients with germ cell tumors of the gonads and extragonadal sites: correlation between endodermal sinus (yolk sac) tumor and raised serum AFP. Cancer 1980;46:380.
29. Truong LD, Harris L, Mattioli C, et al. Endodermal sinus tumor of the mediastinum: a report of seven cases and review of the literature. Cancer 1986;58:730.
30. Teilum G, Albrechtsen R, Norgaard-Pedersen B. Immunofluorescent localization of alpha-fetoprotein synthesis in endodermal sinus tumor (yolk sac tumor). Acta Pathol Microbiol Scand 1974;82:568.
31. Nichols CR, Saxman S, Williams SD, et al. Primary mediastinal nonseminomatous germ cell tumors: a modern single institution experience. Cancer 1990;65:1641.
32. Dulmet EM, Macchiarini P, Suc B, Verley JM. Germ cell tumors of the mediastinum: a 30-year experience. Cancer 1993;72:1894.
33. Takei Y, Pearl GS. Ultrastructural study of intracranial yolk sac tumor with special reference to the oncologic phylogeny of germ cell tumors. Cancer 1981;48:2038.
34. Collins DH, Pugh RCB. Classification and frequency of testicular tumours. Br J Urol 1964;36(Suppl):1.

35. Hartley AL, Birch JM, Kelsey AM, et al. Are germ cell tumors part of the Li-Fraumeni cancer family syndrome? Cancer Genet Cytogenet 1989;42:221.
36. Murty VV, Dmitrovsky E, Bosl GJ, et al. Nonrandom chromosome abnormalities in testicular and ovarian germ cell tumor lines. Cancer Genet Cytogenet 1990;50:67.
37. Andrews PW, Oosterhuis JW, Damjanov I. Cell lines from human germ cell tumors. In: Robertson EJ, ed. Teratocarcinomas and embryonic stem cells: a practical approach. Oxford: IRL Press, 1987:207.
38. Matzuk MM, Finegold MJ, Su J-GJ, Hsueh AJW, Bradley A. α-Inhibin is a tumor-suppressor gene with gonadal specificity in mice. Nature 1992;360:313.
39. Marsden HB, Birth JH, Swindell R. Germ cell tumors of childhood: a review of 137 cases. J Clin Pathol 1981;34:872.
40. Margo CE, Folberg R, Zimmerman LE, Sesterhenn IA. Endodermal sinus tumor (yolk sac tumor) of the orbit. Ophthalmology 1983;90:1426.
41. Young R, Scully RE. Endodermal sinus tumor of the vagina: a report of nine cases and review of the literature. Gynecol Oncol 1984;18:380.
42. Hawkins EP, Finegold MJ, Hawkins HK, et al. Nongerminomatous malignant germ cell tumors in children: a review of 89 cases from the Pediatric Oncology Group, 1971-1984. Cancer 1986;58:2579.
43. Holt LP, Melcher DH, Colquhoun J. Extragonadal choriocarcinoma in the male. Postgrad Med J 1965;41:134.
44. Hart WR. Primary endodermal sinus (yolk sac) tumor of the liver: first reported case. Cancer 1975;35:1453.
45. Lewis BD, Hurt RD, Payne WS, et al. Benign teratomas of the mediastinum. J Thorac Cardiovasc Surg 1983;86:727.
46. Knapp RH, Hurt RD, Payne WS, et al. Malignant germ cell tumors of the mediastinum. J Thorac Cardiovasc Surg 1985;89:82.
47. Uchiyama M, Kantoff PW, Kaplan WD. Gallium-67 citrate imaging in extragonadal and gonadal seminomas: relationship to radiologic findings. J Nucl Med 1994;35:1624.
48. Koide O, Watanabe Y, Sato K. A pathological survey of intracranial germinoma and pinealoma in Japan. Cancer 1980;45:2119.
49. Stachura I, Mendelow H. Endodermal sinus tumor originating in the region of the pineal gland. Cancer 1980;45:2131.
50. Shibamoto Y, Abe M, Yamashita J, et al. Treatment results of intracranial germinoma as a function of the irradiated volume. Int J Radiat Oncol Biol Phys 1988;15:285.
51. Packer RJ, Sutton LN, Rosenstock JG, et al. Pineal region tumors of childhood. Pediatrics 1984;74:97.
52. Wara WM, Jenken DT, Evans A, et al. Tumors of the pineal and suprasellar region: Children's Cancer Study Group treatment results. Cancer 1979;43:698.
53. Loeffler JS, Mauch P. Tumors in the pineal region. In: Williams CJ, Krikorian JG, Green MR, Raghavan D, eds. Textbook of uncommon cancer. New York: John Wiley, 1988:693.
54. de Bruin TWA, Slater RM, Defferrari R, et al. Isochromosome 12p-positive pineal germ cell tumor. Cancer Res 1994;54:1542.
55. Sung DI, Harisiadis L, Chang CH. Midline pineal tumors and suprasellar germinomas: highly curable by irradiation. Radiology 1978;128:745.
56. Rich TA, Cassady JR, Strand RD, Winston KR. Radiation therapy for pineal and suprasellar germ cell tumors. Cancer 1985;55:932.
57. Edwards M, Davis RL, Laurent JP. Tumor markers and cytologic features of cerebrospinal fluid. Cancer 1985;56:1773.
58. Conway LW. Stereotaxic diagnosis and treatment of intracranial tumors including an initial experience with cryosurgery for pinealomas. J Neurosurg 1973;28:483.
59. Spiegel AM, DiChiro G, Gorden P, et al. Diagnosis of radiosensitive hypothalamic tumors without craniotomy. Ann Intern Med 1976;85:290.
60. Griffin BR, Griffin TW, Tong DYK, et al. Pineal region tumors: results of radiation therapy and indications for elective spinal irradiation. Int J Radiat Oncol Biol Phys 1981;7:605.
61. Gay JC, Janco RL, Lukens JN. Systemic metastases in primary intracranial germinoma: case report and literature review. Cancer 1985;55:2688.
62. Bloom HJG. Intracranial tumors: response and resistance to therapeutic endeavors, 1970-1980. Int J Radiat Oncol Biol Phys 1982;8:1083.
63. Jennings MT, Gelman R, Hochberg F. Intracranial germ-cell tumors: natural history and pathogenesis. J Neurosurg 1985;63:155.
64. Jooma R, Kendall BE. Diagnosis and management of pineal tumors. J Neurosurg 1983;58:654.
65. Haimovic IC, Sharer L, Hyman RA, Beresford HR. Metastasis of intracranial germinoma through a ventriculoperitoneal shunt. Cancer 1981;48:1033.
66. Bamberg M, Metz K, Alberti W, Heckemann R, Schulz U. Endodermal sinus tumor of the pineal region: metastases through a ventriculoperitoneal shunt. Cancer 1984;54:903.
67. Linstadt D, Wara WM, Edwards MSB, Hudgins RJ, Sheline GE. Radiotherapy of primary intracranial germinomas: the case against routine craniospinal irradiation. Int J Radiation Oncol Biol Phys 1988;15:291.
68. Dearnaley DP, A'hern RP, Whittaker S, Bloom HJG. Pineal and CNS germ cell tumors: Royal Marsden Hospital experience 1962-1987. Int J Radiat Oncol Biol Phys 1990;18:773.
69. Eberts TJ, Ransburg RC. Primary intracranial endodermal sinus tumor. J Neurosurg 1979;50:246.
70. Packer RJ, Sutton LN, Rorke LB, et al. Intracranial embryonal cell carcinoma. Cancer 1984;54:520.
71. Rustin GJS, Newlands ES, Bagshawe KD, Begent RHJ, Crawford SM. Successful management of metastatic and primary germ cell tumors in the brain. Cancer 1986;57:2108.
72. Kobayashi T, Yoshida J, Ishiyama J, et al. Combination chemotherapy with cisplatin and etoposide for malignant intracranial germ-cell tumors. J Neurosurg 1989;70:676.
73. Sakai N, Yamada H, Andoh T, Nishimura Y, Niikawa S. Long-term survival in malignant intracranial germ-cell tumors: a report of two cases and a review of the literature. Child Nerv Syst 1993;9:431.
74. Altman RP, Randolph JG, Lilly JR. Sacrococcygeal teratoma: American Academy of Pediatrics Surgical Section Survey, 1973. J Pediatr Surg 1974;9:389.
75. Schey WL, Shkolnik A, White H. Clinical and radiographic considerations of sacrococcygeal teratomas: an analysis of 26 new cases and review of the literature. Radiology 1977;125:189.
76. Noseworthy J, Lack EE, Kozakewich HPW, Vawter GF, Welch KJ. Sacrococcygeal germ cell tumors in childhood: an updated experience with 118 patients. J Pediatr Surg 1981;16:358.
77. Raney RB, Chatten J, Littman P, et al. Treatment strategies for infants with malignant sacrococcygeal teratoma. J Pediatr Surg 1981;16:573.
78. Whalen TV, Mahour GH, Landing BH, Woolley MM. Sacrococcygeal teratomas in infants and children. Am J Surg 1985;150:373.
79. Greco FA, Vaughn WK, Hainsworth JD. Advanced poorly differentiated carcinoma of unknown primary site: recognition of a treatable syndrome. Ann Intern Med 1986;104:547.
80. Hainsworth JD, Greco FA. Poorly differentiated carcinoma and poorly differentiated adenocarcinoma of unknown primary tumor site. Semin Oncol 1993;20:279.
81. Woods RL, Fox RM, Tattersall MHN, et al. Metastatic adenocarcinomas of unknown primary sites: a randomized study of two combination chemotherapy regimens. N Engl J Med 1980;303:87.
82. Garrow GC, Greco FA, Hainsworth JD. Poorly differentiated neuroendocrine carcinoma of unknown primary tumor site. Semin Oncol 1993;20:287.
83. Braunstein GD, Vaitukaitis JL, Carbone PP, Ross GT. Ectopic production of human chorionic gonadotropin by neoplasms. Ann Intern Med 1973;78:39.
84. Iseki M, Suzuki T, Koizumi Y, et al. Alpha-fetoprotein-producing pancreatoblastoma: a case report. Cancer 1986;57:1833.
85. Hainsworth JD, Wright EP, Gray GF, Greco FA. Poorly differentiated carcinoma of unknown primary site: correlation of light microscopic findings with response to cisplatin-based combination chemotherapy. J Clin Oncol 1987;5:1275.
86. Nichols CR, Hoffman R, Einhorn LH, et al. Hematologic malignancies associated with primary mediastinal germ-cell tumors. Ann Intern Med 1985;102:603.
87. DeMent SH, Eggleston SC, Spivac JL. Association between mediastinal germ cell tumors and hematologic malignancies: report of two cases and review of the literature. Am J Surg Pathol 1985;9:23.
88. Nichols CR, Roth BJ, Heerema N, Griep J, Tricot G. Hematologic neoplasias associated with primary mediastinal germ-cell tumors. N Engl J Med 1990;322:1425.
89. Garnick MB, Griffin JD. Idiopathic thrombocytopenia in association with extragonadal germ cell cancer. Ann Intern Med 1983;98:926.
90. Helman LJ, Ozols RF, Longo DL. Thrombocytopenia and extragonadal germ-cell neoplasm. (Letter) Ann Intern Med 1984;101:280.
91. Landanyi M, Roy I. Mediastinal germ cell tumors and histiocytosis. Hum Pathol 1988;19:586.

92. Larsen M, Evans WK, Shepherd FA, et al. Acute lymphoblastic leukemia: possible origin from a mediastinal germ cell tumor. Cancer 1984; 53:441.
93. Landanyi M, Samaniego F, Reuter VE, et al. Cytogenetic and immuno-histochemical evidence for the germ cell origin of a subset of acute leukemias associated with mediastinal germ cell tumors. J Natl Cancer Inst 1990;82:2217.
94. Orazi A, Neiman RS, Ulbright TM, et al. Hematopoietic precursor cells within the yolk sac tumor component are the source of secondary hematopoietic malignancies in patients with mediastinal germ cell tumors. Cancer 1993;71:3873.
95. Manivel C, Wich MR, Abenoza P, Rosai J. The occurrence of sarcomatous components in primary mediastinal germ cell tumors. Am J Surg Pathol 1986;10:711.
96. Ulbright TM, Loehrer PJ, Roth LM, et al. The development of non-germ cell malignancies within germ cell tumors. Cancer 1984;54: 1824.
97. Gonzalez-Vela JL, Savage PD, Manivel JC, Torkelson JL, Kennedy BJ. Poor prognosis of mediastinal germ cell cancers containing sarcomatous components. Cancer 1990;66:1114.
98. Klinefelter HFJ, Reifenstein ECJ, Albright F. Syndrome characterized by gynecomastia, aspermatogenesis without α-leydigism and increased excretion of follicle-stimulating hormone. J Clin Endocrinol 1942;2:615.
99. Jackson AW, Muldal S, Ockey CH, et al. Carcinoma of male breast in association with Klinefelter's syndrome. Br Med J 1965;1:223.
100. Curry WA, McKay CE, Richardson RL, et al. Klinefelter's syndrome and mediastinal germ cell neoplasms. J Urol 1981;125:127.
101. McNeil MM, Leong ASY, Sage RE, et al. Primary mediastinal embryonal carcinoma associated with Klinefelter's syndrome. Cancer 1981;47:343.
102. Mann BD, Sparkes RS, Kern DH, et al. Chromosomal abnormalities of a mediastinal embryonal cell carcinoma in a patient with 47,XXY Klinefelter syndrome: evidence for a premeiotic origin of a germ cell tumor. Cancer Genet Cytogenet 1983;8:191.
103. Nichols CR, Heerema NA, Palmer C, et al. Klinefelter's syndrome associated with mediastinal germ cell neoplasms. J Clin Oncol 1987; 5:1290.
104. Arens R, Marcus D, Engelberg S, et al. Cerebral germinomas and Klinefelter syndrome: a review. Cancer 1988;61:1228.
105. Penchansky L, Krause JR. Acute leukemia following a malignant teratoma in a child with Klinefelter's syndrome: case report and review of secondary leukemias in children following treatment of a primary neoplasm. Cancer 1982;50:684.
106. Dexeus FH, Logothetis CJ, Chong C, et al. Genetic abnormalities in men with germ cell tumors. J Urol 1988;140:80.
107. Einhorn LH, Donohue J. Cis-diamminedichloroplatinum, vinblastine, and bleomycin combination chemotherapy in disseminated testicular cancer. Ann Intern Med 1977;87:293.
108. Samuels ML, Johnson DE, Holoye PY. Continuous intravenous bleomycin (NS-125066) therapy with vinblastine (NSC-49842) in stage II testicular neoplasia. Cancer Chemother Rep 1975;59:563.
109. Birch R, Williams S, Cone A, et al. Prognostic factors for favorable outcome in disseminated germ cell tumors. J Clin Oncol 1986;4:400.
110. Mead GM, Stenning SP, Parkinson MC, et al. The second Medical Research Council study of prognostic factors in nonseminomatous germ cell tumors. J Clin Oncol 1992;10:85.
111. Feun LG, Samson MK, Stephens RL. Vinblastine (VLB), bleomycin (BLEO), cis-diamminedichloroplatinum (DDP) in disseminated extragonadal germ cell tumors: a Southwest Oncology Group study. Cancer 1980;45:2543.
112. Logothetis CJ, Samuels ML, Selig DE, et al. Chemotherapy of extragonadal germ cell tumors. J Clin Oncol 1985;3:316.
113. Hainsworth JD, Einhorn LH, Williams SD, Stewart M, Greco FA. Advanced extragonadal germ-cell tumors: successful treatment with combination chemotherapy. Ann Intern Med 1982;97:7.
114. Childs WJ, Goldstraw P, Nicholls JE, Dearnaley DP. Horwich A. Primary malignant mediastinal germ cell tumors: improved prognosis with platinum-based chemotherapy and surgery. Br J Cancer 1993; 67:1098.
115. Motzer RJ, Bosl GJ, Geller NL, et al. Advanced seminoma: the role of chemotherapy and adjunctive surgery. Ann Intern Med 1988;108: 513.
116. Hurt RD, Bruckman JE, Farrow GM, et al. Primary anterior mediastinal seminoma. Cancer 1982;49:1658.
117. Schantz A, Sewall W, Castleman B. Mediastinal germinoma: a study of 21 cases with an excellent prognosis. Cancer 1972;30:1189.
118. Jain KK, Bosl GJ, Bains MS, Whitmore WF, Golbey RB. The treatment of extragonadal seminoma. J Clin Oncol 1984;2:820.
119. Loehrer PJ, Birch R, Williams SD, Greco FA, Einhorn LH. Chemotherapy of metastatic seminoma: the Southeastern Cancer Study Group experience. J Clin Oncol 1987;5:1212.
120. Delgado FG, Tjulandin SA, Garin AM. Long term results of treatment in patients with extragonadal germ cell tumors. Eur J Cancer 1993; 29A:1002.
121. Motzer RJ, Bosl GJ, Heelan R, et al. Residual mass: an indication for further therapy in patients with advanced seminoma following systemic chemotherapy. J Clin Oncol 1987;5:1064.
122. Schultz SM, Einhorn LH, Conces DJ, Williams SD, Loehrer PJ. Management of postchemotherapy residual mass in patients with advanced seminoma: Indiana University experience. J Clin Oncol 1989;7:1497.
123. Rao YTR, Medini E, Haselow RE, Jones TK, Levitt SH. Pineal and ectopic pineal tumors: the role of radiation therapy. Cancer 1981;48: 708.
124. Economou JS, Trump DL, Holes EC, Eggleston JE. Management of primary germ cell tumors of the mediastinum. J Thorac Cardiovasc Surg 1982;83:643.
125. Kuzur ME, Cobleigh MA, Greco FA, Einhorn LH, Oldham RK. Endodermal sinus tumor of the mediastinum. Cancer 1982;50:766.
126. Nichols CR, Williams SD, Loehrer PJ, et al. Randomized study of cisplatin dose intensity in poor-risk germ cell tumors: a Southeastern Cancer Study Group and Southwest Oncology Group protocol. J Clin Oncol 1991;9:1163.
127. Kersh CR, Constable WC, Hahn SS, et al. Primary malignant extragonadal germ cell tumors: an analysis of the effect of radiotherapy. Cancer 1990;65:2681.
128. Motzer RJ, Geller NL, Tan C, et al. Salvage chemotherapy for patients with germ cell tumors. Cancer 1991;67:1305.
129. Saxman SB, Nichols CR, Einhorn LH. Salvage chemotherapy in patients with extragonadal nonseminomatous germ cell tumors: the Indiana University experience.
130. Kay PH, Wells FC, Goldstraw PA. A multidisciplinary approach to primary nonseminomatous germ cell tumors of the mediastinum. Ann Thorac Surg 1987;44:578.
131. Wright CD, Kesler KA, Nichols CR, et al. Primary mediastinal nonseminomatous germ cell tumors: results of a multimodality approach. J Thorac Cardiovasc Surg 1990;99:210.
132. Dartevelle P, Chapelier A, Pastorino U, et al. Long-term follow-up after prosthetic replacement of the superior vena cava combined with resection of mediastinal-pulmonary malignant tumors. J Thorac Cardiovasc Surg 1991;102:259.
133. Pinkerton CR, Pritchard J, Spitz L. High complete response rate in children with advanced germ cell tumors using cisplatin-containing combination chemotherapy. J Clin Oncol 1986;4:194.
134. Ablin AR, Krailo MD, Ramsay NKC, et al. Results of treatment of malignant germ cell tumors in 93 children: a report from the Children's Cancer Study Group. J Clin Oncol 1991;9:1782.
135. Roth BJ, Greist A, Kublis PS, Williams SD, Einhorn LH. Cisplatin-based combination chemotherapy for disseminated germ cell tumors: long-term follow-up. J Clin Oncol 1988;6:1239.
136. Droz JP, Kramar A, Nichols C, et al. Second line chemotherapy with ifosfamide, cisplatin and either etoposide or vinblastine in recurrent germ cell cancer: assignment of prognostic groups (Abstract). Proc Am Soc Clin Oncol 1993;12:229.
137. Nichols CR, Tricot G, Williams SD, et al. Dose-intensive chemotherapy in refractory germ cell cancer: a phase I/II trial of high-dose carboplatin and etoposide with autologous bone marrow transplantation. J Clin Oncol 1989;7:932.

PART V

Renal Cancer

Principles and Practice of Genitourinary Oncology, edited by Derek Raghavan, Howard I. Scher, Steven A. Leibel, and Paul H. Lange. Lippincott-Raven Publishers, Philadelphia, © 1997.

CHAPTER 73

Anatomy of the Kidney, Adrenal, and Upper Retroperitoneum

John F. Redman

The genitourinary oncologic surgeon has two primary reasons for a thorough knowledge of the coverings and organs of the upper retroperitoneum: (1) to interpret diagnostic imaging; and (2) to effect surgical exposure. Nowhere in urology are the requirements so great for a thorough knowledge of anatomy than for the understanding of diagnostic images and the accomplishment of the extensive surgery demanded in the treatment of genitourinary neoplasms. This chapter, therefore, covers the osteomuscular abdominal and thoracic body wall, soft tissue relationships, the retroperitoneal connective tissue of the upper abdomen, and the anatomy of the kidneys, adrenal glands, and upper urinary collecting structures.

UPPER ABDOMINAL AND THORACIC OSTEOMUSCULAR WALL

The radical extirpation of renal and adrenal neoplasms is performed by various surgical approaches that, when considered as a whole, cut across almost every aspect of the upper abdomen and chest, both anteriorly and posteriorly. For this reason, a comprehensive coverage of the anatomy encountered in cancer surgery of the upper urinary tract and adrenal gland should include that of both the upper abdomen and back and lower chest, which, for discussion, are interrelated.

Skeletal Anatomy

For consideration are the lower ribs, the lower thoracic and lumbar vertebrae, and the upper bony pelvis. The bony skeleton can be seen as an aid to understanding the spatial relationships of the adrenal and kidneys with the overlying bone and also to understanding the attachments of muscles and aponeuroses. The uppermost abdominal contents, except for a narrow V shape, are encircled by the lower ribs, and the space between the lower ribs and upper pelvis is narrow. Two useful basics for understanding are that the lower two ribs are free of any anterior bony attachments, and the iliac crest has three ridges—an outer, an intermediate, and an inner ridge—from which the abdominal wall musculature originates.

Muscular Anatomy

Although overlap is considerable, in this discussion the musculature that covers the upper abdomen is divided into three groups: anterolateral, posterior and thoracic.

Anterolateral Muscles

Three muscles are anterolateral—the external oblique, the internal oblique, and the transversus abdominis, and one muscle, the rectus abdominis, is strictly anterior (Fig. 73-1).

The external oblique muscle arises from the anterior outer surface of the lower fifth through 12th ribs interdigitating with the origins of the serratus anterior muscle. The external oblique extends as far cranially as the lower aspect of the pectoral muscles and therefore is also a muscle of the thorax (see Fig. 73-1*A*).

The fibers pass obliquely and medially to insert on the outer edge of the iliac crest. Between the anterior axillary line and the edge of the rectus abdominis, the external oblique muscle is represented by a broad, flat aponeurosis that passes over the rectus muscle to meld with the contralateral aponeurosis. The aponeurosis is free of the underlying aponeurosis of the internal oblique to almost the midbelly of the rectus, but then it fuses with that structure to form the anterior rectus sheath. From the lower border of the 12th rib to the iliac crest, the external oblique muscle is represented by a free border.

The internal oblique, which is strictly a muscle of the abdomen, arises from the outer costal portions of the seventh through 12th ribs (see Fig. 73-1*B*). The fibers pass obliquely and laterally to insert on the lateral two thirds of the inguinal ligament and the intermediate line of the iliac crest. From the 12th rib to near the iliac crest, the lateral aspect of the internal oblique has a free border, but it inserts caudally by a short aponeurosis

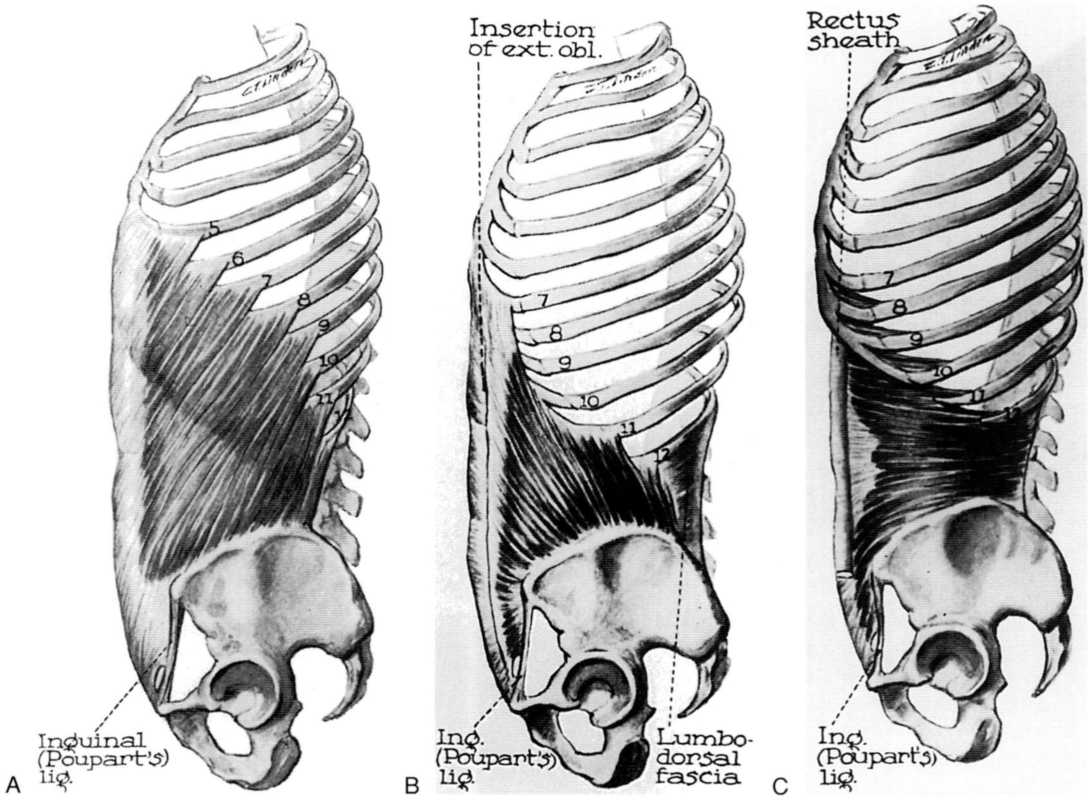

FIG. 73-1. (**A**) External oblique muscle. (**B**) Internal oblique muscle. (**C**) Transversus abdominis muscle. Ing. lig., inguinal ligament. (Thorek P. Anatomy in surgery, 2nd ed. Philadelphia, JB Lippincott, 1962:362.)

into the posterior lamina of the lumbodorsal fascia. Medially, roughly underlying the edge of the aponeurosis of the external oblique muscle, is the aponeurosis of the internal oblique that, at the edge of the rectus abdominis, divides and contributes equally to both the anterior and posterior rectus sheaths.

The transversus abdominis muscle also is a muscle of the abdomen (see Fig. 73-1*C*). It arises from the inner aspects of the costal margins of the eighth through 12th ribs and inserts on the inner lip of the iliac crest. It is characterized by both an anterior and a posterior aponeurosis. The posterior aponeurosis roughly parallels that of the overlying oblique muscles and forms, with a contribution from the internal oblique aponeurosis, the posterior rectus sheath. The posterior, or lateral, aponeurosis is contiguous with the anterior lamina of the lumbodorsal fascia, extending from the 12th rib to the iliac crest.

The rectus abdominis muscles, which are also muscles of the chest and abdomen, insert on the cartilage of the fifth through seventh ribs and xyphoid process and insert by an aponeurosis to the pubic ramus. These muscles are characterized by three or more segmental aponeurotic bands called tendinous intersections. The rectus muscles are covered anteriorly and posteriorly by the rectus sheath.

Posterior Muscles

The posterior muscles may be divided, for discussion, into superficial, intermediate, and deep groups (Fig. 73-2). The superficial group, in addition to the external oblique, includes the latissimus dorsi muscle, which is a large, flat, triangular muscle. It extends by its broad aponeurosis from the posterior lamina of the lumbodorsal fascia, and the spinous processes of the lumbar vertebra and sacrum and the iliac crest, craniolaterally over the expanse of the lower back, to insert on the humerus by a narrow tendon. The intermediate group, in addition to the internal oblique, includes the serratus posterior inferior and the sacrospinalis (erector spinae) muscles. The serratus posterior inferior consists of a short group of muscles that extend cranially and medially from the spinous processes of the lumbar vertebrae, pass dorsal to the sacrospinalis muscle, and insert on the lower, outer borders of the last four ribs just lateral to their angles. The sacrospinalis muscle lies in the groove formed by the spinous and transverse processes of the lumbar and thoracic vertebrae and is covered dorsally and ventrally by the posterior and anterior layers of the lumbodorsal fascia. The deep group of posterior muscles includes the transversus abdominis, the quadratus lumborum, and the psoas. The quadratus muscle arises from an aponeurosis from the inner lip of the iliac crest and the transverse processes of the lumbar vertebrae and inserts on the caudal margin of the 12th rib; it is separated from the sacrospinalis muscle by the anterior layer of the lumbodorsal fascia. Some anatomists refer to the transversalis fascia, which covers the ventrum of the quadratus, as the anterior layer of the lumbodorsal fascia, with the dorsal covering of fascia termed the middle layer. Just lateral to the quadratus is the

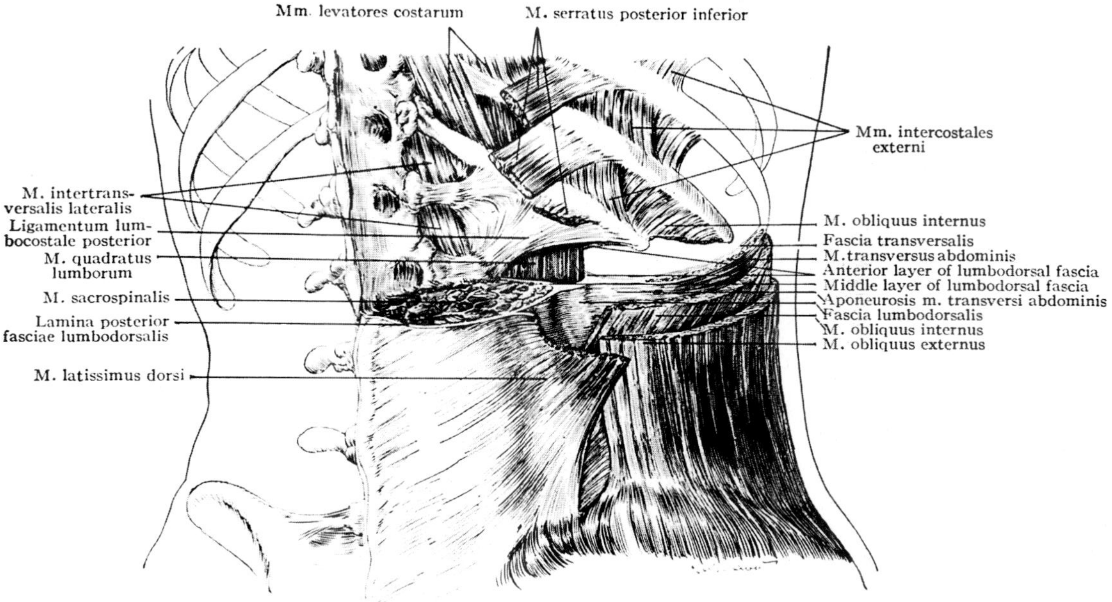

FIG. 73-2. Posterior abdominal wall musculature (After Kelly, Burnham. In: McVay C. Anson & McVay surgical anatomy, 6th ed. Philadelphia, WB Saunders, 1989.)

cranial aspect of the psoas muscle. The psoas may be considered a lumbar extension of the iliac muscle with which it melds in the pelvis to form the iliopsoas muscle, which inserts on the lesser trochanter of the femur. The cranial aspects arise from the bodies of the T12-L5 vertebra, with the muscle lying in the groove formed by the body of the vertebral bodies and the transverse processes.

Thoracic Muscles

The thoracic muscles include the superficial muscles previously described—rectus abdominis, external oblique, latissimus dorsi, and serratus posterior inferior, but it also includes the intercostal muscles and the diaphragm.

The diaphragm is both a muscle of the abdomen and of the chest. It arises from the periphery of the caudal aspect of the inner aspect of the thorax and inserts into a broad, central aponeurosis known as the central tendon of the diaphragm. The peripheral origin has three parts: (1) a sternal portion arising from the posterior aspect of the xyphoid; (2) a costal part arising from the inner aspects of the lower six ribs and their cartilage; (3) and a lumbar part, known as the medial and lateral lumbocostal arcs or arcuate ligaments, where this aponeurotic portion of the diaphragm crosses over the psoas and the quadratus lumborum muscles, respectively. The left and right crura also give origin to the diaphragm. The right crus arises from the upper three lumbar vertebrae, whereas the shorter left crus arises from the upper two. The muscle fibers meld over the aorta to form the medial lumbocostal arc. Other than the hiatus for the aorta, the diaphragm is penetrated by the vena cava on the right and by the esophagus in the midline. In the caudal aspect of the chest, the intercostal muscles are represented primarily by external and inner intercostal muscles, which roughly correspond to the external and internal oblique muscles of the abdomen. An innermost intercostal muscle may also be present. The fibers of the external intercostal muscle pass obliquely down and at the level of the cartilage are replaced by the external intercostal membrane. Likewise, the fibers of the internal intercostal muscle pass obliquely upward and at the angle of the ribs are replaced by the internal intercostal membrane. Along the subcostal groove of the ribs, ventral to the inner intercostal muscle and dorsal to the innermost intercostal muscle, are the intercostal artery, vein, and nerve. On the caudal aspects of the ribs, from the transverse processes to the angle, may be found the levator costorum muscle, and extending from the transverse process to the caudal margins of the ribs is found the lateral costotransverse ligament. Supporting the 12th rib is a similar ligament, the posterior lumbodorsal ligament.

RETROPERITONEAL CONNECTIVE TISSUE

Important in understanding the retroperitoneum is knowledge of the retroperitoneal connective tissue. A useful concept is to think of the retroperitoneal connective tissue as divided into three strata: an outer, an inner, and an intermediate (Fig. 73-3). The outer stratum is synonymous with the transversalis fascia, the contiguous covering of the inner aspect of the osteomuscular wall of the abdomen. The inner stratum is the supporting connective tissue of the peritoneum, and the intermediate stratum is represented by all the fat-laden connective tissue between. The outer stratum, or transversalis fascia, is contiguous with the fascia of the transversus abdominis, diaphragm, quadratus lumborum, and psoas muscles and covers the anterior spinous ligament covering the ventral aspect of the vertebral bodies. The cleavage plane between the transversalis and underlying intermediate stratum is not so distinct at the intersections of the quadratus and transversus abdominis muscles and near the midline ventrally. The inner stratum is scarcely discernible

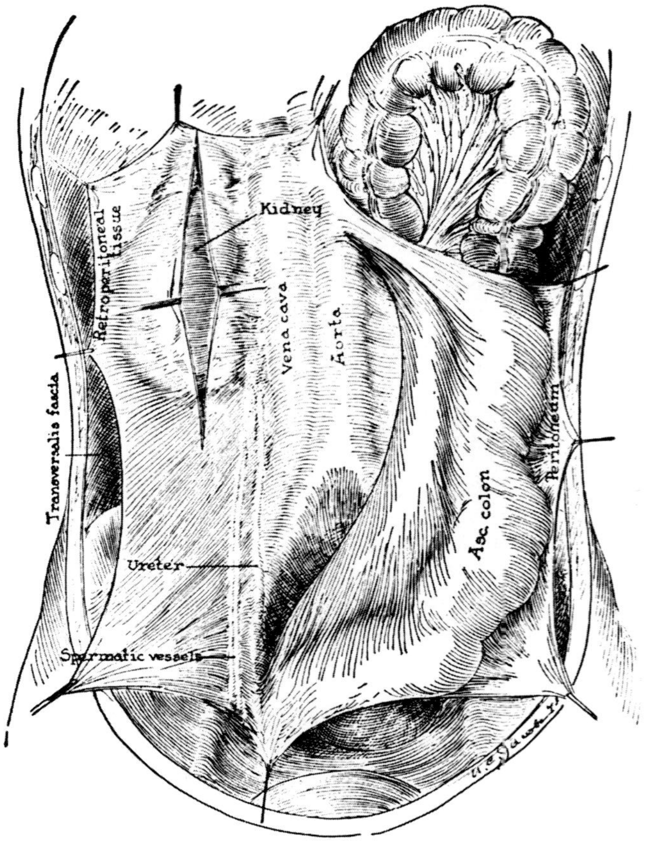

FIG. 73-3. Kidney and ureter contained within the intermediate stratum of retroperitoneal connective tissue. Note the development of a fusion fascial plane to separate the colon and mesentery from the underlying intermediate stratum. (Tobin CE. The renal fascia and its relation to the transversalis fascia. Anat Rec 1944;89:306.)

from the peritoneum, which it supports, but it may, nonetheless, be dissected free from the intermediate stratum with relative ease. Of importance is knowledge of a fusion fascial plane formed when the serosa of formerly overlying serosal surfaces disappears, leaving only apposed inner stratum. A potential cleavage plane is thus formed and is found between the ascending and descending colon and their mesenteries and the underlying intermediate stratum. A similar potential plane is also found posterior to the duodenum and pancreas.

The intermediate stratum is unique because of its specializations and condensations, the most notable in the upper retroperitoneum being Gerota's fascia. The intermediate stratum, like packing material, can be separated dorsally from the osteomuscular wall and ventrally from the colon and its mesentery, leaving only a fat-laden layer containing the kidney, adrenal gland, ureter, and gonadal vessels. The condensations formed are a perirenal fascia (Gerota's fascia) and a periureteric sheath. The Gerota's fascia forming anterior and posterior layers fuses laterally, the lateral conal fascia, forming an envelope around the kidney and contiguous across the ventrum of the great vessels with the Gerota's fascia of the contralateral kidney. Cranially, Gerota's fascia cones down as it covers the adrenal gland, but caudally it is open as it fans around the gonadal vessels and ureter. The fat between the kidneys and Gerota's fascia is termed perirenal fat, whereas that external to Gerota's fascia is pararenal fat.

PERITONEUM

Whether a surgeon works intra- or extraperitoneally, knowledge of the peritoneal attachments and reflections is important. A key anatomic point in extraperitoneal dissections of the upper abdomen is that the peritoneum is densely adherent to the diaphragm with minimal intervening intermediate stratum, and, therefore, sharp dissection is usually required for full freeing of the peritoneal envelope. Within the abdominal cavity, the peritoneal reflection forms folds and so-called ligaments that form convenient starting points for dissection to free and elevate the intraabdominal organs to gain access to the retroperitoneum.

On the lateral aspects of the ascending and descending colon, the line of fusion of the colonic serosa with the parietal peritoneum is known as the white line of Toldt. On the right side, the peritoneal reflection resembles a triangle, with the base represented by the border of the ascending colon, the apex being the duodenal-jejunal junction, the cranial side being the attachment of the transverse mesocolon, and the medial side the root of the small bowel mesentery. With an incision along these lines of peritoneal reflection, all the ascending colon, the right side of the transverse mesocolon, and all the small bowel and duodenum may be retracted away from the intermediate stratum of retroperitoneal connective tissue covering the lower pole of the kidney, right ureter, and gonadal vessels. On the left side, traction on the transverse colon and descending colon brings into clear view peritoneal reflections, termed the phrenicocolic and splenorenal ligaments. Undue or sharp traction on these peritoneal reflections is a common cause of splenic laceration. An incision of the peritoneal reflection on the lateral aspect of the descending colon, the phrenicocolic ligament, and the attachment of the left side of the transverse mesocolon allows medial reflection of the descending colon and its mesentery, to expose the middle and lower pole of the left kidney, the ureter, and the caudal margin of the pancreas. If the peritoneal reflection on the left side is further incised cranial to the phrenicocolic ligament, the following "ligaments" are incised: the splenorenal, the gastrosplenic, and the gastrophrenic, which allows for reflection of the spleen, the pancreas and stomach from the left side of the retroperitoneum exposing the upper pole of the left kidney, the adrenal gland, and the crus of the diaphragm. The liver may be similarly reflected by incising the peritoneal reflections, beginning at the distinct right and left triangular ligaments, respectively, with incision continued along the cranial and caudal coronary ligaments. The reflection of the right lobe of the liver is particularly dramatic, giving full visualization of the upper pole of the right kidney and adrenal gland and the inferior vena cava to the level of the hepatic veins at the diaphragm.

VASCULATURE OF UPPER RETROPERITONEUM

The vasculature of the upper retroperitoneum, although large and impressive, is not nearly as complex as that of the pelvis (Fig. 73-4).

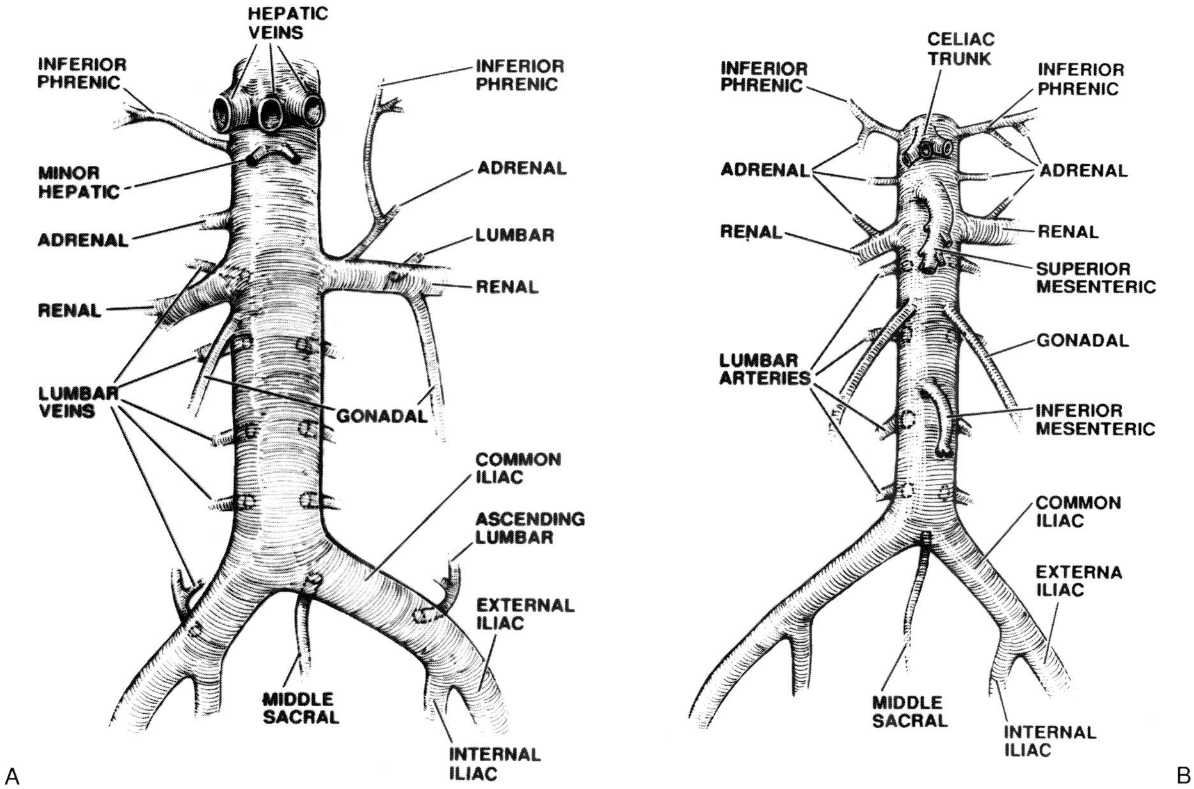

FIG. 73-4. Inferior vena cava (**A**) and aorta (**B**) with major tributaries and branches. At variance with the illustration, the inferior phrenic veins usually drain into the inferior vena cava cranial to the hepatic veins, the left adrenal vein is usually found just opposite the gonadal vein, and a lumbar vein is usually found on the posterior and ventral side of the left renal vein medial to the gonadal. (Kabalin JN. In: Walsh PC, Retik AB, Stamey TA, Vaughan ED Jr, eds. Campbell's urology, 6th ed, vol 1. Philadelphia, WB Saunders, 1992.)

Arteries

At approximately the level of the 12th lumbar vertebra, the aorta emerges in the midline from beneath the median lumbocostal arc of the diaphragm and immediately in the ventral midline, or just to either side, gives origin to the inferior phrenic arteries. To urologists, the inferior phrenic arteries are significant because they give origin to the superior suprarenal arteries as they pass in close proximity to the cranial aspects of the adrenal glands. The second branch of the abdominal aorta in the midline is the large celiac trunk. The celiac trunk almost immediately trifurcates into a large hepatic artery on the right, the large splenic artery on the left, and the smaller midline left gastric artery. Just caudal to the origin of the celiac trunk are the paired middle suprarenal arteries, which arise opposite each other from the lateral aspects of the aorta. Just caudal to the origin of the middle suprarenal arteries is the midline origin of the superior mesenteric artery, and just caudal to the superior mesenteric artery, at the level of the second vertebral body, is the lateral origin of each renal artery. In the short distance of three vertebral bodies, T12-L2, are the origins of all the vasculature of the viscera of the upper abdomen and retroperitoneum, except the descending colon. All arteries are subject to variations and anomalies, particularly the renal arteries, which may be multiple and may arise anywhere from the L1-L3 vertebral body level. Just below the origin of the renal arteries are the paired midline origins of the gonadal arteries. From the dorsolateral aspect of the aorta emanate approximately four pairs of equally spaced lumbar arteries that subsequently pass dorsal to the psoas musculature.

Veins

As compared with the venous system of the pelvis, the venous drainage of the upper abdomen is much less complex. The primary vein is the inferior vena cava, which lies immediately lateral to the right side of the aorta. Its tributaries are considered from cranial to caudal. Immediately distal to the vena caval hiatus and the diaphragm, the inferior vena cava receives on its ventrolateral aspects the paired inferior phrenic veins. The left inferior phrenic vein is of interest to the urologist because it receives the left superior, middle, and inferior suprarenal veins and is contiguous with the left adrenal vein, which drains into the left phrenic vein, usually just opposite the left gonadal vein. Immediately caudal to the inferior phrenic veins is the site of entrance of three large hepatic veins into the ventrum of the vena cava. Other than a few, small, short hepatic veins in the midline, no veins enter the vena cava behind the liver. At the caudal edge of the liver is the right adrenal vein on the right lateral aspect of the vena cava. At the level of the second lumbar body, just below the origin of the superior mesenteric artery, the renal veins enter the inferior vena cava, with the left renal vein passing ventral to the aorta. A lumbar vein, as well as the left gonadal vein, may drain directly into the left renal vein on its caudal and dorsal aspect, just lateral to the aorta. The right gonadal vein enters the inferior vena cava on its ventrolateral aspect at an oblique angle.

The lumbar veins and plexuses are of interest to urologists because these vessels may assume prominence with compression or invasion of the inferior vena cava. Like the lumbar arteries, the veins are paired and segmental and drain into the inferior vena cava on its dorsal aspect. The veins communicate with the ascending lumbar veins, which run parallel to the vertebral bodies just ventral to the transverse processes, and also with the lumbar azygos vein, which courses anterior to the vertebral bodies. The left ascending lumbar vein continues cranially above the diaphragm on the left as the hemiazygos vein and on right as the azygos vein. The veins are subject to considerable variation and anomalies, which include accessory renal veins, venous collars, and duplications of the vena cava.

LYMPHATICS OF THE UPPER RETROPERITONEUM

Of most interest to urologists are the lymphatics related to the kidney and testis (Fig. 73-5). The renal lymphatic drainage of the kidney emerges as three or four anterior and posterior collecting ducts, respectively, which drain into 20 to 30 lymph nodes, primarily distributed as periaortic chains on either side of the aorta. In addition are periaortic and retroaortic nodes and nodes distributed along the inferior vena cava. The ultimate drainage of these lymph nodes is into the cysterna chyli, which is a large, fusiform lymphatic channel located on the left aspect of the ventrum of the L1-L2 vertebral bodies, or into the continuance of the cisterna, the thoracic duct itself.

The lymphatic drainage of the testes follows the course of the gonadal vessels. The majority of the lymphatic drainage from the right testis terminates in the right paraaortic node chain, also frequently termed the interaortocaval nodes. Lymph nodes receiving lymphatic drainage from the right testis, however, may extend from the level of the right renal vein caudally to the level of the bifurcation of the aorta and both pericaval and left paraaortal groups. The left testicular lymphatics primarily drain to the left paraaortic chain, with extensions of drainage above the left renal hilum and right paraaortic chain (interaortocaval nodes), but with little drainage to the right paracaval nodes.

NERVE STRUCTURES OF THE UPPER ABDOMEN AND RETROPERITONEUM

Innervation of the Anterior Abdominal Wall

The somatic innervation of the anterolateral wall is by the ventral rami of the lower seven thoracic and first lumbar spinal

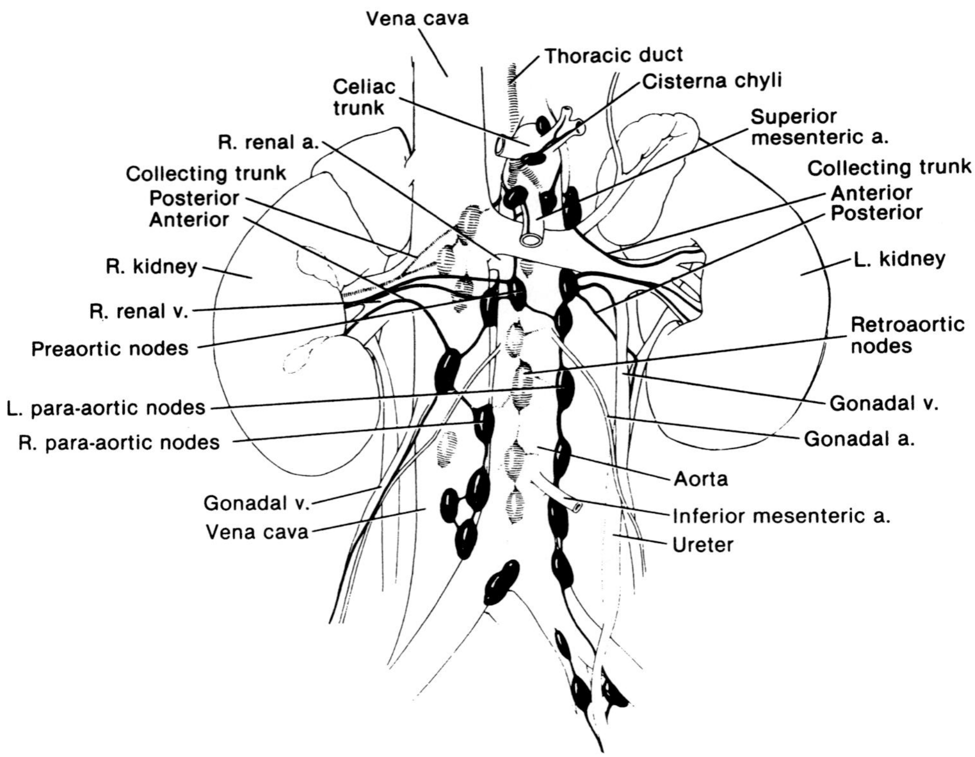

FIG. 73-5. Retroperitoneal lymphatics. (Hinman F. Atlas of urosurgical anatomy. Philadelphia, WB Saunders, 1993.)

nerves. In the intercostal space, the sixth through 11th intercostal nerves run in the costal groove on the caudal aspect of each rib, accompanied by the vascular bundle. At the approximate level of the axillary line, they divide into anterior and lateral cutaneous branches. The anterior branch continues between the internal intercostal and innermost intercostal muscles until it emerges at the level of the costal margin to pass between the internal oblique and transversus abdominis muscles. At the lateral margin of the posterior rectus sheath, it penetrates the sheath, and at the midbelly of the rectus muscle, it penetrates the muscle and subsequently the anterior rectus sheath, to appear on the anterior abdominal wall. The nerves then divide, giving off medial and lateral branches. Innervation is provided to all muscles through which these nerves pass. The lateral cutaneous branch passes abruptly through the internal oblique and transversus abdominis muscles and emerges roughly between the anterior slips of the serratus anterior muscle and more caudally, at the lateral margin of the latissimus dorsi muscle. At the point of emergence, the nerve gives off posterior and anterior branches that pass over the external oblique muscle. The anterior branch passes medially, with the branches of the seventh and eighth nerves coursing upward, the ninth passing horizontally, and those of the tenth and 11th passing obliquely downward. The 12th intercostal nerve passes laterally and obliquely under the lateral lumbocostal arc, crosses the psoas muscle, and penetrates the posterior aponeurosis of the transversus abdominis muscle before dividing into anterior and lateral cutaneous branches. The lateral cutaneous branch is encountered at the anterior axillary line just cranial to the iliac crest.

Innervation of the Posterior Abdominal Wall

The latissimus dorsi muscle is innervated by the lateral cutaneous branches of the T8-T12 ventral rami of the thoracic spinal nerves.

Somatic Innervation of the Deep Posterior Abdominal Wall and Diaphragm Encountered From Within the Abdomen

Innervation of the diaphragm is by the right and left phrenic nerves, which, for the most part, are only encountered by urologists by their branches as they course from medial to lateral just cranial to the medial and lateral lumbocostal arcs.

The 12th intercostal nerve has been described. The remainder of the somatic nerves encountered in the upper retroperitoneum are branches of the lumbar plexus. The ventral ramus of the first lumbar nerve divides into upper and lower branches, the iliohypogastric and iliolumbar nerves, respectively. Both emerge from the dorsal aspect of the psoas muscle as it passes under the medial lumbocostal arc of the diaphragm and course obliquely downward over the quadratus lumborum muscle. These nerves, which are located on the surface of the transversalis fascia, are a helpful aid in dissecting the transversalis fascia from the underlying intermediate stratum. Just above the iliac crest, the iliohypogastric nerve penetrates the posterior aponeurosis of the transversus abdominis muscle, with the ilioinguinal nerve continuing over that muscle before penetrating it in the area of the anterior axillary line. At the level of the L2 innerspace, the genitofemoral nerve, composed of elements of the anterior division of the first and second lumbar spinal nerves, emerges from the ventral midline and courses caudally the length of the abdominal and pelvic portion of the psoas, then dividing into genital and femoral branches. At the level of L3, the lateral femoral cutaneous nerve, composed of elements of the posterior division of both the L2 and L3 spinal nerves, emerges from the dorsolateral margin of the psoas and courses obliquely and caudally over the medial caudal border of the quadratus and iliacus muscles.

Autonomic Innervation of the Upper Retroperitoneum

In the retroperitoneum of the upper abdomen, the autonomic nervous system is represented by nerves of the sympathetic division. These nerves are, with practice, increasingly recognizable by the surgeon. The sympathetic trunk may be identified along the ventral sides of the bodies of the lumbar vertebrae. Equally spaced sympathetic fibers enter the ganglia from the more dorsal spinal nerves by the gray and white rami communicantes. The left sympathetic trunk parallels the left side of the aorta, and the right trunk lies under the dorsal midline of the inferior vena cava. Passing between the aorta and the vena cava on the right and over the aorta on the left are the lumbar splanchnic nerves, which pass from the sympathetic ganglia to coalesce over the ventrum of the aorta, forming the intermesenteric or aortic plexus. Similarly, over the ventral midline of the aorta surrounding the origins of the major tributaries, are the following ganglia, named according to the associated vessels: the celiac ganglia, which forms from the greater, lesser, and least thoracic splanchnic nerves coursing over the crura of the diaphragm; and the superior mesenteric, aorticorenal, and inferior mesenteric ganglia.

ORGANS

The organs of the retroperitoneum, other than the duodenum and pancreas, are the kidneys and their collecting structures and the adrenal glands. These organs are described with specific emphasis on their gross structure, relationships, vasculature, lymphatic drainage, and innervation.

Renal Anatomy

The kidneys are large, bean-shaped organs measuring 10 to 12 cm in length, 5 to 7 cm in width, and 3 to 4 cm in depth, with smaller dimensions in females. The kidneys are generally similar in shape, although the convex border of the left kidney may be thicker, the so-called "dromedary hump." The renal surface, which is covered by an easily strippable fibrous capsule, is generally smooth, but it may be irregular from varying degrees of persistent fetal lobulations. When viewed medially, the contour of the kidney has a centrally depressed aperture, the renal hilum, which widens to become the renal sinus.

Relationships

Relationships of the kidney are usually considered only in regard to the structures surrounding the kidney, although the orientation of the kidney to the surrounding structures, particularly the osteomuscular wall, is important. Although anatomic illustrations frequently depict the kidneys projecting laterally from the great vessels like two doorknobs, the kidneys actually lie in a deep hollow on either side of the vertebral bodies and the psoas muscles (Fig. 73-6). The kidneys, therefore, are located a considerable distance dorsal to the great vessels, which course over the ventrum of the vertebral bodies. Considered another way, the transverse axis of the kidney lies 30 degrees from the coronal plane (Fig. 73-7). Other rotational axes to be considered in the relationships of the kidney are the coronal or frontal axis, in which the upper poles of the kidney tilt medially 15 degrees from ventral, and from a sagittal or lateral projection, the upper pole tilts dorsally approximately 10 degrees from vertical.

The posterior aspect of the kidney, surrounded by thickened perinephric and paranephric fat, is related at its upper pole to the diaphragm and lower ribs (Fig. 73-8). In the midkidney and lower pole regions, from medial to lateral to the psoas muscle, the kidney lies over the quadratus lumborum and posterior aponeurosis of the transversus abdominis muscles. Anteriorly, the kidneys are overlain by the intraperitoneal contents, the duodenum, pancreas, liver, and adrenal glands. The perinephric fat and paranephric fat are scant anteriorly, and therefore the kidneys are easily seen from within the abdominal cavity, through the colonic mesenteries. On the right side, the kidney is covered cranially by the bare area of the liver and the intraperitoneal portion of the liver. Medially, the right adrenal gland may partially cover the surface of the kidney, but it frequently is separate. The medial and caudal aspects of the kidney, laterally, are covered by the ascending and transverse colon (hepatic flexure) and their mesenteries and, medially, by the second portion of the duodenum, which covers the hilum, upper ureter, and medial aspect of the lower pole of the kidney. On the left side, anteriorly, the kidney is overlain cranially and laterally by the spleen

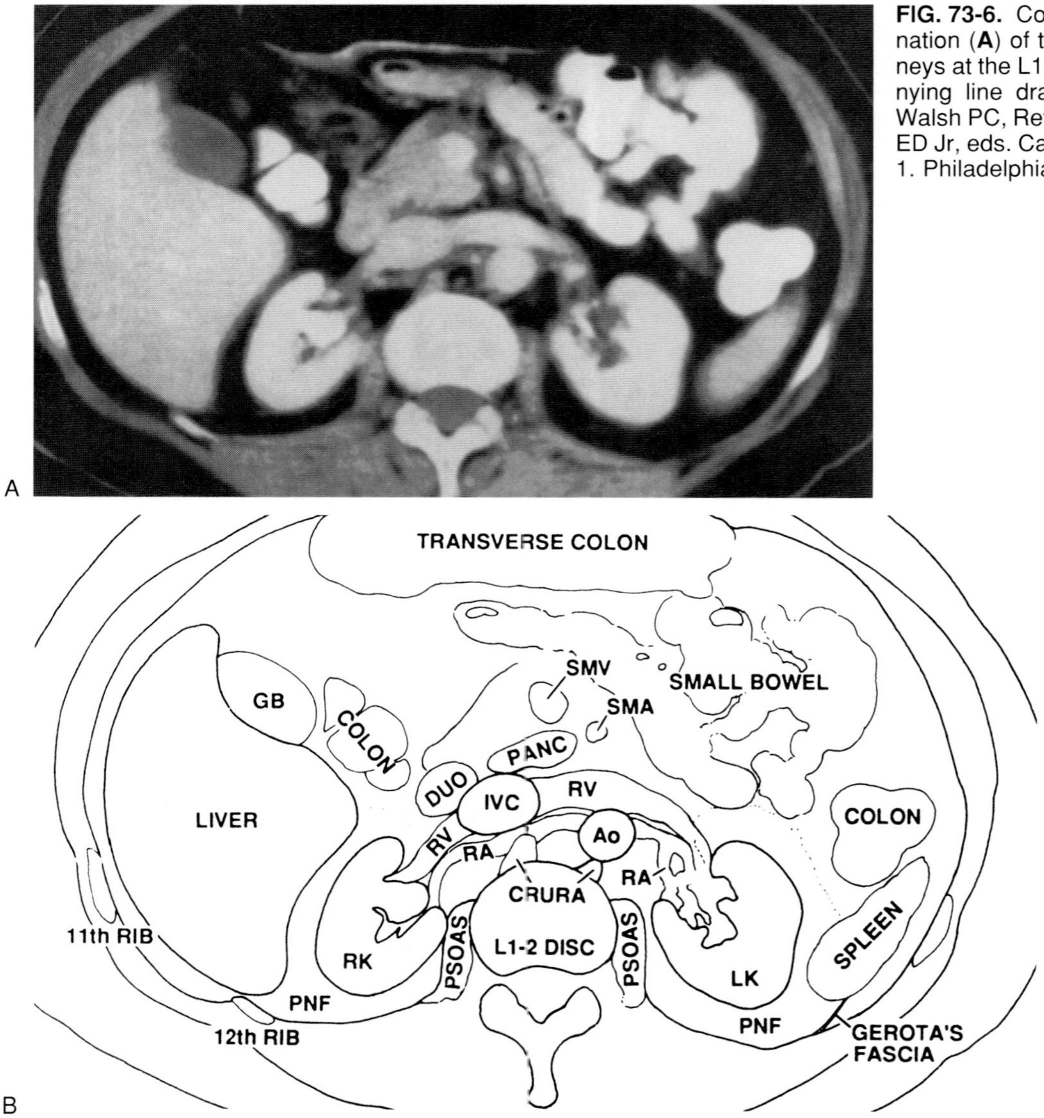

FIG. 73-6. Computed tomographic examination (**A**) of the upper abdomen and kidneys at the L1-L2 disc level with accompanying line drawing (**B**). (Kabalin JN. In: Walsh PC, Retik AB, Stamey TA, Vaughan ED Jr, eds. Campbell's urology, 6th ed, vol 1. Philadelphia, WB Saunders, 1992.)

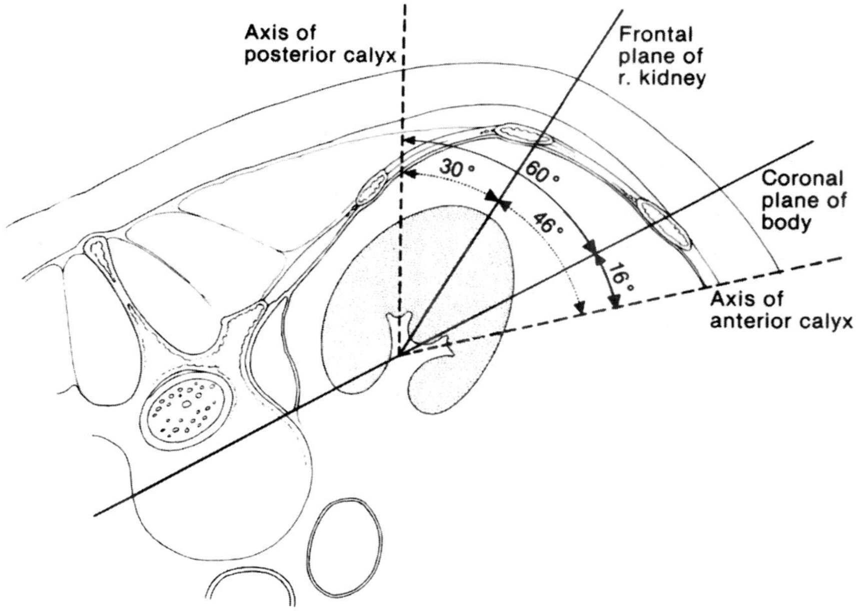

FIG. 73-7. Radiologic orientation for endourology, right kidney. (Hinman F. Atlas of urosurgical anatomy. Philadelphia, WB Saunders, 1993.)

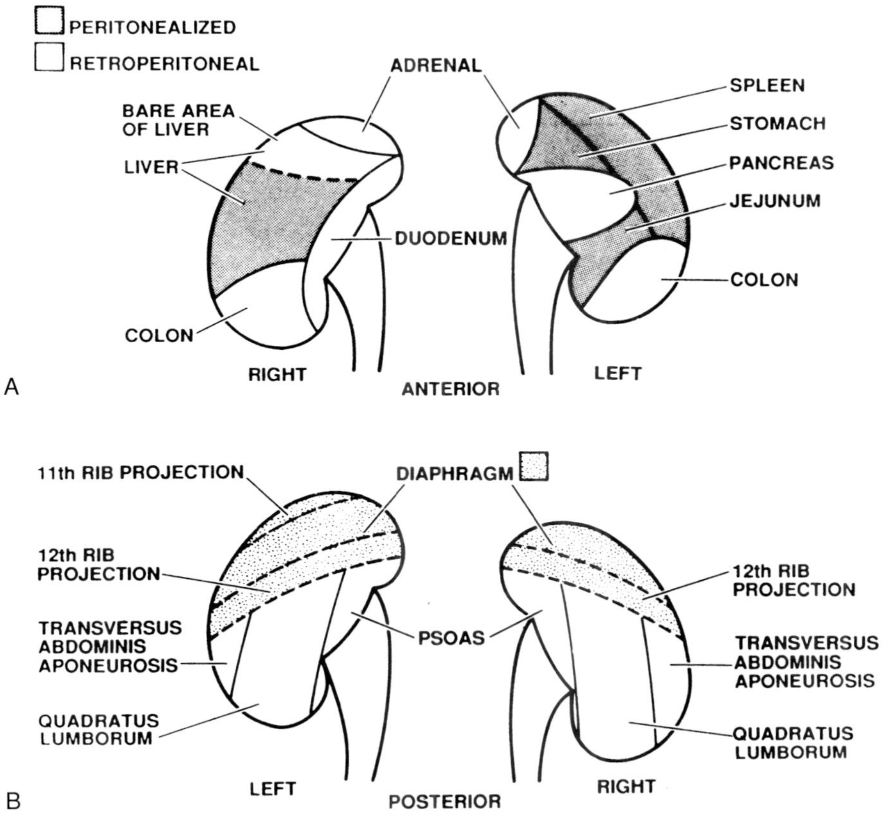

FIG. 73-8. Anatomic relations of the kidneys. (**A**) Anterior relations to abdominal organs. (**B**) Posterior relations to the muscle of posterior body wall and ribs. (Kabalin JN. In: Walsh PC, Retik AB, Stamey TA, Vaughan ED Jr, eds. Campbell's urology, 6th ed, vol 1. Philadelphia, WB Saunders, 1992.)

and is crossed transversely by the splenic artery. The left adrenal gland frequently covers the cranialmost anterior and medial aspects of the kidney. The hilum and medial midportion of the kidney are overlain by the tail of the pancreas, whereas the remainder of the kidney is covered by the descending and transverse colon (splenic flexure) and their mesenteries.

Vasculature

Arteries

The renal arterial vasculature is subject to considerable variation from its origins on the aorta to its intrarenal distribution. The renal arteries are usually single vessels of equal caliber, and, in 75% of cases, they arise from the lateral aorta at the level of the second lumbar vertebral body. Although the right kidney is usually lower than the left, the renal artery may arise at a slightly higher position. Accessory renal arteries, if of significant size, usually arise from the aorta and pass to the cortex of the lower pole of the kidney. Accessory vessels to the upper pole usually arise from the main renal artery. Tumors may cause capsular arteries to achieve added size and significance. These arteries usually originate as separate vessels from the adrenal, renal, and gonadal vessels anywhere from the origin of the renal artery to within the hilum. The renal artery divides into anterior and posterior divisions, with the anterior division supplying the anterior portion of the upper and lower poles or 75% of the kidney. The posterior division supplies the remaining posterior portion. The anterior division gives rise to variable segmental arteries that, as end arteries, supply distinct renal segments: the apical, upper, middle, and lower (Fig. 73-9). Within the parenchyma of the kidney, the segmental renal arteries give rise to interlobular arteries, which course in the renal columns between the renal pyramids, which, in turn, divide into arcuate arteries that cross over the bases of the pyramids within the renal cortex. On transverse section, as in partial nephrectomy, the transected lumina of the arcuate arteries appear as an equally spaced rosette of vessels around the pyramids.

Veins

The renal veins proper drain into the inferior vena cava at approximately the L1-L2 vertebral body level. The renal venous drainage is similar bilaterally in that, within the kidney, the veins intercommunicate, and ligation of an even large branch of a renal vein is of no consequence. In many other respects, however, differences in the right and left renal venous system are considerable. On the right, the renal vein is short, with virtually no tributaries. The left renal vein is long, coursing from the vena cava across the aorta to the left kidney. The most common tributaries are the gonadal and adrenal veins, which frequently enter just opposite each other on the caudal and cranial aspects of the renal vein, respectively. At times, the left renal vein receives the inferior phrenic veins, and commonly just lateral to the aorta on its dorsal aspect, it receives a lumbar vein. Lumbar veins may be large and may form an important collateral vasculature by virtue of their communications with the ascending lumbar veins and lumbar azygos veins. Because of the potential for adequate collateral venous drainage by lumbar, gonadal, and adrenal veins, the left renal vein may be ligated with impunity at its origin, a maneuver intolerable for the right kidney.

Lymphatics

The lymphatics of the renal parenchyma and the renal capsular lymphatics ultimately drain to the same trunk along the renal vasculature. Three or four anterior and posterior lymphatic trunks drain the anterior and posterior aspect of the kidneys, respectively. The lymphatic drainage from the left kidney is primarily to left paraaortic nodes, with communication to paraaortic and retroaortic nodes. The right renal lymphatic trunk

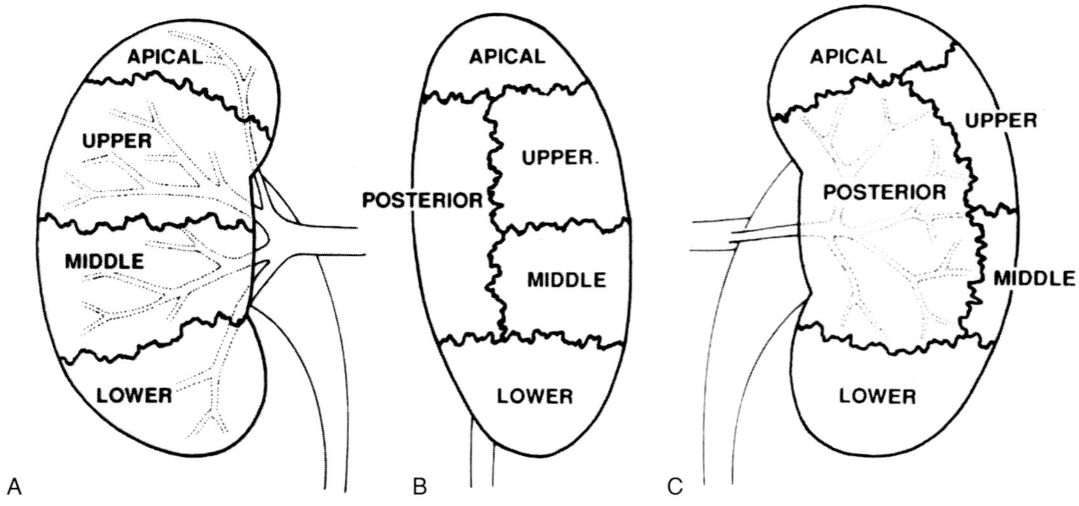

FIG. 73-9. Schematic illustrations of segmental vasculature of kidney. (**A**) Anterior view. (**B**) Lateral view. (**C**) Posterior view. (Kabalin JN. In: Walsh PC, Retik AB, Stamey TA, Vaughan ED Jr, eds. Campbell's urology, 6th ed, vol 1. Philadelphia, WB Saunders, 1992.)

drains to the right paraaortic (intraortocaval) nodes, with communication with anterior and posterior vena caval nodes.

Innervation

Autonomic innervation to the kidney is by the celiac and aortorenal ganglia, with contributions from the second lumbar sympathetic ganglia. Innervation to the celiac and aortorenal ganglia is by the greater, lesser, and least thoracic splanchnic nerves. Ultimately, innervation passes through the renal plexus located over the ventrum of the renal arteries in the renal sinus.

Renal Collecting Structures and Upper Ureter

The renal collecting structures consist of the minor calyces, the infundibula, the major calyces, and the renal pelvis. To allay confusion regarding the use of the term calyx, which means cup, as either major or minor, Hinman has suggested that the collecting structures receiving a papilla be termed a calyceal cup drained by a calyceal neck; the cup and the neck are termed a minor calyx. Consequently, the joining of the two calyceal necks into a common collecting structure is termed an infundibulum, and a total of two or more minor calyces draining into an infundibulum is termed a major calyx. The infundibula of major calyces subsequently drain into the renal pelvis, with the transition to ureter called the ureteropelvic junction.

Relationships

The first portions of the renal collecting structures to be visualized are the renal pelvis and, on occasion, the infundibula, as they emerge from the renal sinus dorsal to the renal vasculature, which courses on its cranial aspect. The ureteropelvic junction is usually located at the lateral aspect of the psoas muscle at the level of the L2-L3 innerspace. The course of the upper ureter parallels the vertebral column, coursing over the ventrum of the psoas muscle. The ureter, encased in the ureteric sheath, a specialization of the intermediate stratum, and the intermediate stratum, itself, is overlain on the right side by the second part of the duodenum cranially and more distally by the mesentery of the ascending colon. On the left side, it is overlain at the renal pelvic level by the tail of the pancreas and caudally by the mesentery of the descending colon. Within the intermediate stratum, each ureter is crossed obliquely and ventrally by the gonadal vessels.

Vasculature

The upper ureter and the renal pelvis are vascularized by arteries from three primary sources: the renal artery, the gonadal artery, and the aorta. The ureteral vasculature, because of anastomoses, gives latitude in ureteral mobilization.

Lymphatics

The lymphatics of the ureter and the renal pelvis follow the renal vasculature, so the renal collecting structures and pelvis drain by lymphatics of the kidney, and that portion of the ureter supplied by the gonadal arteries is like the lymphatic drainage of the testis.

Innervation

The upper ureteral innervation is by autonomic nerves, the superior and middle ureteral nerves, which derive from the renal and aortic plexus, respectively.

Adrenal Anatomy

The adrenal or suprarenal glands are usually described as cadmium yellow, a bright orange yellow distinct from from the surrounding fat. The glands differ from right to left, with the right adrenal triangular, as opposed to the ''palm-leaf'' shape of the left. The glands are thin and are easily fractured, to disclose a brownish medulla. On cross-section, they have a flattened,

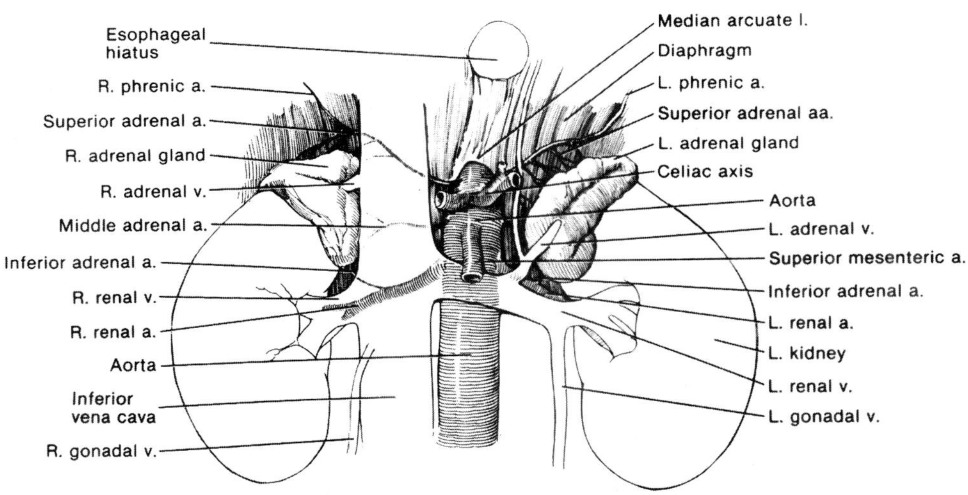

FIG. 73-10. Adrenal vasculature and relationships. (Hinman F. Atlas of urosurgical anatomy. Philadelphia, WB Saunders, 1993.)

triangular appearance, with the apex of the triangle a long posterior ridge termed the alar crest, which slopes laterally on each side to form the alae of the adrenal gland.

Relationships

The adrenal glands are contained within Gerota's fascia and are located just cranial to the kidneys. On the right side, the adrenal gland lies decidedly cranial to the kidney itself, with the base of its triangular body lying alongside the lateral aspect of the inferior vena cava. Ventrally, it is covered by the caudal margin of the right lobe of the liver, and dorsally, it lies on the diaphragm just cranial to the medial lumbocostal arc and medial to the right crus of the diaphragm. On the left, the adrenal gland is more intimately related to the cranial aspect of the kidney; it frequently drapes over the ventral aspect of the cranialmost part of the upper pole. Medially, it lies against the lateral aspect of the aorta. Ventrally, it is overlain by the tail of the pancreas, and dorsally the relationships with the diaphragm are like that of the right adrenal gland.

Vasculature

Arteries

The adrenal glands are vascularized by three suprarenal arteries: superior, middle, and inferior (Fig. 73-10). The arteries are distinctive in that they, in toto, surround the margins of the glands, with sparing of the lateralmost aspects. The superior suprarenal arteries are actually multiple arteries, which arise from the inferior phrenic arteries that course above the superiomedial aspect of the glands. These arteries, in turn, branch further before entering the gland. The middle suprarenal artery arises from the aorta, with multiple branches entering the caudal medial aspects of the gland. The inferior suprarenal artery arising from the renal artery parallels the caudal aspects of the adrenal and gives off multiple branches that enter the gland. Variations of origins of the suprarenal arteries may occur.

Veins

The adrenal glands are drained by a single vein. The right adrenal vein is short, emerging from the midportion of the medial aspect of the gland, and enters the medial dorsolateral aspect of the inferior vena cava almost immediately. The left adrenal gland is generally longer than the right. It emerges from the most caudal and medial aspect of the gland and is joined by the left inferior phrenic vein before entering the cranial aspect of the left renal vein directly opposite the gonadal vein. The left inferior phrenic also drains into the inferior vena cava at the level of the diaphragm just cranial to the left hepatic vein. Thus, the left adrenal vein may be ligated with impunity distal to the entrance of the inferior phrenic vein.

Lymphatics

The adrenal cortex is drained by lymphatics that accompany the arteries, whereas medially, lymphatic drainage is by channels that course along the adrenal veins.

Innervation

Innervation to the adrenal medulla is by the greater thoracic splanchnic nerves, which emerge from the diaphragmatic crura.

BIBLIOGRAPHY

Gillenwater JY, Grayhack JT, Howards SS, Duckett JW, eds. Adult and pediatric urology, 2nd ed, vol 1. St Louis, Mosby-Year Book, 1991.

Hinman F. Atlas of urosurgical anatomy. Philadelphia, WB Saunders, 1993.

Kabalin JN. In: Walsh PC, Retik AB, Stamey TA, Vaughan ED Jr. eds. Campbell's urology, 6th ed, vol 1. Philadelphia, WB Saunders, 1992.

Principles and Practice of Genitourinary Oncology, edited by Derek Raghavan, Howard I. Scher, Steven A. Leibel, and Paul H. Lange. Lippincott-Raven Publishers, Philadelphia, © 1997.

CHAPTER 74

Experimental Models of Renal Cancer

David M. Nanus and Cheryl L. Walker

Advances in molecular biology have improved our understanding of normal genitourinary tract development and have identified numerous genetic events in the multistep process of malignant transformation.[1–6] Many of the alterations associated with neoplasia have been correlated with other biologic characteristics, such as tumor stage or differentiation status, resulting in the generation of genetic models of tumorigenesis.[7] The ideal tumor model in which to assess the genetic defects of a specific tumor type is an in vivo human model of premalignant, malignant, and metastatic cancer. The biologic characteristics of renal cell carcinoma (RCC) preclude the development of a human model based on analyses of tumor specimens because of the following: (1) a premalignant RCC lesion has not been identified; (2) most tumors are locally advanced or metastatic at the time of presentation; and (3) these heterogeneous tumors contain significant amounts of stroma and lymphocytic infiltrate, making molecular analyses imprecise.[8] Thus, molecular studies of RCC have been most often performed using human renal cell culture models in vitro or as xenografts in athymic mice, or using animal models of RCC.

CELL CULTURE MODELS FOR HUMAN RCC

RCC Cell Lines and Xenografts

A human RCC cell line was first established in continuous culture in 1962, and over 100 different characterized RCC cell lines have been derived from both primary and metastatic RCCs.[9–11] The biologic phenotype of cultured RCC cells typically includes a sustained and essentially unlimited growth capacity, a lack of contact inhibition and anchorage dependence, a capacity to form tumors in athymic mice, and an aneuploid karyotype including nonrandom chromosomal abnormalities.[9,10] The antigenic phenotype of RCCs, as determined by monoclonal antibodies generated against cell surface glycoproteins, glycolipids, and blood group antigens of RCCs, provides a series of phenotypic markers that characterize RCCs.[12–14] Many of these monoclonal antibodies also react with the proximal tubule portion of the human nephron and thus confirm earlier studies indicating that more than 90% of RCCs derive from epithelial cells of the proximal tubule.[15,16] Studies have revealed that many of these kidney-related antigens are cell-surface peptidases,[17–19] the primary function of which in the brush border of kidney proximal tubule cells is to hydrolyze peptides to recycle or excrete amino acids,[20] but which may also regulate autocrine and paracrine signals by proteolytic inactivation of specific mitogenic peptides.[21,22]

Established RCC cell lines have frequently been analyzed for molecular defects (see Chap. 75). Their greatest utility has been to screen combinations of chemotherapeutic and biologic agents for antiproliferative activity, however.[23–26] Short-term cultures of renal cancer cells derived from fresh tumor specimens have similarly been used to screen drugs,[27] but inhibitory effects in vitro have not been shown to predict a response in vivo (i.e., in patients). RCC xenografts in athymic mice in which the tumor cells are injected into the flank of the animal have also been used to determine drug sensitivities and their potential clinical applicability.[25,28,29] These studies are designed to simulate systemic administration of drug. Naito and Fidler and their colleagues noted that RCC cells implanted into murine organs other than the kidney do not metastasize,[30,31] and these investigators developed a model of orthotopic injection of RCC cells directly into renal subcapsule.[32] This model has also been used to study the antitumor and antimetastatic activity of various cytokines and other agents and to study the processes of invasion and metastases (see Chap. 2).[33]

Gene Therapy

Technologic advances in delivering genes into mammalian cells have facilitated studies into the feasibility of introducing cytokine genes into human tumor cells as a form of antitumor therapy.[34] That immunologic therapies can induce tumor regression in advanced RCC has made RCC an attractive model in which to explore the effects of gene transfer. Genes expressing interleukin-2, interferon alpha, and interferon gamma have been successfully introduced into RCC cell lines.[35,36] Local tumor formation after subcutaneous injection into athymic mice of tumor cells expressing these cytokine proteins was not affected by interferon gamma secretion, but it was significantly inhibited by release of interleukin-2 and interferon alpha.[35,36] Cytokine genes have also been introduced into cultured tumor cells derived from primary nephrectomy specimens (see Chap. 10).[37]

In Vitro Transformation

The ability to obtain short-term cultures of human kidney cells from fresh nephrectomy specimens allows a direct comparison of the normal and malignant renal phenotypes,[10] and it provides an opportunity to study transformation-related events in vitro.[38] Normal human kidney cells exhibit a biologic phenotype characteristic of other short-term cultures of nonmalignant human epithelial cells. In culture, the normal kidney cell shows the following characteristics: (1) a limited proliferative capacity, which is marked by rapid growth up to passage 2, then followed by a sharp decline in growth capacity and eventual senescence by passage 4 or 5 (i.e., by eight to ten generations); (2) contact inhibition on confluence; (3) anchorage-dependent growth; (4) an inability to form tumors on injection into athymic mice; (5) a diploid karyotype; and (6) the absence of nonrandom chromosomal abnormalities. In addition, as shown by immunophenotyping with RCC-generated monoclonal antibodies, over 90% of cultured normal human kidney cells are derived from the proximal tubule derivation and represent the true progenitor cell of RCCs.[39] Therefore, the in vitro human renal cell culture system has been used to study the effects of carcinogens and specific genes on the normal renal cell phenotype.

The introduction of the SV40 DNA tumor virus into normal human kidney cells results in an altered morphology and increased life span, but not in neoplastic transformation.[38,40] Infected cells enter a crisis phase, which is usually followed by senescence and cell death.[40] Infrequently, some cells survive this phase to yield an immortal but still nontumorigenic human kidney cell line.[40] Similarly, immortalized, nontumorigenic human kidney cells have been obtained by insertion of the human papilloma virus 16 *E6/E7* genes,[41] as well as by treatment with nickel.[42] Complete neoplastic transformation can be achieved in these immortalized, nontumorigenic human cells by introducing a second transforming oncogene such as *HRAS* (formerly known as Ha-ras).[41,42] Single-step transformation of proximal tubules cells is rare, but it has been achieved using a *RAS* (formerly known as v-ras) or *SRC* (formerly known as v-src) oncogene.[43,44] These transformed cells possess a characteristic RCC phenotype, including altered morphology, increased growth capacity, loss of contact inhibition, tumorigenicity, and nonrandom chromosomal defects. Furthermore, cytogenetic analysis of one cell line revealed a deletion of chromosome 3p14-21,[44] the most common nonrandom chromosomal abnormality observed in human RCC.[45] Thus, the in vitro proximal tubule cell model provides a valuable experimental system by which to analyze the effects of oncogenes on the normal functioning of the proximal tubule cell, and it may provide clues to the role of these genes in the pathogenesis of RCC.

ANIMAL MODELS OF RCC

As the utility of immunologic agents such as interferons and interleukins in the treatment of RCC increased (see Chap. 84), investigators realized that studying the effects of cytokines on a human tumor in an immunosuppressed rodent does not take into consideration the indirect, immune-mediated antitumor effects of these agents on RCC cells. Furthermore, xenograft models do not facilitate investigations into the early genetic events in renal carcinogenesis. In contrast, high-incidence animal tumor models offer many opportunities for investigational studies into cancer therapeutics and prevention as well as mechanistic studies to explore the underlying causes of tumor development. With many animal models, researchers can obtain tumors at all stages of development, from early preneoplastic lesions to advanced-stage disease. This easy access allows investigators to determine when during the process of tumor development specific molecular alterations or histologic characteristics first appear. The ability to stage relevant tumor associated changes can facilitate the process of identifying targets for preventive and therapeutic strategies. Both normal kidney and tumor-derived cells can be readily established from rodents in tissue culture, thereby making possible in vitro studies with both normal and transformed cells. Moreover, preclinical studies to identify therapeutic agents in animal models have been valuable in developing many chemotherapeutic agents in use today, as well as facilitating novel methods of gene therapy.

An ideal renal tumor model should arise spontaneously and should have the histologic characteristics of an adenocarcinoma, a predictable growth rate, the capacity to metastasize, and the ability to grow and metastasize without hormonal dependence, as is the case in the majority of human renal cancers.[46] For RCC, both spontaneous and inducible models of tumor development fulfill most or all of these criteria. Spontaneous kidney tumors develop with a high frequency in Eker rats and Long-Evans ''cinnamon'' rats, whereas chemical carcinogens and estrogens have been used to induce RCC in rats and hamsters. Experimentally induced mouse tumor models can be used to reproducibly generate tumor material in syngeneic hosts. One important caveat for using data generated from animal models is how closely tumor development in a particular model system recapitulates the human disease. One way for investigators to determine the relevance of an animal model to its cognate human tumor is to identify molecular alterations present in the animal tumor and to compare this information with similar data available for the human disease. If the pathways to tumor development in the two species are the same, then this resemblance would be reflected in a degree of similarity between molecular alterations in the tumors of both species. Such information can be obtained from cytogenetic data on specific chromosome alterations present in tumor cells, as well as from molecular data on mutations in relevant genes such as oncogenes and tumor suppressor genes. In the examples detailed later, in addition to general data on the animal model, information on the relationship of each specific animal model with human RCC is also discussed (Table 74-1).

Eker Rat

The best characterized animal model for RCC is the Eker rat model in which a line of Long-Evans rats carries a genetic alteration in a tumor susceptibility gene, resulting in a predisposition for the development of RCC.[47] Spontaneous RCC develops in 100% of animals carrying one defective copy of this gene, whereas rats that inherit two normal alleles show no increase in these tumors over the background incidence in Long-Evans rats,

TABLE 74-1. *Human and experimental animal models of renal cell carcinoma*

	Cell type of origin	Inducing agent	Characteristic cytogenetic abnormalities	Gene alterations
Human	Proximal tubule epithelial cells	Spontaneous	Deletion 3p (nonpapillary) Duplication 7,17 (papillary)	von Hippel-Lindau (*VHL*) tumor suppressor gene frequently mutated *P53* infrequent/late *RAS* infrequent *TGFA* overexpressed
Eker rat	Proximal tubule epithelial cells	Spontaneous Chemical carcinogens	Monosomy 5 Deletion 6q24	*P53* infrequent *RAS* infrequent *TGFA* overexpressed Tsc–2 tumor suppressor gene mutated
Syrian hamster	Interstitial stem cell	Estrogens	Unknown	Unknown

which is less than 0.5%.[48] Inheritance of two mutant alleles is lethal, resulting in death of affected embryos early in gestation.[49,50] The requirement for at least one normal allele of this gene for normal development suggests that the affected gene plays an important role in embryonic as well as tumor development.

The cell type of origin of RCC in the Eker rat is the same as in human tumors: epithelial cells of the proximal tubule.[51] Renal tumors develop in adult rats carrying the Eker mutation by 12 months of age.[51] Tumors are bilateral and multifocal, as would be expected in a hereditary syndrome in which the susceptibility mutation occurs in the germ line and is thus present in all cells of the kidney. The cytologic, architectural, and histologic aspects of these tumors are similar to their human counterparts, being nonpapillary, solid, or cystic tumors arising in the renal cortex.[51] One significant difference in the rat tumors is a lack of glycogen accumulation in the tumor cells, resulting in a chromophilic appearance, rather than the clear cell histologic pattern typically seen in human tumors. Tumors progress from early preneoplastic lesions to adenomas and malignant carcinomas that are locally invasive, but they do not appear to metastasize to distant sites.[52] The lack of distant metastases is typical of other types of rat renal epithelial tumors that occur sporadically in other strains or that are induced by carcinogens (J. Everitt, personal communication, July, 1995), a finding suggesting that species-specific differences between rats and humans can modulate the biology of end-stage renal disease.

The gene responsible for inherited predisposition to tumor development in the Eker rat has been cloned.[53] The Eker mutation resides in the rat homologue of the human tuberous sclerosis (*TSC*) gene,[54] which is located on rat chromosome 10.[53] In humans, tuberous sclerosis is inherited in an autosomal dominant fashion and predisposes patients to several types of lesions including renal hamartomas and RCCs.[55] In addition to the predisposing tumor susceptibility gene, additional tumor suppressor genes appear to be involved in tumor development and progression in the rat model, as evidenced by specific loss of all or portions of rat chromosomes 4, 5, and 6 in Eker rat tumors and tumor-derived cell lines.[56] The von Hippel-Lindau tumor suppressor gene, known to be mutated or deleted in both hereditary and spontaneous human RCC, is not mutated in Eker rat tumors.[56a] Alterations in other genes, such as *P53* and *RAS* oncogenes, are only infrequently found in Eker rat tumors and cell lines, a finding similar to observations in human RCC.[57,58] In addition, Eker rat tumors overexpress transforming growth factor alpha (TGF-α), which is also overexpressed in human RCC.[59]

Thus, at the molecular level, tumor development in the Eker rat model has many similarities to the human disease (see Table 74-1). This model may therefore be particularly useful for mechanistic and therapeutic studies of primary RCC. One significant limitation however, appears to be the lack of distant metastases in this animal model, thus limiting its usefulness in studies on this aspect of RCC.

LEC Rat

In addition to the Eker rat, another line of Long-Evans rats develops spontaneous RCC. The LEC Long-Evans cinnamon rat, named for its cinnamon coat color, has historically been used as a model for hereditary hepatitis.[60] More recently, however, investigators reported that these animals develop spontaneous RCC between 1 and 2 years of age.[61] The underlying defect responsible for the development of hepatitis, hepatocellular carcinoma, and RCC is not known, but these animals do exhibit copper toxicity because of an abnormal accumulation of this metal in several organs. Thus, the development of RCC in these animals may possibly result from the systemic effects of copper accumulation.

Renca

The Renca adenocarcinoma of BALB/c mice arose spontaneously and is characterized by intrarenal growth in syngeneic mice and spontaneous metastases from the intrarenal implant to regional lymph nodes, lung, liver, spleen, and other organs.[62,63] Immunogenicity in this model is low, thereby allowing the study of the immune system in response to transplanted Renca cells.[64,65] Accordingly, the Renca model has been primarily used to study the antitumor and immunologic activity of chemotherapeutic and biologic agents and to determine their potential usefulness in the treatment of human RCC. In this model, the primary tumor is implanted in the orthotopic site of the kidney, and animals can be treated at advanced growth stages, before and after nephrectomy. Antitumor agents studied in this model include cyclophosphamide, doxorubicin, cytokine-inducing synthetic flavonoid compounds,[66,67] interleukin-2,[68] interferons,[69] and interleukin-1.[70] Most cytokines are ineffective as single agents, whereas combinations are more likely to cause significant tumor regression. The Renca model has also facilitated immunologic and molecular analyses of the immune system in response to tumor implantation. For example, T cells from mice bearing Renca exhibit a decrease in the phosphorylation of nuclear transcription factors necessary for T-cell activation.[71] A similar defect has been observed in tumor-infiltrating T cells from human RCC.[72] Renca can also help to decipher the mechanism of a specific biologic agent, as shown in studies with murine interleukin-12, which demonstrated complete disappearance of tumor in animals with established Renca metastases and indicated that the antitumor effect of interleukin-12 is mediated through T cells.[73] One disadvantage of the Renca model is that the tumors are all propagated from a single BALB/c murine tumor. Whether this lineage is representative of RCC in general or whether the spectrum of molecular alterations present in this one cell line is similar to that observed in human RCC has yet to be established.

Carcinogen-induced Tumors

Many types of chemical carcinogens have produced tumors in the kidneys of experimental animals. As reviewed by Hard[74] and, more recently, by Rangel and Pontes,[75] experimental protocols are available for inducing renal epithelial cancers, mesenchymal tumors, and embryonic nephroblastomas. The epithelial tumors include cortical adenomas, adenocarcinomas and carcinomas, and renal pelvic tumors such as papillomas, transitional cell carcinomas, and squamous cell carcinomas.[76] Compounds as diverse as nitrosoamines, polycyclic hydrocarbons, mycotoxins, heavy metals, and alkyl halides[75,76] can be used to induce renal tumors with a high incidence, in some cases up to 100%. The cell type of origin for the induced tumors is determined by the specific carcinogen, with epithelial tumors induced in both the proximal and distal segments of the nephron by several carcinogens.[76–78] Site-specific induction of tumors presumably reflects the cell type within the nephron in which the carcinogen is metabolized and activated.

Single-dose regimens as well as those requiring repeated or continuous carcinogen exposure have been described. In some cases, such as with the carcinogen dimethylnitrosamine (DMN), depending on the age of the animal at the time of administration, a single carcinogenic dose can induce mesenchymal (immature rats) or epithelial tumors (adult rats).[74] In contrast to the RCCs that arise spontaneously in the Eker rat model, DMN-induced tumors have been reported to metastasize with a high frequency.[79] This phenomenon may be due to a fundamental difference in the biology of DMN-induced versus spontaneous tumors, or it may simply mean that induction in this model occurs early in the animal's life cycle and may allow tumors sufficient time to acquire additional genetic alterations required for metastatic potential.

Although the protocols for inducing renal tumors with chemical carcinogens are well described, little is known regarding the molecular alterations induced in the resulting tumor cells. Neither cytogenetic nor molecular data have been analyzed in any systematic way to evaluate the degree of similarity between carcinogen-induced rodent tumors and their human counterparts. Although investigators reported that carcinogen-induced rat renal epithelial tumors and mesenchymal tumors had a high frequency of *P53* mutations,[80] this finding was later attributed to the presence of the rat *P53* pseudogene, which confounded the sequencing analysis. We now know, at least for DMN, that *P53* alterations do not occur with any significant frequency in the carcinogen-induced tumors.[58]

Virus-induced Renal Tumors

A virally induced renal tumor occurs in the leopard frog *Rana pipiens*. First described in 1934 by Lucké,[81] these lesions are generally referred to as Lucké tumors. These tumors are caused by the herpes-like Lucké tumor virus (LTV) and arise from proximal tubule cells of infected animals,[82] although other portions of the nephron may become infected as well.[83] Lucké tumors occur in the wild in the northern United States and Canada and affect a significant proportion (3% to 9%) of frogs in these regions. Viral transmission of the disease occurs in the spring, when virus-infected cells lyse and virus is released into the environment, presumably infecting frog embryos at that time.[84] The number of adult frogs carrying this virus has been in decline, and in a 1977 collection of frogs, none of 685 frogs harvested carried tumors.[85]

Syrian Hamster Model

In male Syrian hamsters, administration of estrogens such as diethylstilbestrol (DES) induces renal tumors with high frequency.[86–88] This model has been used as a paradigm for hormonally induced cancers for nearly half a century. The tumors display diverse histologic appearances and express markers consistent with both epithelial and mesenchymal origins. Accordingly, the cell type of origin of these tumors has been the subject of controversy, although more recent data indicate that these tumors arise from an interstitial stem cell that expresses estrogen receptors.[89–93] A transplantable cell line derived from these tumors produces tumors in syngeneic animals within 2 to 3 weeks and requires estrogen supplementation for growth.[94] Estrogen withdrawal results in an increase in apoptosis and regression of tumors produced by this cell line, a finding suggesting that modulation of apoptosis is one of the mechanisms by which estrogens induce the growth of renal tumors in this animal model.[95] Although the estrogen-induced renal tumor model has given many valuable insights into mechanisms of hormonal carcinogenesis, the cell type of origin, the lack of data on relevant molecular alterations that occur during tumor development, and the lack of evidence for a role of estrogens in the development of human RCC limit the utility of this model for studies relating to the human disease.

Transgenic Mice

Transgenic mice carrying viral oncogenes have been reported to develop renal lesions. Mice carrying the *SV40* early region as a transgene develop polycystic kidneys and focal neoplasia.[96] The human BK papovavirus T antigen carried as a transgene also leads to the development of renal lesions in transgenic mice.[97] These mice exhibit thymic abnormalities and unilateral or bilateral kidney tumors. Tumors are adenocarcinomas and can become large.

Transgenic animals in which the expression of exogenous trangenes have been targeted to the kidney have also been described. Using a gamma-glutamyltranspeptidase (GGT) promoter specific for the proximal tubule cells of the kidney,[98] the *RAS* oncogene has been targeted to these cells.[99] Expression of the transgene resulted in renal hyperplasia and polycystic kidneys in affected animals. The absence of frank renal neoplasms in these mice is consistent with the lack of involvement of *RAS* in the genesis of RCC in rodents and humans. Other studies to generate knockout mice in which the *VHL* tumor suppressor gene has been inactivated are in progress in several laboratories, including those that originally cloned this gene, but data on the effects of loss of function of this gene have not been generated.

In Vitro Transformation Systems

In vitro transformation of rodent kidney epithelial cells has been described in at least two model systems. The first, developed by Walker and Ginsler, uses primary rat kidney epithelial (RTE) cells in a quantitative assay to measure transformation induced by chemical carcinogens.[100] In this assay, RTE cells are plated at clonal density and are exposed to carcinogen 24 hours after plating. Four to 6 weeks later, untreated control cultures of cells have senesced and have sloughed off the dish, whereas in carcinogen-exposed dishes, proliferating foci of transformed cells can be identified. These foci give rise to cells with indefinite proliferative capacity (immortal), and these cell lines have the ability to produce tumors when they are injected into nude mice.[100] Cells transformed in this assay have characteristics similar to those isolated from spontaneous rat tumors such as loss of chromosome 5 and 6 and low-frequency *P53* mutations, (C. Walker, unpublished observations, August, 1995), a finding suggesting that in vitro transformation may be a good method for recapitulating the events occurring during transformation of kidney epithelial cells in vivo.

The second transformation model uses SV40-transformed rat kidney epithelial cells. Immortal cell lines have been isolated from clones of rat proximal tubule epithelial cells transfected with the SV40 large T antigen[101] that exhibit altered patterns of growth factor expression. Whereas normal kidney epithelial cells express fibroblast growth factor-1 (FGF-1; acidic FGF), expression of this growth factor is suppressed in the SV40-transformed cells. These cells do express FGF-3 and vascular-endothelial growth factor, which act as autocrine growth factors in the transformed cell lines.[102] These cell lines may therefore serve as useful models for studying growth factors that play a role in transformation of kidney epithelial cells.

CONCLUSIONS

Both animal and human models of RCC provide experimental systems in which to investigate the genetic alterations in the various stages of human RCC. Moreover, these models provide valuable reagents with which to determine the role of specific genes in the pathogenesis of RCC and to test the efficacy of individual biologic response modifiers alone or in combination with chemotherapeutic drugs to mediate antitumor responses.

REFERENCES

1. Chaganti RS, Rogriguez E, Bosl GJ. Cytogenetics of male germ-cell tumros. Urol Clin North Am 1993;20:55.
2. Coffey DS. The molecular biology of the prostate. In: Lepor H, Lawson RK, eds. Prostate diseases. Philadelphia, WB Saunders, 1993.
3. Linehan WM, Gnarra JR, Lerman MI, Latif F, Zbar B. Genetic basis of renal cell cancer. Important Adv Oncol 1993;47.
4. Reznikoff CA, Kao C, Messing EM, Newton M, Swaminathan S. A molecular genetic model of human bladder carcinogenesis. Semin Cancer Biol 1993;4:143.
5. Cordon-Cardo C, Dalbagni G, Sarkis AS, Reuter VE. Genetic alterations associated with bladder cancer. Important Adv Oncol 1994;71.
6. Coppes MJ, Haber D, Grundy PE. Genetic events in the development of Wilms' tumor. N Eng J Med 1994;331:586.
7. Fearon ER, Vogelstein B. A genetic model for colorectal tumorigenesis. Cell 1990;61:759.
8. Linehan M, Miller E, Anglard P, Merino M, Zbar B. Improved detection of allele loss in renal cell carcinomas after removal of leukocytes by immunologic selection. J Natl Cancer Inst 1989;81:287.
9. Ebert T, Bander NH. Kidney-derived cell lines. Semin Urol 1989;7:247.
10. Ebert T, Bander NH, Finstad CL, Ramsawak RD, Old LJ. Establishment and characterization of human renal cancer and normal kidney cell lines. Cancer Res 1990;50:5531.
11. Anglard P, Trahan E, Liu, et al. Molecular and cellular characterization of human renal cell carcinoma cell lines. Cancer Res 1992;52:348.
12. Finstad CL, Cordon Cardo C, Bander NH, Whitmore WF, Melamed MR, Old LJ. Specificity analysis of mouse monoclonal antibodies defining cell surface antigens of human renal cancer. Proc Natl Acad Sci USA 1985;82:2955.
13. Cordon Cardo C, Reuter VE, Finstad CL, et al. Blood group-related antigens in human kidney: modulation of Lewis determinants in renal cell carcinoma. Cancer Res 1989;49:212.
14. Vessella RL, Moon TD, Chiou RK, et al. Monoclonal antibodies to human renal cell carcinoma: recognition of shared and restricted tissue antigens. Cancer Res 1985;45:6131.
15. Bander NH, Cordon Cardo C, Finstad CL, et al. Immunohistologic dissection of the human kidney using monoclonal antibodies. J Urol 1985;133:502.
16. Cordon Cardo C, Finstad CL, Bander NH, Melamed MR. Immunoanatomic distribution of cytostructural and tissue-associated antigens in the human urinary tract. Am J Pathol 1987;126:269.
17. Look AT, Ashmun RA, Shapiro LH, Peiper SC. Human myeloid plasma membrane glycoprotein CD13 (gp150) is identical to aminopeptidase N. J Clin Invest 1989;83:1299.
18. Nanus DM, Engelstein D, Gastl GA, et al. Molecular cloning of the human kidney differentiation antigen gp160: human aminopeptidase A. Proc Natl Acad Sci USA 1993;90:7069.
19. Morrison ME, Vijayasaradhi S, Engelstein D, Albino AP, Houghton AH. A marker for neoplastic progression of human melanocytes is a cell surface ectopeptidase. J Exp Med 1993;177:1135.
20. Danielsen EM, Noren O, Sjostrom H, Ingram J, Kenny AJ. Proteins of the kidney microvillar membrane. Biochem J 1980;189:591.
21. Ahmad S, Ward PE. Role of aminopeptidase activity in the regulation of the pressor activity of circulating angiotensins. J Pharmacol Exp Ther 1989;252:643.
22. Kenny AJ, O'Hare MJ, Gusterson BA. Cell-surface peptidases as modulators of growth and differentiation. Lancet 1989;2:785.
23. Lai T, Ferro MA, Kaisary AV, Smith PJ, Symes MO. Testing the chemosensitivity of renal carcinoma in vitro. Br J Urol 1989;64:25.
24. Nygren P, Larsson R. Differential in vitro sensitivity of human tumor and normal cells to chemotherapeutic agents and resistance modulators. Int J Cancer 1991;48:598.
25. Nanus DM, Pfeffer LM, Bander NH, Bahri S, Albino AP. Antiproliferative and antitumor effects of alpha interferon in renal cell carcinomas: correlation with the expression of a kidney associated differentiation glycoprotein. Cancer Res 1990;50:4190.
26. Safrit JT, Belldegrun A, Bonavida B. Sensitivity of human renal cell carcinoma lines to TNF, adriamycin, and combinations: role of TNF mRNA induction in overcoming resistance. J Urol 1993;149:1202.
27. Mickisch G, Fajta S, Keilhauer G, Schlick E, Tschada R, Alken P.

Chemosensitivity testing of primary human renal cell carcinoma by a tetrazolium based microculture assay. Urol Res 1990;18:131.
28. Beniers AJ, Peelen WP, Hendriks BT, Schalken JA, Romijn JC, Debruyne FM. In vitro antiproliferative efficacy of interferon-alpha, -gamma and tumor necrosis factor on two human renal tumor xenografts. Urol Res 1988;16:309.
29. Shirahama T, Kayajima T, Ohi Y. The antitumor effects of IFN-beta against human renal cell carcinoma in athymic nude mice. In Vivo 1989;3:345.
30. Naito S, von Eschenbach AC, Giavazzi R, Fidler IJ. Growth and metastases of tumor cells isolated from a human renal cell carcinoma implanted into different organs of nude mice. Cancer Res 1986;46: 4109.
31. Naito S, yon Eschenbach AC, Fidler IJ. Different growth pattern and biologic behavior of human renal cell carcinoma implanted into different organs of nude mice. J Natl Cancer Inst 1987;78:377.
32. Fidler IJ, Naito S, Pathak S. Orthotopic implantation is essential for the selection, growth, and metastasis of human renal cell cancer in nude mice. Cancer Metastasis Rev 1990;9:149.
33. Fidler IJ. The biology of renal cancer metastasis. Semin Urol 1992; 10:3.
34. Mulligan RC. The basic science of gene therapy. Science 1993;260: 926.
35. Gastl G, Finstad CL, Guarini A, et al. Retroviral vector-mediated lymphokine gene transfer into humna renal cancer cells. Cancer Res 1992;52:6229.
36. Belldegrun A, Tso CL, Sakata T, et al. Human renal carcinoma line transfected with interleukin-2 and/or interferon alpha gene(s): implications for live cancer vaccines. J Natl Cancer Inst 1993;85:207.
37. Schendel DJ, Gansbacher B. Tumor-specific lysis of human renal cell carcinomas by tumor-infiltrating lymphocytes: modulation of recognition through retroviral transduction of tumor cells with interleukin 2 complementary DNA and exogenous alpha interferon treatment. Cancer Res 1993;53:4020.
38. Nanus DM, Albino AP. Oncogene-induced transformation of human kidney proximal tubule cells. In: Klein EA, Bukowski RM, Finke JH, eds. Renal cell carcinoma: immunotherapy and cellular biology. New York, Marcel Dekker, 1993:53.
39. Bander NH. Monoclonal antibodies in urologic oncology. Cancer 1987;60:658.
40. Abcouwer S, Robinson PS, Goochee CF, Crow MT. Generation of human embryonic kidney cells with extended in vitro life span through viral oncogene transfection. Biotechnology 1989;7:939.
41. Ryan MJ, Johnson G, Kirk J, Fuerstenberg SM, Zager RA, Torok-Storb B. HK-2: an immortalized proximal tubule epithelial cell line from normal adult human kidney. Kidney Int 1994;45:48.
42. Haugen A, Ryberg D, Hansteen IL, Amstad P. Neoplastic transformation of a human kidney epithelial cell line transfected with v-Ha-ras oncogene. Int J Cancer 1990;3:572.
43. Nanus DM, Ebrahim SA, Bander NH, et al. Transformation of human kidney proximal tubule cells by ras-containing retroviruses. Implications for tumor progression. J Exp Med 1989;169:953.
44. Nanus DM, Lynch SA, Rao PH, Anderson SM, Jhanwar SC, Albino AP. Transformation of human kidney proximal tubule cells by a src-containing retrovirus. Oncogene 1991;6:2105.
45. Presti JC, Jr., Rao PH, Chen Q, et al. Histopathologic, cytogenetic, and molecular characterization of renal cortical tumors. Cancer Res 1991;51:1544.
46. Rangel MC, Pontes E. Animal models of renal cell carcinoma. Semin Urol 1989;7:237.
47. Eker R, Mossige J. A dominant gene for renal adenomas in the rat. Nature 1961;189:858.
48. Solleveld HA, Boorman GA. Spontaneous renal lesions in five rat strains. Toxicol Pathol 1986;14:168.
49. Eker R, Mossige J, Johannessen JV, Aars H. Hereditary renal adenomas and adenocarcinomas in rats. Diagn Histopathol 1981;4:99.
50. Hino O, Klein-Szanto AJP, Freed JJ, et al. Spontaneous and radiation-induced renal tumors in the Eker rat model of dominantly inherited cancer. Proc Natl Acad Sci USA 1993;90:327.
51. Everitt J, Goldsworthy T, Wolf D, Walker C. Hereditary renal cell carcinoma in the Eker rat: a rodent familial cancer syndrome. J Urol 1992;148:1932.
52. Everitt J, Walker C, Goldsworthy T, Wolf D. Altered expression of transforming growth factor-alpha is an early event in renal cell tumor development (submitted).
53. Yueng RS, Xiao G-H, Jin F, Lee W-C, Testa JR, Knudson AG. Predisposition to renal carcinoma in the Eker rat is determined by germline mutation of the tuberous sclerosis 2(TSC2) gene. Proc Natl Acad Sci 1994;91:11413.
54. The European Chromosome 16 Tuberous Sclerosis Consortium. Identification and characterization of the tuberous sclerosis gene on chromosome 16. Cell 1993;75:1305.
55. Gomez MR. Tuberous sclerosis, 2nd ed. New York, Raven Press, 1988.
56. Funaki K, Everitt J, Oshimura M, Freed JJ, Knudson AG, Walker C. Hereditary renal cell carcinoma in the rat associated with nonrandom loss of chromosomes 5 and 6. Cancer Res 1991;51:4415.
56a. Walker C, Ahn Y-T, Everitt J, Yuan X. Renal cell carcinoma development in the rat independent of alterations at the VHL gene locus. Mol Carcinog 1996;15:154.
57. Recio L, Lane SC, Ginsler J, Walker C. Analysis of ras DNA sequences in rat renal cell carcinoma. Mol Carcinog 1991;4:350.
58. Horesovsky G, Recio L, Everitt J, Goldsworthy T, Wolf D, Walker C. p53 status in spontaneous and dimethylnitrosamine-induced renal cell tumors from rats. Mol Carcinog 1995;12:236.
59. Walker C, Everitt J, Freed JJ, Knudson AG, Whiteley LO. Altered expression of transforming growth factor-alpha in hereditary rat renal cell carcinoma. Cancer Res 1991;51:2973.
60. Sawaki M, Enomoto K, Takahashi H, Nakajima Y, Mori M. Phenotype of preneoplastic and neoplastic liver lesions during spontaneous liver carcinogenesis of LEC rats. Carcinogenesis 1990;11:1857.
61. Izumi K, Kitaura K, Chone Y, et al. Spontaneous renal cell tumors in Long-Evans Cinnamon rats. Jpn J Cancer Res 1994;85:563.
62. Murphy GP, Hrushevsky WJ. A murine renal cell carcinoma. J Natl Cancer Inst 1973;50:1013.
63. Salup R, Herberman RB, Wiltrout RH. Role of natural killer activity in development of spontaneous metastases in urine renal cancer. J Urol 1985;134:1236.
64. Salup RR, Herberman RB, Wiltrout RH. Role of natural killer activity in development of spontaneous metastases in murine renal cancer. J Urol 1985;6:1236.
65. Salup RR, Sicker DC, Ballou BT, Flack CE, Wolmark N, Hakala TR. Improved lymphocyte cytotoxicity against murine renal cell carcinoma. J Urol 1992;2:491.
66. Mace KF, Hornun RL, Wiltrout RH, Young HA. Correlation between in vivo induction of cytokine gene expression by flavone acetic acid and strict dose dependency and therapeutic efficacy against murine renal cancer. Cancer Res 1990;6:1742.
67. Hornung RL, Back TC, Zaharko DS, Urba WJ, Longo DL, Wiltrout RH. Augmentation of natural killer activity, induction of IFN and development tumor immunity during the successful treatment of established murine renal cancer using flavone acetic acid and IL-2. J Immunol 1988;10:3671.
68. Oya M. Antitumor effect of interleukin-2 entrapped in liposomes on murine renal cell carcinoma. Keio J Med 1994;1:37.
69. Sayer TJ, Wiltrout TA, McCormick K, Husted C, Wiltrout RH. Antitumor effects of alpha-interferon and gamma-interferon on a murine renal cancer (Renca) in vitro and in vivo. Cancer Res 1990;17:5414.
70. Futami H, Jansen R, MacPhee MJ, et al. Chemoprotective effects of recombinant human IL-1 alpha in cyclophosphamide-treated normal and tumor-bearing mice: protection from acute toxicity, hematologyic effects, development of late mortality, and enhanced therapeutic efficacy. J Immunol 1990;12:4121.
71. Ghosh P, Sica A, Young HA, et al. Alterations in NF kappa B/Rel family proteins in splenic T-cells from tumor-bearing mice and reversal following therapy. Cancer Res 1994;11:2969.
72. Finke JH, Zea AH, Stanley J, et al. Loss of T-cell receptor chain and p56 inT-cell infiltrating human renal cell carcinoma. Cancer Res 1993; 53:5613.
73. Brunda MJ, Luistro L, Warrier RR, et al. Antitumor and antimetastatic activity of interleukin 12 against murine tumors. J Exp Med 1993;4: 1223.
74. Hard GC. Experimental models for the sequential analysis of chemically-induced renal carcinogenesis. Toxicol Pathol 1986;14:112.
75. Rangel MC, Pontes JE. Animal models of renal cell carcinoma. Semin Urol 1989;7:237.

76. Hard GC. Renal carcinogenesis, rat. In: Jones TC, Mohr U, Hunt RD, eds. Urinary system. Berlin, Springer-Verlag, 1986:45.
77. Dees JH, Heatfield BM, Trump BF. Adenocarcinoma of the kidney. IV. Electron microscopic study of the development of renal adenocarcinomas induced in rats by N-(4′-fluoro-4-biphenylyl)acetamide. J Natl Cancer Inst 1980;64:1547.
78. Bannasch P. Sequential cellular changes during chemical carcinogenesis. J Cancer Res Clin Oncol 1984;108:11.
79. Hard GC. High frequency, single-dose model of renal adenoma/carcinoma induction using dimethylnitrosamine in Crl:(W)BR rats. Carcinogenesis 1984;5:1047.
80. Ohgaki H, Hard GC, Hirota N, Maekawa A, Takahashi M, Kleihues P. Selective mutation of codons 204 and 213 of the p53 gene in rat tumors induced by alkylating N-nitroso compounds. Cancer Res 1992;52:2995.
81. Lucké B. A neoplastic disease of the kidney of the frog, Rana pipiens. Am J Cancer 1934;20:352.
82. Rafferty KA Jr. Kidney tumors of the leopard frog: a review. Cancer Res 1964;24:169.
83. Rafferty KA Jr. In: Oncogenesis and herpes viruses, vol 2. Lyon, International Agency for Research on Cancer, 1972:159.
84. McKinnell RG, Elis VL, Dapkus DC. Early replication of herpes viruses in naturally occurring frog tumors. Cancer Res 1972;32:1729.
85. McKinnell RG, Gorham E, Martin FB. Reduced prevalence of the Lucke renal adeoncarcinoma in populations of Rana pipiens in Minnesota. J Natl Cancer Inst 1979;63:821.
86. Matthews VS, Kirkman H, Bacon RL. Kidney damage in the golden hamster following chronic administration of diethylstilbestrol and sesame oil. Proc Soc Exp Biol Med 1947;66:195.
87. Kirkman H, Bacon RL. Malignant renal tumors in male hamsters (Circetus auratus) treated with estrogen. Cancer Res 1950;10:122.
88. Kirkman H, Robbins M. Estrogen-induced tumors of the kidney. Vb. Histology and histogenesis in the Syrian hamster. Natl Cancer Inst Monogr 1959;1:93.
89. Cortes-Vizcaino V, Llombart-Bosch A. Estrogen and progesterone receptors in the diethylstilbestrol-induced kidney neoplasms of the Syrian golden hamster: correlation with histopathology and tumoral stages. Carcinogenesis 1993;14:1215.
90. Oberley TD, Gonzalez A, Lauchner LJ, Oberley L, Li JJ. Characterization of early kidney lesions in estrogen-induced tumors in the Syrian hamster. Cancer Res 1991;51:1922.
91. Bhat HK, Hacker H-J, Bannasch P, Thompson EA, Liehr JG. Localization of estrogen receptors in interstitial cells of hamster kidney and in estradiol-induced renal tumors as evidence of the mesenchymal origin of this neoplasm. Cancer Res 1993;53:5447.
92. Goldfarb S, Pugh TD. Morphology and anatomic localization of renal microneoplasms and proximal tubule dysplasias induced by four different estrogens in the hamster. Cancer Res 1990;50:113.
93. Gonzales A, Oberley TD, Li JJ. Morphological and immunohistochemical studies of the estrogen-induced Syrian hamster renal tumor: probable cell of origin. Cancer Res 1989;49:1020.
94. Sirbasku DA, Kirkland WL. Control of cell growth. IV. Growth properties of a new cell line established from an estrogen-dependent kidney tumor of the Syrian hamster. Endocrinology 1976;98:1260.
95. Bursch W, Liehr JG, Sirbasku DA, Putz B, Taper H, Schulte-Hermann R. Control of cell death (apoptosis) by diethylstilbestrol in an estrogen-dependent kidney tumor. Carcinogenesis 1991;12:855.
96. Kelley KA, Agarwal N, Reeders S, Herrup K. Renal cyst formation and multifocal neoplasia in transgenic mice carrying the simian virus 40 early region. J Am Soc Nephrol 1991;2:84.
97. Dalrymple S, Beemon KL. BK virus T antigens induce kidney carcinomas and thymoproliferative disorders in transgenic mice. J Virol 1990;64:1182.
98. Sepulveda AR, Carter BZ, Habib GM, Lebovitz RM, Lieberman MW. The mouse gamma-glutamyl transpeptidase gene is transcribed from at least five separate promoters. J Biol Chem 1994;269:10699.
99. Schaffner DL, Barrios R, Massey C, et al. Targeting of the ras T24 oncogene to the proximal convoluted tubules in transgenic mice results in hyperplasia and polycystic kidneys. Am J Pathol 1993;142:1051.
100. Walker C, Ginsler J. Development of a quantitative in vitro transformation assay for kidney epithelial cells. Carcinogenesis 1992;1:25.
101. Zhang G, Stvens JL. Altered growth regulation of rat kidney proximal tubule epithelial cells transformed in vitro by SV40 viral DNA: fibroblast growth factors (heparin-binding growth factors) are potent inducers of anchorage-independent growth. Mol Carcinog 1991;4:220.
102. Zhang G, Sato JD, Herley MT, et al. Stable and temperature-sensitive transformation of rat kidney epithelial cells suppresses expression of acidic fibroblast growth factor 1 but activates secretion of fibroblast growth factor 3 (int-2) and vascular endothelial growth factor. Cell Growth Differ 1994;5:349.

Principles and Practice of Genitourinary Oncology, edited by Derek Raghavan, Howard I. Scher, Steven A. Leibel, and Paul H. Lange. Lippincott-Raven Publishers, Philadelphia, © 1997.

CHAPTER 75

The Molecular Genetics of Renal Cell Carcinoma

Gladys M. Glenn, James R. Gnarra, Peter L. Choyke, McClellan M. Walther, Berton Zbar, and W. Marston Linehan

Renal cell carcinoma (RCC) is the major malignant renal parenchymal neoplasm in adults. About 25,000 cases of kidney cancer are diagnosed and more than 10,000 deaths are reported each year in the United States.[1] Both sporadic and familial forms of RCC occur, and the distinction between them should be made when planning therapeutic strategies and overall risk management. Sporadic cases generally are diagnosed during the fifth to seventh decades of life and most often are large, unifocal, and late-stage tumors diagnosed after the onset of symptoms including hematuria, flank pain, and abdominal mass. The male-to-female ratio is 2:1. Causes include cigarette smoking, asbestos exposure, and long-term kidney dialysis.[1] By contrast, familial RCC develops after autosomal dominant inheritance of a predisposing trait. The onset of disease is generally at a younger age, and tumors are often multifocal and bilateral. The most prevalent familial form of RCC may prove to be that occurring in the multisystemic tumor syndrome called von Hippel-Lindau disease (VHL), in which many affected family members develop clear cell RCC.[2–5]

In both sporadic and hereditary RCC, alterations of specific genes and loss of heterozygosity (LOH) of specific loci have been associated with certain histopathologic and cytologic types.[6–8] Correlations of disease features with associated molecular genetic abnormalities is proving useful in clarifying diagnoses before treatment and in case-management planning. For example, RCC is most commonly of the clear cell type (about 68% to 80% of all RCCs).[6,9–11] Clear cell RCC is also the predominant type of renal neoplasm in patients with VHL.[2,6,12] Therefore, this multisystemic familial syndrome should be considered in the differential diagnosis of clear cell RCC. In addition to RCC, patients with VHL develop multiple primary tumors of other organs and require extensive and specific extrarenal evaluations. Thus, a single patient with RCC may be the proband for a family with many at-risk relatives to be screened for occult tumors of the kidneys and other organs.

Most RCCs are believed to be of proximal tubular epithelial origin.[13] In addition to the commonly occurring clear cell RCCs, most of which are characterized by a compact or solid growth pattern,[9] the World Health Organization pathologic typing[11] lists granular cell and the less common spindle cell types. Current hypotheses suggest that less common subtypes arise more distally in the nephron.[14] These subtypes include collecting duct carcinoma, a subtype of RCC shown to have prominent tubulopapillary features,[15] and papillary cystadenocarcinoma.[14] A hereditary form of the less common sporadic papillary RCC has been described as hereditary papillary RCC (HPRCC).[16] Unlike clear cell RCC, which is associated with *VHL* on the short arm of chromosome 3 (i.e., 3p), HPRCC does *not* link to chromosome 3p.[16] Non–chromosome 3 karyotypic abnormalities have been reported for papillary RCC.[17] These findings remain consistent with the possibility that a common genetic basis will be found underlying sporadic and familial forms of papillary RCC.

TUMOR SUPPRESSOR GENES IN CANCER

Two categories of genetic changes that cause abnormal cell proliferation and lead to malignant transformation are oncogene amplification or activation and tumor suppressor gene loss or inactivation. A detailed discussion of the principles and techniques of molecular biology is included in Chapter 1. The concept of a tumor suppressor gene implies that cells contain genes capable of inhibiting tumorigenesis. Evidence supporting this concept was suggested previously when investigators demonstrated that normal cells fused with cancer cells suppressed malignancy.[18,19] Knudson advanced the concept by proposing the two-mutation theory of cancer based on epidemiologic studies of Wilms' tumor and retinoblastoma.[20–22] The theory postulates that mutations occurring in the same tumor suppressor gene on two homologous chromosomes in a cell are associated with tumor initiation in a susceptible organ. The two mutations, also called "two hits," may consist of one germline and one acquired (i.e., somatic) mutation; or, alternatively, both mutations (both "hits") may occur somatically (Fig. 75-1). This "two-hit" theory of Knudson explained inactivation of normal, that is, wild-type tumor suppressor genes and proposed the mecha-

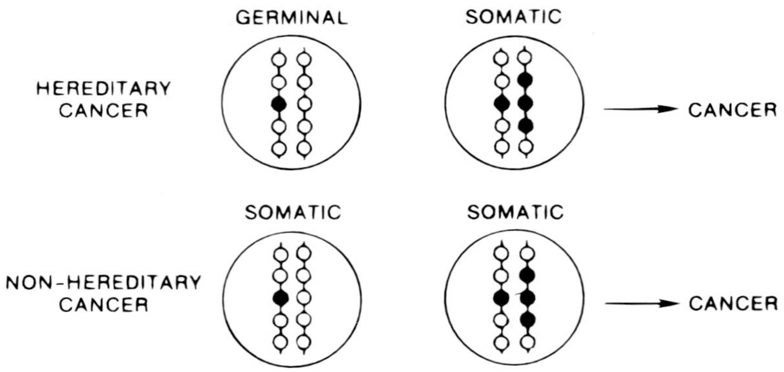

FIG. 75-1. Two-mutation theory of cancer. Each cell contains a pair of homologous chromosomes; *solid circles* indicate sites of mutations. The first mutation usually is a structural change in a specific cancer gene (*single solid circle*). The second mutation usually involves a much larger region of the chromosome by mitotic errors (*multiple solid circles*). (Zbar B. Chromosomal deletions in lung cancer and renal cancer. In: Rosenberg SA, DeVita VT Jr, Hellman S, eds. Important advances in oncology. Philadelphia, JB Lippincott, 1989:41.)

nism for common genetic defects underlying a growing number of sporadic and hereditary cancers.

The *VHL* gene is a model for tumor suppressor genes. What is known of the molecular genetics of RCC is derived mainly from studies of chromosome 3p and the *VHL* gene. As predicted by Knudson's tumor suppressor gene hypothesis, inactivation of both copies of the *VHL* gene has been described in sporadic and hereditary RCCs.[6,7,23] In hereditary RCC, because the total cell pool has the germline mutation, all cells in the kidney have half the genetic alteration needed for neoplastic conversion. Thus, the total renal cell pool is at high risk for developing neoplasms, and this feature explains the clinical features of multifocal, bilateral tumors and the early age of onset seen in hereditary RCC. These disease features should raise suspicion of a hereditary basis for RCC when assessing individuals without a known family history.

FAMILIAL RENAL CELL CARCINOMAS

Of the three major types of hereditary RCC, two are well defined and one has only recently been reported: (1) familial clear cell RCC, some with mixed granular cells, occurring in VHL[2–5,12,24]; (2) familial clear cell RCC without other signs of VHL[25,26]; and (3) HPRCC[16,27] (Table 75-1). The mode of transmission in the two well-described types of familial RCC is autosomal dominant and seems likely to be the inheritance pattern for HPRCC.[16] Germline abnormalities of chromosome 3p have been demonstrated in the two nonpapillary forms of inherited RCC,[23,25,26] whereas HPRCC does not show linkage to chromosome 3.[16]

TABLE 75-1. *Hereditary types of renal cell carcinoma*

Hereditary renal cell carcinomas	Investigators
Familial renal cell carcinoma	Cohen et al, 1979,[25] Kovacs et al, 1989,[26] and Pathak et al, 1982[73]
Renal cell carcinoma associated with Von Hipple-Lindau Disease	Glenn et al, 1990[2] and Melmon and Rosen, 1964[5]
Hereditary papillary renal cell carcinoma	Zbar et al, 1994[16] and Zbar et al, 1995[27]

Von Hippel-Lindau Disease

From an 1864 case illustration[28] to 1926, investigators have published reports of patients with various combinations of retinal, central nervous system (CNS), and visceral lesions including renal cysts culminating in the first description of a hereditary entity by von Hippel in 1904[29] and Lindau in 1926.[30] One hundred years after the earliest reports, Melmon and Rosen[5] described Lindau's disease as an entity in their literature review and report of a large kindred. Interest in VHL was renewed when researchers theorized that the study of hereditary forms of RCC, such as that occurring in VHL, may lead to knowledge of mechanisms underlying sporadic RCC.[2] As the technical methods to analyze DNA have improved, molecular genetic research of VHL and of chromosome 3p has intensified. Additional knowledge of clinical features of VHL has accompanied the progress in understanding the molecular genetics of VHL and RCC.

Clinical Features

VHL is a multiple tumor syndrome in which RCC is the major malignant tumor. The trait is dominantly inherited equally in males and females. The incidence of VHL has been estimated as 1 in 35,000 to 40,000 live births. The median actuarial life expectancy has been reported as 49 years, with RCC being the second most common cause of death after CNS disease and its complications.[2,31,32]

The benign and malignant tumors associated with VHL include retinal angiomas, hemangioblastomas of the brain and spine, RCCs, pheochromocytomas, pancreatic islet cell tumors, endolymphatic sac tumors, and epididymal cystadenomas.[2–5,24] VHL-associated tumors most often develop as multiple bilateral tumors and have an age-related penetrance that is almost complete by age 65 years.[2,4,31–33] Occasionally, obligate carriers of the gene who have not manifested clinical findings have transmitted the trait to offspring who develop the full syndrome.

In general, eye lesions are detected earliest, and ophthalmic examinations should begin in infancy. In asymptomatic children, hemangioblastomas of the brain and spine are usually not detected before age 11 years.[34] Pheochromocytomas have been reported ranging from ages 15 to 41 years,[2] but they have been observed in an 8-year-old member of a VHL family that had a high frequency of pheochromocytomas.[35]

RCC has been reported in 28% to 55% of family members

who have a diagnosis of VHL.[2,36] The clinician must recognize that a much higher prevalence of RCC can occur in certain families in which RCC is one of the visceral tumors expressed.[35,37,38] Although RCC typically manifests symptomatically at a mean age of 39 years,[2] presymptomatic renal imaging tests have revealed solid renal masses in some affected individuals as early as their late teen years or early twenties.[39]

Histopathologically, RCC in VHL consists predominantly of clear cells and less often of mixed clear cells and granular cells.[2,6,12] Poston and associates[12] characterized renal pathologic features in VHL by examining 161 lesions from 15 partial nephrectomies and 1 radical nephrectomy. In malignant lesions, 53% had only clear cell cytologic features, 45.5% had clear cells with scattered granular cells, and 1.5% had mixed clear cell, granular cell, and sarcomatoid features. RCC was found in 21% of cystic lesions and in 91% of solid tumors.[12] Solomon and Schwartz[36] examined 7 kidney specimens from 4 patients with VHL and described the cystic lesions found as a histopathologic continuum ranging from benign cysts to malignant cysts that harbored RCC. Choyke and associates[40] studied the natural history of renal lesions in VHL by a serial study of computed tomographic scans of 228 lesions in 28 patients. Complex cysts and solid masses contained neoplastic tissue in lesions that enlarged and were removed before attaining a size of 3 cm. Of 168 cysts, 71% remained unchanged, 20% enlarged, and 9% became smaller or involuted, whereas 2 cysts in 2 patients transformed to solid tumors over 5 years. Many of these cysts contained foci of malignant cells.[40]

Periodic clinical testing to monitor for occult disease in family members at risk can lead to presymptomatic diagnosis, early-stage detection, and potentially better outcome from treatment.

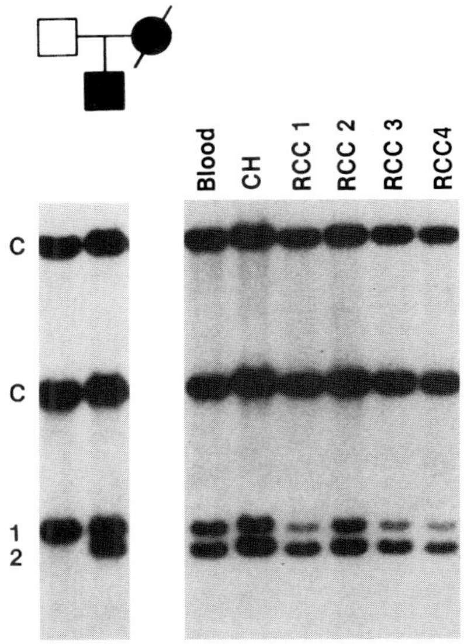

FIG. 75-2. Southern hybridization is used to demonstrate loss of allele from the parent without von Hippel-Lindau (VHL) disease (1) from the cerebellar hemangioblastoma (CH) and from four separate renal cell carcinomas (RCC) from a single patient. DNA in lanes from left to right: 1, patient's father's peripheral blood cells; 2 and 3, patient's peripheral blood cells; 4 to 8, patient's VHL tumors showing decreased band intensities of allele 1 (from unaffected father), but no decrease in allele 2 (presumed from affected mother). Two constant bands (C) are present. (Glenn GM, Choyke PL, Zbar B, Linehan WM. Von Hippel-Lindau disease: clinical review and molecular genetics. Probl Urol 1990;4:312.)

Tumor Suppressor Genes and Development of Neoplasms

Evidence that Knudson's tumor suppressor gene hypothesis was applicable to VHL was reported in 1989 by Tory and colleagues.[41] Polymorphic DNA markers were localized to the region of the suspected *VHL* disease gene to analyze tumors from patients with VHL, including 11 RCCs, 1 pheochromocytoma, and 1 cerebellar and 2 spinal hemangioblastomas. In the tumor cells, these investigators found that the allele inherited from the affected parent (i.e., the deranged copy inherited and present in all cells) was retained, whereas the normal or wild-type allele from the unaffected parent was lost. A similar demonstration is illustrated in Figure 75-2. This meant the tumor cells lacked a functionally normal copy of the *VHL* gene. Demonstration of loss of the wild-type allele in tumor tissue from patients with VHL, that is, persons with germline mutations, supported the hypothesis of a tumor suppressor gene on chromosome 3 associated with the development of kidney cancer in this familial syndrome.

Chromosome 3 Linkage Analysis and VHL *Gene Localization*

After the demonstration of *VHL* as a tumor suppressor gene, researchers prepared for chromosome 3 mapping and tumor suppressor gene cloning by isolating and regionally localizing 2000 single-copy DNA fragments on chromosome 3.[42] This process was followed by a series of linkage analyses used along with additional major research toward the goal of localizing and identifying the *VHL* gene.[35,39,43–46] Linkage analysis is based on the concept of coinheritance of genetic elements. It is a powerful method of tracking disease genes in families. Blood samples are collected from affected and unaffected family members, and the peripheral blood lymphocytes are used as the constitutional source of DNA. The DNA polymorphism results are analyzed using computer programs that consider such factors as age-related penetrance estimates. Complete concordance is first shown between inheritance of a disease gene and a polymorphic DNA probe. Inheritance of the disease is then said to be linked to the same genetic locus as the DNA probe.[47]

Hosoe and associates[43] used multipoint linkage analyses to study 25 families with VHL. This analysis and others[35,39,44–46,48,49] narrowed the *VHL* gene location to a 6- to 8-centimorgan interval at chromosome 3p25-26. Linkage analyses also were used to establish that two distinct VHL family phenotypes were linked to the same *VHL* locus. In a large multigenerational family with VHL, over half the affected members had pheochromoctomas, but no affected member had RCC. This distinct phenotype linked to the same *VHL* locus as that of typical VHL with RCC. This finding suggested that certain mutations at the *VHL* locus are associated with distinct tissue specificities.[35]

An important clinical application of linkage analysis is in presymptomatic diagnoses. This use was demonstrated in a pro-

TABLE 75-2. *Results of clinical examination in asymptomatic individuals predicted by DNA analysis to be carriers of the* VHL *Gene*

Subject	Age, y	Risk of being carrier	Results of clinical examinations
2302	10	0.997	Retinal angiomas
2734	13	0.960	Pancreatic cysts
2655	14	0.997	Pancreatic cysts
2832	20	0.913	Hemangioblastomas of the spinal cord, pancreatic cysts
2651	22	0.956	Retinal angiomas, hemangioblastomas of the cerebellum and spinal cord, renal-cell carcinoma, pancreatic cysts
2707	26	0.958	Retinal angioma, hemangioblastoma of the cerebellum and spinal cord, renal cyst
2760	27	0.960	Retinal angioma, pancreatic cysts
2399	28	0.929	Retinal angiomas, hemangioblastomas of the spinal cord, renal-cell carcinoma, pancreatic cysts
2672	30	0.897	Retinal angiomas, hemangioblastomas of the cerebellum and spinal cord, renal tumor and renal cysts, pancreatic cysts

Glenn GM, Linehan WM, Hosoe S, et al. Screening for von Hippel-Lindau disease by DNA polymorphism analysis. JAMA 1992;267:1226. Copyright 1992, American Medical Association. With permission.

spective blind comparison of DNA polymorphism analysis with a comprehensive clinical screening examination of 48 individuals at risk for VHL. Nine of these asymptomatic individuals were predicted by DNA analysis to be carriers of the *VHL* gene, and all 9 had occult VHL-associated tumors or cysts on clinical examinations (Table 75-2).[39] Maher and associates[45] confirmed the lack of heterogeneity at the *VHL* gene locus by reanalyzing previous linkage studies and by analyzing an additional 23 asymptomatic subjects from 14 families.

Identification of the VHL *Gene*

A critical turning point in the identification and cloning of the *VHL* gene was reached when Yao and colleagues,[50] using pulse field gel electrophoresis, found homozygous deletions in individuals from three kindreds. The constitutional deletions from these three VHL kindreds were found to be nested such that the smallest region of overlap was identified as being most likely to contain the *VHL* gene. Latif and associates[51] cloned the area in yeast artificial chromosomes and cosmid contigs. One of the cosmids mapped to this commonly deleted region. cDNA libraries were screened with evolutionarily conserved restriction fragments. Two unrelated cDNAs were isolated from this cosmid and analyzed. One of the cDNAs was demonstrated as a highly conserved, single-copy gene, and mutations were identified in 13% (28 of 221) of VHL kindred's germline DNA. The finding of mutations in this gene within the constitutional tissue of individuals affected with VHL identified this as the *VHL* gene[23] (Fig. 75-3).

A search for known proteins similar to one that would be encoded by these exons identified a surface membrane protein found in the procyclic surface membrane protein of *Trypanosoma brucei*.[6,23]

Familial Clear Cell Renal Carcinoma

Members of a few families who inherit certain constitutional balanced translocations involving chromosome 3p have been described. This familial RCC is reported as having clear cell histologic features, but these families have no clinical evidence of VHL.[25,26] Affected individuals develop bilateral and multifocal RCC tumors occurring at a younger age than sporadic RCC.[25,52] Inheritance of the trait is through autosomal dominant transmission.

Two translocations reported are t(3;8)[25] and t(3;6).[26] The exact genetic locus and molecular alterations responsible for RCC resulting from chromosome 3p translocations are still under investigation. To some researchers, the breakpoint locations at 3p13 and 3p14.2 have suggested a gene location proximal to the *VHL* gene. The *VHL* gene has been demonstrated to be mutated and lost in one of two renal tumors from a patient with familial RCC and constitutional translocation t(3;8)(p14;q24), however.[6,52] The inherited derivative of chromosome 8 carrying the portion of chromosome 3 distal to the breakpoint was deleted in the tumor, whereas the nontranslocated chromosome 3 was retained. Because the mutated *VHL* allele was in the single wild-type allele remaining from chromosome 3p,[6,52] this provided the second-hit target needed for tumorigenesis. A breakpoint in a 3;8 translocation disrupting a gene (*HRCA1*) has been reported,[53] but whether this gene is associated with the pathogenesis of RCC is unknown. A detailed genetic and physical map of the chromosome 3p region surrounding the familial RCC chromosomal translocation t(3;8)(p14.2;q24.1) breakpoint has been reported and will aid in further investigations and in understanding this region.[54]

Hereditary Papillary Renal Cell Carcinoma

The third type of inherited RCC is HPRCC, which has not shown linkage to 3p[16,27] Papillary RCC, which is seen in 10% of sporadic RCC tumors and differs from previously recognized hereditary cancer syndromes, was reported in 40 affected individuals from 10 families.[16,27] RCC was designated as being of the papillary type if at least 50% of the tumor had a tubulopapillary growth pattern.[16] A papillary growth pattern was defined as the presence of malignant epithelial cells arranged around a central fibrovascular core. Variations of histologic patterns were found within tumors and among family members. Affected individuals had a male-to-female ratio of 1.86:1.00 overall,[27] whereas in one large family, the ratio was 8:1.[16] The median

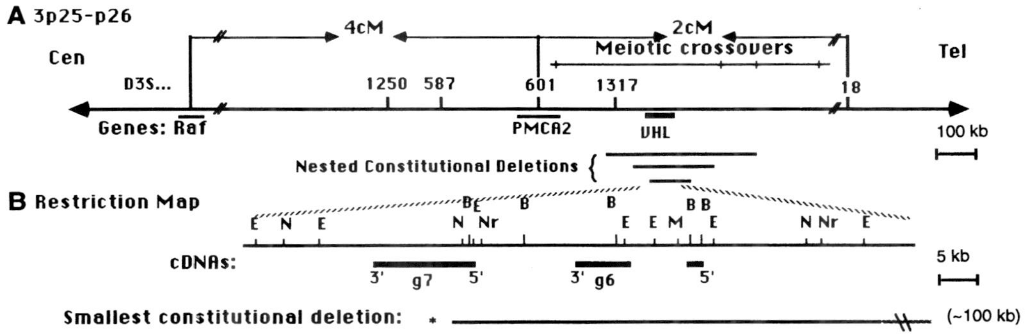

FIG. 75-3. (**A**) Genetic and physical map of the chromosome 3p region encompassing the von Hippel-Lindau (*VHL*) gene. Genetic and physical distances between markers are in centimorgans (cM) and kilobases (kb). The *VHL* locus was positioned on the map by multipoint linkage analysis and meiotic mapping. Locations of selected crossovers are indicated by short vertical lines, and positions of nested deletions discovered in constitutional DNA of three unrelated patients with VHL are shown under the map. Cen, centromere; Tel, telomere. (**B**) Restriction map of cos 3, cos 11, and phage p191 detailing the positions of g6 and g7 cDNAs isolated by screening a teratocarcinoma cDNA library with conserved fragments from cos 11. Orientation of cDNAs was done by sequencing and restriction mapping to the contig. The beginning of the smallest constitutional deletion is indicated by an asterisk and line. Restriction sites: B, Bam HI; E, Eco R1; N, Not 1; Nr, Nru 1; M, Mlu 1. (Latif F, Tory K, Gnarra J, et al. Identification of the von Hippel-Lindau disease tumor suppressor gene. Science 1993;260:1317. Copyright AAAS. With permission.)

age at diagnosis was 45 years, and the median survival age was 52 years. Inheritance appears to be through an autosomal dominant trait. Late age of onset or death from other diseases in some affected family members may contribute to the appearance of incomplete penetrance. The investigators concluded that the predisposition to papillary RCC may be inherited, and therefore, HPRCC is a distinct class of inherited cancer.[27] The clinicopathologic features of HPRCC are defined as multiple bilateral papillary RCC in individuals without a family history, or one or more papillary RCCs in an individual with a family history (Fig. 75-4).[27]

Unlike previously recognized heredity RCC syndromes, HPRCC was not found to be linked to polymorphic markers on chromosome 3p, and no LOH was found at 3p loci in renal tumors. These results suggest that an RCC gene not localized to 3p predisposes patients to this histologically and morphologically distinct form of RCC.[16] Further investigations are warranted to search for genomic alterations associated with the origin of this form of RCC characterized predominantly by a tubulopapillary growth pattern.

SPORADIC RENAL CELL CARCINOMAS

Sporadic RCC is usually unifocal at the primary tumor stage, although an incidence of 7% multicentricity has been reported.[55] Affected persons have an older age of onset, are diagnosed at a late stage because of the absence of early symptoms or signs, and as a result often have poor outcomes from treatment.

To determine whether the *VHL* gene is associated with sporadic RCC, Gnarra and associates[6] and Shuin and colleagues[7] evaluated tumors and cell lines derived from tumors obtained from patients with sporadic case histories. Mutations in the *VHL* gene[6,7,23] and in the locus now identified as containing the *VHL* gene were described in many sporadic RCCs.[56–60] Although additional mutations outside the region of the *VHL* gene were found in advanced disease, whether these mutations are the cause or the effect of disease progression is not known.

The following nonfamilial RCCs described appear be the sporadic counterparts to the hereditary RCCs reviewed earlier. Increasing evidence indicates that sporadic tumors have abnormalities in the same genes as familial tumors.

Sporadic Clear Cell Renal Carcinoma and the VHL *Gene*

Clear cell or mixed clear cell histologic features comprise 80% of RCCs.[61] As in its hereditary counterpart, this phenotype is composed of clear cells most often in a solid or compact growth pattern,[9] and it also is referred to as nonpapillary RCC.[17] Allelic loss at chromosome 3p previously was shown to be characteristic of clear cell RCC.[62] Gnarra and coworkers[6] analyzed the *VHL* gene for mutations in 108 patients with sporadic renal carcinomas. *VHL* somatic mutations were identified in 57% (56 of 98) of the clear cell RCCs analyzed, and of these, 98% had LOH.[7]

The *VHL* tumor suppressor gene in nonfamilial cases is reported to be apparently involved in renal cell carcinogenesis.[6] Shuin and associates[7] found somatic mutations of *VHL* in 22 of 39 (56%) primary human clear cell RCCs, with LOH at *VHL* in 16 of 19 (84%) of informative clear cell RCCs. *VHL* mutations are seen in both localized and advanced RCCs, a finding indicating that *VHL* somatic mutations may occur early in tumorigenesis.[63] Restriction fragment length polymorphism, performed previously,[57,59] demonstrated that almost 90% of clear cell RCCs had chromosome 3p LOH. More recently, deletion analysis of the *VHL* gene was reported by Gnarra and colleagues.[6] When results were combined, 98% (78 of 80) of the

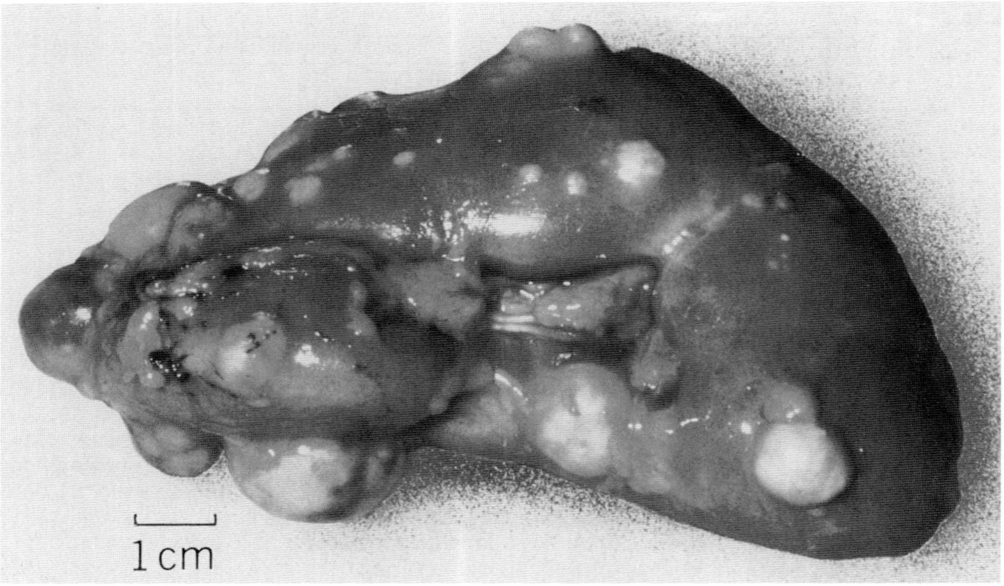

FIG. 75-4. Left kidney demonstrates multiple, discrete tumor nodules of varying size. Tumor nodules in the right kidney were removed by a nephron-sparing procedure. (Zbar B, Tory K, Merino M, et al. Hereditary papillary renal cell carcinoma. J Urol 1994;151:561.)

nonpapillary RCCs examined had chromosome 3p or *VHL* LOH; that is, they were reduced to homozygosity. *VHL* mutations were also demonstrated in 41 cell lines and 15 tumors from patients with sporadic RCC. The types of mutations detected included frameshifts, loss of splice acceptors and new splice acceptors, codon changes, and nonsense mutations,[6,23] the significance of which is being investigated.[37]

The question remains whether the *VHL* gene is rate limiting in RCCs, in particular of the clear cell type. Somatic *VHL* gene mutations in nonfamilial cases appear highly specific for renal tumorigenesis and occur only rarely in other malignant diseases.[6,7] Coupling of the mutational inactivation of one *VHL* allele with the deletion of the second allele strongly implicates the *VHL* gene in renal carcinogenesis.[6] In addition to mutational inactivation of the *VHL* gene, loss of tumor suppressor function associated with methylation of gene sequences has been shown in about 20% of clear cell RCCs analyzed.[64]

Given the broad range of tissue in which VHL mRNA is expressed, as demonstrated in brain, kidney, adrenal, prostate, and lung,[23] and given that VHL affects multiple tissues of varying embryonic origin, a survey of *VHL* mutations in nonrenal cancers was done.[6] No *VHL* mutations were detected in 119 nonrenal tumors tested from 11 different tissues (pheochromocytomas, small cell lung cancer (SCLC), non–SCLC, mesotheliomas, and cancers of the breast, ovary, cervix, prostate, colon, thyroid, and bladder). Some of the tumors tested are known to contain 3p deletions; therefore, other tumor suppressor genes may reside elsewhere on chromosome 3p that are functional in those tumor types. Susceptibility to the development of specific VHL-associated tumors also appears to be controlled by the type of *VHL* mutation, however.[37] For example, no pheochromocytomas were found in patients with germline *VHL* deletions or nonsense mutations that may result in loss of VHL protein expression. Pheochrocytomas were found only when missense *VHL* germline mutations occurred without loss of VHL protein expression.[6,37]

Sporadic Papillary Renal Cell Carcinoma

Papillary RCC is another subtype of RCC with both sporadic and hereditary forms. Renal tumors with papillary growth patterns are reported as comprising 8% to 14% of RCCs.[9,61,65,66] Histologically, the tumors have a complex tubulopapillary architecture. The papillae are lined by cuboidal or columnar cells with basophilic cytoplasm. The stroma of the papillae are filled with what appear to be clear cells, but they are actually macrophages. Reports indicate a more favorable prognosis in patients with papillary RCC, perhaps as a result of the host's inflammatory response.[66]

Investigations are continuing to search for the gene responsible for this papillary form of RCC. Cytogenetic differences between papillary and nonpapillary RCC have been reported.[67–69] Specific karyotypic changes of chromosomes 7, 17, and Y were found in papillary RCC. Loss of the short arm of chromosome 3, although characteristic of nonpapillary RCC, is *not* present in sporadic papillary RCC. The data of Zbar and associates[16] supported nonlinkage to chromosome 3 in a report of a large family with HPRCC, which is suggested as representing the hereditary counterpart of sporadic papillary RCC.

A specific chromosome abnormality, t(X;1) (p11;q21), has been described for a subgroup of papillary RCC. Somatic translocation between chromosomes (1;X) was demonstrated in 4 men with papillary RCC.[70] Fluorescence in situ hybridization and somatic cell hybridization techniques were used to demonstrate that the Xp11 translocation breakpoint in papillary RCC was unique and different from a nearby locus involved in synovial sarcoma. The yeast artificial chromosome that spans this

X;1 translocation provides a starting point from which the breakpoint and the genes may be isolated and characterized.[71] De Jong and associates[72] reported a similar translocation in a 2-year-old child with RCC, thus increasing the interest of researchers in this chromosomal region.

CONCLUSIONS AND FUTURE DIRECTIONS

A major mechanism in the development of nonpapillary clear cell RCC, the most common type of RCC in adults appears to be inactivation of the *VHL* tumor suppressor gene. This mechanism applies to both hereditary and sporadic RCCs. The specificity of the mechanism is demonstrated by the observation that *VHL* mutations were found in 57% of clear cell RCCs, but they were not present in papillary RCCs, sporadic pheochromocytomas, and ten other major types of malignant tumors tested.[6]

Whether malignant transformation is due to loss of protein function or to dominant negative effects has not been determined. VHL protein identification and isolation will permit biochemical investigations of renal cell carcinogenesis. Understanding the fundamental role of the *VHL* gene in the etiology of RCC should lead to a better understanding of renal epithelial cell growth.

Papillary or tubulopapillary RCC appears to have a different genetic mechanism and has been reported to result from a hereditary predisposition and also to occur sporadically. Data suggest that the gene that leads to development of renal cell tumors of this type is not located on chromosome 3p. Clinicians should be alert for multifocal and bilateral renal tumors with papillary morphologic features because such tumors may be due to an inherited disorder for which at-risk family members should be screened.

Current and increasing knowledge of the molecular genetics of RCC continues to provide opportunities for clinical trials to test various interventions that may interfere with malignant transformation. Clinical applications will continue to accrue from this growing body of knowledge, not only for purposes of diagnosis and for use as prognostic indicators, but also for treatment and prevention strategies. For example, prognostic information obtainable from molecular genetics may include information on the biologic aggressiveness of a tumor, the intensity of follow-up testing required for monitoring, and the need for screening other family members. The goal of future investigations should be to determine whether RCCs of different molecular bases and morphologic types are correlated with different clinical patterns that clinicians may use in management of patients.

Significant benefit is already accruing to members of families with VHL through application of these advances to presymptomatic diagnosis, thereby reducing financial and emotional burdens within families.

Note Added in Proof

Since this work was written, Duan and colleagues and Kibel and colleagues have demonstrated that a transcription elongation factor, Elongin, is negatively regulated by the VHL gene protein (Science 269, 1995). The VHL protein has been shown to tightly and specifically bind Elongin B and C subunits and to inhibit Elongin (SIII) transcriptional activity in vitro. Further studies are under way to determine the role of the VHL protein in this transcriptional regulatory pathway.

REFERENCES

1. Linehan WM, Shipley WU, Parkinson DR. Cancer of the kidney and ureter. In: de Vita VT, et al, eds. Cancer: principles and practice of Oncology, 4th ed. Philadelphia, JB Lippicott, 1993:1023.
2. Glenn GM, Choyke PL, Zbar B, Linehan WM. Von Hippel-Lindau disease: clinical review and molecular genetics. Probl Urol 1990;4:312.
3. Choyke PL, Glenn GM, Walther MM, Patronas NJ, Linehan WM, Zbar B. Von Hippel-Lindau disease: genetic, clinical and imaging features. Radiology 1995;194:629.
4. Lamiell JM, Salazar FG, Hsia YE. Von Hippel-Lindau disease affecting 43 members of a single kindred. Medicine 1989;68:1.
5. Melmon KL, Rosen SW. Lindau's disease: review of the literature and study of a large kindred. Am J Med 1964;36:595.
6. Gnarra JR, Tory K, Weng Y, et al. Mutation of the VHL tumour suppressor gene in renal carcinoma. Nat Genet 1994;7:85.
7. Shuin T, Kondo K, Torigoe S, et al. Frequent somatic mutations and loss of heterozygosity of the von Hippel-Lindau tumor suppressor gene in primary human renal cellcarcinomas. Cancer Res 1994;54:2852.
8. Van Der Haut AH, Van Den Berg E, Van Der Vlies P, et al. Loss of heterozygosity at the short arm of chromosome 3 in renal-cell cancer correlates with cytologica l tumor type. Int J Cancer 1993;53:353.
9. Theones W, Storkel ST, Rumpelt HJ. Histopathology and classification of renal cell tumors (adenomas, oncocytomas, and carcinomas): the basic cytological and histopathological elements and their use for diagnostics. Pathol Res Pract 1986;181:125.
10. O'Toole KM, Brown M, Hoffmann P. Pathology of benign and malignant kidney tumors. Urol Clin North Am 1993;20:193.
11. Mostofi FK, ed. Histologic typing of kidney tumours. In: International histological classification of tumours. No 25. Geneva, World Health Organization, 1981.
12. Poston CD, Jaffe GS, Lubensky IA, et al. Characterization of the renal pathology of a familial form of renal cell carcinoma associated with von Hippel-Lindau disease: clinical and molecular genetic implications. J Urol 1995;153:22.
13. Holthofer H: Immunohistology of renal cell carcinoma. Eur Urol 1990; 18(Suppl):15.
14. Fromowitz FB, Bard RH. Clinical implications of pathologic subtypes in renal cell carcinoma in humans. Semin Urol 1990;8:31.
15. Kennedy SM, Merino MJ, Linehan WM, et al. Collecting duct carcinoma of the kidney. Hum Pathol 1990;21:449.
16. Zbar B, Tory K, Merino M, et al. Hereditary papillary renal cell carcinoma. J Urol 1994;151:561.
17. Kovacs G. Molecular cytogenetics of renal cell tumors. Adv Cancer Res 1993;62:89.
18. Harris H, Miller OJ, Klein G, et al. Suppression of malignancy by cell fusion. Nature 1969;223:363.
19. Stanbridge EJ. Suppression of malignancy in human cells. Nature 1976; 260:17.
20. Knudson AG Jr. Mutation and cancer: statistical study of retinoblastoma. Proc Natl Acad Sci USA 1971;68:820.
21. Knudson AG. Hereditary cancer, oncogenes, and antioncogenes. Cancer Res 1985;45:1437.
22. Knudson AG. Genetics of human cancer. Annu Rev Genet 1986;20: 231.
23. Latif F, Tory K, Gnarra J, et al. Identification of the von Hippel-Lindau disease tumor suppressor gene. Science 1993;260:1317.
24. Maher ER, Yates JRW, Harries R, et al. Clinical features and natural history of von Hippel-Lindau disease. Q J Med 1990;77:1151.
25. Cohen AJ, Li FP, Berg S, et al. Hereditary renal-cell carcinoma associated with a chromosomal translocation. N Eng J Med 1979;301:592.
26. Kovacs G, Brusa P, de Riese W. Tissue-specific expression of a constitutional 3;6 translocation: development of multiple bilateral renal-cell carcinomas. Int J Cancer 1989;43:422.
27. Zbar B, Glenn GM, Lubensky I, et al. Hereditary papillary renal cell carcinoma: clinical studies in 10 families. J Urol 1995;153:907.
28. Galezowski J. Traité iconographique d'ophthalmoscopie. Paris, Bailliere et fils, 1886.

29. Von Hippel E. Uber sine sehr seltene erkrankung der netzhaut. von Graefes Arch Ophthalmol 1904;59:83.
30. Lindau A. Studien uber kleinhirncysten: bau, pathogenese und beziehungen zur angiomatosis retinae. Acta Pathol Microbiol Scand 1926; (Suppl) 1:1.
31. Maher ER, Iselius L, Yates JRW, et al. Von Hippel-Lindau disease: a genetic study. J Med Genet 1991;28:443.
32. McKusick VA. Mendelian inheritance in man, 10th ed. Baltimore, Johns Hopkins University Press, 1992;1145.
33. Linehan WM, Gnarra JR, Lerman MI, Zbar B. Genetic basis of renal cancer. In: de Vita VT, et al, eds. Important advances in oncology. Philadelphia, JB Lippincott, 1993;47.
34. Filling-Katz MR, Choyke PL, Oldfield E, et al. Central nervous system involvement in von Hippel-Lindau disease. Neurology 1991;41:41.
35. Glenn GM, Daniel LN, Choyke P, et al. Von Hippel-Lindau disease: distinct phenotypes suggest more than one mutant allele at the VHL locus. Hum Genet 1991;87:207.
36. Solomon D, Schwartz A. Renal pathology in von Hippel-Lindau disease. Hum Pathol 1988;19:1072.
37. Chen F, Kishida T, Yao M, et al. Germ line mutations in the von Hippel-Lindau disease tumor suppressor gene: correlations with phenotype. Hum Mutat 1995;5:66.
38. Neumann HPH, Wiestler OD. Clustering of features of von Hippel-Lindau disease: evidence of a complex genetic locus. Lancet 1991;337: 1052.
39. Glenn GM, Linehan WM, Hosoe S, et al. Screening for von Hippel-Lindau disease by DNA polymorphism analysis. JAMA 1992;267: 1226.
40. Choyke PL, Glenn GM, Walther MM, et al. The natural history of renal lesions in von Hippel-Lindau disease: a serial CT study in 28 patients. AJR Am J Roentgenol 1992;159:1229.
41. Tory K, Brauch, Linehan WM, et al. Specific genetic change in tumors associated with von Hipppel-Lindau disease. J Natl Cancer Inst 1989; 81:1097.
42. Lerman MI, Latif F, Glenn GM, et al. Isolation and regional localization of a large collection (2,000) of single copy DNA fragments on human chromosome 3 for mapping and cloning tumor suppressor genes. Hum Genet 1991;86:567.
43. Hosoe S, Brauch H, Latif F, et al. Localization of the von Hippel-Lindau disease gene to a small region of chromosome 3. Genomics 1990;8:634.
44. Maher ER, Bentley E, Yates JRW, et al. Mapping of the von Hippel-Lindau disease gene to a small region of chromosome 3p by genetic linkage analysis. Genomics 1991;10:957.
45. Maher ER, Bentley E, Payne SJ, et al. Presymptomatic diagnosis of von Hippel-Lindau disease with flanking DNA markers. J Med Genet 1992;29:902.
46. Tory K, Latif F, Modi W, et al. A genetic linkage map of 96 loci on the short arm of human chromosome 3. Genomics 1992;13:275
47. Ott J. Analysis of human genetic linkage. Baltimore, Johns Hopkins University Press, 1985.
48. Seizinger BR, Rouleau GA, Ozelius LJ, et al. Von Hippel-Lindau disease maps to the region of chromosome 3 associated with renal cell carcinoma. Nature 1988;332:268.
49. Seizinger BR, Smith DI, Filling-Katz MR, et al. Genetic flanking markers refine diagnostic criteria and provide new insights into the genetics of von Hippel-Lindau disease. Proc Natl Acad Sci USA 1991;88:2864.
50. Yao M, Latif F, Kuzmin I, et al. Von Hippel-Lindau disease: identification of deletion mutations by pulsed field gel electrophoresis. Hum Genet 1993;92:605.
51. Latif F, Duh F-M, Gnarra J, et al. Von Hippel-Lindau syndrome: cloning and identification of the plasma membrane Ca + + transporting ATPase isoform 2 gene that resides in the von Hippel-Lindau gene region. Cancer Res 1993;53:861.
52. Li FP, Decker HJH, Zbar B, et al. Clinical and genetic studies of renal cell carcinomas in a family with a constitutional chromosome 3;8 translocation. Ann Intern Med 1993;118:106.
53. Boldog FL, Gemmill RM, Wilke CM, et al. Positional cloning of the hereditary renal cell carcinoma 3;8 chromosome translocation breakpoint. Proc Natl Acad Sci USA 1993;90:8509.
54. LaForgia S, Lasota J, Latif F, et al. Detailed genetic and physical map of the 3p chromosome region surrounding the familial renal cell carcinoma chromosome translocation, t(3;8)(p14.2;q24.1). Cancer Res 1993;53:3118.
55. Cheng WS, Farrow GM, Zincke H: The incidence of multicentricity in renal cell carcinoma. J Urol 1991;146:1221.
56. Kovacs G, Frisch S. Clonal chromosome abnormalities in tumor cells from patients with sporadic renal cell carcinomas. Cancer Res 1989; 49:651.
57. Anglard P, Brauch H, Weiss GH, et al. Molecular analysis of genetic changes in the origin and development of renal cell carcinoma. Cancer Res 1991;51:1071.
58. Yamakawa K, Morita R, Takahashi E, Hori T, Ishikawa J, Nakamura Y. detailed deletion mapping of the short arm of chromosome 3 in sporadic renal cell carcinoma. Cancer Res 1991;51:4707.
59. Anglard R, Trahan E, Liu S, et al. Molecular and cellular characterization of human renal cell carcinoma cell lines. Cancer Res 1992;52:348.
60. Gnarra JR, Glenn FM, Latif F, et al. Molecular genetic studies of sporadic and familial renal cell carcinoma. Urol Clin North Am 1993;20: 207.
61. Farrow GM. Diseases of the kidney. In: Urological pathology. Philadelphia, WB Saunders, 1989;409.
62. Ogawa O, Kakehi Y, Ogawa K, Koshiba M, Sugiyama T, Yoshida O. Allelic loss at chromosome 3p characterizes clear cell phenotype of renal cell carcinoma. Cancer Res 1991;51:949.
63. Reiter RE, Anglard P, Liu S, Gnarra JR, Linehan WM. Chromosome 17p deletions and p53 mutations in renal cell carcinoma. Cancer Res 1993;53:3092.
64. Herman JG, Latif F, Weng Y, et al. Silencing of the VHL tumor suppressor gene by DNA methylation in renal carcinoma. Proc Natl Acad Sci 1994;91:9700.
65. Theones W, Storkel ST, Rumpelt HJ, Moll R. Cytomorphological typing of renal cell carcinoma: a new approach. Eur Urol 1990;18(Suppl 2):6.
66. Mancilla-Jimenez R, Stanley RJ, Blath RA. Papillary renal cell carcinoma: a clinical radiologic and pathologic study of 34 cases. Cancer 1976;38:2469.
67. Kovacs F, Wilkens L, Papp T, De Piese W. Differentiation between papillary and non papillary renal cell carcinoma by DNA analysis. J Natl Cancer Inst 1989;81:527.
68. Kovacs G. Papillary renal cell carcinoma: a morphologic and cytogenetic study of 11 cases. Am J Pathol 1989;134:27.
69. Kovacs G, Fuzesi L, Emanuel A, Kung H-F. Cytogenetics of papillary renal cell tumors. Genes Chromosom Cancer 1991;3:249.
70. Meloni AM, Dobbs RM, Pontes JE, Sandberg AA. Translocation (X; 1) in papillary renal cell carcinoma: a new cytogenetic subtype. Cancer Genet Cytogenet 1993;65:1.
71. Suijkerbuij RF, Meloni AM, Sinke RJ, et al. Identification of a yeast artificial chromosome that spans the human papillary renal cell carcinoma associated t(X;1) breakpoint in Xp11.2. Cancer Genet Cytogenet 1993;71:164.
72. De Jong B, Molenaar IM, Leeuw JA, Idenburg VIS, Oosterhuis JW. Cytogenetics of a renal adenocarcinoma in a 2-year old child. Cancer Genet Cytogenet 1986;21:165.
73. Pathak S, Strong LC, Ferrell RE, Trindade A. Familial renal cell carcinoma with a 3;11 chromosome translocation limited to tumor cells. Science 1982;217:939.

Principles and Practice of Genitourinary Oncology, edited by Derek Raghavan, Howard I. Scher, Steven A. Leibel, and Paul H. Lange. Lippincott-Raven Publishers, Philadelphia, © 1997.

CHAPTER 76

Epidemiology and Etiology of Renal Cell Carcinoma

William J. Ellis

Cancer of the kidney and renal pelvis is expected to be diagnosed in 30,600 people and account for 12,000 deaths in 1996.[1] Adenocarcinoma of the kidney or renal cell carcinoma (RCC) is the most common tumor in the adult kidney, accounting for 80% to 90% of the primary tumors in in that organ.[2] This tumor arises from proximal tubular cells. The abundant clear cytoplasm in the cells of many of these neoplasms led early physicians to mistakenly believe that this tumor arose from the adrenal gland; thus the term hypernephroma was used to describe this lesion.

Hereditary forms of RCC exist. This trait is transmitted in an autosomal dominant fashion. The familial form of the disease is commonly seen in patients with the von Hippel-Lindau syndrome and is seen less commonly in patients with autosomal dominant (adult) polycystic kidney disease and tuberous sclerosis.[3–7] As compared with von Hippel-Lindau patients, those with adult polycystic kidney disease or tuberous sclerosis tend to develop disease at a younger age and often develop disease in both kidneys. The hereditary form of RCC appears to be associated with deletions on the short arm of chromosome 3.[8] The genetics of RCC are discussed in detail in Chapter 75.

RCC is most common in men, with a male-to-female ratio of approximately 2:1.[9] The disease is rare in children and young adults. Eighty percent of cases occur between the ages of 40 and 69 years, with a peak incidence in the sixth decade of life.[2] A recent analysis of the Connecticut Tumor Registry suggested that RCC is increasing in incidence.[10] Katz and colleagues[10] compared the incidence of RCC during the periods 1935 to 1939 and 1985 to 1989 and found the incidence in women increased from 0.7/100,000 to 4.2/100,000, and the incidence in men increased from 1.6/100,00 to 9.6/100,000.

Worldwide, the highest rates of RCC are found in Denmark and Sweden, and the lowest rates are found in Yugoslavia, Venezuela, and Japan.[9] This may be the result of genetic factors or, as discussed later, dietary factors. In the United States, there does not appear to be an increased incidence of the disease in African Americans compared with Caucasians, with age adjusted incidence rates of 1 and 0.9 in African American men and women, respectively.[11]

The risk factor with the strongest association to RCC is cigarette smoking (Table 76-1). This is not surprising, because smokers are known to have higher rates of urothelial carcinoma, and presumably the renal tubules are bathed in the same carcinogens as the urothelium.[12,13] Yamasaki and Ames[14] have shown that the urine concentrate of smokers is mutagenic in a dose-response fashion. Numerous cohort and smaller case-control studies have suggested an increased relative risk (RR) of RCC of 1.5 to 2.5 in smokers compared with nonsmokers.[6, 13, 15–23] In the largest study to date, McLaughlin and colleagues[24] studied a group of 250,000 U.S. veterans, comparing smoking habits with development of RCC. They found a dose-response relation between the number of cigarettes per day and the risk of kidney cancer. The RR varied from 1.31 for one to nine cigarettes to 2.06 for 40 or more cigarettes daily. They estimated that one fifth of all renal cancer deaths could be attributed to cigarette smoking. In another study of smokers, Yu and colleagues[22] estimated that 43% of RCC cases in Los Angeles–area men could be attributed to smoking cigarettes. They found no association between RCC and cigar or pipe smoking. The effect of smoking is noted across cultural lines as well. McLaughlin and colleagues[25] found an RR of 2.3 for renal carcinoma among smokers in Shanghai.

Most urologists are aware of the association between analgesic abuse and transitional cell carcinomas of the renal pelvis; an association between analgesic use and RCC has also been noted. Armstrong and colleagues[20] reported a 10.5-fold greater incidence of renal adenocarcinoma in persons using analgesics on a daily basis compared to those who stated they never used analgesics, yet these researchers felt the relation between analgesics and renal cancer was noncausal, because the analgesic use was often of short duration and possibly caused by symptomatic tumors. McLaughlin and colleagues[6] compared long-term users of analgesics (>36 months) with those who denied use of analgesics and found a trend toward higher incidence of carcinoma in the long-term analgesic users, with RRs of 2.2 in men and 2.5 in women. Most patients admitted to taking both phenacetin and acetaminophen, and the investigators were not able to distinguish which medication produced the observed

TABLE 76-1. *Postulated renal cell carcinoma risk factors*

Risk factor	Relative risk
Smoking	1.5–2.5
Analgesics	2–3
Diuretics	2–6
Cadmium exposure	1.5–2.5
Asbestos exposure	2
Dietary protein consumption	1.5–2
Coffee consumption	1–2
Obesity	1.5–3

effect. In a case-control study of 360 patients with renal adenocarcinoma and 985 control patients, McCredie and colleagues[26] found analgesics containing phenacetin but not aspirin to be significantly associated with RCC. In a follow-up study, McCredie and colleagues[27] compared the incidence of analgesic nephropathy with the incidence of RCC in two territories in Australia. Although the incidence of end-stage renal disease as a result of analgesic nephropathy began to decrease in the mid to late 1970s as a result of the withdrawal of phenacetin from the market, there was not a parallel decrease in the incidence of renal cancers. Reported renal parenchymal cancer incidence rates actually increased. These studies suggest that a relation exists between analgesic use, particularly use of phenacetin, and RCC, but the data are inconsistent.

Another class of medications that appears to be associated with increased incidence of RCC is diuretics. A Danish cohort study by Mellemgaard and colleagues[28] evaluated 192,133 people who were hospitalized with a diagnosis of hypertension, heart failure, or edema between 1977 and 1978 and were presumed to be receiving diuretics. These researchers noted that the risk of RCC was more than doubled in this cohort compared with the standard mortality index. Yu and associates[22] found diuretic use to be associated with RCC with an RR of 4 when controlled for hypertension. These findings were not noted in men, in whom the RR of diuretic use was 1. The reason for this is not clear, although many of the female patients were taking the diuretics for weight control. These women had a RR of 6, compared with 1.7 for those with hypertension McLaughlin[29] reported similar findings with no association between diuretic use and RCC in men but a RR of 1.9 in women. When the reason for diuretic use was examined in women, there was no increase in RCC in women taking diuretics for hypertension, but a RR of 5.3 was noted in those without hypertension. This association persisted after controlling for body mass index. It was postulated that diuretics induce tumor formation through their action on the renal tubular cells. A subsequent study of women by the same group examined the medical records of 191 cases and 191 controls for prescription diuretics.[30] Controlling for hypertension, obesity, and smoking, they found a RR of 2.9 for development of renal cancer in women taking diuretics. Those women who had been taking prescription diuretics for 10 or more years had an RR of 3.5. These data suggest a causal relation between diuretic use and the subsequent development of RCC. The relation is strongest in women taking diuretics for weight loss rather than for hypertension. Whether the type or dose of diuretic differs between women taking these medications for weight loss and those taking diuretics for hypertension is unclear. It is possible that other medications used by women seeking to lose weight, such as amphetamines, may induce RCC in their own right or potentiate the ability of diuretics to induce the renal tumors.

OCCUPATIONAL EXPOSURE TO CARCINOGENS

A number of occupational exposures have been proposed to cause renal cancer. Cadmium can induce tumor formation in rats, although kidney tumors have not been reported.[31] Kolonel[21] found a relation between occupational (RR, 2.5) and dietary (RR, 1.5) cadmium exposure and renal cancer risk. He noted a RR with smoking of only 1.2. He also noted an apparent synergistic relation between cigarette smoking and occupational cadmium exposure that produced an RR of 4.4. This synergistic effect led him to postulate that something in addition to cadmium in cigarettes was responsible for the excess incidence of RCC in smokers.

Exposure to aromatic hydrocarbons and petroleum products have also been considered risk factors for RCC. Aromatic hydrocarbons can induce renal carcinomas in rodents.[32] In a study of coke oven workers, Redmond and colleagues[33] noted an RR of developing RCC of 7.5. This risk increased with duration of exposure to the coke ovens. Gasoline exposure has also been suspected of inducing RCC since an excess of renal tumors was noted in rats following long-term exposure to gasoline vapors.[34] However, as reviewed by McLaughlin,[35] there appears to be no association between gasoline exposure and RCC.

Although lead is a potent renal carcinogen in rats, studies of lead workers have generally not shown an increased risk of renal cancer in humans.[11,36,37] However, one occupational group—newspaper pressmen—was noted to have a threefold higher incidence of renal cancers than expected.[38]

Asbestos exposure may be associated with increased risk of renal carcinoma. A study of 17,800 asbestos insulation workers found deaths from renal carcinoma to occur at more twice the expected rate.[39] Enterline and colleagues[40] followed a cohort of 1074 men who were retired from an asbestos company until 88% of the men had died. They found a significant increase in deaths as a result of renal carcinoma over expected rates. A case-control study by Maclure[41] found that men with renal adenocarcinoma were nearly twice as likely to have been moderately or heavily exposed to asbestos than were controls. Asbestos exposure is generally considered to be associated with respiratory and gastrointestinal malignancies. The mechanism that causes an association between asbestos exposure and renal carcinoma is unclear. Some have suggested that asbestos can be ingested and secreted in the urine.[42]

DIET

The impact of diet on RCC risk is becoming manifest. Epidemiologists have previously noted an apparent association between geographic regions with high renal cancer mortality and high per capita protein and fat consumption.[19,43] Several studies have suggested that increased consumption of meat or milk may be associated with RCC.[6,25,26,44] A more recent population-based case-control study by Chow and associates[45] evaluated dietary risk factors for RCC in the state of Minnesota. They noted significant increases in the risk of RCC in those people with high consumption of red meats, high-protein foods, and staples (e.g., grains, breads, potatoes). The common denominator in these categories was protein. When adjusted for age, gender, caloric intake, body mass index, and cigarette smoking, an RR of 1.4 and 1.9 were noted for the third and fourth quartiles of protein intake. Surprisingly, no difference was noted between animal and vegetable protein in this study. Most epidemiologic studies of nonrenal malignancies have correlated the incidence of cancer incidence with animal, but not vegetable, protein intake. The animal fat consumed with the protein is implicated as the cancer-inducing agent. The mechanism by which protein alone induces carcinogenesis is unclear, although high protein intake is thought to produce renal tubular damage.

Coffee consumption was implicated in the etiology of RCC by Yu and colleagues,[22] who found that women who drank coffee daily had an RR of developing renal carcinoma of 2.3. However, they were unable to show an increased risk among male coffee drinkers. The increased risk in female coffee drinkers was not associated with increased use of artificial sweeteners. A subsequent study by Chow and colleagues[45] found no increased risk of renal cancer among coffee drinkers.

OBESITY

Obesity is another factor consistently linked to RCC. This association has been examined by several case-control studies, which demonstrate an increased risk for women[6,19,46] or for both men and women.[22,44,47] In a hospital-based case-control study, Goodman and colleagues[47] found men and women in the upper tertile of the of body mass index had odds ratios of 2.7 and 2.4, respectively, compared with the lowest tertile. Maclure and Willet[44] found odds ratios of 1.7 for both men and women in the highest quintile of relative weight. A cohort study by Mellemgaard and colleagues[46] has recently confirmed the association for women but not men. They observed that an obese women had an RR of 2.67 of developing renal carcinoma but an RR of only 0.8 of developing urothelial carcinoma. These studies suggest that obesity is the true risk factor for RCC.

ACQUIRED RENAL CYSTIC DISEASE

Another group of patients at high risk of developing renal adenocarcinomas are those with end-stage renal disease, who are prone to development of acquired cystic kidney disease. This sequela is noted in 35% to 50% of patients on hemodialysis but may develop in end-stage kidneys of patients on peritoneal dialysis or, occasionally, in patients who are not receiving dialysis.[48–50] The prevalence of acquired cystic disease increases with the length of time on dialysis.[50] Investigators have estimated that between 5% and 9% of patients with acquired cystic disease develop renal cancer.[49,51] Most of the cancers are small and are discovered incidentally at autopsy. Brennan and coworkers[52] estimate the risk of RCC in patients with acquired renal cystic disease to be 30-fold higher than that in the general population. These cancers appear to arise from the cysts themselves, because coexisting papillary hyperplasia of the cyst epithelium is found in nearly every case of renal cancer in patients with acquired cystic disease.[51]

RENAL ADENOMA

Small renal tumors (<3 cm in diameter) are found incidentally in 7% to 23% of autopsies.[2] Because these lesions rarely metastasize, they are often referred to as renal adenomas. However, size alone is inadequate to predict tumor behavior, and such a designation is improper. A complete discussion of the controversies surrounding the distinction between renal adenoma and carcinoma is provided in Chapter 77.

CONCLUSIONS

RCC is increasing in incidence in the United States. The risk factor consistently associated with this tumor is smoking. Substantial evidence also exists associating diet, analgesic use, diuretic use, and obesity with this disease. However, the exact relation of these factors to renal carcinoma is poorly defined. The environmental exposures most frequently linked to renal carcinoma are asbestos, cadmium, and hydrocarbons, yet these associations cannot be shown consistently. The integration of molecular genetics with epidemiologic studies may better define these relations.

REFERENCES

1. Parker SL, Tong T, Boldon S, Cancer Statistics, 1996. CA Cancer J Clin, 1996;46:5.
2. Peterson RO. Kidney. In: Petersen RO, ed. Urologic pathology. Philadelphia: JB Lippincott, 1986:1.
3. Malek RS, Greene LF. Urologic aspects of Hippel-Lindau syndrome. J Urol 1971;106:800.
4. Green JS, Bowmer ME, Johnson GJ. von Hippel-Lindau disease in a Newfoundland kindred. Can Med Assoc J 1986;134:133.
5. Lauritson JG. Lindau's disease: a study of one family through six generations. Acta Chir Scand 1973;139:482.
6. McLaughlin JK, Mandel JS, Blot WJ, et al. A population-based case-control study of renal cell carcinoma. J Natl Cancer Inst 1984;72:275.
7. Washeka R, Hanna M. Malignant renal tumors in tuberous sclerosis. Urology 1991;37:340.
8. Reiter R, Zbar B, Linehan M. Molecular genetic studies of renal cell carcinoma: potential biologic and clinical significance for genitourinary malignancy. In: Walsh P, Retik A, Stamey T, Vaughan E, eds. Campbell's urology, update 7. Philadelphia: WB Saunders, 1993:1.
9. Kantor AF. Epidemiology of renal cell carcinoma in Connecticut. J Natl Cancer Inst 1976;57:415.
10. Katz DL, Zheng T, Holford TT, Flannery J. Time trends in the incidence of renal carcinoma: analysis of the Connecticut Tumor Registry data, 1935-89. Int J Cancer 1994;58:57.
11. Paganini-Hill A, Ross RK, Henderson BE. Epidemiology of renal cancer. In: Skinner D, Leskovsky G, eds. Diagnosis and management of genitourinary cancer. Philadelphia: WB Saunders, 1988:32.
12. Cole P, Monson RR, Haning H, Friedell GH. Smoking and cancer of the lower urinary tract. N Engl J Med 1971;284:129.
13. Doll R, Peto R. Mortality in relation to smoking: 20 years observations on male British doctors. Br Med J 1976;2:1525.
14. Yamasaki E, Ames BN. Concentration of mutagens from urine by absorption with the nonpolar resin XAD-2: cigarette smokers have mutagenic urine. Proc Natl Acad Sci U S A 1977;74:3555.
15. Hammond EC, Horn D. Smoking and death rates: report on 44 months of follow-up of 187, 783 men. II. Death rates by cause. JAMA 1958; 166:1294.
16. Kahn HA. The Dorn study of smoking and mortality among United States veterans: report on 81/2 years of observation. NCI Monogr 1966; 19:1.
17. Weir JM, Dunn JE Jr. Smoking and mortality: a prospective study. Cancer 1970;25:105.

18. Bennington JL, Laubscher FA. Epidemologic studies on carcinoma of the kidney. I. Association of renal adenocarcinoma with smoking. Cancer 1968;21:1069.
19. Wynder EL, Mabuchi K, Whitmore W. Epidemiology of adenocarcinoma of the kidney. J Natl Cancer Inst 1974;53:1619.
20. Armstrong B, Garrod A, Doll R. A retrospective study of renal cancer with special reference to coffee and animal protein consumption. Br J Cancer 1976;33:127.
21. Kolonel LN. Association of cadmium with renal cancer. Cancer 1976; 37:1782.
22. Yu MC, Mack TM, Hanisch R, Cicioni C, Henderson BE. Cigarette smoking, obesity, diuretic use and coffee consumption as risk factors for renal cell carcinoma. J Natl Cancer Inst 1986;77:351.
23. Hirayama T. Changing patterns in Japan with special reference to the decrease in stomach cancer mortality. In: Hiatt HH, Watson JD, Windston JA, eds. Origins of human cancer, book A. New York: Cold Spring Harbor Laboratories, 1977.
24. McLaughlin JK, Hrubec Z, Heineman EF, Blot WJ, Fraumeni JF Jr. Renal cancer and cigarette smoking in a 26-year followup of U.S. veterans. Public Health Rep 1990;105:535.
25. McLaughlin JK, Gao YT, Gao RN, et al. Risk factors for renal-cell cancer in Shanghai, China. Int J Cancer 1992;52:562.
26. McCredie M, Ford JM, Stewart JH. Risk factors for cancer of the renal parenchyma. Int J Cancer 1988;42:13.
27. McCredie M, Stewart JH, Mathew TH, Disney AP. The effect of withdrawal of phenacetin-containing analgesics on the incidence of kidney and urothelial cancer and renal failure. Clin Nephrol 1989;31:35.
28. Mellemgaard A, Moller H, Olsen JH. Diuretics may increase risk of renal cell carcinoma. Cancer Causes Control 1992;3:309.
29. McLaughlin J. Diuretics and renal cell cancer. (Letter) J Natl Cancer Inst 1988;80:378.
30. Finkle WD, McLaughlin JK, Rasgon SA, Yeoh HH. Increased risk of renal cell cancer among women using diuretics in the United States. Cancer Causes Control 1993;4:555.
31. Heath JC, Daniel MR. The production of malignant tumours by cadmium in the rat. Br J Cancer 1964;18:124.
32. Guerin M, Chouroulinkow I, Riviere MR. Experimental kidney tumors. In: Rouiller C, Muller RF, eds. The kidney, vol. 2. New York: Academic Press, 1969:199.
33. Redmond CK, Cikocco A, Lloyd JW, et al. Long-term mortality study of steelworkers. IV. Mortality from malignant neoplasms among coke oven workers. J Occup Med 1972;14:621.
34. MacFarland HN, Ulrich C, Holdsworth C, Kitchen D. A chronic inhalation study with unleaded gasoline vapor. J Am Coll Toxicol 1984;3: 231.
35. McLaughlin JK. Renal cell cancer and exposure to gasoline: a review. Environ Health Perspect 1993;101:111.
36. Boyland E, Dukes CE, Grover PL, Mitchley BC. The induction of renal tumours by feeding lead acetate to rats. Br J Cancer 1962;16:283.
37. Van Esch GJ, Kroes R. The induction of renal tumours by feeding basic lead acetate to mice and hamsters. Br J Cancer 1979;23:765.
38. Paganini-Hill A, Glazer E, Henderson BE, Ross RK. Cause-specific mortality among newspaper web pressmen. J Occup Med 1980;22:542.
39. Selikoff IJ, Hammond EC, Seidman H. Mortality experience of insulation workers in the United States and Canada 1943-1976. Ann NY Acad Sci 1979;330:91.
40. Enterline PE, Hartley JS, Henderson V. Asbestos and cancer: a cohort followed up to death. Br J Ind Med 1987;44:396.
41. Maclure M. Asbestos and renal adenocarcinoma: a case-control study. Environ Res 1987;42:353.
42. Cook PM, Olson GF. Ingested mineral fibers: elimination in human urine. Science 1979;204:195.
43. Armstrong B, Doll R. Environmental factors and cancer incidence and mortality in different countries with special reference to dietary practices. Int J Cancer 1975;15:617.
44. Maclure M, Willet W. A case control study of diet and risk of renal adenocarcinoma. Epidemiology 1990;1:430.
45. Chow WH, Gridley G, McLaughlin JK, et al. Protein intake and risk of renal cell cancer. J Natl Cancer Inst 1994;86:1131.
46. Mellemgaard A, Moller H, Olsen JH, Henson OM. Increased risk of renal carcinomå among obese women. J Natl Cancer Inst 1991;83: 1581.
47. Goodman M, Morgenstern H, Wynder E. A case-control study of factors affecting the development of renal cell cancer. Am J Epidemiol 1986;124:926.
48. Chung-Park M, Parveen T, Lam M. Acquired cystic disease of the kidneys and renal cell carcinoma in chronic renal insufficiency without dialysis treatment. Nephron 1989;53:157.
49. Bretan PN Jr, Busch MP, Hricak H, Williams RD. Chronic renal failure: a significant risk factor in the development of acquired renal cysts and renal cell carcinoma. Cancer 1986;57:1871.
50. Matson MA, Cohen EP. Acquired cystic kidney disease: occurrence, prevalence, and renal cancer. Medicine (Baltimore) 1990;69:217.
51. Hughson MD, Buchwald D, Fox M. Renal neoplasia and acquired cystic kidney disease in patients receiving long-term dialysis. Arch Pathol Lab Med 1986;110:592.
52. Brennan JF, Stilmanat MM, Babayan RK, Siroky MB. Acquired renal cystic disease: implications for the urologist. Br J Urol 1991;57:342.

Principles and Practice of Genitourinary Oncology, edited by Derek Raghavan, Howard I. Scher, Steven A. Leibel, and Paul H. Lange. Lippincott-Raven Publishers, Philadelphia, © 1997.

CHAPTER 77

Pathology of Renal Cancers

Lawrence D. True and David Grignon

Although this chapter focuses on malignancies, benign tumors are discussed when relevant to the differential pathologic diagnosis. Because an accurate pathologic diagnosis evolves from an accurate differential diagnosis, charts are provided that list the differential diagnostic considerations of tumors based on both gross and microscopic features. Furthermore, because accurate distinction of poorly differentiated tumors is best done by characterizing antigens expressed by the tumor cells, the immunohistochemical profiles of selected tumors is provided. Information is given concerning the genetic features of renal cell carcinomas.

EPITHELIAL NEOPLASMS

Principles of Pathologic Classification

The classification of renal epithelial tumors has traditionally been based on the cytologic and architectural patterns of growth. This approach is generally used in North America (see Table 77-1). Thoenes and colleagues[1] have proposed a system that is based on the cytoplasmic features of cells; this system has gained acceptance in Europe. Kovacs[2] presented a scheme based on cytogenetic features. These schemes are summarized in Table 77-2.

An assumption of these classifications is that cells in a given tumor have a common phenotype; however, many tumors belie this assumption. Some renal cell carcinomas are composed of mixtures of clear cells, granular cells, and spindle cells, and mixed collecting duct–transitional cell carcinomas have been reported.[3] The proportion of cells of different histologic type comprising tumors may be prognostically important.[4]

Renal Cell Carcinoma, Usual Type

More than 90% of solid epithelial renal tumors are of the usual type. Although most cases occur sporadically, a small percentage of cases have a hereditary association (e.g., von Hippel-Lindau disease, tuberous sclerosis, adult polycystic kidney disease). Hereditary tumors tend to be multifocal and bilateral, in contrast with sporadic tumors, which tend to have a single focus and be unilateral. However, the histology of hereditary and sporadic tumors is identical. Both sporadic and familial tumors have similar cytogenetic changes, the most frequent of which are deletions within 3p. The von Hippel-Lindau locus has been mapped to 3p25. In addition, most renal carcinomas have deletions within 3p12-14.2.[5–9] Fluorescent in situ hybridization has demonstrated ploidy heterogeneity within tumors.[10]

Renal cell carcinomas have a highly variable gross appearance. Typically, they are large, lobulated masses that distort the kidney and bulge into perinephric fat (Fig. 77-1), which is not necessarily indicative of extracapsular invasion. A fibrous pseudocapsule gives these tumors a sharply circumscribed appearance. The cut surface is variegated yellow (indicating either necrosis or the high lipid content of clear tumor cells or macrophages) to red-brown (indicating a granular cell component). Necrosis, hemorrhage, cystic change, and fibrosis are frequent. Some cystic tumors resemble a multilocular cyst. Gross invasion of the renal vein or vena cava occurs in as many as 40% of cases.[11]

Histologically, the usual renal cell carcinoma is composed predominantly of clear, lipid-rich cells (Fig. 77-2). Variable numbers of eosinophilic (granular) and, rarely, spindle cells may be present. Tumors composed predominantly of spindle cells are classified as sarcomatoid carcinomas (discussed later). The ratios of cell types may be of prognostic value[4]; an increased proportion of spindle cells portends a poorer prognosis. Typically, tumor cells grow as sheets or confluent nests with a prominent sinusoidal vascular pattern. Other patterns (e.g., tubular, alveolar, papillary) may be present.

The most common grading scheme is a four-point system based on nuclear features.[12] Grade 1 nuclei are small, round, and hyperchromatic, without observable nucleoli. Grade 2 nuclei are large, with an open chromatin pattern and small nucleoli. Grade 3 nuclei have large, prominent nucleoli. Grade 4 nuclei are large and pleomorphic with marked atypia and hyperchromasia. Nuclear grade, which correlates with mitotic activity, has significant prognostic power, independent of tumor stage. The grade assigned is that of the highest grade within the tumor, even if it is only focal. Nuclear morphometry is potentially a more reliable way of grading renal carcinomas.[13]

Pathologic staging of resection specimens, using the TNM system of the Union Internationale Contre le Cancre, is based

TABLE 77-1. *Histologic classification of kidney tumors according to the modified WHO scheme*

Epithelial tumors of renal parenchyma
- Adenoma, including oncocytoma
- Carcinoma
  - Usual renal cell carcinoma
  - Other histologic types

Epithelial tumors of renal pelvis
- Transitional cell papilloma
- Transitional cell carcinoma
- Squamous cell carcinoma
- Adenocarcinoma
- Undifferentiated carcinoma

Nephroblastic tumors
- Nephroblastoma (Wilms' tumor)
- Mesoblastic nephroma
- Multilocular cystic nephroma (multilocular cyst)

Nonepithelial tumors
- Benign
  - Angiomyolipoma
  - Fibroma
  - Hemangioma
  - Others, including leiomyoma, lipoma, and neurilemmoma
- Malignant
  - Sarcoma

Miscellaneous tumors
- Juxtaglomerular cell tumor
- Others, including neuroblastoma, carcinoid, and teratoma

Secondary (metastatic) tumors, including lymphoma

Unclassified tumors

Tumor-like lesions
- Renal blastema, persistent or massive
- Renal dysgenesis
- Cysts
- Xanthogranulomatous pyelonephritis
- Malakoplakia
- Others

Mostofi FK. Histological typing of kidney tumours. World Health Organization, Geneva, 1981.

TABLE 77-2. *Classification schemes of renal epithelial tumors*

WHO (Mostofi, 1981)	Thoenes et al, 1986[1]	Kovacs, 1993[2]
Adenoma	Renal cell carcinoma	Papillary tumor
Renal cell carcinoma	Clear cell	Adenoma
Clear cell	Chromophil	Carcinoma
Granular cell	Eosinophil	Nonpapillary carcinoma
Spindle cell	Basophil	Chromophobe carcinoma
Others	Chromophobe	Oncocytoma
Collecting duct	Typical	
Chromophobe cell	Eosinophil	
	Collecting duct	
	Oncocytoma	

on both gross and microscopic findings. Gross data include tumor size (the size threshold distinguishing T1 and T2 tumors is 2.5 cm in greatest dimension), invasion of perinephric tissues, involvement of extrarenal organs (e.g., lymph nodes, adrenal gland), and invasion of the renal vein, vena cava, or both. Microscopic invasion of vessels is irrelevant for staging. Invasion of perinephric fat requires histologic confirmation that tumor cells extend beyond the kidney parenchyma and the tumor pseudocapsule, if present.

Stage is the best predictor of tumor behavior.[11] Markers of cell proliferation, including mitotic activity, expression of proliferating cell nuclear antigen or the Ki-67 epitope, and S-phase fraction of cells, determined by flow cytometry, correlate with grade and survival but do not consistently provide prognostic information of value beyond that provided by stage and grade.[14–16]

Adenoma

The distinction between adenoma and carcinoma is an unresolved but significant issue, because many small lesions are

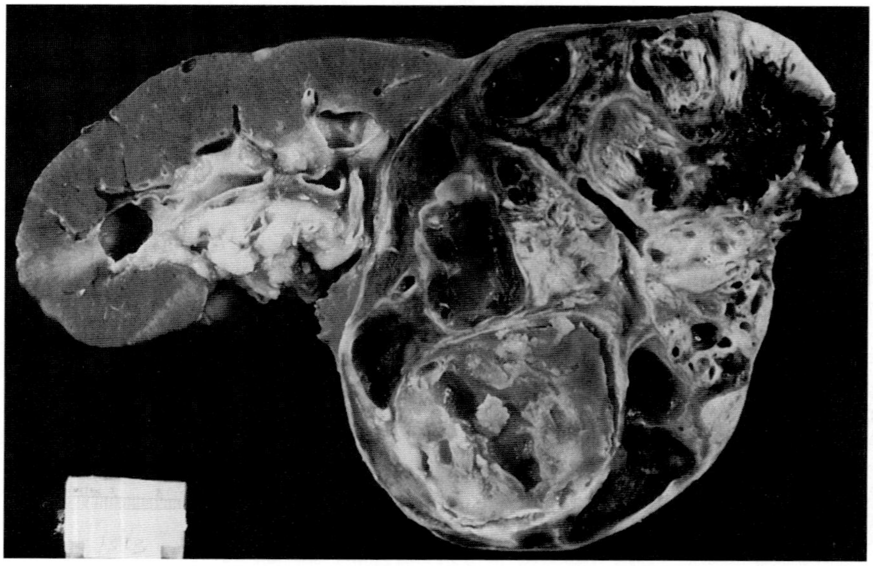

FIG. 77-1. The typical gross appearance of renal cell carcinoma is a large tumor mass with cystic areas admixed with bridging bands of fibrous tissue, and more solid areas of renal cell carcinoma, which are multifocally yellow as a result of the clear cell component of this tumor.

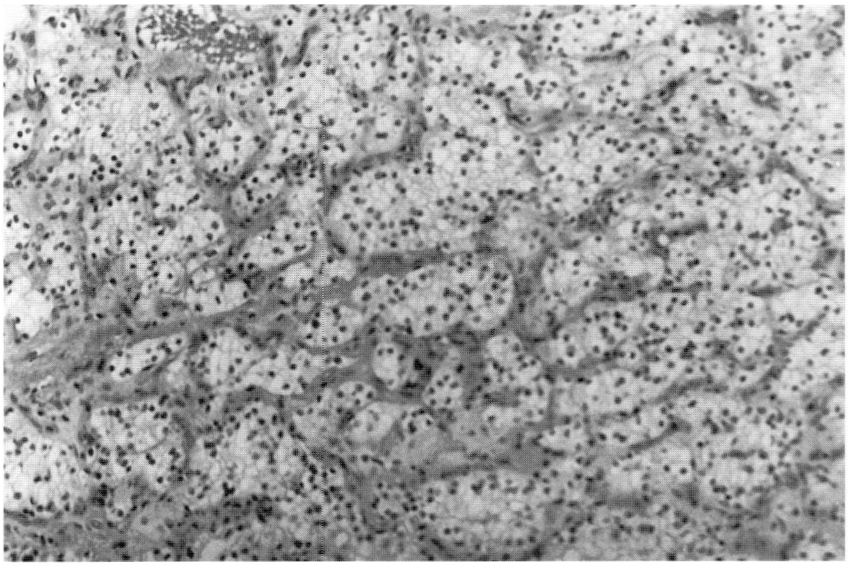

FIG. 77-2. The most common histologic pattern of clear cell—type renal cell carcinoma consists of cells with a clear cytoplasm as a result of the high content of lipid, which is extracted during tissue processing. Note the fine network of capillaries between the nests of tumor cells. This tumor is classified as Fuhrman's grade 2 because of the small nuclei and infrequent nucleoli.

being detected with increasingly sensitive techniques. In a large autopsy series, small cortical epithelial lesions were found in 21% of patients; frequency increased with age, from 10% in 21- to 40-year-old patients to 40% in 70- to 90-year-old patients.[17] Adenomas have other clinical associations. Those with a papillary histology are often multiple and are associated with papillary carcinoma.[18] Many patients with acquired cystic disease develop adenomas. Papillary adenomas have characteristic cytogenetic changes: trisomy 7 and 17 and loss of the Y chromosome.[18]

Grossly, the adenoma is sharply circumscribed and yellow-tan to gray; it protrudes from the cortical surface. Histologically, the tumor has a tubulopapillary architecture and lacks a capsule, merging with adjacent renal parenchyma. Cells have an eosinophilic to basophilic cytoplasm and small, uniform nuclei (Fig. 77-3). When clear tumor cells are present, the tumor should be regarded as a carcinoma, regardless of size.

Investigators have used different pathologic criteria to distinguish adenoma from carcinoma. Size is not a sufficiently specific criterion, because small tumors (as small as 0.5 cm in diameter) have metastasized.[19] Some authors restrict the diagnosis of adenoma to small lesions composed of closely packed tubules and papillae with small, uniform cuboidal cells having nuclei of uniform size and shape and virtually absent mitoses.[20] Others recommend diagnosing such tumors as "small renal epithelial neoplasms of low malignant potential."[21] Adenoma should not be diagnosed by fine needle aspiration biopsy, because sampling may not be representative.

Papillary Renal Cell Carcinoma

As many as 10% of renal cell carcinomas are papillary variants; according to Kovacs and Kovacs'[18] criteria, more than

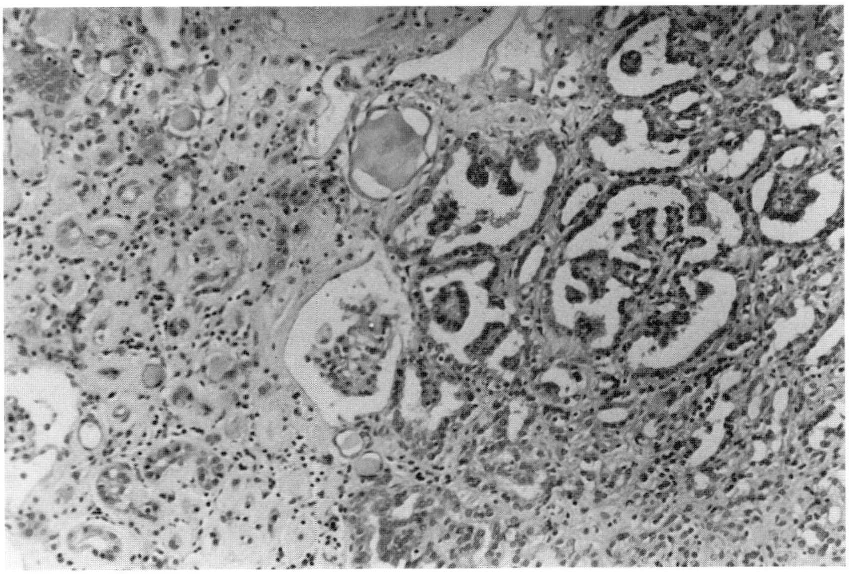

FIG. 77-3. A typical adenoma is not encapsulated and has a complex papillary tubular architecture of cells with scanty basophilic cytoplasm and a high nuclear–cytoplasmic ratio but minimal nuclear atypia. No mitoses are seen.

75% of the tumor must have a papillary architecture. The cells are typically chromophilic (either eosinophilic or basophilic); clear cells are rare. Tumors that meet these pathologic criteria have specific cytogenetic changes: trisomy or tetrasomy of 7 and 17 and loss of the Y chromosome.[2] Papillary adenomas have the same cytogenetic changes. No abnormalities of 3p have been found in these lesions. In addition, abnormalities of chromosomes 12, 16, and 20 may be found and may mark the development of malignancy.[2]

Grossly, papillary renal cell carcinoma is well circumscribed, brown, soft, and friable, with central cystic change. The cystic change is often not a result of necrosis, which is uncommon. These tumors are often multifocal and are associated with small, papillary adenomas. The predominant histologic pattern is papillary; small cuboidal or columnar cells of low cytologic grade line fibrovascular stalks which contain foamy histiocytes. Psammoma bodies may be present. Although these tumors have been associated with a better prognosis than the usual renal cell carcinoma, at least some of these tumors may behave aggressively.[22,23]

Oncocytoma

Oncocytoma, first reported in 1976, accounts for fewer than 5% of solid renal tumors in adults.[24] The most controversial aspect of this tumor concerns its malignant potential. The debate has been confused by the use of different pathologic criteria.[24–27] In studies using strict criteria, renal oncocytomas behaved in a uniformly benign nature. Cytogenetic studies also support distinguishing this tumor from the usual renal cell carcinoma. The most frequent abnormality associated with oncocytoma is trisomy 17. Abnormalities in mitochondrial DNA have been found; 3p deletions are not present.[28]

Grossly, the oncocytoma is a sharply circumscribed, nonencapsulated tumor with a central stellate scar, which may be inconspicuous in small tumors (Fig. 77-4). Oncocytomas are a uniform tan-brown or mahogany brown. Histologically, oncocytomas are composed of a pure population of round or cuboidal cells with coarse, granular, eosinophilic cytoplasm (Fig. 77-5). These cytoplasmic features are the result of abundant mitochondria. An organoid growth pattern is typical, particularly in association with the scar. Solid, alveolar, or tubular patterns may be seen. Nuclei are round and of uniform size, with small, central nucleoli. Scattered cells with enlarged, atypical hyperchromatic nuclei are often present; this is considered a degenerative feature. Mitoses are not seen. According to some authors, the finding of even a single mitosis excludes the diagnosis of oncocytoma. Extension into perinephric fat has been found in rare tumors that had a benign clinical course.[27]

Oncocytomas, by definition, are not graded. The possibility that a subset of oncocytomas with a high nuclear grade has malignant potential has been raised.[26] However, the study on which this observation is based failed to apply strict criteria to defining oncocytomas; the category ''pink cell (or, granular, eosinophilic cell) tumors'' of the kidney includes not only oncocytoma but also chromophobe cell carcinoma and eosinophilic papillary renal cell carcinoma.

The minimal diagnostic criteria for oncocytoma include a characteristic gross appearance, a pure population of oncocytes, and the absence of mitoses. To satisfy these criteria, sampling should be thorough; at least one block of tissue per centimeter of maximum tumor dimension should be analyzed. The diagnosis should probably not be made either by frozen section or fine needle aspiration biopsy because of sampling limitations.

Cystic Renal Carcinoma

Cystic renal lesions have a variety of associations with renal cell carcinoma. Cystic degeneration is not uncommon in renal cell carcinoma; as many as 15% of renal cell carcinomas are radiographically cystic.[29] Usually, the presence of cystic change presents a greater problem to the radiologist than to the pathologist. However, in some cases, the identification of diagnostic tumor tissue may be problematic because of the paucity of tumor cells, which may be of low grade.

Cystic renal carcinomas are characterized by variably sized, noncommunicating cysts separated by irregular, thick, fibrous

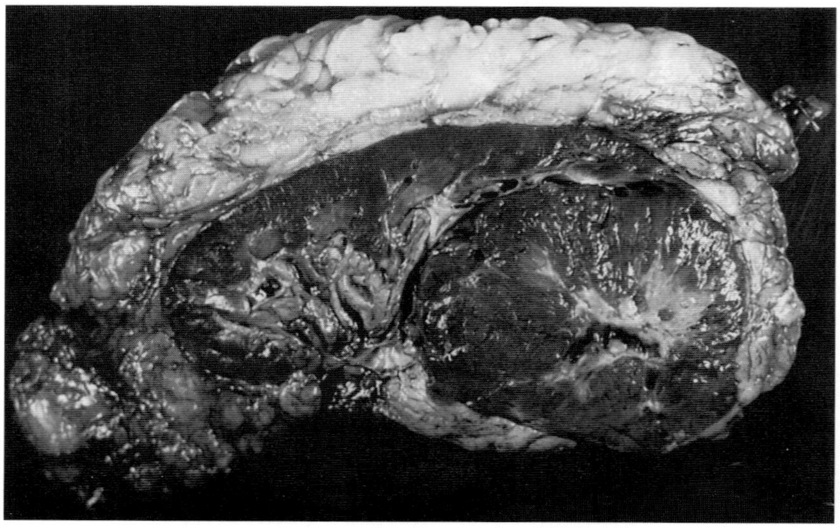

FIG. 77-4. The typical oncocytoma is a round, circumscribed, tan-to-brown mass with a central stellate scar.

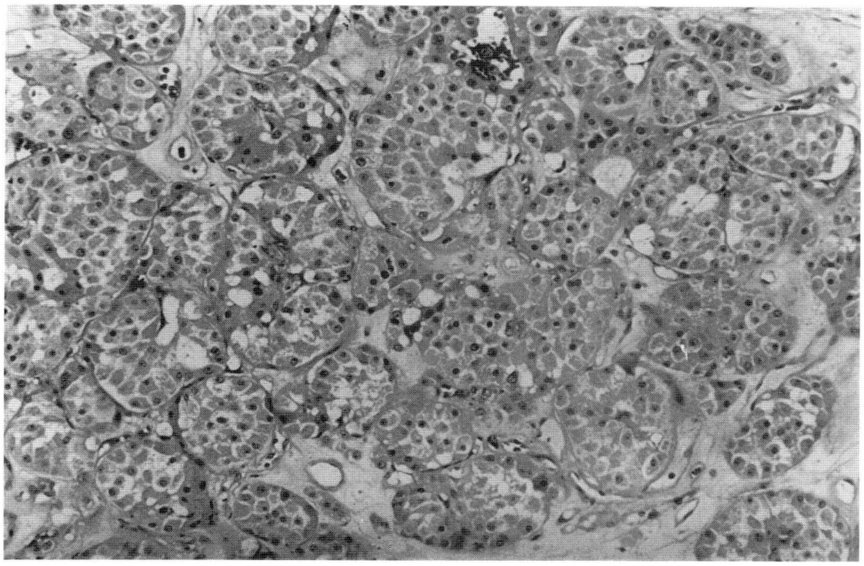

FIG. 77-5. Oncocytoma tumor cells form small nests in a fibrous, variably edematous, myxoid stroma. The brown color of the gross tumor and the granular eosinophilia seen microscopically result from the high content of mitochondria. Typical oncocytoma cells have large nuclei with prominent nucleoli.

septae. The septae usually show marked hyalinization and may contain calcifications or foci of ossification. The tumor cells that line the cysts may be markedly attenuated or absent. Nests of tumor cells can be found within the septae; these are most often of the clear cell type. A unilocular variant has a thick irregular fibrous wall and a lining of tumor cells which may be clear or granular. Characteristically, there are papillary excrescenses; the papillae are covered by clear or granular cells.

In cases resulting from cystic necrosis of a previously solid tumor, the cyst contains hemorrhage and necrotic tissue. The cyst wall is thickened and irregular. These cases may be difficult to diagnose because an epithelial lining is often absent. Any cystic mass in the kidney that contains hemorrhagic or necrotic material should be suspected to be malignant and should be extensively sampled.

Carcinomas may arise in benign cystic disease of the kidney, including acquired cystic disease, adult polycystic kidney disease, and simple unilocular cortical cysts.[30,31] Tumors in simple cysts are typically small, solid, yellow nodules within the cyst wall. Histologically, most such tumors are composed of clear cells and have a low nuclear grade. The prognosis with these lesions is good.

Collecting Duct (Bellini's Duct) Carcinoma

This rare epithelial tumor, which was first recognized in 1976, tends to occur at a younger age than the usual renal cell carcinoma.[22,32,33] Many patients have a family history of cancer.[33] Collecting duct tumors are located in the medulla, are gray-white, and show an infiltrative growth pattern. Necrosis is frequent. Histologically, collecting duct carcinomas typically have a mixed papillary and infiltrative tubular architecture. There is pronounced stromal desmoplasia. Often, tumor cells diffusely invade renal parenchyma, trapping normal renal structures. Nuclear atypia is marked and mitoses are frequent. Dysplasia or carcinoma in situ may be found in the collecting ducts. Tumors have also been described in which this pattern is associated with a transitional cell carcinoma.[3] The common embryologic derivation of the collecting duct and renal pelvis is a histogenetic basis for this event. A sarcomatoid variant has also been described.[34] These tumors have a very aggressive course. Of 18 patients, 10 died of metastatic disease within 2 years; the median survival was 22 months.[33]

Recently, Davis and colleagues[35] have reported as ''renal medullary carcinoma'' a highly malignant tumor that occurs almost exclusively in individuals with sickle cell disease or trait and that shares the following pathologic features with collecting duct carcinoma: desmoplastic stroma, marked nuclear atypia, in situ neoplasia in the calyceal epithelium, and a medullary location. The authors consider it different, however, from collecting duct carcinoma because of its distinctive histologic features, including a reticular, yolk sac–like histology. General acceptance of renal medullary carcinoma as a new tumor type awaits confirmatory reports.

Chromophobe Cell Carcinoma

Chromophobe cell carcinoma, first reported in 1985, represents fewer than 5% of renal cell carcinomas.[36,37] This tumor warrants distinction from other variants because of its unique morphology and cytogenetic features and the possibility of misdiagnosing it as an oncocytoma. Many cases of ''malignant oncocytoma'' actually represent chromophobe cell carcinoma. Cytogenetically, there is loss of chromosomes 1, 2, 6, 10, 13, 17, 21 and of sex chromosomes; no loss of 3p has been found.[38]

Grossly, the tumor is circumscribed and tan to brown. Areas of necrosis and hemorrhage may be found. No central scar, which is characteristic of oncocytoma, is seen. Microscopically, there are two patterns. In the classic type, the cells are voluminous, with a finely reticular, pale, eosinophilic cytoplasm, which tends to condense along the cell membrane, producing a perinuclear halo. The eosinophilic type is characterized by smaller cells with a denser, finely granular, eosinophilic cytoplasm and a less conspicuous perinuclear halo.

These tumor cells grow in a solid pattern with a capillary-rich stroma. Histochemical staining with Hale's colloidal iron shows intense blue cytoplasmic reactivity; this result is not seen in usual renal cell carcinoma or in oncocytoma. Nuclei vary from small, round, and hyperchromatic to large with clumped chromatin and prominent nucleoli. Ultrastructurally, the cells contain abundant microvesicles and variable numbers of mitochondria. The reported cases of chromophobe cell carcinoma behaved in a manner similar to that of usual renal cell carcinoma.[37]

Sarcomatoid Renal Cell Carcinoma

As many as 5% of renal tumors in adults are sarcomatoid renal cell carcinomas. Although their clinical presentation is similar to that of usual renal cell carcinoma, sarcomatoid renal cell carcinomas often are of higher stage at diagnosis.[39,40]

Grossly, this tumor is often a gray-white, infiltrating mass that is often contiguous with a usual renal cell carcinoma. Histologically, sarcomatoid renal cell carcinoma is composed of malignant spindle cells that can mimic virtually any histologic type of sarcoma.[4] Tumor cells are often arranged as poorly formed, interlacing fascicles. Cytologically bizarre tumor cells and atypical mitoses are frequent. Although osteoid or chondroid material may be present, a diagnosis of osteosarcoma or chondrosarcoma should not be made. When no epithelial component can be found, evidence of epithelial differentiation should be sought by special studies (e.g., immunohistochemical localization of keratin to tumor cells, ultrastructural identification of desmosomes).[41] Because sarcomatoid differentiation of carcinoma is more common than pure sarcoma of the kidney, malignant spindle cell tumors of the kidney should be presumed to be carcinomas until proven otherwise. Clinically, these tumors are highly malignant. In one series, the 5-year survival rate was 19%. Adjuvant chemotherapy may improve survival.[40]

Transitional Cell Carcinoma

Approximately 5% of primary renal tumors are transitional cell carcinomas. These tumors originate in renal pelvic urothelium. The histology and biology of transitional cell carcinomas of the kidney are similar to that of transitional cell tumors in the urinary bladder.[42] Most transitional cell carcinomas are low-grade, noninvasive papillary neoplasms; invasive, high-grade tumors are less frequent. Rarely, these tumors have other histologic components, including, in order of frequency, squamous, glandular, and sarcomatoid elements. Because of their low cytologic grade and the difficulty of visualizing and biopsying the renal pelves and calyces, these tumors can be clinically and pathologically challenging to diagnose. As in the bladder, tumor stage is of greatest prognostic power.[43] Low grade and absence of aneuploid or tetraploid cell populations are independent predictors of a good prognosis for low-stage tumors.[44] For tumors that abut renal parenchyma, distinguishing intraductal extension of tumor from renal parenchymal invasion probably is also of prognostic importance.[45]

Infrequently, renal transitional cell carcinomas grow as solid masses that infiltrate the renal parenchyma and lack a papillary component (Fig. 77-6). The differential diagnosis of such a diffusely infiltrative tumor includes lymphoma and renal cell carcinoma. Immunohistochemical characterization of the tumor can help make the distinction. Transitional cell carcinomas are characterized by expression of high-molecular-weight keratins and of keratin 20.[46]

As in the urinary bladder, squamous cell carcinoma and adenocarcinoma of the renal pelvis occur, although rarely. More often, squamous and glandular differentiation occur as components of a transitional cell carcinoma. Pure squamous cell carcinoma has distinctive clinical associations (i.e., renal calculi and a history of recurrent upper urinary tract infections). These tumors have the same histology as their counterparts in the bladder. Patterns of adenocarcinoma of urothelium include papillary, glandular, and mucinous with signet ring formation. Differentiation from metastatic carcinoma can be difficult but can be aided by immunohistochemical studies. The prognosis associated with these tumors is poor.

Neuroendocrine Neoplasms

Primary neuroendocrine tumors of the kidney are very rare. Fewer than one dozen cases of intrarenal neuroblastoma and

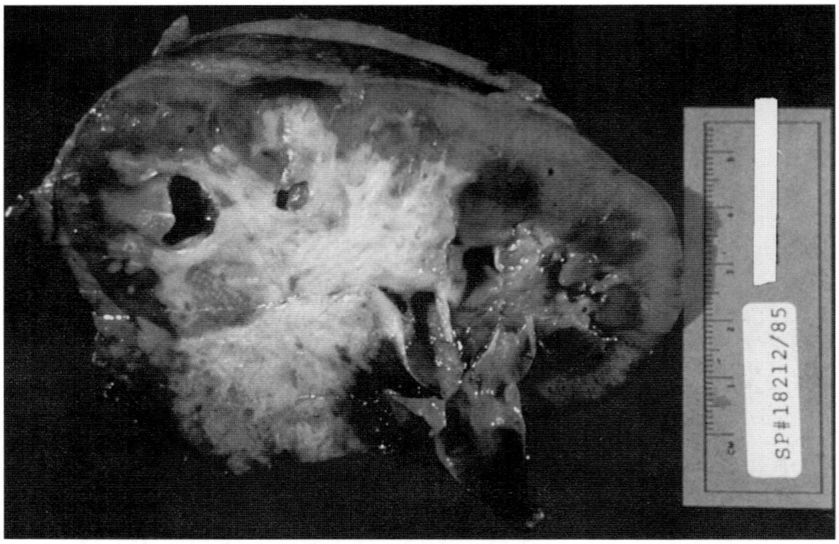

FIG. 77-6. Transitional cell carcinoma has only a minimal component in the collecting system. It diffusely infiltrates renal parenchyma as an irregular, white-to-tan mass.

pheochromocytoma have been reported in adults.[47,48] Carcinoid tumors of the kidney are sometimes hormonally active and have caused Cushing's syndrome[49] and hyperglucagonemia.[50] Grossly, carcinoids are usually well circumscribed, solid, and tan. Rarely, carcinoid is a component of cystic teratoma.[51] Although typically following a benign course, some carcinoids have had a lethal course.[52]

Small cell undifferentiated carcinoma of the kidney is white to tan, with an infiltrative margin. Histologically, this lesion is composed of sheets of tumor cells that have scanty cytoplasm, a fine chromatin pattern, and inconspicuous nucleoli. Because the histology is identical with that of small cell carcinoma of other sites (e.g., lung), the possibility of the tumor being a metastasis should be excluded clinically. The association of small cell undifferentiated carcinoma of the kidney with the renal pelvis[53] and with concurrent transitional cell carcinoma of the pelvis[54] raises the possibility that these tumors originate in transitional epithelium. Differentiation from other diffusely infiltrative, small cell undifferentiated tumors can be made by immunohistochemistry. These tumors are highly malignant; most patients die of tumor within 1 year of diagnosis.[55,56]

All of these neoplasms have a neuroendocrine phenotype. Neurosecretory granules can be found ultrastructurally, and immunoreactive neuron-specific enolase, chromogranin, and synaptophysin can be localized to tumor cells.

Juxtaglomerular Cell Tumor (Reninoma)

Patients with this rare tumor of juxtaglomerular cells, which are the normal site of renin synthesis, present clinically with severe hypertension as a result of abnormal renin secretion. The tumor can be difficult to localize when small; some of these lesions are smaller than 0.3 cm in size.[57] The histology is varied, although localization of immunoreactive renin to tumor cells and ultrastructural identification of distinctive rhomboidal crystals confirm the diagnosis. Not all cases of hyperreninemia-associated hypertension are caused by renal reninomas; examples of renin-secreting renal carcinoma have been reported.[58] Reninomas are not malignant.

NONEPITHELIAL AND MULTILINEAGE NEOPLASMS

Angiomyolipoma

Angiomyolipoma is a benign hamartoma composed of varying ratios of smooth muscle, fat, and blood vessels. About 50% of angiomyolipomas occur in patients with tuberous sclerosis; conversely, between 50% and 80% of patients with tuberous sclerosis develop one or more angiomyolipomas. Most patients with multifocal angiomyolipoma have tuberous sclerosis; however, in sporadic cases, the tumor is usually unilateral and unifocal.

Grossly, the tumor is circumscribed and not encapsulated. It is usually variegated yellow (because of adipocytes) and tan (because of smooth muscle cells). Areas of hemorrhage and, less frequently, necrosis can be seen.

The classic angiomyolipoma is composed of three cell types: smooth muscle cells, which grow as sheets of generally eosinophilic cells that do not form fascicles; adipose tissue; and thick-walled, dysmorphic blood vessels (Fig. 77-7). An abundant adipocyte component imparts a distinctive radiologic and gross appearance; however, in some cases the adipocyte component is sparse or even absent. The diagnosis of these angiomyolipomas can be difficult, both radiologically and pathologically.[59] The diagnosis is based on recognition of the distinctive blood vessels, which have a media that is histologically continuous with the spindle cell component of the tumor.

Angiomyolipomas can have atypical features: hemorrhage, necrosis, macroscopic invasion of the renal vein, and cell and nuclear pleomorphism; tumors with these features are benign. Some patients with renal angiomyolipoma have the same lesion in other abdominal organs (e.g., renal hilar lymph nodes, spleen, liver).[60] These discontiguous foci do not represent metastases of a renal angiomyolipoma but are separate benign masses that are thought to be manifestations of multifocality of this hamartomatous process. Rare patients with angiomyolipomas have a lymphangioleiomyomatosis syndrome characterized by extrarenal tumors in the lung.[61] Virtually all angiomyolipomas have a

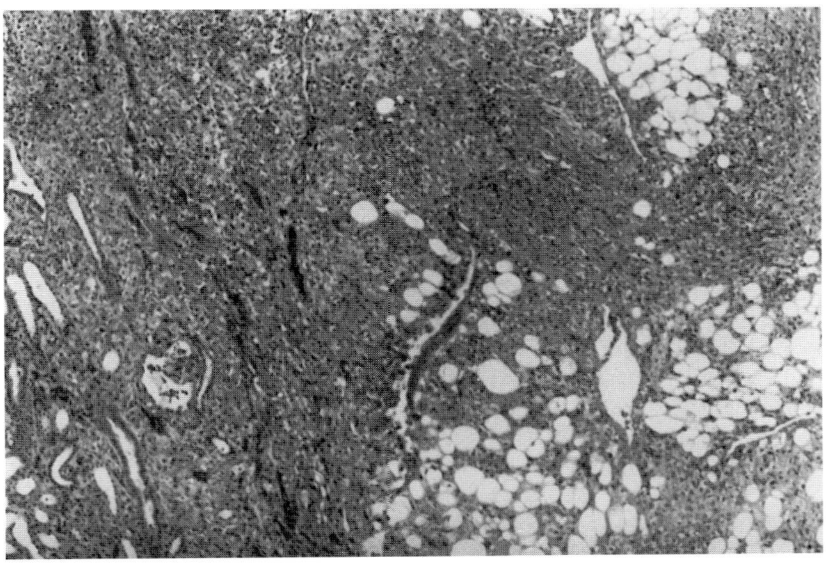

FIG. 77-7. Angiomyolipoma is composed of smooth muscle cells, which grow as sheets of generally eosinophilic cells that do not form orderly fascicles, histologically mature adipose tissue, and thick-walled blood vessels that lack a distinct adventitia.

TABLE 77-3. *Immunohistochemical profile of tumors involving the kidney*

	Intermediate filaments*	Membrane antigen	Specific protein
PRIMARY TUMORS			
Renal cell carcinoma	Keratin (LMW)/vimentin	EMA	
Clear cell type	Keratins (8/18)		
Non–clear cell types	Keratins (7/19)		
Collecting duct carcinoma type	HMW keratins		
Neuroendocrine tumors	Keratin (LMW), neurofilament	CD57	Neuron-specific enolase, chromogranin, synaptophysin
Transitional cell carcinoma	Keratin (HMW, 20)	EMA	
Rhabdoid tumor	Keratin (LMW)/vimentin		
Lymphoma	Vimentin	CD45	Immunoglobulins
Angiomyolipoma	Vimentin/desmin		Muscle actin, S100, HMB45
Smooth muscle tumor	Vimentin/desmin		Muscle actin
Adipocyte tumor	Vimentin		S100
METASTATIC TUMORS			
Melanoma	Vimentin/focal keratin		S100, HMB45 antigen
Adrenal cortical carcinoma	Vimentin		

EMA, epithelial membrane antigen; HMW, high molecular weight; LMW, low molecular weight; S100, S100 protein.

* The number in parentheses after keratin refers to specific keratins, based upon the Moll nomenclature of keratins.

benign course. There is one report of a histologically malignant spindle cell component arising from typical angiomyolipoma,[62] and cases of concurrent renal cell carcinoma and angiomyolipoma have been reported.[63] Thus, not all renal masses in patients with previously diagnosed angiomyolipoma are benign.

Tumors in the differential histopathologic diagnosis include benign and malignant tumors of smooth muscle and adipocyte origin (e.g., leiomyoma, leiomyosarcoma, lipoma, liposarcoma), and sarcomatoid carcinomas of the kidney of either renal cell or transitional cell origin.[64] Immunohistochemistry can help establish the correct diagnosis (Table 77-3). A subset (<1%) of actin-expressing spindle cells demonstrate HMB45 immunoreactivity, which can help distinguish angiomyolipoma from all other spindle cell renal tumors.[65]

Other Stromal Cell Tumors

Leiomyomas and lipomas of renal origin are quite rare; many cases are probably angiomyolipomas in which one cell type predominates.[66] Pathologically, smooth muscle tumors are white to tan masses composed of spindle cells. Predicting behavior using histologic features can be difficult. Most authors reporting leiomyomas of the kidney have stressed the absence of mitoses and nuclear pleomorphism. Large size, the presence of necrosis, nuclear pleomorphism, or one or more mitoses per 10 high-power fields is indicative of malignancy. However, there are low-grade leiomyosarcomas with a low mitotic rate (<2 per 10 high-power fields) that have metastasized.

Of renal sarcomas, leiomyosarcomas are the most common.[67] Other primary renal sarcomas include, in decreasing order of frequency, fibrosarcoma, malignant fibrous histiocytoma, hemangiopericytoma, and liposarcoma.[68] In general, sarcomas of the kidney have the same histology as their soft tissue counterparts. Sarcomatoid carcinomas should be considered in the differential pathologic diagnosis, as well as secondary involvement of the kidney by a retroperitoneal sarcoma.[69]

Lymphoproliferative Disease and Lymphoma

Lymphoma in the kidney is usually a manifestation of systemic non-Hodgkin's lymphoma; 35% of patients who die of lymphoma have lymphomatous involvement of the kidney, as either a mass lesion or a diffuse infiltrate of renal parenchyma, compromising renal function and producing uremia. Usually, renal involvement is not recognized antemortem.

Grossly, lymphomas are well circumscribed, nonencapsulated, and white (Fig. 77-8). When the kidney is the site where the lymphoma is brought to clinical attention, it may mistakenly be managed as a primary renal tumor. The possibility of lymphoma is raised by finding numerous, atypical lymphocytes in a fine needle aspiration biopsy specimen. However, diagnosis of lymphoma by cytology is problematic, because lymphoid cells are present in many diseases affecting the kidney. Some subtypes of lymphoma (e.g., large cell) are sufficiently distinctive that they can be recognized cytologically. However, most subtypes can only be suspected by the pathologist on the basis of large numbers of variably atypical lymphoid cells.

The evidence that some lymphomas are limited to the kidney is anecdotal. Most old cases of putative primary renal lymphoma should be disregarded for several reasons: tumors were understaged by imaging studies before computed tomography was used, immunohistochemical confirmation that these were lymphomas and not carcinomas was not obtained, and many patients had disseminated lymphoma at autopsy.[70] Rare patients who underwent nephrectomy for lymphoma that was diagnosed preoperatively were disease-free after 2 to 6 years of follow-up.[71]

Lymphoma is one of few kidney lesions for which an attempt

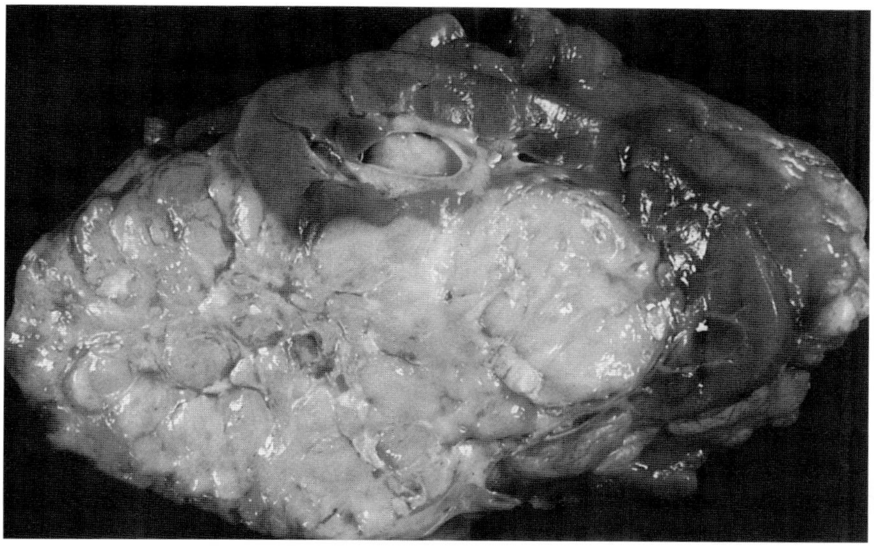

FIG. 77-8. This multinodular, confluent lymphoma is white as a result of the high cellularity of the tumor.

at diagnosis by fine needle aspiration cytology might be appropriate, particularly if the clinical context is unusual for a renal cell carcinoma (e.g., a young, immunocompromised patient with multifocal renal masses). If a diagnosis of lymphoma is made, disease should be sought elsewhere under the assumption that lymphoma is a systemic disease. Rarely does lymphoma involve only the kidney and has nephrectomy been curative. Otherwise, renal lymphoma is treated as a component of a systemic lymphoma (i.e., by a nonsurgical approach).[70,72]

Polyclonal lymphoproliferative disease rarely complicates immunosuppressive therapy of transplant patients; fewer than 3% of renal allograft recipients develop this lesion. Polyclonal lymphoproliferative disease is characterized by proliferation of lymphocytes of predominantly B-cell origin; these may form a mass. Histologically differentiating a lymphoproliferative lesion from rejection or infection can be difficult. Although this lesion can be successfully treated by decreasing the dose of immunosuppressive therapy and resecting the lymphoproliferative lesions, 50% of patients die, some as a result of progression of the disease to monoclonal lymphoma.[73]

Nephroblastic and Undifferentiated Multipotential Tumors

Wilms' tumor and rhabdoid tumor occur most commonly in young children and rarely occur in adults.[74,75] Pathologically, these are typically fleshy, white, nonencapsulated, infiltrative tumors composed of undifferentiated cells. In Wilms' tumors, the undifferentiated blastema cells are admixed with tubules and glomeruloid structures. The prognosis of these tumors in adults is similar to that of tumors with the same histology in children. The typical Wilms' tumor has a favorable prognosis; in significant contrast, the prognosis for patients with clear cell sarcoma or rhabdoid tumor is poor.

Tumors that may be histogenetically related to Wilms' tumor but are benign are mesoblastic nephroma and multilocular cystic nephroma.[76,77] Mesoblastic nephroma is a solid, white tumor composed of spindle cells. The differential diagnosis includes solid spindle cell tumors (i.e., smooth muscle tumors and sarcomatoid carcinomas). Terminology for benign multilocular cystic nephroma is uncertain; some authors use this term interchangeably with multilocular cyst, whereas others recognize these as two distinct entities. The term cystic nephroma includes both entities.[76] Multilocular cyst has a distinctive bimodal age distribution; 50% of cases occur before 2 years of age, and 40% of cases occur between the ages of 40 and 69 years. Grossly, multilocular cysts are unilateral, solitary, and surrounded by a thick fibrous capsule. The septae contain only mature connective tissue without epithelial elements.[78] The cysts are lined by a single layer of eosinophilic epithelial cells that have a hobnail morphology. Clear cells may be seen in some cases.

Rare cases of cystic teratoma, some with carcinoid tumor, of the kidney have been reported. This tumor has malignant potential.[51]

METASTATIC TUMOR

Fewer than 5% of cancers that present clinically as possible primary renal tumors are of metastatic origin.[79] Only rarely is diagnosing a metastatic tumor a problem, because most patients with metastasis in the kidney have a known primary. The most common primary sites are cutaneous melanoma, lung, kidney (from a contralateral renal cell carcinoma), breast, and esophagus. Rarely, metastatic tumor may not form a mass but may instead occur as microscopic glomerular disease that can be diagnosed in a needle core biopsy specimen.[80] A time interval of as long as 37 years has been reported between resection of a primary tumor and appearance of a renal metastasis.[81]

Distinction between a primary renal cell tumor and a metastasis can be made by light microscopy in some cases. However, the histology of many metastatic carcinomas may be indistinguishable from that of one of the histologic variants of renal cell carcinoma. Immunohistochemistry can help in the diagnosis of some metastatic tumors by identifying specific antigens: thyroglobulin in thyroid carcinoma and prostate specific antigen in prostate carcinoma. Contiguous invasion of the kidney by an adrenal cortical carcinoma can be difficult to distinguish from a primary renal tumor because the cells composing adrenal cortical tumors can grow as sheets and cords of clear to faintly eosinophilic cells, often of low nuclear grade.

As discussed previously, lymphoma is conventionally regarded as metastatic when it presents clinically in the kidney, even if the kidney appears to be the sole focus of tumor in the patient. Sarcomas that are primary in the kidney are less common than sarcomas of retroperitoneal origin that invade the kidney and are histologically indistinguishable from primary renal sarcomas.[69]

TUMORLIKE LESIONS

Xanthogranulomatous Pyelonephritis and Malakoplakia

Xanthogranulomatous pyelonephritis and malakoplakia of the kidney are chronic inflammatory processes that produce mass lesions which may extend into perinephric fat and should be distinguished from cancer. At the gross level, the lesion forms one or more poorly demarcated, infiltrative masses which have a variegated yellow to tan surface.[82,83] Histologically, these diseases are composed of variable numbers of inflammatory cells of different types. The presence of lipid-rich, foamy macrophages imparts a yellow color, which is the basis for the term xanthogranulomatous; these macrophages can be mistaken for low-grade clear cells of a renal cell carcinoma. Xanthogranulomatous pyelonephritis and malakoplakia may represent the same process, clinically and pathologically, but for the fact that histiocytes in malakoplakia have calcified, basophilic cytoplasmic bodies (i.e., Michaelis-Gutmann bodies).[84,85] These unusual lesions apparently are rare sequelae of recurrent bacterial infection of the lower urinary tract, kidney, or both. Michaelis-Gutmann bodies have ultrastructural features of gram-negative bacilli; bacteria that cause cystitis (i.e., *Escherichia coli* and *Proteus* sp) have been associated with these lesions. These diseases cannot be diagnosed with accuracy by biopsy, either cytologically or in a tissue sample, because the histologic features are nonspecific.

Nonneoplastic Cystic Lesions

A variety of cystic lesions, ranging from simple unilocular cysts to renal dysplasia (or renal dysgenesis), can be virtually impossible to distinguish from cystic renal neoplasms by clinical and radiologic criteria. Histologically, the distinction between nonneoplastic cystic lesions and carcinoma is readily made. Renal dysplasia is usually restricted to childhood as either a diffuse or segmental renal process. Histologically, renal dysplasia consists of cysts of varying sizes and an intervening stroma containing dysmorphic renal cortical tissue admixed with immature stroma and cartilage. Cystic lesions that have neoplastic connotations are found in patients with von Hippel Lindau syndrome[86] and in those with acquired cystic disease on long-term dialysis.[31,87] Rarely, carcinoma has been found in simple cysts.[88]

TABLE 77-5. *Differential diagnosis based on gross appearance of primary renal tumor*

Tan-brown	Oncocytoma Chromophobe cell carcinoma Granular renal cell carcinoma Angiomyolipoma (fat-poor) Leiomyoma or leiomyosarcoma
Cystic	Cystic renal cell carcinoma Cystic necrosis of a renal cell carcinoma Multilocular cystic nephroma Papillary carcinoma
White	Sarcomatoid renal cell carcinoma Collecting duct carcinoma Infiltrative transitional cell carcinoma Small cell carcinoma Lymphoma Mesoblastic nephroma Sarcoma
Yellow variegated	Renal cell carcinoma (solid) Angiomyolipoma (fat-rich) Lipoma Xanthogranulomatous pyelonephritis Malakoplakia

ISSUES IN HISTOLOGIC PATHOLOGY

Cytologic Diagnosis of Renal Lesions

Although primary renal neoplasms have been diagnosed with accuracy using fine needle aspiration biopsy, especially when the cells are immunohistochemically characterized,[89] wide-

TABLE 77-4. *Cytogenetic abnormalities in renal cell carcinomas*

Renal cell carcinoma in general	Deletion and mutations in 3p. Some show loss of heterozygosity for 17p. Some have deletions in 5q, 6q, and 10q. Increased numbers of loci with LOH, loss 6q, 8p, 9, and 14q, or both correlate with higher grade and with apparent tumor progression.
Hereditary renal cell carcinoma	Some families have a t(3;8) translocation. Patients with von Hippel-Lindau syndrome have mutations in 3p.
Renal cell carcinoma, papillary variant	Trisomy or tetrasomy of 7 and 17; loss of Y chromosome; abnormalities of 12, 16, 20. Some have a t(x;1) translocation. No 3p abnormality reported.
Papillary adenoma	Trisomy or tetrasomy of 7 and 17; loss of Y chromosome.
Oncocytoma	Trisomy 17. Some tumors are 44X, -Y, -1. No 3p abnormality reported.
Chromophobe cell carcinoma	Loss of chromosomes 1, 2, 6, 10, 13, 17, 21, and X(Y). No 3p abnormality reported.

TABLE 77-6. *Differential diagnosis based on microscopy of primary renal tumor*

Eosinophilic cell	Oncocytoma Granular cell variant of renal cell carcinoma Chromophobe cell variant of renal cell carcinoma
Spindle cell	Sarcomatoid variant of usual renal cell carcinoma and subtypes Leiomyosarcoma or leiomyoma Angiomyolipoma Sarcomatoid variant of transitional cell carcinoma Mesoblastic nephroma
Large cell	Renal cell carcinoma and variants Collecting duct carcinoma Transitional cell carcinoma Clear cell sarcoma Lymphoma, large cell subtypes Adrenal cortical carcinoma Metastatic large cell carcinoma
Small cell	Small cell carcinoma of kidney Neuroblastoma Lymphoma Wilms' tumor (blastematous component) Rhabdoid tumor

spread use of cytology for definitive characterization of renal neoplasms can be problematic. Sampling errors can lead to misdiagnosis of lesions such as granular cell tumors (oncocytoma versus granular cell component of renal cell carcinoma), spindle cell tumors (benign angiomyolipoma versus sarcomatoid carcinoma versus sarcoma), small cortical tumors (adenoma versus carcinoma), and cystic tumors. The frequency of needle tract seeding is less than 0.01%; no case of seeding has had significant clinical consequences.[90]

Transitional cell carcinomas can be diagnosed with accuracy, when they are of high-grade,[91] by urine cytology. However, low-grade transitional cell carcinomas may exhibit too little cytologic atypia to be diagnosed with accuracy. Tumors of renal parenchyma (i.e., renal cell carcinomas and primary sarcomas) virtually never shed cells into the urine.

Special Pathology Techniques

The diagnosis of poorly differentiated and undifferentiated tumors may require characterization of tumor cell differentiation by ultrastructural analysis or by immunohistochemistry (see Table 77-3). With rare exceptions, monoclonal antibodies are of sufficient specificity and sensitivity when used in an immunohistochemical procedure on formalin-fixed, paraffin-embedded tissue that ultrastructural analyses need only rarely be used to diagnose these tumors.[91,92] Because some antibodies react better with antigens fixed in chemicals other than formalin, samples of tumors should be routinely fixed both in formalin and in a denaturing fixative such as Carnoy's solution, which contains an alcohol rather than formaldehyde.

In the future, the behavior of kidney tumors and their responsiveness to specific therapies may be predicted by use of immunohistochemistry to characterize their function. The proliferative rates of tumors can be assessed both by determining the fraction of cells in the S-phase of the cell cycle using either flow or image cytometry and by determining the percentage of cells that express the proliferation-associated antigens Ki-67 and proliferating cell nuclear antigen. Potentially productive areas of investigation include characterizing genetic abnormalities in kidney cancers. Much of the available genetic characterization has been based on classic cytogenetic analyses (see Table 77-4).[1] In addition, chromosomal characterizations of some tumors has been based on interphase nuclear hybridization analysis.[10]

Pitfalls in Pathologic Diagnosis

An accurate pathologic diagnosis originates from a differential diagnosis that is restricted by clinical and radiologic findings and by the gross (Table 77-5) and microscopic (Table 77-6) features of the lesion. In addition, bearing in mind possible pitfalls (Table 77-7) will help the pathologist avoid errors in pathologic diagnosis.

TABLE 77-7. *Pathologic pitfalls*

Overdiagnosing a small, basophilic cell epithelial neoplasm (adenoma) as an adenocarcinoma
Underdiagnosing a small clear cell epithelial neoplasm as an adenoma
Underdiagnosing a chromophobe cell carcinoma, which can appear oncocytic, as an oncocytoma
Grading an oncocytoma (by definition, oncocytomas are not graded)
Misdiagnosing a sarcomatoid carcinoma as a renal cell carcinoma, a transitional cell carcinoma, or a sarcoma
Misdiagnosing rare primary renal tumors such as small cell carcinoma and mucinous adenocarcinoma as metastatic carcinoma
Underdiagnosing a cystic renal cell carcinoma as a benign unilocular or multilocular cyst
Not considering the wide spectrum of diagnostic possibilities for small cell undifferentiated tumors, which include poorly differentiated transitional cell carcinoma, small cell carcinoma, Wilms' tumor (blastema predominant), rhabdoid tumor, and lymphoma
Misdiagnosing tumors that may have a pseudorhabdoid appearance, including renal and transitional cell carcinoma and adrenal cortical carcinoma, as a rhabdoid tumor
Misdiagnosing adipocyte-rich or muscle cell–rich angiomyolipomas as intrarenal lipoma or intrarenal leiomyoma, respectively
Misdiagnosing muscle-rich angiomyolipoma as leiomyosarcoma or sarcomatoid renal cell carcinoma
Not considering use of fine needle aspiration biopsy to evaluate the possibility that multifocal renal tumor in an immunocompromised patient may be a lymphoma; conversely, a specific diagnosis often cannot be made, because many renal mass lesions contain lymphocytes, which may appear atypical, even in reactive conditions
Metastases of tumors to the kidney may resemble primary renal cell tumors
Mischaracterizing a tumor by insufficient sampling, which can lead to errors in tumor classification, DNA ploidy analysis, and chromosomal analysis

REFERENCES

1. Thoenes W, Storkel S, Rumpelt HJ, et al. Histopathology and classification of renal cell tumors (adenomas, oncocytomas, and carcinomas). Pathol Res Pract 1986;181:125.
2. Kovacs G. Molecular differential pathology of renal cell tumours. Histopathology 1993;2:1.
3. Aizawa S, Kikuchi Y, Suzuki M, Furusato M. Renal cell carcinoma of lower nephron origin. Acta Pathol Jpn 1987;37:567
4. Ro JY, Ayala AG, Sella A, et al. Sarcomatoid renal cell carcinoma: clinicopathologic. Cancer 1987;59:516.
5. Meloni AM, Bridge J, Sandberg AA. Reviews on chromosome studies in urological tumors. I. Renal tumors. J Urol 1992;148:253.
6. Gnarra JR, Tory K, Weng Y, et al. Mutations of the VHL tumour suppressor gene in renal carcinoma. Nat Genet 1994;7:85.
7. Foster K, Crossey PA, Cairns P, et al. Molecular genetic investigation of sporadic renal cell carcinoma: analysis of allele loss on chromosomes 3p, 5q, 11p, 17, and 22. Br J Cancer 1994;69:230.
8. Lubinski J, Hadaczek P, Podolski J, et al. Common regions of deletion in chromosome regions 3p12 and 3p14.2 in primary celar cell renal carcinomas. Cancer Res 1994;54:3710.
9. Kovacs G. The value of molecular genetic analysis in the diagnosis and prognosis of renal cell tumours. World J Urol 1994;12:64.
10. el Naggar AK, van Dekken HD, Ensign LG, Pathak S. Interphase cytogenetics in paraffin-embedded sections for renal cortical neoplasms. Correlation with cytogenetic and flow cytometric DNA ploidy analyses. Cancer Genet Cytogenet 1994;73:134.
11. Hermanek P, Schrott KM. Evaluation of the new tumor, nodes and metastases classification of renal cell carcinoma. J Urol 1990;144:238.
12. Fuhrman SA, Lasky LC, Limas C. Prognostic significance of morphologic parameters in renal cell carcinoma. Am J Surg Pathol 1982;6: 655.
13. van der Poel HG, Schaafsma HE, Voolis GP, et al. Quantitative light microscopy in urological oncology. J Urol 1992;148:1.
14. de Riese WTW, Crabtree WN, Allhoff EP, et al. Prognostic significance of KI-67 immunostaining in nonmetastatic renal cell carcinoma. J Clin Oncol 1993;11:1804.
15. Grignon DJ, Ayala AG, El-Naggar AK, et al. Renal cell carcinoma: a clinicopathological and DNA flow cytometric analysis of 103 cases. Cancer 1989;64:2133.
16. Grignon DJ, Abdel-Malek M, Mertens W, et al. Prognostic significance of cellular proliferation in renal cell carcinoma: a comparison of synthesis-phase fraction and PCNA index. Mod Pathol 1995;8:18.
17. Eble J, Warfel K. Early human renal cortical epithelial neoplasia. (Abstract) Mod Pathol 1991;4:45A.
18. Kovacs G, Kovacs A. Parenchymal abnormalities associated with papillary renal cell tumors: a morphologic study. J Urol Pathol 1993;1:301.
19. Aizawa S, Suzuki M, Kikuchi Y, et al. Clinicopathological study on small renal cell carcinomas with metastases. Acta Pathol Jpn 1987;37: 947.
20. Murphy WM, Beckwith JB, Farrow GM. Tumors of the kidney, bladder, and related Urinary Structures. Atlas of tumor pathology, series 3, fasc. 11. Washington DC: Armed Forces Institute of Pathology, 1994;132.
21. Epstein JI. Differential diagnosis in pathology: urologic disorders. New York: Igaku-Shoin, 1992.
22. Mancilla-Jimenez R, Stanley RJ, Blath RA. Papillary renal cell carcinoma: a clinical, radiologic, and pathologic study of 34 cases. Cancer 1976;38:2469.
23. Mydlo JH, Bard RH. Analysis of papillary renal adenocarcinoma. Urology 1987;30:529.
24. Morra MN, Das S. Renal oncocytoma: a review of histogenesis, histopathology, diagnosis and treatment. J Urol 1993;150:295.
25. Licht MR, Novick AC, Tubbs RR, et al. Renal oncocytoma: clinical and biological correlates. J Urol 1993;150:1380,
26. Lieber MM, Tomera K, Farrow GM. Renal oncocytoma. J Urol 1981; 125:481.
27. Davis CJ Jr, Mostofi FK, Sesterhenn I, Ho CK. Renal oncocytoma: clinicopathological study of 166 patients. J Urogenital Pathol 1991;1: 41.
28. Kovacs G, Welter C, Wilkens L, et al. Renal oncocytoma: a phenotypic and genotypic entity of renal parenchymal tumors. Am J Pathol 1989; 134:967.
29. Hartman DS, Davis CJ Jr, Johns T, Goldman SM. Cystic renal cell carcinoma. Urology 1986;28:145.
30. Gregoire JR, Torres VE, Holley KE, Farrow GM. Renal epithelial hyperplastic and neoplastic proliferation in autosomal polycystic kidney disease. Am J Kidney Dis 1987;9:27.
31. Hughson MD, Buchwald D, Fox M. Renal neoplasia and acquired cystic kidney disease in patients receiving long-term dialysis. Arch Pathol Lab Med 1986;110:592.
32. Rumpelt HJ, Storkel S, Moll R, et al. Bellini duct carcinoma: further evidence for this rare variant of renal cell carcinoma. Histopathology 1991;18:115.
33. Dimpoulos MA, Logothetic CJ, Markowitz A, et al. Collecting duct carcinoma of the kidney. Br J Urol 1993;71:388.
34. Baer SC, Ro JY, Ordonez NG, et al. Sarcomatoid collecting duct carcinoma: a clinicopathologic and immunohistochemical study of five cases. Hum Pathol 1992;24:1017.
35. Davis CJ Jr, Mostofi FK, Sesterhenn IA. Renal medullary carcinoma: the seventh sickle cell nephropathy. Am J Surg Pathol 1995;19:1.
36. Bonsib SM, Lager DJ. Chromophobe cell carcinoma: analysis of five cases. Am J Surg Pathol 1990;14:260.
37. Thoenes W, Storkel S, Rumpelt HJ, et al. Chromophobe cell renal carcinoma and its variants: a report on 32 cases. J Pathol 1988;155: 277.
38. Speicher MR, Schoell B, Du Manoir S, et al. Specific loss of chromosomes 1, 2, 6, 10, 13, 17, and 21 in chromophobe renal cell carcinomas revealed by comparative genomic hybridization. Am J Pathol 1994; 145(2):356.
39. Bonsib SM, Fischer J, Plattner S, Fallon B. Sarcomatoid renal tumors: clinicopathologic correlation of three cases. Cancer 1987;59:527.
40. Sella A, Logothetis CJ, Ro JY, et al. Sarcomatoid renal cell carcinoma: a treatable entity. Cancer 1987;60:1313.
41. DeLong WD, Grignon DJ, Eberwein P, et al. Sarcomatoid renal cell carcinoma: an immunohistochemical study of 18 cases. Arch Pathol Lab Med 1993;117:636.
42. Balslev E, Fischer S. Transitional cell carcinoma of the renal collecting tubules (renal urothelioma). Acta Pathol Microbiol Immunol Scand 1983;91:419.
43. Guinan P, Vogelzang NJ, Randazzo R, et al. Renal pelvis cancer: a review of 611 patients treated in Illinois 1975-1985: Cancer Incidence and End Results Committee. Urology 1992;40:393.
44. Blute ML, Tsushima K, Farrow GM, Therneau TM, Lieber MM. Transitional cell carcinoma of the renal pelvis: nuclear deoxyribonucleic acid ploidy studied by flow cytometry. J Urol 1988;140:944.
45. Fujimoto H, Tobisu K, Sakamoto M, et al. Intraductal tumor involvement and renal parenchymal invasion of transitional cell carcinoma in the renal pelvis. J Urol 1995;153:57.
46. Moll R, Lowe A, Laufer J, Franke WW. Cytokeratin 20 in human carcinomas: a new histodiagnostic marker detected by monoclonal antibodies. Am J Pathol 1992;140:427.
47. Gohji K, Nakonishi T, Hara I, et al. Two cases of primary neuroblastoma of the kidney in adults. J Urol 1987;137:966.
48. Rothwell DL, Vorstman B, Patton I, et al. Intrarenal pheochromocytoma. Urology 1983;21:175.
49. Hannah J, Lippe B, Lai-Goldman M, et al. Oncocytic carcinoid of the kidney associated with periodic Cushing's syndrome. Cancer 1988;61: 2136.
50. Bloom SR. An enteroglucagon tumour. Gut 1972;13:520.
51. Fetissof F, Benatre A, Dubois MP, et al. Carcinoid tumor occurring in a teratoid malformation of the kidney: an immunohistochemical study. Cancer 1984;54:2305.
52. Cauley JE, Almagro UA, Jacobs SC. Primary renal carcinoid tumor. Urology 1988;32:564.
53. Mills SE, Weiss MA, Swanson PE, Wick MR. Small cell undifferentiated carcinoma of the renal pelvis. Surg Pathol 1988;1:83.
54. Guillou L, Duvoisin B, Chobaz C, Chapuiz Z, Costa J. Combined small-cell and transitional cell carcinoma of the renal pelvis. Arch Pathol Lab Med 1993;117:239.
55. Capella C, Eusebi V, Rosai J. Primary oat cell carcinoma of the kidney. Am J Surg Pathol 1984;8:855.
56. Tetu B, Ro JY, Ayala AG, et al. Small cell carcinoma of the kidney. Cancer 1987;60:1809.
57. Mimran A, Leckie BJ, Fourcade JC, et al. Blood pressure, renin-angiotensin system and urinary kallikrein in a case of juxtaglomerular cell tumor. Am J Med 1978;65:527.

58. Steffens J, Bock R, Braedel HU, et al. Renin-producing renal cell carcinoma. Eur Urol 1990;18:56.
59. Hartwick RWJ, Srigley J, Shaw P. Uncommon histologic patterns mimicking malignancy in angiomyolipoma. (Abstract) Lab Invest 1989;60: 39A.
60. Brecher ME, Gill WB, Straus FH. Angiomyolipoma with lymph node involvement: a long-term follow-up study. Hum Pathol 1986;17:962.
61. Lack EE, Dolan MF, Finisio J, et al. Pulmonary and extrapulmonary lymphangioleiomyomatosis with bilateral renal angiomyolipomas, multifocal lymphangioleiomyomatosis, and a glial polyp of the endocervix. Am J Surg Pathol 1986;10:650.
62. Ferry JA, Malt RA, Young RH. Renal angiomyolipoma with sarcomatous transformation and pulmonary metastases. Am J Surg Pathol 1991;15:1083.
63. Taylor RS, Joseph DB, Kohaut EC, et al. Renal angiomyolipoma associated with lymph node involvement and renal cell carcinoma in patients with tuberous sclerosis. J Urol 1989;141:930.
64. Hruban RH, Bhagavdan BS, Epstein JL. Massive retroperitoneal angiomyolipoma: a lesion that may be confused with well differentiated liposarcoma. Am J Clin Pathol 1989;92:805.
65. Sturtz CL, Dabbs DJ. Angiomyolipomas: the nature and expression of the HMB45 antigen. Mod Pathol 1994;7:842.
66. Peterson RO. Urologic pathology, 2nd ed. Philadelphia: JB Lippincott, 1992:58.
67. Srivinas V, Sogani PC, Hadju SI, et al. Sarcomas of the kidney. J Urol 1984;132:12.
68. Murphy WM, Beckwith JB, Farrow GM. Tumors of the kidney, bladder, and related urinary structures. Atlas of tumor pathology, series 3, fasc. 11. Washington DC: Armed Forces Institute of Pathology, 1994: 161.
69. Mayes DS, Fechner RE, Gillenwater JY. Renal liposarcoma. Am J Surg Pathol 1990;14:268.
70. Kandel LB, McCullough DL, Harrison LH, et al. Primary renal lymphoma. Does it exist?. Cancer 1987;60:386.
71. Siegel SW, Risius B, Tubbs R, et al. Bilateral solid renal masses in a young man. J Urol 1986;135:327.
72. Osborne BM, Brenner M, Weitzner S, et al. Malignant lymphoma presenting as a renal mass: four cases. Am J Surg Pathol 1987;11:375.
73. Cohen JI. Epstein-Barr virus lymphoproliferative disease associated with acquired immunodeficiency. Medicine 1991;70:137.
74. Huser J, Grignon DJ, Ro JY, et al. Adult Wilms' tumor: a clinicopathologic study of 11 cases. Mod Pathol 1990;3:321.
75. Lowe W, Weiss RM, Todd MB, True LD. Malignant rhabdoid tumor of the kidney in an adult. J Urol 1990;143:110.
76. Joshi VV, Beckwith JB. Multilocular cyst of the kidney (cystic nephroma) and cystic, partially differentiated nephroblastoma: terminology and criteria for diagnosis. Cancer 1989;64:466.
77. Trillo AA. Adult variant of congenital mesoblastic nephroma. Arch Pathol Lab Med 1990;114:533.
78. Powell T, Shackman R, Johnson HD. Multilocular cysts of the kidney. Br J Urol 1951;23:141.
79. Mazeman E, Wemeau L, Lemaitre G, Kozyreff P. Les tumeurs secondaires du rein. J Urol Nephrol (Paris) 1976;82:145.
80. Melato M, Laurino L, Bianchi P, et al. Intraglomerular metastases: a possibly maldiagnosed entity. Zentralb Allgemein Pathol 1991;137:90.
81. Johnson MW, Morettin LB, Sarles HE, Zaharopoulous P. Follicular carcinoma of the thyroid metastatic to the kidney 37 years after resection of the primary tumor. J Urol 1982;127:114.
82. Gelister JSK, Jarmulowicz M, Doanld J, et al. Renal inflammatory pseudotumor. Br J Urol 1990;65:548.
83. Case reports of the Massachusetts General Hospital. (Case 2-1995). N Engl J Med 1995;332:174.
84. Murphy WM, Beckwith JB, Farrow GM. Tumors of the kidney, bladder, and related urinary structures. Atlas of tumor pathology, series 3, fasc. 11. Washington DC: Armed Forces Institute of Pathology, 1994; 179.
85. Esparza AR, McKay DB, Cronan JJ, Chazan JA. Renal parenchymal malakoplakia: histologic spectrum and its relationship to megalocytic interstitial nephritis and xanthogranulomatous pyelonephritis. Am J Surg Pathol 1989;13:225.
86. Kragel PJ, Walther MM, Pestaner JP, Filling Katz MR. Simple renal cysts, atypical renal cysts, and renal cell carcinoma in von Hippel-Lindau disease: a lectin and immunohistochemical study in six patients. Mod Pathol 1991;4:210.
87. Takahashi S, Shirai T, Ogawa K, et al. Renal cell adenomas and carcinomas in hemodialysis patients: relationship between hemodialysis period and development of lesions. Acta Pathol Jpn 1993;43:674.
88. Ljungberg B, Holmberg G, Sjodin J-G, et al. Renal cell carcinoma in a renal cyst: a case report and review of the literature. J Urol 1990; 143:797.
89. Domagala W, Lubinski J, Weber K, Osborn M. Intermediate filament typing of tumor cells in fine needle aspirates by means of monoclonal antibodies. Acta Cytol 1986;30:214.
90. Smith EH. Complications of percutaneous abdominal fine-needle biopsy. Radiology 1991;178:253.
91. Yazdi HM. Genitourinary cytology. Clin Lab Med 1991;11:369.
92. True LD, ed. Diagnostic immunohistopathology. London: Gower/ Mosby, 1990.

Principles and Practice of Genitourinary Oncology, edited by Derek Raghavan, Howard I. Scher, Steven A. Leibel, and Paul H. Lange. Lippincott-Raven Publishers, Philadelphia, © 1997.

CHAPTER 78

Renal Cell Carcinoma

Tumor Markers

James M. Kozlowski

In 1996, carcinomas of the renal parenchyma will account for over 30,000 new cancer cases and be responsible for more than 18,000 cancer deaths.[1] Overt evidence of metastatic disease is demonstrable in over 30% of patients with renal cell carcinoma (RCC) at the time of initial presentation.[2] Furthermore, metastatic disease develops metachronously in about 50% of patients who have undergone a "curative" radical nephrectomy.[2–4] In general, the outlook for both groups of patients is dismal. A 10% 1-year survival rate is anticipated for patients presenting with synchronous metastases (average survival is 4 months). Patients with a delayed onset of systemic relapse can anticipate a median survival of approximately 11 months.[5–8]

Radical nephrectomy and nephron-sparing surgery play a preeminent role in the management of putatively organ-confined disease. In addition, aggressive surgical therapy has been associated with 5-year survival rates of 35% to 50% in patients with RCC who present with or who develop apparently solitary metastatic lesions.[8] With respect to the latter phenomenon, studies by Skinner and associates,[3] Tolia and Whitmore,[9] O'Dea and associates,[10] and Middleton[11] have cited an incidence of 3.6%, 3.2%, 2.5%, and 1.6%, respectively.

Unfortunately, the majority of these patients harbor subclinical, multifocal, micrometastatic disease and ultimately succumb to the uncontrolled proliferation of RCC despite aggressive systemic therapy. For example, partial and complete response rates of 17% and 4%, respectively, have been associated with the use of high-dose interleukin-2 (IL-2). Most impressive is that these responses are generally durable, and 40% of such patients maintain the achieved response for at least 2 years.[12] Once again, most patients do not benefit from these toxic therapies, and most responders ultimately manifest evidence of disease progression. The nature of RCC is extremely variable and unpredictable. Indeed, 20% to 30% of such patients exhibit the phenomenon of disease stabilization.[6,8] This finding implies that some primary tumors and established metastatic foci may fail to exhibit evidence of sustained growth or metastatic potential for many years. Obviously, the perceived benefits of any systemic therapy for RCC must be viewed within this context.

The availability of sensitive and specific markers of RCC tumor activity would be advantageous for several reasons. The presence of secretory or degradation products measurable in the serum or urine would possibly facilitate the detection of low-stage, organ-confined RCC in both the general population and in those cohorts at high risk for developing RCC (patients with von Hippel-Lindau disease and those receiving hemodialysis). In addition, such easily assayable markers could permit the early detection of local recurrence or systemic relapse and could provide a means of prompt assessment of the antitumor activity of administered systemic therapies. RCC-associated monoclonal antibodies (MABs) could be used to detect antigens shed or secreted into blood, urine, or renal cystic fluid.[13] Radioimmunoscintigraphy using RCC-reactive MABs could possibly facilitate the localization of metastatic disease and the evaluation of complex cystic renal masses.[14] Finally, MABs capable of targeting RCC foci in vivo could provide the delivery vehicle for potentially effective therapy by linkage to chemotherapeutic agents, radionuclides, or toxins.[13]

No highly sensitive and specific markers of RCC tumor activity capable of fulfilling all the previously enumerated functions are available. Certain biologic markers have been evaluated with respect to their ability to detect RCC tumor activity and have proved unreliable because of unacceptably low sensitivity and specificity profiles. These markers include renin,[15] erythropoietin,[15] lipid-associated sialic acid,[16] carcinoembryonic antigen,[17] fibrinogen,[18] haptoglobin,[19] and C-reactive protein.[20] More recent investigations have defined a diverse array of biologic markers that hold much greater promise with respect to their ability to detect RCC-related tumor activity and include the following: (1) serum ferritin (SF); (2) nephrocalcin (NC); (3) γ-enolase; (4) aldolase; (5) S-100a$_0$ protein; (6) interleukin-6 (IL-6) and other cytokines; (7) basic fibroblast growth factor (bFGF) and other angiogenic peptides; (8) parathyroid-related protein (PRP); and (9) RCC-reactive MABs. The remainder of this chapter provides a brief overview of each of these areas.

SERUM FERRITIN

Ferritin is an intracellular iron-storage protein whose main function is to sequester iron in a nontoxic form and to release it to iron pools when required for metabolic activity.[21,22] Apoferritin is the protein component of ferritin and is composed of a variable number of polypeptide subunits responsible for the different isomeric forms of ferritin.[23] The basic isoferritins are predominantly located in the liver and spleen and are found in greatest concentration in those cells involved in iron storage (macrophages and hepatocytes).[24] Acidic isoferritins have been found in most mammalian cells, with substantial concentrations in the normal heart, pancreas, placenta, and kidney.[21,24] With respect to the kidney, immunocytochemical studies have demonstrated that acidic isoferritin is confined to the proximal tubular cells of the maturing fetal nephron and the adult kidney.[23]

Although the SF concentration generally reflects the magnitude of available iron stores in the body, in the following conditions, for example, SF is disproportionately elevated: (1) various infections and inflammatory disorders; (2) anemia of chronic disease; (3) hepatic disease or damage; and (4) certain neoplastic conditions such as Hodgkin's disease, acute lymphatic leukemia, hepatoma, and carcinomas of the breast, stomach, pancreas, and kidney.[21,24] That the acidic isoferritins are preferentially expressed in these malignant conditions helps to explain their alternative designation as the oncofetal ferritins.[24]

In 1987, Flemming used polyclonal antiferritin antisera to perform an immunocytochemical localization of ferritin in 18 nephroblastomas, 4 renal sarcomas, 26 RCCs, and 8 renal oncocytomas.[23] Ferritin was located within the neoplastic cells of 54% of RCCs and 63% of renal oncocytomas. Ferritin was not seen in the other tumor types. Although stromal macrophages also contain ferritin, these studies tend to support the contention that the ''ferritinemia'' of cancer patients is directly related to the production and release of ferritin by tumor cells.[23]

Esen and associates analyzed SF levels in 32 patients with RCC using a ferritin radioimmunoassay. Serum samples were evaluated before and after nephrectomy in this cohort. The mean SF concentration was significantly higher in patients with RCC than in age- and sex-matched controls (259.10 ng/mL versus 61.30 ng/mL, $P = .001$).[21] In addition, the SF levels rose proportionately and significantly with advancing tumor stage. Indeed, SF was elevated in 33%, 80%, 100%, and 93% of patients with stages I, II, III, and IV, respectively. In this study, the mean preoperative SF level for patients with stage I-II disease was 132.27 ng/mL, and only this cohort exhibited a statistically significant diminution in this parameter after nephrectomy (mean = 77.39 ng/mL). In contrast, patients with stage III-IV disease had a mean preoperative SF level of 361.42 ng/mL. These patients did not demonstrate a significant diminution in this marker after nephrectomy. Concomitant immunohistochemical studies demonstrated a marked increase in intracellular ferritin content in the RCC tissues when compared with normal parenchyma. In the latter, only proximal tubular cells demonstrated ferritin content.

Ferritin appears to constitute more than an inert marker of RCC tumor activity. For example, iron is required for the proliferation of normal and neoplastic cells. Moreover, proteins involved with iron metabolism (ferritin and transferrin) may favorably modulate those iron supplies available to malignant cells and may enhance their growth potential.[25] Further, a tumor-derived acidic ferritin appears to possess a distinct immunosuppressive effect, particularly with respect to inhibiting the activation of T lymphocytes.[22] Indeed, this same phenomenon has been associated with the acidic ferritins derived from the placenta, and investigators have suggested that the high serum levels of placental ferritin during pregnancy may be responsible for suppression of the immune system of the mother, thus insuring ''immune tolerance'' of the maturing fetus.[22] In this respect, acidic or oncofetal ferritin may facilitate both neoplastic progression and embryonic development through its inhibition of the host immune system.[22]

NEPHROCALCIN

NC is a glycoprotein derived from the cells of the proximal tubule and thick ascending limb.[26] NC is present in mammalian urine, and its major function is that of a urinary calcium oxalate monohydrate crystal growth inhibitor.[27] Patients with a history of calcium oxalate stones generally have decreased urinary NC activity, which is otherwise detectable at stable levels in healthy controls.[28] The specific elution pattern of urinary NC in healthy adults has been thoroughly described and demonstrates the presence of approximately 5 isomers whose generation is contingent on differences in the phosphorylation of the NC molecule.[29]

Nakagawa and associates used polyclonal antibodies specific to NC and measured urinary and serum NC levels by an enzyme-linked immunosorbent assay (ELISA) in 19 patients with newly diagnosed (localized) RCC and 21 controls.[26] The mean level of urinary NC in the patients with RCC was 0.241 ± 0.341 μg NC/mg creatinine. In contrast, the average urinary NC level in the controls was 0.022 ± 0.012 μg NC/mg creatinine ($P = .0112$). Only 4 of 19 patients with RCC had urinary NC levels within the control range. No obvious correlation was seen between the urinary NC levels demonstrated and such factors as tumor stage, tumor size, tumor histotype, or tumor grade. The serum and urinary NC concentrations were closely correlated. In previous studies, this group had demonstrated elevated urinary NC levels in patients with RCC with documented metastatic disease.[27] This latter observation suggests that NC maybe a useful tumor marker even when RCC tissue is not contact with the urothelial system. Furthermore, the NC isolated from RCC cells demonstrates a distinctly abnormal elution pattern characterized by the following: (1) increased amounts of isomer 1; (2) low phosphate content; and (3) larger amounts of carbohydrate residues.[26,27]

NC, unlike γ-enolase and aldolase, appears to be kidney-specific.[26] Another distinction between NC and these other markers (discussed later) is that NC has been localized to RCC of all grades and histologic types.[26] These observations, coupled with the apparent close correlation between urinary and serum levels, suggest that NC maybe a unique and important marker of RCC tumor activity.

γ-ENOLASE

Enolases are glycolytic enzymes that catalyze the reaction pathway between 2-phosphoglycerate and phosphoenolpyruvate.[30] These enzymes are dimers composed of α, β, and γ, subunits. Five distinct isozymes have been recognized ($\alpha\alpha$, $\beta\beta$, $\gamma\gamma$, $\alpha\beta$, and $\alpha\gamma$), with each dimer having an approximate molecular weight of 100,000.[31] The α subunit appears to be ubiquitously distributed, whereas the β subunit is preferentially expressed in striated muscle and heart.[31] With respect to γ-enolase, high levels have been found in neuronal and neuroendocrine cells. For this reason, γ-enolase is alternatively designated neuron-specific enolase.[32–34]

Haimoto and associates used immunohistochemical techniques to determine the localization of enolase isozymes in normal renal tubules.[30] In that study, the $\alpha\alpha$ dimer was found preferentially in the proximal tubules, whereas the $\gamma\gamma$ form was located in the loops of Henle. Finally, the medullary collecting ducts and macula densa exhibited the $\alpha\alpha$, $\gamma\gamma$, or $\alpha\gamma$ isozymes. The reason for the preferential expression of γ-enolase in the loops of Henle may be that this isozyme is more stable in the presence of chloride ions that undergo active transepithelial transport in that segment of the nephron.[30,35]

Haimoto and associates detected evidence of γ-enolase expression in all 36 RCCs subjected to immunohistochemical analysis.[36] Using a corroborative immunoassay, these same investigators demonstrated that the levels of γ-enolase in the normal cortex were 16.8 ± 3.7 ng/mg protein. In contrast, the levels expressed in RCC were approximately 55-fold higher (928 ± 554 ng/mg protein) than those documented in normal cortical tissue. In this same study, serum γ-enolase levels were elevated in 49% (20 of 41) of patients with RCC. The sera of 100 healthy adults were analyzed for γ-enolase activity, and a mean value of 3.1 ± 0.9 ng/mL was documented. Similarly, in the 41 patients with RCC, the mean serum γ-enolase concentration was 9.1 ± 11.0 ng/mL. The values in excess of 6 ng/mL were considered elevated and were consequently documented in 20 of 41 patients.[30]

The preceding observations were expanded in the study conducted by Kusama and associates.[37] In that study, all 13 RCCs tested demonstrated strong immunohistochemical reactivity for neuron-specific enolase. Serum γ-enolase levels were also measured in these patients by means of radioimmunoassay, with 10 ng/mL designated as the upper limit of normal. A mean value of 24.7 ± 33.2 ng/mL was detected. In all, the γ-enolase levels were elevated in 65% (11 of 17) patients. Six of 7 of the patients with stage I disease exhibited normal serum levels. In contrast, all the patients (10 of 10) with stage II-IV disease had elevated γ-enolase serum levels. These results suggested that neuron-specific enolase activity is correlated with tumor volume and may be most useful as an indicator of advanced-stage RCC.

The preceding observations validated the findings of Takashi and associates.[31] These investigators demonstrated that tissue γ-enolase levels were 34 times higher in RCC than in the healthy renal cortex. Similarly, 51% (53 of 103) of patients with RCC had serum γ-enolase levels higher than 6 ng/mL. The mean serum γ-enolase level in RCC was 8.0 ± 5.7 ng/mL, in contrast to a value of 3.1 ± 0.9 ng/mL noted in healthy subjects. Patients with stage III-IV tumors had higher mean serum γ-enolase levels (9.9 ± 6.8 ng/mL) those with stage I-II neoplasms (5.8 ± 3.0 ng/mL). Positive serum detection rates of 34% and 22% were noted in patients with stage I and stage II disease, respectively. In contrast, positive detection rates of 80%, 61%, and 61%, were noted in patients with stage III, stage IV, and recurrent disease, respectively. Complete surgical excision was associated with a significant reduction in serum γ-enolase levels. Finally, 7 of 8 patients whose values normalized after nephrectomy had increased values at the time of systemic relapse. No apparent relationship was noted between serum γ-enolase levels and the site of metastatic disease. Although patients with granular cell histotypes demonstrated higher serum γ-enolase levels than those with clear cell tumors, these results were not statistically significant.

γ-Enolase is not a tumor marker specific for RCC. Nonetheless, it is avidly expressed by most such tumors at the tissue level, and elevated serum levels are frequently demonstrable in patients with advanced-stage disease.

ALDOLASE

Fructose-1, 6-bisphosphate aldolase is a tetrameric enzyme involved in the anaerobic glycolytic pathway.[38] It is composed of three immunologically distinct subunits (A, B, and C).[39] Aldolase A and C are the predominant isozymes expressed in the fetal kidney.[40] In contrast, aldolase B represents 94.1% of total aldolase content in the normal adult kidney, with A and C isozymes contributing 5.8% and 0.1%, respectively.[38,41] Aldolase B is localized predominantly in the proximal tubules of the nephron.

Previous studies have demonstrated altered expression of aldolase isozymes during carcinogenesis, and most have demonstrated reversion to the fetal isozymes (A and C) during this process.[42,43] In concert with these observations, Zhu and associates analyzed RCC tissues by means of sensitive enzyme immunoassays capable of discriminating the various aldolase isozymes and demonstrated that these tumor tissues contained 97.6% of A isozyme, with B and C isozymes contributing 1.7% and 0.7%, respectively.[38] Furthermore, these investigators noted that the concentrations of aldolases A and C in RCC exceeded the concentrations documented in normal renal cortex tenfold and fivefold, respectively. This quantitative analysis by enzyme immunoassay was further correlated with immunohistochemical studies that demonstrated the presence of aldolases A and C in all ten RCC specimens subjected to this analysis. Conversely, aldolase B was only faintly expressed in 20% of these specimens.[38]

These same investigators determined the serum levels of aldolase A in patients with RCC (n = 40), patients with benign urogenital diseases (n = 48), and in patients with prostatic, testicular, and urothelial cancers (n = 34).[38] The average serum aldolase A level in normal controls was 198 ± 51 ng/mL. The upper limit of normal for serum for aldolase A was established at 300 ng/mL. The mean serum aldolase A level in patients with RCC was 472 ± 258 ng/mL. Using these parameters, elevated serum aldolase A levels were detected in 75%, 6.3%, and 21%, of patients with RCC, benign urologic diseases, and non-RCC malignant diseases, respectively. When stratified by tumor stage, elevated serum aldolase levels were noted in 53% (9 of 17) of patients with stage I disease. All patients with stage II (4 of 4) and stage III (7 of 7) disease demonstrated elevated levels. Finally, 83% (10 of 12) patients with stage IV RCC demonstrated elevated serum levels of this "fetal" isozyme.

Aldolase is apparently similar to γ-enolase in several respects. First, neither marker is specific for RCC. Nonetheless, both markers appear to be consistently elevated in patients with advanced-stage disease. Finally, both markers are expressed in low concentrations in the healthy kidney cortex, but both isozymes undergo a resurgence of expression during carcinogenesis. The latter observation legitimizes their designation as ''oncofetal'' tumor markers.

S-100A$_0$ PROTEIN

The S-100 protein family consists of dimers composed of two subunits, α and β. Three isoforms have been identified and include the following: (1) S-100a$_0$, $\alpha\alpha$; (2) S-100a, $\alpha\beta$: and (3) S-100b, $\beta\beta$.[44] The S-100a$_0$ isoform is expressed in particularly high concentrations in the heart, skeletal muscle, kidney, cartilage tissue, and brain.[44] The S-100a$_0$ protein is preferentially localized in the proximal tubules of the normal adult kidney. The α antigen is not expressed in the epithelial cells of the distal and collecting tubules.

Using a sandwich enzyme immunoassay system for S-100a$_0$ protein,[45] Kato[44] and Kimura[45] and their associates demonstrated that the average content of S-100a$_0$ in RCC was fourfold higher than that expressed in normal kidney tissue (650 ng/mg protein versus 160 ng/mg protein, respectively). When serum S-100a$_0$ levels were measured in healthy adults (n = 40), all patients exhibited levels less than 0.3 ng/mL. Indeed, 78% of healthy controls exhibited serum levels less than 0.2 ng/mL, the lowest limit of detectability for their assay.[44] Elevated levels of S-100a$_0$ (>0.5 ng/mL) were detected in 53% (17 of 32) of patients with RCC at the time of diagnosis. Serial determinations were also made in 13 patients at various times during their clinical course, and the S-100a$_0$ levels diminished after nephrectomy, but they increased at the time of clinically documented relapse. Unfortunately, a detailed subset analysis of these patients (i.e., tumor stage, tumor grade, and histologic type) was not reported.

The ultimate utility of S-100a$_0$ as a tumor marker for RCC will depend on the outcome of larger and more rigorously designed clinical trials. Elevations of this marker are not unique to RCC, but have also been detected in patients with lung cancer (30%), breast cancer (20%), and chronic nephritis (15%).[44] In chronic nephritis, obstruction of the proximal tubules as a component of the inflammatory process probably accounts for the increased serum level of S-100a$_0$ protein.

INTERLEUKIN-6 AND OTHER CYTOKINES

IL-6 is a pleiotropic cytokine whose synonyms include interferon beta$_2$, hepatocyte-stimulating factor, and B-cell stimulatory factor-2.[46] The gene for human IL-6 is located on the short arm of chromosome 7 p15-p21, consists of five exons and four introns, and is homologous with the gene for granulocyte colony-stimulating factor (G-CSF).[46] The IL-6 gene transcribes a 1.3-kb mRNA that is subsequently translated into a 212-amino acid (26-kd) precursor protein. The final 184-amino acid protein is obtained after removal of a 28-amino acid signal peptide. Before secretion, IL-6 is glycosylated, and this posttranslational modification apparently may play an important role in the pharmacokinetics of IL-6, as well as in tissue-specific functions.[46]

Disturbances of homeostasis, including infection, tissue injury, immunologic disorders, and neoplastic growth, are the major catalysts of IL-6 production. Endothelial cells, fibroblasts, and monocytes and macrophages constitute the major sources of IL-6 during elicitation of the acute-phase response.[46] Both interleukin-1 (IL-1) and tumor necrosis factor-alpha (TNF-α) stimulate the synthesis of IL-6, whereas steroid hormones tend to be inhibitory. The interaction of IL-6 with its numerous target cells is contingent on the expression of the IL-6-receptor by those target cells. The IL-6-receptor cDNA transcribes a protein of 468 amino acids that contains a signal peptide (19 amino acids) and a domain resembling that of the immunoglobulin superfamily (90 amino acids).[46] The molecular weight of the IL-6 receptor protein is approximately 80 kd.

The liver, a particularly sensitive target organ for IL-6, is largely responsible for the induction of acute-phase proteins by that organ.[47] These proteins include the following: (1) C-reactive protein; (2) serum amyloid A; (3) haptoglobin; (4) alpha$_1$-antichymotrypsin; (5) fibrinogen; (6) alpha$_1$-antitrypsin; and (8) alpha$_2$-macroglobulin.[46]

IL-6 also plays an obligatory role in the terminal differentiation of B cells into immunoglobulin-secreting cells.[46,47] IL-6 induces the proliferation of the pluripotential hematopoietic stem cells in synergy with IL-3, IL-4, granulocyte-macrophage colony-stimulating factor (GM-CSF), and macrophage colony stimulating factor (M-CSF).[46] Finally, IL-6 is an endogenous pyrogen, along with IL-1, TNF-α, and interferon beta.[46]

IL-6 is constituitively produced by many human nonhematopoietic tumor cell lines, most notably RCC.[48–50] Gastl and associates demonstrated in vitro secretion of IL-6 (>20 pg/mL/72 hours) in a total of 94% (17 of 18) of the RCC cell lines tested.[48] These observations are not limited to RCC cell lines. Studies conducted by Takenawa and associates documented of IL-6 gene expression by Northern blot analysis in over 50% (22 of 43) of fresh primary RCC tissues. In addition, these same investigators used DNA-polymerase chain reaction and detected the presence IL-6 receptor transcripts in all RCC tissues (43) and cell lines (7).[49] These observations contrast with analyses performed in normal kidney tissues that reveal that mesangial cells, but not tubular epithelial cells, produce IL-6.[49,50] Some studies have suggested that IL-6 may function as an autocrine growth factor in RCC.[51] This perception remains controversial, however.[52] IL-6 has also promoted tumor-cell motility in vitro.[53] Compelling evidence also indicates that IL-6 plays a major role in many paraneoplastic syndromes observed in RCC patients including fever, erythrocytosis, leucocytosis, amyloidosis, and increased acute-phase proteins.[49] Finally, some observations suggest that IL-6 is an etiologic factor in the hepatic dysfunction syndrome (Stauffer's syndrome).[54–55]

Several studies have suggested that IL-6 expression in RCC, at both tissue and serum levels, is an adverse prognostic variable. In the study performed by Takenawa and associates, clinical and pathologic data were available in 24 of 43 patients with RCC.[49] These investigators performed a subset analysis based on the ratio of tumor to normal tissue of IL-6 gene expression (i.e., ≤1.0 or >1.0). Patients exhibiting high-level expression of IL-6 (>1.0) had a significantly greater incidence of both lymph node metastasis and substantially greater levels of serum C-reactive protein. These investigators did not observe any significant difference in tumor size, tumor grade, or distant metastasis.

Tsukamoto and associates used an ELISA assay for IL-6 and analyzed the serum levels in 71 patients with RCC.[47] Because none of the controls exhibited IL-6 serum levels higher than

10 pg/mL, this value was established as the upper limit of normal. Using this parameter definition, 25.3% of the patients with RCC had elevated IL-6 levels. In this study, the likelihood of abnormal IL-6 levels closely correlated with advancing tumor stage. Contrary to the observations of Takenawa and associates,[49] these investigators did not document any obvious relationship between nodal status and abnormal serum IL-6 levels; however, abnormal IL-6 expression did roughly correlate with tumor grade, because patients with grade 1, grade 2, and grade 3 disease had abnormal IL-6 levels in 6.3%, 27.9%, and 46.2% of cases, respectively. Moreover, the 5-year disease-specific survival was significantly greater in those patients with stage M0 disease who manifested normal serum IL-6 levels. These findings were further validated by Blay and associates, who observed that patients with elevated IL-6 serum levels exhibited a poor response to systemic IL-2 therapy and generally manifested a shorter survival interval when compared with patients with RCC who had normal or undetectable levels of this cytokine.[56]

Other cytokines have also been identified in RCC cell lines and tissues. For example, G-CSF has been identified as a secretory product in the RCC cell line BA1119 and may be responsible for the striking polymorphonuclear leukocytosis documented in nude mice bearing this xenograft.[54,55] G-CSF production may contribute to similar paraneoplastic findings in patients with RCC. Moreover, the sequence homology shared between IL-6 and G-CSF is important.[46]

Similarly, Gastl and associates detected IL-10 secretion (>40 pg/mL/72 hours) in 22% of RCC cell lines (4 of 18) cultivated in vitro.[48] IL-10 is generally coexpressed with IL-6 in both lymphoid cells and cells of the macrophage lineage.[57] Both cytokines appear to contain homologous noncoding region sequences associated with transcriptional regulation.[58] IL-10 is capable of inhibiting numerous aspects of the immune system, including: antigen presentation, cytokine production, macrophage activation, and antigen-specific T-cell proliferation.[48,57,59] Although the ultimate importance of IL-10 with respect to a human RCC remains to be elucidated, investigators have suggested that IL-6 and IL-10 represent major elements of an important cytokine network operative within the microenvironment of some solid tumors.[48]

BASIC FIBROBLAST GROWTH FACTOR AND OTHER ANGIOGENIC PROTEINS

Hypervascularity is a prototypic trait demonstrable in over 85% of RCCs. The production of angiogenic growth factors by RCC tumor cells is postulated to be responsible for this feature.[60] Indeed, strong evidence suggests that the angiogenesis exhibited by RCCs in vivo may involve the cooperative interaction of three specific angiogenic factors: (1) bFGF; (2) vascular endothelial growth factor (VEGF); and (3) placenta growth factor (PlGF).[61] The potential importance of each of these proteins is briefly summarized in this section.

bFGF is a member of the heparin-binding growth factor family, which includes acidic fibroblast growth factor, bFGF, int-2, hst-1, FGF-5, hst-2/FGF-6, and keratinocyte growth factor.[61,62] The gene for bFGF is located on chromosome 4, appears to be interrupted by at least 2 introns, extends over 40 kb, and transcribes two to five mRNA species that ultimately translate a protein containing 157 amino acids with a molecular weight of 17,500.[62–64] bFGF contains four cysteine residues, two of which are conserved among all members of the heparin-binding growth factor family.[65] bFGF has been identified in virtually in all organs, solid tissues, tumors, and cultured cells subjected to vigorous characterization.[62] Similarly, receptors for bFGF have been identified in numerous cultured cells, including endothelial cells, baby hamster kidney cells, and fibroblasts, including those of prostatic origin.[62,66] Two receptors with molecular weights of 125,000 and 145,000 have been identified. Members of the heparin-binding growth factor family appear to have overlapping receptor affinity. That receptor-expression is downregulated by the production of endogenous bFGF is suggested by the observed inverse relationship between the receptor density per cell and the latter's content of bFGF.[67] bFGF mRNA lacks a definitive signal sequence. For this reason, the release of bFGF into the surrounding milieu does not occur through normal secretory pathways. Indeed, no definite mechanism for bFGF release has been identified other than as a consequence of cell death.[62]

bFGF demonstrates a diverse array of biologic activity, including the following: (1) induction during embryonic development; (2) increased cell growth and migration; (3) induction of plasminogen activator and type IV collagenase; and (4) rapid neovascularization.[62,66,68–70] These bFGF-related activities appear to be directly related to binding of bFGF to extracellular matrix components (heparin sulfate proteoglycans and glycosaminoglycans) after the release of bFGF as a consequence of cell death. The sequestration of bFGF within basement membrane and extracellular matrix provides a continuous reservoir of this angiogenic protein that permits the sustained occupancy of the bFGF receptor that appears to be required for long-term stimulation.[62,71] Moreover, the bFGF-glycosaminoglycan complexes are highly soluble and possess an increased radius of diffusion.[72] This matrix-bound bFGF is biologically active and is protected against proteolytic degradation.[73] One characteristic of an invasive neoplasm is the induction of heparanases and proteases that facilitate the degradation of the extracellular matrix.[71] Once elaborated, these matrix-degrading enzymes ease the release of bFGF-glycosaminoglycan complexes possessing mitogenic and angiogenic properties that facilitate local tumor progression and invasion.[71]

The literature is replete with observations supportive of bFGF's role as a marker of RCC tumor activity. Mydlo and associates characterized an angiogenic, heparin-binding growth factor similar to bFGF from tissue extracts of RCC specimens and a RCC cell line (A-498).[74] The potential importance of bFGF as a marker of RCC tumor activity was further suggested by the observations of Chodak and associates, who identified increased levels of FBF-like activity in the urine of 100% (7 of 7) of patients with RCC.[75] In fact, these investigators demonstrated more than 20 ng bFGF of urine production hourly in this cohort. Similar levels of bFGF activity were appreciated in only 6% (2 of 32) of the urine samples from the control group.[75]

In 1991, Fujimoto and associates used a sandwich enzyme immunoassay to monitor the serum levels of bFGF patients with RCC.[76] These investigators detected elevated bFGF serum levels (>30 pg/mL) in 52% (16 of 31) of patients with RCC.

Elevated bFGF serum levels were detected in 0%, 38%, and 73%, of patients with stage pT2a, pT2b, and pT3 disease, respectively. Only 20% of patients without evidence of venous involvement demonstrated bFGF serum levels higher than 30 pg/mL. In contrast, approximately 80% of patients with either renal vein or inferior venacaval involvement had elevated bFGF serum levels. When bFGF was correlated with tumor grade, only 27% of patients with grade I neoplasms had elevated bFGF serum levels, whereas 78% and 71% of patients with grade II and grade III tumors exhibited such elevations, respectively. No statistically significant difference was seen in serum bFGF levels between clear cell and granular cell neoplasms. Although a good correlation existed between the serum levels of bFGF and tumor grade and stage, the daily urinary output of bFGF was not associated with either parameter.[76]

The preceding studies provide compelling evidence of the role of bFGF as a marker of RCC tumor activity. In 1993, Nanus and associates attempted to identify the site of bFGF activity within RCC tumor tissue. Using immunohistochemical staining, these investigators analyzed renal tumor specimens that had been surgically removed from 62 patients (stage I, 1; stage II, 23; stage III, 19; stage IV, 17) and demonstrated bFGF expression in blood vessel walls, extracellular matrix, and tumor cell cytoplasm in 98%, 87%, and 16% of cases, respectively.[60] In this study, no statistically significant correlation was found between bFGF expression and tumor stage, grade, or histotype. The cytoplasmic expression of bFGF was associated with a shorter survival time, however, and the risk of death was 3.5 times higher than in patients with bFGF expression in blood vessel walls or the extracellular matrix. These investigators postulate that bFGF expression within the RCC tumor cells themselves contributes to the ability of such neoplasms to propagate within a given metastatic site, given their ability to produce this angiogenic protein constitutively.[60]

VEGF, which is structurally related to platelet-derived growth factor, is a secreted angiogenic mitogen that stimulates endothelial cell proliferation in vitro and exhibits angiogenic activity in vivo.[61,77–79] Four different molecular species are generated by alternative splicing of mRNA.[80] With respect to these species, $VEGF_{121}$ and $VEGF_{165}$ are secreted proteins, whereas $VEGF_{189}$ $VEGF_{206}$ bind to the cell surface and basement membrane.[81] VEGF also acts as a vascular permeability factor that promotes the formation of an extravascular fibrin gell that enhances both tumor and endothelial cell growth by providing an optimal growth substrate.[61] Using Northern blot analysis, Takahashi and associates demonstrated that 96% (26 of 27) of hypervascular RCC tissues exhibited three- to 13-fold elevations of VEGF mRNA, compared with adjacent normal kidney tissue.[61] No statistically significant relationship was seen between the level of VEGF mRNA and tumor histotype, grade, or stage.

PlGF, like VEGF, is a secreted angiogenic factor originally isolated from human placenta and choriocarcinoma cells.[61,82,83] PlGF, which shares 53% homology with VEGF, is a dimeric, glycosylated protein that induces the proliferation of endothelial cells in vitro. Takahashi and associates, again using Northern analysis, noted that the mRNA for PlGF was expressed in 91% (21 of 23) of hypervascular RCC tissues. PlGF mRNA was not detected in adjacent normal kidney tissue.[61] Although the exact role of PlGF in RCC angiogenesis remains to be elucidated, investigators have proposed that VEGF and PlGF constitute sensitive markers of RCC tumor activity, particularly during the incipient stage of tumor development.[61]

PARATHYROID-RELATED PROTEIN

Hypercalcemia has been observed in 3% to 16.8% of patients with RCC.[84] In this respect, RCC counts for about 3% of all cases of hypercalcemia of malignancy.[85] Most instances of paraneoplastic hypercalcemia associated with RCC are attributable to the elaboration of a novel PRP by the tumor cells.[86] The human gene for PRP is located on chromosome 12, consists of multiple exons, and through alternative splicing generates three nRNA transcripts that enode for three PRPs that possess 139, 141, and 173 amino acids, respectively.[87] These proteins share a common ''prepro'' sequence (amino acids −36 to −1) and are otherwise identical through residue 139.[87] The PRPs exhibit sequence homology with parathyroid hormone from amino acid 1 to 13.[86] The 36-amino acid parathyroid hormone-like amino terminus of the mature PRP peptide is responsible for the hypercalcemic effect.[87] PRPs are constitutively expressed in certain nonmalignant tissues, including lactating breast, pituitary, placenta, bone, uterus, central nervous system, and epidermis. In addition, PRPs are expressed in the fetal liver, kidney, and parathyroid tissue.[87] Complex posttranslational processing appears to account for the tissue specificity of PRPs.[87] Under homeostatic conditions, PRP may play an instrumental role in the autocrine or paracrine regulation of smooth muscle relaxation, transepithelial calcium transport, and fetal and adult growth and development.[87]

The syndrome of hormonal hypercalcemia of malignancy (SHHM) has been traditionally characterized by an elevated serum calcium level (total calcium >10.5 mg/dL; ionized calcium >2.7 mEq/L), raised urinary excretion of cyclic adenosine monophosphate (cAMP), and phosphaturia.[88] More recently, two region-specific immunoassays have been developed to measure PRP in the plasma and involve immunoradiometric assays of either the large N-terminal (1-74) peptide, or the C-terminal (109-138) peptide.[86] In the study by Burtis and associates, undetectable concentrations of these peptides were noted in 60 normal control subjects. In contrast, patients exhibiting evidence of SHHM had elevated levels of both N-terminal and C-terminal peptides.[86] This study included 2 patients with RCC with humoral hypercalcemia. The plasma concentrations of immunoreactive PRPs closely correlated with urinary cAMP levels.

PRP expression may constitute more than a useful marker for SHHM in patients with RCC. Burton and associates conducted in vitro studies using the PRP expressing a human RCC cell line, SKRC-1.[88] These investigators observed that the growth of this cell line was significantly inhibited the presence of polyclonal PRP antiserum. Tumor cell proliferation was also significantly inhibited by the competitive parathyroid hormone antagonist PTH (3-34) NH_2.[88] They emphasized that PRPs are not expressed in the normal adult kidney, whereas evidence of such expression can be found in the developing tubules of the human fetal kidney. These investigators postulated that PRP expression in RCC represents yet another example of reexpression of this transformed or ''oncofetal'' phenotype.[88]

The study conducted by Fahn and associates demonstrated that the development of SHHM in patients with RCC constitutes an adverse prognostic feature.[84] These investigators detected evidence of hypercalcemia in 9.2% (20 of 218) of patients with RCC. Although hypercalcemia was noted in only 3% of patients with stage I disease, an incidence of 5.9%, 14.1%, and 18.9% was detected in patients with stage II, stage III, and stage IV disease, respectively. They did not observe any significant correlation between tumor histotype and the development of SHHM. They did, however, note a statistically significant difference in survival between hypercalcemic and eucalcemic patients with stage IV RCC (excluding patients with bone metastasis), with a median survival of 45 days in the hypercalcemic group, compared with 286 days in the eucalcemic cohort ($P <$ .005).[84]

MONOCLONAL ANTIBODIES

A large panel of MABs has been identified that recognize differentiated antigens expressed in the normal kidney,[13,89–95] as well as those that react with unique RCC-restricted antigens.[14,96–99] Despite the existence of an impressive library of murine MABs, clinical studies designed to assess the utility of these probes for the diagnosis and treatment of RCC remain in the early stages of development.[100] Important variables influencing both the sensitivity and the specificity of such MAB-dependent techniques include the following: (1) cross-reactivity of the MAB with normal tissues; (2) the inherent ability of MAB to reach antigen-positive tissues; (3) the saturability of normal tissue antigen sites; (4) the intensity and heterogeneity of epitome expression; (5) the adequacy of tumor vascularization; (6) tumor location and volume; and (7) the presence or absence of circulating antigen.[14,100] The most rigorously characterized MABs include gp160, which is a human kidney differentiation antigen, and G250, which is an RCC-associated cell-surface antigen. The remainder of this section is devoted to a brief overview of the respective MABs.

The gp160 antigen is a cell-surface differentiation-related glycoprotein (160 kd) expressed by epithelial cells of the glomerulus and proximal tubule of the human nephron. In addition, approximately 80% of RCCs exhibit gp160 expression.[91,101] Nanus and associates demonstrated that gp160 expression closely correlated with resistance of RCC cell lines to the antiproliferative effects of interferon alpha.[102] Indeed, the proliferation of 7 gp160-positive RCC cell lines was not significantly inhibited by concentrations of interferon alpha as high as 3000 units/mL. Conversely, 8 of 9 gp160-negative cell lines were inhibited by interferon alpha. These in vitro findings were further validated by in vivo studies using athymic nude mice. The latter confirmed the interferon resistance of gp160-positive RCC xenografts.[102] Molecular cloning has subsequently confirmed that gp160 cDNA has a 78% homology to the murine BP-1/6C3 antigen, which is a B-lymphocyte differentiation protein exhibiting aminopeptidase (APA) activity. Furthermore, enzymatic assays performed on human RCC cell lines demonstrated perfect concordance between gp160 expression and APA activity.[101] Human APA catalyzes the removal of amino-terminal acidic residues from unblocked oligopeptides and may play a role in the catabolic pathway of the renin-angiotensin system by facilitating the removal of the aspartyl residue of angiotensin II to yield angiotensin III.[101] The exact mechanism by which human APA (i.e., gp160-positive) renders RCCs resistant to the antiproliferative effects of interferon alpha requires further study.

G250 is a cell-surface antigen that appears to be uniformly expressed by clear cell RCCs. Other RCC tumor histotypes and neoplasms derived from other organ sites do not express G250. With respect to normal tissues, G250 expression appears to be restricted to the bile duct epithelium and the gastric mucosal cells.[14,96]

Three clinical studies using athymic nude mice bearing RCC xenografts[96,103] and ex vivo perfusion experiments using RCC-bearing kidneys[104] suggested that iodine-131 (^{131}I)-MAB G250 could be used as an imaging agent. Oosterwijk and associates reported the results of a phase I/II clinical trial involving 16 patients with RCC who were administered ^{131}I-labeled monoclonal antibody G250 7 to 8 days before surgery.[14] Clear tumor images were observed in 13 patients, 1 of whom had a G250-negative tumor. The smallest lesion visualized was 8 mm in diameter. The fraction of injected ^{131}I-MAB G250 dose per gram of tumor approached levels as high as 0.02% to 0.12%. These results suggested that the use of MAB G250 has both diagnostic and therapeutic potential. Despite these encouraging results, several problems were highlighted in this study. First, poorly understood microenvironmental or macroenvironmental factors appear to account for the heterogeneous uptake of the ^{131}I-MAB G250, even though the tumors possessed an adequate vascular supply and demonstrated strong or homogeneous G250 expression using immunohistochemical techniques.[14] Second, about 25% of RCCs do not express the G250 antigen. To circumvent this problem of antigenic heterogeneity, Oosterwijk and associates propose to create an MAB cocktail that would incorporate both G250 and a second monoclonal antibody, MAB F31. F31 appears to be a renal differentiation antigen more uniformally expressed by RCC.[14,93]

The results of these and similar studies using other RCC-associated MABs[105] suggest that further improvements in radioimmunoscintigraphy may facilitate the identification of recurrent or metastatic RCC and the evaluation of complex cystic renal masses.[14] Similarly, RCC-associated and RCC-specific MABs constitute a theoretically attractive delivery vehicle for potentially effective therapy by complexing these antibodies to chemotherapeutic agents, radionuclides, or toxins.[13]

CONCLUSIONS

None of the markers of RCC tumor activity discussed in this chapter are sufficiently sensitive or specific to render them uniformally reliable barometers of RCC biologic activity. Further studies will be needed to determine which of these parameters should constitute a select panel of RCC tumor markers to facilitate the following: (1) the detection of low-stage, organ-confined RCC; (2) prompt identification of local recurrence or systemic relapse; (3) the early evaluation of treatment efficacy after the administration of systemic therapies; and (4) the development of novel therapies utilizing a "cocktail" of MABs complexed with appropriate cytotoxic agents. The identification of DNA sequence deletions involving the short arm of chromosome 3 in both sporadic and familial RCC by means of restriction length fragment polymorphism analysis suggests that additional insights derived through molecular epidemiology may provide highly specific markers of RCC tumor activity.[106]

ACKNOWLEDGMENT

I wish to reiterate my indebtedness to both Sharon Lang and Rose DeLeon for their invaluable assistance in the research and preparation of this manuscript.

REFERENCES

1. Parker SL, Tong T, Bolden S, Wing PA. Cancer statistics, 1996. CA Cancer J Clin 1996;65:5.
2. Lokich J, Harrison JH. Renal cell carcinoma: natural history and chemotherapeutic experience. J Urol 1975;114:371.
3. Skinner DG, Colvin RD, Vermillion CD, Pfister RC, Leadbetter WF. Diagnosis and management of renal cell carcinoma: a clinical and pathological study of 309 cases. Cancer 1971;28:1165.
4. Swanson DA, Orovan WL, Johnson DE, Giacco G. Osseous metastases secondary to renal cell carcinoma. Urology 1981;18:556.
5. deKernion JB. Treatment of advanced renal cell carcinoma: traditional methods and innovative approaches. J Urol 1983;130:2.
6. deKernion JB, Ramming KP, Smith RB. The natural history of metastatic renal cell carcinoma: computer analysis. J Urol 1978;120:148.
7. Droz JP, Ray A, Mahjoubi M, Philippot I, Bouleuc C, Kramar A. Prognostic factors in metastatic renal cell carcinoma. In: Klein EA, Bukowski RM, Finke JH, eds. Renal cell carcinoma: immunotherapy and cellular biology. New York, Marcel Dekker, 1993.
8. Maldazys JD, deKernion JB. Prognostic factors in metastatic renal carcinoma. J Urol 1986;136:376.
9. Tolia BM, Whitmore WF Jr. Solitary metastases from renal cell carcinoma. J Urol 1975;114:836.
10. O'Dea MJ, Zincke H, Utz DC, Bernatz PE. The treatment of renal cell carcinoma with solitary metastases. J Urol 1978;120:540.
11. Middleton RG. Surgery for metastatic renal cell carcinoma. J Urol 1967;97:973.
12. Sznol M, Thurn A, Parkinson DR. Overview of interleukin-2 trials in patients with renal cell carcinoma. In: Klein EA, Bukowski RM, Finke JH, eds. Renal cell carcinoma: immunotherapy and cell biology. New York, Marcel Dekker, 1993:171.
13. Vessilla RL, Moon TD, Chiou RK, et al. Monoclonal antibodies to human renal cell carcinoma: recognition of shared and restricted tissue antigens. Cancer Res 1985;45:6131.
14. Oosterwijk E, Bander NH, Divgi CR, et al. Antibody localization in human renal cell carcinoma: phase 1 study of monoclonal antibody G250. J Clin Oncol 1993;11:738.
15. Nseyo UO, Williams PD, Murphy GP. Clinical significance of erythropoietin levels in renal carcinoma. Urology 1986;28:301.
16. Echenique JE, Graham SD Jr. Significance of lipid-associated sialic acid and CA 19-9 as tumor markers for renal cell carcinoma. Urology 1988;32:397.
17. Chu TM, Shukla SK, Mittleman AO, Murphy GP. Plasma carcinoembyonic antigen in renal cell carcinoma patients. J Urol 1974;111:742.
18. Sufrin G, Mink I, Fitzpatrick J, Moore R, Murphy GP. Coagulation factors in renal cell carcinoma. J Urol 1978;119:727.
19. Babaian RJ, Swanson DA. Serum haptoglobin: a non-specific tumor marker for renal cell carcinoma. South Med J 1982;75:1345.
20. Richards B, Robinson MR, Pidcock NB, Cooper EH. Serum protein profiles in carcinoma of the kidney. Eur Urol 1982;8:32.
21. Esen A, Ozen H, Ayhan A, Ergen A, Tasar C, Remzi F. Serum ferritin: tumor marker for renal cell carcinoma. J Urol 1991;145:1134.
22. Moroz C, Bessler H. Ferritin as a marker of malignancy. In: deSousa M, Brock JH, eds. Iron in immunity, cancer and inflamation. New York, John Wiley & Sons, 1989:283.
23. Fleming S. Immunocytochemical localization of ferritin in the kidney and renal tumors. Eur Urol 1987;13:407.
24. Mufti GJ, Hamblin TJ, Stevens J. Basic isoferritin and hypercalcemia in renal cell carcinoma. J Clin Pathol 1982;35:1008.
25. Cazzola M, Bergamaschi G, Dezza L, Arosio P. Manipulations of cellular iron metabolism for modulating normal and malignant cell proliferation: achievements and prospects. Blood 1990;75:1903.
26. Nakagawa Y, Netzer M, Michaels EK, Suzuki F, Ito H. Nephrocalcin in patients with renal cell carcinoma. J Urol 1994;152:29.
27. Nakagawa Y, Sirivongs D, Novy MB, et al. Nephrocalcin: biosynthysis by human renal carcinoma cells in vitro and in vivo. Cancer Res 1992;52:1573.
28. Nakagawa Y, Abram V, Parks JH, Lau HS, Kawooya JK, Coe FL. Urine glycoprotein crystal growth inhibitors: evidence for a molecular abnormality in calcium oxalate nephrolithiasis. J Clin Invest 1985; 76:1455.
29. Nakagawa Y, Otsuki T, Coe FL. Elucidation of multiple forms of nephrocalcin by ^{31}P-NMR spectrometer. FEBS Lett 1989;250:187.
30. Haimoto H, Takasi M, Koshikawa T, Asai J, Kato K. Enolase isozymes in renal tubules and renal cell carcinoma. Am J Pathol 1986; 124:488.
31. Takashi M, Haimoto H, Tanaka J, Murase T, Kato K. Evaluation of gamma-enolase as a tumor marker for renal cell carcinoma. J Urol 1989;141:830.
32. Rider CC, Taylor CB. Evidence of a new form of enolase in rat brain. Biochem Biophys Res Commun 1975;66:814.
33. Schmechel D, Marangos PJ, Brightman M. Neuron-specific enolase is a molecular marker for peripheral and central neuroendocrine cells. Nature 1978;276:834.
34. Wharton J, Polak JM, Cole GA, Marangos PJ, Pearse AGE. Neuron-specific enolase as an immunocytochemical marker for the diffuse neuroendocrine system in human fetal lung. J Histochem Cytochem 1981;29:1359.
35. Marangos PJ, Parma AM, Goodwin FK. Functional properties of neuronal and glial isoenzymes of brain enolase. J Neurochem 1978;31: 727.
36. Haimoto H, Takahashi Y, Koshikawa T, Nagura H, Kato K. Immunohistochemical localization of gamma-enolase in normal human tissues other than nervous and neuroendocrine tissues. Lab Invest 1985;52: 257.
37. Kusama K, Asano M, Moro I, et al. Tumor markers in human renal cell carcinoma. Tumor Biol 1991;12:189.
38. Zhu Y, Takashi M, Miyake K, Kato K. An immunochemical and immunohistochemical study of aldolase isozymes in renal cell carcinoma. J Urol 1991;146:468.
39. Penhoet E, Rutter WJ. Catalytic and immunochemical properties of homomeric and heteromeric combinations of aldolase subunits. J Biol Chem 1971;246:318.
40. Kellen JA, Chan A, Caplan B, Malkin A. Aldolase isoenzyme patterns during human ontogeny and in lung, kidney and breast cancer. Enzyme 1980;25:228.
41. Haimoto H, Kurobe N, Hosoda S, Kato K. Sensitive enzyme immunoassay for human aldolase B. Clin Chim Acta 1989;181:27.
42. Schapira F, Reuber MD, Hatzfeld A. Resurgence of two fetal-type of aldolases (A and C) in some fast growing hepatomas. Biochem Biophys Res Commun 1970;40:321.
43. Schapira F, Hatzfeld A, Reuber MD. Fetal pattern of aldolase in transplantable hepatomas. Cancer Res 1971;31:1224.
44. Kato K, Haimoto H, Ariyoshi Y, Horisawa M, Washida H, Kimura S. High levels of S-100a$_0$ ($\alpha\alpha$) protein in tumor tissues and in serum of patients with renal cell carcinoma. Jpn J Cancer Res 1985;76:856.
45. Kimura S, Kato K, Semba R, Isobe T. Regional distribution of S-100a$_0$ ($\alpha\alpha$) S-100a ($\alpha\beta$) and S-100b ($\beta\beta$) in the bovine central nervous tissue determined with a sensitive enzyme immunoassay system. Neurochem Int 1984;6:513.
46. Heinrich PC, Castell JV, Andus T. Interleukin-6 and the acute phase response. Biochem J 1990;265:621.
47. Tsukamoto T, Kumamoto Y, Miyao N, Masumori N, Takahashi A, Yanase M. Interleukin-6 in renal cell carcinoma. J Urol 1992;148: 1778.
48. Gastl GA, Abrams JS, Nanus DM, et al. Interleukin-10 production by human carcinoma cell lines and its relationship to interleukin-6 expression. Int J Cancer 1993;55:96.
49. Takenawa J, Kaneko Y, Fukumuto M, et al. Enhanced expression of interleukin-6 in primary human renal cell carcinomas. J Natl Cancer Inst 1991;83:1668.
50. Fukatsu A, Matsuo S, Tamai H, et al. Distribution of interleukin-6 in normal and diseased human kidney. Lab Invest 1991;65:61.
51. Miki S, Iwano M, Miki Y, et al. Interleukin-6 (IL-6) functions as an in vitro autocrine growth factor in renal cell carcinomas. FEBS Lett 1989;250:607.
52. Mule JJ, McIntosch JK, Jablons DM, Rosenberg SA. Anti tumor activity of recombinant interleukin-6 in mice. J Exp Med 1990;171:629.
53. Tamm I, Cardinale I, Krueger J, Murphy JS, May LT, Seghal PB.

Interleukin-6 decreases cell-cell association and increases motility of ductal breast-carcinoma cells. J Exp Med 1989;170:1649.
54. Sherwood ER, Keer HN, Fike W, Smith D, Kozlowski JM. The role of colony stimulating factor(s) in the pathogenesis of nephrogenic hepatic dysfunction (Stauffers) syndrome. Presented at the annual meeting of American Urological Association, Boston, 1984:254A. Abstract 368.
55. Nelson JB, Sutkowski DM, Kozlowski JM. Role of interleukins 6 and 8 in the production of nephrogenic hepatic dysfunction. Proc 84th Annual Meeting Am Assoc for Cancer Res, Orlando, FL, 1993;34: 58. (Abstract 342).
56. Blay J-Y, Negrier S, Combaret V, et al. Serum level of interleukin-6 as a prognosis factor in metastatic renal cell carcinoma. Cancer Res 1992;52:3317.
57. deWaal-Malefyt R, Abrams J, Benet B, Figdor C, deVries J. IL-10 inhibits cytokine synthesis by human monocytes: an autoregulatory role of IL-10 produced by monocytes. J Exp Med 1991;174:1209.
58. Kim JM, Brannan CI, Copeland NG, Jenkins NA, Kahn TA, Moore K. Structure of the mouse interleukin-10 gene and chromosomal localization of the mouse and human genes. J Immunol 1992;148:3618.
59. deWaal-Malefyt R, Haanen J, Spits H, et al. Interleukin-10 (IL-10) and viral IL-10 strongly reduce antigen-presenting human T-cell proliferation by diminishing the antigen-presenting capacity of monocytes via down-regulation of class-II major histocompatability complex expression. J Exp Med 1991;174:915.
60. Nanus DM, Schmitz-Dräger BJ, Motzer RJ, et al. Expression of basic fibroblast growth factor in primary human renal tumors: correlation with poor survival. J Natl Cancer Inst 1993;85:1597.
61. Takahashi A, Saskai H, Kim SJ, et al. Markedly increased amounts of messenger RNAs for vascular endothelial growth factor and placenta growth factor in renal cell carcinoma associated with angiogenesis. Cancer Res 1994;54:4233.
62. Rifkin DB, Moscatelli D. Recent developments in the cell biology or basic fibroblast growth factor. J Cell Biol 1989;109:1.
63. Mergia AER, Abraham JA, Fiddes JC, Shows TB. The genes for basic and acidic fibroblast growth factors are on different human chromosomes. Biochem Biophys Res Commun 1986;138:644.
64. Abraham JA, Whang JL, Tumolo A, et al. Human basic fibroblast growth factor: nucleotide sequence and genomic organization. EMBO J 1986;5:2523.
65. Yoshida T, Miyagawa K, Odagiri H, et al. Genomic sequence of hst, a transforming gene encoding a protein homologous to fibroblast growth factor and the int-2 encoded protein. Proc Natl Acad Sci USA 1987;84:7305.
66. Sherwood ER, Fong C-J, Lee C, Kozlowski JM. Basic fibroblast growth factor: a potential mediator of stromal growth in the human prostate. Endocrinology 1992;130:2955.
67. Moscatelli D. High and low infinity binding sites for basic fibroblast growth factor on cultured cells: absence of a role for low affinity binding in the stimulation of plasminogen activator production by bovine capillary endothelial cells. J Cell Physiol 1987;131:123.
68. Gospodarowicz D, Ferrara N, Schweigerer L, Neufeld G. Structual characterization and biological functions of fibroblast growth factor. Endocr Rev 1987;8:95.
69. Moscatelli D, Presta M, Rifkin DB. Purification of a factor from human placenta that stimulates capillary and endothelial cell protease production, DNA synthesis, and migration. Proc Natl Acad Sci USA 1986;83:2091.
70. Presta M, Moscatelli D, Joseph-Silverstein J, Rifkin DB. Purification from a human hepatoma cell line of a basic fibroblast growth factor-like molecule that stimulates capillary and enothelial cell plasminogen activator production, DNA synthesis, and migration. Mol Cell Biol 1986;6:4060.
71. Folkman J, Kalgsbrun M, Sasse J, Wadzinski M, Ingber D, Volodasky I. Heparin-binding angiogenic protein—basic fibroblast growth factor—is stored within basement membrane. Am J Pathol 1988;130: 393.
72. Flaumenhaft R, Moscatelli D, Rifkin DB. Heparin and heparan sulfate increase the radius of diffusion and action of basic fibroblast growth factor. J Cell Biol 1990;111:1651.
73. Flaumenhaft R, Moscatelli D, Saksela O, Rifkin DB. Role of extracellular matrix in the action of basic fibroblast growth factor: matrix is a source of growth factor for long-term stimulation of plasminogen activator production and DNA synthesis. J Cell Physiol 1989;140:75.
74. Mydlo JH, Heston WDW, Fair WR. Characterization of a heparin-binding growth factor from adenocarcinoma or the kidney. J Urol 1988;140:1575.
75. Chodak GW, Hospelhorn V, Judge SM, Mayforth R, Koeppen H, Sasse J. Increased levels of fibroblast growth factor-like activity in urine from patients with bladder or kidney cancer. Cancer Res 1988; 48:2083.
76. Fujimoto K, Ichimori Y, Kakizoe T, et al. Increased serum levels of basic fibroblast growth factor in patients with renal cell carcinoma. Biochem Biophys Res Commun 1991;180:386.
77. Leung DW, Cachianes G, Kuang W-J, Goeddel DV, Ferrara N. Vascular endothelial growth factor is a secreted angiogenic mitogen. Science 1989;246:1306.
78. Keck PJ, Hauser SD, Krivi G, et al. Vascular permeability factor: an endothelial cell mitogen related to PDGF. Science 1989;246:1309.
79. Plouët J, Schilling J, Gospodarowicz D. Isolation and characterization of a newly identified endothelial cell mitogen produced by AtT-20 cells. EMBO J 1989;8:3801.
80. Tischer E, Mitchell R, Hartman T, et al. The human gene for vascular endothelial growth factor: multiple protein forms are encoded through alternative exon splicing. J Biol Chem 1991;266:11947.
81. Houck KA, Leung DW, Rowland AM, Winer J, Ferrara N. Dual regulation of vascular endothelial growth factor bioavailability by genetic and proteolytic mechanisms. J Biol Chem 1992;267:26031.
82. Maglione D, Guerriero V, Viglietto G, Delli-Bovi P, Persico MG. Isolation of a human placenta cDNA coding for a protein related to the vascular permeability factor. Proc Natl Acad Sci 1991;88:9267.
83. Maglione D, Guerriero V, Viglietto G, et al. Two alternative mRNAs coding for the angiogenic factor, placenta growth factor (PlGF), are transcribed from a single gene of chromosome 14. Oncogene 1993; 8:925.
84. Fahn H-J, Lee Y-H, Chen M-T, Huang J-H, Chen K-K, Chang LS. The incidence and prognostic significance of humoral hypercalcemia in renal cell carcinoma. J Urol 1991;145:248.
85. Mundy GR, Martin TJ. The hypercalcemia of malignancy: pathogenesis and management. Metabolism 1982;31:1247.
86. Burtis WJ, Brady TG, Orloff JJ, et al. Immunochemical characterization of circulating parathyroid hormone-related protein in patients with humoral hypercalcemia of cancer. N Engl J Med 1990;322:1106.
87. Yang KH, dePapp AE, Soifer NE, et al. Parathyroid hormone-related protein: evidence for isoform- and tissue-specific posttranslational processing. Biochemistry 1994;33:7460.
88. Burton PBJ, Moniz C, Knight DE. Parathyroid hormone related peptide can function as an autocrine growth factor in human renal cell carcinoma. Biochem Biophys Res Commun 1990;167:1134.
89. OOsterwijk E, Ruiter DJ, Wakka JC, et al. Immunohistochemical analysis of monoclonal antibodies to renal antigens: application in the diagnosis in the renal cell carcinoma. Am J Pathol 1986;123:301.
90. Luner SJ, Ghose T, Chatterjee S. Monoclonal antibodies to kidney and tumor-associated surface antigens of human renal cell carcinoma. Cancer Res 1986;46:5816.
91. Ueda R, Ogata SI, Morrissey DM, et al. Cell surface antigens of human renal cancer defined by mouse monoclonal antibodies: identification of tissue-specific kidney glycoproteins. Proc Natl Acad Sci USA 1981;78:5122.
92. Finstad CL, Cordon-Cardo C, Bander NH, et al. Specificity analysis of mouse monoclonal antibodies detecting cell surface antigens of human renal cancer. Proc Natl Acad Sci USA 1985;82:2995.
93. Bander NH, Finstad C, Cordon-Cardo C, et al. Analysis of a mouse monoclonal antibody that reacts with a specific region of the human proximal tubule and subsets renal cell carcinomas. Cancer Res 1989; 49:6774.
94. Tagliabue E, Canevari S, Menard S, et al. Human renal antigen defined by a murine monoclonal antibody. J Natl Cancer Inst 1984;73:363.
95. Yoshida SO, Imam A. Monoclonal antibody to a proximal nephrogenic renal antigen: immunohistochemical analysis of formalin-fixed, paraffin-embedded human renal cell carcinomas. Cancer Res 1989; 49:1802.
96. OOsterwijk E, Ruiter DJ, Hoedemaeker PJ, et al. Monoclonal antibody G250 recognizes a determinant present in renal cell carcinoma and absent from normal kidney. Int J Cancer 1986;38:489.
97. Schärfe T, Becht E, Kaltwasser R, et al. Tumor-specific monoclonal antibodies for renal cell carcinoma. Eur Urol 1985;11:117.
98. Kochevar J. A renal cell carcinoma neoplastic antigen detectable by immunohistochemistry is defined by a murine monoclonal antibody. Cancer 1987;60:2031.

99. Wahlström T, Närvänen A, Suni J, et al. Mr 75,000 protein, a tumor marker in renal cell carcinoma, reacting with antibodies to a synthetic peptide based on a cloned human endogenous retroviral nucleotide sequence. Int J Cancer 1985;36:379.
100. Bander NH. Monoclonal antibodies to renal cancer antigens. Eur Urol 1990;18:10.
101. Nus DM, Engelstein D, Gastl GA, et al. Molecular cloning of the human kidney differentiation antigen gp 160: human aminopeptidase A. Proc Natl Acad Sci USA 1993;90:7069.
102. Nanus DM, Pfeffer LM, Bander NH, Bahri S, Albino AP. Antiproliferative and antitumor effects of α-interferon in renal cell carcinomas: correlation with the expression of a kidney-associated differentiation glycoprotein. Cancer Res 1990;50:4190.
103. Van Dijk J, Zegveld STh, Fleuren GJ, et al. Localization of monoclonal antibody G250 and bispecific monoclonal antibody CD3/G250 in renal cell carcinoma xenografts: relative effects of size and affinity. Int J Cancer 1991;48:738.
104. Van Dijk J, Oosterwijk E, Van Kroonenburgh MJPG, et al. Perfusion of tumor-bearing kidneys is a model for scintigraphic screening of monoclonal antibodies. J Nucl Med 1988;29:1078.
105. Vessella RL. Radioimmunoconjugates in renal cell carcinoma. In: Debruyne FMS, Bukowski RM, Pontes JE, et al, eds. Immunotherapy of renal cell carcinoma. Heidelberg, Springer Verlag, 1991:38.
106. Zbar B, Brauch H, Talmadge C, Linehan M. Loss of alleles of loci on the short arm of chromosome 3 in renal cell carcinoma. Nature 1987;327:721.

Principles and Practice of Genitourinary Oncology, edited by Derek Raghavan, Howard I. Scher, Steven A. Leibel, and Paul H. Lange. Lippincott-Raven Publishers, Philadelphia, © 1997.

CHAPTER 79

Renal Cell Carcinoma

Clinical Diagnosis and Prognosis

David P. Wood Jr. and James E. Montie

Each year, approximately 27,000 new cases of renal cell carcinoma are diagnosed in the United States, and 11,000 patients die of the disease.[1] Historically, 30% of patients with renal cell carcinoma already have metastatic disease by the time they are seen by a physician, and 40% of patients with clinically localized disease develop distant metastases despite eradication of the primary tumor.[2–4] Several factors contribute to our inability to diagnose renal cell carcinoma early enough to allow most patients to be cured; these factors include the location of the kidneys, the unusual signs and symptoms produced by renal cell carcinoma, and the occasionally unpredictable nature of the disease. Before the advent of computed tomography (CT) scans and ultrasonography, unless the classic triad of flank pain, abdominal mass, and hematuria was present, renal cell carcinoma often was unrecognized until distant metastases were identified. Only 10% of patients have these signs and symptoms. With the increasing use of CT scans and ultrasonography to image the abdomen for a variety of nonurologic reasons, however, many ''incidental'' tumors are now identified in the kidneys of otherwise healthy patients. Konnak and Grossman[5] found that only 13% of renal cell carcinomas at their institution from 1961 to 1973 were identified incidentally, compared with 38% between 1980 and 1984. The biologic significance of these small tumors is unclear, but pathologically they are often renal cell carcinomas, and in some cases they can produce distant metastases. Although many renal cell carcinomas are now diagnosed incidentally, clinicians should appreciate the signs and symptoms of this disease. Any patient with these manifestations should be evaluated with an intravenous pyelogram, abdominal CT scan, or ultrasonographic examination.

The prognosis for renal cell carcinoma is confounded by the occasionally unpredictable nature and immunologic responsiveness of this tumor. Spontaneous tumor regression has been reported, and the tumor can grow to large proportions and invade venous structures without the development of metastatic lesions. Conversely, metastatic lesions can develop from small tumors less than 3 cm in diameter. These features have limited our ability to devise an effective staging system that accurately predicts the patient's prognosis.

In this chapter, we discuss the signs and symptoms of renal cell carcinoma, the evaluation of the incidentally recognized renal mass, the current American Joint Commission on Cancer (AJCC) staging system for renal cell carcinoma, and the prognosis for each of these stages.

SIGNS AND SYMPTOMS

The signs and symptoms produced by renal cell carcinoma can be classified into three groups: (1) those caused by local tumor growth; (2) those caused by metastatic development; and (3) those caused by systemic manifestations of the disease (Table 79-1).

TABLE 79-1. *Signs and symptoms related to renal cell carcinoma*

LOCAL SIGNS AND SYMPTOMS
Flank pain
Abdominal mass
Hematuria
Varicocele
SIGNS AND SYMPTOMS RESULTING FROM METASTASIS
Hemoptysis
Bone pain
Liver dysfunction
SYSTEMIC MANIFESTATIONS
Stauffer's syndrome
Hypercalcemia
Anemia
Fever
Nonspecific gastrointestinal complaints

Local Signs and Symptoms

Approximately 40% of patients with renal cell carcinoma have hematuria at the time of presentation, but as more tumors are identified incidentally, fewer patients are presenting with hematuria.[6] The cause of this hematuria is the vascular and infiltrative nature of the disease. Renal cell carcinoma forms in the cortex of the kidney and develops an extensive network of neovascular tumor vessels. These tumor vessels are friable and, as the tumor grows, can break into the collecting system. Hematuria is usually seen only when the tumor is large. It is a rare sign in small tumors unless they are located in the central portion of the kidney.

Flank pain, another constituent of the classic triad, is a presenting symptom in fewer than 20% of cases.[6] This pain may be caused by irritation of the renal capsule as the tumor expands. When the tumor becomes advanced, it may encroach on the psoas and quadratus lumborum muscles, resulting in severe back pain. This pain, in general, is unrelenting and is exacerbated by leg lifting or positional movements. Severe back pain often heralds the presence of unresectable disease.

Abdominal masses are rare in renal cell carcinoma, but they can be present, particularly in thin patients. When these patients are relaxed, the kidney can be readily palpated. Conversely, obese patients often do not notice an enlarging abdominal mass, which can be palpated on directed physical examination.

Occasionally, a left varicocele is present in a patient with a renal tumor on the left side of the body. This varicocele is often recent in onset. The classic sign that the varicocele is caused by renal cell carcinoma is that it does not decompress with recumbency. The cause of the varicocele is tumor invasion into the renal vein, resulting in relative obstruction of the left spermatic vein as it enters the left renal vein or from increased outflow through the spermatic vein as collateral circulation.

An occasional finding is nonspecific gastrointestinal complaints. Patients may complain of early satiety, nausea, and weight loss. Acute abdominal pain can result from hemorrhage into the renal cell carcinoma and can lead to a paranephric hematoma.

Signs and Symptoms Resulting From Metastatic Development

The most common sites of metastatic formation from renal cell carcinoma are the lungs, bone, and liver.[7] Because most metastases occur in the lung, recognition and management of pulmonary metastasis are critical. Most metastases can be seen on a plain chest radiograph. Rarely is a chest CT scan required to identify metastatic lesions (see Chap. 80). In general, pulmonary metastases do not produce any distinctive signs or symptoms, although endobronchial lesions can cause hemoptysis and bronchial obstruction. Additionally, pleural lesions can cause pleuritic chest pain mimicking pneumonia. If pleural metastases are extensive, then restrictive airway disease can evolve.*

Bony metastases from renal cell carcinoma are generally lytic, painful, and vascular, and they may present as pathologic fractures. Orthopedic surgeons are commonly confronted with a vascular tumor when they evaluate a pathologic fracture from an unknown primary site. If time permits, an abdominal CT scan is warranted in patients with such a fracture to determine whether a renal cell carcinoma is present. This is important information because of the highly vascular nature of renal cell carcinomas and the possible need for tumor embolization before repair of the pathologic fracture.

Liver metastasis is usually a late occurrence in patients with renal cell carcinoma, although it can cause significant jaundice and liver dysfunction. Most liver metastases are identified during the abdominal CT scan routinely used in staging renal cell carcinoma. Other entities that can mimic liver metastases are hepatic hemangiomas or cysts. The most difficult diagnostic question is whether the patient has a hemangioma of the liver or a renal cell metastasis. A radiolabeled blood cell study or a dynamic CT scan of the liver can help to differentiate between these two diagnoses.

Systemic Manifestations

A well-known manifestation of renal cell carcinoma is Stauffer's syndrome.[8] First described in 1961 as a reversible hepatic dysfunction in patients with renal cell carcinoma, this syndrome is found in approximately 15% of patients.[9,10] Classically, patients have elevations in serum alkaline phosphatase level, prothrombin time, bilirubin level, and alpha$_2$-globulin level.[8] Although the cause of Stauffer's syndrome is undetermined, some researchers have suggested the production of some type of biologic response modifier. These serum abnormalities return to normal after nephrectomy, and the presence of this syndrome has not been documented as an adverse factor in the overall prognosis of the patient. An isolated elevation of the alkaline phosphatase level in the absence of either hepatic metastasis or elevated liver enzymes should warrant a bone scan to evaluate the patient for evidence of bony metastasis.

Renal cell carcinoma produces substances that can cause systemic symptoms, including fever, anemia, and hypercalcemia. The high fevers occasionally seen in patients with renal cell carcinoma are probably caused by a pyrogen or another type of growth factor.[9] Approximately 10% of patients have high fevers, often occurring at a particular time of day.

Hypercalcemia, the most common endocrinologic manifestation of renal cell carcinoma, generally occurs only when metastatic disease is present.[11] Patients complain of lethargy, mental deterioration, and oliguria. Recognition of hypercalcemia is extremely important because of the life-threatening nature of this disorder. Reduction in the size of the primary tumor is rarely required, but nephrectomy may be beneficial in selected patients with refractory disease if a large primary tumor is present.

The most common systemic manifestation of renal cell carcinoma is anemia.[12] Approximately 20% to 30% of patients are anemic at the time of initial presentation. Anemia is associated with a low serum iron-binding capacity; however, hematuria or bleeding into the tumor itself can also cause anemia. The anemia usually resolves after nephrectomy. Occasionally, these tumors are associated with erythropoietin production and consequent polycythemia.

Renal cell carcinoma is fascinating because of its varied modes of presentation. Urologists and internists must be acutely

*Editor's note: Metastatic cancer of unknown primary site is one of the commonest malignant diseases in Western society. After investigation, renal cell carcinoma is frequently shown to be the tumor of origin.

aware of the signs and symptoms of this disease if delay in diagnosis is to be prevented. All physicians must be cognizant of the unusual metastatic sites of renal cell carcinoma, including the prostate, vagina, thyroid, and retina.[7] Masses in these locations, particularly if they have an abnormal histologic pattern, signal the possibility of metastatic renal cell carcinoma and warrant further investigation.

EVALUATION OF THE INCIDENTAL RENAL MASS

Because an abdominal ultrasonogram or CT scan is obtained for a variety of illnesses, the number of kidneys visualized radiographically has increased. Both ultrasonography and CT can identify masses 1 cm or larger in diameter, a property that makes these tests much more sensitive than intravenous urography (see Chap. 80). Most of these incidental renal masses are simple renal cysts that need no further therapy; however, 2% to 4% of these lesions are solid or of an indeterminant nature, but only 50% of these are renal cell carcinoma.[13] Therefore, advocating a radical nephrectomy for all patients with an incidental solid renal mass is inappropriate. When evaluating an incidental renal mass, the clinician must keep in mind the differential diagnosis. Table 79-2 lists the common incidental renal masses.

The algorithm for the evaluation of a renal mass identified by an intravenous urogram is seen in Figure 79-1. If the renal mass has all the characteristics of a simple cyst, then an ultrasonographic examination is sufficient to confirm that the mass is indeed a cyst. If the results of the intravenous urogram suggest that the renal mass is solid, however, particularly if the mass is deforming the architecture of the kidney, then a CT scan with contrast is necessary. A CT scan can determine whether the mass is solid, whether it enhances with contrast, and whether the mass has any fat suggestive of an angiomyolipoma. Studies have reported renal cell carcinomas containing a significant amount of fat, however, thus mimicking an angiomyolipoma.[14]

TABLE 79-2. *Differential diagnosis of incidental renal masses*

Renal cyst
Simple
Complex
Renal cell carcinoma
Oncocytoma
Angiomyolipoma
Other
Lymphoma
Sarcoma
Hematoma

If the mass appears to be a complex cyst, then aspiration of the lesion is reasonable. If the fluid is clear and the results of cytologic study are negative, then it is rational to stop at that point. The concern always exists, however, that a small amount of renal cell carcinoma may be present in the cyst wall but may go undetected by aspiration. If the mass appears to be solid and has no fat content, then the diagnosis is either renal cell carcinoma or oncocytoma. Although other infiltrating lesions such as lymphoma, sarcoma, or metastatic lesions are possible, they are rare.

The "spoke wheel" arterial pattern characteristic of an oncocytoma can be seen on an angiogram. This pattern, as well as the central scar of an oncocytoma occasionally seen on a CT scan, is nonspecific, however, because renal cell carcinomas can have central necrosis (Fig. 79-2). In our experience, angiography has not allowed accurate discrimination between a renal cell carcinoma and an oncocytoma. A biopsy of the solid mass may be helpful; however, distinguishing between an oncocytoma and an "oncocytic" renal cell carcinoma is difficult on the basis of cytologic features alone.[15] Therefore, we recommend resection of an indeterminant renal lesion unless it is clearly an angiomyolipoma or a complex cyst. The decision for treatment must also consider several other factors, however, including the patient's age and overall health status.

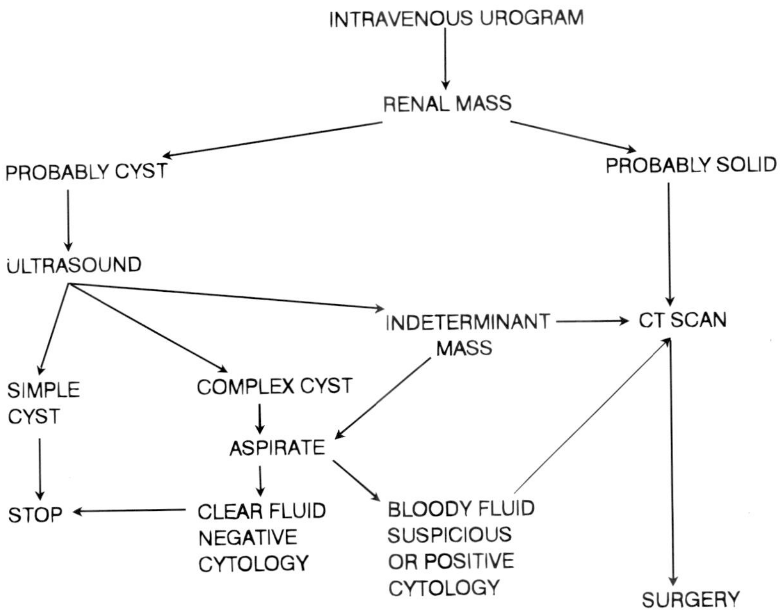

FIG. 79-1. Algorithm for the evaluation of an incidental renal mass found on an intraveneous urogram. CT, computed tomography.

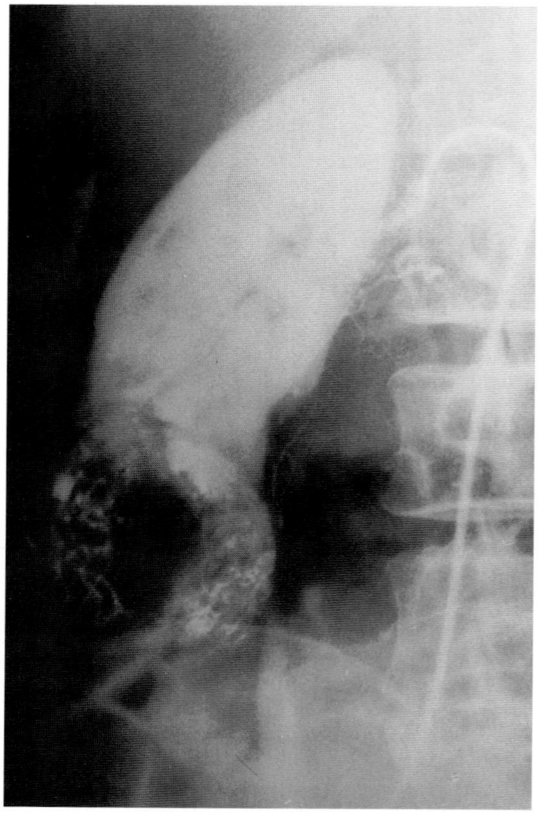

FIG. 79-2. Right renal angiogram showing central necrosis in a renal cell carcinoma. (Montie JE, Levin HS. Detection and diagnosis of renal cell carcinoma. In: Montie JE, Pontes JE, Bukowski RM, eds. Clinical management of renal cell cancer. Chicago, Year Book, 1990:6.)

STAGING

The optimal staging system for renal cell carcinoma is controversial. If a staging system is to be effective, each stage must predict a different survival rate. In 1969, Robson and associates created a staging system that was quickly accepted and is still used by many urologists.[16] The Robson classification is seen in Table 79-3.

This staging system was effective, but several studies have shown that the prognosis for patients with only renal vein involvement is closer to that for patients with perinephric fat involvement than for those with lymphatic metastasis.[2] The tumor node metastasis (TNM) system was introduced by the International Union Against Cancer (Union Internationale Contre le Cancer; UICC) in 1953 and has subsequently been modified several times. The AJCC published the *Manual for Staging Cancer* in 1977. In 1987, the UICC and AJCC agreed on the TNM staging system for all tumors. The current AJCC staging system for renal cancer is seen in Table 79-4.[17] The principal difference between the current TNM classification and the previous classification is the inclusion of the T3C category, which is vena caval thrombus extension above the diaphragm. In an

TABLE 79-3. *Robson classification of renal cell carcinoma*

Stage	Criteria
1	Confinement to kidneys
2	Perirenal fat involvement, but confinement to Gerota's fascia
3	Extrarenal involvement
	3A Gross right ventricular or vena caval involvement
	3B Lymphatic involvement
	3C Vascular and lymphatic involvement
4	Invasion into adjacent organs or distant metastasis

TABLE 79-4. *Current American Joint Committee on Cancer recommendations for staging*

PRIMARY TUMOR (T)	
TX	Primary tumor cannot be assessed
T0	No evidence of primary tumor
T1	Tumor $\leq$ 2.5 cm in greatest dimension limited to kidney
T2	Tumor $>$ 2.5 cm in greatest dimension limited to kidney
T3	Tumor extends into major veins or invades adrenal gland or perinephric tissues but not beyond Gerota's fascia
T3a	Tumor invades adrenal gland or perinephric tissues but not beyond Gerota's fascia
T3b	Tumor grossly extends into renal vein or vena cava below the level of the diaphragm
T3c	Tumor grossly extends into the vena cava above the diaphragm
T4	Tumor invades beyond Gerota's fascia
REGIONAL LYMPH NODES (N)	
NX	Regional lymph nodes cannot be assessed
N0	No regional lymph nodes metastasis
N1	Metastasis in a single lymph node, $\leq$ 2 cm in greatest dimension
N2	Metastasis in a single lymph node, $>$ 2 cm but not $>$ 5 cm in greatest dimension, or multiple lymph nodes, none $>$ 5 cm in greatest dimension
N3	Metastasis in a lymph node $>$ 5 cm in greatest dimension
DISTANT METASTASIS (M)	
MX	Presence of distant metastasis cannot be assessed
M0	No distant metastasis
M1	Distant metastasis

STAGE GROUPING			
Stage I	T1	N0	M0
Stage II	T2	N0	M0
Stage III	T1	N1	M0
	T2	N1	M0
	T3a	N0	M0
	T3a	N1	M0
	T3b	N0	M0
	T3b	N1	M0
	T3c	N0	M0
	T3c	N1	M0
Stage IV	T4	Any N	M0
	Any T	N2	M0
	Any T	N3	M0
	Any T	Any N	M1

Data from American Joint Committee on Cancer. Staging Manual, 4th ed. Philadelphia, JB Lippincott, 1992.

effort to simplify the staging system in 1983, vena caval involvement was included in the category of renal vein invasion. Because some studies have suggested that the extent of inferior vena caval thrombus involvement has an adverse impact on survival, the T3C category was reinstated.[18,19]

The classification of a tumor when the thrombus invades the wall of the renal vein or vena cava is unclear. In 1991, Hatcher and colleagues evaluated a group of patients with renal vein or vena caval involvement.[20] They found a 69% 5-year survival rate for patients with a free-floating tumor thrombus, compared with a 26% 5-year survival rate if actual invasion into the wall of the vein had occurred. Whether this direct invasion should be categorized as T4 (invasion into adjacent organs) is unclear, but, at least in this preliminary study, the survival rate appeared to be closer to that of patients with a T4 tumor than to that of patients with a free-floating thrombus.

Methods

The imaging modalities used to stage renal cell carcinoma fall into three main groups: (1) evaluation of the primary tumor; (2) evaluation of the vena caval thrombus; and (3) evaluation for metastatic disease. A complete description of these techniques is found in Chapter 80. Many studies may be performed in the staging of renal cell carcinoma; however, only rare patients require more than one or two of these tests. Limiting the number of diagnostic tests will become increasingly important as health care reform restricts the use of multiple imaging modalities.

Primary Tumor Staging

Historically, the intravenous pyelogram has been the most common imaging test used to evaluate the kidneys for renal cell carcinoma. Because of the increasing use of ultrasonography in the evaluation of abdominal pain, however, this test is surpassing the intravenous pyelogram in the detection of renal masses. Ultrasonography can identify renal masses as small as 1 to 3 cm in diameter.[21] If a mass has the radiologic characteristics of a simple cyst, the chance that the mass is truly a simple renal cyst is 98%.[22] Likewise, if a mass is solid and appears to be within the renal parenchyma, the differential diagnosis includes angiomyolipoma, oncocytoma, and renal cell carcinoma. Because fat is highly echogenic, angiomyolipomas containing a significant amount of fat can be detected by ultrasonography. Nevertheless, ultrasonography is usually inadequate to allow ready discernment among these three most common solid renal masses.

Intravenous Urography

Intravenous urography with tomography is still recommended for the initial evaluation of a patient with either renal colic or hematuria. The advantage of an intravenous urogram is that it evaluates the function of the renal cortex and the collecting system. An intravenous urogram cannot enable the clinician to discern small renal masses adequately and to determine whether they are cystic or solid, however. Therefore, we recommend that ultrasonography or a CT scan be performed if the intravenous urogram indicates the presence of any renal mass (see the previous section of this chapter on the evaluation of the incidental renal mass).

Computed Tomography

A CT scan of the abdomen with contrast medium is the primary test for diagnosing renal cell carcinoma. This test provides the information needed to evaluate the primary tumor, including the functionality of both renal units, the location and architecture of the mass, the vascularity of the mass, the presence of regional lymphadenopathy or invasion into adjacent organs, and the presence of a venous thrombus. A CT scan can be misleading in identifying mesenteric or liver invasion, however. As seen in Figure 79-3, because of volume averaging, the renal tumor appears to have invaded the liver. In most cases, however, the peritoneum remains intact between the two organs and separates the renal mass from the adjacent organs. Therefore, unless the patient exhibits manifestations of liver, mesenteric, or skeletal muscle involvement, such as grossly elevated liver enzymes, obstructive jaundice, small bowel obstruction, or unrelenting back pain aggravated by manipulation of the psoas muscle, the tumor has probably not invaded these organs.

The role of angiography has lessened over the years; this test is important only if renal bench surgery or a complex partial nephrectomy is planned, or if a large tumor is present. We do not routinely perform angiography before partial nephrectomy unless the tumor is large and centrally located. Although angiomyolipoma, oncocytoma, and renal cell carcinoma have classic arterial patterns, angiography does not allow accurate discrimination among these entities because of the significant overlap in their radiologic findings. Finally, angiography is of limited use in determining whether incidental renal masses are true carcinomas. Often, these masses are so small that they do not have sufficient tumor vascularity to allow identification by routine angiography.

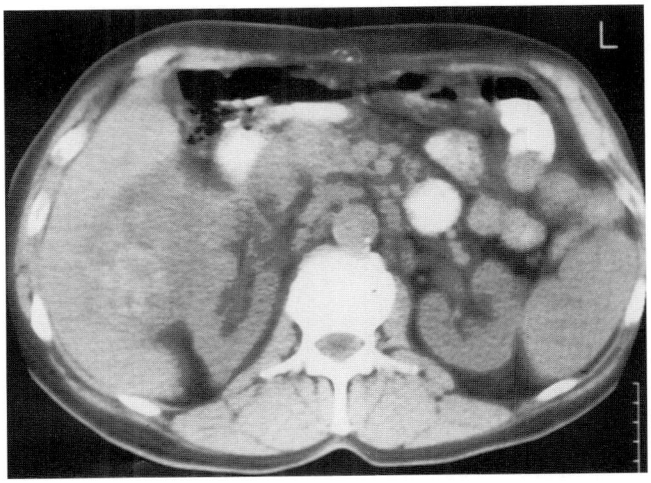

FIG. 79-3. A computed tomographic scan showing renal cell carcinoma with apparent direct liver invasion. On histologic examination, the tumor was confined to the kidney.

Caval Thrombus Evaluation

If the results of CT scan or ultrasonography suggest a renal vein or vena caval thrombus, further evaluation is warranted. The clinician must determine the presence and extent of the venous thrombus before surgery is performed. The following findings should prompt further testing: a filling defect in or enlargement of the renal vein or vena cava as seen on CT scan; a large, medially located renal tumor; and signs and symptoms of vena caval obstruction, including lower extremity vascular congestion or the new onset of a varicocele. The two techniques primarily used to evaluate the presence and extent of a caval thrombus are inferior venacavography and magnetic resonance imaging (MRI) (see Chap. 80). We use MRI to evaluate the caval thrombus because this test can permit accurate and noninvasive determination of the extent of the thrombus. No testing method allows an accurate determination of the presence of actual invasion into the renal vein or vena cava, however. Indicators of vessel wall invasion include absence of flow around the thrombus and obliteration of tissues surrounding the renal vein or vena cava (Fig. 79-4)

PROGNOSIS

As stated earlier, if a staging system is to be effective, the prognosis must be different for each stage. A significant improvement in survival for patients with renal cell carcinoma will depend on progress in earlier detection of small renal lesions, chemotherapy, immunotherapy, and possibly gene therapy. Until then, perifascial surgical extirpation of the involved kidney with early ligation of the arterial and venous blood supply is the mainstay of therapy. To discuss the prognosis of patients with renal cell carcinoma, we first must evaluate the natural history of the disease and the known prognostic factors.

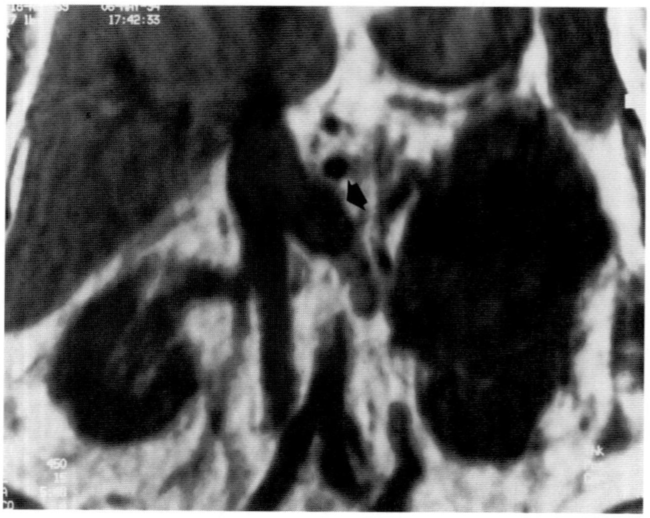

FIG. 79-4. A magnetic resonance imaging scan showing a large vena cava thrombus from a left-sided renal cell carcinoma. Lack of blood flow and an indistinct renal vein border (*arrow*) indicate possible invasion of the renal vein wall by tumor thrombus. Surgical resetion confirmed that the tumor thrombus had invaded the wall of the renal vein.

TABLE 79-5. *Seven important prognostic factors in renal cell carcinoma*

Distant metastasis
Regional lymphatic involvement
Renal vein involvement
Local extension of the cancer outside the renal parenchyma
Local tumor extension to adjacent organs
Size of the primary tumor
Histologic grade of the tumor

Natural History

Renal cell carcinoma is one of the few tumors that can grow to immense size and extend into vascular channels without metastasizing. Reports of metastases originating from tumors smaller than 3 cm in diameter have been published,[23,24] however, a finding that contributes to the widely held view that renal cell carcinoma has an unpredictable natural history. Despite these idiosyncrasies, some generalities about the natural history of this tumor can be stated. First, approximately 90% of patients with symptomatic localized renal cell carcinoma die if the disease is left untreated.[25] Second, no curative therapy exists for metastatic renal cell carcinoma. Third, although spontaneous regression of metastatic renal cell carcinoma has been reported, it is rare. In a review of the literature, Davis and associates found only three cases of histologically confirmed metastatic renal cell carcinoma undergoing spontaneous regression; all were pulmonary metastases.[26] Such findings strengthen the concept that biologic and immunologic factors play a significant role in the eventual outcome of patients with renal cell carcinoma.

Prognostic Factors

Seven factors that are important in determining the prognosis of patients with renal cell carcinoma are listed in Table 79-5. The stage of the renal tumor is the most important prognostic factor. As seen in Table 79-6, the 5-year survival rate for patients with T1-T3, N0, M0 disease is between 59% and 92%, compared with 15% for patients with N1-3M0 disease.[27] No significant survival difference is noted between patients with T1 and T2, N0, M0 tumors: 91% versus 92% 5-year survival, respectively. If T1 and T2 tumors are combined, the difference in the 5-year survival between T1-T2 tumors and T3 tumors is significant: 91% versus 64% respectively. Additionally, the presence of a tumor thrombus worsens the 5-year survival; pa-

TABLE 79-6. *Survival results for patients undergoing radical nephrectomy*

Stage	No. of patients	5-Year survival (%)
T1N0, NxM0	10	91 ± 34
T2N0, NxM0	268	92 ± 7
T3aN0, NxM0	165	77 ± 12
T3bN0, NxM0	202	59 ± 10
T4N(any)M0	210	15 ± 6

tients with extension into Gerota's fascia had a 77% 5-year survival rate, compared with 59% if renal vein involvement was present.

The size and grade of the primary tumor are also independent prognostic factors in renal cell carcinomas. Tumors less than 5 cm and more than 5 cm in diameter have 90% and 75% 5-year survival rates, respectively.[28] No survival difference was noted between patients with tumors that were larger than 5 to 10 cm in diameter and those with tumors larger than 10 cm in diameter. Low-grade tumors are associated with improved survival in all stages of disease, but this impact is most pronounced in patients with organ-confined disease.[28,29] In patients with T1 and T2 tumors, the 5-year survival rate for grade 1-2 and grade 3-4 tumors was 90% and 70%, respectively (P = .01). Grade was less important in patients with metastatic disease, partly because most of these patients had high-grade tumors.

What has been clearly shown is the importance of lymph node metastases in patients with renal cell carcinoma.[30] Reports have noted a 30% to 40% 5-year survival rate in patients with regional lymphatic metastasis who undergo radical nephrectomy plus extensive retroperitoneal lymphadenectomy, including the original description of a radical nephrectomy by Robson in 1963.[31] The use of extended lymphadenectomy has been popularized by Giuliani and associates, who reported a 50% 5-year survival rate for patients with node-positive disease.[32] Conversely, studies that did not include extensive lymph node dissection reported an 11% to 21% 5-year survival rate for patients with nodal metastases.[2,33,34] This discrepancy may be explained by the volume of disease present. Robson found that patients with only microscopic lymph node involvement did significantly better than patients with grossly involved lymph nodes.[35] Additionally, Giuliani and associates reported a 36% 5-year survival rate for patients with cancerous involvement in more than two lymph nodes, versus a 63% 5-year survival rate for those with involvement in only one or two lymph nodes.[32]

CONCLUSIONS

Renal cell carcinoma is unpredictable and can have many different manifestations. Therefore, both primary care physicians and urologists must be acutely aware of the varying presentations of this disease. Because of the increasing number of incidentally identified lesions, the number of patients with symptomatic lesions is bound to decrease. Judicious use of imaging modalities is necessary for the evaluation of these incidental tumors, particularly in this era of cost containment.

REFERENCES

1. Boring CC, Squires TS, Tong T, Montgomery S. Cancer statistics 1994. CA Cancer J Clin 1994:44:7.
2. Skinner DG, Colvin RB, Vermillion CD, Pfister RC, Leadbetter WF. Diagnosis and management of renal cell carcinoma: a clinical and pathologic study of 309 cases. Cancer 1971;28:1165.
3. NcNichols DW, Segura JW, DeWeerd JH. Renal cell carcinoma: long-term survival and late recurrence. J Urol 1981;126:17.
4. Middleton RG. Surgery for metastatic renal cell carcinoma. J Urol 1967;97:973.
5. Konnak JW, Grossman HB. Renal cell carcinoma as incidental finding. J Urol 1985;134:1094.
6. deKernion JB, Belldegrun A. In: Walsh PC, Retik AB, Stamey TA, Vaughan ED Jr, eds. Campbell's urology, 6th ed. Philadelphia, WB Saunders, 1992:1053.
7. Saitoh H. Distant metastasis of renal adenocarcinoma. Cancer 1981; 48:1487.
8. Stauffer MH. Nephrogenic hepatosplenomegaly. Gastroenterology 1961;40:694. Abstract.
9. Gibbons RP, Montie JE, Correa RJ. Manifestations of renal cell carcinoma. Urology 1976;8:201.
10. Fletcher MS, Packham DA, Pryor JP, et al. Hepatic dysfunction in renal carcinoma. Br J Urol 1981;53:533.
11. Burt ME, Brenan MF. Incidence of hypercalcemia and malignant neoplasm. Arch Surg 1980;115:704.
12. Loughlin KR, Gittes RF, Partridge D, et al. The relationship of lactoferrin to the anemia of renal cell carcinoma. Cancer 1987;59:566.
13. Aso Y, Homma Y. Survey on incidental renal cell carcinoma in Japan. J Urol 1992;147:340.
14. Hélénon O, Chrétien Y, Paraf F, Melki P, Denys, Moreau JF. Renal cell carcinoma containing fat: demonstration with CT. Radiology 1993; 188:429.
15. Lieber MM, Tomera KM, Farrow GM. Renal oncocytoma. J Urol 1981; 125:481.
16. Robson CJ, Churchill BM, Anderson W. The results of radical nephrectomy for renal cell carcinoma. J Urol 1969;101:297.
17. American Joint Committee on Cancer: Manual for staging of cancer, 4th ed. Philadelphia, JB Lippincott, 1992.
18. Selli C, Hinshaw WM, Woodard BH, Paulson DF. Stratification of risk factors in renal cell carcinoma. Cancer 1983;52:899.
19. Siminovitch JMP, Montie JE, Straffon RA. Prognostic indicators in renal adenocarcinoma. J Urol 1983;130:20.
20. Hatcher PA, Anderson EE, Paulson DF, Carson CC, Robertson JE. Surgical management and prognosis of renal cell carcinoma invading the vena cava. J Urol 1991;145:20.
21. McClennan BL. Computed tomography in the diagnosis and staging of renal cell carcinoma. Semin Urol 1985;3:111.
22. Dalton D, Neiman H, Grayhack JT. The natural history of simple renal cysts: a preliminary study. J Urol 1986;135:905.
23. Hajdu SI, Thomas AG. Renal cell carcinoma at autopsy. J Urol 1967; 97:978.
24. Bell ET. A classification of renal tumors with observation on the frequency of the various types. J Urol 1938;39:238.
25. Riches EW, Griffiths IH, Thackray AC. New growths of the kidney and ureter. Br J Urol 1951;23:297.
26. Davis SD, Koizumi JH, Pitts WR. Spontaneous regression of pulmonary metastasis from renal cell carcinoma. Urology 1989;33:141.
27. Hermanek P, Schrott KM. Evaluation of the new tumor, nodes and metastases classification of renal cell carcinoma. J Urol 1990;144:238.
28. Gelb AB, Shibuya RB, Weiss LM, Medeiros LJ. Stage I renal cell carcinoma. Am J Surg Pathol 1993;17:275.
29. Nurmi MJ. Prognostic factors in renal carcinoma: an evaluation of operative findings. Br J Urol 1984;56:270.
30. Wood DP Jr. Role of lymphadenectomy in renal cell carcinoma. Urol Clin North Am 1991;18:421.
31. Robson CJ. Radical nephrectomy for renal cell carcinoma. J Urol 1963; 89:37.
32. Giuliani L, Giberti C, Martorana G, Rovida S. Radical extensive surgery for renal cell carcinoma: long-term results and prognostic factors. J Urol 1990;143:468.
33. Siminovitch JP, Montie JE, Straffon RA. Lymphadenectomy in renal adenocarcinoma. J Urol 1982;127:1090.
34. Flocks RH, Kadesky MC. Malignant neoplasms of the kidney: an analysis of 353 patients followed five years or more. J Urol 1958;79:196.
35. Robson CJ. Results of radical thoraco-abdominal nephrectomy in the treatment of renal cell carcinoma. Prog Clin Biol Res 1982;100:481.

Principles and Practice of Genitourinary Oncology, edited by Derek Raghavan, Howard I. Scher, Steven A. Leibel, and Paul H. Lange. Lippincott-Raven Publishers, Philadelphia, © 1997.

CHAPTER 80

Imaging of Renal Cancer

Howard P. Forman and Bruce L. McClennan

The imaging evaluation of renal cell carcinoma has evolved in the past two decades.[1] Once limited to urography and angiography, the radiologist can now call on ultrasonography (including gray scale, duplex Doppler, and color Doppler), computed tomography (CT) (including helical or spiral technique), radionuclide imaging, and magnetic resonance imaging (MRI) in an attempt to improve detection and preoperative staging of tumors. These newer techniques have been successful and present a myriad of imaging appearances that mirror the variation in the pathologic appearance of renal tumors.

In the past 2 decades, in large part because of the introduction of high-resolution, cross-sectional, and multiplanar imaging, the average size of renal cancers at the time of detection has decreased substantially. Over 25% of tumors detected in the mid-1980s were smaller than 3 cm in diameter, compared with only 5% in the mid-1970s, according to reports from the largest such series.[2] The smaller cancers were detected incidentally in most cases, generally by CT and ultrasonography.

Although imaging tests were previously relegated to detection, with only poor success at staging, newer imaging methods allow highly accurate staging of the primary tumor as well evaluation of metastatic disease and postoperative follow-up, to detect recurrent disease. Each available modality has a role to play in screening and detection, staging, or follow-up. In each case, the clinician must be aware of the various pitfalls and variations in appearance to avoid false-positive and false-negative results.

The goal of the imaging examination should be to detect cancers in symptomatic patients and to stage the tumor accurately. With regard to renal cell carcinoma, such staging must pay close attention to perinephric extent, renal vascular involvement, lymphadenopathy, additional primary tumors, and metastatic disease. Most often, one examination suffices in staging patients. Frequently, however, additional studies may be required to resolve a diagnostic dilemma.

In this chapter, each modality is evaluated with specific attention to strengths, weaknesses, and important pitfalls in diagnosis. Although many alternative imaging techniques are available and are only occasionally used at some institutions, we dedicate the majority of this chapter to generally available techniques in mainstream use. These techniques include excretory urography, CT, ultrasonography, MRI, angiography and venography, radionuclide bone scintigraphy, and plain film radiography.

EXCRETORY UROGRAPHY

Whereas modern cross-sectional imaging studies detect renal cancers in patients without symptoms or signs referable to the urinary tract, excretory urography has been, and generally continues to be, used to evaluate patients with suspicious signs or symptoms such as hematuria. Although this technique cannot usually enable the clinician to determine the nature of a renal mass, and thus warrants follow-up imaging with ultrasound, CT, or MRI, occasionally imaging features suggest the diagnosis of renal cell carcinoma (Table 80-1).

Radiographically detectable calcification in a mass always raises the suspicion of malignancy.[3] This sign is seen in 8% to 20% of renal cell carcinomas and in 1% of simple renal cysts.[4–6] When calcification can be identified on urography as being central, malignancy is even more strongly suggested. When calcification is perceived as peripheral, however, 20% of these masses are still malignant.[3]

When ureteral notching is seen in the presence of a urographically detected mass, thrombosis of the renal vein is suggested.[7]

In all cases, cross-sectional imaging is necessary to evaluate the primary tumor to discriminate between a cyst and a solid mass.

COMPUTED TOMOGRAPHY

The typical CT appearance of renal cell carcinoma has been well described.[3,7] The examination should always begin with unenhanced scans, followed by contrast enhancement with collimation based on the size of the mass (if known). If the mass

TABLE 80-1. *Urographic features of renal cell carcinoma*

Mass effect
Deforms or expands the renal contour
Amputates, effaces, or distorts the collecting system
Opacifies similar to renal parenchyma on tomography
Calcification
Poor, delayed, or absent visualization
Ureteral notching

is small and the detection of fat is important to establish the diagnosis of an angiomyolipoma, then thin sections (<2 mm) are required. In most other cases, 5-mm sections at 5-mm intervals are generally used. The mass is generally identified on precontrast studies as isodense (similar attenuation) with renal parenchyma, although hemorrhage and calcification make the mass hyperdense (increase in attenuation).

When intravenous contrast is administered, contrast enhancement of part or all of the tumor is usually noted. With smaller and lower-grade tumors, contrast enhancement is generally uniform, whereas larger and necrotic tumors may have no central enhancement and can appear cystic but should not be confused with simple cysts.[8–10]

Although much has been written about the benign oncocytoma, no specific CT or other imaging signs allow a reliable preoperative diagnosis.[11–13] Radiologic features described as typical for oncocytoma include a solid mass with homogeneous enhancement, sharp margination, central, stellate scar, and, at angiography, a spoke-wheel, vascular pattern.[12] Some investigators suggest that when typical features are present, fine-needle biopsy may be indicated preoperatively.[13]

CT is an accurate technique for staging renal cell carcinoma, with reported accuracies of 71% to 91% compared with pathologic staging[3,14] (Fig. 80-1). CT scanning has a positive predictive value of more than 96% for malignant renal tumors when the typical features are present.[15] CT can detect enlarged lymph nodes in the parahilar and paraaortic regions; lymph nodes larger than 2 cm are nearly always involved with tumor, and those smaller than 1 cm are generally uninvolved. Lymph nodes larger than 1 cm and smaller than 2 cm are considered indeterminate, but they are viewed with suspicion.[3,16] A report noted that nodal status was accurately staged in 90% of cases by CT.[17]

Evaluation of venous invasion is important in staging renal cell carcinoma. CT is excellent in the evaluation of renal vein and inferior vena caval involvement. Previous reports noted that the evaluation of the cephalad extent of tumor thrombus was limited by the transaxial nature of CT imaging.[18] With the introduction of spiral (helical) CT and the ability to perform multiplanar reformations in the coronal and sagittal planes, this problem may be overcome. CT is also useful to identify venous anomalies (retroaortic or circumaortic renal veins) that may alter the surgical approach.[19]

Because of the known propensity of renal cell carcinoma to lead to vascular metastases to the liver, precontrast scans should first be obtained because postcontrast studies may mask liver metastases.[3] CT can occasionally identify lytic bony metastases involving the lower thoracic, lumbar, and sacral spine as well as the bony pelvis. Uncommon patterns of metastatic disease

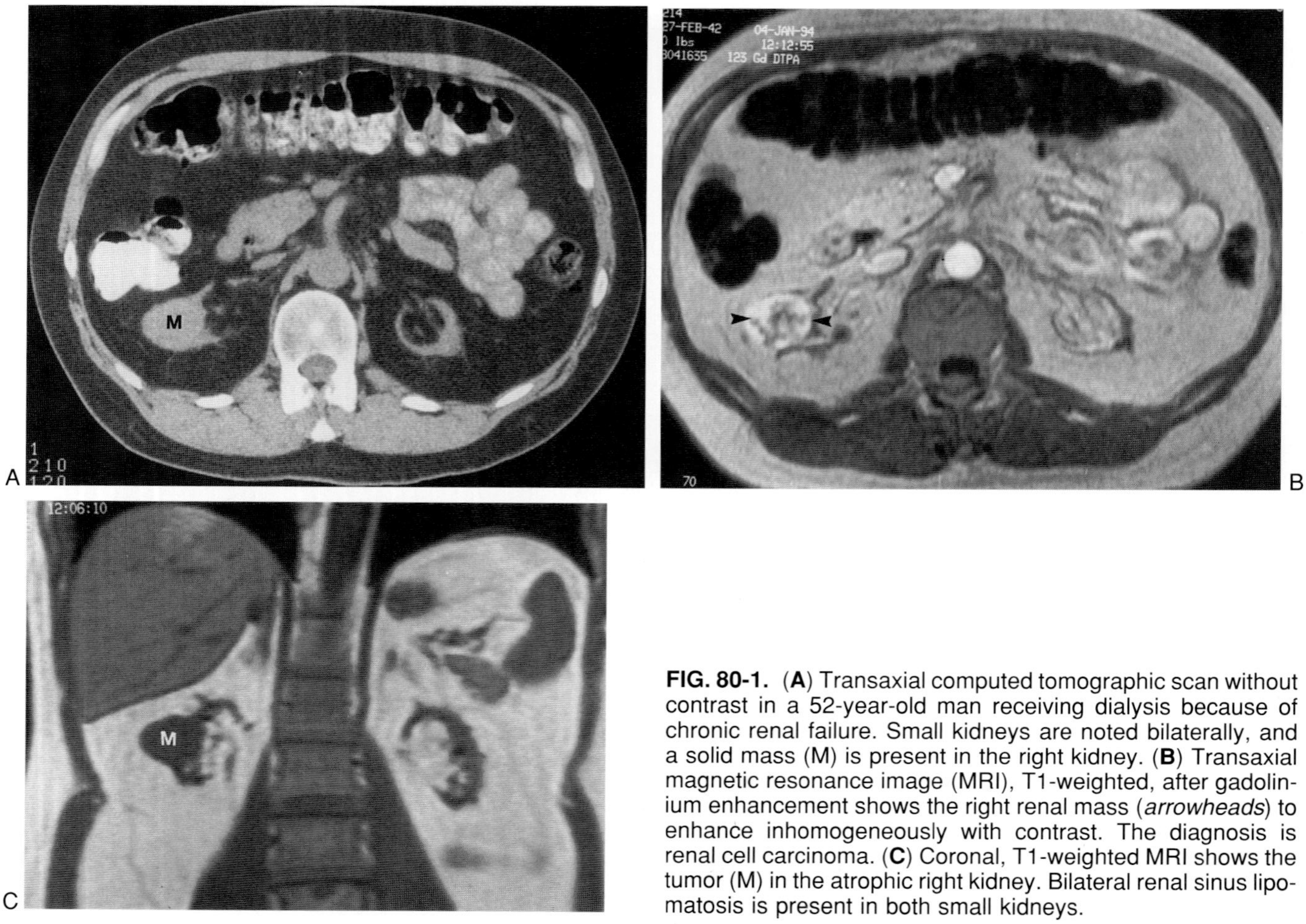

FIG. 80-1. (**A**) Transaxial computed tomographic scan without contrast in a 52-year-old man receiving dialysis because of chronic renal failure. Small kidneys are noted bilaterally, and a solid mass (M) is present in the right kidney. (**B**) Transaxial magnetic resonance image (MRI), T1-weighted, after gadolinium enhancement shows the right renal mass (*arrowheads*) to enhance inhomogeneously with contrast. The diagnosis is renal cell carcinoma. (**C**) Coronal, T1-weighted MRI shows the tumor (M) in the atrophic right kidney. Bilateral renal sinus lipomatosis is present in both small kidneys.

may be noted, such as diffuse peritoneal metastases causing an omental cake.[20]

Cystic masses in the kidney are generally easy to identify as either benign cysts or neoplasms, but a clear-cut discrimination may be difficult to make.[21–25] The Bosniak classification system[9] is useful in allowing categorization of cystic lesions of the kidney into four categories, in which category 1 represents benign simple cysts and category 4 indicates obvious cystic neoplasms. Category 2 lesions are those that generally have a single complicating feature, such as single septum, but can be reliably diagnosed as benign, whereas category 3 lesions are those with either large soft tissue components or other atypical features warranting further workup and typically surgery. This classification scheme has proved successful in some prospective evaluations.[25]

Regarding the CT diagnosis of angiomyolipoma, historically, the diagnosis has been ensured if fat is found within the tumor on CT. Although some reports in the literature seem to defy this rule,[26–29] most imaging centers continue to regard the presence of fat within a renal mass as evidence of benignity. Those reports showed actual ossification and some myeloid material within a complex renal mass (tumor).[26–29]

Three-dimensional spiral (helical) CT imaging of renal tumors has been described and promises to be helpful in planning partial nephrectomy while conserving normal renal tissue.[30,31] This imaging technique is available in many major medical centers and rivals MRI for its ability to depict anatomy in multiple planes and dimensions (Fig. 80-2).

ULTRASONOGRAPHY

Ultrasound has a substantial responsibility for the incidental detection of renal cell carcinomas.[32–33] In one series,[32] 48% of newly diagnosed renal cell carcinomas were detected on abdominal ultrasound performed for a nonurologic indication. In a large screening series[33] using abdominal ultrasonography, 54% of the renal cancers detected were in patients without microscopic or gross hematuria or clinical symptoms of renal cell carcinoma. The trend toward smaller tumors has not yet had a positive impact on survival, although future studies will likely show a benefit.

As with CT, ultrasonography has been used for many years in the diagnosis and, to a lesser extent, staging of renal cell carcinoma. In 1980, Coleman and her colleagues[34] described the gray-scale sonographic features of renal cell carcinoma and showed that these tumors varied in echogenicity from hypoechoic to hyperechoic. In this and subsequent series, most renal cell carcinomas were shown to be hypoechoic or isoechoic to normal renal parenchyma.[35–36] More recent reports have shown that, particularly with more commonly encountered small renal cancer (≤3 cm), most renal cell carcinomas are, in fact, hyperechoic.[10,37] In some of these cases, the echogenicity of the tumor was as echoic as renal sinus fat and thus mimicked the classic ultrasound appearance of angiomyolipoma. In one series, 13% of all tumors and 32% of small tumors (≤3 cm in size) had this appearance.[37] Although Yamashita and colleagues[38] have described signs of intratumoral cysts and an anechoic rim in

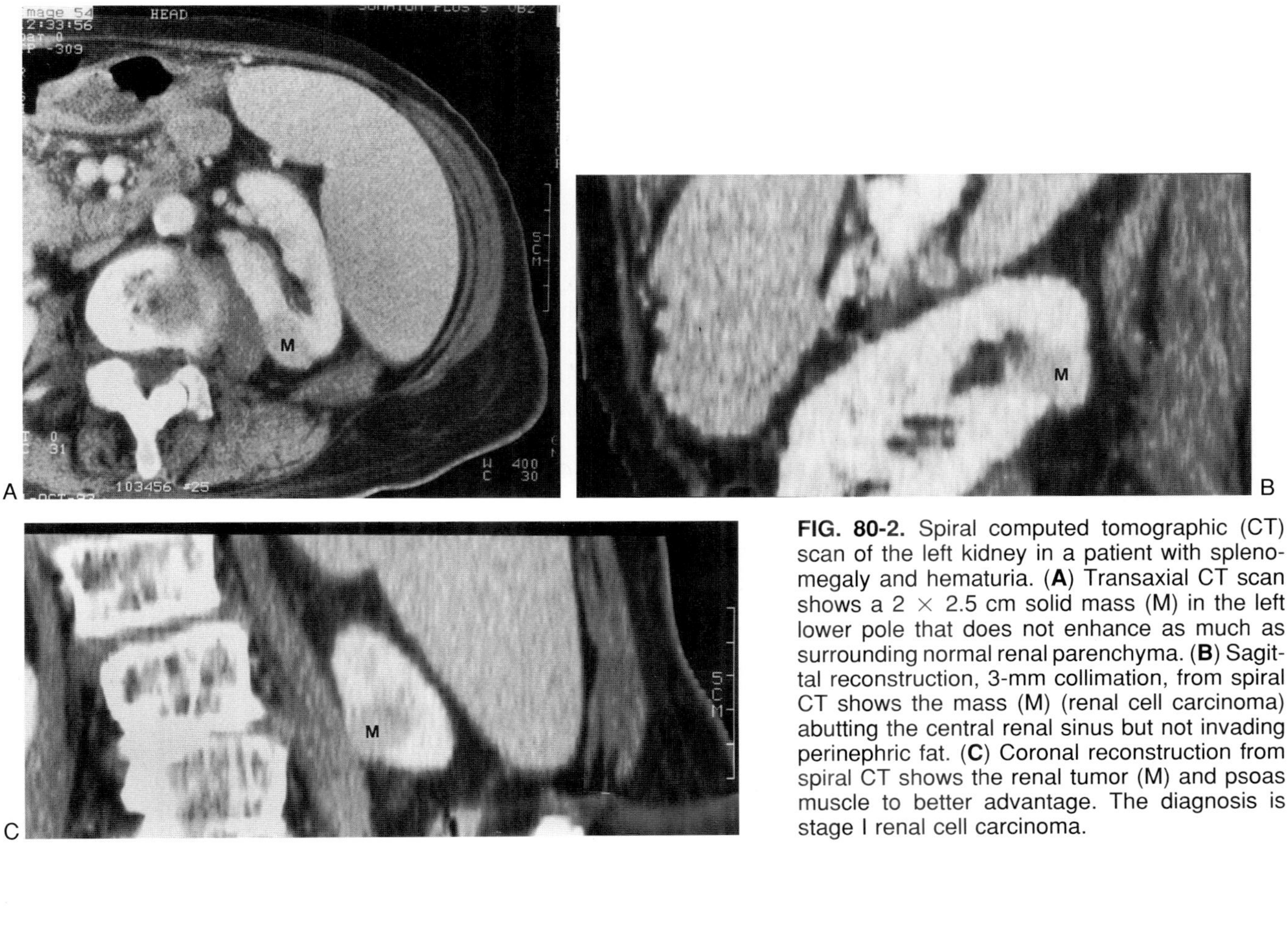

FIG. 80-2. Spiral computed tomographic (CT) scan of the left kidney in a patient with splenomegaly and hematuria. (**A**) Transaxial CT scan shows a 2 × 2.5 cm solid mass (M) in the left lower pole that does not enhance as much as surrounding normal renal parenchyma. (**B**) Sagittal reconstruction, 3-mm collimation, from spiral CT shows the mass (M) (renal cell carcinoma) abutting the central renal sinus but not invading perinephric fat. (**C**) Coronal reconstruction from spiral CT shows the renal tumor (M) and psoas muscle to better advantage. The diagnosis is stage I renal cell carcinoma.

such cancers, angiomyolipomas have no similar specific features on ultrasound, and therefore all solid masses in the kidney detected on ultrasound examination should be further evaluated with CT and MRI.

Although ultrasound is excellent for screening the renal parenchyma for solid tumors and particularly good for differentiating simple benign cysts from solid tumors, it has many limitations. First, isoechoic renal parenchymal tumors that are nondeforming of the renal contour (capsule) are sonographically occult. Thus, in the setting of high clinical suspicion of a renal tumor, CT should be obtained even in the presence of a normal-appearing renal ultrasound scan.[36] Second, ultrasonography is insensitive to the evaluation of retroperitoneal lymph nodes.[39] Similarly, in patients with corpulent body habitus, renal vascular involvement is difficult to assess even with duplex or color Doppler sonography (Fig. 80-3).

Despite these limitations, ultrasound does play a role in staging renal cell carcinoma. Specifically, when CT is equivocal, Doppler ultrasonography can help to assess the renal vein and inferior vena cava in many patients. Further, ultrasound, with its real-time capability, can assess the extent of thrombus in the inferior vena cava at the level of the right atrium, a critical area to image. Reports have demonstrated the use of color Doppler techniques to differentiate bland thrombus from tumor thrombus by showing color flow in tumor thrombus.[1] The potential utility of Doppler evaluation of renal masses to differentiate benign from malignant may make ultrasound evaluation of renal masses more valuable and cost-effective.

MAGNETIC RESONANCE IMAGING

With over a decade of clinical experience available, MRI has proved to be an effective problem solver as well as a primary imaging technique in the evaluation of renal cancers in selected cases. In general, MRI offers information at least comparable to that obtained by high-quality contrast-enhanced CT.[7,40–44]

In certain subpopulations, however, the slightly higher cost of MRI is warranted, particularly in patients in whom iodinated contrast material is contraindicated because of allergy or renal insufficiency. MRI also offers an exquisite ability to demonstrate renal parenchymal and vascular abnormalities in multiple planes. This feature is particularly helpful when the organ of origin, the invasion of adjacent organs, or the level of inferior vena cava thrombus is an issue. Spiral CT may supplant this particular indication, and the body of literature on this application is growing (Fig. 80-4).

MRI is best performed with gadopentate dimeglumine or another contrast medium, which causes enhancement of renal parenchyma and, selectively, of vascular renal tumors on T1-weighted sequences, analogous to iodinated contrast used for CT. Many investigators recommend increasing the visibility of lesions with the use of fat-saturation sequences, which null the

A

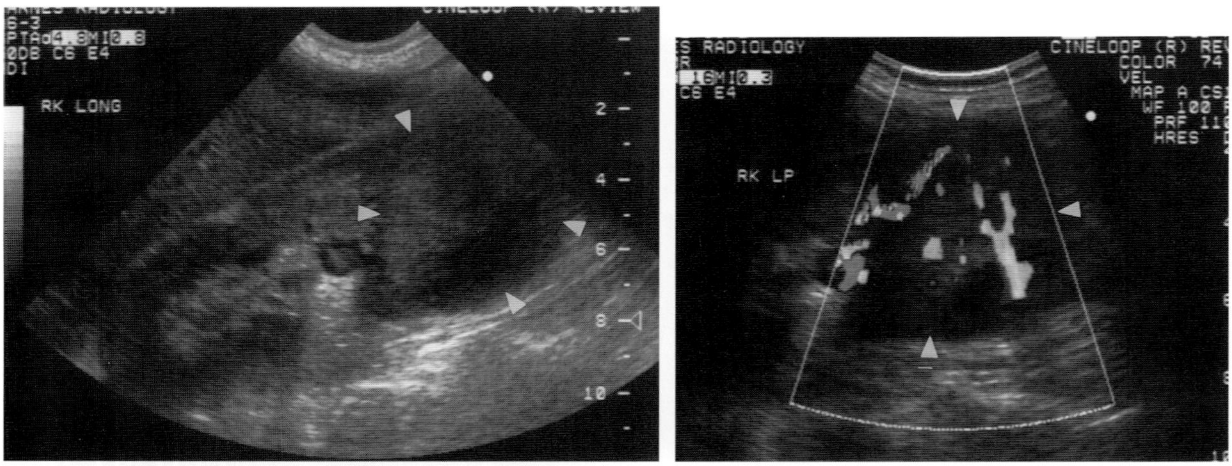

B

C

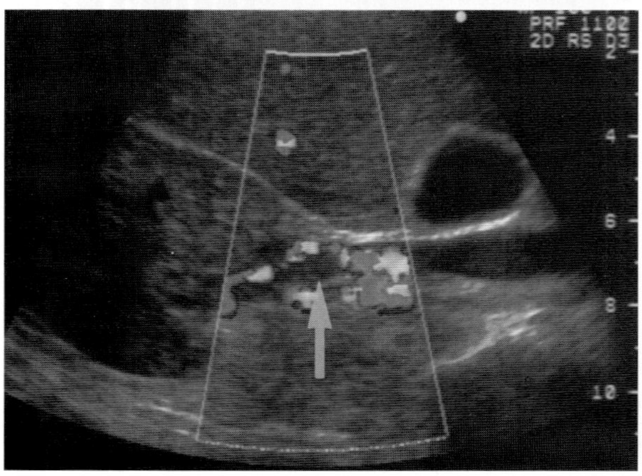

FIG. 80-3. (**A**) Large right lower pole solid mass (*arrowheads*) on a longitudinal sonogram. A computed tomographic scan also showed the mass, but not the right renal vein. (**B**) Longitudinal view of right kidney with color Doppler ultrasound shows flow within the mass (*arrowheads*) confirming the diagnosis of renal cell carcinoma. (**C**) Transverse view through the right kidney and tumor at the level of the right renal vein. Flow around thrombus (*arrow*) in the renal vein is indicated by colored areas (red and blue) within the vein. (See Color Figure 80-3.)

A
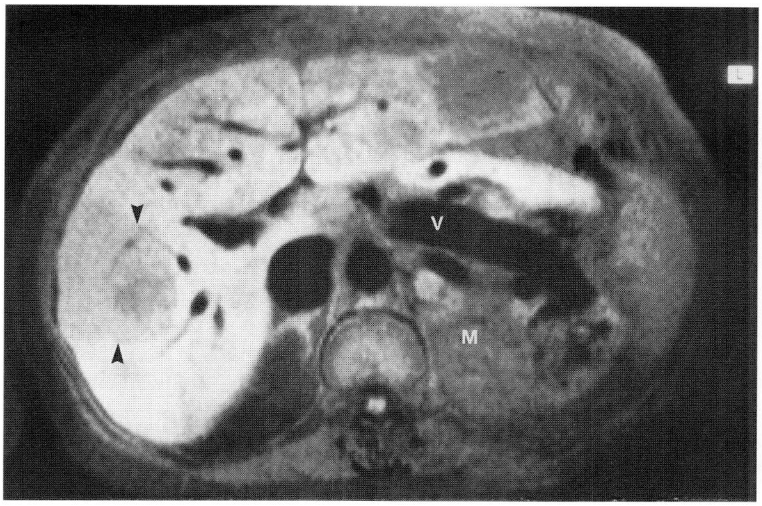

B
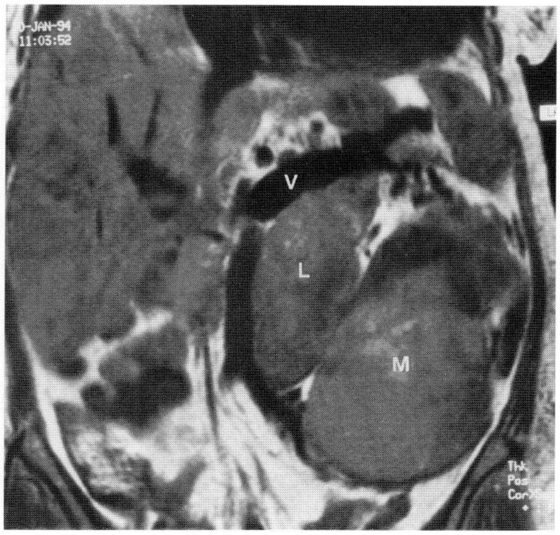

C
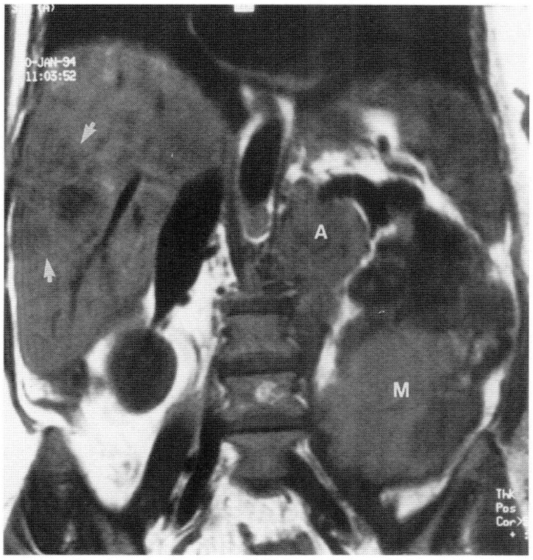

FIG. 80-4. (**A**) Magnetic resonance image (MRI), transaxial projection, with fat saturation technique shows top of a large left renal cell carcinoma (M) and a large, patent left renal vein (V). A large metastasis to the liver is noted (*arrowheads*); other metastasis are also evident. (**B**) Coronal MRI, T1-weighted, shows a large left renal cell carcinoma (M) and a perihilar lymph node mass (L). The renal vein (V) is draped over the lymph node mass and renal tumor. (**C**) Coronal MRI, T1-weighted, shows a large left renal cell carcinoma (M) and a large adrenal metastasis (A). Liver metastases are again noted (*arrows*). The diagnosis is stage IV renal cell carcinoma with local and distant metastates; the renal vein is patent.

high-signal appearance of fat surrounding the kidneys and allow better detection of perinephric extension of tumor.[41,45,46] At present, gadolinium-enhanced MRI is an effective method for characterizing renal lesions in patients with renal insufficiency and subsequently a contraindication to radiopaque contrast media.[47] Gadolinium does not appear to have any nephrotoxic sequelae in such patients.

The use of gradient-recalled echo sequences has improved the sensitivity and specificity of MRI in the detection of renal vein and inferior vena caval involvement by tumor thrombus.[48] In the largest series published,[48] vena caval involvement was correctly identified in 100% of patients, and renal vein involvement was identified correctly in 88%. Right atrial involvement was correctly identified in 4 of 5 patients. Other investigators have confirmed this high level of efficacy and have reported that the need for inferior vena cavography no longer exists.[43]

VASCULAR RADIOLOGY

Invasive vascular techniques in the diagnostic workup of renal cell carcinoma have largely been replaced by less invasive cross-sectional imaging modalities (CT, MRI, and ultrasound). Despite these advances, some knowledge of arteriography, venography (renal and inferior vena caval), and embolization techniques is important.

Angiography can be useful in identifying tumor vascularity and in discriminating this appearance of renal cell carcinomas from the often typical features of microaneurysms seen in many angiomyolipomas. Angiography can also enable the clinician to assess renal venous involvement by tumors during the late angiographic phase.[3] In the largest published series from 1968, angiography was 97% accurate in diagnosis.[49] Although angiography can be useful to delineate vascular anatomy, its overall sensitivity and specificity, even in high-risk populations such as those with von Hippel-Lindau disease, are insufficient to warrant its routine use.[50]

Evaluation of renal venous involvement by tumor is a critical part of the workup of patients with renal cell carcinoma. Venous involvement can be suggested by angiography,[51] and some investigators have suggested indications for venacavography in this population.[52,53] In the past, this study was performed in all patients unless the renal vein was well visualized and normal at angiography or the tumor was peripheral and did not extend to the renal hilus.[52] Most of these reports appeared before the introduction of newer imaging techniques, and thus venacavography is now rarely performed.

Embolization of renal cell carcinoma was, until recently, an accepted approach in patients who were not considered candidates for surgery or in whom limitation of perioperative blood loss was paramount.[3] One report[54] suggests that the efficacy of this procedure is unproved, particularly for reducing blood loss during surgery.

EVALUATION OF METASTATIC DISEASE

Evaluation of metastatic disease is important in the evaluation of patients with carcinoma, particularly in patients with renal cell carcinoma.[55] Patients with renal cell carcinoma have derived some survival benefit when solitary synchronous or metachronous metastases are detected and are resected.[3] The impact of imaging, therefore, is critical. If imaging is insensitive to the detection of metastases, then these lesions may be missed in a potentially curable or treatable stage. Similarly, a solitary metastasis may be detected when multiple metastases are actually present, and surgery may be tried when it is not indicated. Thus, in patients with known renal cell carcinoma, workup for metastatic disease to the lungs and liver should be routine and based on the best available technologies. Recommendations for imaging of pulmonary metastatic disease vary, but they generally include high-quality standard radiography of the chest. If the chest radiograph shows multiple pulmonary metastases, no further workup is required. If a solitary metastasis, equivocal pulmonary nodule, or no pulmonary nodule is identified, the clinician should proceed to CT of the chest.[3,56,57]

To evaluate a patient for liver metastasis, high-quality pre- and postcontrast CT of the liver should be performed. Typically,

TABLE 80-2. *Imaging methods for evaluation of renal cell carcinoma*

Method	Capability	Benefit-to-cost ratio	Routine recommendation
NONINVASIVE			
Chest radiography	Limited usefulness; CT may be required for detection of metastases	High	Yes, in conjunction with CT
Skeletal radiography	Limited usefulness except to confirm positive bone scan for metastases or to evaluate skeletal pain (focal)	Low	No
Ultrasound (Doppler and color flow)	Useful to exclude simple cysts; limited staging information available; less sensitive and less specific than CT for tumor extent; Doppler may be of use for vascular invasion	Fair	Not usually
NEARLY NONINVASIVE			
Excretory urography	Most widely used screening test; limited ability for precise staging	High	Yes, although management usually affected by cross-sectional imaging only
Radionuclide bone scans	Best screening test for skeletal metastases	High	No, unless symptomatic
CT	Useful test for TNM staging information; requires IV contrast media	High	Yes, unless iodinated contrast contraindicated
MRI	Equivalent accuracy for tumor staging with CT; comparable use but fair for tumor detection; expensive; limited availability	Medium	As an alternative to CT when contrast contraindicated or CT equivocal
INVASIVE			
Angiography (including digital studies)			
Arteriography	Limited diagnostic and staging information compared with CT and MRI; arteriography may be required for embolization or surgical planning	Low	No
Venography	Useful if ultrasound, CT, or MRI indeterminate for renal vein or vena cava involvement	Low	No
Biopsy (CT, ultrasound)	Percutaneous biopsy requires ultrasound, CT, or fluoroscopy; open biopsy rarely needed; not necessary for T-stage confirmation; may be useful to confirm metastases and determine resectability	Low	No

CT, computed tomography; *MRI,* magnetic resonance imaging.

this imaging is best done during staging of the primary tumor, thus avoiding the need to administer a separate dose of contrast. MRI shows nearly equal or perhaps better efficacy at detecting metastatic disease to the liver and can be used in patients with contrast allergy or other contraindication or when MRI is used to evaluate an equivocal finding on another study.[58]

Although 32% of patients with metastatic renal cell carcinoma have involvement of bone,[59] most investigators have recommended the use of preoperative skeletal scintigraphy only when symptoms are present.[58,60,61] In this setting, additional plain radiographs may be obtained when a suspicious solitary lesion is seen on a bone scan. In addition, plain radiographs may be indicated to assess the orthopedic significance of strategically located metastasis prone to complication.

CONCLUSIONS

Diagnostic imaging of renal cell carcinoma has advanced dramatically with the introduction of cross-sectional imaging. The ability to stage the primary tumor accurately allows for better preoperative planning and appropriate management. Algorithms for the workup and management of renal cell carcinoma are presented elsewhere in this text. We have presented the most current knowledge of the most commonly used imaging modalities for the diagnosis and staging of renal cell carcinoma. Table 80-2 summarizes the salient points of this chapter and includes a statement regarding the cost and benefit of each modality.

REFERENCES

1. McClennan BL, Deyoe LA. The imaging evaluation of renal cell carcinoma: diagnosis and staging. Radiol Clin North Am 1994;32:55.
2. Smith SJ, Bosniak MA, Megibow AJ, Hulnick DH, Horii SC, Raghavendra BN. Renal cell carcinoma: earlier discovery and increased detection. Radiology 1989;170:699.
3. Levine E. Malignant renal parenchymal tumors in adults. In: Pollack HM, ed. Clinical urography: an atlas and textbook of urological imaging. Philadelphia, WB Saunders, 1990:1216.
4. Daniel WW, Hartman GW, Witten DM, Farrow GM, Kelalis PP. Calcified renal masses: a review of ten years' experience at the Mayo Clinic. Radiology 1972;103:503.
5. Weyman PJ, McClennan BL, Lee JKT, Stanley RJ, Sagel SS. Computed tomography of calcified renal masses. AJR Am J Roentgenol 1982;138:1095.
6. Sniderman KW, Krieger JN, Seligson GR, Sos TA. The radiologic and clinical aspects of calcified hypernephroma. Radiology 1979;131:31.
7. Davidson AJ, Hartman DS. Diagnostic set: large, unifocal, unilateral. In: Davidson AJ, Hartman DS, eds. Radiology of the kidney and urinary tract, 2nd ed. Philadelphia, WB Saunders, 1994:327.
8. Zagoria RJ, Wolfman NT, Karstaedt N, Hinn GC, Dyer RB, Chen YM. CT features of renal cell carcinoma with emphasis on relation to tumor size. Invest Radiol 1990;25:261.
9. Bosniak MA. The small (≤3.0 cm) renal parenchymal tumor: detection, diagnosis, and controversies. Radiology 1991;179:307.
10. Yamashita Y, Takahashi M, Watanabe O, et al. Small renal cell carcinoma: pathologic and radiologic correlation. Radiology 1992;184:493.
11. Davidson AJ, Hayes WS, Hartman DS, McCarthy WF, Davis CJ. Renal oncocytoma and carcinoma: failure of differentiation with CT. Radiology 1993;186:693.
12. Palmer WE, Chew FS. Renal oncocytoma. AJR Am J Roentgenol 1991;156:1144.
13. Tikkakoski T, Päivänsalo M, Alanen A, et al. Radiologic findings in renal oncocytoma. Acta Radiol 1991;32:363.
14. Miles KA, London NJM, Lavelle JM, Messios N, Smart JG. CT staging of renal carcinoma: a prospective comparison of three dynamic computed tomography techniques. Eur J Radiol 1991;13:37.
15. Johnson CD, Dunnick NR, Cohan RH, Illescas FF. Renal adenocarcinoma: CT staging of 100 tumors. AJR Am J Roentgenol 1987;148:59.
16. Levine E, Lee KR, Weigel J. Preoperative determination of abdominal extent of renal cell carcinoma by computed tomography. Radiology 1979;132:395.
17. Dinney CPN, Awad SA, Gajewski JB, et al. Analysis of imaging modalities, staging systems, and prognostic indicators for renal cell carcinoma. Urology 1992;39:122.
18. Didier D, Racle A, Etievent JP, Weill F. Tumor thrombus of the inferior vena cava secondary to malignant abdominal neoplasms: US and CT evaluation. Radiology 1987;162:83.
19. Fritzsche PJ, Millar C. Multimodality approach to staging renal cell carcinoma. Urol Radiol 1992;14:3.
20. Tartar VM, Heiken JP, McClennan BL. Renal cell carcinoma presenting with diffuse peritoneal metastases: CT findings. J Comput Assist Tomogr 1991;15:450.
21. Hartman DS, Weatherby E, Laskin WB, Brody JM, Corse W, Baluch JD. Cystic renal cell carcinoma: CT findings simulating a benign hyperdense cyst. AJR Am J Roentgenol 1992;159:1235.
22. Parikh PU, Korobkin M, McClennan BL, Platt JF, Weingarten BJ. CT of parapelvic cystic renal cell carcinoma. J Comput Assist Tomogr 1992;16:586.
23. Munechika H, Kitanosono T, Sato S, et al. Bilateral multiple renal adenocarcinomas in a patient with acquired renal cystic disease: correlation of imaging with pathological study. Urol Radiol 1992;13:146.
24. Bosniak MA. Difficulties in classifying cystic lesions of the kidney. Urol Radiol 1991;13:91.
25. Aronson S, Frazier HA, Baluch JD, Hartman DS, Christenson PJ. Cystic renal masses: usefulness of the Bosniak classification. Urol Radiol 1991;13:83.
26. Radin DR, Chandrasoma P. CT demonstration of fat density in renal cell carcinoma. Acta Radiol 1992;33:365.
27. Strotzer M, Lehner KB, Becker K. Detection of fat in a renal cell carcinoma mimicking angiomyolipoma. Radiology 1993;188:427.
28. Helenon O, Chretien Y, Paraf F, Melki P, Denys A, Moreau JF. Renal cell carcinoma containing fat: demonstration with CT. Radiology 1993;188:429.
29. Davidson AJ, Davis CJ. Fat in renal adenocarcinoma: never say never. Radiology 1993;188:316.
30. Chernoff DM, Silverman SG, Kikinis R, et al. Three-dimension imaging and display of renal tumors using spiral CT: a potential aid to partial nephrectomy. Urology 1994;43:125.
31. Silverman SG, Lee BY, Seltzer SE, Bloom DA, Corless CL, Adams DF. Small (≤3 cm) renal masses: correlation of spiral CT features and pathologic findings. AJR Am J Roentgenol 1994;163:597.
32. Porena M, Vespasiani G, Rosi P, et al. Incidentally detected renal cell carcinoma: role of ultrasonography. JCU J Clin Ultrasound 1992;20:395.
33. Tosaka A, Ohya K, Yamada K, et al. Incidence and properties of renal masses and asymptomatic renal cell carcinoma detected by abdominal ultrasonography. J Urol 1990;1097.
34. Coleman BG, Arger PH, Mulhern CB, Pollack HM, Banner MP, Arenson RL. Gray-scale sonographic spectrum of hypernephromas. Radiology 1980;137:757.
35. Hartman DS, Goldman SM, Friedman AC, et al. Angiomyolipoma: ultrasonic-pathologic correlation. Radiology 1981;139:451.
36. Charboneau JW, Hattery RR, Ernst EC, et al. Spectrum of sonographic findings in 125 renal masses other than benign simple cyst. AJR 1983;140:87.
37. Forman HP, Middleton WD, Melson GL, McClennan BL. Hyperechoic renal cell carcinomas: increase in detection at US. Radiology 1993;188:431.
38. Yamashita Y, Ueno S, Makita O, et al. Hyperechoic renal tumors: anechoic rim and intratumoral cysts in US differentiation of renal cell carcinoma from angiomyolipoma. Radiology 1993;188:179.
39. Levine E, Maklad NF, Rosenthal SJ, et al. Comparison of computed tomography and ultrasound in abdominal staging of renal cancer. Urology 1980;16:317.
40. Kuijpers D, Kruyt RH, Oudkerk M. Renal masses: value of duplex Doppler ultrasound in the differential diagnosis. J Urol 1994;151:326.
41. Semelka RC, Hricak H, Stevens SK, Finegold R, Tomei E, Carroll

PR. Combined gadolinium-enhanced and fat saturation MR imaging of renal masses. Radiology 1991;178:803.
42. Dunnick NR. Renal lesions: great strides in imaging. Radiology 1992; 182:305.
43. Kabala JE, Gillatt DA, Persad RA, Penry JB, Gingell JC, Chadwick D. Magnetic resonance imaging in the staging of renal cell carcinoma. Br J Radiol 1991;64:683.
44. Fein AB, Lee JKT, Balfe DM, et al. Diagnosis and staging of renal cell carcinoma: a comparison of MR imaging and CT. AJR Am J Roentgenol 1987;148:749.
45. Semelka RC, Shoenut JP, Kroeker MA, MacMahon RG, Greenberg HM. Renal lesions: controlled comparison between CT and 1.5T MR imaging with nonenhanced and gadolinium-enhanced fat-suppressed spin-echo and breath-hold FLASH techniques. Radiology 1992;182: 425.
46. Rominger MB, Kenney PJ, Morgan DE, Bernreuter WK, Listinsky JJ. Gadolinium enhanced MR imaging of renal masses. Radiographics 1992;12:1097.
47. Rofsky NM, Weinreb JC, Bosniak MA, Libes RB, Birnbaum BA. Renal lesion characterization with gadolinium-enhanced MR imaging: efficacy and safety in patients with renal insufficiency. Radiology 1991; 180:85.
48. Roubidoux MA, Dunnick NR, Sostman HD, Leder RA. Renal carcinoma: detection with gradient echo MR imaging. Radiology 1992;182: 269.
49. Watson RC, Fleming RJ, Evans JA. Arteriography in the diagnosis of renal carcinoma: review of 100 cases. Radiology 1968;91:888.
50. Miller DL, Choyke PL, McClellan M, et al. Von Hippel-Lindau disease: inadequacy of angiography for identification of renal cancers. Radiology 1991;179:833.
51. Ferris EJ, Bosniak MA, O'Connor JF. An angiographic sign demonstrating extension of renal carcinoma into the renal vein and vena cava. AJR Am J Roentgenol 1968;102:384.
52. Madayag MA, Ambos MA, Lefleur RS, Bosniak MA. Involvement of the inferior vena cava in patients with renal cell carcinoma. Radiology 1979;133:321.
53. Palmer J, Barry B, Williams R, Briscoe P. Diagnosis of venous extension in renal cell carcinoma: the value of routine inferior venacavography. Australas Radiol 1975;19:265.
54. Lanigan D, Jurriaans E, Hammonds JC, Wells IP, Choa RG. The current status of embolization in renal cell carcinoma: a survey of local and national practice. Clin Radiol 1992;46:176.
55. Neves RJ, Zincke H, Taylor WF. Metastatic renal cell cancer and radical nephrectomy: identification of prognostic factors and patient survival. J Urol 1988;139:1173.
56. McClennan BL. Oncologic Imaging of renal and adrenal carcinoma: diagnosis, staging and follow-up. Categorical course on imaging of cancers. Reston, VA, American College of Radiology, 1992.
57. Coppage L, Shaw C, Curtis AM. Metastatic disease to the chest in patients with extrathoracic malignancy. J Thorac Imaging 1987;2:24.
58. Amendola MA, King LR, Pollack HM, Gefter W, Kressel HY, Wein AJ. Staging of renal carcinoma using magnetic resonance imaging at 1.5 Tesla. Cancer 1990;66:40.
59. Bennington JL, Beckwith JB. Atlas of tumor pathology, 2nd series, Fascicle 12. Tumors of the kidney, renal pelvis and ureter. Washington DC, Armed Forces Institute of Pathology, 1975:93.
60. Rosen PR, Murphy KG. Bone scintigraphy in the initial staging of patients with renal cell carcinoma: concise communication. J Nucl Med 1984;25:289.
61. Swanson DA, Orovan WL, Johnson DE, Giacco G. Osseous metastases secondary to renal cell carcinoma. Urology 1981;18:556.

Principles and Practice of Genitourinary Oncology, edited by Derek Raghavan, Howard I. Scher, Steven A. Leibel, and Paul H. Lange. Lippincott-Raven Publishers, Philadelphia, © 1997.

CHAPTER 81

Surgery for Renal Cell Carcinoma

Overview

James E. Montie

Surgery for cancer is simple. If the cancer is confined to an anatomic area and if part or all of that organ with the cancer is removed, treatment will be successful. Next case.

Unfortunately, real-life situations in surgery are not so clear-cut. The intent and limitations of the craft of surgery must remain in focus, however. If a cancer is already metastatic at the time of diagnosis, whether it has been identified or not, any operation on the primary tumor will not cure the patient. The type of operation used must focus on local issues: local recurrence rate, complications, and morbidity. If surgeons do not keep this concept paramount, the trap is laid for either inadequate or excessive surgery. Surgeons must continuously reevaluate operations with the intent of doing enough but not too much. We must also acknowledge the goal of performing the smallest operation possible that will eliminate the cancer and have the fewest complications. Diagnostic practices may change that identify smaller cancers more amenable to a lesser operation with comparable results. Adjuvant treatments may become available that control micrometastatic disease and make an even more extensive operation to resect a large primary tumor appropriate. Neoadjuvant treatments may require resection of residual local disease after chemotherapy or radiotherapy. Thus, the character of clinical problems changes, and the operations required for optimal treatment may change as well.

Surgeons must commonly make decisions about the preferred operation with inadequate data to make judgments. Data on the survival or local failure rate to compare operations in similar patients are often not available. All we can do is act on the information available, remaining open to new ideas and approaches. Prospective trials, although desirable, may not be available or may be difficult to accomplish.

Surgery for renal cell carcinoma faces may of the foregoing issues. First, abdominal ultrasound and computed tomography detect small asymptomatic cancers. Is a radical nephrectomy required in all these cases? Second, improvements in surgical techniques, such as cardiopulmonary bypass with hypothermic circulatory arrest, allow an incredibly large and complicated cancer with an inferior vena cava (IVC) tumor thrombus to be grossly resected. Is such a procedure going to have a realistic hope of curing the patient or alleviating suffering? Finally, some patients with renal cancer have occult lymph node metastases in nodes not directly adjacent to the renal hilum. Is a bigger operation to remove more regional lymph nodes going to result in longer survival? Earlier chapters written by international experts have addressed many of the specific problems associated with renal cell carcinoma. The following summary is one perspective on several aspects of surgery for renal cell carcinoma; the opinions may be defensible now, but they may be proved wrong as additional data or new treatments become available.

PARTIAL NEPHRECTOMY

The indications for partial nephrectomy for renal cell carcinoma depend on a balance of the risks versus the benefits. Removal of only a portion of an organ, rather than the entire organ, seems attractive intuitively; patients are often immediately attracted to this possibility. For other cancers, organ preservation may have clear benefits, such as partial mastectomy versus total mastectomy for a cosmetic benefit in treating breast cancer or lobectomy versus pneumonectomy for a functional benefit in treating lung cancer. What are the benefits of a partial nephrectomy for renal cell carcinoma? If the other kidney is abnormal or absent, the patient may benefit tremendously from preservation of renal function and avoidance of dialysis. A better appreciation of the use of partial nephrectomy for renal cell carcinoma in a solitary or impaired kidney should be viewed as a major advance in the last 20 years in urologic surgery.[1–3] What is the benefit of partial nephrectomy if the contralateral kidney is normal? This question is much more difficult to answer; in the short term, the risk of deterioration of total renal function is low.[4,5] In the long term, that is, more than 20 years after surgery, data are not available on the risk of loss of renal function after unilateral nephrectomy. The pathologic entity of glomerulosclerosis, presumably related to hyperfiltration injury, may or may not become an important factor.[4,5] If the risk of renal deterioration is negligible, should we consider partial nephrectomy for renal cell carcinoma for the so-called "elective" indication? The downside of partial nephrectomy is the risk of local recurrence in the kidney (albeit low, but undeniably higher than if the entire kidney is removed) and a possibly slightly higher complication rate.[1,6,7]

Early experience with partial nephrectomy was dominated by interest in ex vivo resections ("bench" surgery).[2] As surgeons became more comfortable with intrarenal and hilar dissections, they realized that many cancers previously believed to require an ex vivo resection could actually be managed more safely and as effectively in situ. An ex vivo resection increases the risk of postoperative temporary renal dysfunction, vascular complications, ureteral ischemia, and urinary leakage; the operations commonly take 10 to 12 hours, and thus, the attendant risk from the surgery increases. The indications for ex vivo resection are limited to tumors that truly require a microvascular anastamosis or are so large that total nephrectomy is needed to provide exposure of the hilar vasculature for dissection of the early branches of the main renal vessels. These two indications compromise a minority of cases now requiring a partial nephrectomy.[3] When necessary and feasible, however, ex vivo partial nephrectomy may provide a substantial benefit for the patient in spite of the increased complexity and danger of the procedure.

Partial nephrectomy for a small incidental renal mass, which may or may not be a renal cell carcinoma, is used more commonly, and preliminary data are favorable.[8–11] Some of the tumors found are, in fact, benign. We must be cognizant that the rules for successful partial nephrectomy are strict, and the expected standard for results of this operation are extraordinarily high. A few local recurrences of cancer in the kidney that may ultimately lead to metastases cannot be tolerated in this setting. To avoid potentially harming patients, the conditions appropriate for offering a partial nephrectomy, such as size and a margin of normal tissue, must be carefully followed.

INFERIOR VENA CAVA THROMBUS RESECTION

The unique propensity for renal cell carcinoma to propagate as a tumor thrombus in the main renal vein and IVC presents a specific surgical challenge. The refinements of a surgical approach, well described by Marsh and Lange, allow a tumor to be removed with a degree of safety not available using techniques that did not afford such complete control during IVC thrombus extraction.[12]

If the thrombus is below the main hepatic veins, a clamp can be placed on the vena cava above the thrombus but below the hepatic veins, to provide complete control of the infrahepatic IVC. If an infrahepatic thrombus does not allow placement of a vascular clamp above the cephalic extent of the thrombus, but the thrombus is free-floating and does not occlude the IVC, extraction using a balloon catheter can be the simplest procedure (if everything goes well). Caution must be used with this approach, however, because fragments of tumor can be left behind, and the occlusive clamp on the IVC must be properly and quickly placed on the cavotomy to allow complete repair of the IVC without compromise of the lumen.

A third level of complexity is required for resection of an intrahepatic IVC thrombus that may not extract easily.[13] Control of all IVC tributaries requires more dissection around the IVC, often difficult because of enlargement of thin-walled venous collateral vessels associated with IVC occlusion. Occlusion of the porta hepatis (Pringle maneuver) can be done safely for only 30 to 40 minutes. Occlusion of the suprahepatic IVC can cause profound hypotension in some patients because of impairment of venous return; a venovenous extracorporeal bypass obviates this problem but requires systemic heparinization.[14] Anticoagulation is undesirable because of the large dissection required around the cancer, with frequent small venous collateral vessels that are tedious to control. Nevertheless, this approach is valuable and avoids the potential complications of cardiopulmonary bypass.[13,15]

If the thrombus extends above the diaphragm into the right atrium, cardiopulmonary bypass is needed to provide optimal control of intraoperative events.[12] All dissection of the kidney must be completed and hemostasis ensured before initiating cardiopulmonary bypass. The risks of cardiac bypass by itself are low, and pump time is generally less than 1 hour. Rarely, associated severe coronary artery occlusive disease can be corrected concurrently to increase the safety of the procedure. Cardiac bypass is suitable for a thrombus that extends to the heart but is likely to be extracted easily. The last level of complexity is needed for a large thrombus extending into the heart associated with enlargement and complete occlusion of the IVC. The thrombus may be adherent to the IVC wall and may need to be removed piecemeal. The technique of cardiac bypass and deep hypothermic circulatory arrest provides unsurpassed exposure to resect the thrombus and to repair or resect the IVC.[16] The danger of the operation is increased, however, primarily because of coagulation abnormalities associated with deep hypothermia. Although the operation is effective when needed, it should only be used when simpler options appear unworkable.

Patients requiring such an extensive surgical procedure represent a spectrum of renal cell cancer from those with an isolated free-floating thrombus, which is associated with an approximately 50% 5-year survival, to those with concomitant perinephric fat extension, regional node metastases, or direct invasion of the IVC wall, who may only have a 10% to 20% survival rate. The ability to resect larger primary tumors than previously possible only emphasizes the desperate need for an effective systemic therapy to cure the patient. In spite of recent studies, biologic response modified (BMR) therapy provides durable complete responses in only a small fraction of patients with established metastatic renal cell carcinoma; data are not available on the value of BMR therapy as adjuvant treatment, partially because of substantial toxicity associated with high-dose interleukin-2. Thus, we may have approached a plateau in renal cell carcinoma therapy; even though a larger operation may successfully extirpate the primary tumor, the overall treatment commonly fails because of the overwhelming risk of metastatic disease. This circumstance is particularly applicable to the large IVC thrombus from renal cell carcinoma in which extensive venous tumor propagation or invasion can be surgically treated, but the survival rate may be only minimally altered.

LYMPHADENECTOMY

Regional lymphadenectomy is an integral part of the surgical therapy for most primary cancers. Lymphadenectomy has prognostic value for essentially all epithelial cancers; therapeutic value is more difficult to quantify. The role of regional lymphadenectomy for renal cell carcinoma is particularly ambiguous for several reasons. The regional lymphatic drainage of the kidney is less precisely defined than that of many other solid organs.[17] Most of the regional lymph nodes from the kidney are in the hilum around the main renal artery and vein; however, periaortic nodes from the left and precaval, retrocaval, or interaortocaval nodes on the right may be part of the first-echelon nodal drainage. If lymphadenectomy is to be beneficial therapeutically, it should ideally encompass all regional nodes.[18] Unfortunately, this dissection of periaortic, retrocaval, and interaortocaval nodes may be particularly tedious in patients with renal cell carcinoma because of expansion of thin-walled, collateral venous drainage channels around the great vessels. The larger the cancer, the more likely the involvement of regional lymph nodes, but also the more likely these collateral venous channels are to be enlarged and the less attractive additional dissection becomes. In the United States, lymph node dissection is commonly limited primarily to the renal hilar area of the ipsilateral great vessel.[19] Treatment failure in the retroperitoneum secondary to unresected regional lymph nodes is occasionally noted but has not been well quantified.[19] Excellent results have been reported from Europe with a more thorough retroperitoneal lymph node dissection.[20,21] Patients who may benefit most may be those with micrometastases rather than those with enlarged, metastatic disease. Justification of lymphadenectomy for prognostic reasons is weak because no additional adjuvant therapy that may improve survival in higher-risk patients is available for renal cell carcinoma. Until results of a randomized trial from Europe are available on the value of lymphadenectomy, or until effective adjuvant treatment exits, extensive lymph node dissection will probably not be commonly included with total nephrectomy in the United States.

PERSPECTIVE

Twenty years ago, a hot topic of debate in renal cell carcinoma was the use of adjunctive nephrectomy in the hope of a spontaneous regression of metastatic disease; this does not work. Ten years ago, angioinfarction and nephrectomy were used to induce regression of metastatic disease; this does not work. Five years ago, it was thought that nephrectomy was necessary for an optimal response for BMR therapy. This appears unnecessary. Thus, perhaps nephrectomy in metastatic renal cell carcinoma should be reserved for the highly unusual patient with recalcitrant symptoms from a resectable primary tumor or for those patients achieving a complete response of metastatic disease from systemic treatment. Additional patients appropriate for surgery may be those entering immunotherapy protocols requiring renal tissue or tumor-infiltrating lymphocytes for preparation of immunotherapy.

The discussion has addressed the issue that surgery for renal cell carcinoma must be dynamic. Procedures appropriate *now* may be inappropriate or unnecessary in the future. The goal of continuous improvement needs to apply to our operations as well as to other aspects of care.

REFERENCES

1. Licht MR, Novick AC. Nephron sparing surgery for renal cell carcinoma. J Urol 1993;149:1.
2. Stormont TJ, Bilhartz DL, Zincke H. Pitfalls of "bench surgery" and autotransplantation for renal cell carcinoma. Mayo Clin Proc 1992;67:621.
3. Montie JE. "Bench surgery" for renal cell carcinoma: a proper niche. Mayo Clin Proc 1992;67:701. Editorial.
4. Steckler RE, Riehle RA Jr, Vaughan ED Jr. Hyperfiltration-induced renal injury in normal man: myth or reality. J Urol 1990;144:1323.
5. Lent V, Harth J. Nephropathy in remnant kidneys: pathological proteinuria after unilateral nephrectomy. J Urol 1994;152:312.
6. Zincke H, Blute ML. Renal tumors. J Urol 1994;152:43. Editorial.
7. Campbell SC, Novick AC, Streem SB, Klein E, Licht M. Complications of nephron sparing surgery for renal tumors. J Urol 1994;151:1177.
8. Moll V, Becht E, Ziegler M. Kidney preserving surgery in renal cell tumors: indications, techniques and results in 152 patients. J Urol 1993;150:319.
9. Herr HW. Partial nephrectomy for renal cell carcinoma with a normal opposite kidney. Cancer 1994;73:160.
10. Thrasher JB, Robertson JE, Paulson DF. Expanding indications for conservative renal surgery in renal cell carcinoma. Urol 1994;43:160.
11. Licht MR, Novick AC, Goormastic M. Nephron sparing surgery in incidental versus suspected renal cell carcinoma. J Urol 1994;152:39.
12. Montie JE, El Ammar R, Pontes JE, et al. Renal cell carcinoma with inferior vena cava tumor thrombi. Surg Gynecol Obstet 1991;173:107.
13. Boyd SD, Skinner DG, Lieskovsky G. Renal cell carcinoma with vena caval extension: operative management. Recent Results Cancer Res 1993;126:105.
14. Janosko EO, Powell CS, Spence PA, Hodges WE, Lust RM. Surgical management of renal cell carcinoma with extensive intracaval involvement using a venous bypass system suitable for rapid conversion to total cardiopulmonary bypass. J Urol 1991;145:555.
15. Marsh CL, Lange PH. Application of liver transplant and organ procurement techniques to difficult upper abdominal urological cases. J Urol 1994;151:1652.
16. Novick AC, Kaye MC, Cosgrove DM, et al. Experience with cardiopulmonary bypass and deep hypothermic circulatory arrest in the management of retroperitoneal tumors with large vena caval thrombi. Ann Surg 1990;212:472.
17. Marshall FF, Powell KC. Lymphadenectomy for renal cell carcinoma: anatomical and therapeutic considerations. J Urol 1982;128:677.
18. Montie JE. Lymphadenectomy for renal cell carcinoma. Semin Urol 1989;7:181.
19. Phillips E, Messing EM. Role of lymphadenectomy in the treatment of renal cell carcinoma. Urology 1993;41:9.
20. Giuliani L, Giberti C, Martorana G, Rovida S. Radical extensive surgery for renal cell carcinoma: long-term results and prognostic factors. J Urol 1990;143:468.
21. Herrlinger A, Schrott KM, Schott G, Sigel A. What are the benefits of extended dissection of the regional renal lymph nodes in the therapy of renal cell carcinoma? J Urol 1991;146:1224.

Principles and Practice of Genitourinary Oncology, edited by Derek Raghavan, Howard I. Scher, Steven A. Leibel, and Paul H. Lange. Lippincott-Raven Publishers, Philadelphia, © 1997.

CHAPTER 82

Classical Surgical Approaches to Renal Cell Carcinoma

Christopher Lee Marsh

This chapter reviews the history of surgery as treatment for renal cell carcinoma (RCC) as well as the operative aspects, including indications for surgery, various surgical approaches and the classic technique, adjunctive techniques available for addressing difficult cases, results of surgical therapy, and techniques being developed for future consideration.

HISTORY OF SURGICAL RESECTION FOR RENAL TUMORS

Study of the early history of surgery for Grawitz's tumors, now called RCC, reveals stages of learning in which we are only a part of a continuum. Transperitoneal ligation of the renal vessels was described by Walker in 1905.[1] In 1908, Burg[2] described 25 cases of renal tumors removed using a simple nephrectomy and flank incision below the 12th rib but with early ligation of the vessels. Stevens in 1923[3] and Vivian in 1926[4] advised more "radical surgery" but without describing a descriptive technique. In 1925, Cabot[5] described a variety of surgical incisions, including the classic oblique and the high transverse incision with thoracoabdominal extension across the 10th and 11th rib. In 1929 Judd and Hand[6] from the Mayo Clinic reported their experience removing hypernephromas using a lumbar extraperitoneal approach. In 10% of their cases, clamps were left on the renal pedicle for vascular control for 3 to 4 days. They also advocated removal of the renal vein thrombus, early ligation of the renal pedicle, and removal of the capsule and perinephric tissue, but only 10% of patients lived 10 years after nephrectomy for renal tumors. In 1935, Bergendal[7] reported the experience from the Surgical Clinic of Lund with an operative mortality of 6.6%; previous reported mortality rates were 7.7% to 22.2%. Beer's[8] 1937 report describes the milking of the renal vein tumor thrombus back into the vein for ligation and control of the inferior vena cava (IVC) with sponge forceps if a venacavotomy is performed. In 1939, Priestley[9] from the Mayo Clinic reported his experience using a posterior lumbar incision for simple nephrectomy. He advised preventing rupture of the tumor and noted that some early postoperative deaths were probably related to dislodgment of the renal vein thrombus into the vena cava at the time of surgery.

In 1949, Chute[10] reported the use of a thoracoabdominal incision in 39 cases as a more radical approach for nephrectomy; this followed a 1948 case report by Mortensen[11] who advocated removal of perirenal fascia and fat, early ligature of vessels, and avoidance of trauma to renal substance using this approach. Lessons learned from World War II, including "intratracheal anesthesia," allowed the safe use of this incision. In 1952, Foley and colleagues[12] provided detailed anatomic description of radical nephrectomy using a flank approach across the 11th and 12th ribs.

Robson's[13] 1969 report is considered a sentinel paper because of the improved results reported with the combined use of radical nephrectomy using the thoracoabdominal transpleural/transperitoneal approach and early ligation of the artery first, followed by the vein, and removal of the kidney, tumor, fascia, and lymph nodes en block.

These reports show how the guiding principles of surgical resection of RCC were developed. Good exposure, via a variety of incisions, and wide surgical resection using "Halstead's principles" of resection were recognized as critical elements of successful surgical treatment of RCC. The key elements continue to be adequate exposure; ability to control and ligate vascular structures early; en block removal of kidney, tumor, and fascia; capacity to assess and possibly resect adjacent organs and nodes; and potential to extend the incision to accomplish surgical goals.

INDICATIONS FOR RADICAL NEPHRECTOMY

As many as 40% of tumors are locally advanced or have distant metastases on initial diagnosis.[14,15] Increasing incidental discovery through ultrasonography, computed tomography, and bone scans has decreased the percentage of patients initially presenting with metastatic disease, thereby lowering the stage of presentation and resulting in improved overall 5-year survival rates.[16,17]

Currently, locally confined or locally advanced disease without extensive regional or distant metastasis are the accepted indications for radical nephrectomy. "Locally confined disease" ranges from small, incidentally discovered tumors to large tumors with IVC involvement. Many studies have clearly documented that nephrectomy in patients with multiple distant metastasis does not improve survival rates when used as the sole therapy.[18–21] Some studies support aggressive surgical intervention with low-volume or single-site metastatic disease, which can be treated with irradiation or surgical excision.[22–24] An example of such a case would be a patient with a single pulmonary or osseous metastasis that can be resected at the time of or following radical nephrectomy.

There is controversy about the role of surgery in patients with metastatic disease who will receive immunotherapy. Two schools of thought exist: surgical debulking by removal of the primary tumor, followed by immunotherapy and surgical resection of any single confined focus, and immediate immunotherapy followed by surgical resection of the tumor in any patient who appears to have evidence of response to immunotherapy. The downside to preemptive surgical resection is that up to 40% of patients may not be able to receive immunotherapy because of complications of surgery, disease progression, or both.[25] Therefore, the selection of the patient and the therapeutic course may be important in acquiring patients in both treatment courses.

SURGICAL APPROACHES

Urologists surgically resecting RCC have used a variety of surgical approaches and incision types, including the Turner-Warwick 11th-rib approach, subcostal incision, midline abdominal incision, chevron incision, and paramedian incisions.[26]

In the early 1900s, the standard surgical technique for removing renal tumors was through a flank (primarily extraperitoneal) approach, possibly because of the decreased surgical morbidity compared with anterior transperitoneal approach, considering the type of anesthesia at that time. A flank approach has the advantage of staying extraperitoneal with early recovery of bowel function and is still popular for small renal tumors and partial nephrectomies. Disadvantages to this approach, however, are that it may require rib resection, risks entry to the pleural cavity, and provides limited exposure to the midline vessels and abdomen.

The thoracoabdominal approach as described by Chute and colleagues [10] and by Robson[13] expanded the surgical exposure to renal tumors and may be the most widely used approach.[27] The advantage of the thoracoabdominal incision includes the ability to palpate the ipsilateral lung cavity and resect solitary pulmonary metastases, but this is less important in the age of sensitive radiologic evaluation.

The anterior approaches, such as the chevron, midline, and bilateral subcostal incisions, with or without cephalad extension up to the xiphoid, provide exposure to the abdominal structures, vessels, and most of the retroperitoneal structures, which is important for large and complex tumors with tumor thrombus IVC extension.[28] These approaches provide good exposure and flexibility for incision extension, which may be important when there is a good chance of requiring vascular bypass, whereas a thoracoabdominal approach may be preferable when there is a large upper pole tumor that does not require surgery in distant areas simultaneously, such as cardiac bypass, contralateral pneumonectomy, or extended regional lymph node dissection.[10,11,27,29–31] Figure 82-1, provides examples of several commonly used incisions. Other unique and less common approaches include Nagumatso's incision, modified paramedian incision, and transverse S incision.[30,32] The choice of incision depends on such factors as the location of the lesion, size of the lesion, need to access and resect adjacent structures, patients body habitus, surgeon's preference, and anesthesiologist's needs.

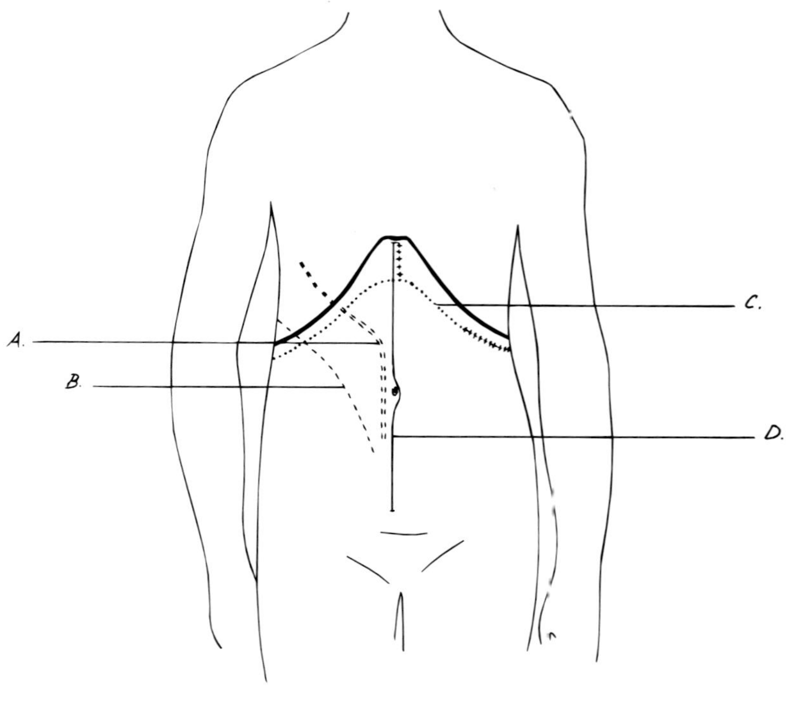

FIG. 82-1. Types of surgical incisions for approaching renal cell carcinomas: (**A**) thoracoabdominal, (**B**) flank, (**C**) chevron, or bilateral subcostal, and (**D**) midline and/or incision extension.

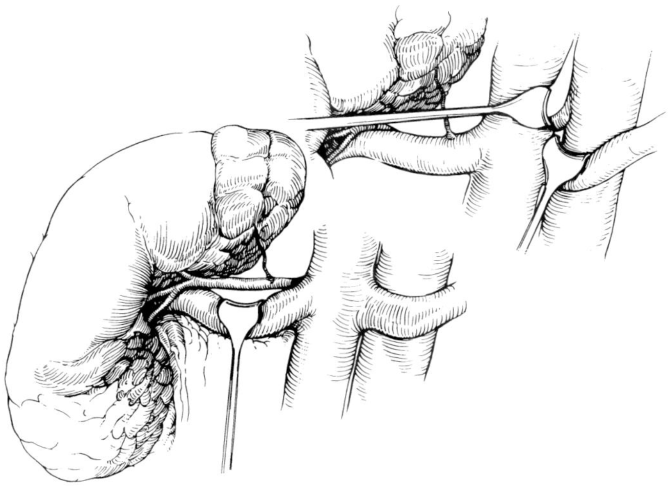

FIG. 82-2. Exposure and early ligation of the artery and vein during radical nephrectomy. (From Pontes JE. Stewart's operative urology, 2nd ed. Baltimore: Williams & Wilkins, 1989: 100.)

SURGICAL TECHNIQUE FOR RADICAL NEPHRECTOMY

The transabdominal approach to renal tumors requires mobilization of the ipsilateral colon from the splenic or hepatic flexure to the pelvic brim. Once the colon and small bowel is reflected, the retroperitoneum is entered, exposing the perirenal fat and Gerota's fascia, in which lies the kidney, adrenal, tumor, renal vessels, perihilar lymph nodes, and ureter. The en block radical nephrectomy includes all of these structures as well as the ipsilateral adrenal. Winter and colleagues[33] evaluated adrenal metastasis of RCC and determined that there was ipsilateral adrenal involvement in 8 of 138 cases; this figure concurs with prior studies reporting the incidence of adrenal metastasis at between 1.2% and 10%.[13] The dissection for the radical nephrectomy begins medially along the aorta or IVC, ligating lymph chains and isolating the renal vessels. The renal artery is identified and ligated early, followed by the renal vein, and the ureter is divided caudally (Fig. 82-2). The remaining circumferential dissection consists of ligating the remaining small lymphatic and adrenal arterial or venous attachments. On the right side, because of the direct drainage of the adrenal vein to the IVC, the surgeon must be careful that the vein is not avulsed, which will cause undue hemorrhage.

LYMPH NODE SPREAD OF TUMOR

Many researchers are responsible for our understanding of the lymphatic drainage of the kidneys.[34–41] Their excellent work has provided detailed information on the various lymphatic channels that drain from the kidneys to the retroperitoneal lymph nodes and beyond. The right kidney is drained by three lymph channels: the posterior, anterior, and middle channels. The posterior channel exits the renal hilum superior and posterior to the vessels and enters the postcaval lymph nodes, the anterior caval lymph nodes, the L1-L3 interaortocaval nodes, and the upper lateral caval nodes. The anterior lymphatic vessels exit anterior to the renal vessels and drain medially to the precaval nodes and occasionally to the posterior caval lymphatics. They may also cross the IVC and end in the upper inter aortocaval nodes. The middle lymphatic drainage courses between the artery and vein and joins the posterior and anterior lymphatic change. Thus, the regional nodes for the right kidney consist of the lateral caval nodes, the precaval nodes, the postcaval nodes, and the interaortocaval nodes.

The drainage of the left renal lymphatic nodes are similar, although there are two drainage systems: the anterior and posterior. The anterior lymph system is anterior to the renal vein and drains inferiorly or superiorly along the aorta with interconnections to the posterior lymphatic channel. The posterior channel leaves the renal hilum posterior to the renal vessels and courses to the left crus of the diaphragm, draining into the inferior or superior branches. These channels course through the diaphragmatic nodes and diaphragm into the thoracic posterior aortic lymph nodes. The inferior lymphatics connect at the left lateral lumbar nodes between the lower pole of the kidney and the renal vein; thus, the regional lymphatic drainage of the left kidney includes the preaortic, postaortic, and left lateral lumbar lymph nodes, to the left crus of the diaphragm and then to the L2-L3 diaphragmatic nodes. When the caval or aortic lymph nodes are involved with tumor, the subsequent drainage is altered to the thoracic duct, to the common iliac and sacral nodes, and occasionally to right crus of the diaphragm.

REGIONAL LYMPHADENECTOMY

The lymphatic drainage and the extent of the regional or extended lymphadenectomy is indicated in Figure 82-3. This figure shows the areas of lymph node spread for right- and left-sided tumors and the area of regional lymphadenectomy taken from the work by Marshall and Powell[40] and Pizzocaro.[41] The lymphadenectomy for a left-sided tumor includes the preaortic and postaortic lymph nodes, the left lateral lumbar nodes, and the left diaphragmatic nodes, covering the area from the diaphragm to the bifurcation of the aorta and above and below the aorta. A right-sided lymphadenectomy includes the precaval, postcaval, and lateral caval nodes, as well as the interaortocaval nodes from the bifurcation of the IVC up to the crus of the

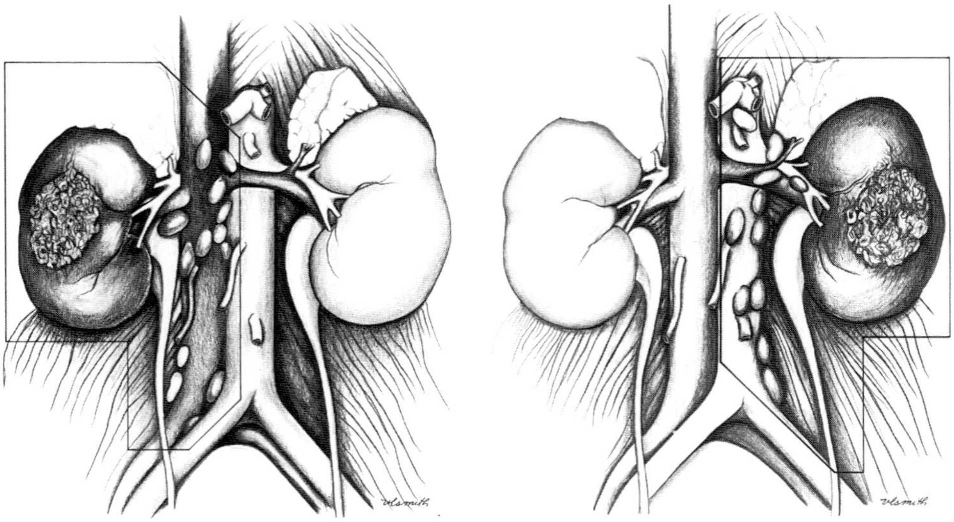

FIG. 82-3. Location of the area of lymph node spread and surgical resection for extended lymphadenectomy. (**A**) Right–sided tumor. (**B**) Left–sided tumor. (Adapted from Marshall FF, Powell KC. Lymphadenectomy for renal cell carcinoma: anatomical and therapeutic considerations. J Urol 1982;128:677; and Pizzocaro G. Lymphadenectomy in renal adenocarcinoma. In: deKernion JB, Pavone-Macalusco M, eds. Tumors of the kidney. Baltimore: Williams & Wilkins, 1986:75.)

diaphragm. The superior, inferior, and medial connections of these resected lymph node chains are ligated to prevent lymphocele formation. If there appears to be significant nodal involvement by tumor within the described area, then it is unlikely that extending the dissection will have any therapeutic benefit.

ROLE OF ANGIOINFARCTION OF RENAL TUMORS

Percutaneous transcatheter angioinfarction of local or metastatic tumor pathology has been used since the late 1960s for various indications in the urinary tract.[42] Angioinfarction has been used for the following indications[43–52]:

- to palliate pain from metastatic tumor to bone
- to control severe hematuria
- to provide preoperative angioinfarction of resectable tumors and to decrease operative blood loss
- to improve operative tissue planes
- to assure control of renal vessels
- to decrease IVC tumor thrombus size
- to improve patients' clinical status
- as adjunctive therapy in patients with metastatic disease to induce an immune response, which may allow spontaneous regression of metastases
- to increase patient survival

In 1969, Lalli and colleagues[53] reported the use of Sephadex as an agent for angioinfarcting dog kidneys. The types of materials and methods that have been used for intra arterial embolization include muscle suspension, Gelfoam (Upjohn), balloon catheter (e.g., Swan-Ganz catheters), isobutyl 2-cyanoacrylate, Gianturco-Anderson-Wallace stainless-steel coils, methylcellulose microcapsules of mitomycin or actinomycin D, and radioactive particles (I^{125} or radioactive gold seeds).[48,54–63] The most commonly used material for intraarterial embolization is absolute ethanol.

Early studies in dogs documented the potential safety and efficacy of angioinfarction.[53,57] Subsequent clinical studies elaborated some of the postinfarction complications and syndromes. Almost all patients experience postinfarction syndrome, which can begin immediately postinfarction and last for days and consists of pain, fever, nausea, vomiting, abdominal pain, hiccups, and hematuria.[44,46,63] This syndrome can be effectively controlled with appropriate medications. Other infrequent but significant complications with angioinfarction include inadvertent embolization of other organs such as the colon, permanent renal failure secondary to the intravenous contrast load, parenchymal organ abscess, and fatal pulmonary tumor thrombus embolus.[64,65]

The theoretical advantages and uses for angioinfarction are not consistently substantiated by clinical studies. Early reports noted stabilization of metastatic disease,[54] and Swanson and colleagues[44] noted a 28% to 36% overall response rate, which may be greater in patients with low-volume pulmonary metastases. Wallace and colleagues[46] noted a 36% response rate in patients with metastases undergoing embolization, delayed nephrectomy, and postoperative hormonal therapy. Patients with pulmonary metastases may have a survival advantage with this procedure, and Wallace and colleagues[46] suggested at least 4- to 5-day interval between embolization and nephrectomy. However, several excellent reports have found no significant increase in patient survival, which calls into question the routine use of angioinfarction.[49,66,67]

SPECIAL CIRCUMSTANCES

The following section is a brief overview of techniques used for the aggressive surgical resection of complex tumors. It must be remembered that the clinical situation dictates when to use these techniques, and that in general, local and distant metastatic disease is not curable by surgery alone, unlike locally confined disease, in which surgery is the mainstay of therapy.

Large renal tumors present unique challenges to the surgeon; the following techniques may allow removal of tumors initially considered unresectable. Adequate exposure is critical; the approach or incision must be chosen with the patient's anatomy and surgical plan in mind.

Liver mobilization and rotation is performed to provide exposure to the right retroperitoneum for approaching large renal tumors with or without IVC tumor thrombus.[29] The right and left coronary (triangular) ligaments are incised, and the right lobe of the liver is mobilized posteriorly. The liver rotation and IVC exposure allows direct surgery on the intrahepatic portion of the IVC tumor thrombus.

Spleen and pancreas mobilization is performed to provide exposure to the left retroperitoneum for large, left, upper pole renal tumors.[68] The pancreas and spleen are mobilized by reflecting the stomach and incising the posterior peritoneal attachments circumferentially around the spleen and pancreas. The spleen is used as a handle to dissect and elevate the tail and body of the pancreas in a "no-touch" technique. The distal pancreas and spleen can be folded over to the patient's right side, providing excellent exposure from the diaphragm down.

Tumor thrombus extensions of RCC into the renal vein occur in approximately 21% of patients, with IVC tumor thrombus occurring in 4% of patients.[69,70] IVC tumor thrombus extension is categorized by levels, as depicted in Figure 82-4. Preoperative computed tomography or magnetic resonance scans provide information regarding the magnitude of liver involvement, IVC tumor thrombus extension, and invasion into the IVC wall.[71–74] Accordingly, once an IVC tumor thrombus is identified, the placement of right heart lines such as Swan-Ganz catheters should not be taken lightly, especially in level III or IV thrombi, because there maybe a risk of inducing pulmonary thromboembolism.

Intraoperative evaluation of tumor thrombus is useful in gaining additional information about tumor extension, which may guide the surgeon in choosing options such as the need for cardiac arrest, IVC resection and reconstruction with a pericardial patch, or partial liver resection.[75–77] Additionally, ultrasonography is particularly useful in partial nephrectomies for determining the extent of tumor, ruling out tumor multicentricity, and evaluating renal cysts for unsuspected tumor foci.[78,79] Transesophageal echocardiography can be used to gain information regarding the intraatrial extent and intraoperative behavior of an IVC tumor thrombus and cardiac function.[80]

Prevention of intraoperative tumor thromboembolism is assured by early placement of an Adams-DeWeise clip, partial occluding clamp, or a Rummel tourniquet on the suprathrombus IVC prior to manipulating the liver, tumor, or IVC when there is a thrombus floating in the IVC. Alternatively, suprarenal placement of a Greenfield filter has been reported to prevent pulmonary embolism in patients with IVC tumor thrombi.[81] Intraoperative thromboembolism can be lethal and requires emergent cardiopulmonary bypass and pulmonary artery thrombectomy.[82–84] A study by Henriksson and colleagues[85] on performing preoperative and postoperative pulmonary scintigraphy found a 36% incidence of new pulmonary defects postoperatively.

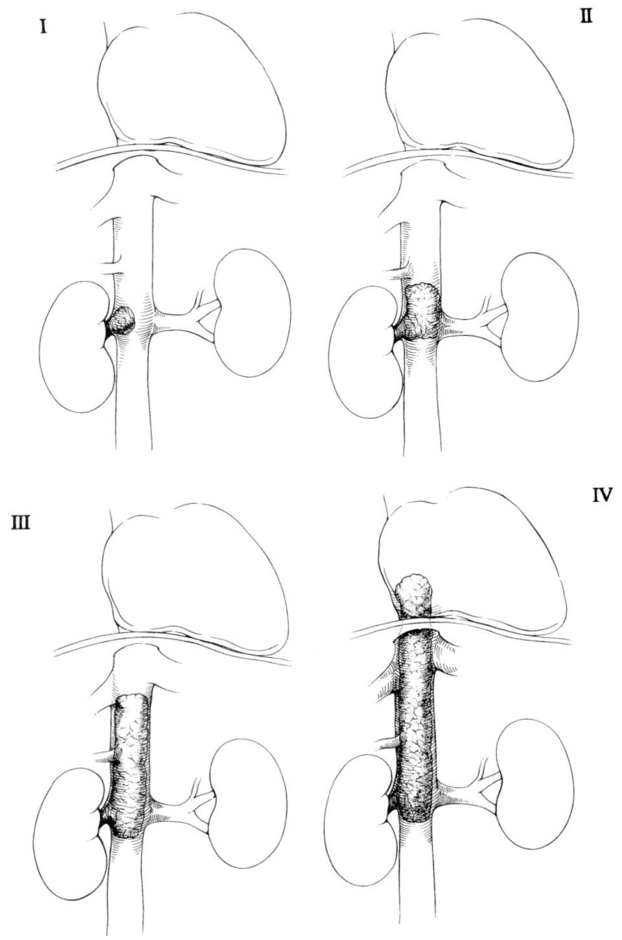

FIG. 82-4. Levels of inferior vena cava tumor thrombi. (From Novick A. Stewart's operative urology, 2nd ed. Baltimore: Williams & Wilkins, 1989:105.)

Methods of Venous Control of the Inferior Vena Cava

Control of the IVC is necessary for removal of a IVC tumor thrombus. The radical nephrectomy is performed up to the point of ligating the renal artery and isolating the renal vein and tumor thrombus. The IVC is controlled intraabdominally by placing a Rummel tourniquet around the infrarenal IVC, the contralateral renal vein, and the suprathrombus IVC. If the thrombus is below the liver, placement of a Rummel tourniquet or vascular clamp below the caudate lobe is sufficient. If the thrombus is intrahepatic, the IVC is controlled within the pericardium. The Pringle's maneuver, vascular occlusion of the porta hepatis, is used to decrease blood flow into the liver and thus blood effluxing out of the hepatic veins, which is important when extracting tumor thrombus from the intrahepatic IVC and reconstructing the IVC.[86] There have been reports of splenic rupture with the Pringle maneuver as a result of the sudden increase in portal pressure, although other measures can be used to decrease portal pressures.[87] Complex tumor thrombi above the level of the caudate lobe may require the use of bypass to allow complete resection. The choice of bypass type or cardiac arrest depends on many factors, including: the extent of IVC tumor thrombus, the

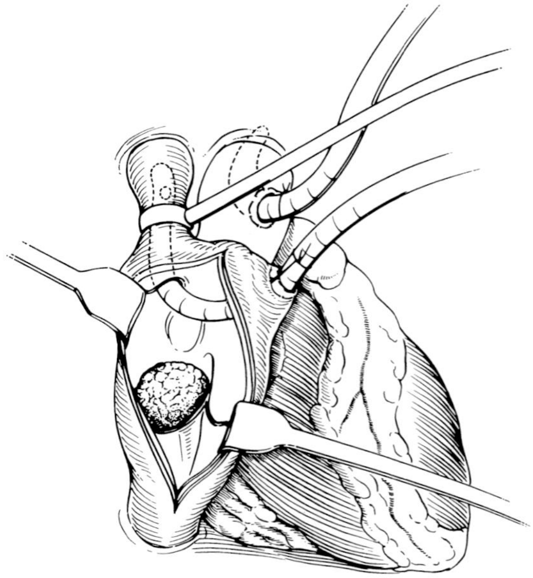

FIG. 82-5. Intraoperative intraatrial exposure provided by cardiac bypass or arrest. (From Novick A. Stewart's operative urology, 2nd ed. Baltimore: Williams & Wilkins, 1989:112.)

patency of the IVC, the extent of surgical resection necessary for the nephrectomy, the amount of IVC invasion requiring resection and reconstruction, cardiac function including cardiac disease, and the surgeon's experience.

Venovenous bypass is a method of providing circulatory isolation of the intra abdominal IVC. It provides the necessary blood return to the heart to ensure intraoperative cardiac stability and avoids the additional time, incisions, coagulopathy, and risks of cardiac bypass.[29,88–90] Venovenous bypass can be used successfully when the tumor thrombus is below the level of the diaphragm, there is no caudal infrarenal IVC thrombosis, and the patient cannot tolerate total clamping of the IVC. The bypass tubes shunt blood between the saphenous and axillary veins.

Cardiac bypass has been used for operative bypass of coronary artery disease for years. The operative mortality was originally as high as 10%, but it has decreased significantly, even in elderly patients.[91–94] The potential complications of cardiac bypass or arrest include: bleeding from post pump coagulopathy, renal failure, sternal wound infections, and neurologic sequelae.[95–100] Cardiac bypass, with or without circulatory arrest, is advisable when the tumor thrombus extends into the right atrium or invades the IVC wall or hepatic veins, which would require extensive resection and reconstruction.[101–103] The use of cardiac bypass to address the intraatrial tumor thrombus is an advance beyond finger or Foley balloon embolectomy.[101,102] The patient is placed on bypass, the IVC is controlled as described previously, the atrium is opened, and the tumor thrombus is dissected free cephalad and delivered down into the abdominal IVC for extraction en block (Fig. 82-5).

Total circulatory arrest is a relatively new procedure that has been reported in urologic literature since the 1980s for level III and IV tumor thrombi in the right atrium. The patient undergoes cardiopulmonary bypass and induction of deep hypothermia in conjunction with total cardiac and circulatory arrest and temporary total body exsanguination.[104,105] This creates a bloodless field for excision of the IVC tumor thrombus and IVC reconstruction. Up to 60 minutes of cold ischemia time is possible. This modality provides excellent visibility, and there have been numerous reports by various centers indicating success with this technique without significant postoperative morbidity or mortality in a very select group of patients.[106,107]

Inferior Vena Cava Reconstruction

The work by Clayman and colleagues[108] has nicely delineated the renal collateral circulation to each kidney (Fig. 82-6). There is commonly collateral circulation to the left kidney, which allows the left renal vein to be ligated with relative safety.[108] The right renal vein lacks collateral circulation and thus requires venous reconstruction to maintain outflow in circumstances of IVC tumor thrombus obstruction.

The objectives of IVC resection and reconstruction are to remove the intraluminal tumor thrombus, resect any tumor-invasive component in the IVC wall, prevent future thromboembolism, and obtain adequate cardiac venous return from the lower extremities and remaining kidney in patients without collateral venous return. The IVC with complete caudal thrombosis does not usually require reconstruction because venous drainage is maintained by collateral circulation, and the IVC can actually be resected, clipped, or oversewn without sequelae.[109–112] If there is venous return from the IVC but there is intraluminal nontumor thrombus, an Adams-DeWeise clip may be placed to prevent pulmonary thromboembolism. Defatted pericardium is the material most commonly used for IVC reconstruction, al-

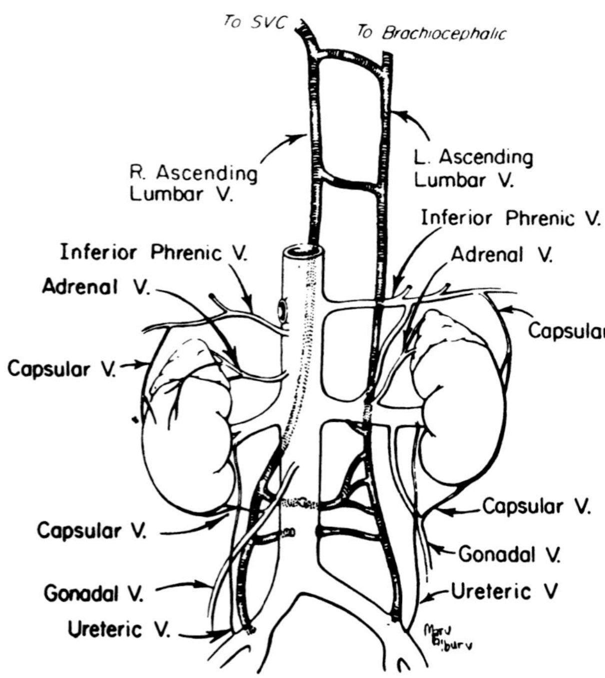

FIG. 82-6. Inferior vena cava and renal collateral circulation. SVC, superior vena cava. (From Clayman RV, Gonzales R, Fraley EE. Renal cell cancer invading the inferior vena cava: clinical review and anatomical approach. J Urol 1980; 123:157.)

though spiral saphenous grafts, Dacron, bovine pericardium, and polytetrafluoroethylene grafts have occasionally been used to patch the IVC or provide renal vein extension. There is minimal data on long-term patency rates using nonautogenous material.[113–115]

A pericardial window is made by incising the diaphragm from the midline medial down toward the vena caval foramen, thereby gaining an anterior abdominal entrance to the pericardium. This midline approach avoids the phrenic nerves and allows control of the supradiaphragmatic IVC and procurement of pericardium.[29]

Adjacent Structure Involvement and Local Recurrence

Although invasion of adjacent organ structures is associated with poor patient survival rates, it is occasionally justifiable to resect locally invasive tumor in patients who have no evidence of metastatic disease. Usually, local invasion is suggested on preoperative radiographic studies, but occasionally, clinical symptoms such as pain, sepsis, or gastrointestinal hemorrhage, which is associated with erosion of the tumor into the gastrointestinal tract, may be the presenting signs of other organ involvement. Rarely, a large, left upper pole renal tumor invades the tail of the pancreas or spleen and it may be necessary to resect the involved portion. Resection can be performed by mobilizing the spleen and exposing the body and tail of the pancreas. The distal pancreas–spleen segment, tumor, and kidney can be removed en block. There should be no evidence of proximal pancreatic duct dilation or obstruction, and the patient should receive prophylactic postoperative pneumococcal vaccination because of the splenectomy. Tumor may infrequently invade portions of the bowel such as the second portion of the duodenum, small bowel, or colon. Partial duodenal resections can be performed, reconstructing the duodenum with an ileal patch or Roux-en-Y procedure. Occasionally, a large, right-sided tumor may invade a portion of the liver, which can be treated by tumor enucleation, angioinfarction of the involved segment with a resection of the demarcated zone of infarction, or a formal right lobe resection. Posterior psoas muscle invasion is handled by resection of the anterior one third of the psoas muscle; with deeper resection, there is an increased risk of injury to the underlying femoral nerve.

Renal Fossa Recurrence

The chance of local recurrence increases if there is incomplete resection of tumor, tumor spill, positive tumor margins, or nodal involvement.[22] In patients without evidence of metastatic disease, wide local excision of the recurrent lesion should be considered. The excision may require resection of adjacent bowel, psoas muscle, and remaining lymph nodes. Frydenberg and colleagues[116] used preoperative (4500 to 5040 cGy) as well as intraoperative radiotherapy (1000 to 2500 cGy) as an adjunct to maximal surgical resection with good results. This approach may be successful, but they suggested that the ideal patient should not have prior chemotherapy or radiotherapy to the site before the combined therapy attempt.

RESULTS OF SURGICAL EXTIRPATION

Results by Stage

Postoperative pathologic analysis is important for determining true pathologic stage. Tumor size, grade, and stage provide valuable information on the patient's prognosis.[117–123] Adverse findings include nodal or metastatic disease, microscopic venous infiltration, and adjacent organ involvement.[124,125] Early reports suggested that renal vein tumor extension was associated with a poor prognosis,[119,126–127] but data by Skinner and colleagues[125] reveal that results of renal vein extension alone are comparable to those with stage I tumors. Table 82-1 provides the 5- and 10-year survival rates to be expected by surgical therapy alone and by tumor stage. The best survival rates are

TABLE 82-1. *Comparison of expected survival for surgery by cancer stage*

		Five-year survival		Ten-year survival	
Investigators/year	Stage	No. of patients	Percent	No. of patients	Percent
Robson et al, 1969[176]	I	14	64	6	67
	II	24	42	13	38
	III				
	IV				
Skinner et al, 1971[125]	I	59/91	65	34/61	56
	II	8/17	47	2/10	20
	III	51/100	51	25/68	37
	IV				
Middleton and Preslo, 1973[177]	I	25/35	71	7/10	70
	III local LN	2/3	67	1/3	33
	Renal V	7/14	50		
	LN and RV	1/4	25		
Giuliani et al, 1990[178]	RV	16	0		0
	IVC	38	5		0
	+LN	20	52		26
	T3	21	70		34

IVC, inferior vena cava; LN, lymph node; RV, renal vein.

seen with locally confined disease (i.e., negative for tumor spill, nodal disease, metastatic disease, invasion of the perinephric fat, vein extension, and residual tumor).[119,124,127–129]

Results of Simple versus Radical Nephrectomy

Resection of RCC has evolved from simple nephrectomy to a radical nephrectomy. The historical data of several series comparing simple nephrectomy with radical nephrectomy in various eras is shown in Table 82-2. Comparing the series of Robson and colleagues,[130] using radical nephrectomy, to prior reports in which a simple nephrectomy was the standard[13] shows that there is an improvement in the 5- and 10-year survival rates with radical nephrectomy. However, concurrent advances in anesthesia, surgery, and patient care could be responsible for the improvement seen with the more recent radical surgical approach. Skinner and colleagues'[125] retrospective review revealed an increase in survival with radical nephrectomy for stage I and II, but not stage III disease. This could be the result of selection, because the radical approach was chosen for stage III tumors.[125] Middleton[14] also showed a substantial improvement in 5- and 10-year survival rates with radical nephrectomy. Since that time, radical nephrectomy has become the standard of care, especially because 29% of renal tumors have perinephric fat or nodal involvement.[125] A simple nephrectomy could be as adequate as radical nephrectomy in low-stage, low-grade, and low-volume disease when the 5-year survival rates with nephron-sparing surgery in low-volume disease are considered.[131–133] This may explain the results of early studies, in which there are components of patient and therapy selection.

Results With Radiotherapy

Radiotherapy has been used, alone or as an adjunct to surgical resection, throughout the middle of this century. Table 82-3 provides a summary of reports comparing surgical resection to surgery combined with preoperative or postoperative irradiation. Early results by Riches[134] suggested improved results with nephrectomy with x-ray therapy, with 5-year survival rates of 49% compared with 30% for nephrectomy alone. Rafla[135] noted improved 5-year survival rates with radiotherapy, with a decrease in local recurrence rates. Bloom[136] noted improved 3-year survival rates in patients with renal vein or capsule involvement. However, other reports by Bloom,[136] Finney[137] and van der Werf-Messing[138] have not confirmed a substantial survival benefit with the addition of radiotherapy. Because RCC is a radioresistant tumor, it not surprising that the data do not provide compelling evidence that there is enhancement of survival with the use of radiotherapy. Interestingly, the van der Werf-Messing data[138] revealed that more cases were downstaged with the use of radiotherapy, decreasing the inoperability from 30% to 14% in patients receiving preoperative irradiation; and Rafla noted a decrease in the local recurrence rates from 25% to 7%.[135] Today radiotherapy is not used as an adjunct to radical nephrectomy in locally confined disease, although radiotherapy clearly has a role in the palliation of metastatic disease, therapy for or cure of single-site metastasis, and control of local recurrence of tumor in the renal fossa.[116]

Results With Regional (Extended) Lymphadenectomy

The use of regional, or extended, lymphadenectomy is a controversial issue. Some surgeons advocate only radical nephrectomy, whereas others advocate the routine use of extended lymphadenectomy. Clearly, lymphadenectomy stages the patient's disease, which helps predict expected long-term survival. Table 82-4 summarizes and compares the reported results of type of lymphadenectomy (none or incidental to regional or extended) to survival rates. The incidence of lymph node involvement varies by series from as low as 4% to as high as 29%. The 5-year survival rate for patients who have had lymphadenectomy ranges from 11% to 66% depending on era, stage, and type of lymphadenectomy. Evidence for improvement in survival with lymphadenectomy emerge from reports by Peters and colleagues[139] and Herrlinger and colleagues[140] that show a 10% or higher improvement in survival rates. However, the data by Novick and colleagues[133] and Zinke and colleagues[141] on performing nephron-sparing surgery for low-volume RCC reveal that 5-year survival rates are as good as those with radical

TABLE 82-2. *Comparison of radical and simple nephrectomy by eras*

			Five-year survival				Ten-year survival			
			Simple		Radical		Simple		Radical	
Investigators	Era (years)	Stage	No. of patients	Percent	No. of patients	Percent	No. of patients	Percent	No. of patients	Percent
Hand, 1932[179]	1901–1923	I–III	44/193	22.8			24/193	12.4		
Bergendal[7]	1901–1932	I–III	57	40.4			40	30		
Libertino et al, 1987[198]	1910–1936	I–III	137/357	38.4			69/253	27.3		
Foot[180]	1926–1949	I–III	33/85	38			9/40	22.5		
Riches et al, 1951[188]	1932–1952	I–III	165	35			104	18		
Throckmorton[182]	1922–1953	I–III	22/42	36.3			14	14.5		
Throckmorton, 1955[182]	1926–1950	I–III	56	48.2			39	23		
Myers[127]	1940–1955	I–III	254/508	50			183/508	36		
Robson[176]	1949–1964	I–III			41/79	52			18/37	49
Kaufman[184]	1966	I–III			37/79	47			27/79	34
Middleton[177]	1950–1967	I–III			36/61	59			8/20	40
Rafla, 1970[135]	1935–1965	I	28/45	62	30/44	68	20/39	51	13/20	65
		II	2/5	40	6/12	50	1/4	25	1/6	17
		III	13/24	54	37/75	49	9/24	38	15/43	35

TABLE 82-3. *Comparison of surgery to surgery plus radiotherapy*

			Five-year survival						Ten-year survival					
			Surgery alone		Preoperative Irradiation plus surgery		Surgery plus postoperative Irradiation		Surgery alone		Preoperative Irradiation plus surgery		Surgery plus postoperative Irradiation	
Investigators	Era (years)	Radiotherapy dose (cGy)	No. of patients	Per-cent	No. of patients	Per-cent	No. of patients	Per-cent	No. of patients	Per-cent	No. of patients	Per-cent	No. of patients	Per-cent
Hand, 1932[179]	1901–1923	None	44/193	22.8					24/193	12.4				
Bixler et al, 1944[186]	1924–1940	2200–2500	4/8	50			11/36	31	1/2	50			3/11	27
Foot et al, 1951[180]	1926–1949	None	33/85	38					9/40	22.5				
Chateris, 1951[187]	1951		29	28			14	36						
Flocks and Kadesky, 1958[183]	1926–1958	7000	27/56	48	13/25	52	21/40	52	9/39	23	7/14	50	9/27	33
Riches et al, 1981[188]	1935–1950	3000–6150	105/345	30	4/15	27	26/53	49	30/177	17	1/10	10	4/15	27
Bratherton and Chin, 1964[189]	1964	3000	10/35	29			9/21	43	4/15	26			3/9	33
Peeling et al, 1969[190]	1940–1965	None	50/96	52			17/68	25						
Cox et al, 1970[191]	1941–1968	3000–5000	26/58	45			9/28	32	5/46	11			2/24	8.3
Rafla, 1970[135]	1955–1964	4500–6000	35/94	37	0/1	0	46/81	56	13/68	19	0/1	0	16/47	34
Skinner et al, 1989[185]	1935–1965	None	109/190	57			9/18	50	61/139	44				
van der Werf-Messing and Van Gilse, 1971[185]	1965–1972	3000	62	28	64	28								
Finney, 1973[137]	1973	None	12/27	44			11/30	37						

TABLE 82-4. *Type of lymphadenectomy and survival*

Investigators	Era (years)	No. of cases	Positive lymph nodes (%)	Stage	Five-year survival: Incidental/none, No. of patients	Five-year survival: Incidental/none, Percent	Five-year survival: Regional/extended, No. of patients	Five-year survival: Regional/extended, Percent	Ten-year survival: Incidental/none, No. of patients	Ten-year survival: Incidental/none, Percent	Ten-year survival: Regional/extended, No. of patients	Ten-year survival: Regional/extended, Percent	Operative mortality (%)
Flocks and Kadesky, 1958[183]	1926–1958	133	16	III	3	14			2	16.6			
Skinner et al, 1989[185]	1935–1965	108	26.8	III			3/9	33			1/7	14	3
Robson et al, 1969[176]	1949–1964	87	22.7	III			10/24	42			5/13	38	
Middleton, 1967[14]	1950–1967	61	11.5	III			36/61	59			8/20	40	4.9
Waters and Richie, 1979[69]	1957–1977	67	24	III			8	12.3					2
Petkovic, 1959[192]	1959	100	22	I–III				0–5				0	22.7
Peters and Brown, 1980[139]	1963–1979	31	41.9	III		25.69		43.75					
Siminovitch et al, 1982[193]	1968–1978	102	9	II–III			reg. 8/21	38					
					1/5	20	ext. 4/11	36					
Herrlinger et al, 1991[140]	1970–1986	511	10	I–III (all)		58		66		39		54	inc. 3.8
			17	I		70		90		54		80	ext. 1
				II		55		80		54		80	
				III		37		40		28		37	
Giuliani et al. 1990[178]	1970–1987	200	10	III				52				26	5.5

nephrectomy alone. Their results suggest that in low-volume tumors, the chance of having positive microscopic disease for which a lymphadenectomy is therapeutic is small.

The available data reveal that 10% to 25% of patients may have nodal disease, and those who undergo extended lymphadenectomy may have a 10% improvement in 5-year survival rates. Sensitive radiologic evaluation, which can accurately stage the patient by tumor volume and determine whether the tumor is locally confined, combined with low-morbidity surgery, affords the surgeon an opportunity to provide a component of therapeutic survival advantage by resecting microscopic and macroscopic nodal disease.

Surgery for Locally Advanced or Tumor Involving the Inferior Vena Cava

In general, contiguous involvement of adjacent structures with tumor is associated overall poor prognosis. In cases without distant metastases, extensive regional disease resection of adjacent structures or single solitary metastatic lesions can provide 5-year survival rates of 8% to 29%.[125] Angervall and Wahlqvist[142] evaluated their experience in 45 patients with pelvic wall involvement, tumor thrombus in the renal vein, or spread within the renal fascia and found that these findings did not influence prognosis.

Table 82-5 provides a comparison of survival rates by IVC level, degree of resection, and nodal and metastatic status. The 5-year patient survival rates for a selected group of patients with IVC tumor extension alone (negative metastasis, nodes, or caval wall invasion) range from 20% to 69%.[143] Incomplete resection of tumor thrombus, increasing level of tumor thrombus extension, nodal involvement, or metastatic disease significantly decreases patient survival rates, but the data argue for an aggressive stance in this unusual circumstance.

Surgery for Metastatic Disease

Adjunctive nephrectomy in patients with metastatic disease, especially large-volume metastasis or metastases to multiple sites, does not improve patient survival rates; the 1-year survival rate in such patients is dismal (10%).[69,122,144] Several studies have noted an improvement in survival with adjunctive nephrectomy in patients with selected low-volume disease (e.g., single-site osseous or pulmonary metastasis) or in patients in whom these sites can be excised. Swanson and colleagues[23] noted an improvement in survival rate with adjunctive nephrectomy only in patients with a solitary bone metastasis; metastases to multiple sites were associated with with 1-, 3-, and 5-year survival rates of 74%, 52%, and 15%, respectively. The reported incidence of a solitary metastasis varies depending on the study, ranging from a low of 1.6% to a high of 30%.[14,23,24,70]

The 5-year survival rates with an ''excised or radiated solitary'' metastatic lesion is as high as 30%.[14,22,23,125,145,146] Katzenstein and colleagues[145] reported on 44 cases of metastatic RCC to the lung. Their data supported surgical resection of unilateral lung lesions, with a mean survival rate of 38 months. Adverse prognostic features included multiple lung lesions and positive bronchial lymph nodes; improved survival was associated with extensive necrosis of the tumor and lung metastasis more than 2 years following nephrectomy.[145,147] However, Johnson and colleagues[144] found no improvement with pulmonary resection. deKernion and colleagues[22] also noted improved survival in patients (5-year survival rate, >20%) when the disease was confined to the lungs, the metastatic focus was excised, and there was absence of local recurrence or a longer disease-free interval after primary nephrectomy.

Montie and colleagues[146] reported a 1-year survival rate of 36% in patients with osseous metastases versus 18% for metastases in other sites in patients receiving adjunctive nephrectomy. Smith and colleagues[148] found that palliative orthopedic procedures for symptoms of metastatic osseous disease were effective in providing functional improvement and relief of pain in patients. Swanson and colleagues[23] found that the median disease-free interval from diagnosis of RCC to osseous metastasis was 8.5 months; 80% of patients developed metastasis within 3 years. Badalament and colleagues[149] reported a 1-year survival rate of 36% after local excision and radiotherapy for cerebral metastases discovered more than 1 year following excision of the primary lesion versus 19% in those discovered less than 1 year following excision.

O'dea and colleagues[24] noted that patients with a single metastatic lesion tend to do poorly, but for those who present with a single metastasis after nephrectomy, surgical resection seems to improve results (5-year survival, 50%), with occasional long-term survival.[24] Conversely, others have found only transient stabilization of disease or no benefit with excision of a solitary metastasis.[20]

Adjunctive nephrectomy for induction of spontaneous regression of metastasis is not justified. Spontaneous regression is rarely seen, with a reported incidence from 0.3% to 8% depending on definition, evaluation, and follow-up. Although Fairlamb[150] reported that 50% of patients died of tumor as long as 15 years following adjunctive nephrectomy, for most, the regression was short lived.[146,151,152] Complete regression has been reported in 12% of patients treated with medroxyprogesterone acetate.[146] The morbidity and mortality associated with nephrectomy is low, but in patients with poor performance status (e.g., those presenting with metastatic disease), it could be as high as 6%.[150] Adjunctive nephrectomy appears to be justified only for palliation of symptoms such as pain and hematuria or hemorrhage, as an adjunct to planned chemotherapeutic or immunotherapeutic regimens, and as part of an aggressive surgical approach with radical nephrectomy and excision or irradiation of single-site metastasis.

Hajdu and Thomas[153] evaluated causes of death in patients with RCC and found that death from tumor occurred in only 50%, and in 20%, a second primary malignancy was the cause of death. Interestingly, Hellsten and colleagues[154] in a postmortem study found that cardiovascular disease was the leading cause of death in 44% of RCC patients.

Renal fossa recurrence rarely occurs, but deKernion and colleagues[22] found that 86% of patients with recurrence died within 1 year. Others have found that a 36% 3-year survival rate can be achieved with wide surgical resection, with or without adjunctive radiotherapy.[116,155] Late recurrence is unusual but has been known to occur from 10 to 30 years after treatment.[156,157]

All of this data seems to suggest that an aggressive stance

TABLE 82-5. *Comparison of level of inferior vena cava involvement and resection to survival**

Investigators/year published	Sosa et al, 1984[194]	Schefft et al, 1978[195]	Neves and Zincke, 1987[196]	Sogani et al, 1983[197]	Cherrie et al, 1982[117]	Giulani et al, 1990[178]	Libertino et al, 1987[198]
Study time span	1950–1981	1956–1976	1962–1984	1965–1981	1970–1980	1970–1987	1971–1985
Total cases	24	21	54	16	27	54	44
IVC LEVEL							
I							
1 y							
3 y							
5 y							
II							
1 y							
3 y							
5 y							
III/IV							
1 y							
3 y							
5 y							
METASTASES							
(V + M0)							
1 y			80%				
3 y		50% 14–120 mo	75%	50% 34–199 mo	45% 12–84 mo		
5 y			55%			5%	69%
(V+M+)							
1 y		0%	50%	12% 10–28 mo			
3 y			20%		5% 2 y	22% 2 y	0%
5 y			12%		0%	0% 5 y	
THROMBUS RESECTION							
Incomplete			17% 5 y				
Complete			68% 5 y				
OVERALL SURVIVAL RATE							
1 y							
3 y	46% 2 y						
5 y							44%
Operative mortality	16%	19%	9.3%	6.2%	11%		4.5%

* When available, subgroup survival data is shown. IVC, inferior vena cava; M+, metastasis; V+, vein positive.

is warranted in selected patients to provide not only appropriate terminal medical care, but that surgery can provide genuine palliation to prolonged survival.

FUTURE OF SURGERY IN RENAL CELL CARCINOMA

Surgery and Systemic Therapy

Areas of future refinement include how best to combine surgical resection with flow cytometric data, angioinfarction capabilities, and immunotherapeutic protocols for locally advanced, regional, and metastatic disease. There have been numerous reports using cytotoxic immunotherapeutic protocols with biologic response modifiers for advanced disease.[158–162] A review of data from several institutions noted improved response of pulmonary metastasis to interferon therapy in patients who had nephrectomy prior to systemic therapy.[163] Accordingly, most protocols involve debulking the primary tumor to maximize the systemic response, with objective response rates of 20% to 31%.[159,164–167] However, data exist that suggest that surgery may interfere with the immune response to biologic response modifiers, and several studies have documented that medical or tumor-related complications developing after surgery can prevent the use of immunotherapy.[162,168,169] Along these lines, Fleishmann and colleagues[170] suggested prenephrectomy systemic therapy followed by selective abdominal cytoreductive surgery in patients who have had a response to systemic therapy as evident by regression of peripheral metastasis. Reports suggest that patients with an isolated metastatic focus downstaged by immunotherapy or who have an isolated recurrence after a complete response should be aggressively surgically resected.[147,171,172]

These data emphasize that there are many options regarding the role and timing of various adjunctive therapies, and close collaboration between the oncologist and surgeon is indispensable. An aggressive surgical and medical posture is essential in selected patients.

TABLE 82-5. *Continued.*

Kearney et al, 1981[109]	Pritchett et al, 1986[199]	Hatcher et al, 1991[200]	Skinner et al, 1989[185]	Vaislic et al, 1986[201]	Hedderich et al, 1987[202]	Novick et al, 1990[203]	Burt, 1991[89]
1972–1979	1972–1983	1972–1987	1972–1988	1973–1983	1977–1986	1984–1989	1985–1991
24	25	44	53	18	13	39	17
	50%						
	42%						
	42%		35%				
	60%						
	50%				65% 7–52 mo		
	17%		18%				
	33%						
	0%				90% 7–64 mo		
	0%		0%				
					(− nodes)		100%
100% 3–69 mo				71% 1 mo–10 y	88% 7–64 mo	63.9%	65%
	33%	42%	57%	75%			
	0%			0%	(+ nodes)		50%
0% 5–24 mo					75% 7–52 mo	10.9%	25%
							0%
		<18%	0%				
0%	0% <6 mo	0% 5 y	8% 1 y				
19% 6–69 mo	36% 5 yr	57% 5 y	34%				
17% 6–69 mo			56%				
			34%		85% 7–64 mo		
			25%				50%
4%	4%	6.8%	13%	0%	0%	4.7%	23.5%

Laparoscopic Surgery for Cancer

The use of laparoscopic surgery is rapidly expanding, and this procedure is being applied to removal of kidneys for benign and malignant disease.[173] The techniques, technology, and indications associated with laparoscopy for cancer are being evaluated and developed, but it its to early to know whether this procedure is a viable option for treating low-volume, low-stage, and low-grade RCCs.[174] The anticipated results of this technology are good, based on data from stage I tumors and nephron-sparing surgery, with a predicted decrease in patient morbidity and mortality.[175]

Radical nephrectomy is the mainstay of therapy for locally confined RCC. Extended lymphadenectomy may augment and predict survival in selected patients, such as those with large-volume disease. Radiotherapy, aggressive surgical resection of locally confined disease, adjunctive surgery in the presence of metastasis, and chemotherapy or immunotherapy are clearly advantageous in certain circumstances and continue to be explored. Surgery will continue to evolve toward safer complex techniques and to less invasive procedures that hopefully will continue to improve patient outcome.

REFERENCES

1. Walker G. Transperitoneal ligation of the renal vessels. JAMA 1905; 45:1647.
2. Berg AA. Malignant hypernephroma of the kidney, its clinical course and diagnosis, with a description of the author's method of radical operative cure. Surg Gynecol Obstet 1913;17:463.
3. Stevens WE. Diagnosis and surgical treatment of malignant tumors of the kidney. J Urol 1923;10:121.
4. Vivian CS. Hypernephroma. S W Med 1926;10:7.
5. Cabot H. The operative approach for malignant tumors of the kidney. J Urol 1925;14:261.
6. Judd ES, Hand JR. Hypernephroma. J Urol 1929;22:10.
7. Bergendal S. To the clinical study and prognosis of tumors of the kidney: a study of 94 nephrectomized cases. Acta Chir Scand 1935; 77:563.
8. Beer E. Some aspects of malignant tumors of the kidney. Surg Gynecol Obstet 1937;65:433.
9. Priestley JT. Survival following removal of malignant renal neoplasms. JAMA 1939;113:902.
10. Chute R, Soutter L, Kerr WS. The value of the thoracoabdominal incision in the removal of kidney tumors. N Engl J Med 1949;241: 951.
11. Mortensen H. Transthoracic nephrectomy. J Urol 1948;60:855.
12. Foley FB, Mulvaney WP, Richardson EJ, Victor I. Radical nephrectomy for neoplasm. J Urol 1952;68:39.

13. Robson CJ. Radical nephrectomy for renal cell carcinoma. J Urol 1963;89:37.
14. Middleton RG. Surgery for metastatic renal cell carcinoma. J Urol 1967;97:973.
15. Mostofi FK. Pathology and spread of renal cell carcinoma. Boston: Little, Brown & Company, 1967:41.
16. Nakano E, Iwasaki A, Seguchi T, et al. Incidentally diagnosed renal cell carcinoma. Eur Urol 1992;21:294.
17. Konnak JW, Grossman HB. Renal cell carcinoma as an incidental finding. J Urol 1985;134:1094.
18. Patel NP, Lavengood RW. Renal cell carcinoma: natural history and results of treatment. J Urol 1978;119:722.
19. Nacey JN, Delahunt B. Renal cell carcinoma. I. Clinical indicators of prognosis. N Z Med J 1986;99:531.
20. Dineen MK, Pastore RD, Emrich LJ, Huben RP. Results of surgical treatment of renal cell carcinoma with solitary metastasis. J Urol 1988; 140:277.
21. Dinney CP, Awad SA, Gajewski JB, et al. Analysis of imaging modalities, staging systems, and prognostic indicators for renal cell carcinoma. Urology 1992;39:122.
22. deKernion JB, Ramming KP, Smith RB. The natural history of metastatic renal cell carcinoma: a computer analysis. J Urol 1978;120:148.
23. Swanson DA, Orovan WL, Johnson DE, Giacco G. Osseous metastases secondary to renal cell carcinoma. Urology 1981;18:556.
24. O'dea MJ, Zincke H, Utz DC, Bernatz PE. The treatment of renal cell carcinoma with solitary metastasis. J Urol 1978;120:540.
25. Walther MM, Alexander RB, Weiss GH, et al. Cytoreductive surgery prior to interleukin-2-based therapy in patients with metastatic renal cell carcinoma. Urology 1993;42:250.
26. Turner Warwick RT. The supracostal approach to the renal area. Br J Urol 1965;37:671.
27. Steiner MS, Naslund MJ, Stutzman RE. A modified thoracoabdominal approach for retroperitoneal lymphadenectomy. J Urol 1993;149:23.
28. Thomalla JV, Friend PJ. Modified cruciate incision for transabdominal radical nephrectomy. J Urol 1991;145:1245.
29. Marsh CL, Lange PH. Application of liver transplantation and organ procurement techniques to difficult upper abdominal urological cases. J Urol 1994;151:1652.
30. Srougi M. Transverse "S" laparotomy for radical nephrectomy and upper retroperitoneal access. J Urol 1994;152:139.
31. Novick AC, Montie JE. The kidneys, adrenal glands, and retroperitoneum. In: Novick AC, Streem SB, Pontes JE, eds. Stewart's operative urology, vol. 1, 2nd ed. Baltimore: Williams & Wilkins, 1989:104.
32. Sugao H, Matsuda M, Nakano E, Seguchi T, Sonoda T. Comparison of lumbar flank approach and transperitoneal approach for radical nephrectomy. Urol Int 1991;46:43.
33. Winter P, Miersch WD, Vogel J, Jaeger N. On the necessity of adrenal extirpation combined with radical nephrectomy. J Urol 1990;144:842.
34. Poirer P, Cuneo B, Delamere G. The lymphatics. London: Archibald Constable & Company, Ltd., 1903.
35. Parker AE. Studies on the main posterior lymph channels of the abdomen and their connections with the lymphatics of the genito-urinary system. Am J Anat 1971;56:409.
36. Cockett ATK, Roberts AP, Moore RS. Evidence for two intrarenal lymphatic networks. Invest Urol 1970;7:266.
37. Cockett ATK. Lymphatic network of kidney. I. Anatomic and Physiologic Considerations. Urology 1977;11:125.
38. Peirce EC. Renal lymphatics. Anat Rec 1944;90:315.
39. Threefoot SA, Kent WT, Hatchett BF. Lymphaticovenous and lymphaticolymphatic communications demonstrated by plastic corrosion models of rats and by post-mortem lymphangiography in man. J Lab Clin Med 1963;61:9.
40. Marshall FF, Powell KC. Lymphadenectomy for renal cell carcinoma: anatomical and therapeutic considerations. J Urol 1982;128:677.
41. Pizzocaro G. Lymphadenectomy in renal adenocarcinoma. In: deKernion JB, Pavone-Macalusco M, eds. Tumors of the kidney. Baltimore: Williams & Wilkins, 1986:75.
42. McLean GK, Meranze SG. Embolization techniques in the urinary tract. Urol Clin North Am 1985;12:743.
43. Feldman F, Casarella WJ, Dick HM, Hollander BA. Selective intraarterial embolization of bone tumors. Radiology 1975;123:130.
44. Swanson DA, Johnson DE, von Eschenbach AC, Chuang VP, Wallace S. Angioinfarction plus nephrectomy for metastatic renal cell carcinoma: an update. J Urol 1983;130:449.
45. Craven WM, Redmond PL, Kumpe DA, Durham JD, Wettlauffer JN. Planned delayed nephrectomy after ethanol embolization of renal carcinoma. J Urol 1991;146:704.
46. Wallace S, Chaung VP, Swanson D, et al. Embolization of renal carcinoma. Radiology 1981;138:563.
47. Wallace S, Granmayeh M, DeSantos LA, et al. Arterial occlusion of pelvic bone tumors. Cancer 1979;43:322.
48. Singsaas MW, Chopp RT, Mendez R. Preoperative renal embolization as adjunct to radical nephrectomy. Urology 1979;14:1.
49. Gottesman JE, Crawford ED, Grossman HB, Scardino P, McCracken JD. Infarction-nephrectomy for metastatic renal carcinoma. Urology 1985;25:248.
50. Bakal CW, Cynamon J, Lakritz PS, Sprayregen S. Value of preoperative renal artery embolization in reducing blood transfusion requirements during nephrectomy for renal cell carcinoma. J Vasc Interv Radiol 1993;4:727.
51. Kaisary AV, Williams G, Riddle PR. The role of preoperative embolization in renal cell carcinoma. J Urol 1984;131:641.
52. Varma J, Huben RP, Wajsman Z, Pontes JE. Therapeutic embolization of pelvic metastases of renal cell carcinoma. J Urol 1984;131:647.
53. Lalli AF, Peterson N, Bookstein JJ. Roentgen-guided infarctions of kidneys and lungs: a potential therapeutic technique. Radiology 1969; 93:434.
54. Almgard LE, Fernstrom I, Haverling M, Ljungqvist A. Treatment of renal adenocarcinoma by embolic occlusion of the renal circulation. Br J Urol 1973;45:474.
55. Sato K, Kato T. Arterial chemoembolization using microencapsulated anticancer drugs. Gan To Kagaku Ryoho 1990;17:1105.
56. Klimberg I, Hunter P, Hawkins IF, Drylie DM, Wajsman Z. Preoperative angioinfarction of localized renal cell carcinoma using absolute ethanol. J Urol 1985;133:21.
57. Ellman BA, Green CE, Eigenbrodt E, Garriott JC, Curry TS. Renal infarction with absolute ethanol. Invest Radiol 1980;1:318.
58. Turner RD, Rand RW, Bentson JR, Mosso JA. Ferromagnetic silicone necrosis of hypernephromas by selective vascular occlusion to the tumor: a new technique. J Urol 1975;113:455.
59. Dotter CT, Goldman ML, Rosch J. Instant selective arterial occlusion with isobutyl 2-cyanoacrylate. Radiology 1975;114:227.
60. Kato T, Nemoto R, Mori H, Takahashi M, Harada M. Arterial chemoembolization with mitomycin C microcapsules in the treatment of primary or secondary carcinoma of the kidney, liver, bone and intrapelvic organs. Cancer 1981;48:674.
61. Wiley AL, Wirtanen GW, Ansfield FJ, Ramirez G. Combined intraarterial actinomycin D and radiation therapy for surgically unresectable hypernephroma. J Urol 1975;114:198.
62. Mee AD, Heap SW. Pre-operative balloon occlusion of the renal artery for radical nephrectomy. Br J Urol 1978;50:153.
63. Leinonen A. Embolization of renal carcinoma. Ann Clin Res 1985; 17:299.
64. Jennings SB, Austenfeld MS, Basham K. Fatal pulmonary embolus from ischemic necrosis of intracaval tumor thrombosis: a case report. J Urol 1993;150:1492.
65. Cox GG, Lee KR, Price HI, Gunter K, Noble MJ, Mebust WK. Colonic infarction following ethanol embolization of renal cell carcinoma. Radiology 1982;145:343.
66. Kurth KH, Debruyne FM, Hall RR, et al. Embolization and postinfarction nephrectomy in patients with primary metastatic renal adenocarcinoma. Eur Urol 1987;13:251.
67. Mebust WK, Weigel JW, Lee KR, Cox GG, Jewell WR, Krishnan EC. Renal cell carcinoma: angioinfarction. J Urol 1984;131:231.
68. Marsh CL. Enhancing exposure of the left upper retroperitoneum. Contemp Urol 1994;6:15.
69. Waters WB, Richie JP. Aggressive surgical approach to renal cell carcinoma: review of 130 cases. J Urol 1979;122:306.
70. Maldazys JD, deKernion JB. Prognostic factors in metastatic renal carcinoma. J Urol 1986;136:376.
71. Lim DJ, Carter MF. Computerized tomography in the preoperative staging for pulmonary metastases in patients with renal cell carcinoma. J Urol 1993;150:1112.
72. Rahoumi A, Mathieu D, Berger JF, Montazel JL, Chopin DK, Vasile N. Fast magnetic resonance imaging in the evaluation of tumoral obstructions of the inferior vena cava. J Urol 1992;148:14.
73. Goldfarb DA, Novick AC, Lorig R, et al. Magnetic resonance imaging for assessment of vena caval tumor thrombi: a comparative study

with venocavography and computerized tomography scanning. J Urol 1990;144:1100.
74. Gohji K, Yamashita C, Ueno K, Simogaki H, Kamidono S. Preoperative computerized tomography detection of extensive invasion of the inferior vena cava by renal call carcinoma: possible indication for resection with partial cardiopulmonary bypass and patch grafting. J Urol 1994;152:1993.
75. Didier D, Racle A, Etievent JP, Weill F. Tumor thrombus of the inferior vena cava secondary to malignant abdominal neoplasms: US and CT evaluation. Radiology 1987;162:83.
76. Komatsu H, Yoh T, Murakami K, et al. Renal cell carcinoma with intracaval tumor thrombus extending to the diaphragm: ultrasonography and surgical management. J Urol 1985;134:122.
77. Long JP, Choyke PL, Shawker TA, et al. Intraoperative ultrasound in the evaluation of tumor involvement of the inferior vena cava. J Urol 1993;150:13.
78. Marshall FF, Holdford SS, Hamper UM. Intraoperative sonography of renal tumors. J Urol 1992;148:1393.
79. Walther MM, Choyke PL, Hayes W, Shawker TH, Alexander RB, Linehan WM. Evaluation of color Doppler intraoperative ultrasound in parenchymal sparing renal surgery. J Urol 1994;152:1984.
80. Treiger BFG, Humphrey LS, Peterson CV, et al. Transesophageal echocardiology in renal cell carcinoma: an accurate diagnostic technique for intracaval neoplastic extensions. J Urol 1991;145:1138.
81. Brenner DW, Brenner CJ, Scott J, Wehberg K, Granger JP, Schellhammer PF. Suprarenal Greenfield filter placement to prevent pulmonary embolus in patients with vena caval tumor thrombi. J Urol 1992; 147:19.
82. Judd ES, Scholl AJ. Thrombosis and embolism resulting from renal tumors. JAMA 1924;82:75.
83. Markham NI, Doyle PT. Prolonged survival following emergency pulmonary tumor embolectomy and subsequent nephrectomy. Br J Urol 1987;59:484.
84. Milne B, Cervenko FW, Morales A, Salerno TA. Massive intraoperative pulmonary tumor embolus from renal cell carcinoma. Anesthesiology 1981;54:253.
85. Henriksson C, Aldenborg F, Lindberg S, Pettersson S. Pulmonary embolism in renal cell carcinoma with vena cava extension. Scand J Urol Nephrol 1988;22:215.
86. Abdelsayed MA, Bissada NK, Finkbeiner AE, Redman JF. Renal tumors involving the inferior vena cava: plan for management. J Urol 1978;120:153.
87. Baniel J, Bihrle R, Wahle GR, Foster RS. Splenic rupture during occlusion of the porta hepatis in resection of tumors with vena caval extension. J Urol 1994;151:992.
88. Attwood S, Land DM, Goiti J, Grant J. Venous bypass for surgical resection of renal carcinoma invading the vena cava: a new approach. Br J Urol 1988;61:402.
89. Burt M. Inferior vena caval involvement by renal cell carcinoma. Use of venovenous bypass as adjunct during resection. Urol Clin North Am 1991;18:437.
90. Janosko EO, Powell CS, Spence PA, Hodges WE, Lust RM. Surgical management of renal cell carcinoma with extensive intracaval involvement using a venous bypass system suitable for rapid conversion to total cardiopulmonary bypass. J Urol 1991;145:555.
91. Spiess BD. Cardiac anesthesia risk management. Hemorrhage, coagulation, and transfusion: a risk-benefit analysis. J Cardiothorac Vasc Anesth 1994;8:19.
92. Horton DA, Hicks RG, O'Brien HD. Operative mortality after coronary artery surgery: a seven-year experience of 1500 consecutive operations. Med J Aust 1986;144:508.
93. Montague NT, Kouchoukos NT, Wilson TA, et al. Morbidity and mortality of coronary bypass grafting in patients 70 years of age and older. Ann Thorac Surg 1985;39:552.
94. Rich MW, Keller AJ, Schechtman KB, Marshall WGJ, Kouchoukos NT. Morbidity and mortality of coronary bypass surgery in patients 75 years of age or older. Ann Thorac Surg 1988;46:638.
95. Woodman RC, Harker LA. Bleeding complications associated with cardiopulmonary bypass. Blood 1990;76:1680.
96. Wong DH. Perioperative stroke. Part II. Cardiac surgery and cardiogenic embolic stroke. Can J Anaesth 1991;38:471.
97. Mills SA. Cerebral injury and cardiac operations. Ann Thorac Surg 1993;56:S86.
98. Mills SA, Prough DS. Neuropsychiatric complications following cardiac surgery. Semin Thorac Cardiovasc Surg 1991;3:39.
99. Ley SJ. Myocardial depression after cardiac surgery: pharmacologic and mechanical support. AACN Clin Issues Crit Care Nurs 1993;4: 293.
100. Tucker LA. Post-pump delirium. Intens Crit Care Nurs 1993;9:269.
101. Wilkinson CJ, Kimovec MA, Uejima T. Cardiopulmonary bypass in patients with malignant renal neoplasms. Br J Anaesth 1986;58:461.
102. Novick AC, Cosgrove DM. Surgical approach for removal of renal cell carcinoma extending into the vena cava and the right atrium. J Urol 1980;123:947.
103. Turini D, Selli C, Barbanti G, Beneforti P, Calamai G. Removal of renal cell carcinoma extending to the supradiaphragmatic vena cava with the aid of cardiopulmonary bypass. Urol Int 1986;31:303.
104. Marshall FF, Reitz BA, Diamond DA. A new technique for management of renal cell carcinoma involving the right atrium: hypothermia and cardiac arrest. J Urol 1984;131:103.
105. Krane RJ, deVere White R, Davis Z, Sterling R, Dobnik DB, McCormick JR. Removal of renal cell carcinoma extending into the right atrium using cardiopulmonary bypass, profound hypothermia and circulatory arrest. J Urol 1984;131:945.
106. Montie JE, Jackson CL, Cosgrove DM, Streem SB, Novick AC, Pontes JE. Resection of large inferior vena caval thrombi from renal cell carcinoma with the use of circulatory arrest. J Urol 1988;139:25.
107. Marshall FF, Dietrick DD, Baumgartner WA, Reitz BA. Surgical management of renal cell carcinoma with intracaval neoplastic extension above the hepatic veins. J Urol 1988;139:1166.
108. Clayman RV, Gonzalez R, Fraley EE. Renal cell cancer invading the inferior vena cava: clinical review and anatomical approach. J Urol 1980;123:157.
109. Kearney GP, Waters WB, Klein LA, Richie JP, Gittes RF. Results of inferior vena cava resection for renal cell carcinoma. J Urol 1981; 125:769.
110. Cole AT, Julian WA, Fried FA. Aggressive surgery for renal cell carcinoma with vena cava tumor thrombus. Urology 1975;6:227.
111. Caplan BB, Halasz NA, Bloomer WE. Resection and ligation of the suprarenal inferior vena cava. J Urol 1964;92:25.
112. Duckett JW, Lifland JH, Peters PC. Resection of the inferior vena cava for adjacent malignant diseases. Surg Gynecol Obstet 1973;136: 711.
113. Cochran JL, Noble MJ, Weigel JW, Mebust WK, Lin F, Lee KR. Inferior vena cava replacement after resection of left renal tumor in canine model. Urology 1984;24:262.
114. Chan EL, Bardin JA, Bernstein EF. Inferior vena cava bypass: experimental evaluation of externally supported grafts and initial clinical application. J Vasc Surg 1984;1:675.
115. Marshall FF, Reitz BA. Supradiaphragmatic renal cell carcinoma tumor thrombus: indications for vena caval reconstruction with pericardium. J Urol 1985;133:266.
116. Frydenberg M, Gunderson L, Hahn G, Fieck J, Zincke H. Preoperative external beam radiotherapy followed by cytoreductive surgery and intraoperative radiotherapy for locally advanced primary or recurrent renal malignancies. J Urol 1994;152:15.
117. Cherrie RJ, Goldman DG, Lindner A, deKernion JB. Prognostic implications of vena caval extension of renal cell carcinoma. J Urol 1982; 128:910.
118. Wei CH, Chen A, Tseng HH, Tu YC, Yen CY. Simultaneous renal cell carcinoma and angiomyolipoma in a kidney: a case report and literature review. Chung Hua I Hsueh Tsa Chih 1990;45:126.
119. Bottiger LE. Prognosis in renal carcinoma. Cancer 1970;26:780.
120. Eker R, Nesland JM, Andersen A, Johannessen JV. Prognostic factors in renal cell carcinoma. Histol Histopathol 1986;1:255.
121. Fuhrman SA, Lasky LC, Limas C. Prognostic significance of morphologic parameters in renal cell carcinoma. Am J Surg Pathol 1982;6: 655.
122. Frank W, Stuhldreher D, Saffrin R, Shott S, Guinan P. Stage IV renal cell carcinoma. J Urol 1994;152:1998.
123. Targonski PV, Frank W, Stuhldreher D, Guinan PD. Value of tumor size in predicting survival from renal cell carcinoma among tumors, nodes and metastases stage 1 and stage 2 patients. J Urol 1994;152: 1389.
124. Mrstik CH, Salamon J, Weber R, Stogermayer F. Microscopic venous infiltration as predictor of relapse in renal cell carcinoma. J Urol 1992; 148:271.

125. Skinner DG, Colvin RB, Vermillion CD, Pfister RC, Leadbetter WF. Diagnosis and management of renal cell carcinoma: a clinical and pathologic study of 309 cases. Cancer 1971;28:1165.
126. Dick VS, Flint LD. The prognosis of renal tumors. Surg Clin North Am 1951;31:633.
127. Myers GH, Fehrenbaker LG, Kelalis PP. Prognostic significance of renal vein invasion by hypernephroma. J Urol 1968;100:420.
128. McDonald JR, Priestley JT. Malignant tumors of the kidney; surgical and prognostic significance of tumor thrombosis of the renal vein. Surg Gynecol Obstet 1943;77:295.
129. Beare JB, McDonald JR. Involvement of the renal capsule surgically removed hypernephroma: a gross and histopathologic study. J Urol 1949;61:857.
130. Robson CJ, Churchill BM, Anderson W. The results of radical nephrectomy for renal cell carcinoma. Trans Am Assoc Genitourin Surg 1968;60:122.
131. Frydenberg M, Malek RS, Zincke H. Conservative renal surgery for renal cell carcinoma in von Hippel-Lindau's disease. J Urol 1993; 149:461.
132. Malek RS, Utz DC, Culp OS. Hypernephroma in the solitary kidney: experience with 20 cases and review of the literature. J Urol 1976; 116:553.
133. Novick AC, Streem S, Montie JE, et al. Conservative surgery for renal cell carcinoma: a single-center experience with 100 patients. J Urol 1989;141:835.
134. Riches E. The place of radiotherapy in the management of parenchymal carcinoma of the kidney. J Urol 1966;95:313.
135. Rafla S. Renal cell carcinoma. Natural history and results of treatment. Cancer 1970;25:26.
136. Bloom HJG. Adjuvant therapy for adenocarcinoma of the kidney: present position and prospects. Br J Urol 1973;45:237.
137. Finney R. The value of radiotherapy in the treatment of hypernephroma: a clinical trial. Br J Urol 1973;45:258.
138. Van Der Werf-Messing B. Carcinoma of the kidney. Cancer 1973; 32:1056.
139. Peters PC, Brown GL. The role of lymphadenectomy in the management of renal cell carcinoma. Urol Clin North Am 1980;7:705.
140. Herrlinger A, Schrott KM, Schott G, Sigel A. What are the benefits of extended dissection of the regional renal lymph nodes in the therapy of renal cell carcinoma? J Urol 1991;146:1224.
141. Zincke H, Engen DE, Henning KM, McDonald MW. Treatment of renal cell carcinoma by in situ partial nephrectomy and extracorporeal operation with autotransplantation. Mayo Clin Proc 1985;60:651.
142. Angervall L, Wahlqvist L. Follow-up and prognosis of renal carcinoma in a series operated by perifascial nephrectomy combined with adrenalectomy and retroperitoneal lymphadenectomy. Eur Urol 1978; 4:13.
143. Skinner DG, Pfister RF, Colvin R. Extension of renal cell carcinoma into the vena cava: the rationale for aggressive surgical management. J Urol 1972;107:711.
144. Johnson DE, Kaesler KE, Samuels ML. Is nephrectomy justified in patients with metastatic renal carcinoma? J Urol 1975;114:27.
145. Katzenstein AL, Purvis R, Gmelich J, Askin F. Pulmonary resection for metastatic renal adenocarcinoma. Cancer 1978;41:712.
146. Montie JE, Stewart BH, Straffon RA, Banowsky LHW, Hewitt CB, Montague DK. The role of adjunctive nephrectomy in patients with metastatic renal cell carcinoma. J Urol 1977;117:272.
147. Pogrebniak HW, Haas G, Linehan M, Rosenberg SA, Pass HI. Renal cell carcinoma: resection of solitary and multiple metastases. Ann Thorac Surg 1992;54:33.
148. Smith EM, Kursh ED, Makley J, Resnick MI. Treatment of osseous metastases secondary to renal cell carcinoma. J Urol 1992;148:784.
149. Badalament RA, Gluck RW, Wong GY, et al. Surgical treatment of brain metastases from renal cell carcinoma. Urology 1990;36:112.
150. Fairlamb DJ. Spontaneous regression of metastases of renal cancer: a report of two cases including the first recorded regression following irradiation of a dominant metastasis and review of the world literature. Cancer 1981;47:2102.
151. Freed SZ, Halperin JP, Gordon M. Idiopathic regression of metastases from renal cell carcinoma. J Urol 1977;118:538.
152. Van Der Werf-Messing B, Van Gilse HA. Hormonal treatment of metastases of renal carcinoma. Br J Urol 1971;25:423.
153. Hajdu ST, Thomas AG. Renal cell carcinomata autopsy. J Urol 1967; 97:978.
154. Hellsten S, Berge T, Wehlin L. Unrecognized renal cell carcinoma: clinical and pathological aspects. Scand J Urol 1981;8:273.
155. Esrig D, Ahlering TE, Lieskovsky G, Skinner DG. Experience with fossa recurrence of renal cell carcinoma. J Urol 1992;147:1491.
156. McNichols DW, Segura JW, DeWeerd JH. Renal cell carcinoma: long-term survival and late recurrence. J Urol 1981;126:17.
157. Kradjian RM, Bennington JL. Renal carcinoma recurrent 31 years after nephrectomy. Arch Surg 1965;90:192.
158. Minasian LM, Motzer RJ, Gluck L, Mazumdar M, Vlamis V, Krown SE. Interferon alfa-2a in advanced renal cell carcinoma: treatment results and survival in 159 patients with long-term follow-up. J Clin Oncol 1993;11:1368.
159. Ellerhorst JA, Kilbourn RG, Amato RJ, Zukiwski AA, Jones E, Logothetis CJ. Phase II trial of low dose interferon in metastatic renal cell carcinoma. J Urol 1994;152:841.
160. Fujioka T, Yoshida N, Hasegawa M, Ishikura K, Suzuki Y, Kubo T. Interleukin-2 expanded tumor-infiltrating lymphocytes and their response to preoperative interferon in patients with renal cell carcinoma. J Urol 1994;152:852.
161. Osband ME, Lavin PT, Babayan RK, et al. Effect of autolymphocyte therapy on survival and quality of life in patients with metastatic renal-cell carcinoma. Lancet 1990;335:994.
162. Rackley R, Novick A, Klein E, Bukowski R, McLain D, Goldfarb D. The impact of adjuvant nephrectomy on multimodality treatment of metastatic renal cell carcinoma. J Urol 1994;152:1399.
163. Muss HB. Interferon therapy for renal cell carcinoma. Semin Oncol 1987;14:36.
164. Krown SE. Interferon treatment of renal cell carcinoma. Cancer 1987; 59:647.
165. Rosenberg SA, Lotxe MT, Muul LM, et al. A progress report on the treatment of 157 patients with advanced cancer using lymphokine-activated killer cells and interleukin-2 or high-dose interleukin-2 alone. N Engl J Med 1987;316:889.
166. Bloom HJ, Wallace DM. Hormones and the kidney: possible therapeutic role of testosterone in a patient with regression of metastases from renal adenocarcinoma. Br Med J 1964;2:476
167. Belldegrun A, Pierce W, Kaboo R, et al. Interferon-alpha primed tumor-infiltrating lymphocytes combined with interleukin-2 and interferon-alpha as therapy for metastatic renal cell carcinoma. J Urol 1993;150:1384.
168. Eggermont AMM, Steller EP, Sugarbaker PH. Laparotomy enhances intraperitoneal tumor growth abrogates the antitumor effects of interleukin-2 and lymphokine-activated killer cells. Surgery 1987;102: 71.
169. Robertson CN, Linehan WM, Pass HI, et al. Preparative cytoreductive surgery in patients with metastatic renal cell carcinoma treated with adoptive immunotherapy with interleukin-2 or interleukin- plus lymphokine activated killer cells. J Urol 1990;144:614.
170. Fleishman JD, Kim B. Interleukin-2 immunotherapy followed by resection of residual renal cell carcinoma. J Urol 1991;145:938.
171. Long JP, Walther MM, Alexander RB, Linehan WM, Rosenberg SA. The management of isolated renal recurrence of renal cell carcinoma following complete response to interleukin-2 based immunotherapy. J Urol 1993;150:176.
172. Sherry RM, Pass HI, Rosenberg SA, Yang JC. Surgical resection of metastatic renal cell carcinoma and melanoma after response to interleukin-2-based immunotherapy. Cancer 1992;69:1850.
173. Rassweiler JJ, Henkel TO, Potempa DM, Coptcoat M, Alken P. The technique of transperitoneal laparoscopic nephrectomy, adrenalectomy and nephroureterectomy. Eur Urol 1993;23:425.
174. Ono Y, Sahashi M, Yamada S, Ohshima S. Laparoscopic nephrectomy without morcellation for renal cell carcinoma: report of initial 2 cases. J Urol 1993;150:1222.
175. Marberger M, Pugh RCB, Auvert J, et al. Conservative surgery of renal carcinoma: the EIRSS experience. Br J Urol 1981;53:528.
176. Robson CJ, Churchill BM, Anderson W. The results of radical nephrectomy for renal cell carcinoma. J Urol 1969;101:297.
177. Middleton RG, Presto AJ. Radical thoracoabdominal nephrectomy for renal cell carcinoma. J Urol 1973;110:36.
178. Giuliani L, Giberti C, Martorana G, Rovida S. Radical extensive surgery for renal cell carcinoma: long-term results and prognostic factors. J Urol 1990;143:468.
179. Hand JR. Carcinoma of the kidney: the degree of malignancy in relation to factors nearing on prognosis. J Urol 1932;2:199.

180. Foot NC, Humphreys GA, Whitmore WF. Renal tumors: pathology and prognosis in 295 cases. J Urol 1951;66:190.
181. Humphreys GA, Foot NC. Survival of patients (235) following nephrectomy for renal cell and transitional cell tumors of the kidney. J Urol 1960;83:815.
182. Throckmorton MA. Prognosis in hypernephroma: review of the literature and report of 42 cases. J Urol 1955;73:773.
183. Flocks RH, Kadesky MC. Malignant neoplasms of the kidney: an analysis of 353 patients followed five years or more. J Urol 1958;79: 196.
184. Kaufman JJ, Mims MM. Tumor of the kidney. Chicago: Year Book Medical, 1966:2.
185. Skinner DG, Pritchett TR, Lieskovsky G, Boyd SD, Stiles QR. Vena caval involvement by renal cell carcinoma: Surgical resection provides meaningful long-term survival. Ann Surg 1989;210:387.
186. Bixler LC, Stenstrom KW, Creevy CD. Malignant tumors of the kidney: review of 117 cases. Radiology 1944;42:329.
187. Charteris AA. Radiotherapy in the treatment of kidney tumors. Br J Urol 1951;23:361.
188. Riches EW, Griffiths IH, Thackray AC. New growths of the kidney and ureter. Br J Urol 1951;23:297.
189. Bratherton DG, Chir B. The place of radiotherapy in the treatment of hypernephroma. Br J Radiol 1964;37:141.
190. Peeling WB, Mantell BS, Shepheard BGF. Post-operative irradiation in the treatment of renal cell carcinoma. Br J Urol 1969;41:23.
191. Cox CE, Lacy SS, Montgomery WG, Boyce WH. Renal adenocarcinoma: 28-year review, with emphasis on rationale and feasibility of preoperative radiotherapy. J Urol 1970;104:53.
192. Petkovic SD. An anatomical classification of renal tumors in the adult as a basis for prognosis. J Urol 1959;81:618.
193. Siminovitch JP, Montie JE, Straffon RA. Lymphadenectomy in renal adenocarcinoma. J Urol 1982;127:1090
194. Sosa RE, Muecke EC, Vaughan ED, McCarron JP. Renal cell carcinoma extending into the inferior vena cava: the prognostic significance of the level of vena caval involvement. J Urol 1984;132:1097.
195. Schefft P, Novick AC, Straffon RA, Stewart BH. Surgery for renal cell carcinoma extending into the inferior vena cava. J Urol 1978; 120:28.
196. Neves RJ, Zincke H. Surgical treatment of renal cancer with vena cava extension. Br J Urol 1987;59:390.
197. Sogani PC, Herr HW, Bains MS. Renal cell carcinoma extending into the inferior vena cava. J Urol 1983;130:660.
198. Liebertino JA, Zinman L, Watkins E. Long-term results of resection of renal cell cancer with extension into inferior vena cava. J Urol 1987;137:21.
199. Pritchett TR, Lieskovsky G, Skinner DG. Extension of renal cell carcinoma into the vena cava: clinical review and surgical approach. J Urol 1986;135:460.
200. Hatcher PA, Anderson EE, Paulson DF, Carson CC, Robertson JE. Surgical management and prognosis of renal cell carcinoma invading the vena cava. J Urol 1991;145:20.
201. Vaislic CD, Puel P, Grondin P, et al. Cancer of the kidney invading the vena cava and heart. J Thorac Cardiovasc Surg 1986;91:604.
202. Hedderich GS, O'Connor RJ, Reid EC, Mulder DS. Caval tumor thrombus complicating renal cell carcinoma: a surgical challenge. Surgery 1987;102:614.
203. Novick AC, Kaye MC, Cosgrove DM, et al. Experience with cardiopulmonary bypass and deep hypothermic circulatory arrest in the management of retroperitoneal tumors with large vena caval thrombi. Ann Surg 1990;212:472.

Principles and Practice of Genitourinary Oncology, edited by Derek Raghavan, Howard I. Scher, Steven A. Leibel, and Paul H. Lange. Lippincott-Raven Publishers, Philadelphia, © 1997.

CHAPTER 83

Nephron-Sparing Surgery for Renal Cell Carcinoma

Andrew C. Novick

Nephron-sparing surgery for the treatment of a renal tumor was first described by Czerny in 1890.[1] High morbidity rates limited its application, however. In 1950, Vermooten suggested that peripheral encapsulated renal neoplasms could be excised locally while leaving a margin of normal parenchyma around the tumor.[2] Robson and associates then established radical nephrectomy as the standard curative operation for localized renal cell carcinoma (RCC) with their report of 66% and 64% overall survival for stage I and II tumors, respectively.[3] These results demonstrated significantly improved survival rates compared with patients treated with perifascial nephrectomy. Robson and associates attributed these improved survival results to early ligation of the renal vessels to decrease hematologic spread of tumor, removal of the perinephric fat, removal of the ipsilateral adrenal gland, and excision of all regional lymph nodes to control local tumor dissemination. Controversy exists concerning the need for some of these practices in all patients. Performance of a perifascial nephrectomy is of undoubted importance in preventing postoperative local tumor recurrence because approximately 25% of localized RCCs manifest perinephric fat involvement. Preliminary renal arterial ligation remains an accepted practice; however, in large tumors with abundant collateral vascular supply, complete preliminary control of the arterial circulation is not always attainable. Removal of the ipsilateral adrenal gland is not routinely necessary unless the entire kidney or adjacent upper portion of the kidney is involved with RCC.[4] Finally, the need for a complete regional lymphadenectomy in all cases is unresolved, and urologists disagree about this aspect of radical nephrectomy.

Interest in nephron-sparing surgery for RCC has been stimulated by advances in renal imaging, experience with renal vascular surgery for other conditions, improved methods of preventing ischemic renal damage, the growing incidence of incidentally discovered low-stage RCC, and good long-term survival in patients undergoing this form of treatment. Nephron-sparing surgery entails complete local resection of a renal tumor while leaving the largest possible amount of normal functioning parenchyma in the involved kidney. Extended experience has established that nephron-sparing surgery can be performed safely with low morbidity, good preservation of renal function, and long-term cure in many patients.[5] Nephron-sparing surgery for RCC is primarily indicated when preservation of functioning renal parenchyma is important.

CURRENT INDICATIONS

The accepted indications for nephron-sparing surgery include situations in which radical nephrectomy would render the patient anephric, with a subsequent immediate need for dialysis. This indication encompasses patients with bilateral synchronous RCC or RCC involving a solitary functioning kidney. The latter circumstance may be the result of unilateral renal agenesis, prior removal of the contralateral kidney, or irreversible impairment of contralateral renal function by a benign disorder.

In patients with bilateral synchronous RCC, my philosophy has been to attempt to preserve as much functioning renal tissue as possible. This entails performing bilateral nephron-sparing operations when feasible, usually as staged procedures with the less involved side done first. When a large tumor on one side precludes partial nephrectomy, a radical nephrectomy is performed on the more involved side, with a contralateral partial nephrectomy. In such cases, partial nephrectomy is performed first as a separate procedure. This sequence obviates temporary dialysis in the immediate postoperative period if acute tubular necrosis follows the partial nephrectomy. It also provides the most flexibility in planning the procedure on the opposite side, and my colleagues and I occasionally have performed a partial rather than a radical nephrectomy on the second side to avoid dialysis when the initial procedure resulted in a renal remnant of borderline size.

Patients with RCC involving a functionally or anatomically solitary kidney do not have the luxury of a functioning contralateral kidney to protect against ischemic acute tubular necrosis. These patients must be advised about the potential need for temporary or permanent dialysis postoperatively, which, in my experience, has occurred in 8% and 4% of cases, respectively.[6] A functioning renal remnant of at least 20% of one normal kidney is necessary to avoid end-stage renal failure.

Another accepted indication for nephron-sparing surgery is represented by patients with unilateral RCC and a functioning opposite kidney that is affected by a condition that may threaten its future function. Examples of these conditions include renal artery stenosis,[7] hydronephrosis, chronic pyelonephritis, ureteral reflux, calculus disease, or systemic diseases such as diabetes and nephrosclerosis.

OPERATIVE CONSIDERATIONS

Evaluation of patients with RCC for nephron-sparing surgery should include preoperative testing to rule out locally extensive or metastatic disease. For most patients, preoperative renal arteriography to delineate the intrarenal vasculature aids in excising the tumor with minimal blood loss and damage to adjacent normal parenchyma. This test can be deferred in patients with small peripheral tumors. Selective renal venography is performed in patients with large or centrally located tumors to evaluate for intrarenal venous thrombosis secondary to malignancy. Preoperative hydration and mannitol administration are important adjuncts to ensure optimal renal perfusion at operation.

Performing partial nephrectomy for RCC is usually possible in situ by using an operative approach that optimizes exposure of the kidney and by combining meticulous surgical technique with an understanding of the renal vascular anatomy in relation to the tumor.[8] I use an extraperitoneal flank incision through the bed of the 11th or 12th rib for almost all these operations; I occasionally use a thoracoabdominal incision for large tumors involving the upper portion of the kidney. These incisions allow the surgeon to operate on the mobilized kidney almost at skin level and provide excellent exposure of the peripheral renal vessels. With an anterior subcostal incision, the kidney is invariably located in the depth of the wound, and the surgical exposure is simply not as good.

The kidney is mobilized within Gerota's fascia while the perirenal fat around the tumor is left intact. For small peripheral renal tumors, control of the renal artery may not be necessary. In most cases, however, partial nephrectomy is most effectively performed after temporary renal arterial occlusion. This measure not only limits intraoperative bleeding, but, by reducing renal tissue turgor, it also improves access to intrarenal structures. In most cases, I believe that it is important to leave the renal vein patent throughout the operation. This measure decreases intraoperative renal ischemia and, by allowing venous backbleeding, facilitates hemostasis by enabling identification of small transected renal veins. In patients with centrally located tumors, I do occlude the renal vein temporarily to minimize intraoperative bleeding from transected major venous branches.

When the renal circulation is temporarily interrupted, in situ renal hypothermia is used to protect against postischemic renal injury. Surface cooling of the kidney with ice slush allows up to 3 hours of safe ischemia without permanent renal injury.[9] An important caveat with this method is to keep the entire kidney covered with ice slush for 10 to 15 minutes immediately after occluding the renal artery and before commencing the partial nephrectomy. This amount of time is needed to obtain core renal cooling to a temperature (15° to 20°C) that optimizes in situ renal preservation. During excision of the tumor, invariably large portions of the kidney are no longer covered with ice slush and, in the absence of adequate prior renal cooling, rapid rewarming and ischemic renal injury can occur. Cooling by perfusion of the kidney with a cold solution instilled by the renal artery is not recommended because of the theoretic risk of tumor dissemination. Mannitol is given intravenously 5 to 10 minutes before arterial occlusion. This regimen has been shown to aid in preventing ischemic renal damage by decreasing intracellular edema and intrarenal resistance, by increasing renal plasma flow, and by inducing an osmotic diuresis on restoration of the renal circulation.[10] Systemic or regional anticoagulation to prevent intrarenal vascular thrombosis is not necessary.

Several surgical techniques are available for performing in situ partial nephrectomy in patients with RCC. These include the following: (1) polar segmental nephrectomy; (2) wedge resection; and (3) transverse resection. All these techniques require adherence to basic principles of early vascular control, avoidance of ischemic renal damage, complete tumor excision with free margins, precise closure of the collecting system, careful hemostasis, and closure or coverage of the renal defect with adjacent fat, fascia, peritoneum, or Oxycel. Before commencing the renal resection, any enlarged or suspicious regional lymph nodes are excised for staging purposes. The value of partial nephrectomy for RCC with lymph node involvement is not established.

Polar segmental nephrectomy is indicated for tumors confined to the upper or lower pole of the kidney. A transverse resection is done to remove large tumors that extensively involve the upper or lower portion of the kidney (Fig. 83-1).

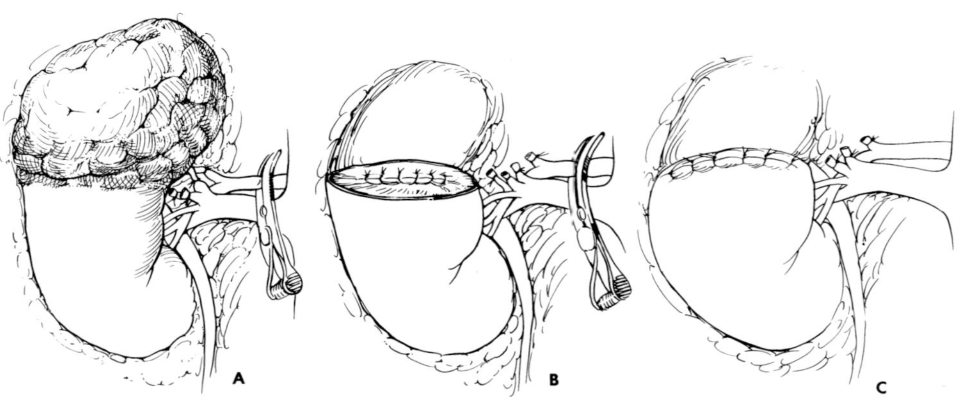

FIG. 83-1. (**A** to **C**) The technique of transverse resection for a tumor involving the upper half of the kidney.

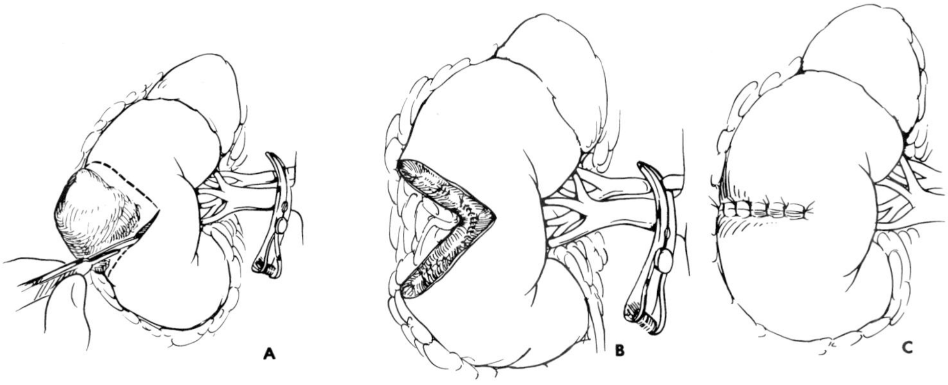

FIG. 83-2. (**A** to **C**) The technique of wedge resection for a tumor on the midlateral aspect of the kidney.

Wedge resection is appropriate for excising tumors that are not confined to the upper or lower moieties of the kidney (Fig. 83-2).

Whichever technique is used, the tumor is removed with at least a 1-cm surrounding margin of grossly normal renal parenchyma. Intraoperative ultrasound is helpful for accurate tumor localization, particularly for intrarenal lesions that are not visible or palpable from the external surface of the kidney.[11] In excising the tumor, the renal parenchyma is divided by a combination of sharp and blunt dissection. Intrarenal vessels that are identified during the resection are directly suture-ligated at that time, while they are most visible. When the tumor resection is complete, the collecting system is closed with interrupted 4-0 chromic sutures. Remaining transected blood vessels on the renal surface are secured with figure-of-eight 4-0 chromic sutures. Immediately after excision of the tumor, biopsies of the remaining portion of the kidney are done to verify complete tumor excision. Such biopsies do not usually demonstrate residual tumor, but, if so, additional renal tissue must be excised.

If possible, the renal defect created by the excision is closed as an additional hemostatic measure. This closure is done by approximating the transected cortical margins with interrupted 3-0 chromic sutures, with care taken to avoid tension on the suture line or distortion of blood vessels supplying the kidney. A retroperitoneal Penrose drain is always left in place for at least 7 days. An intraoperative ureteral stent is placed only when major reconstruction of the intrarenal collecting system has been performed.

Extracorporeal Partial Nephrectomy

Extracorporeal nephron-sparing surgery for RCC with autotransplantation of the renal remnant was initially described by several surgeons.[12,13] This surgical technique allows for the successful excision of large, complex tumors involving the renal hilus. Reconstruction of kidneys with RCC as well as renal artery disease may be facilitated with this approach. Although an occasional large hypervascular, centrally located tumor can only be excised with extracorporeal surgery, such cases are uncommon. Disadvantages of extracorporeal surgery include longer operative time, with the need for vascular and ureteral anastomoses, and an increased risk of temporary and permanent postoperative renal failure[6]; the latter presumably reflects a more severe intraoperative ischemic insult to the kidney. My experience suggests that extracorporeal surgery is rarely necessary during nephron-sparing surgery for RCC, and almost all cases can be managed satisfactorily in situ.

Enucleation

Enucleation of a renal tumor involves circumferential incision of the parenchyma around the tumor, followed by blunt shelling out of the mass along the plane outside its pseudocapsule. The ability to perform this procedure successfully depends on the structural integrity of the pseudocapsule of compressed parenchyma that separates the tumor from normal kidney. The advantage of this procedure is the ability to remove tumors simply and rapidly at any location on the kidney, often with no vascular occlusion and with maximum preservation of normal renal parenchyma.

Initial reports indicated satisfactory short-term clinical results after enucleation with good rates of patient survival and a low rate of local tumor recurrence.[14–17] More recent studies have suggested a higher risk of leaving residual malignant disease in the kidney when enucleation is performed, however.[18–21] These later reports include several careful histopathologic studies that demonstrated frequent microscopic tumor penetration of the pseudocapsule that surrounds the neoplasm. These data indicate that the surgeon cannot always ensure complete tumor encapsulation preoperatively. Local recurrence of tumor in the treated kidney is a grave complication of nephron-sparing surgery for RCC, and every attempt should be made to prevent it. Therefore, I believe that a surrounding margin of normal parenchyma should be removed with the tumor whenever possible. This procedure provides an added margin of safety against the development of local tumor recurrence and, in most cases, does not appreciably increase the technical difficulty of the operation.

CLINICAL RESULTS

Surgical Complications

Most reports of nephron-sparing surgery for RCC have focused on the issue of cancer control through analysis of patient survival and tumor recurrence rates. Nephron-sparing surgery may be technically challenging, however, and the morbidity of this approach is also important. One study detailed the incidence and clinical outcome of technical or renal-related complications occurring after 259 nephron-sparing operations for RCC at the Cleveland Clinic.[6] In the overall series, local or renal-related complications occurred after 78 operations (30.1%). The incidence of complications was lower for operations performed after 1988 (22% versus 37%, $P = .009$) and lower for incidentally detected versus suspected tumors (22% versus 37%, $P = .009$).

The most common complications were urinary fistula formation and acute renal failure. A urinary fistula occurred after 45 of 259 operations (17%). Significant predisposing factors for a urinary fistula included central tumor location ($P = .001$), tumor size larger than 4 cm ($P = .001$), the need for major reconstruction of the collecting system ($P = .001$), and ex vivo surgery ($P = .001$). Only one urinary fistula required open operative repair, whereas the remainder resolved either spontaneously (n = 30) or with endoscopic management (n = 14).

Acute renal failure occurred after 30 of 115 operations (26%) performed on a solitary kidney. Significant predisposing factors for acute renal failure were tumor size larger than 7 cm ($P = .008$), more than 50% parenchymal excision ($P = .001$), longer than 60-minute ischemia time ($P = .035$), and ex vivo surgery ($P = .001$). Acute renal failure resolved completely in 25 patients, of whom 9 (8%) required temporary dialysis; 5 patients (4%) required permanent dialysis.

Overall, only 8 complications (3.1%) required repeat open surgery for treatment, whereas all other complications resolved with noninterventive or endourologic management. Surgical complications contributed to an adverse clinical outcome in only 7 patients (2.9%). These data indicate that nephron-sparing surgery can be performed safely with preservation of renal function in most patients with RCC.

Survival

Many reports of excellent long-term cancer-free survival rates with nephron-sparing surgery for localized RCC have been published (Table 83-1).[22–36] Mean disease-specific survival in these studies has ranged from 57% to 100%, with many surgeons reporting long-term disease-specific survival rates of 90% or more. Zincke and associates compared their patients who had undergone partial nephrectomy with a matched group of patients who had undergone radical nephrectomy and showed equivalent 5-year disease-specific survival rates of 87% and 93%, respectively.[37]

One study reviewed the outcome of nephron-sparing surgery in 216 patients with sporadic RCC treated at the Cleveland Clinic.[38] Patients with RCC and von Hippel-Lindau disease were excluded from this study. Specific indications for nephron-sparing surgery included bilateral synchronous RCC (n = 47), RCC in a solitary functioning kidney (n = 95), and associated azotemia or medical or urologic disease (n = 57). In 17 patients, nephron-sparing surgery was performed for unilateral RCC with a normal opposite kidney.

A majority (83%) of the 216 patients in this study had pathologic T1-2 or T3a tumors. The mean postoperative follow-up interval was 53 months. The 5-year cancer-specific survival rate for the entire series of patients was 87%. The corresponding survival rates for patients with T1-2 and T3a tumors were 94% and 79%, respectively. I also found improved 5-year cancer-specific survival rates in patients with unilateral RCC (95%), compared with synchronous (85%) or asynchronous (73%) bilateral RCC. Postoperative local tumor recurrence developed in 9 of 216 patients, for an overall incidence of 4%. These results attest to the efficacy of nephron-sparing surgery for properly selected patients with low-stage RCC when the need exists to preserve functioning renal parenchyma.

Local Tumor Recurrence

The principal disadvantage of nephron-sparing surgery for RCC is the risk of postoperative local tumor recurrence, the rate of which has ranged from 1.4% to 10% (Table 83-2).[39,40] Such local recurrence may occasionally be the result of incomplete resection of the primary lesion, but, more likely, it is due to unrecognized additional lesions elsewhere within the treated kidney as a manifestation of multicentric RCC. The overall low local recurrence rates observed after nephron-sparing surgery are no doubt a consequence of patient selection, because large or locally advanced tumors generally are not considered amenable to this approach. The importance of patient selection was

TABLE 83-1. *Results of nephron-sparing surgery for renal cell carcinoma*

Investigators	No. of patients	Disease-specific survival (%)	Follow-up
Jacobs et al, 1980[22]	51	84.4	5 y
Marberger et al, 1981[23]	72	77.8	36–142 mo
Gislason et al, 1981[24]	4	100	Mean 40 mo
Bennett et al, 1982[25]	7	71.4	Mean 44.6 mo
Palmer, 1983[26]	7	57	62–85 mo
Marshall and Walsh, 1984[27]	10	90	Mean 24.5 mo
Bazeed et al, 1986[28]	51	96	Mean 35.8 mo
Carini et al, 1988[29]	35	88.6	Mean 45.8 mo
Novick et al, 1989[30]	100	84	5 y
Gohji et al, 1990[31]	21	100	1–76 mo
Morgan and Zincke, 1990[32]	104	88.9	5 y
Van Poppel et al, 1991[33]	31	93.5	Mean 41 mo
Provet et al, 1991[34]	44	88	Mean 36 mo
Steinbach et al, 1991[35]	106	93	3–4.5 y
Selli et al, 1991[36]	57	89.5	Mean 46.2 mo

TABLE 83-2. *Local recurrence after nephron-sparing surgery for sporadic renal cell carcinoma*

Investigators	No. of patients	No. LR (%)	Isolated LR	LR with metastases	Follow-up
Licht et al, 1994[38]	216	9 (4)	3	6	Mean 50 mo
Moll et al, 1993[39]	143	2 (1.4)	2	0	3 y
Steinbach et al, 1992[40]	140	5 (3.6)	5	0	3–4.5 y
Morgan and Zincke, 1990[32]	104	6 (5.7)	5	1	5 y
Marberger et al, 1981[23]	72	6 (8.3)	3	3	36–142 mo
Jacobs et al, 1980[22]	61	6 (10)	5	1	5 y
Provet et al, 1991[34]	44	1 (2.3)	Not specified	Not specified	Mean 36 mo
Carini et al, 1988[29]	36	1 (2.8)	1	0	Mean 46 mo

LR, Local recurrence.

underscored in a study from the Cleveland Clinic in which the local recurrence rate was much higher for patients with larger symptomatic tumors (6.7%), compared with patients with smaller incidentally discovered tumors (1.1%).[38]

As shown in Table 83-2, local recurrence after nephron-sparing surgery for RCC has been an isolated event in the majority of cases (24 of 35 = 69%). My experience at the Cleveland Clinic has been disparate in this regard.[38] My colleagues and I have found local recurrence after nephron-sparing surgery for sporadic RCC to be an ominous finding, because most of our patients have had disseminated disease or soon develop it. Patients who develop a local recurrence with no signs of metastasis may be considered for secondary surgical treatment.[41,42] In some cases, another partial nephrectomy can be done with preservation of renal function. If this operation is not technically possible, total nephrectomy with initiation of long-term dialysis and subsequent renal allotransplantation is an alternative.

MANAGEMENT OF RENAL CELL CARCINOMA WITH COEXISTENT RENAL ARTERY DISEASE

Occasionally, renal cell carcinoma and renal artery disease are found within the same patient. When RCC and renal artery disease coexist in the same kidney, with a normal contralateral kidney, radical nephrectomy is the treatment of choice. Involvement of all functioning parenchyma by these two conditions poses a more challenging therapeutic dilemma. In such patients, renal function may be compromised by vascular disease, and efforts to achieve maximal tumor control must be balanced with the need to preserve renal parenchyma.

My colleagues and I reviewed our experience in the management of 34 patients with coexistent RCC and renal artery disease affecting all of the functioning renal parenchyma.[7] These patients represented four distinct categories: (1) a solitary kidney with RCC and renal artery disease (n = 5); (2) bilateral RCC and coexistent renal artery disease (n = 5); (3) unilateral RCC and contralateral renal artery disease (n = 13); and (4) unilateral RCC and bilateral renal artery disease (n = 11). Atherosclerosis was the cause of renal artery disease in 30 of these patients (88%). A total of 23 patients (68%) presented with azotemia, and 11 patients (32%) presented with hypertension.

All patients underwent complete surgical excision of RCC. A nephron-sparing operation was performed in 30 patients (88%), and bilateral renal cancer operations were staged. Eight patients underwent simultaneous partial (n = 6) or radical (n = 2) nephrectomy and surgical renal revascularization. No operative deaths occurred. Postoperatively, renal function was preserved in 33 patients, and 1 patient required long-term dialysis. At a mean follow-up of 47 months, 23 patients (68%) were alive with no evidence of malignancy, and 2 were alive with recurrent RCC. Three patients died of metastatic RCC, whereas 6 died of unrelated causes. All the latter 6 patients were free of RCC at death. Nephron-sparing surgery combined occasionally with renal arterial reconstruction can yield gratifying results in this complex patient population.

ADVANCED RENAL CELL CARCINOMA

Few studies have examined the role of nephron-sparing surgery in patients with locally extensive or metastatic RCC. Angermeier and colleagues reviewed 9 patients who underwent nephron-sparing surgery for RCC with venous involvement in a solitary functioning kidney.[43] In all cases, resection of the tumor and preservation of renal function were achieved. A total of 5 patients were alive without disease at a mean follow-up of 33.2 months, whereas 4 died of metastatic RCC, including 2 who also had local tumor recurrence in the renal remnant. These data suggest an increased incidence of postoperative tumor recurrence when nephron-sparing surgery is done for localized RCC with venous involvement.

Small numbers of patients from other studies show poor survival and nephron-sparing surgery for RCC with lymph node involvement or metastatic disease. Marberger and associates reported on 3 patients with metastatic disease at the time of nephron-sparing surgery; these patients all died 3 to 43 months postoperatively.[23] Of 4 patients with lymph node involvement, 3 also died of metastatic disease shortly after surgery. In the study by Bazeed and colleagues, 2 patients with metastatic disease died of their malignant disease soon after nephron-sparing surgery.[28] Similarly, Morgan and Zincke reported on 6 patients with metastatic RCC, of whom 4 died of their malignant disease.[32] My colleagues and I reported a 42% 5-year disease-specific survival rate in 6 patients who underwent nephron-sparing surgery and resection of a solitary metastasis.[30] Use of nephron-sparing surgery in patients with advanced RCC may have wider application in the future if effective systemic therapy for RCC becomes available.

RENAL CELL CARCINOMA IN VON HIPPEL-LINDAU DISEASE

Renal cell carcinoma in von Hippel-Lindau disease differs from its sporadic counterpart in that the diagnosis is made at a younger age, and patients usually have multiple bilateral renal tumors.[44–46] Although these lesions are generally low-stage tumors, they are capable of progression with metastasis and represent a frequent cause of death in patients with von Hippel-Lindau disease. In one large study of 152 patients with von Hippel-Lindau disease, RCC was the leading cause of death, and life-table analysis indicated that RCC would eventually develop in most long-term survivors.[47]

Histopathologically, RCC in these patients is characterized by both solid tumors and renal cysts that contain either frank RCC or a lining of hyperplastic clear cells representing incipient RCC.[48,49] Therefore, adequate surgical treatment of localized RCC in von Hippel-Lindau disease requires excision of all solid and cystic renal lesions.

The surgical options in patients with bilateral RCC and von Hippel-Lindau disease consist of bilateral nephrectomy or a nephron-sparing operation to avoid end-stage renal failure. Although the early results of nephron-sparing surgery were promising,[49] subsequent studies suggested a high incidence of postoperative tumor recurrence in the remaining portion of the kidney.[50,51] Most of these local recurrences were probably a manifestation of residual microscopic RCC that was not removed at the time of the original nephron-sparing operation.

A multicenter study has further delineated the outcome after surgical treatment of RCC in 65 patients with von Hippel-Lindau disease who were managed at 8 medical centers in the United States.[52] RCC was present bilaterally and unilaterally in 54 and 11 patients, respectively. Only 1 patient presented with metastatic disease. Radical nephrectomy and nephron-sparing surgery were performed in 16 and 49 patients, respectively. The mean posttreatment follow-up interval was 68 months.

The 5-year and 10-year cancer-specific survival rates for all patients were 95% and 77%, respectively. The corresponding rates for patients treated with nephron-sparing surgery were 100% and 81%, respectively. In the second group, 25 patients (51%) developed postoperative local tumor recurrence, although only 2 of these patients had concomitant metastatic disease; survival free of local recurrence was 71% at 5 years, but it was only 15% at 10 years.

End-stage renal failure occurred in 15 patients (23%). Six patients underwent renal transplantation, of whom 5 are currently alive with satisfactory renal function and no evidence of malignancy. Nine patients were managed with long-term dialysis, of whom 6 are currently alive and tumor-free.

The results of this study indicate that nephron-sparing surgery can provide effective initial treatment for patients with RCC and von Hippel-Lindau disease. These patients must be followed-up closely because most eventually develop locally recurrent RCC. When removal of all renal tissue is necessary to achieve control of malignancy, renal transplantation can provide satisfactory replacement therapy for end-stage renal disease.

NORMAL CONTRALATERAL KIDNEY

The number of solid renal masses detected incidentally in individuals with no urologic symptoms has increased in recent years. This increase has occurred because of the widespread use of abdominal ultrasound, computed tomographic scanning, and magnetic resonance imaging as screening modalities in patients with nonspecific or unrelated symptoms. Many of these incidentally detected solid renal masses ultimately prove to be RCC.[53–55] Controversy exists concerning the management of small or incidentally detected unilateral solid renal masses with characteristics indicative of RCC when the opposite kidney is normal. Although radical nephrectomy is the standard treatment for localized RCC with a normal contralateral kidney, interest in the use of nephron-sparing surgery in this setting is growing.

One review article detailed the outcome of nephron-sparing surgery in 241 reported patients with unilateral localized RCC and a normal opposite kidney.[5] The mean cancer-specific survival rate was 95% at approximately 3 years of follow-up, and only 2 cases of postoperative tumor recurrence were reported. Significantly, the mean tumor size in most reports was less than 3.5 cm. Patient selection on the basis of small tumor size has been a significant factor accounting for the favorable outcome after nephron-sparing surgery in these studies.

In one study from our center, my colleagues and I reviewed the outcome of nephron-sparing surgery in 216 patients with sporadic RCC.[38] Our findings confirmed that extended cancer-free survival was significantly improved in patients with small (<4 cm) tumors compared with larger ones. Other factors associated with significantly improved survival were unilateral renal involvement, low pathologic tumor stage, and the presence of a single tumor. This study also highlighted that these favorable characteristics are more likely to be present in patients with incidentally detected RCCs, compared with patients with suspected RCCs. These data suggest that nephron-sparing surgery may be an acceptable therapeutic approach in patients who present with a single, small (<4 cm), unilateral RCC and a normal opposite kidney. To test this hypothesis, the outcome after radical nephrectomy versus nephron-sparing surgery for patients in this category was evaluated in a subsequent study.

From 1975 to 1992, 88 patients with a single, small (<4 cm), localized, unilateral, sporadic RCC were treated with either radical nephrectomy (n = 42) or nephron-sparing surgery (n = 46).[56] The mean postoperative follow-up interval was 48 months. The radical and nephron-sparing surgical groups were well matched for patient age, sex, renal function, diabetes, hypertension, tumor size, tumor location, and tumor stage. All patients in both groups had low-pathologic-stage RCC. No difference was noted between the two groups in terms of the mean hospital stay, the requirement for blood transfusions, or the occurrence of surgical complications. No difference was reported in the mean preoperative and postoperative serum creatinine levels for patients in the nephron-sparing surgery group. The mean postoperative serum creatinine level was significantly higher than the mean preoperative level for patients in the radical nephrectomy group ($P < .001$), however. A single patient in each group developed recurrent RCC postoperatively. The cancer-specific 5-year survival rate for patients in the radical nephrectomy and nephron-sparing surgical groups was 97% and 100%, respectively. The results of this study suggest that radical nephrectomy and nephron-sparing surgery each provide safe and effective curative treatment for patients with a single, small, unilateral localized RCC.* Moreover, the long-term renal functional advantage of nephron-sparing surgery in this setting is not established.

*Editor's note: This study, however, was not a randomized clinical trial and may be subject to selection bias.

POSTOPERATIVE LONG-TERM RENAL FUNCTION

Data suggest that patients with less than one kidney are at higher risk for developing proteinuria, glomerular damage, and impaired renal function as a result of glomerular hyperfiltration.[57,58] In one study, long-term renal function was evaluated in 14 patients with a solitary kidney who underwent partial nephrectomy for localized malignant disease.[59] Preoperatively, these patients had no clinical or histopathologic evidence of primary renal disease. Postoperative renal function remained stable in 12 patients, whereas 2 developed end-stage renal failure. A total of 9 patients had proteinuria that was low grade in 4 (<750 mg/day) and moderate to severe in 5 (930 to 6740 mg/day). A statistically significant association was found between more proteinuria and a lesser amount of remaining renal tissue, as well as a longer follow-up interval. A renal biopsy done in 4 patients with moderate to severe proteinuria showed focal segmental or global glomerulosclerosis.

These data suggest that patients with a greater than 50% reduction in overall renal mass are at increased risk for proteinuria, glomerulopathy, and progressive renal failure. Structural or functional renal damage in such cases is usually antedated by the appearance of proteinuria. Therefore, the follow-up of patients after nephron-sparing surgery should include a 24-hour urinary protein determination, in addition to a serum creatinine level and glomerular filtration rate. Patients who have proteinuria (>150 mg/day) may be treated with a low-protein diet and a converting-enzyme inhibitor agent, which in experimental studies have prevented glomerulopathy caused by reduced renal mass.[60,61]

REFERENCES

1. Czerny HE. Cited by Herczel E. Ueber nierenexstirpation. Beitr Klin Chir 1890;6:485.
2. Vermooten V. Indications for conservative surgery in certain renal tumors: a study based on the growth pattern of the clear cell carcinoma. J Urol 1950;64:200.
3. Robson CJ, Churchill BM, Anderson W. The results of radical nephrectomy for renal cell carcinoma. J Urol 1969;101:297.
4. Sagalowsky AI, Kadesky KT, Ewalt DM, et al. Factors influencing adrenal metastasis in renal cell carcinoma. J Urol 1994;151:1118.
5. Licht MR, Novick AC. Nephron-sparing surgery for renal cell carcinoma. J Urol 1993;145:1.
6. Campbell SC, Novick AC, Streem SB, Klein E, Licht M. Complications of nephron-sparing surgery for renal tumors. J Urol 1994;151:1177.
7. Campbell SC, Novick AC, Streem SB, Klein EA. Management of renal cell carcinoma with coexistent renal artery disease. J Urol 1993;150:808.
8. Novick AC. Partial nephrectomy for renal cell carcinoma. Urol Clin North Am 1987;14:419.
9. Novick AC. Renal hypothermia: in vivo and ex vivo. Urol Clin North Am 1983;10:637.
10. Nosowsky EE, Kaufman JJ. The protective action of mannitol in renal artery occlusion. J Urol 1963;89:295.
11. Assimos DG, Boyce WH, Woodruff RD, Harrison LH, McCullough DL Kroovand RL. Intraoperative renal ultrasonography: a useful adjunct to partial nephrectomy. J Urol 1991;146:1218.
12. Calne RY. Treatment of bilateral hypernephromas by nephrectomy, excision of tumor, and autotransplantation. Lancet 1973;2:1164.
13. Gittes RF, McCullough DL. Bench surgery for tumor in a solitary kidney. J Urol 1975;113:12.
14. Graham SD Jr, Glen JF. Enucleative surgery for renal malignancy. J Urol 1979;122:546.
15. Carini M, Selli C, Muraro GB, Trippitelli A, Masini G, Turini D. Conservative surgical treatment of renal cell carcinoma. J Urol 1988;140:725.
16. Jaeger N, Weissbach L, Vahlensieck W. Value of enucleation of tumor in solitary kidneys. Eur Urol 1985;11:369.
17. Novick AC, Zincke H, Neves RJ, Topley HM. Surgical enucleation for renal cell carcinoma. J Urol 1986;135:235.
18. Smith RB, deKernion JB, Ehrlich RM, Skinner DG, Kaufman JJ. Bilateral renal cell carcinoma and renal cell carcinoma in the solitary kidney. J Urol 1984;132:450.
19. Rosenthal CL, Kraft R, Zingg EJ. Organ-preserving surgery in renal cell carcinoma: tumor enucleation versus partial kidney resection. Eur Urol 1984;10:222.
20. Marshall FF, Taxy JB, Fishman EK, Chang R. The feasibility of surgical enucleation for renal cell carcinoma. J Urol 1986;135:231.
21. Blackley SK, Ladaga L, Woolfitt RA, Schellhammer PF. Ex situ study of the effectiveness of enucleation in patients with renal cell carcinoma. J Urol 1988;140:6.
22. Jacobs SC, Berg SI, Lawson RK. Synchronous bilateral renal cell carcinoma: total surgical excision. Cancer 1980;46:2341.
23. Marberger M, Puch RCB, Auvert J, et al. Conservative surgery of renal carcinoma: the EIRSS experience. Br J Urol 1981;53:528.
24. Gislason T, Purcell MH, Hawatmeh IS, Gregory JG. Aggressive management of bilateral renal cell carcinoma. J Urol 1981;126:686.
25. Bennett AH, Lempert N, Rivard DJ, Harrison JH. Surgical options in solitary and bilateral renal carcinoma: a report of 7 cases. Br J Urol 1982;54:480.
26. Palmer JM. Role of partial nephrectomy in solitary or bilateral renal tumors. JAMA 1983;249:2357.
27. Marshall FF, Walsh PC. In situ management of renal tumors: renal cell carcinoma and transitional cell carcinoma. J Urol 1984;131:1045.
28. Bazeed MA, Scharfe T, Becht E, Jurincic C, Alkin P, Turoff JW. Conservative surgery of renal cell carcinoma. Eur Urol 1986;12:238.
29. Carini M, Selli C, Barbanti G, Lapini A, Turini D, Costantini A. Conservative surgical treatment of renal cell carcinoma: clinical experience and reappraisal of indications. J Urol 1988;140:725.
30. Novick AC, Streem SB, Montie JE, et al. Conservative surgery for renal cell carcinoma: a single-center experience with 100 patients. J Urol 1989;141:835.
31. Gohji K, Kamidono S, Yamanaka N. Renal carcinoma in a solitary kidney. Br J Urol 1990;66:248.
32. Morgan WR, Zincke H. Progression and survival after renal-conserving surgery for renal cell carcinoma: experience in 104 patients and extended follow up. J Urol 1990;144:852.
33. Van Poppel H, Claes H, Willemen P, Oyen R, Baert L. Is there ia place for conservative surgery in the treatment of renal carcinoma? Br J Urol 1991;67:129.
34. Provet J, Tessler A, Brown J, Golimbu M, Bosniak M, Morales P. Partial nephrectomy for renal cell carcinoma: indications, results and implications. J Urol 1991;145:472.
35. Steinbach F, Stockle AM, Riedmiller H, Weingartner K, Hohenfellner R. Tumor enucleation of renal cell carcinoma: operative technique, DNA cytometry, results, complications. Prog Clin Biol Res 1991;370:1.
36. Selli C, Lapini A, Carini M. Conservative surgery of kidney tumors. Prog Clin Biol Res 1991;370:9.
37. Zincke H, Engen DE, Henning KM, McDonald MW. Treatment of renal cell carcinoma by in situ partial nephrectomy and extracorporeal operation with autotransplantation. Mayo Clin Proc 1985;60:651.
38. Licht MR, Novick AC, Goormastic M. Nephron-sparing surgery in incidental versus suspected renal cell carcinoma. J Urol 1994;152:39.
39. Moll V, Becht E, Ziegler M. Kidney preserving surgery in renal cell tumors: indications, techniques and results in 152 patients. J Urol 1993;150:319.
40. Steinbach F, Stockle M, Muller SC, et al. Conservative surgery of renal cell tumors in 140 patients: 21 years of experience. J Urol 1992;148:24.
41. Novick AC, Straffon RA. Management of locally recurrent renal cell carcinoma after partial nephrectomy. J Urol 1987;138:607.
42. Gittes RF, Blute RD, Jr. Repeat bench surgery on a solitary kidney. J Urol 1982;127:530.
43. Angermeier KW, Novick AC, Streem SB, Montie JE. Nephron-sparing surgery for renal cell carcinoma with venous involvement. J Urol 1990;144:1352.

44. Richards RD, Mebust WK, Schimke RN. A prospective study of von Hippel-Lindau disease. J Urol 1973;110:27.
45. Christoferson LA, Gustafson MB, Peterson AG. von Hippel-Lindau's disease. JAMA 1961;178:280.
46. Horton WA, Wong V, Eldridge R. von Hippel Lindau disease: clinical and pathological manifestations in nine families with 50 affected members. Arch Intern Med 1976;136:769.
47. Maher ER, Yates JRW, Harris R, et al. Clinical features and natural history of Hippel-Lindau disease. Q J Med 1990;238:1151.
48. Loughlin KR, Gittes RF. Urologic management of patients with von Hippel-Lindau's disease. J Urol 1986;136:789.
49. Spencer WF, Novick AC, Montie JE, Streem SB, Levin HS. Surgical treatment of localized renal cell carcinoma in von Hippel-Lindau's disease. J Urol 1988;139:507.
50. Novick AC, Streem BS. Long-term follow up after nephron sparing surgery for renal cell carcinoma in von Hippel Lindau disease. J Urol 1992;147:1488.
51. Frydenberg M, Malek RS, Zincke H. Conservative renal surgery for renal cell carcinoma in von Hippel Lindau's disease. J Urol 1993;149: 461.
52. Steinbach F, Novick AC, Zincke H, et al. Treatment of renal cell carcinoma in von Hippel Lindau disease: a multi-center study. J Urol 1995; 153:1812.
53. Konnak JW, Grossman HB. Renal cell carcinoma as an incidental finding. J Urol 1985;134:1094.
54. Smith SJ, Bosniak MA, Megibow AJ, Hulnick DH, Horii SC, Raghavendra BN. Renal cell carcinoma: earlier discovery and increased detection. Radiology 1989;170:699.
55. Ritchie AWS, deKernion JB. Incidental renal neoplasms: incidence Los Angeles County, treatment and prognosis. Prog Clin Biol Res 1988; 269:347.
56. Butler B, Novick AC, Miller D, Campbell SC, Licht MR. Management of small unilateral renal cell carcinomas: Radical versus nephron-sparing surgery. Urology 1995;45:34.
57. Solomon LR, Mallick NP, Lawler W. Progressive renal failure in a remnant kidney. Br Med J 1985;291:1610.
58. Foster MH, Sant GR, Donohoe JF, Harrington JT. Prolonged survival with a remnant kidney. Am J Kidney Dis 1991;17:261.
59. Novick AC, Gephardt G, Guz B, Steinmuller D, Tubbs RR. Long-term follow-up after partial removal of a solitary kidney. New Engl J Med 1991;325:1058.
60. Brenner BM. Hemodynamically mediated glomerular injury and progressive nature of kidney disease. Kidney Int 1983;23:647.
61. Meyer TW, Anderson S, Rennke HG, Brenner BM. Converting enzyme inhibitor therapy limits progressive glomerular injury in rats with renal insufficiency. Am J Med 1985;79(Suppl 3C):31.

Principles and Practice of Genitourinary Oncology, edited by Derek Raghavan, Howard I. Scher, Steven A. Leibel, and Paul H. Lange. Lippincott-Raven Publishers, Philadelphia, © 1997.

CHAPTER 84

Systemic Immunotherapy for Genitourinary Neoplasms

Mitchell H. Sokoloff, Robert A. Figlin, Jean B. de Kernion, and Arie S. Belldegrun

Despite advances in prevention and early detection, refinement in surgical technique, and improvements in adjuvant radio- and chemotherapy, the ability to cure cancer remains elusive in many patients. The continuing challenge of cancer treatment is the successful management and eradication of metastatic disease. Over the past decade, it has become increasingly apparent that effector cells of the immune system play an important role in the recognition and elimination of neoplastic cells. Recently, therefore, cancer therapies have been directed at modulating and exploiting the components of the immune system. Specific molecules (i.e., cytokines) have been targeted because of their involvement in the initiation and maintenance of immune surveillance and response. Early clinical studies with systemic cytokine infusions demonstrated tumor regression, but usually at the cost of substantial toxicity and side effects. Refinements have included the concept of adoptive immunotherapy using lymphokine-activated killer (LAK) and tumor-infiltrating lymphocyte (TIL) cells, with the intent to increase the amount of tumor regression while reducing toxicity. Current research focuses on utilizing gene therapy as a mechanism by which the immune response to neoplastic tissue can be modulated and improved.

Renal cell carcinoma and bladder cancer are prime examples of diseases where immunotherapy holds promise for achieving improved cure rates. Metastatic renal cell carcinoma has a poor prognosis, with an average survival of only 6 to 12 months from the time of diagnosis. Recent developments in immunotherapy, however, have resulted in an improved outlook. The incidence of bladder cancer is on the rise, yet the mortality peaked in the mid 1980s and continues to decline. Nonetheless, the number of patients with recurrent or progressing superficial bladder tumors after treatment with transurethral resection and established intravesical chemotherapy protocols remains at 50% of those treated. It is in this patient population where innovation in traditional treatment methods is most needed and immunotherapy can fill the void. Investigations into applying immuno- and gene therapy for the treatment of metastatic prostate cancer have been initiated, and early results appear promising (although it is too soon for definitive conclusions).

This chapter explores the role of immunotherapy in the treatment of advanced genitourinary neoplasms. Principles of immunotherapy will be discussed, along with reviews of the most current immunotherapeutic applications to the treatment of renal cell, bladder, and prostate cancers. Future treatment modalities will also be outlined.

OVERVIEW: HUMORAL AND CELLULAR IMMUNOLOGIC EFFECTOR CELLS*

Although immune responses have traditionally been divided into two categories—humoral, mediated by antibody-secreting B-lymphocytes, and cellular, mediated by T-lymphocytes—they involve interactions from both cell types, with additional support from a third, the antigen-presenting cell (APC). After initial MHC-restricted activation by APCs, T-lymphocytes act through either direct contact with target cells, or via secreted cytokines, agents that augment target cell behavior through a variety of mechanisms.

Initially, T-lymphocytes were divided into T8 (CD8+) and T4 (CD4+) elements, based on specific surface molecules that appeared to influence their behavior. CD8+ cells were determined to be cytotoxic, and were therefore named cytolytic T lymphocytes. They secrete a limited spectrum of cytokines, such an interleukin 3 (IL3), interferon γ (IFNγ), and granulocyte–monocyte colony–stimulating factor (GM-CSF). CD4+ elements can now be further divided functionally, by the cytokines they secrete, into Th_1 cells, which produce IL2, IL3, IFNγ, lymphotoxin, and GM-CSF, and Th_2, which produce GM-CSF, IL3, IL4, IL5, IL6, and IL10. These cytokines have widespread effects on APCs, B lymphocytes, and other T lymphocytes, and are discussed later in this chapter.

Once activated by antigen, cytokines, or APCs, B lympho-

* For a thorough review of the principles of immunology, please refer to William Paul's text *Fundamental Immunology*. (New York: Raven Press, 1993).

cytes proliferate into plasma cells, which subsequently produce antibodies. "Monoclonal antibodies" are laboratory-designed antibodies produced with specific characteristics and in high quantity. They have come to play a significant role in medical research. Currently, however, monoclonal antibodies have had little utility in the treatment of genitourinary neoplasms. When renal, prostate, or bladder tumor-specific peptides can be identified, isolated, and characterized, monoclonal antibodies to that antigen can be produced, attached to cytotoxic agents, and perhaps used to directly target and destroy those tumor cells. At this time, however, this is mostly conjecture. T lymphocytes, on the other hand, maintain a primary role in current immunotherapeutic protocols for advanced genitourinary cancers, and will be discussed further throughout this chapter.

FUNDAMENTALS OF IMMUNOTHERAPY

The immune system contributes to the surveillance and destruction of tumor cells.[1] Multiple cellular and humoral immune effectors inhibit tumor proliferation. Cellular mediators with antitumor activity killer (MHC-restricted cytotoxic T cells (Tc), natural killer (NK) cells, and lymphokine-activated killer (LAK) cells. The goal of immunotherapy in the treatment of advanced cancers is to sensitize these immune effector cells to tumor antigen and produce a cytolytic response directed at the sites of tumor with minimal systemic toxicity. The application of immunotherapy is limited to *immunogenic* malignancies, those tumors which are known to be vulnerable to immune-mediated cytotoxicity. Renal cell carcinoma and bladder cancer are both immunogenic, and therefore should be responsive to immunotherapy. Preliminary in vitro data suggest that prostate cancer cells can also respond to immunomodulation by cytokines.[2,3,4] Modern immunotherapy can be applied to neoplastic disease in one of several manners: (1) by systemic or locoregional infusion of immunostimulatory agents; (2) by passively transferring immune cells with antitumor reactivity (such as LAK or TIL cells) to the tumor-bearing host to attack sites of cancerous cells (*adoptive immunotherapy*); or (3) by vaccination with tumor cells transformed with genes or other immune stimulators to promote the generation of immune lymphoid cells with anti-tumor activity, or systemic or locoregional transfection of tumor cells with genetic material that can either induce tumor cell differentiation, cause direct cytolytic activity, produce regional cytokine secretion, or enhance MHC receptor expression ("gene therapy"). This latter method is referred to as *active immunotherapy* and intensive investigation is currently underway.

Adoptive Immunotherapy

Adoptive immunotherapy involves the in vitro growth, expansion, and immune-modification of lymphoid cells (NK and T cells) prior to reinfusion back into the host.[5,6,7] One such example is TIL therapy, which has been shown to cause regression of bulky tumors in a variety of animal tumor models and in humans. TILs are lymphoid cells isolated from fresh solid tumors upon co-culturing a tumor-cell suspension with the cytokine interleukin-2. After expansion of these cells in culture, which usually takes 3 to 4 weeks, TILs are reinfused into the patient in the hope that these cytotoxic T lymphocytes will recognize, home to, and destroy tumor deposits throughout the body.[6,8] Our own data at UCLA using TILs in patients with advanced renal cell carcinoma resulted in a response rate of 34% (see below).

Active Immunotherapy

Active or specific immunotherapy refers to the immunization of a patient with agents that will increase the host immunologic response against the tumor. The first report dates to 1971 when a patient with metastatic renal cell carcinoma was cured after receiving serum obtained from a relative, also with renal cell carcinoma, but in remission.[9] Current research is concentrated on creating tumor vaccines. During the intervening 20 years, the study of immunotherapy has introduced systemic cytokine treatment modalities as well as the adoptive immunotherapeutic techniques of LAK cells and TILs into the war against cancer.

Tumor vaccine protocols utilize the ability of cytokines to increase tumor cell immunogenicity, thereby increasing the ability of the host immune system to recognize and destroy cancer foci. Autologous tumor cells are transfected in vitro with cytokine producing genes. These transfected cells, now producing cytokines and expressing increased MHC class I antigens, are retransplanted into the host where they stimulate a tumor-specific immune response. Cytokine production occurs only at the implant site, thereby producing a strong antitumor response without systemic toxicity. The stimulated immune effector agents can then diffuse throughout the host to hunt down and destroy other tumor foci and provide immunological memory to the host. Studies in animals with subcutaneously placed vaccines have demonstrated potent, specific, and long-lasting antitumor immunity with protection upon rechallenge with tumor.[10,11]

Another approach to modulating the host immune response is by increasing the tumor's immunogenicity in vivo by systemic or intralesional injections of genetic elements that will transfect tumor cells and either enhance MHC class I expression, stimulate regional cytokine production, or introduce foreign antigenic material.[12] Such genetic material includes cytokine, suicide, and suppressor genes. This modality of gene therapy is currently under investigation, and is so far limited by technical difficulties involving efficient and safe gene delivery systems.

Cytokines

Cytokines are important elements in the antitumor response: they are soluble factors that are responsible for communication between cells of the immune system. In addition to direct tumoricidal effects, they also activate effector components of the immune system.[1,13–19] The introduction of cytokine genes into tumor cells has been repeatedly proven to enhance antitumor immune responses in both in vitro and in vivo studies. The following are the cytokines which have shown the most promise in genitourinary neoplasms. Tumor necrosis factor-α (TNF-α) has direct effects on neoplastic cells resulting in cell death. Interferon-α (IFN-α) induces a marked increase in the surface expression of class I MHC antigens in addition to direct antitumor activity. It also up-regulates adhesion molecule expression on the surface of tumor cells, aiding the immune response. Interferon-γ (IFN-γ) induces a marked increase in the surface expression of class I and II MHC antigens. Interleukin-2 (IL-2) is produced by activated T cells and causes proliferation of cytotoxic T (Tc), natural killer (NK), and LAK cells capable of lysing autologous, syngeneic, or allogeneic tumor cells, but not normal cells. IL-2 has no direct antitumor effect, but secretion of IL-2 from tumor cells abrogates tumorigenicity by stimulating the activation and proliferation of immune effector cells.[20]

IMMUNOTHERAPY FOR METASTATIC RENAL CELL CARCINOMA

In 1996, 30,600 Americans will be diagnosed with renal cell carcinoma, accounting for 2 percent of all adult malignancies.[21] Surgically unresectable disease has a poor outcome, as no successful radio- or chemotherapy strategies have been devised.[22] The natural history of renal cell carcinoma is not always predictable, and spontaneous regression of metastases after nephrectomy does occur, albeit rarely (less than 1%). Early observations of spontaneous regression, along with the discovery of circulating humoral and cellular elements in such patients, delayed growth of metastatic lesions, and varying tumor doubling times, suggested involvement of the immune system in the natural host response to this neoplasm.[23] Since then, renal cell carcinoma has become a paradigm for the immunotherapeutic approach to treating solid organ malignancies.

Initial approaches to immunotherapy utilized nonspecific immune stimulators, such as bacillus Calmette-Guérin, or xenogeneic RNA-treated lymphocytes (probably a stimulator of interferon production). Despite initial enthusiasm,[24–26] this approach ultimately yielded no significant improvement in prognosis.[27] Several studies with BCG showed some initial benefit although larger randomized studies were not performed.[28–30] A similar situation holds for *Corynebacterium parvum*[31] and transfer factor,[32] two other nonspecific agents no longer in vogue. One third of the patients enrolled in a pilot study to assess the antitumor activity of 1,2-benzopyrene responsed to treatment, yet subsequent phase II studies with this nonspecific agent were associated with only a 6% response rate. These nonspecific agents are now mainly of historical interest with regards to treating renal cell carcinoma.

Biologic Therapy with Cytokines

The isolation, identification, and molecular cloning of IL-2 revolutionized the field of cancer immunotherapy and significantly altered the treatment of metastic renal cell carcinoma.[33,34] Since then, other immunostimulatory cytokines have been identified and purified. With the advent of recombinant DNA technology, the ability to produce large quantities of these cytokines has resulted in their wide-spread use and, in a relatively short period of time, these agents have become an accepted treatment for metastatic disease. To date, most studies investigating the use of cytokines in the treatment of metastatic renal cell carcinoma have used IFN-α, IL-2, combinations of these cytokines, or adoptive immunotherapy with TILs or LAK cells. The role of a new generation of cytokines such as IL-4, IL-7, IL-12, and GM-CSF is currently under investigation.

Interferon Alpha and Gamma

Research at UCLA in the early 1980s was the among the first to demonstrate the effectiveness of IFN-α in the treatment of metastatic renal cell carcinoma.[35] Independent studies at the same time confirmed the regression of metastatic disease with objective response rates of 16% to 26% lasting an average of 8 to 10 months.[36,37] These numbers have not changed significantly in the past decade, despite numerous phase II trials and attempts at modifying doses and dosing schedules.[38–49] Table 84-1 summarizes the major studies of the past decade, demonstrating a reproducible response rate of 15–20 percent and a response duration of 8 to 10 months. Responses appear independent of the preparation and dosing used. Improved response rates of 30% and durable clinical responses lasting more than 27 months can be seen in a select subset of patients treated with IFN-α.[45,47] These patients have had a prior nephrectomy, no previous chemotherapy or radiation therapy, good to excellent performance status, and primarily pulmonary metastases. (Lung metastases appear more responsive to IFN-α therapy than those of other viscera.[43] At UCLA, survival rates increased from 49 to 115 weeks in IFN-α treated patients with these favorable prognostic variables.[47]

Side effects of IBN-α treatment include fever, chills, myalgia, anorexia, and headache. These are usually associated with the initial dosing and often improve spontaneously with continued administration of the drug. Reversible hematologic and hepatic changes are occasionally noted, but they, too, usually resolve without necessitating changes in dosing.[50,51]

Combining accessory agents with IFN-α has been investigated as a means of increasing responsiveness and decreasing

TABLE 84-1. *Phase II trials of interferon-alpha for the treatment of metastatic renal cell cancer*

Investigators	Patients	Response
DeKernion et al, 1983[35]	43	16.5%
Quesada et al, 1983[36]	19	26%
Neidart et al, 1984[41]	33	15%
Figlin et al, 1985[48]	23	13%*
Quesada et al, 1985[37]	50	26%
Kirkwood et al, 1985[38]	30	23%
Umeda and Niijima, 1986[40]	226	17.7%
Fossa et al, 1986[57]	18	33%*
Muss et al, 1987[45]	97	7%†
Creagan et al, 1987[49]	29	34%‡
Sarna et al, 1987[47]	43	14%§
	22	14%*
Figlin et al, 1989[39]	18	26%
Minasian et al, 1993[44]	159	10%*
Total	651	20%

* Addition of vinblastine (0.15 mg/kg).

† Select subpopulation (+ prior nephrectomy, − prior chemotherapy, − bone mets) had 23% response rate.

‡ Aspirin, 600 mg PO qid.

§ Select subpopulation (+ prior nephrectomy, − prior chemotherapy, − bone mets) had 24% response rate.

TABLE 84-2. *Phase II trials of interferon-beta and gamma for the treatment renal cell cancer*

Investigators	Patients	Response
Rinehart et al, 1986[62]	18	17%*
Rinehart et al, 1986[64]	13	0%
Quesada et al, 1987[63]	33	7%
Aulitzky et al, 1989[65]	22	27%
Ellerhorst et al, 1994[61]	35	15%
Total	121	14%

* Interferon-beta

toxicity. In one study, the addition of aspirin increased response rates to 34%, but few changes in constitutional symptoms (the reason for adding aspirin to the treatment protocol) occurred.[49] In vitro, the administration of 5-FU increases the susceptibility of renal cell carcinoma to LAK cells, and the combined administration of 5-FU and IFN for the treatment of bladder cancer has also shown promise.[52–54] Several studies have investigated using different combinations of IFN-α and chemotherapeutic agents to treat renal cell carcinoma, and have demonstrated a favorable response rate. At the M. D. Anderson Cancer Center, Houston, Texas, combinations of IFN-α, mitomycin C, and 5-FU were found to be synergistic and improved the response rate to 35%.[55] With the combination of IL-2, IFN-α, and 5-FU, the response rate increased to 45 percent with only moderate toxicity.[56] The addition of other agents, such as vinblastine,[48,57] doxorubicin,[58] and BCNU[59] do not appear to alter the response rate or the duration of the response, yet results in increased fatigue, hepatotoxicity, and myelosuppression.[60]

Several studies investigating the use of IFN-γ in the treatment of metastatic renal cell carcinoma are summarized in Table 84-2. The response rates and duration of response were favorable, but no better than those of IFN-α or IL-2.[61–65] The toxicities are similar, and consist primarily of malaise, fever, anorexia, and headache. As discussed earlier, IFN-α upregulates expression of MHC class I antigens while IFN-γ increases both class I and II expression. Because these two cytokines have different roles in stimulating the immune response, there is speculation that a treatment approach combining both IFN-α and IFN-γ would be complementary, and thus more effective. In vitro studies do demonstrate synergistic activity between IFN-α and IFN-γ, although with a significantly added toxity.[66] Preliminary clinical trials have failed to show any additive effects, and toxicity was significant.[67–69]

Interleukin-2

IL-2 was the first cytokine demonstrated to mediate antitumor effects via the host immune system. Unlike TNF, IL-2 has no demonstrable direct and antitumor effect, but activates immune effector cells which then target neoplastic lesions.[20] In vitro and in vivo studies demonstrate that IL-2 can generate LAK cells, enhance NH cell function, augment alloantigen responsiveness, stimulate growth Tc cells, and mediate the regression of large tumor burdens.[70] The first large studies investigating the therapeutic role of IL-2 in metastatic renal cell carcinoma were undertaken at the National Cancer Institute (NCI).[71] One hundred and thirty-two patients were treated with IL-2 alone or co-administered with LAK cells. The overall response rate was 18% (IL-2 alone) and 35% (IL-2 and LAK cells). Other researchers have confirmed these results[72,73] and, when combined with further studies comprising a total of 255 patients treated with IL-2, an overall objective response rate of 15% and a duration of almost 2 years was demonstrated.[74] This data was used by the United States Food and Drug Adminstration in 1992 when IL-2 was approved for the treatment of metastatic renal cell carcinoma. Rosenberg has summarized his experienced with high dose IL-2 therapy and metastatic renal cell carcinoma, noting a 20% overall response rate.[75] Table 84-3 summarizes the major clinical investigations of IL-2 on metastatic renal cell carcinoma. These studies have identified certain patient characteristics associated with a better response to IL-2 therapy: good to excellent performance scores and either lung, lymph node, or small-volume extrahepatic abdominal disease.

The use of IL-2 is associated with significant side effects, the most serious of which is a prerenal azotemia with resultant hypotension, pulmonary edema, renal failure, and fluid retention. Myocardial infarction, gastrointestinal bleeding and perforation, and death may also occur. (Although the mortality from IL-2 therapy was initially set at 1.5% to 4%,[90,91] more recent data show reduced toxicity as more experience is gained with this treatment modality.[75] At UCLA we have not experienced any deaths in our series.) These major toxicities are dose-related and result from increased membrane permeability and subsequent fluid and colloid loss into viscera and soft tissue.[76–80] Other common side effects include fever, chills, anorexia, gastrointestinal upset, mental status changes, tachyarrythmias, and third spacing of fluids. These are reversible and usually resolve within 72 hours of discontinuing therapy.

To prevent these severe but largely reversible toxicities, alternative infusion schedules and dosing regimens have been devised. Several studies have compared continuous versus bolus IL-2 administration.[72,81–83] Results demonstrate similar response rates of 15% to 20% and equivalent side effects between the two groups, although continuous infusion of IL-2 requires less total drug.

Other researchers have focused on low-dose IL-2 therapy, especially since many metastic renal cell carcinoma patients are not candidates for high-dose treatment given their age, concomitant disease states, and overall incapacity. The results are inconsistent: although all studies associated the lower dose with decreased toxicity, some demonstrated similar efficacy between high- and low-dose IL-2 therapy,[84,85] while others[86] failed to

TABLE 84-3. *Phase II trials of interleukin-2 for the treatment of metastatic renal cell cancer*

Investigators	Patients	Response
West et al, 1987[72]	40	32%
Fisher et al, 1988[73]	35	16%
Rosenberg et al, 1989[91]	54	22%
Bukowski et al, 1990[81]	41	12%
Geertsen et al, 1992[82]	30	20%
Weiss et al, 1992[83]	94	18%
Rosenberg et al, 1992[71]	60	18%
Atkins et al, 1993[218]	71	17%
Rosenberg et al, 1994[75]	143	20%
Total	568	20%

TABLE 84-4. *Phase II trials of combination cytokine therapy for metastatic renal cell cancer*

Investigators	Patients	Response
Rosenberg et al, 1989[89]	35	31%*
Mittleman et al, 1990[219]	18	22%
Kirchner et al, 1990[220]	17	29%
Atzpodien et al, 1990[221]	17	36%
Atzpodien et al, 1990[93]	14	35%
Hirsch et al, 1990[94]	15	40%
Bukowski et al, 1990[222]	20	15%
Thomas et al, 1992[223]	34	6%
Spencer et al, 1992[224]	22	5%
Budd et al, 1992[225]	21	10%
Figlin et al, 1992[92]	52	25%
Sznol et al, 1992[226]	42	19%*
Rosenberg, 1992[71]	41	34%
Ilson et al, 1992[227]	34	12%
Lipton et al, 1993[228]	39	33%
Atkins et al, 1993[218]	28	11%
Bermann et al, 1993[229]	30	30%
Vogelzang et al, 1993[90]	42	12%
Total	521	22%

* Includes lymphocyte-activated killer cells.

observe any objective response with low-dose treatment. Further studies using low-dose IL-2 either via continuous infusion or subcutaneous administration are currently underway.

Combination Therapy: IL-2 and IFN-α

Combining IL-2 infusion with other cytokines has also been investigated as a means of reducing toxicity. After in vitro studies demonstrated a synergistic activity of IL-2 with IFN-α,[87,88] the first human trials were undertaken at the NCI. Patients with metastatic renal cell carcinoma had a 31% response rate to this treatment.[89] Since then, other studies have investigated this combined approach, with an emphasis on outpatient, low-dose regimens. The results are listed in Table 84-4. These studies show a wide range of response rates with an average of 22%, depending on patient selection and study assessment parameters. Since 1988, 52 patients at UCLA have been treated with combination IL-2 and IFN-α, with results comparing favorably to those achieved with high-dose IL-2 alone: the response rate was 25%, the median duration of response was 23 months, and the median duration of survival was 34 months or more.[92] Similar studies have confirmed these findings.[93,94] These phase II protocols demonstrate that combination IL-2/IFN-α can be administered to patients with metastatic renal cell carcinoma successfully and safely on an outpatient basis with results similar to that of high-dose IL-2 alone. The main adverse effects of combination therapy—fever, chills, nausea, anorexia, and hypotension—are less severe than those of high-dose IL-2 alone and are easily treated on a symptomatic basis.

Adoptive Immunotherapy for Metastatic Renal Cell Carcinoma

Autolymphocyte Therapy

The theoretical basis of autolymphocyte therapy (ALT) relies on activation of memory T-lymphocytes (mT cells) in patients with metastatic cancer. These are T cells that have been exposed in vivo to tumor antigens and have the potential for mediating tumor regression following nonspecific activation.[95] Activation is performed by incubating mT cells (from peripheral blood) with anti-T cell receptor (CD-3) antibodies, thus triggering a clonal proliferation of effector cells.[96,97] In 1990, Osband and colleagues reported a 21% response rate in 90 patients with metastatic renal cell carcinoma, achieving a significant survival advantage (21 months versus 8.5 months) with only mild toxicity.[98] Further studies are currently in progress,[99,100] but randomized trials comparing ALT to IL-2 have not been performed.[101]

Lymphokine-Activated Killer Cellular Therapy

Lymphokine-activated killer (LAK) cells are generated by cultivating peripheral blood cells with IL-2 for 3 to 4 days and represent the nonspecific arm of immune effector cells that mediate tumorilysis in a non-MHC restricted fashion.[102] After initial studies[103,104] demonstrated that IL-2 plus LAK therapy resulted in the regression of established animal tumor models for melanoma, renal cell, sarcoma, colon adenocarcinoma, and bladder carcinoma, clinical studies were begun.[71] LAK cells are infused into the patient along with IL-2 in either high or low doses. Side effects are related to the dose of IL-2 administered and responsiveness is related to patient performance profiles. A number of large phase II clinical trials are listed in Table 84-5, response rates for the treatment of metastatic renal cell carcinoma ranged from 9% to 33%. The combined response rate of all published trials is 23.5% as summarized by Sznol.[90] A single randomized study has compared IL-2 alone to IL-2 combined with LAK cells, without any demonstration of superiority of IL-2/LAK over IL-2 alone.[105] This study was, however, associated with a higher percentage of complete clinical remissions in the LAK/IL-2 groups.

Tumor Infiltrating Lymphocyte (TIL) Cellular Therapy

The most intriguing new application of IL-2 therapy is in conjunction with tumor infiltrating lymphocytes. Whereas LAK cells are mainly NK cells, TILs are activated cytotoxic T cells, which show greater specificity in their targets. Specific immune reactivity, however, is more clearly seen in TILs obtained from patients with malignant melanoma rather than renal cell carci-

TABLE 84-5. *Phase II trials of combination interleukin-2 and lymphocyte-activated killer cells for the treatment of metastatic renal cell cancer*

Investigators	Patients	Response
Rosenberg et al[105]	72	35%
Parkinson et al[230]	47	9%
Dillman et al[231]	50	14%
Palmer et al[232]	102	18%
Weiss et al[83]	94	17%
Foon et al[233]	23	26%
Thompson et al[84]	42	33%
Sznol et al[226]	40	20%
Total	470	23.5%

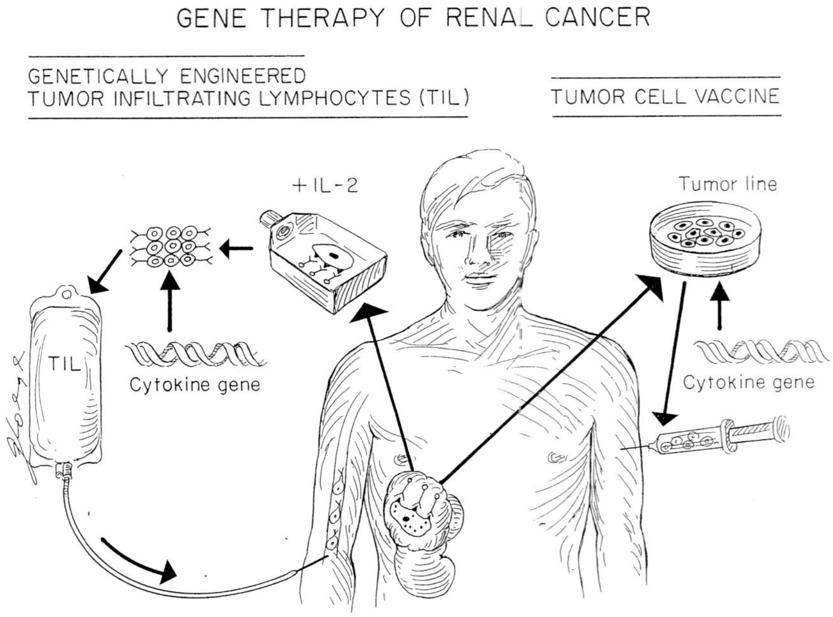

FIG. 84-1. Gene therapy of renal cancer. Genetically engineered tumor-infiltrating lymphocytes (TILs) are produced (*left*) by the mechanical and enzymatic digestion of nephrectomy specimens under sterile conditions, to obtain single-cell suspensions of lymphoid and tumor cells. By culturing with IL-2, lymphoid populations are expanded. After 5 to 6 weeks in culture, 10^{10} TILs are produced and are returned to patient along with IL-2. "Tumor vaccine" is produced (*right*) by isolating tumor cells from the primary lesion and transfecting them ex vivo with cytosine-producing genes to increase immunogenicity. The transfected cells are then reimplanted to the host to stimulate an immune response.

noma, although specific TIL clones from renal cell carcinoma have been characterized.[106,107] When given with IL-2, TILs are capable of eradicating advanced and bulky tumors against which LAK cells have been unsuccessful. TILs are isolated from solid tumors and are grown by preparing a single cell suspension of tumor tissue and then culturing these cells with IL-2. After in vitro expansion with IL-2, TILs are reinfused back to the patient in the hope that they will home to tumor deposits and destroy the neoplastic tissue while leaving normal tissue unscathed. On a cellular basis, TILs are 50- to 100-fold more potent than LAK cells in mediating tumor regression.[6,108] The preparation of TILs is schematically diagrammed in Figure 84-1.[78] Under sterile conditions, radical nephrectomy specimens are mechanically and enzymatically disrupted to obtain single cell suspensions of both lymphoid and tumor cells. Cells are expanded ex vivo by culturing the TILs with IL-2. This produces a TIL population with antitumor specificity. After 5 to 6 weeks in culture, 10^{10} to 10^{11} TILs are produced and then infused into the patient along with IL-2.

Few clinical studies have been undertaken with TIL immunotherapy. The UCLA experience includes 48 patients with a response rate of 33%, an average response duration of 14 months, and an mean survival of 22 months.[92] Bukowski and coworkers, summarized the Cleveland Clinic series, which involved two individual trials.[109] The first study, with TILs retrieved from metastatic sites, yielded no clinical responses. The second trial involved harvesting TILs from the primary tumor site (as done at UCLA) with a response rate of 25%. Survival is increased in patients with good to excellent performance status, prior nephrectomy, less metastic sites, and no prior cytotoxic therapy.[110] We have increased our efficacy to 40% by enhancing the proportion of CD8+ cells in our TIL population.[111] Additionally, a recent report has documented that a preimmunotherapy reduction in circulating CD8+ cells is associated with an improved response to immunotherapy in patients with metastatic cell carcinoma.[112] A multicenter randomized trial comparing the results of nephrectomy and IL-2 versus nephrectomy, IL-2, and CD8+/TILs is soon to begin.

Vaccine and Gene Therapies for Metastatic Renal Cell Carcinoma

An important new strategy to overcome the poor immunogenicity of some neoplastic lesions is to insert cytokine genes directly into tumor cells. Animal studies of this technique have demonstrated prevention of tumor growth, decreased metastatic spread, and prolonged immunologic memory, resulting in the rejection of subsequent tumor challenges.[113–120] This treatment strategy is the "tumor vaccine" alluded to earlier in the chapter; it is schematically diagrammed in Figure 84-1. At UCLA we have transfected the genes for IL-2 and IFN-α into human renal cell carcinoma cell lines. When these cells are implanted subcutantously into nude mice, cytokine secretion from these cells prevents tumor growth locally and is more effective than systemic IL-2 and IFN-α administration.[92,121] The local production of high concentrations of cytokine may directly alter tumor properties associated with invasion and metastasis. Another approach to cytokine gene therapy is the direct transfection of TILs with cytokine genes. The rationale is that the TILs will traffic directly to tumor deposits, concentrate at these sites, and secrete high levels of cytotoxic cytokines with minimal systemic toxicity. Preliminary studies, including the use of double-gene marking approaches to evaluate the homing properties of renal TILs vs PBLs, are currently underway.[122,123]

The past two decades have witnessed impressive advancements in the application of immunotherapy to renal cell carcinoma. At UCLA we have seen a progressive increase in responses to treatment as therapy has evolved from systemic IFN-α administration (16%), to combination IFN-α/IL-2 use (25%), to the current method of bulk TILs (33%) and CD8+/TILs (40%). We have identified patient characteristics that predict improved responsiveness to therapy, and have established treatment protocols that decreased toxicity. The most encouraging results have been the improved rates of complete clinical response, most of which are durable and long-lasting. Our current focus is on creating tumor vaccines and furthering systemic gene therapy modalities.

Further refinements in the treatment of renal cell carcinoma with immunotherapy are still needed, yet there is no doubt that current immunotherapeutic protocol produce changes in the natural history of renal cell carcinoma and cause significant and lasting remissions in select patients.

The Role of Surgery in Metastatic Renal Cell Carcinoma

When diagnosed with renal cell carcinoma, approximately 30% of patients already have metastatic lesions.[22] These lesions are usually multifocal, either within the same organ or to multiple sites. Occasionally (in approximately 1% to 3% of cases) patients do present with a solitary metastasis; the 5-year survival after excision of such a lesion is approximately 25%.[124,125] In a study at our institution, aggressive therapy of solitary skeletal, CNS, and soft tissue lesions produced significant palliation of symptoms.[126] This is a select group of patients, however, and only those patients with a definite solitary lesion and no lymphatic involvement have any prospect of benefiting from surgical management. Patients therefore must be carefully chosen. The most favorable lesions for resection are solitary pulmonary masses, which occasionally appear more than one year after removal of the primary tumor.[127] Unfortunately, a metastatic lesion identified at the time of diagnosis of renal cell carcinoma is seldom an isolated tumor, and more clinically evident lesions invariably appear shortly after surgical excision.

In the past, nephrectomy was advocated in the treatment of metastatic disease as a method of both reducing the growth of the primary lesions and possibly triggering a spontaneous regression of metastatic disease. Unfortunately, this can be expected to occur in less than 1% of cases, the remissions are extremely short-lived, and the mortality rate from surgery can be significant.[128–130] This concept has been abandoned as it is now clear that nephrectomy itself seldom, if ever, has any influence on metastatic disease. Therefore, the routine use of "adjunctive nephrectomy" is unwarranted. Palliation of symptoms is, however, a reasonable rationale for nephrectomy in the face of metastases, provided that the primary tumor can be completely removed without undue morbidity. Patients with paraneoplastic syndromes will occasionally benefit from palliative nephrectomy, especially if the metastatic sites are not large. Repeated hemorrhage and tumor pain can also frequently be effectively ameliorated by nephrectomy.

The advent of immunotherapy for renal cell carcinoma has once again raised the issue of the role of surgery in patients with metastatic disease. Studies performed at UCLA[126,131,132] and elsewhere[40,44,133,134] have documented improved response rates to immunotherapy when given in conjunction with removal of the diseased kidney. Our data indicate that even when considering all the various prognostic factors, patients who received immunotherapy (primarily with interferons) had a better response rate and survival when nephrectomy was performed prior to treatment. Nonetheless, whether nephrectomy is best performed before or after immunotherapy is debatable, and a randomized study is being performed which may resolve this question.

Other than for palliation, at UCLA our current philosophy is to perform adjunctive nephrectomies in patients with metastatic renal cell carcinoma only in conjunction with immunotherapy, either (1) to obtain tissue for TILs and other experimental protocols, or (2) to reduce tumor load in very large primary tumors, which are either symptomatic or have a probability of becoming symptomatic in the near future. Conversely, patients with small primary masses and/or multiple small metastatic lesions are first given immunotherapy. Those patients whose metastases respond to the treatment are then subsequently selected for a nephrectomy.

IMMUNOTHERAPY FOR BLADDER CANCER

In 1996, 52,900 new cases of bladder cancer will be diagnosed in the United States, accounting for 4% of all adult malignancies and ranking as the third most prevalent visceral neoplasm.[21,135] In the past ten years there has been a 36% increase in the number of cases of bladder cancer diagnosed, although during the same period there has been an 8% decline in mortality. Thirty percent of newly diagnosed bladder tumors are invasive. While many of these patients can be made disease-free with surgery, approximately 10,000 will die this year alone. Surgery (radical cystectomy) produces significant morbidity and cures less than 50% of patients with locally advanced tumor, and in patients with positive lymph nodes at time of surgery, the prognosis is poor.[136]

Seventy percent of presenting bladder tumors, therefore, are superficial. The natural history of individual bladder tumors is unpredictable due to the heterogeneity of this neoplasm. While superficial papillary tumors are easily resected by transurethral procedures (TUR), there is a 30% to 90% recurrence rate after surgery.[137–142] Risk factors for recurrence include the presence of multiple lesions, high-grade tumors, and a history of previous recurrences. Likewise, the presence of carcinoma in situ (CIS) predicts a worse outcome. Prevention of invasion and recurrence by superficial tumors and the amelioration of CIS is paramount in the treatment of bladder cancer, given the morbidity and mortality of advanced disease. BCG has had a dramatic role in the treatment of noninvasive bladder cancer and is recommended for recurrence prophylaxis after successful TUR, treatment of residual tumor in patients too debilitated for or after incomplete TUR, and for primary treatment of CIS.[143] Despite the impressive success of BCG treatment, an average of 20% of patients treated with combined TUR and BCG fail therapy and will either develop recurrent tumors or progress to invasive disease.[144–148] For these patients, treatment options are limited.

Some patients with superficial transitional cell cancer of the bladder can be treated with intravesical chemotherapy: the most widely used agents include thiotepa, epodyl, mitomycin-C, and adriamycin.[149,150] Their effectivenesses are very comparable and are generally considered equal: papillary tumors have a 30% to 60% response rate whereas CIS has a 55% to 66% response rate.[136,149,151,152] Chemotherapeutic prophylaxis post-TUR can reduce recurrence rates to 30% to 44%. Although chemotherapy is not as effective as BCG therapy, some BCG failures will respond to chemotherapy. Likewise, some chemotherapy failures will respond to BCG therapy. For the treatment of superficial bladder lesions, however, chemotherapy is current a second-line agent behind BCG.

Although BCG is generally well-tolerated by 90% to 95% of patients, moderate to severe complications do occur and mortality is not negligible.[153] Two to five percent of patients will experience life-threatening complications.[150] To decrease this toxicity, other immunotherapeutic modalities have been introduced. Although most are not as effective as BCG, they do demonstrate some success in treating superficial disease with significantly less morbidity and can therefore by safely used as second line therapies for BCG failures.

Nonspecific Immunotherapy

All forms of intravesical immunotherapy depend on the host's ability to mount an immune response that results in the destruction of bladder cancer cells.[142] To be effective, both chemotherapeutic and immunotherapeutic agents must come into direct contact with the abnormal urothelium. Initial attempts at immunotherapy for bladder cancer were with nonspecific agents. Early experiments with *Corneybacterium parvum* seemed promising, decreasing recurrence rates from 55% to 21%.[154,155] Unfortunately, persistent remissions and enhancement of survival were never documented. Studies by Kagawa[156] utilized OK-432, a nonspecific immunogen derived from *Streptococcus pyrogenes*. Although initial reports boasted a 14.3% tumor regression rate, results were not as encouraging as BCG. Further studies have had inconsistent results.

Bacillus Calmette-Guérin Immunotherapy

BCG was first administered to humans for the treatment of bladder cancer in 1976,[157] and has since become the preferred intravesical therapy for prophylaxis in tumor-free patients, eradicating residual papillary lesions, and treating CIS.[135,144–148,158,159] The ideal preparation, dose, and schedule of BCG therapy has yet to be standardized, although traditionally a 6-week course with weekly 120 mg intravesical administrations has been used.[160] In a recent review, however, this schedule was found to be suboptimal, and the addition of 3 weekly treatments at 3 months was found to increase complete response in CIS from 70% to 82%.[161] Likewise, the exact mechanism of BCG action is unclear, although it is believed to exert its antitumor effect through immune effectors.[3,159–164] There are two hypotheses. The first is that BCG exerts its effect by initiating a tumor-specific immune response involving T cell-dependent agents, including T_H cells, macrophages, IL-2, IFN-α, IFN-γ, and TNF. The other theory is that BCG causes a nonspecific inflammation which results in the sloughing of both normal and neoplastic cells. It has been established that the degree of the immune response correlates directly with the likelihood of a patient remaining disease-free.[142]

Prospective randomized studies have demonstrated the effectiveness of intravesical BCG for prophylaxis in tumor-free patients after TUR, eradicating residual papillary lesions after TUR, treating unresectable tumors, and eliminating CIS. With BCG therapy, recurrence rates for superficial tumors after TUR decrease from 30% to 90% to 0% to 40% (average 20%).[144–149,165] Fifty-eight percent of surgically unresectable tumors respond to BCG.[147,158] BCG instillations also prevent muscle invasion, decreasing tumor extension from 36% to 9% in treated patients.[146] Because 50% to 90% of patients with CIS respond to BCG therapy, it is recommended over cystectomy for the primary treatment of CIS.[147,149,166,167] Not all tumors that fail BCG therapy are destined to become muscle invasive, however. The two risk factors that have the most significant impact on survival are noninvasive involvement of the prostatic urethra at the time of BCG failure and the presence of superficially invasive tumor at the time that BCG therapy was initiated.[137,164,165]

Ninety-five percent of patients treated with intravesical BCG have minor to moderate side effects, including cystitis (91%), hematuria (43%), low grade fevers (28%), malaise (24%), and nausea (8%).[139,153,168] Two to five percent of patients develop severe, potentially life-threatening complications that require intensive treatment. (For a an extensive review of the complications associated with BCG therapy, please refer to the study of 2600 BCG-treated patients by Lamm and colleagues.[153]) Intravesical treatment has its own-associated risks, including urethral and bladder trauma from catheterization, bladder contracture, and urinary tract infection.[169]

In the search for therapies as equally effective as BCG, yet less toxic, other immunotherapeutic agents have been tested. These agents are discussed below.

Keyhole Limpet Hemocyanin

Keyhole limpet hemocyanin (KLH) is a powerful nonspecific immunostimulant that induces both cell-mediated and humoral immune responses.[170] Initial research was performed in 1974 by Olsson, who treated patients after TUR with intracutaneous immunization with KLH.[171] Nineteen patients followed for 204 patient-months had a recurrence rate of 11%, as compared to a recurrence rate of 70% (with a total of 18 tumors) in ten untreated patients. The potential value of KLH therapy was confirmed in 44 patients with superficial tumors status post-TUR.[172] Patients were divided into two intravesical therapy groups, KLH versus mitomycin-C. KLH-treated patients had a 14.2% recurrence rate (follow-up mean 20.7 months) compared to a 39.1% recurrence rate in mitomycin-C–treated patients (mean follow-up 18.3 months). The total response rates (complete and partial remissions) were 95% (KLH) and 69% (mitomycin-C). In another series, 81 patients at high risk for recurrence of superficial lesions were treated with intravesical KLH after TUR. A 20.9% recurrence rate was noted (22.8 month follow-up).[172] Animal studies with intralesional KLH injection have also demonstrated significantly reduced tumor incidence, growth rate and morbidity.[173] In these studies KLH compared favorably to BCG in the inhibition of tumor growth and prolongation of survival. Patients treated with KLH have reported minimal side effects, usually consisting of slight urinary discomfort and occasional low grade fevers, both of which resolve within 24 to 48 hours of treatment. Further studies are needed with KLH to determine its ultimate role in the arsenal of therapies against superficial bladder cancer.[174–177]

Interferon

Cytokines are potent immunoregulatory peptides involved in intracellular communication. Relevant cytokines in the treatment of bladder cancer include IFN-α, IFN-γ, IL-2, and TNF. The antitumor effects of BCG and KLH on bladder tumors are postulated to result from the increased endogenous cytokine secretion that occurs with stimulation of host defense mechanisms by these agents.[138] Therefore, many researchers have attempted to treat bladder cancer with the direct administration of cytokines, instead of via indirect methods.

Interferon was the first cytokine to be used in the treatment of superficial bladder cancer. The mechanism of IFN-mediated antitumor effects is unclear and may include direct inhibition of tumor cell growth as well as enhancement of the tumoricidal capacity of host defense cells via upregulation of MHC antigens.[138] One conclusion is unrefuted: locoregional administration of IFN is superior to systemic administration, because complete regression of bladder tumors occurs more frequently and with fewer adverse effects after intralesional application.[177,178]

Intravesical interferon was initially used for the treatment of unresected lesions. The first protocol involved 16 patients: 8 with CIS, who had no response, and 8 with papillary tumors, who had a 75% response.[179] In another study, intravesical IFN-α was given to 19 patients with high grade intraepithelial tumors (including 18 with CIS) and 16 patients with papillary tumors.[180] In CIS patients, a 32% complete response (duration 18–37 months) and 26% partial response was noted. Of the 16% of patients who had recurrences, all were downgraded from CIS to low-grade cancers. A 25% complete response rate was noted in the 16 patients with papillary tumors, including several patients for whom previous treatments with BCG had failed.

Interferon-α has shown more promise as a prophylactic agent post-TUR. Bartoletti demonstrated a 79% disease-free rate at 98 weeks median follow-up.[181] Glashan used high dose IFN-α and had a 43% complete response and 23% partial response rate, with 90% of the responders disease-free at 6 months and 50% disease-free at 12 months.[182] Six of nine patients who failed previous BCG treatments responded to IFN-α in this study. Other investigators have documented similar success with IFN-α in preventing tumor recurrence, with response rates averaging 55% to 70%.[180,183–187]

IFN-α has also tested well against chemotherapeutic agents. When compared to mitomycin-C, IFN-α was found to be equally effective in preventing the recurrence of superficial tumors.[140] Combining the two agents, however, was more effective than either agent alone, and with minimal toxicity.[170] When compared to epirubicin, IFN-α treated patients had fewer recurrences and longer disease-free survival.[141,186,188] The side effects of IFN-α are extremely mild and consist mainly of low-grade temperatures.

Fewer studies have assessed the role of interferon-β for the treatment of superficial lesions, Niijima demonstrated 25% and 67% response rates, respectively.[189] Migliari showed that IFN-β had an efficacy comparable to that obtained with other chemoprophylactic agents.[190] As with IFN-α, side effects were negligible. When IFN-γ was injected directly into lesions after TUR, 83% of the patients were tumor free for an average of 246 days.[191]

Bropirimine is an oral agent shown to have multiple immunostimulatory properties, including the stimulation of endogenous interferon production. A phase 1 trial of oral bropirimine for the treatment of superficial bladder cancer was reported upon by Sarosdy and colleagues in 1992.[192] With minimal toxicity, approximately one quarter of the patients had complete regression of their tumors, and a total response rate of 33% was achieved. Bropirimine demonstrated increased activity against CIS as compared with papillary transitional cell tumors.

These initial studies with IFN show promise, yet more research is needed to identify the optimal patient population and to establish the most effective preparation, dose, and schedule of interferon therapy for the treatment of bladder cancer.

Interleukin-2 and Tissue Necrosis Factor

Interleukin-2 (IL-2) activates tumor reactive cells, such as NK and LAK cells. The short half-life of systemic IL-2 requires high dosages which results in significant toxicity.[138] Intravesical administration avoids the complications of systemic infusion and has been shown to be effective in several studies. In one protocol, repeated intra- and paralesional injections of IL-2 resulted in a 50% complete response and a 33% partial response rate (greater than 60% tumor reduction).[193] No side effects were noted. In another study, 33% of the patients had complete tumor regression and an additional 33% had a partial response (greater than 50% reduction in tumor mass).[194] Intralesional injections of murine bladder tumors in vivo reduced tumor growth more than with BCG.[138] Less impressive results were reported by Huland,[195] who acheived only a 20% response rate with continuous IL-2 (crude, not recombinant) bladder irrigations after TUR, and Hermann,[196] whose continuous intravesical infusion of combined IL-2/LAK cells in patients with metastic bladder cancer was without responders.

Combining BCG and IL-2 has been suggested as a potentially effective treatment for superficial bladder cancer. In one study, T-antigen positive patients achieved an 81% tumor-free response lasting an average of 28 months.[197] In another study, without pretreatment selection criteria, patients experienced a 85% complete response rate (lasting 13 months).[198] Side effects were self-limited and minor, consisting of low-grade fever, hematuria, and bladder irritability, which generally lasted less than 24 hours.

Two in vivo studies have evaluated the use of TNF in superficial bladder cancer. Hersh demonstrated an 11% partial response rate with intravesical TNF therapy,[199] while Lee,[200] in a murine model, showed that TNF suppressed tumor growth to 48 percent of that of control mice. In vitro studies of TNF combined with IFN-γ on cultured bladder cancer cells have demonstrated powerful antiproliferative effects; this same study, however, noted proliferative effects on tumor cells by IL-2 and GM-CSF.[201]

Tumor Vaccines and Other Future Applications

Future applications of immunotherapy for bladder cancer involve the standardization of BCG therapy, the development of tumor vaccines, and the application of gene therapy techniques to intravesical regimens. Several studies have investigated the effectiveness of tumor vaccines. Conner used IL-2– and IFN-γ–treated murine bladder cells to create a tumor vaccine which not only demonstrated significant impairment of tumor-forming capacity, but successfully prevented tumor rechallenge, proving that long-term immunological memory was established in cured mice.[202] Lamm and coworkers, however, utilizing a BCG-based tumor vaccine in mice, demonstrated that the vaccine was inferior to BCG therapy alone.[203]

At UCLA we have been studying the application of gene therapy to treating superficial bladder tumors. We have used an intravesically-administered adenoviral vector to transfect murine bladder tumors[204] and are currently characterizing the most potent agents to treat superficial lesions, including IFN-α, IFN-γ, GM-CSF, TNF, and *P*53 suppressor gene. Gilboa and associates have recently demonstrated that an IL-2-secreting murine bladder tumor (MBT-2) cell preparation can be used as a tumor vaccine and result in 50 percent cure rates in animals carrying a large tumor burden.[205]

Currently, combined TUR/BCG therapy is the most effective treatment for the majority of patients with superficial bladder cancer. The ultimate therapeutic regimen, however, has yet to be introduced.[150] For the 20% who fail to respond to TUR/BCG therapy, options have been limited and cystectomy is usually inevitable. Immunotherapeutic agents other than BCG have demonstrated promise in the treatment of bladder cancer and are recommended for use in BCG failure patient to achieve a long-standing remission or to delay the need for radical surgery.

The field of immunotherapy for superficial bladder cancer is still in a rudimentary stage. Over the next decade the introduction of novel approaches to its treatment (including tumor vaccines and gene therapy) should significantly improve the prognosis and further decrease the mortality of this common disease.

IMMUNOTHERAPY FOR PROSTATE CANCER

As longevity increases, prostate cancer presents a growing problem in the United States and other Western countries. In 1994 in the United States, 132,000 new cases of prostate cancer were diagnosed and 36,000 men died from the disease.[1,206] Prostate cancer has become the most frequently diagnosed malignancy in men, and it is estimated that in the next decade there will be a 37% increase in prostate cancer deaths and a 90% increase in number of cases diagnosed.[207] The optimal approach to the diagnosis and management of prostate cancer remains controversial throughout the medical, political, and economic communities. While advances in the detection and treatment of localized prostate cancer have become established,[208] minimal progress has been made in the treatment of advanced disease.

The 1941 landmark publication on prostate cancer by Huggins and Hodges[209] established androgen ablation as the mainstay treatment for newly diagnosed metastatic disease. Oral estrogens have since been replaced by luteinizing-hormone releasing hormone as the primary pharmacologic agent, yet 60% to 80% of men with advanced prostate cancer respond to either chemical or surgical castration.[210] Unfortunately, the durability of this treatment is short-lived and the tumor usually becomes hormone insensitive within 2 to 4 years. Once this occurs, the prognosis is bleak and median survival approaches 6 to 8 months.

Since the 1970's several new modalities of salvage therapy have been introduced.[210–212] With the possible exception of suramine,[213,214] none shows much promise. At the present time no effective or dependable, palliative or curative treatment exists for hormone refractory cancer of the prostate. With this current stasis of the traditional interventional therapies, immunotherapy offers an innovative and promising approach to the treatment of stage D-3 prostate cancer.

Immunotherapy and Prostate Cancer

Recent studies suggest that prostate cancer can be modulated by immune manipulations.[2,4,215,216] If this preliminary data is confirmed, new therapeutic modalities can be applied to treat prostate cancer, such as direct cytokine delivery and tumor vaccine production. Extensive research is currently focused on cytokines and the growth factors involved in the proliferation of prostate cancer cells. In vitro studies have demonstrated that numerous cytokines such as IL-2 and -4, IFN-α, IFN-γ, TNF-α, G-CSF, and GM-CSF, can generate immune responses against prostate tumor cells.[10,11,217]

Sanda and associates have recently described the use of a GM-CSF transduced retroviral tumor vaccine in a rat model, with subsequent tumor formation, reduction in tumor size, and regression of established tumors with a 30% cure rate.[11] Prolonged survival rates were noted in all treated animals, including those with residual tumors. The use of vaccine and gene therapies for treating prostate cancer is still in its early development. Its ultimate success will depend upon a comprehensive investigation of prostate cancer biology and a careful evaluation of potentially effective interventions.

CONCLUSION

Other than the application of BCG instillation in the treatment of superficial bladder cancer, immunotherapy is in its infancy. Yet even the specifics of BCG therapy, including such fundamental issues as the mechanism of action and the optimal dose and schedule of administration, have not been fully elucidated. Surgical treatment of genitourinary tumors, although very successful in ameliorating localized tumor, has little role in the therapy of advanced disease. Likewise, chemotherapy has been extremely disappointing in the application to metastatic renal cell, bladder, and prostate cancer. Immunotherapy holds promise as a viable treatment method for advanced disease. Obviously, continued research and clinical trials are needed to better define the optimal agents for treating advanced genitourinary tumors. This chapter has given an overview of the current status of immunotherapy as applied to these neoplasms. Exciting new treatment modalities, including the development of gene therapy and the creation of tumor vaccines, will further refine the indications and applications of immunotherapy.

REFERENCES

1. Nabel GJ, et al. Immunotherapy for malignancy by in vivo gene transfer into tumors. Hum Gene Ther 1992;3:399.
2. Haas GP, Solomon D, Rosenberg SA. Tumor infiltrating lymphocytes

from nonrenal urological malignancies. Cancer Immunol Immunother 1990;30:342.
3. Morales A, Nickel JC. Immunotherapy for superficial bladder cancer: a developmental and clinical overview. Urol Clin North Am 1992; 19:549.
4. Tso CL, Taneja S, et al. Modulation of cellular and molecular characteristics in prostate cancer cell lines by treatment with cytokines. Presented at AACR Annual Meeting, San Francisco, CA, 1994.
5. Belldegrun A, Figlin R, deKernion J. Immunotherapy for renal cell carcinoma. Semin Urol 1992;10:23.
6. Rosenberg SA, Spiess P, Lafreniere R. A new approach to the adoptive immunotherapy of cancer with tumor-infiltrating lymphocytes. Science 1986;233:1318.
7. Belldegrun A, et al. Human renal carinoma line transfected with interleukin-2 and/or interferon-gamma genes: implications for live cancer vaccines. J Natl Cancer Inst 1993;85:207.
8. Spiess PJ, Yang JC, Rosenberg SA. In vivo anti-tumor activity of tumor-infiltrating lymphocytes expanded in recombinant interleukin-2. J Natl Cancer Inst 1987;79:1067.
9. Horn HJG. Hormone-induced and spontaneous regression of metastatic renal cancer. Cancer 1973;32:1066.
10. Pardoll D. Immunotherapy with cytokine gene-transduced tumor cells the next wave in gene therapy for cancer. Curr Opin Oncol 1992;4: 1124.
11. Sanda MG, et al. Demonstration of a rational strategy for human prostate cancer gene therapy. J Urol 1994;151:622.
12. Pardoll DM. New strategies for enhancing the immunogenicity of tumors. Curr Opin Immunol 1993;5:719.
13. Gansbacher B, Rosenthal FM, Zier K. Retroviral vector-mediated cytokine gene transfer into tumor cells. Cancer Invest 1993;11:345.
14. Hill ADK, et al. Cytokines in tumour therapy. Br J Surg 1992;79: 990.
15. Talmadge JE. Development of immunotherapeutic strategies for the treatment of malignant neoplasma. Biotherapy 1992;4:215.
16. Weidmann E, et al. Rapid cytokine release in cancer patients treated with interleukin-2. J Immunol 1992;12:123.
17. Tomita Y, et al. Interferon-gamma but not tumor necrosis for factor alpha decreases susceptibility of human renal cell cancer lines to lymphokine-activated killer cells. Cancer Immunol Immunother 1992;35: 381.
18. Ogasawar M, Rosenberg SA. Enhanced expression of HLA molecules and stimulation of autologous human tumor infiltrating lymphocytes following transduction of melanoma cells with gamma-interferon genes. Cancer Res 1993;35:3561.
19. Zier B, et al. Retroviral gene transfer induced constitutive expression of interleukin-2 or interferon-gamma in irradiated human melanoma cells. Blood 1992;80:2817.
20. Smith KA. Interleukin-2: inception, impact, and implications. Science 1988;240:1169.
21. Parker SL, Tong T, Bolden S, Wingo PA. Cancer Statistics, 1996. CA Cancer J Clin 1996;65:5.
22. deKernion JB, Belldegrun A. Renal tumors. In: Walsh PC, et al. eds. Campbell's urology. Philadelphia: WB Saunders, 1993:1053.
23. deKernion JB. Renal tumors. In: Skinner DG, ed. Genitourinary cancer. Philadelphia: WB Saunders, 1978.
24. deKernion JB, Ramming KP. The therapy of renal adenocarcinoma with immune RNA. Invest Urol 1980;17:378.
25. Richie JP, et al. In vivo and in vitro effects of xenogeneic immune ribonucleic acid in patients with advanced renal cell carcinoma: a phase I study. J Urol 1981;126:24.
26. Steele G, et al. Results of oncogenic I-RNA therapy in patients with metastatic renal cell carcinoma. Cancer 1981;47:1286.
27. Ramming KP, deKernion JB. Immune RNA therapy for renal cell carcinoma: survival and immunologic monitoring. Ann Surg 1977; 186:549.
28. Minton JP, et al. Immunotherapy of human kidney cancer. Proc Am Soc Clin Oncol 1976;17:301.
29. Montie JD, et al. A critical review of immunotherapy of disseminated renal adenocarcinoma. J Surg Oncol 1982;21:5.
30. Morales A, et al. Cytoreductive surgery and systemic BCG therapy in metastatic renal cancer: a phase II trial. J Urol 1982;127:230.
31. McCune CS, Schapira DV, Henshaw EC. Specific immunotherapy of advanced renal carcinoma: evidence for polyclonality of metastases. Cancer 1981;47:1984.
32. Bukowski RM, et al. Immunotherapy of metastatic renal cell carcinoma. Proc Am Soc Clin Oncol 1979;20:402.
33. Morgan DA, Ruscetti FW, Gallo R. Selective in vitro growth of T lymphocytes from normal human bone marrow. Science 1976;193: 1007.
34. Duckett T, Figlin RA, Belldegrun A. Biological response modifiers in metastatic renal cell carcinoma. Curr Opin Urol 1992;2:339.
35. deKernion J, et al. The treatment of renal cell carcinoma with human leukocyte alpha-interferon. J Urol 1983;130:1063.
36. Quesada JR, et al. Renal cell carcinoma: antitumor effects of alpha-interferon. Cancer Res 1983;43:940.
37. Quesada JR, et al. Phase II study of interferon alpha in metastatic renal cell carcinoma. J Clin Oncol 1985;3:1086.
38. Kirkwood JM, et al. Randomized study of low and high doses of leukocyte alpha-interferon in metastatic renal cell carcinoma. Cancer Res 1985;45:863.
39. Figlin RA, deKernion JB, et al. Recombinant interferon alpha-2a in metastatic renal cell carcinoma. J Clin Oncol 1988;6:1604.
40. Umeda T, et al. Phase II study of alpha interferon on renal cell carcinoma: summary of three collaborative trials. Cancer 1986;58:1231.
41. Neidhart JA, et al. Interferon-alpha treatment of renal cancer. Cancer Res 1984;44:4140.
42. Vugrin D, Hood L, Laszlo J. A phase II trial of high dose human lymphoblastoid alpha interferon in patients with advanced renal carcinoma. J Biol Resp Mod 1986;5:309.
43. Vugrin D, Hood L, Taylor W, Laszlo J. Phase II study of human lymphoblastoid interferon in patients with advanced renal carcinoma. Cancer Treat Rep 1985;69:817.
44. Minasian LM, et al. Interferon alfa-2a in advanced renal cell carcinoma. J Clin Oncol 1993;11:1368.
45. Muss HB, et al. Recombinant alfa interferon in renal cell carcinoma: a randomized trial of two routes of administration. J Clin Oncol 1987; 5:286.
46. Neidhart JA. Interferon therapy for the treatment of renal cancer. Cancer 1986;57(Suppl 8):1696.
47. Sarna G, Figlin R, deKernion JB. Interferon in renal cell carcinoma. Cancer 1987;59:610.
48. Figlin RA, deKernion JB, Maldazys J, Sarna G. Treatment of renal cell carcinoma with alpha interferon and vinblastine in combination: a phase I–II trial. Cancer Treat Rep 1985;69:263.
49. Creagan ET, et al. An evaluation of recombinant leukocyte-A interferon with aspirin in patients with metastatic renal cell cancer. Cancer 1988;61:1787.
50. Jones GJ, Itri LM. Safety and tolerance of recombinant interferon 2a in cancer patients. Cancer 1986;57:1709.
51. Taguchi T. Clinical studies of recombinant interferon alfa-2a in cancer patients. Cancer 1986;57:1705.
52. Logothetis C, et al. 5-Fluorouracil and interferon-alpha in chemotherapy-refractory bladder carcinoma. Anticancer Resh 1994;14:1265.
53. Logothetis C. Treatment of chemotherapy-refractory metastatic urothelial tumors. Urol Clin North Am 1992;19:775.
54. Tomita Y, et al. 5-Fluorouracil increases susceptibility of renal cell cancer cell lines to lymphokine-activated killer cells. Cancer Lett 1993;75:27.
55. Sella A, et al. Phase II study of interferon-alpha and chemotherapy (5-FU and mitomycin-C) in metastatic renal cell carcinoma. J Urol 1992;147:573.
56. Sella A, Zukiwski A, et al. Interleukin-2 with interferon-alpha and 5-flourouricil in patients with metastatic renal cell cancer. Proc Am Soc Clin Oncol 1994;13:237.
57. Fossa SD, et al. Recombinant interferon alfa-2a with and without vinblastine in metastatic renal cell carcinoma. Cancer 1986;57:1700.
58. Muss HB, et al. Interferon and doxorubicin in renal cell carcinoma. Cancer Treat Rep 1985;69:721.
59. Creagan ET, et al. Phase I study of recombinant leukocyte a human interferon combined with BCNU in selected patients with advanced cancer. J Clin Oncol 1986;4:408.
60. Homma Y, Aso Y. Effect of alpha-interferon alone and combined with other anti-neoplastic agents on renal cell carcinoma determined by the tetrazolium microculture assay. Eur Urol 1994;25:164.
61. Ellenhorst JA, et al. Phase II trial of low dose gamma-interferon in metastatic renal cell carcinoma. J Urol 1994;152:841.
62. Rinehart J, et al. Phase I/II trial of human recombinant beta-interferon serine in patients with renal cell carcinoma. Cancer Res 1986;46:5364.

63. Quesada JR, et al. Phase II studies of recombinant human interferon gamma in metastic renal cell carcinoma. J Biol Resp Mod 1987;6:20.
64. Rinehart JJ, et al. Phase I/II trial of recombinant human interferon gamma in renal cell carcinoma. J Biol Resp Mod 1986;5:300.
65. Aulitzski W, et al. Successful treatment of metastatic renal cell carcinoma with a biologically active dose of recombinant interferon-gamma. J Clin Oncol 1989;7:1875.
66. Sayers TS, et al. Anti-tumor effects of alpha-interferon and gamma interferon in a murine renal cell carcinoma in vitro and in vivo. Cancer Rese 1990;20:5414.
67. Geboers AD, et al. Alpha and gamma interferon in the treatment of advanced renal cell carcinoma. Semin Surg Oncol 1988;4:191.
68. Nair SG, et al. Phase I/II trial of recombinant interferons alpha and gamma in patients with metastic renal cell carcinoma. Proc Am Soc Clin Oncol 1988;7:126.
69. Ernstoff MS, et al. A phase Ia trial of sequential administration of recombinant DNA-produced interferons. J Clin Oncol 1990;8:1637.
70. Rosenberg SA. Immunotherapy of cancer using IL-2. Immunol Today 1988;9:58.
71. Rosenberg SA. The immunology and gene therapy of cancer. Cancer Res 1991;51(18S):5074.
72. West WH, et al. Constant-infusion recombinant interleukin-2 in adoptive immunotherapy of advanced cancer. N Engl J Med 1987;316:898.
73. Fisher RI. Metastatic renal cancer treated with interleukin-2 and lymphokine-activated killer cells. Ann Intern Med 1988;108:518.
74. FDA Biological Response Modifiers Advisory Committee Hearings, Washington, DC, 1992.
75. Rosenberg SA, Yang JC, Topaliam SL, et al. Treatment of 283 consecutive patients with metastatic melanoma or renal cell cancer using high-dose bolus interleukin-2. JAMA 1994;271:907.
76. Rosenstein M, Ettinghausen SE, Rosenberg SA. Extravasation of intravascular fluid mediated by the systemic administration of recombinant interleukin-2. J Immunol 1986;137:1735.
77. Siegel JP, Puri RK. Interleukin-2 toxicity. J Clin Oncol 1991;9:694.
78. Belldegrun A, Pierce WC, Kakoo R, et al. Interferon alpha-primed tumor infiltrating lymphocytes combined with interleukin-2 and interferon-alpha as a therapy for metastatic renal cell carcinoma. J Urol 1993;150:1384.
79. Belldegrun A, Webb DA, Austin HA, et al. Effects of interleukin-2 on renal function in patients receiving immunotherapy for advanced cancer. Ann Intern Med 1987;106:817.
80. Webb ED, Austin HA, Belldegrun A, et al. Metabolic and renal effects of IL-2 immunotherapy for metastatic renal cell carcinoma. Clin Nephrol 1988;30:141.
81. Bukowski RM, et al. Phase II trial of high-dose intermittent interleukin-2 in metastatic renal cell carcinoma. J Natl Cancer Inst 1990;82:143.
82. Geertsen PF, Hermann GG, van der Maase H, Steven K. Treatment of metastatic renal cell carcinoma by continuous intravenous infusion of recombinant interleukin-2: a single center phase II study. J Clin Oncol 1992;10:753.
83. Weiss GR, et al. A randomized phase II trial of continuous infusion interleukin-2 or bolus injection interleukin-2 plus lymphokine-activated killer cells for advanced renal cell carcinoma. J Clin Oncol 1992;19:275.
84. Thompson JA, Shulman KL, Benyunes MC, et al. Prolonged continuous intravenous infusion interleukin-2 and lymphocyte-activated killer cell therapy for metastic renal cell carcinoma. J Clin Oncol 1992;10:960.
85. Buter J, et al. A progress report on the outpatient treatment of patient with advanced renal cell carcinoma using subcutaneous recombinant interleukin-2. Semin Oncol 1993;20(Suppl 9):16.
86. Koretz MJ, et al. Randomized study of interleukin-2 alone vs IL-2 plus lymphokine-activated killer cells for treatment of melanoma and renal cell cancer. Arch Surgery 1991;126:898.
87. Rosenber SA, Schwarz SL, Spiess PJ. Combination immunotherapy for cancer: synergistic antitumor interactions of interleukin-2, alfa interferon, and tumor-infiltrating lymphocytes. J Natl Cancer Inst 1988;80:1393.
88. Brunda MJ, Bellantoni D, Sulich V. In vivo anti-tumor activity of combinations of interferon alpha and interleukin-2 in a murine model. Int J Cancer 1987;40:365.
89. Rosenberg SA, et al. Combination therapy with interleukin-2 and alpha-interferon for the treatment of patients with advanced cancer. J Clinical Oncol 1989;7:1863.
90. Vogelzang NJ, Lipton A, Figlin RA. Subcutaneous IL-2 plus interferon in metastatic renal cell cancer: an outpatient multicenter trial. J Clin Oncol 1993;11:1809.
91. Rosenberg SA, et al. Experience with the use of high-dose interleukin-2 in the treatment of 652 cancer patients. Ann Surg 1989;210:474.
92. Figlin RA, Belldegrun A, Moldawer N, Zeffren J, deKernion J. Concomitant administration of recombinant human interleukin-2 and recombinant interferon alfa-2a: an active outpatient regimen in metastatic renal cell carcinoma. J Clinical Oncol 1992;10:414.
93. Atzpodien J, Korfer A, Palmer PA, et al. Treatment of metastatic renal cell cancer patients with recombinant subcutaneous human interleukin-2 and alpha-interferon. Ann Oncol 1990;1:377.
94. Hirsch M, et al. Phase I study of interleukin-2 and interferon-alpha-2a as outpatient therapy for patients with advanced malignancy. J Clin Oncol 1990;8:1657.
95. Gray D, Sprent J. Immunological memory. Curr Top Microbiol Immunol 1990;159:1.
96. Sawcsuk IS. Autolymphocyte therapy in the treatment of metastatic renal cell carcinoma. Urol Clin North Am 1993;20:297.
97. Herzberg VL, Smith KA. T cell growth without serum. J Immunol 1987;139:998.
98. Osband ME, Lavin PT, Babayan RK, et al. Effect of autolymphocyte therapy on survival and quality of life in patients with metastatic renal cell carcinoma. Lancet 1990;335:994.
99. Lavin PT, Maar R, Franklin M, et al. Autolymphocyte therapy for metastatic renal cell carcinoma: initial clinical results from 335 patients treated in a multi-site clinical practice. Transplant Proc 1992;24:3059.
100. Graham S, Babayan RK, Lamm DL, et al. The use of ex vivo-activated memory T cells (autolymphocyte therapy) in the treatment of metastatic renal cell carcinoma: final results from a randomized controlled multi-site study. Semin Urol 1993;11:27.
101. Pierce WC, Belldegrun A, Figlin RA. Cellular therapy: scientific rationale and clinical results in the treatment of metastatic renal cell carcinoma. Semin Oncol 1995;22(1):74.
102. Grimm EA, Mazumder A, Zhang HZ, et al. Lymphokine-activated killer cell phenomenon. J Exp Med 1993;155:1823.
103. Mule JJ, Shu S, Rosenberg SA. The anti-tumor efficacy of lymphokine-activated killer cells and recombinant interleukin-2 in vivo. J Immunol 1985;135:646.
104. Rosenberg SA, et al. Regression of established pulmonary metastases and subcutaneous tumor mediated by the systemic administration of high dose IL-2. J Exp Med 161:1169.
105. Rosenberg SA, Lotze MT, Yang JC, et al. Prospective randomized trial of high-dose interleukin-2 alone or in conjunction with lymphokine-activated killer cells for the treatment of patients with advanced cancer. J Natl Cancer Inst 1993;85:622.
106. Belldegrun A, Pierce W, Sayah D, et al. Soluble tumor necrosis factor expression in patients with metastatic renal cell carcinoma treated with interleukin-2-based immunotherapy. J Immunother 1993;13:175.
107. Schendel DJ, Gansbacher B, Oberneder R, et al. Tumor-specific lysis of human renal cell carcinomas by tumor-infiltrating lymphocytes. J Immunol 1993;151:4209.
108. Rosenberg SA, et al. Use of tumor-infiltrating lymphocytes and interleukin-2 in the immunotherapy of patients with metastatic melanoma. N Engl J Med 1988;319:1676.
109. Bukowski PM, et al. Clinical results and characterization of tumor-infiltrating lymphocytes with or without recombinant interleukin-2 in human metastatic renal cell carcinoma. Cancer Res 1991;51:4199.
110. Elson PJ, Witte RS, Trump DL. Prognostic factors for survival in patients with recurrent or metastatic renal cell carcinoma. Cancer Res 1988;48:7310.
111. Steger GG, Pierce WC, et al. Patterns in cytokine release of unselected and CD8+ selected renal cell carcinoma tumor-infiltrating lymphocytes. Clin Immol Immunopathol 1994;72:237.
112. Ernstoff MS, Gooding W, Nair S, et al. Immunological effects of treatment with sequential administration of recombinant interferon-gamma and alpha in patients with metasatic renal cell carcinoma during a phase I trial. Cancer Res 1992;52:851.
113. Watanabe Y, Kuribayashi K, Miyatake S, et al. Exogenous expression of mouse interferon-gamma cDNA in mouse neuroblastoma C1300

alpha-inteferon for renal cell carcinoma and melanoma. Eur J Cancer 1992;28A:1047.
224. Spencer WF, Linehan WM, Walter MM, et al. Immunotherapy with interleukin-2 and alpha interferon in patients with metastatic renal cell carcinoma with in situ primary cancers: a pilot study. J Urol 1992; 147:24.
225. Budd GT, et al. Phase I trial of high dose bolus interleukin-2 and interferon-alpha-2a in patients with metastatic malignancy. J Clin Oncol 1992;10:804.
226. Sznol M, Clark JW, Smith JW, et al. Pilot study of interleukin-2 and lymphokine-activated killer cells combined with immunomodulatory doses of chemotherapy and sequenced with interferon alfa-2a in patients with metastatic melanoma and renal cell carcinoma. J Natl Cancer Inst 1992;84:929.
227. Ilson DH, Motzer RJ, Kradin RL, et al. A phase II trial of interleukin-2 and interferon alfa-2a in patients with advanced renal cell carinoma. J Clin Oncol 1992;10:1124.
228. Lipton A, Harvey H, Givant E, et al. Interleukin-2 and interferon alpha-2a outpatient therapy for metastatic renal cell carcinoma. J Immunother 1993;13:122.
229. Bergmann L, et al. Daily alternating administration of high-dose alpha-2b interferon and interleukin-2 bolus infusion in metastatic renal cell cancer. Cancer 1993;72:1733.
230. Parkinson DR, Fisher RI, Rayner AA, et al. Therapy of renal cell carcinoma with interleukin-2 and lymphokine-activated killer cells: phase II experience with a hybrid bolus and continuous infusion interleukin-2 regimen. J Clin Oncol 1990;8:1630.
231. Dillman RO, Church C, et al. Inpatient continuous-infusion interleukin-2 in 788 patients with cancer: the national biotherapy study group experience. Cancer 1993;71:2358.
232. Palmer PA, Vinke J, Ever P, et al. Continuous infusion of recombinant interkleukin-2 with or without autologous lymphocyte-activated killer cells for the treatment of advanced renal cell carcinoma. Eur J Cancer 1992;28A:1038.
233. Foon KA, Walther PJ, Bernstein ZP, et al. Renal cell carcinoma treated with continuous-infusion interleukin-2 with ex-vivo activated killer cells. J Immunother 1992;11:184.

Principles and Practice of Genitourinary Oncology, edited by Derek Raghavan, Howard I. Scher, Steven A. Leibel, and Paul H. Lange. Lippincott-Raven Publishers, Philadelphia, © 1997.

CHAPTER 85

Chemotherapy for Renal Cell Carcinoma

Robert J. Motzer and Nicholas J. Vogelzang

Renal cell carcinoma (RCC) is a frequent cause of cancer mortality, responsible for more than 10,000 deaths per year in the United States.[1] This is the result of a lack of effective systemic treatment for patients with metastatic disease. Advanced RCC is characterized by a high level of resistance to all treatment modalities that have been studied, including cytotoxic agents, hormonal therapy, and biologic response modifiers. Although no single agent consistently shows a response proportion of 20% or higher, interleukin 2 (IL2) and interferon-α (IFNA) have demonstrated a low but reproducible response proportion in the 10% to 20% range, with durable responses of 5% or less.[2] The experience with chemotherapy and hormonal treatment are reviewed in this chapter, along with the general principles of management for patients with advanced RCC.

CHEMOTHERAPY

Investigative efforts with chemotherapeutic agents have been extensive. Prior to 1975, nitrogen mustard,[3] hydroxyurea,[4] lomustine,[5] dacarbazine,[6] and hexamethylmelamine[6] were studied and did not show antitumor activity for RCC. A comprehensive review of the published literature shows that from 1975 through 1994, 80 single agents were studied in 155 trials (Table 85-1). Overall, 143 (4%) responses were achieved in 3951 evaluable patients. No agent has been shown to achieve major responses (complete or partial) in more than 20% of evaluable patients (with a sample size of 14 or more patients). Because of the lack of antitumor activity with conventional agents, the study of new agents remains justifiable in chemotherapy-naive patients.

The two agents that have been reported to have some, albeit minimal, antitumor activity are vinblastine and floxuridine (FUDR). Early studies suggested vinblastine had activity as a single agent, with a 26% response proportion reported in 135 patients.[7] This study served as the basis for the inclusion of vinblastine in trials as a part of combined therapy with IFN or with agents that modulate multidrug resistance (MDR). However, the results of more recent trials with vinblastine showed only nine responses in 135 (6%) evaluable patients (see Table 85-1).[74,90,195–199]

A 20% response proportion was reported with continuous intravenous infusion of FUDR administered according to a circadian schedule.[8] Response proportions ranged from 0% to 14% in seven subsequent trials of FUDR given in a similar fashion; one of these trials included folinic acid.[9–15] Enthusiasm prompted by the first trial resulted in the conduction of a randomized multicenter phase III trial of FUDR administered by flat continuous infusion versus a circadian modified 14-day infusion schedule. The preliminary report of this trial indicated that the response proportion for 82 evaluable patients treated in both arms was 9% (95% confidence interval, 4% to 17%).[16]

In addition to the trials of single agents, many combinations of chemotherapy agents have been studied.[17–25] These have not shown superior antitumor activity over the single agents, and toxicity was generally increased. The lack of antitumor activity for any of the many chemotherapy agents that have been studied emphasizes the need for novel treatment strategies in patients with advanced RCC.

HORMONAL THERAPY

The rationale for the study of hormonal agents in RCC was provided by results obtained in animal models in the 1940s and the low concentrations of progesterone receptors found in human RCC.[26] The animal models showed hormone dependence and responsiveness in renal cancers induced in the Syrian hamster model.[26]

Bloom[26,27] initially reported a 16% to 21% response proportion for medroxyprogesterone (MP) in RCC. In the four trials published since 1980, the response proportion declined to 5% (Table 85-2).[28–31] Other hormonal agents also have been extensively studied. Testosterone and various other androgens achieved an overall 7% response proportion (see Table 85-2). The direct androgen antagonist flutamide was shown to be inactive.[32] The antiestrogens—tamoxifen, nafoxidine, and toremifene—were also studied in multiple trials and found to be relatively inactive, with a 6% response proportion achieved in 318 patients treated in 11 trials.

The addition of hormonal therapy to chemotherapy does not add efficacy; this was evident from the results of single-arm

TABLE 85-1. *Results of chemotherapy for renal cell carcinoma*

Agent	Year and reference	No. of patients	Complete response/ partial response (%)
Acivicin	1988[74]	27	0/1 (4)
Aclacinomycin	1984[75]	15	0/0 (0)
L-Alanosine	1988[74]	36	1/0 (3)
6-Aminonicatinamide	1989[76]	19	1/0 (5)
Ametantrone	1985[77]	25	0/2 (8)
Aminothiazide	1988[74]	46	0/1 (2)
Amonafide	1991[78]	24	0/0 (0)
Amsacrine	1980[79]	16	0/0 (0)
	1980[80]	21	0/0 (0)
	1983[81]	61	0/1 (2)
	1983[82]	42	0/1 (2)
5′-Aza-2-deoxycytidine	1987[83]	12	0/0 (0)
Bisantrene	1982[84]	26	0/0 (0)
	1982[85]	37	0/2 (3)
	1985[86]	20	0/0 (0)
	1985[87]	14	0/0 (0)
	1987[19]	29	1/2 (10)
Bleomycin	1975[88]	15	0/0 (0)
	1976[89]	8	0/3 (37)
	1977[90]	7	0/0 (0)
Carboplatin	1988[91]	19	0/0 (0)
	1990[92]	18	0/0 (0)
Chlorozotocin	1979[93]	21	0/0 (0)
Cisplatin	1978[94]	23	0/0 (0)
	1979[95]	10	0/0 (0)
Cyclophosphamide	1975[96]	10	0/0 (0)
	1979[97]	44	0/2 (4)
	1980[98]	12	0/0 (0)
Plus misonidazole	1986[99]	30	0/1 (3)
Dactinomycin	1981[23]	61	0/1 (2)
10-Deazaaminopterin	1984[100]	12	0/0 (0)
2-Deoxycoformycin (Pentostatin)	1991[101]	18	0/0 (0)
	1992[102]	25	0/0 (0)
4′-Deoxydoxorubicin (Esorubicin)	1986[103]	12	0/0 (0)
	1986[104]	27	0/0 (0)
	1987[105]	24	0/0 (0)
	1989[106]	19	1/1 (10)
	1990[107]	15	0/1 (7)
4-Demethoxydaunorubicin	1985[108]	19	0/0 (0)
Dianhydrogalactitol	1981[97]	53	0/0 (0)
	1982[109]	41	0/1 (2)
Diaziquone	1982[110]	20	0/0 (0)
	1984[111]	29	0/0 (0)
	1986[112]	55	0/1 (2)
	1986[113]	15	0/0 (0)
Dibromodulcitol (Mitolactol)	1981[114]	13	0/1 (8)
	1986[115]	31	1/2 (10)
Didemnin B	1990[116]	21	0/1 (5)
	1992[117]	22	0/0 (0)
Docetaxel	1994[118]	18	0/0 (0)
Doxorubicin	1977[119]	38	0/2 (5)
Echinomycin	1993[120]	47	0/1 (2)
Elliptinium	1985[121]	8	0/0 (0)
	1985[122]	38	2/3 (13)
	1988[123]	14	0/0 (0)
4'-Epi-adriamycin (Epirubicin)	1982[124]	20	0/0 (0)
	1983[125]	19	0/0 (0)
Estramustine	1981[126]	16	0/0 (0)
Etoposide	1979[97]	43	1/0 (2)

TABLE 85-1. *Continued.*

Agent	Year and reference	No. of patients	Complete response/ partial response (%)
Floxurine (circadian)	1990[8]	56	4/7 (20)
	1990[9]	42	3/3 (14)
	1991[10]	14	0/0 (0)
	1991[11]	40	0/4 (10)
	1992[12]	26	0/2 (8)
	1993[13]	28	0/4 (14)
	1993[14]	15	0/1 (7)
Plus folinic acid	1991[15]	15	0/0 (0)
By flat infusion	1991[127]	29	0/0 (0)
	1993[128]	29	1/5 (21)
Fludarabine	1987[129]	30	0/0 (0)
	1989[130]	15	0/0 (0)
5-Fluorouracil	1991[42]	27	0/2 (7)
	1993[43]	35	0/4 (11)
	1994[44]	61	1/2 (5)
Plus folinic acid	1989[45]	14	0/0 (0)
Fosquidone	1992[131]	21	0/0 (0)
Fotemustine	1991[132]	62	1/3 (7)
	1993[133]	16	0/0 (0)
Ftorafur	1993[134]	14	0/0 (0)
Gallium nitrate	1984[135]	10	0/0 (0)
	1987[136]	25	0/1 (4)
Gemcitibine	1992[137]	30	1/2 (10)
	1993[138]	18	0/1 (6)
Hydroxyrea	1981[139]	19	0/1 (5)
ICRF-187	1986[140]	40	0/0 (0)
Ifosfamide	1980[141]	11	0/1 (9)
	1981[142]	10	0/2 (20)
	1987[143]	16	0/0 (0)
	1988[144]	9	0/0 (0)
Liposomal encapsulated doxorubicin	1995[145]	14	0/0 (0)
Lomustine	1977[90]	9	0/0 (0)
	1986[146]	5	0/0 (0)
Lonidamine	1986[147]	25	0/2 (8)
	1991[148]	19	1/1 (10)
LY186641	1993[149]	16	1/0 (6)
Mafosfamide	1992[150]	16	1/0 (6)
Melphalan	1993[151]	8	0/0 (0)
Menogaril	1990[152]	56	0/3 (5)
	1991[153]	15	0/0 (0)
Methodichlorophen	1979[154]	10	0/3 (30)
Methotrexate	1980[20]	8	0/2 (25)
Mitoguazone (methyl-GAG)	1981[155]	25	1/3 (16)
	1981[156]	31	0/0 (0)
	1982[157]	30	0/3 (10)
	1981[158]	14	0/0 (0)
	1983[159]	87	1/3 (4)
Mitomycin	1987[160]	12	0/3 (25)
Mitotane	1981[161]	12	0/0 (0)
Mitoxantrone	1984[162]	20	0/0 (0)
	1984[163]	49	0/0 (0)
	1984[164]	29	0/0 (0)
	1986[165]	48	0/0 (0)
Mitozolomide	1989[166]	17	0/0 (0)
N-methylformamide	1986[167]	16	0/0 (0)
	1989[168]	14	0/0 (0)
Navelbine	1991[169]	14	0/0 (0)
	1993[170]	24	1/0 (4)

(continued)

TABLE 85-1. *Continued.*

Agent	Year and reference	No. of patients	Complete response/ partial response (%)
Paclitaxel	1991[171]	18	0/0 (0)
PALA (sparfosic acid)	1982[172]	15	0/0 (0)
	1983[81]	52	0/2 (4)
PCNU	1984[173]	34	0/1 (3)
	1987[19]	45	0/0 (0)
Pirarubicin	1987[174]	16	0/1 (6)
	1993[175]	34	0/1 (3)
Piperazinedione	1977[176]	23	0/0 (0)
Piroxantrone	1992[177]	32	0/0 (0)
Spirogermanium	1987[178]	26	0/0 (0)
	1984[179]	36	0/0 (0)
Streptozocin	1987[180]	18	0/1 (6)
Sulofenur	1992[181]	18	0/0 (0)
Suramin	1991[182]	10	0/0 (0)
	1992[183]	26	0/1 (4)
Tauromustine	1989[184]	33	0/0 (0)
Taxotere	1993[185]	33	0/2 (6)
Teniposide	1979[186]	12	0/0 (0)
	1984[187]	32	0/3 (9)
	1987[188]	51	0/1 (2)
6-Thioguanine	1991[189]	30	0/2 (7)
Thiotepa	1977[90]	7	0/1 (14)
Topotecan	1994[190]	14	0/0 (0)
Triazinate	1981[23]	59	1/2 (5)
1,2,4-Triglycidyl-urazo	1986[191]	14	0/0 (0)
	1987[192]	16	0/0 (0)
Trimetrexate	1989[193]	14	0/0 (0)
	1992[194]	34	0/1 (3)
Vinblastine	1977[90]	10	0/0 (0)
	1984[195]	19	0/3 (16)
	1984[196]	10	0/0 (0)
	1985[197]	14	0/0 (0)
	1987[198]	21	1/1 (9)
	1988[74]	35	0/3 (9)
	1992[199]	26	1/0 (4)
Vindesine	1977[200]	17	0/0 (0)
	1983[201]	24	0/0 (0)
Yoshi-864*	1982[202]	30	0/2 (6)

* Plus medroxyprogesterone acetate.

phase II trials[25,33–35] as well as a randomized trial that showed no increase in the response proportion when MP combined with IFN was compared with IFN alone.[36] Hormonal therapy has little antitumor effect against RCC; responses are infrequent and generally of short duration. The role of hormones in the treatment of RCC may be best considered as a component of supportive care for the properties of progestins in promoting appetite and weight gain.

COMBINATION THERAPY

Based on the low but reproducible response proportion of immunotherapeutic agents such as IL2 and IFN, combinations of chemotherapy and immunotherapy have been studied in RCC (Table 85-3). The combination that has been most extensively studied is IFN plus vinblastine. The results of 13 studies that included 307 patients showed an overall 24% response rate, which appeared to be somewhat higher than that reported with IFN alone.[2] Three randomized trials have addressed the efficacy of interferon α (IFNA) plus vinblastine versus IFNA alone.[37–39] Although one trial showed a slightly higher response proportion for the combination,[38] none have shown improved survival (compared with survival for patients treated with IFNA alone), and the vinblastine added gastrointestinal and hematologic toxicity.[37]

Combinations of 5-fluorouracil (5-FU) or FUDR with IL2, IFN, or both have been studied. The rationale was based on the single-agent activity of FUDR in RCC and the antitumor effects of IFN and 5-FU, another pyridamole analog, against adenocarcinoma of the colon. Two studies have shown high response rates with a combination of 5-FU, IFN and IL2.[40,41] Although these combinations are promising and warrant further investigation, caution must be exercised in interpreting the results of these studies in the context of standard care of patients with advanced RCC. The antitumor activity of single-agent 5-FU ranged from 0% to 11% in four trials.[42–45] The combination of IL2 and IFN has been extensively studied; response proportions range from 0% to 40%, with an overall response proportion of

TABLE 85-2. *Results of hormonal therapy for renal cell carcinoma*

Agent	Year and reference	No. of patients	Complete response/ partial response (%)
Medroxyprogesterone (or other progestins)	1969[203]	8	0/2 (13)
	1970[204]	15	0/2 (13)
	1971[205]	60	0/9 (15)
	1971[206]	35	0/6 (17)
	1971[207]	21	0/2 (10)
	1973[208]	61	5/2 (11)
	1974[209]	17	0/0 (0)
	1980[210]	23	1/2 (13)
	1981[28]	9	0/0 (0)
	1984[29]	13	0/0 (0)
	1985[30]	18	0/0 (0)
	1986[31]	21	1/2 (14)
Testosterone propionate (or other androgens)	1969[203]	11	0 (0)
	1971[206]	27	0/2 (7)
	1974[209]	23	0 (0)
	1975[32]	20	0 (0)
Flutamide	1984[211]	25	0/1 (4)
Nafoxidine	1979[212]	20	0/1 (5)
	1981[139]	19	2/1 (16)
Tamoxifen	1980[213]	15	0/0 (0)
	1980[214]	12	0/0 (0)
	1981[215]	79	2/3 (6)
	1981[216]	10	0/0 (0)
	1992[217]	34	1/3 (12)
	1993[218]	59	0/1 (2)
	1993[219]	20	1/0 (5)
	1991[148]	25	2/1 (12)
Toremifene	1993[220]	25	0/3 (12)

TABLE 85-3. *Results of selected combination regimens for renal cell carcinoma*

Agents	Author and reference	No. of patients	Complete response/ partial response (%)
Interferon plus vinblastine	1985[221]	23	0/3 (13)
	1986[222]	18	1/7 (44)
	1986[223]	16	0/5 (31)
	1987[224]	24	1/8 (37)
	1987[225]	13	0/3 (23)
	1988[226]	40	1/16 (42)
	1989[227]	18	1/4 (28)
	1989[220]	56	0/9 (16)
	1990[228]	11	0/2 (18)
	1990[229]	22	3/3 (30)
	1990[230]	15	0/1 (7)
	1991[231]	42	1/5 (14)
	1991[232]	9	0/0 (0)
Interferon plus fluorouracil	1992[233]	14	0/0 (0)
	1992[234]	20	0/7 (35)
	1993[235]	21	0/5 (24)
	1994[236]	31	1/6 (23)
Interferon plus floxurine	1991[237]	13	0/4 (31)
	1992[238]*	20	0/0 (0)
	1993[239]	15	1/4 (33)
	1993[240]	11	0/0 (0)
Interleukin 2, interferon, 5-fluorouracil	1993[40]	35	4/13 (49)
	1994[41]	19	3/6 (47)
Inteferon plus 13-cis-retinoic acid	1994[48]†	43	3/7 (30)

* Plus leukovorin.
† Results updated for presentation.

19% in 607 patients.[46] In a randomized phase II trial, increased toxicity was seen with the addition of IFN to IL2 compared with IL2 alone, without an increase in response proportion.[47] Combination therapy generally is associated with additive toxicity; the proportion of patients with grade III/IV stomatitis in one of the trials of IFN, IL2, and 5-FU was 26%, which is most likely attributable to 5-FU.[41] Response proportions vary among clinical trials of cytokines in patients with RCC, which suggests that patient selection plays an important role in the response proportion. Although the response proportion of these regimens is encouraging, their relative efficacy compared to that of IFN or IL2 alone can only be assessed in the context of a randomized phase III trial.

The combination of IFN and 13-cis-retinoic acid (CRA) produced a 30% response proportion in a phase II trial.[48] Several aspects of this study suggested that CRA added efficacy to IFNA:

The response proportion was triple that previously reported from the same center in trials of IFNA alone or in combination with vinblastine (10% in 149 patients).[37]
Durable responses were achieved.
Responses were seen in sites generally considered to be resistant to IFNA, (i.e., bone and primary tumor).

Moreover, in vitro studies suggested that CRA augmented the antitumor effects of IFNA in several renal cancer cell lines and suggested that retinoid effects in renal cancer cells may be mediated through the retinoic acid receptor-β. Therefore, a phase III randomized trial has been initiated to study the relative efficacy of IFN and CRA compared with IFN.

MODULATION OF DRUG RESISTANCE

The observation that RCC is refractory to chemotherapy has prompted studies that attempt to overcome inherent drug resistance. One proposed mechanism of drug resistance is MDR, which is associated with the *MDR1* gene and its protein product, the P-glycoprotein.

RCC has been shown to arise from the renal proximal tubular epithelial cell in more than 85% of cases.[49] Phenotypic markers that characterize proximal tubule cells are commonly found on renal carcinoma cells, an association that may explain the nearly uniform expression of P-glycoprotein on renal carcinoma cells, because this protein is normally present in the luminal membrane of the proximal tubule cell.[49] Expression of P-glycoprotein, a 170-kd phosphoglycoprotein encoded by the *MDR1* gene, is necessary for MDR, which was first recognized in the laboratory, where models exposed to a single drug developed a broad cross-resistance to a group of distinct cytotoxic agents.

The results of phase II trials of MDR reversal agents used in clinical trials against RCC are shown in Table 85-4. The addition of cyclosporin A, dipyridamole, nifedipine, tamoxifen, or quinidine to vinblastine did not result in enhanced antitumor activity. The Cancer and Leukemia Group B has completed a randomized phase II trial of vinblastine alone followed by treatment with vinblastine plus either cyclosporin A or tamoxifen.[50] Sixty-four patients were evaluable to response to vinblastine alone; no responses were seen. Twenty-eight patients received modulators without an observed objective response. The final results of this trial are awaited.

The prototype of MDR reversal agents is verapamil, which since 1981 has been known to substantially reverse MDR in vitro.[51] The clinical application of verapamil, however, has been limited by the profound hypotension, negative inotropic effects, and atrioventricular conduction delays associated with plasma levels of verapamil that in nearly all instances have been lower than those targeted for reversal of resistance.[52–57]

Standard verapamil is a racemic mixture of dextro (d-) and levo (l-) stereoisomers. The l-isomer has a markedly greater effect on the slowing of atrioventricular node conduction compared with the d-isomer.[58] Because both isomers have been shown to be equally effective in reversing drug resistance in vitro,[59,60] the decreased cardiovascular toxicity of the d-isomer (dexverapamil) made this drug an attractive alternative to the standard racemic verapamil preparations for MDR reversal. A trial of dexverapamil and vinblastine was conducted in patients with advanced RCC.[61] Dexverapamil was generally well tolerated; however, no antitumor activity was found in 23 assessable patients, despite the fact that plasma concentrations of dexverapamil and norverapamil were achieved that were in the range that resulted in enhanced cytotoxicity in vitro.[61]

The existence of multiple, redundant mechanisms of resistance has been proposed as one explanation for the lack of antitumor activity observed in clinical trials utilizing MDR modulation in patients with tumors that constitutively express *MDR1*, which includes RCC.[62] The lack of antitumor activity found in these trials emphasizes the need for new insights in overcoming drug resistance in RCC.

OBSERVATION ALONE

Metastatic RCC is characterized by a variability in clinical course. It is one of the few malignancies for which spontaneous regressions are well documented.[63] A prospective phase II trial was conducted in which patients who were referred to a center were identified prospectively and observed. Several patients were noted to have spontaneous regression, and the proportion of patients who remained progression-free for 12 months or more was 12%.[64] This finding has implications both in clinical

TABLE 85-4. *Results of drug resistance reversal agents against renal cell carcinoma*

Agents	Author and reference	No. of patients	Complete response/ partial response (%)
Vinblastine plus cyclosporin A	1991[241]	15	0/0 (0)
Vinblastine plus dipyridamole	1994[242]	15	0/0 (0)
Vinblastine plus nifedipine	1991[243]	14	0/0 (0)
Vinblastine plus quinidine	1991[244]	23	1/0 (4)
Vinblastine plus dexverapamil	1994[61]	23	0/0 (0)
Vinblastine plus cyclosporin A or tamoxifen	1994[50]	28	0/0 (0)

investigations and in patient care. Tumor regressions attributed to an investigational agent must be separated from those that occur as a consequence of natural history. One means of accomplishing this is to include only patients with documented progressive disease in clinical trials. Additionally, responses to systemic therapies for RCC are infrequent and all are associated with some degree of toxicity; therefore, patients who are asymptomatic may be observed until evidence of progression or symptoms, at which time systemic treatment can be initiated.

SURGERY IN PATIENTS WITH METASTATIC DISEASE

In patients with metastatic disease, surgical resection may be considered in selected patients with solitary metastases. Several series have shown a 5-year survival range of 15% to 50%.[65–70] Resection may also include the renal primary tumor in cases of synchronous presentation with a solitary metastasis.

One controversy in the management of patients with RCC is the role of nephrectomy in the setting of metastatic disease. Nephrectomy may be justified when the intent is providing improved quality of life, such as the alleviation of local symptoms. However, a nephrectomy for the purpose of inducing spontaneous regression is not justifiable; the incidence of regression after nephrectomy in nine series of 474 patients was only 0.8%.[71] More controversial is the role of nephrectomy as an adjunct to immunotherapy. Until a benefit for this approach is established in a randomized trial, its use should be considered investigational and not part of standard care.

Based on the lack of antitumor effect with systemic therapy and the relative resistance of RCC to radiotherapy, surgical intervention is an appropriate palliative measure in highly selected instances. These include the resection of solitary brain metastasis, surgery to alleviate spinal cord compression, and repair of pathologic or impending fractures in weight-bearing bones.

CONCLUSIONS

Despite extensive investigations with many different treatment modalities, RCC remains a disease that is highly resistant to systemic therapy. Novel treatment strategies should be studied in RCC. The identification of new agents with better antitumor activity remains the highest clinical investigation priority in this refractory tumor.

Although response proportions with IFN and IL2 are low (10% to 20%), responses have been reproducible and occasionally are durable. As such, these agents represent a direction for continued research. In particular, the combinations of IFN and CRA or 5-FU, with or without IL2, are encouraging, and their relative efficacy must be further investigated in the context of a randomized trial. Moreover, the investigation of new cytokines is warranted. One particularly promising new cytokine is interleukin 12, which is entering phase I and II trials in RCC.[72]

Prognostic factors need to be established to help direct therapy to patients who are most likely to benefit. Although features such as high performance status and lung-only metastasis are predictive of survival and response, more precise pretreatment factors are needed.[37,39] The limitations of prognostic classifications based on clinical factors are well recognized; future efforts should include prognostic factors based on tumor biology. For example, the absence of a kidney-restricted glycoprotein of 160,000 kd (gp160) in renal cancer cells is associated with marked sensitivity in vitro to inhibition of growth by IFN, whereas tumor cells expressing gp160 are resistant to the antiproliferative effects of IFN.[73] Whether this correlates to response in patients treated with IFN is unknown, but it is an example of the potential application of laboratory findings to the management of patients with RCC.

REFERENCES

1. Boring CC, Squires TS, Tong T, Montgomery S. Cancer Statistics, 1994. Ca Cancer J Clin 1994;44:7.
2. Wirth MP. Immunotherapy for metastatic renal cell carcinoma. Urol Clin North Am 1993;20:283.
3. Talley RW, Moorehead EL, Tucker W. Treatment of metastatic hypernephroma. JAMA 1969;207:322.
4. Nevinny HB, Hall TC. Chemotherapy with hydroxyurea (NSC-32065) in renal cell carcinoma. J Clin Pharmacol 1968;8:352.
5. Mittelman A, Albert DJ, Murphy GP. Lomustine treatment of metastatic renal cell carcinoma. JAMA 1973;225:32.
6. Carter SK, Wasserman TH. The chemotherapy of urologic oncology. Cancer 1975;36:729.
7. Hrushesky WJ, Murphy GP. Current status of the therapy of advanced renal carcinoma. J Surg Oncol 1977;9:277.
8. Hrushesky WJ, von Roemeling R, Lanning RM, Rabatin JT. Circadian-shaped infusions of floxuridine for progressive metastatic renal cell carcinoma. J Clin Oncol 1990;8:1504.
9. Damascelli B, Marchiano A, Spreafico C, et al. Circadian continuous chemotherapy of renal cell carcinoma with an implantable, programmable infusion pump. Cancer 1990;66:237.
10. Merrouche Y, Negrier S, Lanier F, et al. Phase II study of continuous circadian infusion FUDR in metastatic renal cell cancer (RCC). (Abstract) Eur J Cancer Clin Oncol 1991;27:S102.
11. Dexeus FH, Logothetis CJ, Sella A, et al. Circadian infusion of floxuridine in patients with metastatic renal cell carcinoma. J Urol 1991; 146:709.
12. Budd GT, Murthy S, Klein E, et al. Time-modified infusion of floxuridine in metastatic renal cell carcinoma (mRCC). (Abstract) Proc Am Assoc Cancer Res 1992;33:220.
13. Conroy T, Geoffrois L, Guillemin F, et al. Simplified chronomodulated continuous infusion of floxuridine in patients with metastatic renal cell carcinoma. Cancer 1993;72:2190.
14. Porter RL, Bakker PJM, Kurth KH, et al. Circadian modulated continuous infusion of FUDR in patients with disseminated renal cell cancer (RCC). Eur J Cancer 1993;29:116.
15. Raminski D, Creaven PJ, Rustum YM, et al. Phase I clinical trial of floxuridine (FUdr) with leucovorin (LV) in patients (PTS) with advanced genitourinary cancer (AGC). (Abstract) Proc Am Soc Clin Oncol 1992;11:206.
16. Bjarnason GA, Hrushesky WJM, Diasio R, et al. Flat versus circadian modified 14 day infusion of FUDR for advanced renal cell cancer (RCC): a phase-III study. (Abstract) Proc Am Soc Clin Oncol 1994; 13:233.
17. Dana BW, Alberts DS. Combination chemoimmunotherapy for advanced renal carcinoma with Adriamycin, bleomycin, vincristine, cyclophosphamide, plus BCG. Cancer Clin Trial 1981;4:205.
18. Droz JP, Theodore C, Ghosn M, et al. Twelve-year experience with chemotherapy in adult metastatic renal cell carcinoma at the Institut Gustave-Roussy. Semin Surg Oncol 1988;4:97.
19. Elson PJ, Earhart RH, Kvols LK, et al. Phase II studies of PCNU and bisantrene in advanced renal cell carcinoma. Cancer Treat Rep 1987; 71:331.
20. Baumgartner G, Heinz R, Arbes H, Lenzhofer R, Pridun N, Schuller J. Methotrexate-citrovorum factor used alone and in combination chemotherapy for advanced hypernephromas. Cancer Treat Rep 1980; 64:41.
21. Jekunen A, Stengard J, Pyrhonen S, et al. Phase II study of vinblastine and doxorubicin in advanced renal cell carcinoma. (Letter) Eur J Cancer 1994;30A:245.

22. Sommer HH, Fossa SD, Lien HH. Combination chemotherapy of advanced renal cell cancer with CCNU and vinblastine. Cancer Chemother Pharmacol 1985;14:277.
23. Hahn RG, Begg CB, Davis T. Phase II study of vinblastine-CCNU, triazinate, and dactinomycin in advanced renal cell cancer. Cancer Treat Rep 1981;65:711.
24. Merrin C, Mittelman A, Fanous N, Walsman Z, Murphy GP. Chemotherapy of advanced renal cell carcinoma with vinblastine and CCNU. J Urol 1975;113:21.
25. Hahn RG, Temkin NR, Savlov ED, et al. Phase II study of vinblastine, methyl-CCNU, and medroxyprogesterone in advanced renal cell cancer. Cancer Treat Rep 1978;62:1093.
26. Bloom HJ. Hormone treatment of renal tumours: experimental and clinical observations. In: Riches E, ed. Tumours of the kidney and ureter. Edinburgh: ES Livingstone, 1964:311.
27. Bloom HJ. Hormone-induced and spontaneous regression of metastatic renal cancer. Cancer 1973;32:1066.
28. Pearson J, Friedman MA, Hoffman PG Jr. Hormone receptors in renal cell carcinoma: their utility as predictors of response to endocrine therapy. Cancer Chemother Pharmacol 1981;6:151.
29. Nakano E, Tada Y, Fujioka H, et al. Hormone receptor in renal cell carcinoma and correlation with clinical response to endocrine therapy. J Urol 1984;132:240.
30. Gottesman JE, Crawford ED, Grossman HB, Scardino P, McCracken JD. Infarction-nephrectomy for metastatic renal carcinoma. Urology 1985;25:248.
31. Samuels ML, Sullivan P, Howe CD. Medroxyprogesterone acetate in the treatment of renal cell carcinoma (hypernephroma). Cancer 1968; 22:525.
32. Morales A, Kiruluta G, Lott S. Hormones in the treatment of metastatic renal cancer. J Urol 1975;114:692.
33. Wada T, Houjou T, Kubo R, Yasutomi M, Kurita T. A combined chemo-endocrine treatment with tegafur, adriamycin, methotrexate and tamoxifen for advanced renal cell carcinoma. Anticancer Res 1993;13:2465.
34. Katakkar SB, Franks CR. Chemo-hormonal therapy for metastatic renal cell carcinoma with adriamycin, hydroxyurea, vinblastine, and medroxyprogesterone acetate. Cancer Treat Rep 1978;62:1379.
35. Vosika GJ, Ryan MJ, Fortuny IA, et al. CCNU, vinblastine, and delalutin therapy in renal cell carcinoma. Med Pediatr Oncol 1978;5:89.
36. Porzsolt F, Messerer D, Hautmann R, et al. Treatment of advanced renal cell cancer with recombinant interferon alpha as a single agent and in combination with medroxyprogesterone acetate. A randomized multicenter trial. J Cancer Res Clin Oncol 1988;114:95.
37. Minasian LM, Motzer RJ, Gluck L, Mazumdar M, Vlamis V, Krown SE. Interferon alfa-2a in advanced renal cell carcinoma: treatment results and survival in 159 patients with long-term follow-up. J Clin Oncol 1993;11:1368.
38. Fossa SD, Raabe N, Moe B. Recombinant interferon-alpha with or without vinblastine in metastatic renal carcinoma: results of a randomised phase II study. Br J Urol 1989;64:468.
39. Neidhart JA, Anderson SA, Harris JE, et al. Vinblastine fails to improve response of renal cancer to interferon alfa-n1: high response rate in patients with pulmonary metastases. J Clin Oncol 1991;9:832.
40. Atzpodien J, Kirchner H, Hanninen EL, Deckert M, Fenner M, Poliwoda H. Interleukin-2 in combination with interferon-alpha and 5-fluorouracil for metastatic renal cell cancer. Eur J Cancer 1993; 29A(Suppl 5):S6.
41. Sella A, Zukiwski A, Robinson E, et al. Interleukin-2 (IL-2) with interferon-alpha (IFN-alpha) and 5-fluorouracil (5-FU) in patients with metastatic renal cell cancer (RCC). (Abstract) Proc Am Soc Clin Oncol 1994;13:237.
42. Schulof R, Lokich J, Wampler G, Schulz J, Ahgren J. Phase II trial of protracted infusional 5-FU (PIF) for metastatic renal cell carcinoma. (Abstract) Proc Am Soc Clin Oncol 1991;10:170.
43. Ahlgren JD, Lokich J, Auerbach M, et al. Protracted infusional 5FU (PIF): a well tolerated regimen in metastatic renal carcinoma (MRC): a Mid-Atlantic Oncology Program (MOAP) study. (Abstract) Proc Am Soc Clin Oncol 1993;12:244.
44. Kish JA, Wolf M, Crawford ED, et al. Evaluation of low dose continuous infusion 5-fluorouracil in patients with advanced and recurrent renal cell carcinoma: a Southwest Oncology Group Study. Cancer 1994;74:916.
45. Zaniboni A, Simoncini E, Marpicati P, Montini E, Ferrari V, Marini G. Phase II trial of 5-fluorouracil and high-dose folinic acid in advanced renal cell cancer. J Chemother 1989;1:350.
46. Vogelzang NJ, Lipton A, Figlin RA. Subcutaneous interleukin-2 plus interferon alfa-2a in metastatic renal cancer: an outpatient multicenter trial. J Clin Oncol 1993;11:1809.
47. Atkins MB, Sparano J, Fisher RI, et al. Randomized phase II trial of high-dose interleukin-2 either alone or in combination with interferon alfa-2b in advanced renal cell carcinoma. J Clin Oncol 1993;11:661.
48. Motzer RJ, Murray-Law T, Schwartz L, Fischer P, Scher HI, Nanus DM. Antitumor activity of interferon alfa-2a and 13-cis-retinoic acid in patients with advanced renal cell carcinoma. (Abstract) Proc Am Soc Clin Oncol 1994;13:232.
49. Cordon-Cardo C, O'Brien JP, Boccia J, Casals D, Bertino JR, Melamed MR. Expression of the multidrug resistance gene product (p-glycoprotein) in human normal and tumor tissues. J Histochem Cytochem 1990;38:1277.
50. Samuels BL, Trump DL, Rosner G, Vogelzang NJ, Schilsky RL. Multidrug resistance modulator in renal cell carcinoma using cyclosporin-A or tamoxifen. (Abstract) Proc Am Soc Clin Oncol 1994;13:252.
51. Tsuruo T, Iida H, Tsukagoshi S, Sakurai Y. Overcoming of vincristine resistance in P388 leukemia in vivo and in vitro through enhanced cytotoxicity of vincristine and vinblastine by verapamil. Cancer Res 1981;41:1967.
52. Ozols RF, Cunnion RE, Klecker RW, et al. Verapamil and adriamycin in the treatment of drug-resistant ovarian cancer patients. J Clin Oncol 1987;5:641.
53. Gore ME, Selby PJ, Millar B, Maitland J, McElwain TJ. The use of verapamil to overcome drug resistance in myeloma. (Abstract) Proc Am Soc Clin Oncol 1988;7:228.
54. Dalton WS, Grogan TM, Meltzer PS, et al. Drug-resistance in multiple myeloma and non-Hodgkin's lymphoma: detection of p-glycoprotein and potential circumvention by addition of verapamil to chemotherapy. J Clin Oncol 1989;7:415.
55. Presant CA, Kennedy PS, Wiseman C, et al. Verapamil reversal of clinical doxorubicin resistance in human cancer. Am J Clin Oncol 1986;9:355.
56. Benson AB, Trump DL, Koeller JM, et al. Phase I study of vinblastine and verapamil given by concurrent iv infusion. Cancer Treat Rep 1985;69:795.
57. Cairo MS, Siegel S, Anas N, Sender L. Clinical trial of continuous infusion verapamil, bolus vinblastine, and continuous infusion VP-16 in drug-resistant pediatric tumors. Cancer Res 1989;49:1063.
58. Echizen H, Brecht T, Niedergesass S, Vogelgesang B, Eichelbaum M. The effect of dextro-, levo-, and racemic verapamil on atrioventricular conduction in humans. Am Heart J 1985;109:210.
59. Mickisch GH, Kossig J, Keilhauer G, Schlick E, Tschada RK, Alken PM. Effects pf calcium antagonists in multidrug resistant primary human renal cell carcinomas. Cancer Res 1990;50:3670.
60. Gruber A, Peterson C, Reizenstein P. D-verapamil and L-verapamil are equally effective in increasing vincristine accumulation in leukemic cells in vitro. Int J Cancer 1988;41:224.
61. Lyn PA, Motzer RJ, O'Brien J, Murray-Law T, Fischer P, Ochoa M. Phase I/II trial of velban (VLB) plus dexverapamil (DEX) for patients (PTS) with advanced renal cell carcinoma (RCC). (Abstract) Proc Am Soc Clin Oncol 1994;13:244.
62. Sikic BI. Modulation of multidrug resistance: at the threshold. J Clin Oncol 1993;11:1629.
63. Vogelzang NJ, Priest ER, Borden L. Spontaneous regression of histologically proved pulmonary metastases from renal cell carcinoma: a case with 5-year followup. J Urol 1992;148:1247.
64. Oliver RT, Nethersell AB, Bottomley JM. Unexplained spontaneous regression and alpha-interferon as treatment for metastatic renal carcinoma. Br J Urol 1989;63:128.
65. Dineen MK, Pastore RD, Emrich LJ. Results of surgical treatment of renal cell carcinoma with solitary metastasis. J Urol 1988;140:277.
66. Golimbu M, Joshi P, Sperber A. Renal cell carcinoma: survival and prognostic factors. Urology 1991;27:291.
67. Klugo RC, Detmers M, Stiles RE. Aggressive versus conservative treatment of stage IV renal cell carcinoma. J Urol 1977;118:244.
68. Maldazys JD, deKernion JB. Prognostic factors in renal cell carcinoma. J Urol 1986;136:376.
69. Middleton RG. Surgery for metastatic renal cell carcinoma. J Urol 1967;97:973.

70. Wagle DG, Scal DR. Renal cell carcinoma: a review. J Surg Oncol 1970;2:23.
71. Couillard DR, deVere R. Surgery of renal cell carcinoma. Urol Clin North Am 1993;20:263.
72. Gately MK. Interleukin-12: a recently discovered cytokine with potential for enhancing cell-mediated immune responses to tumors. Cancer Invest 1993;11(4):500.
73. Nanus DM, Pfeffer LM, Bander NH, Bahri S, Albino AP. Antiproliferative and antitumor effects of alpha-interferon in renal cell carcinomas: correlation with the expression of a kidney-associated differentiation glycoprotein. Cancer Res 1990;50:4190.
74. Elson PJ, Kvols LK, Vogl SE, et al. Phase II trials of 5-day vinblastine infusion (NSC 49842), L-alanosine (NSC 153353), acivicin (NSC 163501), and aminothiadiazole (NSC 4728) in patients with recurrent or metastatic renal cell carcinoma. Invest New Drugs 1988;6:97.
75. Decker DA, Drelichman A, Opipari MI, Al-Sarraf M. Phase II evaluation of aclacinomycin-A (NSC-208734) in adenocarcinoma of the kidney. Am J Clin Oncol 1984;7:527.
76. Cowan DH, Alison RE. Evaluation of 6-aminonicotinamide (NSC-21206) in the treatment of metastatic hypernephroma: part 1. Cancer Chemother Rep 1970;54:175.
77. Hansen M, Clavel M, Zonnenberg BA, Bruntsch U, Knobf MK, Rozencweig M. Phase II study of ametantrone (NSC-287513) in advanced renal cell carcinoma. (Abstract) Proc Am Soc Clin Oncol 1985;4:99.
78. Higano CS, Goodman P, Craig JB, et al. Phase II evaluation of amonafide in renal cell carcinoma: a Southwest Oncology Group study. Invest New Drugs 1991;9:361.
79. Van Echo DA, Markus S, Aisner J, Wiernik PH. Phase II trial of 4′-(9-acridinylamino)methanesulfon-m-anisidide (AMSA) in patients with metastatic renal cell carcinoma. Cancer Treat Rep 1980;64:1009.
80. Schneider RJ, Woodcock TM, Yagoda A. Phase II trial of 4′-(9-acridinylamino)methanesulfon-m-anisidide (AMSA) in patients with metastatic hypernephroma. Cancer Treat Rep 1980;64:183.
81. Earhart RH, Elson PJ, Rosenthal SN, Hahn RG, Slayton RE. Phase II study of PALA and AMSA in advanced renal cell carcinoma. Am J Clin Oncol 1983;6:555.
82. Amrein PC, Coleman M, Richards F, et al. Phase II study of amsacrine in metastatic renal cell carcinoma: a Cancer and Leukemia Group B study. Cancer Treat Rep 1983;67:1043.
83. Abele R, Clavel M, Dodion P, et al. The EORTC early clinical trials cooperative group experience with 5′-aza-deoxycytidine (NSC 127716) in patients with colorectal, head and neck, renal carcinomas, and malignant melanomas. Eur J Cancer Clin Oncol 1987;23:1921.
84. Scher HI, Schwartz S, Yagoda A. Phase II trial of 9,10 antracenedicarboxaldehyde bis(4,5 dihydro-1 H imidazol-2-yl) hydrazone) dichloride (CL 216,942) for metastatic hypernephroma. Cancer Treat Rep 1982;66:1653.
85. Myers JW, Von Hoff DD, Coltman CA. Phase II evaluation of bisantrene in patients with renal cell carcinoma. Cancer Treat Rep 1982; 66:1869.
86. Evans WK, Shepherd FA, Blackstein ME. Phase II evaluation of bisantrene in patients with renal cell carcinoma. Cancer Treat Rep 1985; 69:727.
87. Spicer D, Daniels J, Skinner D, et al. Phase II study of bisantrene administered weekly in patients with advanced renal cell carcinoma. Proc Am Soc Clin Oncol 1985;4:101.
88. Johnson DE, Chalbaud RA, Holoye PY, Samuels ML. Clinical trial of bleomycin (NSC-125066) in the treatment of metastatic renal carcinoma: part 1. Cancer Chemother Rep 1975;59:433.
89. Haas CD, Coltman CA, Gottlieb JA. Phase II evaluation of bleomycin. Cancer 1976;38:8.
90. Hahn DM, Schimpff SC, Ruckdeschel JC, Wiernik PH. Single-agent therapy for renal cell carcinoma: CCNU, vinblastine, thioTEPA, or bleomycin. Cancer Treat Rep 1977;61:1585.
91. Tait N, Abrams J, Egorin MJ, Cohen AE, Eisenberger M, Van Echo DA. Phase II carboplatin (CBDCA) for metastatic renal cell cancer with a standard dose (SD) and a calculated dose (CD) according to renal function. (Abstract) Proc Am Soc Clin Oncol 1988;7:125.
92. Trump DL, Elson P. Evaluation of carboplatin (NSC 241240) in patients with recurrent or metastatic renal cell carcinoma. Invest New Drugs 1990;8:201.
93. Gralla RJ, Yagoda A. Phase II evaluation of chlorozotocin in patients with renal cell carcinoma. Cancer Treat Rep 1979;63:1007.
94. Rodriguez LH, Johnson DE. Clinical trial of cisplatinum (NSC 119875) in metastatic renal cell carcinoma. Urology 1978;11:344.
95. Merrin CE. Treatment of genitourinary tumors with cis-dichlorodiammineplatinum(II): experience in 250 patients. Cancer Treat Rep 1979; 63:1579.
96. Kiruluta G, Morales A, Lott S. Response of renal adenocarcinoma to cyclophosphamide. Urology 1975;6:557.
97. Hahn RG, Bauer M, Wolter J, Creech R, Bennett JM, Wampler G. Phase II study of single-agent therapy with megestrol acetate, VP-16-213, cyclophosphamide, and dianhydrogalactitol in advanced renal cell cancer. Cancer Treat Rep 1979;63:513.
98. Wajsman Z, Beckley S, Madajewicz S. High dose cyclophosphamide in metastatic renal cell cancer. (Abstract) Proc Am Soc Clin Oncol 1980;21:423.
99. Glover D, Trump D, Kvols L, Elson P, Vogl S. Phase II trial of misonidazole (MISO) and cyclophosphamide (CYC) in metastatic renal cell carcinoma. Int J Radiat Oncol Biol Phys 1986;12:1405.
100. Scher HI, Yagoda A, Ahmed T, Hollander P, Watson RC. Phase II trial of 10-deazaaminopterin for advanced hypernephroma. Anticancer Res 1984;4:409.
101. Venner P, Eisenhauer EA, Wierzbicki R, Johnston J. Phase II study of 2′-deoxycoformycin in patients with renal cell carcinoma. A National Cancer Institute of Canada Clinical Trials Group study. Invest New Drugs 1991;9:273.
102. Witte RS, Walsh C, Fisher H, Okem MM, Reding DJ, Trump DL. Evaluation of deoxycoformycin in patients with advanced renal cell carcinoma. An ECOG pilot study. Invest New Drugs 1992;10:49.
103. Braich TA, Salmon SE, Robertone A, et al. Phase II trial of esorubicin (4′deoxydoxorubicin) in cancers of the breast, colon, kidney, lung and melanoma. Invest New Drugs 1986;4:269.
104. van Oosterom AT, Bono AV, Kaye SB, et al. 4′Deoxydoxorubicin in advanced renal cancer: a phase II study in previously untreated patients from the EORTC Genito-Urinary Tract Cancer Cooperative Group. (Letter) Eur J Cancer Clin Oncol 1986;22:1531.
105. Carlson RW, Williams RD, Billingham ME, Kohler M, Torti FM. Phase II trial of esorubicin in the treatment of metastatic carcinoma of the kidney: a study of the Northern California Oncology Group. Cancer Treat Rep 1987;71:767.
106. Hurteloup P, Chollet P, Roche H, et al. Phase II trial of esorubicin in advanced renal carcinoma: Clinical Screening Group of the EROTC. Eur J Cancer Clin Oncol 1989;25:995.
107. Kish JA, Ensley JF, Al-Sarraf M. Phase II evaluation of 4′deoxydoxorubicin in advanced renal cell carcinoma. Am J Clin Oncol 1990;13: 17.
108. Scher HI, Yagoda A, Ahmed T, Budman D, Sordillo P, Watson RC. Phase-II trial of 4-demethoxydaunorubicin (DMDR) for advanced hypernephroma. Cancer Chemother Pharmacol 1985;14:79.
109. Ratanatharathorn V, Baker LH, Balducci L, Talley RW, Hoogstraten B. Phase II trial of dianhydrogalactitol in advanced renal cell carcinoma: a Southwest Oncology Group study. Cancer Treat Rep 1982; 66:1231.
110. Nichols WC, Kvols LK, Richardson RL. A phase II study of aziridinylbenzoquinone (AZQ) in advanced genitourinary (GU) cancer. (Abstract) Proc Am Soc Clin Oncol 1982;1:117.
111. Hansen M, Gallmeier WM, Vermorken J, et al. Phase II trial of diaziquone in advanced renal adenocarcinoma. Cancer Treat Rep 1984; 68:1055.
112. Stephens RL, Kirby R, Crawford ED, Bukowski R, Rivkin SE, O'Bryan RM. High dose AZQ in renal cancer: a Southwest Oncology Group phase II study. Invest New Drugs 1986;4:57.
113. Decker DA, Kish J, Al-Sarraf M, Goldfarb S. Phase II clinical evaluation of AZQ in renal cell carcinoma. Am J Clin Oncol 1986;9:126.
114. Mischler NE, Tormey DC, Klotz J, et al. Phase II study of dibromodulcitol in colorectal, kidney, and other carcinomas. Cancer Clin Trials 1981;4:407.
115. Brubaker LH, Nelson MO Jr, Birch R, Williams S. Treatment of advanced adenocarcinoma of the kidney with mitolactol: a Southeastern Cancer Study Group Trial. Cancer Treat Rep 1986;70:305.
116. Motzer R, Scher H, Bajorin D, Sternberg C, Bosl GJ. Phase II trial of Didemnin B in patients with advanced renal cell carcinoma. Invest New Drugs 1990;8:391.
117. Taylor SA, Goodman P, Crawford ED, Stuckey WJ, Stephens RL, Gaynor ER. Phase II evaluation of didemnin B in advanced adenocar-

cinoma of the kidney: a Southwest Oncology Group study. Invest New Drugs 1992;10:55.
118. Mertens WC, Eisenhauer EA, Jolivet J, Ernst S, Moore M, Muldal A. Docetaxel in advanced renal carcinoma: a phase II trial of the National Cancer Institute of Canada Clinical Trials Group. Ann Oncol 1994;5:185.
119. O'Bryan RM, Baker LH, Gottlieb JE. Dose response evaluation of adriamycin in human neoplasia. Cancer 1977;39:1940.
120. Marshall ME, Wolf MK, Crawford ED, et al. Phase II trial of echinomycin for the treatment of advanced renal cell carcinoma: a Southwest Oncology Group study. Invest New Drugs 1993;11:207.
121. Sternberg CN, Yagoda A, Casper E, Scoppetuolo M, Scher HI. Phase II trial of elliptinium in advanced renal cell carcinoma and carcinoma of the breast. Anticancer Res 1985;5:415.
122. Caille P, Mondesir JM, Droz JP, et al. Phase II trial of elliptinium in advanced renal cell carcinoma. Cancer Treat Rep 1985;69:901.
123. Piot G, Droz JP, Theodore C, Ghosn M, Rouesse J, Amiel JL. Phase II trial with high-dose elliptinium acetate in metastatic renal cell carcinoma. Oncology 1988;45:371.
124. Fossa SD, Wik B, Bae E, Lien HH. Phase II study of 4'-epi-doxorubicin in metastatic renal cancer. Cancer Treat Rep 1982;66:1219.
125. Benedetto P, Ahmed T, Needles B, Watson RC, Yagoda A. Phase II trial of 4'epi-adriamycin for advanced hypernephroma. Am J Clin Oncol 1983;6:553.
126. Swanson DA, Johnson DE. Estramustine phosphate (Emcyt) as treatment for metastatic renal carcinoma. Urology 1981;17:344.
127. Richards III F, Cooper MR, Jackson DV, et al. Continuous 5-day (D) intravenous (IV) FUDR infusion for renal cell carcinoma (RCC): a phase I-II trial of the Piedmont Oncology Association. (Abstract) Proc Am Soc Clin Oncol 1991;10:170.
128. Wilkinson MJ, Frye JW, Small EJ, et al. A phase II study of constant-infusion floxuridine for the treatment of metastatic renal cell carcinoma. Cancer 1993;71:3601.
129. Balducci L, Blumenstein B, Von Hoff DD, et al. Evaluation of fludarabine phosphate in renal cell carcinoma: a Southwest Oncology Group Study. Cancer Treat Rep 1987;71:543.
130. Shevrin DH, Lad TE, Kilton LJ, et al. Phase II trial of fludarabine phosphate in advanced renal cell carcinoma: an Illinois Cancer Council Study. Invest New Drugs 1989;7:251.
131. Kaye SB, Brampton M, Harper P, et al. Phase II trials of fosquidone, (GR63178A), in colorectal, renal and non-small cell lung cancer: CRC Phase II Clinical Trials Committee. Br J Cancer 1992;65:624.
132. Chevallier B, Toussaint C, Kerbrat P, et al. Final report: phase II study of fotemustine in advanced renal cell carcinoma (RCC): an assessment of Elson prognostic factors. (Abstract) Proc Am Soc Clin Oncol 1991;10:180.
133. Lasset C, Merrouche Y, Negrier S, et al. Phase II study of fotemustine as second-line treatment after failure of immunotherapy in metastatic renal cell carcinoma. Cancer Chemother Pharmacol 1993;32:329.
134. Esteban E, Buesa JM, Cueva J, et al. Phase II study of oral ftorafur and uracil in patients with advanced renal cell carcinoma. (Letter) Eur J Cancer 1993;29A:1354.
135. Schwartz S, Yagoda A. Phase I-II trial of gallium nitrate for advanced hypernephroma. Anticancer Res 1984;4:317.
136. Vugrin D, Einhorn LH, Birch R. Phase II trial of gallium nitrate in patients with metastatic renal cell carcinoma. (Abstract) Proc Am Assoc Cancer Res 1987;28:203.
137. Weissbach L, de Mulder P, Osieka R, Ermisch S, Jakse G. Phase II study of Gemcitidine in renal cancer. (Abstract) Proc Am Soc Clin Oncol 1992;11:219.
138. Mertens WC, Eisenhauer EA, Moore M, et al. Gemcitabine in advanced renal cell carcinoma: a phase II study of the National Cancer Institute of Canada Clinical Trials Group. Ann Oncol 1993;4:331.
139. Stolbach LL, Begg CB, Hall T, Horton J. Treatment of renal carcinoma: a phase III randomized trial of oral medroxyprogesterone (Provera), hydroxyurea, and nafoxidine. Cancer Treat Rep 1981;65:689.
140. Brubaker LH, Vogel CL, Einhorn LH, Birch R. Treatment of advanced adenocarcinoma of the kidney with ICRF-187: a Southeastern Cancer Study Group Trial. Cancer Treat Rep 1986;70:915.
141. Fossa SD, Talle K. Treatment of metastatic renal cancer with ifosfamide and mesnum with and without irradiation. Cancer Treat Rep 1980; 64:1103.
142. Heim ME, Fiene R, Schick E, Wolpert E, Queisser W. Central nervous side effects following ifosfamide monotherapy of advanced renal carcinoma. J Cancer Res Clin Oncol 1981;100:113.
143. De Forges A, Droz JP, Ghosn M, Theodore C. Phase II trial of ifosfamide/mesna in metastatic adult renal carcinoma. Cancer Treat Rep 1987; 71:1103.
144. Bodrogi I, Baki M, Sinkovics I, Eckhardt S. Ifosfamide chemotherapy of metastatic renal cell cancer. Semin Surg Oncol 1988;4:95.
145. Murray Law T, Mencel P, Motzer RJ. Phase II trial of liposomal encapsulated doxorubicin in patients with advanced renal cell carcinoma. Invest New Drugs 1994;12:323.
146. Presant CA, Kennedy P, Wiseman C, et al. Pilot phase II trial of amphotericin B and CCNU in renal and colorectal carcinomas. Eur J Cancer Clin Oncol 1986;22:329.
147. Weinerman BH, Eisenhauer EA, Besner JG, Coppin CM, Stewart D, Band PR. Phase II study of lonidamine in patients with metastatic renal cell carcinoma: a National Cancer Institute of Canada Clinical Trials Group Study. Cancer Treat Rep 1986;70:751.
148. Stahl M, Schmoll E, Becker H, et al. Lonidamine versus high-dose tamoxifen in progressive, advanced renal cell carcinoma: results of an ongoing randomized phase II study. Semin Oncol 1991;18:33.
149. Mahjoubi M, Kattan J, Bonnay M, Schmitt H, Droz JP. Phase II trial of LY 186641 in advanced renal cancer. Invest New Drugs 1993;11: 323.
150. Schomburg A, Menzel T, Hadam M, et al. Biologic and therapeutic efficacy of mafosfamide in patients with metastatic renal cell carcinoma. Mol Biother 1992;4:58.
151. Falkson CI. New formulation intravenous melphalan in the treatment of patients with metastatic renal cancer. Invest New Drugs 1993;11: 93.
152. Stephens RL, Goodman P, Crawford ED, et al. Evaluation of menogaril in renal cell carcinoma: a Southwest Oncology Group phase II study (8504). Invest New Drugs 1990;8(Suppl 1):S69.
153. Long HJ, Hauge MD, Therneau TM, Buckner JC, Frytak S, Hahn RG. Phase II evaluation of menogaril in patients with advanced hypernephroma. Invest New Drugs 1991;9:261.
154. Hindmarsh JR, Hall RR, Kulatilake AE. Renal cell carcinoma: a preliminary clinical trial of methodichlorophen (D.D.M.P.). Clin Oncol 1979;5:11.
155. Todd RF, Garnick MB, Canellos GP, et al. Phase I—II trial of methyl-GAG in the treatment of patients with metastatic renal adenocarcinoma. Cancer Treat Rep 1981;65:17.
156. Zeffron J, Yagoda A, Watson RC, et al. Phase II trial of methylgloxal bis-guanylhydrazone in advanced renal cancer. Cancer Treat Rep 1981;65:525.
157. Child JA, Bono AV, Fossa SD, ten Bokkel Huinink WW, De Pauw M, Stoter G. An EORTC phase II study of methyl-glyoxal bis-guanylhydrazone in advanced renal cell cancer. Eur J Cancer Clin Oncol 1982;18:85.
158. Fuks AZ, Van Echo DA, Aisner J. Phase II trial of methyl-G (methylglyoxal bis-guanylhydrazone) in patients with metastatic renal cell carcinoma. Cancer Clin Trial 1981;4:411.
159. Knight WA, Drelichman A, Fabian C, Bukowski RM. Mitoguazone in advanced renal carcinoma: a phase II trial of the Southwest Oncology Group. Cancer Treat Rep 1983;67:1139.
160. Stewart DJ, Futter N, Irvine A, Danjoux C, Moors D. Mitomycin-C and metronidazole in the treatment of advanced renal-cell carcinoma. Am J Clin Oncol 1987;10:520.
161. Hogan TF, Citrin DL, Freeberg BL. A preliminary report of mitotane therapy of advanced renal and prostate cancer. (Letter) Cancer Treat Rep 1981;65:539.
162. DeJager R, Cappelaere P, Armand JP. An EORTC phase II study of mitoxantrone in solid tumors and lymphomas. Eur J Cancer Clin Oncol 1984;28:1369.
163. Taylor SA, Von Hoff DD, Baker LH, Balcerzak SP. Phase II clinical trial of mitoxantrone in patients with advanced renal cell carcinoma: a Southwest Oncology Group study. Cancer Treat Rep 1984;68:919.
164. van Oosterom AT, Fossa SD, Pizzocaro G, et al. Mitoxantrone in advanced renal cancer: a phase II study in previously untreated patients from the EORTC Genito-Urinary Tract Cancer Cooperative Group. Eur J Cancer Clin Oncol 1984;20:1239.
165. Gams RA, Nelson O, Birch R. Phase II evaluation of mitoxantrone in advanced renal cell carcinoma: a Southeastern Cancer Study Group Trial. Cancer Treat Rep 1986;70:921.
166. van Oosterom AT, Stoter G, Bono AV, et al. Mitozolomide in ad-

vanced renal cancer: a phase II study in previously untreated patients from the EORTC Genito-Urinary Tract Cancer Cooperative Group Eur J Cancer Clin Oncol 1989;25:1249; erratum, Eur J Cancer Clin Oncol 1989;25(11):1673.
167. Sternberg CN, Yagoda A, Scher HI, Hollander P. Phase II trial of N-methylformamide for advanced renal cell carcinoma. Cancer Treat Rep 1986;70:681.
168. Abrams JS, Tait N, Silva H, et al. Phase II trial of N-methylformamide in advanced renal cancer. Am J Clin Oncol 1989;12:41.
169. Canobbio L, Boccardo F, Guarneri D, et al. Phase II study of navelbine in advanced renal cell carcinoma. (Letter) Eur J Cancer 1991;27:804.
170. Wilding G, Kirkwood J, Clamon G, et al. Phase II trial of navelbine in metastatic renal cancer. (Abstract) Proc Am Soc Clin Oncol 1993; 12:253.
171. Einzig AI, Gorowski E, Sasloff J, Wiernik PH. Phase II trial of taxol in patients with metastatic renal cell carcinoma. Cancer Invest 1991; 9:133.
172. Natale RB, Yagoda A, Kelsen DP, Gralla RJ, Watson RC. Phase II trial of PALA in hypernephroma and urinary bladder cancer. Cancer Treat Rep 1982;66:2091.
173. Harvey JH, Smith FP, Bowers MW, et al. Phase II trial of PCNU in advanced renal cell carcinoma and malignant mesothelioma. Cancer Treat Rep 1984;68:1049.
174. DeVassal F, Misset JL, Brienza Ŝ, et al. A phase II trial of 4′-O-tetrahydropyranyl-Adriamycin (THP-ADM) in advanced solid tumors. Invest New Drugs 1987;5:123.
175. Roche H, Guiochet N, Kerbrat P, et al. Phase II trials of tetrahydropyranyl-adriamycin (Pirarubicin) on renal and colon carcinoma, melanoma, and soft tissue sarcoma. Am J Clin Oncol 1993;16:137.
176. Pasmantier MW, Coleman M, Kennedy BJ, et al. Piperazinedione in metastatic renal carcinoma. Cancer Treat Rep 1977;61:1731.
177. Allen A, Wolf M, Crawford ED, Davis MP, Natale RB, Barnett ML. Phase II evaluation of piroxantrone in renal cell carcinoma: a Southwest Oncology Group Study. Invest New Drugs 1992;10:129.
178. Saiers JH, Slavik M, Stephens RL, Crawford ED. Therapy for advanced renal cell cancer with spirogermanium: a Southwest Oncology Group Study. Cancer Treat Rep 1987;71:207.
179. Schulman P, Davis RB, Rafla S, Green M, Henderson E. Phase II trial of spirogermanium in advanced renal cell carcinoma: a Cancer and Leukemia Group B study. Cancer Treat Rep 1984;68:1305.
180. Licht JD, Garnick MB. Phase II trial of streptozocin in the treatment of advanced renal cell carcinoma. Cancer Treat Rep 1987;71:97.
181. Weinerman B, Eisenhauer E, Stewart D, et al. Phase II study of sulofenur (LY186641) in measurable metastatic renal cancer. Ann Oncol 1992;3:83.
182. La Rocca RV, Stein CA, Danesi R, Cooper MR, Uhrich M, Myers CE. A pilot study of suramin in the treatment of metastatic renal cell carcinoma. Cancer 1991;67:1509.
183. Motzer RJ, Nanus DM, O'Moore P, et al. Phase II trial of suramin in patients with advanced renal cell carcinoma: treatment results, pharmacokinetics, and tumor growth factor expression. Cancer Res 1992; 52:5775.
184. van Oosterom AT, Droz JP, Fossa ST, et al. TCNU in advanced renal cancer: phase II study in previously untreated patients from the EORTC Genito-Urinary Tract Cancer Cooperative Group. Eur J Cancer Clin Oncol 1989;25:1889.
185. Bruntsch U, Van Oosterom A, Heinrich B. Taxotere (T) in advanced renal cell carcinoma (RCC): a phase II trial of the EORTC Early Clinical Trials Group. Eur J Cancer 1993;29A:233.
186. Hire EA, Samson MK, Fraile RJ, Baker LH. Use of VM-26 as a single agent in the treatment of renal carcinoma. Cancer Clin Trial 1979;2: 293.
187. Pfiefle D, Renter N, Hahn R. Phase II trial of VM-26 in advanced measurable renal cell carcinoma. (Abstract) Proc Am Soc Clin Oncol 1984;3:162.
188. Oishi N, Berenberg J, Blumenstein BA, et al. Teniposide in metastatic renal and bladder cancer: a Southwest Oncology Group Study. Cancer Treat Rep 1987;71:1307.
189. Shevrin D, Kilton L, Lad T, Mullane M, Esparaz B, Knop R. 6-Thioguanine in advanced renal cell carcinoma: an Illinois Cancer Council phase II study. (Abstract) Proc Am Soc Clin Oncol 1991;10: 180.
190. Murray Law T, Ilson DH, Motzer RJ. Phase II trial of topotecan in patients with advanced renal cell carcinoma. Invest New Drugs 1994; 12:143.
191. Bruntsch U, Dodion P, ten Bokkel Huinink WW, et al. Primary resistance of renal adenocarcinoma to 1,2,4-triglycidylurazol (TGU, NSC 332488), a new triexpoxide cytostatic agent—a phase II study of the EORTC early clinical trials group. Eur J Cancer Clin Oncol 1986;22: 697.
192. Wagner H, Possinger K, Bremer K, Donhujsen-Ant R, Peukert M, Queisser W. Phase II trial of 1,2,4-triglycidylurazol in patients with metastasized renal cell carcinoma. Cancer Treat Rep 1987;71:209.
193. Sternberg CN, Yagoda A, Scher H, et al. Phase II trial of trimetrexate in patients with advanced renal cell carcinoma: Clinical Community Oncology Program. Eur J Cancer Clin Oncol 1989;25:753.
194. Witte RS, Elson P, Bryan GT, Trump DL. Trimetrexate in advanced renal cell carcinoma: an ECOG phase II trial. Invest New Drugs 1992; 10:51.
195. Kuebler JP, Hogan TF, Trump DL, Bryan GT. Phase II study of continuous 5-day vinblastine infusion in renal adenocarcinoma. Cancer Treat Rep 1984;68:925.
196. Zeffron J, Yagoda A, Kelsen D, Winn R. Phase I-II trial of a 5-day continuous infusion of vinblastine sulfate. Anticancer Res 1984;4: 411.
197. Tannock IF, Evans WK. Failure of 5-day vinblastine infusion in the treatment of patients with renal cell carcinoma. Cancer Treat Rep 1985;69:227.
198. Crivellari D, Tumolo S, Frustaci S, et al. Phase II study of five-day continuous infusion of vinblastine in patients with metastatic renal-cell carcinoma. Am J Clin Oncol 1987;10:231.
199. Fossa SD, Droz JP, Pavone-Macaluso MM, Debruyne FJ, Vermeylen K, Sylvester R. Vinblastine in metastatic renal cell carcinoma: EORTC phase II trial 30882: the EORTC Genitourinary Group. Eur J Cancer 1992;28A:878.
200. Wong PP, Yagoda A, Currie VE, Young CW. Phase II study of vindesine sulfate in the therapy for advanced renal carcinoma. Cancer Treat Rep 1977;61:1727.
201. Fossa SD, Denis L, van Oosterom AT, De Pauw M, Stoter G. Vindesine in advanced renal cancer: a study of the EORTC Genito-urinary Tract Cancer Cooperative Group. Eur J Cancer Clin Oncol 1983;19: 473.
202. Altman SJ, Stephens RL, Bonnet JD. Yoshi 864 plus medroxyprogesterone acetate in adenocarcinoma of the kidney: a Southwest Oncology Group Study. Cancer Treat Rep 1982;66:1781.
203. Talley RW, Moorhead EI, Tucker WG, San Diego EL, Brennan MJ. Treatment of metastatic hypernephroma. J Am Med Assoc 1969;207: 322.
204. Paine CH, Wright FW, Ellis F. The use of progestogen in the treatment of metastatic carcinoma of the kidney and uterine body. Br J Cancer 1970;24:277.
205. Bloom HJ. Medroxyprogesterone acetate (Provera) in the treatment of metastatic renal cancer. Br J Cancer 1971;25:250.
206. Wagle DG, Murphy GP. Hormonal therapy in advanced renal cell carcinoma. Cancer 1971;28:318.
207. Werf-Messing B, Gilse HA. Hormonal treatment of metastases of renal carcinoma. Br J Cancer 1971;25:423.
208. Talley RW. Chemotherapy of adenocarcinoma of the kidney. Cancer 1973;32:1062.
209. Alberto P, Senn HJ. Hormonal therapy of renal carcinoma alone and in association with cytostatic drugs. Cancer 1974;33:1226.
210. Tirelli U, Frustaci S, Galligioni E, et al. Medical treatment of metastatic renal cell carcinoma. Tumori 1980;66:235.
211. Ahmed T, Benedetto P, Yagoda A, et al. Estrogen, progesterone, and androgen-binding sites in renal cell carcinoma: observations obtained in Phase II trial of flutamide. Cancer 1984;54:477.
212. Feun LG, Drelichman A, Singhakowinta A, Vaitkevicius VK, Oishi N. Phase II study of nafoxidine in the therapy for advanced renal carcinoma. Cancer Treat Rep 1979;63:149.
213. Glick JH, Wein A, Torri S, Alavi J, Harris D, Brodovsky H. Phase II study of tamoxifen in patients with advanced renal cell carcinoma. Cancer Treat Rep 1980;64:343.
214. Ferrazzi E, Salvagno L, Fornasiero A, Cartei G, Fiorentino M. Tamoxifen treatment for advanced renal cell cancer. Tumori 1980;66:601.
215. Al-Sarraf M, Eyre H, Bonnet J, et al. Study of tamoxifen in metastatic renal cell carcinoma and the influence of certain prognostic factors: a Southwest Oncology Group Study. Cancer Treat Rep 1981;65:447.

216. Weiselberg L, Budman D, Vinciguerra V, Schulman P, Degnan TJ. Tamoxifen in unresectable hypernephroma: a phase II trial and review of the literature. Cancer Clin Trial 1981;4:195.
217. Stahl M, Wilke H, Schmoll HJ, et al. A phase II study of high dose tamoxifen in progressive, metastatic renal cell carcinoma. Ann Oncol 1992;3:167.
218. Schomburg A, Kirchner H, Fenner M, Menzel T, Poliwoda H, Atzpodien J. Lack of therapeutic efficacy of tamoxifen in advanced renal cell carcinoma. Eur J Cancer 1993;29A:737.
219. Papac RJ, Keohane MF. Hormonal therapy for metastatic renal cell carcinoma combined androgen and provera followed by high dose tamoxifen. Eur J Cancer 1993;29A:997.
220. Schornagel JH, Verweij T, ten Bokkel Huinink WW, et al. Phase II study of recombinant interferon alpha-2a and vinblastine in advanced renal cell carcinoma. J Urol 1989;142:253.
221. Figlin RA, deKernion JB, Maldazys J, Sarna G. Treatment of renal cell carcinoma with alpha (human leukocyte) interferon and vinblastine in combination: a phase I-II trial. Cancer Treat Rep 1985;69:263.
222. Ceto GL, Franceschi T, Bassetto MA, Molino AM, Capelli C. Phase I/II trial of recombinant alpha-2 interferon (IFN) and vinblastine (VBL) in metastatic renal cell cancer (MRCC). (Abstract) Proc Am Soc Clin Oncol 1986;5:110.
223. Fossa SD, Nesland JM, Melvik JE, et al. Recombinant interferon with or without vinblastine in metastatic renal cell carcinoma. Cancer 1986; 57:1700.
224. Otto U, Schneider A, Conrad S, et al. Treatment of patients with metastatic renal cell carcinoma: results of two clinical phase II studies with alpha-2-interferon plus vinblastine or gamma interferon in 55 patients. (Abstract) J Urol 1987;137:327a.
225. Fossa SD, de Garis ST. Further experience with recombinant alfa-2a with or without vinblastine in metastatic renal cell carcinoma: a progress report. Int J Cancer 1987;1:36.
226. Bergerat JP, Herbrecht R, Dufour P, et al. Combination of recombinant interferon alpha-2a and vinblastine in advanced renal cell cancer. Cancer 1988;62:2320.
227. Rizzo M, Bartoletti R, Selli C, Sicignano A, Criscuolo D. Interferon alpha-2a and vinblastine in the treatment of metastatic renal carcinoma. (Review) Eur Urol 1989;16:271.
228. Palmeri S, Gebbia V, Russo A, Gebbia N, Rausa L. Vinblastine and interferon-alpha-2a regimen in the treatment of metastatic renal cell carcinoma. Tumori 1990;76:64.
229. Kellokumpu-Lehtinen P, Nordman E. Recombinant interferon-alpha 2a and vinblastine in advanced renal cell cancer: a clinical phase I-II study. J Biol Resp Mod 1990;9:439.
230. Trump DL, Ravdin PM, Borden EC, Magers CF, Whisnant JK. Interferon-alpha-n1 and continuous infusion vinblastine for treatment of advanced renal cell carcinoma. J Biol Resp Mod 1990;9:108.
231. Massidda B, Migliari R, Padovani A, et al. Metastatic renal cell cancer treated with recombinant alpha 2a interferon and vinblastine. J Chemother 1991;3:387.
232. Merimsky O, Shnider BI, Chaitchik S. Does vinblastine add to the potency of alpha interferon in the treatment of renal cell carcinoma? Mol Biother 1991;3:34.
233. Murphy BR, Rynard SM, Einhorn LH, Loehrer PJ. A phase II trial of interferon alpha-2A plus fluourouracil in advanced renal cell carcinoma: a Hoosier Oncology Group Study. Invest New Drugs 1995; 10(3):225.
234. Sella A, Logothetis CJ, Fitz K, et al. Phase II study of interferon-alpha and chemotherapy (5-fluorouracil and mitomycin C) in metastatic renal cell cancer. J Urol 1992;147:573.
235. Schuth J, Goldschmidt JW, Tunn UV. Response in patients with metastatic renal cell carcinoma (RCC) during the treatment with alpha interferon in combination with 5-fluorouracil. (Abstract) Eur J Cancer 1993;29:234.
236. Haarstad H, Jacobsen AB, Schjolseth SA, Risberg T, Fossa SD. Interferon-alpha, 5-FU and prednisone in metastatic renal cell carcinoma: a phase II study. Ann Oncol 1994;5:245.
237. Dimopoulous MA, Dexeus FH, Jones E, Amato RJ, Sella A, Logothetis CJ. Evidence for additive anti-tumor activity and toxicity for the combination of FUDR and interferon alpha2B in patients (pts) with metastatic renal cell carcinoma (RCC). (Abstract) Proc Am Assoc Cancer Res 1991;32:186.
238. Stadler WM, Vogelzang NJ, Vokes EE, Charette J, Whitman G. Continuous-infusion fluorodeoxyuridine with leucovorin and high-dose interferon: a phase II study in metastatic renal-cell cancer. Cancer Chemother Pharmacol 1992;31:213.
239. Falcone A, Cianci C, Ricci S, Brunetti I, Bertuccelli M, Conte PF. Alpha-2B-interferon plus floxuridine in metastatic renal cell carcinoma: a phase I-II study. Cancer 1993;72:564.
240. Soori G, Schuloff R, Stark J, et al. Phase II trial of continuous infusion floxuridine and interferon-alpha-2b in advanced renal cancer. Proc Am Soc Clin Oncol 1993;12:236.
241. Rodenburg CJ, Nooter K, Herweijer H. Phase II study of combining vinblastine and cyclosporin-A to circumvent multidrug resistance in renal cell cancer. Ann Oncol 1991;2:305.
242. Murphy BR, Rynard SM, Pennington KL, Grosh W, Loehrer PJ. A phase II trial of vinblastine plus dipyridamole in advanced renal cell carcinoma: a Hoosier Oncology Group Study. Am J Clin Oncol 1994; 17:10.
243. Schwartsmann G, Medina de Cunha F, Silveira LA, et al. Phase II trial of vinblastine plus nifedipine (VN) in patients with advanced renal cell carcinoma (RCC): Brazilian Oncology Trials Group. (Letter) Ann Oncol 1991;2:443.
244. Agarwala S, Bahnson R, Wilson J, Szumowski J, Downs M, Ernstoff M. Evaluation of the combination of vinblastine and quinidine in patients with metastatic renal cell carcinoma. (Abstract) Proc Am Assoc Cancer Res 1991;32:195.

Principles and Practice of Genitourinary Oncology, edited by Derek Raghavan, Howard I. Scher, Steven A. Leibel, and Paul H. Lange. Lippincott-Raven Publishers, Philadelphia, © 1997.

CHAPTER 86

Uncommon Neoplasms of the Kidney

Philip J. Walther

Renal malignancy in the child is almost always Wilms' tumor; in the adult, renal malignancy is predominantly renal cell carcinoma (RCC). Approximately 80% to 90% of primary malignant neoplasms in the adult age group are adenocarcinoma; most of the remainder are tumors of urothelial origin, primarily transitional cell. Of the adenocarcinomas, approximately 8% of these are tumors derived from the distal tubule–collecting duct epithelia. An additional small percentage are renal benign tumors, sarcomas, or symptomatic secondary tumors. Although clinically insignificant, incidental findings of secondary neoplasms of the kidney on autopsy are quite common. RCCs of proximal tubular origin and urothelial cell carcinomas are discussed in other chapters; this chapter examines the remaining—the uncommon—tumors of the kidney.

TUMORS OF EPITHELIAL ORIGIN

In the many decades of practical surgical pathology experience, it has been difficult to develop a consistent pathologic grading system for RCC with prognostic reliability. Arner and colleagues[1], using a database of 197 cases, attempted to devise such a grading system, incorporating gross, histopathologic (i.e., architectural), and cytologic features. Skinner and colleagues[2] and Fuhrman and colleagues[3] have proposed grading schemes based solely on cytologic features, particularly nuclear characteristics. Although these later systems were designed to be simpler in the hope of achieving greater reproducibility with acceptable prognostic correlation, a substantial number of cases are not easily stratified using these systems.[4] Moreover, the issue of subtypes of RCC is only just undergoing substantial acceptance, and these subtypes have not been incorporated into these systems.

Historically, the practicing surgical pathologist generally referred to RCC in an all-inclusive fashion. Although allusions to cytologic variants may have been described, differentiation of the histologic morphology has not received common attention. Efforts to reassess this large cohort of patients for pathologic subtypes has gained momentum, substantiated in principle by cytogenetic analyses of tumors corresponding to such histiotypes. Fromowitz and Bard[5] have published a synopsis of these attempts at pathologic subtyping. In their categorization, the histologic subgroups include typical, sarcomatoid, adenoma, papillary, chromophobe, oncocytoma, and collecting duct carcinomas (CDCs). It now appears more clear-cut that the three latter tumors are distinct both cytogenetically and immunologically from those of proximal tubular origin; therefore it is appropriate to classify these lesions as histologically unique neoplasias. Because of the rarity of presentation of chromophobe, oncocytoma, and CDCs and their apparent separate cell of origin (i.e., collecting duct–distal tubule) as opposed to typical adenocarcinoma of the kidney, they are included in this discussion. Attention is focussed on the cytogenetic studies that seek to differentiate these tumors from "typical" RCC; although submission of fresh tumor specimens for karyotypic analysis is not presently part of the surgical pathologic characterization of specimens, such information will probably allow easier histologic typing of tumors that are difficult to characterize histopathologically and is destined to become part of the standard surgical pathologic protocol in the near future.

Collecting Duct Carcinomas

Within the microenvironment of the kidney, the highly differentiated and immunologically distinct proximal tubule, the distal tubule, and collecting duct epithelial cells have been recognized histologically, and specific physiologic functions have been ascribed to each. However, there has been substantial controversy regarding the cell of origin of renal carcinomas; most investigators considered the majority of renal carcinomas as products of proximal convoluted tubule dedifferentiation. Conversely, it had been speculated that there might also be tumors arising from the epithelium of the collecting ducts, which are often referred to as the ducts of Bellini. Cromie and colleagues[6] first described a renal malignancy grossly involving the renal pelvis and extending to the cortical surface that contained marked variation in histopathologic pattern, from a papillary tubular infiltrative pattern more typical of a renal carcinoma to areas of solid and papillary foci within the renal pelvis more suggestive of a transitional cell carcinoma. However, Fleming and Lewi,[7] in a report of six cases, systematized the diagnostic criteria for CDC. Both gross and microscopic criteria are important elements required for the diagnosis of CDC and include the following features: a medial location in close proximity to the collecting system within the organ, both a mixed solid and tubular papillary histologic pattern, and an infiltrating tubular component eliciting a substantial desmoplastic reaction surrounding the tumor. The variable histologic pattern with emphasis on cytologic anaplasia is the most prominent feature in the tubular-solid components of the tumor. The stem cell of origin appears to be distal collecting duct epithelia; immunohistochemical studies demonstrate positive staining with antibodies most commonly associated with the distal nephron such as high-molecular-weight keratin, soy bean agglutinin, and peanut agglutinin.[7,8]

Clinical Characteristics, Prognosis, and Therapeutic Management

Approximately 25 cases of CDC have been reported comprehensively in the literature. To put this tumor in perspective by incidence in an institutional setting, Theones and colleagues,[9] in a survey of nearly 800 renal carcinomas reviewed at their institution, diagnosed CDCs in only 0.9% of cases. The most comprehensive clinical experience reported is by Dimopoulos and colleagues[10] from the M.D. Anderson Cancer Institute. In this study, 12 patients were systematically evaluated. One of the more striking aspects is the relatively young age of diagnosis (median, 43 years; range, 16 to 62 years). There was generally a striking family history of associated malignancies seen in patients with this histiotype. However, to my knowledge, no familial cases of this histiotype have been reported. Six patients had a positive family history of cancer in more than one family member: lung primary (one small cell; three adenocarcinoma), gastrointestinal tract origin (one pancreatic; two adenocarcinoma); and female reproductive (one uterine, one ovarian, one cervical). Utilizing the grading criteria of Fuhrman and colleagues,[3] all tumors were high grade: grade 3 in four patients and grade 4 in four of eight patients. In the six cases in which tumors were subjected for ploidy analysis, five were aneuploid.

The prognosis of such patients is dismal. In the four patients in this study without metastasis at the time of diagnosis, radical nephrectomy was performed; in all cases, the tumor recurred within 1 year. This is similar to the outcomes seen in a six-case study reported by Kennedy and colleagues.[8] In that study, two patients had cervical adenopathy at diagnosis; of the four with localized disease, all relapsed with 24 months.

The results of chemotherapy for CDC are, not surprisingly, highly disappointing, although results are highly anecdotal in nature. Using a combination of 5-fluorouracil, interferon-α, and mitomycin, stabilization was noted for 16 months in a single case. A minor response was also seen in one patient treated with MVAC; it was presumed initially that this was an atypical transitional cell carcinoma. The experience in treating such patients with biologic response modifiers is intriguing, because it might be suggested that the immunogenicity of this tumor could be substantially different from RCC of proximal tubule origin. Six patients have been treated with a combination of interleukin 2 and interferon-α. One of these patients with extensive nodal involvement had a dramatic response after neoadjuvant immunotherapy followed by nephrectomy with node dissection; less than 5% of the tumor was still viable, and the patient remained tumor-free for 30 months. No other patients received objective stabilization of their tumors. My experience with chemotherapy for CDC is highly anecdotal. In the one patient that I have seen, a 22-year-old woman, the disease remained resistant to high-dose interleukin 2 therapy as well as interferon-α and 5-fluorouracil therapy. In the M.D. Anderson Hospital experience, the median survival was 22 months (range, 4 to 65 months).

Cytogenetic Characterization

Some of the most exciting work being performed in the field of renal malignancy is cytogenetic characterization, which seeks to correlate patterns with subtypes of renal carcinoma. Fuzesi and colleagues[11] reported the first cytogenetic characterization of three cases of CDC. Each of the three tumors showed monosomies for chromosomes 1, 6, 14, 15, and 22. These results are striking because they constitute a marked difference from the cytogenetic alterations associated with cortical papillary renal malignancies, which generally show trisomies of chromosome 17 and trisomy or tetrasomies of chromosome 7, and also the nonpapillary renal carcinomas, which characteristically demonstrate deletions of the short arm of chromosome 3.

Two cases have been subjected to limited allelotyping to evaluate genomic sites of allelic deletion (i.e., loss of heterozygosity [LOH]) of tumor suppressor genes.[12] These researchers noted no *P53* LOH; in one case, LOH was seen in 18q in the region of the tumor suppressor gene *DCC*. However, in both cases, LOH was noted in the retinoblastoma (*RB1*) locus. This was striking in that this phenomenon was seen in only 1 of 47 tumors of proximal tubule origin (including several sarcomatoid variants) in their study, suggesting some relation with aggressiveness of the rare clinical variant, CDC.

Chromophobe Carcinomas

Chromophobe carcinoma has become one of the more controversial variants of renal carcinoma. First described by Thoenes and colleagues,[13] these tumors comprise about 4% of kidney adenocarcinomas.[9] Its appellation is a reflection of the lack of affinity of these cells for routine histologic stains. These tumors are found in the renal medulla and are usually beige to gray-white, as opposed to the gray-white character of CDCs or the mahogany red color of oncocytoma. Although routine histopathology shows a large cell with pale, finely reticular, mildly eosinophilic cytoplasm with prominent, distinct cell borders, Hale's colloidal iron staining is generally intense. Clear cells of typical renal carcinoma do not stain in this manner. Ultrastructural examination is generally required to confirm the diagnosis. The most characteristic finding is the presence of numerous "studded" intracytoplasmic microvesicles, mirroring the intercalated cell of the normal renal collecting duct epithelia.

Immunohistochemical analysis of cytoskeletal protein content demonstrates a striking contrast from typical renal carcinomas; although cytokeratin 18 is uniformly present in large amounts and cytokeratins 7 and 19 to a varying degree (i.e., similar to typical RCC), no vimentin can be detected in these tumors immunohistochemically.[14] Moreover, these tumors express carbonic anhydrase in large amounts, whereas oncocytomas do not[15]; likewise, band 3 protein, the erythrocyte anion exchanger protein, which is expressed in oncocytomas,[15,16] is not detected in such tumors. Finally, γ-glutamyltransferase, a protein associated with the proximal tubule, is not seen in chromophobe carcinomas.[17]

Cytogenetic Analysis

Limited work has been performed cytogenetically with chromophobe carcinomas. Crotty and colleagues[18] analyzed a single case in which a clone demonstrating loss of the Y chromosome and an interstitial deletion of part of the chromosome 11p arm was seen. In contrast, Kovacs and Kovacs[19] reported a loss of chromosomes in these tumors, and frequent loss of one allele of 3p, 5q, and 17, as opposed to the 3p allelic loss and frequent trisomy of 7 and 17 described in typical RCC.[20] Substantial alterations in the mitochondrial DNA have also been seen.[20]

Clinical Outcome

Few studies on clinical outcomes have been reported for chromophobe carcinomas. Metastasis appears to be infrequent, and a 92% 5-year survival has been reported.[14]

Oncocytoma

The term oncocytoma is a most unfortunate one because of the blurring in its etymologic derivation. Hamperl[21] coined the term "oncocyte" and used it in several publications on oncocytosis and oncocytomas. Although the root *onco* denotes "tumor or volume" and the Greek word *onkoustai* means "to swell," less classically versed clinicians have inferred the meaning of cancer from this term. Initially, Hamperl[21] used the term to describe only transformed epithelial cells in certain organs which characteristically showed enlarged, homogeneous, dense cytoplasm filled with acidophilic granules; the term was first applied oncologically to describe an adenolymphoma of the salivary gland. Since that time, multiple reports have described these neoplasms in other organs such as the lacrimal glands, bronchial mucus glands, parathyroid and adrenal glands, pancreas, and kidney. Although other terms such as oxyphilic adenoma, mitochondrioma, or proximal tubule adenoma with oncocytic features have all been used to allude to this entity, oncocytoma seems to have remained the predominant designation of this renal carcinoma subtype.

Histopathologic Characteristics

Klein and Valensi[22] focused interest on the diagnosis of renal oncocytoma by recognition of four specimens that they interpreted as oncocytomas. Moreover, in a retrospective institutional review of renal neoplasms, an additional nine cases were identified, indicating that this entity was not that uncommon but had been interpreted inclusively as a RCC prior to that time. As a result of a new perception of this variant histiotype after that report, more than 600 cases of renal oncocytoma have been reported in the medical literature. In a survey by Thoenes and colleagues[9] of nearly 800 primary renal epithelial neoplasms, oncocytoma was seen in 5% of specimens. Differences between oncocytoma and typical RCCs are summarized in Table 86-1.

TABLE 86-1. *Important differences between renal oncocytoma and renal adenocarcinoma*

Oncocytoma	Typical adenocarcinoma
GROSS PATHOLOGY	
Well circumscribed	Often show local invasion
Uniform ruddy tan to mahogany brown color	Orange, yellow color
Rare hemorrhage or necrosis	Frequent hemorrhage or necrosis within tumor
Stellate scar on cross section	
HISTOPATHOLOGY	
Classic picture is large uniform cells with eosinophilic granular cytoplasm	Clear or granular cell patterns; often nuclear pleomorphism; large round to polygonal cells
Architecture: solid nests, alveolar, or tubular, but not papillary	Architecture: acinar, tubular, or occasional small component of papillary pattern
ULTRASTRUCTURE	
"Choking" appearance of prominent mitochondrial proliferation with few other organelles	Prominence of Golgi's apparatus and endoplasmic reticulum
PLOIDY	
Primarily diploid	Variable
CYTOGENETICS	
Loss of Y chromosome	Deletion of chromosome 3p
Abnormalities of chromosome 1	Rearrangement of chromosome 5q
Translocation involving 9 and 11	Loss of chromosome 14q sequences

Oncocytomas have a characteristic pattern on gross examination. Tumors are usually highly regular, well-circumscribed lesions with an encapsulated appearance; on bisection, the characteristic uniform ruddy tan to mahogany brown color is classically found (see Chap. 77). Except in the largest lesions, little or no evidence of necrosis or hemorrhage is seen.[5] Occasionally a central stellate scar is observed. This gross pathologic character is in marked contrast to RCCs, which commonly show frequent areas of necrosis or hemorrhage and typically are orange-yellow. The characteristic microscopic feature of renal oncocytoma is a highly regular, homogeneous cytoplasm with marked eosinophilia. Ultrastructurally, this phenomenon is accounted for by the extraordinary preponderance of mitochondria as the dominant cellular organelle.

Efforts to ascertain the ontogeny of renal oncocytoma have focussed on seeking both immunocytochemical and ultrastructural correlates with well-defined, normal, differentiated renal epithelia from different zones of the kidney. Although some researchers had considered oncocytoma a tumor of proximal tubule origin,[22] histochemical and immunohistochemical studies suggest that renal oncocytomas are not of proximal tubular origin but share antigenic epitopes with the distal convoluted tubule and collecting duct.[23–25] Moreover, Storkel and colleagues[26] found that the vast majority of oncocytomas (9 of 10 specimens) demonstrated immunoreactivity specific for the band 3 protein, which in the normal kidney is limited to the intercalated cell, which is a specialized cell that represents nearly 50% of the cortical collecting duct epithelium. Similarly, another protein, carbonic anhydrase C, which is also limited to this highly differentiated intercalated cell, was detectable in 6 of 10 tumors.[26] From interpretation of ultrastructural studies of oncocytomas, it has been concluded that these tumors are derived from distal tubular origin.[27]

Histopathology and Malignant Potential

One of the more controversial aspects of the clinical phenomenon of renal oncocytoma is its putative malignant potential. Although it was originally considered to be invariably benign, there has been substantial controversy regarding its potential for malignancy, particularly in cases in which more pleomorphic histopathologic patterns have been seen in the tumor. One of the controversies relates to the appropriateness of grading oncocytomas. A series from the Mayo Clinic[28] used a three-grade system in a survey of 90 tumors diagnosed as oncocytoma. Of the 28 patients with grade 2 tumors, two specimens contained tumor within regional lymph nodes, and four patients died of metastatic disease.

The clinical cohort from which such outcome analyses are derived is established by the histopathologic definitions. Criticisms of the Mayo Clinic study[28] have focused on the fact that the six cases in question were assigned a grade 2 classification but no other pathologic data were described; moreover, sampling of the tumors was limited in several instances, which may have precluded recognition of more aggressive histiotypes in other areas of the tumor. Fromowitz and Bard[5] pointedly state that tumors with oncocytic features but containing atypical histopathologic features, which Lieber and colleagues[28] considered a major reason justifying the need to assign a grade 2 or 3 designation to such tumors, should not be interpreted as oncocytomas. Petersen[29] has also questioned the relevance of this grading system, because there appears to be such a poor correlation with clinical outcomes. Moreover, Petersen[29] points out the marked deficiencies in the medical literature regarding correlation of histopathology with clinical outcomes; many cases of oncocytoma that have been reported were in fact autopsy surveys, studies with meager follow-up, or reports in which absence of adequate gross pathologic staging information was available. As a result, Petersen[29] emphasizes that conclusions have been prematurely drawn regarding the natural history of this tumor when a cohort of only 21 patients has been thoroughly examined.

Ploidy

The presence of a nondiploid amount of DNA per cancer cell (i.e., aneuploidy) has been correlated with adverse clinicopathologic features and outcomes in many organ sites and histiotypes. This is perhaps a reflection of the genetic instability inherent in tumor progression.[30] It is not surprising that ploidy status has been evaluated in renal oncocytomas; the inclusion of a more diverse histiotypic picture may alter the conclusions of such studies. In the Mayo Clinic experience,[31] 39% of oncocytomas had a tetraploid peak, whereas 11% were distinctly aneuploid. However, essentially all other investigators have found a uniformly diploid pattern in such tumors.[32–35]

Cytogenetic Studies

Numerous studies have been reported in which cytogenetic analyses of numerous specimens have been performed. Because these tumors are noted ultrastructurally for intracellular proliferation of mitochondria, the report that mitochondrial DNA rearrangement or deletion occurred in these tumors is noteworthy.[36] This alteration of mitochondrial DNA associated with renal oncocytomas appears to be, in at least six tumors, an alteration in the cytochrome C oxidase subunit in 1 gene,[37] which might disrupt efficient aerobic respiration in such cells. Because oncocytes are considered by many to be "degenerative or senescent" cells,[38] this molecular finding is provocative. Other abnormalities in the genomic DNA have been noted. Chromosome 1 deletions are not uncommon.[18,39] Loss of the Y chromosome is frequently seen, but because this tumor often occurs in women, it seems unlikely that this cytogenetic abnormality is uniquely and directly related. Relatively balanced translocations involving chromosomes 9, 11, and 20 have been reported[40,41]; genes for nuclear coding for certain mitochondrial proteins are present on chromosome 11. However, not every oncocytoma shows a karyotypic abnormality; therefore, the significance of these gross chromosomal abnormalities is uncertain.

Conversely, one of the most important observations is that LOH or deletion of the short arm of chromosome 3, which is thought to be characteristic of typical clear cell carcinomas,[42,43] is not seen in oncocytoma.[12,18,44] The trisomy of chromosome 17 and the polysomy of 7 seen in chromophilic and papillary variants is not noted in oncocytoma. Perhaps such cytogenetic fingerprinting will help the pathologist to better assess the biologic potential of the oncocytic tumors, which have been difficult to categorize when atypical changes are evident.

Clinical Characteristics

Numerous retrospective reviews of renal oncocytoma have been published in the biomedical literature, as summarized in a recent review.[45] It is relevant to note that numerous instances of bilateral lesions have been reported.[45] Because oncocytoma has only an extremely remote likelihood of metastasizing, it must be inferred from this information that these are multifocal lesions. Unfortunately, to my knowledge, no synchronous lesions have been analyzed cytogenetically to assess clonality or discern a common cytogenetic characteristic.

Another important clinical factor is coincident occurrence of oncocytoma with RCC.[33,46,47] A recent report of oncocytomas noted that 10% of oncocytomas have an associated RCC elsewhere, and that multiple oncocytomas were seen at least 15% of the time.[33] Consequently, it is imperative to recognize that sampling of one lesion does not define the pathology for the other lesions.

Diagnostic Imaging

It is commonly believed that oncocytoma is nearly always a tumor of benign clinical natural history; as a result, it is not surprising that advocacy of renal-sparing surgery has been made in these circumstances. However, it is important to make the diagnosis prior to surgery; awaiting the results of frozen-section specimens after performing an arduous partial nephrectomy is not cost-effective and may be associated with patient morbidity. There has been some evidence of radiologic criteria suggestive of oncocytoma, but it appears that these characteristics are not pathognomonic (see Chap. 80). Although intravenous pyelography (IVP) has been the mainstay of diagnosis historically, computed tomography (CT) has become one of the more common techniques for diagnosis of asymptomatic renal masses. IVP is of little help in differentiating renal oncocytoma from other renal masses. Ultrasonography also fails to differentiate among these lesions. Goiney and colleagues[48] reported on the sonographic characteristics of a 14-case series of oncocytoma. They concluded that oncocytomas tend to be homogeneous, isoechoic, well-marginated masses if smaller than 6 cm. However, three patients in their series had masses that were larger than 8 cm and contained areas of central necrosis or calcification; these could not be distinguished from renal carcinoma. In only one of the large lesions could an area consistent with a central scar be identified.

Angiography historically played a substantial role in the diagnostic workup of renal masses but has somewhat diminished in importance with the advent of CT and magnetic resonance (MR) imaging. The term ''spoke-wheel'' was coined by Weiner and Bernstein[49] on the basis of angiographic features in two oncocytomas and has received substantial attention as a pathognomonic sign of oncocytoma. Moreover, in this anecdotal experience, they described the angiographic characteristic of oncocytoma as having a dense parenchymal blush but lacking the more typical angiographic features seen in renal carcinoma (i.e., contrast puddling, arteriovenous shunting, and renal vein invasion). Others in small anecdotal series initially corroborated these findings.[50–52] However, these phenomena occur only rarely, and subsequent studies have confirmed that; many of the features ascribed to oncocytoma have since been seen in typical renal carcinomas.[53,54] Moreover, other researchers have evaluated the angiographic pattern of oncocytoma; none of these reports match the previously described angiographic findings. Giuffre and Gulliver[55] reported a series of seven cases, none of which correlated with the original description. Moreover, microaneurysms, thought to be exclusively associated with carcinomas, have been seen in renal oncocytoma.[55–58]

The use of CT for imaging renal oncocytoma has also been extensively scrutinized. Wojtowicz and colleagues[59] were among the first to report on a CT image of renal oncocytoma, but they concluded that the findings were nonspecific. Others with more extensive experience have also concluded that characteristics seen on CT are not pathognomonic of oncocytoma, although more typically, a distinct margin, smooth contour, occasional stellate scar formation, and homogenous appearance on contrast-enhanced CT scan can be seen.[60–63] Most recently, Davidson and colleagues[64] reviewed CT scans from 53 oncocytoma patients compared with a cohort of 63 adenocarcinomas, seeking to assess the hypothesis that differences between adenocarcinoma and oncocytoma would become more apparent with larger tumors. In this study, of oncocytomas larger than 3 cm, only 67% exhibited criteria for oncocytoma, whereas 33% fulfilled the criteria for adenocarcinoma. Among adenocarcinomas larger than 3 cm, 84% fulfilled criteria for malignancy, but 16% were incorrectly predicted to be oncocytomas. It was their conclusion that CT provided little value in differentiating between these tumors.[65] The case of a pathologically confirmed oncocytoma depicted in Figure 86-1 demonstrates the problems in interpreting such imaging studies; whereas one section of the CT image of tumor was very suggestive of oncocytoma, other sections revealed morphology more consistent with RCC.

State-of-the-art MR images of oncocytomas have been evaluated, although far less experience exists with this imaging modality than with CT.[65–68] Remark and colleagues[67] described different signal intensities that could be useful in evaluating renal oncocytomas in the absence or presence of the so-called central scar. However, Defossez and colleagues,[68] using recent MR technology to evaluate a small series of three patients with oncocytoma, described the imaging characteristics of oncocytoma only in nonspecific terms that they did not consider pathognomonic. Moreover, the scar sign of renal carcinoma, which can be documented by MR, has also been seen in RCC.[65]

There has been some controversy regarding whether radionuclide imaging might have potential to differentiate renal oncocytoma from renal carcinoma. Lautin and colleagues[69] showed no uptake of radionuclide in four oncocytomas using ^{99m}Tc-glucoheptanate, or ^{131}I-iodohipporate in one patient. Similar results have been reported by others.[54,57,70] However, Choudhri and colleagues[71] reported that ^{99m}Tc-diethylenetriaminepentaacetic acid (DTPA) could recognize a highly vascular oncocytoma. Recently, Larcos and colleagues[72] described two cases in which vascular renal masses were identified that showed persistent DTPA uptake. Based on this anecdotal experience, these authors postulated that the persistence of DTPA activity with failure to accumulate ^{131}I-hippuran or ^{99m}Tc-glucoheptnate could be indicative of oncocytoma. It should be noted that this approach has not been evaluated in a critical fashion by comparing large cohorts of oncocytomas versus adenocarcinomas; such diagnostic interpretations must be considered premature and uncorroborated.

The use of aspiration biopsy in renal oncocytoma has been anecdotally reported in a small number of cases,[73–75] including one in which a grade II oncocytoma was ultimately diagnosed. However, it is my opinion that the controversies regarding the histopathologic definition of oncocytoma are substantial enough that the potential sampling error associated with aspirate biopsy renders this modality of limited practical value as a parameter on which to base clinical decisions.

Management

The biologic potential of oncocytoma is extremely favorable for the patient, but expectations of using an expectant management approach as opposed to surgery, as is often used for angiomyolipoma (vide infra) are inappropriate, because there is no pathognomonic diagnostic maneuver that is 100% specific (as in angiomyolipoma) or cost-effective. The mode or extent of the surgical intervention is controversial, because most reports

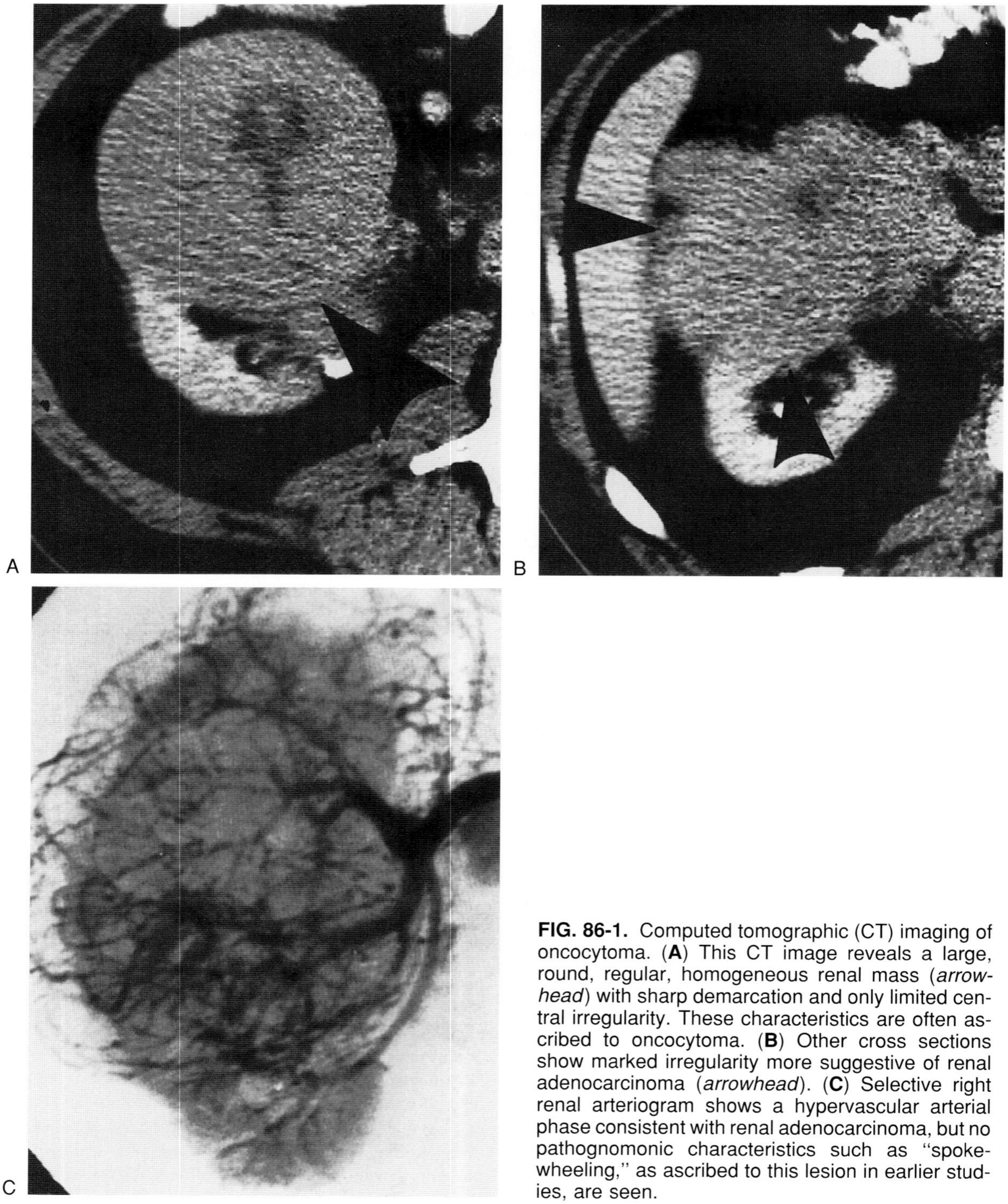

FIG. 86-1. Computed tomographic (CT) imaging of oncocytoma. (**A**) This CT image reveals a large, round, regular, homogeneous renal mass (*arrowhead*) with sharp demarcation and only limited central irregularity. These characteristics are often ascribed to oncocytoma. (**B**) Other cross sections show marked irregularity more suggestive of renal adenocarcinoma (*arrowhead*). (**C**) Selective right renal arteriogram shows a hypervascular arterial phase consistent with renal adenocarcinoma, but no pathognomonic characteristics such as "spoke-wheeling," as ascribed to this lesion in earlier studies, are seen.

regarding the biologic potential of this rare tumor allude to the possibility that nephron-sparing surgery should be entertained. From my perspective, this is an intraoperative decision that a surgeon should be prepared for when there are lesions with suggestive radiographic characteristics. Aspiration biopsy is not appropriate; the preponderant number of lesions are not oncocytoma, it is expensive, it is associated with a defined risk of morbidity, and it could be associated with tracking (i.e., seeding of disease from a RCC radiographically mimicking oncocytoma).

Excellent survival has been reported in retrospective reviews of patients with normal contralateral kidneys whose RCC was extirpated nonsystematically by partial nephrectomy.[76–78] However, the use of nephron-sparing surgery for RCC is considered controversial.[79] Although this approach has never withstood the test of randomized trial, the use of partial nephrectomy for small or clearly exophytic lesions has its adherents. In the case of lesions that are consistent with the classic radiographic appearance of oncocytoma and are small (<4 cm), polar, or exophytic, it seems appropriate to contemplate partial nephrectomy. Licht and colleagues[80] have defined criteria derived by retrospective review of their institutional experience in which partial nephrectomy for sporadic incidental lesions is appropriate with nearly uniform survival. Consequently, use of partial nephrectomy for small lesions when oncocytoma is suspected radiographically is not beyond the emerging standard of care. Using a frozen section of the resected lesion post–partial nephrectomy to gain some assessment of the biologic potential of the lesion, the surgeon can decide whether to proceed to full nephrectomy if an undesirable histiotype is uncovered or if a RCC of proximal tubular origin is revealed that the surgeon is uncomfortable with managing by partial nephrectomy alone. In large lesions such as the one depicted in Figure 86-1, full nephrectomy appears warranted.

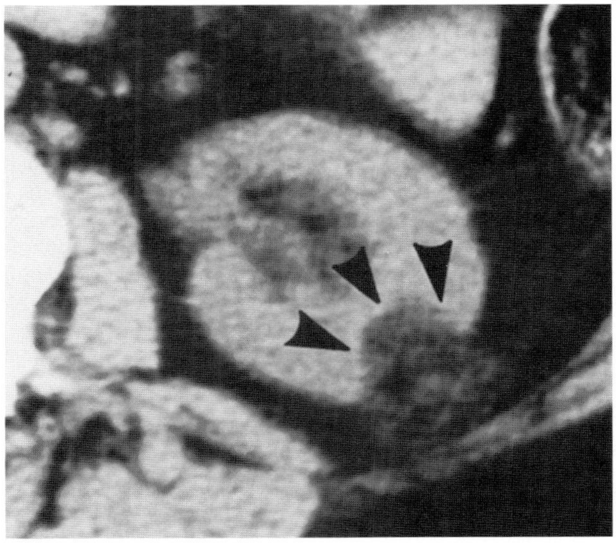

FIG. 86-2. This incidentally found solitary angiomyolipoma (*arrowheads*) shows the characteristic inhomogenous consistency with areas of very low (below water) attenuation coefficients (indicating fat) in a patient not demonstrating tuberous sclerosis. This lesion has not progressed in 10 years of monitoring.

TUMORS OF HAMARTOMATOUS ORIGIN

Angiomyolipoma

The nomenclature of angiomyolipoma was first introduced by Morgan and associates[81] in 1951 to describe a renal tumor that contained aberrant vasculature of a thick-walled nature with variable amounts of intermixed tissue of smooth muscle, adipose tissue, or both. Such mixed tumors associated with the cerebral and cutaneous manifestations of Bourneville's disease (tuberous sclerosis) had already been recognized. Because relatively little attention had been given to comprehensive descriptions of the complex histopathology of such tumors, it is likely that substantial numbers of these lesions were incorrectly interpreted earlier in this century as leiomyomas, leiomyosarcomas, or lipomas.

Although there is still some controversy regarding the origin of such tumors, the tumor's mixed cellular constitution is generally considered strong evidence of this lesion being a hamartoma of the kidney or mesenchymoma. More than 300 cases of such tumors have been reported, and the majority of these patients show no clinical evidence of the associated neurologic condition of tubular sclerosis.

Clinical Features

Angiomyolipoma occurs in the absence of tuberous sclerosis most frequently in women between the ages of 35 to 60 years. Such cases often present with flank pain and hematuria, and occasionally, massive hemorrhage necessitating emergent surgery has been reported.[82] Most symptomatic cases tend to be large single lesions, whereas lesions associated with tuberous sclerosis are multiple but usually asymptomatic and found incidentally during complete radiologic examination of a patient with the neurologic manifestations of tuberous sclerosis. Prior to the advent of CT, such lesions represented a therapeutic diagnostic dilemma, because such masses are characteristically hypervascular lesions that share many characteristics with renal cell carcinoma. With the development of CT, identification of zones of extremely low density (reflecting adipose tissue) within the masses allows the diagnosis of angiomyolipoma to be made pathognomonically in the vast majority of cases.[83] Small lesions such as the one in Figure 86-2 can be monitored expectantly.

Pathologic Characteristics

The cut surfaces of angiomyolipomas have a markedly variable appearance depending on the relative proportions of the three components of such lesions. Strikingly, however, they are not encapsulated, and some show local infiltration into the adjacent renal tissue. Hemorrhage and necrosis can often be seen, as can focal cystic deterioration. When hemorrhage occurs, it can be massive, with extension into the adjacent tissue. Histologically, such tumors demonstrate a mixture of both smooth muscle cells with poor organization and markedly prominent thick-walled blood vessels. Occasional mitoses in the smooth muscle component sometimes result in a misdiagnosis of leiomyosarcoma.

The clinical behavior of angiomyolipoma has been the focus of considerable attention. No clearly defined evidence of distant metastatic disease has ever been reported. Nevertheless, numerous reports of dissemination of angiomyolipomatous tissue to adjacent lymph nodes has been described. Such events have been interpreted as evidence of multicentricity of this hamartomatous condition.[84–88] A recent study by Ro and colleagues[89] has reported diploid DNA histograms in both the renal and lymph node tissues of three patients, demonstrating constancy of this benign cytogenetic characteristic in these multicentric sites.

Management

Patients who present with flank pain and hematuria usually have substantial lesions. In the absence of tuberous sclerosis, nephrectomy is curative and is important in the presence of massive hemorrhage. Selective angioinfarction or nephron-sparing surgery has more commonly been used since the ability to make the diagnosis preoperatively.[90] Nevertheless, it is relevant to recognize that examples of coincident renal AML and renal carcinoma within the same kidney have been reported[91]; therefore each lesion must be carefully evaluated. Treatment management of angiomyolipoma includes the following:

Asymptomatic single lesions: expectant management with CT evaluation every 1 to 2 years to determine the trend of enlargement.
Large multiple lesions in tubular sclerosis: careful monitoring using CT. Evidence of growth suggests the need for exploration.
Symptomatic hematuria: renal-sparing surgery (i.e., partial nephrectomy), if anatomically possible.
Massive life-threatening hemorrhage with retroperitoneal hematoma: selective angioinfarction with follow-up renal-sparing surgery or total nephrectomy if necessary.

TUMORS OF MESENCHYMAL ORIGIN

Tumors of mesenchymal origin, both benign and malignant, are extremely rare. As noted in Table 86-2, only approximately 500 cases have been reported. Specific tumors that have some unique significance by clinical characteristics or incidence are discussed in the following sections.

Table 86-2. *Mesenchymal neoplasms of the kidney*

Tumor type	No. of patients
BENIGN	
Hemangioma	163
Leiomyoma	28
Juxtaglomerular cell tumor	29
Lymphangioma	25
Lipoma	19
Schwannoma	4
Capsuloma	5
	273
MALIGNANT	
Leiomyosarcoma	111
Fibrosarcoma	29
Hemangiopericytoma	18
Malignant fibrocystic cytoma	21
Liposarcoma	16
Osteosarcoma	13
Rhabdomyosarcoma	13
Leiomyosarcoma of renal vein	11
Angiosarcoma	8
Chondrosarcoma	4
Malignant schwannoma	2
Malignant capsular tumors	9
	255

Compiled from data collected by Peterson RO. Urologic pathology; 2nd ed. Philadelphia: JB Lippincott, 1992 132.

Juxtaglomerular Cell Tumor

The presentation of a patient with severe systemic hypertension caused by a renin-secreting tumor was first classically described by Robertson and colleagues.[92] In this case, the cause of the hypertension associated with hypokalemia was discovered to be of renal origin only after a subtotal adrenalectomy failed to satisfactorily control the patient's blood pressure. Ultimately, a nephrectomy was performed and provided satisfactory control of the hypertension; the resected specimen contained a 3-cm tumor interpreted as a hemangiopericytoma of the juxtaglomerular apparatus. Because of the paraneoplastic consequences of the renin-secreting tumor, this syndrome is a favorite discussion of many renal endocrinologists. However, the actual incidence of this commonly referred to clinical disorder is limited to approximately 30 cases. More than 80% of such cases occur in patients younger than 30 years of age, with nearly a 3 to 1 female predominance. The hypereninemic state is associated with secondary aldosteronism. Selected renal vein renin level determinations have been helpful in lateralization of the tumor in most of the early patients studied, and arteriography has demonstrated that these lesions are hypervascular. CT is more commonly used in the more recently reported cases. Although these tumors range in size from 3 mm to 8 cm, the vast majority are approximately 1 to 5 cm. All cases have been clinically benign. Surgical treatment has been curative for the vast majority of all preoperative hypertensive states caused by juxtaglomerular cell tumor.

Hemangioma

These benign vascular neoplasms have been diagnosed in patients in the pediatric age group through those in their late seventies. Most commonly, diagnosis is made in the third decade of life as a result of intermittent hematuria. Angiographically, hemangiomas can appear hypovascular or even normal.[93–95] The management of such tumors must be individualized. The presence of recurrent hematuria lateralized to the involved kidney would suggest that nephrectomy[96] or partial nephrectomy may be of help. Reports of selective angioinfarction of such lesions have been described in the literature only anecdotally,[97] probably because of an inability of make the diagnosis reliably prior to surgical exploration.

Capsulomas

Benign tumors of mesenchymal origin derived from the renal capsule are common incidental findings at the time of necropsy. Colvin[98] described an incidence of capsulomas of 5.5% in more than 2000 consecutive autopsies. Clinically significant renal capsular tumors are rare in the literature, but of those reported, substantial histiotypic diversity is seen, including leiomyomas, fibromas, neurofibromas, schwannomas, and lipomas. Malignant neoplasms originating from the renal capsule include malignant fibrous histiocytoma,[99] leiomyosarcoma,[100] liposarcoma, and hemangiopericytoma.[101] (See also Chap. 99.)

Leiomyosarcoma

The most frequently encountered primary sarcoma of the kidney is leiomyosarcoma. The most comprehensive literature reviews of this malignancy have been published by Bazaz-Malik and Gupta,[102] Loomis[103] and Niceta and colleagues.[104] A small subset of these patients have tumors that derive from the renal vein or renal pelvis. These tumors occur predominantly in patients in the fifth and sixth decades of life at a 2-to-1 female-to-male ratio. The most common clinical presentation is that of a flank mass without hematuria.

Diagnostically, no characteristic angiographic features have been reported for leiomyosarcoma.[105] Microscopic features of these tumors include evidence of common renal and perirenal infiltration with vascular invasion. Metastasis by hematogenous routes to the liver and lung are particularly common. Regional lymph node involvement is a rare phenomenon.[104] The principal therapy historically used for this tumor is radical nephrectomy. Incidental anecdotal reports of radiotherapy and chemotherapy have been reported.[106] Only isolated cases of patients living for longer than 5 years with this malignancy have been published.[107]

Liposarcoma

There are approximately 45 reports of renal liposarcoma in the literature; however, this is an extremely difficult diagnosis to make. Some of these reported tumors may very well be angiomyolipomas that were incorrectly diagnosed. On gross pathology, distinction between actual renal involvement and perinephric origin is a difficult; however, many reports have failed to give any attention to this distinction. Many renal liposarcomas may in reality be perirenal liposarcomas arising in the fat within Gerota's fascia.[108] Figure 86-3 shows such a neoplasm of indeterminant origin.

Most cases of liposarcoma appear to occur in young and middle-aged adults with a female predominance. These tumors tend to be large, fatty masses. They are apparently well demarcated but commonly replace much of the renal parenchyma and extend through the capsule. Management of liposarcomas is usually by radical nephrectomy, with resection of adjacent organs if possible. The outcome in patients with these tumors is poor.

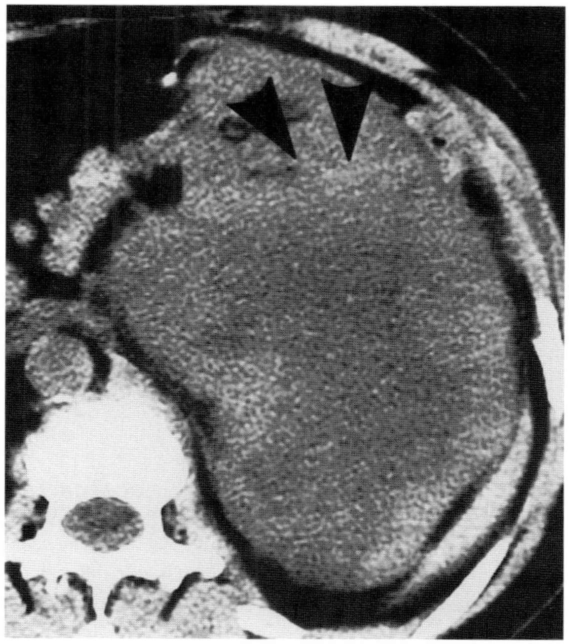

FIG. 86-3. Perirenal liposarcoma of kidney (*arrowheads*). The difficulty of defining the difference between liposarcoma deriving from renal parenchymal mesenchyme versus liposarcoma deriving from perinephric adipose tissue is demonstrated in this computed tomographic scan, which suggests intimate continuous extension of tumor from renal parenchyma. The arteriogram (not shown) failed to reveal any renovascular vascular source, and the gross pathology defined a plane separating parenchyma and tumor, suggesting a perirenal rather than renal origin for this tumor.

SECONDARY HEMATOPOIETIC NEOPLASMS

Lymphoma

Primary renal lymphoma starting within the kidney is a distinctly rare phenomenon.[109,110] Conversely, renal lymphomatous involvement is an extremely common and well-documented entity at autopsy[111]; 34% of patients dying of malignant lymphoma had evidence of renal involvement.[111] Nearly three fourths of these cases had bilateral involvement at autopsy, but only 14% of those with renal involvement were diagnosed prior to death. The vast majority of these cases were asymptomatic. Uremia was seen in only 0.5% of the total group. Non-Hodgkin's lymphoma appears to be more likely to involve the kidney than does Hodgkin's disease.[111,112]

Lymphomatous infiltration of the kidney may be nodular or diffuse in distribution. Occasionally, it can present in the form of a single mass effect, which historically has been difficult to differentiate from renal carcinoma using older imaging systems. With the development of CT, the coexistent involvement of retroperitoneal lymph nodes usually suggests the diagnosis.

Clinical Management

Although two reports in the literature demonstrate examples in which primary renal lymphoma occurring without evidence of systemic disease and managed by nephrectomy resulted in disease-free intervals of 1[113] and 5 years,[114] such examples are extremely rare. CT-guided biopsy in cases in which there is a high suspicion of lymphoma should establish the diagnosis, for example, situations in which both kidneys show irregularity or when there is retroperitoneal adenopathy that is out of proportion to the size of the renal lesion. In cases in which renal function has been compromised, radiotherapy and chemotherapy have resulted in a dramatic improvement in renal function.[115–118] Generally, maximal sparing of renal function should be the goal to allow maximal systemic chemotherapy.

Leukemia

Leukemic infiltration of the kidney is an extraordinarily rare diagnosis made antemortem. The incidence of uremia attributable to leukemic infiltrations is rare.[119] The extent of leukemic infiltration does not appear to be the crucial element in the degree of impairment in renal function.[119,120]

Plasmacytoma

So-called myeloma kidney is a recognized entity reflecting renal involvement in multiple myeloma, which is a common condition. In most cases, microscopic infiltration of the renal interstitial spaces occurs by the malignant plasma cells; this can be associated with evidence of renal amyloid.[121] The various plasma cell disorders contain an uncommon subset of extraosseous plasmacytomas; most involve the upper respiratory tract and oral cavity. Rare examples of isolated lesions within the kidney have been reported. Documented cases with various degrees of certitude appear to be limited to fewer than 20. Most of these patients are men in the sixth and seventh decades of life, and most patients have a renal mass. Painless hematuria has been reported in at least one case. Monoclonal immunoglobulin components have been identified (i.e., Bence-Jones protein) and documented in the urine of at least three patients.[122–124] The radiologic appearance of these isolated lesions is rather nonspecific. The lesions are hypervascular with palisading tumor vessels.[125,126] Extensive imaging with intravenous contrast is considered contraindicated in cases of multiple myeloma because of the threat to renal function.

Management

Because it is common for occult disseminated disease to be present, usually in bone or liver, surgical intervention appears unwarranted in the vast majority of plasmacytoma patients. Even in the absence of defined accessory lesions, most oncologists consider systemic chemotherapy the most appropriate initial approach.

SECONDARY EPITHELIAL NEOPLASMS

The frequency of metastatic deposits involving the kidney at necropsy is high. Only the liver, lungs, adrenal glands, and brain show a higher incidence of such lesions.[127] Of the available series defining secondary epithelial neoplasms,[128–132] it appears that the compiled incidence approaches 10%. There is substantial variance in frequency of renal involvement among studies, based on the primary organ and histiotype of such tumors (Table 86-3). Lung, breast, and melanoma are the most common neoplasms to secondarily involve the kidney. Nevertheless, the antemortem diagnosis for metastatic tumor is distinctly uncommon. Approximately 40 cases have been reported in the literature; in 10 of these cases, the symptomatic renal metastasis was the first manifestation of disease.[133–138] Most patients with clinically diagnosed renal metastases present with hematuria. Radiologic examination of the kidney typically demonstrates single or multiple solid tumors which generally are described as hypovascular or avascular in nature.[139–141] The histiotype does influence the angiographic appearance; in the anecdotal experience of Herzberg and colleagues[142] with a secondary breast metastasis, a substantial degree of angiographic hypervascularity was noted, creating a continued uncertainty regarding the diagnosis of primary RCC. The extent of disease, in terms of both tumor burden and multiplicity of organs involved, in most patients is extensive; therefore, palliative management is usually considered the highest priority. In the experience of Walther and colleagues,[143] selective angioinfarction can be markedly helpful in achieving palliation in patients with substantial hematuria.

Occasionally, certain subsets of patients may benefit from surgical intervention. Patients with adenoid cystic carcinoma

TABLE 86-3. *Secondary epithelial neoplasms of the kidney: autopsy experience*

Site	Willis, 1967[129] (%)	Bracken et al, 1979[130] (%)
Lung	15	18
Breast	16	8
Melanoma	25	36
Esophagus	6	10
Stomach	0	6
Colon or rectum	5	14
Pancreas	0	16
Testis		23

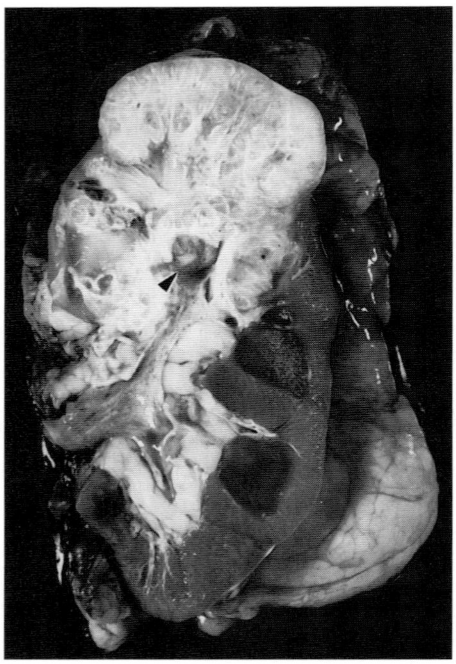

FIG. 86-4. Symptomatic secondary renal neoplasm. This isolated solitary metastasis of solitary adenoid cystic breast cancer found 12 years after mastectomy was successfully managed by nephrectomy without further systemic recurrence. (From the case reported by Herzberg AJ, Bossen EH, Walther PJ. Adenoid cystic carcinoma of the breast metastatic to the kidney: a clinically symptomatic lesion requiring intervention. Cancer 1991;68:1015.)

of the breast, for example, have a characteristically different natural history of disease, with long intervals between systemic, often solitary metastases. One such case occurred in a patient who presented with gross hematuria 12 years after primary mastectomy and 6 years after a resection of an isolated pulmonary metastasis.[142] An angiogram demonstrated a moderately hypervascular mass; nephrectomy demonstrated evidence of adenoid cystic carcinoma—the only demonstrable evidence of disease in this patient (Fig. 86-4). The patient has remained symptom-free for more than 4 years without further recurrence. Nevertheless, in most cases palliative nephrectomy must be undertaken with a substantial degree of conservatism. Maintenance of maximal renal function to allow full-dose chemotherapy may be desirable. If previous hematuria has been troublesome and a thrombocytopenic chemotherapeutic regimen is contemplated, palliative nephrectomy may be warranted.

REFERENCES

1. Arner O, Blanck C, von Schreeb T. Renal adenocarcinoma: morphology-grading of malignancy-prognosis: a study of 197 patients. Acta Chir Scand 1965;(Suppl 346):1.
2. Skinner DG, Colvin RB, Vermillion CD, Pfister RC, Leadbetter WF. Diagnosis and management of renal cell carcinoma: a clinical and pathologic study of 309 cases. Cancer 1971;28:1165.
3. Fuhrman SA, Lasky LC, Limas C. Prognostic significance of morphologic parameters in renal cell carcinoma. Am J Surg Pathol 1982;6: 655.
4. Petersen RO. Urologic pathology, 2nd ed. Philadelphia: JB Lippincott, 1992:96.
5. Fromowitz FB, Bard RH. Clinical implications of pathologic subtypes in renal cell carcinoma. Semin Urol 1990;8:31.
6. Cromie WJ, Davis CJ, DeTure FA. Atypical carcinoma of kidney: possibly originating from collecting duct epithelium. Urology 1979; 13:315.
7. Fleming S, Lewi HJ. Collecting duct carcinoma of the kidney. Histopathology 1986;10:1131.
8. Kennedy SM, Merino MJ, Linehan WM, Roberts JR, Robertson CN, Neumann RD. Collecting duct carcinoma of the kidney. Hum Pathol 1990;21:449.
9. Thoenes W, Storkel S, Rumpelt HJ, Moll R. Cytomorphological typing of renal cell carcinoma: a new approach. Eur Urol 1990;18(Suppl 2):6.
10. Dimopoulos MA, Logothetis CJ, Markowitz A, Sella A, Amato R, Ro J. Collecting duct carcinoma of the kidney. Br J Urol 1993;71: 388.
11. Fuzesi L, Cober M, Mittermayer C. Collecting duct carcinoma: cytogenetic characterization. Histopathology 1992;21:155.
12. Brooks JD, Bova GS, Marshall FF, Isaacs WB. Tumor suppressor gene allelic loss in human renal cancers. J Urol 1993;150:1278.
13. Thoenes W, Storkel S, Rumpelt HJ. Human chromophobe cell renal carcinoma. Virchows Arch B Cell Pathol 1985;48:207.
14. Thoenes W, Storkel S, Rumpelt HJ, Moll R, Baum HP, Werner S. Chromophobe cell renal carcinoma and its variants: a report on 32 cases. J Pathol 1988;155:277.
15. Storkel S, Steart PV, Drenckhahn D, Thoenes W. The human chromophobe cell renal carcinoma: its probable relation to intercalated cells of the collecting duct. Virchows Arch B Cell Pathol 1989;56:237.
16. Bonsib SM, Bromley C. Immunocytochemical analysis of band 3 protein in renal cell carcinoma, nephroblastoma, and oncocytoma. Arch Pathol Lab Med 1994;118:702.
17. Fischer P, Storkel S, Haase W, Scherberich JE. Differential diagnosis of histogenetically distinct human epithelial renal tumours with a monoclonal antibody against gamma-glutamyltransferase. Cancer Immunol Immunother 1991;33:382.
18. Crotty TB, Lawrence KM, Moertel CA, et al. Cytogenetic analysis of six renal oncocytomas and a chromophobe cell renal carcinoma: evidence that -Y, -1 may be a characteristic anomaly in renal oncocytomas. Cancer Genet Cytogenet 1992;61:61.
19. Kovacs A, Kovacs G. Low chromosome number in chromophobe renal cell carcinomas. Genes Chromosomes Cancer 1992;4:267.
20. Kovacs A, Storkel S, Thoenes W, Kovacs G. Mitochondrial and chromosomal DNA alterations in human chromophobe renal cell carcinomas. J Pathol 1992;167:273.
21. Hamperl H. Benign and malignant oncocytoma. Cancer 1962;15: 1019.
22. Klein MJ, Valensi QJ. Proximal tubular adenomas of kidney with so-called oncocytic features: a clinicopathologic study of 13 cases of a rarely reported neoplasm. Cancer 1976;38:906.
23. Holthofer H. Renal oncocytoma: immuno- and carbohydrate histochemical characterization. Virchows Arch A Pathol Anat Histopathol 1987;410:509.
24. Ulrich W, Horvat R, Krisch K. Lectin histochemistry of kidney tumours and its pathomorphological relevance. Histopathology 1985; 9:1037.
25. Cohen C, McCue PA, Derose PB. Histogenesis of renal cell carcinoma and renal oncocytoma: an immunohistochemical study. Cancer 1988; 62:1946.
26. Storkel S, Pannen B, Thoenes W, Steart PV, Wagner S, Drenckhahn D. Intercalated cells as a probable source for the development of renal oncocytoma. Virchows Arch B Cell Pathol 1988;56:185.
27. Eble JN, Hull MT. Morphologic features of renal oncocytoma: a light and electron microscopic study. Hum Pathol 1984;15:1054.
28. Lieber MM, Tomera KM, Farrow GM. Renal oncocytoma. J Urol 1981;125:481.
29. Petersen RO. Urologic pathology, 2nd ed. Philadelphia: JB Lippincott, 1992:75.
30. Friedlander ML, Hedley DW, Taylor IW. Clinical and biological significance of aneuploidy in human tumours. J Clin Pathol 1984;37: 961.
31. Rainwater LM, Farrow GM, Lieber MM. Flow cytometry of renal oncocytoma: common occurrence of deoxyribonucleic acid polyploidy and aneuploidy. J Urol 1986;135:1167.
32. Eble JN, Sledge G. Cellular deoxyribonucleic acid content of renal oncocytomas: flow cytometric analysis of paraffin-embedded tissues from eight tumors. J Urol 1986;136:522.
33. Licht MR, Novick AC, Tubbs RR, Klein EA, Levin HS, Streem SB. Renal oncocytoma: clinical and biological correlates. J Urol 1993; 150:1380.
34. Hartwick RW, el-Naggar AK, Ro JY, et al. Renal oncocytoma and granular renal cell carcinoma: a comparative clinicopathologic and DNA flow cytometric study. Am J Clin Pathol 1992;98:587.
35. Veloso JD, Solis OG, Barada JH, Fisher HA, Ross JS. DNA ploidy of oncocytic-granular renal cell carcinomas and renal oncocytomas by image analysis. Arch Pathol Lab Med 1992;116:154.
36. Kovacs G, Welter C, Wilkens L, Blin N, Deriese W. Renal oncocytoma: a phenotypic and genotypic entity of renal parenchymal tumors. Am J Pathol 1989;134:967.
37. Welter C, Kovacs G, Seitz G, Blin N. Alteration of mitochondrial DNA in human oncocytomas. Genes Chromosom Cancer 1989;1:79.
38. Chang A, Harawi SJ. Oncocytes, oncocytosis, and oncocytic tumors. Pathol Annu 1992;27(Pt 1):263.
39. Psihramis KE, Dal Cin P, Dretler SP, Prout GR Jr, Sandberg AA. Further evidence that renal oncocytoma has malignant potential. J Urol 1988;139:585.
40. Walter TA, Pennington RD, Decker HJ, Sandberg AA. Translocation t(9;11)(p23;q12): a primary chromosomal change in renal oncocytoma. J Urol 1989;142:117.
41. Fuzesi L, Gunawan B, Braun S, Boeckmann W. Renal oncocytoma with a translocation t(9;11)(p23;q13). J Urol 1994;152:471.
42. Zbar B, Brauch H, Talmadge C, Linehan M. Loss of alleles of loci on the short arm of chromosome 3 in renal cell carcinoma. Nature 1987;327:721.
43. Kovacs G, Erlandsson R, Boldog F, et al. Consistent chromosome 3p deletion and loss of heterozygosity in renal cell carcinoma. Proc Natl Acad Sci USA 1988;85:1571.
44. Brauch H, Tory K, Linehan WM, Weaver DJ, Lovell MA, Zbar B. Molecular analysis of the short arm of chromosome 3 in five renal oncocytomas. J Urol 1990;143:622.
45. Morra MN, Das S. Renal oncocytoma: a review of histogenesis, histopathology, diagnosis and treatment. J Urol 1993;150:295.
46. Lehmann HD, Blessing MH. Renal oncocytoma (pathology, preoperative diagnosis, therapy). Prog Clin Biol Res 1982;100:589.

47. Kavoussi LR, Torrence RJ, Catalona WJ. Renal oncocytoma with synchronous contralateral renal cell carcinoma. J Urol 1985;134:1193.
48. Goiney RC, Goldenberg L, Cooperberg PL, et al. Renal oncocytoma: sonographic analysis of 14 cases. AJR Am J Roentgenol 1984;143:1001.
49. Weiner SN, Bernstein RG. Renal oncocytoma: angiographic features of two cases. Radiology 1977;125:633.
50. Sos TA, Gray GF Jr, Baltaxe HA. The angiographic appearance of benign renal oxyphilic adenoma. Am J Roentgenol 1976;127:717.
51. Ambos MA, Bosniak MA, Valensi QJ, Madayag MA, Lefleur RS. Angiographic patterns in renal oncocytomas. Radiology 1978;129:615.
52. Barth KH, Menon M. Renal oncocytoma. Further diagnostic observations. Diagn Imaging 1980;49:259.
53. Jander HP. Renal oncocytoma: a nonentity. Radiology 1979;130:815.
54. Bonavita JA, Pollack HM, Banner MP. Renal oncocytoma: further observations and literature review. Urol Radiol 1980;2:229.
55. Giuffre BM, Gulliver DJ. Renal oncocytoma. Australas Radiol 1984;28:120.
56. Pearse HD, Houghton DC. Renal oncocytoma. Urology 1979;13:74.
57. Johnson JR, Thurman AE, Metter JB, Bannayan GA. Oncocytoma of kidney. Urology 1979;14:181.
58. Slasky BS, Bron KM. Aneurysms in renal oncocytoma. Urology 1982;20:552.
59. Wojtowicz J, Karwowski A, Konkiewicz J, Lukaszewski B. Case report. Renal oncocytoma. J Comput Assist Tomogr 1979;3:124.
60. Levine E, Huntrakoon M. Computed tomography of renal oncocytoma. AJR Am J Roentgenol 1983;141:741.
61. Cohan RH, Dunnick NR, Degesys GE, Korobkin M. Computed tomography of renal oncocytoma. J Comput Assist Tomogr 1984;8:284.
62. Quinn MJ, Hartman DS, Friedman AC, et al. Renal oncocytoma: new observations. Radiology 1984;153:49.
63. Jasinski RW, Amendola MA, Glazer GM, Bree RL, Gikas PW. Computed tomography of renal oncocytomas. Comput Radiol 1985;9:307.
64. Davidson AJ, Hayes WS, Hartman DS, McCarthy WF, Davis CJ Jr. Renal oncocytoma and carcinoma: failure of differentiation with CT. Radiology 1993;186:693.
65. Ball DS, Friedman AC, Hartman DS, Radecki PD, Caroline DF. Scar sign of renal oncocytoma: magnetic resonance imaging appearance and lack of specificity. Urol Radiol 1986;8:46.
66. Sohn HK, Kim SY, Seo HS. MR imaging of a renal oncocytoma. J Comput Assist Tomogr 1987;11:1085.
67. Remark RR, Berquist TH, Lieber MM, Charboneau JW, Hartman GW. Magnetic resonance imaging of renal oncocytoma. Urology 1988;31:176.
68. Defossez SM, Yoder IC, Papanicolaou N, Rosen BR, McGovern F. Nonspecific magnetic resonance appearance of renal oncocytomas: report of 3 cases and review of the literature. J Urol 1991;145:552.
69. Lautin EM, Gordon PM, Friedman AC, et al. Radionuclide imaging and computed tomography in renal oncocytoma. Radiology 1981;138:185.
70. Lee VW, Allard J, Foster J, Sheahan K, Franklin P. Functional oncocytoma of the kidney: evaluation by dual tracer scintigraphy. J Nucl Med 1987;28:1911.
71. Choudhri AH, Patel PR, Cunningham DA. Uptake of ^{99m}Tc-DTPA by a renal oncocytoma. Eur J Nucl Med 1987;13:311.
72. Larcos G, Mullan BP, Forstrom LA. Scintigraphic findings of renal oncocytoma. Clin Nucl Med 1993;18:884.
73. Rodriguez CA, Buskop A, Johnson J, Fromowitz F, Koss LG. Renal oncocytoma: preoperative diagnosis by aspiration biopsy. Acta Cytol 1980;24:355.
74. Nguyen GK, Amy RW, Tsang S. Fine needle aspiration biopsy cytology of renal oncocytoma. Acta Cytol 1985;29:33.
75. Alanen KA, Tyrkko JE, Nurmi MJ. Aspiration biopsy cytology of renal oncocytoma. Acta Cytol 1985;29:859.
76. Morgan WR, Zincke H. Progression and survival after renal-conserving surgery for renal cell carcinoma: experience in 104 patients and extended followup. J Urol 1990;144:852.
77. Provet J, Tessler A, Brown J, Golimbu M, Bosniak M, Morales P. Partial nephrectomy for renal cell carcinoma: indications, results and implications. J Urol 1991;145:472.
78. Steinbach F, Stockle M, Muller SC, et al. Conservative surgery of renal cell tumors in 140 patients: 21 years of experience. J Urol 1992;148:24.
79. Novick AC. Renal-sparing surgery for renal cell carcinoma. Urol Clin North Am 1993;20:277.
80. Licht MR, Novick AC, Goormastic M. Nephron sparing surgery in incidental versus suspected renal cell carcinoma. J Urol 1994;152:39.
81. Morgan GS, Straumfjord JV, Hall EJ. Angiomyolipoma of the kidney. J Urol 1951;65:525.
82. Vasko JS, Brockman SK, Bomar RL. Renal angiomyolipoma: a rare cause of spontaneous massive retroperitoneal hemorrhage. Ann Surg 1965;161:577.
83. Bosniak MA, Problem P. Angiomyolipoma (hamartoma) of the kidney: a preoperative diagnosis is possible in virtually every case. Urol Radiol 1981;3:135.
84. Bloom DA, Scardino PT, Ehrlich RM, Waisman J. The significance of lymph nodal involvement in renal angiomyolipoma. J Urol 1982;128:1292.
85. Hulbert JC, Graf R. Involvement of the spleen by renal angiomyolipoma: metastasis or multicentricity? J Urol 1983;130:328.
86. Chawla K, Silber L, Alexander LL. Renal angiomyolipoma with retroperitoneal adenopathy. J Natl Med Assoc 1983;75:431.
87. Manabe T, Tasaka Y, Amano M, Okunobo T. Regional lymph node involvement in benign renal angiomyolipoma. Acta Pathol Jpn 1984;34:889.
88. Dao AH, Pinto AC, Kirchner FK, Halter SA. Massive nodal involvement in a case of renal angiomyolipoma. Arch Pathol Lab Med 1984;108:612.
89. Ro JY, Ayala AG, el-Naggar A, Grignon DJ, Hogan SF, Howard DR. Angiomyolipoma of kidney with lymph node involvement. DNA flow cytometric analysis. Arch Pathol Lab Med 1990;114:65.
90. Oesterling JE, Fishman EK, Goldman SM, Marshall FF, Problem P. The management of renal angiomyolipoma. J Urol 1986;135:1121.
91. Huang J-K, Ho DM, Wang J-H, et al. Coincidental angiomyolipoma and renal cell carcinoma: report of 1 case and review of literature. J Urol 1988;140:1516.
92. Robertson PW, Klidjian A, Harding LK, Walters G, Lee MR, Robb-Smith AH. Hypertension due to a renin-secreting renal tumour. Am J Med 1967;43:963.
93. Cubillo E, Hesker AE, Stanley RJ. Cavernous hemangioma of the kidney: an angiographic-pathologic correlation. J Can Assoc Radiol 1973;24:254.
94. Ekelund L, Gothlin J. Renal hemangiomas. AJR Am J Roentgenol 1975;125:788.
95. Gordon R, Rosenmann E, Barzilay B, Siew F. Correlation of selective angiography and pathology in cavernous hemangioma of the kidney. J Urol 1976;115:608.
96. Yazaki T, Takahashi S, Ogawa Y, Kanoh S, Kitagawa R. Large renal hemangioma necessitating nephrectomy. Urology 1985;25:302.
97. Pinet A, Lyonnet D. Embolization of benign non tumoral diseases of the kidney. Semaine des Hopitaux 1982;58:159.
98. Colvin SH Jr. Certain capsular and subcapsular mixed tumors of the kidney herein called "capsuloma." J Urol 1942;48:585.
99. Osamura RY, Watanabe K, Yoneyama K, Hayashi T. Malignant fibrous histiocytoma of the renal capsule: light and electron microscopic study of a rare tumor. Virchows Arch A Pathol Anat Histol 1978;380:327.
100. Ng WD, Chan KW, Chan YT. Primary leiomyosarcoma of renal capsule. J Urol 1985;133:834.
101. Myerson D, Rosenfield AT, Itzchak Y. Renal capsular tumors: the angiographic features. J Urol 1979;121:238.
102. Bazaz-Malik G, Gupta DN. Leiomyosarcoma of kidney: report of a case and review of the literature. J Urol 1966;95:754.
103. Loomis RC. Primary leiomyosarcoma of the kidney: report of a case and review of the literature. J Urol 1972;107:557.
104. Niceta P, Lavengood RW Jr, Fernandes M, Tozzo PJ. Leiomyosarcoma of kidney: review of the literature. Urology 1974;3:270.
105. Ziter FM Jr, Wieche DR, McAndrews JF. Renal leiomyosarcoma: a case report with angiographic findings. J Urol 1971;105:776.
106. Srinivas V, Sogani PC, Hajdu SI, Whitmore WF Jr. Sarcomas of the kidney. J Urol 1984;132:13.
107. Tetelman MM, Lisa JR. Leiomyosarcoma of the kidney: report of 2 cases. J Urol 1945;54:224.
108. Graff J, Funke PJ, Ruhl GH. The so-called liposarcoma of the kidney: a case report and review of the literature. Urologe A 1986;25:43.

109. Betta PG, Bottero G, Cosimi MF, Musante F. Primary renal lymphoma. Eur Urol 1986;12:352.
110. Kandel LB, McCullough DL, Harrison LH, Woodruff RD, Ahl ET Jr, Munitz HA. Primary renal lymphoma. Does it exist? Cancer 1987; 60:386.
111. Richmond J, Sherman RS, Diamond HD, Craver LF. Renal lesions associated with malignant lymphomas. Am J Med 1962;32:184.
112. Farrow GM, Harrison EG Jr, Utz DC. Sarcomas and sarcomatoid and mixed malignant tumors of the kidney in adults. II. Cancer 1968;22: 551.
113. Knoepp LF. Lymphosarcoma of kidney. Surgery 1956;39:510.
114. Silber SJ, Chang CY. Primary lymphoma of kidney. J Urol 1973;110: 282.
115. Ellman L, Davis J, Lichtenstein NS. Uremia due to occult lymphomatous infiltration of the kidneys. Cancer 1974;33:203.
116. Kanfer A, Vandewalle A, Morel-Maroger L, Feintuch MJ, Sraer JD, Roland J. Acute renal insufficiency due to lymphomatous infiltration of the kidneys: report of six cases. Cancer 1976;38:2588.
117. Coggins CH. Renal failure in lymphoma. Kidney Int 1980;17:847.
118. Randolph VL, Hall W, Bramson W. Renal failure due to lymphomatous infiltration of the kidneys. Cancer 1983;52:1120.
119. Sternby NH. Studies in enlargement of leukaemic kidneys. Acta Haematol (Basel) 1955;14:354.
120. Boggs DR, Wintrobe MM, Cartwright GE. The acute leukemias: analysis of 322 cases and review of the literature. Med 1962;41:163.
121. Hayes DW, Bennett WA, Heck FJ. Extramedullary lesions in multiple myeloma: Review of literature and pathologic studies. Arch Pathol Lab Med 1952;53:262.
122. Catalona WJ, Biles JD. Therapeutic considerations in renal plasmacytoma. J Urol 1974;111:582.
123. Morris SA, Vaughan ED Jr, Makoui C. Renal plasmacytoma. Urology 1977;9:303.
124. Kandel LB, Harrison LH, Woodruff RD, Williams CD, Ahl ET Jr. Renal plasmacytoma: a case report and summary of reported cases. J Urol 1984;132:1167.
125. Solomito VL, Grise J. Angiographic findings in renal (extramedullary) plasmacytoma: case report. Radiology 1972;102:559.
126. Siemers PT, Coel MN. Solitary renal plasmacytoma with palisading tumor vascularity. Radiology 1977;123:597.
127. Olsson CA, Moyer JD, Laferte RO. Pulmonary cancer metastatic to the kidney: a common renal neoplasm. J Urol 1971;105:492.
128. Klinger ME. Secondary tumors of the genitourinary tract. J Urol 1951; 65:144.
129. Willis RA. Metastases. In: Pathology of tumours, 4th ed. London: Butterworth, 1967:174.
130. Bracken RB, Chica G, Johnson DE, Luna M. Secondary renal neoplasms: an autopsy study. South Med J 1979;72:806.
131. Pascal RR. Renal manifestations of extrarenal neoplasms. Hum Pathol 1980;11:7.
132. Petersen RO. Urologic pathology, 2nd ed. Philadelphia: JB Lippincott, 1992:132.
133. Payne RA. Metastatic renal tumors. Br J Surg 1960;48:310.
134. Newsam JE, Tulloch WS. Metastatic tumours in the kidney. Br J Urol 1966;38:1.
135. Patrick CE, Norton JH, Dacso MR. Choriocarcinoma in kidney: case report. J Urol 1967;97:444.
136. Roy JB, Walton KN. Secondary tumors of the kidney. J Urol 1970; 103:411.
137. Marsan RE, Baker DA, Morin ME. Esophageal carcinoma presenting as a primary renal tumor. J Urol 1979;121:90.
138. Grise P, Botto H, Camey M. Esophageal cancer metastatic to kidney: report of 2 cases. J Urol 1987;137:274.
139. Bosniak MA, Stern W, Lopez F, Tehranian N, O'Connor SJ. Metastatic neoplasm to the kidney: a report of four cases studied with angiography and nephrotomography. Radiology 1969;92:989.
140. Schreck WR, Holmes JH. Ultrasound as a diagnostic aid for renal neoplasms and cysts. J Urol 1970;103:281.
141. Weiner SN. Intraluminal renal vein thrombus secondary to metastatic disease to the kidney: a case report. J Urol 1982;128:372.
142. Herzberg AJ, Bossen EH, Walther PJ. Adenoid cystic carcinoma of the breast metastatic to the kidney: a clinically symptomatic lesion requiring intervention. Cancer 1991;68:1015.
143. Walther PJ, Marks LS, Stern D, Smith RB. Renal metastasis of adenocarcinoma of the lung: massive hematuria managed by therapeutic embolization. J Urol 1979;122:398.

PART VI

Cancer of the Penis

Principles and Practice of Genitourinary Oncology, edited by Derek Raghavan, Howard I. Scher, Steven A. Leibel, and Paul H. Lange. Lippincott-Raven Publishers, Philadelphia, © 1997.

CHAPTER 87

Anatomy of the Penis and Groin

Douglas E. Johnson and Anthony J. Costello

All urologic surgeons must have clear and precise knowledge of the anatomy of the penis and groin if they are to understand the pathologic processes affecting these areas and to provide their patients with the treatment needed. A few decades ago, one needed only to memorize a few operative procedures, but today's treatment options include reconstruction, prosthetic insertion, and cancer surgical procedures, making thorough familiarity with the anatomy of these areas essential. We offer the following as an overview, but encourage the reader to seek additional information from the ever-expanding number of good anatomic texts.[1–4]

ANATOMY OF THE PENIS

The penis is composed of three tubular structures, each individually encased by the tunica albuginea, a thick fibromuscular sheath (Fig. 87-1). Dorsally (uppermost) are paired corpora cavernosa (erectile bodies) that attach to the pubic arch by crural elongations. Fibromuscular trabeculae arising from the tunica albuginea penetrate the corporal bodies, dividing them into cavernous spaces and creating a spongy appearance. These cavernous spaces become engorged with blood during sexual arousal, thus producing a penile erection. Below (ventrally) is the corpus spongiosum, through which runs the urethra. The tunica albuginea of the corpus spongiosum is thinner and more elastic than that surrounding the corpora cavernosa. Buck's fascia (deep layer of the superficial abdominal fascia) encloses the penile structures; the corpora cavernosa occupy one compartment and the corpus spongiosum another. Because the fascial coverings are thus separate, the corpus spongiosum can readily be dissected free of its attachments to the cavernosal bodies from the perineal membrane to the glans penis, an arrangement that allows the urologic surgeon to perform a urethrectomy with ease. The ischiocavernosus and bulbospongiosus muscles lie above Buck's fascia but beneath both the superficial penile and Colles fascia (Fig. 87-2).

Blood Supply

The penis is supplied by two arterial systems: *superficial*, from the external pudendal arteries, and *deep*, from the internal pudendal arteries. The superficial blood supply lies above Buck's fascia and consists of paired superficial penile arteries that divide into dorsolateral and ventrolateral branches. Most of the blood to the penis, however, arises from the internal pudendal arteries (anterior branches of the hypogastric arteries), which bifurcate to form the perineal artery and the penile artery. The penile artery pierces the urogenital diaphragm along the medial margin of the inferior ischial ramus and divides into three branches: the bulbourethral artery, the cavernous artery, and the deep dorsal artery.[5] The bulbourethral artery, usually short and of large caliber, pierces Buck's fascia and enters the bulbospongiosum. The dorsal artery drains along the dorsum of the penis and produces three to ten circumflex branches that course around the lateral surface of the corpora. Its terminal branch supplies the glans penis. The cavernosal artery enters the corpus cavernosa and runs the length of the penile shaft, generating the small vessels (helicine arteries) that constitute the erectile apparatus.

The penis is drained by three venous systems: *superficial*, *intermediate*, and *deep*.[6–8] The superficial veins located in the dartos fascia on the dorsal lateral aspects of the penis join at the penile base to form a single superficial vein that, most frequently, enters the left saphenous vein. The intermediate system consists of the deep dorsal and circumflex veins, located below Buck's fascia; they originate from the small veins within the erectile spaces and those emerging from the glans penis. The deep drainage system consists of the small crural and cavernosal veins, which empty into either the deep dorsal vein or the periprostatic plexus. The veins of these three systems have variable communications with each other.

Lymphatics

The glans penis is drained by three lymphatic networks: one in the skin, one in the mucosa, and one beneath the mucosa. The trunks of all three drain to the frenulum, where they may communicate with lymphatic vessels from the urethra. From the frenulum, the lymphatic vessels ascend circumferentially around the coronal sulcus, forming one to four major collecting trunks dorsally that run proximally beside the deep dorsal veins to the suspensory ligament of the penis (Fig. 87-3). At the level

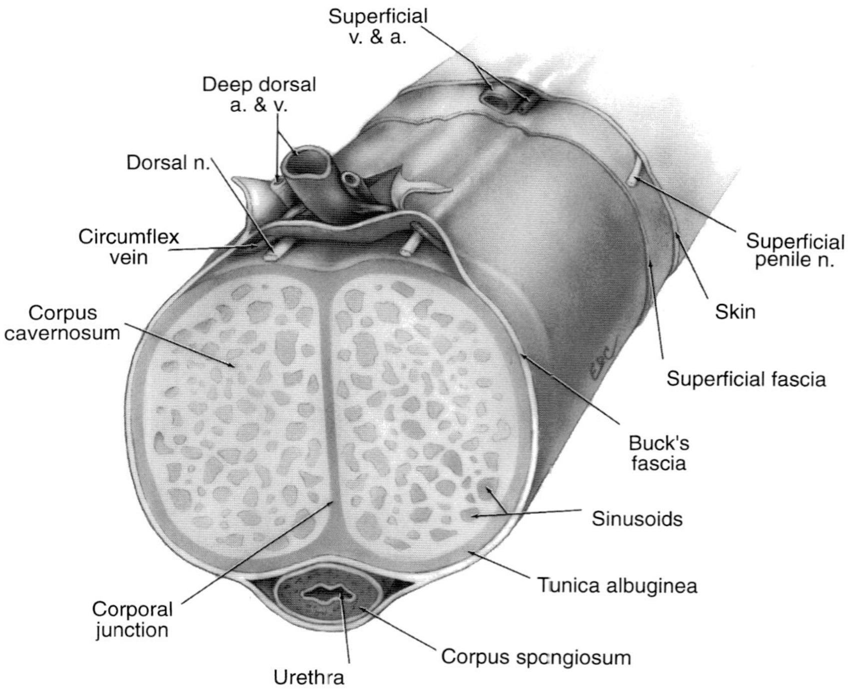

FIG. 87-1. Structural layers of the penis.

of the suspensory ligament, these lymphatic channels form anastomoses with each other, creating the presymphyseal plexus, which drains to the superficial inguinal nodes (see the section later in this chapter on superficial inguinal lymph nodes).

The lymphatics of the prepuce (both inner and outer surfaces) and the penile skin converge on the dorsum of the penis and form several trunks that run to the base of the penis, where they desiccate and drain to the superficial inguinal nodes. These anastomoses place patients at risk for bilateral regional nodal involvement.

Innervation

The penis is supplied with both somatic and autonomic nerves. The somatic nervous supply comes from the spinal nerves S2-S4 by way of the pudendal nerve. The first branch of the pudendal nerve, called the dorsal nerve of the penis, runs over the surface of the obturator internus muscle and under the levator ani on the medial side of the internal pudendal vessels and penetrates the urogenital diaphragm to reach the dorsum of the penis. The dorsal nerves continue along their respective dorsolateral penile surfaces, lateral to the dorsal artery. The main cutaneous nerve supply of the penis and scrotum originates from branches of these dorsal nerves.

Penile autonomic innervation arises from the pelvic plexus, which is derived from fibers originating from the parasympathetic nerves (S2-S4) and the sympathetic nerves (T1-L2). Beyond the prostate, the parasympathetic nerves (cavernosus nerves) run adjacent to the membranous urethra, pierce the urogenitial diaphragm, and enter the corpora cavernosa.

ANATOMY OF THE GROIN

The inguinal lymph nodes are usually the first barrier against the lymphatic spread of cancer metastasizing from the skin of the lower extremity and from the scrotum, labia majora and minora, perineum, perianal region, umbilicus, infraumbilical part of the abdominal wall, penis, and glans clitoris. In addition, the inguinal nodes may be the recipients of metastases from primary tumors in a variety of sites in both men and women: prostate, urinary bladder, testis, epididymis, spermatic cord, ureter, kidney, and urethra.[9] As early as 1830, Cooper recommended groin lymphadenectomy for patients with scrotal carcinoma when the nodes were obviously involved.[10] In 1886, MacCormac treated five cases of penile cancer by penectomy and bilateral inguinal lymphadenectomy.[11] Since the turn of this century, groin dissections have become an integral component of urologic surgical management of these malignant diseases; the urologist, therefore, must be thoroughly familiar with inguinal anatomy and with the pattern of lymphatic drainage before performing a groin dissection.

Femoral Triangle (Scarpa's Triangle)

To understand the anatomy of the groin, one must know the anatomic landmarks that form the femoral triangle and the various anatomic relationships within its boundaries (Fig. 87-4). The inguinal ligament forms the base of the triangle, curving slightly from the anterior superior iliac spine to the pubic tubercle. The apex points distally. The sartorius muscle laterally and the adductor longus muscle medially form the triangle's sides. The floor of the triangle is formed, from lateral to medial, by

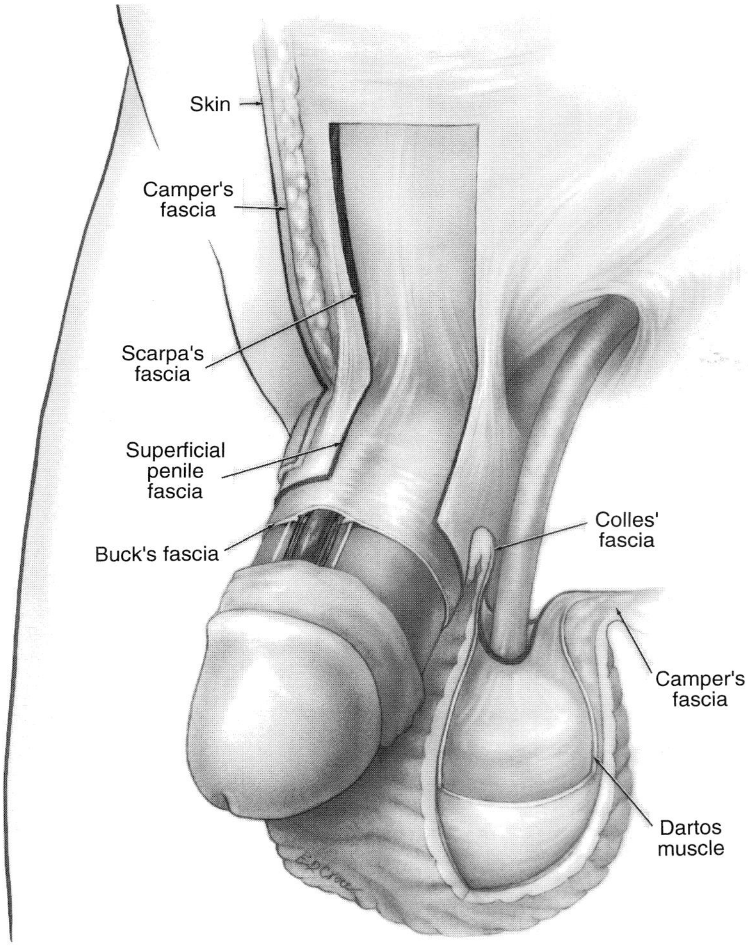

FIG. 87-2. Superficial and deep penile fascia.

the iliacus, psoas major, pectineus, and, sometimes, a small part of the adductor brevis muscles. The fascia lata covers the triangle, leaving a small opening (fossa ovalis) through which the greater saphenous vein runs as it runs toward the underlying femoral vein (Fig. 87-5).

The femoral vessels pass from the near middle of the base of the triangle to its apex. For the first 4 cm, these vessels are surrounded by the funnel-shaped femoral sheath, formed by extensions of the abdominal fasciae that pass under the inguinal ligament. The sheath is divided by two vertical partitions that form a lateral compartment containing the femoral artery, an intermediate compartment containing the femoral vein, and a smaller medial compartment (femoral canal) that contains fatty areolar tissue and in which lies the node of Cloquet or Rosenmüller. Reportedly, the femoral canal exits only in humans, for whom it serves a protective function; when a human stands upright, the femoral vein expands suddenly, and the canal then protects the vein from the sharp edge of the lacunar ligament.[12] The femoral nerve lies behind the fascia iliaca and outside the femoral sheath. In the proximal part of the femoral triangle, the femoral vein lies medial to the femoral artery, but distally it usually becomes more posterior. Occasionally, however, the femoral vein lies in a medial position throughout the length of the femoral triangle.

The femoral artery is the continuation of the external iliac artery. It begins immediately distal to the inguinal ligament, passes distally along the anterior medial thigh, and becomes the popliteal artery as it passes through an opening in the adductor magnus muscle at the junction of the middle and lower thirds of the thigh. Within the femoral triangle, the femoral artery spawns several branches, both superficial and deep. The most important named branches include the superficial epigastric artery, the superficial iliac circumflex artery, the superficial external pudendal artery, the deep external pudendal artery, and the deep femoral artery (profunda femoris) (Fig. 87-6). Other branches of the femoral artery supply the sartorius, vastus medialis, and adductores muscles.

The three superficial arteries arise from the femoral artery about 1 cm below the inguinal ligament and near each other. The superficial epigastric artery then passes through the femoral sheath, crosses superficial to the inguinal ligament, and ascends almost to the umbilicus. The superficial iliac circumflex artery, the smallest of the cutaneous branches, pierces the fascia lata and runs laterally, parallel to the inguinal ligament to the crest

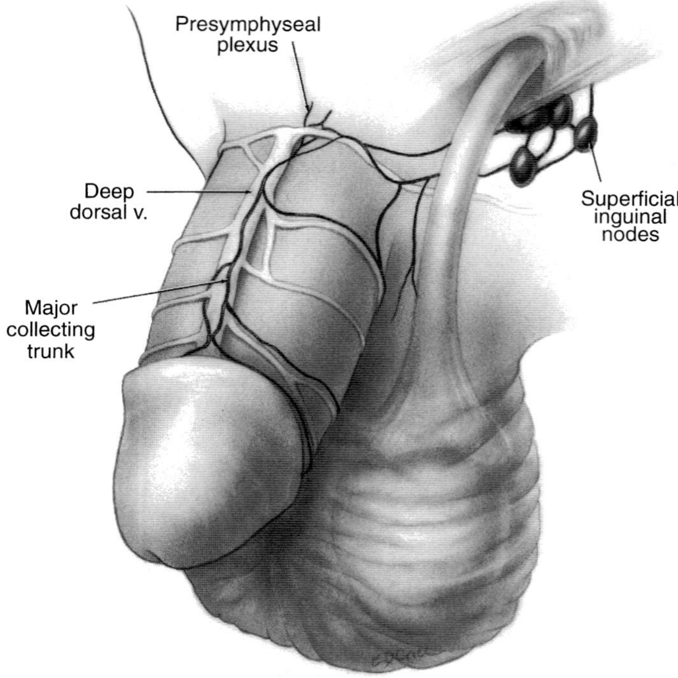

FIG. 87-3. Lymphatic drainage of the penis.

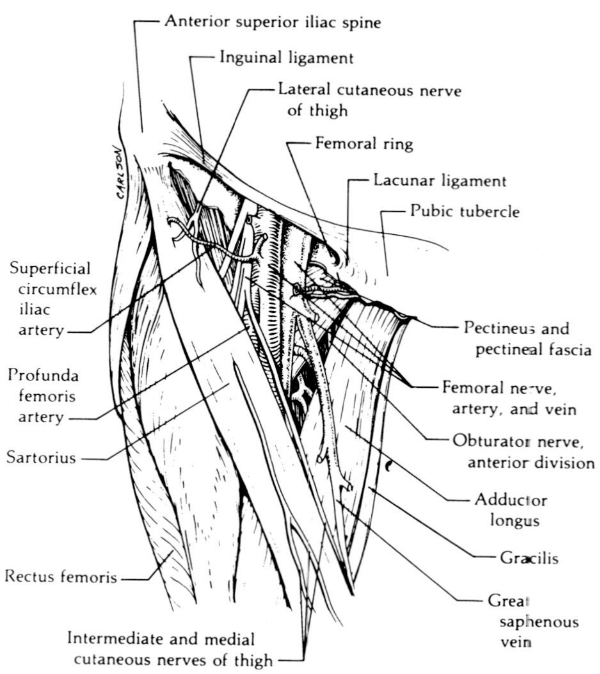

FIG. 87-4. Femoral triangle. (Johnson DE, Ames FC. Groin dissection. Chicago, Year Book, 1985:5.)

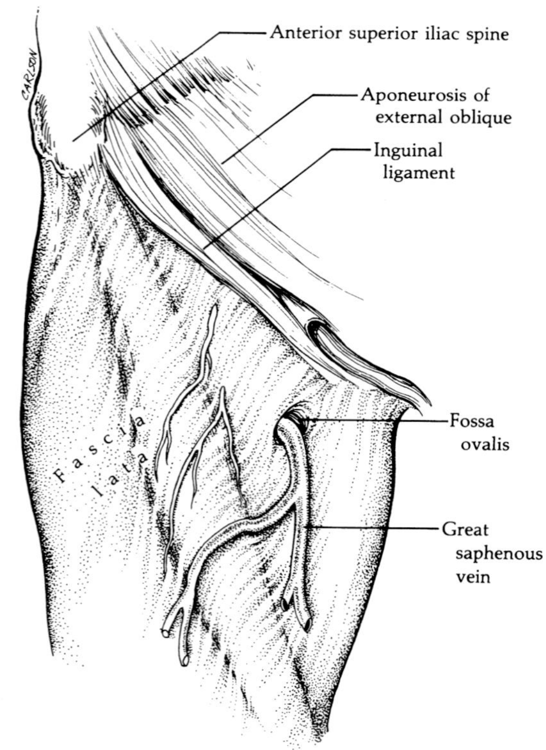

FIG. 87-5. Fossa ovalis. (Johnson DE, Ames FC. Groin dissection. Chicago, Year Book, 1985:7.)

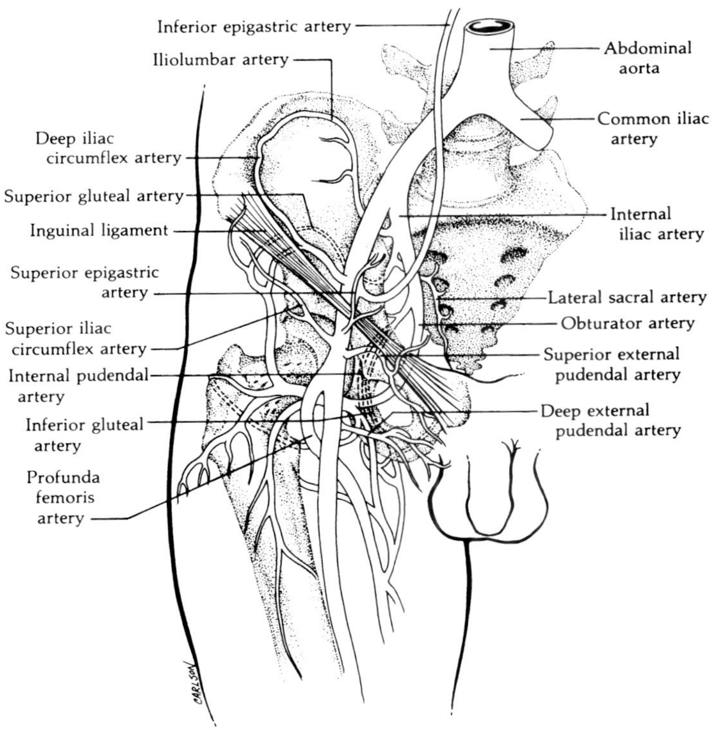

FIG. 87-6. Major arteries of the pelvis and groin. (Johnson DE, Ames FC. Groin dissection. Chicago, Year Book, 1985:8.)

of the ilium. The superficial external pudendal artery arises on the medial side of the femoral artery; after piercing the femoral sheath, it runs medially across the spermatic cord in men or the round ligament in women. The deep external pudendal artery arises more deeply than the three superficial vessels and procedes medially across the pectineus and adductor longus muscles. The deep femoral artery is a large vessel of varied origin. In about 75% of adults, it arises from the lateral and posterior part of the femoral artery 2.25 to 5 cm below the inguinal ligament. It can, however, originate anywhere from above the inguinal ligament (from the external iliac artery) to more than 5 cm below the inguinal ligament. It may also arise from the medial side or from the back of the femoral artery. Nevertheless, this vessel usually lies lateral to the femoral artery and then runs posterior to it and the femoral vein to the medial side of the femur, passing distally posterior to the adductor longus muscle.

The femoral vein accompanies the femoral artery through the proximal two thirds of the thigh. In the distal part of its course, it lies lateral to the artery; more proximally, it is deep to the artery; and at the inguinal ligament it lies medial to the artery and in the same plane. It receives numerous muscular tributaries, and about 4 cm below the inguinal ligament it is joined by the deep femoral vein. About 3 cm below the inguinal ligament, the greater saphenous vein passes through the fossa ovalis to enter the femoral vein (see Fig. 87-5).

Inguinal Lymph Nodes

Because different investigators have developed two sets of terminology to identify and describe the various groups of inguinal lymph nodes, clinicians have become the victims of unnecessary confusion. Some investigators have chosen to separate the inguinal nodes into two groups by a horizontal line that crosses the thigh at the point where the greater saphenous vein enters the femoral vein. Those lymph nodes above the line are termed "superficial inguinal" and those below "subinguinal."[13–15] The subinguinal group has been further subdivided into two sets: the superficial nodes (those external to the fascia lata) and the deep nodes (those beneath the fascia lata and close to the femoral vessels). This arbitrary and anatomically incorrect division is cumbersome to use in clinical practice. Consequently, we prefer the divisions originally suggested by Rouvière,[16] namely, that the inguinal nodes are of two types: superficial and deep.

Superficial Inguinal Nodes

Each extremity contains an average of eight superficial inguinal nodes, although the number varies from four to 25. Normally, in the absence of infection or malignancy, their size varies inversely with their number. These lymph nodes, along with the saphenous vein and its tributaries, lie within subcutaneous fatty tissue surrounded by the two-layered superficial fascia of the thigh. The deep membranous layer of the superficial fascia can be separated easily from the immediately underlying fascia lata.

Almost all the superficial lymphatics of the extremity, scrotum, labia majora and minora, penis, preputium clitoridis, abdominal wall below the umbilical line, perineum, and anus below the dentate margin drain into the superficial inguinal nodes. Originally, this group of nodes was believed to be bounded above by the inguinal ligament (Poupart's ligament), below by the intersection of the sartorius and adductor muscles, laterally by a vertical line dropped from the anterior superior iliac spine, and medially by a similar line originating at the spine of the pubis.[17] After performing 450 anatomic dissections, however, Daseler and associates[18] reported that these boundaries were inaccurate. Their research showed that the superficial inguinal nodes were in *all* cases located within the confines of a quadrilateral area bounded as follows: superiorly, by a line 12 cm long parallel to, and 1 cm above, the inguinal ligament and beginning medially just above the pubic tubercle; medially, by a line 15 cm long dropped perpendicularly downward from the pubic tubercle; laterally, by a similar line 20 cm long dropped from the lateral limit of the superior boundary; and inferiorly, by a transverse line 11 cm long connecting the lower limits of the lateral and medial borders (Fig. 87-7).

Quenu, as cited by Rouvière,[16] divided the superficial inguinal nodes into five groups, named by their relationship with the point where the greater saphenous vein joins the femoral vein. By drawing an almost horizontal line through this junction, he divided the nodes into superior and inferior groups. Although early anatomists found none of these glands above the inguinal ligament, Daseler and associates[18] occasionally identified a lymph node above the level of the inguinal ligament, but never by more than 1 cm. By dropping another, almost vertical line downward following the greater saphenous vein and prolonging it upward to the inguinal ligament, each superior and inferior group was divided into medial and lateral subgroups, forming four subsets: superolateral, superomedial, inferolateral, and inferomedial. In addition, Quenu distinguished a central, or fifth, zone in front of the greater saphenous vein, in which a few nodes can occasionally be found (Fig. 87-8).

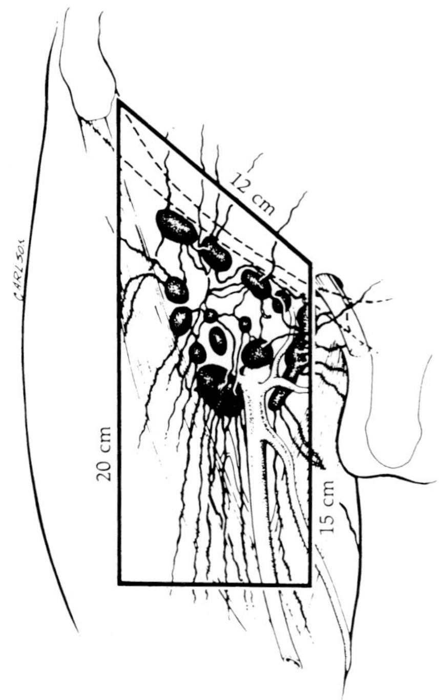

FIG. 87-7. Boundaries of the superficial inguinal nodes as described by Daseler and associates.[18] (Johnson DE, Ames FC. Groin dissection. Chicago, Year Book, 1985:15.)

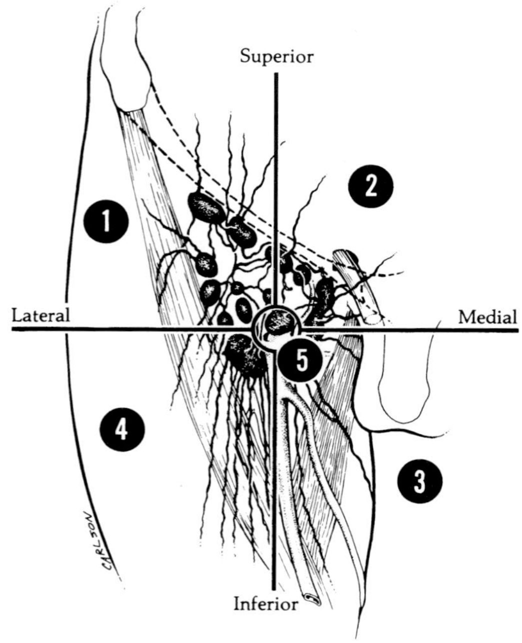

FIG. 87-8. Zonal anatomy of the superficial inguinal nodes. (Johnson DE, Ames FC. Groin dissection. Chicago, Year Book, 1985:16.)

Superolateral Group

These nodes usually form an oblique line parallel to and just below the inguinal ligament,[16,18] following the course of the superficial iliac circumflex blood vessels. They are frequently elongated and tend to be arranged in chain-like fashion. The nodes receive their afferent lymphatics from the skin of the upper gluteal region, the lateral posterior abdomen below the level of the umbilicus, and occasionally the penile skin or preputium clitoridis.

Superomedial Group

These nodes are usually circular or rounded and are less numerous than those of the superolateral group. They receive afferent cutaneous lymphatics from the umbilical and infraumbilical portions of the abdomen, perineum, cutaneous anal area, scrotum, penile skin, preputium clitoridis, vulva, and portions of the external genital organs.

Within the superomedial group of nodes, Cabanas[19,20] identified the important *sentinel lymph node,* the first filter in the penile lymphatic pathway. For 8 years, Cabanas studied in detail lymphangiograms, anatomic dissections, and microscopic reports of 100 patients, including 80 with penile carcinoma, 10 with inflammatory diseases of the penis, and 10 normal volunteers. He concluded that a specific lymph node center (the sentinel lymph node) is located medial to and above the epigastric-saphenous junction and is the first site of metastasis from penile cancer. This lymph node is associated with the superficial epigastric vein, and its location never varies by more than 1 cm (the superficial epigastric vein is absent in less than 2% of cases). Although Cabanas did find that, occasionally, the superficial epigastric group contained more than one lymph node, the true sentinel lymph node was always identified by its larger size and more medial location.

Inferomedial Group

Lymph nodes are most frequently absent (38% of the time) from this quadrant, and only 24% of humans have more than one node.[18] When they are present, the lymph nodes are usually elongated, and their long axis extends vertically. They receive afferent lymphatics predominantly from the skin of the perineum and cutaneous anal area, scrotum, vulva, medial aspect of the thigh, leg, and foot and rarely from the glans penis, glans clitoridis, penile skin, and preputium clitoridis.

Inferolateral Group

Glands in this group may be either rounded or oval. They are usually grouped around the lateral accessory saphenous vein and the termination of the superficial iliac circumflex vein. Their afferent lymphatics originate in the skin of the anterior, lateral, and posterior surfaces of the thigh, leg, and foot, in the skin of the caudal portion of the gluteal region, and occasionally in the skin of the perineum.

Central Group

Although Daseler and colleagues[18] labeled the contents of this area a "group," they actually found only a single lymph node, and that in only 15% of the patients they examined. When present, this lymph node was located in front of the termination of the greater saphenous vein. Its afferent lymphatics may come directly from the skin of the scrotum, penis, or vulva or by channels from any of the other zones.

Some superficial inguinal lymph nodes communicate directly with others. Rouvière[16] found that the majority of nodes belonging to a given group are interconnected, and, in general, efferent vessels extend from inferior to superior nodes on the same side. Efferent trunks leaving the superficial inguinal nodes proceed either to the deep inguinal nodes or, more frequently, directly to the external iliac group of lymph nodes. In the latter situation, efferent trunks may pass by one of three routes: through the femoral canal; in front of the femoral vessels and the femoral sheath; or through the interstices between the inguinal ligament and the fascia that covers the iliospsoas muscle, lateral to and some distance away from the femoral vessels.

An additional lymph node should be evaluated along with the superficial inguinal group—the prepubic node, occasionally present in the subcutaneous tissue anterior to the pubic symphysis. Although Cabanas[19] did not opacify the prepubic lymph node in any of his 43 patients who underwent penile lymphangiograms, this node, when present, can carry metastases from the penis or clitoris and then drain into the superficial inguinal lymph nodes. This finding was emphasized in 1 of our (DEJ) patients with penile cancer who underwent sentinel lymph node biopsy. Although his lymph nodes were deemed to be negative, he later was found to have an isolated metastasis in a prepubic lymph node.

Deep Inguinal Nodes

Efferent trunks from the superficial inguinal nodes drain to the deep inguinal nodes or directly to the external iliac nodes. The deep inguinal nodes, located under the fascia and medial to the femoral vein, are small and of varied numbers. Although anatomists have described upward of six to eight deep inguinal nodes, most people have only one to three.[15] Whenever several nodes are present, they are medial or anteromedial to the femoral vein. Most frequently, however, only one deep inguinal lymph node is present: the node of Cloquet or Rosenmüller. It is located in the femoral canal between the femoral vein and the lacunar ligament.

Although many texts decribe lymphatics from the glans penis or corporal bodies draining directly to the external iliac nodes, Cabanas[19] failed to identify any such communications on injecting the dorsal penile lymphatics. Similarly, clinical studies by Cabanas[19] and by Puras and associates[21] failed to demonstrate any incidence of pelvic lymph node involvement without previous metastasis to the inguinal lymph nodes. These findings strongly support the premise that direct drainage to the pelvic nodes, skipping the superficial inguinal nodes, rarely, if ever, occurs.

CONCLUSIONS

The anatomy of the penis has important implications for the diagnosis and treatment of penile and urethral cancer, Peyronie's disease, impotence, and genitourinary trauma. In addition, because the lymphatics of the penis, scrotum, and anterior urethra (in men and women) drain primarily to the superficial inguinal lymph nodes, especially the superomedial group, where the sentinel lymph node is located and where inguinal metastases from other urologic sites (testis, spermatic cord, bladder, prostate, kidney, and ureter) occasionally occur, every urologist must be familiar with the regional anatomy of the penis and groin.

REFERENCES

1. Goss CM, ed. Gray's anatomy, 29th ed. Philadelphia, Lea & Febiger, 1973.
2. Hollingshead WH. Anatomy for surgeons, vol 2. The thorax, abdomen and pelvis. New York, Hoeber-Harper, 1956.
3. Grant JC. Grant's atlas of anatomy, 5th ed. Baltimore, Williams & Wilkins, 1992.
4. Last RJ. Anatomy: region and applied, 5th ed. Edinburgh, Churchill Livingstone, 1973.
5. Breza J, Aboseif SR, Orvis BR, Lue TF, Tanagho EA. Detailed anatomy of penile neurovascular structures: surgical significance. J Urol 1989; 141:437.
6. Paick J, Lue TE. Anatomy of the penis. In: Hashmat AJ, Das S, eds. The penis. Philadelphia, Lea & Feibger, 1993:12.
7. Aboseif SR, Breza J, Lue TF, Tanagho E. Penile venous drainage in erectile dysfunction: anatomical, radiological and functional considerations. Br J Urol 1989;64:183.
8. Devine CJ Jr, Jordan GH, Schlossberg SM. Surgery of the penis and urethra. In: Walsh PC, Retik AB, Stamey TA, Vaughan ED Jr, eds. Campbell's urology, 6th ed. Philadelphia, WB Saunders, 1992:2957.

9. Zaren HA, Copeland EM, III. Inguinal node metastases. Cancer 1978; 41:919.
10. Cooper A, ed. Observations on the structure of diseases of the testis, 2nd ed. London, J Churchill, 1841:13.
11. MacCormac W. Five cases of amputation of the penis for epithelioma. Br Med J 1886;1:343.
12. Keith A. On the origin and nature of hernia. Br J Surg 1923–1924;11: 455.
13. Crawford ED, Dancshgaki F. Management of regional lymphatic drainage in carcinoma of the penis. Urol Clin North Am 1992;19:305.
14. Gray DB, Bailey HA. A new technic for radical ilioinguinal lymph node dissection. Ann Surg 1957;145:873.
15. Sedgwick CE. Regional lymphatic dissection for malignancy of extremity: radical groin dissection; radical axillary dissection Surg Clin North Am 1956;36:785.
16. Rouvière HA, ed. Anatomy of the human lymphatic system (trans, Tobias MJ). Ann Arbor, MI, Edwards Bros, 1938.
17. Ashley FL, Anson BJ. Hypogastric artery in American whites and negroes. Am J Phys Anthropol 1941;28:381.
18. Daseler EH, Anson BJ, Reimann AF. Radical excision of the inguinal and iliac lymph glands: a study based on 450 anatomical dissections and upon supportive clinical observations. Surg Gynecol Obstet 1948; 87:679.
19. Cabanas RM. An approach for the treatment of penile carcinoma. Cancer 1977;39:456.
20. Cabanas RM. Anatomy and biopsy of sentinel lymph nodes. Urol Clin North Am 1992;19:267.
21. Puras A, Gonzales-Florez B, Rodriguez R. Treatment of carcinoma of the penis. In: Stevenson HG, ed. Proceedings of the Kimbrough urologic seminar. Utica, NY, Bradock Press, 1979;12:143.

Principles and Practice of Genitourinary Oncology, edited by Derek Raghavan, Howard I. Scher, Steven A. Leibel, and Paul H. Lange. Lippincott-Raven Publishers, Philadelphia, © 1997.

CHAPTER 88

Biology of Penile Cancer

Robert P. Huben

Penile cancer is an uncommon malignant disease in the United States, but it is the most common cancer of the genitourinary system in some developing countries. The biologic significance of the study of penile cancer is not simply a matter of numbers, however. The remarkable advances made in the field of molecular biology in the past decade have drastically altered our concepts of the process of malignant transformation in penile cancer. Growing evidence indicates that the development of penile cancer is associated with infection with the human papillomavirus (HPV), and some of the steps by which the viral genes interact with those of the infected human cell are being elucidated. The intriguing parallels in the clinical course and histologic characteristics of penile cancer in men and cancer of the cervix in women appears to reflect common mechanisms of oncogenesis. Convincing epidemiologic evidence and results of basic scientific research also indicate that both penile cancer and cervical cancer are sexually transmissible, a finding with important social and medical implications. Finally, information on the cellular and molecular mechanisms of viral oncogenesis that may be obtained in the study of penile cancer may have application to our understanding of other viral-cellular interactions such as those occurring with the human immunodeficiency virus.

Our understanding of penile cancer is based on convincing epidemiologic data and on new findings from research. The purpose of this chapter is to review some of the developments and conclusions that have emerged from both these areas and to integrate these findings.

INCIDENCE AND EPIDEMIOLOGY

Penile cancer is uncommon in the United States, accounting for less than 1% of all malignant diseases in American men, with an incidence rate of 1 case per 100,000 men.[1,2] This translates into 750 to 1000 cases of penile cancer annually in the United States, a number that has remained remarkably constant for the past 50 years.[3,4]

Worldwide, the incidence of penile cancer in a particular area or population is clearly influenced by cultural or religious practices and hygienic standards. The disease is rare in developed countries; the incidence is higher in developing countries such as India, Mexico, and China, and it is particularly high in the Hindu populations in Bali.[5] Although the incidence of penile cancer has been stable in the United States, other areas with high rates of penile cancer have seen declining rates as socioeconomic conditions have improved.[3]

The role of racial or ethnic influences in the development of penile cancer is unclear, but such issues are undoubtedly influenced by socioeconomic factors, availability of medical care and reporting practices, and cultural biases.[6] A higher incidence of penile cancer in African-American men in the United States has been reported in several studies, but environmental conditions and a lower rate of neonatal circumcision in African-Americans have been suggested as confounding factors.[3,4] When an ethnic group emigrates from an area of high incidence to one of lower incidence, the risk of developing penile cancer appears to decrease.[7] An increase in the incidence of penile cancer with advancing age has been reported in all populations studied.[3,4] Penile cancer has been reported to have an earlier age of onset and to occur in a higher proportion of younger patients in areas of high incidence of the disease.[7]

Since the classic report of Wolbarst in 1932, irrefutable evidence has indicated that neonatal circumcision is completely effective in preventing the development of penile cancer.[8] Wolbarst was also the first to emphasize the importance of circumcision in the neonatal period, because circumcision in later life affords significantly less protection from penile cancers.

Circumcision rates for newborn American males have shown several interesting trends over the past several decades, as influenced by medical opinion, religious and cultural factors, funding issues, and social trends. In the non-Jewish population in the United States, circumcision did not become a widespread practice until the 1940s, and in the 1950s, 85% to 90% of male infants in the United States were circumcised annually.[1,2] Circumcision remained the norm in the United States until the late 1960s, when an anticircumcision movement began to grow and expand into the 1970s. In 1971, the Commission on the Fetus and Newborn of the American Academy of Pediatrics (AAP) took a strong position against routine circumcision after evaluating the potential benefits of the procedure and the perceived potential for physical and psychologic harm.[9] The "back to nature" movement of the time also rallied around the circumcision issue and denounced the procedure as "unnatural" and "mutilating." As emphasized in a subsequent task force statement by the AAP in 1975, conscientious penile hygiene was held to be necessary and sufficient in preventing penile cancer, although no epidemiologic evidence supports this contention.[10] The rate of circumcision fell from 85% to 70% between 1978 and 1984, and data indicate that the current rate of circumcision among newborns in the United States is about 60%.[2] The AAP has softened its position on circumcision in recent years, however, as evidence of a demonstrable benefit from routine circumcision has gathered.[11] The major benefits cited are in the prevention of urinary tract infection in infant boys and of sexually transmitted diseases in young men, rather than the prevention of penile cancer.[12–16] Beyond the medical and social aspects of the neonatal circumcision issue is the growing focus on funding or reimbursement policies and their potential impact on national health care policy.

The low incidence of penile cancer, particularly in industrialized nations, suggests that factors other than the presence of a foreskin are important in the development of penile cancer. Chronic irritation, infectious agents, and chemicals have all been proposed as etiologic agents.[3,4] Phimosis, which is congenital in about 2% to 3% of uncircumcised men, is a common finding in men with penile cancer and has been reported in up to 50% of men with penile cancer in some series.[3,4]

Uncircumcised men appear to be more susceptible to sexually transmitted diseases that disrupt epithelial surfaces, such as genital herpes, syphilis, condyloma acuminatum, and chancroid.[17–19] Genital ulceration in men may also be an important risk factor in the transmission of the human immunodeficiency virus, a finding with profound implications for the neonatal circumcision issue.[20–23] Although a history of syphilis and gonorrhea has been reported frequently in men with penile cancer, no evidence suggests that these diseases contribute directly to the development of penile cancer.[3,4] The experimental data suggesting a causative role for smegma in the pathogenesis of penile cancer are dated and are largely of historic interest.[24]

An article by Maden and associates illustrates some risk factors conventionally been associated with the development of penile cancer and their relative significance.[25] In a study of 110 men with penile cancer and 355 control subjects, the risk of penile cancer was 3.2 times greater among men who had never been circumcised relative to men circumcised at birth and 3.0 times greater among men who had been circumcised after the neonatal period. For current smokers, the risk was 2.8 times that of men who had never smoked. The risk among men reporting a history of genital warts was 5.9 times that of men reporting no such history. Relative risks associated with a reported history of penile rash or penile tear were 9.4 and 3.9, respectively. Among men not circumcised at birth, the relative risk associated with the presence of smegma was 2.1, and that of difficulty in retracting the foreskin was 3.5. Finally, 28% of case subjects reported 30 or more sexual partners, compared with only 10% of control subjects.

HUMAN PAPILLOMAVIRUS AND BENIGN AND MALIGNANT LESIONS OF THE PENIS

One of the most fascinating topics of research in the study of penile cancer is the association of HPV with both benign and malignant lesions of the penis. The papillomavirus is a double-stranded DNA icosahedron containing approximately 8000 base pairs.[26] The use of two nucleic acid-based assays, polymerase chain reaction (PCR) and in situ hybridization (ISH), has helped to define the association of HPV infection with the subsequent development of premalignant and malignant lesions of the penis.[27] A detailed discussion of the principles and techniques of molecular biology is included in Chapter 1. PCR is a highly sensitive technique that amplifies a specific DNA sequence, and it has been adapted to detect HPV in paraffin-embedded tissue samples.[28–31] ISH may also be used for localization of HPV in fixed tissues.[27] Such advances in molecular biology have led to the development of specific HPV probes that characterize new viral types that differ by more than 50% from the defined viral genomes.[32] More than 65 types of HPV have been identified.[27] The HPVs that infect the anogenital area can be separated into two distinct groups on the basis of their association with recognized clinical entities.[33] The first group, including HPV-6 and HPV-11, is generally associated with benign condylomata, which are not associated with the subsequent development of penile cancer and are referred to as "low-risk" viruses.[33,34] The "high-risk" group, including HPV-16 and HPV-18, is associated with premalignant and malignant lesions of the cervix and penis.[33–35] Cloned viral genomes from high-risk but not low-risk HPVs have been shown to transform cells in culture, a finding suggesting that these papillomavirus types may play an etiologic role in the development of these tumors.[34] The link between HPV infection and penile cancer has become more apparent as detection techniques for HPV have become progressively more refined. In an examination of 30 specimens of penile cancer from 23 patients by PCR and ISH assays, the HPV-16 genome was found in 15 patients (65%), HPV-30 was found in 3 (13%), and HPV-6 or HPV-11 was found in 2 (9%).[28] These HPV types were not detected in any of 20 nonneoplastic adult penile foreskins by PCR. In a similar study from Japan, 70 of 111 untreated penile carcinomas, or 63%, were positive for HPV DNA by PCR; subtypes were HPV-16 in 68 cases and HPV-18 in 2.[36] These investigators demonstrated HPV-16 in a lymph node metastasis of penile cancer, the same HPV type as found in the primary tumors. These investigators were also able to demonstrate localization of HPV DNA in the nuclei of carcinoma cells by ISH.

The role of HPV infection in various pathologic conditions of the penis was examined in a study by Sarkar and associates.[37] The spectrum of lesions studied included 15 cases of carcinoma in situ of the penis (7 bowenoid and 8 nonbowenoid), 11 invasive squamous carcinomas, 1 verrucous carcinoma, 2 cases of verrucous hyperplasia, 1 urethral adenocarcinoma, and 1 solitary papilloma. Viral DNA was not detected in any of the nonbowenoid specimens of carcinoma in situ, the verrucous carcinoma, the adenocarcinoma, or the papilloma of the penis. Specific sequences of HPV type 6–11 and 18 were not detected in any of the specimens examined; however, all 7 of the bowenoid forms of carcinoma in situ were positive for HPV-16 DNA. HPV-16 was also detected in 9 of 11 invasive squamous carcinomas and in both cases of verrucous hyperplasia. This study confirms the strong association of the presence of HPV-16 DNA and the bowenoid forms of intraepithelial neoplasia characteristic of carcinomas in situ of both the cervix and the penis as well as invasive carcinomas of these organs.[38–42]

Further evidence has been gathered regarding the molecular

basis of HPV infection, cell transformation, and the development of penile and cervical carcinomas. Transfection of normal HPV-negative keratinocytes derived from human foreskin or cervical epithelium with high-risk but not low-risk genomes immortalizes but does not transform these cells.[34] The immortalizing properties of high-risk HPV types are destroyed only by mutations in E6 and E7, which are two transforming proteins encoded by HPV.[43] The proteins coded by E6 and E7 are termed transforming proteins or oncoproteins.[34]

The E7 oncoprotein is a 98-amino acid nuclear protein that shares amino acid-sequence homology and certain biologic properties with adenovirus and SV40 transforming proteins.[34,44] One of these properties is the ability of the E7 oncoprotein to bind to certain proteins in cells that have been transformed by these viruses, particularly the retinoplastoma tumor suppressor protein, pRB.[45] Moreover, the presence of serum antibodies to HPV-16 E7 correlates both with the presence and the stage of cervical cancer.[46]

The E6 oncoprotein is a 158-amino acid protein that can form complexes with the cellular tumor suppressor protein, P53, which was originally classified as an oncogene.[34] The P53 protein is a 53-kd nuclear phosphoprotein encoded by a gene mapped to the short arm of chromosome 17.[47–49] The following evidence has been cited to suggest that P53 is a tumor suppressor protein or ''antioncogene'': (1) abnormalities on the short arm of chromosome 17 in the region of P53 and loss of heterozygosity in the P53 region have been demonstrated in various human cancers; (2) sporadic mutations in the *P53* gene are among the most frequent genetic alterations detected in human malignancies, and corresponding mutant P53 proteins have been identified in many of these tumors; and (3) some tumor-associated DNA viruses such as subtypes of HPV, SV40, and adenovirus produce proteins that bind to wild-type P53 protein, apparently rendering it ''ineffective'' in tumor suppression.[33,50–53] Studies suggest that P53 expression correlates with abnormal cell proliferation and increasing grade of certain carcinomas, including prostate cancer.[54–59] Although investigators have suggested that P53 expression is an early event in neoplastic transformation, the demonstration of P53 protein overexpression is not necessarily indicative of malignancy.[34] In the study by Walts and associates of squamous lesions of the anogenital area, immunoreactivity for P53 was seen in 81% of benign and low-grade squamous intraepithelial lesions, in 73% of high-grade lesions, and in 86% of infiltrating squamous carcinomas.[33]

As pointed out by Holly and Palefsky, the association of penile cancer with a sexually transmitted agent has important implications for public health that extend beyond the affected individuals.[60] Population-based studies have shown a clear geographic correlation between penile and cervical cancers, as well as the association of these malignant diseases between husbands and wives.[61–63] These studies have also confirmed the importance of HPV subtype in the development of various penile and cervical lesions. A study of 500 patients confirmed the different molecular origins of benign and malignant genital lesions: 33% of the partners of women with cervical intraepithelial changes but only 4% of the partners of women with condylomata acuminata were shown to have premalignant penile lesions.[64] In 60% of these cases, HPV-16 and HPV-33 were demonstrated, whereas benign lesions such as condylomata were associated with HPV-6, HPV-11, and HPV-42. These data clearly suggest that cervical cancer and cervical premalignant changes are related to genital HPV infections in male sex partners, and premalignant and malignant penile lesions are associated with HPV infection in female sex partners. In the epidemiologic study by Maden and associates, 28% of patients with a history of penile cancer reported having 30 or more sexual partners, compared with only 10% of control subjects.[25] Men with HPV-positive tumors by PCR in this series were also more likely to report a greater number of sexual partners.

The incidence of cervical cancer is much higher in the United States than the incidence of penile cancer, however.[65,66] An anatomic or hormonal basis may exist for this difference in infection rates.[67] Investigators have suggested that the cervical transition zone may serve as ''fertile soil'' for infection with HPV, and hormonal factors have been shown to influence infectivity.[34,68] To suggest that factors found in epidemiologic studies to be associated with the development of penile cancer, such as the uncircumcised state or poor hygiene, may be related to an increased risk of HPV infection that these conditions may impart seems reasonable.

What implications does this finding raise regarding the sexual partners of patients with known cervical or penile cancer? Because of the unpredictable incubation time and variable clinical appearance of genital HPV infection, surveillance alone appears to be a weak strategy for the prevention of anogenital warts and premalignant intraepithelial changes. The use of condoms should be strongly recommended when one of the sexual partners has a history of either condyloma or premalignant changes. For women, routine screening by cervical cytologic examination should be performed to identify early atypia. No clinical correlate exists in men. Investigators have suggested that the male sex partners of women who have been treated for HPV infection be screened to identify and treat a potential viral reservoir.[34] The treatment of subclinical infections remains a dilemma.[34]

In summary, advances and techniques in molecular biology have shown an ever-increasing association between infection with certain HPV subtypes and the development of both penile and cervical cancer. This finding may explain the strong association of premalignant and malignant changes of the penis or cervix in men or women with a large number of sexual partners. Common epidemiologic factors in men that are associated with a higher incidence of penile cancer, such as phimosis or chronic inflammation of the penis, may actually indicate a higher risk of HPV infection and subsequent malignant cellular transformation. Some of the processes in the development of penile cancer are shown in Figure 88-1.

CONCLUSIONS

Both the available epidemiologic data and molecular biologic studies indicate that penile cancer is a sexually transmissible disease, and infection with the HPV virus, particularly HPV-16 and HPV-18, is the cause of this disease. Infection with this virus is also the predominant cause of cervical cancer in women, a disease that shares many clinical, as well as molecular, characteristics with penile cancer. The risk of HPV infection and subsequent malignant transformation is higher in women than in men because of various host factors. Neonatal circumcision prevents the development of penile cancer by preventing HPV

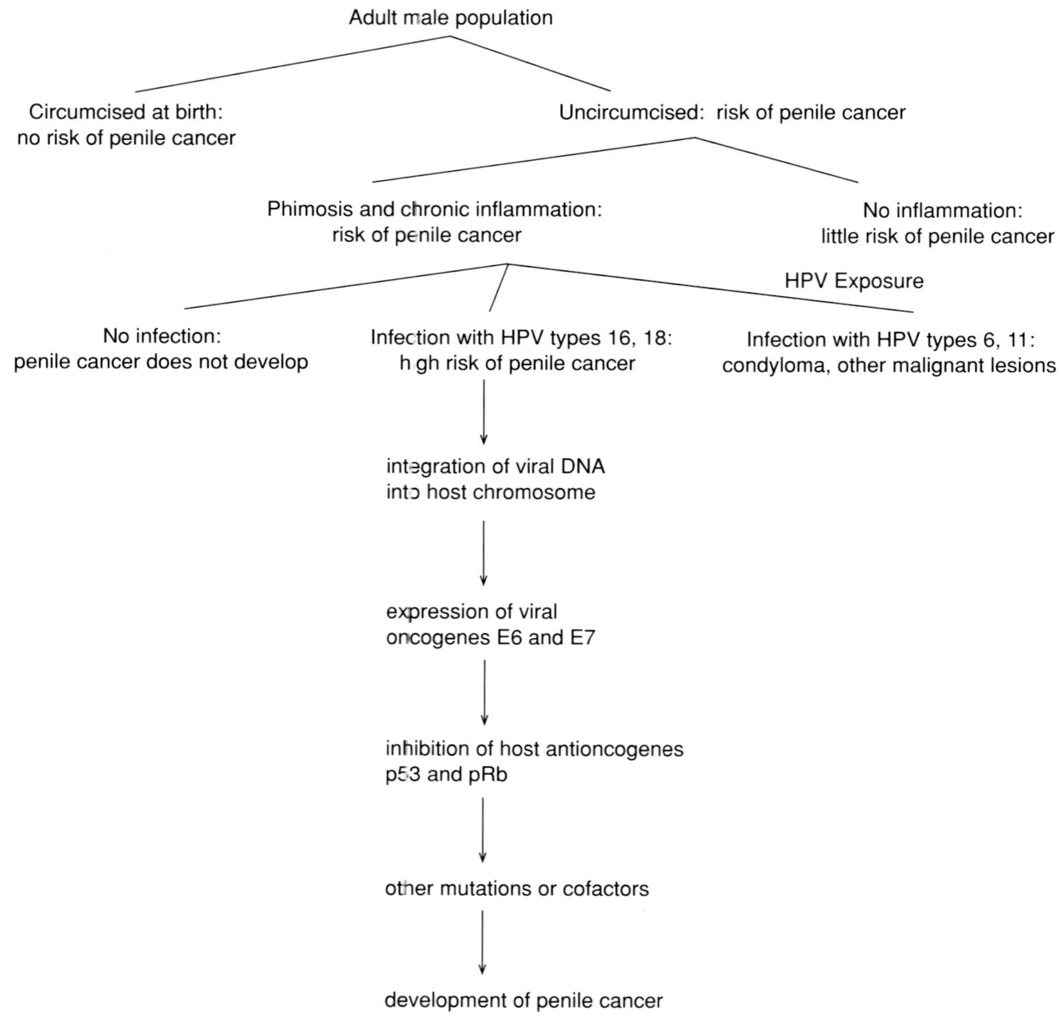

FIG. 88-1. Possible steps in the development of penile cancer. HPV, human papilloma virus.

infection and may also decrease the risk of contracting other sexually transmitted diseases. Although growing evidence shows a public health benefit from routine neonatal circumcision, cultural factors will likely determine both the rate of implementation of this procedure and its potential benefit for a particular population.

REFERENCES

1. Schoen EJ. The relationship between circumcision and cancer of the penis. CA Cancer J Clin 1991;41:306.
2. Schoen EJ. The status of circumcision of newborns. N Engl J Med 1990;322:1308.
3. Sufrin G, Huben R. Benign and malignant lesions of the penis. In: Gillenwater JY, Grayhack JT, Howards SS, Duckett JW, eds. Adult and pediatric urology, 2nd ed. St Louis, Mosby-Year Book, 1991:1643.
4. Schellhammer PF, Jordan GH, Schlossberg SM. Tumors of the penis. In: Walsh PC, Retik AB, Stamey TA, Vaughan ED Jr, eds. Campbell's urology, 6th ed. Philadelphia, WB Saunders, 1992:1264.
5. Boon ME, Susanti I, Tasche MJ, et al. Human papillmomavirus (HPV)-associated male and female genital carcinomas in a Hindu population: the male as vector and victim. Cancer 1989;64:559.
6. Hall NEL, Schottenfeld D. Penis. In: Schottenfeld D, Fraumens JF Jr, eds. Cancer epidemiology and prevention. Philadelphia, WB Saunders, 1982;964.
7. Waterhouse J, Shanmugaratnam K, Muir C, et al. Cancer incidence in five continents. IARC Sci Publ 1982;4:750.
8. Wolbarst AL. Circumcision and penile cancer. Lancet 1932;1:150.
9. American Academy of Pediatrics Committee on the Fetus and Newborn. Standards and recommendations for hospital care of newborn infants, 5th ed. Evanston, IL, American Academy of Pediatrics, 1971: 110.
10. Thompson HC, King LR, Knox E, Korones SB. Report of the ad hoc task force on circumcision. Pediatrics 1975;56:610.
11. Task Force on Circumcision. Report of the Task Force on Circumcision. Pediatrics 1989;84:388.
12. Wiswell TE, Enzenauer RW, Holton ME, Cornish JD, Hankins CT. Declining frequency of circumcision: implications for changes in the absolute incidence and male female sex ratio of urinary tract infections in early infancy. Pediatrics 1987;79:338.
13. Wiswell TE, Miller GM, Gelston HM Jr, Jones SK, Clemmings AF. Effect of circumcision status on periurethral bacterial flora during the first year of life. J Pediatr 1988;113:442.
14. Eden CS, Eriksson B, Hanson LA, et al. Adhesion to normal human uroepithelial cells of Escherichia coli from children with various forms of urinary tract infection. J Pediatr 1978;93:398.
15. Fussell EN, Kaack BM, Cherry R, Roberts JA. Adherence of bacteria to human foreskins. J Urol 1988;140:997.

16. Wiswell TE, Smith FR, Bass JW. Decreased incidence of urinary tract infections in circumcised male infants. Pediatrics 1985;75:901.
17. Wilson RA. Circumcision and venereal disease. Can Med Assoc J 1947; 56:54.
18. Parker SW, Stewart AJ, Wren MN, Gollow MM, Straton JAY. Circumcision and sexually transmitted disease. Med J Aust 1983;2:288.
19. Taylor PK, Rodin P. Herpes genitalis and circumcision. Br J Vener Dis 1975;51:274.
20. Quinn TC, Glasser D, Cannon RO, et al. Human immunodeficiency virus infection among patients attending clinics for sexually transmitted diseases. N Engl J Med 1988;318:197.
21. Stamm WE, Handsfield HH, Rompalo Am, Ashley RL, Roberts PL, Corey L. The association between genital ulcer disease and acquisition of HIV infection in homosexual men. JAMA 1988;260:1429.
22. Handsfield HH. Heterosexual transmission of human immunodeficiency virus. JAMA 1988;260:1943.
23. Cameron DW, Simonsen JN, D'Costa LJ, et al. Female to male transmission of human immunodeficiency virus type 1: risk factors for seroconversion in men. Lancet 1989;2:403.
24. Plaut A, Kohn-Speyer AC. The carcinogenic action of smegma. Science 47;105:391.
25. Maden C, Sherman KJ, Beckmann AM, et al. History of circumcision, medical conditions, and sexual activity and risk of penile cancer. J Natl Cancer Inst 1993;85:19.
26. Haye KR, et al. Cytological screening to detect subclinical anal human papillomavirus (HPV) infection in homosexual men attending genitourinary medicine clinic. Genitourin Med 1988;64:378.
27. Siegel JF, Mellinger BC. Human papillomavirus in the male patient. Urol Clinic North Am 1992;19:83.
28. Varma VA, Sanchez-Lanier M, Unger ER, et al. Association of human papillomavirus with penile carcinoma: a study using polymerase chain reaction and in situ hybridization. Hum Pathol 1991;22:908.
29. Shibata DK, Arnheim N, Martin WJ. Detection of human papillomavirus in paraffin-embedded tissue using the polymerase chain reaction. J Exp Med 1988;167:225.
30. Mullis KB, Faloona FA. Specific synthesis of DNA in vitro via a polymerase-catalyzed chain reaction. Methods Enzymol 1987;155:335.
31. Shibata DK, Arnheim N, Martin WJ. Detection of human papillomavirus in normal and dysplastic tissue by the polymerase chain reaction. Lab Invest 1988;59:555.
32. Howley PM, et al. The human papillomaviruses. Am J Med 1988;85: 155.
33. Walts AE, Koeffler HP, Said JW. Localization of p53 protein and human papillomavirus in anogenital squamous lesions. Hum Pathol 1993;24:1238.
34. Werness BA. Cervical cancer: search for an infectious etiology. Contemp Oncol 1994;45.
35. Strohmeyer TG, Slamon DJ. Proto-oncogenes and tumor suppressor genes in human urological malignancies. J Urol 1994;151:1479.
36. Iwasawa A, Kumamoto Y, Fujinaga K. Detection of human papillomavirus deoxyribonucleic acid in penile carcinoma by polymerase chain reaction and in situ hybridization. J Urol 1993;149:59.
37. Sarkar FH, Miles BJ, Plieth DH, Crissman JD. Detection of human papillomavirus in squamous neoplasm of the penis. J Urol 1992;147: 389.
38. Brescia RJ, Jenson AB, Lancaster WD, Kurman RJ. The role of human papillomaviruses with pathogenesis and histologic classification of precancerous lesions of the cervix. Hum Pathol 1986;17:552.
39. zar Hausen H. Papillomaviruses in human cancer. Cancer 1987;59: 1692.
40. Tase T, Okagaki T, Clark BA, Twiggs LB, Ostrow RS, Faras AJ. Human papillomavirus DNA in adenocarcinoma in situ, microinvasive adenocarcinoma of the uterine cervix, and coexisting cervical squamous intraepithelial neoplasia. Int J Gynecol Pathol 1969;8:8.
41. Sarkar FH, Crissman JD. Detection of human papilloma virus DNA sequences by polymerase chain reaction. Biotechniques 1990;9:180.
42. Ikenberg H, Gissman L, Gross G, Grussendorf-Conen EI, zurHausen H. Human papillomavirus type-16-related DNA in genital Bowen's disease and in bowenoid papulosis. Int J Cancer 1983;32:563.
43. Werness BA, Levine AJ, Howley PM. Association of human papillomavirus types 16 and 18 E6 proteins with p53. Science 1990;248:76.
44. Schlegel R, Phelps WC, Zhang YL, et al. Quantitative keratinocyte assay detects two biological activities of human papillomavirus DNA and identifies viral types associated with cervical carcinoma. EMBO J 1988;7:3181.
45. Munger K, Phelps WC, Bubb V, et al. The E6 and E7 genes of the human papillomavirus type 16 together are necessary and sufficient for transformation of primary human keratinocytes. J Virol 1989;63: 4417.
46. Galloway DA. Serological assays for the detection of HPV antibodies. In: Munoz N, Bosch FX, Shah KV, et al, eds. The epidemiology of cervical cancer and human papillomavirus. Lyon, Scientific Publications, 1992:147.
47. Lamb P, Crawford L. Characterization of the human p53 gene. Mol Cell Biol 1986;6:1379.
48. Isobe M, Emanuel BS, Givol D, et al. Localization of gene for human p53 tumor antigen to band 17p13. Nature 1986;320:84.
49. Miller C, Mohandas T, Wolf D, et al. Human p53 gene localized to short arm of chromosome 17. Nature 1986;3319:783.
50. Nigro HM, Baker SJ, Preisinger AC, et al. Mutations in the p53 gene occur in diverse human tumour types. Nature 1989;342:705.
51. Harris AL. Mutant p53: the commonest genetic abnormality in human cancer? J Pathol 1990;162:5.
52. Fujita M, Inoue M, Tanizawa O, et al. Alterations of the p53 gene in human primary cervical carcinoma with and without papillomavirus infection. Cancer Res 1992;52:5323.
53. Scheffner M, Takahashi T, Huibregtse JM, et al. Interaction of the human papillomavirus type 16 E6 oncoprotein with wild-type and mutant human p53 proteins. J Virol 1992;66:5100.
54. Hudson JB, Bedell MA, McCance DJ, et al. Immortalization and altered differentiation of human keratinocytes in vitro by the E6 and E7 open reading frames of human papillomavirus type 18. J Virol 1990;64:519.
55. Crook T, Morgenstern JP, Crawford L, et al. Continued expression of HPV-16 E7 protein is required for maintenance of the transformed phenotype of cells co-transformed by HPV-16 plus EJ ras. EMBO J 1989;8:513.
56. Munger K, Werness BA, Dyson N, et al. Complex formation of human papillomavirus E7 proteins with the retinoblastoma tumor suppressor gene product. EMBO J 1989;8:4099.
57. Scheffner M, Werness BA, Huibregtse JM, et al. The E6 oncoprotein encoded by human papillomavirus types 16 and 18 promotes the degradation of p53. Cell 1990;63:1129.
58. Hubbert NL, Sedman SA, Schiller JT. Human papillomavirus type 16 E6 increases the degradation rate of p53 in human keratinocytes. J Virol 1992;66:6237.
59. Liang XH, Volkmann M, Klein R, et al. Colocalization of the tumor suppressor protein p53 and human papillomavirus E6 protein in human cervical carcinoma cell lines. Oncogene 1993;8:2645.
60. Holly EA, Palefsky JM. Factors related to risk of penile cancer: new evidence from a study in the pacific northwest. J Natl Cancer Inst 1993; 85:2.
61. Skegg DCG, et al. Importance of the male factor in cancer of the cervix. Lancet 1982;2:581.
62. Smith PG, et al. Mortality of wives of men dying of cancer of the penis. Br J Cancer 1980;41:422.
63. Deeley TJ. Cancer of the cervix uteri: an epidemiological survey. Clin Radiol 1976;27:43.
64. Barrasso R, DeBrux J, Croissant O, et al. High prevalence of papillomavirus-associated penile intraepithelial neoplasia in sexual partners of women with cervical intraepithelial neoplasia. N Engl J Med 1987; 317:916.
65. Hellberg D, Valentin J, Eklund T, et al. Penile cancer: is there an epidemiological role for smoking and sexual behaviour? Br Med J 1987;295:1306.
66. Gupta J, Pilotti S, Rilke F, et al. Association of human papillomavirus type 16 with neoplastic lesions of the vulva and other genital sites by in-situ hybridization. Am J Pathol 1987;27:206.
67. Martinez I. Relationships of squamous cell carcinoma of the cervix uteri to squamous cell carcinoma of the penis among Puerto Rican women married to men with penile carcinoma. Cancer 1969;24:777.
68. Graham S, et al. Genital cancer in wives of penile cancer patients. Cancer 1979;44:1870.

Principles and Practice of Genitourinary Oncology, edited by Derek Raghavan, Howard I. Scher, Steven A. Leibel, and Paul H. Lange. Lippincott-Raven Publishers, Philadelphia, © 1997.

CHAPTER 89

Pathology of Penile Cancer

Alberto G. Ayala and Jae Y. Ro

The incidence of malignant neoplasms of the penis is approximately 1 in 100,000 males, accounting for less than 0.5% of all neoplasms in males in Western countries.[1] In certain countries such as Uganda, Brazil, Jamaica, Mexico, and Haiti, penile cancer is far more common, representing 10% to 12% of all malignant diseases in males.[1–4] The most frequently occurring malignant neoplasm is squamous carcinoma, which accounts for more than 95% of cases. Nonsquamous malignant lesions of the penis are rare and account for less than 5% of penile cancers. Sarcomas are the most common nonsquamous type of penile cancers, but they are rare. Less common primary tumors include melanoma and basal cell carcinoma. Because of the close relationship between penile squamous carcinoma and lesions caused by the human papilloma virus (HPV), condyloma is included in this discussion.

CONDYLOMA

Condyloma acuminatum, the most common tumor-like lesion of the penis, is caused by HPV.[5,6] The incidence of condyloma is about 5% in adults between the ages of 20 and 40 years.[7,8] Most of these lesions are sexually transmitted. Men whose partners have HPV-related cervical lesions have a higher-than-average incidence of penile condyloma, and autoinfections are common.[9,10] The incubation period for penile condyloma varies from several weeks to months or even years.[11]

Condylomata are commonly located on the corona of the glans, fossa navicularis of the urethra, or penile meatus, and the scrotal skin and perineum are also commonly involved.[11] Grossly, the lesions are either flat or papillary, with a cauliflower-like appearance. Histologically, they are characterized by a papillomatous proliferation of squamous epithelium that is associated with hyperkeratosis, parakeratosis, and koilocytosis.[12] Cytologic atypia is usually minimal, but mitoses may be found in the basal layer. Treatment with podophyllin or laser beam can cause bizarre cytologic changes.[13]

HPV can be demonstrated by in situ hybridization or by immunohistochemical methods.[14–17] HPV-6 and HPV-11 are commonly involved in nondysplastic genital warts, and HPV-16 and HPV-18 are frequently associated with dysplastic condylomas.[14–16] Although spontaneous regression of the lesions may occur, they usually persist in approximately one half the cases. HPV-16 and HPV-18 have been demonstrated in approximately 50% of penile squamous carcinomas. HPV infections may also play a role in the development of squamous carcinoma of the penis, which has a multifactorial etiology.

Management is usually with topical podophyllin or laser beam, and most patients have a good response to treatment.[17]

PREMALIGNANT LESIONS

Premalignant intraepithelial lesions of the penis having carcinoma in situ as common denominators but different clinical presentations have been classified as erythroplasia of Queyrat, Bowen's disease, and bowenoid papulosis.[18,19] Because controversy exists about whether these lesions are the same or represent different clinical entities, some investigators recommend that these terms be replaced by the term intraepithelial neoplasia or carcinoma in situ.[20]

Erythroplasia of Queyrat

In 1911, Queyrat[21] used the term erythroplasia to describe a bright red, well-defined, barely raised, glistening, velvety, and persistent plaque that involved the glans penis and the prepuce.

Erythroplasia of Queyrat occurs most commonly in uncircumcised men in the fifth and sixth decades of life and is rare or does not occur in circumcised patients. Clinically, it exhibits a shiny, elevated, reddish, velvety, erythematous plaque that is usually located on the glans penis or the prepuce,[22,23] but it may also involve the urethral meatus, the frenulum, or the neck of the penis. It usually presents as a solitary lesion, but multiple lesions may also occur.[22] The clinical differential diagnosis includes chronic circumscribed balanitis, inflammatory processes, and penile manifestations of benign dermatoses such as drug eruption, psoriasis, and lichen planus.[22,23]

Histologically, erythroplasia of Queyrat is a carcinoma in situ; the epithelium shows loss of polarity, proliferation of large atypical cells, dyskeratosis, multinucleated cells, and numerous normal and abnormal mitoses. The underlying stroma shows a bandlike infiltration of chronic inflammatory cells, and vascular proliferation provides the reddish discoloration typical of the gross appearance.

About 10% of patients with erythroplasia of Queyrat develop invasive squamous carcinoma, and 2% develop distant metastases.[22]

Bowen's Disease

First described in 1912, Bowen's disease is a squamous carcinoma in situ that arises in sun-exposed or sun-protected skin.[24] In the penis, the term Bowen's disease has been used when the squamous carcinoma in situ does not exhibit red discoloration or when it involves the shaft.[18–20,25]

Because one third of patients with extrapenile Bowen's disease develop cutaneous or extracutaneous malignant disease and patients with erythroplasia of Queyrat do not,[22] investigators have argued about keeping the two entities separate under different terminology.[22,26–28] More recent studies on Bowen's disease, however, have cast doubt on whether it is associated with internal malignant diseases.

Bowen's disease most often occurs in men in the fourth and fifth decades of life, about one decade earlier than the occurrence of erythroplasia of Queyrat.[25] Grossly, the lesion exhibits a crusted, sharply demarcated scaly plaque or plaques, and rarely it is papillomatous.[29] Histologically, this carcinoma in situ is similar to erythroplasia of Queyrat, but some minor differences have been reported,[19] including involvement of the pilosebaceous apparatus and hyperkeratosis, which does not occur in erythroplasia of Queyrat.[20,22,30]

Bowen's disease progresses to invasive disease in approximately 5% to 10% of cases.

Bowenoid Papulosis

In 1978, Wade and associates[31] introduced the term bowenoid papulosis to describe a dysplastic lesion of the epithelium that involved the penile shaft or the perineum in young men (average age 29.5 years).[30] The lesion histologically resembles squamous carcinoma in situ, but it is multicentric and has an indolent clinical course.[30,32] Lesions are commonly located on the penile shaft, and are characterized by light brown to gray papules that range in size from 2 to 10 mm and that may coalesce to form plaques.[30] Today, most researchers regard bowenoid papulosis as the male counterpart of the multifocal vulvovaginal dysplasia that occurs in young women.[33]

Histologically, bowenoid papulosis is characterized by a dysplastic proliferation of the epithelium and is often found with hyperkeratosis, parakeratosis, irregular acanthosis, and papillomatosis (Fig. 89-1).[30] Keratinocytes in the upper layers of the epithelium are usually more mature than those observed in Bowen's disease or erythroplasia of Queyrat. Patterson and associates[30] noted that the atypical keratinocytes in bowenoid papulosis involve the upper parts of the sweat glands, whereas pilosebaceous units are usually spared. This pattern is reversed in Bowen's disease.

Because HPV DNA has been demonstrated in several bowenoid papulosis lesions,[34,35] this disorder has been thought to be of viral origin. Hormonal and immunologic factors may also play important etiologic roles, however.[30]

The clinical course of bowenoid papulosis is different from that of Bowen's disease or erythroplasia of Queyrat. Spontaneous regression of the lesions has been reported in certain cases, but progression to invasive carcinoma or the development of systemic malignant diseases has not been observed.[36] The diagnosis of bowenoid papulosis should be heavily based on clinical presentation, rather than on pure histologic examination. In all reported cases, the lesions either responded to conservative treatment (local excision, topical podophyllin, or laser beam) or regressed spontaneously.[30,37]

SQUAMOUS CARCINOMA

Squamous carcinoma is the most common malignant disease of the penis. Various factors have been associated with an in-

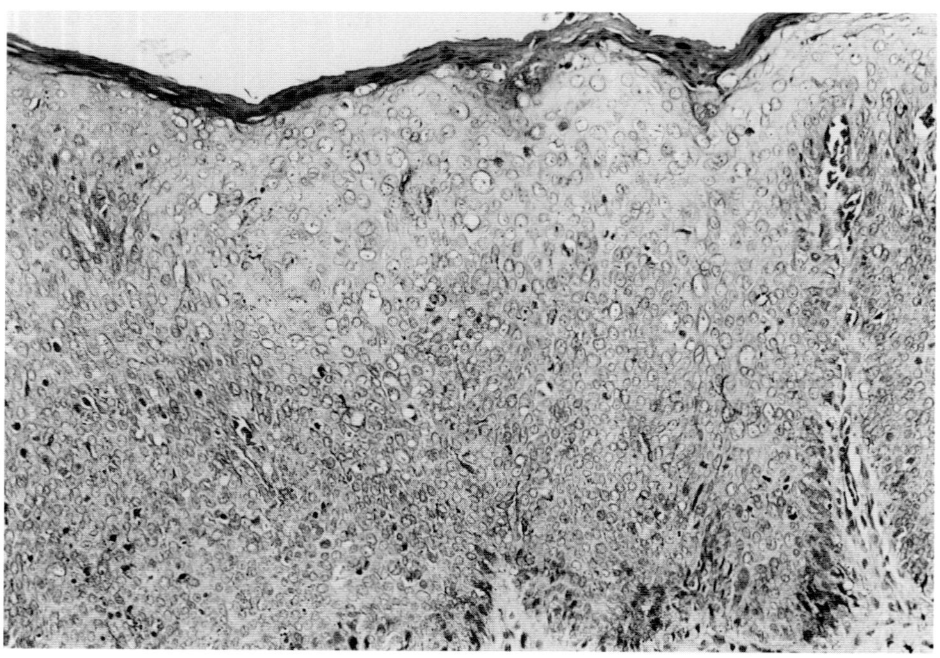

FIG. 89-1. Squamous carcinoma in situ. This illustration shows marked cellular atypia involving the entire thickness of the surface epithelium. This pattern may be seen in erythroplasia of Queyrat, in Bowen's disease, and in bowenoid papulosis. The specimen is from a patient with bowenoid papulosis.

creased risk of developing squamous carcinoma of the penis.[38–63] These factors are discussed in detail in Chapter 88.

The majority of lesions develop in the glans or the prepuce,[1,63] but lesions can also arise from the preputial sac or the coronal sulcus. The penile shaft and the urethral meatus are rare sites of carcinoma.[59–63]

Grossly, penile carcinomas show two types of growth: fungating and exophytic or ulcerating and infiltrative. Exophytic penile carcinoma forms a large polypoid mass that may be secondarily ulcerated (Fig. 89-2) and is usually well differentiated.

Ulcerating penile carcinoma tends to originate on the glans penis and is moderately to poorly differentiated. It can invade deeply, reaching the corpora cavernosa (Fig. 89-3), and may permeate the lymphatic system. The ulcerating tumor has a higher incidence of metastasizing to the lymph nodes than does the fungating tumor.

Histologically, squamous carcinoma of the penis is not different from squamous carcinoma of other sites, and it is graded according to its degree of differentiation. Most squamous carcinomas are low grade at the time of biopsy. Well-differentiated squamous carcinomas show downward, finger-like projections of atypical squamous cells that originate from a thickened, hyperkeratotic, papillomatous epidermis. Concentrically arranged masses of cells often surround accumulations of anucleate keratin known as keratin pearls. Intercellular bridges may be prominent. The cellular atypia of well-differentiated lesions is limited and consists of nuclear enlargement and pleomorphism and the presence of one or more prominent nucleoli. Mitotic figures can be identified, but they are rare. Individual cells may be become dyskeratotic and appear to be deeply eosinophilic. Usually, the dermis along the tumor margin contains a dense lymphocytic or mixed inflammatory infiltrate. High-grade (grade 3) squamous carcinomas show little or no keratin pearls, but they have marked nuclear pleomorphism and hyperchromasia and may have areas of necrosis. Mitoses are usually numerous, and deep invasion is usually seen. Moderately differentiated carcinoma (grade 2) shows histologic differentiation between grade 1 and grade 3 tumors and greater nuclear atypia, increased mitotic activity, and fewer keratin pearls than grade I tumors.

Maiche and colleagues[65] proposed a scoring system of 1 to 4 for the histologic grading of these lesions on the basis of four criteria: (1) the degree of keratinization; (2) the number of mitotic cells per high-power field (× 400); (3) the presence of cellular atypia; and (4) the presence of inflammatory cells. These investigators reported that the new scoring system was practical and showed a correlation between histologic grade and stage.[65] In the work of these investigators, patients with stage I and II diseases were more frequently found to have grade 1 and 2 tumors than were patients with stage III and IV diseases. The highest proportion of poorly differentiated grade 4 tumors was found in patients with stage IV disease. Maiche and colleagues[65] also found that histologic grade appeared to be a valuable prognostic factor. The 5- and 10-year relative survival rates were highest among patients with grade 1 tumors and lowest among those with grade 4 tumors. No significant difference in survival rate was noted between patients with grade 2 tumors and those with grade 3 tumors.[65]

Cubilla and coworkers[66] divided 66 cases of penile cancers into four categories: superficially spreading epidermoid carcinoma; vertically growing carcinoma; verrucous carcinoma (discussed separately); and multicentric carcinoma. Superficially spreading carcinoma was found most frequently; inguinal lymph node metastases were found in 82% of patients with vertically growing carcinoma, in 42% of those with superficially spreading carcinoma, and in 33% of those with multicentric carcinoma.

Little information is available on the use of DNA flow cytometric analysis in penile cancers because these tumors are rare.[67–70] Yu and associates[67] reported that patients with DNA diploid cancers had a better survival rate than patients with aneuploid cancers, and tumors with a low S-phase fraction were associated with a favorable outcome. Tumor invasiveness was also related to DNA ploidy.[67] The overall incidence of aneuploidy increased as the stage of disease increased. Yu and colleagues[67] reported that all patients who were alive and well had diploid tumors, whereas 80% of the patients who died of cancer had aneuploid DNA content in their tumors. Gustafson and associates[68] reported similar results; they found that low-grade malignant tumors were predominantly diploid and high-grade malignant tumors were not. Death from cancer was observed in only 1 of 14 patients with diploid tumors, in contrast to 4 of 12 patients with nondiploid tumors.[68] Therefore, a better prognosis can be made by considering both tumor grade and

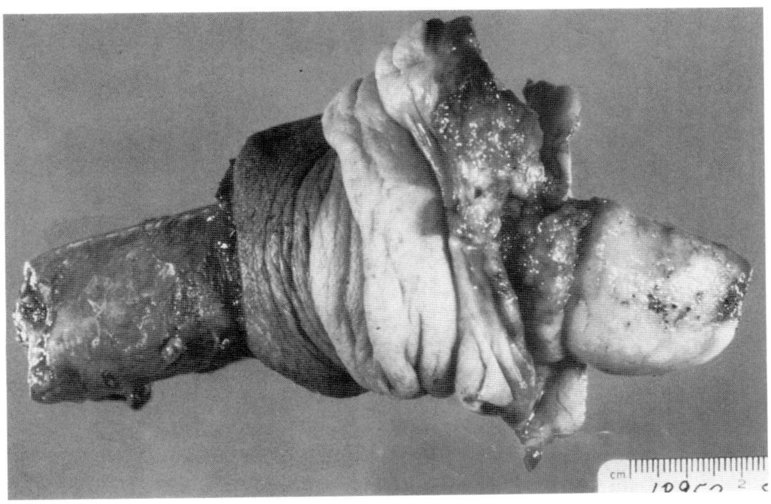

FIG. 89-2. This radical penectomy specimen shows a large carcinoma involving the prepuce extending to the glans penis.

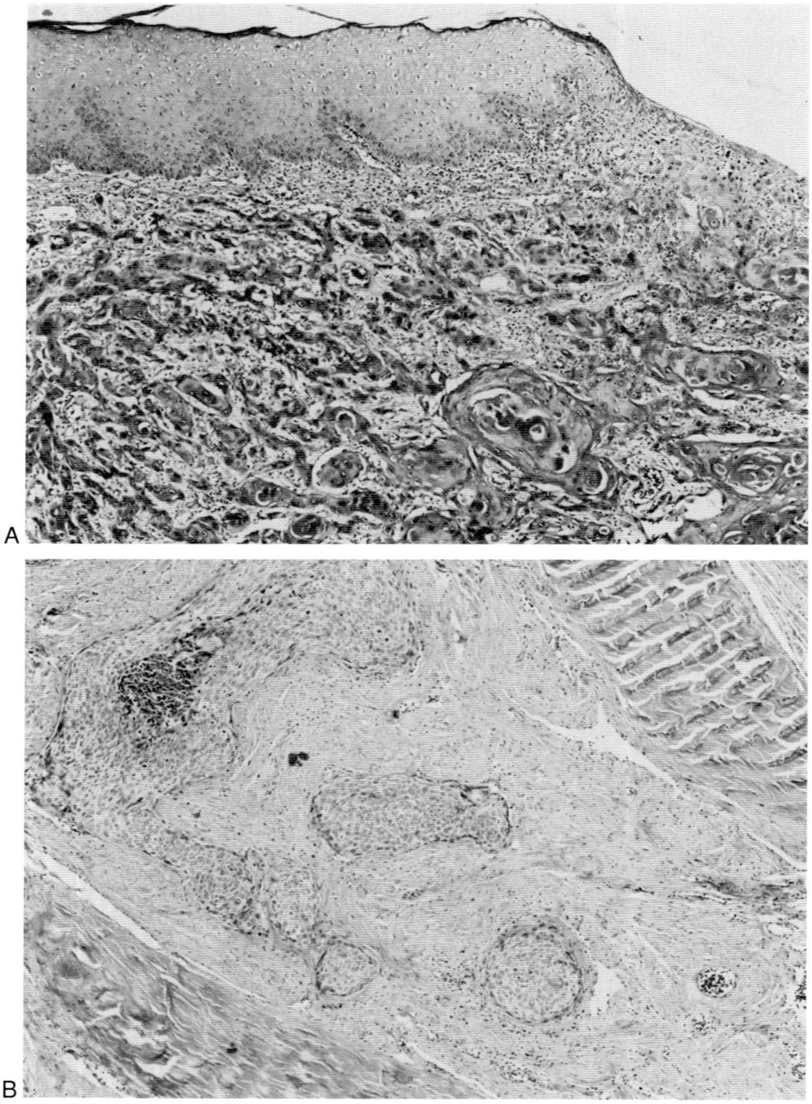

FIG. 89-3. (**A**) Histologically, squamous carcinoma arises from the surface epithelium and invades the subjacent stroma. (**B**) The corpus cavernosum is invaded.

ploidy than by considering tumor grade alone. This finding may be of particular value in a large series of patients with moderately differentiated tumors.

Penile cancer initially spreads locally, destroying the prepuce and the penile shaft.[1] Urethral involvement usually occurs secondary to fistula formation. Buck's fascia, which has rich elastic fibers, forms an initial barrier against tumor invasion. With progressive tumor growth, however, Buck's fascia and the corpus cavernosum are penetrated. Despite the rich vascularity of the corpus cavernosum, hematogenous spread is rare. Distant metastasis most commonly occurs by lymphatic spread; the inguinal lymph nodes are generally the first involved. The lymphatics of the penis form richly anastomosing channels that cross the midline along the shaft and at the penile base. Therefore, cross-inguinal lymph node metastasis may occur. The presence and number of lymph nodes involved with a metastatic tumor correlate with prognosis,[71] but infection of the primary tumor can cause inguinal lymph node enlargement without tumor metastases; therefore, sentinel node biopsy is commonly performed to stage the tumor correctly.

The extent of penile shaft involvement and the type of growth pattern of squamous carcinoma have been correlated with the frequency of lymph node metastases. Patients with tumors that involve the shaft and have an ulcerating and infiltrative growth pattern have a greater incidence of lymph node involvement. The size of the primary tumor, the grade, and the length of the delay in diagnosis have not correlated with the incidence of lymph node metastasis.[58,63] Palpable inguinal lymphadenopathy is present at diagnosis in 58% of patients.[1] Of these patients, 45% have cancer in the lymph nodes, and the remainder have inflammatory lymphadenopathy secondary to infection of the primary tumor. About 20% of nonpalpable lymph nodes contain metastases.[1] Presenting symptoms attributable to distant metastasis in the absence of regional lymph node metastasis are unusual. Hematogenous dissemination is rare. Fewer than 2% of patients with penile carcinoma show distant visceral metastases at the time of diagnosis; however, hepatic, pulmonary, and osseous metastases can occur in untreated cases.[72,73]

Almost 50% of tumors originating in the shaft of the penis are poorly differentiated, whereas only 10% of tumors located in

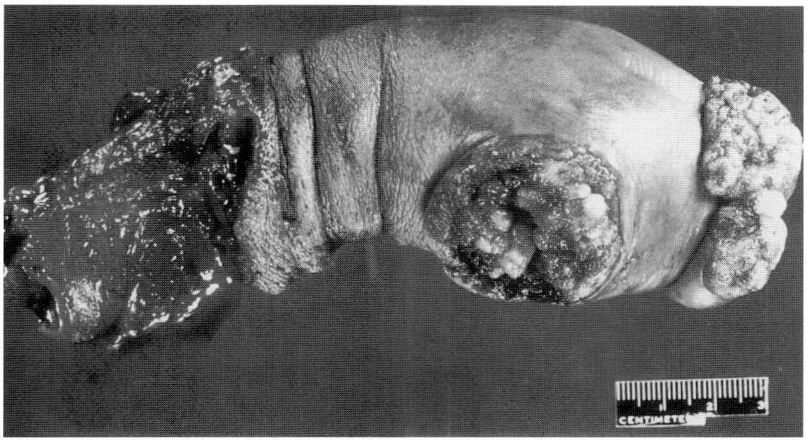

FIG. 89-4. Gross specimen of a verrucous carcinoma. This lesion arises from the prepuce and, burrowing through the adjacent corpus spongiosum, emerges from the side of the shaft of the penis.

the prepuce are of this high grade.[74] This phenomenon evidently reflects differences in the growth pattern of carcinomas at different sites, which may also have some affect on the prognosis.

The most widely used clinical staging systems include one proposed by Jackson[75] and one by the American Joint Committee on Cancer.[76]

Histologic differentiation and disease stage are the most reliable prognostic factors of penile carcinomas. The most important prognostic factor is the stage. Patients with a higher stage of cancer have a worse outcome than patients with a lower stage of cancer, and survival time is shorter for patients who have inguinal or iliac node involvement or distant metastases. Histologic grading is another important prognostic factor. Histologic grade correlates well with the clinical stage. Patients with poorly differentiated tumors tend to have advanced disease and a poor prognosis. Patients with well-differentiated tumors have a favorable prognosis, and more than 80% are long-term survivors.

The philosophy of treatment of penile cancer[77–84] remains controversial, as discussed in other chapters in this section. Accurate histopathologic classification and staging remain essential for successful management, however.

VERRUCOUS CARCINOMA

Since its first description in the oral cavity, verrucous carcinoma has been recognized in various organs, including the larynx, vulva, vagina, anus, and penis. Verrucous carcinoma of the penis accounts for 5% to 16% of malignant penile tumors[85] and is commonly seen in middle-aged men.[85–91] Typically, it is a large, fungating, frequently ulcerated, warty lesion that burrows through the normal tissues (Fig. 89-4). Most of these lesions start on the coronal sulcus and spread to the glans and the preputial skin.

Microscopically, verrucous carcinoma is a well-differentiated squamous carcinoma with an exophytic papillary growth pattern and knobby pushing borders (Fig. 89-5). No cytologic atypia is visible, and the rare mitoses are confined to the deeper portion of the tumor.[90]

These tumors grow locally and do not metastasize. If verrucous carcinoma is not treated adequately, multiple recurrences can occur. The differential diagnosis includes condyloma acuminatum, giant condyloma of Buschke-Löwenstein, and well-differentiated keratinizing squamous carcinoma. When a lesion is

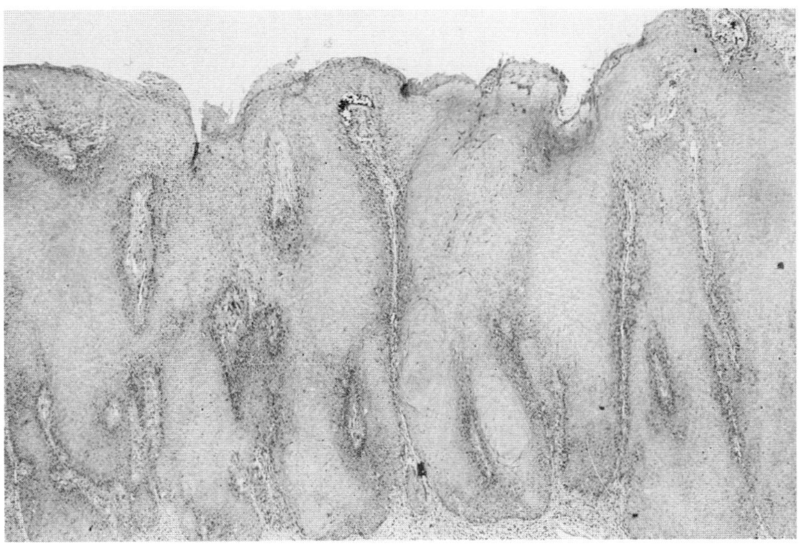

FIG. 89-5. Histologically, verrucous carcinoma exibits an acanthotic papillomatous growth pattern with knobby advancing edges. Although the epithelium is acanthotic, it shows no nuclear atypia.

small, to differentiate condyloma acuminatum from verrucous carcinoma is only of academic interest because the management of both lesions is conservative. When the lesion is large, giant condyloma of Buschke-Löwenstein enters into the differential diagnosis. Most authorities consider giant condyloma of Buschke-Löwenstein and verrucous carcinoma to be the same entity,[90,91] but even for those who believe otherwise, separating the two is clinically unimportant because they are managed the same way conservatively.

Squamous carcinoma, however, must be differentiated from verrucous carcinoma because it has different clinical course and is managed differently.[3,90,91] The lack of cytologic atypia, mitoses, and an infiltrative growth pattern differentiate verrucous carcinoma from well-differentiated squamous carcinoma.

About 25% of verrucous carcinomas show microscopic foci of cellular anaplasia, high mitotic activity, and invasion of the stroma.[85,90] These tumors have been designated as hybrid squamous-verrucous carcinoma (Fig. 89-6).[85,90–92] The hybrid squamous-verrucous carcinoma and pure verrucous carcinoma show no significant differences with regard to patient age, tumor location, or clinical outcome, but the number of reported cases of hybrid squamous-verrucous carcinomas is limited.[85,90] DNA ploidy and cell-cycle analysis done by Masih and associates[90] showed that both the pure and hybrid verrucous carcinomas have uniform diploid cell populations with similar proliferation activity.

Clinical outcome for patients with verrucous carcinoma correlates with the type of treatment. Partial or radical penectomy has resulted in a 33% recurrence rate, whereas local excision has resulted in an 80% recurrence rate.[85,90,91] Therefore, partial and, if necessary, total penectomy are recommended to avoid the high recurrence rate associated with local excision. Radiotherapy should be avoided because it has been associated with dedifferentiation of verrucous carcinoma.[85,90,91]

SPINDLE CELL SQUAMOUS CARCINOMA

Only a few cases of spindle cell squamous carcinoma of the penis have been reported.[93,94] These lesions are usually polypoid and histologically are composed predominantly of spindle

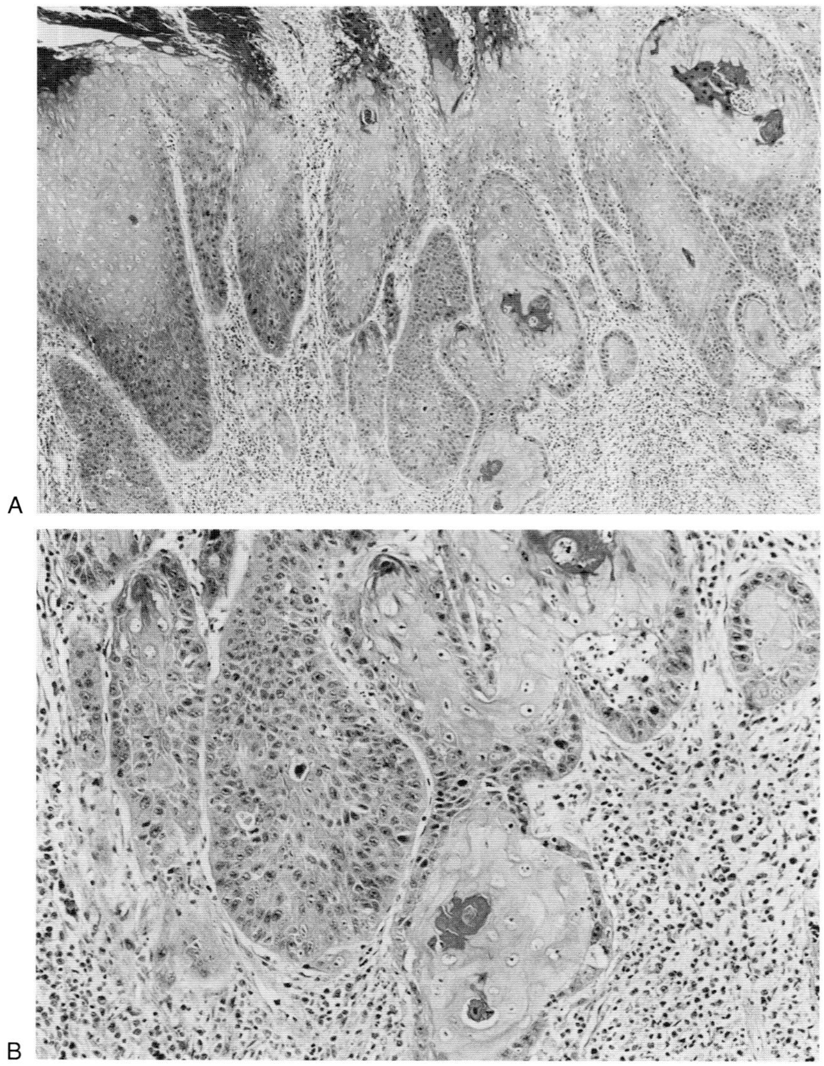

FIG. 89-6. Hybrid verrucous carcinoma. (**A**) The typical acanthotic papillomatous growth is present in this tumor, but a change of the cytologic features to those of a higher-grade carcinoma in the lower half is noted and can be seen better in (**B**) the higher-power illustration.

cells with focal areas of squamous differentiation. Marked nuclear pleomorphism and increased mitoses are common in the spindle component. The prognostic significance of this variant remains unclear because few cases have been reported.

BASAL CELL CARCINOMA

Basal cell carcinoma rarely occurs in the penis or scrotum.[94–98] The shaft (56%), followed by the glans (30%) and the prepuce (14%) are the usual areas of involvement.[97,98] Most reported patients have been white and range in age from 37 to 79 years.[97,98] Histologically, basal cell carcinoma shows the same basaloid morphology as basal cell tumors of the skin. The clinical course is indolent, and local excision is sufficient to cure it.

MALIGNANT MELANOMA

Primary malignant melanoma of the penis is rare, with fewer than 100 cases reported in the literature; it accounts for approximately 1% of all penile cancers.[99–103] Most reported cases have occurred in white men in their fifth and sixth decades of life.[104] In contrast to squamous carcinomas, penile malignant melanomas are rare in black men. In the majority of cases, the melanomas affect the glans.[18] Occasional lesions may occur on the prepuce and the shaft.

Clinically, a black, brown, or blue papule or an ulcerated plaque is present in the penis. The histologic findings in penile melanomas are similar to those of malignant melanomas arising in any other mucosa or skin sites.[18]

The prognosis of penile malignant melanomas depends on the depth of invasion and the stage. Stage I melanoma is confined to the penis, stage II melanoma metastasizes to the lymph nodes, and stage III melanoma involves distant metastases. Penile melanomas with a thickness of 0.75 mm or less have an excellent prognosis. Those with a depth of invasion of 1.5 mm or greater carry an extremely poor prognosis because of the high frequency of metastasis.[18] Overall, half of these patients show lymph node metastases at the time of diagnosis.[18]

Studies[99,102] recommend prophylactic superficial lymph node dissection as an adjunct to penectomy only for lesions thicker than 1.5 mm in patients with stage I melanoma. Bilateral inguinal lymph node dissection remains routine for patients with stage II melanomas.

Malignant melanoma of soft parts (clear cell sarcoma) is an uncommon neoplasm found predominantly in the tendons and aponeuroses of the extremities. Although unusual, the penis has also been reported to be a site of malignant melanoma of soft parts.[105]

SARCOMAS

Sarcomas of the penis are rare, representing fewer than 5% of all malignant penile tumors. The peak occurrence of penile sarcoma is in the fifth and sixth decades of life, except for rhabdomyosarcoma, which occurs in children and in young men. Sarcomas are most frequently located on the penile shaft, except for Kaposi's sarcoma, which is most commonly located on the glans penis.

Vascular tumors, including Kaposi's sarcoma, epithelioid hemangioendothelioma, and angiosarcoma, are the most common penile sarcomas. Sarcomas of myogenic, neurogenic, and fibrous origin can also occur.[106] The histologic features of these lesions are similar to those of sarcomas arising at other locations.

Kaposi's sarcoma of the penis is recognized more frequently in patients exposed to the human immunodeficiency virus.[107–109] The penis is rarely the first area of involvement of this disease, however. Kaposi's sarcoma usually involves the skin of the shaft or the glans penis. Around 20% of patients who have acquired immunodeficiency syndrome (AIDS) and Kaposi's sarcoma have lesions on the penis, and as many as 3% of patients with AIDS initially present with penile Kaposi's sarcoma. Local excision can be effective for small, localized lesions, but radiotherapy may be required.[110,111]

The majority of the vascular sarcomas are hemangioendotheliomas, but they are rare, with only 35 cases reported.[112] Hemangioendotheliomas are indolent, but high-grade angiosarcomas metastasize to lymph nodes or to distant sites such as lung, liver, and bone. Most vascular tumors of the penis display a low-grade morphology, with anastomosing networks of irregularly shaped vascular spaces lined by plump, often piled-up, endothelial cells, and all are in the category of epithelioid-histiocytoid hemangioendothelioma.[113,114] High-grade angiosarcomas display solid or anastomosing masses of anaplastic tumor cells with numerous mitoses and associated hemorrhage and necrosis.

Leiomyosarcoma of the penis frequently occurs in the fifth to seventh decades of life. Superficial leiomyosarcomas are believed to arise from smooth muscle of the glans penis or from smooth muscle of the dermis of the shaft, and subcutaneous nodules usually form. Patients with superficial lesions tend to do well with local excision, but the tumor may recur locally. The less common deep type of leiomyosarcoma arises from the smooth muscle of the corpus cavernosum and tends to metastasize early or to invade the urethra. Deep lesions carry a poor prognosis despite radical surgery because of their tendency to metastasize to distant sites.[115,116]

Fibrosarcomas can be superficial or deep and usually present as a slow-growing, firm, nontender mass on the dorsum of the penile shaft or on the glans. Fibrosarcoma shares many clinical and gross features with leiomyosarcoma.[117] Malignant fibrous histiocytoma has rarely been reported in the penis, with only 2 cases reported in the literature, 1 of which was an inflammatory type of malignant fibrous histiocytoma.[118,119]

Rhabdomyosarcoma has been reported in the penis, particularly on the shaft near the root. Most rhabdomyosarcomas occur in children and are embryonal rhabdomyosarcomas.[120,121]

Eight cases of epithelioid sarcomas involving the penis have been reported.[122,123] The patients' ages at diagnosis ranged from 23 to 43 years (mean age 32 years). They present as single or multiple, firm, slowly growing, painless, subcutaneous nodules. The masses may produce surface ulceration and may cause erectile pain or dysuria. Radical excision is the preferred method of treatment, although local excision combined with radiotherapy has been used with success.[122,123] Epithelioid sarcoma is a slow-growing but aggressive tumor in the penis, as it is elsewhere in the body. Regardless of the therapy used, as many as

80% of the lesions may recur locally. Metastases to the lung have been reported in 2 cases of penile lesions, but most reports had no long-term follow-up.

Other soft-tissue sarcomas, including hemangiopericytoma and malignant schwannomas, have been reported in the penis. Benign tumors such as hemangioma, lymphangioma, glomus tumor, neurofibroma, schwannoma, and granular cell tumor have also been reported in the penis. Reported cases have been approximately equally divided between benign and malignant lesions.[74]

Primary lymphoma of the penis is rare, with only 6 reported cases. Investigators have suggested that this presentation is merely the manifestation of occult nodal disease or a complication of late nodal lymphoma because the penis has no lymphoid tissue.[124,125]

METASTATIC TUMORS

Metastatic disease to the penis is rare and usually represents a late manifestation of systemic metastasis. In 1985, Powell and associates[126] reviewed the literature and found only 219 cases. In a 1989 review, Perez-Mesa and Oxenhandler[127] reported only 6 additional cases. In all reported series, the most common primary site was the prostate, followed by the rectosigmoid colon, bladder, and kidney.[128–130] Less common primary sites include the testes, ureters, and nonpelvic organs such as the lung, pancreas, nasopharynx, and bone.[126–132]

The most common location of metastatic tumors is the corpus cavernosum.[128] Clinically, the disease presents as multiple, palpable, painless nodules that may involve the skin and that may ulcerate, mimicking a syphilitic chancre. In half the patients, diffuse involvement of the corpus cavernosum occurs, causing priapism.[128] Hematuria and dysuria can be seen. In most cases, penile metastases occur at the end stage of a known primary tumor and pose no diagnostic difficulty. In some cases, however, the penis can be the first metastatic site.[133,134]

Five modes of metastasis to the penis have been described: (1) retrograde venous dissemination, which is thought to be the most common pathway; (2) retrograde lymphatic dissemination; (3) arterial dissemination; (4) direct extension; and (5) perineural tumor infiltration.[126,127]

The prognosis for patients with metastasis to the penis is poor. Paquin and Rowland[135] reported that 95% of patients died within weeks to months of diagnosis. Similarly, Mukamel and associates[136] reported that 71% of patients died within 6 months of diagnosis. Treatment for these patients should be supportive and systemic. Mukamel and colleagues[136] suggested, however, that total penectomy may be indicated for relief of pain or of severe urinary symptoms if metastases are confined to the penis without extension to the pelvis or pelvic diaphragm.

REFERENCES

1. Sufrin G, Huben R. Benign and malignant lesions of the penis. In: Gillenwater JY, Grayhack JT, Howards SS, Duckett JW, eds. Adult and pediatric urology. Chicago, Year Book, 1987:1448.
2. Persky L, deKernion J. Carcinoma of the penis. CA Cancer J Clin 1986;36:258.
3. Dodge OG, Linsell CA. Carcinoma of the penis in Uganda and Kenya Africans. Cancer 1963;16:1255.
4. Riveros M, Lebron R. Geographic pathology of cancer of penis. Cancer 1963;16:798.
5. Rosenberg SK, Reid R. Sexually transmitted papilloma viral infections in the male. I. Anatomic distribution and clinical features. Urology 1987;29:488.
6. Chuang T-Y. Condyloma acuminatum (genital warts): an epidemiologic view. J Am Acad Dermatol 1987;16:376.
7. Chuang T-Y, Perry HO, Kurland LT, Ilstrup DM. Condyloma acuminatum in Rochester, Minn, 1950–1978. I. Epidemiology and clinical features. Arch Dermatol 1984;120:469.
8. Syrjanen K, Syrjanen S. Epidemiology of human papillomavirus infections and genital neoplasia. Scand J Infect Dis Suppl 1990;69:7.
9. Barrasso R, De Brux J, Croissant O, Orth G. High prevalence of papilloma virus-associated penile intraepithelial neoplasia in sexual partners of women with cervical intraepithelial neoplasia. N Engl J Med 1987;317:916.
10. Schackner L, Hankin DE. Assessing child abuse in childhood condyloma acuminatum. J Am Acad Dermatol 1985;123:157.
11. Oriel JD. Natural history of genital warts. Br J Vener Dis 1971;47:1.
12. Margolis S. Genital warts and molluscum contagiosum. Urol Clin North Am 1984;11:163.
13. Goette DK. Review of erythroplasia of Queyrat and its treatment. Urology 1976;8:311.
14. Del Mistro A, Braunstein JD, Halwer M, Koss LG. Identification of human papilloma virus types in male urethral condylomata acuminata by in-situ hybridization. Hum Pathol 1987;18:936.
15. O'Brien WM, Jenson AB, Lancaster WD, Maxted WC. Human papillomavirus typing of penile condyloma. J Urol 1989;141:863.
16. Nuovo GJ, Hochman HA, Eliezri HA, Lastarria D, Comite SL, Silvers DN. Detection of human papillomavirus DNA in penile lesions histologically negative for condylomata: analysis by in-situ hybridization and the polymerase chain reaction. Am J Surg Pathol 1990;14:829.
17. Weaver MG, Abdul-Karim FM, Dale G, Sorensen K, Huang YT. Detection and localization of human papillomavirus in penile condylomas and squamous cell carcinomas using in-situ hybridization with biotinylated DNA viral probes. Mod Pathol 1989;2:94.
18. Hewan-Lowe K, Moreland A, Finnerty DP. Penis and scrotum, tumors and related disorders. In: Someren A, ed. Urologic pathology with clinical and radiologic correlations. New York, Macmillan, 1990:640.
19. Rosai J. Penis and scrotum. In: Rosai J, ed. Ackerman's surgical pathology, 8th ed. St. Louis, Mosby, 1996:1305.
20. Kaye V, Zhang G, Dehner LP, Fraley EE. Carcinoma in situ of penis: is distinction between erythroplasia of Queyrat and Bowen's disease relevant? Urology 1990;36:479.
21. Queyrat L. Erytroplasie du gland. Bull Soc Fr Dermatol Syphilol 1911;22:378.
22. Graham JH, Helwig EB. Erythroplasia of Queyrat: a clinicopathologic and histochemical study. Cancer 1973;32:1396.
23. Anderson L, Johnson G, Brehmer-Anderson E. Erythroplasia of Queyrat-carcinoma in situ. Scand J Urol Nephrol 1967;1:303.
24. Bowen JT. Precursor dermatoses: a study of two cases of chronic atypical epithelial proliferation. J Cutan Dis 1912;30:241.
25. Mostofi FK, Price EB Jr. Tumors of the penis and scrotum. In: Atlas of tumor pathology: tumors of the male genital system. Washington, DC, Armed Forces Institute of Pathology, 1973:295.
26. Graham JH, Helwig EB. Bowen's disease and its relationship to systemic cancer. Arch Dermatol 1961;83:738.
27. Chuang TY, Tse J, Reizner GT. Bowen's disease (squamous cell carcinoma in-situ) as a skin marker for internal malignancy: a case control study. Am J Prev Med 1990;6:238.
28. Callen JP, Headington JT. Bowen's and non-Bowen's squamous intraepithelial neoplasia of the skin: Relationship to internal malignancy. Arch Dermatol 1980;116:422.
29. Haneke E. Skin diseases and tumors of the penis. Urol Int 1982;37:172.
30. Patterson JW, Kao GF, Graham JH, Helwig EB. Bowenoid papulosis: a clinicopathologic study with ultrastructural observations. Cancer 1986;57:823.
31. Wade TR, Kopf AW, Ackerman AB. Bowenoid papulosis of the penis. Cancer 1978;42:1890.
32. Taylor DR Jr, South DA. Bowenoid papulosis: a review. Cutis 1981;27:92.
33. Chesney TMcC, WM Murphy. Diseases of the penis and scrotum. In:

WM Murphy, ed. Urological pathology. Philadelphia, WB Saunders, 1989:380.
34. Zachow KR, Ostrow RS, Bender M, et al. Detection of human papillomavirus DNA in anogenital neoplasias. Nature 1982;300:771.
35. Zelickson AS, Prawer SE. Bowenoid papulosis of the penis, demonstration of intranuclear viral-like particles. Am J Dermatopathol 1980; 2:305.
36. Barnes RD, Sarembock LA, Abratt RP, Pontin AR. Carcinoma of penis. J R Coll Surg Edinb 1989;34:44.
37. Eisen RF, Bhawan J, Cahn TH. Spontaneous regression of bowenoid papulosis of the penis. Cutis 1983;32:269.
38. Brinton LA, Li JY, Rong SD, et al. Risk factors for penile cancer: results from a case-control study in China. Int J Cancer 1991;47:504.
39. Bissada NK, Morcos RR, El-Senoussi M. Post-circumcision carcinoma of the penis: clinical aspects. J Urol 1986;135:283.
40. Leiter E, Lefkovitis AM. Circumcision and penile cancer. NY State J Med 1975;75:1520.
41. Dagher R, Selzer ML, Lapides J. Carcinoma of the penis and the anti-circumcision crusade. J Urol 1980;110:79.
42. Apt A. Circumcision and penile cancer. Acta Med Scand 1965;174: 493.
43. Jensen MS. Cancer of the penis in Denmark 1942 to 1962 (511 Cases). Danish Med Bull 1977;24:66.
44. Reddy CRRM, Devendranath V, Pratap S. Carcinoma of penis-role of phimosis. Urology 1984;24:85.
45. Koutsky LA, Wolner-Hanssen P. Genital papillomavirus infections: current knowledge and future prospects. Obstet Gynecol Clin North Am 1989;16:541.
46. Loning T, Riviere A, Henke RP, Von Preyss S, Dorner A. Penile/anal condylomas and squamous cell cancer: a HPV DNA hybridization study. Virchows Arch A Pathol Anat Histopathol 1988;413:491.
47. McCance DJ, Kalache A, Ashdown K, et al. Human papillomavirus types 16 and 18 in carcinomas of penis from Brazil. Int J Cancer 1986;37:55.
48 Broker TR, Chin MT, Dong G, et al. Papillomavirus transcriptional regulation in human genital neoplasia. In: Proceedings of the Annual Meeting of the American Association for Cancer Research, Washington, DC. 1990;31:488.
49. Masih AS, Stoler MH, Farrow GM, Johansson SL. Human papillomavirus in penile squamous cell lesions: a comparison of an isotopic RNA and two commercial nonisotopic DNA in situ hybridization methods. Arch Pathol Lab Med 1993;117:302.
50. Scinicariello F, Rady P, Saltzstein D, Orihuela E, Tyring SK. Human papillomavirus 16 exhibits a similar integration pattern in primary squamous cell carcinoma of the penis and in its metastasis. Cancer 1992;70:2143.
51. Sarkar FH, Miles BJ, Plieth DM, Crissman JD. Detection of human papillomavirus in squamous neoplasm of the penis. J Urol 1992;147: 389.
52. Wiener JS, Effert PJ, Humphrey PA, Yu L, Liu ET, Walther PJ. Prevalence of human papillomavirus types 16 and 18 in squamous cell carcinoma of the penis: a retrospective analysis of primary and metastatic lesions by differential polymerase chain reaction. Int J Cancer 1992;50:694.
53. Rosemberg SK, Herman G, Elfont E. Sexually transmitted papillomaviral infection in the males. VII. Is cancer of penis sexually transmitted? Urology 1991;37:437.
54. Graham S, Priore R, Graham M, Browne R, Burnett W, West D. Genital cancer in wives of penile cancer patients. Cancer 1979;44: 1870.
55. Maiche AG, Pyrhonen S. Risk of cervical cancer among wives of men with carcinoma of the penis. Acta Oncol 1990;29:569.
56. Stern RS, Members of the Photochemotherapy Follow-up Study. Genital tumors among men with psoriasis exposed to psoralens and ultraviolet A radiation (PUVA) and ultraviolet B radiation. N Engl J Med 1990;332:1093.
57. Droller MJ. Carcinoma of penis: an overview. Urol Clin North Am 1980;7:783.
58. Fraley EE, Zhang G, Sazama R, Lange PH. Cancer of the penis: prognosis and treatment plans. Cancer 1985;55:1618.
59. Jones WG, Hamers H, Van Den Bogaert W. Penis cancer: a review by the joint radiotherapy committee of the European organisation for research and treatment of cancer (EORTC) genitourinary and radiotherapy groups. J Surg Oncol 1989;40:227.
60. Fossa SD, Hall KS, Johannessen NB, Urnes T, Kaalhus O. Cancer of the penis. Eur Urol 1987;13:372.
61. Narayana AS, Olney LE, Loening SA, Weimar GW, Culp DA. Carcinoma of the penis. Cancer 1982;49:2185.
62. Merrin CE. Cancer of the penis. Cancer 1980;45:1973.
63. Burgers JK, Badalament RA, Drago JR. Penile cancer: clinical presentation, diagnosis, and staging. Urol Clin North Am 1992;19:247.
64. Derrick FC Jr, Lynch K M Jr, Kretkowski RC, Yarbrough W. Epidermoid carcinoma of the penis: computer analysis of 87 cases. J Urol 1973;110:303.
65. Maiche AG, Pyrhonen S, Karkinen M. Histological grading of squamous cell carcinoma of the penis: a new grading system. Br J Urol 1991;67:522.
66. Cubilla AL, Barreto J, Caballero C, Ayala G, Riveros M. Pathologic features of epidermoid carcinoma of the penis: a prospective study of 66 cases. Am J Surg Pathol 1993;17:753.
67. Yu DS, Chang SY, Ma CP. DNA ploidy, S-phase fraction and cytomorphometry in relation to survival of human penile cancer. Urol Int 1992;48:265.
68. Gustafson O, Tribukait B, Nyman CR, Borgstrom E. DNA pattern and histopathology of penis: a prospective study. Scand J Urol Nephrol Suppl 1988;110:219.
69. Hoofnagle RF, Mahin EJ, Lamm DL, Kandzari S. Deoxyribonucleic acid flow cytometry of squamous cell carcinoma of the penis. J Urol 1990;143:352A.
70. Pettaway CA, Stewart D, Vuitch F, Savino D, Ewalt D, McConnell JD. Penile squamous carcinoma: DNA flow cytometry versus histopathology for prognosis. J Urol 1991;145:367A.
71. Pow-Sang JE, Benavente V, Pow-Sang JM, Pow-Sang M. Bilateral inguinal lymph node dissection in the management of cancer of the penis. Semin Surg Oncol 1990;6:241.
72. Schellhammer PF, Jordan GH, Schlossberg SM. Tumors of the penis. In: Walsh PC, Retik AB, Stamey TA, Vaughan ED Jr, eds. Campbell's urology, 6th ed. Philadelphia, WB Saunders, 1992:1264.
73. Johnson DE, Fuerst DE, Ayala AG. Cancer of the penis: experience with 153 cases. Urology 1973;1:404.
74. Nitti VW, Macchia RJ. Neoplasms of the Penis. In: Hashmat AI, Das S, eds. The Penis. Philadelphia, Lea & Febiger, 1993:269.
75. Jackson SM. The treatment of carcinoma of the penis. Br J Surg 1966; 53:33.
76. Beahrs OH, Henson DE, Hutter RVP, Kennedy BJ. American Joint Committee on Cancer manual for staging of cancer, 4th ed. Philadelphia, JB Lippincott, 1992:191.
77. Johnson DE, Lo RK. Management of regional lymph nodes in penile carcinoma: five year results following therapeutic groin dissections. Urology 1984;24:308.
78. Ornellas AA, Seixas ALC, de Moraes JR. Analysis of 200 lymphadenectomies in patients with penile carcinoma. J Urol 1991;146:330.
79. Srinivas V, Joshi A, Agarwal B, Mundhada U, Shah A, Phadke AG. Penile cancer: the sentinel lymph node controversy. Urol Int 1991; 47:108.
80. Horenblas S, van Tinteren H, Delemarre JFM, Moonen LMF, Lustig V, van Waardenburg EW. Squamous cell carcinoma of the penis. III. Treatment of regional lymph nodes. J Urol 1993;149:492.
81. Young MJ, Reda DJ, Waters WB. Penile carcinoma: a twenty-five-year experience. Urology 1991;38:529.
82. Caballero C, Cubilla AL, Barreto J, Riveros M. Factores patologicos relacionados con metastasis inguinal en carcinomas epidermoide del glande peneal. Pathologia 1991;24:1137.
83. Maiche AG, Pyrhonen S. Clinical staging of cancer of the penis: By size? By localization? Or by depth of infiltration? Eur Urol 1990;18: 16.
84. Fraley EE, Zhang G, Manivel C, Niehans GA. The role of ilioinguinal lymphadenectomy and significance of histological differentiation in treatment of carcinoma of the penis. J Urol 1989;142:1478.
85. Johnson DE, Lo RK, Srigley J, Ayala AG. Verrucous carcinoma of the penis. J Urol 1985;133:216.
86. McKee PH, Lowe D, Haigh RJ. Penile verrucous carcinoma. Histopathology 1983;7:897.
87. Kraus FT, Perez-Mesa C. Verrucous carcinoma: clinical and pathologic study of 105 cases involving oral cavity, larynx, and genitalia. Cancer 1966;19:26.
88. Yeager JK, Findlay RF, McAleer IM. Penile verrucous carcinoma. Arch Dermatol 1990;126:1208.

89. Blessing K, McLaren K, Lessells A. Viral etiology for verrucous carcinoma. Histopathology 1986;10:1101.
90. Masih AS, Stoler MH, Farrow GM, Wooldridge TN, Johansson SL. Penile verrucous carcinoma: a clinicopathologic, human papillomavirus typing and flow cytometric analysis. Mod Pathol 1992;5:48.
91. Noel JC, Vandenbossche M, Peny MO, et al. Verrucous carcinoma of the penis: importance of human papillomavirus typing for diagnosis and therapeutic decision. Eur Urol 1992;22:83.
92. Medina JE, Dichtel W, Luna MA. Verrucous-squamous carcinomas of the oral cavity: a clinicopathologic study of 104 cases. Arch Otolaryngol 1984;110:437.
93. Manglani KS, Manaligod JR, Biswamay R. Spindle cell carcinoma of the glans penis: a light and electron microscopic study. Cancer 1980;46:2266.
94. Wood EW, Gardner WA Jr, Brown FM. Spindle cell squamous carcinoma of the penis. J Urol 1972;107:990.
95. Rahbari H, Mehregan AH. Basal cell epitheliomas in usual and unusual sites. J Cutan Pathol 1979;6:425.
96. Hall TC, Britt DB, Woodhead DM. Basal cell carcinoma of the penis. J Urol 1968;99:314.
97. McGregor DH, Tanimura A, Weigel JW. Basal cell carcinoma of penis. Urology 1982;20:320.
98. Goldminz D, Scott G, Klaus S. Penile basal cell carcinoma: report of a case and review of the literature. J Am Acad Dermatol 1989;20:1094.
99. Stillwell TJ, Zincke H, Gaffey TA, Woods JE. Malignant melanoma of the penis. J Urol 1988;140:72.
100. Oldbring J, Mikulowski P. Malignant melanoma of the penis and male urethra: report of nine cases and review of the literature. Cancer 1987;59:581.
101. Begun FP, Grossman HB, Diokno AC, Sogani PC. Malignant melanoma of the penis and male urethra. J Urol 1984;132:123.
102. Manivel JC, Fraley EE. Malignant melanoma of the penis and male urethra: 4 case reports and literature review. J Urol 1988;139:813.
103. Johnson DE, Ayala AG. Primary melanoma of the penis. Urology 1973;2:174.
104. Konigsberg HA, Gray GF. Benign melanosis and malignant melanoma of penis and male urethra. Urology 1976;7:323.
105. Saw D, Tse CH, Chan J, Wyatt CY, Ng ABP, Poon YF. Clear cell sarcoma of the penis. Hum Pathol 1986;17:423.
106. Dehner LP, Smith BH. Soft tissue tumors of the penis: a clinicopathologic study of 46 cases. Cancer 1970;25:1431.
107. Casado M, Jimenez F, Borbujo J, Almagro M. Spontaneous healing of Kaposi's angiosarcoma of the penis. J Urol 1988;139:1313.
108. Lowe FC, Lattimer G, Metroka CE. Kaposi's sarcoma of the penis in patients with acquired immunodeficiency syndrome. J Urol 1989;142:1475.
109. Bayne P, Wise G. Kaposi's sarcoma of penis and genitalia: a disease of our times. Urology 1988;31:22.
110. Vapnek JM, Quivey JM, Carroll PR. Acquired immunodeficiency syndrome-related Kaposi's sarcoma of the male genitalia: management with radiation therapy. J Urol 1991;146:333.
111. Lands RH, Ange D, Hartman DL. Radiation therapy for classic Kaposi's sarcoma presenting only on the glans penis. J Urol 1992;147:468.
112. Rasbridge SA, Parry JRW. Angiosarcoma of the penis. Br J Urol 1989;63:440.
113. Weiss SW, Enzinger FM. Epithelioid hemangioendothelioma: a vascular tumor often mistaken for a carcinoma. Cancer 1982;50:970.
114. Deutsch M, Lee RLS, Mercado R. Hemangioendothelioma of the penis with late appearing metastases: report of a case with review of the literature. J Surg Oncol 1973;5:27.
115. Isa SS, Almaraz R, Magovern J. Leiomyosarcoma of the penis: case report and review of the literature. Cancer 1984;54:939.
116. Valadez RA, Waters WB. Leiomyosarcoma of penis. Urology 1986;27:265.
117. Wilson LS, Lockhart JL, Bergman H, Politano VA. Fibrosarocma of the penis: case report and review of the literature. J Urol 1983;129:606.
118. Parsons MA, Fox M. Malignant fibrous histiocytoma of the penis. Eur Urol 1988;14:75.
119. Fletcher CDM, Lowe D. Inflammatory fibrous histiocytoma. Histopathology 1984;8:1079.
120. Dalkin B, Zaontz MR. Rhabdomyosarcoma of the penis in children. J Urol 1989;141:908.
121. Pak K, Sakaguchi N, Takayama H, Tomoyoshi T. Rhabdomyosarcoma of the penis. J Urol 1986;136:438.
122. Huang DJ, Stanisic TH, Hansen KK. Epithelioid sarcoma of the penis. J Urol 1992;147:1370.
123. Gower RL, Pambakian H, Fletcher CDM. Epithelioid sarcoma of the penis: a rare tumour to be distinguished from squamous carcinoma. Br J Urol 1987;59:592.
124. Gonzalez-Campora R, Nogales FF, Lerma E, Navarro A, Matilla A. Lymphoma of the penis. J Urol 1981;126:270.
125. Yu GSM, Nseyo UO, Carson JW. Primary penile lymphoma in a patient with Peyronie's disease. J Urol 1989;142:1076.
126. Powell BL, Craig JB, Muss HB. Secondary malignancies of the penis and epididymis: a case report and review of the literature. J Clin Oncol 1985;3:110.
127. Perez-Mesa C, Oxenhandler R. Metastatic tumors of the penis. J Surg Oncol 1989;42:11.
128. Haddad FS. Penile metastases secondary to bladder cancer: review of the literature. Urol Int 1984;39:125.
129. Robey EL, Schellhammer PF. Four cases of metastases to the penis and review of the literature. J Urol 1984;132:992.
130. Khubchandani M. Metachronous metastasis to the penis from carcinoma of the rectum: report of a case. Dis Colon Rectum 1986;29:52.
131. Hashimoto H, Saga Y, Watabe Y, Sasaki M, Tokunaka S, Yachiku S. Case report: secondary penile carcinoma. Urol Int 1989;44:56.
132. Ordonez NG, Ayala AG, Bracken RB. Renal cell carcinoma metastatic to penis. Urology 1982;19:417.
133. Adjiman S, Flam TA, Zerbib M, Debre B, Steg A. Delayed nonurothelial metastatic lesions to the penis: a report of two cases. Eur Urol 1989;16:391.
134. Powell FC, Venencie PY, Winkelmann RK. Metastatic prostate carcinoma manifesting as penile nodules. Arch Dermatol 1984;20:1604.
135. Paquin AJ, Rowland SI. Secondary carcinoma of the penis: a review of the literature and a report of nine new cases. Cancer 1956;9:626.
136. Mukamel E, Farrer J, Smith RB, deKernion JB. Metastatic carcinoma to penis: when is total penectomy indicated? Urology 1987;29:15.

Principles and Practice of Genitourinary Oncology, edited by Derek Raghavan, Howard I. Scher, Steven A. Leibel, and Paul H. Lange. Lippincott-Raven Publishers, Philadelphia, © 1997.

CHAPTER 90

Clinical Presentation and Staging of Penile Cancer

Robert B. Huben

Penile cancer is a malignant process that varies in its initial manifestations, growth characteristics, and natural history. Despite the presence of an early visible lesion in most cases, a significant delay in the diagnosis of penile cancer often occurs, as reflected by an unacceptably high incidence of metastatic disease at diagnosis. Delays of a year or more between initial signs or symptoms and presentation for medical attention are frequently reported in patients with penile cancer, for reasons that are often difficult to fathom. Regardless of the reasons for this delay, appropriate categorization of the stage of the primary lesion and of the status of the regional lymph nodes is the major determinant of both prognosis and optimal management of the disease.

The purpose of this chapter is to examine the various ways in which penile cancer may manifest, to evaluate the staging modalities used to determine the extent of disease, and to review the staging classifications that guide subsequent therapy.

THE PRIMARY LESION

Early penile cancer has no characteristic appearance, so the need for a high index of suspicion of penile cancer in a patient with a persistent penile lesion must be reiterated. Penile cancer can mimic various inflammatory or infectious processes that involve the glans or prepuce, particularly when phimosis exists, and patients commonly have a history of treatment with one or more topical agents before the diagnosis of penile cancer is established. Patients may sometimes report temporary improvement of the primary lesion after the use of topical antiinflammatory or antifungal agents, as may occur when the lesion has an inflammatory or infectious component, but this apparent response may lull the patient into assuming that the lesion is not a cause for concern.

The earliest appreciable lesion of penile cancer may be a small nodule, a papillary growth, or an ulcer on the glans or prepuce.[1–5] In a review of larger series of penile cancer, the site of apparent origin of the primary lesion was the glans in 48%, the prepuce in 21%, both glans and prepuce in 9%, and the coronal sulcus in 6%.[6] Only 2% of tumors were reported to arise from the shaft of the penis, whereas the remaining 14% invaded the penile shaft from more distal sites. These investigators also reported a 0.7% incidence of occult penile cancer in prepuces at circumcision in adults.[7]

As the primary lesion grows, it develops one of two typical growth patterns: exophytic or ulcerating.[7,8] Exophytic or papillary tumors generally have a better prognosis than flat or ulcerative lesions, because the latter tend to infiltrate more deeply and are less differentiated than exophytic tumors.[2,4] The diverse growth patterns of primary penile cancers are shown in Figures 90-1 through 90-4.

Some of the important characteristics of the primary lesion in penile cancer that should be observed and recorded are the tumor configuration, size, and location. For lesions of the foreskin or skin of the penis, fixation of the lesion to the underlying Buck's fascia can be assessed by trying to rotate the involved skin around the corporal bodies. Infiltration of the glans or corporal bodies may be felt as woody induration of these tissues, and the corporal bodies should be palpated carefully to determine the proximal extent of the tumor. The inguinal areas are palpated bilaterally to assess the status of the local lymph nodes, and any hard or enlarged nodes should be measured and mapped on the patient's records for comparison with the findings of subsequent examination. A ''50% rule'' applies to the presence and significance of palpable inguinal lymph nodes; that is, nodes are palpable in 50% of cases, and 50% of these nodes are subsequently shown to have tumor involvement, the remainder being inflammatory.[9–12] In contrast, up to 30% of patients without clinical lymphadenopathy have histologic evidence of tumor in nodes after resection, although this percentage varies significantly with the severity of the primary tumor (see Chaps. 93 and 94).

Certain radiologic techniques have been used to evaluate the extent and invasiveness of the primary lesion in penile cancer. Cavernosography has been reported to be useful in evaluating the corporal bodies for tumor invasion, but the invasive nature of the procedure and occasional reports of impotence resulting from corporal fibrosis associated with contrast injection have hindered the use of this procedure in patients with questionable

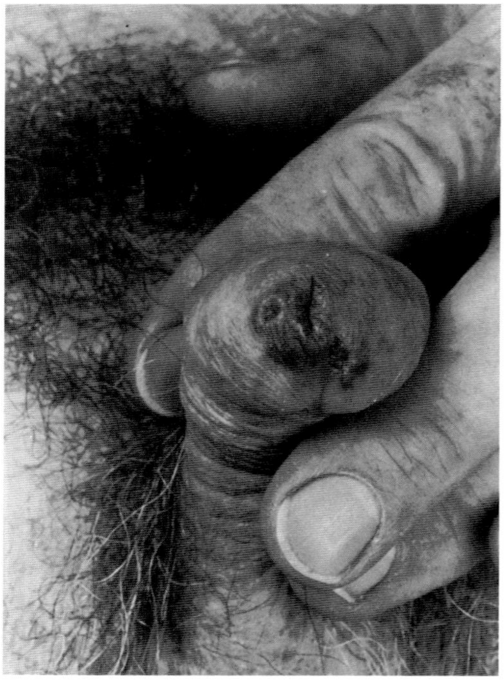

FIG. 90-1. Early ulcerative cancer of the glans penis.

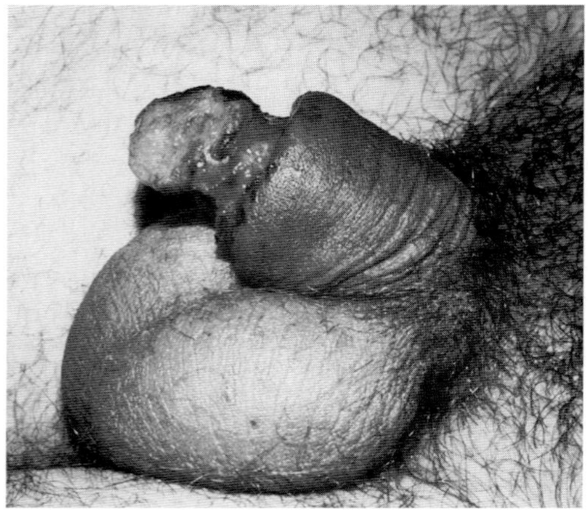

FIG. 90-3. Advanced ulcerative penile cancer with extensive tissue erosion.

corporal invasion, the clinical group most likely to benefit from cavernosography.[13—15] The procedure may be useful, however, in determining the proximal extent of corporal involvement with more obviously invasive lesions.[15] Ultrasonography has also been used to assess the proximal extent of corporal involvement in invasive penile cancers.[16] Although this technique has had limited reported use in this manner, its ease of application, non-invasiveness, and low cost may make ultrasonography a useful diagnostic study in staging penile cancer. Computed tomography (CT) has not been shown to have any practical use in staging the primary lesion in penile cancer, because it does not enable the clinician to distinguish tumor from adjacent corporal tissue.[17]

Several reports have suggested that magnetic resonance imaging (MRI) has promise in determining the extent and stage of the primary lesion.[18,19] Advantages include superior tissue contrast and imaging in multiple planes. Studies of the normal penis have shown that the tunica albuginea enveloping the cor-

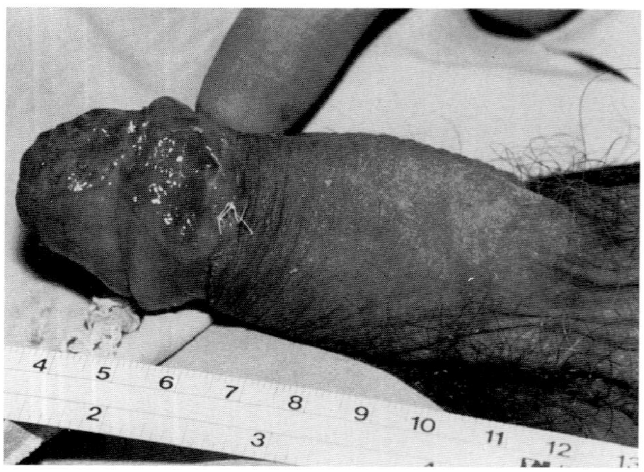

FIG. 90-2. More extensive ulcerative penile cancer. Biopsy showed well-differentiated squamous cell cancer with invasion of the corpus cavernosum. Note the previous biopsy site at the proximal edge of the lesion.

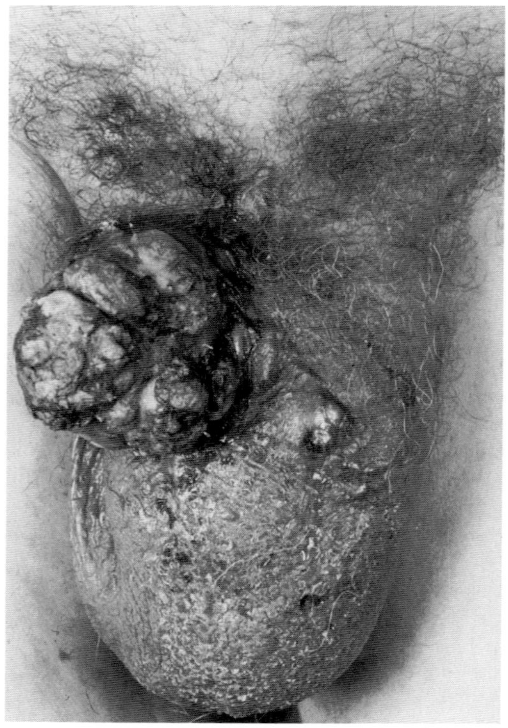

FIG. 90-4. Advanced exophytic or papillary penile cancer. Biopsy revealed well-differentiated squamous cell cancer.

pora has low signal intensity, and the contrast between the tunica and the corpora is increased on T2 (transverse)-weighted images.[19,20] Buck's fascia is indistinguishable from the tunica on T2-weighted images, but the two may appear as separate structures on T1 (longitudinal)-weighted images.[20] In the imaging of urethral tumors, MRI can show interruption of the normally low-density tunica albuginea of the corpus spongiosum or invasion into the corpora cavernosa, a discriminating ability with obvious application to the staging of penile cancer as well.[20]

ASSESSMENT OF THE INGUINAL LYMPH NODES

In addition to careful examination, certain techniques have been used to evaluate the inguinal lymph nodes, the primary metastatic site for penile cancer, in patients with no or equivocal evidence of nodal spread. Lymphangiography was the first diagnostic test to be applied with some frequency, but it has largely been supplanted by newer techniques.[21,22] In the series of Wajsman and associates, pedal lymphangiography was shown to have a diagnostic accuracy of 81.5%, with a false-negative rate of 18.5% and a false-positive rate of 0% when subsequent surgical findings were correlated with radiographic findings.[23] Because of its invasive nature and the emergence of newer techniques, lymphangiography as a routine staging procedure for penile cancer has few proponents. Ultrasonography has also had limited use in assessing nodal status in patients with penile cancer, although it has some real and potential advantages as a diagnostic study in this clinical situation.[20]

CT is the most popular imaging technique for the detection of lymphadenopathy.[17,20] Identification and evaluation of the pelvic nodes may be more difficult than assessment of the para-aortic nodes, because of the relative scarcity of fat enveloping the pelvic nodes and their oblique orientation.[24] Furthermore, CT can only detect nonspecific lymph node enlargement, and thus it has the same limitations that have limited the role of routine CT in the assessment of clinically localized prostate and bladder cancers. Nonetheless, this study is done routinely to determine the status of the pelvic nodes even in the absence of inguinal adenopathy, although the yield is generally recognized as low in this situation.[24] Examples of positive CT studies are shown in Figures 90-5 and 90-6.

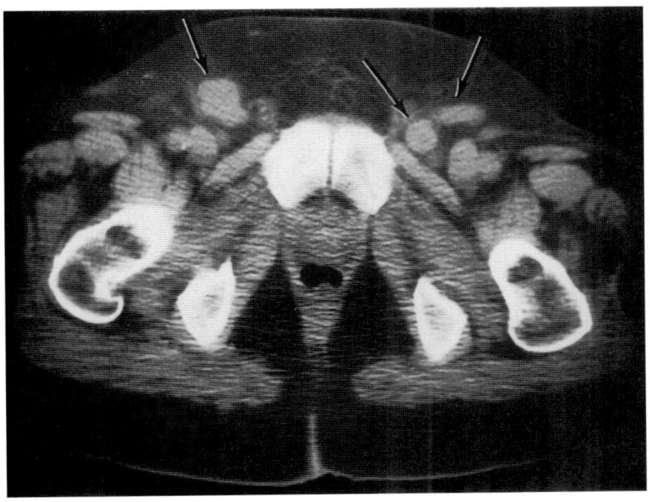

FIG. 90-5. Computed tomographic scan of the pelvis showing bilateral inguinal adenopathy (*arrows*) in a patient with penile cancer.

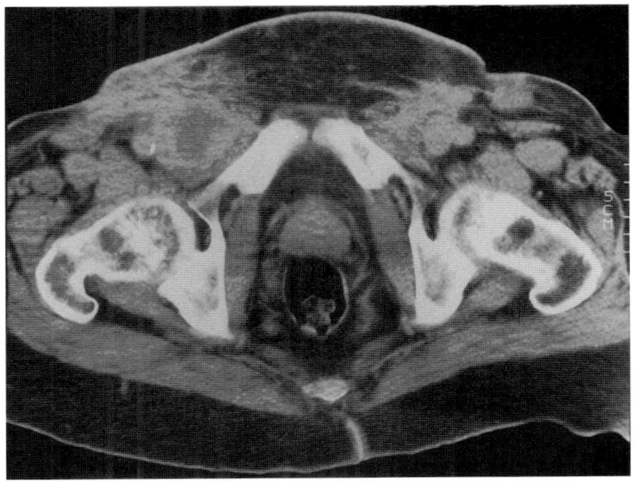

FIG. 90-6. Computed tomogroaphic scan of the pelvis demonstrating massive bilateral inguinal adenopathy from penile cancer.

MRI may also be used to assess the status of both inguinal and pelvic lymph nodes in patients with penile cancer, although experience with this modality is limited.[17,20] Although it has the advantage of scanning in multiple planes, MRI also depends on enlargement of the lymph nodes in defining abnormality, and does not enable the clinician to discriminate tumor from other causes of nodal enlargement.[20] For these reasons, MRI imaging does not appear to offer any clear advantage over CT in the evaluation of patients with penile cancer.

Little question exists that the diagnostic accuracy of many of these modalities, including lymphangiography, ultrasonography, and CT, could be enhanced by the use of fine-needle aspiration.[25–27] The staging of patients with penile cancer appears to be an ideal application of this technique, because the lymph nodes are readily accessible and aspiration of the inguinal nodes can be done under direct vision. An ideal use of fine-needle aspiration would be in the patient who has negative or equivocal lymph nodes at diagnosis and who has significant contraindications to inguinal node dissection, such as obesity, previous pelvic surgery, or a history of cardiac or thromboembolic disease. Negative results of fine-needle aspiration of the inguinal lymph nodes would be reassuring when observation of the inguinal area is contemplated. For reasons that are not clear, however, fine-needle aspiration appears to be underused in the United States in the evaluation of patients with penile cancer, and perhaps this may be true for the evaluation of other genitourinary cancers as well. Although the actual technique of fine-needle aspiration is uncomplicated, the procedure does require a skilled cytopathologist and, more important, confidence in the results of aspiration and a willingness to direct subsequent therapy on the basis of cytopathologic findings. With further advances in imaging techniques, fine-needle aspiration may play more of a role in patients with penile cancer in the future. Although MRI-directed biopsies can be performed in women with breast cancer, this technique has not yet been applied to patients with other diseases in other locations.

An additional technique to assess the status of the inguinal lymph nodes in patients with penile cancer is sentinel node biopsy, as proposed by Cabanas in 1977.[9] Based on previous lymphangiographic studies, Cabanas defined the sentinel node as the primary site of metastasis for penile carcinoma, and this lymph node is located on the anteromedial aspect of the superficial epigastric vein medial to and above the epigastric-saphenous junction. In his original series, Cabanas reported that inguinal lymph node metastases were absent in patients with negative sentinel lymph node biopsy. Eighty percent of patients with a positive sentinel node had no other nodal involvement, whereas regional spread was documented in the remaining 20%. Despite this remarkable consistency in the original report, several case reports have been published of patients who have developed deep inguinal and iliac lymph node metastases despite a negative sentinel node biopsy.[28–31] Other series, however, have also confirmed Cabanas' initial report.[7] As in the case of fine-needle aspiration, a negative sentinel node biopsy may be reassuring when inguinal node dissection would pose a significant risk to a particular patient, thereby making observation the preferred approach.

Evaluation for distant metastases can usually be limited to chest radiography and possibly a bone scan. The diagnostic yield is generally low, because only about 5% of patients with penile cancer have distant metastases at the time of diagnosis.[4,10,32] Results of routine laboratory tests are generally normal in patients with penile cancer, although anemia may exist in patients with more advanced disease. Hypercalcemia is frequently associated with penile cancer in more advanced stages, and in one series, about 20% of patients developed hypercalcemia during the course of their disease.[33–36] Hypercalcemia is usually a late-stage phenomenon indicative of a dire prognosis.

STAGING CLASSIFICATIONS

Staging systems for a particular malignant disease are intended to define the extent of the disease according to its usual mode of progression in an effort to determine optimal therapy and to facilitate comparison of therapies according to the designated stages. More specifically, a staging system must facilitate assessment of the extent of the primary lesion, the status of the regional nodes, and evidence of distant metastases. Although no staging classification is universally accepted for penile cancer, the classification system that was the first to be widely used and is still used to some extent is that of Jackson, which was first reported in 1966 (Table 90-1).[37] Although this classification is useful, it has certain failings. This classification is geographic, in that tumors are staged according to location, but not according to either size or depth of invasion, which are recognized as critical factors in determining both therapy and prognosis. The grouping of locally advanced, bulky regional, and distant metastases within stage IV in this classification is also misleading and makes it difficult to determine prognosis according to this particular stage, because this stage may represent varying states of disease. For practical purposes, the Jackson classification system should be considered only for historic purposes.

TABLE 90-1. *Jackson classification of carcinoma of the penis*

Stage	Criteria
I	Tumors confined to glans, prepuce, or both
II	Tumors extending onto shaft of penis
III	Tumors with operable inguinal metastasis
IV	Tumors involving adjacent structures; tumors associated with inoperable inguinal metastasis or distant metastasis

Data from Jackson SM. The treatment of carcinoma of the penis. Br J Surg 1966;53:33.

The TNM classification has gained widespread acceptance internationally, and although it has some limitations, this system appears to have more practical value in classifying the extent of penile cancers.[38] The TNM classification currently proposed for staging penile cancer is shown in Table 90-2.[39,40] A comparison between the TNM classification and the Jackson classification is shown in Table 90-3.[40] The current TNM staging system has been adopted by both the International Union Against Cancer (Union Internationale Contre le Cancer) and the American Joint Committee on Cancer.[39,40] Although the primary tumor is not classified by size in the TNM classification, tumors are stratified on the basis of depth of invasion, which is more important than size in determining therapy for the primary tumor. Because the management of regional nodal involvement is primarily surgical, a classification based in part on surgical resectability would be helpful, but the N categories in the TNM classi-

TABLE 90-2. *TNM classification of penile cancer*

PRIMARY TUMOR (T)	
TX	Primary tumor cannot be assessed
T0	No evidence of primary tumor
Tis	Carcinoma in situ
Ta	Noninvasive verrucous carcinoma
T1	Tumor invades subepithelial connective tissue
T2	Tumor invades the corpus spongiosum or cavernosum
T3	Tumor invades the urethra or prostate
T4	Tumor invades other adjacent structures
REGIONAL LYMPH NODES (N)	
NX	Regional lymph nodes cannot be assessed
N0	No regional lymph node metastasis
N1	Metastasis in a single superficial inguinal lymph node
N2	Metastasis in multiple or bilateral superficial inguinal lymph nodes
N3	Metastasis in deep inguinal or pelvic lymph nodes, unilateral or bilateral
DISTANT METASTASIS (M)	
MX	Presence of distant metastasis cannot be assessed
M0	No distant metastasis
M1	Distant metastasis

Data from Harmer MH. TNM classification of malignant tumours, 3rd ed. Geneva, International Union Against Cancer (Union Internationale Contre le Cancer), 1978; and American Joint Committee on Cancer. Manual for Staging of Cancer, 4th ed. Philadelphia, JB Lippincott, 1992.

TABLE 90-3. *Comparison of Jackson and TNM classifications*

Jackson stage	TNM stage		
0	Tis	N0	M0
	Ta	N0	M0
I	T1	N0	M0
II	T1	N1	M0
	T2	N0	M0
	T3	N1	M0
III	T1	N2	M0
	T2	N2	M0
	T3	N0	M0
	T3	N1	M0
	T3	N2	M0
IV	T4	Any N	M0
	Any T	N3	M0
	Any T	Any N	M1

fication appear to be adequate otherwise. The ultimate test of any staging system is whether the designations have significant prognostic and therapeutic implications, and widespread acceptance of a common staging system would be critically important. Use of the existing TNM classification is recommended for this reason.

CONCLUSIONS

As previously discussed, several modalities exist for evaluating the extent of penile cancer once the diagnosis is made, although careful physical examination remains the most important and informative method. Moreover, incisional or excisional biopsy is the diagnostic and staging procedure of choice in patients with known or suspected penile cancer. The extent to which the patient is evaluated for nodal metastases depends not only on apparent physical findings, but also on the extent to which a reason to perform, or not perform, lymphadenectomy is sought. That is, further diagnostic and staging procedures are meaningless if a decision has already been made to recommend that a patient undergo groin dissection.

When such a decision is predicated on the results of further diagnostic procedures, ultrasonography, CT, and MRI are of potential benefit as staging studies. Percutaneous fine-needle aspiration is a safe and reliable indicator of the presence or absence of inguinal nodal metastasis, if the clinician is willing to make subsequent therapeutic decisions on the basis of the results of the procedure. Delays in diagnosis of penile cancer, often resulting from the patient's reluctance to seek medical attention, continue to be a serious problem in the management of this disease.

REFERENCES

1. Bassett JW. Carcinoma of the penis. Cancer 1975;5:530.
2. Dean AL. Epithelioma of the penis. J Urol 1935;33:252.
3. Grabstald H. Carcinoma of the penis. J Contin Ed Urol 1979;18:15.
4. Beggs JH and Spratt JS Jr. Epidermoid carcinoma of the penis. J Urol 1986;135:283.
5. Colon JE. Carcinoma of the penis. J Urol 1931;25:461.
6. Sufrin G, Huben R. Benign and malignant lesions of the penis. In: Gillenwater JY, ed. Adult and pediatric urology. Chicago, Year Book, 1987:1462.
7. Sufrin G, Huben R. Benign and malignant lesions of the penis. In: Gillenwater JY, ed. Adult and pediatric urology, 2nd ed. Chicago, Year Book, 1991:1643.
8. Buddington WT, Kickham CJE, Smith WE: An assessment of malignant disease of the penis. J Urol 1963;89:442.
9. Cabanas RM. An approach for the treatment of penile carcinoma. Cancer 1977;59:456.
10. Derrick FC Jr, Lynch KM Jr, Kretkowski RC, et al. Epidermoid carcinoma of the penis: computer analysis of 87 cases. J Urol 1975;110:303.
11. El-Dimiry MIM, Oliver RTD, Hope-Stone HF, et al. Reappraisal of role of radiotherapy and surgery in the management of carcinoma of the penis. Br J Urol 1984;56:724.
12. Hardner GJ, Bhanalaph T, Murphy GP, et al. Carcinoma of the penis: analysis of therapy in 100 consecutive cases. J Urol 1972;108:428.
13. Escribanl G, Allona A, Burgos FJ, et al. Cavernosography in diagnosis of metastatic tumors of the penis: 5 new cases and a review of the literature. J Urol 1987;138:1174.
14. Hadded FS, Kovac A, Kivirand A, et al. Cavernosonography in diagnosis of penile metastases secondary to bladder cancer. Urology 1985;26:585.
15. Raghavaiah NV. Corpus cavernosogram in the evaluation of carcinoma of the penis. J Urol 1978;120:423.
16. Yamashita T, Ogawa A. Ultrasound in penile cancer. Urol Radiol 1989;11:174.
17. Burgers JK, Badalament RA, Drago JR. Penile cancer: clinical presentation, diagnosis, and staging. Urol Clin North Am 1992;19:247.
18. Hricak H, Marotti M, Gilbert TJ, et al. Normal penile anatomy and abnormal penile conditions: evaluation with MR imaging. Radiology 1988;169:683.
19. Satragno L, Martinoli C, Cittadini G. Magnetic resonance imaging of the penis: normal anatomy. Magn Reson Imaging 198;7:95.
20. Vaprek JM, Hricale H, Carroll PR. Recent advances in imaging studies for staging of penile and urethral carcinoma. Urol Clin North Am 1992;19:257.
21. Riveros M, Garcia R, Cabanas R. Lymphadenography of the dorsal lymphatics of the penis: technique and results. Cancer 1967;20:2026.
22. Castellino RA. Lymphography. In: Pollack HM, et al, eds. Clinical urography. Philadelphia, WB Saunders, 1990:504.
23. Wajsman Z, Moore RH, Merrin CE, et al: Surgical treatment of penile cancer: a follow-up report. Cancer 1977;40:1697.
24. Jing B, Wallace S, Zornoza J. Metastases to retroperitoneal and pelvic lymph nodes: computed tomography and lymphangiography. Radiol Clin North Am 1982;20:511.
25. Luciani L, Piscioli F, Scappini P, et al. Value and role of percutaneous regional node aspiration cytology in the management of penile carcinoma. Eur Urol 1984;10:294.
26. Scappini P, Piscioli F, Pusiol T, et al. Penile cancer: aspiration biopsy cytology for staging. Cancer 1986;58:1526.
27. Melicow MM, Ganem EJ. Cancerous and precancerous lesions of the penis: a clinical and pathological study based on 23 cases. J Urol 1946;55:486.
28. Perinetti E, Crane DB, Catalona WJ. Unreliability of sentinel lymph node biopsy for staging penile carcinoma. J Urol 1980;124:734.
29. Wespes E, Simon J, Schulman CC. Cabanas approach: is sentinel node biopsy reliable for staging penile carcinoma? Urology 1986;28:278.
30. Fowler JE Jr. Sentinel lymph node biopsy for staging penile cancer. Urology 1984;23:352.
31. Catalona WJ. Surgical staging of genitourinary tumors. Cancer 1987;60:459.
32. Horenblas S, van Tinteren H, Delemarre JFM, Moonen LMF, Lustig V, Kroger R. Squamous cell carcinoma of the penis: accuracy of tumor, nodes and metastasis classification system, and tole of lymphangiography, computerized tomography scan and fine needle aspiration cytology. J Urol 1991;146:1279.
33. Schellhammer PF, Jordan GH, Schlossberg SM. Tumors of the penis. In: Walsh PC, Retik AB, Stamey TA, Vaughan ED Jr, eds. Campbell's urology, 6th ed. Philadelphia, WB Saunders, 1992:1264.
34. Anderson EE, Glenn JF. Penile malignancy and hypercalcemia. JAMA 1965;192:128.
35. Rudd FV, Rott RK, Skoglund RW, Ansell JS. Tumor-induced hypercalcemia. J Urol 1972;107:986.

36. Sklaroff RB, Yagoda A. Penile cancer: natural history and therapy. In: Chemotherapy and urological malignancy. New York, Springer-Verlag, 1982:98.
37. Jackson SM. The treatment of carcinoma of the penis. Br J Surg 1966; 53:33.
38. Horenblas S, van Tinteren H. Squamous cell carcinoma of the penis. IV. Prognostic factors of survival: analysis of tumor, nodes and metastasis classification system. J Urol 1994;151:1239.
39. Harmer MH. TNM classification of malignant tumours, 3rd ed. Geneva, International Union Against Cancer, 1978.
40. American Joint Committee on Cancer. Manual for Staging of Cancer, 4th ed. Philadelphia, JB Lippincott, 1992:191.

Principles and Practice of Genitourinary Oncology, edited by Derek Raghavan, Howard I. Scher, Steven A. Leibel, and Paul H. Lange. Lippincott-Raven Publishers, Philadelphia, © 1997.

CHAPTER 91

Organ-Sparing Dermatologic Surgical Approaches to Cancer of the Penis

Peter B. Odland

For all forms of cancer, long-term survival is a major treatment consideration. An equally important concept to consider is the effect of selected therapy on the patient's quality of life. For cancer of the penis, the issue of quality of life is measured in terms of functional and psychological morbidity,[1–3] both of which depend on the modality selected for treatment of the primary lesion.

Squamous cell carcinoma (SCC) accounts for 95% of cancer of the penis[4]; however, primary cancer can arise from any cell type. Although exceedingly rare, cancer from distant sites can metastasize to the penis as well. This discussion focuses on SCC.

Guidelines for care of cutaneous SCC are well established.[5] Local control of SCC of the penis has included excisional techniques, partial or total amputation,[6–10] radiotherapy,[3,11–13] laser ablation,[14–16] liquid nitrogen cryosurgery,[17] and topical[18] and systemic[19] chemotherapy as single therapy[20] or in various combinations.[21,22]

Organ-sparing dermatologic surgical techniques are gaining acceptance for local control of this tumor. In this chapter, use of these surgical techniques for local control, with an emphasis on Mohs micrographic surgery (MMS), is discussed.

MMS was first described in the 1930s by a general surgeon at the University of Wisconsin, Frederic E. Mohs. As a well-established form of margin-controlled surgery, the technique has been producing results unmatched by other modalities of treatment for cutaneous SCC.[23–26] In an exhaustive review of the literature, Rowe and associates[26] demonstrated that MMS produces better results for cutaneous SCC than all other modalities (Table 91-1).

For treatment of penile SCC, MMS produces impressive long-term cure rates and compares favorably with the more disfiguring technique of partial penectomy.[27] What is most impressive about the data from the report by Mohs and colleagues is that many patients were being retreated after prior treatments had failed. In that sense, the cases seen by Mohs and coworkers were arguably more difficult than those encountered by Horenblas and associates (Table 91-2).[11]

CLINICAL PRESENTATION

Primary SCC of the penis arises distally (including glans, prepuce, and coronal sulcus) in 84% of patients and accounts for 95% of all penile cancers.[4,28] The tumor is usually painless, exophytic, erythematous, and indurated, and it may be ulcerated.[29] The patient's medical history may reveal that the lesion arose from within a pruritic or burning erythematous plaque or ulceration (SCC in situ)[4] or from an otherwise benign precursor lesion.[30–32] Regional adenopathy can be associated with infection or metastasis[33] which complicates proper clinical staging.

The most important prognostic factor for penile SCC is the clinical stage at presentation, and the most reliable indicator of survival is the presence or absence of nodal involvement at presentation.[4] Not to be overlooked are factors that influence prognosis as described for cutaneous SCC,[26] including tumor size, depth of penetration, histologic grade, and host immune status. The diagnosis must be confirmed by biopsy, a procedure often delayed for various reasons.[4,34] Such a delay in the biopsy of a lesion clinically suspected of being penile carcinoma is not inconsequential.

STAGING

Historically, staging schemes have varied enough from report to report to make comparison of data difficult to interpret.[11,35–38] Only recently have attempts been made to standardize the classification systems for staging penile SCC. Histologic grading is at least as important in understanding the nature of a particular lesion as is staging.[35,39,40] This feature of penile tumors is often unclear from data in the literature, but it represents a reliable risk factor for local recurrence and metastasis for cutaneous SCC,[5,26] and it must be addressed when formulating a treatment plan.

ORGAN-SPARING SURGICAL TECHNIQUES

Organ-sparing surgical techniques include laser ablation, circumcision, wedge resections, frozen section-guided ellipse ex-

TABLE 91-1. *Local recurrence rates for cutaneous squamous cell carcinoma (SCC) (more than 5 years' follow-up)*

Lesion	Non-Mohs modalities % (total)	MMS % (total)
Primary Cutaneous SCC	7.9 (366)	3.1 (2065)
Primary Lip SCC	10.5 (7022)	2.3 (952)
Primary Ear SCC	18.7 (214)	5.3 (337)
Locally Recurrent SCC	23.3 (34)	10.0 (151)

MMS, Mohs micrographic surgery.

Data from Rowe DE, Carroll RJ, Day CL. Prognostic factors for local recurrence, metastasis, and survival rates in squamnous cell carcinoma of the skin, ear, lip: implications for treatment modality selection. J Am Acad Dermatol 1992;26:976.

cisions, and MMS. Local recurrence after penis-conserving therapy ranges from 6% to 50%.[11,27,41] Lasers have been used effectively to treat various precursor lesions and early penile SCC. Because standard wedge resections and circumcision are associated with higher recurrence rates,[6,11,37] frozen section-controlled excisions (standard and Mohs) have been favored as organ-sparing techniques. An important distinction must be made here (one that is critical for surgeons to understand): standard excision and MMS are significantly and fundamentally different regarding, among other aspects, the way in which the surgical specimens are pathologically processed (see later). This difference is profoundly important and has serious implications regarding the quality of the margin control.

Mohs Surgery

Of the modalities described for treatment of cancer of the penis, MMS is embraced by a growing contingent of specialists treating penile SCC.[6,16,42] The application of MMS to in situ and minimally invasive, wel-differentiated penile SCC is advocated as the superior treatment option. Several series have demonstrated the combined cure rates and tissue-sparing nature to be better overall than with other tissue sparing modalities.[27,43–46] Furthermore, micrographic surgeons and urologists have successfully combined MMS and lymphadenectomy for more advanced tumors.[27,43,44,47] Such an interdisciplinary approach to the treatment of difficult cutaneous neoplasms has also been described in the oculoplastic literature,[48] as well as in the literature of otolaryngology and head and neck surgery.[49]

As Mohs demonstrated, these tumors tend to grow in a contiguous fashion and often send out "silent extensions."[50] That these irregular outgrowths may not be detected when tumors are treated by non-Mohs techniques undoubtedly accounts for the higher local recurrence rates for these other treatment modalities.

Historically, MMS was performed with the fixed tissue technique, then known as chemosurgery, described later. This method is still used in some instances. Because it is painful and less expeditious, however, it has largely been replaced by the fresh tissue technique.[23,25,27,32,34,46,51]

Fresh Tissue Technique

MMS is a specialized surgical technique commonly used by specially trained physicians for the treatment of malignant neoplasms of the skin and mucosa. The Mohs technique couples high cure rates (highest of any treatment modality) with maximal normal tissue conservation by orienting the tissue in a way that allows for histologic evaluation of virtually 100% of the surgical margin (Fig. 91-1).

This outpatient procedure is done using local anesthesia (with or without mild sedation). The overall procedure is composed of a series of excisions and pathologic tissue processing described as stages. All stages begin with establishing effective sedation and anesthesia. In stage one, the clinically evident tumor is surgically debulked. A beveled incision is made circumferentially around this defect to produce a uniformly thin (1- to 3-mm) saucer-like layer of tissue, which is placed in a container such that meticulous orientation to the cutaneous defect can be maintained. A two-dimensional diagram, "the Mohs map," drawn of the specimen relates its orientation to the surgical defect. When hemostasis is adequate, the wound is dressed, and the patient is guided to a waiting area or recovery room while the tissue is processed. In the adjacent Mohs laboratory, the saucer-like specimen is subdivided, numbered, and color-coded. These steps are recorded on the Mohs map. (Cutting smaller specimens allows the beveled edges of the specimen to fall into the same horizontal plane as the deeper tissues. Furthermore, because several sections of the smaller specimens fit onto a standard microscope slide, effectively adding a third dimension, interpretive accuracy is enhanced.) These prepared specimens are handed to a specially trained histologic technician. While maintaining meticulous orientation of the specimens, the technician prepares horizontally oriented frozen sections. Each section is microscopically reviewed by the Mohs surgeon, who is trained in the interpretation of horizontally oriented pathology specimens.

TABLE 91-2. *Local recurrence rates for penile carcinoma (more than 5 years' follow-up)*

Investigators	No. of patients	Tumor stages	Treatment	Local cure (%)
Mohs	31	Jackson I-III	MMS	94
Horenblas	51	T1-T3, N0, M0	Non-Mohs*	82

* Laser, circumcision, radiotherapy.
MMS, Mohs micrographic surgery.

Data from Horenblas S, van Tinteren H, Delemarra JF, Boon TA, Moonen LM, Lustig V. Squamous cell carcinoma of the penis. II. Treatment of the primary tumor. J Urol 1992;147:1533; and Mohs FE, Snow SN, Larson PO. Mohs micrographic surgery for penile tumors. Penile Urethral Sciotal Cancer 1992;19:291.

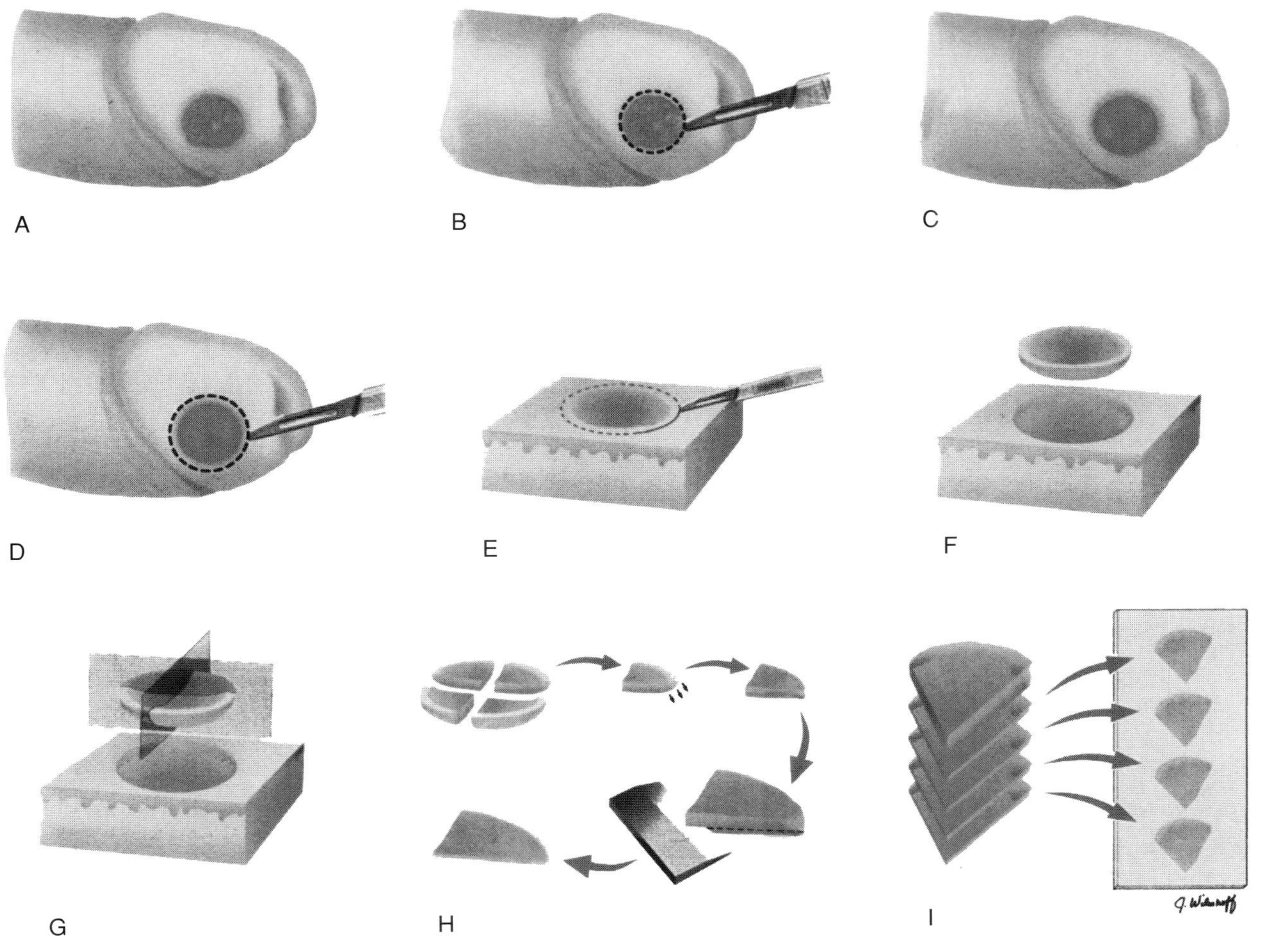

FIG. 91-1. (**A** to **I**) Fresh tissue technique of the Mohs surgical procedure.

When microscopic examination reveals tumor in one or more of the subdivided specimens, a corresponding mark is drawn on the Mohs map. So marked, the Mohs map is used to outline residual tumor precisely within the surgical defect for subsequent Mohs stages. Subsequent stages are performed as outlined previously until all specimens processed are free of tumor. In this way, essentially only the malignant tissue is removed, whereas the surrounding normal tissues are spared.

The concept of orienting the tissue specimens horizontally, which allows for review of 100% of the surgical margin, is unique and is what sets MMS apart from all other techniques of skin cancer removal. In addition, the Mohs surgeon performs the excision and interprets the pathologic specimens, thereby further enhancing maintenance of appropriate orientation of tissues.

Fixed Tissue Technique

Although the fixed tissue technique has been elegantly described in detail previously,[23,43,46] a brief discussion is warranted here. The fixed tissue technique is similar to the fresh tissue technique. The greatest differences are that the tissue is pretreated in vivo at each stage with a fixative paste and the entire process can take many days.

With the surgical field under local anesthesia, an excision to debulk the gross tumor is performed. After adequate hemostasis, a chemical fixative (zinc chloride paste) is applied to this cutaneous wound. An occlusive dressing is applied, and the fixative is allowed to penetrate the tissues for approximately 24 hours. The patient is usually discharged home. When the patient returns the next day, a saucerized specimen is excised, and frozen sections are processed horizontally as in the fresh tissue technique. The entire process is repeated until all margins are clear. For extensive tumors, the fixed tissue technique requires several days for complete removal of all cancerous cells. The final cutaneous defect heals by secondary intention over the ensuing days to weeks. The functional and cosmetic outcome in most cases is entirely acceptable.

Standard Excisional Techniques

In general, 5 mm has been recommended for adequate margins, as well as removing "the deeper tissue layers" in carcinoma in situ.[16] Other surgeons advise that such tissue-sparing techniques should be combined with multiple deep and lateral frozen section biopsies to establish adequate surgical margins.[6]

In contrast to MMS, other excisional techniques rely on standard methods of tissue processing: a surgeon removes the tumor and passes it off to another physician, a pathologist. The pathologist then processes the tissue by one of several techniques, all of which orient the tissue specimens vertically. This orientation has been shown to allow for surveillance of less than 1% of the surgical margins.[52] For example, one commonly used technique removes samples from the tissue block that are analogous to slices from a loaf of bread. From these ''slices,'' the pathologist must determine the status of the margins of the entire tissue block, but must do so without actually having the opportunity to review the entire surgical margin. Because the inherent risk of leaving residual tumor within the defect is greater with these standard techniques, surgeons must remove larger amounts of normal tissue to decrease chances of recurrence and spread of the skin cancer. This procedure generally results in larger cutaneous surgical defects than in MMS, a significant factor in the treatment of penile carcinoma.

Lasers

The energy from a laser beam is absorbed by light-absorbing substances (chromophores) in the tissues. On absorption, the beam is converted to thermal, mechanical, or chemical energy. As the light energy is converted, the chromophores (and therefor the associated target tissues) are disrupted, leading to their ultimate destruction. For example, water is the chromophore for the carbon dioxide laser. Because water is a major component of human tissues, vaporization occurs when the tissues are exposed to the energy of a carbon dioxide laser, and every tissue in its path is destroyed.

Lasers can be used effectively for many clinical disorders. Several laser systems are used in the treatment of malignant cutaneous neoplasms. The carbon dioxide and the Nd:YAG (neodymium: yttrium-aluminum-garnet) lasers have been used successfully for ablation of noninvasive and precursor forms of carcinoma of the penis,[14–16] and promising investigations are using newer generations of photodynamic systems.

Reports of successful treatment with the Nd:YAG and carbon dioxide lasers for early lesions, including precursor lesions, in situ SCC, and early invasive SCC, have demonstrated the effectiveness of these techniques. Cure rates range from 67% to 100% for follow-up periods of up to 2 years.[14–16] In one retrospective study,[11] Nd:YAG laser treatment compared favorably (local recurrence rates of 10% for T1; 32% for T2) with penis-conserving techniques, including circumcision, local excision, and radiotherapy for early, histologically well-differentiated and moderately well-differentiated primary penile carcinomas less than 3.5 cm. None of their patients with T1 tumors treated with laser died of penile SCC. Follow-up periods should be long, as with all forms of treatment. Most local recurrences develop within 2 years.[11] Determination of adequate margins can be estimated with preoperative (frozen section) scout biopsies.[14] Wounds formed from destructive laser techniques necessarily heal by secondary intention, which is surprisingly well tolerated by patients. The cosmetic results are generally reported to be excellent.

Use of lasers for destruction of malignant cutaneous lesions makes some experienced oncologic surgeons uneasy because surgical specimens for margin analysis are nonexistent. As such, success with lasers is perhaps more operator-dependent than with other surgical techniques. Special training is advised, and most hospitals require documentation of supervised instruction before extending operating privileges to physicians for laser procedures.

COMMENTS AND RECOMMENDATIONS

Few would disagree that treatment of SCC of the penis should combine high cure rates with minimal sacrifice of normal, uninvolved tissue. Historically, the highest local cure rates achieved for this lesion have been presented by Frederic Mohs.

One concern of surgeons treating this lesion in T1-T4, N0, M0 stage or less is the uncertainty about clinically undetected, in-transit disease. This uncertainty has compelled surgeons to perform total or partial penectomy even if the patient has no clinical evidence for disease extension. A valid question remains regarding the need for such disfiguring surgery in these cases. Mohs has written that it is unnecessary, but it is done with such regularity because of misunderstanding the mode of spread of these tumors. His conviction is that these tumors metastasize through embolization rather than through direct lymphatic permeation.[46] As such, local control of the tumor is a critical component for successful treatment.

Although MMS is described as a tissue-conserving modality, the technique offers the greatest certainty of elimination of the primary tumor because of the way in which the tissues are processed. For all Mohs' cases of penile SCC through 1992 for which he used MMS, the cure rate for local disease was 94% (see Table 91-2). Because of these outstanding results, it is reasonable to consider his recommendations to use MMS for all lesions except those involving just the distal two thirds of the prepuce, in which circumcision produces equal local control, and Jackson stage IV (inoperable) tumors.

The issue of regional metastasis can be regarded as the other critical component for long-term cure of disease. Excising the primary tumor with an exacting, organ-sparing technique (i.e., MMS) and performing a regional lymphadenectomy are not mutually exclusive.

No organ-sparing treatment can prevent metastasis that has occurred before initial treatment. Local recurrence of a tumor is associated with a significantly higher risk of metastasis of cutaneous SCC, however,[5,26] so control of local diseases can clearly alter the outcome, a finding that further supports the use of MMS. For a unifocal tumor, such as the contiguously enlarging SCC, MMS should theoretically produce a 100% cure rate.[24]

Based on the compelling data presented by Mohs, the favorable early results presented by other micrographic surgeons,[44,45] and the thoughtful series and reviews in the urologic literature,[11,37] the following recommendations for treatment of primary penile SCC are proposed (Table 91-3). A critical component of successful treatment is ongoing, interdisciplinary cooperation between the urologic and the micrographic surgeons. For lesions treated with partial or total penectomy, the intraoperative frozen sections should be processed by the horizontal technique, as used for MMS. This procedure assures the surgeon that all the margins of resection are clear. Ideally, this specimen should be handled by the Mohs laboratory and the surgeon cooperating with the urologic surgeon. Postoperatively, the patient should be followed-up for recurrence regularly and carefully every 3 months after treatment by the micrographic

TABLE 91-3. *Treatment of primary penile squamous cell carcinoma (<3.5 cm diameter)*

Jackson (UICC) stage	Well differentiated	Moderately well differentiated	Poorly differentiated
I (Tis, T1-2, N0, M0)	MMS	MMS	MMS
II (T3-4, N0, M0)	MMS	MMS	PP/MMS
III T1-4, N1-3, M0	PP/MMS	PP/MMS	TP/MMS

MMS, Mohs micrographic surgery; *PP,* partial penectomy with horizontal (Mohs) tissue processing; *TP,* total penectomy with horizontal (Mohs) tissue processing.

surgeon and by the urologist for 6 years. Any suspicious lesions must undergo biopsy immediately, and if recurrence is identified, total penectomy should be considered. This approach seems a prudent form of management of this disease until prospective trials further clarify the issues that currently obscure definitive therapeutic decisions.

Horizontal orientation of tissue specimens is time-consuming and cumbersome compared with standard surgical pathologic techniques, and indeed, in certain instances in oncologic surgery, micrographic surgery cannot play a role (i.e., tumors that are surgically unresectable).[24]

Issues of tissue sparing and control of local disease are imperative for cure and are not mutually exclusive. As this claim is substantiated in the future by controlled, prospective investigations for penile SCC, the true value and effectiveness of the organ-sparing surgical modality, MMS, will become apparent. Meanwhile, to propose an interdisciplinary, combined MMS and urologic approach is reasonable, as described in Table 91-3.

REFERENCES

1. Narayana AS, Olney LE, Loening SA, Weimar GW, Gulp DA. Carcinoma of the penis: analysis of 219 cases. Cancer 1982;49:2185.
2. Lai CS, Chou CK, Yang CC, Lin SD. Immediate reconstruction of the penis with an iliac flap. Br J Plast Surg 1990;43:621.
3. Gerbaulet A, Lambin P. Radiation therapy of cancer of the penis: indications, advantages, and pitfalls. Penile Urethral Scrotal Cancer 1992; 19:325.
4. Burgers JD, Badalament RA, Drago JR. Penile cancer: clinical presentation, diagnosis, and staging. Penile Urethral Scrotal Cancer 1992;19: 247.
5. Johnson TM, Rowe DE, Nelson BR, Swanson NA. Squamous cell carcinoma of the skin (excluding lip and oral mucosa). J Am Acad Dermatol 1992;26:467.
6. Bissada NK. Conservative extripative treatment of cancer of the penis. Penile Urethral Scrotal Cancer 1992;19:283.
7. Young MJ, Reda DJ, Waters WB. Penile carcinoma: a twenty-five year experience. Urology 1991;38:529.
8. Das S. Penile amputations for the management of primary carcinoma of the penis. Penile Urethral Scrotal Cancer 1992;19:277.
9. Hunter MR, Rodriquez P. Squamous cell carcinoma of the penis. Bol Asoc Med P R 1990;82:416.
10. Rotolo JE, Lynch JH. Penile cancer: curable with early detection. Hosp Pract 1991;32:131.
11. Horenblas S, van Tinteren H, Delemarra JF, Boon TA, Moonen LM, Lustig V. Squamous cell carcinoma of the penis. II. Treatment of the primary tumor. J Urol 1992;147:1533.
12. Krieg RM, Luk KH. Carcinoma of penis: review of cases treated by surgery and radiation therapy 1960–1977. Urology 1981;18:149.
13. Daly NJ, Douchez J, Combes PF. Treatment of carcinoma of the penis by iridium 192 wire implant. Int J Radiat Oncol Biol Phys 1982;8: 1239.
14. Malek RS. Laser treatment of premalignant and malignant squamous cell lesions of the penis. Lasers Surg Med 1992;12:246.
15. Greenbaum SS, Glougau R, Stegman SJ, Tromovitch TA. Carbon dioxide laser treatment of erythroplasia of Queyrat. J Dermatol Surg Oncol 1989;15:747.
16. Gerber GS. Carcinoma in situ of the penis. J Dermatol Surg Oncol 1994;20:829.
17. Sonnex TS, Ralfs IG, DeLanza MP, Dawber RPR. Treatment of erythroplasia of Queyrat with liquid nitrogen crysourgery. Br J Dermatol 1982;106:581.
18. Tolia BM, Castro VL, Mouded IM, Newman HR. Bowen's disease of shaft of penis: successful treatment with 5-fluorouracil. Urology 1976; 7:617.
19. Ichikawa T, Nakano I, Hirokawa I. Bleomycin treatment of the tumors of penis and scrotum. J Urol 1989;102:699.
20. Jorgensen SJ, Ohlsen AS, Andersen I. Cancer of the penis treated with bleomycin. Ugeskr Laeger 1971;133:335.
21. Pedrick TJ, Wheeler W, Riemenschneider H. Combined modality therapy for locally advanced penile squamous cell carcinoma. Am J Clin Oncol 1993;16:501.
22. Modig H, Duchek M, Sjodin JG. Carcinoma of the penis: treatment by surgery or combined bleoycin and radiation therapy. Acta Oncol 1993;32:653.
23. Swanson NA. Mohs surgery: technique indications, applications, and the future. Arch Dermatol 1983;119:761.
24. Hruza GJ. Mohs micrographic surgery local recurrences. J Dermatol Surg Oncol 1994;20:573.
25. Tromovitch TA, Stegman SJ. Microscopic-controlled excision of cutaneous tumors: chemosurgery, fresh tissue technique. Am Cancer Soc 1978;41:653.
26. Rowe DE, Carroll RJ, Day CL. Prognostic factors for local recurrence, metastasis, and survival rates in squamous cell carcinoma of the skin, ear, lip: implications for treatment modality selection. J Am Acad Dermatol 1992;26:976.
27. Mohs FE, Snow SN, Larson PO. Mohs micrographic surgery for penile tumors. Penile Urethral Scrotal Cancer 1992;19:291.
28. Lucia MS, Miller GJ. Histopathology of malignant lesions of the penis. Penile Urethral Scrotal Cancer 1992;19:227.
29. Johnson RA. Disease and disorders of the anogenitalia of males. In: Fitzpatrick TB, Eisen AZ, Wolff K, Freedberg IM, Austen KF, eds. Dermatology in General Medicine, 4th ed, vol 1. New York, McGraw-Hill, 1993:1417.
30. Bart RS, Kopf AW. Tumor conference No. 18: squamous-cell carcinoma arising in balanitis xerotica obliterans. J Dermatol Surg Oncol 1978;4:556.
31. Rosemberg SK, Herman G, Elfont E. Sexually transmitted papillomaviral infection in the male. VII. Is cancer of penis sexually transmitted? Urology 1991;37:437.
32. Leal-Khouri S, Hruza GJ. Squamous cell carcinoma developing within lichen planus of the penis. J Dermatol Surg Oncol 1994;20:272.
33. Lubke WL, Thompson IM. The case for inguinal lymph node dissection in the treatment of T2-T4, N0 penile cancer. Semin Urol 1993;11:80.
34. Moritz DL, Lynch WS. Extensive Bowen's disease of the penile shaft treated with fresh tissue mohs micrographic surgery in two separate operations. J Dermatol Surg Oncol 1991;17:374.
35. Jackson SM. The treatment of carcinoma of the penis. Br J Surg 1966; 53:33.
36. Horenblas S, Tinteren HV. Squamous cell carcinoma of the penis. IV. Prognostic factors of survival: analysis of tumor, nodes and metastasis classification system. J Urol 1994;151:1239.
37. Fraley EE, Zhang G, Sazama R, Lange PH. Cancer of the penis: prognosis and treatment plans. Cancer 1985;55:1618.
38. Maiche AG, Pyrhonen S. Clinical staging of cancer of the penis: by

size? by localization? or by depth of infiltration? Eur Urol 1990;18: 16.
39. Maiche AG, Pyrhonen S, Karkinen M. Histological grading of squamous call carcinoma of the penis: a new scoring system Br J Urol 1991;67:522.
40. Cubilla AL, Barreto J, Caballero C, Ayala G, Riveros M. Pathologic features of epidermoid carcinoma of the penis: a prospective study of 66 cases. Am J Surg Pathol 1993;17:753.
41. Horenblas S, Newling DWW. Local recurrent (tumour) after penis-conserving therapy: a plea for long-term follow-up. Br J Urol 1993; 72:976.
42. Drake LA, Ceilley RI, Cornelison RL, et al. Guidelines of care for cutaneous squamous cell carcinoma. J Am Acad Dermatol 1993;28: 628.
43. Mohs FE, Snow SN, Messing EM, Kuglitsch ME. Microscopically controlled surgery in the treatment of carcinoma of the penis. J Urol 1985;133:961.
44. Brown MD, Zachary CB, Grekin RC, Swanson NA. Penile tumors: their management by Mohs micrographic surgery. J Dermatol Surg Oncol 1987;13:1163.
45. Mikhail GR. Cancers of the genitalia and the perineum: Mohs micrographic surgery. Philadelphia, WB Saunders, 1991:237.
46. Mohs FE. Carcinoma of the penis and scrotum. In: Chemosurgery: microscopically controlled surgery for skin cancer. Springfield, IL, Charles C Thomas, 1978:210.
47. Gelabert MA, Arango O, Alcaraz A, Vesa J, Umbert B, Llad'o. Micrographic surgery and inguinal lymphadenectomy: elective therapy in carcinoma of the penis (stage I and II). Actas Urol Esp 1991;15:568.
49. Anderson RL, Ceilley RI. A multispecialty approach to the excision and reconstruction of eyelid tumors. Trans Am Acad Ophthalmol Otolaryngol 1978;85:1150.
49. Baker SR, Swanson NA, Grekin RC. An interdisciplinary approach to the management of basal cell carcinoma of the head and neck. J Dermatol Surg Oncol 1987;13:1095.
50. Mohs FE. Modes of spread of cancer. In: Chemosurgery: microscopically controlled surgery for skin cancer. Springfield, IL, Charles C Thomas, 1978:256.
51. Bernstein G, Forgaard DM, Miller JE. Carcinoma in situ of the glans penis and distal urethra. J Dermatol Surg Oncol 1986;12:450.
52. Abide JM, Nahai F, Bennett RG. The meaning of surgical margins. Plast Reconstr Surg 1984;73:492.

Principles and Practice of Genitourinary Oncology, edited by Derek Raghavan, Howard I. Scher, Steven A. Leibel, and Paul H. Lange. Lippincott-Raven Publishers, Philadelphia, © 1997.

CHAPTER 92

Surgical Management of Penile Cancer

The Primary Tumor

Robert Huben

> "But if a Cancer should infect the Penis, the morbid Parts are, in that Case, to be immediately divided from the rest, to prevent the Disorder from spreading into the adjacent sound Parts, to the Destruction of the Patient."
>
> *Heister's Surgery*, 1739[1]

Successful management of the primary lesion of penile cancer requires total removal of the lesion, with adequate tumor-free margins, with the least possible cosmetic and functional loss. Although some early lesions may be amenable to more conservative measures such as local excision, invasive or advanced penile cancer usually requires partial or complete penectomy to achieve the goal of tumor eradication.[2] Surgery therefore remains an important element in the management of penile cancer, although its role in the treatment of early lesions has been lessened significantly by the emergence of newer approaches to local control, such as the use of topical agents, Mohs chemosurgery, and laser therapy.[2–4] Irradiation is considered by some to be an alternative approach for certain invasive lesions (see Chap. 93). However, partial or total penectomy remains the procedure of choice in bulky, exophytic penile cancers, which continue to be evident at diagnosis in many cases. In one large, cumulative series of patients with newly diagnosed penile cancer, 248 (47%) of 526 patients had stage T2 (invasion of corpus spongiosum or cavernosum) or more advanced penile cancer at presentation.[5] Until earlier diagnosis of penile cancer, resulting from a high index of suspicion and prompt medical attention on the part of patient and physician alike, becomes the norm, more radical surgical procedures for penile cancer remain necessary in the treatment of the primary lesion.

HISTORY OF SURGERY FOR PENILE CANCER

The evolution of various surgical procedures employed in the treatment of penile cancer was recently reviewed by Crawford and Dawkins.[3] Celsus reported on the use of amputation and cautery in the first century A.D., and cancer of the penis was described in the writings of the Egyptians, Hebrews, Persians, and Indians. Heister, in 1739, described a crude method of penile amputation in which a hollow tube of silver or lead was passed through the urethra beyond the penile lesion, after which a suture was secured tightly behind the lesion, causing the distal penis to slough off.[1] The first detailed description of an operation for penile cancer was by Thiersch in 1875. In 1912, Gibson described total penectomy by complete removal of the corpora and transection of the corpus spongiosum at the pubic symphysis, which was then brought out the anterior wall of the scrotum. In the early 1920s, Barringer and Dean described partial amputation of the penis 1.5 cm proximal to the lesion and also recommended irradiation of the groin area.[6] In 1931, Young reported the results of partial penectomy and unilateral groin dissection for penile cancer; in this technique, the femoral nodes as well as the inguinal nodes were removed.[7,8] The basic techniques of partial and total penectomy have remained largely the same since that time.

LOCAL EXCISION OF THE PRIMARY LESION

Incisional or excisional biopsy is indicated to confirm the diagnosis of penile cancer if the disease is suspected. Smaller lesions (those 1 cm or less) which are noninvasive (stage T1 or less) and which are located on the shaft of the penis may be amenable to wide local excision. Local excision has been associated with recurrence rates approaching 50%, however, and it is clearly inadequate treatment for invasive lesions of the glans or shaft (stage T2 or greater).[9–11] Larger lesions and those located on the glans are managed by wedge biopsy before a decision about definitive therapy. I strongly recommend biopsy as a separate procedure rather than as a step toward a more radical operation. It is only after as much as possible is known about both the diagnosis and the stage that reasonable treatment options can adequately be discussed with the patient. A simple wedge biopsy is usually adequate, and it is important to include a portion of the margin or edge of the lesion, because the malignant potential of a lesion can be assessed by observing the cellular interaction of the tumor with normal adjacent tissue and the nature and extent of invasion. Similarly, a biopsy must also be deep enough to determine the lesion's depth of penetration of underlying tissue layers. Wedge biopsies can usually be performed under local anesthesia, except in cases in which retraction of the foreskin or other manipulation is associated with marked discomfort. Occasionally, a dorsal slit may be necessary to adequately expose a lesion on the glans for biopsy. Circumcision may be performed at a later time, depending on the results of the biopsy and the extent of the primary lesion on adequate exposure.

Circumcision appears to have a fairly limited role as the sole treatment of penile cancer, because recurrence rates of 32% to 50% have been reported.[12–14] For superficial lesions limited to the foreskin, however, circumcision would appear to be an ideal form of management. The high recurrence rate associated with circumcision as definitive management of lesions involving the foreskin undoubtedly reflects poor patient selection rather than an inherent flaw in this procedure as a mode of treatment. Careful attention to the margins is necessary when circumcision is performed, and it is helpful to mark the specimen clearly to assist the pathologist in examining the most critical margins, which may be less obvious in the attenuated and distorted pathologic specimen. A patient with severe phimosis and chronic balanoposthitis who undergoes circumcision may have an occult cancer with tumor present at the surgical margins.[2] The authors of this report recommend external beam irradiation of approximately 5000 cGy over 5 weeks to eradicate any remaining malignancy, after postoperative edema and induration have resolved.

If wedge biopsy of a lesion on the glans indicates carcinoma in situ, either topical therapy with 5-fluorouracil or Mohs chemosurgery appears to provide appropriate therapy.[2–4] Partial penectomy is indicated for more extensive lesions involving the glans. Partial penectomy for invasive penile cancers in the absence of inguinal metastases is associated with 5-year survival rates of 70% to 80%.[9,15]

A recommendation for partial or complete amputation of the penis is abhorrent to most patients and undoubtedly leads a significant number to choose less radical and less effective alternatives. It is sometimes difficult to comprehend the patients' distress at this suggestion, considering the appearance of many of these lesions. Although loss of sexual function is usually the main concern, this apprehension may seem paradoxical in patients with large, fungating lesions that obviously have made normal sexual intercourse impossible for some time.

In the decision regarding partial versus total penectomy, it is not always true that "something is better than nothing." Partial penectomy must ensure an adequate penile length for voiding in the upright position. If the penile stump is too short, it may be engulfed by the groin fat pad, and the patient ends up dribbling down both legs when he tries to void. In most circumstances, however, the choice between a partial and total penectomy is clearly mandated by the extent of the primary lesion.

Because of the small number of cases in most series, it is difficult to obtain more than anecdotal information regarding sexual function after partial penectomy. Most patients report that they maintain erectile capability in the remaining portion of the penis after partial penectomy, although some men seem to lose interest in sex because of frustration or embarrassment regarding the size of the remaining penis. A major factor in the patient's ability to function sexually after partial penectomy is the stability of the relationship with his sexual partner. For patients who require a partial penectomy based on the extent of their primary lesion but who are reluctant to undergo this operation because of the effects on sexual function, the possibility of penile reconstruction may be suggested, as discussed later. However, penile reconstruction is indicated only in carefully selected and highly motivated patients and should not be suggested as a remedy for the consequences of partial penectomy if it is unrealistic because of the patient's age, poor prognosis, or interest.

TECHNIQUE OF PARTIAL PENECTOMY

The technique of partial penectomy is outlined in Fig. 92-1. The anatomy of the penis is discussed in detail in Chapter 87.

Broad-spectrum antibiotic therapy is initiated the evening before surgery and again 1 hour before operation in an effort to reduce gross bacterial contamination of the primary lesion and to prevent bacterial seeding into the bloodstream during manipulation of the lesion at the time of surgery. Some authors recommend the use of cleansing enemas the evening before surgery or the morning of the procedure in an effort to decrease postoperative contamination of the operative site. The epidural route is an ideal form of anesthesia for performing partial penectomy, although a general anesthetic may be more appropriate for some patients because of the nature of the procedure being done. The patient is placed in the supine position, unless there is a possibility that a total penectomy may be necessary based on intraoperative findings, in which case a dorsal lithotomy position is more appropriate. After the lower abdomen, perineum, and genitalia have been prepared and draped, a sterile condom or small surgical glove is passed over the primary lesion on the penis and secured snugly with a heavy silk suture. This maneuver is intended to eliminate gross contamination of the operative site from the heavily colonized lesion. A 1.3-cm Penrose drain is passed around the base of the penis and secured snugly with a clamp to control intraoperative bleeding.

A circumferential skin incision is made 2.0 cm proximal to the most cephalad extension of the primary lesion. Some authors recommend the formation of a dorsal skin flap at this point of the operation; however, this procedure is unnecessary from a cosmetic standpoint because of the relative laxity of the penile skin, and it could compromise the dorsal margin. The smaller subcutaneous veins can be cauterized and the larger veins, particularly on the dorsal surface of the penis, ligated with 3-0 polyglycolic acid (PGA) sutures. I prefer to use absorbable sutures throughout the course of this operation because of the risk of infection in the postoperative period and the problems that nonabsorbable sutures can promote in this circumstance. Buck's fascia is incised at the same level, and a plane can then be developed between the dorsal veins and arteries and the underlying corporal bodies. The vessels are doubly clamped and ligated with 2-0 or 3-0 PGA sutures. The corporal bodies are then transected about 0.5 cm proximal to the skin incision to allow for tension-free reapproximation of the penile skin at the completion of the procedure. The penile skin is ordinarily fairly lax and redundant, unless there is invasion of the dermal lymphatics by the tumor, so excessive shortening of the corporal bodies should be avoided. The corpus spongiosum should not

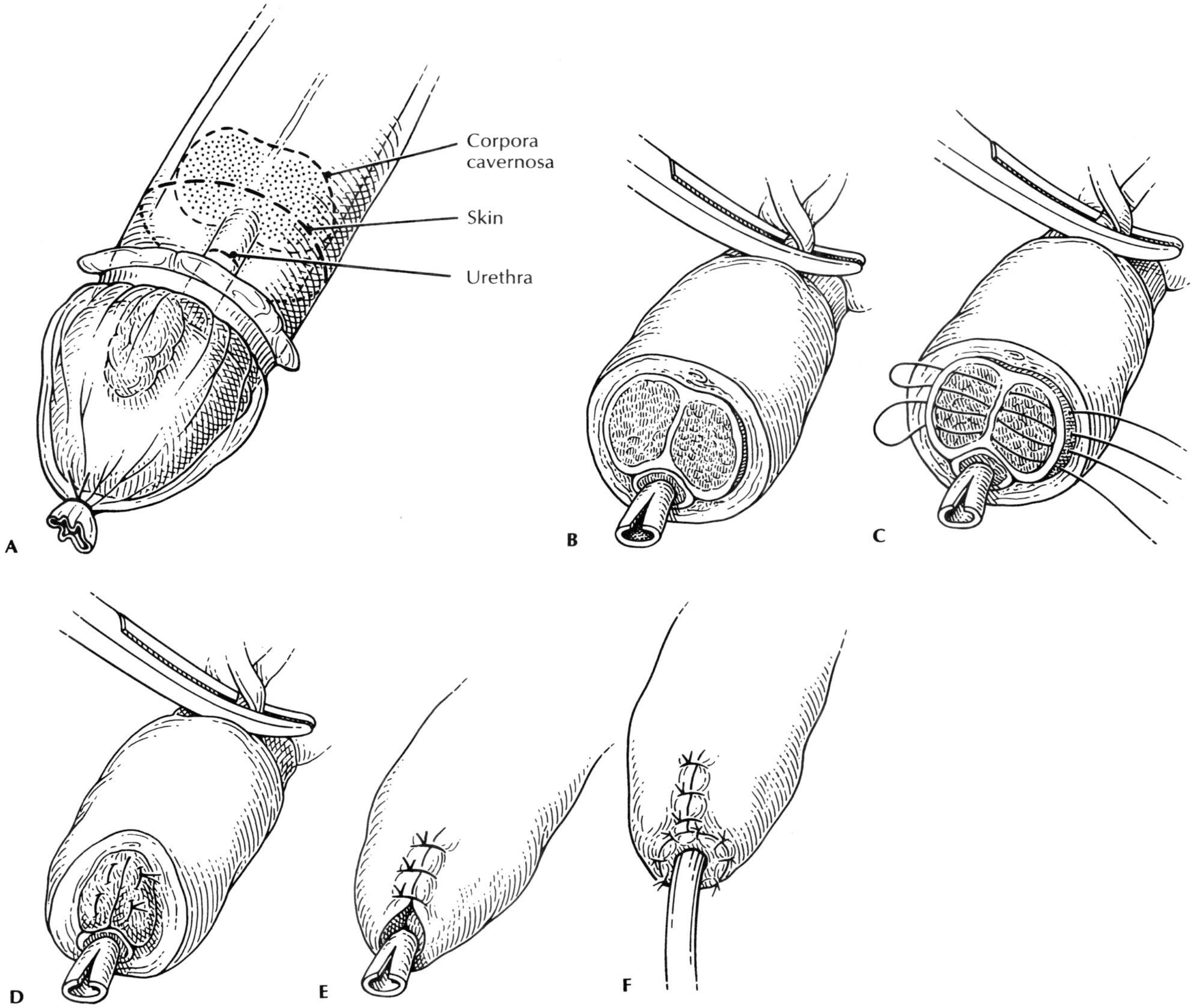

FIG. 92-1. Partial penectomy. (**A**) A circumferential skin incision is made 2 cm proximal to the tumor margin. (**B**) A soft rubber drain serves as a tourniquet, and the corpora cavernosa are amputated 0.5 to 1.0 cm proximal to the original skin incision. Additional urethral length allows spatulation. (**C** and **D**) The corpora cavernosa are closed with 2-0 polyglycolic acid. (**E**) The dorsal shaft skin is closed longitudinally with 3-0 polyglycolic acid, down to the urethral stump. (**F**) The spatulated urethra is approximated to the shaft skin with 3-0 polyglycolic acid.

be transected at this stage. The profunda arteries within each corporal body are usually readily identifiable centrally and can be ligated with 4-0 PGA figure-of-eight sutures. To facilitate subsequent urethral spatulation, the corpus spongiosum is mobilized for a length of about 1 cm distal to the level of the transection of the corporal bodies and transected at that level. The surgical specimen is then removed from the operative field, and the pathologist is requested to confirm the presence of tumor-free margins by frozen section histologic examination.

Although some authors suggest that a better cosmetic and functional effect can be obtained by closing the corporal bodies in a horizontal fashion, a stronger closure is made by closing the corporal bodies vertically, using 2-0 PGA sutures that incorporate the tunica laterally and are reinforced by inclusion of the intercavernosal septum. The tourniquet at the base of the penis is then released, and any obvious bleeding points are secured. This is an important step in the prevention of postoperative hemorrhage and hematoma formation.

The skin is closed vertically, beginning on the dorsal surface of the penis. Closure is carried down to the level of the transected corpus spongiosum. The urethra and encircling corpus spongiosum are spatulated ventrally, and the urethra is mobilized and approximated to the adjacent penile skin with 3-0 PGA sutures. An 6-mm Foley catheter is passed through the neomeatus into the bladder, and the operative site is wrapped with nonadhesive gauze. A pressure dressing is applied and is removed on the following day. The Foley catheter can usually be removed on the second or third postoperative day.

Complications of partial penectomy include infection and hemorrhage with resultant hematoma of the penile remnant.

This is best avoided by meticulous attention to hemostasis after the tourniquet is removed from the base of the penis intraoperatively and by use of a pressure dressing postoperatively. Infections can result from contamination from the primary lesion itself or from the bacterial flora of the perineum. I advocate use of intravenous antibiotics in the perioperative period and continuation postoperatively of an oral antibiotic that has good activity against most skin flora, such as an oral cephalosporin.

Stenosis of the neomeatus is a very common occurrence after partial penectomy. Although a fairly wide spatulation of the distal urethral remnant helps obviate this development, the trauma of daily activity to tissues that are ordinarily unexposed to such insult appears to promote scarring and subsequent narrowing of the neomeatus. This problem usually can be managed by intermittent self-catheterization with a small red rubber catheter or coudé catheter two to three times per week.

TECHNIQUE OF TOTAL PENECTOMY

If total penectomy is deemed the most appropriate method of managing a locally advanced primary lesion, preoperative and perioperative antibiotics are given and the patient is placed in a modified lithotomy position after administration of epidural or general anesthesia. If feasible, a Foley catheter is passed into the bladder, and the primary lesion is again covered with a sterile condom or surgical glove. An elliptical or diamond-shaped incision is made around the base of the penis (Fig. 92-2). For lesions involving the base of the penis, the incision should be carried widely enough to allow a 2-cm margin of uninvolved tissue. The incision is carried down through the subcutaneous fat layer. Usually, several large veins can be observed passing through the subcutaneous fat toward the base of the penis. These vessels can be ligated with 3-0 PGA sutures. In addition, several large lymphatic channels can usually be recognized at this point, and these vessels should be ligated or clipped, if feasible.

Dorsally, the penis is attached to the anterior abdominal wall by a thickening of Scarpa's fascia in the midline known as the fundiform ligament and to the pubic symphysis by an extension of Buck's fascia termed the suspensory ligament. The dorsal arteries of the penis (which arise from the internal pudendal artery) and the dorsal vein of the penis are isolated at the penile base and ligated with sutures of 2-0 PGA. Attention is then directed ventrally, where the corpus spongiosum and urethra are isolated in the ventral midline 1 to 2 cm distal to the base of the penis. The corpus spongiosum and urethra are divided at this point, and the proximal portions are mobilized with blunt and sharp dissection as much as possible. This facilitates further mobilization of the urethra for the formation of a perineal urethrostomy at a subsequent stage.

With further blunt and sharp dissection, the corpora cavernosa are dissected down to their origin from the ischial rami of the symphysis, clamped, and ligated with a suture ligature of 1-0 PGA. The surgical specimen is removed at this point and sent for frozen section examination and confirmation of negative margins. Small bleeding vessels at the base of the penis can be controlled with interrupted figure-of-eight sutures of 3-0 PGA.

Proper positioning of the perineal urethrostomy is facilitated by passing a urethral sound through the transected urethra and corpus spongiosum and cutting down the sound to expose the urethra and corpus spongiosum in the midline approximately halfway between the base of the scrotum and the anus. A 1.5- to 2.0-cm circular piece of skin is excised at this point, and the distal urethra and corpus spongiosum are mobilized completely and brought out through the opening that has been created. The excess length of corpus spongiosum and urethra is transected without tension, and the end of the remaining urethra is spatulated at the 12 o'clock position for approximately 1 cm. The spatulated urethra is then sutured to the perineal skin with simple interrupted sutures of 3-0 PGA. Dorsal spatulation facilitates forward flow of urine when the patient voids in the sitting position. Similarly, the initial diamond-shaped incision made at the base of the penis is closed with interrupted 3-0 PGA.

Despite excision of a wide circle of perineal skin and lengthy spatulation of the most distal segment of urethra, stricture of the perineal urethrostomy frequently occurs. Consequently, the patient may need to dilate the urethrostomy on a regular basis. Because stricture is so common, I routinely perform a "Y-V plasty" of the perineal urethrostomy at the time of total penectomy (Fig. 92-3). The urethra and encircling corpus spongiosum that have been transected near the base of the penis are again mobilized and brought through the perineum in the usual fashion. A V-shaped incision is made at the 12 o'clock position, and the redundant urethra is excised without tension and spatulated for a distance of 1 cm. The apex of the V is brought to the apex of the spatulated urethra and sutured with interrupted simple sutures of 3-0 PGA. The remaining portion of the urethral edge is sutured to the perineal skin with similar interrupted sutures. A Foley catheter is then placed through the urethrostomy and left indwelling for 5 to 7 days. A pressure dressing is applied to the primary incision. Parenteral antibiotics are continued for the next 24 hours, and the patient is sent home with oral antibiotics for another 7 days.

If stricture of the perineal urethrostomy occurs, initial management is by intermittent dilation with a small red rubber catheter or coudé catheter. Usually these strictures are difficult to manage in this fashion, and an initial or repeat Y-V plasty may be necessary. Bleeding and wound infections after total penectomy occur less frequently than after partial penectomy. Prolonged drainage of lymph fluid from the penectomy site may occasionally be encountered; it is best avoided by ligation of the larger lymph vessels that are exposed at the base of the penis early in the procedure. Such drainage usually resolves with conservative management.

PHALLIC RECONSTRUCTION AFTER TOTAL PENECTOMY FOR PENILE CANCER

A number of techniques have been described for reconstruction of the penis after total amputation, and such procedures may be considered in selected patients with a history of penile cancer. Borgoras was the first to report penile reconstruction, in 1936; he used tubed abdominal flaps with ribbed cartilage for rigidity. Among the imaginative techniques that have been used over the years are local tubed pedicle flaps and skin flaps, muscle and myocutaneous flaps, local fasciocutaneous flaps, and, more recently, sensate fasciocutaneous microvascular free flaps.[16] Jordan and associates reported the results of a small series of patients who underwent total phallic reconstruction with insertion of a penile prosthesis; the procedure met with

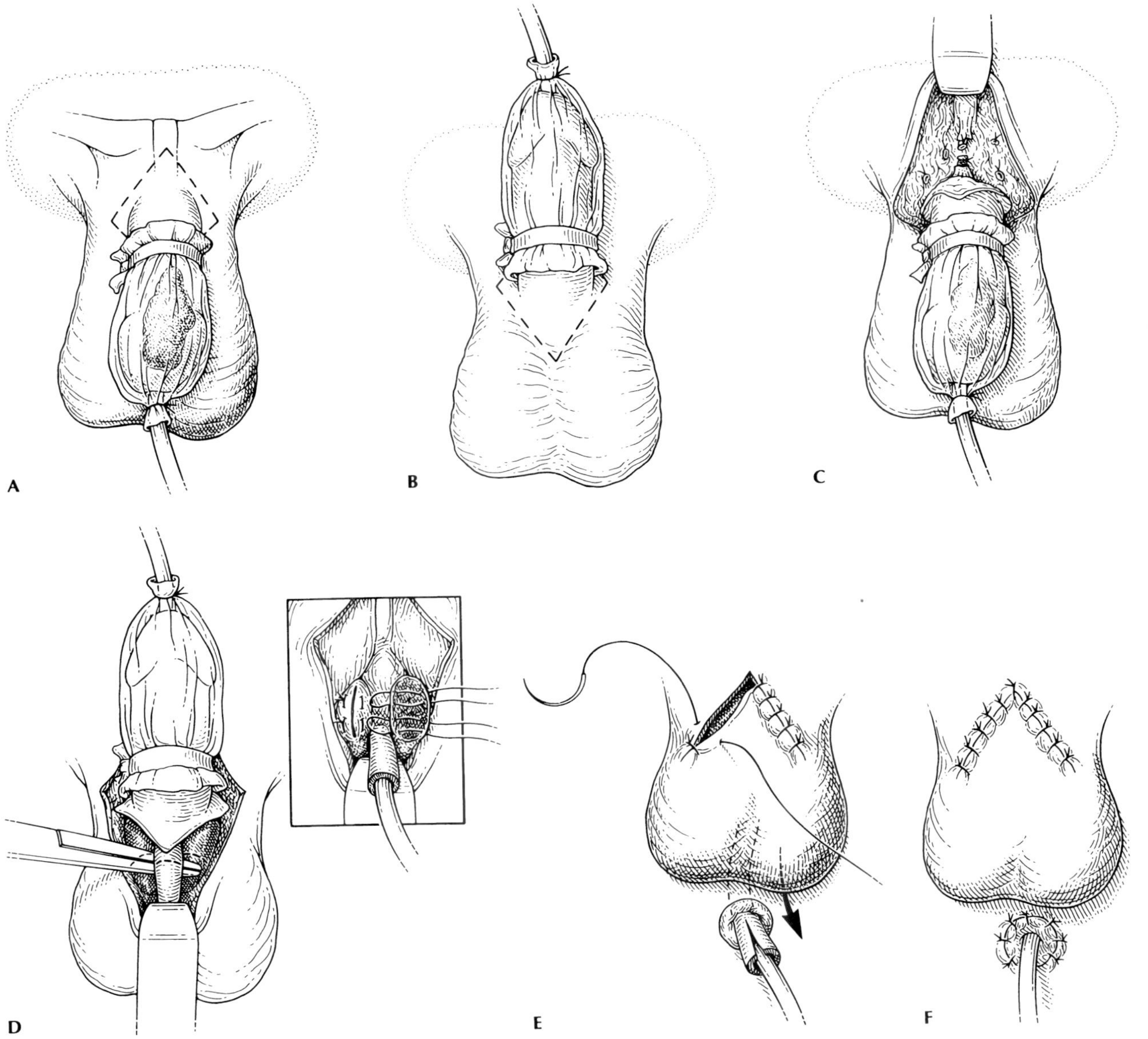

FIG. 92-2. Total penectomy. (**A** and **B**) A diamond-shaped incision is made around the base of the penis. (**C**) The dissection is extended superiorly through the subcutaneous fat, lymphatic vessels, and superficial veins to the surface of the pubis. The suspensory ligament of the penis is divided, and the vessels are transected between ligatures. (**D**) Cephalad deflection of the penis allows ventral isolation of the urethra. Proximal crural amputation and division of the urethra are accomplished. The corpora are closed (*inset*) with 3-0 polyglycolic acid. (**E** and **F**) Adequate bulbar urethral length is achieved, and a perineal urethrostomy is created. The diamond-shaped defect is closed.

success in a high percentage of patients.[17] These surgical techniques and results are briefly reviewed.

A fasciocutaneous forearm free flap is the usual tissue donor site. The forearm flap is elevated on either the radial or ulnar artery and is transferred to the recipient site by microsurgical anastomosis to either the inferior epigastric vessels or, through a vein interposition graft, to the superficial femoral artery. The medial or lateral antebrachial nerves are included in the flap for coaptation to the dorsal nerves of the penis. Reinnervation of the flap after phalloplasty usually takes 4 to 9 months, and insertion of the prosthesis is delayed until the neophallus has regained sensation. The urethra that was created by tubularization of the free forearm flap should also be stable, and the patient should be voiding with a good stream, with no evidence of urinary tract infection.[18]

An incision is made in the base of the phallus, and a space is developed in the folded plane of the phallic flap by blunt dissection. Care must be taken during this phase of the procedure to avoid injury to the urethra, the vascular anastomoses, and the nerves. A second incision is made over the ischial tuber-

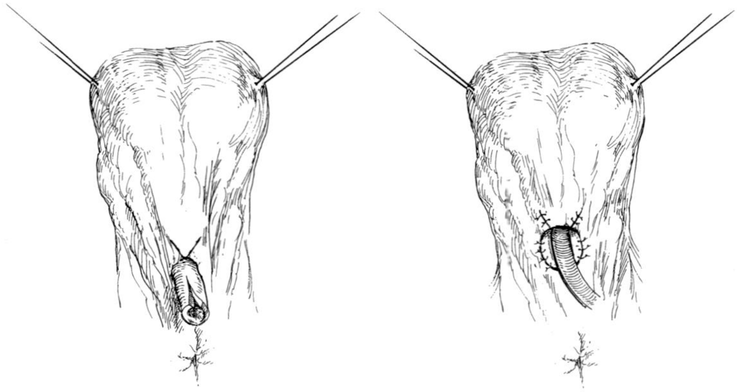

A B **FIG. 92-3.** Technique of Y-V plasty of perineal urethrostomy. (**A**) V-shaped incision of perineal skin at 12 o'clock position; spatulation of urethra. (**B**) Completed Y-V plasty.

osity, and a space is developed from the suprapubic region to the ischial tuberosity along the inferior pubic ramus.

A neotunica is fashioned from vascular stretch polytetrafluoroethylene. The distal end is closed, and the shaft of the neotunica is formed from struts of polytetrafluoroethylene. In patients who have undergone total penectomy, the remnants of crura of the corpora are dilated and used to secure the proximal portion of the prosthesis. If an inflatable prosthesis is used, the reservoir is inserted in its usual preperitoneal location. One or sometimes two cylinders are then secured within the neotunica and fixed to one or both ischial tuberosities. Drains are used for a full 48 hours, and broad-spectrum antibiotics are given for 72 hours, followed by 14 days of oral cephalosporin therapy.

Of 8 patients who underwent either total phalloplasty or free flap penile reconstruction with prosthetic implantation in the Norfolk series, 4 patients developed infections that required explantation, and 2 of those patients had subsequent successful reimplantation. The 6 patients with implants in place have been monitored for up to 3 years. Because there were 8 patients who underwent 10 attempts at implantation, of which 6 were successful, a 60% success rate was reported by the authors, including all of the last four implantations performed.[17]

SUMMARY

In the management of penile cancer, partial or total penectomy is a radical solution for a life-threatening problem, and these procedures remain the standard of therapy for invasive lesions (stage T2 or greater) despite their mutilating nature. The understandable reluctance to accept surgical management of advanced penile cancers continues to motivate patients to seek less radical but also less effective treatment alternatives. Although an important goal in the management of penile cancer is to cause the least possible cosmetic and functional impairments, inadequate management of the primary lesion undoubtedly compromises the potential curability of this disease. Although penile cancer is uncommon in the United States, the high incidence of invasive lesions at diagnosis, regardless of the cause of delay in diagnosis or treatment, suggests that partial and total penectomy will continue to be necessary to treat advanced penile cancers until equally effective and less destructive alternatives are developed. The role of local excision will probably lessen progressively in the future, because comparable cure rates with less aggressive forms of management such as Mohs chemosurgery and laser therapy appear to be available already.

In carefully selected and highly motivated patients who have undergone partial or total penectomy for the treatment of penile cancer, reconstructive surgery has become a more viable option as surgical techniques for reconstruction have improved significantly. However, the patient's age, general medical condition, prognosis, and motivation are all critical factors in making such a recommendation, and it is unfair to suggest reconstruction as a future option unless there is a realistic likelihood that such an option is a valid one. Although partial or total penectomy is a drastic measure for control of penile cancer, it is important for the patient to realize the life-threatening nature of the disease and the fact that prognosis worsens significantly if the initial method of management of the primary lesion is unsuccessful.

REFERENCES

1. Heister L. Of a cancer of the penis. In: Heister L. Heister's surgery. Germany, Helmstadt, 1739. Chapter 132, Sect 3, Part 2.
2. Johnson DE, Lo RK. Tumors of the penis, urethra and scrotum. In: deKernion JB, Paulson DF, eds. Genitourinary cancer management. Philadelphia, Lea & Febiger, 1987:219.
3. Crawford ED, Dawkins CA. Cancer of the penis. In: Skinner DG, Lieskovsky G, eds. Diagnosis and management of genitourinary cancer. Philadelphia, WB Saunders, 1988:549.
4. Mohs FE, Snow SN, Messing EM, Kuglitsch ME: Microscopically controlled surgery in the treatment of carcinoma of the penis. J Urol 1985;133:961.
5. Fair WR, Fuks ZY, Scher HI. Cancer of the urethra and penis. In: DeVita VT Jr, Hellman S, Rosenberg SA, eds. Cancer principles and practice of oncology, 4th ed. Philadelphia, JB Lippincott, 1993:4.
6. Barringer BS, Dean AL Jr. Epithelioma of the penis. J Urol 1924;11:497.
7. Young HH. A radical operation for the cure of cancer of the penis. J Urol 1931;26:285.
8. Lewis LG. Young's radical operation for the cure of cancer of the penis: a report of 34 cases. J Urol 1931;26:295.
9. Schellhammer PF, Jordan GH, Schlossberg SM. Tumors of the penis. In: Walsh PC, Retik AB, Stamey TA, Vaughan ED JR, eds. Campbell's urology, 6th ed. Philadelphia, WB Saunders, 1992:1264.
10. Staubitz WJ, Lent MH, Oberkircher OJ. Carcinoma of the penis. Cancer 1955;8:371.
11. Hanash KA, Furlow WL, Utz DC, et al. Carcinoma of the penis: a clinicopathologic study. J Urol 1970;104:291.
12. Hardner GJ, Bhanalaph T, Murphy GP, et al. Carcinoma of the penis: analysis of therapy in 100 consecutive cases. J Urol 1972;108:428.
13. Bassett JW. Carcinoma of the penis. Cancer 1975;5:530.

14. Beggs JH, Spratt JS Jr. Epidermoid carcinoma of the penis. J Urol 1986;135:283.
15. Schellhammer PF. Carcinoma of the penis. In: Seidmon EJ, Hanno PM, eds. Current urologic therapy. Philadelphia, WB Saunders, 1990: 458.
16. Gilbert DA, Williams MW, Horton CE, et al. Phallic reinnervation via the pudendal nerve. J Urol 1988;140:295.
17. Jordan GH, Alter GJ, Gilbert DA, Horton CE, Devine CJ Jr. Penile prosthesis implantation in total phalloplasty. J Urol 1994;152:410.
18. Benderev TV. Preservation of penile length in penile cancer and trauma by use of a pedicled flap. J Urol 1988;140:145.

BIBLIOGRAPHY

Andriole GL, Catalona WJ. Partial and total penectomy. In: Fowler EJ Jr, ed. Mastery of surgery: urologic surgery. Boston, Little, Brown, 1992: 415.

Bissada NK. Conservative extirpative treatment of cancer of the penis. Urol Clin North Am 1992;19:283.

Borgoras NA. Uber die volle plastische Wiederherslellung eines zum Kortus fahigen Penis (Peniplasticon totalis). Zentralb Chir 1936:1271.

Das S. Penile amputations for the management of primary carcinoma of the penis. Urol Clin North Am 1992;19:277.

Gilbert DA, Horton CE, Terzis JK, Devine CJ Jr, Winslow BH, Devine PC. New concepts in phallic reconstruction. Ann Plast Surg 1987;18: 128.

Gilbert DA, Jordan GH, Devine CJ Jr, Winslow BH. Microsurgical forearm ''cricket bat-transformer'' phalloplasty. Plast Reconstr Surg 1992;90: 711.

Grabstald H, Hilaris B, Henchike U, Whitmore WF Jr. Cancer of the female urethra. JAMA 1966;197:835.

Ritter DW. Primary malignancy of the female urethra. West J Surg Obstet Gynecol 1953;51:420.

Sufrin G, Huben R. Benign and malignant lesions of the penis. In: Gillenwater JY, Grayhack JT, Howards SS, Duckett JW, eds. Adult and pediatric urology, 2nd ed. St Louis, Mosby–Year Book, 1991:1643.

White JM. Carcinoma of the penis. In: Glenn JF, ed. Urologic surgery, 4th ed. Philadelphia, JB Lippincott, 1991:831.

Principles and Practice of Genitourinary Oncology, edited by Derek Raghavan, Howard I. Scher, Steven A. Leibel, and Paul H. Lange. Lippincott-Raven Publishers, Philadelphia, © 1997.

CHAPTER 93

Radiotherapy for Cancer of the Penis

Robert H. Sagerman and Gary L. Whipple

Penile cancer accounts for only 0.5% of all male cancers in North America,[1] but it is far more common elsewhere.[2,3] It is usually classified as well or moderately differentiated squamous cell cancer. The underlying philosophy of the treatment of penile cancer should be based on achieving tumor control with preservation of anatomic form and function. Therapeutic decisions are based on the size, location, and depth of infiltration of the primary lesion and the presence or absence of clinically detectable lymphadenopathy, which may or may not represent metastatic disease. Distant metastases beyond the inguinal or pelvic nodes are rare at the time of diagnosis. In addition, personal and cultural preferences must always be considered. This chapter reviews the results of irradiation and present a logical radiotherapeutic approach to the primary lesion, the inguinopelvic lymph nodes, and postsurgical recurrence. The radiotherapeutic results are similar to those of surgery. The prognosis for cure falls drastically with clinical involvement of the inguinal nodes and is extremely poor with more remote metastases.

PATHOLOGY

The most common malignant penile tumor is squamous cell carcinoma, usually described as well or moderately differentiated. Increasing degrees of anaplasia have been correlated with more advanced disease and poorer prognosis.[4–8] Marcial and colleagues[5] reported the 5-year survival rate among 216 patients to be 64% in those with grade I lesions, 40% in grade II, and 25% in grade III. Long-term cure was achieved in 87% of well differentiated tumors and 62% of moderately or poorly differentiated tumors in the classic study of Ekstrom and Edsmyr.[6] Others, however, have not found cell differentiation to correlate with survival.[9,10]

Basal cell carcinoma has been noted rarely in series dealing with penile cancer[9]; a recent paper documented only the twelfth reported case.[11] Local excision has usually been curative,[12] although a good result may be expected with radiotherapy in cases in which surgery is contraindicated or refused. Malignant melanoma is similarly uncommon[13] and often has spread to the inguinal nodes by the time of diagnosis; radiotherapy is typically used only for palliative or adjuvant care after primary resection in this setting.

Soft tissue tumors, typically of smooth muscle, peripheral nerve, or vascular origin, are also rare, and about half are malignant.[14] Those occurring on the shaft, as opposed to the glans, are more likely to be malignant.

One case of primary lymphoma of the penis, which arose in a patient with Peyronie's disease, has been reported. Most lymphomas of the penis have been secondary.[15]

Two premalignant conditions, Bowen's disease and erythroplasia of Queyrat, are treatable with radiotherapy.[16,17] Bowen's disease is a squamous cell carcinoma in situ that typically appears as a red plaque on the skin of the penile shaft and inguinal region. An association between Bowen's disease and concurrent visceral malignancy has not been confirmed by case-controlled studies.[18] Erythroplasia of Queyrat is a red, velvety lesion that involves the mucocutaneous areas of the glans and prepuce and almost always occurs in uncircumcised men.[12]

Cancer metastatic to the penis is uncommon. The most frequent primary sites of such metastases are the bladder, prostate, colorectum, and kidney.[19] Most patients have evidence of metastatic disease elsewhere at the time of penile metastasis.[20]

STAGING AND PROGNOSIS

The most important correlates of survival in penile cancer are the presence of regional lymph node metastases and the extent of the primary tumor.[5,6,9,21,22] Several staging systems have been used to quantify these factors, the most common being the system proposed by Jackson[23] and the TNM system of the International Union Against Cancer (UICC).[24,25] The use of different staging systems has led to some difficulty in quantifying results from the various studies. The more commonly used Jackson system stratifies patients according to the anatomic extent of the tumor and the operability of nodes. However, patients within a single Jackson stage can have significantly different tumor burdens, which can obscure the results of therapy reported for that stage. Fraley and colleagues,[22] in a surgical series, noted that patients within Jackson stage I, who could be subclassified as having Tcis, T1, or T2 lesions by the TNM UICC system, had very dissimilar outcomes. In addition, the TNM UICC staging system has undergone several revisions. Some studies have classified patients with the use of a TNM system based on lesion size alone,[24] whereas the current system[25] is based on the degree of invasion into the penis and neighboring structures. Comparisons of studies, with their different staging systems and variety of treatment philosophies, must be undertaken with a careful examination of patient characteristics. For additional discussion on staging, see Chapter 90.

SURGICAL TREATMENT

Surgery for the primary penile lesion is the most commonly used form of local therapy, and it is the method against which other treatments are compared (see Chap. 92). A variety of methods, including penile-sparing procedures such as circumcision, local excision, Mohs micrographic surgery, partial amputation, and the more radical total penectomy, are used. In general, local control with penile-conserving procedures ranges from 8% to 50%,[26] with salvage amputation successful after most failures. A recent compilation of data from numerous surgical studies[27] reported local control rates for circumcision, local excision, and partial or radical amputation to be 70%, 56%, and 89%, respectively. Five-year survival rates for each treatment group were 60%, 82%, and 50%, respectively. These figures are crude numbers that do not categorize patients according to stage of disease. This same summary also noted that among patients who were clinically negative for groin involvement at diagnosis, 14% eventually developed metastatic inguinal adenopathy (see Chaps. 92 and 94 for further details and correlations with the extent of the primary tumor).

RADIOTHERAPY IN THE MANAGEMENT OF PENILE CANCER

The principal advantage of radiotherapy in the management of cancer lies in the potential for an organ-sparing cure, with maintenance of function. The functional and psychological consequences of undergoing penectomy, whether total or partial, can be devastating, particularly in younger patients, and the psychological need for normal urinary and sexual function should not be underestimated in the elderly. An intact penis was even required for full religious participation by the Holy Writ: "[He] that hath his privy member cut off shall not enter into the assembly of the Lord" (Deuteronomy 23:1).[28] Hanash and colleagues[29] reported on 3 patients who committed suicide after penile amputation. The prospect of losing a part or all of this organ can be a cause of considerable distress in patients with this disease.[30]

An organ-sparing cancer treatment cannot be considered worthwhile unless its results, either alone or with salvage therapy, are equivalent to those obtained with the more radical treatment. There have been no randomized, prospective studies comparing radiotherapy with surgery for penile cancer, and it is unlikely that there will be; precise comparisons are therefore difficult. Given its rarity and lack of consistent treatment through the years, penile cancer lends itself poorly to strict scientific comparisons. A review of the literature indicates that a significant number of patients treated with radiotherapy enjoy long-term survival with the penile structure and function intact. In patients who have local recurrence after radiotherapy, surgical salvage results in survival rates equal to those obtained by primary surgical treatment.[31–33] This finding underscores the need for close follow-up and interdisciplinary cooperation.

MANAGEMENT OF THE PRIMARY TUMOR

Most penile cancers occur in the prepuce, glans penis, or coronal ridge. Before radiotherapy is initiated, circumcision should be performed, both to assess the extent of the tumor and to minimize the morbidity associated with radiotherapy (eg, swelling, secondary infection, moist desquamation). Infection, which can occur secondary to tumor, should be treated because it increases radioresistance.[34] Fibrosis of the foreskin can occur as a late complication, causing an inability to retract the foreskin and impeding sexual function.[35] In addition, follow-up care is better facilitated by the absence of the foreskin, which allows for a more thorough tactile and visual examination.

Historically, a number of different radiotherapeutic methods have been used to treat the primary lesion, including superficial x-rays, teleradium sources, electron beams, megavoltage gamma and x-rays, and interstitial and contact brachytherapy. External beam irradiation and interstitial implants with iridium-192 (^{192}Ir) sources are used most commonly.

EXTERNAL BEAM RADIOTHERAPY: TECHNICAL ASPECTS

The principal advantages of external beam radiotherapy are that it is widely available, is simple to perform in a reproducible manner, facilitates homogeneity of dose, allows for treatment of the entire shaft if necessary, and minimizes radiation exposure to the staff. Several devices have been designed to achieve a homogeneous dose. Most consist of a plastic box containing tissue-equivalent material, with a central opening through which the penis is inserted. Most use a molded wax bolus[16,33,36–38] and treat the patient in the supine position. Sagerman and associates[31] have made use of a water-filled container into which the penis is suspended, the patient being treated in the prone position, which allows better coverage of the base of the shaft while sparing the skin of the perineum and groin (Fig. 93-1). This is especially useful in the obese patient and in the patient with a short penis.

Another unique device[39] consists of a Perspex tube which is placed over the penis and attached to a Perspex plate resting on the skin. The Perspex tube is connected to a vacuum pump which, when activated, fixes the position of the penis with negative pressure. A Perspex block can then be placed around the tube to serve as bolus. The patient can be treated either prone or supine, and the penis is reproducibly positioned without being squeezed by the bolus.

A wide variety of machine energies have been used in the past, and most have achieved similar results, which would be expected given the typically superficial extent of the disease and the diameter of the penis. Modern studies, reflecting the technology available in most radiotherapy departments, have used cobalt-60 (^{60}Co) or 4-MV photons with appropriate bolus. Most series have treated patients to total doses of 50 to 60 Gy in fractions of 2 to 3.5 Gy through parallel opposed fields. Although it is probable that smaller daily doses reduce the inci-

A

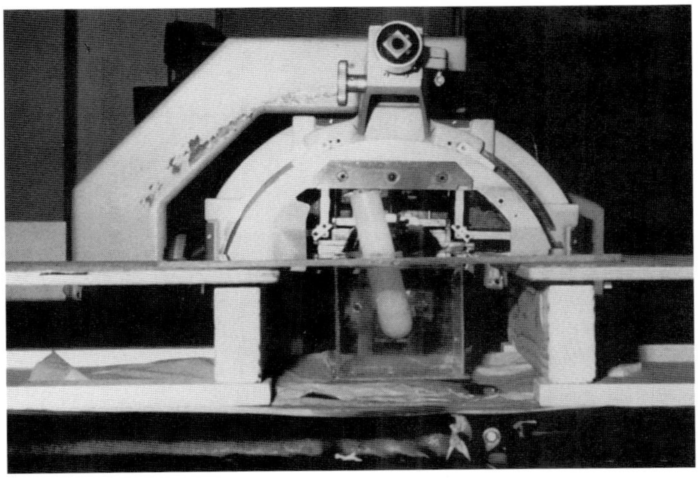

B

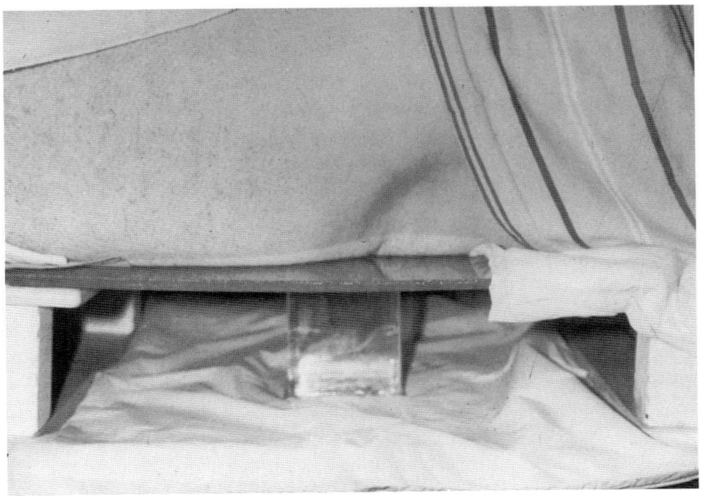

FIG. 93-1. (**A**) Plexiglas water bath, used as tissue-equivalent bolus, with cobalt-60 teletherapy unit in the background. (Sagerman RH, Yu WS, Chung CT, Puranik A. External beam irradiation of carcinoma of the penis. Radiology 1984;152:183.) (**B**) A patient, in the prone position, with the penis suspended in the water bath, is treated with opposed lateral fields.

dence of late complications, such as necrosis and urethral stenosis, this has not been definitively established, and complications most often reflect the size and location of the lesion and depth of invasion. Nevertheless, it would seem prudent that daily doses in the range of 1.8 to 2.5 Gy should be used if preservation of penile form and function are important.

RESULTS OF EXTERNAL BEAM RADIOTHERAPY

Early authors, such as Dean,[40] Lederman,[41] Knudsen and Brennhovd[42] and Zausner,[43] employed a variety of treatments and were among the first to document penis-sparing cures using teleradium, contact radium, radium needles, and superficial x-rays. Murrell and Williams[4] noted control of the primary lesion in 48 (52%) of 92 patients treated with 250 peak kilovolt (kVp) x-rays. This group included patients who were either clinically negative for groin involvement or had adenopathy categorized as operable. Amputation carried out for those with persistent (27%) or recurrent (21%) disease resulted in an overall control rate of 73% and a crude 3-year survival rate of 58%, which compared favorably with the rate in a smaller group treated with surgery in the same institution.

In a classic study by Engelstad,[44] complete and durable destruction of the primary tumor was achieved in 30 of 64 patients. Of 34 patients who presented with no evidence of metastatic disease, 31 (89%) were alive and symptom free at 3 years; surgical salvage was required in 14 patients. These results were roughly equivalent to those of contemporary surgical studies by Ekstrom and Edsmyr,[6] who achieved a 5-year survival rate of 90%, and by Staubitz and associates,[9] who reported a 3-year rate of 89% after surgery for patients with stage I disease.

Modern practitioners, using megavoltage equipment, have usually achieved results equal to or superior to those noted in the earlier studies. Reported results from modern studies are listed in Table 93-1.

Krieg and Luc[32] noted local control in 9 of 12 patients treated with a cesium-137 (^{137}Cs) unit to a tumor dose of 50 to 65 Gy. Surgical salvage was successful in 2 of the 3 failures, producing local control in a total 11 of 12 patients. Three patients, who presented with clinically positive inguinal nodes, received megavoltage irradiation with a ^{60}Co source, and control was achieved in 2. Overall, 10 of the 12 patients survived disease free. These results compared favorably with surgical results from the same institution, in which local control was achieved in 15 of 17 patients, with 13 of 17 surviving disease free.

Duncan and Jackson[36] compared the results of external beam radiotherapy at the Christie Hospital (Manchester, England)

TABLE 93-1. *External beam radiotherapy for penile cancer*

Investigators	Local control by stage			Penile preservation*	3-Year survival rate (%)		
	I	I/II	II		I	I/II	II
Duncan and Jackson, 1972[36]	18/20		—	16/20	90		—
McLean et al, 1993[16]	11/15		0/2	—	79†		—
Sagerman et al, 1984[31]	6/9		2/3	8/15	78		67
Kaushal and Sharma, 1987[33]		13/16		13/16		93	
Grabstald and Kelly, 1980[47]	9/10		—	9/10‡	90		—
Almgard and Edsmyr, 1973[46]	10/16		—	—§	88		—
Haile and Delclos, 1980[45]		18/20‖		16/20		—	
Newaishy and Decley, 1968[37]		18/28		—	90		37
Pointon, 1975[48]	27/32		—	27/32	78		—
Englestad, 1948[44]		29/58		30/64	89		68
Krieg and Luk, 1981[32]	5/7		4/4	9/12	—		—
Modig et al, 1993[58]		20/25		20/25		80†	
TOTAL	86/109		6/9	148/413			
TOTAL %	79%		67%	69%			
Stage I + II		190/265 (72%)					

* Includes stages I, II, and III.
† 5-Year survival rate.
‡ One patient had a new penile primary appear 8 years post RT and was treated with amputation.
§ Five patients underwent local excision for local recurrence without functional outcome specified.
‖ Includes patients treated by external beam and brachytherapy; results were not subdivided.

with Jackson's previously published series[23] from the same institution, in which radium mold therapy was used. Twenty patients with Jackson stage I penile cancer were treated with ^{60}Co teletherapy or a 4-MV linear accelerator to a tumor dose of 50 to 57 Gy over 22 days. Local control was achieved in 18, with surgical salvage required in 2 for recurrence. The overall survival rate at 3 years was 90%, which was comparable to the rate achieved by these authors with brachytherapy, but with a greater percentage of patients (80% versus 47%) retaining an intact penis. Haile and Delclos[45] reported similar results among 20 patients who were treated with external beam irradiation or brachytherapy at the M. D. Anderson Cancer Center; local control was achieved in 18 of 20 cases with radiotherapy alone and surgical salvage was successful in both instances of recurrence.

Almgard and Edsmyr[46] achieved local control in 10 of 16 patients treated with superficial x-rays alone, and local radical excision produced long-term control (10 to 30 years) in 5 of the 6 who had recurrence of penile cancer. Seventeen others underwent penectomy for recurrence after radiotherapy, with 16 being free of disease at 5 to 32 years. Kelly and colleagues[17] made use of a single direct electron beam, with the penile shaft within the 90% isodose curve, to treat 10 patients with primary tumors less than 3 cm in diameter. One patient required bilateral inguinal node dissection for metastatic disease. In their initial report, all patients were alive and disease free. In a follow-up report published 6 years later,[47] 1 patient had developed a new primary penile lesion 8 years after radiotherapy and was successfully salvaged with penectomy.

Sagerman and associates[31] reported on 15 patients with disease localized to the penis who were treated with 250 kVp x-rays or ^{60}Co to tumor doses ranging from 45 Gy (15 fractions in 3 weeks) to 64 Gy (32 fractions in 6.5 weeks). Control was achieved in 6 of 9 patients with Jackson stage I cancer and in 2 of 3 patients with stage II disease, with irradiation alone (Fig. 93-2*A* and 93-2*C*). Two patients with stage I disease and 1 patient with stage II disease were successfully salvaged with surgery. Three patients who presented with stage IV disease but clinically negative groin involvement were also treated as described, with 1 patient disease free more than 5 years after treatment. Only 1 patient, of those initially free of inguinal disease, went on to develop inguinal adenopathy. Nine patients received palliative inguinal irradiation, and in-field control of disease was achieved in 4. However, no member of this group survived longer than 18 months after radiotherapy.

Kaushal and Sharma[33] treated 12 patients with Jackson stage I tumors and 4 with stage II tumors to 55 Gy (25 fractions in 5 weeks), with local control and preservation of the organ achieved in 13 patients. Two patients had persistent disease, and 1 had a late recurrence; all were salvaged with partial penectomy, but the long-term local control rate was not specified. Pointon[48] reported local control in 27 of 32 patients given a tumor dose of 52.5 to 55 Gy (16 fractions in 22 days) with a 4-MV linear accelerator. All patients presented without inguinal adenopathy, but 3 later developed metastatic inguinal disease. Partial amputation for recurrence was carried out in 5 cases, with only 3 patients overall succumbing to disease.

Kearsley and associates[49] reported 1 patient with a locally advanced carcinoma and ulcerating inguinal lymph node who was alive and free of disease 26 years after being treated with irradiation alone (40 Gy in 15 fractions). This outcome is remarkable, given the low dose and the universally poor outcome of patients with stage IV disease.

Cancer metastatic to the penis is rare; in more than two thirds of patients, it is part of a widespread process, and it usually occurs secondary to primary cancers of the prostate, bladder, colorectum, or kidney.[20,50–53] These patients are often symptomatic, complaining of pain, swelling, priapism, and alterations in voiding.[54] Although more than 300 cases have been reported, Ben-Yosef and Kapp[19] found only 59 in which treat-

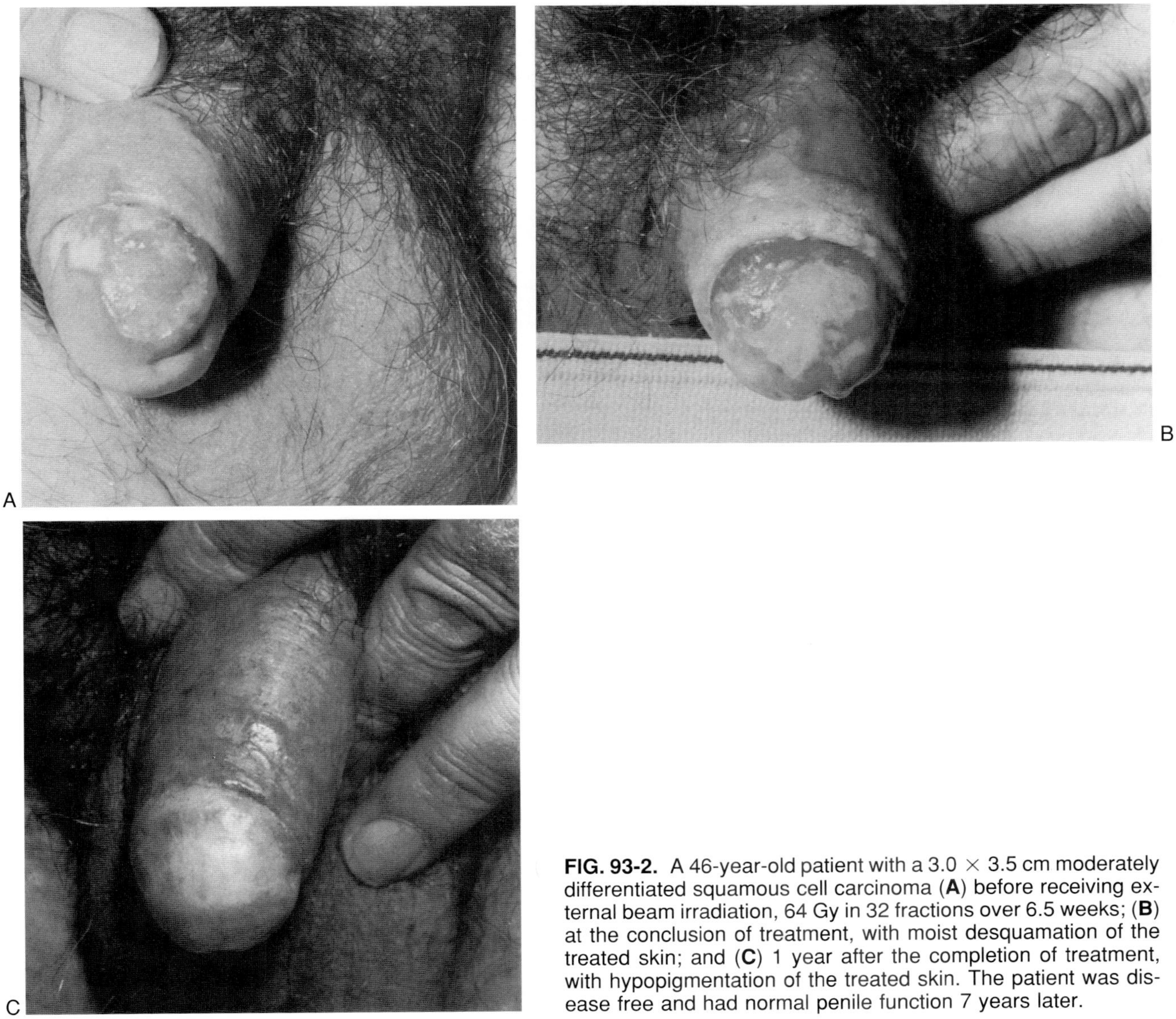

FIG. 93-2. A 46-year-old patient with a 3.0 × 3.5 cm moderately differentiated squamous cell carcinoma (**A**) before receiving external beam irradiation, 64 Gy in 32 fractions over 6.5 weeks; (**B**) at the conclusion of treatment, with moist desquamation of the treated skin; and (**C**) 1 year after the completion of treatment, with hypopigmentation of the treated skin. The patient was disease free and had normal penile function 7 years later.

ment or outcome was specified. Surgery (either penectomy or excision) and radiotherapy yielded similar results, with median survivals times of 9 months and 6 months, respectively, but with good symptomatic relief for the duration of life. The authors' own experience with 4 patients suggested a possible advantage to hyperthermia in conjunction with irradiation.[19] Hormonal therapy or chemotherapy may be useful, and careful consideration of each patient's situation dictates the irradiation technique and dose and fractionation scheme to be employed, from 30 Gy in 10 fractions to 60 Gy in 30 fractions.

Bowen's disease and erythroplasia of Queyrat, which are typically treated with local excision or topical 5-fluorouracil, may respond well to irradiation. McLean and colleagues[16] reported a complete response with no local recurrences in a group of 11 patients treated with external beam radiotherapy. Depending on the extent of tumor, patients were irradiated with a direct orthovoltage or 13-MeV electron field, or with parallel opposed fields using a ^{60}Co unit. A variety of doses, from a single fraction of 15 Gy for a terminally ill patient to 60 Gy in 30 fractions, were used. A dose of 45 to 50 Gy given over 5 weeks has been recommended for these preinvasive lesions.[55]

CHEMORADIOTHERAPY

There is limited experience in combining radiation and chemotherapy to treat penile cancer. Bleomycin has been the most commonly used agent and has been demonstrated to have a synergistic effect.[56] Edsmyr and associates[57] analyzed 42 patients treated to 45 Gy in 33 days or 58 Gy in 38 days with superficial x-rays, combined with a total dose of 225 mg of bleomycin, with similar results in the two groups. A complete response was noted in 39 of 42 patients at the primary site, with surgical salvage successful in 2. Six of 8 patients who underwent inguinal lymph node dissection and were given 45 Gy by megavoltage irradiation to the groin postoperatively, achieved disease-free survival. Urethral stenosis occurred in 17% of patients, which is within the range noted in other studies in which chemotherapy was not used. Modig and coworkers[58] reported local control in 20 of 25 patients with clinically negative groin involvement who were treated with megavoltage irradiation to a dose of 56 to 58 Gy with concurrent bleomycin chemotherapy. All 5 patients who had recurrence were successfully salvaged with partial amputation.

Abratt[59] reported a case in which a patient with bilateral ulcerative inguinal adenopathy was treated in split-course fashion to 56 Gy with concurrent methotrexate and bleomycin. The patient was alive and clinically disease free 63 months after completion of treatment.

REACTIONS AND COMPLICATIONS OF EXTERNAL BEAM RADIOTHERAPY

Almost all patients given external beam irradiation to the penis experience erythema, swelling of the penis, and dry or moist desquamation (Fig. 93-2*B*). Although uncomfortable, these reactions usually resolve within weeks after completion of radiotherapy. Proper hygiene and judicious use of topical corticosteroids aid in healing and overall patient comfort.

The most common late reactions are atrophy, thinning, and telangiectasia of the penile skin; these reactions occur in most patients but are usually asymptomatic. Urethral strictures have been reported to occur in 0% to 30% of patients, with the average cumulative occurrence from these studies being 17.3%.[4,6,16,31–33,36,37,44–48,58] Most strictures occur at the meatus and respond well to urethral dilatation, which may have to be repeated. This incidence compares favorably with that seen after penectomy.[4]

Radionecrosis of the penis has been reported to occur in 0% to 20% of cases, with the average cumulative incidence being 7.7%.[4,6,16,31–33,36,37,44–48,58] Although amputation may be required on occasion, most lesions labeled as necroses present as small ulcerations that respond to conservative measures or local excision.[31,45,46] The likelihood of both urethral stenosis and necrosis is increased in those with extensively invasive tumors. For patients undergoing external beam radiotherapy, the likelihood of requiring amputation for a complication is approximately 3%.[4,6,16,31–33,36,37,44–48,58]

Although inguinal radiotherapy may cause edema of the legs, lymphedema usually occurs if irradiation is given after lymphadenectomy for extensive lymphadenopathy or lymphatic recurrence.[4,37] In most circumstances, there are sufficient deep lymphatic channels so that edema does not occur unless there is pelvic nodal involvement or high-dose (>55-Gy) pelvic radiotherapy is given.

Sexual function after radiotherapy has been reported in few studies. Most patients who have been monitored continuously and queried report satisfactory sexual function, with impotence noted occasionally (Fig. 93-3).[32,46,48]

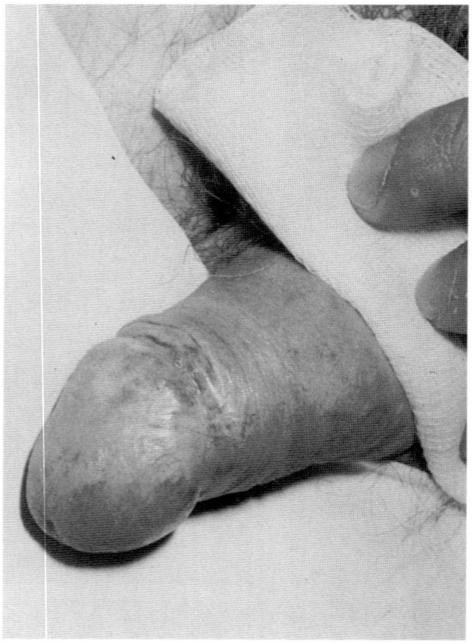

FIG. 93-3. A 53-year-old patient, who presented with a 3.0 × 2.5 cm squamous cell carcinoma of the glans and shaft, 8 years after external beam therapy, 55 Gy in 11 fractions over 5.5 weeks. Normal penile function was preserved, and the patient remained disease free until death from intercurrent disease 12 years later.

PENILE CANCER: BRACHYTHERAPY

Although external beam irradiation is more commonly employed, brachytherapy is still used frequently in Europe and has been shown to have equal merit to surgery in many studies. Two types of brachytherapy are used: (1) contact brachytherapy, in which the radioactive source is placed in contact with the tissues to be irradiated; and (2) interstitial brachytherapy, in which the radioactive sources are placed inside the tumor bed. Of the two, interstitial brachytherapy is used more often.

Under general or spinal anesthesia, a Foley catheter is inserted and is left in place for the duration of treatment. A Plexiglas template is placed on each side of the penis, and holes are drilled in a pattern to match the desired arrangement of the implant. Angiocatheters[60] or hypodermic needles,[61] which are to be used as vectors for insertion of the radioactive sources, are inserted in one or more parallel planes through the tumor bed, oriented perpendicular to the axis of the penis (Fig. 93-4). The vectors may be spaced with some variation, but usually an intersource distance of 10 to 22 mm is used.[35,60,61] One end of the vector is sealed with lead, after which the radioactive source is inserted and the other end is sealed. A small sponge placed at the penile base is used to elevate the penis and distance the testicles from the radioactive sources.[35] A variety of radioactive sources have been used throughout the years including ^{60}Co, radium-226 (^{226}Ra), tantalum-182 (^{182}Ta), and gold-190 (^{190}Au), but ^{192}Ir is now most common. Recent studies using ^{192}Ir wires have typically delivered total doses of 60 to 65 Gy to the reference isodose curve, according to the Paris System of dosimetry.[35,60–62] Low-dose rate sources deliver approximately 50 to 60 cGy per hour at the reference isodose level.

Contact brachytherapy involves the use of a surface mold containing radioactive sources, which is worn over the penis. A cylindrical plastic mold is fitted to the penis, and an outer mold is constructed to slide over the inner mold. After the patient is comfortable removing and replacing the outer mold, it

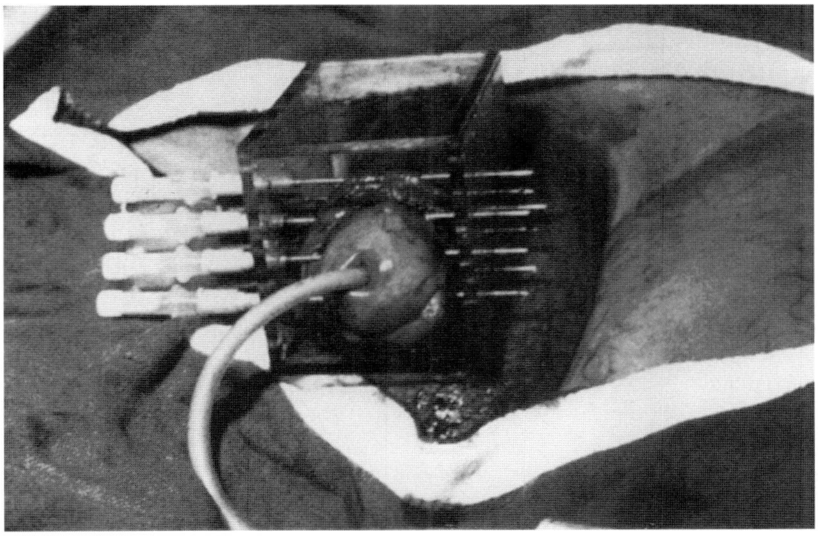

FIG. 93-4. Interstitial implant. Angiocatheters are directed through a custom Plexiglas template and later afterloaded with iridium-192 sources. (Delannes M, Malavaud B, Douchez J, Bonnet J, Daly NJ. Iridium-192 interstitial therapy for squamous cell carcinoma of the penis. Int J Radiat Oncol Biol Phys 1992; 24:479, with permission from Elsevier Science Ltd, Kidlington, UK.)

is then loaded with the radioactive sources. The applicator mold can be removed if the patient wishes to urinate or otherwise remove it, and it is kept in a lead container at the bedside. Typically, it is left in place for 10 to 12 hours per day over a 7- to 8-day period.[7,63] Meticulous recordkeeping is a must for this type of therapy. Early-stage tumors that are confined to the glans or prepuce, without invasion of the corpora,[8] are suitable for this form of treatment.[7,63] The aim is to treat the tumor with a margin 2 cm proximal to the tumor and 1 cm distal to the tip of the penis.[63] A dose of 60 Gy is given to the tumor, with the urethral dose limited to 50 Gy.[7,63] The gonads receive approximately 8 to 16 Gy.

Penile cancer has typically been staged by either the Jackson[23] or UICC[24,25] systems, neither of which is helpful to the radiation oncologist in choosing the method of treatment. Two general features[35,61,62] are considered contraindications to brachytherapy: tumor size greater than 4 cm and major invasion of the corpora cavernosa (>1 cm invasion).[35] It may be difficult to gain an adequate margin for lesions of the proximal shaft.

BRACHYTHERAPY RESULTS

A comparison of brachytherapy with either surgical or external beam radiotherapy is difficult because no randomized, prospective studies have been performed. In general, brachytherapy with surgical salvage in the event of failure has been shown to produce results equivalent to those of primary surgery, the principal advantages being sparing of the organ and the psychological sequelae that accompany penectomy, and the much shorter treatment time than that required for external beam irradiation. Results of studies using both interstitial and contact brachytherapy are listed in Table 93-2.

In Jackson's classic series,[23] patients were treated with either

TABLE 93-2. *Brachytherapy for penile cancer*

Investigators	Local control by stage			Penile preservation	5-Year survival rate (%)		
	I	I/II	II		I	I/II	II
Daly et al, 1982[62,*]	6/6		14/14	18/20		58%†	
Delannes et al, 1992[60,*]		41/45		42/51†		72%†	
El-Demiry et al, 1984[8]	18/23		1/4	19/27	89%		75%
Gueda et al, 1989[65,*]	7/9		5/5	12/14		79%	
Hope-Stone, 1975[63,*]		15/23		—		83%	
Jackson, 1966[23]		31/79‡		20/45†§	66%	55%	80%‡
Mazeron et al, 1984[61,*]	8/9		21/27	37/50†	7/8		14/23
Salaverria and Hope-Stone, 1979[7]	12/13		4/6	—	9/9		4/5
TOTAL	51/60		45/56	148/207			
TOTAL %	85%		80%	71%			
Stage I + II		183/263 (70%)					

* Numerical staging corresponds to T stage (ie, stage I = T1).

† Includes data on patients with T3 lesions.

‡ Ten patients with stage III or IV disease are included in the denominator. Data include 12 patients treated with external beam therapy and 67 treated with brachytherapy; no separation of those with advanced disease or external beam treatment was made by the author.

§ Based on those surviving 5 years only.

^{226}Ra or ^{60}Co molds, with treatment failures undergoing total or partial amputation. Overall and disease-free survival rates for patients with stage I disease who underwent brachytherapy with surgical salvage were 66% and 86%, versus 70% and 81% for the primary surgical group, respectively. Seven of 11 patients with stage II cancer and 4 of 7 with stage III disease who underwent initial brachytherapy had continuous local control, versus 8 of 12 with stage II and 3 of 7 with stage III in the primary surgical group. Overall, radiation cured the primary growth in 49% of cases without surgical salvage. Metastatic disease in the inguinal nodes developed in 14 (20%) of 69 patients treated with irradiation and 3 (8%) of 37 treated with surgery. Jackson's statistical analysis, however, did not show this difference to be of significance. Overall, 10% of the radiotherapy group and 8% of the surgical group died from metastatic disease.

Hope-Stone[63] reviewed the results for 23 patients from the London Hospital who were treated by mold therapy with ^{226}Ra needles or ^{182}Ta or ^{192}Ir wires. Primary tumor control was achieved in 15 patients with mold therapy alone, with salvage surgery bringing the 5-year survival rate to 83%. The stage of disease at presentation, however, was not specified.

Salaverria and associates[7] retrospectively compared stage I and II patients treated with either an ^{192}Ir mold or partial amputation. The mold technique, performed as described previously, achieved a crude 5-year survival rate of 12 (92%) of 13 patients, after correcting for death secondary to intercurrent disease. Of the 13 patients, 3 developed recurrences requiring partial amputation, which was successful in 2. In comparison, stage I patients treated with partial amputation had a 77% crude 5-year survival rate.

Interstitial implantation with ^{192}Ir wire, described by Pierquin and colleagues,[64] has also produced excellent results. Mazeron and associates[61] reported on 50 patients with UICC-staged T1 to T3 lesions who received a mean dose of 65 Gy. Conservation of the penis was achieved in 39 (78%). Control of the primary lesion was achieved in 8 of 9 T1 lesions, 21 of 27 T2 lesions and 10 of 14 T3 lesions with brachytherapy alone. Nine of the 11 brachytherapy failures underwent salvage surgery, which was successful in 4, producing final local control rates of 100% (9/9), 96% (26/27), and 79% (11/14) for T1, T2, and T3 lesions, respectively. Actuarial survival rates were 70% at 3 years, 63% at 5 years, and 55% at 8 years, with penile preservation in 97%, 87%, and 75% of those patients who were without disease at the respective time intervals.

Daly and coworkers[62] achieved similar results in a group of 22 patients who received a median dose of 60 Gy from interstitial ^{192}Ir. Local control was achieved in 6 of 6 patients with T1 lesions, 14 of 14 with T2 lesions, and 1 of 2 T3 lesions treated with interstitial therapy alone. In the 1 patient with a T3 lesion in whom the tumor recurred, partial amputation proved to be definitive. There were no metastases seen in the 18 patients who originally had clinically negative nodes. Actuarial survival rates were 81% at 3 years and 58% at 5 years.

Delannes and colleagues[60] analyzed 51 patients who were treated to a mean of 60 Gy with ^{192}Ir, of whom 43 had no clinically positive lymph nodes at presentation. Tumor control at the primary site was achieved in 36 (92%) of 39 patients with T1 or T2, N0 disease and in 2 of 6 with T3 disease, with 6 of the 7 failures successfully salvaged by partial or total penectomy. Two patients who were clinically N0 at presentation had recurrence in the lymph nodes, which ultimately led to their deaths. The actuarial survival rates were 72% at 5 years and 62% at 10 years; correction for death from intercurrent disease produced a 5- and 10-year survival rate of 85%.

Others have shown similar excellent results. Gueda and associates[65] documented local control in 14 of 16 patients with T1 to T3 tumors treated with ^{192}Ir wires. Penile amputation produced definitive local control in the 2 who had recurrence of their cancer. Suchaud and coworkers[66] reported local control in 42 of 53 patients treated with interstitial radiotherapy, with successful surgical salvage in 10 of 11 who had recurrences.

REACTIONS AND COMPLICATIONS OF BRACHYTHERAPY

Brachytherapy produces erythema and edema of the subcutaneous tissues and urethral mucositis in almost all patients. The reactions, which are uncomfortable, appear within a few days of the completion of treatment and usually subside within several weeks.[18]

The most frequently reported late complications are minor and include telangiectasia, dyschromia, and superficial sclerosis. Urethral stenosis is reported variably in 0% to 45% of cases, with an average occurrence rate of approximately 16%.[7,8,60–62,67] Stenosis usually occurs at the meatus and responds well to repeated simple instrumental dilatation; plastic reconstruction may be required in more severe cases. This complication is more frequent in T3 tumors that invade the urethra.[35]

The most severe complication is necrosis, which typically occurs within 18 months after completion of treatment, is associated with trauma or sexual intercourse, and can be difficult to differentiate from recurrence. Necrosis of varying degrees has been reported in 0% to 23% of cases treated with brachytherapy, with an average occurrence of approximately 6%.[7,8,60–62,65,67] Multivariate analysis showed the initial stage of disease, the presence of a tumor more than 40 mm in size, the volume of the implant, and the number of implant planes to be significantly related to the probability of necrosis.[60] Overall, approximately 6% of patients treated with brachytherapy have required amputation for complications.[7,23,60–62,65]

TREATMENT OF REGIONAL LYMPHATICS

Two sets of lymphatics drain the penis. The lymphatic drainage of the prepuce and penile skin converge into larger trunks on the dorsum of the penis, coursing to the base, and terminating bilaterally in the superficial inguinal nodes. Those of the glans and corpora run along the dorsal vein of the penis, eventually terminating bilaterally in the superficial and deep inguinal nodes.[68]

Several factors are important to consider in evaluating patients with penile cancer with regard to the regional lymph nodes and their treatment. First, metastases to the regional lymphatics occur by embolization rather than by a stepwise permeation, usually late in the disease. The exception to this may be in those with poorly differentiated tumors.[5] Second, although 30% to 60% of patients may present with palpable lymph nodes in the groin,[5,6,21,36,69] the false-positive rate as determined by pathologic review of lymphadenectomy specimens is approximately 50%.[5,6,21] This high rate of false-positive nodes is secondary to the high rate of lymphadenitis incident to the local infections that often occur with penile tumors. Considering these factors, a course of antibiotics and 4 to 6 weeks of observation are often recommended after treatment of the primary lesion. Third, approximately 10% to 20% of those with clinically negative groin involvement harbor metastatic disease.[6,16,46,70]

Experience with radiotherapy to control metastatic adenopathy is limited in penile cancer. It is known, however, that squamous cell carcinoma metastatic to lymph nodes, both gross and microscopic, is controllable with radiotherapy. A recent compilation of data[37] compared survival rates in patients who underwent lymphadenectomy or radiotherapy for either prophylactic or therapeutic treatment of the groin. Overall survival rates for all patients, including those with clinically positive and clinically negative groin involvement, were 64% for surgery and 44% for radiotherapy at 3 years, and 50% and 44% at 5 years, respectively. For patients with clinical involvement of the groin, the 3-year survival rates for the surgery and radiotherapy groups were 52% and 27%, with the 5-year rate again roughly equivalent at 34% and 30%, respectively. A strict comparison of these results is difficult, however, for three reasons. First, some surgical studies have included only histologically proven cases in the survival data. Second, some older radiotherapy studies,[4,6,37,44,46] which included large numbers of patients, used low doses of 30 to 40 Gy. Third, patient selection factors are often not specified.

Elective irradiation of clinically uninvolved groins, known to be of benefit for squamous cell cancers at other sites (eg, head and neck cancers,[71] cervical cancers[72]), is of uncertain benefit for penile cancer. Both Englestad[44] and Ekstrom and Edsmyr[6] showed a 5-year survival rate of approximately 90% in groups of patients with stage I disease who received prophylactic irradiation. Given the relatively low rate of metastasis after treatment of the primary lesion, however, prophylactic radiotherapy should not generally be used for all node-negative patients. Patients who present with extensive or poorly differentiated tumors, which have been shown to have an increased rate of metastasis, may benefit from elective groin irradiation. In that instance, a dose of 50 Gy over 5 weeks is recommended.

Treatment of involved regional lymph nodes has resulted in long-term control and cure in a number of patients. In the Narayana[73] series, 2 of 16 patients with histologically proven metastases were cured, and 3 died of unknown causes. Staubitz and colleagues[9] documented survival at 5 years in 5 of 19 patients given irradiation to the groin. El-Demiry and associates[8] documented 5-year survival in 2 of 8 patients after groin irradiation. No description of the radiotherapy technique or dose was specified in these studies. Krieg and Luk[32] controlled disease in 2 of 3 patients given doses of 50.9 to 70 Gy. Others[55,58] have reported long-term survival in patients with advanced adenopathy who were treated with radiotherapy alone or in combination with chemotherapy.

If irradiation of the regional lymph nodes is undertaken, both the inguinal and pelvic nodes should be treated. Megavoltage x-rays, using parallel opposed, anterior and posterior, shaped fields, should be used. Because of the anterior position of the inguinal nodes, weighted photon beams, with or without bolus over the inguinal areas, may be required. Alternatively, an anterior electron beam can be used for a portion of the treatment to bring the inguinal dose to a therapeutic level. In patients with unresectable or recurrent lymph node disease, a dose of 65 to 70 Gy is recommended.[55]

SUMMARY

Penile cancer carries a severe psychological impact. Careful analysis of the available literature suggests that tumor control and survival are similar for surgery and for radiotherapy. It is, therefore, surprising that the surgical approach is favored today when cure with preservation of form and function has become a basic tenet in cancer therapy. This goal is more feasible with radiotherapy, which must be accomplished with a meticulous technique at a full cancericidal dose; bilateral groin and pelvic irradiation can be performed, if indicated, and the roles of surgery and radiotherapy must be carefully defined. Altered fractionation schemes and three-dimensional treatment planning may improve the therapeutic ratio. Combined-modality therapy using hyperthermia and chemotherapy remain to be explored. The development of effective systemic treatment (chemotherapy) is mandatory for the control of systemic metastases. Careful staging with the use of modern radiographic techniques is essential for comparison of results. Finally, the psychosocial aspects of penile cancer must be studied so that these men can be better served.

REFERENCES

1. Burgers JK, Badalament RA, Drago JR. Penile cancer: clinical presentation, diagnosis and staging. Urol Clin North Am 1992;19:247.
2. Persky L. Epidemiology of cancer of the penis: recent results. Cancer Res 1977;60:97.
3. Riveros M, Lebron R. Geographical pathology of cancer of the penis. Cancer 1963;16:798.
4. Murrell DS, Williams JL. Radiotherapy in the treatment of carcinoma of the penis. Br J Urol 1965;37:211.
5. Marcial VA, Figueroa-Colon J, Marcial-Rojas RA, et al. Carcinoma of the penis. Radiology 1962;79:211.
6. Ekstrom T, Edsmyr FF. Cancer of the penis: a clinical study of 229 cases. Acta Chir Scand 1958;115:25.
7. Salaverria JC, Hope-Stone HF, Paris AMI, Blandy JP. Conservative treatment of carcinoma of the penis. Br J Urol 1979;51:32.
8. El-Demiry MIM, Oliver RTD, Hope-Stone HF, Blandy JP. Reappraisal of the role of radiotherapy and surgery in the management of carcinoma of the penis. Br J Urol 1984;56:724.
9. Staubitz WJ, Melbourne HL, Oberkircher OJ. Carcinoma of the penis. Cancer 1955;8:371.
10. Hardner GJ, Bhanalaph T, Murphy GP, Albert DJ, Moore RH. Carcinoma of the penis: an analysis of therapy in 100 consecutive cases. J Urol 1972;108:428.
11. Sulaiman MZC, Polacarz SV, Partington PE. Basal cell carcinoma of penis: case report. Genitourin Med 1989;64:128.
12. Schellhammer PF, Jordan GH, Schlossberg SM. Tumors of the penis. In: Walsh PC, Retik AB, Stamey TA, Vaughan ED Jr, eds. Campbell's urology. Philadelphia, WB Saunders, 1992:1264.
13. Kherzi AA, Dounis A, Roberts JBM. Primary malignant melanoma of the penis: two cases and review of the literature. Br J Urol 1979;51:147.
14. Dehner LP, Smith BH. Soft tissue tumors of the penis: a clinicopathologic study of 46 cases. Cancer 1970;25:1431.
15. Yu GSM, Nseyo UO, Carson JW. Primary penile lymphoma in a patient with Peyronie's disease. J Urol 1989;142:1076.
16. McLean M, Ahmed MA, Warde P, Bissett R, Panzarella T, Gospardowicz M. The results of primary radiation in the management of squamous cell carcinoma of the penis. Int J Radiat Oncol Biol Phys 1993;25:623.
17. Kelly CD, Arthur K, Rogoff E, Grabstald H. Radiation therapy of penile cancer. Urology 1974;4:571.

18. Epstein E. Association of Bowen's disease with visceral cancer. Arch Dermatol 1960;82:349.
19. Ben-Yosef R, Kapp DS. Cancer metastatic to the penis: treatment with hyperthermia and radiation therapy and review of the literature. J Urol 1992;148:67.
20. Powell BL, Craig JB, Muss HB. Secondary malignancies of the penis and epididymis: a case report and review of the literature. J Clin Oncol 1985;3:110.
21. Beggs JH, Spratt JS. Epidermoid carcinoma of the penis. J Urol 1986; 135:283.
22. Fraley EE, Zhang G, Sazama R, et al. Cancer of the penis: prognosis and treatment plans. Cancer 1985;55:1618.
23. Jackson SM. The treatment of carcinoma of the penis. Br J Surg 1966; 53:33.
24. TNM classification of tumors, 4th ed. Geneva, International Union Against Cancer (UICC), 1979.
25. TNM classification of tumors, 5th ed. Geneva, International Union Against Cancer (UICC), 1987.
26. Horenblas S, van Tinteren H, Delemarre JFM, Boon TA, Moonen LMF, Lustig V. Squamous cell carcinoma of the penis: II. Treatment of the primary tumor. J Urol 1992;147:1533.
27. Sufrin G, Huben R. Benign and malignant lesion of the penis. In: Gillenwater JY, Grayhack JT, Howards SS, Duckett JW, eds. Adult and pediatric urology, 2nd ed. St Louis, CV Mosby, 1991:1664.
28. Naegeli FD. Epithelioma of the penis. J Urol 1941;45:202.
29. Hanash KA, Furlow WL, Utz DC, Harrison EG. Carcinoma of the penis: a clinicopathologic study. J Urol 1970;104:291.
30. Mount BM. Psychological impact of urologic cancer. Cancer 1980;45: 1980.
31. Sagerman RH, Yu WS, Chung CT, Puranik A. External beam irradiation of carcinoma of the penis. Radiology 1984;152:183.
32. Krieg RM, Luk KH. Carcinoma of the penis: review of the cases treated by surgery and radiation therapy, 1960–1977. Urology 1981;16:145.
33. Kaushal V, Sharma SC. Carcinoma of the penis: a 12 year review. Acta Oncol 1987;26:413.
34. Lederman M. Radium treatment of cancer of the penis. Br J Radiol 1940;156:393.
35. Gerbaulet A, Lambin P. Radiation therapy of cancer of the penis: indications, advantages and pitfalls. Urol Clin North Am 1992;19:325.
36. Duncan W, Jackson SM. The treatment of early cancer of the penis with megavoltage x-rays. Clin Radiol 1972;23:246.
37. Newaishy GA, Deeley TJ. Radiotherapy in the treatment of carcinoma of the penis. Br J Radiol 1968;41:519.
38. Vaeth JM, Green JP, Lowy RO. Radiation therapy of carcinoma of the penis. AJR Am J Roentgenol 1970;108:130.
39. Franzen L, Henricksson R, Karlsson NO, Lofroth PO, Nilsson MA. A technical device for irradiation of the penis. Acta Oncol 1987;26:77.
40. Dean AL. Epithelioma of the penis. J Urol 1935;33:252.
41. Lederman M. Radiotherapy of cancer of the penis. Br J Urol 1953;25: 224.
42. Knudsen OS, Brennhovd IO. Radiotherapy in the treatment of carcinoma of the penis. Acta Chir Scand 1967;133:69.
43. Zausner J. Penile carcinoma. Radiology 1940;50:786.
44. Engelstad RB. Treatment of cancer of the penis at the Norwegian Radium Hospital. AJR Am J Roentgenol 1948;60:801.
45. Haile K, Delclos L. The place of radiation therapy in the treatment of carcinoma of the distal penis. Cancer 1980;45:1980.
46. Almgard LE, Edsmyr F. Radiotherapy in treatment of patients with carcinoma of the penis. Scand J Urol Nephrol 1973;7:1.
47. Grabstald H, Kelly CD. Radiation therapy of penile cancer: six to ten year followup. Urology 1980;15:575.
48. Pointon RCS. External beam therapy. Proc R Soc Med 1975;68:779.
49. Kearsly JH, Roberts SJ, Kynastron B. Curative radiotherapy for stage IV carcinoma of the penis. Med J Aust 1986;145:474.
50. Hashimoto H, Saga Y, Watabe Y, Sasaki M, Tokunaka S, Yachiku S. Case report: secondary penile carcinoma. Urol Int 1989;44:56.
51. Haddad FS. Penile metastases secondary to bladder cancer: review of the literature. Urol Int 1984;39:125.
52. Haddad FS, Manne RK. Prostatic tumors with penile secondaries: review of the literature with a case report. Urol Int 1986;41:465.
53. Haddad FS, Manne RK. Involvement of the penis by rectocolic adenocarcinoma. Dis Colon Rectum 1987;30:123.
54. Robey EL, Schellhammer PF. Four cases of metastases to the penis and a review of the literature. J Urol 1984;132:992.
55. Perez CA, Pilepich MV. Penis and male urethra. In: Perez CA, Brady LW, eds. Principles and practices of radiation oncology. Philadelphia, JB Lippincott, 1992:1135.
56. Shrieve DC, Harris JW. Effects of bleomycin and irradiation on euoxic and hypoxic cells. Int J Radiat Oncol Biol Phys 1979;5:1495.
57. Edsmyr F, Andersson L, Esposti PL. Combined bleomycin and radiation therapy in carcinoma of the penis. Cancer 1985;56:1257.
58. Modig H, Duchek M, Sjodin JG. Carcinoma of the penis: treatment by surgery or combined bleomycin and radiation therapy. Acta Oncol 1993;32:653.
59. Abratt RP. The treatment of bilateral ulcerated lymph node metastases from carcinoma of the penis: a case report. Cancer 1984;54:1720.
60. Delannes M, Malavaud B, Douchez J, Bonnet J, Daly NJ. Iridium-192 interstitial therapy for squamous cell carcinoma of the penis. Int J Radiat Oncol Biol Phys 1992;24:479.
61. Mazeron JJ, Langlois D, Lobo PA, et al. Interstitial radiation therapy for carcinoma of the penis using iridium-192 wires: the Henri Hondor experience (1970–1979). Int J Radiat Oncol Biol Phys 1984;10:1891.
62. Daly NJ, Douchez J, Combes PF. Treatment of carcinoma of the penis by iridium 192 wire implant. Int J Radiat Oncol Biol Phys 1982;8: 1239.
63. Hope-Stone H. Carcinoma of the penis. Proc R Soc Med 1975;68:777.
64. Pierquin B, Bunescu U, Jomain J. L'endocurietherapie des cancers de la verge traitee par l'iridium 192: technique et resultats. J Urol (Paris) 1970;76:1.
65. Gueda F, Craven-Bartle J, Carles J. Interstitial radiotherapy using iridium 192 wires for carcinoma of the penis. Bull Cancer Radiother 1991;78:141.
66. Suchaud JP, Kantor G, Richaud P. Curietherapie des cancers de la verge: analyse d'une serie 53 cas. J Urol 1989;95:27.
67. Cox R. Radiotherapy in malignant disease of the testicle and penis. J Urol 1954;260:350.
68. Crawford ED, Daneshgari F. Management of regional lymphatic drainage in carcinoma of the penis. Urol Clin North Am 1992;19:305.
69. Cabanas RM. An approach for the treatment of penile carcinoma. Cancer 1977;39:456.
70. Catalona WJ. Modified inguinal lymphadenectomy for carcinoma of the penis with preservation of the saphenous veins: technique and preliminary results. J Urol 1988;140:306.
71. Sagerman RH, Chung CT, King Ga, Dalal P, Yu WS. High dose preoperative irradiation of the lower neck and supraclavicular fossae. AJR Am J Roentgenol 1979;132:357.
72. Rutledge FN, Fletcher GH. Transperitoneal pelvic lymphadenectomy following supervoltage irradiation for squamous cell carcinoma of the cervix. Am J Obstet Gynecol 1958;76:321.
73. Narayana AS, Olney LE, Loening SA: Carcinoma of the penis: analysis of 219 patients. Cancer 1982;49:2185.

Principles and Practice of Genitourinary Oncology, edited by Derek Raghavan, Howard I. Scher, Steven A. Leibel, and Paul H. Lange. Lippincott-Raven Publishers, Philadelphia, © 1997.

CHAPTER 94

Cancer of the Penis

Regional Therapy and Lymphadenectomy

W. Scott McDougal

Cancer of the penis is one of the few diseases that, when metastatic to regional lymph nodes, can be cured by regional lymphadenectomy. The most efficacious therapy for both localized and regional metastatic disease is surgical excision, because chemotherapy and irradiation are only modestly effective. Primary malignancies of the penis include squamous cell carcinoma, basal cell carcinoma, malignant melanoma, Paget's disease, and sarcoma. For the purposes of this chapter, only the treatment of squamous cell carcinoma of the penis is discussed. This histologic type constitutes more than 95% of primary lesions and can be classified as either poor, moderately, or well differentiated. The differentiation is important for prognosis as well as for determining appropriate treatment options; on occasion, histologic grade of the primary lesion is the sole basis on which regional therapy is determined.

Survival and the likelihood of regional spread are correlated with the degree of differentiation of the primary tumor and the depth of its invasion. The prognostic significance of tumor classification (Figs. 94-1 and 94-2) can be seen by the reported progression rate to regional lymphatic involvement: 82% if primary lesions are poorly differentiated, 46% if moderately differentiated, and 24% if well differentiated.[1] In one reported series, all patients who had poorly differentiated primary tumors developed regional nodal metastases.[2] Moreover, the local recurrence rate was much higher if primary lesions were poorly differentiated.[1,3] Patients with poorly differentiated primary tumors have a 5-year survival rate of 47%, but for those with well differentiated lesions, the rate is 79%.[4] The depth of invasion is also important in determining the likelihood of regional and distant spread. Lesions that do not invade the substance of the corpus spongiosum or the corpus cavernosum have a 5% to 11% rate of progression to regional disease.[5,6] These superficial penile lesions have a 92% survival rate at 3 years.[5] In our series, 19 patients with superficial disease were studied; none developed metastases over a 5-year period.[7] In Fraley's series,[2] all those with superficial disease showed no progression of disease and none underwent regional lymphadenectomy. On the other hand, if the tumor involves the corpora, 61% to 75% of patients have regional lymphatic involvement.[1,7]

Whatever staging system is to be used, differentiation of the primary lesion and its depth of invasion must be an integral part. The TNM system does not address both of these issues simultaneously, nor does it provide a useful classification for determining the necessity of regional therapy. Therefore, a modification of the Jackson system has been made to reflect current therapy. With this modification, appropriate determination of stage allows a reasonably certain prediction of the likelihood of positive regional lymph node involvement. With this determination, a more rational approach to local or regional therapy may be made. The modified staging system is outlined in Table 94-1. Stage 1 consists of lesions that are superficial, in which there is no subcutaneous tissue invasion, no invasion of the corpora cavernosa, corpus spongiosum, or scrotum, and no palpable regional lymphadenopathy. Histologically, the tumor is well differentiated. The survival rate in this stage with local therapy alone is 95% to 100%. Stage 2A disease includes all of those tumors that are locally invasive, with no invasion of the corpora spongiosum or corpora cavernosum. There is no regional lymph node involvement, and the tumor is well or moderately differentiated. With local therapy alone, the 5-year survival rate in this group is 95%. Stage 2B disease includes all tumors that are invasive into the corpora spongiosum or corpora cavernosa and all poorly differentiated tumors irrespective of the depth of invasion. There is no palpable regional lymphadenopathy. The 5-year survival rate in this group of patients ranges from 40% to 90%, depending on the initial form of therapy with respect to the regional lymph nodes. Stage 3 disease includes all patients with palpably positive regional lymph nodes that are surgically resectable. The 5-year survival rate ranges from 30 to 70%. Stage 4 disease includes any of the following: inoperable lymph nodes, positive pelvic lymph nodes and distant metastases. The 5-year survival rate is less than 5%. Table 94-2 depicts the disease-free survival rates for 52 patients treated at our facility. Notice that for stages 2B and 3 disease, an immediate lymphadenectomy was performed.

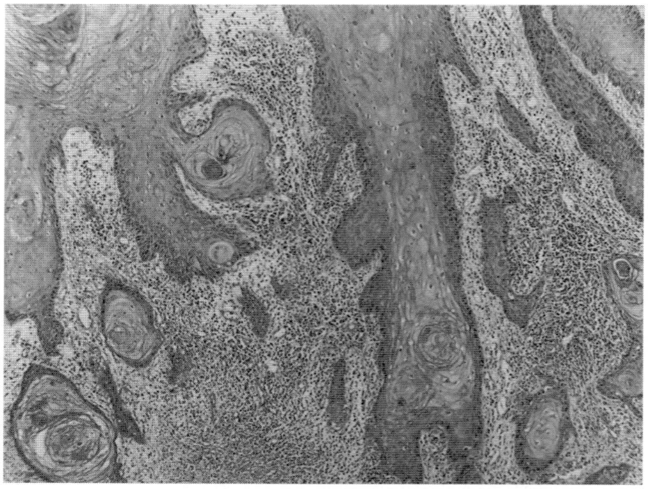

FIG. 94-1. Well differentiated squamous cell carcinoma of the penis. Nests of focally keratinizing squamous epithelium penetrate the submucosa in an irregular fashion. (H&E stain; original magnification ×150.)

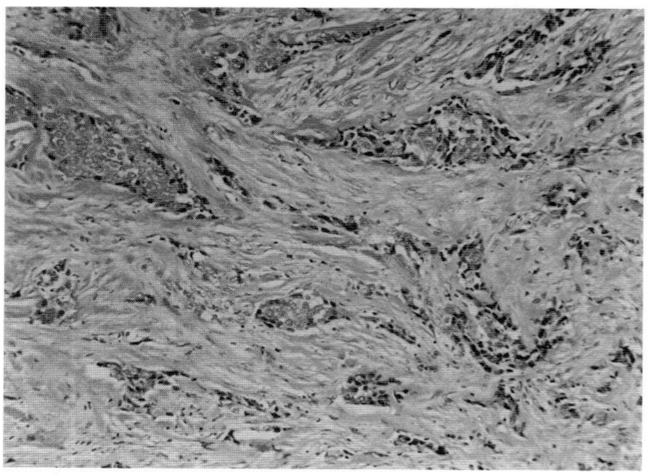

FIG. 94-2. Poorly differentiated squamous cell carcinoma of the penis. Nests and clusters of poorly differentiated squamous cells infiltrate in a desmoplastic stroma. (H&E stain; original magnification ×150.)

TABLE 94-1. *Proposed staging system for penile carcinoma*

Stage 1	Superficial; does not extend into the subcutaneous tissue; well differentiated.
Stage 2A	Locally invasive without involvement of the corpora spongiosum or corpora cavernosum; well or moderately differentiated.
Stage 2B	Invasion to the corpus spongiosum or corpus cavernosum, or poorly differentiated.
Stage 3	Palpable inguinal nodes that persist after 6 weeks of antibiotic therapy.
Stage 4	Inoperable groin nodes, iliac node involvement, distant metastases.

TABLE 94-2. *Survival according to modified staging system*

Stage	Disease-free survival rate*
1	100%
2A	100%
2B†	90%
3†	70%

* Includes patients who lived 5 years without disease or who died of other causes in less than 5 years and at the time of death had no evidence of metastatic disease.

† All patients had a regional lymphadenectomy shortly after treatment of the primary lesion.

TREATMENT: REGIONAL LYMPHADENECTOMY

Very few would argue for a regional lymphadenectomy in patients with stage 1 disease. Local excision alone carries with it a 95% to 100% cure rate. Conversely, few would argue with the necessity for a regional lymphadenectomy in stage 3 disease. The 5-year survival rate without lymphadenectomy in this group approaches zero,[7] and with lymphadenectomy it ranges between 30% and 70%.[4] In patients with an invasive primary lesion who have palpably negative regional lymph nodes (stage 2), however, there is controversy as to whether to proceed with a regional lymphadenectomy immediately or to carefully monitor the patient and, if nodes appear, to perform a delayed lymphadenectomy at that time. In those patients in whom a delayed lymphadenectomy is performed, 8% to 42% survive 5 years.[3,7] If a regional lymphadenectomy is done in a patient with nonpalpable nodes and microscopic metastases are found pathologically, 84% survive 5 years.[7] The cure rate therefore is much better if regional disease is removed when microscopic rather than palpable.[7]

If those patients without palpable adenopathy who have microscopic nodal metastases could be identified, they would certainly benefit from a lymphadenectomy. A false-positive prediction, however, would lead to performance of a lymphadenectomy with no survival benefit at a cost of increased morbidity. Some have suggested that a biopsy of regional nodes could provide a basis for making this decision. However, the experience of many is that lymph node biopsy carries a false-negative rate of at least 50%,[7,8] and some have reported progression to positive nodes shortly after a negative node biopsy.[9] Cabanas proposed that a sentinel node biopsy would be helpful, but the lack of full follow-up on some of the patients in that study[10] and the experience of many others suggest that this type of biopsy has a high rate of false-negative results as well.[11] Therefore, the use of regional biopsy to predict the presence of regional nodal disease does not appear appropriate.

In the clinical staging system proposed here, patients with stage 2A disease have a very low incidence of regional nodal involvement, but 38% to 66% of patients with stage 2B disease have microscopic regional lymph node involvement.[5,7] It has previously been stated that only 20% of patients with nonpalpable groin adenopathy have micrometastases; however, those series lumped together stages 1, 2A, and 2B. The chance of nodal metastasis is exceedingly small in stages 1 and 2A, and the inclusion of these cases with 2B cases skews the numbers downward.[7] It appears advisable to perform a regional lymphadenectomy in patients with stage 2B disease, because the likelihood of pathologically positive nodes is high and, in my opinion, offsets the risk of morbidity to those who would undergo the procedure for no benefit (ie, those with negative nodes). Moreover, complications of groin dissection are much less in those receiving a groin dissection for microscopic disease compared with delayed dissection for nodes that are palpably positive at a later date.[2] Another argument for proceeding with regional lymphadenectomy in those with a high likelihood of microscopic metastases, rather than waiting to see whether palpable nodes develop, is the experience reported by Uehling, in which the most common cause of treatment failure was progression to inoperable nodes in 22% of the patients monitored.[12] If, on lymphadenectomy, the lymph nodes are found to be negative, there is an 87% to 100% survival rate.[3,4] In one series, all patients with only one positive node survived 5 years.[4] Fifty percent to 84% of patients with one to two positive nodes survive 5 years.[7,13] If the regional adenopathy extends to the iliac nodes, survival is limited, with only an occasional survival past 5 years having been reported.[14] Iliac nodes are rarely positive unless inguinal nodes are positive.[4,15]

Seventy percent of patients with stage 3 disease, in whom nodes are palpably positive, are found to have pathologically positive nodes.[3] The morbidity of lymphadenectomy is well justified in patients with palpable adenopathy that persists during 6 weeks of antibiotic therapy after excision of the primary lesion. Because there is also such a high probability of regional spread in 2B disease, it is my practice to perform a bilateral regional lymphadenectomy in all patients with stages 2B or stage 3 disease. If the nodes are positive, an iliac lymphadenectomy is also performed on the same side, realizing that, if these nodes are also positive, the possibility of survival for as long as 5 years is very poor.

EXTENT OF REGIONAL LYMPHADENECTOMY

The prepuce and skin drain to the superficial inguinal nodes, whereas the corpora and glans drain to the deep inguinal and iliac nodes. Because there is considerable crossover of lymphatics, if one groin is involved, the opposite groin is also involved 60% of the time.[15] Moreover, superficial inguinal nodes may be bypassed with direct spread to the deep inguinal nodes if the corpora is involved. Finally, iliac nodes are unlikely to be involved unless the groin nodes are also involved.[4,15] Recurrences after a groin dissection portend a very poor prognosis and are very difficult to manage.[4] With these facts in mind, it has been my practice in performing a regional lymphadenectomy to perform the procedure bilaterally and to include both superficial and deep nodes. This reduces the risk of local groin recurrence in comparison with a superficial dissection. Some have suggested that only a superficial node dissection need be performed initially, and that deep dissection should be performed only if the superficial nodes are positive. The thought is that this approach reduces postoperative morbidity. However, some of the lymphatics from the penis drain directly to the deep nodes, bypassing the superficial group; failure to remove the deep fascia carries with it the risk of leaving superficial nodes behind. For these reasons, I prefer to perform both a superficial and a deep dissection, preserving the saphenous vein if possible. If the groin nodes are positive, then an iliac node dissection is performed en bloc on that side.

TECHNIQUE OF LYMPHADENECTOMY

The classic ilioinguinal lymphadenectomy is a removal of the superficial and deep inguinal nodes in continuity with the iliac nodes. (The anatomy of the inguinal region is detailed in Chapter 87.) Unless the groin nodes are positive, the iliac nodes are not routinely removed. Preoperatively, the patient is hydrated, a mechanical bowel cleansing is performed, and the lower extremities are wrapped with pneumatic compression stockings. I prefer to perform the dissection in both groins simultaneously through an oblique-transverse incision 4 cm below and parallel to the inguinal ligament. Others prefer a vertical incision that follows the contour of the skin crease for several centimeters when it is crossed. If the nodes are attached to the dermis, an ellipse of overlying skin is removed. Skin flaps are developed deep to the superficial fascia, care being taken not to make them too thin. The flaps extend to 2 cm above the inguinal ligament cephalad, the junction of the adductor longus and sartorius caudad, the lateral border of the sartorius laterally, and the medial border of the adductor longus medially. The medial dissection extends to the pubic tubercle cephalad.

The dissection begins at the inguinal ligament. After the tissue is freed from the ligament for 2 cm above its reflection, lateral and medial dissection is carried to a line perpendicular to the anterior superior iliac spine laterally and the pubic tubercle medially. The saphenous vein can be preserved by careful dissection, although its five branches at the fossa ovalis must be sacrificed. My preference is to define the lateral, medial, and inferior limits of dissection at this point by exposing the lateral border of the sartorius, the medial aspect of the adductor longus, and the junction of the two inferiorly. Care must be taken not to displace either of the above muscles during the definition of their coaptation, for this may result in carrying the dissection too far caudad. After the limits of the groin dissection have been defined, attention is turned to exposure of the femoral vessels. The femoral vein is best identified by tracing the saphenous vein through the fossa ovalis to the femoral vein. The deep fascia overlying the femoral vessels may be dense and must be incised to expose the femoral artery and vein. Several small, superficial arteries may be encountered and should be ligated close to their origin from the femoral artery. These include the superficial epigastric artery, the superficial circumflex iliac artery, and the superficial external pudendal artery. All originate 1 to 3 cm below the inguinal ligament. Removal of the fascia overlying the vessels ensures that no superficial nodes are left behind. Removal of the tissue medial to the femoral vein with the fascia includes both superficial and deep nodes in the specimen. Both vein and artery should be cleared to their adventia. The nodal package is dissected and left attached to the pedicle entering the empty space medial to the femoral vein. All vessels are tied with 4-0 silk and ligated. Subsequently, if an iliac node dissection is indicated, the nodes are dissected through a lower midline extraperitoneal incision from the hypogastric artery cephalad to the inguinal specimen caudad, from the obturator nerve dorsally to the external iliac artery ventrally, and from the bladder wall medially to the psoas muscle and genitofemoral nerve anteriorly and laterally. The tissue specimen may then

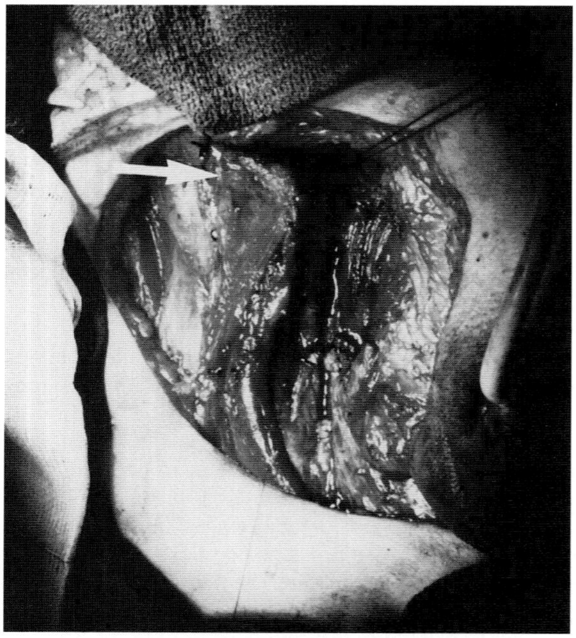

FIG. 94-3. The sartorius (*arrow*) has been mobilized off the anterior superior iliac spine and is sutured to the inguinal ligament to cover the vessels.

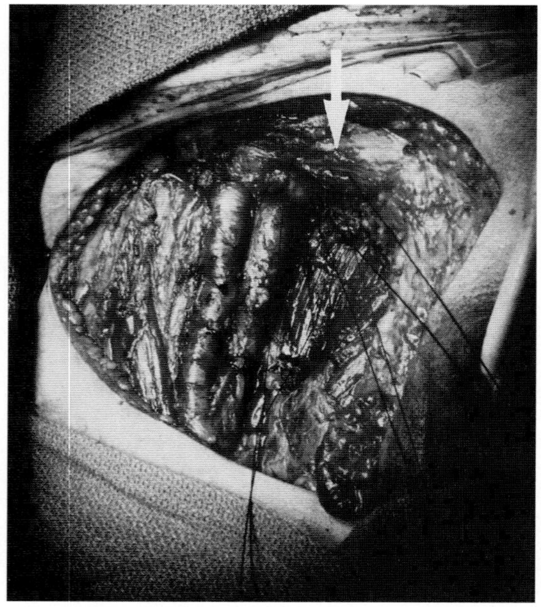

FIG. 94-4. Large amounts of soft tissue may have to be sacrificed. Notice that the lateral boarder of the adductor longus, a portion of the pectineus, and a segment of the inguinal ligament (*arrow*) have been removed.

be removed en bloc by carrying the dissection through the empty space.

The sartorius is transposed over the femoral vessels and sutured to the inguinal ligament (Fig. 94-3). The sartorius can be detached off the anterior superior iliac spine by sharp dissection with a Mayo scissors. It is rotated medially and is sutured to the fascia of the inguinal ligament. The wounds are drained with a Jackson-Pratt closed drain, and dressings are applied. The legs are kept in thigh-length stockings and thigh-length pneumatic compression boots, and the patient is kept at bed rest for 4 to 5 days. I do not use prophylactic heparinization either in the preoperative or postoperative period. If a wound seroma develops, it is aspirated periodically. The patient is ambulated on the fifth postoperative day, and elastic stockings are then worn for the ensuing 3 months.

Special Circumstances Involving Groin Dissection

Occasionally, patients who have recurrent disease in a previously dissected groin or local tissue necrosis because of extensive tumor involvement or irradiation require a palliative groin dissection. On rare occasions, particularly if a recurrence occurs in a previously dissected groin, the procedure may be curative. Under these circumstances, a more extensive dissection is required, in which large portions of skin, muscle, fascia, nerve, or vessels are removed. Groin and abdominal wall skin with the inguinal fascia may be sacrificed if need be. Similarly, the adductor longus and sartorius and portions of the iliacus, pectineus, and rectus femoris may require removal (Fig. 94-4). The femoral artery, if involved, can be removed and replaced with a prosthetic graft. The graft is anastomosed to the external iliac artery and communicates with the superficial femoral artery and the profundus femoris artery. Many of these patients have significant arteriosclerotic peripheral vascular disease, particularly in the superficial femoral artery, making anastomosis distal to both vessels desirable. The femoral nerve may also be sacrificed if necessary. If it is taken above the inguinal ligament, the patient will loose extension of the leg at the knee and have some difficulty with gait, but usually he will be able to ambulate without the need for a brace. Also, a sensory loss of the medial thigh and leg and the dorsum of the foot occurs. If the femoral nerve requires sacrifice below the inguinal ligament, a lesser degree of morbidity occurs. Occasionally, a neuroma develops at the cut end of the nerve. This can be exceedingly painful and is most troublesome to treat.

Every effort should be made to preserve the femoral vein, because prosthetic replacement is usually not successful and thrombosis is the inevitable sequela. This results in very troublesome leg swelling and can cause significant morbidity.

These dissections are often so extensive that it is not possible to achieve wound closure with the local tissues. Appropriate transfer of skin, fascia, and muscle can be accomplished with the vertical rectus abdominis myocutaneous flap. It is usually preferable to obtain the flap from the contralateral side--particularly if the dissection has extended above the inguinal ligament. The flap is based on the inferior epigastric vessels, and mobilizing it from the contralateral side assures its vascular integrity. The flap is technically easy to harvest and provides excellent muscle, fascia, and skin coverage. If only soft tissue is required, only the muscle need be transferred. Alternatively, a myocutaneous fascia lata flap may be used. If only skin and subcutaneous tissue coverage is needed, I have found it useful to elevate the entire abdominal wall, including skin and subcutaneous tis-

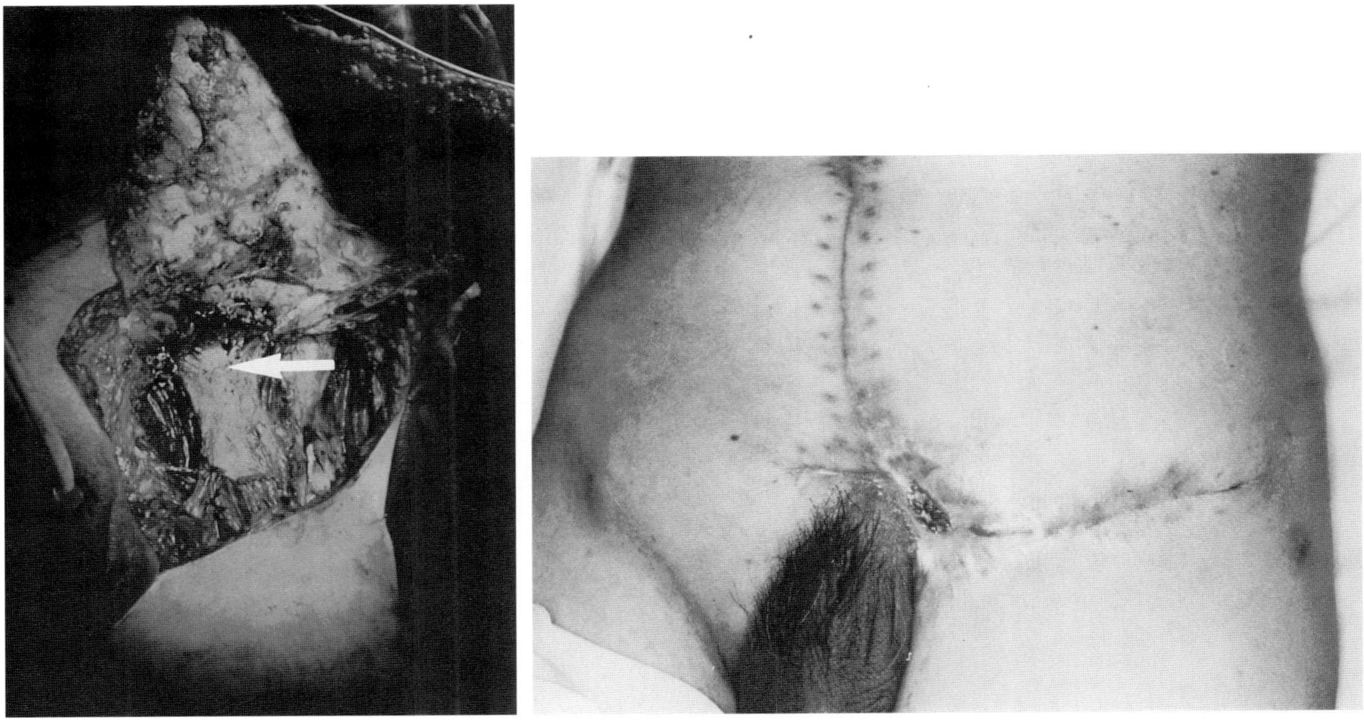

A B

FIG. 94-5. (**A**) If only skin and subcutaneous tissue are required for coverage, a large abdominal flap may be rotated into the wound. Notice that the vessels have been covered with the sartorius muscle (*arrow*). Notice too the elevation of the abdominal flap (*above arrow*). (**B**) Appearance of the rotated flap 3 weeks after operation. The 2-cm loss of skin at the tip filled with granulations over the ensuing 4 weeks. Complete wound coverage was achieved without grafting.

sue, and rotate this tissue into the wound (Fig. 94-5). This results in excellent coverage with little morbidity.

Complications of Groin Dissection

Complications of groin dissection include major flap necrosis in 5%, wound infections in 15%, significant lymphedema of the legs and or scrotum in 16%, and lymphocele formation in 9%.[16] Minor would problems, such as loss of skin edges, occur in 30% but usually heal spontaneously without the need for intervention. Wound seromas occur in 20% to 80% and require periodic aspiration in the immediate postoperative period. A minor degree of lymphedema may occur in as many as 50% of patients.[15] Thrombophlebitis sometimes occurs. This complication, like the others, is more common if the extensive dissections are performed as described in the section on special circumstances.

SUMMARY

Patients with a high likelihood of regional lymph node spread should undergo regional lymphadenectomy. Patients with palpable adenopathy after removal of the primary lesion and administration of antibiotics have a high likelihood of positive nodal involvement (stage 3). Those individuals with poorly differentiated squamous cell carcinoma in the primary lesion or invasion into the corpora cavernosa or spongiosum also have a high likelihood of regional spread (stage 2B) and should undergo regional lymphadenectomy. Limited disease, if microscopically found in the nodes and removed initially, has an excellent 5-year survival probability. Waiting for several years to allow for lymphadenopathy to become apparent before performing a regional lymphadenectomy significantly reduces the 5-year survival rate.

REFERENCES

1. Horenblas S, VanTinteren H, Delemarre JFM, Moonen LMF, Lustig V, vanWaardenburg EW. Squamous cell carcinoma of the penis: III. Treatment of regional nodes. J Urol 1993;149:492.
2. Fraley EE, Zhang G, Manivel C, Niehans GA. The role of ileoinguinal lymphadenectomy and significance of histological differentiation in treatment of carcinoma of the penis. J Urol 1989;142:1478.
3. Ornellas AA, Seixas ALC, Marota A, Wisnescky A, Campos F, deMoraes JR. Surgical treatment of invasive squamous cell carcinoma of the penis: retrospective analysis of 350 cases. J Urol 1994;151:1244.
4. Horenblas S, VanTinteren H. Squamous cell carcinoma of the penis: IV. Prognostic factors of survival: analysis of tumor, nodes and metastasis classification system. J Urol 1994;151:1239.
5. deKernion JB, Tynberg P, Persky L, Fegen JP. Carcinoma of the penis. Cancer 1973;32:1256.
6. Hardner GJ, Bhanalaph T, Murphy GP. Carcinoma of the penis: analysis of therapy in 100 consecutive cases. J Urol 1972;108:428.
7. McDougal WS, Kirchner FK Jr, Edwards RH, Killion LT. Treatment

of carcinoma of the penis: the case for primary lymphadenectomy. J Urol 1986;136:38.

8. Fegen P, Persky L. Squamous cell carcinoma of the penis: its treatment with special reference to radical node dissection. Arch Surg 1969;99: 117.
9. Srinivas V, Joshi A, Agarwal B, Mundhada U, Shah A, Phadke AG. Penile cancer: the sentinel lymph node controversy. Urol Int 1991;47: 108.
10. Cabanas RM. An approach for the treatment of penile cancer. Cancer 1977;39:456.
11. Perinetti E, Crane DB, Catalona WJ. Unreliability of sentinel lymph node biopsy for staging penile carcinoma. J Urol 1980;124:734.
12. Uehling DT. Staging laparotomy for carcinoma of penis. J Urol 1973; 110:213.
13. Srinivas V, Morse MJ, Herr HW, Sogani PC, Whitmore WF Jr. Penile cancer: relation of extent of nodal metastasis to survival. J Urol 1987; 137:880.
14. Baker BH, Spratt JS, Perez-Mesa C, et al. Carcinoma of the penis. J Urol 1976;116:458.
15. Ayyappan K, Ananthakrishnan N, Sankaran V. Can regional lymph node involvement be predicted in patients with carcinoma of the penis. Br J Urol 1994;73:549.
16. Ornellas AA, Seixas ALC, deMoraes JR. Analyses of 200 lymphadenectomies in patients with penile carcinoma. J Urol 1991;146:330.

Principles and Practice of Genitourinary Oncology, edited by Derek Raghavan, Howard I. Scher, Steven A. Leibel, and Paul H. Lange. Lippincott-Raven Publishers, Philadelphia, © 1997.

CHAPTER 95

Chemotherapy for Cancer of the Penis

Giorgio Pizzocaro, Nicola Nicolai, and Luigi Piva

Chemotherapy has a moderate efficacy against squamous cell carcinoma of the penis. Some drugs demonstrated to be effective to some extent, mainly bleomycin, methotrexate and cisplatin, have been clinically tested as single agents or in multidrug schedules. Nonetheless, paucity of experiences, heterogeneity in treatment schedules and patient selection, and generally poor results make difficult a reliable evaluation of the impact of chemotherapy on squamous cell carcinoma of the penis. More recent results in some homogeneous series allowed the definition of the modern role of chemotherapy in squamous cell carcinoma of the penis: as systemic therapy in the rare cases of distant metastases, as primary (neoadjuvant) chemotherapy for fixed inguinal nodes, and as adjuvant therapy after radical resection of nodal metastases. Furthermore, systemic chemotherapy may play a role in organ-sparing combined-treatment modalities in selected cases. Feasibility of chemotherapy, both in terms of easy administration and of acceptable toxicity, represents an important aspect of its use in this disease, which often occurs in elderly patients.

SINGLE-AGENT CHEMOTHERAPY

Bleomycin, methotrexate, and cisplatin represent the most studied single agents in the treatment of squamous cell carcinoma of the penis.[1–3] Experiences are reported in Table 95-1.

Bleomycin represents one of the first drugs employed for the treatment of squamous cell carcinoma of the penis. Complete and partial responses with bleomycin alone were observed in at least one third of cases, as reported by different papers in the 1970s and carefully summarized by Eisenberger.[4] Bleomycin was employed at a level very close to the maximum tolerated dose, and side effects such as skin rashes, fever, chills, and pulmonary interstitial fibrosis were reported. In the series of 14 patients treated by Ahmed and associates,[3] three objective responses were recorded, all belonging to the group of eight patients with inguinal metastases only, whereas none of the six patients who had pelvic or distant metastases responded. Responses were independent of previous chemotherapy. The authors reported two cases of severe pulmonary toxicity, with one death.

Methotrexate has been reported as the most effective single agent for squamous cell carcinoma of the penis by different authors.[3,5,6] Ahmed and associates,[3] extending the previous experience of Sklaroff and Yagoda,[7] reported 8 major responses (complete plus partial) among 13 patients treated with different doses. Responses did not depend on metastatic sites. Five patients had been pretreated: all three who received cisplatin responded, but neither of the two who had been pretreated with bleomycin responded. Conversely, there was no remission in any of the five patients who received bleomycin following methotrexate, and two responses were achieved among the nine patients who were secondarily treated with cisplatin. Methotrexate administration was rarely associated with life-threatening toxicity[4]: Ahmed and associates[3] reported severe granulocytopenia in only two patients, one of whom died of sepsis. Hepatic and renal toxicities were always reversible.

Cisplatin, which is generally effective in squamous cell carcinoma at any site, induced objective responses (complete and partial) in only 15% to 26% of patients with advanced squamous cell carcinoma of the penis. Ahmed and associates[3] reported 3 (25%) partial responses in 12 patients adequately treated. All responses were achieved in patients previously treated with bleomycin (1 case) or methotrexate (2 cases), independent of where metastases occurred. The largest phase II study on single-agent cisplatin in squamous cell carcinoma of the penis was performed by the Southwest Oncology Group (SWOG).[8] Only four (15%) partial responses of short duration were achieved among 26 chemotherapy-naive patients with advanced disease. The SWOG study reported nausea and vomiting, hearing loss, and kidney disfunction in most cases, but no patient suffered severe myelotoxicity. The SWOG results were the poorest in the literature, and the authors concluded that single-agent cisplatin could not be recommended as treatment for squamous cell carcinoma of the penis.

MULTIDRUG CHEMOTHERAPY

Observations about the efficacy of combination chemotherapy in squamous cell carcinoma of the head and neck promoted the use of such regimens in cancer of the penis as well. The Al-Sarraf regimen,[9] consisting of the administration of cisplatin 100 mg/m^2 intravenously on day 1 followed by 24-hour continu-

TABLE 95-1. *Most important experiences with single-agent bleomycin, methotrexate, and cisplatin therapy in squamous cell carcinoma of the penis*

Investigators	Schedule	No. of patients	Jackson's stage	CR plus PR (%)	Response duration (range in mo)
BLEOMYCIN					
Ichikawa, 1977[1]	15 mg/m² 2–3 wk	24	NA	50	NA
Kyalwazi et al, 1974[2]	15–30 mg/m² 1–2 per wk	15	I–IV	45	NA
Ahmed et al, 1984[3]	3–30 U/m² per week	14	III and IV	21	2–4
METHOTREXATE					
Sklaroff and Yaguda, 1980[7]	250–1500 mg/m² q 2 wk	8	III and IV	38	2–11
Ahmed et al, 1984[3]	250–1500 mg/m² q 2–4 wk	13	III and IV	61	2–31
CISPLATIN					
Gagliaro et al, 1991[8]	50 mg/m² 1, 8 q 4 wk	26	III and IV	4 (15)	1–3
Ahmed et al, 1984[3]	70–120 mg/m² q 3 wk	12	III and IV	3 (23)	2–8

CR, complete remission; NA, not available; PR, partial remission.

ous intravenous infusion of 5-fluorouracil 1000 mg/m² daily for 4 days, is the most commonly used combination chemotherapy in advanced squamous cell carcinoma of the penis.

Hussein and associates[10] administered four cycles of this cisplatin and 5-fluorouracil combination (PF) to six patients with recurrent or unresectable metastases from squamous cell carcinoma of the penis, or of the urethra (1 case). One patient also had bone metastases. Five (83%) objective responses were achieved, four of which were partial and one complete. The complete response occurred in the patient with urethral cancer. Two (33%) patients were able to undergo radical resection, with histologic evidence of residual disease in both cases. One of these patients relapsed and was treated with further PF chemotherapy in combination with radiotherapy: he was rendered disease-free and remained alive at 32 months. The other operated patient received adjuvant radiotherapy and survived for 26 months. The patients whose disease remained unresectable received radiotherapy and survived from 6 to 20 months. Toxicity was reported to be moderate and reversible in all cases, without need for interruption of therapy.

Shammas and associates[11] submitted eight patients with metastatic squamous cell carcinoma of the penis to the same therapy: two had resectable disease and four had unresectable inguinal nodes only; the remaining two patients had both inguinal and distant metastases. Two of the six patients with unresectable disease were rendered disease-free with subsequent surgery, alone or in combination with radiotherapy. Both of these patients were alive and disease-free at 32 and 57 months. Of the two patients with resectable inguinal metastases, one progressed, was maintained on chemotherapy, and died at 28 months; the other patient had stable disease, underwent radiotherapy, and died at 8 months. The remaining four patients survived from 2+ to 12 months. Toxicity was significant in this series; only three patients could complete the three courses of therapy. The authors of this study related the poor tolerability to the old age of the patients.

Dexeus and associates[12] used a combination of methotrexate, bleomycin, and cisplatin (Table 95-2) in 14 chemotherapy-naive patients with unresectable squamous cell carcinoma of the genitourinary tract; 12 of these patients had unresectable inguinal metastases from penile cancer. Three patients received cisplatin and bleomycin intraarterially. Of the 14 patients, 10 (72%) responded. Two (14%) achieved a complete remission, which lasted 6 and 24+ months. Only three of eight partial responders were submitted to surgery; one of them was able to undergo radical resection. The median duration of response was 6 months. Toxicity was moderately severe in this series. Five patients developed lung fibrosis, which was clearly symptomatic in two of them. Other important side effects were represented by two cases of granulocytopenic infection and one case of peripheral neuropathy.

Kattan and associates[13] reported relatively poor results in 14 chemotherapy-naive patients who were treated with several cisplatin-based chemotherapy combinations for advanced squamous cell carcinoma of the penis. Cisplatin was given with 5-fluorouracil in four patients, methotrexate and bleomycin were given in four patients, methotrexate alone was given in three patients, and adriamycin, bleomycin or epirubicin were each given in one case. Six patients had distant metastases, six had unresectable inguinal nodes, and two had local, resectable disease. Among 13 evaluable cases, only 2 with unresectable inguinal nodes responded: 1 achieved a complete remission and was alive and disease-free 12 months following complementary ra-

TABLE 95-2. *Methotrexate, bleomycin, and cisplatin combination chemotherapy according to Dexeus et al[12]*

Methotrexate	200 mg/m² IV on days 1, 15 and 22, followed by folinic acid rescue, 25 mg PO, (IV) every 6 h for 12 doses after each administration
INTRAVENOUS SCHEDULE	
Bleomycin	10 mg/m² daily on days 2 through 6 as a 24-h IV infusion
Cisplatin	20 mg/m² daily IV on days 2 through 6
INTRAARTERIAL SCHEDULE (EXTERNAL OR INTERNAL ILIAC ARTERY)	
Cisplatin	100 mg/m² on day 2 as a 6-h intraarterial infusion
Bleomycin	20 mg/m² on day 2 as a 24-h intraarterial infusion
To be repeated every 28 days	

diotherapy, the other achieved a partial response, refused any further treatment, and died of progressive disease 9 months later. Both patients with resectable disease did not achieve any response and died at 15 and 26 months. Median survival for patients who progressed was 7.6 months.

The good results achieved with a combination of low-dose vincristine, bleomycin, and methotrexate (VBM) in advanced squamous cell carcinoma of the head and neck[14] induced us to use this easily administered combination in patients with squamous cell carcinoma of the penis in the following dosage schedule:

- vincristine, 1 mg intravenously on day 1
- bleomycin, 15 mg intramuscularly 6 and 12 hours after vincristine
- methotrexate, 30 mg orally on day 3

This regimen was repeated for 12 weeks. In elderly patients and in patients with chronic bronchitis, only the first dose of bleomycin is administered, and methotrexate is then given on day 2. A first series of 5 patients with fixed inguinal nodes and 12 patients with radically resected inguinal metastases were submitted to either primary or adjuvant VBM chemotherapy. Three of the five unresectable patients achieved partial remission and could undergo surgery; only 1 of the 12 patients who received adjuvant VBM relapsed after a median follow-up of 42 months.[15] Updated results are awaited.

COMBINED TREATMENT MODALITIES

Chemotherapy entered combined treatment modalities of squamous cell carcinoma of the penis in an attempt to improve the results of surgery or radiotherapy, and some successful results allowed oncologists to design new therapeutic strategies. These new strategies focused on organ-sparing treatments in selected patients with organ-confined disease and on the improvement of cure rates in patients with metastatic disease.

Chemotherapy in Conservative Treatment of Primary Tumor for Organ-Confined Disease

Some reports explored the combination of chemotherapy and radiotherapy, mainly relying on the synergism between bleomycin and irradiation. Edsmyr and associates[16] submitted 42 patients with T1-T2 squamous cell carcinoma of the penis to radiotherapy (4500 to 5800 cGy to the whole penis by opposed fields with a conventional x-ray device over 5 to 6 weeks) combined with bleomycin 15 mg intramuscularly on days 3 to 5 of weeks 1, 3, and 5. Complete remission was achieved in 39 (93%) cases, and four patients required a salvage amputation. The overall 5-year survival was 77%, and conservatively treated patients maintained both normal micturition and sexual function if they were normal before therapy. No major side effects were recorded, and in particular, no pulmonary fibrosis occurred. Perez-Tamayo and associates[17] were not able to repeat such excellent results with the same combination therapy in 10 patients with T1-T2 squamous cell carcinoma of the penis. Only four patients were rendered disease-free; two were alive at 3 and 12 years, the other two died from a second cancer after 16 and 19 months. Of the remaining six patients, two underwent salvage amputation, three died of progressive disease, and one died secondary to severe treatment complications.

More recently, Modig and associates[18] reported a series of 25 patients with T1, N0 squamous cell carcinoma of the penis who were treated with a combination of irradiation and bleomycin. Radiotherapy to the whole penis was given from two opposed portals with a daily dose of 1.8 Gy up to a total dose of 56 to 58 Gy over a period of 6 weeks. The patients received 2.5 mg (13 cases) or 5 mg (12 cases) of bleomycin intramuscularly 1 hour before each treatment. The total dose of bleomycin was of 70 to 140 mg. Five (20%) patients had a local recurrence between 5 and 48 months (median, 12 months) after treatment, and they underwent partial amputation. After a minimum follow-up of 8 years, no patient had died of disease. The combination of irradiation and bleomycin was well tolerated, and patients who entered treatment with sexual activity retained this ability. Minor reversible local reactions occurred, but these healed in 3 to 6 months. One patient had a late stricture of the urethral meatus which required repeated meatotomy operations. The authors reported no difference in survival rate between this series and a previous series of 19 T1, N0 patients who underwent surgery.

At our institution (National Cancer Institute, Milan), 27 patients with strictly exophytic T1, N0 squamous cell carcinoma of the penis were selected to enter a program of primary (neoadjuvant) VBM chemotherapy followed by CO_2 laser excision of the glans penis surface and circumcision between 1981 and 1990.[18,19] The CO_2 laser excision was carried out to a depth of 2.5 mm and permitted a histologic evaluation of the resected specimen in all cases.[19–21] Patients were seen every 4 weeks in the outpatient department during chemotherapy, which was administered at home with the cooperation of their family doctors. Twelve weekly courses were to be administered, but some complete responders were operated on after 8 weeks. Elderly patients received only one weekly dose of bleomycin, and methotrexate was administered on the day 2. Twelve (44%) patients achieved a pathologic complete remission and 9 had an incomplete response, for an overall response rate of 78%. Seventeen of the 21 responsive patients remained disease-free following CO_2 laser excisional surgery, and 4 had a recurrence. Recurrences were cured conservatively in three cases, and only one patient needed a partial amputation. Of the six poorly responsive patients, two were cured conservatively and four required penile amputation. Overall, 23 (85%) of the 27 selected patients could avoided penile amputation. After a minimum follow-up of 4 years, no patient had died of the disease, and two patients died disease-free of unrelated causes. Skin rashes occurred in 5 (19%) patients, and only one patient had to withdraw from bleomycin therapy because of early lung fibrosis, which was revealed by the second monthly chest x-ray film. Cosmetic results of laser CO_2 surgery were excellent. Normal micturition and sexual function were preserved in all patients undergoing the conservative approach.

Chemotherapy for Nodal Involvement

Radical surgical excision of nodal metastases represents the therapeutic milestone for nodal metastases from squamous cell carcinoma of the penis. Chemotherapy is used in the adjuvant setting, to improve the disease-free survival after radical dissection, or in the neoadjuvant setting to induce resectability of fixed inguinal nodes.[22,23]

Adjuvant Chemotherapy After Radical Resection of Nodal Metastases

Adjuvant chemotherapy after resection of nodal metastases has been reported in few heterogeneous series in which concomitant groin irradiation was often used. Between 1979 and 1990, 25 consecutive patients with radically resected inguinal metastases from squamous cell carcinoma of the penis were to receive 12 weekly courses of adjuvant VBM at our institution.[24] All patients underwent radical inguinopelvic lymph node dissection, and pelvic nodes were involved in 7 cases. Only four (16%) patients relapsed, with a 5-year disease-free actuarial survival of 82%. This finding compares favorably with a previous series of 31 patients submitted to radical inguinopelvic lymph-node dissection alone, whose 5-year disease-free survival was only 37%. A more accurate analysis of these two series allowed the identification of some risk factors in patients with metastatic nodes.[24] In the series of 31 patients who did not receive adjuvant chemotherapy, bilateral nodal involvement, extracapsular spread, nodes larger than 2 cm, pelvic nodal involvement, and more than one involved node were associated with a poor prognosis, whereas in the series of 25 patients treated with adjuvant VBM, only bilaterality of metastases remained significantly associated with poor prognosis ($P = .006$). In particular, all four relapses occurred in the eight patients with bilateral nodal involvement. None of the nine patients who had intranodal metastases suffered any relapse, regardless of adjuvant chemotherapy. This small subset of patients seems to have no need for adjuvant chemotherapy, whereas patients with bilateral nodal involvement probably require a more aggressive adjuvant regimen.

Neoadjuvant Chemotherapy for Fixed Inguinal Nodes

Historically, primary chemotherapy often meant palliation for unresectable metastases from squamous cell carcinoma of the penis, and it has been often associated with radiotherapy. Nonetheless, important results have been obtained with primary chemotherapy in recent reports.[10–13] By combining the experiences of Hussein and colleagues,[10] Shammas and associates,[11] Dexeus and coworkers,[12] and Kattan and colleagues,[13] it is possible to consider a population of 29 patients who have been treated with various cisplatin-based combination chemotherapies for primary or recurrent fixed inguinal metastases from squamous cell carcinoma of the penis. Objective responses were achieved in 19 (66%) cases, of whom 11 (38%) could be radically resected: 5 patients (17%) were reported to be alive and disease-free at 12, 24, 32, 32, and 57 months.[10–13]

The potential advantage of neoadjuvant chemotherapy in patients with resectable inguinal metastases was evaluated by Fisher and associates[25] in five patients with Jackson's stage III squamous cell carcinoma of the penis. Two courses of PF combination chemotherapy were administered before inguinopelvic dissection. One patient who was unresponsive to the first cycle refused any further treatment and died of progressive disease. Four patients achieved an objective remission and underwent surgery: two had no viable tumor in the specimen and two had residual disease. One of these patients received postoperative radiotherapy. No relapses were recorded after a follow-up of 6 to 40 months.

Since 1979, 16 consecutive patients with fixed nodal metastases from squamous cell carcinoma of the penis have been treated with neoadjuvant chemotherapy at our institution.[24] The first 13 patients received 12 weekly courses of VBM combination chemotherapy, and the last three were to be treated with four courses of PF. Seven of the first 13 cases achieved a partial remission and underwent surgery, but only five could be radically resected. Two of the five radically resected patients are alive and disease-free after 5 and 13 years, respectively. They represent 15% of the 13 patients treated with neoadjuvant VBM. The three patients who relapsed survived 16, 27, and 32 months. Of the eight patients who were not rendered disease-free, five died of progressive disease between 11 and 32 months, and the last three were able to receive PF as second-line therapy.

Of the six patients treated with PF, three of whom were previously treated with VBM and three of whom were chemotherapy-naive, five achieved a partial remission and underwent surgery, which was radical in four patients. Three (50%) of the four radically resected patients were alive and disease-free after 3, 8, and 10 years. The remaining three patients survived 3 to 10 months. Overall, nine (56%) patients could be radically resected following primary chemotherapy, and five (31%) have probably been cured. Cisplatin-based chemotherapy is preferred over VBM as first-line treatment for patients with fixed inguinal nodes.

Chemotherapy for Distant Metastases

No really effective treatment is available for distant metastases from squamous cell carcinoma of the penis. The few patients with distant metastases reported in the aforementioned experiences[10–13] usually had very poor outcomes. Kattan and associates[13] submitted to cisplatin-based chemotherapy 6 patients with distant metastases among a series of 14 patients with advanced disease; 1 patient was reported to be alive and disease-free 84 months after resection of inguinal metastases and irradiation of a solitary bone metastasis.

Six patients with distant metastases from squamous cell carcinoma of the penis were observed at our institution between 1979 and 1990. Only two were chemotherapy-naive, and both of these patients received the VBM regimen. One did not respond, and the other achieved complete remission that lasted 6 months.

CONCLUSIONS

The history of chemotherapy for squamous cell carcinoma of the penis was one of failure for a long time; only recently has it become possible to verify the reproducible efficacy of some combination regimens and to suggest a more rational use of chemotherapy in multimodality treatments.

In selected cases with organ-confined disease, the combination of chemotherapy with radiotherapy or minimally invasive surgery can avoid the heavy psychosocial consequences of amputation of the penis in approximately 80% of patients.[14–16] The relatively poor prognosis of patients with radically resected nodal metastases has been transformed into a 5-year expected disease-free survival of approximately 80% with VBM adjuvant chemotherapy in our experience.[24] Only patients with bilateral nodal involvement probably require a more aggressive adjuvant treatment.

Unresectable nodal metastases from squamous cell carcinoma of the penis is a challenging issue. Nonetheless, combination chemotherapy[9–12,25] seems to be able to produce major responses in approximately 60% of patients, resectability in about 50%, and durable disease-free survivals in 15% to 30% of cases. Of the three reported regimens, VBM is the easiest to administer but probably is also the weakest. The two cisplatin-containing regimens seem to be more effective, and the methotrexate-bleomycin-cisplatin combination seems to be the most toxic. We believe that the PF regimen is advisable as first-line therapy in patients with fixed inguinal nodes or advanced disease.

Occasional patients treated in the neoadjuvant setting for "resectable" nodal metastases progressed to unresectability during the therapy, and no patient with metastatic disease was cured by chemotherapy alone. Radical surgery remains the milestone to achieve definite cure in patients with nodal metastases from squamous cell carcinoma of the penis, whereas combination chemotherapy is expected to improve the cure rate.

Distant metastases may occasionally benefit from chemotherapy, especially if a radical local treatment can be performed.[13] Promising results have been reported with the combination of retinoids and interferon in advanced squamous cell carcinoma of the skin,[27] but no experience with this treatment regimen has been yet reported in advanced squamous cell carcinoma of the penis.

REFERENCES

1. Ichikawa T. Chemotherapy of penis carcinoma. Recent Results Cancer Res 1977;140:60.
2. Kyalwazi SK, Bhams D, Harrison NW. Carcinoma of the penis and bleomycin chemotherapy in Uganda. Br J Urol 1974;689:46.
3. Ahmed T, Sklaroff R, Yagoda A. Sequential trials of methotrexate, cisplatin and bleomycin for penile cancer. J Urol 1984;465:132.
4. Eisenberger MA. Chemotherapy for carcinomas of the penis and urethra. Urol Clin North Am 1992;333:19.
5. Horenblas S, ten Bokkel Hunink WW, van Halteren H, van Tinteren. Squamous cell carcinoma of the penis: the role of chemotherapy. J Urol (in press).
6. Garnick MB, Skarin AT, Steele GD. Metastatic carcinoma of the penis: complete remission after high dose methotrexate chemotherapy. J Urol 1979;265:122.
7. Sklaroff RB, Yagoda A. Methotrexate in the treatment of penile carcinoma. Cancer 1980;214:45.
8. Gagliano RG, Blumenstein BA, Crawford ED, Stephens RL, Coltman CA, Costanzi JJ. Cis-diamminedichloroplatinum in the treatment of advanced epidermoid carcinoma of the penis: a Southwest Oncology Group Study. J Urol 1989;66:141.
9. Al-Sarraf M. Head and neck cancer: chemotherapy concepts. Semin Oncol 1988;70:15.
10. Hussein AM, Benedetto P, Sridar KS. Chemotherapy with Cisplatin and 5-fluorouracil for penile and urethral squamous cell carcinomas. Cancer 1990;433:65.
11. Shammas FV, Ous S, Fossa SD. Cisplatin and 5-fluorouracil in advanced cancer of the penis. J Urol 1992;630:147.
12. Dexeus FH, Logothetis CJ, Sella A, et al. Combination chemotherapy with methotrexate, bleomycin and cisplatin for advanced squamous cell carcinoma of the male genital tract. J Urol 1991;1284:146.
13. Kattan J, Culine S, Droz JP, et al. Penile cancer chemotherapy: twelve years' experience at Institut Gustave-Roussy. Urology 1993;559:42.
14. Molinari R, Mattavelli F, Cantu' G, Chiesa F, Costa L, Tancini G. Results of a low-dose combination chemotherapy with vincristine, bleomycin and methotrexate in the palliative treatment of head and neck squamous cell carcinoma. Eur J Cancer 1980;469:16.
15. Pizzocaro G, Piva L. Adjuvant and neoadjuvant vincristine, bleomycin, and methotrexate for inguinal metastases from squamous cell carcinoma of the penis. Acta Oncol 1988;823:27.
16. Edsmyr F, Anderson L, Espositi PL. Combined bleomycin and radiotherapy in carcinoma of the penis. Cancer 1985;1257:56.
17. Perez-Tamayo C, Wijnmaalen A, Pomp J, van der Werf Messing B. Combined approach to squamous cell carcinoma of the penis (SCP). (Abstract 428) Proc Am Soc Cancer Oncol 1987;(6);109.
18. Modig H, Duchek M, Sjodin AG. Carcinoma of the penis: treatment by surgery or combined bleomycin and radiation therapy. Acta Urol Ital 1993;32(6):653.
19. Bandieramonte G, Lepera P, Moglia D, Faustini M, Pizzocaro G. Neoadjuvant chemotherapy and conservative surgery for exophytic T1 N0 carcinoma of the penis. (Abstract 178) 4th International Congress on Anticancer Chemotherapy, Paris, 1993.
20. Bandieramonte G, Lepera P, Marchesini R, Andreola S, Pizzocaro G. Laser microsurgery for superficial lesions of the penis. J Urol 1987; 315:138.
21. Bandieramonte G, Pizzocaro G, Lepera P, et al. Excisional laser surgery for in situ and initially invasive neoplasia of the penis. In: Giuliani L, Puppo P eds. Urology 1992. Monduzzi: Genova, 1992:649.
22. Maiche AG. Adjuvant treatment using bleomycin in squamous cell carcinoma of penis: study of 19 cases. Br J Urol 1983;542:55.
23. Fossa SD, Hall KS, Johannesses NB, Urnes T, Kaalhus O. Cancer of the penis. Eur Urol 1987;372:13.
24. Pizzocaro G, Piva L, Faustini M, Nicolai N. Indications for lymphadenectomy and adjuvant or neoadjuvant chemotherapy for lymph-node metastases from squamous cell carcinoma of the penis. (Abstract 294) XIth Congress of the European Association of Urology, Berlin, 1994.
25. Fisher HAG, Barada JH, Horton J, von Roemeling R. Neoadjuvant therapy with cisplatin and 5-fluorouracil for stage III squamous cell carcinoma of the penis. (Abstract 653) J Urol 1990;143:352A.
26. Jones WG, Fossa SD, Harmers H, van der Bogaert W. Penis cancer: a review by the Joint Committee of the European Organization for Research and Treatment of Cancer (EORTC), Genito-urinary and Radiotherapy Groups. J Surg Oncol 1989;227:40.
27. Lippman SM, Parkinson DR, Itri LM, et al. 13-Cis-retinoic acid and interferon-2a: effective combination therapy for advanced squamous cell carcinoma of the skin. J Natl Cancer Inst 1992;235:84.

PART VII

Adrenal Cancer

Principles and Practice of Genitourinary Oncology, edited by Derek Raghavan, Howard I. Scher, Steven A. Leibel, and Paul H. Lange. Lippincott-Raven Publishers, Philadelphia, © 1997.

CHAPTER 96

Adrenal Cancer

Endocrinology, Diagnosis, and Clinical Staging

Melissa D. Katz and Julianne Imperato-McGinley

ADRENOCORTICAL CARCINOMA

Incidence

Adrenocortical carcinoma is a rare malignancy with an estimated annual incidence of 0.5 to 2.0 cases per million.[1] The tumors most often present during the first decade in children[2] and during the fourth and fifth decades in adults. A slight female preponderance is noted in several recent series, with a female-to-male ratio varying between 1.1:1 and 2.5:1.[1,3–5] However, Søreide and colleagues[6] found that 58% of 99 patients (18 diagnosed at autopsy) with adrenocortical carcinoma in Norway's Cancer Registry between 1970 and 1984 were male.

Henley and colleagues[5] noted that, in the Mayo Clinic series of 62 patients, the incidence was greater in females younger than 40 years of age but equal in older individuals. In three studies, the mean age at diagnosis was 5 to 10 years older for males,[1,4,5] although Pommier and Brennan, in their review of 73 cases at Memorial Sloan-Kettering Cancer Center, reported the mean age at diagnosis to be 37 years for men and 43 years for women.[3] Women are more likely to have functional adrenal tumors, and men tend to harbor nonfunctional neoplasms. Henley and colleagues[5] reported on 62 patients and Icard and associates[1] described 156 patients with functional adrenal tumors, among whom the female-to-male ratio was approximately 3:1.

Pathogenesis

Speculation regarding the possibility that certain benign adrenocortical conditions may predispose to the development of malignancy remains anecdotal. Untreated congenital adrenal hyperplasia has been associated with the occurrence of adrenal adenomas and carcinomas in adulthood.[7–9] This finding may merely be fortuitous given the extremely low incidence. Whether a malignant lesion can develop from earlier hyperplastic adrenal tissue, and the possible mechanism involved, are not known.

The loss of an allele during oncogenesis, known as loss of heterozygosity (LOH), has been demonstrated on chromosomes 11p, 13q, and 17p in adrenocortical carcinomas but not in adenomas or hyperplastic lesions.[10] Beckwith-Wiedemann syndrome is a rare polymalformation syndrome associated with several malignancies, including adrenocortical carcinoma in 15% of patients.[11,12] LOH at locus 11p15.5 has been observed in adrenal tumors in patients with this syndrome and has been suggested as a predisposing event.[11,12] Furthermore, a recent study of sporadic adrenocortical tumors found that overexpression of insulin-like growth factor-II (IGF2) occurs more frequently in malignant neoplasms and is correlated with rearrangements that include LOH at the 11p15.5 locus, to which the *IGF2* gene also maps.[13] It has been suggested that the 11p15.5 region may contain a tumor suppressor gene; possibly the *H19* gene,2 which maps to this locus and is expressed during development.[13,14]

Clinical Characteristics

The average time between the onset of symptoms and the diagnosis of adrenocortical carcinoma is approximately 9 months.[1,5,15] Patients with nonfunctional tumors can present with pain, nonspecific gastrointestinal complaints, weight loss, fatigue, hematuria, and abdominal mass.[1,3–6] Fever secondary to tumor necrosis may be the initial complaint.[16] Anemia can be a consequence of hemorrhage into the tumor.[16]

Clinically functional tumors cause signs and symptoms of hormone excess, which can be manifested as Cushing's syndrome, virilization, feminization, or hypertension. The functional status of adrenocortical carcinoma by clinical presentation is summarized from five recent series in Table 96-1. The majority of tumors appear to be functional, with hypercortisolemia presenting as Cushing's syndrome the most prevalent manifestation.

TABLE 96-1. *Functional status of adrenocortical carcinoma by clinical presentation*

	Henley et al[5] 1960–1980 (n = 62)	Icard et al[1] 1978–1991 (n = 156)	Pommier and Brennan[3] 1980–1991 (n = 73)	Søreide et al[6] 1970–1984 (n = 81*)	Venkatesh et al[4] 1944–1987 (n = 110)
FUNCTIONAL	58%	52%	60%	32%	35.5%
Cushing's	24%	37%	50%	58%	14.5%
Virilization	5%	22%	34%	27%	N/A
Cushing's and virilization	19%†	23%	11%		N/A
Feminization	2%	2%	2%	8%	N/A
Hypertension	6%	10%	2%	6%	N/A
NONFUNCTIONAL	42%	48%	40%	42%	64.5%

N/A, not available.
* Eighteen patients diagnosed at autopsy not included; symptoms not reported for 26% of those included.
† Reported as "mixed" endocrine function.

Glucocorticoid excess exerts numerous metabolic effects, including the common signs of Cushing's syndrome: violaceous striae, moon facies, truncal obesity, buffalo hump, and supraclavicular fat pads secondary to the central redistribution of fat (Table 96-2). The metabolic abnormalities include glucose intolerance or frank diabetes mellitus caused by increased gluconeogenesis and insulin resistance. Patients can have proximal muscle weakness and wasting in addition to easy bruisability caused by skin atrophy. Lower back pain occur as a result of secondary to osteoporosis and compression fractures. Hypokalemia, hypertension, and lower extremity edema may result from the inherent mineralocorticoid activity of excess glucocorticoid production. The hypertension may also be related to the potentiation of the catecholamine effect on the vasculature. Hypercortisolism can have central nervous system effects and cause mood and behavioral changes. Impotence in men and menstrual irregularities in women may result from suppression of the secretion of gonadotropin or sex steroid hormones, or both, as a result of excessive glucocorticoid synthesis. Virilization, caused by excess androgen production, can occur in conjunction with Cushing's syndrome in females with adrenocortical carcinoma. Hyperpigmentation results mainly from increased levels of adrenocorticotropic hormone (ACTH), which contains α-melanocyte–stimulating hormone within its structure. Immunosuppression from glucocorticoid excess is responsible for oral candidiasis and dermatologic mycoses. In children, generalized weight gain coincident with forestalled growth should raise the suspicion of Cushing's syndrome; malignancy is the most common cause in this population.[17]

Precocious puberty in a male or female child requires an investigation for a virilizing or feminizing adrenocortical neoplasm, respectively.[17,18] Postpubertal females presenting with virilization and postpubertal males experiencing feminizing changes such as gynecomastia should be evaluated for a sex steroid–producing adrenal malignancy[19,20] (see Table 96-2).

Aldosterone-producing tumors and deoxycorticosterone-producing (DOC-producing) tumors can cause hypertension and hypokalemic alkalosis. The symptoms are usually more severe patients with aldosterone-producing carcinomas than in those with adenomas. The former diagnosis should be considered in patients with aldosteronomas requiring increasing doses of spironolactone. Muscle cramps, polyuria, nocturia, headache, and weakness are also associated with these rare tumors (see Table 96-2). Isolated aldosterone excess is unusual; elevated levels of cortisol and other adrenocortical hormones are usually produced in these carcinomas as well.[21–25]

Endocrinology and Diagnosis

Biochemical documentation of steroid excess is the initial step in the evaluation of suspected functional adrenocortical tumors. Steroid production, especially by the Δ^4 pathway, may be inefficient in the malignant adrenal gland, and Δ^5 precursor compounds such as Δ^5-pregnenolone and Δ^5-dehydroepiandrosterone (Δ^5-DHEA) can accumulate[26] (Fig. 96-1). Δ^5-DHEA and other Δ^5 compounds however, can be peripherally converted to Δ^4 compounds.

Sakai and associates[27] recently analyzed messenger RNA (mRNA) concentration of 3β-hydroxysteroid dehydrogenase (3β-HSD) in patients with adrenocortical carcinoma. He found decreased 3β-HSD activity and suggested this as a reason for the elevated Δ^5-DHEA.[27] Virilizing tumors that secrete androgen precursors such as Δ^5-DHEA, as opposed to Δ^5-dehydroepiandrosterone sulfate (Δ^5-DHEAS) are more likely to be malignant, because such tumors have been shown to be inefficient at sulfation.[28]

Bertagna and Orth[26] noted that urinary 17-hydrocorticosteroid (17-OHCS) levels were often relatively lower than expected in comparison with urinary 17-ketosteroid (17-KS) levels in patients with adrenocortical carcinoma and attributed this to the relative inefficiency by which the tumor forms cortisol from its precursor hormones. They also proposed that a 24-hour urinary 17-KS excretion greater than 20 mg/g creatinine strongly implies the diagnosis of carcinoma, and lower values are suggestive of an adenoma.[26]

Lipsett and Wilson[29] studied steroid synthesis and metabolism in adrenocortical carcinoma and determined that elevated levels of 11-deoxycortisol and its urinary metabolite tetrahydrodeoxycortisol (THS) are secondary to the relative inability of the tumor to 11β-hydroxylate the precursor 11-deoxycortisol to cortisol (see Fig. 96-1). THS is the major urinary 17-OHCS excreted in adrenocortical carcinoma, and the documentation of high levels may signal the presence of a very large tumor mass.[30]

Normal plasma pregnenolone with elevated 17-hydroxypreg-

TABLE 96-2. *Clinical manifestations of adrenal hormone excess*

GLUCOCORTICOIDS
Truncal obesity
Facial plethora
Violaceous striae
Hyperpigmentation
Buffalo hump
Supraclavicular fat
Hypertension
Glucose intolerance
Proximal myopathy
Leg edema
Easy bruisability
Poor wound healing
Osteoporosis
Acne
Behavioral changes
Oligomenorrhea or amenorrhea
Impotence
Lack of growth
MINERALOCORTICOIDS
Hypertension
Hypokalemic alkalosis
Hypernatremia
Muscle cramps
Polydipsia
Headache
Palpations
ANDROGENS
Hirsutism
Clitoromegaly
Oligomenorrhea or amenorrhea
Temporal balding
Acne
Breast atrophy
Decreased libido
Deepening of voice
Precocious puberty
ESTROGENS
Gynecomastia
Testicular atrophy
Decreased libido
Precocious puberty
CATECHOLAMINES
Palpations
Headache
Diaphoresis
Nausea
Pallor
Tremor
Anxiety
Abdominal pain
Chest pain
Weakness
Constipation
Postparoxysmal flushing

nenolone has been found in patients with hypercortisolism secondary to a glucocorticoid-producing adrenocortical carcinoma.[31] Lack of suppression of both pregnenolone and 17-hydroxypregnenolone in response to high-dose dexamethasone (2 mg orally, every 6 hours for 2 days) has been proposed as a means of assessing the presence of residual carcinoma postoperatively.[31] The increased formation of 17α-progesterone, resulting in increased urinary pregnanetriol, is another abnormality of steroidogenesis associated with adrenocortical carcinoma.[29]

Lesions that produce solely testosterone are usually benign adrenal adenomas.[32] Conversely, most feminizing adrenal tumors are malignant, and they usually produce elevated levels of several hormones in addition to estrogens. Δ^4-Androstenedione, a weak androgen that may be secreted in excess by feminizing adrenal lesions, can be converted either peripherally or by the tumor itself to testosterone by the enzyme 17β-hydroxysteroid dehydrogenase (17β-HSD) or to estrone by aromatization.[20,33]

As mentioned, adrenal tumors that make aldosterone or 11-DOC have substantial mineralocorticoid activity. Likewise, tumors with defects in 11β-hydroxylation can cause hypermineralocorticoidism in the absence of hypercortisolism by increasing circulating DOC levels.[34,35]

Biochemical Evaluation

Glucocorticoid-Producing Tumors

The diagnosis of Cushing's syndrome requires documentation of hypercortisolism in the setting of an abnormal pituitary-adrenal axis (Fig. 96-2). The normal diurnal variation of cortisol secretion is disrupted, and therefore a 10 P.M. to midnight plasma cortisol level may be inappropriately elevated. Measurement of 24-hour urinary free cortisol (UFC) is the best screening test for Cushing's syndrome; depending on the assay used, the normal value should be less than 90 to 100 μg/day. If a high-pressure liquid chromatography assay is used, the upper limit of normal is approximately 50 μg/day. Quantification of 24-hour urinary 17-OHCS is optional, but it may be useful in conjunction with the finding of elevated 24-hour urinary 17-KS.[26]

The 1-mg overnight dexamethasone suppression test should also be used to screen for Cushing's syndrome. After oral administration of 1 mg dexamethasone at 11 P.M. the previous day, the 8 A.M. cortisol level should be suppressed to 5 mg/dL or less. False-positive results may occur in patients taking rifampin, phenytoin, or oral contraceptives and in patients with depression. False-negative results are less frequent but may have more severe consequences if this screening test is used exclusively.

After hypercortisolism has been demonstrated, it is necessary to determine whether the cortisol excess is ACTH-dependent, indicating a pituitary or ectopic origin, or ACTH-independent, implying a primary adrenal origin. The low-dose (2-mg) dexamethasone suppression test involves a 0.5-mg oral dose every 6 hours for 2 days. Twenty-four hour UFC and 17-OHCS are measured on the second day. Plasma cortisol and ACTH are measured 6 hours after the fourth dose, which is the morning of day 3. Failure to suppress UFC and 17-OHCS to less than 50% of baseline confirms the diagnosis of Cushing's syndrome.

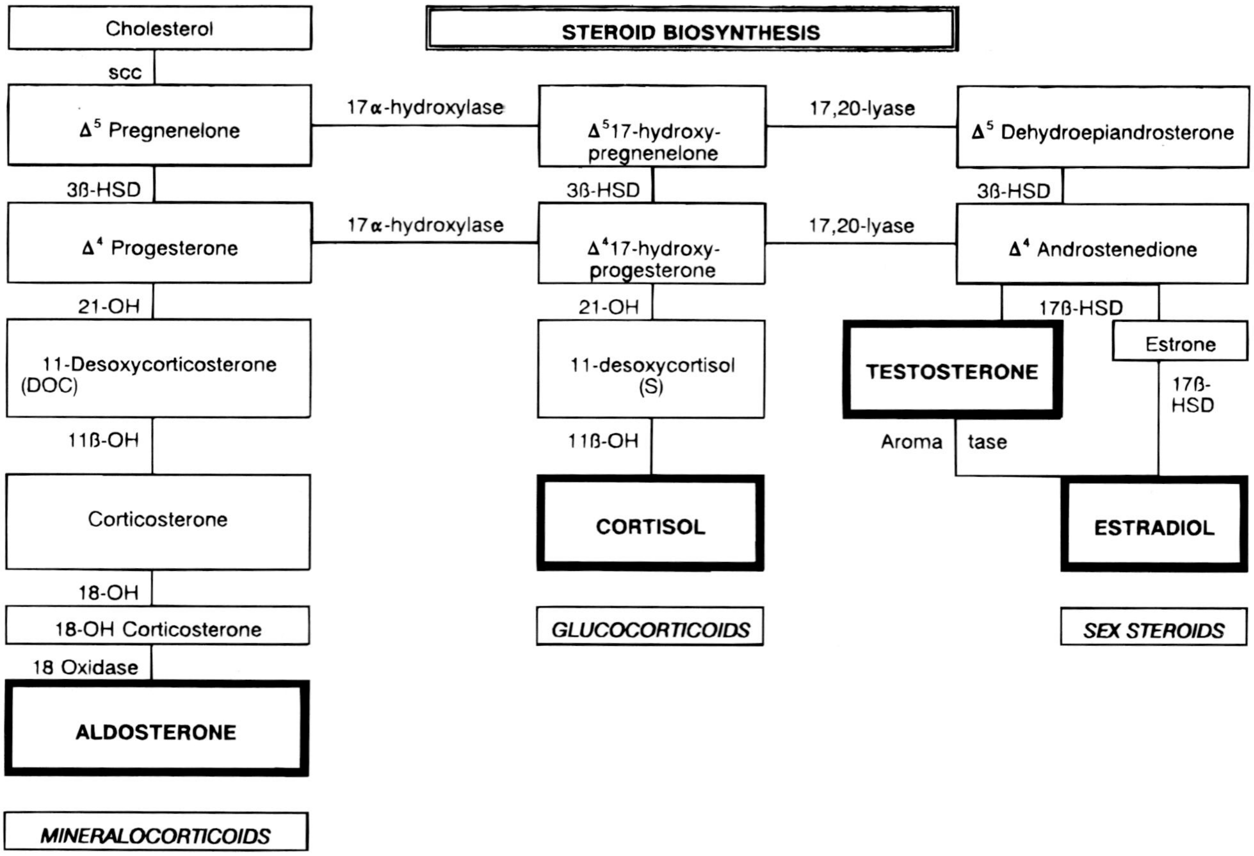

FIG. 96-1. Steroid biosynthesis. scc, side chain cleavage; OH, hydroxylase; HSD, hydroxysteroid dehydrogenase.

After low-dose testing, it is imperative to proceed with the high-dose (8-mg) dexamethasone suppression test in order to differentiate a pituitary from an ectopic or adrenal source of hypercortisolemia. In the classic protocol, 2 mg of dexamethasone is administered orally every 6 hours, for a total of four doses. Alternatively, a single 8-mg dose of dexamethasone can be administered at 11 P.M. in a rapid overnight test, as has been described in a single study.[36] The theory behind high-dose dexamethasone testing is that cortisol production by an ACTH-producing pituitary adenoma is partly suppressed, but autonomous glucocorticoid production from a tumor remains virtually unchanged, with low to unmeasurable ACTH. In the ectopic ACTH syndrome, the pituitary secretion of ACTH is suppressed, but the ectopic production of ACTH is usually extremely high and escapes negative feedback regulation. Lack of suppression of plasma cortisol, 24-hour UFC, and 17-OHCS to less than 50% of baseline usually implies an adrenal or ectopic source. It has been suggested that specificity may be increased if the diagnostic criteria used for suppression of UFC and 17-OHCS are 90% and 64%, respectively.[37]

Large bioactive portions of ACTH may be produced by ectopic tumors and escape detection by the more specific immunoradiometric assay, therefore requiring a radioimmunoassay for detection.[38] Rarely, an increased ACTH level and lack of suppression with high-dose dexamethasone indicate an ACTH-producing pheochromocytoma.[39]

Confirmed ACTH-independent Cushing's syndrome necessitates a radiologic evaluation of the adrenal glands (see later discussion). In occult cases, it can be difficult to distinguish the cause of ACTH-dependent Cushing's syndrome. Imaging of the pituitary and chest, an ovine corticotropin-releasing hormone stimulation test,[40] and bilateral inferior petrosal sinus sampling with corticotropin-releasing hormone stimulation testing[41] can aid in differentiating a pituitary from an ectopic source such as small cell lung cancer, carcinoid tumor, and medullary thyroid carcinoma (MTC).

Sex Hormone–Producing Tumors

Excess androgen and estrogen secretion in adrenocortical carcinoma can occur with or without hypercortisolemia. Therefore, biochemical investigation of a patient presenting with virilization should include plasma cortisol, 24-hour UFC, and 17-OHCS, in addition to 17-KS and plasma determinations of the androgens, testosterone, Δ^4-androstenedione, DHEA, and DHEAS. In cases of feminization, plasma 17β-estradiol, estrone, and urinary estrogens should be measured in addition. Suppression of cortisol with dexamethasone testing, as described for glucocorticoid-producing tumors, should be performed in all patients with sex hormone–producing tumors to ascertain the possible coexistence of Cushing's syndrome.

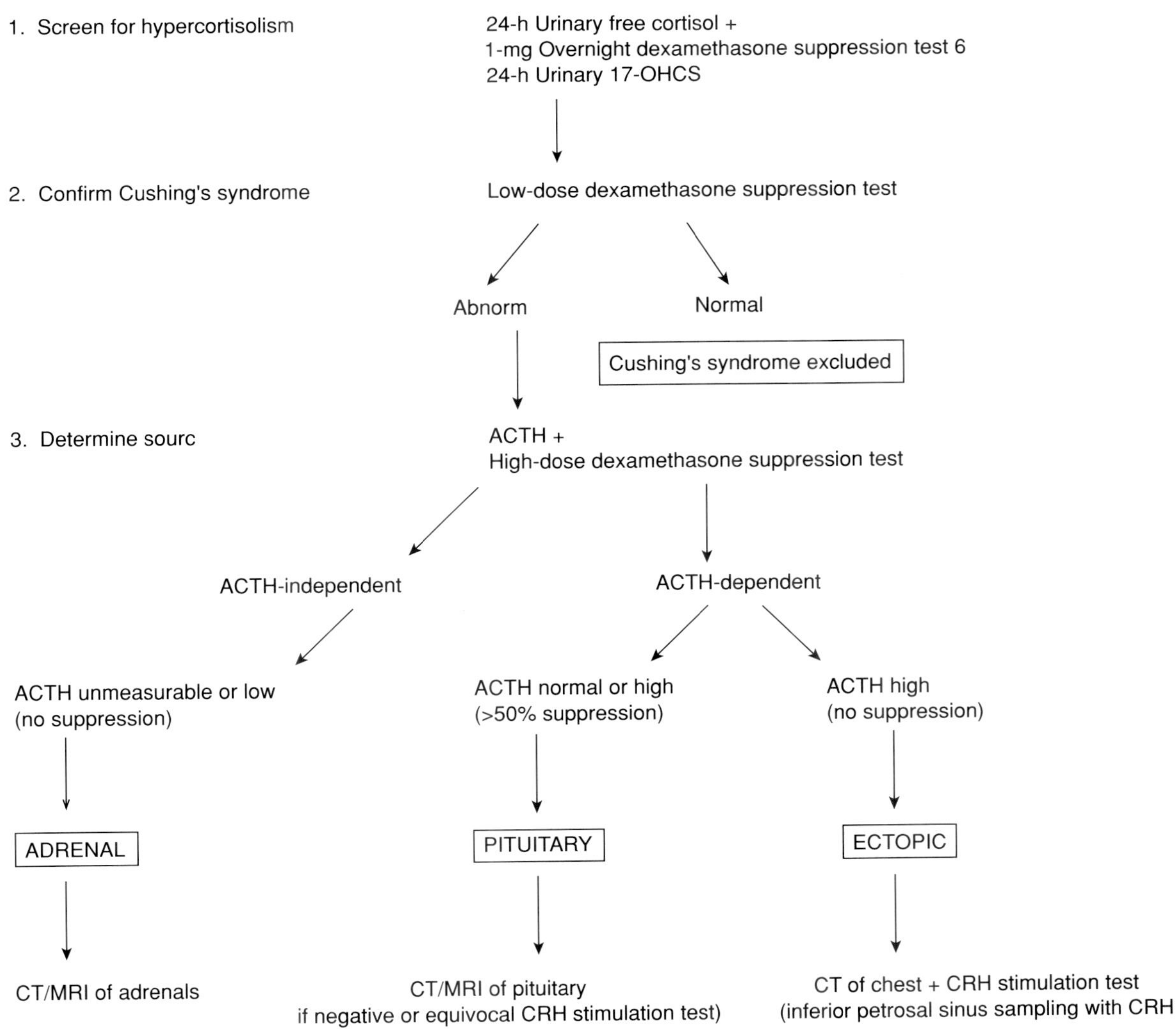

FIG. 96-2. Evaluation of Cushing's syndrome. 17-OHCS, 17-hydroxycorticosteroids; ACTH, adrenocorticotropic hormone; CT, computed tomography; MRI, magnetic resonance imaging; CRH, corticotropin-releasing hormone.

Mineralocorticoid-Producing Tumors

Aldosterone-secreting adrenocortical carcinomas are an extremely rare cause of primary hyperaldosteronism[21–25]; aldosterone-producing adenomas and idiopathic hyperaldosteronism are far more common. DOC-producing adenomas and, even more rarely, carcinomas[34,35] can also cause hypertension, hypokalemia, hypernatremia, and elevated urinary potassium.

To determine the cause of hypermineralocorticoidism, plasma aldosterone and renin should be measured after the patient has spent 3 hours in an upright position. A aldosterone-to-renin ratio greater than 25 with a low renin value supports the diagnosis of primary hyperaldosteronism. In patients with low renin, the lack of suppression of aldosterone during the saline suppression test, in which isotonic saline is infused at 300 to 500 mL/hour for 4 hours, is strong evidence for primary hyperaldosteronism. Likewise, the captopril suppression test, involving 25 mg of oral captopril with lack of suppression of aldosterone and failure of renin to increase at 2 hours, is an alternative test for patients who cannot tolerate volume expansion.

In general, much higher basal aldosterone levels are found with a carcinoma than with an adenoma. Carcinomas also lack the circadian secretion of aldosterone and stimulation by ACTH.[21] In DOC-secreting carcinomas, DOC levels are elevated with low aldosterone and renin levels.

Radiologic Localization

Adrenal imaging with computed tomography is a very sensitive test for locating adrenal masses larger than 1 cm, but it is not specific in identifying the type of lesion. Magnetic resonance imaging is capable of differentiating certain lesions on T2-weighted images. An adrenal-to-liver signal ratio of less than 1.2 is characteristic of adenomas, a ratio of 1.4 to 2.7 is seen with carcinomas, and a ratio higher than 3.4 is seen with pheochromocytomas.[42] Nonetheless, magnetic resonance imaging is unable to definitively discern the cause of up to 30% of adrenal masses visualized, especially metastases and aldosterone-producing tumors.[42,43]

In a study of 119 adrenal masses, ^{131}I-6β-iodomethylnorcholesterol (NP-59) scintigraphy was found to be 76% sensitive and 100% specific in differentiating benign from malignant lesions,[44] because malignant lesions usually do not take up the radionuclide. This scan is limited by its inability to detect lesions smaller than 2.0 cm.[43,44]

Pathology and Prognostic Factors

A slight predilection for the left adrenal gland has been described in patients with adrenocortical carcinoma. Venkatesh and colleagues[4] reported that 71 of 110 patients had tumors of the left gland; similar figures were reported by Icard and associates[1] (79 of 156 patients) and by Søreide and associates[6] (51 of 99 patients). Bilateral carcinoma at presentation was reported in 4 of 110 patients by Venkatesh and colleagues[4] and in 4 of the 99 cases of Søreide and colleagues.[6]

The diagnosis of malignancy in an adrenal cortical tumor can be difficult in the absence of metastases. An immunohistologic comparison between 10 adrenocortical adenomas and 10 carcinomas revealed no differences.[45] A broad trabecular and alveolar pattern with prominent vasculature has been described in aldosterone-producing adrenocortical carcinoma.[24] Calcifications are thought to be representative of malignancy in mineralocorticoid-producing tumors.[22,23]

Radiologic evidence of central necrosis and vena cava involvement is very suggestive of carcinoma.[46] Hough and colleagues,[47] in a study of 41 patients, identified weight loss, histologic presence of fibrous bands, tumor necrosis, mass, vascular invasion, and a diffuse growth pattern as indicative of metastatic potential. Any adrenocortical tumor that weighs more than 500 g should be considered highly suspicious for malignancy. Van Slooten and associates[48] found that mitotic activity and tumor weight, the mean value of which was 1210 g in 42 metastatic adrenocortical tumors, were the best distinguishing characteristics.

The presence of more than 20 mitoses per 50 high-powered fields correlated with a poorer prognosis in 42 patients studied by Weiss and coworkers.[49] Age older than 35 years has also been associated with a less favorable outcome.[1] Only one study has shown a difference in prognosis based on the functional status of the tumor. Icard and associates[1] found that, among 156 cases, those tumors that were androgen-secreting, precursor-secreting or nonfunctional had a better prognosis than mainly cortisol-secreting tumors.

Clinical Staging

The staging criteria applicable to adrenocortical carcinoma are those of Macfarlane,[50] as modified by Sullivan[51] (Table 96-3). As depicted in Table 96-4, the majority of patients are diagnosed with advanced disease.

TABLE 96-3. *Staging criteria for adrenocortical carcinoma*

Symbol	Description
T1	Tumor ≤5 cm, no invasion
T2	Tumor >5 cm, no invasion
T3	Tumor any size, locally invading to but not involving adjacent organs
T4	Tumor any size, locally invading adjacent organs
N0	No regional positive nodes
N1	Positive regional nodes
M0	No distant metastatic disease
M1	Distant metastatic disease
TNM stage	**Components**
I	T1N0M0
II	T2N0M0
III	T1 or T2N1M0, T3N0M0
IV	Any T, any N M1, T3N1, T4

T, tumor; N, nodes; M, metastases.

Criteria developed from: Macfarlane DA. Cancer of the adrenal cortex: the natural history, prognosis and treatment in a study of fifty-five cases. Ann R Coll Surg Engl 23:155, 1958; Sullivan M, Boileau M, Hodges CV. Adrenal cortical carcinoma. J Urol 120:660, 1978; Henley DJ, van Heerden JA, Grant CS. Adrenal cortical carcinoma; a continuing challenge. Surgery 94:926, 1983.

PHEOCHROMOCYTOMA

Incidence and Associated Syndromes

Pheochromocytoma has been estimated to occur in 0.1% to 0.5% of hypertensive patients.[52] Adult men and women are equally affected[52,53]; among children it occurs slightly more often in boys.[53] Most cases are diagnosed in the third to fifth decades; children, however, comprise about 10% of patients with this diagnosis. Characteristics of childhood pheochromocytoma in comparison with adult disease include increased bilaterality (20% versus 10%), multiple tumors (30% versus 10%), and extraadrenal involvement (30% versus 10%).[53] Extraadrenal tumors originate from sympathetic ganglia chromaffin cells, whereas adrenal tumors arise from medullary chromaffin tissue. It is generally believed that more than 13% of pheochromocytomas are malignant.[54]

Pheochromocytoma is familial in about 10% of patients, and it occurs in the multiple endocrine neoplasia (MEN) type 2A and type 2B syndromes. MEN2A, or Sipple syndrome, consists of hyperparathyroidism, MTC, and pheochromocytoma. Approximately 50% of patients with MEN2A develop pheochromocytoma, which is often bilateral and rarely extraadrenal. Epinephrine is usually the predominant catecholamine secreted, and the hypertension tends to be episodic. MEN2B includes mucosal neuromas, MTC, thickened corneal nerves, gastrointestinal ganglioneuromas, a marfanoid habitus, and pheochromocytoma. The genes for both MEN2A and MEN2B are located on chromosome 10 near the centromere.[55–59] The neuroectodermal syndromes of von Recklinghausen's neurofibromatosis,

TABLE 96-4. *Stage at diagnosis of adrenocortical carcinoma*

	Henley et al[5] 1960–1980 (n = 62)	Icard et al[1] 1978–1991 (n = 156)	Pommier and Brennan[3] 1980–1991 (n = 73)	Søreide et al[6] 1970–1984 (n = 81*)	Venkatesh et al[4] 1944–1987 (n = 110)
STAGE					
I	2%	5%	4%	—	—
II	32%	48%	32%	30%†	26%‡
III	13%	25%	29%	18%	27%§
IV	53%	22%	35%	52%	38%‖
METASTASES					
Liver	22%	53%	47%	55%	64%
Lungs	13%	41%	43%	35%	73%
Nodes	8%	—	25%	—	26%
Bone	3%	23%	15%	—	21%
Peritoneum	5%	16%¶	9%**	—	26%

* Includes 18 patients diagnosed at autopsy.
† Stages I and II combined.
‡ Localized disease.
§ Regional disease.
¶ Other including peritoneum.
‖ Metastatic disease.
** Omentum included.

von Hippel-Lindau syndrome, Sturge-Weber syndrome and tuberous sclerosis are also associated with pheochromocytoma, although different genes are involved.

Pathogenesis

LOH in locations other than chromosome 10 has been observed in MEN2A, MEN2B, and sporadic pheochromocytoma.[60,61] Allelic losses on chromosomes 1p,[61] 3p (von Hippel-Lindau locus), 17p, and 22q have been identified in pheochromocytoma.[60] In addition, urinary metanephrine excretion is greater in tumors with LOH of 1p, and larger tumor size correlated with LOH on 1p, 3p and 17p.[60]

The *MEN2A* and *MEN2B* genes have been mapped to the pericentromeric portion of chromosome 10 that includes the *RET* protooncogene.[55–57,62–66] Recently, *RET* protooncogene mutations have also been found in association with familial medullary thyroid carcinoma (FMTC),[62,63,64] and Hirschsprung's disease.[67,68] It is thought that a single amino acid substitution at the *RET* locus may be responsible for the development of MTC in the syndromes that include this malignancy (ie, MEN2A, MEN2B, and FMTC).[62–66,69] In contrast, deletions and premature stop codons have been found at the *RET* protooncogene site in Hirschsprung's disease.[67,68,69]

Additional investigations of the pathogenesis of adrenal tumors have revealed the overexpression of P53 protein.[70] This was found in one sporadic malignant pheochromocytoma and in four of five sporadic benign pheochromocytomas, in addition to 11 of 15 functional adrenal adenomas.[70] A consequence of *P53* gene mutations is loss of inhibition of guanine synthesis, which facilitates tumor growth and hormone expression.[70] In a study of DNA from 10 pheochromocytomas, *RAS* oncogene mutations were not identified.[71]

Clinical Characteristics

Sudden catecholamine release can result in a paroxysm most commonly characterized by headache, perspiration, and palpitations. Other manifestations include nausea, emesis, chest pain, tremors, pallor, anxiety, abdominal pain, constipation, and post-paroxysmal flushing (see Table 96-2). Paroxysms can be provoked by physical activity, pregnancy, micturition (particularly in pheochromocytomas of the bladder wall), straining at stool, or abdominal palpation. Tricyclic antidepressants, opiates, phenothiazines, metoclopramide, glucagon, and intravenous contrast agents can cause catecholamine release and precipitate episodes.[72,73] The duration of the paroxysm is variable, but it can be as long as 45 minutes.

Hypertension in pheochromocytoma may be sustained, resembling essential hypertension, or there may be superimposed paroxysms in addition to the sustained hypertension. Tumors that predominantly produce norepinephrine often cause sustained hypertension, whereas paradoxic hypertension is associated with the release of epinephrine along with norepinephrine. Exclusive epinephrine secretion can cause hypotension.[74] Orthostatic hypotension is not unusual; it is secondary to hypovolemia and a diminished vasoconstrictor response caused by the tachyphalactic effect of excessive catecholamines on the catecholamine receptor.

Increased myocardial oxygen demand from elevated catecholamines can precipitate coronary spasm and myocardial infarction. Catecholamine-induced dilated cardiomyopathy is more common in children than in adults; it can lead to congestive heart failure, which may be reversible with appropriate treatment.[74,75] Thromboses, renal failure, myocarditis, arrhythmias, and pulmonary edema are additional complications of pheochromocytoma.

The hypermetabolic state induced by pheochromocytoma can

cause fever[76] and weight loss. Impaired glucose homeostasis is caused by decreased insulin release.[77] Hypercalcemia may be associated with hyperparathyroidism in MEN2A or MEN2B, or it may occur as an isolated phenomenon, perhaps related to a humoral factor elaborated by the tumor.[78] Polycythemia can occur secondary to an erythropoietin-like factor produced by the pheochromocytoma or because of hypovolemia resulting from sustained vasoconstriction.[52] Cholelithiasis has been reported in 10% to 20% of patients.[53]

Endocrinology and Diagnosis

The conversion of norepinephrine to epinephrine requires phenylethanolamine-*N*-methyl transferase, which is induced by cortisol produced by the surrounding adrenal cortex[52] (Fig. 96-3). Therefore, pheochromocytomas that secrete primarily epinephrine are more likely to be adrenal, whereas norepinephrine-producing tumors may be either adrenal or extraadrenal. Most pheochromocytomas produce both catecholamines, with 50% to 70% manufacturing epinephrine and 75% to 85% norepinephrine. Tumors that predominantly make epinephrine are generally associated with MEN2 syndromes.[79]

Higher levels of plasma and urinary catecholamines are commonly produced by small tumors with rapid catecholamine secretion. In contrast, large tumors often contain enzymes that metabolize the catecholamines, thereby yielding higher urinary levels of metabolites.[74] As a consequence, they grow to a larger size before causing symptoms. The metabolite normetanephrine is derived from norepinephrine by the enzyme catechol-*o*-methyl transferase, and metanephrine is the metabolite of epinephrine by the same enzyme. Vanillylmandelic acid is the common end product (see Fig. 96-3).

Biochemical Evaluation

Biochemical confirmation of excess catecholamine production is essential to the diagnosis of pheochromocytoma. Twenty-four hour urinary determinations of free unconjugated catecholamines and the catecholamine metabolites metanephrine and normetanephrine should be obtained. Vanillylmandelic acid

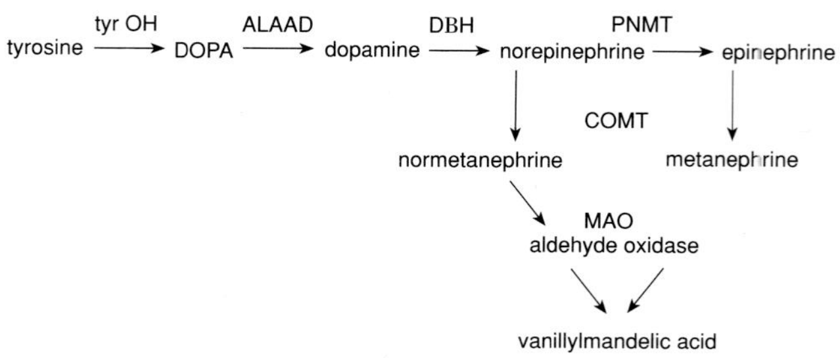

FIG. 96-3. Catecholamine synthesis and metabolism. TYR, tyrosine; OH, hydroxylase; DOPA, dihydrophenylalanine; ALAAD, aromatic L-amino acid decarboxylase; DA, dopamine; DβH, dopamine-β-hydroxylase; NE, norepinephrine; PNMT, phenylethanolamine-*N*-methyl transferase; EPI, epinephrine; COMT, catechol-*o*-methyl transferase; MAO, monoamine oxidase; VMA, vanillylmandelic acid.

is the least sensitive 24-hour urinary test, and false elevations can result from the ingestion of foods such as nuts, chocolate, and bananas. Determination of urinary free catecholamines by high-pressure liquid chromatography is a very sensitive test.[79,80] Fractionation of urinary catecholamines may indicate whether it is likely that the tumor is adrenal. The upper limit of normal for total urinary metanephrines is 1.3 mg/day; levels in pheochromocytoma frequently exceed 3 mg/day.[80] It is of utmost importance that the 24-hour urine sample be accurately collected; urinary creatinine should always be measured to determine the adequacy of the collection.

Plasma catecholamines (total and fractionated norepinephrine and epinephrine) should be measured after the patient has been at rest for a minimum of 30 minutes after the insertion of a catheter. Exogenous xanthines and smoking should be avoided before testing. Catecholamine levels greater than 2000 pg/mL are indicative of pheochromocytoma.[52,53,74,79,80] The combination of elevated plasma catecholamines and increased 24-hour urinary total metanephrines was found to have a 100% positive predictive value in a study of 78 pheochromocytomas and 27 paragangliomas at the Cleveland Clinic.[81]

Chromogranin A, a protein that is stored and released in conjunction with catecholamines, is increased in patients with pheochromocytoma. It is, however, also produced by other neuroendocrine tumors and therefore is not specific.[82]

Equivocal results of baseline plasma and urinary tests require further evaluation, which is best obtained by collecting samples during a paroxysm. Urine can be collected for 4 hours after an attack and quantitated per milligram of creatinine. Provocative agents such as glucagon, histamine, and tyramine can precipitate hypertensive crises and are not recommended. The clonidine suppression test is based on the assumption that catecholamines from an autonomous source do not respond to pharmacologic suppression of the sympathetic nervous system.[83] According to this test, the usefulness of which is controversial, plasma catecholamines in patients without pheochromocytoma should decrease to less than 500 pg/mL 3 hours after ingestion of 0.3 mg of oral clonidine.

Radiologic Localization

Computed tomography and magnetic resonance imaging are both excellent techniques for imaging adrenal masses. As previously stated, however, their ability to distinguish cause is not always optimal. In a review of 78 patients with pheochromocytoma and 27 patients with paraganglioma, computed tomography was 98% sensitive and 69% specific, whereas magnetic resonance imaging was 100% sensitive and 67% specific.[81] ^{131}I-metaiodobenzylguanidine (^{131}I-MIBG) scintigraphy was found in the same study to be 78% sensitive and 100% specific.[81] Functional extraadrenal or multiple pheochromocytomas, as may occur with familial, recurrent, or metastatic disease, can be localized with ^{131}I-MIBG scintigraphy.[84,85] There is, however, a 10% false-negative rate, which is thought to be caused largely by inconsistencies in tumor uptake of radioisotope.[84,85]

Malignant Pheochromocytoma

Because definitive pathologic criteria for malignancy do not exist for pheochromocytoma, careful clinical, biochemical, and radiologic follow-up is essential. Malignant tumors metastasize, most often to the retroperitoneum, bones, lungs, and liver. Extraadrenal lesions have an increased frequency of malignancy.[86]

Schlumberger and colleagues[87] reported on 20 patients with malignant pheochromocytoma. Eleven had evidence of metastatic disease at initial presentation, 7 developed metastases at 10 to 30 months, 2 at 9 years, and 2 at 28 years. A high frequency of bone marrow involvement was found. Vascular invasion by tumor was considered to support a diagnosis of malignant disease. Immunohistochemical analysis revealed elevated levels of neuron-specific enolase, which is usually normal in benign pheochromocytoma. Increased levels of dopamine and its metabolites, homovanillic acid and methoxytyramine, were thought to be related to cellular dedifferentiation and were a negative prognostic factor.[87]

Nine benign and 11 malignant pheochromocytomas were evaluated by Helman and associates[88] for neuropeptide Y mRNA expression. Neuropeptide Y is normally found in the adrenal medulla and in sympathetic nerves. All of the benign tumors but only four of the malignant tumors studied expressed neuropeptide Y mRNA, suggesting that absence of neuropeptide Y may be indicative of malignancy.[88]

DNA ploidy studies of nuclei from 62 pheochromocytomas were performed by flow cytometry and correlated with clinical course.[89] Eight of 26 patients with tetraploid and polyploid peaks and 7 of 18 patients with aneuploid peaks had malignant tumors. The lesions of all 18 patients with normal DNA proved to be clinically benign.[89] A retrospective analysis by the Cleveland Clinic of 78 patients with pheochromocytoma and 27 patients with paraganglioma concluded that two predictive factors of subsequent malignancy were a size greater than 5 cm and an extraadrenal location.[81]

INCIDENTAL ADRENAL MASS

The evaluation and treatment of asymptomatic adrenal masses is controversial. The prevalence of adrenocortical carcinoma and pheochromocytoma among incidental adrenal masses is 58 and 6500 per 100,000, respectively.[90] Adrenal masses that have endocrine activity should be resected. Absolute surgical removal has been advocated by various authors for nonfunctional adrenal masses that measure as much as 3.5 cm,[91] 5 cm,[16,46] or 6 cm[92,93] in diameter. Although no consensus exists, resection should be strongly considered for any adrenal mass larger than 5 cm.

In any adrenal lesion, despite lack of clinical signs and symptoms, true biologic inactivity must be documented. Screening should be individualized and clinically directed but should include the following: (1) electrolytes with particular attention to potassium, (2) 24-hour urine for metanephrines and catecholamines, (3) 24-hour urine for cortisol, (4) plasma renin, aldosterone, and DOC levels in hypertensive patients, and (5) 17-KS, androgens, and estrogens.

It has been suggested that a 1-mg overnight dexamethasone suppression test should be part of the screening criteria for an incidental adrenal mass.[93] Subtle cortisol-producing tumors were identified in 8 (12%) of 68[93] patients in one study and in 6 (5%) of 122[94] patients in another study of incidental adrenal masses and preclinical Cushing's syndrome.

Noninvasive studies, including the functional nuclear medicine scans described, should also be considered. Fine-needle biopsy entails multiple risks, especially in pheochromocytoma. This procedure should be judiciously used; it probably should be reserved for patients with possible metastatic disease.

In patients with a nonfunctional adrenal mass measuring 3.5 to 5 cm who do not have a prior history of malignancy, hormonal and radiologic follow-up is essential at 3 months,[90] then at 6 months, and yearly thereafter if unchanged. Careful hormonal evaluation is warranted, because initially inactive tumors can become hormonally active.[95] In patients with a known nonadrenal malignancy, close observation and potentially aggressive management are recommended.

REFERENCES

1. Icard P, Chapuis Y, Andreassian B, Bernard A, Proye C. Adrenocortical carcinoma in surgically treated patients: a retrospective study on 156 cases by the French Association of Endocrine Surgery. Surgery 1992; 112:972.
2. Neblett WW, Frexes-Steed M, Scott HW. Experience with adrenocortical neoplasms in childhood. Am Surg 1987;53:117.
3. Pommier RF, Brennan MF. An eleven-year experience with adrenocortical carcinoma. Surgery 1992;112:963.
4. Venkatesh S, Hickey RC, Sellin RV, Fernandez, JF, Samaan NA. Adrenal cortical carcinoma. Cancer 1989;64:765.
5. Henley DJ, van Heerden JA, Grant CS, Carney JA, Carpenter PC. Adrenal cortical carcinoma: a continuing challenge. Surgery 1983;94: 926.
6. Søreide JA, Brabrand K, Thoresen Sø. Adrenal cortical carcinoma in Norway, 1970–1984. World J Surg 1992;16:663.
7. Hamwi GJ, Serbin RA, Kruger FA. Does adrenocortical hyperplasia result in adrenocortical carcinoma? N Engl J Med 1957;257:1153.
8. van Seters AP, van Aalderen, Moolenaar AJ, Gorsiro MCB, van Roon F, Backer ET. Adrenocortical tumour in untreated congenital adrenocortical hyperplasia associated with inadequate ACTH suppressibility. Clin Endocrinol (Oxf) 1981;14:325.
9. Shimshi M, Ross F, Goodman A, Gabrilove JL. Virilizing adrenocortical tumor superimposed on congenital adrenocortical hyperplasia. Am J Med 1992;93:338.
10. Yano T, Linehan M, Anglard P, et al. Genetic changes in human adrenocortical carcinomas. J Natl Cancer Inst 1989;81:518.
11. Henry I, Grandjouan S, Couillin P, et al. Tumor-specific loss of 11p15.5 alleles in del11p13 Wilms tumor and in familial adrenocortical carcinoma. Proc Natl Acad Sci U S A 1989;86:3247.
12. Henry I, Jeanpierre M, Couillin P, et al. Molecular definition of the 11p15.5 region involved in Beckwith-Wiedemann syndrome and probably in predisposition to adrenocortical carcinoma. Hum Genet 1989; 81:273.
13. Gicquel C, Bertagna X, Schneid H, et al. Rearrangements at the 11p15 locus and overexpression of insulin-like growth factor-II gene in sporadic adrenocortical tumors. J Clin Endocrinol Metab 1994;78:1444.
14. Hao Y, Crenshaw T, Moulton T, Newcomb E, Tycko B. Tumour-suppressor activity of *H19* RNA. Nature 1993;365,764.
15. Luton JP, Cerdas S, Billaud L, et al. Clinical features of adrenocortical carcinoma, prognostic factors, and the effect of mitotane therapy. N Engl J Med 1990;322:1195.
16. Pommier RF, Brennan MF. Management of adrenal neoplasms. Curr Probl Surg 1991;28:661.
17. Cagle PT, Hough AJ, Pysher TJ, et al. Comparison of adrenal cortical tumors in children and adults. Cancer 1986;57:2235.
18. Wohltmann H, Mathur RS, Williamson HO, Wesley E, Moody L, Landgrebe S. Sexual precocity in a female infant due to feminizing adrenal carcinoma. J Clin Endocrinol Metab 1980;50:186.
19. Gabrilove JL, Sharma DC, Wotiz HH, Dorfman RI. Feminizing adrenocortical tumors in the male: a review of 52 cases including a case report. Medicine (Baltimore) 1965;44:37.
20. Gabrilove JL, Nicolis GL, Hausknecht RU, Wotiz HH. Feminizing adrenocortical carcinoma in a man. Cancer 1970;25:153.
21. Arteaga E, Biglieri EG, Kater CE, Lopez, JM, Schambelan M. Aldoste-

rone-producing adrenocortical carcinoma: preoperative recognition and course in three cases. Ann Intern Med 1984;101:316.
22. Farge D, Chatellier G, Pagny JY, Jeunemaitre X, Plouin PF, Corvol P. Isolated clinical syndrome of primary aldosteronism in four patients with adrenocortical carcinoma. Am J Med 1987;83:635.
23. Greathouse DJ, McDermott MT, Kidd GS, Hofeldt FD. Pure primary hyperaldosteronism due to adrenal cortical carcinoma. Am J Med 1984; 76:1132.
24. Scott HW, Sussman CR, Page DL, Thompson NW, Gross MD, Lloyd R. Primary hyperaldosteronism caused by adrenocortical carcinoma. World J Surg 1986;10:646.
25. Slee PHThJ, Schaberg A, van Brummelen P. Carcinoma of the adrenal cortex causing primary hyperaldosteronism: a case report and review of the literature. Cancer 1983;51:2341.
26. Bertagna C, Orth DN. Clinical and laboratory findings and results of therapy in 58 patients with adrenocortical tumors admitted to a single medical center (1951 to 1978). Am J Med 1981;71:855
27. Sakai Y, Yanase T, Hara T, Takayanagi R, Haji M, Nawata H. Mechanism of abnormal production of adrenal androgens in patients with adrenocortical adenomas and carcinomas. J Clin Endocrinol Metab 1994;78:36.
28. Imperato-McGinley J, Young IS, Huang T, Dreyfus JC Reckler JM, Peterson RE. Testosterone secreting adrenal cortical adenomas. Int J Gynaecol Obstet 1981;19:421.
29. Lipsett MB, Wilson H. Adrenocortical cancer: steroid biosynthesis and metabolism evaluated by urinary metabolites. J Clin Endocrinol Metab 1962;22:906.
30. Lipsett MB, Hertz R, Ross GT. Clinical and pathophysiologic aspects of adrenocortical carcinoma. Am J Med 1963;35:374.
31. McKenna TJ, Miller RB, Liddle GW. Plasma pregnenolone and 17-OH-pregnenolone in patients with adrenal tumors, ACTH excess, or idiopathic hirsutism. J Clin Endocrinol Metab 1977;44:231.
32. Gabrilove JL, Seman AT, Sabet R, Mitty HA, Nicolis GL. Virilizing adrenal adenoma with studies on the steroid content of the adrenal venous effluent and a review of the literature. Endocr Rev 1981;2: 4622.
33. McKenna TJ, O'Connell Y, Cunningham S, McCabe M, Culliton M. Steroidogenesis in an estrogen-producing adrenal tumor in a young woman: comparison with steroid profiles associated with cortisol- and androgen-producing tumors. J Clin Endocrinol Metab 1990;70:228.
34. Irony I, Biglieri EG, Perloff D, Rubinoff H. Pathophysiology of deoxycorticosterone-secreting adrenal tumors. J Clin Endocrinol Metab 1987; 65:836.
35. Kelly WF, O'Hare MJ, Loizou S, Davies D, Laing I. Hypermineralocorticism without excessive aldosterone secretion: an adrenal carcinoma producing deoxycorticosterone. Clin Endocrinol (Oxf) 1982;17:353.
36. Dichek HL, Nieman LK, Oldfield EH, Pass HI, Malley JD, Cutler GB. A comparison of the standard high dose dexamethasone suppression test and the overnight 8-mg dexamethasone suppression test for the differential diagnosis of adrenocorticotropin-dependent Cushing's syndrome. J Clin Endocrinol Metab 1994;78:418.
37. Flack MR, Oldfield EH, Cutler GB, et al. Urine free cortisol in the high-dose dexamethasone suppression test for the differential diagnosis of the Cushing syndrome. Ann Intern Med 1992;116:211.
38. Raff H, Findling JW. A new immunoradiometric assay for corticotropin evaluated in normal subjects and patients with Cushing's syndrome. Clin Chem 1989;35:596.
39. Spark RF, Connolly PB, Gluckin DS, White R, Sacks B, Landsberg L. ACTH secretion from a functioning pheochromocytoma. N Engl J Med 1979;301:416.
40. Nieman LK, Chrousos GP, Oldfield EH, Avgerinos PC, Cutler GB, Loriaux DL. The ovine corticotropin-releasing hormone stimulation test and the dexamethasone suppression test in the differential diagnosis of Cushing's syndrome. Ann Intern Med 1986;105:862.
41. Oldfield EH, Doppman JL, Nieman LK, et al. Petrosal sinus sampling with and without corticotropin-releasing hormone for the differential diagnosis of Cushing's syndrome. N Engl J Med 1991;325:8997.
42. Reinig JW, Doppman JL, Dwyer AJ, Frank J. MRI of indeterminate adrenal masses. AJR Am J Roentgenol 1986;147:493.
43. Chang A, Glazer HS, Lee JKT, Ling D, Heiken JP. Adrenal gland: MR imaging. Radiology 1987;163:123.
44. Gross MD, Shapiro B, Bouffard A, et al. Distinguishing benign from malignant euadrenal masses. Ann Intern Med 1988;109:613.
45. Wick MR, Cherwitz DL, McGlennen RC, Dehner LP. Adrenocortical carcinoma: an immunohistochemical comparison with renal cell carcinoma. Am J Pathol 1986;122:343.
46. Brennan MF. Adrenocortical carcinoma. CA Cancer J Clin 1987;37: 349.
47. Hough AJ, Hollifield JW, Page DL, Hartmann WH. Prognostic factors in adrenal cortical tumors: a mathematical analysis of clinical and morphologic data. Am J Clin Pathol 1979;72:390.
48. Van Slooten H, Schaberg A, Smeenk D, Moolenaar AJ. Morphologic characteristics of benign and malignant adrenocortical tumors. Cancer 1985;55:766.
49. Weiss LM, Medeiros LJ, Vickery AL. Pathologic features of prognostic significance in adrenocortical carcinoma. Am J Surg Pathol 1989;13: 202.
50. MacFarlane DA. Cancer of the adrenal cortex: the natural history, prognosis and treatment in a study of fifty-five cases. Ann R Coll Surg Engl 1958;23;155.
51. Sullivan M, Boileau M, Hodges CV. Adrenal cortical carcinoma. J Urol 1978;120:660.
52. Shapiro B, Fig LM. Management of pheochromocytoma. Endocrinol Metab Clin North Am 1989;18:443.
53. Samaan NA, Hickey RC. Pheochromocytoma. Semin Oncol 1987;14: 297.
54. Averbuch SD, Steakley CS, Young RC, et al. Malignant pheochromocytoma: effective treatment with a combination of cyclophosphamide, vincristine, and dacarbazine. Ann Intern Med 1988;109:267.
55. Lairmore TC, Dou S, Howe Jr, et al. A 1.5-megabase yeast artificial chromosome contig from human chromosome 10q11.2 connecting three genetic loci (*RET, D10S94,* and *D10S102*) closely linked to the *MEN2A* locus. Proc Natl Acad Sci U S A 1993;90:492.
56. Gardner E, Papi L, Easton DF, et al. Genetic linkage studies map the multiple endocrine neoplasia type 2 loci to a small interval on chromosome 10q11.2. Hum Mol Genet 1993;2:241.
57. Mole SE, Mulligan LM, Healey CS, Ponder BAJ, Tunnacliffe A. Localisation of the gene for multiple endocrine neoplasia type 2A to a 480 kb region in chromosome band 10q11.2. Hum Mol Genet 1993;2:247.
58. Norum RA, Lafreniere RG, O'Neal LW, et al. Linkage of the multiple endocrine neoplasia type 2B gene (MEN2B) to chromosome 10 markers linked to MEN2A. Genomics 1990;8:313.
59. Lairmore TC, Howe JR, Korte JA, et al. Familial medullary thyroid carcinoma and multiple endocrine neoplasia type 2B map to the same region of chromosome 10 as multiple endocrine neoplasia type 2A. Genomics 1991;9:181.
60. Khosla S, Patel VM, Hay ID, et al. Loss of heterozygosity suggests multiple genetic alterations in pheochromocytomas and medullary thyroid carcinomas. J Clin Invest 1991;87:1691.
61. Moley JF, Brother MB, Fong CT, et al. Consistent association of 1p loss of heterozygosity with pheochromocytomas from patients with multiple endocrine neoplasia type 2 syndromes. Cancer Res 1992;52: 770.
62. Mulligan LM, Kwok JBJ Healey CS, et al. Germ-line mutations of the *RET* proto-oncogene in multiple endocrine neoplasia type 2A. Nature 1993;363:458.
63. Donis-Keller H, Dou S, Chi D, et al. Mutations in the *RET* proto-oncogene are associated with MEN 2A and FMTC. Hum Mol Genet 1993;2:851.
64. Mulligan LM, Eng C, Healey CS, et al. Specific mutations of the *RET* proto-oncogene are related to disease phenotype in MEN 2A and FMTC. Nat Genet 1994;6:70.
65. Hofstra RMW, Landsvater RM, Ceccherini I, et al. A mutation in the *RET* proto-oncogene associated with multiple endocrine neoplasia type 2B and sporadic medullary thyroid carcinoma. Nature 1994;367:375.
66. Carlson KM, Dou S, Chi D, et al. Single missense mutation in the tyrosine kinase catalytic domain of the *RET* protooncogene is associated with multiple endocrine neoplasia type 2B. Proc Natl Acad Sci U S A 1994;91:1579.
67. Romeo G, Ronchetto P, Lou Y, et al. Point mutations affecting the tyrosine kinase domain of the *RET* proto-oncogene in Hirschsprung's disease. Nature 1994;367:377.
68. Edery P, Lyonnet S, Mulligan LM, et al. Mutations of the *RET* proto-oncogene in Hirschsprung's disease. Nature 1994;367:378.
69. Van Heyningen V. One gene: four syndromes. Nature 1994;367:319.
70. Lin SR, Lee YJ, Tsai JH. Mutations of the *p53* gene in human functional adrenal neoplasms . J Clin Endocrinol Metab 1994;78:483.
71. Moley JF, Brother MB, Wells SA, Spengler BA, Biedler JL, Brodeur

GM. Low frequency of *ras* gene mutations in neuroblastomas, pheochromocytomas and medullary thyroid cancers. Cancer Res 1991;51: 1596.
72. Raisanen J, Shapiro B, Glazer GM, Desai S, Sisson JC. Plasma catecholamines in pheochromocytoma: effect of urographic contrast media. AJR Am J Roentgenol 1984;143:43.
73. Radin DR, Ralls PW, Boswell WD, Colletti PM, Lapin SA, Halls JM. Pheochromocytoma: detection by unenhanced CT. AJR Am J Roentgenol 1986;146:741.
74. Bravo EL. Pheochromocytoma: new concepts and future trends. Kidney Int 1991;40:544.
75. Imperato-McGinley J, Gautier T, Ehlers K, Zullo MA, Goldstein DS, Vaughan ED. Reversibility of catecholamine-induced dilated cardiomyopathy in a child with a pheochromocytoma. N Engl J Med 1987; 316:793.
76. Gordon DL, Atamian SD, Brooks MH, et al. Fever in pheochromocytoma. Arch Intern Med 1992;152:1269.
77. Stenström G, Sjöström L, Smith U. Diabetes mellitus in pheochromocytoma: fasting blood glucose levels before and after surgery in 60 patients with pheochromocytoma. Acta Endocrinol (Copenh) 1984;106: 511.
78. Stewart AF, Hoecker JL, Mallette LE, et al. Hypercalcemia in pheochromocytoma: evidence for a novel mechanism. Ann Intern Med 1985; 102:776.
79. Sheps SG, Jiang NS, Klee GG. Diagnostic evaluation of pheochromocytoma. Endocrinol Metab Clin North Am 1988;17:397.
80. Gifford RW, Manger WM, Bravo EL. Pheochromocytoma. Endocrinol Metab Clin North Am 1994;23:387.
81. Bravo EL, Nie KR, Gifford RW. Impact of modern technology on the diagnosis and prognosis of pheochromocytoma. 76th Annual Meeting of the Endocrine Society, Anaheim, California, June 15–18, 1994, p 285. Abstract 339.
82. O'Connor DT, Deftos LJ. Secretion of chromogranin A by peptide-producing endocrine neoplasms. N Engl J Med 1986;314:1145.
83. Bravo EL, Tarazi RC, Fouad FM, Vidt DG, Gifford RW. Clonidine-suppression test: a useful aid in the diagnosis of pheochromocytoma. N Engl J Med 1981;305:623.
84. Chatal JF, Charbonnel B. Comparison of iodobenzylguanidine imaging with computed tomography in locating pheochromocytoma. J Clin Endocrinol Metab 1985;61:769.
85. Velchik MG, Alavi A, Kressel HY, Engelman K. Localization of pheochromocytoma: MIBG, CT, and MRI correlation. J Nucl Med 1989; 30:328.
86. Van Heerden JA, Sheps SG, Hamberger B, Sheedy PF, Poston JG, ReMine WH. Pheochromocytoma: current status and changing trends. Surgery 1982;91:367.
87. Schlumberger M, Gicquel C, Lumbroso J, et al. Malignant pheochromocytoma: clinical, biological, histologic and therapeutic data in a series of 20 patients with distant metastases. J Endocrinol Invest 1992; 15:631.
88. Helman LJ, Cohen PS, Averbuch SD, Cooper MJ, Keiser HR, Israel MA. Neuropeptide Y expression distinguishes malignant from benign pheochromocytoma. J Clin Oncol 1989;7:1720.
89. Hosaka Y, Rainwater LM, Grant CS, Farrow GM, van Heerden JA, Lieber MM. Pheochromocytoma: nuclear deoxyribonucleic acid patterns studied by flow cytometry. Surgery 1986;100:1003.
90. Ross NS, Aron DC. Hormonal evaluation of the patient with an incidentally discovered adrenal mass. N Engl J Med 1990;323:1401.
91. Katz RL, Shirkhoda A. Diagnostic approach to incidental adrenal nodules in the cancer patient. Cancer 1985;55:1995.
92. Copeland PM. The incidentally discovered adrenal mass. Ann Intern Med 1983;98:940.
93. Reincke M, Nieke J, Krestin GP, Saeger W, Allolio B, Winkelmann W. Preclinical Cushing's syndrome in adrenal "incidentalomas": comparison with adrenal Cushing's syndrome. J Clin Endocrinol Metab 1992;75:826.
94. McLeod MK, Thompson NW, Gross MD, Bondeson AG, Bondeson L. Sub-clinical Cushing's syndrome in patients with adrenal gland incidentalomas. Am Surg 1990;56:398.
95. Jockenhövel F, Kuck W, Hauffa B, et al. Conservative and surgical management of incidentally discovered adrenal tumors (incidentalomas). J Endocrinol Invest 1992;15:331.

Principles and Practice of Genitourinary Oncology, edited by Derek Raghavan, Howard I. Scher, Steven A. Leibel, and Paul H. Lange. Lippincott-Raven Publishers, Philadelphia, © 1997.

CHAPTER 97

Surgical Management of Adrenal Tumors

Michael O. Koch and Joseph A. Smith, Jr.

Tumors of the adrenal gland include a variety of benign and malignant lesions. Because of their location, they rarely are detectable because of symptomatic local growth or by physical examination. Most often, adrenal cancers are either detected because they are functionally active or diagnosed incidentally.

Adrenal cancer, whether adrenocortical carcinoma or a pheochromocytoma, requires surgical excision. Although adjuvant therapies exist and can have some palliative benefit, there is no curative therapy for unresectable adrenal cancers.

As with most surgical procedures, the operative approach is dictated partly by the preference and experience of the operating surgeon. However, there are anatomic and functional peculiarities of adrenal cancers that demand particular attention to surgical details and knowledge of appropriate incisions and surgical approaches.

PHEOCHROMOCYTOMA

Pheochromocytoma is a relatively uncommon and treacherous tumor that occurs in 1 to 2 per 100,000 adults. It represents one of the curable forms of hypertension, however, and it occurs in 0.1% to 2% of the hypertensive population.[1–4]

Pheochromocytomas are unique neoplasms because their treatment and management spans medicine and surgery, adult and pediatric care, and medical specialties from cardiology to oncology to genetics. Moreover, the effects of sustained catecholamine excess causes significant changes in virtually all organs, further complicating the care of these patients. No other neoplasm requires such a breadth of experience and knowledge for diagnosis and management.

Clinical Features

The most prominent presenting features of pheochromocytoma are related to catecholamine excess. Hypertension is seen in 30% to 65% of patients[5] and can occur in either a sustained or a paroxysmal form. The form of hypertension has important clinical implications: patients with paroxysmal hypertension are more likely to become normotensive after excision of the tumor.[6] Other symptoms caused by catecholamine excess include headache, palpitations, tremor, nervousness, weakness, and weight loss. In patients with large nonfunctional paragangliomas, pain or a palpable mass may be the primary presenting feature (Fig. 97-1). Finally, some patients present with clinical conditions produced by chronic catecholamine excess, such as cardiomyopathy or myocardial infarction, azotemia, encephalopathy, cerebrovascular accidents, and rarely, glucose intolerance. Many of these conditions are reversible with the elimination of the source of catecholamine production or pharmacologic blockade.[7–10]

Pheochromocytomas are seen in nonfamilial and familial variants. The familial forms of pheochromocytoma account for 5% to 10% of patients and are seen in two types of hereditary syndromes. Sipple's syndrome, or multiple endocrine neoplasia type II (MEN2), is the hereditary syndrome most strongly associated with pheochromocytoma. This has an autosomal dominant pattern of inheritance and has been classified into two forms: MEN2A, which includes the association of medullary carcinoma of the thyroid, parathyroid adenomas, and pheochromocytoma, and MEN2B, which is the same syndrome as MEN2A with the additional association of multiple mucosal neuromas, thickened corneal nerves, intestinal ganglioneuromatosis, and a marfanoid habitus. The MEN2 syndromes are thought to occur as the result of an abnormality of a genetic locus on chromosome 10.

The other hereditary syndromes associated with pheochromocytomas are the neuroectodermal dysplasias. These dysplasias include von Recklinghausen's disease (neurofibromatosis), tuberous sclerosis, Sturge-Weber syndrome, and von Hippel-Lindau disease. These are caused by separate genetic abnormalities, for example, the von Hippel-Lindau gene is located on the short arm of chromosome 3.[11] Pheochromocytomas associated with MEN2 and, possibly, the neuroectodermal dysplasias present unique management problems in that they are frequently bilateral and multifocal.

Preoperative Preparation

The major strides that have been made in the surgical management of pheochromocytoma are in large part a result of the preoperative preparation of these patients. Chronic catecholamine excess results in contraction of extracellular fluid vol-

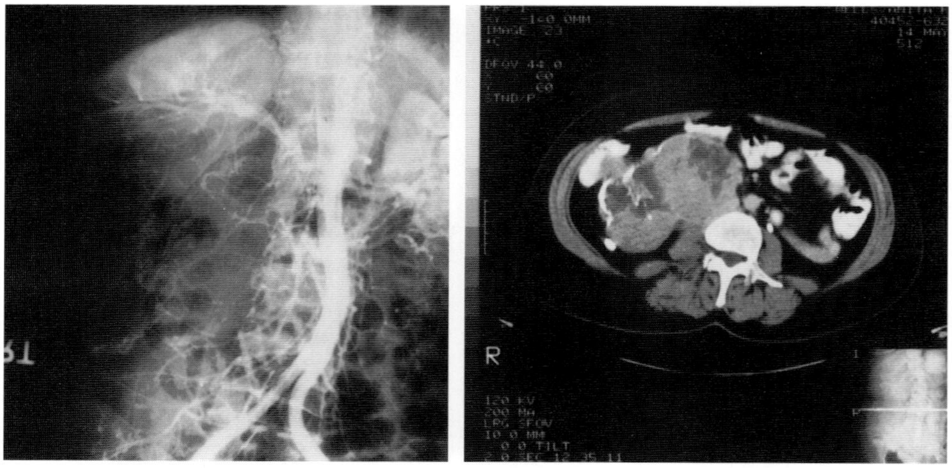

A B

FIG. 97-1. Large nonfunctional retroperitoneal paraganglioma. Notice the displacement of the kidney and aorta on both the arteriogram (**A**) and on computed tomography (**B**). Arteriography demonstrates the neovascular nature of this lesion.

ume. Consequently, the primary goal of preoperative preparation is to control the hypertension and reestablish a normal extracellular fluid volume. If this is not done, the sudden elimination of the source of catecholamines results in cardiovascular collapse.

Most centers favor preoperative preparation with phenoxybenzamine, which irreversibly binds to α-receptors. This drug should be given in daily divided doses of 20 to 200 mg, with an initial starting dose of 10 to 30 mg/day increased by 10 to 20 mg/day until the blood pressure stabilizes and the patient shows evidence of orthostasis. Some authors have advocated the routine use of β-blockade with propranolol. Most, however, recommend that its use be restricted to those patients with cardiac arrhythmias as a prominent presenting feature. The risk of β-blockade is that, after excision of the pheochromocytoma, any chronotropic cardiac response that would normally occur because of a decrease in systemic vascular resistance will be ablated. In addition, β-blockade can have a dramatic paradoxic effect on the patient's blood pressure. β-Stimulation of the peripheral vasculature causes vasodilatation. Blockade of β-receptors without complete α-blockade allows unopposed vasoconstriction by the catecholamines produced by the tumor. Consequently, β-blockade should never be considered until full α-blockade is achieved.

In addition to the use of phenoxybenzamine and propranolol, metyrosine may be used.[12] Metyrosine inhibits tyrosine hydroxylase, which converts tyrosine to dihydroxyphenylalanine. This is the rate-limiting step in catecholamine synthesis. Although the routine use of metyrosine is not widely accepted, nonrandomized studies suggest that it may result in better intraoperative blood pressure control, less blood loss, and a decreased need for intraoperative fluid replacement. However, metyrosine has significant side effects, including central nervous system depression, vivid dreams, behavior disturbances, and diarrhea. Metyrosine is usually administered in doses of 250 mg to 500 mg three times daily. It may have its greatest usefulness in the setting of malignant pheochromocytoma.

Some institutions recommend the use of selective α_1-blockers, such as prazosin, and claim results equal to those reported with phenoxybenzamine.[13] In contrast to phenoxybenzamine, prazosin does not irreversibly bind to the α-receptor, and the α-blocking effects can be overcome by high intraoperative levels of catecholamines.[14] Anecdotal reports suggest that it is not as effective as phenoxybenzamine. Labetalol and similar medications, which have both α- and β-blocking activity, have also been purported to be useful in the management of these patients.[15] The β-blocking effects of labetalol are 4 to 16 times more potent that its α-blocking effects. Consequently, these drugs have been associated with a paradoxic hypertensive response in which the vasodilatory β-effects are blocked but the vasoconstrictive α-effects are unchecked as the α-blocking effects of labetalol are overcome with a sudden catecholamine surge.[16,17]

Perioperative hypertensive crisis can be effectively controlled with intravenous phentolamine or nitroprusside, and norepinephrine can be administered for hypotension. Intraoperative anesthetic management of the patient undergoing surgical resection of a pheochromocytoma should be directed at control of the cardiovascular system. Monitoring of the blood pressure with an arterial cannula and of central filling pressures, usually with a Swann-Gantz catheter, should be strongly considered. Because of the uncertain volume status of these patients, the assessment of central filling pressures can be difficult without invasive monitoring. Moreover, large swings in intraoperative blood pressure, which can occur as a result of catecholamine excess or sudden loss of catecholamines, can make the assessment of volume status difficult.

Surgical Approaches

Most commonly, pheochromocytomas are approached through a thoracoabdominal or transverse transperitoneal (chevron) incision. Although standard flank or posterior approaches are used for benign adenomas and occasionally for adrenocortical cancer, they do not lend themselves to intraoperative examination of the entire abdomen, as is advisable for patients with pheochromocytomas. This is particularly the case for children, patients with MEN2 syndromes, and patients with neuroectodermal dysplasias, who are more prone to multifocal disease.

The standard thoracoabdominal approach involves placing the patient up 30° on the ipsilateral side. The arm is usually supported over the head on an ether screen or other arm support

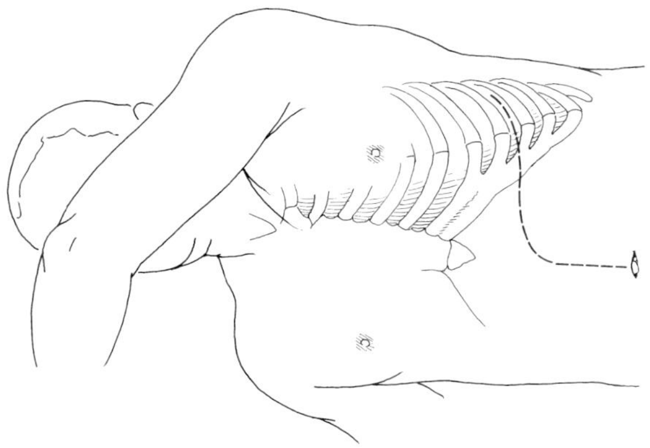

FIG. 97-2. Patient positioning and incision for thoracoabdominal approach to a large adrenal mass. The incision can be extended inferiorly for extremely large tumors.

(Fig. 97-2). The incision is extended through the intercostal cartilage between the ninth and tenth (or eighth and ninth) ribs and medially to a point midway between the umbilicus and the xyphoid process. For very large tumors, this incision can be extended down in the midline toward the umbilicus. The peritoneum is entered first, and the liver is palpated for evidence of metastatic disease. Intercostal muscles are then divided, taking care to identify the pleura as it is encountered. If the pleura is not identified, it is easy to inadvertently divide the diaphragm in an inappropriate location. After the diaphragm is initially divided, the diaphragmatic incision should be extended posterolaterally, leaving approximately 3 to 4 cm of diaphragm attached laterally for later closure. It is advisable to keep the incision lateral, however, so as to denervate as little of the diaphragmatic muscle as possible. A deep diaphragmatic incision should be made to allow cephalad retraction of the liver or spleen.

On the right, the dissection is begun by incising the peritoneal reflection lateral to the ascending colon, well past the hepatocolic ligament (Fig. 97-3). The colon and duodenum are reflected medially to expose the anterior surface of the inferior vena cava. The liver can be more completely mobilized by dividing the falciform ligament between clamps and then using electrocautery to completely divide the falciform and coronary ligaments all the way back to the bare area of the liver. In addition, it facilitates cephalad retraction of the liver to divide the right triangular ligament of the liver between the liver and the diaphragm. With large adrenal masses it may be necessary to further mobilize the liver. The peritoneum should be incised as it reflects off of the liver to the anterior surface of the adrenal mass. The liver can then be dissected bluntly off the anterior surface of the mass. Usually, inferior hepatic veins run between the caudate lobe of the liver and the vena cava. With cephalad retraction of the liver, these can be avulsed, and bleeding can be significant. By incision of the peritoneum between the liver and vena cava in this location, these veins can be identified, ligated with suture, and divided if necessary for adequate surgical exposure. After the adrenal gland is properly exposed, it is best to ligate the adrenal vein that drains into the posterolateral aspect of the vena cava. This vein can be exposed by medial rotation of the vena cava, either with the hand or with a surgical sponge stick. The vein should be doubly ligated with silk suture and divided. The anesthesiologist should be warned before the adrenal vein is ligated, because a precipitous drop in blood pressure may occur.

The adrenal gland is then dissected circumferentially. The technique for this is frequently referred to as "dissecting the patient from the adrenal gland." Traction should be applied to the surrounding structures, not to the adrenal gland. Palpation of the tumor itself should be avoided in order to minimize catecholamine surges. It is best to start superiorly and laterally. By dissection around the tumor in this location, a clear plane down to the psoas fascia can usually be developed with minimal difficulty. Inferior retraction of the kidney facilitates exposure of the adrenal mass and allows exposure of the mass without palpation of the tumor itself (Fig. 97-4). Multiple small arteries from the inferior phrenic artery, capsular renal arteries, and renal artery can be controlled either with small ties or with surgical clips. Pheochromocytomas are frequently quite vascular, and hemostasis is of the essence in order to carry out a meticulous dissection. The last attachments that should be taken are between the superior pole of the kidney and the adrenal mass. If the adrenal tumor is adherent in this location, the surgeon can proceed with an intracapsular dissection; this is usually free and is usually a relatively bloodless field. If there is some question of contiguous extension to the kidney, however, the kidney should be removed en bloc with the adrenal.

With left adrenal tumors, the dissection is begun by taking down the peritoneal attachments to the left colon, well past the splenic flexure. Failure to do this past the splenic flexure may result in avulsion of a small portion of the splenic capsule from the intact spleen by pulling forces on the lienocolic ligament.

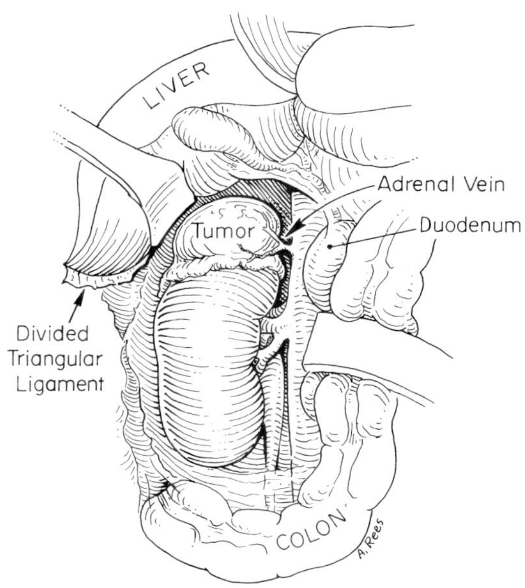

FIG. 97-3. Right radical adrenalectomy. The peritoneum between the right posterior lobe of the liver and adrenal, and the right triangular ligament of the liver, have been incised in order to retract the liver cephalad. The duodenum is fully kocherized in order to expose the anterior surface of the inferior vena cava. The short right adrenal vein exits the inferior vena cava posterolaterally to enter the right adrenal gland.

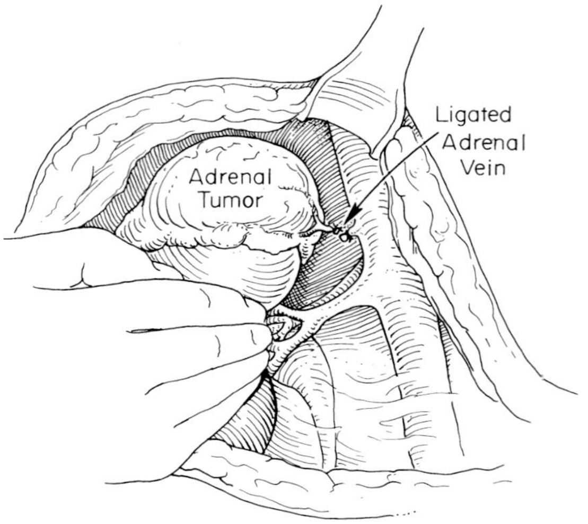

FIG. 97-4. Inferior traction on the adjacent kidney allows exposure of the superior attachments to the adrenal gland without actual palpation of the tumor. The attachments between the adrenal gland and kidney should be divided last.

The spleen can be reflected upward into the thorax with a thoracoabdominal incision after a plane is developed between the adrenal gland and the tail of the pancreas and splenic artery and vein (Fig. 97-5). At this point, the main adrenal vein draining into the renal vein can easily be identified and ligated between silk sutures. As with a right-sided pheochromocytoma, the superior and lateral attachments are taken first, followed by those to the superior pole of the kidney. Small surgical clips are often useful to secure hemostasis from the multiple small feeding arteries. The diaphragmatic incision is usually closed

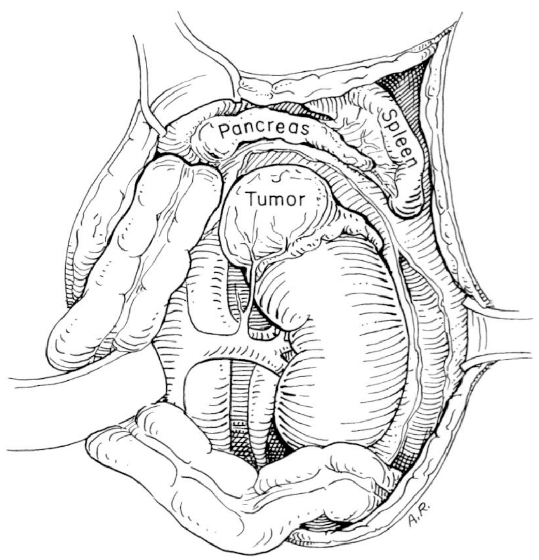

FIG. 97-5. Left radical adrenalectomy. The left colon has been fully mobilized to expose the anterior surface of the aorta. The peritoneum has been incised superiorly between the adrenal tumor and the spleen and tail of pancreas, so that these organs can be retracted superiorly. The left adrenal vein is seen emptying into the left renal vein.

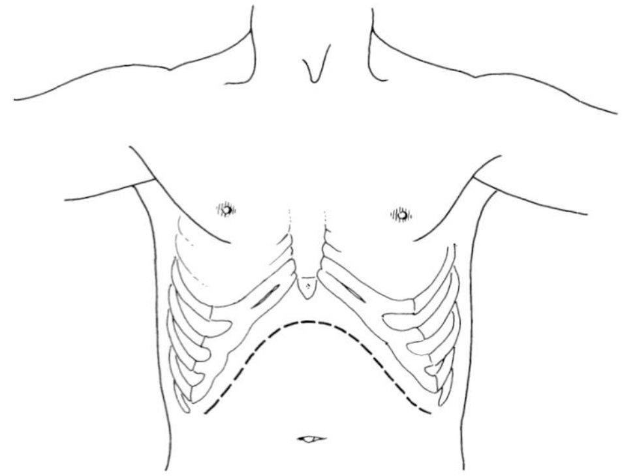

FIG. 97-6. A unilateral or bilateral subcostal (chevron) incision provides excellent exposure for small- to intermediate-sized tumors. It does not provide good exposure below the level of the aortic bifurcation, however. This incision provides the best surgical exposure if the back is slightly hyperextended and a self-retaining fixed retractor is used to lift the costal margin anteriorly and superiorly.

with vertical mattress sutures of 2-0 silk, and a chest tube is placed. The remainder of the wound is closed according to the surgeon's preference; usually, no drains are placed. Chest tube drainage is usually required only for 24 to 48 hours.

With a chevron or anterior transabdominal approach, the incision can usually be confined to the side of the tumor (Fig. 97-6). This still allows palpation along the great vessels for the detection of multifocal disease and the assessment of metastases. This incision does not lend itself to lower abdominal exposure, however. Bilateral exposure is a particular concern in the patient whose blood pressure does not normalize intraoperatively after adrenalectomy. Exposure with an anterior approach is facilitated by a self-retaining upper arm retractor or other retractor system that is fixed to the operative table. In patients with suspected malignant pheochromocytomas, en bloc dissections may include the ipsilateral kidney, a portion of the liver, the spleen, or even the tail of the pancreas (Fig. 97-7). It is imperative that all gross tissue be excised even in the setting of metastatic pheochromocytoma, because debulking of tumor tissue may have an important role in control of symptomatic disease.

Recently, there has been some enthusiasm for the use of a laparoscopic approach to adrenal tumors, including some pheochromocytomas. This has been accomplished with both a retroperitoneal and a transperitoneal approach. At present, the limited experience with this technique does not support a recommendation for its routine use in patients with pheochromocytomas.

Pheochromocytoma in Children

Pheochromocytomas in children are somewhat different from those in adults in that the hypertension is usually quite severe, and associated physiologic changes from chronic catecholamine excess are seen in most patients.[18] These changes include congestive heart failure, encephalopathy and even death. In a review of 71 cases of pheochromocytoma in children, Hume reported the frequent association of headaches, nausea, and

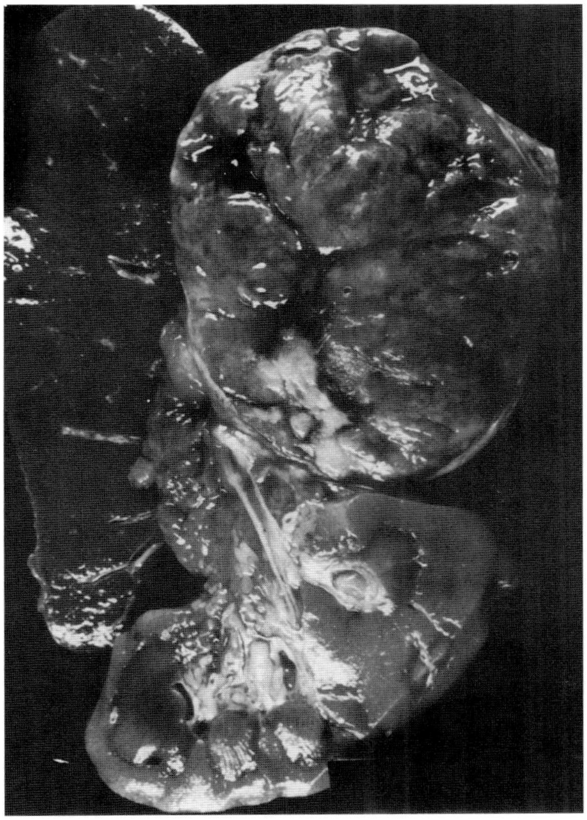

FIG. 97-7. En bloc resection of a malignant pheochromocytoma involving the renal hilum, tail of pancreas, and spleen.

vomiting in children.[19] More than half of children have visual complaints, and 70% present with funduscopic changes caused by accelerated hypertension. Most important in terms of planning surgical management is that almost half of the tumors seen in children are bilateral, multiple, or extraadrenal. The incidence of malignancy appears to be less than in adults, at approximately 2.5%. In a series of 100 children with pheochromocytoma, the single most important cause of death during the intraoperative and early postoperative period was an additional, undiscovered pheochromocytoma.[20] The overall operative mortality in this collected series was 22%. Because of the high incidence of multifocal disease, the general consensus is that transperitoneal exposure, including careful exploration of both adrenals, the periaortic area, and the retroperitoneal space, is essential. In children, a bilateral subcostal incision provides good exposure of all intraabdominal sites. One explanation for the higher incidence of multifocality in children may be the more frequent finding of a familial form of the disease in this setting.

Hereditary Pheochromocytoma

In the setting of MEN2A or MEN2B, there is a much higher incidence of multifocal disease. The most common problem with these patients, however, is medullary carcinoma of the thyroid, which accounts for the greatest percentage of deaths in most kindreds. In one series of 18 patients with medullary carcinoma of the thyroid, 15 had metastases at the time of surgery[21]; 8 of the 18 had pheochromocytomas, and 6 of these 8 had bilateral involvement. As with childhood pheochromocytoma, the incidence of malignant lesions appears to be less than in sporadic pheochromocytoma. Because of the high likelihood of development of bilateral tumors, some authors advocate bilateral adrenalectomy in all cases.[22,23] Others argue against routine bilateral adrenalectomy because of the associated risk of Addisonian crisis.

Lairmore and colleagues[24] reported on an extensive series of patients with MEN2 syndromes in which 23 patients with unilateral pheochromocytoma and a macroscopically normal contralateral adrenal gland underwent unilateral adrenalectomy. A pheochromocytoma developed in the remaining adrenal gland in 52% of patients; the mean duration between the initial adrenalectomy and the development of the new tumor was 12 years. Forty-three patients had both adrenal glands removed and 10 (23%) of these experienced at least one episode of acute adrenal insufficiency, including 1 patient who died of an Addisonian crisis.[24] Because of the low potential for malignancy of pheochromocytoma in these patients and the availability of radiographic studies such as ^{131}I-metaiodobenzylguanidine (^{131}I-MIBG) scintigraphy scans for surveillance, bilateral adrenalectomy need not be routinely performed. Moreover, medullary carcinoma of the thyroid accounts for the greatest percentage of deaths in these patients, and, consequently, bilateral adrenalectomy may not have a beneficial impact on survival. In those patients who did undergo bilateral adrenalectomy, microscopic nodular adrenal medullary hyperplasia was present in virtually all cases.[24]

Some authors have suggested that the size of the ipsilateral adrenal tumor be used as a criterion for bilateral adrenalectomy in the MEN2 syndromes. Tibblin and associates[25] reported on 13 patients with MEN2A with a mean follow-up of 7.4 years after unilateral adrenalectomy. In 8 of 9 patients in whom a contralateral pheochromocytoma did not develop, the presenting tumors were less than 5 cm is size; in the 4 patients with contralateral pheochromocytoma, the initial tumor was more than 5 cm. ^{131}I-MIBG scanning in this setting may lead to many false-positive results. Jansson and associates[26] studied ^{131}I-MIBG scans in 16 patients with MEN2 who did not have symptoms of pheochromocytoma, including a large subset of patients who had undergone previous unilateral adrenalectomy. Of 8 patients with a remaining unilateral adrenal gland, 7 had accumulation of the radionuclide. At exploration, only 2 of these were found to have pheochromocytomas, each less than 2 cm in diameter. All of these patients were normotensive and lacked symptoms referable to a pheochromocytoma and, hence, the clinical significance of the these lesions seemed minimal.

Prognosis in Pheochromocytoma

The 36-year experience of Vanderbilt University Medical Center with management of patients with pheochromocytoma was summarized by Scott and colleagues in 1987.[5] Sixty-three patients underwent excision of a pheochromocytoma; 11 (16%) patients had malignant disease, and 52 (84%) had benign disease with prolonged follow-up. In the group of 63 patients who underwent surgical excision of the tumor, there was a single perioperative death (1.5%). Of the 52 patients who underwent excision of tumors for benign disease, hypertension resolved in 40 (77%) and remained present in 12 (23%). All patients showed biochemical evidence of correction of their state of catecholamine excess. Of the 11 patients with metastatic pheochromocytoma, 3 had metastases at presentation and survived a mean of 2 years. Of the 8 patients who had apparent confined but malignant disease at presentation, mean survival time was 8 years, with the longest survivor living 17 years after presentation. This particular patient had undergone resection of an extensive tumor involving the splenic and renal vessels. Because of the long survival times that can be achieved even with regionally advanced disease, surgical resection is the standard of care whenever it is feasible. Because of the untoward effects of chronic catecholamine excess, resection of all tumor, even in patients with metastatic disease, should be considered if feasible.[27] The significant duration of survival of patients with metastatic disease supports this approach.

ADRENOCORTICAL CARCINOMA

Adrenal carcinomas can be functional or nonfunctional. Tumors may produce multiple compounds and may cause Cushing's syndrome, feminization in males, virilization in females, or hyperaldosteronism. Functional tumors can carry a worse prognosis than nonfunctioning lesions,[28] but the frequency with which adrenal cancers are reported to produce functional metabolites depends partially on the sensitivity and thoroughness of the assays used.[29]

Because adrenal carcinomas often attain a large size before diagnosis, they usually are associated with a poor prognosis. More recently, however, the frequent use of diagnostic abdominal ultrasonography and computed tomographic scanning has led to an increased incidental diagnosis of solid adrenal masses.[30,31] In some circumstances, this has allowed earlier diagnosis of adrenal cancer. More often, incidentally detected adrenal masses are benign but create dilemmas regarding appropriate diagnosis and satisfactory methods for exclusion of malignancy.

Most diagnosed adrenal malignancies are larger than 6 cm in size.[32,33] It is generally agreed that solid lesions exceeding 6 cm in size should be removed surgically. At the other end of the spectrum, solid adrenal masses of less than a few centimeters in size probably do not require surgical exploration or treatment if they are nonfunctioning.[34] The management of intermediate-sized (3- to 6-cm) nonfunctioning adrenal masses is controversial.[35–37] Although the substantial majority of these lesions are benign, some adrenal carcinomas may be detected incidentally when of this size. All functioning adrenal tumors should be excised.

Surgical Approach

The primary factors that influence the surgical approach to adrenal carcinoma are the anatomy and location of the adrenal gland, the tumor size, and the surgeon's experience. Avoidance of intraoperative manipulation or traction on the tumor is of less importance with carcinomas than with pheochromocytomas, where tumor metabolites may be introduced into the circulation and precipitate a hypertensive crisis. However, because of the relatively inaccessible location of the adrenal gland, the vascular and friable nature of the glandular tissue, and the short adrenal vein, especially on the right, adequate intraoperative exposure is essential.

For large adrenal cancers, a thoracoabdominal incision provides the optimal surgical exposure. This can be achieved by making an incision between the eighth and ninth (or ninth and tenth) ribs with division of the diaphragm and pleura. A flank incision with or without rib resection is adequate for some smaller tumors. A dorsal lumbotomy approach is usually reserved for benign lesions, but modified posterior incisions have been described for adrenal cancer.[38] An anterior approach through either a chevron or subcostal incision has the advantage of allowing intraoperative exploration and palpation or direct examination of the contralateral adrenal gland, if required.[39] However, a search for multiple tumors, as may be indicated with pheochromocytomas, is unnecessary with adrenal cancer.

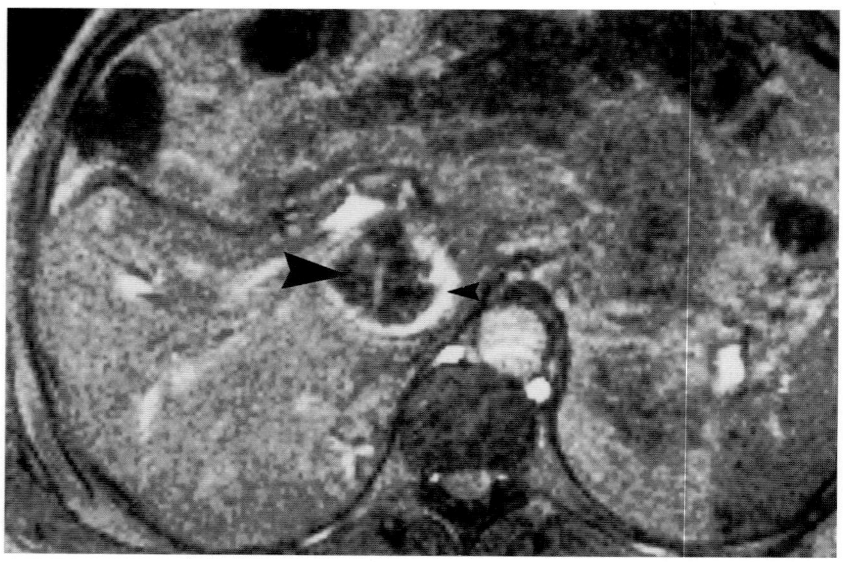

FIG. 97-8. Magnetic resonance imaging study of adrenocortical carcinoma with extension of tumor thrombus into retrohepatic inferior vena cava. Notice flow in vena cava (*small arrow*) around the tumor thrombus (*large arrow*).

As described in the previous section, the key surgical principles involve adequate mobilization of the splenic flexure of the colon and avoidance of traction on the splenic capsule on the left side. On the right, mobilization of the liver may be required for adequate exposure. The short right adrenal vein may be obscured by a large tumor, and access to the posterior lateral inferior vena cava where the vein enters, may be difficult. The arterial supply is usually multiple and variable.

Large tumors may require en bloc resection of adjacent organs for complete extirpation. On the left side, splenic resection may be required. An adequate plane between the tumor and the upper pole of the kidney can usually be developed. Resection of the capsule of the upper pole of the kidney, partial nephrectomy, or en bloc nephrectomy should be performed as needed to allow complete excision of the tumor.

Management of Venous Invasion

Direct invasion of the venous drainage of the adrenal gland can occur with adrenal carcinomas, as it can with renal cell carcinomas. Because of the short vein on the right, extension into the inferior vena cava is seen. On the left, the tumor may invade the renal vein by way of the adrenal vein and, in some circumstances, extend into the inferior vena cava.

Preoperative identification of the extent of venous invasion is essential for planning of the surgical procedure. Magnetic resonance imaging is usually the least invasive method to assess the proximal extent of an inferior vena caval tumor thrombus[40] (Fig. 97-8). Inferior vena cavography may also be used. The most important determination is whether the thrombus extends proximal to the intrahepatic portion of the inferior vena cava. Tumor thrombus below that region can usually be removed through a direct abdominal or thoracoabdominal approach. The vena cava is secured both proximally and distally, and a vena cavotomy incision is performed. The thrombus usually can be extracted en bloc with the tumor, followed by primary closure of the inferior vena cava. Coronary bypass may be required for tumors that extend proximal to the intrahepatic portion of the inferior vena cava. The thrombus may be adherent at the ostium of the adrenal vein, but usually it can be freely removed at other points. Complete obstruction of the inferior vena cava by tumor or direct invasion of the wall of the inferior vena cava portend a poor prognosis and, sometimes, an unresectable tumor.

Staging and Prognosis

Adrenocortical carcinoma is usually staged according to the criteria of Macfarlane[41] (Table 97-1). Except for organ-confined disease, survival for as long as 5 years is rare. Consequently, the most effective therapy is complete surgical excision. Patients with metastases at the time of presentation or with unresectable disease rarely live beyond 1 year, and untreated patients have an average survival time of only 3 months. Even with what appears to be local or regional spread, however, an aggressive surgical approach is usually advocated because it currently offers the only possibility of prolonged survival. Patients with a postoperative disease-free interval of longer than 2 years have an excellent prognosis.[42]

TABLE 97-1. *Staging of adrenocortical carcinoma*

Stage	Description	5-Year survival rate
I	<5 cm	100%
II	>5 cm	80%
III	Local/regional spread or positive nodes	11%
IV	Local/regional spread and positive nodes or distant metastases	0%

From Macfarlane DA. Cancer of the adrenal cortex: the natural history, prognosis and treatment in a study of fifty-five cases. Ann R Coll Surg Engl 1958;23:155.

REFERENCES

1. Van Way CW III, Scott HW Jr, Page DL, Rhamy RK. Pheochromocytoma. Curr Probl Surg 1974;(June):1.
2. Chong GC, ReMine WH, van Heerdeu JA, Sheps SG, Harrison E. Current management of pheochromocytoma. Ann Surg 1974;179:740.
3. Sheps SG, Jrang N-S, Klee GG. Diagnostic evaluation of pheochromocytoma. Endocrinol Metab Clin North Am 1988;17:397.
4. Samaan NA, Hickey RC, Shutts PE. Diagnosis, localization, and management of pheochromocytoma: pitfalls and follow-up in 41 patients. Cancer 1988;62:2451.
5. Scott HW, Van Way CW III, Gray GF, Sussman CR. Pheochromocytoma. In: HW Scott, ed. Surgery of the adrenal glands. Philadelphia, JB Lippincott, 1990:187.
6. Pruszczyk P, Januszewicz W, Feltynowski T, et al. Long-term follow-up after surgical removal of pheochromocytoma: observations in 61 patients. Clin and Exper Hyper—Theory and Practice 1991;A13:1179.
7. Hicks RJ, Wood B, Kalff V, Anderson ST, Kelly MJ. Normalization of left ventricular ejection fraction following resection of pheochromocytoma in a patient with dilated cardiomyopathy. Clin Nucl Med 1991; 16:413.
8. Krentz AJ, Hale PJ, Horrocks PM, et al. Metabolic effects of pharmacological adrenergic blockade in pheochromocytoma. Clin Endocrinol (Oxf) 1991;34:139.
9. Schuiki ER, Jenni R, Amarin FW, Ziegler WH. A reversible form of apical left ventricular hypertrophy associated with pheochromocytoma. J Am Soc Echocardiography 1993;6:327.
10. Hamada N, Algamatsu A, Joh T. A case of pheochromocytoma complicated with acute renal failure and cardiomyopathy. Jpn Circ J 1993; 57:84.
11. Tory K, Brauch H, Linehan WM, et al. Specific genetic change in tumors associated with von Hippel-Lindau disease. J Natl Cancer Inst 1989;81:1097.
12. Perry RR, Keiser HR, Norton JA, et al. Surgical management of pheochromocytoma with the use of metyrosine. Ann Surg 1990;212:621.
13. Havlik RJ, Cahow CE, Kinder BK. Advances in the diagnosis and treatment of pheochromocytoma. Arch Surg 1988;123:626.
14. Nicholson JP, Vaughn ED, Pickering TG, et al. Pheochromocytomas and prazosin. Ann Intern Med 1983;99:477.
15. Chung PC, Sum DC. Preliminary experience using fixed dose labetalol in surgical resection of pheochromocytoma. Ma Tsui Hsueh Tsa Chi 1993;31:211.
16. Briggs RSJ, Birtwell AJ, Pohl JEF. Hypertensive response to labetalol in pheochromocytoma. Lancet 1978:1045.
17. Yamaguchi T, Irisawa C, Watanabe H, Kawamura S, Nakada T. Failure of blood pressure control by a new combined alpha and beta-blocking agent (amosulalol) in a patient with pheochromocytoma. Int Urol Nephrol 1991;23:209.
18. Stockpole RH, Melicow MM, Uson AC. Pheochromocytoma in children. J Pediatr 1963;63:315.
19. Hume DM. Pheochromocytoma in the adult and in the child. Am J Surg 1960;99:458.
20. Revillon Y, Daher P, Jan D, et al. Pheochromocytoma in children: 15 cases. J Pediatr Surg 1992;27:910.
21. Vasen HFA, Van Der Feltz M, Raue F, et al. The natural course of

multiple endocrineoplasia type IIB: a study of 18 cases. Arch Intern Med 1992;152:1250.
22. Lipps CJM, Minder WH, Leo JR, Alleman A, Hackeng WHL. Evidence of multicentric origin of the multiple endocrineoplasia syndrome type IIA (Sipple syndrome) in a large family in the Netherlands Am J Med 1978;64:569.
23. Van Heerden JA, Sixemore GW, Carney JA, Grant CS, Remine WH, Sheps SG. Surgical management of the adrenal glands and multiple endocrineoplasia type II syndrome. World J Surg 1984;8:612.
24. Lairmore TC, Ball DW, Baylin SB, Wells SA. Management of pheochromocytoma in patients with multiple endocrineoplasia type II syndromes. Ann Surg 1993;217:595.
25. Tibblin S, Dymling JF, Ingemansson S, et al. Unilateral vs. bilateral adrenalectomy in multiple endocrineoplasia IIa. World J Surg 1983;7:201.
26. Jansson S, Tisell LE, Fjalling M, et al. Early diagnosis of and surgical strategy for adrenal medullary disease in MENII gene carrier. Surgery 1988;103:11.
27. Whalen RK, Althausen AF, Daniels GH. Extra-adrenal pheochromocytoma. J Urol 1992;147:1.
28. Lewinsky BS, Grigor KM, Symington T, Nelville AM. The clinical and pathologic features of ''non-hormonal'' adrenocortical tumors: Report of 20 new cases and review of the literature. Cancer 1974;33:778.
29. Luton JP, Cerdas S, Billaud L, et al. Clinical features of adrenocortical carcinoma, prognostic factors, and the effect of mitotane therapy. N Engl J Med 1990;322:1195.
30. Belldegrun A, deKernion JB. What to do about the incidentally found adrenal mass. World J Urol 1989;7:117.
31. Belldegrun A, Hussain S, Seltzer SE, Loughlin KR, Gittes RF, Richie JP. The incidentally discovered adrenal mass: a therapeutic dilemma. BWH experience 1976–1983. Surg Gynecol Obstet 1986;163:203.
32. Bertagna C, Orth DN. Clinical and laboratory findings and results of therapy in 58 patients with adrenocortical tumors admitted to a single medical center (1951 to 1978). Am J Med 1981;71:855.
33. Sullivan M, Boileau M, Hodges CV. Adrenal cortical carcinoma. J Urol 1978;120:660.
34. Ross NS, Aron DC. Hormonal evaluation of the patient with an incidentally discovered adrenal mass. N Engl J Med 1990;323:1401.
35. Glazer HS, Weyman PJ, Sagal SS, Levitt RG, McClennan RL. Nonfunctioning adrenal masses: incidental discovery on computed tomography. AJR Am J Roentgenol 1982;139:81.
36. Prinz RA, Brooks MH, Churchill R, et al. Incidental asymptomatic adrenal masses detected by computed tomographic scanning: is operation required? JAMA 1982;248:701.
37. Copeland PM. The incidentally discovered adrenal mass. Ann Intern Med 1983;98:940.
38. Vaughan ED Jr, Phillips H. Modified posterior approach for right adrenalectomy. Surg Gynecol Obstet 1987;165:453.
39. Bloom LS, Libertino JA. Surgical management of Cushing's syndrome. Urol Clin North Am 1989;16:547.
40. Long JP, Choyke PL, Shawker TA, et al. Intraoperative ultrasound in the evaluation of tumor involvement of the inferior vena cava. J Urol 1993;150:13.
41. Macfarlane DA. Cancer of the adrenal cortex: the natural history, prognosis and treatment in a study of fifty-five cases. Ann R Coll Surg Engl 1958;23:155.
42. King DR, Rack EE. Adrenocortical carcinoma: a clinical and pathologic study of 119 cases. Cancer 1979;44:239.

Principles and Practice of Genitourinary Oncology, edited by Derek Raghavan, Howard I. Scher, Steven A. Leibel, and Paul H. Lange. Lippincott-Raven Publishers, Philadelphia, © 1997.

CHAPTER 98

Nonsurgical Treatment of Adrenocortical Cancer

Gabriel P. Haas, Jeffery Triest, J. Edson Pontes, and Donald L. Trump

Adrenal cortical carcinoma (ACC) is an exceedingly rare tumor; 78 to 130 new cases are diagnosed annually in the United States.[1,2] Prognosis of patients diagnosed with ACC is poor.[1–8] Patients typically die from complications caused by locally recurrent or metastatic disease.[3,4] Median survival for patients with ACC is less than 3 years; patients with unresectable disease have a mean survival of 3 months.[5] The stage of the tumor at initial surgery is the most significant prognostic variable.[2] Tumor necrosis, vascular invasion, nuclear mitoses, pleomorphism, and involvement of the zona reticularis have been reported to be poor prognostic signs.[6] Age or gender of the patient and size, grade, or functional status of the tumor have no consistent influence on survival.[3–11]

Surgical cure is possible with T1/T2 lesions. For disease spread beyond the adrenal, the duration of median and mean survival is 1.7 and 2.3 years, respectively.[2] Anecdotal cases of long-term survival after surgical resection of locally invasive disease have been reported. Investigators from the Cleveland Clinic reported the 5-year survival of 44% for patients with T1/T2 disease, 12.5% for patients with T3/T4 or N+ disease, and 5.5% for patients with metastatic disease.[12] Five-year survival for advanced or metastatic disease is typically less than 15% if complete resection of tumor cannot be achieved. Almost all patients with stage T3 disease or higher will have recurrent or metastatic disease within 5 years of resection. Aggressive surgical resection of locally recurrent or metastatic adrenal cortical cancer has been recommended; however, even with aggressive intervention, the 5-year survival in these patients is only 10% to 20%.

The infrequent nature of this neoplasm makes it particularly difficult to study novel treatment modalities. A few large institutions or cooperative groups, such as the Genitourinary Committee of the Southwest Oncology Group, have been successful in carrying out innovative clinical trials.

ADJUVANT THERAPY

Because ACC has a poor prognosis, effective adjuvant therapy has been sought to supplement aggressive surgical care. Radiotherapy is useful in the palliation of painful bony metastases; however, it has not been effective in preventing local recurrence or prolonging patient survival.[7–9] Drugs that block the synthesis of steroids, such as metyrapone, aminoglutethamide, and ketoconazole, or those that block the action of androgens, mineralocorticoids, or glucocorticoids in their target tissue, may be of clinical benefit in controlling the endocrine manifestations of the tumors; however, none have been reported to inhibit tumor growth.[7] No single agent or combined-modality approach has demonstrated any survival benefit in an adjuvant setting.[12]

MITOTANE

Mitotane (1,1-dichloro-2-(o-chlorophenyl)-2-(p-chlorophenyl)-ethane) was recognized early in its development to cause necrosis of the adrenal gland. It is one of the few drugs with demonstrated activity in patients with metastatic ACC.[13] Mitotane (op-DDD), an analog of the insecticide DDT, is the treatment of choice for metastatic disease and effects an objective regression in tumor size in 35% of patients.[14] In one series, eight patients treated with mitotane had objective tumor regression compared with no response in patients not treated with the drug, leading to the suggestion that mitotane is beneficial in at least some patients.[7] Tumor regression in this and many other studies is not associated with clear prolongation of survival.[13,14] Large doses of mitotane, ranging from 1 to 16 g/day, are used in the treatment of patients with metastatic disease.[13,15] The usual approach to therapy is to initiate treatment at 0.5 to 1 g/day and escalate to tolerance. Long-term administration of op-DDD at doses higher than 3 g/day results in adrenal cortical atrophy. Early in therapy there is a need for both glucocorticoid and mineralocorticoid replacement.[13,15] Hydrocortisone replacement is given at doses of 25 to 35 mg/day.[13]

The toxicity of mitotane is related to its method of metabolism and storage. Mitotane stimulates liver lysosomal enzymes and alters cortisol metabolism.[15] Because of it high fat solubility, op-DDD is deposited in subcutaneous fat, liver, brain, and

TABLE 98-1. *Side effects of mitotane therapy*

Side effect	Percent of patients affected
Anorexia, nausea	88
Diarrhea	38
Vomiting	23
Decreased memory	50
Rash	23
Gynecomastia in men	50
Arthralgia	19
Leukopenia	7

Adapted from Schteingart DE, Mutazedi A, Noonan RA, Thompson NW. Treatment of adrenal carcinomas. Arch Surg 1982;117:1142.

both normal and malignant adrenal tissue.[14,15] The side effect profile of mitotane is listed in Table 98-1.

Late occurrence of central nervous system toxicity may be the result of the accumulation of op-DDD and may manifest itself as incapacitating depression.[15] The toxicity profile of mitotane leads to poor patient compliance, even in the presence of objective tumor response.[14] Toxicities are, however, reversible with discontinuation of the drug.

In an attempt to minimize the toxic side effects of mitotane and to improve its therapeutic efficacy, combinations with other drugs have been tried. One such drug is streptozocin, a nitrosourea active in pancreatic islet cell and carcinoid tumors. This drug was found to be concentrated in mice adrenal cortex, and when combined with mitotane in the treatment of metastatic ACC, it effected an objective tumor regression in two of three patients and allowed surgical resection to occur in those with otherwise inoperable disease.[15] Additional combinations with op-DDD are expected. No significant survival benefit has been gained through the use of op-DDD, and its use in an adjuvant setting remains controversial.[2,7,12,14–16]

CYTOTOXIC THERAPY

Because of the rarity of ACC, there is little information regarding the activity of conventional neoplastic agents in its treatment.[17] Anecdotal reports of tumor regression in response to single-agent chemotherapy or combinations of chemotherapeutic agents are present in the literature. Responses have been noted in single patients given carmustine (BCNU), porfiromycin, doxorubicin, peptichemio, cisplatin, and combined therapies such as doxorubicin and cyclophosphamide or bleomycin; 5-fluorouracil (5-FU) with mitotane or methotrexate; and cyclophosphamide, vincristine, semustine, and bleomycin (COMB).[17–21] Responses were graded as partial or complete, with the majority of positive results involving regression of metastatic lesions in the lungs, liver, and retroperitoneum. One of the advantages of antineoplastic agents is their potential synergy when used in combination. Cisplatin and etoposide (VP16) are such a synergistic combination and have shown some antitumor activity against ACC. The use of this combination has been suggested for patients who are refractory to or are unable to tolerate mitotane.[17] The Eastern Cooperative Oncology Group reported a 19% (3 of 19 patients) response rate with adriamycin when used as initial therapy but no responses (0 of 15 patients) in prior mitotane failures.[21] Major side effects of cytotoxic agents are myelosuppression and hepatotoxicity. Because mitotane is free of these detrimental effects, its use in combination with classic chemotherapies has been suggested.[17] A phase II Southwest Oncology Group clinical trial of mitotane and cisplatin in inoperable, residual, recurrent, or metastatic adrenal cancer showed a 30% objective response in 37 patients (1 complete and 10 partial responses) with a median survival of 12 months.[22] However, the toxicity of the combination was moderate to severe, with gastrointestinal, renal, and neurologic side effects resulting in discontinuation of the therapy in 47% of patients.[22] Whether the addition of mitotane increased the effectiveness of cisplatin is unclear from this experience, but the combination appeared to have increased toxicity. The combination of mitotane, cisplatin, and VP16 is under investigation by the Southwest Oncology Group. Preliminary data suggest that responses may be seen with this regimen, however, at the price of significant toxicity, leading to dose reduction.

SURAMIN

Suramin is a polysulfonated naphthylurea that has been used as treatment for Rhodesian and Gambian trypanosomiasis and *Onchocerca volvulus* since the early 1920s.[23,24] Suramin has many biologic effects. It is a potent reverse transcriptase inhibitor, and it suppresses the growth of human immunodeficiency virus in vitro.[23,25] Suramin also inhibits a number of cellular enzymes, including DNA polymerases and ornithine decarboxylase.[23] Suramin is structurally similar to the highly sulfated glycoaminoglycans such as heparan and dermatin sulfate. This structural analogy explains why Suramin effectively blocks iduronate sulfatase, the key enzyme in the desulfation and eventual degradation of the sulfated glycosaminoglycans. In addition, Suramin binds to and inactivates a wide range of tumor growth factors that share little structural similarity to one another other than the fact that they bind to heparin.[24] Suramin causes selective adrenal cortical necrosis when administered to cynomolgus monkeys.[23] With the exception of the kidneys, accumulation in the adrenal glands is 3 to 20 times higher than that in a variety of organs evaluated, including lung, muscle, liver, brain, spleen, and large bowel.[23]

Suramin is extensively protein bound and has no detectable metabolism. Clearance of the drug appears to be predominantly renal elimination of free rather than protein-bound species.[22] The half-life of Suramin is 45 to 50 days.

By inhibiting iduronate sulfatase, Suramin causes accumulation of the sulfated glycoaminoglycans heparin and dermatin sulfate, which alter and interfere with tumor angiogenesis, possibly explaining Suramin's apparent anticancer activity.[23,24]

During early use for the treatment of trypanosomiasis in the 1930s, and consequently during clinical trails for AIDS, Suramin was recognized to be toxic for the adrenal glands.[25,26] Based on these clinical experiences and preclinical studies demonstrating the inhibition of adrenocortical carcinoma cell line colony formation by Suramin,[23] the first clinical trial for patients with adrenocortical cancer was initiated at the National Cancer Institute.[23,24,27] Of 17 patients, 2 partial responses, 2 minor responses, and 5 instances of stable disease for 3 to 10 months were observed.[23]

In trials using Suramin in the treatment of bulky ACC, administration of a cumulative dose of at least 10 g reaching a steady-state plasma Suramin level of at least 150 μg/mL may be necessary for both inhibition of malignant steroid hormone production and objective tumor regression.[23] The most serious side effects related to Suramin administration are the development of coagulopathy and severe polyneuropathy characterized by flaccid extremity paralysis, elevated cerebrospinal fluid protein levels, and respiratory muscle compromise requiring mechanical ventilation.[23] Progressive polyradiculopathy resembling Guillain-Barré syndrome may develop. Febrile episodes and documented sepsis can be attributed to the immunosuppressive effect of Suramin.[23] Additional side effects of Suramin include reversible renal insufficiency, thrombocytopenia, and vortex keratopathy presenting as a foreign-body sensation in one or both eyes.[23]

A close temporal correlation between the development of anticoagulation and measurable tumor shrinkage may exist.[24] Prothrombin time is usually allowed to increase to 17.5 to 18 seconds before discontinuing the drug.[23] Patients are given hydrocortisone to present adrenal insufficiency.

The ability of patients to achieve partial responses with Suramin indicate that the drug does have some activity against surgically unresectable disease. The ability of Suramin to decrease pathologic steroid hormone production also suggests a role in the treatment of nonmalignant conditions of the adrenal cortical and in the hormonal treatment of other malignancies.[23] Recent efforts in a variety of tumor systems resulted in pharmacokinetically based administration of Suramin. Jodrell[28] used intermittent short infusions of Suramin to optimize plasma drug concentrations, and Reyno and colleagues[29] developed a fixed-dose regimen to maintain concentrations in the 150 to 250 mcg/mL range. There is continued active interest in Suramin using modified and presumably improved dosage regimens.

GOSSYPOL

Gossypol, a spermatotoxin, has been used as a male contraceptive in China. The drug is a plant extract derived from crude cotton seed oil.[30] Early testing with this agent suggested it had an inhibitory effect on tumor growth, particularly human adrenal cortical tumors in nude mice. In a human trial, 21 patients with metastatic ACC were treated with oral Gossypol at doses ranging from 30 to 70 mg/day. The drug was fairly well tolerated by patients. Three patients succumbed to the disease prior to achieving adequate blood levels to be included in the analysis. Another three patients achieved partial tumor responses (17%) with durations ranging from several months to more than 1 year.[30] The partial responses were seen in patients whose disease was refractory to other forms of chemotherapy. The side effects of Gossypol include xerostomia, intermittent nausea, transient elevation of hepatic enzymes, dry skin, fatigue, vomiting, transient ileus, minor hair thinning, and aggravation of preexisting gynecomastia.[30] Suggested modes of action of Gossypol in the treatment of malignancies involve its ability to uncouple oxidative phosphorylation, destroy mitochondria, and decrease intracellular adenosine triphosphate.[30] Another potential mechanism of action is its ability to inhibit endothelium-derived relaxing factor (nitrous oxide), which is required for blood vessel dilatation. This interferes with tumor blood supply and may lead to necrosis.[30] Although the partial response rate of metastatic ACC to oral gossypol is low, it is comparable to the other medical therapies available. The precise role of this drug remains to be determined.

TABLE 98-2. *Response to therapy*

Agent	Chief toxicity	CR plus PR (%)
Mitotane	Gastrointestinal	35
Cytotoxic agents	Myelosuppression Hepatotoxicity	30
Suramin	Coagulopathy Neuropathy	12
Gossypol	Gastrointestinal	17

CONCLUSIONS

The treatment of advanced ACC continues to remain an enigma, with practically no complete responses and only few partial responses of limited duration seen. Despite interest in several investigational agents, none has proven to be clearly superior to mitotane (Table 98-2). Mitotane continues to be the mainstay of therapy; however, its effectiveness limited by significant dose-related toxicity. The addition of platinum-based cytotoxic agents may prove to be of further benefit in the future.

REFERENCES

1. Venkatesh S, Hickey RC, Sellin RV, Fernandez JF, Samaan NA. Adrenal cortical carcinoma. Cancer 1989;64:765.
2. Cohn K, Gottesman L, Brennan M. Adrenocortical carcinoma. Surgery 1986;100:1170.
3. Icard P, Chapuis Y, Andreassian B, Bernard A, Proye C. Adrenocortical carcinoma in surgically treated patients: a retrospective study on 156 cases by the French Association of Endocrine Surgery. Surgery 1992; 112:972.
4. Hough AJ, Hollifield JW, Page DL, Hartmann WH. Prognostic factors in adrenal cortical tumors: a mathematical analysis of clinical and morphologic data. Am J Clin Pathol 1979;72:390.
5. Eriksson B, Oberg K, Curstedt, T, et al. Treatment of hormone-producing adrenocortical cancer with o,p′DDD and streptozocin. Cancer 1987; 59:1398.
6. Weiss LM, Medeiros LJ, Vickery AL. Pathologic features of prognostic significance in adrenocortical carcinoma. Am J Surg Pathol 2989;13: 202.
7. Luton JP, Cerdas S, Billaud L, et al. Clinical features of adrenocortical carcinoma, prognostic factors, and the effect of mitotane therapy. N Engl J Med 1990;322:1195.
8. Nader S, Hickey RC, Sellin RV, Samaan NA. Adrenal cortical carcinoma: a study of 77 cases. Cancer 1983;52:707.
9. Didolkar MS, Bescher RA, Elias EG, Moore RH. Natural history of adrenal cortical carcinoma: a clinicopathologic study of 42 patients. Cancer 1981;47:2153.
10. Henley DJ, van Heerden JA, Grant CS, Carney JA, Carpenter PC. Adrenal cortical carcinoma: a continuing challenge. Surgery 1983;94: 926.
11. Richie JP, Gittes RF. Carcinoma of the adrenal cortex. Cancer 1980; 45:1957.
12. Bodie B, Novick AC, Pontes JE, et al. The Cleveland clinic experience with adrenal cortical carcinoma. J Urol 1989;141:257.
13. Schteingart DE, Motazedi A, Noonan RA, Thompson NW. Treatment of adrenal carcinomas. Arch Surg 1982;117:1142.

14. Boven E, Vermorken JB, van Slooten H, Pinedo HM. Complete response of metastasized adrenal cortical carcinoma with o,p′-DDD. Cancer 1994;53:26.
15. Jarabak J, Rice K. Metastatic adrenal cortical carcinoma: prolonged regression with mitotane therapy. JAMA 1981;15:246.
16. Vassilopoulou-Sellin R, Guinee VF, Klein MJ, et al. Impact of adjuvant mitotane on the clinical course of patients with adrenocortical cancer: M.D. Anderson Cancer Center. (Abstract 547) Proc Am Soc Clin Oncol 1993;12:189.
17. Johnson DH, Greco FA. Treatment of metastatic adrenal cortical carcinoma with cisplatin and etoposide (VP-16). Cancer 1986;58:2198.
18. Haq MM, Legha SS, Samaan NA, Bodey GP, Burgess MA. Cytotoxic chemotherapy in adrenal cortical carcinoma. Cancer Treat Rep 1980; 64:909.
19. Schlumberger M, Ostronoff M, Bellaiche M, Rougier P, Droz JP, Parmentier C. 5-Fluorouracil, doxorubicin, and cisplatin regimen in adrenal cortical carcinoma. Cancer 1988;61:1492.
20. van Slooten H, van Oosterom AT. CAP (cyclophosphamide, doxorubicin and cisplatin) regimen in adrenal cortical carcinoma. Cancer Treat Rep 1983;67:377.
21. Decker RA, Elson P, Hogan TF, et al. Eastern Cooperative Oncology Group Study 1879: mitotane and adriamycin in patients with advanced adrenocortical carcinoma. Surgery 1991;110:1006.
22. Bukowski RM, Wolfe M, Levine HS, et al. Phase II trial of mitotane and cisplatin in patients with adrenal carcinoma: a Southwest Oncology Group study. J Clin Oncol 1993;11:161.
23. LaRocca F, Stein CA, Danesi R, Jamis-Dow CA, Weiss GH, Myers E. Suramin in adrenal cancer: modulation of steroid hormone production, cytotoxicity in vitro, and clinical antitumor effect. J Clin Endocrinol Metab 1990;71:496.
24. Stein CA, LaRocca RV, Thomas R, McAtee TN, Myers CE. Suramin: An anticancer drug with a unique mechanism of action. J Clin Oncol 1989;7:499.
25. Levine AM, Gill PS, Cohen J, et al. Suramin antiviral therapy in the acquired immunodeficiency syndrome. Ann Intern Med 1986;105:32.
26. Wells HG, Humphreys EM, Work EG. Significance of the increased frequency of selected cortical necrosis of adrenal as a cause of Addison's disease. JAMA 1937;109:490.
27. Stein CA. Suramin: a novel antineoplastic agent with multiple potential mechanisms of action. Cancer Res 1993;53:2239.
28. Jodrell DI. Suramin: development of a population pharmacokinetic model and its use with intermittent short infusions to control plasma drug concentration in patients with prostate cancer. J Clin Oncol 1994; 12:166.
29. Reyno LM, Egorin MJ, Eisenberger MA, et al. Development and validation of a pharmacokinetically based fixed dosing scheme for Suramin. Proc Am Soc Clin Oncol 1993;12:135.
30. Flack GR, Pyle RG, Mullen NM, et al. Oral gossypol in the treatment of metastatic adrenal cancer. J Clin Endocrinol Metab 1993;76:1019.

SECTION VIII

Genitourinary Sarcomas

Principles and Practice of Genitourinary Oncology, edited by Derek Raghavan, Howard I. Scher, Steven A. Leibel, and Paul H. Lange. Lippincott-Raven Publishers, Philadelphia, © 1997.

CHAPTER 99

Genitourinary Sarcomas

Ellis G. Levine, John S. J. Brooks, James Spellman, and Satish Velagapudi

In 1996, it is estimated that 6400 new cases of sarcoma will be diagnosed in the United States and 3700 deaths will occur from this malignancy.[1] Of this uncommon disorder, genitourinary sarcomas constitute only 5%. Experience has been accumulated over years, almost exclusively from single institutions. Consistent approaches to the description, assessment, and treatment of sarcomas at different genitourinary sites have not been discernible because of the substantial advances in clinical medicine that have occurred over the lengthy interval during which these cases have been culled. Nonetheless, traditionally favored approaches are reviewed in this chapter; following a review of the pathology of genitourinary sarcomas, anatomic sites are discussed in the following order: prostate, paratesticular structures, penis, kidney and ureter, and bladder. Because many other chapters in this book are devoted to pediatric sarcomas of the genitourinary tract (see Chaps. 100–102), this chapter focuses on adult genitourinary sarcomas.

PATHOLOGY

For this chapter on adult sarcomas, the definition of adult is an age of 20 years or older, which eliminates most childhood sarcomas, including rhabdomyosarcoma of various genitourinary sites. The inclusion of childhood disease has confounded statistics relating to survival in genitourinary sarcomas of the adult. Regarding relative incidence, the paratesticular region is the one genitourinary area most commonly affected by sarcomas, followed by the bladder, prostate, kidney, and ureter; sarcomas of the testis, penis, and urethra are the least common sites affected (Table 99-1). As a cautionary note, clinicians should not consider carcinosarcomas with true sarcomas; they have a poorer prognosis than sarcomas and typically are highly aggressive lesions.

Whether genitourinary sarcomas behave in a manner similar to other soft tissue sarcomas is an issue of some controversy. Factors such as size, resectability, and tumor grade do impact on the outcome of patients with genitourinary sarcomas of the solid organs (i.e., kidney, prostate, and testis), as they do elsewhere. However, we believe that bladder and paratesticular sarcomas sometimes have different natural histories as a result of the presence of pedunculated bladder tumors, making segmental resection and favorable outcome possible regardless of size and grade, and the propensity for paratesticular lesions to extend into the pelvic retroperitoneum, making resection difficult and recurrence common regardless of grade.

Renal Sarcomas

Like other solid organs, the kidney is an extremely uncommon site for primary sarcoma.[2–17] Renal sarcomas account for only 1% of all renal primary malignancies.[5,6] There is a slight male predominance and a very wide age range associated with these lesions.[15] Primary renal sarcomas are high-stage, notoriously lethal tumors; more than 80% of patients die of disease, the majority within 2 years of diagnosis.[6,15]

Clinicians should realize that conditions that mimic sarcoma occur more frequently in this area and should retain a healthy skepticism of a diagnosis of renal sarcoma. The major mimics are sarcomatoid renal or transitional cell carcinomas, which may resemble leiomyosarcoma or malignant fibrous histiocytoma[4,6,13,16,17]; angiomyolipoma, which may exhibit prominent atypia resulting in a misdiagnosis as either leiomyosarcoma[5,6] or liposarcomas[8]; and perirenal retroperitoneal sarcomas masquerading as primary parenchymal disease.[6] For example, any liposarcoma should be considered as retroperitoneal in origin; those present in the literature as primary renal liposarcomas are probably not primary tumors. Criteria should be restricted to those lesions arising in the renal pelvis, where the adipose tissue resides.

The most common renal sarcoma is leiomyosarcoma[2,5,6,14] which accounts for 50% to 75% of cases. There are about 150 cases in the literature; interestingly, no firm criteria for diagnosis have been established. Smooth muscle tumors in other sites such as the uterus are judged to be malignant on the basis of a specific mitotic rate, but no such figure is available for kidney tumors. Conservatively, any mitoses in a primary renal smooth muscle tumor indicate that the treatment approach should be directed toward a potentially aggressive lesion.

Although rare liposarcomas of the kidney have been reported,[9,11] proof of renal origin is difficult in the absence of a complete resection. Perhaps because of the high incidence of

TABLE 99-1. *Relative incidence and histologic types of adult genitourinary sarcomas*

Site	Relative frequency	Most common	Other types
Kidney	4	Leiomyosarcoma Malignant fibrous histiocytoma	Liposarcoma Rhabdomyosarcoma Angiosarcoma Osteosarcoma Hemangiopericytoma
Uterer	5	Leiomyosarcoma	
Bladder	2	Leiomyosarcoma	
Prostate	3	Leiomyosarcoma	Phyllodes tumor Rhabdomyosarcoma Angiosarcoma Rhabdoid sarcoma Malignant fibrous histiocytoma
Seminal vesicle	5	Leiomyosarcoma	Angiosarcoma
Testis	5		
Germ cell associated		Rhabdomyosarcoma	Angiosarcoma
Pure sarcoma		Leiomyosarcoma (scrotum)	Osteosarcoma
Penis	5	Leiomyosarcoma	Epithelioid sarcoma Kaposi's sarcoma
Paratesticular	1	Liposarcoma Leiomyosarcoma	Malignant fibrous histiocytoma Malignant peripheral nerve sheath

the low-grade, well-differentiated variant, renal liposarcomas have an overall better prognosis than do other sarcoma types.

Malignant fibrous histiocytoma is a high-grade sarcoma that also may rarely occur in the kidney.[5,6,12] There is a high male predominance (3 : 1) and an occasional presentation with fever of unknown origin. The differential diagnosis includes xanthogranulomatous pyelonephritis because of the high content of histiocytes in both lesions. Fibrosarcomas that have been reported in the past are probably actually examples of malignant fibrous histiocytoma.

Other uncommon histologies that may be seen in the kidney are rhabdomyosarcoma,[7] malignant hemangiopericytoma,[5] angiosarcoma,[6] Kaposi's sarcoma,[3] and osteosarcoma.[10]

Ureteral Sarcomas

Ureteral sarcomas are extraordinarily rare tumors; of the few reported, most have been leiomyosarcomas.[6]

Bladder Sarcomas

Although the bladder is the commonest site for sarcoma when compared with the prostate and kidney, it is also the commonest location for reactive pseudosarcomas and other sarcoma mimics.[18–26] Fibromyxoid pseudosarcoma has a characteristic presentation; a sizable (2- to 5-cm) polypoid nodule arises within 1 to 3 months after a surgical procedure such as transurethral endoscopic resection of the bladder or transurethral endoscopic resection of the prostate.[21–24] A proliferation of spindle myofibroblasts is mingled with scattered inflammatory cells in a loose edematous stroma; this picture is easily mistaken for leiomyosarcoma morphologically. Additionally, immunohistochemical markers of muscle differentiation such as desmin and actin are frequently positive, as they are in smooth muscle tumors. Thus, confusion commonly occurs. In this type of postoperative clinical setting, there should be considerable skepticism about a sarcoma diagnosis. Indeed, the presence of this and other pseudosarcomatous proliferations of the bladder makes a diagnosis of spindle cell lesions of the bladder difficult for the general pathologist and signifies the need for a second opinion on the pathology slides when the clinician has any question about a diagnosis of a bladder sarcoma.

Spindle cell transformation of transitional cell carcinoma mimicking sarcoma is also a phenomenon of which clinicians should be aware.[18,25] Spindle cell transformation may be seen in a primary carcinoma or perhaps more commonly in a recurrence of transitional cell carcinoma. Paravesicular sarcomas, if they cannot be clearly assigned an origin from the bladder wall or rectum, should be considered retroperitoneal tumors and be treated accordingly.

The manner of presentation of sarcoma in the bladder is important.[27–43] For example, pedunculated sarcomas,[31] which bulge into the intravesicular space, have an effect on the surgical approach to management. Judging from pedunculated sarcomas in other sites such as the pleural space (malignant solitary fibrous tumors) and the cervical esophagus, pedunculated sarcomas are associated with a better prognosis because of the frequent lack of invasion of the base of the polyp into the surrounding tissues. The presumed better prognosis of pedunculated sarcomas may also be the result of the fact that they present earlier than the average tumor because of erosion of the mucosa with hematuria or obstructive symptoms. Unfortunately, most studies of bladder sarcomas fail to mention whether the tumor was predominantly intramural or pedunculated. We have seen several pedunculated leiomyosarcomas of the bladder treated successfully by segmental resection without recurrence.

As is true in many genitourinary sites, leiomyosarcoma is the most common malignant mesenchymal tumor, arising in the urinary bladder from either the muscularis mucosa or the detrusor muscle proper (Fig. 99-1).[31,34,36,40,41] Men tend to outnumber women, and these patients generally are in their sixth or seventh decade of life. Gross hematuria is the most frequent

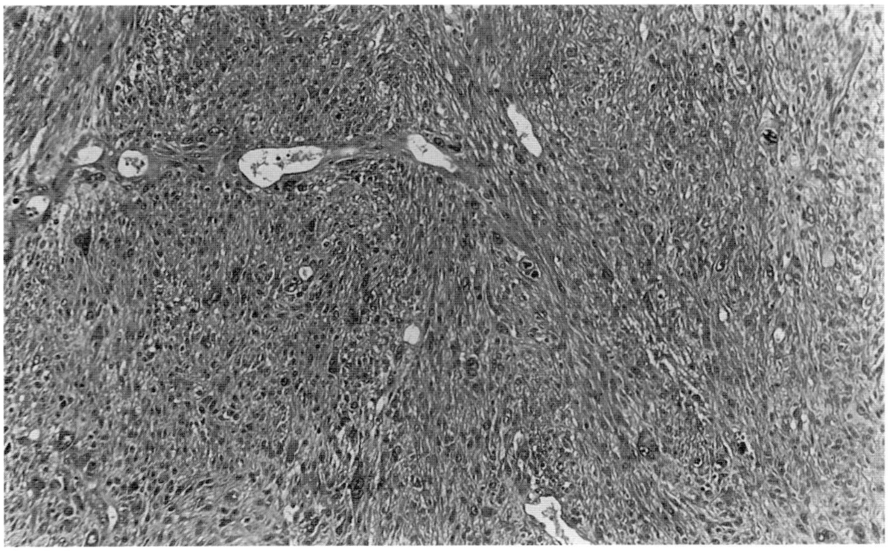

FIG. 99-1. This leiomyosarcoma of the bladder appeared as a polypoid and pedunculated lesion in a 40-year-old woman. Fascicles of spindle cells are noted parallel and perpendicular to the plane of section, pleomorphic nuclei are present, and atypical mitoses can be seen (*center and upper right*). The patient was alive and without disease after segmental resection 3 years postdiagnosis. Original magnification × 100.

presenting complaint, followed by decreasing force of urinary stream and dysuria.[31] The bladder dome is the most common site of origin.[31] Perhaps because of a low-pressure effect, some tumors grow into the bladder lumen as large pedunculated neoplasms. Strict criteria for the diagnosis of malignancy in a bladder smooth muscle tumor are lacking. Most tumors have necrosis, pleomorphism, and a high mitotic rate that enable their differentiation from leiomyoma. When necrosis is absent, the diagnosis depends on the presence of any consistent mitotic activity (e.g., 1/10 high-power fields), especially when the tumor has an infiltrating border into the surrounding muscle. In the series by Mills and colleagues,[31] tumors that had mitotic rates of 1 per 10 high-power fields or fewer did not metastasize; tumors with rates of 3 to 6 per 10 high-power fields did well, with only 1 death in 5 cases; and tumors with rates of more than 10 per 10 high-power fields were uniformly fatal. Interestingly, 8 of 9 patients who underwent partial cystectomy were alive without disease 8 months to 11 years after diagnosis. When predominantly serosal, bladder leiomyosarcomas may infiltrate surrounding structures such as the rectum and prostate. The overall 5-year survival has been estimated to be 24% by Peterson,[34] based on a literature review of mostly older reports. In more recent summaries such as that by Walker and associates,[41] the prognosis of these tumors is considerably better; the majority are low-grade tumors that recur without metastases.

Other sarcomas involving the bladder are angiosarcoma,[27,32,37,42] osteosarcoma,[28,43] adult rhabdomyosarcoma,[29,38] myxoid malignant fibrous histiocytoma,[33] and malignant mesenchymoma[39]; these other histologies may also present as polypoid or pedunculated intravescicular tumors.

Prostatic Sarcomas

Primary prostatic sarcomas[44–59] account for only 0.1% to 0.2% of all prostatic malignancies. Whereas rhabdomyosarcoma is the most common mesenchymal malignancy in childhood, leiomyosarcoma is the commonest adult prostatic sarcoma.[44,49,52,54,55,59] Leiomyosarcomas are typically found in patients who are between 40 and 70 years of age and may reach huge dimensions (24 cm). The average size of these lesions is 5 cm. Despite local excision, multiple recurrences are the rule, leading to a mean survival of 3 to 4 years. Because stromal hyperplasia of the prostate may be composed of smooth muscle proliferation, diagnosis of prostatic leiomyosarcoma on transurethral resection specimens may be difficult[59]; attention must be paid to the presence and quantity of mitoses.

Cystosarcoma phyllodes, more appropriately termed phyllodes tumor, may be found in the prostate[48,58] as it is in the breast. It should be considered a sarcomatous lesion, because the associated benign glands are likely reactive to growth factors secreted by the mesenchymal component. Additionally, although there are no large series delineating the distinction between benign and malignant tumors in the prostate as there are in the breast, it seems appropriate to apply the same criteria for malignancy. These criteria include high mitotic rate, presence of necrosis, and so-called stromal overgrowth, wherein the glandular elements are no longer found in a broad area of the tumor. With such criteria in place, the defined malignant phylloides tumors are more aggressive than their benign counterparts.

Other types of primary prostatic sarcoma include adult rhabdomyosarcoma,[45,51] rhabdoid sarcoma,[46] malignant "schwannoma" (i.e., malignant peripheral nerve sheath tumor),[44] angiosarcoma,[44] carcinosarcoma,[50,57] and malignant fibrous histiocytoma.[44,56]

Seminal Vesicle Sarcomas

Only 10 to 20 cases of primary sarcoma of the seminal vesicle have been reported,[60–63] and most are not well-documented cases. Leiomyosarcomas[62] and angiosarcomas[60,63] predominate. Despite the relatively small size of the angiosarcomas (<5 cm), local nodal metastases and distant metastases are the rule, and patients die of the disease within months. This kind of highly aggressive course is similar to that of angiosarcoma elsewhere in the body. Fibrosarcoma, neurofibrosarcoma, phyllodes tumor,[62] and undifferentiated sarcoma have also been reported.[63]

Testicular Sarcomas

In comparison with paratesticular sarcomas, truly intratesticular sarcomas are far less common. Additionally, the majority of testicular sarcomas are, in reality, an element of germ cell neoplasia.[64–69] Rhabdomyosarcoma,[64,66,69] primitive neuroectodermal tumor,[67] angiosarcoma,[65,68] and other tumors may be found in association with seminoma, spermatocytic seminoma,[69] and nonseminomatous germ cell tumors, including yolk sac tumor[66] and teratoma.[65] Even initially diagnosed pure sarcoma should be suspected of having germ cell origin. Clinicians should be cognizant of this fact and inquire about proper sampling of a tumor diagnosed as a pure testicular sarcoma.

Pure testicular sarcomas have been reported and include osteosarcoma and fibrosarcoma.[70–75] If treated early, these cases are associated with a favorable outcome. Leiomyosarcoma characteristically occurs on the scrotum,[71,72,74] where it presumably arises from the dartos muscle or erector pili muscles. Malignant schwannoma may also arise in the scrotum.[73]

Carcinosarcoma and malignant mixed müllerian tumors analogous to those seen in the female genital tract may arise from the epididymis.

Paratesticular Sarcomas

If rhabdomyosarcoma, most of which occur in childhood,[76–79] is eliminated, the most common type of paratesticular sarcoma in the adult is the well-differentiated liposarcoma.[80–82] Their location is usually listed as either inguinal or groin. This common tumor is not found frequently in most series of ''paratesticular'' sarcomas, probably because of the nonuniformity of site designation.[80,83] Most paratesticular well-differentiated liposarcomas occur in middle-aged or elderly persons and present as a mass lesion. Some are undoubtedly mistaken for inflammatory pseudotumors (i.e., ''inflammatory liposarcoma'') and fibrous pseudotumors because of the overgrowth of a fibrous-appearing nodule in some liposarcomas. Care should be taken to examine the adipose tissue surrounding such lesions, where atypical lipoblasts may be identified (Fig. 99-2). The typical natural history of this tumor is one of repeated recurrences over a long period of time (2 to 5 years between recurrences). Indeed, recurrence of an ''inflammatory pseudotumor'' should alert the physician to the possibility of a well-differentiated liposarcoma. After a period of time or even initially, these tumors may extend under the inguinal ligament and into the pelvic retroperitoneum; the workup should include evaluation of this possibility. Nonetheless, because of their low grade and indolent nature, an attempt at resection should be made, even if it is incomplete. The well-differentiated liposarcoma does not metastasize unless so-called dedifferentiation—a highly cellular and mitotically active region resembling malignant fibrous histiocytoma—is noted. The designation ''atypical lipoma'' or ''atypical lipomatous tumor'' describes the same lesion occurring on the extremities, precisely because of its nonmetastatic nature.

Leiomyosarcoma is the second most common paratesticular sarcoma and is often listed as the most common in articles on ''paratesticular'' sarcomas.[80,83] Most leiomyosarcomas in this area present as masses in middle-aged persons. This tumor can metastasize to regional lymph nodes, and any resection attempt should include at least clinical and perhaps pathologic assessment of the inguinal and retroperitoneal node-bearing areas. The same precaution should be taken with malignant fibrous histiocytomas of the paratesticular region.[84] Identifying a leiomyosarcoma in this site on frozen-section specimens at the time of operation can be very difficult, because of problems finding mitoses if the lesion is rightly recognized as a smooth muscle tumor and because of diagnostic consideration of similar spindled lesions such as the fibrous pseudotumor[85] and granulomatous inflammation. Thus, if a lesion is large, an incisional biopsy may be warranted, with a final therapeutic operation awaiting a permanent histologic diagnosis.

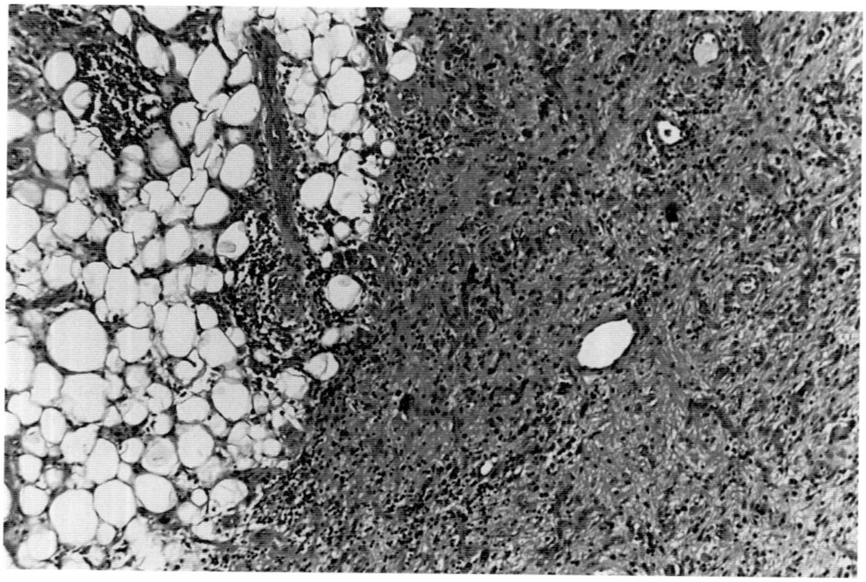

FIG. 99-2. Inflammatory, well-differentiated liposarcoma of the paratesticular area. Fat and fibrous tissue with prominent infiltration by lymphocytes prompted an initial diagnosis of inflammatory pseudotumor; however, the presence of several enlarged and pleomorphic nuclei strongly suggested liposarcoma, and lipoblasts were seen elsewhere. The fact that the tumor recurred within 1 year is more consistent with a diagnosis of liposarcoma. Original magnification ×100.

Other tumors occurring in this region include paraganglioma,[86] neurogenic sarcoma (malignant peripheral nerve sheath tumor),[87] malignant mesenchymoma,[88] adult rhabdomyosarcoma,[82,87] and malignant fibrous histiocytoma.[84]

Penile Sarcomas

Leiomyosarcoma is the most common type of sarcoma of the penis.[89–91] In most instances, it arises from the smooth muscle of the vascular plexus, the corpus cavernosum, and attains considerable size. Smaller, more superficial tumors apparently originate from erector pili muscles of the skin along the shaft; these lesions may be present for many years and, presumably because of their small size and superficial location, may be cured by excision in a manner similar to that for cutaneous sarcomas occurring elsewhere.

Kaposi's sarcoma may present on the penis as the initial manifestation of acquired immunodeficiency syndrome (AIDS) and may appear as a nonhealing ulcer.[92,93]

When epithelioid sarcoma involves the penis,[94] it may present as priapism. Nestled among the ligamentous attachment near the pubic bone, a population of spindled and epithelioid cells is found in a dense fibrous stroma. The lesion may mimic a granulomatous process or fibromatosis.

Other malignancies such as osteosarcoma,[95] angiosarcoma,[96] and malignant fibrous histiocytoma[97] may occur on the glans penis.

PROSTATIC SARCOMAS

Prostatic sarcomas comprise approximately 0.1% to 0.2% of all prostatic malignancies.[52,98] When all ages are considered, 40 to 50 years is the median age at diagnosis.[49] However, up to one third of prostatic sarcomas—almost exclusively rhabdomyosarcomas—occur in the pediatric age group.

The relative frequencies at which specific histologies of prostatic sarcoma are found do not parallel those in other areas of the body. The majority of prostate sarcomas are myosarcomas—leiomyosarcomas and rhabdomyosarcomas—although several other histologies have been described.[49,54]

A few of the sarcoma types in adults are relatively unique to the prostate and deserve special consideration. Ten to 15 cases of cystosarcoma phyllodes have been well characterized in the literature.[58,99] The age range for this lesion is broad, from the fourth to the eighth decade of life. Cystosarcoma phyllodes resembles its namesake in the female breast both pathologically and clinically. Specifically, these lesions are characterized by slow growth, local invasion of surrounding tissues, and an uncommon tendency to metastasize. Although the majority of described cases of cystosarcoma phyllodes have manifested this relatively benign behavior, these lesions can be aggressive and produce rapid death.[100] The pathologic characteristics that tend to separate benign from aggressive lesions include degrees of cellularity, nuclear pleomorphism, and mitotic activity.

Another lesion that is relatively unique to the prostate is carcinosarcoma. Fewer than 25 cases have been reported.[50,101,102] The pathologic criteria that constitute carcinosarcoma have been debated over the decades; today, the diagnosis requires unequivocal demonstration of adenocarcinoma mixed with malignant mesenchymal components of leiomyosarcoma, rhabdomyosarcoma, osteosarcoma, chondrosarcoma, or angiosarcoma. Theories of the genesis of carcinosarcoma have also been actively debated; the postulate that the separate components of adenocarcinoma and sarcoma originate from prostatic ductal stem cells capable of divergent differentiation appears to hold sway.[50] Cases have been diagnosed among patients between the fifth and eighth decade of life. Carcinosarcoma has also been reported among patients with a previous diagnosis of adenocarcinoma of the prostate who have received either external beam radiotherapy or brachytherapy; the scarcity of such descriptions implies that sarcoma arising from a previously irradiated prostate gland is rare.[102] The metastatic pattern parallels that of sarcomas more closely than does that of prostatic adenocarcinomas.[103] Mean survival among the few patients with this disorder is 21 months; median survival is approximately 1 year.[57,104]

Rhabdomyosarcoma of the prostate does occur in adults and is probably even more uncommon than the literature suggests. In a Finnish study involving a collection of 880 cases of soft tissue sarcoma among adults older than 40 years, 25 were originally identified as rhabdomyosarcomas. However, when these 25 cases were retrospectively evaluated by histology, immunochemistry, and electron microscopy and strict criteria for the diagnosis of striated muscle differentiation were employed, only 2 of the 25 cases were convincingly demonstrated to be rhabdomyosarcoma. Both of these tumors arose in the urogenital region, one in the prostate and the other in the bladder.[105] These tumors are characterized by their rapid growth; large pelvic and abdominal masses, bilateral ureteral obstruction, or both are not uncommon. Diagnosis is usually established by transurethral or transrectal biopsy or by fine needle aspiration. Common sites of spread are lungs, bone, liver, serosal surfaces, and regional lymph nodes. Although a combined-modality therapy has contributed to significant gains in the treatment of the pediatric population, the prognosis generally remains poor in the few adults treated using this approach.[106]

Among the more typical pathologic subtypes of prostatic sarcoma (e.g., leiomyosarcoma), signs and symptoms tend to be uniform.[52,54] Most common are difficulty in urination or urinary retention, hematuria (microscopic much greater than gross), pyuria, dysuria, and nocturia. The differential diagnosis of an abnormal prostate examination in the setting of prostatic sarcoma typically includes benign prostatic hypertrophy, cysts or abscesses of the prostate, cysts or neoplasms of the seminal vesicles and of müllerian duct remnants, tuberculosis prostatitis, sarcomas or transitional cell carcinomas of the bladder invading the prostate, and metastatic lesions to the prostate. Tissue diagnosis has been made by conventional means (i.e., by aspiration, punch, or open biopsy, or some combination of these).

The radiographic assessment of prostatic sarcomas also demonstrates no distinctive findings, although this assessment remains critical to determining extent of disease and monitoring response. An intravenous pyelogram or cystography typically shows a mass elevating or displacing the bladder.[107] Ultrasonography is also useful when tumor extends into the bladder because of the optimal acoustic window that the bladder represents. However, computed tomography (CT) or magnetic resonance (MR) imaging represent preferred modalities because of their ability to better delineate spread of disease outside of the prostate. MR has been performed in relatively few cases of prostatic sarcoma,[108] but by extrapolation from the radiographic assessment of sarcoma in other locations, it is presumed to represent the modality of choice. MR has proven superior to CT for the evaluation of soft tissue neoplasms because of its ability to differentiate tumor from muscle, neurovasculature, fat, and bone.[109]

There have been few formal attempts to evaluate prognostic factors among the more common histologies of prostatic sarcoma. The staging system of the American Joint Commission on Cancer (AJCC) for sarcoma recognizes four elements of importance; patients fare poorly when they have tumors of high grade (many mitotic figures), tumors of large size (>5 cm), the presence of lymph node metastases, or the presence of distant metastases. Although this staging system has been formulated based largely on information from extremity sarcomas, this same prognostic information has been found to be of importance in retroperitoneal and visceral sarcomas as well.[110–113] Size is of lesser prognostic importance among nonextremity sarcomas not easily accessible to examination, probably because of their almost universal large volume at the time of discovery.[114,115] Conversely, complete surgical resection of retroperitoneal and visceral sarcomas, especially those of low grade, is associated with longer survival.[116,117] The location of the tumor itself (i.e., extremity versus retroperitoneal or visceral) may confer a worse prognosis.[112,113] It is unclear whether the influence of location is secondary to the difficulty in achieving negative margins, the evolution of the malignancy's biologic characteristics over the probably long period of growth predating its discovery, or both. In a study of 43 adults with genitourinary sarcoma seen at the Memorial Sloan-Kettering Cancer Center (MSKCC) between 1982 and 1989, those with stage III disease, defined as high-grade malignancies larger than 5 cm, and those with grade IV (metastatic) disease had a combined 3-year relapse-free survival rate of only 26%.[118] Those patients not fulfilling these criteria and therefore of lower stage had 3-year disease-free survival rates greater than 85%. However, patients with prostatic or seminal vesicle sarcoma comprised only 12 of these 43 patients.

Upon our literature review of cases of prostatic sarcoma containing sufficient clinical detail, a minimal recurrence rate of 40% to 50% was found; most cases reported only short follow-up. The initial recurrences were equally divided between local and distant sites, a pattern that parallels that of other nonextremity sarcomas.[119,120] Furthermore, the metastatic spread pattern was also similar to that of nonextremity sarcomas. Specifically, the lung was less often affected as a recurrence site than the regional area.

Not surprisingly, there are no consistent treatment approaches to prostatic sarcoma because of its infrequency. Surgery alone or surgery combined with radiotherapy have been the most commonly used therapies, although radiotherapy alone has been employed. The role of these modalities in prolonging survival is uncertain—some of the longest survivors of prostatic sarcoma have had metastatic disease for several years[121,122]; however, the palliative benefit of these modalities is likely to be considerable.

Among nonextremity sarcomas other than prostatic malignancies, patients who undergo complete resection of their malignancy, usually defined as negative margins or microscopically positive margins, have routinely had longer survivals than patients who did not achieve this surgical result.[110–112] Therefore, based on the data from other nonextremity sarcomas, it appears reasonable to approach high-grade prostatic sarcomas with aggressive surgery. Complete resection of all gross disease should be the primary goal, because lesser resections do not appear to measurably prolong survival. For recurrences, a similar policy can be considered whether the recurrence is local or distant; additional studies of nonextremity sarcomas have shown that complete resection of recurrences also results in a more favorable survival.[113,119] Given the morbidity associated with these procedures, resection should be attempted only if the surgeon feels that all gross disease can be successfully removed. The use of radiotherapy as an adjunctive treatment following complete resection, because of the common presence of microscopic residual disease, should also be considered. There are few data in nonextremity sarcoma to support this practice, but sarcomas are known to be moderately radiosensitive, and 60 to 70 Gy can usually be delivered to the prostate region with acceptable toxicity. Surgery alone for low-grade lesions appears acceptable if clear margins can be obtained. The role of chemotherapy as adjuvant treatment or for treatment of metastatic disease is discussed later.

Rhabdomyosarcoma, an uncommon lesion in adults, should be treated in parallel with the evolving and highly successful treatments for genitourinary rhabdomyosarcoma of children. However, adults should be expected to fare generally worse.[106]

Any neoplasm of the seminal vesicle is even more rare than adult prostatic sarcoma; fewer than 100 cases have been reported.[123] Furthermore, most of the malignant neoplasms reported have been carcinomas rather than sarcomas; however, of the latter, histologies appear similar to those of the prostate gland.[61,63] Limited experience dictates that malignant sarcomas of the seminal vesicle be handled in a manner similar to that for those of the prostate.

PARATESTICULAR AND TESTICULAR SARCOMAS

Paratesticular sarcomas refer to those that involve the epididymis, scrotal tunics, and spermatic cord. Because these structures are in contiguity with each other, determination of the exact origin of sarcomas in this area is not always possible. As a result, this region is often considered as a whole for descriptive purposes. Most paratesticular sarcomas, however, appear to arise from the spermatic cord. Approximately 30% of the tumors involving the cord are malignant in nature[124–126]; of these malignancies, 90% are sarcomas. Because the contents of the spermatic cord embryonically originate from mesodermal tissues, the predominance of sarcomas is not surprising.

Among adults, no one histology seems to predominate, although liposarcoma and leiomyosarcoma are perhaps more common than others.[125–127] Among children, as in other areas of the genitourinary tract, the most commonly reported pathology is rhabdomyosarcoma.

Signs and symptoms include a slowly enlarging mass that is distinct from the testis and often unassociated with pain.[82] The paratesticular mass may be associated with an inguinal hernia.[128] Among reported cases, the masses were present for a median of 1 to 3 months (range, 1 week to >6 years) before presentation. The period of time during which the mass has been present is not a reliable predictor of tumor behavior.[129]

Radiographically, ultrasonography has been used to differentiate a paratesticular mass from the testis and to demonstrate scrotal extension.[127] CT of the pelvis has also been performed for purposes of staging; however, the sensitivity and specificity of this method of staging is unknown.

Because of the limited number of cases reported at any one center and usually over a period of several years, estimating prognosis of paratesticular sarcomas has been difficult. In one of the largest collections of cases, Catton and colleagues[80] reviewed 21 patients older than 16 years of age who were seen with a diagnosis of paratesticular sarcoma between 1958 and 1987 at the Princess Margaret Hospital in Toronto. Fourteen patients had primary disease, and seven had recurrent tumors. The median age of these 21 patients was 49 years. Among the 14 patients with a primary sarcoma, 9 presented with interscrotal tumor, 4 with a mass in the groin, and 1 with lesions in both sites. Histologies among these 14 patients were 5 rhabdomyosarcomas, 6 leiomyosarcomas, 2 malignant fibrous histiocytomas, and 1 liposarcoma. The actuarial survival of these 14 patients was 58% at 5 years; follow-up extended from 20 to 237 months with a median of 60 months. Thirteen of the 14 patients were treated with radical orchiectomy as the definitive procedure. Six of these 14 ultimately relapsed at a median of 8 months: 2 in the scrotum, 2 in the retroperitoneal lymph nodes, and 2 in the lungs. Adjuvant therapy varied; some patients received low-dose irradiation and few received adjuvant chemotherapy. Maguire and colleagues[128] suggested that survival among patients with paratesticular sarcoma may be better than that with sarcoma in other sites because of the exposed location of the tumor.

As the data in the Catton study reveal,[80] recurrences of paratesticular sarcoma can be both local and distant. Further local excision, with or without the use of radiotherapy, has resulted in long-term success, especially for low-grade lesions.[130] Metastatic sites in the lung, liver, bone, and bowel have been described.[131]

The traditional approach to treatment of paratesticular sarcoma has been orchiectomy with high ligation of the spermatic cord.[75,80,82,128,132] The role of retroperitoneal lymph node dissection has been debated over the years. Because lymph node spread probably correlates with aggressive disease, hematogenous spread, or both, retroperitoneal lymph node dissection (RPLND) should be used with great prudence.

When attempts have been made to delineate the specific site of origin of paratesticular and testicular sarcomas, the spermatic cord is easily the most common site. Average age of patients, with the exception of those with rhabdomyosarcoma, is 53 years. Approximately one third of spermatic cord tumors are malignant, and as stated previously, 90% of these are sarcomas. In regard to the epididymis, approximately 25% of the tumors are malignant, and 40% to 50% of these are sarcomas; fibrosarcomas seem to be most common.[124] Average age among those with sarcoma of the epididymis is 40 years. In the testis, sarcomatous transformation of testicular germ cell tumors occasionally occurs and is usually associated with an aggressive clinical course. Among these cases, other germ cell elements are readily apparent, but in rare instances, pure testicular sarcomas have been reported.[75,133] Whether primary sarcomas of the testis truly arise from mesenchymal tissue or, alternatively, represent unrecognized variants of germ cell malignancies is uncertain. Of interest in this regard, Fuzesi and colleagues[133] described a case of primary chondrosarcoma of the testis that contained an isochromosome of the short arm of chromosome 12 [i(12p)] on cytogenetic analysis. In this specific case, because i(12p) is a specific chromosomal abnormality in testicular germ cell tumors, strong evidence for the germ cell origin of the tumor cells was manifest.

PENILE SARCOMA

Sarcomas of the penis are rare. A variety of histologic types has been described.[90,134] No one histologic type appears to predominate, although the collection of cases over several years in the setting of evolving histologic classifications may partly account for this fact. Leiomyosarcomas are perhaps the most common type of penile sarcoma. Reports of penile sarcoma have increased as a result of Kaposi's sarcoma among the AIDS population.

Signs and symptoms of penile sarcoma include pain, edema and swelling, irritative or obstructive symptoms on urination, painful erection, and appearance of a mass.[135] The penile shaft is the most commonly affected site.[90] Duration of symptoms range from as short as 3 days to as long as 12 years.[90] Penile sarcoma is predominantly a malignancy of adults, although a few children have been reported to have this condition. Adult cases occur across a broad age range (21 to 83 years).[90]

Excluding both classic and AIDS-related Kaposi's sarcoma, partial or radical penectomy is the preferred therapeutic approach.[135] Not only are cases few, but follow-up is too brief or insufficiently detailed to justify conclusions regarding the efficacy of treatment. Of note, among a collection of 17 cases of penile sarcoma collected by Dehner and Smith[90] in which sufficient follow-up was available, many patients were alive and well several years following primary treatment which in many cases consisted of excision alone, therapy that is presently considered inadequate. The seemingly favorable prognosis of penile sarcomas may be associated with easy accessibility and earlier detectability, as has been speculated for sarcomas in the paratesticular location. Although radiotherapy has been applied in a few of these cases, its role is currently unknown.

Classic Kaposi's sarcoma has been approached in a different manner. These lesions have been treated with electrocautery, partial or total penectomy, or low-dose radiotherapy.[136] Radiotherapy at low doses is the preferred approach, because classic Kaposi's sarcoma is an indolent disease associated with long survival and a propensity to spread outside the area of treatment. AIDS-associated Kaposi's sarcoma has also responded well to low-dose irradiation,[137] which again represents the treatment of choice. Although autopsy information has shown that AIDS-associated Kaposi's sarcoma can involve many sites in the genitourinary tract, these sites rarely become clinically manifest.[92,138]

SARCOMAS OF THE KIDNEY AND URETER

Primary renal sarcomas constitute approximately 1% of malignant tumors of the kidney.[7,10,15,139–152] As the incidence of human immunodeficiency virus (HIV) infection increases, more reports of genitourinary sarcomas may be seen. Adjiman and colleagues[141] identified four patients with tumors of the genitourinary system and HIV infection. Of these four, one patient had a renal angiosarcoma.

Because most ureteral tumors are of urothelial origin, malignant mesenchymal tumors of the ureter are equally uncommon and represent approximately 1% of all tumors of the upper urinary tract.[153–155] Sarcomas of the ureter have also been noted in association with other malignant histologies; four cases of carcinosarcoma of the ureter have been recorded.[156–159] These cases behave clinically as sarcomas rather than adenocarcinomas.

Among the larger series of patients with renal sarcoma, median age has ranged from 52 to 65 years.[15,139,140,154] Approximately 25% are diagnosed before the age of 40 years, and 50% are diagnosed after the age of 60 years. Among patients with renal cell and transitional cell carcinomas, only 4% and 2% present when they are younger than 40 years of age, and 59% and 77% present when they are older than 60 years of age, respectively.

There seems to be a slight preponderance of male patients with renal sarcoma, ranging from 1.25 : 1 to 1.5 : 1 in previously cited series.[15,139,140] This ratio is somewhat lower than that in renal cell carcinoma, in which males account for approximately 70% of cases.[160] In a review of 14 cases of primary leiomyosarcoma of the ureter, Gislason and Arnarson[161] noted a female-to-male ratio of 11 : 3, which contrasts with the male dominance seen in transitional cell carcinoma of the ureter.[162]

Pain and a palpable mass are the most common presenting complaints.[7,10,15,139–152] The pain is usually localized to the flank but may be located in the epigastrium, simulating other disease processes such as cholecystitis. Gross hematuria may or may not be present. Fatigue, malaise, and weight loss are less commonly reported. The signs and symptoms of patients with sarcoma of the ureter are not distinctive from patients harboring renal sarcoma (Table 99-2).[153–158,161,163,164]

Plain abdominal x-ray films are rarely helpful in making a diagnosis of a renal malignancy. However, in cases of primary osteogenic sarcoma of the kidney, a calcified mass may be appreciated.[10,147,148] Intravenous pyelography, although neither sensitive nor specific, is often used as an initial test in evaluating signs and symptoms of a potential urologic nature. Excretory urography often demonstrates distortions or nonvisualization of the collecting system. Excretory urography also allows for confirmation of a functional contralateral kidney. This knowledge is mandatory, because the treatment of renal sarcoma usually necessitates nephrectomy.[114] MR and contrast-enhanced CT help define the extent of the tumor and its relation to vital vascular structures,[162] as well as delineate extracapsular spread and invasion of adjacent organs. Ultrasonography may also clarify the relation of the tumor to the inferior vena cava and aorta. Furthermore, cystic and necrotic masses may be aspirated under ultrasonographic guidance and the aspirate examined for evidence of malignancy. If concerns remain regarding the potential involvement of the inferior vena cava by tumor, an inferior venacavogram should be obtained.[162] A chest x-ray film or chest CT is obtained for the evaluation of metastatic disease. There is an equal likelihood of spread to either the liver or the lungs. Accordingly, some investigators suggest obtaining a preoperative CT of both the chest and liver to rule out the presence of metastases.[165]

TABLE 99-2. *Presenting signs and symptoms in patients with sarcoma of the kidney*

Sign or Symptom	No. of patients
Pain	41
Palpable mass	33
Gross hematuria	19
Weight loss	12
Anorexia	8
Fatigue	4
Malaise	Not stated
None	5
Hypoglycemia	1

Patient data from references 1 through 3 and 6 through 19.

Angiography is seldom used in the evaluation of retroperitoneal tumors but has historically been a standard part of the evaluation of the patient with a renal mass. Frija and associates[166] reported the angiographic findings of five histologically confirmed cases of sarcoma of the kidney. The arteriographic appearances were variable and seemed neither to relate to histologic type nor to be fundamentally different from those with adenocarcinoma of the kidney. A hypovascular mass was the most consistent finding. Shirkhoda and Lewis[167] examined the angiographic features of seven patients with renal sarcoma. Two were hypervascular, showing areas of neovascularity, whereas the other five were hypovascular or avascular. The two hypervascular tumors were leiomyosarcomas. Granmayeh and colleagues[168] reviewed the angiograms of seven patients with renal sarcoma of various histology. Only one tumor was hypervascular. All others, including leiomyosarcoma, were hypovascular.

The radiologic workup of a ureteral lesion is much the same as that for a renal mass. Excretory urography should be part of the initial examination. The tract above the tumor may show hydronephrosis or complete obstruction, or it may be completely normal.[154,157–159,161,163,164] Cystoscopy and retrograde pyelography may be of some use in making the diagnosis of ureteral sarcoma. Retrograde pyelograms help to delineate the distal extent of the tumor. Brushings, biopsy specimens, or urinary sediment may be obtained through the cystoscope; however, because most mesenchymal tumors do not involve the urothelium, such attempts may prove to be fruitless. Abdominal and pelvic CT scans should be obtained for staging information and for determining extension of the tumor outside the ureter.[162] Chest x-ray films, CT scans, or both, as well as CT scans of the abdomen, are obtained to rule out metastatic disease.

The staging of renal and ureteral sarcomas has not been addressed, and no formal evaluation of prognostic factors has been undertaken. There is no convincing evidence that genitourinary sarcomas that are not easily accessible to examination behave differently than other retroperitoneal sarcomas (see Prostatic Sarcomas). Not surprisingly, most renal sarcomas are found to be 10 cm or larger at laparotomy. In contrast, many ureteral sarcomas are smaller than 10 cm on pathologic examination. This discordance probably relates to early symptoms produced by ureteral obstruction. Grignon and colleagues[169] reviewed the DNA flow cytometry of 17 cases of primary sarcoma of the kidney. Ploidy pattern and outcome or time to death were not found to correlate with the results of DNA analysis. From the limited information available, prognosis does not appear to be much different from that for retroperitoneal sarcomas; 5-year survivals are in the range of 20% to 30%.

When approaching the diagnosis of a renal mass, the surgeon must be able to distinguish between renal cell carcinoma, sarcoma, transitional cell carcinoma, adrenal tumors, lymphoma, and metastatic disease.[170] A formal open biopsy should be performed. Needle biopsy is discouraged, because insufficient material is obtained to make an accurate diagnosis. Rydholm[171] has been able to demonstrate a high degree of accuracy in diagnosing soft tissue sarcomas of the extremity through fine needle aspiration cytology. Open biopsy must be performed with extreme care, because tumor spillage in the peritoneal space can have dire consequences.[165] The biopsy site should be isolated by laparotomy pads and sufficient viable tumor sent for pathologic examination. Vigilance is required to ensure adequate hemostasis, and the tumor capsule at the biopsy site should be reapproximated before wound closure. If the clinical impression, radiologic survey, and frozen section examination all point to the same diagnosis, the surgeon may proceed with a definitive procedure at the time of biopsy. However, if discrepancies arise, the surgeon should await review of the remaining sections by the pathologist.[114,171]

Surgical considerations for renal sarcoma parallel those of prostatic sarcomas (discussed previously). The mainstay of therapy for soft tissue sarcomas at any location is surgical extirpation with a wide margin of normal tissue. Complete resection can be accomplished in 40% to 78% of patients with retroperitoneal sarcoma.[113,115,165,172,173] Resectability is not related to histopathologic findings or grade but may be related to the site of the lesion. In one study, tumors in a lateral position in the retroperitoneum were easiest to remove.[115] In reviewing the MSKCC experience with primary and recurrent retroperitoneal sarcomas, Jaques and colleagues[113] determined that 83% of patients with a complete resection required resection of adjacent organs. Patients who achieved complete resection survived significantly longer than patients who underwent a lesser procedure. Criteria of unresectability were vascular involvement in 43%, peritoneal implants in 28%, distant metastases in 19%, and extensive disease in 17%. Other researchers have also demonstrated that complete resection of all visible disease, especially among patients with low-grade tumors, potentially leads to a lengthy survival.[174] It remains the responsibility of the surgeon to demonstrate unresectability through involvement of structures that cannot be removed or replaced. Armed with the knowledge that microscopic margins do not impact on survival, the surgeon must persist in his or her dissection to remove all gross tumor and provide the patient with an opportunity for a prolonged, quality existence.[115]

The experience with retroperitoneal sarcomas appears to be applicable to renal sarcomas. In a series of 21 patients with primary sarcoma of the kidney (47% leiomyosarcoma) reviewed by Volgelzang and colleagues,[15] 14 had tumor localized to the kidney. Eighteen patients underwent radical nephrectomy, two had biopsy only, and one patient received no treatment. Of patients who underwent resection, six, all of whom had disease localized to the kidney and five of whom had leiomyosarcoma, were NED (no evidence of disease) after at least 3 years of follow-up; two patients were NED after 11 and 12 years of follow-up. All other patients died of retroperitoneal or distant site recurrences within 18 months of diagnosis. Srinivas and colleagues [140] reported five patients with primary renal sarcoma confined to the kidney and nine patients with disease infiltrating adjacent organs, all but one of whom underwent nephrectomy. Among the former five, two patients were alive without recurrence at 120 and 144 months; the other three had recurrences and died at 14, 18, and 90 months postresection. Among the latter nine patients, 8 experienced recurrences and died within 3 years; one died of an intercurrent illness at 16 months.

Treatment of sarcomatous tumors of the ureter follows the same principles as that for sarcomas of the kidney. Nephroureterectomy is the standard resection. In the largest reported series, Roemer and associates[154] reviewed the results of therapy in nine patients with leiomyosarcoma of the ureter who were found to be free of intraabdominal spread at the time of laparotomy. The extent of disease beyond the confines of the ureter was not cited. At time of last follow-up, three patients were found to be free of disease at 5 months, 14 months, and 5 years postresection. All other patients had recurrent disease or died of intracurrent illness, often within 2 years. Other investigators[161,164] describe patients with ureteral sarcoma who were alive without recurrence at least 2 years following resection; one patient required both a nephroureterectomy and partial resection of the involved vena cava to achieve this result.

The use of adjuvant radiotherapy in the treatment of retroperitoneal sarcomas remains unproven[115,172] but can be selectively considered in anatomic areas such as the renal bed, where high doses can be delivered with tolerable toxicity. Unfortunately, because of the propensity of sarcomas to disseminate to distant sites, radiotherapy is unlikely to profoundly influence survival rates. A randomized controlled trial does not seem feasible because of the small number of patients.

BLADDER SARCOMA

Sarcoma accounts for less than 1% of all malignant bladder tumors. Although there are reports of surgicopathologic studies and many case reports of bladder sarcomas in the medical literature, no single institution has had sufficient numbers to define strategies for diagnosis, staging, prognosis, and treatment outcome. Shortcomings in defining optimal strategies include the rarity of these lesions, the diversity of histologic type, the tumor extent, and the varied responsiveness to chemotherapy and radiotherapy. Discussion of this topic is based on the experience of several institutions.[35,118,175–178]

The etiology of most soft tissue sarcomas is unknown. There is an increased incidence of sarcomas in the field of previous radiotherapy at a frequency of 1 in approximately 2500 who survive for at least 5 years.[179] Jacobsen and Mellemgaard[180] noted a threefold increased risk of sarcoma in the irradiated field among 6187 men with testicular cancer (seminoma) treated with radiotherapy. The interval between testicular cancer and the sarcoma varied from 5 to 34 years. Sarcomas have also been reported after treatment with chemotherapy, especially following the use of long-term cyclophosphamide.[40,181] However, the infrequency of these reports suggest that chemotherapeutic induction of sarcoma is rare, unrelated, or represents monophasic differentiation of other more common bladder histologies. Foreign bodies have also been implicated in the development of bladder sarcoma after latent periods of up to 40 years. Historically, long-term indwelling Foley catheters have been associated with the genesis of squamous cell and transitional cell carcinomas, but sarcomas also must be included among the differential diagnoses.

In reviewing the MSKCC experience from 1920 to 1984,

Morse and Whitmore[175] reported 31 adult cases of bladder sarcoma. The most common histologic type was leiomyosarcoma (17 patients) followed by rhabdomyosarcoma (12 patients), although the accuracy of the latter diagnosis among adults has been questioned.[105] In a subsequent report from MSKCC, Russo and associates[118] reported 10 adult patients with bladder sarcomas over a 7-year period from 1982 to 1989; once again, leiomyosarcoma (6 patients) was most common, followed by adult rhabdomyosarcoma (3 patients). In several other series,[35,176,177] leiomyosarcoma has been the most common bladder sarcoma.

Although formal evaluations of prognostic factors are few, not surprisingly, high histologic grade appears to be associated with a worse prognosis. High-grade sarcomas are poorly differentiated, hypervascular, hypercellular, and possess minimal stroma.

Because of the low incidence of adult bladder sarcomas, the urologic community continues to stage them according to the TNM system of the AJCC or the Jewett-Strong-Marshall system.[175] Although staging by conventional means is convenient, it probably has little or no clinical relevance with these tumors.

The most common symptom of bladder sarcoma is gross hematuria.[35,118,175,177] Frequently, patients complain of irritative symptoms and, more occasionally, urinary retention.[35,175] Intravenous urography may show a filling defect in the bladder. The cystoscopic appearance of bladder sarcoma is that of a sessile or widely pedunculated lesion. Although Patterson and Barrett[178] noted a higher incidence of bladder sarcomas in the region of the trigone, no predominant location for bladder sarcoma has been noted in other series.[35,118,175–177]

Diagnosis is made by transurethral resection of the bladder mass. Needle biopsies are usually inadequate to assess grade, vascularity, cellularity, and degree of differentiation. As in other anatomic locations in which the two most commonly reported histologies of bladder sarcoma appear, rhabdomyosarcoma has been associated with more widespread disease than has leiomyosarcoma.[175] In the MSKCC series previously cited,[175] 6 of 12 patients with rhabdomyosarcoma had distant or nodal metastasis, involvement of adjacent pelvic viscera, or both. Six of 17 patients with leiomyosarcoma had locally advanced disease (T4), and none had clinically apparent distant metastases.

Local extent is best determined by both bimanual examination under anesthesia and CT or MR imaging. For high-grade lesions, CT of the chest may also be indicated. The most common metastatic sites are lung, liver, and bone; therefore, a bone scan is also justifiable in the setting of bony pain.

Treatment recommendations for patients with bladder sarcoma are based on information obtained over many years from a small number of cases managed with diverse treatment regimens.[35,118,175,177] In general, management is based on primary surgical resection with the occasional addition of chemotherapy or radiotherapy. Treatment approaches used in centers with the largest published experience have been reviewed.[35,118,175–177]

Reviewing MSKCC records over the 64-year period from 1920 to 1984, Morse and Whitmore[175] found 31 cases of bladder sarcoma. Seventeen of these were leiomyosarcomas and 12 were rhabdomyosarcoma. The three surgical approaches used were transureteral resection (TUR), full-thickness partial cystectomy, and radical cystectomy. Unlike the situation in transitional cell carcinomas of the bladder, TURs were deemed appropriate in only a small number of cases. Only 4 of 31 patients were primarily treated with TUR, and in 2 of these, palliation was the goal.

In the MSKCC experience,[175] only three patients had tumors amenable to segmental resection. Two of three patients had a small leiomyosarcoma in the dome of the bladder. Full-thickness partial cystectomy is appropriate in selected patients with sarcomas of the bladder. Segmental resection is feasible when the tumor is solitary and random bladder biopsy specimens are negative. Both preservation of functional bladder capacity and a tumor-free circumferential margin of at least 2 cm are considered important.

Radical cystectomy was performed in 19 patients (12 leiomyosarcoma, 5 rhabdomyosarcoma, 2 both), 4 of whom had preoperative radiotherapy. Combination chemotherapy and radiotherapy were used on the basis of lesion size, metastatic burden, degree of aggressiveness, and surgical resectability. Overall results of treatment were much better for those with leiomyosarcoma than those with rhabdomyosarcoma. Of the 17 patients treated for leiomyosarcoma, 5 died of disease. Four patients have survived longer than 5 years, and the remainder are alive at a lesser duration of follow-up. Of 12 patients treated for rhabdomyosarcoma, 8 died of disease and only 2 have survived for more than 5 years.

In a later series from MSKCC, Russo and colleagues[118] reported 10 patients with bladder sarcoma, 8 of which were high grade and 2 low grade. The histologic diagnosis was leiomyosarcoma in six, rhabdomyosarcoma in three, and mesenchymoma in one. Nine patients underwent resection of primary tumor with negative margins; of these, two with small (2-cm) leiomyosarcomas, one high grade and one low grade, underwent complete transurethral resection only and are both disease-free after 7 years of follow-up. Of the 10 patients in this series, 8 remain alive without evidence of disease. The three patients with rhabdomyosarcoma have done well with aggressive trimodality therapy. All five cases of resectable leiomyosarcoma remained free of disease with or without the use of adjuvant chemotherapy.

Swartz and associates[176] from the M.D. Anderson Cancer Center reported 10 patients with leiomyosarcoma of the bladder. Four patients alive without disease for more than 5 years had been treated with segmental resection. An additional patient who had recurrence was treated with radical cystectomy, radiotherapy, and combination chemoimmunotherapy and was alive without disease at 10 years.

Reporting on their experience over the 10-year period from 1974 to 1984, Alhering and colleagues[177] identified seven patients with leiomyosarcoma of the bladder of unknown grade. For patients with nonbulky leiomyosarcoma, aggressive surgical resection with nodal dissection was performed. Patients with positive surgical margins or nodes were treated with adjuvant radiotherapy and chemotherapy. Patients with bulky disease were treated with preoperative chemotherapy with or without radiotherapy, followed by an exenterative operation. Of seven patients treated using this protocol, six were alive with a mean follow-up of 56 months.

In a Mayo Clinic series, Patterson and Barrett[178] reported five cases of leiomyosarcoma of the bladder seen during the 20-year period from 1958 to 1978. Segmental resection was curative in selected cases, but radical cystectomy was warranted in larger lesions. In a subsequent series from the Mayo Clinic, Sen and colleagues[35] reported five patients with leiomyosarcoma and three patients with rhabdomyosarcoma over the 10-year period from 1970 to 1980. Most of these patients were treated with radical cystectomy, and an occasional patient received preoperative radiotherapy. Three patients were alive without any evidence of disease at a mean follow-up of 5 years.[35]

As previously stated, agreement regarding treatment recommendations for bladder sarcoma cannot easily be found in this collected experience. However, because previous experience with genitourinary and other nonextremity sarcomas has suggested that neither radiotherapy, chemotherapy, nor lymph node dissection has major benefit, surgery that is appropriately aggressive for the clinical findings continues to be the therapy of choice. Rhabdomyosarcoma is an exception; it should be treated based on the lessons learned in the pediatric population (see Chaps. 100–102); however, adults have not fared as well with these approaches.[106]

CHEMOTHERAPY AS ADJUVANT TREATMENT AND FOR THE TREATMENT OF METASTATIC DISEASE

All the sites of genitourinary sarcoma discussed previously were treated sporadically with adjuvant chemotherapy. Traditionally, adult sarcomas have been treated as a group with little distinction between histopathologies because of their similar biologic behavior. Adjuvant therapy is usually reserved for malignancies of advanced grade or stage.

Among the 12 randomized controlled trials reported, only 2 have shown a survival benefit for adjuvant chemotherapy, which is usually doxorubicin-based. In fact, in three trials, survival on the observation arm was longer than that on the chemotherapy arm.[182] A meta-analysis of outcome among randomized trials of adjuvant chemotherapy conducted by Jones and colleagues[183] was published in abstract form. These trials included 1400 patients. The authors concluded that overall survival was increased by 9% among patients receiving adjuvant chemotherapy; both distant and local recurrences were also reduced. Even if these preliminary findings are accepted, optimism regarding this approach must be tempered by the considerable side effects experienced by patients on these regimens. For example, as many as 10% of doxorubicin-treated patients have suffered clinical congestive heart failure.

With the use of standard regimens, the benefit of adjuvant therapy is modest or nonexistent. In this setting, it is both reasonable and ethical to consider only either randomized controlled or investigational trials for treatment of these patients to better define the role of adjuvant chemotherapy.

With regard to metastatic disease, three chemotherapeutic drugs are associated with modest response rates. These include doxorubicin and ifosfamide (20% to 25% response rates in previously untreated patients) and DTIC (17% response rates in pretreated patients). Although combination chemotherapy has been associated with higher response rates, these responses have not translated into longer survival and have been associated with increased, and at times unacceptable, toxicity.[184] However, of the 5% to 10% of patients with metastatic disease who achieve complete responses with or without the use of extirpative surgery, approximately one third of these achieve long-term disease-free survival.[185,186] No second-line (salvage) therapies have been shown to be effective.

Treatment of metastatic disease is worthy of consideration because select patients benefit greatly. However, because the overwhelming majority of patients do not, it is not unreasonable to withhold therapy for patients with poor performance status or to discontinue therapy among patients achieving a suboptimal response or suffering unacceptable toxicity. The use of doxorubicin alone at doses of 60 mg/m^2 or higher or in combination with DTIC or ifosfamide, all constitute acceptable regimens.

A number of new strategies have been tried or are in progress for sarcomas of the abdominal and pelvic cavity. Response rates associated with neoadjuvant therapy appear better than those achieved in the setting of metastatic disease; these data infer that the primary tumor may be more chemoresponsive.[184] The potential of neoadjuvant therapy to allow resectability in previously unresectable cases or to maximize the potential of clear margins is under investigation. Intraperitoneal chemotherapy in the early postoperative period is also being used investigationally.[116] The use of intraoperative radiotherapy combined with external beam irradiation has also been explored in resectable adult retroperitoneal soft tissue sarcomas. In a trial including only 35 patients randomized to both intraoperative and external beam irradiation versus external beam irradiation alone, survival times were similar, although less toxicity was experienced with the approach using intraoperative therapy.[187]

Although the use of biologic response modifiers has, in general, been disappointing in soft tissue sarcomas, one particular therapy employing muramyl tripeptide phosphatidylethanolamine (MTP-PE), a synthetic analog of the bacterial cell wall component muramyl dipeptide, appears promising.[188] Increase in the cytotoxic activity of monocytes by this agent appears to be its mode of action. Early results using MTP-PE in animal models of sarcoma have been encouraging.

REFERENCES

1. Parker SL, Tong T, Bolden S, Wingo PA. Cancer Statistics, 1996. CA Cancer J Clin 1996;65:5.
2. Ball ABS, Fisher C. Leiomyosarcoma of the renal vein: a report of two cases. Eur Urol 1990;18:150.
3. Butkus DE, Kirchner KA, Neill J, Raju S. Kaposi's sarcoma in a transplanted kidney. Transplantation 1989;48:146.
4. Farrow GM, Harrison EG, Utz DC. Sarcomas and sarcomatoid and mixed malignant tumors of the kidney in adults. Cancer 1968;22:556.
5. Grignon DJ, Ayala AG, Ro JY, el-Naggar A, Papadopoulos NJ. Primary sarcomas of the kidney: a clinicopathologic and DNA flow cytometric study of 17 cases. Cancer 1990;65:1611.
6. Grignon DJ, Ro JY, Ayala AG. Mesenchymal tumors of the kidney. In: Elbe JN, ed. Tumors and tumor-like conditions of the kidneys and ureters. New York: Churchill Livingston, 1990:123.
7. Grignon DJ, McIsaac GP, Armstrong RF, Wyatt JK. Primary rhabdomyosarcoma of the kidney: a light microscopic, immunohistochemical, and electron microscopic study. Cancer 1988;62:2027.
8. Hruban RH, Bhagavan BS, Epstein JI. Massive retroperitoneal angiomyolipoma: a lesion that may be confused with well-differentiated liposarcoma. Am J Clin Pathol 1989;92:805.
9. Mayes DC, Fechner RE, Gillenwater JY. Renal liposarcoma. Am J Surg Pathol 1990;14:268.
10. O'Malley FP, Grignon DJ, Shepherd RR, Harker LA. Primary osteosarcoma of the kidney: report of a case studied by immunohistochemistry, electron microscopy, and DNA flow cytometry. Arch Pathol Lab Med 1991;115:1262.
11. Sasagawa I, Suzuki K, Ishizaki M, Takahashi H, Taguma Y, Nakamura K. Liposarcoma of the renal capsule. Urol Int 1992;48:223.

12. Schneider JA, König H, Hertel E. Malignant fibrous histiocytoma of the renal capsule. Br J Urol 1992;69:435.
13. Suster S, Robinson MJ. Spindle cell carcinoma of the renal pelvis: immunohistochemical and ultrastructural study of a case demonstrating coexpression of keratin and vimentin intermediate filaments. Arch Pathol Lab Med 1989;113:404.
14. Thirumavalavan VS, Kennedy CL, Al-Rufaie HK. Leiomyosarcoma of kidney. Br J Urol 1991;68:659.
15. Vogelzang NJ, Fremgen AM, Guinan PD, Chmiel JS, Sylvester JL, Sener SF. Primary renal sarcoma in adults: a natural history and management study by the American Cancer Society, Illinois Division. Cancer 1993;71:804.
16. Wick MR, Perrone TL, Burke BA. Sarcomatoid transitional cell carcinomas of the renal pelvis: an ultrastructural and immunohistochemical study. Arch Pathol Lab Med 1985;109:55.
17. Young RH, Dunn J, Dickersin GR. An unusual oncocytic renal tumor with sarcomatoid foci and osteogenic differentiation. Arch Pathol Lab Med 1988;112:937.
18. Chasko SB, Keuhnelian JG, Gutowski WT III, Gray GF. Spindle cell cancer of bladder during cyclophosphamide therapy for Wegener's granulomatosis. Am J Surg Pathol 1980;4:191.
19. Das S, Upton JD, Amar AD. Nodular fasciitis of the bladder. J Urol 1988;140:1532.
20. Dietrick DD, Kabalin JN, Daniels GF Jr, Epstein AB, Fielding IM. Inflammatory pseudotumor of bladder. J Urol 1992;148:141.
21. Proppe KH, Scully RE, Rosai J. Postoperative spindle cell nodules of genitourinary tract resembling sarcomas: a report of eight cases. Am J Surg Pathol 1984;8:101.
22. Ro JY, Ayala AG, Ordonez NG, Swanson DE, Babaian RJ. Pseudosarcomatous fibromyxoid tumor of the urinary bladder. Am J Clin Pathol 1986;86:583.
23. Roth JA. Pseudosarcomatous tumors of the lower urinary tract. Am J Clin Pathol 1992;98:271.
24. Wick MR, Brown BA, Young RH, Mills SE. Spindle-cell proliferations of the urinary tract: an immunohistochemical study. Am J Surg Pathol 1988;12:379.
25. Young RH, Wick MR. Transitional cell carcinoma of the urinary bladder with pseudosarcomatous stroma. Am J Clin Pathol 1988;90:216.
26. Young RH. Carcinosarcoma of the urinary bladder. Cancer 1987;59:1333.
27. Aragona F, Ostardo E, Prayer-Galetti T, Piazza R, Capitanio G. Angiosarcoma of the bladder: a case report with regard to histologic and immunohistochemical findings. Eur Urol 1991;20:161.
28. Berenson RJ, Flynn S, Freiha FS, Kempson RL, Torti FM. Primary osteogenic sarcoma of the bladder: case report and review of the literature. Cancer 1986;57:350.
29. Boyle ET Jr, Reiman HM, Kramer SA, Kelalis PP, Rainwater LM, Lieber MM. Embryonal rhabdomyosarcoma of bladder and prostate: nuclear DNA patterns studied by flow cytometry. J Urol 1988;140:1119.
30. Leestma JE, Price EB. Paraganglioma of the urinary bladder. Cancer 1971;28:1063.
31. Mills SE, Bova GS, Wick MR, Young RH. Leiomyosarcoma of the urinary bladder: a clinicopathologic and immunohistochemical study of 15 cases. Am J Surg Pathol 1989;13:480.
32. Morgan MA, Moutos DM, Pippitt CH Jr, Suda RR, Smith JJ, Thurnau GR. Vaginal and bladder angiosarcoma after therapeutic irradiation. South Med J 1989;82:1434.
33. Oesterling JE, Epstein JI, Brendler CB. Myxoid malignant fibrous histiocytoma of the bladder. Cancer 1990;66:1836.
34. Peterson RO. Urologic pathology. Philadelphia: JB Lippincott, 1986.
35. Sen SE, Malek RS, Farrow GM, Lieber MM. Sarcoma and carcinosarcoma of the bladder in adults. J Urol 1985;133:29.
36. Souto CA, Monteiro SA. Bladder sarcoma: the presentation of three cases. Hospital (Rio J) 1968;73:1603.
37. Stroup RM, Chang YC. Angiosarcoma of the bladder: a case report. J Urol 1987;137:984.
38. Taylor RE, Busuttil A. Case report: adult rhabdomyosarcoma of bladder: complete response to radiation therapy. J Urol 1989;142:1321.
39. Terada Y, Saito I, Morohoshi T, Niijima T. Malignant mesenchymoma of the bladder. Cancer 1987;60:858.
40. Thrasher JB, Miller GJ, Wettlaufer JN. Bladder leiomyosarcoma following cyclophosphamide therapy for lupus nephritis. J Urol 1990;143:119.
41. Walker AN, Mills, SE, Young RH. Mesenchymal and miscellaneous other primary tumors of the urinary bladder. In: Young RH, ed. Pathology of the urinary bladder. New York: Churchill Livingston, 1989:139.
42. Wasmer JM, Block NL, Politano VA, Tejada F. Penile angiosarcoma presenting in bladder. Urology 1981;18:179.
43. Young RH, Rosenberg AE. Osteosarcoma of the urinary bladder: report of a case and review of the literature. Cancer 1987;59:174.
44. Ahlering TE, Weintraub P, Skinner DG. Management of adult sarcomas of the bladder and prostate. J Urol 1988;140:1397.
45. Bos SD, Slaa ET. An adult man with a rhabdomyosarcoma of the prostate: a case report. Scand J Urol Nephrol 1991;25:329.
46. Ekfors R, Aho H, Kekomaki M. Malignant rhabdoid tumor of the prostatic region: immunohistological and ultrastructural evidence for epithelial origin. Virchows Arch [A] 1985;406:381.
47. Mackenzie AR, Whitmore WF Jr, Melamed MR. Myosarcomas of the bladder and prostate. Cancer 1968;22:833.
48. Manivel C, Shenoy BV, Wick MR, Dehner LP. Cystosarcoma phyllodes of the prostate. A pathologic and immunohistochemical study. Arch Pathol Lab Med 1986;110:534.
49. Narayana AS, Loening S, Weimar GW, Culp DA. Sarcoma of the bladder and prostate. J Urol 1978;119:72.
50. Nazeer T, Barada JH, Fisher HAG, Ross JS. Prostatic carcinosarcoma: case report and review of literature. J Urol 1991;146:1370.
51. Palmer MA, Viswanath S, Desmond AD. Adult prostatic rhabdomyosarcoma. Br J Urol 1993;71:489.
52. Schmidt JD, Welch MJ. Sarcoma of the prostate. Cancer 1976;37:1908.
53. Scully JM, Uno JM, McIntyre M, Mosely S. Radiation-induced prostatic sarcoma: a case report. J Urol 1990;144:746.
54. Smith BH, Dehner LP. Sarcoma of the prostate gland. Am J Clin Pathol 1972;58:43.
55. Tannenbaum M. Sarcomas of the prostate gland. Urology 1975;5:810.
56. Tungekar MF, Al Adnani MS. Sarcomas of the bladder and prostate: the role of immunohistochemistry and ultrastructure in diagnosis. Eur Urol 1986;12:180.
57. Wick MR, Young RH, Malvesta R, Beebe DS, Hansen JJ, Dehner LP. Prostatic carcinosarcomas: clinical, histologic, and immunohistochemical data on two cases, with a review of the literature. Am J Clin Pathol 1989;92:131.
58. Young JF, Jensen PE, Wiley CA. Malignant phyllodes tumor of the prostate: a case report with immunohistochemical and ultrastructural studies. Arch Pathol Lab Med 1992;116:296.
59. Yum M, Miller JC, Agrawal BL. Leiomyosarcoma arising in atypical fibromuscular hyperplasia (phyllodes tumor) of the prostate with distant metastasis. Cancer 1991;68:910.
60. Chiou R, Limas C, Lange PH. Hemangiosarcoma of the seminal vesicle: case report and literature review. J Urol 1985;134:371.
61. Fain JS, Cosnow I, King BF, Zincke H, Bostwick DG. Cystosarcoma phyllodes of the seminal vesicle. Cancer 193;71:2055.
62. Schned AR, Ledbetter JS, Selikowitz SM. Primary leiomyosarcoma of the seminal vesicle. Cancer 1986;57:2202.
63. Lamont JS, Hesketh PJ, de las Morenas A, Babayan RK. Primary angiosarcoma of the seminal vesicle. J Urol 1991;146:165.
64. Ahlgren AD, Simrell CR, Triche TJ, Ozols R, Barsky SH. Sarcoma arising in a residual testicular teratoma after cytoreductive chemotherapy. Cancer 1984;54:2015.
65. Hughes DF, Allen DC, O'Neill JJ. Angiosarcoma arising in a testicular teratoma. Histopathology 1991;18:81.
66. Michael H, Ulbright TM, Brodhecker CA. The pluripotential nature of the mesenchyme-like component of yolk sac tumor. Arch Pathol Lab Med 1989;113:1115.
67. Navarro S, Noguera R, Peydro-Olaya A, Pellin A, Llombart-Bosch A. Primitive neuroectodermal tumor of the testis: report of a new case with cytogenetic and cell culture analysis. Prog Surg Pathol 1990;11:137.
68. Ulbright TM, Clark SA, Einhorn LH. Angiosarcoma associated with germ cell tumors. Hum Pathol 1985;16:268.
69. Floyd C, Ayala AG, Logothetis CJ, Silva EG. Spermatocytic seminoma with associated sarcoma of testis. Cancer 1988;61:409.
70. Hargreaves HK, Scully RE, Richie JP. Benign hemangioendothelioma of the testis: case report with electron microscopic documentation and review of the literature. Am J Clin Pathol 1982;77:637.

71. Moon TD, Sarma DP, Rodriguez FH. Leiomyosarcoma of the scrotum. J Am Acad Dermatol 1989;20:290.
72. Newman PL, Fletcher CDM. Smooth muscle tumours of the external genitalia: clinicopathological analysis of a series. Histopathology 1991;18:523.
73. Safak M, Baltaci S, Yaman S, Uluoglu Ö, Eryilmaz Y. Intrascrotal extratesticular malignant schwannoma. Eur Urol 1992;21:340.
74. Yachia D, Auslaender L. Primary leiomyosarcoma of the testis. J Urol 1989;141:955.
75. Zukerberg LR, Young RH. Primary testicular sarcoma: a report of two cases. Hum Pathol 1990;21:932.
76. Blyth B, Mandell J, Bauer SB, et al. Paratesticular rhabdomyosarcoma: results of therapy in 18 cases. J Urol 1990;144:1450.
77. Nistal M, Fachal C, Paniagua R. Testicular carcinoma in situ associated with rhabdomyosarcoma of the spermatic cord. J Urol 1989;142:358.
78. Raney RB Jr, Tefft M, Lawrence W Jr, et al. Paratesticular sarcoma in childhood and adolescence: a report from the Intergroup Rhabdomyosarcoma Studies I and II, 1973–1983. Cancer 1987;60:2337.
79. Tanimura H, Furuta M. Rhabdomyosarcoma of the spermatic cord. Cancer 1968;22:1215.
80. Catton CN, Cummings BJ, Fornasier V, O'Sullivan B, Quirt I, Warr D. Adult paratesticular sarcomas: a review of 21 cases. J Urol 1991;146:342.
81. Goodman FR, Staunton MD, Rees HC. Liposarcoma of the spermatic cord. J R Soc Med 1991;84:499.
82. Sonksen J, Hansen EF, Colstrup H. Liposarcoma of the spermatic cord: case report. Scand J Urol Nephrol 1991;25:239.
83. Abell MR, Holtz F. Testicular and paratesticular neoplasms in patients 60 years of age and older. Cancer 1968;21:852.
84. Sclama AO, Berger BW, Cherry JM, Young JD. Malignant fibrous histiocytoma of the spermatic cord: the role of retroperitoneal lymphadenectomy in management. J Urol 1983;130:577.
85. Watson RA, Harper BN. Paratesticular fibrous pseudotumor in a patient with Gorlin's syndrome: nevoid basal cell carcinoma syndrome. J Urol 1992;148:1254.
86. Bacchi CE, Schmidt RA, Brandao M, Scapulatempo R, Costa JCM, Schmitt FC. Paraganglioma of the spermatic cord: report of a case with immunohistochemical and ultrastructural studies. Arch Pathol Lab Med 1990;114:899.
87. Banks E, Yum M, Brodhecker C, Goheen M. A malignant peripheral nerve sheath tumor in association with a paratesticular ganglioneuroma. Cancer 1989;64:1738.
88. Stein BS, Petersen RO, Conger KB. Malignant mesenchymoma of the spermatic cord. J Urol 1984;131:551.
89. Bakken CL, Hanna EA, Seybold HM. Leiomyosarcoma of the penis. J Urol 1968;99:769.
90. Dehner LP, Smith BH. Soft tissue tumors of the penis: a clinicopathologic study of 46 cases. Cancer 1970;25:1431.
91. Newman PL, Fletcher CD. Smooth muscle tumours of the external genitalia: clinicopathological analysis of a series. Histopathology 1991;18:523.
92. Angulo JC, Lopez JI, Unda-Urzaiz M, Larrinaga JR, Zubiaur CL, Flores NC. Kaposi's sarcoma of the penis as an initial urological manifestation of AIDS: a report of two cases. Urol Int 1991;46:235.
93. Schmidt ME, Yalisove BL, Parenti DM, Elgart ML, Williams CM. Rapidly progressive penile ulcer: an unusual manifestation of Kaposi's sarcoma. J Am Acad Dermatol 1992;27:267.
94. Iossifides I, Ayala AG, Johnson DE. Epithelioid sarcoma of penis. Urology 1979;14:190.
95. Edwards AT, Somerville JJF. Primary osteosarcoma of penis. Br J Urol 1990;66:552.
96. Prescott RJ, Mainwaring AR. Irradiation-induced penile angiosarcoma. Postgrad Med J 1990;66:576.
97. Moran CA, Kaneko M. Malignant fibrous histiocytoma of the glans penis. Am J Dermatopathol 1990;12:182.
98. Christoffersen J. Leiomyosarcoma of the prostate. Acta Chir Scand Suppl 1973;433:75.
99. Kevwitch MK, Walloch JL, Waters WB, Flanigan RC. Prostatic cystic epithelial-stromal tumors: a report of 2 new cases. J Urol 1993;149:860.
100. Yokota T, Yamashita Y, Okuzono, et al. Malignant cystosarcoma phyllodes of prostate. Acta Pathol Jpn 1984;34:663.
101. Quay SC, Proppe KH. Carcinosarcoma of the prostate: case report and review of the literature. J Urol 1981;125:436.
102. Lauwers GY, Schevchuk M, Armenakas N, Reuter VE. Carcinosarcoma of the prostate. Am J Surg Pathol 1993;17:342.
103. Hokamura K, Kurozumi T, Tanaka K, Yamaguchi A. Carcinosarcoma of the prostate. Acta Pathol Jpn 1985;35:481.
104. Zenklusen HR, Weymuth G, Rist M, Mihatsch MJ. Carcinosarcoma of the prostate in combination with adenocarcinoma of the prostate and adenocarcinoma of the seminal vesicles. Cancer 1990;66:998.
105. Miettinen M. Rhabdomyosarcoma in patients older than 40 years of age. Cancer 1988;62:2060.
106. Waring PM, Newland RC. Prostatic embryonal rhabdomyosarcoma in adults. Cancer 1992;69:755.
107. King DG, Finney RP. Embryonal rhabdomyosarcoma of the prostate. J Urol 1977;117:88.
108. Bartolozzi C, Selli C, Olmastroni M, Menchi I, DiCandio G. Rhabdomyosarcoma of the prostate: MR findings. Am J Roentgenol 1988;150:1333.
109. Tehranzadeh J, Mnaymneh W, Ghavam C, Morillo G, Murphy BJ. Comparison of CT and MR imaging in musculoskeletal neoplasm. J Comput Assist Tomogr 1989;13:466.
110. Farhood AI, Hajdu SI, Shiu MH, Strong EW. Soft tissue sarcomas of the head and neck in adults. Am J Surg 1990;160:365.
111. Meijer S, Peretz T, Gaynor JJ, Tan C, Hajdu SI, Brennan MF. Primary colorectal sarcoma. Arch Surg 1990;125:1163.
112. Glenn J, Sindelar WF, Kinsella T, et al. Results of multimodality therapy of resectable soft-tissue sarcomas of the retroperitoneum. Surgery 1985;97:316.
113. Jacques DP, Coit DG, Hajdu SI, Brennan MF. Management of primary and recurrent soft-tissue sarcoma of the retroperitoneum. Ann Surg 1990;212:519.
114. Jacques DP, Coit DG, Brennan MF. Soft tissue sarcoma of the retroperitoneum. In: Shiu MH, Brennan MF, eds. Surgical management of soft tissue sarcoma. Philadelphia: Lea & Febiger, 1989:157.
115. Bevilacqua RG, Rogatko A, Hajdu SI, Brennan MF. Management of primary and recurrent soft-tissue sarcomas. Arch Surg 1991;126:328.
116. Fern ndez-Trigo V, Sugarbaker PH. Sarcomas involving the abdominal and pelvic cavity. Tumori 1993;79:77.
117. Rossi CR, Nitti D, Foletto M, et al. Management of primary sarcomas of the retroperitoneum. Eur J Surg Oncol 1993;19:355.
118. Russo P, Brady MS, Conlon K, et al. Adult urological sarcoma. J Urol 1992;147:1032.
119. Potter DA, Glenn J, Kinsella, T, et al. Patterns of recurrence in patients with high-grade soft-tissue sarcomas. J Clin Oncol 1985;3:353.
120. Fortner JG, Martin S, Hajdu S, Turnbull A. Primary sarcoma of the retroperitoneum. Semin Oncol 1981;8:180.
121. Mottola A, Selli C, Carini M, Natali A, Gambacorta G. Leiomyosarcoma of the prostate. Eur Urol 1985;11:131.
122. Witherow R, Molland E, Oliver T, Hind C. Leiomyosarcoma of prostate and superficial soft tissue. Urology 1980;15:513.
123. Benson RC Jr, Clark WR, Farrow GM. Carcinoma of the seminal vesicle. J Urol 1984;132:483.
124. Beccia DJ, Krane RJ, Olsson CA. Clinical management of non-testicular intrascrotal tumors. J Urol 1976;116:476.
125. Sogani PC, Grabstald H, Whitmore WF Jr. Spermatic cord sarcoma in adults. J Urol 1978;120:301.
126. Hartwick RWJ, Srigley JR, Burns B, McCaughey WTE. A clinicopathologic review of 112 paratesticular tumors. (Abstract) Lab Invest 1987;56:30A.
127. Cardenosa G, Papanicolaou N, Fung CY, et al. Spermatic cord sarcomas: sonographic and CT features. Urol Radiol 1990;12:163.
128. Maguire BM, Lewis SB, Cooke SL. Malignant fibrous histiocytoma: review and case report. Aust N Z J Surg 1991;61:636.
129. Malek RS, Utz DC, Farrow GM. Malignant tumors of the spermatic cord. Cancer 1972;29:1109.
130. Lewis P, Salaman RA, Aubrey DA. Liposarcoma of the spermatic cord. Br J Clin Pract 1990;44:795.
131. Grey LF, Sorial RF, Shaw W. Spermatic cord sarcoma. Urology 1986;27:28.
132. Minervini R, Morelli G, Benvenuti S, Sepich CA, Cecchi M. Leiomyosarcoma of the spermatic cord: report of a case. Acta Urol Belg 1992;60:97.
133. Fuzesi L, Rixen H, Kirschner-Hermanns R. Cytogenetic findings in

a metastasizing primary testicular chondrosarcoma. Am J Surg Pathol 1993;17:738.
134. Edwards AT, Somerville JJF. Primary osteosarcoma of penis. Br J Urol 1990;66:552.
135. Huang DJ, Stanisic TH, Hansen KK. Epithelioid sarcoma of the penis. J Urol 1992;147:1370.
136. Lands RH, Ange D, Hartman DL. Radiation therapy for classic Kaposi's sarcoma presenting only on the glans penis. J Urol 1992; 147:468.
137. Vapnek JM, Quivey JM, Carroll PR. Acquired immunodeficiency syndrome-related Kaposi's sarcoma of the male genitalia: management with radiation therapy. J Urol 1991;146:333.
138. Miles BJ, Melser M, Farah R, Markowitz N, Fisher E. The urological manifestations of the acquired immunodeficiency syndrome. J Urol 1989;142:771.
139. Farrow GM, Harrison EG, Utz DC, ReMine WH. Sarcomas and sarcomatoid and mixed malignant tumors of the kidney in adults: I. Cancer 1968;22:545.
140. Srinivas V, Sogani PC, Hajdu SI, Whitmore WF. Sarcomas of the kidney. J Urol 1984;132:13.
141. Adjiman S, Zerbib M, Flam T, Brochard M, Desligneres S, Boissonnas A, Debre B, Steg A. Genitourinary tumors and HIV1 infection. Eur Urol 1990;18:61.
142. Ah-Chong AK, Yip AWC. Primary osteogenic sarcoma of the kidney presenting as staghorn calculus. Br J Urol 1993;71:233.
143. Gupta OP, Dube MK. Rare primary renal sarcoma. Br J Urol 1971; 43:546.
144. Klein B, Falkson G, Simson IW, Stevens K, DeVilliers FJ, Keogan PG, Thatcher CJ. Granulocytic sarcoma of the kidney in a patient with acute myelomonocytic leukaemia: a case report. South Am Med J 1986;70:696.
145. Mead JH, Herrera GA, Kaufman MF, Herz JH. Case report of a primary cystic sarcoma of the kidney, demonstrating fibrohistiocytic, osteoid, and cartilaginous components (malignant mesenchymoma). Cancer 1982;50:2211.
146. Micolonghi TS, Liang D, Schwattz S. Primary osteogenic sarcoma of the kidney. J Urol 1984;131:1164.
147. Moon TD, Dexter DF, Morales A. Synchronous independent primary osteosarcoma and adenocarcinoma of kidney. Urology 1983;21:608.
148. Mortensen PHG. Primary osteogenic sarcoma of the kidney. Br J Urol 1989;63:101.
149. Ogawa K, Nakashima Y, Kim Y-C, et al. Unusual renal sarcoma in a young adult: its similarities to clear cell sarcoma of the kidney. J Urol 1987;137:730.
150. Taccagni G, Terreni MR, Leone BE, Cantaboni A. Nondifferentiated-type small cell sarcoma of kidney in a young woman. Ultrastruct Pathol 1991;15:291.
151. Williams JP, Savage PT. Liposarcoma of kidney. Br J Surg 1958;46: 225.
152. Yokose T, Fukuda H, Ogiwara A, Sakai K, Saitoh K. Myxoid leiomyosarcoma of the kidney accompanying ipsilateral ureteral transitional cell carcinoma: a case report with cytological, immunohistochemical, and ultrastructural study. Jpn Soc Pathol 1991;41:694.
153. Abeshouse BS. Primary benign and malignant tumors of the ureter: a review of the literature and report of one benign and twelve malignant tumors. Am J Surg 1956;91:237.
154. Roemer CE, Pfister RC, Brodsky G, Sacknoff EJ. Primary leiomyosarcoma of the ureter. Urology 1980;16:492.
155. Werth DD, Weigel JW, Mebust WK. Primary neoplasms of the ureter. J Urol 1981;125:628.
156. Renner MJ. Primary malignant tumors of the ureter. Surg Gynecol Obstet 1931;52:793.
157. Byard RW, Bell MEA, Alkan MK. Primary carcinosarcoma: a rare cause of unilateral ureteral obstruction. J Urol 1987;137:732.
158. Fleming S. Carcinosarcoma (mixed mesodermal tumor) of the ureter. J Urol 1987;138:1234.
159. Orsatti G, Corgan FJ, Goldberg SA. Carcinoma of urothelial organs: sequential involvement of urinary bladder, ureter, and renal pelvis. Urology 1993;41:289.
160. Natale R. Tumors of the kidney, ureter, and bladder. In: Kelley WN, ed. Internal medicine. Philadelphia: JB Lippincott, 1989:805.
161. Gislason T, Arnarson OO. Primary ureteral sarcoma. Scand J Urol Nephrol 1984;18:253.
162. Linehan WM, Shipley WU, Longo DL. Cancer of the kidney and ureter. In: DeVita VT Jr, Hellman S, Rosenberg SA, eds. Cancer: principles and practice of oncology. Philadelphia: JB Lippincott, 1989:979.
163. Rushton HG, Sens MA, Garvin AJ, Turner WR. Primary leiomyosarcoma of the ureter: a case report with electron microscopy. J Urol 1983;129:1045.
164. Madgar I, Goldwasser B, Czerniak A, Many M. Leiomyosarcoma of the ureter. Eur Urol 1988;14:487.
165. Storm FK, Mahvi DM. Diagnosis and management of retroperitoneal soft-tissue sarcoma. Ann Surg 1991;214:2.
166. Frija G, Dana A, Dhamelincourt AM, Affre J, Bismuth V, Michel JR. Manifestations radiologiques des sarcomes primitifs du rein chez l'adulte. J Radiol 1979;60:613.
167. Shirkhoda A, Lewis E. Renal sarcoma and sarcomatoid renal cell carcinoma: CT and angiographic features. Radiology 1987;162:353.
168. Granmayeh M, Wallace S, Barrett AF, Fisher R, Heslep JH. Sarcoma of the kidney: angiographic features. Am J Roentgenol 1977;129:107.
169. Grignon DJ, Ayala AG, Ro JY, El-Naggar A, Papadopoulos NJ. Primary sarcomas of the kidney: a clinicopathologic and DNA flow cytometric study of 17 cases. Cancer 1990;65:1611.
170. Pack GT, Tabah EJ. Primary retroperitoneal tumors: a study of 120 cases. Surg Gynecol Obstet 1954;99:209.
171. Rydholm A, Gustafson P, Rooser B, et al. Limb-sparing surgery without radiotherapy based on anatomic location of soft tissue sarcoma. J Clin Oncol 1991;9:1757.
172. Karakousis CP, Velez AF, Emrich LJ. Management of retroperitoneal sarcomas and patient survival. Am J Surg 1985;150:376.
173. Brennan MF, Shiu MH. Presentation, demographics, and prognostic factors of soft tissue sarcoma. In: Shiu MH, Brennan MF, eds. Surgical management of soft tissue sarcoma. Philadelphia: Lea & Febiger, 1989:45.
174. Karakousis CP, Blumenson LE, Canavese G, Rao U. Surgery for disseminated abdominal sarcoma. Am J Surg 1992;163:560.
175. Morse MJ, Whitmore WF. Genitourinary sarcomas in adults. In: Shiu MH, Brennan MF, eds. Surgical management of soft tissue sarcomas. Philadelphia: Lea & Febiger, 1989:189.
176. Swartz DA, Johnson DE, Ayala AG, Watkins DL. Bladder leiomyosarcoma: a review of 10 cases with 5 year followup. J Urol 1985; 133:200.
177. Ahlering TE, Weintraub P, Skinner DG. Management of adult sarcomas of the bladder and prostate. J Urol 1988;140:1397.
178. Patterson DE, Barrett DM. Leiomyosarcoma of urinary bladder. Urology 1983;21:367.
179. Robinson E, Neugut AI, Wylie P. Clinical aspects of the postirradiation sarcomas. J Natl Cancer Inst 1988;80:233.
180. Jacobsen GK, Mellemgaard A, Engelholm SA, Moller H. Increased incidence of sarcoma in patients treated for testicular seminoma. Eur J Cancer 1993;29:664.
181. Hajdu SI. Pathology of soft tissue tumors. Philadelphia: Lea & Febiger, 1979.
182. Mazanet R, Antman KH. Adjuvant therapy for sarcomas. Semin Oncol 1991;18:603.
183. Jones GW, Chouinard E, Patel M. Adjuvant adriamycin (doxorubicin) in adult patients with soft tissue sarcomas: a systematic overview and quantitative meta-analysis. (Abstract) Clin Invest Med 1991;14:A772.
184. Verweij J, Pinedo HM. Changing concepts in the systemic treatment of locally advanced or metastatic soft tissue sarcomas. In: Verweij J, Pinedo HM, Suit HD, eds. Multidisciplinary treatment of soft tissue sarcomas. Boston: Kluwer Academic Publishers, 1993:107.
185. Elias AD. Chemotherapy for soft-tissue sarcomas. Clin Orthop 1993; 289:94.
186. Yap BS, Sincovics JG, Burgess MA, Benjamin RS, Bodey GP. The curability of advanced soft tissue sarcomas in adults with chemotherapy. (Abstract) Proc Am Soc Clin Oncol 1983;239.
187. Kinsella TJ, Sindelar WF, Lack E, Glatstein E, Rosenberg SA. Preliminary results of a randomized study of adjuvant radiation therapy in resectable adult retroperitoneal soft tissue sarcomas. J Clin Oncol 1988;6:18.
188. Mertens WC, Bramwell VHC. Adjuvant chemotherapy of soft tissue sarcomas. In: Verweij J, Pinedo HM, Suit HD, eds. Multidisciplinary treatment of soft tissue sarcomas. Kluwer Academic, 1993:117.

SECTION IX

Pediatric Rhabdomyosarcomas and Soft Tissue Sarcomas

Principles and Practice of Genitourinary Oncology, edited by Derek Raghavan, Howard I. Scher, Steven A. Leibel, and Paul H. Lange. Lippincott-Raven Publishers, Philadelphia, © 1997.

CHAPTER 100

Pathology of Genitourinary Rhabdomyosarcoma in Children and Adolescents

William A. Newton, Jr., and Ala B. Hamoudi

Although rhabdomyosarcoma (RMS) accounts for about one tenth of all malignancies in children and adolescents, it occurs in the genitourinary (GU) organs more frequently than in any other body system (Fig. 100-1). The most commonly involved GU organs are bladder, prostate, and paratesticular tissues, but all sites are at risk (Fig. 100-2). The histology of these tumors differs in subtype from those seen elsewhere in the body; histologically, they are predominantly of cell subtypes that are associated with a better prognosis, but they include those that predict poor outcome as well.[1] The differential diagnosis of this group of tumors includes other soft tissue tumors, both benign and malignant. RMS in GU sites usually remains localized, except for spread to local lymph nodes from paratesticular tumors[2–4] (Fig. 100-3). The survival rate for patients with these tumors has improved significantly with the combined use of surgery, radiation, and chemotherapy. This improvement has been accompanied by an increased rate of preservation of normal organ structure and function.[5–8] Biopsies of primary tumor sites after initial chemotherapy have demonstrated that the cancer cells can be eliminated by effective therapy, but they very often show the presence of maturing RMS cells, whose malignant potential has been difficult to predict but appears to be negligible.

HISTOLOGY OF RHABDOMYOSARCOMA SUBTYPES

The subtypes of soft tissue sarcoma that were eligible for entry into Intergroup Rhabdomyosarcoma Study I (IRS-I) included all of the subtypes in the Horn and Enterline classification system,[9] including embryonal RMS, alveolar RMS, botryoid variant of embryonal RMS, and pleomorphic RMS. Other specific sarcoma entities were excluded from these studies. Each tumor was classified for study purposes by the IRS Pathology Committee. Some were so poorly preserved or inadequate in amount that a precise diagnosis was not possible. If such a lesion met other criteria that established it as a sarcoma, it was classified as "sarcoma, not otherwise specified." Tumors that were too poorly preserved or too small to be thus classified were designated ineligible for study analysis. Tumors that consisted of primitive cells without differentiation were classified as undifferentiated sarcoma, or UDS (Fig. 100-4). Several specific sarcomas have been identified recently that previously had been classified as UDS. Lesions from patients entered in IRS-III and the pilot IRS-IV that were classified as UDS have been restudied using a battery of immunohistochemical (IHC) antibodies. One third of 51 such tumors have been reclassified as extraosseous Ewing's sarcoma (EOE), peripheral neuroectodermal tumor (PNET), intraabdominal desmoplastic small cell tumor, ectomesenchymoma, or rhabdoid tumor of soft tissue; the remainder were left classified as UDS (Bruce Pawel, IRS data, 1994).

It is possible to categorize all but the residual group of UDS lesions into histologic subgroups using classic histologic methods, aided by IHC studies and, to a lesser extent, by ultrastructural studies. These subtypes have been shown to have prognostic significance, as is discussed later with relation to the international classification system that has recently been formulated and tested.[10] The morphologic criteria for each major subtype are included here in the order of their frequency. The IRS Pathology Committee review of the histologic classification of bladder and prostate RMS is depicted in Figure 100-5. Almost all of the lesions were classified as embryonal RMS, with only a few designated alveolar RMS. In the bladder, almost half of the embryonal subtypes were subclassified as botryoid variant. This is in contrast to the prostatic site, in which only seven tumors had the characteristic features of a botryoid RMS. In general, botryoid subtypes of embryonal RMS occur only if the tumor can grow into a lumen, as opposed to originating within the substance of an organ. The bladder is the most common site for a botryoid lesion, and it is also seen in vaginal, bile duct, nasopharyngeal, and middle ear sites. Patients with lesions classified as botryoid RMS have one of the highest 5-year survival rates, almost 100%.[10]

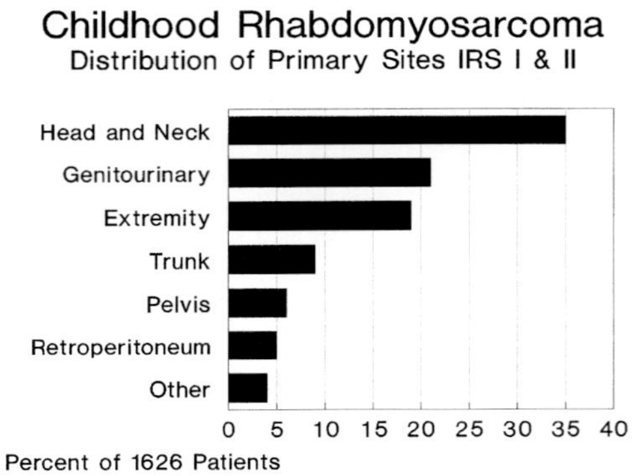

FIG. 100-1. Bar graph illustrating the distribution of the primary sites of childhood rhabdomyosarcoma in 1626 patients eligible for Intergroup Rhabdomyosarcoma Studies I and II.

Embryonal Rhabdomyosarcoma

Embryonal RMS tumors consist of primitive mesenchymal cells that show a spectrum of differentiation of rhabdomyoblasts (Fig. 100-6). The degree of differentiation is approximated by the amount of tumor cell cytoplasmic development. Their cellularity, or the relation of the number of tumor cells to the amount of supporting tissue, varies widely, from a densely cellular tumor to one that is sparsely cellular, with intervening myxoid stroma. The tumor cells and their nuclei tend to be elongated or spindle-shaped, but the less mature cells may be rounded. The most differentiated cells show abundant eosinophilic-staining cytoplasm, which is often fibrillar, forming so called ''strap'' cells. Cross-striations may be present in the most mature cells but are not used as a diagnostic feature. Their nuclei are often irregularly shaped and have a lighter chromatin pattern than that seen in the usual alveolar RMS. The least differentiated cells may have a stellate appearance consisting of small nuclei surrounded by delicate, thin cytoplasmic strands resembling fetal cells. These tumors are often loosely cellular. If differentiation is moderate to marked, these cells are readily identified as RMS. IHC evaluation can be used for confirmation but is of most help in identifying those tumors with the least degrees of myogenic differentiation.

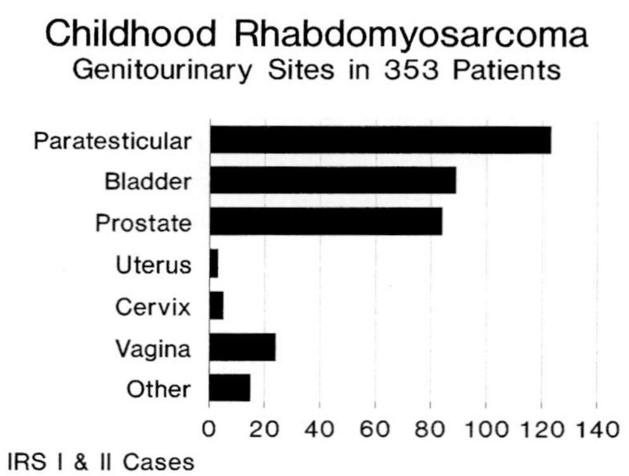

FIG. 100-2. Bar graph illustrating the specific genitourinary system sites in 353 patients eligible for Intergroup Rhabdomyosarcoma Studies I and II.

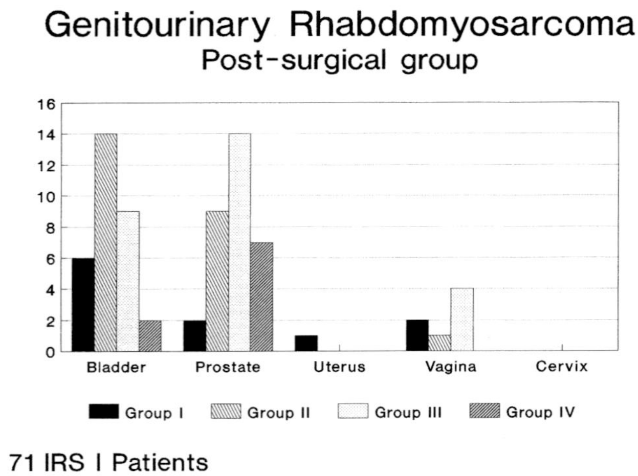

FIG. 100-3. Bar graph illustrating the number of patients in each of four postsurgical groups, out of a total of 71 patients eligible for Intergroup Rhabdomyosarcoma Study I, by tumor site. Group I patients had complete removal of their tumor, group II had microscopic residual, group III had gross tumor residual, and group IV had metastatic disease at diagnosis.

Alveolar Rhabdomyosarcoma

About a fifth of RMS tumors are of the alveolar subtype, and they are clinically most important because of their association with a poor response to therapy. This tumor is characterized by interconnecting strands of anastomosing fibrovascular connective tissue septa, which form spaces that have a pattern simulating that of pulmonary alveoli. The tumor cells lie free in these spaces as relatively similar-appearing, small, round cells that line the septal structures in single file and also fill the ''alveolar'' spaces to varying degrees (Figs. 100-7 and 100-8). The tumors showing the greatest density of tumor cells have been designated as a ''solid'' variant, particularly if the typical lining up of the cells along the septae is not apparent.[11]

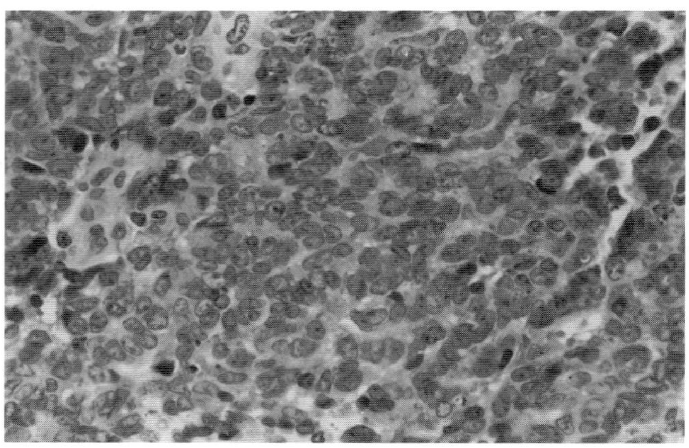

FIG. 100-4. Photomicrograph of undifferentiated sarcoma. The nuclei are larger than those seen in rhabdomyosarcoma, and cytoplasm is present in moderate amounts. These sarcomas demonstrated a negative reaction to immunohistochemical muscle antigens but a positive reaction to vimentin.

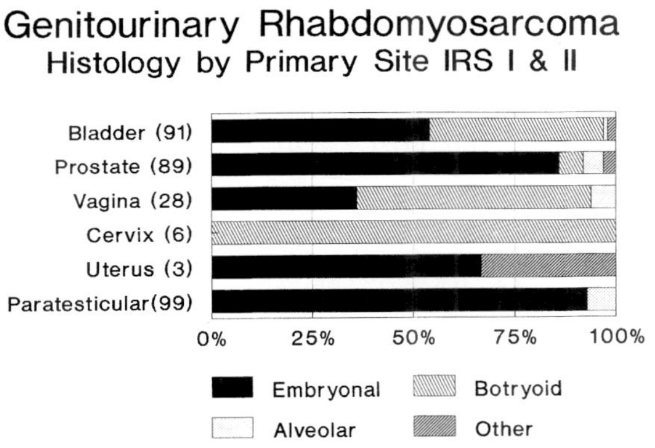

FIG. 100-5. Bar graph illustrating the Intergroup Rhabdomyosarcoma Study Pathology Committee classification of genitourinary rhabdomyosarcoma lesions from 316 patients eligible for Intergroup Rhabdomyosarcoma Studies I and II by site.

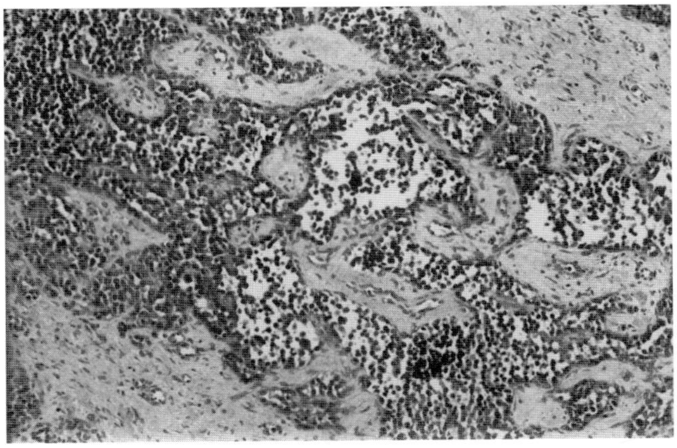

FIG. 100-7. Photomicrograph of an alveolar rhabdomyosarcoma showing the alveolar-like spaces lined by round tumor cells, with varying numbers of single isolated tumor cells. Myogenesis is present.

The individual tumor cells differ from those seen in embryonal RMS in that they are not spindled but are almost always rounded, particularly their nuclei. The nuclei also show a darker staining of the chromatin. On the other hand, the same tendency of these cells to undergo differentiation is observed, with development of varying amounts of cytoplasm with the same appearance as in the embryonal subtype. In general, each tumor tends to have a uniform degree of cytoplasmic differentiation, varying from minimal to marked in extent. Again, IHC evaluation can be used to confirm the RMS nature or to exclude other, non-RMS tumors, particularly those that consist of small round blue cells, such as EOE/PNET, lymphomas, and neuroblastoma.

Botryoid Variant of Embryonal Rhabdomyosarcoma

Patients with embryonal RMS of the botryoid type almost always survive if given current treatment schedules. It is found in most body sites in which the tumor can grow into an open space (eg, bladder, vagina, middle ear, nasopharynx, bile duct). These tumors often have a grape-like appearance grossly: hence, the name. This embryonal RMS subtype is usually sparsely cellular, with abundant myxoid stroma. The tumor cells may be of the more immature stellate type, but they often have an appearance that simulates muscle bundles in miniature. Their cytoplasm tends to be more abundant than that of the usual small RMS cell, often having IHC characteristics of a cell with moderate or marked differentiation. The hallmark of this subtype, however, is the presence of a layer of tumor cells that are condensed together and located immediately below the overlying epithelium, the so-called cambium layer (Fig. 100-9). This feature is essential for the designation of this diagnosis.

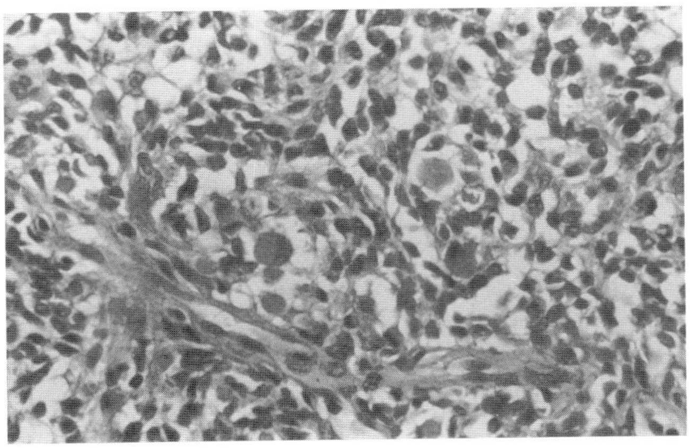

FIG. 100-6. Photomicrograph of embryonal rhabdomyosarcoma showing the tendency toward a spindle shape of both nuclei and cells. There is a varying amount of myogenesis, as evidenced by the amount of their cytoplasm.

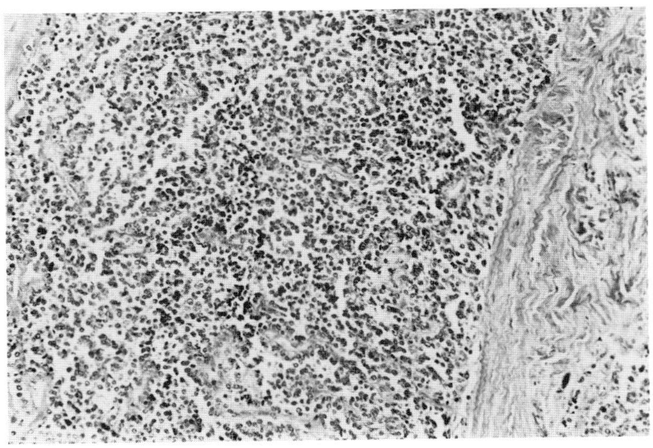

FIG. 100-8. Photomicrograph of an alveolar rhabdomyosarcoma whose features are similar to those of the lesion in Figure 100-6 except that the alveolar-like spaces are partially to completely filled, giving a solid appearance. Survival of patients with this variant is similar to those whose tumor has the classic alveolar features.

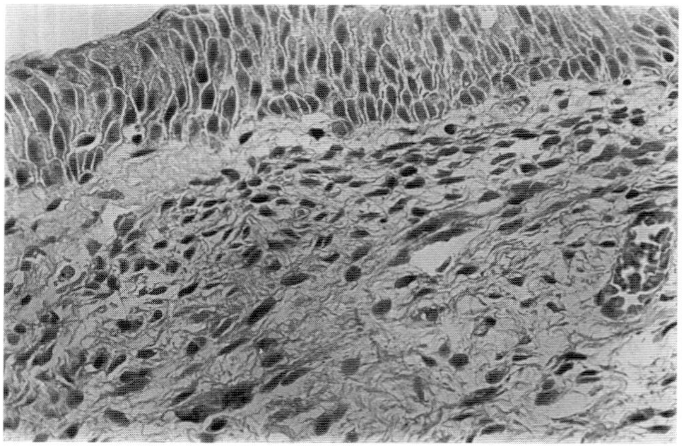

FIG. 100-9. Photomicrograph of a botryoid subtype of embryonal rhabdomyosarcoma. Notice the loose arrangement of the small rhabdomyoblasts in a myxoid stroma and the cambium layer of concentrated tumor cells lying just below the epithelial surface.

Spindle-Cell Rhabdomyosarcoma

Another embryonal RMS subtype of clinical significance is the recently defined spindle-cell subtype.[12,13] This variant is important because it is most often seen in paratesticular RMS lesions, although it can be seen elsewhere in the body, and its identification predicts an unusually good prognosis for survival. It is also found in other sites of the body. It consists almost exclusively of spindle-shaped cells, either in a prominent collagen stroma or in a pattern similar to that of leiomyosarcoma, with only sparse amounts of intercellular collagen. Those with abundant collagen usually display a characteristic storiform pattern (Fig. 100-10).

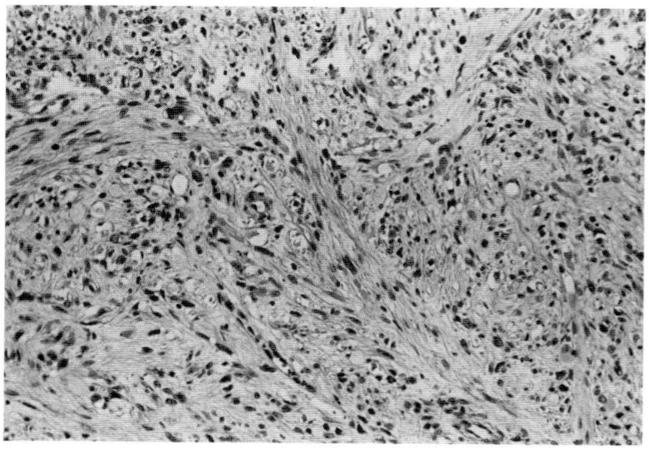

FIG. 100-10. Photomicrograph of spindle cell rhabdomyosarcoma variant of embryonal rhabdomyosarcoma. The spindle-shaped tumor cells predominate but are separated into patterns by cords of dense connective tissue, including a storiform pattern. The collagen-poor variant lacks the prominent collagen component and resembles a leiomyosarcoma.

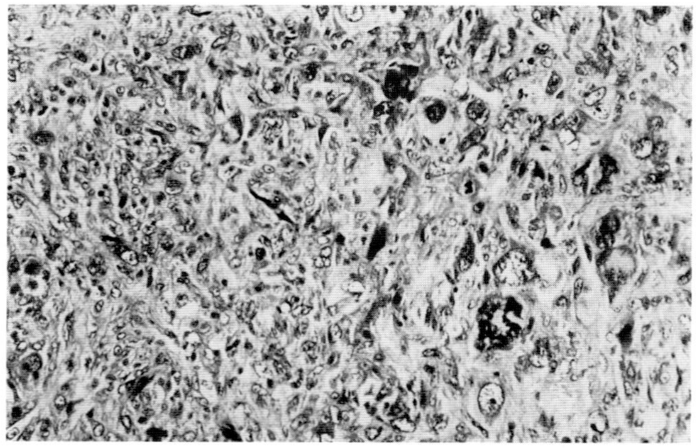

FIG. 100-11. Photomicrograph of an embryonal rhabdomyosarcoma showing the presence of anaplastic tumor cells distributed diffusely throughout the tumor.

Anaplasia

In a study to reevaluate whether the pleomorphic RMS subtype of Horn and Enterline was seen in RMS tumors of children and adolescents, about 3000 tumors from the IRS Pathology Center files were reviewed. About 110 showed the presence of varying numbers of tumor giant cells whose nuclei were three times or more larger than those of the other tumor cells. The nucleus was lobated, but always single, and quite hyperchromatic. The cytoplasm was also increased in amount but did not have unusual features other than size (Fig. 100-11). If these giant cells were present diffusely throughout the tumor or in frequent clumps, survival time of the patient was significantly shorter than for those with embryonal RMS without anaplasia. Patients whose lesion showed only a few such cells had a survival time intermediate between those without anaplasia and those with more numerous anaplastic cells.[14]

IMMUNOHISTOCHEMICAL AND MOLECULAR DIAGNOSTIC STUDIES

Although typical RMS subtypes can readily be diagnosed without additional studies, recently developed IHC antibodies and molecular probes have become increasingly important in identifying the lesions that do not have sufficiently differentiated characteristics. IHC antibodies identify antigens characteristic of myogenic proteins in differentiating rhabdomyoblasts, which also enables an approximation of their maturation level.[15–17] All primitive sarcomas react to vimentin, particularly if the tissue is pretreated by microwave heating. UDS tumors react only to antivimentin. The earliest level of myogenesis is detected by antidesmin. Skeletal muscle–specific actin reacts slightly later in myogenesis (Hiruoki Hojo, IRS data, 1995). Antimyoglobin positivity is seen only in more mature, obviously moderately or markedly differentiated cells. Many of the less differentiated tumors show positive reactions in only a small fraction of the tumor cells.

IHC studies, however, are not completely or consistently dependable. Tissues that are not well preserved either do not react or show a diffuse staining of all of the types of tissue, making the pattern uninterpretable. A recent study of a large number of randomly selected RMS lesions were reacted with a panel of IHC reagents that identify several tissue types: muscle, nerve, epithelium, and MIC2 antigen (Hirouki Hojo, IRS data, 1995). Positive reactions were obtained to each of the nonmuscle antibodies in a small but significant number of the tumors, which were characteristically positive to antimuscle reagents. This suggests a heterogeneous nature of the cell types for some tumors. Molecular analysis recently demonstrated both myogenic and primitive neuroectodermal elements in an RMS tumor.[18] The presence of more than one cell type is known to occur in synovial sarcoma, ectomesenchymoma, and Triton tumors. Nonspecificity may also be an explanation for reactions to nonmuscle antibodies. The MYOD family of myogenic transcription factors are probably responsible for the transcriptional activation of muscle-specific genes.[19]

Molecular probe studies have established specific abnormalities that can be identified to further refine the understanding of several types of soft tissue tumors of children. The two that are most relevant to this discussion are the breakpoints of the chromosomal translocations that are known to occur in most alveolar RMS and EOE/PNET lesions. This knowledge makes possible a new level of preciseness in identification of these lesions. Most alveolar RMS tumors have t(2,13)(q35;q,14) translocation,[20] and the fusion gene has now been cloned.[21,22] In contrast, most embryonal RMS tumors appear to have undergone genetic loss of heterozygosity.[23] Techniques are already available to identify the fusion gene in alveolar RMS by fluorescence in situ hybridization (FISH) and with reverse transcriptase polymerase chain reaction (RTPCR). The differential diagnosis of RMS and EOE/PNET has been enhanced by identification of the fusion gene associated with the t(11,22)(q24•2) translocation found in most EOE-PNET lesions. This can also be identified by either FISH or RTPCR.

PROPOSED INTERNATIONAL CLASSIFICATION FOR RHABDOMYOSARCOMA

Because of the need to develop a single, prognostically significant classification of RMS and other related tumors of children, adolescents, and young adults, a recent study has recently been carried out by the proponents of four existing systems,[9,11,24,25] using 800 lesions of the 999 eligible patients treated as part of Intergroup Rhabdomyosarcoma Study Group II (IRS-II). Each tumor was classified according to each of the four systems by the proponents and by several other pathologists expert in the diagnosis of soft tissue tumors from the United States and Europe. Figure 100-12 presents an approximation of the interrelations of the subtypes of the four systems. The new classification scheme was based largely of the subtypes included in the most commonly used existing system, that described originally by Horn and Enterline.[9]

A study of the survival rates for each subtype of each of the four systems enabled the development of the new system, which was found to be both reproducible and predictive of patient outcome[10,26] (Fig. 100-13). Botryoid RMS and spindle-cell RMS, both being variants of classic embryonal RMS, predicted an excellent outcome. Patients with classic embryonal RMS

Comparison of Four Classification Systems

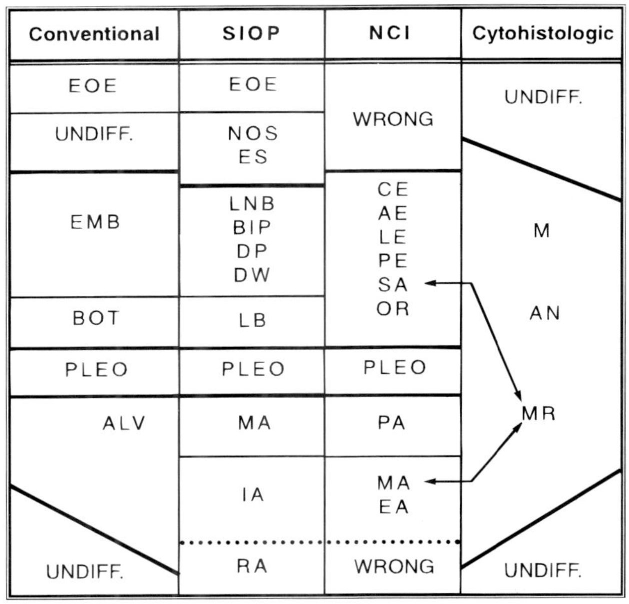

FIG. 100-12. Outline of the subtypes of the four rhabdomyosarcoma (RMS) classification systems studied as a basis for construction of a proposed prognostically significant, reproducible classification, with an approximation of their interrelationships. AE, aggressive embryonal RMS; ALV, alveolar RMS; AN, anaplastic RMS; BIP, biphasic RMS; BOT, botryoid RMS; CE, classic embryonal RMS; DP, dense, poorly differentiated RMS; DW, dense, well differentiated RMS; EA, Ewing's alveolar RMS; EMB, embryonal RMS; EOE, extraosseous Ewing's; ES, embryonal sarcoma; IA, intermediate alveolar RMS; LB, loose botryoid RMS; LE, leiomyomatous embryonal RMS; LNB, loose nonbotryoid RMS; M, mixed RMS; MA, monomorphic alveolar RMS; MA, myogenic alveolar RMS; MR, monomorphic round cell RMS; NCI, National Cancer Institute; NOS, not otherwise specified sarcoma; OR, other RMS; PA, pleomorphic alveolar RMS; PE, pleomorphic embryonal RMS; PLEO, pleomorphic RMS; RA, round cell alveolar RMS; SA, solid alveolar RMS; SIOP, International Society for Pediatric Oncology; Undiff., undifferentiated sarcoma; Wrong, wrong diagnosis.

had an intermediate life expectancy, and patients with alveolar RMS or UDS had a poor prognosis.

The most favorable outcomes were seen in patients whose primary RMS lesion was in the paratesticular area.[13] The botryoid RMS variant, characterized by the presence of a subepithelial cambium layer of tumor cells,[27] was a common type seen in the GU system but was limited to organ sites permitting free growth of the tumor into an open lumen (eg, bladder, vagina). Alveolar RMS had long been thought to be a histologic subtype with an associated poor prognosis for survival, and that suspicion was confirmed in this study. The definition used in this study was that *any* amount of alveolar feature was sufficient for the diagnosis to be made. The so-called solid alveolar variant[11] was included with all other alveolar lesions because there was no significant evidence that it was any more likely to predict a different outcome. Alveolar RMS is found only rarely in RMS tumors in GU sites.

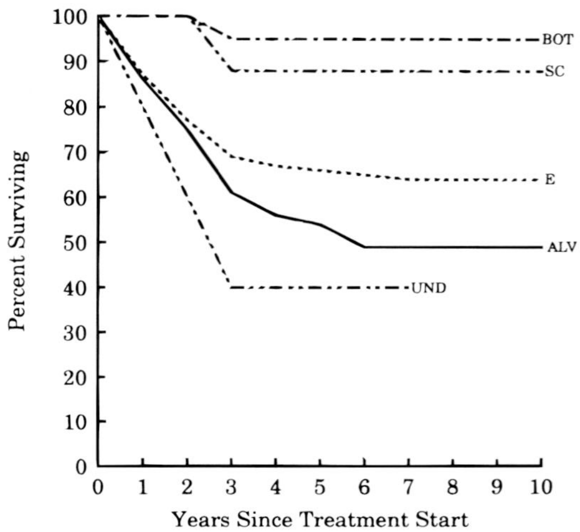

FIG. 100-13. Kaplan-Meier 5-year survival estimates of patients whose lesions were classified by the new international classification of rhabdomyosarcoma (RMS) and related sarcomas of children and adolescents by histologic subtype. BOT, botryoid RMS; SC, spindle cell RMS; E, embryonal RMS; ALV, alveolar RMS; UND, undifferentiated sarcoma.

Lesions that consisted of undifferentiated mesenchymal cells without identifiable histogenic type features were designated as UDS. This group probably will decrease in size as more sophisticated techniques become available to establish their basic cell types. Patients with lesions thus classified also experienced a poor survival rate. The remaining classic embryonal RMS lesions predicted an intermediate survival rate.

Paratesticular Rhabdomyosarcoma

One third of GU RMS tumors occur in paratesticular sites; these account for 8% of all RMS lesions and contribute significantly to the 1.4:1 male predominance of RMS. These tumors do not arise within the testis, but they may invade testicular structures. Patients with primary RMS in this site have a favorable prognosis, as do those with orbital and nonparameningeal head and neck primary sites. The reasons for this are not clear, but factors that have been shown to be important are age at diagnosis, extent of disease, and histology of the primary tumor.[28]

Distant metastases occur only half as often among patients with paratesticular RMS than among all IRS-I and IRS-II patients taken as a whole. However, those who have clinical involvement of retroperitoneal nodes, as determined by computed tomographic (CT) scan, have a 5-year progression-free survival rate of only 69%, compared with 93% for those who do not.[29] Eighty-one percent of 121 patients studied were negative on CT evaluation of the retroperitoneal area for node involvement. Surgical sampling of this CT-negative group showed positive nodal involvement in 14%; in contrast, among those who were CT positive, 94% had histologically confirmed nodal involvement. Patients with no residual disease were given chemotherapy, and those with microscopic or gross residual disease received radiation to the tumor area. Only 2 of these 121 patients developed tumor recurrence.[29]

The histologic characteristics of 173 paratesticular tumors from patients treated in IRS-I through IRS-III were reviewed and reclassified to evaluate a possible role of histology in the favorable prognosis.[13] A third of this patient group were found to have a specific variant of embryonal RMS that was characterized by a spindle shape of the tumor cells. Most of these had an excess of collagen separating the cells, often with a storiform pattern (see Fig. 100-10). The remaining spindle-cell variant contained little or no intercellular collagen and in that way resembled a leiomyosarcoma. The 5-year survival rate of these patients with spindle-cell embryonal RMS was 95%, compared with 80% for patients whose tumor was classic embryonal RMS. In contrast, the survival time of patients with the spindle form of embryonal RMS in lesions elsewhere in the body was not significantly different from that of all those with embryonal RMS taken as a whole. This finding may have resulted from the fact that disease was more extensive in these patients than in those with spindle-cell embryonal RMS in the paratesticular region. Histologically, the cells of the spindle-cell RMS lesions were more differentiated than those of the nonspindle embryonal tumors. These observations have been confirmed by others.[12]

Bladder and Prostate Rhabdomyosarcoma

Tumors of the bladder in children are rare. They accounted for only 0.5% of all cancers diagnosed at Columbus Children's Hospital during a 45-year period. Nineteen out of 22 of these tumors were RMS lesions, and three were epithelial in origin. One of the latter resulted from drug toxicity incident to treatment of cancer. The bladder is one of the more common sites for RMS of the GU tract, but it makes up only 5% of all RMS tumors entered in IRS-I and IRS-II.[1] Clinicians frequently regard the bladder and prostate as a single RMS site, because it is difficult to define the origin of a tumor that arises in the trigone area. In IRS-I, the primary sites were in the bladder trigone (12 patients), in the dome of the bladder (11), in the bladder wall (4), and diffuse or multiple (4). Bladder RMS is usually nonmetastatic; distant metastases were seen in only 2 of 31 IRS-I patients.[30] Patients in this study were not treated with a program designed to maximize bladder salvage. Therefore, the data on extent of disease at diagnosis most accurately represent the true proportions observed in clinical groups, in contrast to later studies, in which most initial surgery was conservative. The postsurgical groupings for these patients were complete excision (6 patients), microscopic residual (14), and gross residual (9), and the sites of distant metastasis included lung (3), pleura (1), bone marrow (1), and liver (1).

Tumor cell anaplasia, another histologic feature that may be seen in lesions of the bladder-prostate or adjacent pelvis, is associated with a poor survival rate.[14] Although seen most often in embryonal RMS, it also occurs in other RMS subtypes. This variant is characterized by the presence of many tumor giant cells whose single nuclei measure more than three times that of the other adjacent tumor cells (see Fig. 100-11). One fifth of all RMS tumors with microscopic anaplasia in these studies were found in GU sites. If anaplasia was seen in only an occasional cell, it was without significance; if it was present in clumps or sheets of cells, the patients had a significantly unfavorable survival prognosis. As an example, 4 of 12 patients with pelvic RMS treated in IRS-III with chemotherapy and radiation died; 3 of them had anaplastic changes in their tumor cells.

Primary Rhabdomyosarcoma Tumors of Vagina, Cervix, and Uterus

Vaginal RMS most often presents as a polypoid mass, with or without hemorrhage. Perhaps because of the freeness of the tumor to grow into an open space, most vaginal lesions have a botryoid histology. In keeping with the data from the classification study, the survival rate for patients with botryoid RMS lesions is excellent, with only 2 tumor-related deaths out of 28 patients treated in IRS-I and IRS-II.[8] One patient died of treatment-induced toxicity. These patients were treated conservatively, with only localized surgical removal.

Primary RMS is relatively rare in the cervix and uterine body in girls. IRS reports have combined the two sites, with a total of 10 patients studied for IRS-I and IRS-II combined.[31] Three have died of tumor, and one of treatment toxicity. The majority of the cervical lesions were a botryoid RMS subtype, whereas the uterine primaries were embryonal RMS or UDS tumors. Brand and colleagues[32] reported 4 new cases and found 17 other instances of sarcoma botryoides of the cervix. The ages of these patients ranged from 5 months to 48 years, with a peak at 14 to 18 years. Eighty percent of these patients were alive with a mean follow-up time of 68 months. Seventy-five percent had a surgically removable tumor; the survival rate in this group was 88%. Of the 5 patients with recurrent disease, 2 had survived. The authors concluded that the extent of surgery should be guided by the initial response to chemotherapy, and that there should be an attempt to conserve the function of the bladder, rectum, vagina, and ovaries.

Daya reported on the consultation files of Scully, citing 13 cases of sarcoma botryoides of the cervix.[33] The ages of these patients ranged from 12 to 26 years. All but one of these patients were alive after 1 to 8 years (average, 3.5 years). Six of the 13 tumors contained mature cartilage. Perone and colleagues[34] reported on a 20-year-old with RMS of the cervix, who had mixed botryoid and alveolar subtypes that also included mature cartilage; this patient died of tumor metastases.

PSEUDOSARCOMA (MYOFIBROBLASTIC) TUMOR OF THE BLADDER

The great majority of malignancies of the GU tract in children are RMS tumors, and the reader is referred to a more detailed discussion[35] for all but one benign lesion, one that has been misdiagnosed as a malignancy, most often embryonal RMS.

Pseudosarcoma (myofibroblastic) tumor of the bladder (PMT) is a benign proliferation of fibroblasts and myofibroblasts that produces tumor formation simulating malignancy.[36–38] One of the common sites for this to occur in children is the bladder. A recent re-review of the IRS pathology files of bladder tumors identified 11 cases that were initially diagnosed as embryonal RMS at the treating institution, and also by the IRS Pathology Committee on their initial review, but were clear examples of this entity based on tumor morphology, IHC studies, and clinical behavior.[38] All 11 patients were living and well free of disease, with only one showing continued growth of the presenting mass. Histologically, the lesion consists of proliferating fibroblasts and myofibroblasts in a loose myxoid stroma (Fig. 100-14), associated with varying degrees of active acute and chronic inflammation. Inflammation is limited to the tumor or extends into the mucosa, which frequently is ulcerated at the site. The IHC profile includes positive reactions to vimentin, desmin, both muscle-specific and smooth muscle actin, and keratin. The age of these patients ranged from 3 to 19 years at diagnosis, and the predominant symptoms were hematuria and dysuria. The tumor sites were usually in the wall or dome of the bladder and ranged from 3 to 9 cm in diameter.

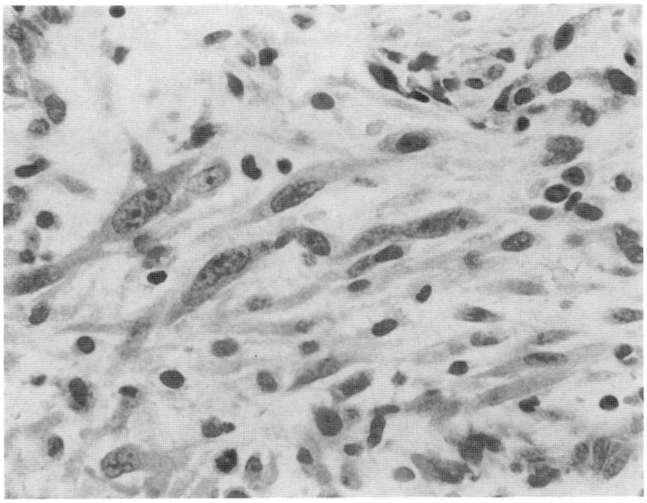

FIG. 100-14. Photomicrograph illustrating the typical proliferating myofibroblasts of pseudosarcomatous myofibroblastic proliferation of the bladder. This lesion was mistaken for an embryonal rhabdomyosarcoma, both by the institutional pathologist and initially by the Intergroup Rhabdomyosarcoma Study Pathology Committee.

POSTTHERAPY MORPHOLOGIC CHANGES

One of the most difficult morphologic problems in the pathology of GU RMS tumors is the determination of the malignant potential of the residual cell population at primary tumor sites after chemotherapy or radiotherapy if the primary was not surgically removed at diagnosis. This is particularly important in sites in which preservation of the normal structures is an important therapeutic goal (eg, bladder, vagina, uterus).

Current studies are evaluating this issue, but no conclusions have been finalized. The initial results of one IRS study showed that almost all primary bladder RMS tumors undergo significant posttherapy changes, with loss of most of the initial malignant cells, leaving a mixture of fibrosis, edema, and often a few residual maturing rhabdomyoblasts (Fig. 100-15). There are no obvious histologic evidences of malignancy (eg, mitotic figures, invasion of adjacent tissue) in these cells, but they are not fully matured to the level of skeletal muscle. Clinical correlations suggest that these residual cells are not likely to have a potential for tumor growth. However, the limited data do not permit prediction of their ultimate cellular behavior. This posttreatment maturation phenomenon has been known for some time.[39–42]

A 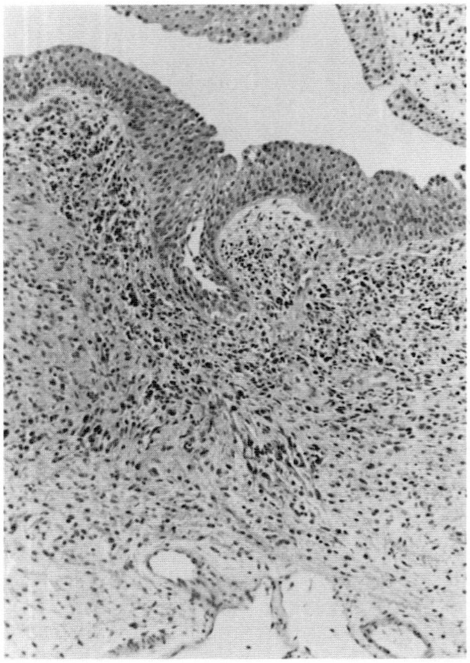 B 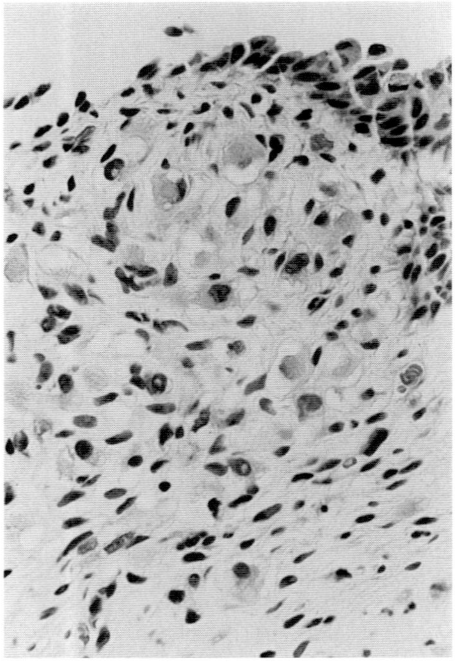

FIG. 100-15. (**A**) Photomicrograph of a typical embryonal rhabdomyosarcoma showing increased cellularity and the predominance of primitive spindle-shaped rhabdomyoblasts. (**B**) Photomicrograph of the same lesion after chemotherapy and radiation. Notice the decrease in cellularity, the change of the tumor cells from primitive, relatively undifferentiated cells to those showing mild to marked maturation (cytoplasmic development).

The maturation process seems to follow the sequence observed in the development of human muscle.[43] It is necessary to extend these studies to all GU sites and to sites elsewhere in the body and to correlate posttreatment biopsy results with clinical outcome. The bladder data suggest that a conservative approach may be taken to enable preservation of normal organ structures.

ACKNOWLEDGMENTS

The authors recognize and express thanks to all investigators—oncologists, surgeons, pathologists, radiotherapists, and many others—who have contributed to the evergrowing database available for study of childhood RMS. The IRS publications relating to the GU system have been used for much of the clinical data in this chapter; we recognize their efforts in making this data available as well.

REFERENCES

1. Newton WA Jr, Soule EH, Hamoudi AB, et al. Histopathology of childhood sarcomas: Intergroup Rhabdomyosarcoma Studies I and II. Clinicopathologic correlation. J Clin Oncol 1988;6:67.
2. Lawrence W Jr, Hays DM, Moon TE. Lymphatic metastasis with childhood rhabdomyosarcoma. Cancer 1977;39:556.
3. Wiener E, Lawrence W, Hays D, et al. When is retroperitoneal node dissection or biopsy necessary in childhood paratesticular rhabdomyosarcoma? J Pediatr Surg 1993;29:171.
4. Hays DM, Raney RB, Lawrence W, et al. Rhabdomyosarcoma of the female urogenital tract. J Pediatr Surg 1981;16:828.
5. Maurer HM, Beltangady M, Gehan EA, et al. The Intergroup Rhabdomyosarcoma Study I: a final report. Cancer 1988;61:209.
6. Maurer HM, Gehan EA, Beltangady M, et al. The Intergroup Rhabdomyosarcoma Study II. Cancer 1993;71:1904.
7. Crist W, Gehan EA, Ragab AH, et al. Intergroup Rhabdomyosarcoma Study III. J Clin Oncol 1994;74:2579.
8. Hays DM, Raney RB, Lawrence W, et al. Primary chemotherapy in the treatment of children with bladder-prostate tumors in the Intergroup Rhabdomyosarcoma Study (IRS-II). J Pediatr Surg 1992;17:812.
9. Horn RC Jr, Enterline HT. Rhabdomyosarcoma: a clinicopathological study and classification of 39 cases. Cancer 1958;11:181.
10. Newton WA Jr, Gehan EA, Webber BL, et al. Classification of rhabdomyosarcoma and related sarcomas: pathologic aspects and proposal for a new classification. An Intergroup Rhabdomyosarcoma Study. Cancer 1995;76:1073.
11. Tsokos M, Webber B, Parham D, et al. Rhabdomyosarcoma: a new classification scheme related to prognosis. Arch Pathol Lab Med 1992; 116:847.
12. Cavazzana AO, Schmidt D, Ninfo V, et al. Spindle cell rhabdomyosarcoma: a prognostically favorable variant of rhabdomyosarcoma. Am J Surg Pathol 1992;16:229.
13. Leuschner I, Newton WA, Schmidt D, et al. Spindle cell variants of embryonal rhabdomyosarcoma in the paratesticular region: a report of the Intergroup Rhabdomyosarcoma Study. Am J Surg Pathol 1993;17: 221.
14. Kodet R, Newton WA, Hamoudi AB, Asmar L, Jacobs DL, Maurer HM. Childhood rhabdomyosarcoma with anaplastic (pleomorphic) features: a report of the Intergroup Rhabdomyosarcoma Study. Am J Surg Pathol 1993;17:443.
15. Tsokos M. The role of immunocytochemistry in the diagnosis of rhabdomyosarcoma. Arch Pathol Lab Med 1986;110:776.
16. Parham DM, Webber B, Holt H, Williams WK, Maurer HM. Immunohistochemical study of childhood rhabdomyosarcoma and related neoplasms: results of an Intergroup Rhabdomyosarcoma Study project. Cancer 1991;67:3072.
17. Parham DM. Immunohistochemistry of childhood sarcomas: old and new markers. Mod Pathol 1993;6:133.
18. Sorensen PHB, Shimada H, Liu XF, Lim JS, Thomas G, Triche TJ. Biphenotypic sarcomas with myogenic and neural differentiation express the Ewing's sarcoma EW/FLII fusion gene. Cancer Res 1995; 55:1385.
19. Dias P, Dilling M, Houghton P. The molecular basis of skeletal muscle differentiation. Semin Diagn Pathol 1994;11:3. Review.
20. Douglass EC, Shapiro DN, Valentine M. Alveolar rhabdomyosarcoma with the t(2,13): cytogenetic findings and clinicopathologic correlations. Med Pediatr Oncol 1993;21:83.
21. Shapiro DM, Sublet J, Li BY. Fusion of PAX3 to a member of the Forkhead family of transcription factors in human alveolar rhabdomyosarcoma. Cancer Res 1993;53:5108.

22. Galili N, Davis RJ, Fredericks WJ. Fusion of a forkhead domain gene to PAX3 in solid tumor alveolar rhabdomyosarcoma. Nat Genet 1993; 5:230.
23. Kufos A, Hansen MF, Copeland NG, Jenkins NA, Lampkin BC, Cavenee WK. Loss of heterozygosity in three embryonal tumors suggests a common pathogenetic mechanism. Nature 1985;316:330.
24. Caillaud JM, Gerard-Marchant R, Marsden HB, et al. Histopathological classification of childhood rhabdomyosarcoma: a report from the International Society of Pediatric Oncology Pathology Panel. Med Pediatr Oncol 1989;17:391.
25. Palmer NF, Sachs N, Foulkes M. Histopathology and prognosis in rhabdomyosarcoma. Proc Int Soc Ped Oncol 1981;1:113. Abstract.
26. Asmar L, Gehan EA, Newton WA, et al. Agreement among and within groups of pathologists in the classification of rhabdomyosarcoma and related childhood sarcomas: report of an international study of four pathology classifications. Cancer 1994;74:2579.
27. Nicholson GWdeP. Studies on tumor formation. London, Butterworth, 1952.
28. Raney RB Jr, Tefft M, Lawrence W Jr, et al. Paratesticular sarcoma in childhood and adolescence: a report from the Intergroup Rhabdomyosarcoma Studies I and II, 1973–1983. Cancer 1987;60:2337.
29. Wiener ES, Lawrence W, Hays D, et al. Retroperitoneal node biopsy in paratesticular rhabdomyosarcoma. J Pediatr Surg 1994;19:171.
30. Hays DM, Raney RB Jr, Lawrence W Jr, Soule EH, Gehan EA, Tefft M. Bladder and prostatic tumors in the Intergroup Rhabdomyosarcoma Study (IRS-I): results of therapy. Cancer 1982;50:1472.
31. Hays DM, Shimada H, Raney RB Jr, et al. Clinical staging and treatment results in rhabdomyosarcoma of the female genital tract among children and adolescents. Cancer 1988;61:1903.
32. Brand E, Berek JS, Nieberg RK, Hacker NF. Rhabdomyosarcoma of the uterine cervix: Sarcoma botryoides. Cancer 1987;60:1552.
33. Daya DA, Scully RE. Sarcoma botryoides of the uterine cervix in young women: a clinicopathological study of 13 cases. Gynecol Oncol 1988; 29:290.
34. Perrone T, Carson LF, Dehner LP. Rhabdomyosarcoma with heterologous cartilage of the uterine cervix: a clinicopathologic and immunohistochemical study of an aggressive neoplasm in a young female. Med Pediatr Oncol 1990;18:72.
35. Klein FA. Unusual bladder tumors in children. In: Broecker FH, Klein FA, eds. Pediatric tumors of the genitourinary tract. New York, Alan R Liss, 1988:177.
36. Albores-Saavedra J, Manivel JC, Essenfeld H, Dehner LP, Drut R, Gould E, et al. Pseudosarcomatous myofibroblastic proliferations in the urinary bladder of children. Cancer 1990;66:1234.
37. Lundgren L, Aldenborg F, Angervall L, Kindbloom L. Pseudomalignant spindle-cell proliferations of the urinary bladder. Hum Pathol 1994;25:181.
38. Hojo H, Newton WA Jr, Hamoudi AB, et al. Pseudosarcomatous myofibroblastic tumors of the urinary bladder in children. Am J Surg Pathol 1995;19:1224–36.
39. Molenaar WM, Oosterhuis JW, Kamps WA. Cytologic ''differentiation'' in childhood rhabdomyosarcomas following polychemotherapy. Hum Pathol 1984;15:973.
40. Schmidt D, Reimann O, Treuner J, Harms D. Cellular differentiation and prognosis in embryonal rhabdomyosarcoma. Virchows Arch A Pathol Anat Histopathol 1986;409:183.
41. d'Amore ESG, Tollot M, Stracca-Pansa V, et al. Therapy associated differentiation in rhabdomyosarcomas. Mod Pathol 1994;7:69.
42. Bale PM, Parsons RE, Stevens MM. Diagnosis and behavior of juvenile rhabdomyosarcoma. Hum Pathol 1983;14:596.
43. Carter RL, Jameson CF, Philip ER, Pinkerton CR. Comparative phenotypes in rhabdomyosarcomas and developing skeletal muscle. Histopathology 1990;17:301.

Principles and Practice of Genitourinary Oncology, edited by Derek Raghavan, Howard I. Scher, Steven A. Leibel, and Paul H. Lange. Lippincott-Raven Publishers, Philadelphia, © 1997.

CHAPTER 101

Clinical Presentation, Diagnosis, and Prognosis of Children with Soft Tissue Sarcoma of the Genitourinary Tract

R. Beverly Raney

Soft tissue sarcomas of the genitourinary (GU) tract are somewhat common in the first two decades of life and account for 20% to 25% of all soft tissue sarcomas occurring in childhood and adolescence. The predominant histologic type of GU sarcoma in young patients is the embryonal rhabdomyosarcoma (RMS), which is divided into a solid subtype and a looser, myxoid subtype that is called botryoid RMS because it simulates a cluster of grapes (see Chap. 100). The botryoid lesions are submucosal in location and usually arise in the bladder or vagina. Occasionally, alveolar RMS can develop in the GU tract, as can undifferentiated sarcoma or other, rarer tumors such as the leiomyosarcoma or malignant rhabdoid tumor.[1]

This chapter outlines the clinical presentation of sarcomas arising in the GU tract, assesses the appropriate diagnostic studies for determining the extent of disease (staging and clinical grouping), and discusses the prognosis for survival. Therapeutic considerations are covered in detail in Chapter 102.

SITES OF OCCURRENCE

The most common sites of primary soft tissue sarcoma of the GU tract are the paratesticular region and prostate, the bladder, and the vulva, vagina, cervix, and uterus. Very infrequently, a sarcoma (other than a Wilms' tumor variant) can arise in the kidney[2] or the ovary.[3] These two sites are not discussed at length here, owing to the rarity of GU sarcomas in these locations. Sarcomas can also arise in the retroperitoneum, pelvis, or perineum contiguous with but outside the GU tract; differentiation of these lesions from primary GU sarcoma is important and is discussed later in this chapter.

Sarcomas can arise in mesenchymal tissues distributed throughout the body. A sarcoma usually presents as a localized, nontender mass that can deviate or infiltrate surrounding structures. If superficial or if critically located, the mass becomes obvious rather early. More deeply situated tumors may be asymptomatic for weeks to months. However, they usually produce symptoms and signs of obstruction of the bladder or rectum or discharge from the orifice of a hollow structure such as the bladder, cervix, or vagina.[4,5]

Paratesticular Region

Patients with paratesticular sarcoma usually have a solid embryonal RMS that presents as an enlarging, nontender, unilateral mass, sometimes associated with a hydrocele. The disease was once thought to have two peaks in incidence by age, but the largest available study, 95 cases from the Intergroup Rhabdomyosarcoma Studies (IRS-I and IRS-II, 1972–1984), showed almost equal frequency in each quinquennium from birth through 20 years of age.[6] In that report, the tumors ranged in size from 0.9 to 19 cm in widest diameter (median, 6.9 cm). Ipsilateral inguinal adenopathy and fixation of the mass to ipsilateral scrotal skin are unusual at diagnosis, but either or both conditions can result from an inappropriate attempt to make the diagnosis by transscrotal biopsy or transscrotal orchidectomy. Some of the larger tumors occur in teenagers, who are more often concerned with privacy and are thus less likely to be observed unclothed than are younger children.

Prostate

Patients with prostatic sarcoma usually have solid embryonal RMS and present with symptoms and signs of urinary retention and strangury (straining while attempting to pass urine), urinary tract infection, constipation resulting from rectal compression, and, rarely, hematuria caused by transurethral growth of the tumor. These tumors can become quite large because they are situated posteriorly and are usually extrinsic to the bladder. The mass should be readily palpable on digital rectal examination and often can also be felt on abdominal palpation. Again, it is not commonly tender. Young people of any age may be affected.[4,5,7,8]

Bladder

Patients with bladder sarcoma may be infants or older children, and they may have either solid or botryoid embryonal RMS. The signs and symptoms vary with location of the primary lesion. Frequently, the bladder trigone is affected; in such cases, the children usually present to their physician with strangury, hematuria, and, occasionally, constipation. A urinary tract infection may be present. Sometimes, portions of whitish, slightly bloody tumor may be passed in the urine. In patients with a lesion in the dome of the bladder or the urachal region, the diagnosis is made after discovery of an abdominal mass. Usually, the tumor produces discomfort because of pressure on surrounding structures.[4,5,7,8]

Vulva and Vagina

Children with vulvovaginal sarcoma most often have solid or botryoid embryonal RMS and are usually younger than 4 years of age at diagnosis. These patients have an odoriferous, often serosanguineous, vaginal discharge and may or may not have difficulty with urination. Fragments of tissue are sometimes extruded from botryoid masses. Occasionally, a vulvar mass may simulate a Bartholin's gland cyst, which is not common in infants. The rectum is usually not involved.[4,5,9–11]

Cervix and Uterus

Patients with cervical or uterine sarcoma may have either solid or botryoid embryonal RMS; these tumors can occur at any age but most commonly affect older girls in the second or third quinquennium of life.[10,12] As with vulvovaginal tumors, a tumor mass may be visible, with or without vaginal discharge. If the tumor occurs in the body of the uterus, it may become quite large before it is detected. If the mass is located in the cervix, hydrometrocolpos can occur in a virginal patient and cause abdominal distention and pain. In postmenarchal women, menstrual flow may become irregular or may even be interrupted if the tumor obstructs the cervix.[10,12]

DIAGNOSIS AND STAGING

Pathologic Diagnosis

Tissue is required for pathologic examination, in order to confirm the diagnosis of soft tissue sarcoma and to determine the subtype of the disease. Embryonal and botryoid RMS make up the overwhelming majority of soft tissue sarcomas in the GU tract in patients younger than 21 years old. Of the 348 GU cases reviewed in IRS-I and IRS-II, 71% were embryonal RMS and 20% were botryoid RMS.[1] Only 2% were alveolar RMS, 2% undifferentiated sarcoma, 4% sarcomas not otherwise specified, and 1% pleomorphic sarcoma (1 patient only). In a review of 173 IRS patients with paratesticular sarcoma, Leuschner and colleagues found that patients with the spindle cell variant of embryonal RMS had a better prognosis than did those with classic embryonal RMS.[13] These forms of RMS and the other, considerably less common, soft tissue sarcomas in the GU tracts of children can usually be differentiated by light microscopy. Sometimes electron microscopy is helpful in doubtful cases. However, most pathologists now also perform immunohistochemical staining with desmin or muscle-specific actin to confirm the myogenic origin of the tumor.[14] More sophisticated laboratory techniques, such as determination of DNA ploidy,[15–17] DNA image analysis,[18] positivity for *MYOD1* and other muscle genes,[19] and cytogenetic studies with or without specific molecular probes[20,21] are becoming available, but they are presently used primarily in research.

Staging

After the diagnosis is confirmed, other investigations should be undertaken to establish the extent of detectable tumor. Two systems are in use in the IRS. The first is the clinical grouping system, which is based on surgical and pathologic findings, results of radiographic imaging, and a sample of bone marrow obtained before treatment with multiple-agent chemotherapy. Table 101-1 shows this system, which has been in use since 1972. The IRS is also using a modified tumor, node, metastasis (TNM) system that is based on site of primary tumor, invasion of or fixation to surrounding tissues, tumor size (widest diameter), presence or absence of regional nodal clinical involvement, and presence or absence of distant metastases as defined in Table 101-1. This system is shown in Table 101-2. Both systems yield information of therapeutic and prognostic importance, and treatment decisions are currently based on the category into which each patient's disease is classified. The decision to use radiotherapy is made according to the patient's clinical group, because the clinical group reflects the degree of residual disease. Group I patients, having no detectable residual tumor, receive chemotherapy but no radiotherapy; all others receive both treatments. Decisions about what chemotherapeutic agents to use are based on the TNM stage. These issues are discussed in detail in Chapter 102.

Diagnostic Imaging

Primary Site

There is some flexibility in the type of diagnostic imaging that can be performed during evaluation of the primary tumor

TABLE 101-1. *Intergroup Rhabdomyosarcoma Study clinical grouping system*

Group I	Localized tumor, completely removed; no tumor cells at margins or in regional lymph nodes
Group II	Localized tumor, grossly removed but with tumor cells at margins, in regional lymph nodes, or both
Group III	Localized tumor sampled by biopsy only or incompletely removed, with visible residual tumor, with or without tumor cells in regional lymph nodes
Group IV	Distant metastases at any site, including tumor cells or implants in the pleural or peritoneal cavity or in the crebrospinal fluid

TABLE 101-2. *IRS modified tumor-node-metastasis (TNM) staging system*

Stage	Description
ntStage 1	Localized tumor arising in the orbit or head and neck (not parameningeal*) or the genitourinary tract (not bladder or prostate); the tumor may be T1 or T2, N0 or N1, and of any size.
Stage 2	Localized tumor at all sites other than those in stage 1; T1 or T2, N0, ≤5 cm in widest diameter.
Stage 3	Localized tumor as in stage 2, T1 or T2, N1 with primary tumor size ≤5 cm in widest diameter, or N0 or N1 with primary tumor size >5 cm.
Stage 4	Any site with distant metastases, T1 or T2, N0 or N1, any size.

T1, tumor confined to anatomic site of origin; T2, tumor extended or fixed to surrounding tissue; N0, no or unknown (NX) clinical involvement of regional lymph nodes; N1, regional nodes clinically involved.

* Parameningeal tumors are those arising in nasopharynx or nasal cavity; paranasal sinuses; middle ear or mastoid; or parapharyngeal area, pterygopalatine, or infratemporal fossa.

in a child with a suspected sarcoma of the GU tract. Three primary modalities are available; in order of increasing cost, difficulty, and diagnostic information, these are ultrasonography, computed tomographic (CT) scanning, and magnetic resonance imaging (MRI).

Ultrasonography is useful for confirming the presence of a solid tumor in a testicular or paratesticular location, and it can also show a mass in any of the other areas of the GU tract. It is particularly helpful if the lesion involves or abuts the bladder, because of the contrast in density between urine and the surrounding solid structures.[22,23] Ultrasonography can also be used to survey the liver and has virtually replaced the intravenous pyelogram for examination of the kidneys and inferior vena cava. However, CT scans are generally more useful for detecting the presence of adenopathy and may also demonstrate the presence of peritoneal or omental metastases.[23,24] Often the most anatomically precise pictures are obtainable by MRI scanning. MRI is particularly useful in defining the extent of pelvic tumors and in indicating whether the tumor has spread into the spinal area through the sacral neural foramina.[25]

It is important to distinguish the exact site of the primary tumor, because it is desirable to preserve the bladder (and prostate or uterus) but also to remove all gross tumor whenever possible. A surgeon can often best visualize a bladder tumor by cystoscopy, or a vaginal or uterine tumor during a pelvic examination. Careful evaluation is needed to exclude the presence of a tumor that is extrinsic to the bladder and arises in the retroperitoneum, pelvis, or perineum, because patients with tumors in these sites have a worse prognosis than do those with GU primary tumors.[26,27]

Distant Metastases

Plain radiographs are useful in assessing the bones and lungs for metastases. The best technique for finding pulmonary metastases is a CT scan. Bones can also be assessed by a radionuclide scan using technetium-99; some physicians believe that the skeletal survey is as good as or better than a scan, but the radionuclide scan requires less radiation exposure.[28] Radionuclide scans with gallium-67[29] or thallium-201[30] may be useful for imaging both the primary site and distant metastases.

PROGNOSIS

The outlook for cure of soft tissue sarcoma in childhood is related to the site of the primary tumor, the extent of disease, the degree of resectability of the tumor (clinical group), and the response to therapy.[31,32] Much progress has been made since the late 1960s and early 1970s, when combined-modality programs for children with GU sarcoma were introduced. Each modality (surgery, radiotherapy, and chemotherapy) has both benefits and risks. Long-term sequelae of the disease and of treatment are major concerns to patients who survive the disease. This section contains information collected from the recent literature relating the site of the primary tumor to the expected outcome. In general, patients with paratesticular and vulvovaginal tumors have the best overall prognosis, followed by those with tumors of the bladder, those with prostate sarcoma, and finally those with uterine sarcomas. Results of therapy from several recent series are reviewed in Chapter 102.

Paratesticular Region

The likelihood of cure is very high, approaching 90%, for all children with localized paratesticular sarcoma.[6] This probably results from several favorable factors that appear to concur in these patients. First, tumors in this region are easily visible and relatively easily removed at radical orchidectomy. The pathologic tumor type is almost always favorable: classic embryonal RMS or the even more favorable variant, spindle-cell embryonal RMS.[13] Usually, distant metastases are not detected. Although regional lymph node metastases occur in about 28% of patients, about 90% of them can be cured with combined chemotherapy and radiotherapy. Although the cure rate in children presenting with hematogenous metastases (group IV) from RMS at all sites is only 30%, the figure was 57% (8 of 14 patients) with group IV paratesticular sarcomas in the IRS-I and IRS-II series.[6]

Long-term sequelae of treatment have been reported primarily from the IRS[33] and from St. Jude Children's Research Hospital.[34] Some patients in both series had early problems with intestinal obstruction related to exploratory laparotomy for retroperitoneal lymph node dissection or sampling, growth problems related to radiotherapy, hemorrhagic cystitis, hypogonadism related to cyclophosphamide with or without radiotherapy, and, occasionally, impotence caused by interruption of autonomic nerves during retroperitoneal lymph node dissection. Because almost all patients are cured, the IRS recommends that clinicians avoid dissection or biopsy of the retroperitoneal lymph nodes altogether and obtain tissue samples only from those patients whose nodes appear enlarged on CT or MRI scans of the retroperitoneum and pelvis. In addition, the IRS treats patients who have stage 1, clinical group I paratesticular sarcoma with only vincristine and actinomycin D, to avoid the deleterious effects of alkylating agents on the bladder and remaining testis.

Prostate

Patients with prostatic sarcoma had a very poor prognosis before the advent of multimodal treatment in the 1970s.[8] The outlook has since improved, and the percentage of patients alive at 3 years after initiation of therapy was 82% in IRS-I and 59% in IRS-II.[35] The difference is probably related to the fact that in IRS-I, about half of the patients underwent total cystectomy at the outset and therefore had clinical group I or II disease. In IRS-II, almost all patients were placed by design in clinical group III, because the goal of IRS-II for these patients was to preserve the bladder, if possible, along with preserving life. However only 21% of IRS-II patients who were alive 3 years after treatment still had the bladder in place. The corresponding figure for IRS-I patients was 22%, if the groups of patients with bladder and prostate lesions were considered together.[35] Preliminary results from IRS-III indicate that a regime of intensified chemotherapy using five drugs (vincristine, actinomycin D, cyclophosphamide, doxorubicin, and cisplatin) and local radiotherapy beginning after 6 weeks of chemotherapy has improved the likelihood of bladder preservation. In 1991, the overall survival rate for 81 patients treated for localized, clinical group III bladder or prostate sarcoma in IRS-III was 90% at 3 years. Of the 73 survivors, 60% retained their bladders.[36] A subsequent analysis has confirmed these results.[37] It therefore appears that bladder preservation is possible for an increasing percentage of these patients.[38–41]

Bladder

In their review of children with bladder and prostate sarcoma, Tefft and Jaffe[8] noted that patients with bladder tumors had a better prognosis than those with prostatic tumors. Prostate tumors tend to be large and clinically silent, they often occur in older children (compared with intrinsic bladder sarcomas), and the patients often present early with hematuria or urethral strangury. As noted, the current objective of treatment is to eliminate the tumor without eliminating the bladder. Especially in the case of a tumor situated away from the bladder trigone, a partial cystectomy can both afford excellent local tumor control and leave a functioning, continent urinary bladder.[42] Inadequate bladder volume as the child grows may be improved by augmentative vesicoplasty, which involves attaching an isolated segment of ileum to the bladder remnant to increase its storage capacity.

The long-term effects in patients with bladder or prostate RMS have been reviewed in 109 5-year survivors from the IRS-I and IRS-II; approximately half of these patients had a permanent urinary diversion. Acceptable renal function and blood pressure levels were preserved in almost all patients. Abnormal follow-up renal imaging studies were more likely in patients with urinary conduits than in patients whose bladders remained in place. Bladder function was considered acceptable in 38 (73%) of the 52 patients for whom follow-up data were available; the other 14 patients had incontinence (9 patients) or frequent urination (5 patients).[43]

Vulva and Vagina

The prognosis of girls with sarcomas in the vulvovaginal region is good, almost as high as that of boys with paratesticular sarcoma.[35] Vulvovaginal tumors are also external and can be diagnosed quickly, before distant metastases become detectable. A substantial proportion of these tumors occur as the favorable botryoid form of embryonal RMS. In IRS-II, the survival rate for girls with vaginal tumors was 85% at 3 years,[35] similar to results of the series from Villejuif, France.[44] Preliminary results from the IRS-III protocol are also encouraging.[37] Fifteen girls with vaginal sarcoma have been followed for several years by the Villejuif group[44]; another report concerned three girls.[45] As expected, patients with extensive surgical procedures have the most deleterious residua (eg, infertility and hormonal problems after hysterectomy and bilateral oophorectomy). Radiotherapy, especially if given to infants, predictably suppresses growth of soft tissues and bone in the treated volume. Stricture of the vaginal orifice, urethra, and rectum may result, along with diminished bladder growth.[45] Because these tumors are surgically accessible and the region can be repaired after growth has occurred, the current trend is to combine chemotherapy and operative management and to avoid radiotherapy.

Cervix and Uterus

There is limited information regarding prognosis of patients with sarcomas of the cervix and uterus, because these tumors are rare in the first two decades of life. The published IRS experience (IRS-I and IRS-II, 1972–1984) suggests that the outlook for these patients is worse than for those with vulvovaginal sarcoma.[12] Perhaps the deeper location of cervical and uterine lesions is responsible for a later diagnosis, with a correspondingly greater chance for metastasis. It is not clear whether patients with small cervical tumors may have a better chance for cure than patients with larger tumors of the corpus uteri; data relating to this possibility are being analyzed by the IRS.[46] Treatment often consists of hysterectomy, and sterility is an expected result. However, the ovaries should be preserved if possible, so that patients will not require long-term replacement steroid therapy.

SUMMARY

The outlook for cure of children and young adults with soft tissue sarcomas of the GU tract has improved considerably in the past 30 years. Treatment efforts were initially directed toward saving lives. As survival rates increased, strategies were formulated with the goal of preservation of organ function as much as possible. Various combinations of all the three effective therapeutic modalities (surgery, radiotherapy, and chemotherapy) provide individual treatment options for these patients. Reports of long-term follow-up at 10 years and beyond will enable the development of further refinements in therapy for children with GU sarcoma.

REFERENCES

1. Newton WA Jr, Soule EH, Hamoudi AB, et al. Histopathology of childhood sarcomas: Intergroup Rhabdomyosarcoma Studies I and II. Clinicopathologic correlation. J Clin Oncol 1988;6:67.
2. Gaboardi F, Carbone M, Bozzola A, Galli L. Rhabdomyosarcoma of the kidney. Arch Esp Urol 1990;43:205.

3. Nunez C, Abboud SL, Lemon NC, Kemp JA. Ovarian rhabdomyosarcoma presenting as leukemia: Case report. Cancer 1983;52:297.
4. Hays DM. Pelvic rhabdomyosarcomas in childhood: diagnosis and concepts of management reviewed. Cancer 1980;45:1810.
5. Shapiro E, Strother D. Pediatric genitourinary rhabdomyosarcoma. J Urol 1992;148:1761.
6. Raney RB Jr, Tefft M, Lawrence W Jr, et al. Paratesticular sarcoma in childhood and adolescence: a report from the Intergroup Rhabdomyosarcoma Studies I and II, 1973–1983. Cancer 1987;60:2337.
7. Clatworthy HW Jr, Braren V, Smith JP. Surgery of bladder and prostatic neoplasms in children. Cancer 1973;32:1157.
8. Tefft M, Jaffe N. Sarcoma of the bladder and prostate in children: rationale for the role of radiation therapy based on a review of the literature and a report of fourteen additional patients. Cancer 1973;32: 1161.
9. Flamant F, Chassagne D, Cosset J-M, Gerbaulet A, Lemerle J. Embryonal rhabdomyosarcoma of the vagina in children: conservative treatment with curietherapy and chemotherapy. Eur J Cancer 1979;15: 527.
10. Hays DM, Shimada H, Raney RB Jr, et al. Sarcomas of the vagina and uterus: the Intergroup Rhabdomyosarcoma Study. J Pediatr Surg 1985; 20:718.
11. McHenry CR, Reynolds M, Raffensperger JG. Vaginal neoplasms in infancy: the combined role of chemotherapy and conservative surgical resection. J Pediatr Surg 1988;23:842.
12. Hays DM, Shimada H, Raney RB Jr, et al. Clinical staging and treatment results in rhabdomyosarcoma of the female genital tract among children and adolescents. Cancer 1988;61:1893.
13. Leuschner I, Newton WA Jr, Schmidt D, et al. Spindle cell variants of embryonal rhabdomyosarcoma in the paratesticular region: a report of the Intergroup Rhabdomyosarcoma Study. Am J Surg Pathol 1993; 17:221.
14. Parham DM, Webber B, Holt H, Williams WK, Maurer H. Immunohistochemical study of childhood rhabdomyosarcomas and related neoplasms: results of an Intergroup Rhabdomyosarcoma Study project. Cancer 1991;67:3072.
15. Shapiro DN, Parham DM, Douglas EC, et al. Relationship of tumor-cell ploidy to histologic subtype and treatment outcome in children and adolescents with unresectable rhabdomyosarcoma. J Clin Oncol 1991; 9:159.
16. Pappo AS, Crist WM, Kuttesch J, et al. Tumor-cell DNA content predicts outcome in children and adolescents with clinical group III embryonal rhabdomyosarcoma. J Clin Oncol 1993;11:1901.
17. Boyle ET, Reiman HM, Kramer SA, Kelalis PP, Rainwater LM, Lieber MM. Embryonal rhabdomyosarcoma of bladder and prostate: nuclear DNA patterns studied by flow cytometry. J Urol 1988;140:1119.
18. Kowal-Vern A, Gonzalez-Crussi F, Turner J, et al. Flow and image cytometric DNA analysis in rhabdomyosarcoma. Cancer Res 1990;50: 6023.
19. Tonin PN, Scrable H, Shimada H, Cavenee WK. Muscle-specific gene expression in rhabdomyosarcoma and stages of human fetal skeletal muscle development. Cancer Res 1991;51:5100.
20. Shapiro DN, Valentine MB, Sublett JE, et al. Chromosomal sublocalization of the 2;13 translocation breakpoint in alveolar rhabdomyosarcoma. Genes Chromosom Cancer 1992;4:241.
21. Whang-Peng J, Knutsen T, Theil K, Horowitz ME, Triche T. Cytogenetic studies in subgroups of rhabdomyosarcoma. Genes Chromosom Cancer 1992;5:299.
22. Bahnson RR, Zaontz MR, Maizels M, Shkolnik AA, Firlit CF. Ultrasonography and diagnosis of pediatric genitourinary rhabdomyosarcoma. Urology 1989;33:64.
23. Finkelstein MS, Sherman NH, Rosenberg HK, Mahboubi S, Raney RB. Correlative imaging of pelvic soft-tissue sarcomas in children. J Am Osteopath Assoc 1993;93:75.
24. Baker ME, Silverman PM, Korobkin M. Computed tomography of prostatic and bladder rhabdomyosarcomas. J Comput Assist Tomogr 1985;9:780.
25. Cohen MD, DeRosa GP, Kleiman M, et al. Magnetic resonance evaluation of disease of the soft tissues in children. Pediatrics 1987;79:696.
26. Crist WM, Raney RB, Tefft M, et al. Soft-tissue sarcomas arising in the retroperitoneal space in children: a report from the Intergroup Rhabdomyosarcoma Study (IRS) committee. Cancer 1985;56:2125.
27. Raney RB Jr, Crist W, Hays D, et al. Soft-tissue sarcoma of the perineal region in childhood: a report from the Intergroup Rhabdomyosarcoma Studies I and II, 1972 through 1984. Cancer 1990;65:2787.
28. Quddus FF, Espinola D, Kramer SS, Leventhal BG. Comparison between x-ray and bone scan detection of bone metastases in patients with rhabdomyosarcoma. Med Pediatr Oncol 1983;11:125.
29. Southee AE, Kaplan WD, Jochelson MS, et al. Gallium imaging in metastatic and recurrent soft-tissue sarcoma. J Nucl Med 1992;33:1594.
30. Nadel HR. Thallium-201 for oncological imaging in children. Semin Nucl Med 1993;23:243.
31. Rodary C, Rey A, Olive D, et al. Prognostic factors in 281 children with nonmetastatic rhabdomyosarcoma (RMS) at diagnosis. Med Pediatr Oncol 1988;16:71.
32. Crist WM, Garnsey L, Beltangady MS, et al. Prognosis in children with rhabdomyosarcoma: a report of the Intergroup Rhabdomyosarcoma Studies I and II. J Clin Oncol 1990;8:443.
33. Heyn R, Raney RB Jr, Hays DM, et al. Late effects of therapy in patients with paratesticular rhabdomyosarcoma. J Clin Oncol 1992;10: 614.
34. Hughes LL, Baruzzi MJ, Ribeiro RC, et al. Paratesticular rhabdomyosarcoma: delayed effects of multimodality therapy and implications for current management. Cancer 1994;73:476.
35. Raney RB Jr, Gehan EA, Hays DM, et al. Primary chemotherapy with or without radiation therapy and/or surgery for children with localized sarcoma of the bladder, prostate, vagina, uterus, and cervix: a comparison of the results in Intergroup Rhabdomyosarcoma Studies I and II. Cancer 1990;66:2072.
36. Hays D, Raney RB, Crist W, et al. Improved survival and bladder preservation among patients with bladder/prostate primary tumors in Intergroup Rhabdomyosarcoma Study III. Proc Am Soc Clin Oncol 1991;10:318. Abstract 1119.
37. Crist W, Gehan EA, Ragab AH, et al. The Intergroup Rhabdomyosarcoma Study III. J Clin Oncol 1995;13:610.
38. Voûte PA, Vos A, de Kraker J, Behrendt H. Rhabdomyosarcomas: chemotherapy and limited supplementary treatment program to avoid mutilation. Monogr Natl Cancer Inst 1981;56:121.
39. Heij HA, Vos A, de Kraker J, Voûte PA. Urogenital rhabdomyosarcoma in children: is a conservative surgical approach justified? J Urol 1993; 150:165.
40. Rivard G, Ortega J, Hittle R, Nitschke R, Karon M. Intensive chemotherapy as primary treatment for rhabdomyosarcoma of the pelvis. Cancer 1975;36:1593.
41. Ortega JA. A therapeutic approach to childhood pelvic rhabdomyosarcoma without pelvic exenteration. J Pediatr 1979;94:205.
42. Hays DM, Lawrence W Jr, Crist WM, et al. Partial cystectomy in the management of rhabdomyosarcoma of the bladder: a report from the Intergroup Rhabdomyosarcoma Study. J Pediatr Surg 1990;25:719.
43. Raney B Jr, Heyn R, Hays DM, et al. Sequelae of treatment in 109 patients followed for 5 to 15 years after diagnosis of sarcoma of the bladder and prostate. Cancer 1993;71:2387.
44. Flamant F, Gerbaulet A, Nihoul-Fekete C, Valteau-Couanet D, Chassagne D, Lemerle J. Long-term sequelae of conservative treatment by surgery, brachytherapy, and chemotherapy for vulval and vaginal rhabdomyosarcoma in children. J Clin Oncol 1990;8:1847.
45. Piver MS, Rose PG. Long-term follow-up and complications of infants with vulvovaginal embryonal rhabdomyosarcoma treated with surgery, radiation therapy, and chemotherapy. Obstet Gynecol 1988;71:435.
46. Corpron CA, Andrassy RJ, Hays DM, et al. Conservative management of uterine rhabdomyosarcomas: a report from the Intergroup Rhabdomyosarcoma Study III and IV pilot. J Pediatr Surg 1995;30:942.

Principles and Practice of Genitourinary Oncology, edited by Derek Raghavan, Howard I. Scher, Steven A. Leibel, and Paul H. Lange. Lippincott-Raven Publishers, Philadelphia, © 1997.

CHAPTER 102

Genitourinary Rhabdomyosarcoma in Children

Principles of Treatment

Richard J. Andrassy, Moody D. Wharam, Jr., and R. Beverly Raney

Radical surgical excision was the first effective treatment for rhabdomyosarcoma (RMS). For pelvic genitourinary tumors, this consisted of total pelvic exenteration. It was later demonstrated that RMS was radiosensitive,[1] but high doses were required for local tumor control. Survival rates remained at less than 10% until the late 1960s, when combination therapy was introduced with the use of chemotherapy and radiotherapy following attempts at complete surgical excision.[2] Later, it was found that survival was significantly enhanced if chemotherapy was routinely administered after surgery.[3]

In 1972 the Intergroup Rhabdomyosarcoma Study (IRS) was established. This trial studied large numbers of patients in a prospective fashion, which led to tremendous advances in chemotherapy and improvement in survival. The modern excellent responses to chemotherapy and radiotherapy have fostered a more conservative surgical approach, and the concepts of delayed surgery and second-look surgery have been advanced. Since this study was begun there has been a progressive increase in survival among children with RMS. During the early years of the IRS (1972 to 1978), radical surgical intervention prior to chemotherapy with or without radiotherapy was considered standard management. Once it was demonstrated that most patients would survive the disease, investigators explored the use of primary chemotherapy and radiotherapy to avoid exenterative surgery for genitourinary RMS.[4,5] A major aim of the protocols in IRS-II (1978 to 1984) for patients with primary tumors in these sites was preservation of a functional distal urinary tract while maintaining the high survival rates achieved in IRS-I.[6] Unfortunately, primary chemotherapy with vincristine, dactinomycin (Actinomycin D), and cyclophosphamide did not obviate the need for radiotherapy or radical surgery for patients with pelvic RMS, and the percentage of patients alive at 3 years was the same in IRS-II as in IRS-I.[7] In IRS-III (1985 to 1992), more intensive chemotherapy was used (vincristine, dactinomycin, and cyclophosphamide [VAC] plus doxorubicin and cisplatin), and radiotherapy was initiated sooner in the treatment course. The intensification of treatment for pelvic RMS in IRS-III has produced an increased rate of functional bladder preservation while maintaining overall survival.[7]

A number of therapeutic and nontherapeutic advances have been made during the IRS studies. Some of these specifically related to the surgical aspects of genitourinary RMS include the following:

- identification of histology, site, and extent of disease as prognostic factors[8]
- reduced need for radical surgery
- increased bladder preservation from 25% to 60% while increasing survival[9]
- partial cystectomy affording comparable survival with satisfactory bladder function[10]
- demonstration of the benefit of primary tumor reexcision for microscopic residual disease after initial nondefinitive excision
- second-look surgery to determine pathologic tumor status while increasing complete response rate and possibly survival[11]
- elimination of routine lymphadenectomy for localized paratesticular RMS[12]
- reduced or eliminated radiotherapy for special groups or sites (e.g., patients with localized vaginal RMS, patients with localized tumors and clear surgical margins postoperatively)

Chemotherapy for children with genitourinary sarcoma has evolved along with chemotherapy for RMS and related tumors at all sites in the first two decades of life. Identification of the active agents vincristine, dactinomycin, and cyclophosphamide (VAC) took place in the 1950s and 1960s as they became available; each was tested in patients with recurrent or unresectable sarcoma so that response rates could be estimated.[13] Later, combinations of these agents with or without newer drugs such as doxorubicin (Adriamycin), cisplatin, ifosfamide, etoposide, and dimethyltriazenoimidazole carboxamide (DTIC) were undertaken, both in previously untreated and in relapsing patients.[13] Heyn and colleagues[3] first showed in 1974 in a randomized study that the addition of vincristine and Actinomycin D therapy for 1 year after complete removal of localized RMS led to a significantly improved relapse-free survival rate of 82%, compared with 47% (P = .02) in similar patients who received no postoperative chemotherapy. Since then, chemotherapeutic regimens containing at least these two drugs have been standard for patients with RMS. At the same time, Wilbur and coworkers[14] demonstrated the efficacy of pulsed doses of VAC in shrinking tumors in patients with inoperable RMS. At the time of that report, 10 of 16 (63%) patients with localized gross residual tumor and 4 of 8 (50%) patients with metastatic disease were alive without evident tumor. Since then, the IRS has been testing various combinations of agents for efficacy in preventing metastases and in reducing bulky residual disease.[6,15–17]

In IRS-II, a primary chemotherapy approach was tested for patients with tumors in special pelvic sites (i.e., bladder, prostate, vagina, cervix, and uterus) in an attempt to preserve the bladder and avoid giving radiotherapy if possible. Unfortunately, this approach proved unsatisfactory. The bladder preservation rate was the same as in IRS-I (~23% at 3 years), and survival was not improved.[6] These disappointing results may be attributed to the low dose intensity of the chemotherapy (one course of VAC every 28 days), the deferral of radiotherapy to week 16 or beyond in many patients, or both. In IRS-III patients were given weekly vincristine for 13 doses, Adriamycin and cisplatin were added, and radiotherapy was reintroduced at week 6 for patients with bladder-prostate (BP) tumors. This approach has given the best results available, with a 3-year survival rate of 90% and a bladder preservation rate of 60% in 82 group III patients.[18] However, none of the IRS protocols[6,15–17] has shown a clear-cut advantage for patients given Adriamycin with or without cisplatin compared with those who received VAC without these other agents; therefore, more intensive combinations of drugs other than Adriamycin and cisplatin are being studied in IRS-IV.

RADIOTHERAPY TECHNIQUE

The components of radiotherapy in children with genitourinary RMS include treatment planning, treatment delivery, and follow-up management. The two principal elements of treatment planning are patient data acquisition and computerized dosimetry planning. Data acquisition occurs at the time of treatment simulation using either a conventional (two-dimensional) diagnostic x-ray unit simulator or a computed tomography (CT)–based (three-dimensional) simulator. Two critical steps precede the simulation procedure. Children 3 years of age or younger usually require sedation or anesthesia to remain motionless for the protracted period required,[19] whereas older children may benefit from desensitization training to reduce anxiety.[20] Reproducible supine immobilization is accomplished with thermoplastic compound body molds, orthogonal laser beam skin markings, or similar methods. When the patient and the tumor volume of interest are properly aligned with the reference point (i.e., isocenter) of the simulator, orthogonal (i.e., 90 degrees anteroposterior and lateral) x-ray films are obtained or multiple CT images that subtend the volume of interest are taken. Intravenous contrast to opacify the bladder and rectal contrast may be required. The body surface contour is mapped at appropriate planes. The tumor extent is drawn on the simulation films based on the initial extent of tumor at diagnosis using all imaging methods and data obtained at operation. Particular attention must be paid to the inferior border for tumors involving the prostate, which may not be clearly defined on images obtained in axial planes.

The data are used by a specially trained medical dosimetrist who employs a computerized treatment planning system to determine the combination of external irradiation beam parameters that will maximize dose to the tumor volume and minimize doses to normal tissues and organs. For BP primary tumors, these normal structures include the rectum, the femoral heads, and the acetabula. In females, the reproductive organs receive essentially the same dose as the bladder primary unless the ovaries have been surgically relocated outside the pelvis. The organs of interest for a paratestis primary site include the lower thoracic and lumbosacral spine, the spinal cord, the kidneys, and the remaining testis.

The typical treatment plan for a BP primary tumor uses a combination of anteroposterior portals, which shield the femoral heads and acetabula, if possible, and opposing lateral portals that spare the posterior wall of the rectum. The typical portals for a group II paratestis primary tumor are anteroposterior opposing fields that cover the paraaortic nodes but do not cover more than a thin medial strip of renal tissue. The peak radiation beam energy is usually 4 or 6 MeV. The computerized treatment plan is typically presented as the radiation dose distribution in an axial plane through the isocenter. Dose is shown as lines of equal, relative dose (i.e., isodose lines); the line that most closely approximates the tumor volume is assigned a value of 100%. The other isodose lines are relative to the 100% (i.e., tumor) isodose line. The plan is designed to avoid areas of dose deposition greater than 105%.

Treatment delivery is performed with the patient in their customized immobilization device on the treatment table of a medical linear accelerator. A peak energy of 4 to 6 MeV is appropriate for most children, but higher energies (i.e., 10 to 15 MeV) may be used for teenagers. Treatment of inguinal and femoral nodes may be done with electron beams of energy appropriate for the depth of the lymph nodes; this method may spare underlying bone and hip joint.

In addition to carefully planned computerized dosimetry, other components of treatment delivery such as focused blocks, transmission filters, and wedge filters should be used where appropriate. Initial and weekly portal verification radiographs should be taken, and in vivo confirmation of treatment dose should be considered. The physician and nurse monitor the acute toxicity of treatment each week.

Radiation dose for the primary tumor is usually 1.8 Gy per daily treatment session, assuming a standard of five treatments (i.e., fractions) are given per week. Total dose is determined by surgicopathologic group; group II tumors receive 41.4 Gy and group III lesions receive 50.4 Gy. Dose to the primary site of a group IV patient corresponds to that which would be required if there were no distant metastases.

Experience at the St. Jude Children's Research Hospital indicates that children with RMS at various sites (group III at diagnosis) can attain local control with a dose of approximately 40 Gy if they achieve a status of response to induction chemotherapy or similar chemotherapy followed by definitive second-look surgery that results in microscopic residual tumor.[21] At the Memorial Sloan-Kettering Cancer Center, seven boys with positive retroperitoneal lymph node dissection (RPLND) for a paratestis primary were locally controlled with a postoperative dose of less than 40 Gy (range, 31 to 36.5 Gy).[22]

Experience with brachytherapy for genitourinary RMS is limited. Twelve patients at the Institut Gustav-Roussy in Paris received induction chemotherapy and conservative surgery with perioperative iridium-192 implantation for BP RMS. Five-year survival without tumor recurrence was 75%, and there were no severe complications. The investigators recommend brachytherapy for primary tumors smaller than 4 cm in maximum diameter.[23]

Posttreatment management includes monitoring for systemic and local relapse. Biopsy of the primary tumor should be done only when there is convincing clinical evidence of local recurrence, because the interpretation of postirradiation biopsy material is difficult and prone to false-positive interpretation.

The current IRS-IV treatment approach for patients with localized tumors in various genitourinary sites is outlined in the following section.

SPECIFIC SITES

Bladder and Prostate Tumors

Presentation, symptoms, and findings in patients with RMS of the bladder or prostate are described in detail in Chapter 101. As previously mentioned, the role of surgical intervention has become more conservative during the past 20 years. Although conservative surgical therapy for bladder tumors has not been as successful as it has for vaginal primaries, the bladder salvage rate has increased,[7,10] and anterior pelvic exenteration is no longer considered the initial therapy for pelvic RMS.[24] The intensification of chemotherapy and earlier use of local radiotherapy for pelvic RMS in IRS-III produced an increased preservation rate of functional bladders while maintaining overall survival. Today, 60% of patients retain a functional bladder at 4 years from diagnosis, and overall survival exceeds 85%.[7]

Before the development of effective adjuvant therapy, the recurrence rate after partial cystectomy for vesical RMS was high. However, partial resection of the bladder wall for primary tumors affecting the dome or sides of the bladder distant from the trigone is recommended either as initial therapy or as a delayed procedure after chemotherapy. This approach was used in 40 patients reported to the IRS with an overall survival of 80%.[7] Of the 32 long-term survivors, 75% of patients have no bladder-related symptoms. Bladder augmentation or substitution has been used in some of these patients to achieve good functional results.[25]

Unfortunately, a large percentage of bladder and prostate tumors arise from the trigonal area or prostate and are not amenable to local or partial resection. Local recurrence is likely to occur if adequate resection is not accomplished. If chemotherapy does not result in adequate shrinkage of the tumor to allow partial resection, then radical cystectomy may be necessary. Pelvic exenteration is also employed for relapsed tumors.[7]

In selected patients, prostatectomy with bladder preservation and urethral reconstruction can be accomplished. Prostatectomy without cystectomy has been performed in selected patients with persistent disease or local relapse[7,26]; however, local relapses occurred in 40% of these patients. The completeness of surgical resection may be difficult to determine by frozen sections, which can be misleading; this often results in local recurrence.[26]

In patients requiring bladder resection for persistent or recurrent disease, a nonrefluxing colon conduit or a continent ileocecal segment with an appendiceal stoma may be preferable to an ileal loop for urinary tract diversion.

Most BP cancer patients initially present with tumors whose complete removal would require total cystectomy. To preserve the bladder and prostate, primary chemotherapy with VAC, VAI (vincristine, dactinomycin, ifosfamide), or VEI (vincristine, etoposide, ifosfamide) is given by random assignment, as in patients with group II or III paratesticular tumors (discussed later). Conventional or twice-daily fractionated radiotherapy is begun at week 6 of chemotherapy.

In BP RMS, bladder function can be preserved and primary tumor controlled with carefully planned radiotherapy, when it is administered by a radiation oncologist who is part of an experienced multidisciplinary team. The data supporting this rationale come from the IRS-III study, which enrolled 81 pediatric BP RMS patients between 1985 and 1990. This study employed conservative surgery (usually biopsy only) and definitive irradiation of the primary tumor at week 6 of a 24-month course of multiagent chemotherapy. The 3-year survival and ''alive with functional bladder'' percentages were 90% and 60%, respectively, compared with 70% and 25% for the prior trial (IRS-II, 1979 to 1984) which placed less emphasis on radiotherapy and used less-aggressive chemotherapy.[18] Data supporting acceptable long-term bladder function with this approach were presented earlier in this chapter in children with BP RMS who were enrolled in the IRS-I and IRS-II protocols (1972 to 1984) who retained their bladder and were followed for 5 to 15 years after treatment. Thirty-eight patients (73%) had satisfactory bladder function; the remainder reported urinary incontinence or frequency.[24]

The indications for radiotherapy are based on the extent of disease at diagnosis (i.e., stage) and the outcome of the initial surgical procedure (i.e., group; see Chap. 101). Patients with BP primary tumors are in stage 2 if the lesions are smaller than 5 cm in maximum tumor diameter and regional lymph nodes are negative and in stage 3 if their primary lesion of any size is node-positive or is larger than 5 cm. For both stage 1 and stage 2 tumors, there must be no imaging evidence of hematogenous dissemination; if present, this puts the patient in stage 4 and group IV. A patient who has a complete cystectomy or cystoprostatectomy with clear margins and without tumor-involved regional nodes is placed in group I, and postoperative radiotherapy is not indicated. A similar or lesser procedure that results in microscopic residual tumor remaining in the operative bed or lymph nodes defines a group II patient, and adjunctive irradiation is required. Major organ-sacrificing procedures are discouraged; therefore, the majority of patients are in group III, having had only biopsy or a conservative procedure that leaves gross residual tumor. Definitive radiotherapy is required for these patients. Group IV patients may have dissemination to one or many organs, typically lung, bone, bone marrow, or supradiaphragmatic lymph nodes. Radiotherapy is indicated for these metastatic sites, except bone marrow. The indication for radiotherapy to the primary site (either BP or paratestis) is governed by the stage and group guidelines that would apply in the absence of dissemination.

PARATESTICULAR RHABDOMYOSARCOMA

Paratesticular RMS accounts for 7% of RMS and 12% of childhood scrotal tumors.[27] Paratesticular RMS arises in the distal portion of the spermatic cord and may invade the testis or surrounding tissues. More than 90% of paratesticular RMS are embryonal in histology and have a good prognosis. The peak age at presentation is between 1 and 5 years.[12,27]

The presenting symptom is often a unilateral, painless scrotal swelling or mass above the testis. On physical examination, a firm mass that is usually distinct from the testis is present. Ultrasonography confirms the solid nature of the lesion.

Radical inguinal orchiectomy is recommended as the initial treatment. A paratesticular mass should be resected by inguinal orchidectomy, with complete resection of the spermatic cord structures to the level of the internal ring (Fig. 102-1). If a prior transcrotal procedure has been performed, this increases the risk of local recurrence and nonregional lymph node spread. If cord elements remain, inguinal exploration with removal of the remaining spermatic cord and a partial hemiscrotectomy including the prior scrotal incision are performed. In a review of 14 hemiscrotectomy specimens at Memorial Sloan-Kettering Cancer Center, 28% had residual tumor.[28]

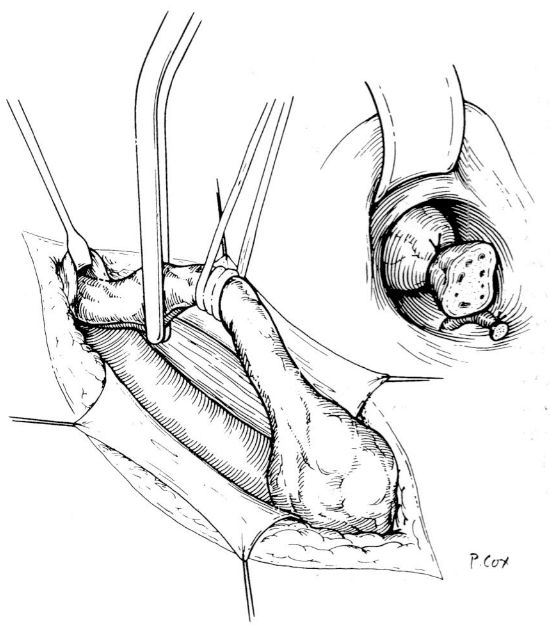

FIG. 102-1. Radical inguinal orchiectomy. After cross-clamping the spermatic cord, the testes is delivered into the operative field. If pathologic examination of the biopsy specimen demonstrates tumor, high inguinal orchiectomy is performed, and microscopic inspection of proximal cord confirms the presence or absence of proximal disease.

Before the advent of effective systemic therapy, surgery alone produced a 50% relapse-free survival at 2 years.[29] With the introduction of multimodal treatment, chemotherapy, and radiotherapy for selected patients, survival rates of 90% are expected.[12] A metastatic evaluation is performed at diagnosis. CT imaging of the retroperitoneum to identify nodal metastases is mandatory, because lymphatic spread is present in 28% to 40% of children.[8,30] The initial use of RPLND for paratesticular RMS was based on the management of non-RMS testicular malignancies and the high incidence of retroperitoneal lymph node involvement. It was felt that RPLND was important for staging the disease and not necessarily as treatment. Unilateral RPLND with sampling of the contralateral nodes is recommended. Patients who have positive lymph nodes receive radiotherapy in the involved areas.

The role of RPLND in paratesticular RMS is controversial.[12,31,32] The fact that grossly involved retroperitoneal nodes can be detected by preoperative imaging studies, that microscopic nodal disease can be effectively treated by chemotherapy, and that there is significant morbidity associated with RPLND are arguments against its routine use. Heyn and colleagues[33] reported a 10% incidence of intestinal obstruction, 8% incidence of ejaculatory dysfunction, and 5% incidence of edema of the lower extremities in patients who had undergone RPLND for paratesticular RMS. This series involved patients reported to the first IRS study, the majority of whom underwent bilateral node dissection. Modified unilateral node dissection is appropriate for staging, and with the addition of nerve-sparing techniques, it may avoid some of the morbidity reported with node dissection.[28,34] It is clear that even with advances in imaging there is a significant false-negative rate (14% for IRS-III patients) associated with CT for identifying involved retroperitoneal lymph nodes in patients with paratesticular RMS.[12] The ability of laparoscopy to identify retroperitoneal nodal disease in this setting remains to be evaluated, but it may offer a less morbid alternative to RPLND.

Olive and colleagues[31] reported 19 children with paratesticular RMS who had no clinical evidence of retroperitoneal nodal involvement. Nodal recurrence developed in two patients (10.5%), but both survived after salvage therapy. A subsequent report of the SIOP experience with 46 children who had completely excised tumors and negative CT or lymphangiogram treated with intensive chemotherapy alone also found that all children survived.[35] However, it should be noted that the vast majority of children received doxorubicin, which has potential for late adverse effects.

In a review of 121 children with paratesticular RMS undergoing RPLND reported to IRS-III, 14% of patients with clinically negative nodes were found to have positive lymph nodes on pathologic evaluation.[12] There were two cases of nodal relapse, one of which had a prior negative RPLND. This suggests a small risk of nodal relapse in these patients if regional radiotherapy and appropriate chemotherapy are administered. The overall 5-year survival for the 98 patients with clinically negative nodes was 96%, but less than 10% of patients received doxorubicin. Although the finding of positive retroperitoneal lymph nodes identified a group of patients with decreased survival, it is recommended that patients with clinically negative nodes undergo treatment with primary chemotherapy alone.[32] An exception may be children older than 10 years of age; this group of patients has a significantly worse prognosis.[12]

Most of patients with paratesticular RMS have stage 1, clinical group I disease after radical orchidectomy. The survival rate is 90% or higher; therefore in IRS-IV, only vincristine and Actinomycin D are given, in three 12-week cycles that comprise 8 weeks of drug administration followed by 4 weeks of rest. Thus, these patients finish chemotherapy at the completion of week 32. Patients with regional nodal involvement and microscopic residual tumor (group II) or gross residual sarcoma (group III) are randomized to receive one of three three-drug combinations—VAC, VAI, or VEI—for 1 year, as well as local radiotherapy.

Late effects of therapy were studied in 86 children with paratesticular RMS treated in IRS-I and IRS-II protocols.[33] Complications were as mentioned previously. Most of these complications could have been prevented by avoiding RPLND. Sequelae from chemotherapeutic drugs, especially alkylating agents (cyclophosphamide), included hemorrhagic cystitis in 33% of patients. Diminished contralateral testicular size was found in 30% of children who received both radiotherapy and cyclophosphamide. Elevated follicle-stimulating hormone levels, azoospermia, or both was present in 50% of patients studied. Current studies attempt to decrease exposure to alkylating agents, radiotherapy, and RPLND, especially in patients with limited disease.

The rationale for radiotherapy for paratesticular RMS is based on the observed 90% relapse-free survival rate at 3 years reported for group II patients in IRS-I and IRS-II trials. Patients in these studies received multimodal therapy, including radiotherapy, for nonbulky iliac and paraaortic lymphadenopathy.[36]

In the absence of distant metastases, a patient with a paratestis primary tumor is usually in stage 1. No radiotherapy is necessary for patients who are group I following resection of the primary lesion. A patient who is group II on the basis of a positive margin of the scrotal skin, epididymis, or spermatic cord should be reoperated promptly to have a hemiscrotectomy or additional exploration of the affected region so that he can be placed in group I and thus avoid the need for irradiation. If retroperitoneal node examination is accomplished and positive nodes are found, the patient is considered group II. If bulky nodes are present and not removed, the patient is considered group III.

Radiotherapy to the retroperitoneal nodes is indicated for both groups. The time to begin irradiation is determined by the patient's group. For the IRS-IV study, group II receives radiotherapy in week 1, group III in week 9, and group IV in week 19.

PATIENTS WITH METASTASES AT DIAGNOSIS

More active agents are needed to try to improve the poor survival expectancy of patients with metastases at diagnosis. Little changed in treatment regimens from IRS-I through IRS-III.[6,15–17] We administer vincristine plus melphalan or ifosfamide plus etoposide by random assignment, followed by VAC and radiotherapy, to all group IV patients. Some centers administer high-dose chemotherapy followed by autologous bone marrow or stem cell reinfusion to ameliorate the associated pancytopenia, but such an approach is experimental and the available data are sparse.

REFERENCES

1. Stobbe GC, Dargeon H. Embryonal rhabdomyosarcoma of the head and neck in children and adolescents. Cancer 1950;3:826.
2. Pinkel D, Pickren J. Rhabdomyosarcoma in children. JAMA 1961;175:293.
3. Heyn RM, Holland R, Newton WA Jr, et al. The role of combined chemotherapy in the treatment of rhabdomyosarcoma in children. Cancer 1974;34:2128.
4. Ortega JA. A therapeutic approach to childhood pelvic rhabdomyosarcoma without pelvic exenteration. J Pediatr 1979;94:205.
5. Voute PA, Vos A, deKraker J, Behrendt H. Rhabdomyosarcomas: chemotherapy and limited supplementary treatment to avoid mutilation. Natl Cancer Inst Monogr 1981;56:121.
6. Raney RB, Gehan EA, Hays DM, et al. Primary chemotherapy with or without radiation therapy and or surgery for children with localized sarcoma of the bladder, prostate, vagina, uterus, and cervix. Cancer 1990;66:2072.
7. Hays DM. Bladder/prostate rhabdomyosarcoma: results of the multi-institutional trials of the Intergroup Rhabdomyosarcoma Study. Semin Surg Oncol 1993;9:520.
8. Lawrence W, Gehan EA, Hays DM, et al. Prognostic significance of staging factors of the UICC staging system in childhood rhabdomyosarcoma: a report from the Intergroup Rhabdomyosarcoma Study (IRS-II). J Clin Oncol 1987;5:46.
9. Hays DM, Raney RB, Lawrence W, et al. Primary chemotherapy in the treatment of children with bladder-prostate tumors in the Intergroup Rhabdomyosarcoma Study (IRS-II). J Pediatr Surg 1982;17:812.
10. Hays DM, Lawrence W, Crist W, et al. Partial cystectomy in the management of rhabdomyosarcoma of the bladder: a report from the Intergroup Rhabdomyosarcoma Study (IRS). J Pediatr Surg 1990;25:719.
11. Hays DM, Raney RB, Crist W, et al. Secondary surgical procedures to evaluate primary tumor status in patients with chemotherapy responsive stage III–IV sarcomas. J Pediatr Surg 1990;25:1100.
12. Wiener ES, Lawrence W, Hays D, et al. Retroperitoneal node biopsy in childhood paratesticular rhabdomyosarcoma. J Pediatr Surg 1994;29:171.
13. Raney RB Jr, Hays DM, Tefft M, Triche TJ. Rhabdomyosarcoma and the undifferentiated sarcomas. In: Pizzo PA, Poplack DG, eds. Principles and practice of pediatric oncology, 2nd ed. Philadelphia: JB Lippincott, 1993:769.
14. Wilbur JR. Combination chemotherapy for embryonal rhabdomyosarcoma. Cancer Chemother Rep 1974;58:281.
15. Maurer HM, Beltangady M, Gehan EA, et al. The Intergroup Rhabdomyosarcoma Study I: a final report. Cancer 1988;61:209.
16. Maurer HM, Gehan EA, Beltangady M, et al. The Intergroup Rhabdomyosarcoma Study II. Cancer 1993;71:1904.
17. Crist W, Gehan EA, Ragab AH, et al. The Intergroup Rhabdomyosarcoma Study III. J Clin Oncol 1995;13:610.
18. Hays D, Raney RB, Crist W, et al. Improved survival and bladder preservation among patients with bladder/prostate primary tumors in Intergroup Rhabdomyosarcoma Study III (IRS). (Abstract 1119) Proc Am Soc Clin Oncol 1991;10:318.
19. Bucholtz JD. Issues concerning the sedation of children for radiation therapy. Oncol Nurs Forum 1992;19:649.
20. Slifer KJ, Bucholtz JD, Cataldo MD. Behavioral training of motion control in young children undergoing radiation treatment without sedation. J Pediatr Oncol Nurs 1994;11:55.
21. Regine WF, Fontanesi J, Bowman L, et al. Evaluation of local control with selective use of low-dose irradiation following induction/preoperative chemotherapy for locally advanced rhabdomyosarcoma. (Abstract 7) Int J Radiat Oncol Biol Phys 1993;27:131.
22. Mandell L, Ghavimi F, Peretz T, et al. Radiocurability of microscopic disease in childhood rhabdomyosarcoma with radiation doses less than 4,000 cGy. J Clin Oncol 1990;8:1536.
23. Haie-Meder C, Flamant F, Revillon Y, et al. Brachytherapy in the multidisciplinary therapy of prostate and/or bladder. Rhabdomyosarcoma in children. (Abstract 0–74) Med Pediatr Oncol 1994;23:188.
24. Raney RB, Heyn D, Hays DM, et al. Sequelae of treatment in 109

patients followed for 5 to 15 years after diagnosis of sarcoma of the bladder and prostate. Cancer 1993;71:2387.

25. Hicks BA, Hensle TW, Burbige KA, Altman PR. Bladder management in children with genitourinary sarcoma. J Pediatr Surg 1993;28:1019.
26. McLorie GA, Abara OE, Churchill BM, et al. Rhabdomyosarcoma of the prostate in childhood: current challenges. J Pediatr Surg 1989;24: 977.
27. Wiener ES. Rhabdomyosarcoma: new dimensions in management. Semin Pediatr Surg 1993;2:47.
28. LaQuaglia M, Ghavimi F, Heller G, et al. Mortality in pediatric paratesticular rhabdomyosarcoma: a multivariate analysis. J Urol 1989;142: 473.
29. Sutow WW, Sullivan MP, Ried HL, et al. Prognosis in childhood rhabdomyosarcoma. Cancer 1970;25:1385.
30. Raney RB, Hays DM, Lawrence W Jr, et al. Paratesticular rhabdomyosarcoma in children. Cancer 1978;42:729.
31. Olive D, Flamant F, Zucker JM, et al. Para-aortic lymphadenectomy is not necessary in the treatment of localized rhabdomyosarcoma. Cancer 1984;54:1283.
32. Rodary C, Flamant F, Maurer H, et al. Initial lymphadenectomy is not necessary in localized and completely resected paratesticular rhabdomyosarcoma. Med Pediatr Oncol 1992;20:430.
33. Heyn R, Raney RB, Hays DM, et al. Late effects of therapy in patients with paratesticular rhabdomyosarcoma: for the Intergroup Rhabdomyosarcoma Study Committee. J Clin Oncol 1992;10:614.
34. Dohohue JP, Foster RS, Rowland RG, et al. Nerve-sparing retroperitoneal lymphadenectomy with preservation of ejaculation. J Urol 1990; 144:287.
35. Olive-Sommelet D. Paratesticular rhabdomyosarcoma: International Society of Pediatric Oncology Protocol. Dial Pediatr Urol 1989;12(11): 4.
36. Raney RB, Tefft M, Lawrence W, et al. Paratesticular sarcoma in childhood and adolescence: a report from the Intergroup Rhabdomyosarcoma Studies I and II, 1973–1983. Cancer 1987;60:2337.

SECTION X

Neuroblastoma

Principles and Practice of Genitourinary Oncology, edited by Derek Raghavan, Howard I. Scher, Steven A. Leibel, and Paul H. Lange. Lippincott-Raven Publishers, Philadelphia, © 1997.

CHAPTER 103

Genetics of Neuroblastoma Tumors

Carol J. Thiele

A genetic basis of cancer is now well established. At each step during tumorigenesis, rare, heritable mutations can occur that contribute to the morphologic and biologic alterations detected in an evolving cancer cell. Support for this type of model in human cancers comes from the elegant studies detailing an increasing number of alterations in protooncogenes and suppressor genes in tissue samples, from benign adenomatous polyposis to advanced-stage colon cancer.[1] A complete discussion of principles and techniques of molecular biology is presented in Chapter 1.

Neuroblastomas (NB), pediatric tumors of embyronal neural crest cells, contain a number of genetic alterations that have been described, some of which have predictive value in terms of patient outcome. Further delineation and analysis of the nature of these genetic alterations may elucidate the mechanisms of tumorigenesis in NB and allow the development of novel and specific therapies. This chapter reviews the genetics and genetic alterations contained in NBs and their biologic and clinical significance.

MEDICAL GENETICS

NBs comprise approximately 9% of all childhood cancers, with an annual incidence of approximately 1 in 10^5 children younger than 15 years of age.[2] The median age at diagnosis is 22 months; more than 88% of cases are diagnosed by the age of 5 years. Some studies indicate a bimodal age distribution, with one peak at approximately 1 year and the second between 2 and 4 years.[3] The ethnic and geographic incidence of NB in the world is relatively uniform, with the exception of tropical Africa and India, where the incidence is markedly lower.[4] Environmental factors have been invoked to account for the unusually high geographic incidence of tumors such as Burkitt's lymphoma, it is conceivable that similar factors could suppress or adversely affect the incidence of NBs.

A 1967 report of familial NB affecting four of five siblings led Knudson and Meadows to formulate a mutation model for neuroblastoma in 1976.[5] This model proposed that all NBs derive from a single cell that is transformed from a normal cell by two mutations: one that arises prezygotically in the germline and a second that arises in a somatic cell of the target tissue. Such a "two-hit" model of tumor development had been hypothesized first to describe the genetics of retinoblastoma tumors[6] and was subsequently verified with the identification of the retinoblastoma gene, *RB1*, which is deleted in all retinoblastomas.

Familial NB accounts for approximately 22% of all cases of NB. Because it follows an autosomal dominant form of inheritance, the probability of tumor occurrence in familial or germline NB would be expected to be high. However, the actual incidence is quite low, possibly because the elaboration of both mutations causes an embryonic lethal condition or because of failure to detect affected parents, who may have occult tumors that spontaneously regress or benign tumors such as ganglioneuromas.[7,8] The majority of NBs arise sporadically. In sporadic cases, germline mutations do not occur, and both mutations arise somatically. NBs occur early in life, and the age-associated incidence suggests that the target cell may differentiate or does not persist into adult life. For sporadic NBs to ensue, both mutations must occur in the cell before it fully differentiates.

Secondary tumors, including pheochromocytoma, brain tumors and leukemia, and renal cell carcinoma, have been found in patients with NB, although their low frequency precludes a genetic link with NB such as has been detected between retinoblastoma and osteosarcoma. Occasionally, NBs have been detected in patients with neurofibromatosis,[9,10] although ganglioneuromas are more frequently associated with this syndrome.[11]

CYTOGENETICS

DNA Ploidy

Fluorescence-activated cell scanning, using DNA intercalating dyes such as propidium iodine, has been used extensively to estimate DNA content and modal chromosome number in both normal and tumor tissues. Studies indicate that the modal chromosome number or DNA index (DI) in NB may be predictive of the response of particular tumors to chemotherapy and eventual outcome.[12–14] Figure 103-1 illustrates DNA histograms representative of those detected in NB patients. NBs with a hyperdiploid or aneuploid DNA content (DI>1) are typically found in the patient population with a favorable outcome (see

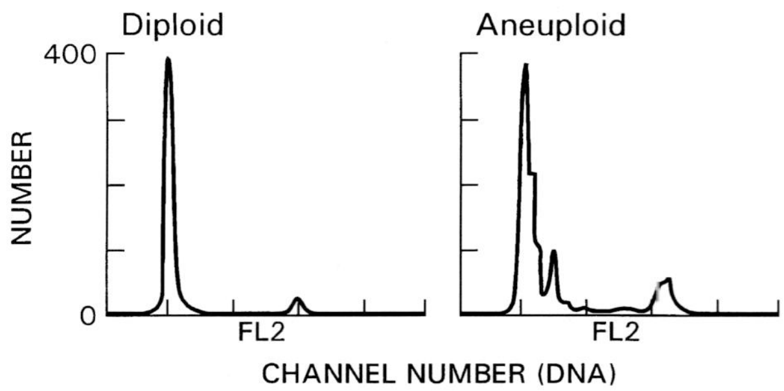

FIG. 103-1. Representative DNA histograms derived from fluorescent activated cell sorter analysis of propidium iodine–stained tumor cells. Left panel is a DNA histogram of tumor cells with a diploid DNA content (DNA index = 1), which is characteristically found in poor-prognosis neuroblastoma tumors. Right panel is a DNA histogram of tumor with an aneuploid DNA content (DNA index > 1), and this is characteristic of tumors from patients with a good prognosis.

Fig. 103-1*B*). In contrast, tumors with a diploid DNA content (DI = 1) are found in those with poor prognosis (see Fig. 103-1*A*). Use of DI and *MYCN* copy number adds significantly to the predictive value of age and stage in the prognosis of NB.[14]

Chromosomal Anomalies

NBs are characterized by three major cytogenetic abnormalities: double minute chromosomes (DMs), homogeneously staining regions (HSRs), and deletions in chromosome 1p.

Double Minute Chromosomes and Homogeneously Staining Regions

Metaphase chromosomal preparations of many NBs contain extra chromosomal DMs or chromosomally integrated HSRs, or both.[15–18] DMs can be visualized in nonbanded metaphase chromosomal spreads; with the advent of banding techniques, researchers have identified HSRs as expanded bands of intermediate-staining chromosomal material (Fig. 103-2*A*). These cytogenetic abnormalities are the consequences of gene amplification and are thought to be alternate forms of the same genetic alteration.[19,20] The mechanisms leading to these genetic alterations are unknown. In 1983, the commonly amplified gene in NB was identified as a homolog of the *MYC* protooncogene and named N-*myc* (now called *MYCN*; see later discussion).[21,22] Amplification of other genes, such as the gene encoding for ornithine decarboxylase, which is located on chromosome 2 near *MYCN*, occurs occasionally in NBs, but these are thought to be bystander events during the amplification of *MYCN*.[23]

Chromosome 1p Deletions

Alterations and deletions of chromosome 1 are found in many neural crest tumors (eg, melanoma, neuroepithelioma, pheochromocytoma) and in other tumors, including breast cancer, Wilms tumor, and colon carcinoma. This implies that several tumor suppressor genes may be located on chromosome 1p. In NB, chromosome 1p deletions are the most consistent nonrandom genetic alteration detected, and they result in chromosome 1p monosomy.[17] Banding studies indicate deletions of variable size but consistently encompassing 1p36 through 1pter[18,24–27] (Fig. 103-3). This has led to the hypothesis that the putative NB suppressor genes are localized to that region.[28,29]

Because a specific chromosomal translocation has not been routinely identified in this region of chromosome 1, it is proposed that the putative NB suppressor gene is deleted in tumors. In order to more precisely map the location of the gene, a panel of specific DNA probes that identify restriction fragment length polymorphisms (RFLPs) on both the short and long arm of chromosome 1 have been used to assess chromosomal deletion or somatic loss of heterozygosity (LOH) in tumor specimens. In this type of analysis, DNA is extracted from the patient's normal and tumor tissues, digested with specific restriction enzymes, and analyzed for the presence of an RFLP by Southern blot analysis or by the single-strand conformation polymor-

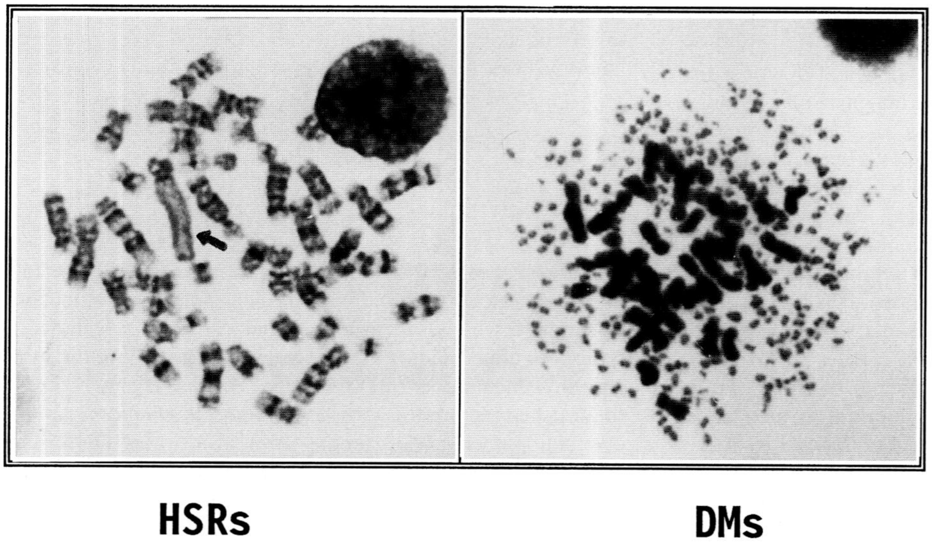

FIG. 103-2. Homogeneously staining regions (HSRs) and double minute chromosomes (DMs) in neuroblastoma tumor cells. (**A**) A metaphase chromosome spread, with a neuroblastoma cell line carrying a chromosome with an HSR (*arrow*). (**B**) A chromosomal spread from another neuroblastoma cell line carrying double minute chromosomes. The amplified gene in both cases is *NMYC*. (Courtesy of B. Spengler, MD, and J. Biedler, PhD).

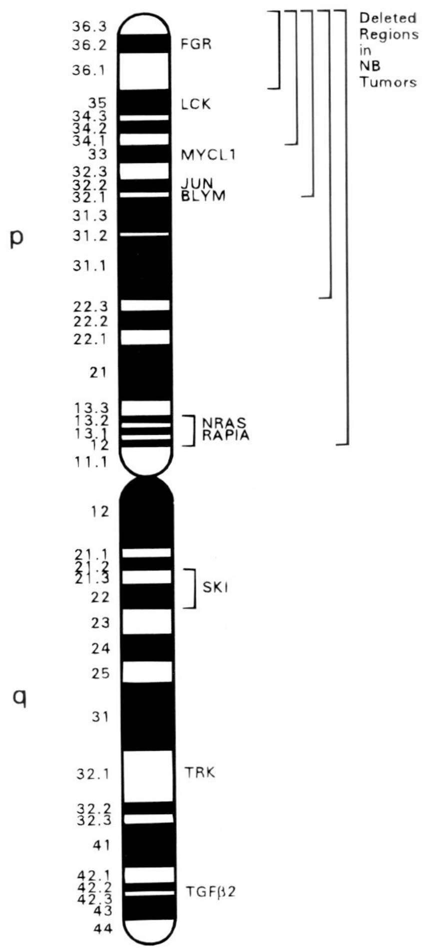

Chromosome 1

FIG. 103-3. Banding pattern of human chromosome 1 with brackets indicating regions of chromosome 1p frequently deleted in neuroblastoma (NB) tumors. The numbers indicate the specific regions and bands to which the genes are assigned.

phism (SSCP) technique, which is based on the polymerase chain reaction (PCR). The presence of an RFLP in the patient's normal DNA indicates that the patient is informative for that locus, and analysis of the tumor tissue DNA indicates the presence or absence of the allele. LOH studies indicate that NBs can be grouped into those whose deletion of 1p encompasses 1p36.3 and/or 1p36.1.[28,29]

If the putative NB tumor suppressor gene follows the classic Knudson two-hit theory, sporadic cases of NB may require two mutations for tumor formation. Because LOH results in the loss of only one allele of a putative suppressor gene, another mutation or alteration is required to functionally suppress the gene and lead to tumor formation. One mechanism postulated to account for functional gene loss without mutation or chromosomal alterations is genomic imprinting. Genomic imprinting is an epigenetic alteration occurring in a cell that results in alterations in expression of parental alleles. Studies of preferential loss of maternal or paternal alleles in chromosomal regions containing suppressor genes indicate that there is a functional difference between maternal and paternal alleles. If one allele is deleted and the other allele is silenced by genomic imprinting, then the locus contains two hits and is essentially null. Hypermethylation or hypomethylation of genes is postulated to be one epigenetic mechanism that occurs either de novo or by germline inheritance that can alter gene expression.[30]

Studies analyzing the parental origin of chromosome 1p36 deletions provide indirect evidence that two putative suppressor genes may reside in the region 1p36.1–2 to 1p36.3.[31–33] In a series of 22 NBs with *MYCN* expression, Cheng and colleagues[32] demonstrated that the deletions of 1p were randomly distributed between the maternal and paternal alleles. In contrast, Caron and colleagues[31] analyzed a series of 53 patients in which 13 of 15 informative patients had preferentially lost the maternal allele. Because Caron's group analyzed a set of NBs that included both single-copy and *MYCN*-amplified tumors and in Cheng's study[32] were analyzed only *MYCN*-amplified tumors, the apparently contradictory results may be caused by differences in the tumor sets analyzed and the DNA probes used. A possible reconciliation of the data would postulate the existence of two putative NB suppressor genes, one that is imprinted and one that is not. Such a situation has been demonstrated in Wilms tumors: the suppressor gene on chromosome 11p15 is imprinted, but the *WT1* suppressor gene at 11p13 is not[34] (see Chap. 111).

Other Genetic Alterations

Fragile sites are gaps, breaks, or rearrangements that nonrandomly occur in the chromosomes of normal cells after treatment with defined chemical agents such as azacytidine, aphidicolin, 5-bromodeoxyuridine (BrdU), or folic acid. Some of these fragile sites are constitutive, whereas others may be inherited. Five common fragile sites have been identified on chromosome 1p; they may to 1p21.2, 1p22, 1p31.2, 1p32, and 1p36.[35] An inducible 1p32 fragile site was detected in at least one parent for 18 of 20 NB patients analyzed.[36] This was a statistical increase over the rate in the control population and raises the issue that a heritable inducibility of a fragile site may predispose to cancer development.

Cytogenetic analyses of NBs indicate additional alterations in chromosomes 11, 14, and 17. Recently, a study found 12 (32%) of 37 informative cases to contain LOH involving 11q13–11q23 or 11p, and 6 (22%) of 27 informative cases to contain LOH on 14q.[37] Alterations of 17q were detected in 23% of 35 NB cell lines examined.[38] The significance of these alterations is unclear. Somatic cell hybrid and microcell fusion studies are two mechanisms that introduce normal chromosomes into tumor cells and assess the ability of the introduced chromosome and putative suppressor genes residing thereon to suppress tumorigenicity. One such study indicated that introduction of the normal chromosome 1 induced senescence or apoptosis, whereas chromosome 17 induced suppression of tumorigenicity, and chromosome 11 induced differentiation but not suppression of tumorigenicity in NB cells.[39] This would indicate a putative suppressor gene on chromosome 17 as well as chromosome 1.

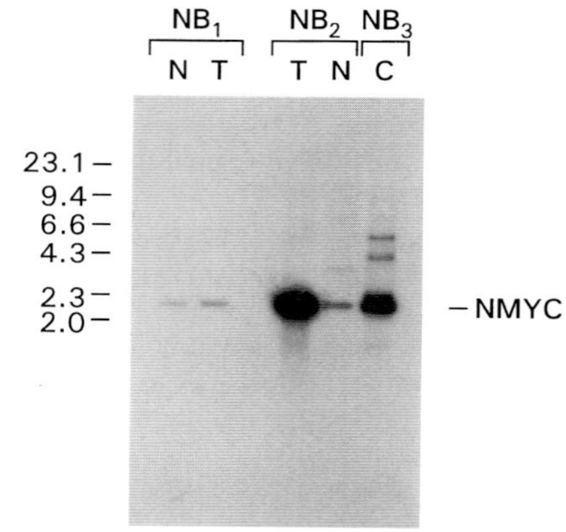

FIG. 103-4. *NMYC* gene amplification. Southern analysis of EcoRI restriction enzyme–digested DNA isolated from neuroblastoma (NB) tumor specimens (T), or normal tissue (N), or an NB cell line (C). NB_1 is an example of a poor-prognosis NB tumor in which the *NMYC* copy number is normal. NB_2 is an example of tumor tissue from a poor-prognosis NB tumor in which the *NMYC* copy number is amplified in the tumor. NB_3 is an NB-derived cell line showing *NMYC* amplification.

SPECIFIC GENE ALTERATIONS

Because of the multistage nature of cancer progression, the alteration of a number of genes, perhaps sequentially, is required to cause a normal cell to be initiated, transit to a promoted state, become fully transformed, and finally progress into a highly metastatic tumor cell. Oncogenes and suppressor genes are two functional classes of normal genes in which mutations leading to gain or enhanced function or loss of function are associated with tumorigenesis. In NB, a number of genes have been identified whose altered structure or function may contribute to tumor development or progression.

Oncogenes

NRAS and *HRAS*

RAS genes are frequently altered in human cancers. A mutated *RAS* gene (*NRAS*) with homology to other members of the *RAS* gene family was the first gene found to be altered in a NB cell line, and it was capable of transforming normal cells.[40] However, analysis of a number of primary tumor samples found that the mutations of codons 12, 13, 59, or 61 were rare events in NBs[41–43] and not characteristic of any clinical stage of the disease. An isolated study indicated that elevated levels of expression of *HRAS* (formerly v-Ha-*ras*) in NBs were associated with a better prognosis.[44]

MYCN

Low-stringency Southern hybridization analysis (see Chap. 1) of *MYC* to NB DNA identified the gene amplified in NB DMs and HSRs to be a relative of *MYC* called *MYCN*.[45] *MYCN* is amplified between 3 to 300 times per haploid genome in a subset of NBs, leading to a 40- to 60-fold increase in the levels of *MYCN* expression in cells (Fig. 103-4). DNA sequence analysis showed *MYCN* was structurally similar to *MYC*, and transfection studies indicated that, like *MYC*, *MYCN* can cooperate with mutated *RAS* genes to transform normal cells.[46] Mutations in the *MYCN* gene have not been identified. Structural and functional studies indicate that the MYCN protein binds a consensus DNA sequence CACGTG; it contains a helix-loop-helix region and is known to form heterodimers with p20/22 Max.[47] These proteins have been implicated in DNA replication, RNA processing, and transcriptional regulation.

MYCN became the first oncogene with proven clinical relevance when it was shown to be amplified in a subset of NBs (stage III and IV) marking poor prognosis tumors.[48] *MYCN* amplification was found to correlate with rapid disease progression. Furthermore, even if found in patients with good prognosis (stage I, II, and IVS disease), the presence of *MYCN* amplification predicted an ultimately fatal outcome. Analysis of simultaneous or sequential tumor samples from patients shows that *MYCN* copy number is unchanged, indicating that the amplification is a stable and intrinsic feature of a subset of NBs. The size of the amplicon or amplification unit varies, and additional bystander genes in the proximity of *MYCN*, such as the gene encoding ornithine decarboxylase, may be coamplified in some NBs.[23] The contribution of these genes is unclear.[48]

TRK

TRK was identified as a transforming gene formed from a hybrid gene between tropomyosin and the tyrosine kinase domain of a receptor tyrosine kinase gene.[49] The normal proto-*TRK*, *TRKA*, encodes the signal-transducing receptor for nerve growth factor.[50,51] Analysis of human NBs demonstrated that NBs offering good prognosis express high levels of *TRKA* relative to tumors associated with poor prognosis.[52] Another member of the *TRK* family of genes, *TRKB*, and its ligand brain-derived neurotrophic factor (BDNF) are expressed in a large number of tumors and cell lines associated with poor prognosis.[53,54] The significance of expression of *TRKB* is unclear in NBs, because it is also expressed in patients with ganglioneuromas and stage IVS NBs, who typically have a good prognosis.[54]

Suppressor Genes

P53

Although mutation of *P53* is the most common gene alteration in human cancers, it is an infrequent occurrence in NBs. Using PCR-based SSCP analysis, one study failed to detect mutation in 38 primary tumors from all stages, with 13 being from advanced-stage tumors.[55] An analysis by SSCP found mutations in only 2% of 86 primary NBs. *MYCN* amplification was not detected in the two cases in which mutations were detected.[56]

NF1

Von Recklinghausen neurofibromatosis (neurofibromatosis type 1, or NF1) is a common genetic disorder in humans, and

TABLE 103-1. *Genetic and clinical subsets of human neuroblastoma*

Feature	Type 1	Type 2	Type 3
Age	≤1 year	>1 year	1–5 years
Stage	I, II, IVS	III, IV	III, IV
MYCN	Normal	Normal	Amplified
DNA ploidy	>50	44–49	44–49
1p Loss of heterozygosity	<50%	25%–50%	80%–90%
TRK expression	High	Low	Absent
14q Loss of heterozygosity	<5%	25%–50%	10%
Survival rate	90%–95%	25%–50%	<10%

Adapted from Brodeur, GM. Molecular pathology of human neuroblastoma. Semin Diagn Pathol. 1994;11:118.

NF1 patients show an increased frequency of nervous system tumors and, occasionally, of NB. Because the genetic defect in NF1 maps to chromosome 17q11.2, involving Lys-1423 of the *NF1* gene, and chromosome 17 can suppress NB tumorigenicity in cell lines, studies have investigated whether *NF1* is altered in NB. No mutations were found in the *NF1* gene by PCR-based SSCP in the Lys-1423 region of the *NF1* gene in 50 NBs that encompassed all stages.[56] However, absent or reduced expression of *NF1* has led some investigators to postulate mutations of *NF1* in some NB cell lines.[57,58] Further studies are needed to elucidate whether mutations in other portions of the *NF1* gene may occur in NB.

MTS1

A putative suppressor gene, multiple tumor suppressor 1 (*MTS1*) encodes the p16 inhibitor of the cell cycle gene, cyclin-dependent kinase 4 (*CDK4*), and is localized to chromosome 9p21. This gene is homozygously deleted in a number of different tumors, including astrocytoma (82%), breast tumors (60%), and melanoma (58%). However, none of 10 NBs tested had alterations in this gene.[59]

SUMMARY

The retrospective analysis of NB tumor tissue banks has enabled genetic alterations to be correlated with clinical tumor progression. Several of these genetic alterations have prognostic significance. Brodeur and colleagues[60] have summarized these findings, noted characteristic occurrences, and developed a schema of clinical and genetic subtypes of neuroblastoma (Table 103-1). It is unknown whether NBs in patients who present with a poor prognosis have evolved from a tumor that at some point would have offered a good prognosis. Early detection of NB by screening of infants for elevated urinary catecholamines should enable researchers to determine whether there is a relation between NBs associated with good and poor prognosis. Stratification of NBs according to their clinical, genetic, and biologic features may enable more effective analysis of treatment protocols. Clearly, the identification of the putative NB suppressor gene or genes will yield new insights into the mechanisms of NB tumorigenesis and may impact the development of new therapies for the treatment of NBs.

REFERENCES

1. Vogelstein B, Fearon ER, Hamilton SR, et al. Genetic alteration during colorectal tumor development. N Engl J Med 1988;319:525.
2. Young JLJ, Ries LG, Silverberg E, et al. Cancer incidence, survival and mortality for children younger than 15 years. Cancer 1986;58:598.
3. Voute PA. Neuroblastoma. In: Sutow WW, Fernbach DJ, Vietti TJ, eds. Clinical pediatric oncology. St Louis, CV Mosby, 1984:559.
4. Miller RW, Fraumeni JF Jr. Neuroblastoma: epidemiologic approach to its origin. Am J Dis Child 1968;115:253.
5. Knudson AGJ, Meadows AT. Developmental genetics of neuroblastoma. J Natl Cancer Inst 1976;57:675.
6. Knudson AG. Mutation and cancer: statistical study of retinoblastoma. Proc Natl Acad Sci U S A 1971;68:8820.
7. Everson TC, Cole WH. Spontaneous regression of neuroblastoma. In: Everson TC, Cole WH, eds. Spontaneous regression of cancer. Philadelphia, WB Saunders, 1966:88.
8. Schwartz AD, Dadash-Zadeh M, Lee H, Swaney JJ. Spontaneous regression of disseminated neuroblastoma. J Pediatr 1974;85:760.
9. Kushner BH, Hajdu SI, Helson L. Synchronous neuroblastoma and von Recklinghausen's disease: a review of the literature. J Clin Oncol 1985; 3:117.
10. Witzleben CL, Landy RA. Disseminated neuroblastoma in a child with von Recklinghausen's disease. Cancer 1974;34:786.
11. Bolande RP. The neurocristopathies: a unifying concept of disease arising in neural crest maldevelopment. Hum Pathol 1974;5:409.
12. Look AT, Hayes FA, Nitschke R, et al. Cellular DNA content as a predictor of response to chemotherapy in infants with unresectable neuroblastoma. N Engl J Med 1984;311:231.
13. Look AT, Hayes FA, Shuster JJ, et al. Clinical relevance of tumor cell ploidy and N-*myc* gene amplification in childhood neuroblastoma: a pediatric oncology group study. J Clin Oncol 1991;9:581.
14. Cohn SL, Rademaker AW, Salwen HR, et al. Analysis of DNA ploidy and proliferative activity in relation to histology and N-*myc* amplification in neuroblastoma. Am J Pathol 1990;136:1043.
15. Cox D, Yuncken C, Spriggs AI. Minute chromatin bodies in malignant tumors of childhood. Lancet 1965;2:55.
16. Biedler JL, Helson L, Spengler BA. Morphology and growth, tumorigenicity, and cytogenetics of human neuroblastoma cells in continuous culture. Cancer Res 1973;33:2643.
17. Brodeur GM, Sekhon GS, Goldstein MN. Chromosomal aberrations in human neuroblastomas. Cancer 1977;40:2256.
18. Brodeur GM, Green AA, Hayes FA, et al. Cytogenetic features of human neuroblastomas and cell lines. Cancer Res 1981;41:4678.
19. Biedler JL, Albrecht AM, Hutchinson DJ. Cytogenetics of mouse leukemia L1210: I. Association of a specific chromosome with dihydrofolate reductase activity in amethopterin-treated sublines. Cancer Res 1965;2:246.
20. Balaban-Malenbaum G, Gilbert F. Double minute chromosomes and the homogenously staining regions in chromosomes of a neuroblastoma cell line. Science 1977;1198:739.
21. Schwab M, Alitalo K, Klempnauer KH, et al. Amplified DNA with limited homology to *myc* cellular oncogene is shared by human neuroblastoma cell lines and a neuroblastoma tumour. Nature 1983;305:245.

22. Kohl N, Kanda N, Schrenk, et al. Transposition and amplification of oncogene-related sequences in human neuroblastomas. Cell 1983;35:359.
23. Winqvist R, Makela TP, Seppanen, et al. Human ornithine decarboxylase sequences map to chromosome regions 2pter—p23 and 7cen–qter, but are not coamplified with the *NMYC* oncogene. Cytogenet Cell Genet 1986;42:133.
24. Gilbert F, Balaban G, Moorhead P, et al. Abnormalities of chromosome 1p in human neuroblastoma tumors and cell lines. Cancer Genet Cytogenet 1982;7:33.
25. Lampert F, Rudolph B, Christiansen H, Franke F. Identical chromosome 1p breakpoint abnormality in both the tumor and the constitutional karyotype of a patient with neuroblastoma. Cancer Genet Cytogenet 1988;34:235.
26. Peter M, Michon J, Vielh P, et al. PCR assay for chromosome 1p deletion in small neuroblastoma samples. Int J Cancer 1992;52:544.
27. White P, Kaufman B, Marshall H, Brodeur G. Use of the single-strand conformation polymorphism technique to detect loss of heterozygosity in neuroblastoma. Genes Chromosom Cancer 1993;7:102.
28. Fong CT, et al. Loss of heterozygosity for chromosome 1 or 14 define a subset of advanced neuroblastomas. Cancer Res 1985;52:1780.
29. Weith A, Martinsson T, Cziepluch C, et al. Neuroblastoma consensus deletion maps to 1p36.1–2. Genes Chromosom Cancer 1989;1:159.
30. Razin A, Cedar H. DNA methylation and genomic imprinting. Cell 1994;77:473.
31. Caron H, van Sluis P, van Hoeve M, et al. Allelic loss of chromosome 1p36 in neuroblastoma is of preferential maternal origin and correlates with N-*myc* amplification. Nat Genet 1993;4:187.
32. Cheng J, Hiemstra J, Schenider S, et al. Preferential amplification of the paternal allele of the N-*myc* gene in human neuroblastomas. Nat Genet 1993;4:191.
33. Hayashi Y, Kanda N, Inaba T, et al. Cytogenetic findings and prognosis in neuroblastoma with emphasis on marker chromosome 1. Cancer 1989;63:126.
34. Gerald WL. The molecular genetics of Wilm's tumor: a paradigm of heterogeneity in tumor development. Cancer Invest 1994;12:350.
35. Melino G, Sansone R. Highly recombinogenic chromosomal sites in the inheritance and progression of pediatric cancer. In: Tonini GP, Sansone R, Thiele CJ, eds. Molecular genetics of pediatric solid tumors. Chur, Switzerland, Harwood Academic Publishers, 1991:65.
36. Vernole P, Tedeschi B, Nicoletti B. Fragile site induction by aphidicolin may be increased in parents of neuroblastoma patients. Cancer Genet Cytogenet 1990;50:35.
37. Srivatsan E, Ying K, Seeger R. Deletion of chromosome 11 and of 14q sequences in neuroblastoma. Genes Chromosom Cancer 1993;7:32.
38. Gilbert F, Balaban G, Moorhead P, Bianchi D, Schlesinger H. Abnormalities of chromosome 1p in human neuroblastoma tumors and cell lines. Cancer Genet Cytogenet 1982;7:33.
39. Bader S, Fasching C, Brodeur G, Stanbridge E. Dissociation of suppression of tumorigenicity and differentiation in vitro effected by transfer of single human chromosomes into human neuroblastoma cells. Cell Growth Differ 1991;2:245.
40. Hall A, Marshall CJ, Spurr NK, Weiss RA. Identification of transforming gene in two human sarcoma cell lines as a new member of the *ras* gene family located on chromosome 1. Nature 1983;303:396.
41. Ballas K, Lyons J, Jannsen JWG, Bartram CR. Incidence of *ras* gene mutations in neuroblastoma. Eur J Pediatr 1988;147:313.
42. Ireland CM. Activated N-*ras* oncogenes in human neuroblastoma. Cancer Res 1989;49:5530.
43. Moley JF, Brother MB, Wells SA, et al. Low frequency of *ras* gene mutations in neuroblastomas, pheochromocytomas and medullary thyroid cancers. Cancer Res 1991;51:596.
44. Tanaka T, Slamon DJ, Shimada H, et al. Expression of Ha-*ras* oncogene products in human neuroblastomas and the significant correlation with a patient's prognosis. Cancer Res 1988;48:1030.
45. Schwab M, Alitalo K, Klempnauer KH, et al. Amplified DNA with limited homology to *myc* cellular oncogene is shared by human neuroblastoma cell lines and a neuroblastoma tumor. Nature 1983;305:245.
46. Schwab M, Varmus HE, Bishop JM. The human N-*myc* gene contributes to tumorigenic conversion of mammalian cells in culture. Nature 1985;316:160.
47. Schwab M. Molecular cytogenetics of human neuroblastoma. Biochim Biophys Acta 1992;1114:43.
48. Brodeur G, Seeger RC, Schwab M, Varmus HE, Bishop JM. Amplification of N-*myc* in untreated human neuroblastomas correlates with advanced disease stage. Science 1984;224:1121.
49. Martin-Zanca D, Oskam R, Mitra G, Copeland T, Barbacid M. Molecular and biochemical characterization of the human *trk* proto-oncogene. Mol Cell Biol 1989;9:24.
50. Klein R, Jing S, Nanduri V, O'Rourke E, Barbacid M. The *trk* proto-oncogene encodes a receptor for nerve growth factor. Cell 1991;65:189.
51. Kaplan D, Hempstead B, Martin-Zanca D, Chao M, Parada L. The *trk* proto-oncogene product: a signal transducing receptor for nerve growth factor. Science 1991;252:554.
52. Nakagawara A, Arima-Nakagawara M, Scavarda N, Azar C, Cantor A, Brodeur G. Association between high levels of expression of the *TRK* gene and favorable outcome in human neuroblastoma. N Engl J Med 1993;328:847.
53. Nakagawara A. Expression and function of *TRK-B* and *BDNF* in human neuroblastoma. Mol Cell Biol 1994;14:759.
54. Kaplan DR, Matsumoto K, Lucarelli E, Thiele CJ. Induction of *TrkB* by retinoic acid mediates biologic responsiveness to BDNF and differentiation of human neuroblastoma cells. Neuron 1993;11:321.
55. Vogan K, Bernstein M, Leclerc J-M, et al. Absence of *p53* gene mutations in primary neuroblastoma. Cancer Res 1993;53:5269.
56. Imamura J, Bartram CR, Berthold F, Harms D, Nakamura H, Koeffler HP. Mutation of the *p53* gene in neuroblastoma and its relationship with N-*myc* amplification. Cancer Res 1993;53:4053.
57. Inge T, Murthy AE, Hannigan GE, et al. Neurofibromatosis type 1 gene mutations in neuroblastoma. Nat Genet 1993;3:62.
58. Johnson MR, Look AT, DeClue JE, Valentine MB, Lowy DR. Inactivation of the *NF1* gene in human melanoma and neuroblastoma cell lines without impaired regulation of *GTP*. Proc Natl Acad Sci U S A 1993;90:5539.
59. Kamb A, Gruis N, Weaver-Feldhaus J, et al. A cell cycle regulator potentially involved in genesis of many tumor types. Science 1994;264:436.
60. Brodeur GM. Molecular pathology of human neuroblastomas. Semin Diagn Pathol 1994;11:10.

Principles and Practice of Genitourinary Oncology, edited by Derek Raghavan, Howard I. Scher, Steven A. Leibel, and Paul H. Lange. Lippincott-Raven Publishers, Philadelphia, © 1997.

CHAPTER 104

Human Neuroblastoma Cell Differentiation

June L. Biedler, Barbara A. Spengler, and Robert A. Ross

TUMORS AND CELL LINES

Neuroblastoma, a tumor of the peripheral autonomic nervous system, is the most common extracranial neoplasm affecting young children. About 8% to 10% of all pediatric cancers are neuroblastomas, corresponding to an incidence of 8 per 1 million newborns per year in the United States. One intriguing and potentially pertinent biologic feature of this tumor is its differentiative diversity. Neuroblastoma presumably arises from cells of the neural crest during the course of their proliferation, migration, and maturation. A fundamental question, which is considered in this chapter, is whether the tumor arises from committed sympathoadrenal progenitor cells or from developmentally earlier, multipotent stem cells.

Other peripheral nervous system tumors grouped with neuroblastoma are the ganglioneuroblastomas and the ganglioneuromas.[1] At one end of the spectrum are the undifferentiated neuroblastomas, which comprise densely packed, small round cells with little, if any, evidence of neuronal differentiation. These are the tumors that tend to be confused with other embryonal tumors such as Ewing's sarcoma or peripheral neuroepithelioma. Ganglioneuroblastomas are heterogeneous tumors consisting of diffuse or focal mixtures of neuroblasts and more mature neuronal cells. At the other end of the spectrum are the ganglioneuromas: benign tumors comprising mature ganglion cells and stromal elements such as Schwann-like cells, which may have the same cellular origin as the ganglion cells or may represent infiltrating normal cells. As noted by Brodeur,[1] there are reported instances of classification of a tumor as immature neuroblastoma at initial biopsy and classification as ganglioneuroma at a subsequent biopsy, usually after treatment. There is some consensus that maturation of malignant neuroblasts may occur, possibly as a result of the primary or secondary effects of chemotherapy or irradiation. Another intriguing and conceivably related feature of neuroblastoma is its capacity to regress or mature spontaneously with disappearance of disease. Even though the overall incidence of spontaneous regression may be no greater than 5%; occurring mainly in infants,[1] this phenomenon likewise implicates both induced and spontaneous neuroblastoma cell differentiation as a potentially important factor in the progression or regression of the disease.

Tumor histology is one of several criteria used to confirm the diagnosis of neuroblastoma, classify disease progression according to a staging system (exemplified by the International Neuroblastoma Staging System proposed in 1988[2]), and determine response to treatment. Other clinical and biologic criteria include site of origin of the primary tumor and extent of dissemination of disease; chromosome ploidy; *MYCN* (formerly N-*myc*) amplification and chromosome 1p deletion status; and the presence of tumor markers such as neuronal-specific enolase, ferritin, and the ganglioside, G_{D2}. Understanding of neuroblastoma at the biologic level has been facilitated greatly by studies of cell lines established in culture. In particular, the human neuroblastoma cell system, as a model for both tumor cell differentiation and normal peripheral nervous system development, has received considerable recent attention and is the focus of this chapter.

NEURAL CREST CELL DIFFERENTIATION

The neural crest is a transient embryonic structure that gives rise to a variety of cells, such as neuronal and glial cells of the peripheral nervous system, endocrine cells of the adrenal medulla and calcitonin-producing cells, melanocytes, and mesectodermal derivatives contributing to skeletal, connective, and muscle tissue of the face and head.[3] Clonal analysis of neural crest cells has demonstrated that the migrating cells exhibit various levels of pluripotency; some cells retain their pluripotency throughout development, whereas others are already committed when they start to migrate.

One of the better understood mammalian systems described in recent years is the sympathoadrenal lineage that yields both neuronal cells and endocrine cells in the rat autonomic nervous system.[4] This cell lineage gives rise primarily to chromaffin cells of the adrenal gland and to autonomic neurons. Committed sympathoadrenal progenitor cells, described as bipotent, transiently express both neuron- and chromaffin-specific markers before differentiating along one or the other pathway. This investigation and others have revealed the extraordinary plasticity of neural crest cells and have provided systems for identifying genes whose products regulate phenotypic expression. A striking example of this plasticity was provided by clonal analysis of cells of early stages in neural crest development.[5] The major findings were that single neural crest cells are multipotent, that the multipotent cells can generate multipotent progeny and are thus self-renewing stem cells, and that they can also generate clonal progeny that give rise to only neurons or glia. The implication is that multipotent stem cells can produce committed neuroblasts or glioblasts. Isolation of mammalian stem cells that can give rise to both neurons and glia is directly relevant to experimental findings obtained with human neuroblastoma cells in culture.

SPONTANEOUS DIFFERENTIATION IN HUMAN NEUROBLASTOMA CELL LINES

Phenotypically Variant Cells

The earliest published attempts to culture human neuroblastoma cells were those of Murray and Stout in 1947.[6] Since the successful establishment of a continuous cell line, NJB, reported in 1968,[7] numerous neuroblastoma lines have been described in the literature. Among the best characterized and most widely used in experimental studies are the cell lines IMR-32[8]; SK-N-SH[9]; LA-N-1 and LA-N-2[10]; NGP[11]; SK-N-BE(2)[12]; GOTO[13]; CHP-234[14]; SMS-KCN, SMS-KCNR, and SMS-KAN[15]; and LA-N-5.[16] A distinguishing feature of most but not all human neuroblastoma cell lines is their neuroblast-like morphology and growth behavior. Cells are usually small and rounded, frequently display neurites (cytoplasmic projections), and show poor substrate attachment, sometimes growing as tight aggregates of floating cells.

With respect to spontaneous morphologic differentiation, our experiences in attempting to establish cell lines are illuminating. Biopsy specimens from 13 patients were placed into culture, and only 4 cell lines were obtained.[9] Failure to establish proliferative cell populations appeared to be a result of the propensity of the cells to differentiate. Usually, there was a progressive increase in number and length of neurite-like processes. Eventually, an extensive neuritic network connected cellular aggregates (pseudoganglia), and no proliferative cells were evident, all indicative of terminal neuronal differentiation. Among the successfully established lines, one (SK-N-MC) was later reclassified as a peripheral neuroepithelioma, based primarily on the presence of a chromosome 11;22 translocation.

Another important observation was that the SK-N-SH line, arising from a bone marrow aspirate obtained from a patient with a large tumor in the upper chest,[9] comprised two distinctly different cell types. In plating experiments, it was possible to obtain pure colonies of one cell type or the other. The major cell component of this line is the neuroblast, termed N. The other prominent cell type, termed S, is a large, highly substrate-adherent cell that lacks cell processes and forms a contiguous monolayer. After SK-N-SH was cloned in order to obtain cell lines that were homogeneously N-type or S-type,[9] a third cell type, termed I, was identified. I-type cells, morphologically intermediate between N and S, are substrate-adherent and may have short neurite-like processes. Table 104-1 lists examples of N-, S-, and I-type clones or purified populations (ie, highly enriched for one cell type) that have been isolated and characterized. SH-IN is a representative I-type clone of SK-N-SH cells. SH-SY5Y represents the neuroblastic population and was cloned and subcloned three times in order to obtain a relatively stable N-type cell line.[12] SH-EP1 is an epithelial-like S-type clone.

Transdifferentiation of N and S Cells

Early observations led us to speculate that the N-type and S-type cells seen in the SK-N-SH line represented morphologic extremes in a spectrum of phenotypic alterations and that the two types of cells could convert from one to the other. It was important, therefore, to obtain evidence that SH-SY5Y and SH-EP1 had a common cellular origin, and this was provided by the finding of chromosome 7 trisomy and the same two structurally abnormal marker chromosomes in both clonal cell lines.[17,44] The finding also that each of the lines had a unique chromosomal marker gave us the opportunity to examine in detail the dynamics of the conversion process.[45] It was demonstrated that SH-SY5Y cells could give rise to cells with a flat, S-type morphology and that SH-EP cells could generate neuroblastic cells. Moreover, consistent, coordinate biochemical changes accompanied the dramatic morphologic changes. Newly arising N-type cells derived from SH-EP expressed TH (tyrosine hydroxylase), AADC (aromatic L-amino acid decarboxylase), and DBH (dopamine-β-hydroxylase), whereas newly arising S cells did not. Thus, for N and S cells derived from the parental SK-N-SH line, bidirectional phenotypic interconversion or transdifferentiation was proven. Another clone isolated from SK-N-SH was intermediate in morphology and hence named SH-IN.[45] It is somewhat unstable in culture, giving rise to both N-type and S-type cells. Biochemically, the I-type SH-IN cells express both N and S cell properties. As discussed in detail in the next section of this chapter, we propose that I cells represent malignant neural crest stem cells. The differentiation and transdifferentiation patterns observed to date (I to N and S; N to S and S to N; and N to a mature neuronal cell) are illustrated in Figure 104-1.

Our initial, rigorous study of SK-N-SH cell variants led to (1) an examination of other neuroblastoma lines for presence of variant cells, (2) a search for additional changes in gene expression involved in the striking alteration of differentiation program between N and S cells, and (3) a search for genes whose expression could contribute mechanistically to the transdifferentiation process.

As noted earlier and shown in Table 104-1, a number of parental cell lines comprise at least two or three variant cell types, identifiable as N, S, and I morphologically and biochemically. In some cell lines, such as LA-N-2 and GOTO, the preponderant cell type is I. Thus, the phenomenon of transdifferentiation is not limited to SK-N-SH, although in most cases it has not been demonstrated rigorously. However, with the use of karyotype analysis, we have confirmed N-S interconversion in clonal sublines of the parental LA-N-1 cell line (unpublished results). It has become clear from detailed studies of N and S cells derived from seven independent cell lines that all of the N–type cells share neuronal cell attributes, whereas all S–type variants lack neuronal properties and share other markers, including a large series of cell surface differentiation antigens.[20,23] Thus, N/S interconversion represents an ordered transition between two neuroectodermal differentiation programs.

TABLE 104-1. *Representative, phenotypically distinct subpopulations of human neuroblastoma cells arising spontaneously or induced by differentiating agents*

Spontaneously arising				
	Phenotypic variants			
Cell line	N	I	S	References
SK-N-SH	SH-SY5Y,-EP5	SH-IN	SH-EP1,-EP12	9,17–24
	SH-N		SH-F	25
SK-N-BE(1)	BE(1)n		BE(1)s	23
SK-N-BE(2)	BE(2)-M17,-88n	BE(2)-C	BE(2)s,-7s	20,23
LA-N-1	LA1-55n,-19n	LA1-22n/i	LA1-5s,-19Bs	20,21,23,24
IMR-32	IMR-32n		IMR-32s	20
CHP-234	CHP-234n		CHP-234s	20
SMS-KCN	KCN-65n, KCNn	KCNn/i	KCN-9s, KCNs	20,23,24
SMS-SAN	SMS-SANn		SMS-SANs	20
NBL-W	NBL-W N		NBL-W S	26
KP-N-SI	4n		SI8s, SI9s	26
KP-N-YN	YN2n		YN1s, YN3s	27

Experimentally induced			
Cell line	Induced phenotype	Inducing agent	References
GOTO	N	RA, IFNγ	28–30
	S	BUdR	28,29
NB-1	Nrl	dbcAMP	29
SK-N-SH	Nrl	BUdR, RA	31
SH-SY5Y	Nrl	RA, TPA, NGF, STP	32–34
SH-IN	N	FSK, dbcAMP, NGF	35,36
	S	RA, BUdR	35
SH-N	Nrl	RA, STP	37
SH-F	Nrl	RA	37
	S	RA	38
BE(2)-C	Nrl	RA	35
	S	BUdR	35
CHP-126	Nrl	dbcAMP	39
	S	RA	39
SMS-SAN	Nrl	dbcAMP, RA	39
SMS-KCNR	Nrl	RA	40
NUB-7	N	dbcAMP	41
	S	RA	41
RT-LN-1	Nrl	RA, dbcAMP	28
	S	BUdR	28
LA-N-5	Nrl	RA, VIP	42
HTLA230	Nrl	RA	43

N, neuroblastic; I, intermediate; S, substrate-adherent; Nrl, neuronal; RA, all-*trans* retinoic acid; IFNγ, gamma-interferon; BUdR, 5-bromo-2′-deoxyuridine; dbcAMP, dibutyryl cyclic adenosine monophosphate; TPA, phorbol 12-myristate 13-acetate; NGF, nerve growth factor; STP, staurosporine; FSK, forskolin; VIP, vasoactive intestinal peptide.

To further examine the possible significance of the N/S interconversion phenomenon in the tumor biology of neuroblastoma, we examined paired sets of N and S cells for their malignant potential.[46] Tumorigenicity testing in nude mice revealed that N–type cells (and most I–type cells as well) are tumorigenic whereas S–type cells are not. Generally, the capacity for anchorage–independent growth (colony–forming capacity in soft agar) mirrored tumorigenicity. Indeed, N and I cells in culture have growth characteristics of transformed cells, and S cells are highly contact–inhibited and tend to have a finite lifespan in vitro. With the exception of SK–N–SH, all of the cell lines tested in this study[46] and in a more recent study (unpublished) have multiple copies of the cellular oncogene, *MYCN*.[47] Differences in tumorigenicity between N (and I) and S cells correlate with marked differences in expression of this gene, as will be described in a later section.

As discussed in a recent review,[48] transdifferentiation—or transition from one differentiated state to another—can occur in a number of different cell types. For example, retinal pigmented epithelial cells of the chick embryo can switch their cell type to that of lens cells. It is noted that there has been a recent expansion of examples of transdifferentiation and that certain prerequisites may be needed in order to avoid ambiguity. The term transdifferentiation appears appropriate for the neuroblastoma model system because the two proposed prerequisites are fulfilled: (1) the differentiation state before and after transdiffer-

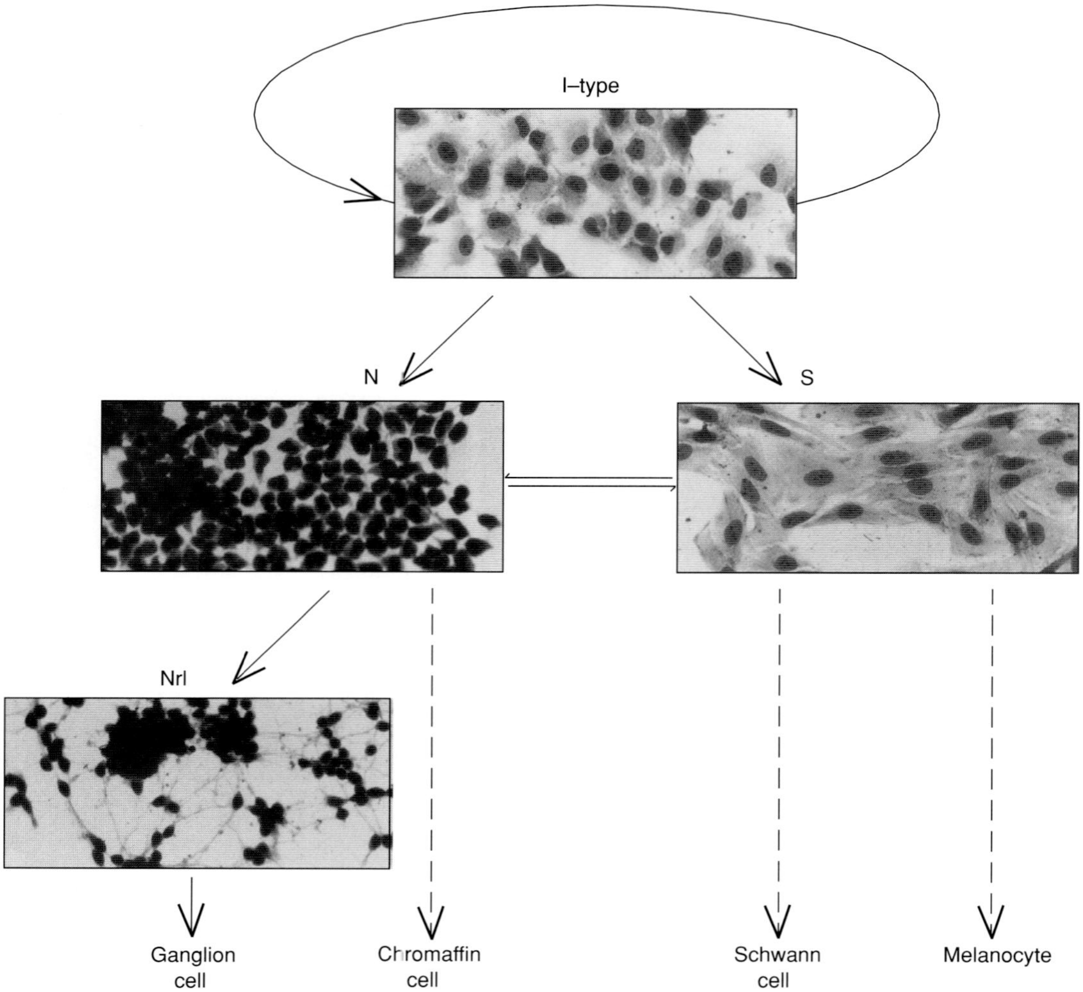

FIG. 104-1. Current understanding of differentiation and transdifferentiation of human neuroblastoma cells in culture. I-type cells represent malignant neural crest stem cells, capable of both self-renewal (*circular arrow*) and differentiation to N or S cells, either spontaneously or after exposure to appropriate inducing agents. N-type cells (neuroblasts) are malignant neuronal precursors, able to progress along the same pathway to a more neuronally differentiated state (Nrl). In the normal neural crest, these precursor cells could give rise to mature ganglion cells or to chromaffin cells of the adrenal medulla (*dashed arrow*). S-type cells are most likely the precursor cells for the nonneuronal differentiation lineage, leading during normal neural crest development to mature Schwann and glial cells or melanocytes. Whereas S cells may express some properties of these more mature cell types, overt differentiation has not been observed in vitro. N and S cells can also transdifferentiate from one to the other phenotype. Such interconversion occurs spontaneously in different neuroblastoma cell lines, but with a variable and generally low frequency. Whether N or S cells can revert to I-type cells or whether N-S transdifferentiation involves a transient I-cell stage is not known.

entiation can be reliably distinguished by molecular biologic evidence as well as by morphologic criteria, and (2) the ancestor-descendent relation between cells before and after the switch can be clearly confirmed.[48]

Biochemical Characteristics of Cell Variants

A major feature of neuroblastoma cell lines and of N-type and I-type subpopulations is the presence of enzymes involved in the biosynthesis of the catecholamines dopamine and norepinephrine and of acetylcholine. A systematic study of 13 cell lines revealed that all had properties of noradrenergic neurons, and 10 expressed all of the enzymes required for norepinephrine synthesis (ie, TH, AADC, and DBH).[49] None of the lines had detectable phenylethanolamine-*N*-methyl transferase activity, a trait expressed by adrenal chromaffin cells and adrenergic neurons. Five cell lines had readily detectable choline acetyltransferase activity as well as TH, AADC, and DBH. The presence of enzymes for the biosynthesis of both catecholamines and acetylcholine is consistent with the origin of neuroblastoma from embryonic neural crest cells that would normally give rise to both adrenergic and cholinergic neurons of the peripheral nervous system.[3,4] In other studies it was found that N-type and I-type populations derived from SK-N-BE (2), SK-N-SH, LA-N-1, and SMS-KCN lines expressed both TH and DBH activities, whereas their S-type counterparts did not.[17,18] The study by Ross and colleagues[18] provided the first convincing evidence that S cells do not have neuronal properties and are likely, therefore, to represent some other neural crest cell lineage (see next section).

N- and I-type cell variants have additional neuronal-specific protein markers. Cytoskeletal proteins, in particular intermediate filament proteins, are commonly used to characterize cell type. For example, the three neurofilament proteins (70, 150, and 200 kd) are coexpressed only in neuronal cells. These proteins, to varying degrees, are present in all N and I cells but are not found in S-type cells. Similarly, β-tubulin, important for microtubular transport in neurites and axons, is abundant in N- and I-type cells. Chromogranin A is a protein localized to the large, dense core vesicles of adrenal chromaffin cells and sympathetic neurons and has been found in human neuroblastoma tumors.[50] It is present in N-type and I-type human variants but not in S cells, a finding consistent with the neuroendocrine character of these malignant sympathoadrenal precursor cells.

Based in part on findings of chromogranin A in the developing adrenal medulla, it has been proposed that neuroblastoma is a cancer of adrenal chromaffin cells.[51] Two pieces of evidence do not support this hypothesis. First, only 50% of human neuroblastoma tumors arise in proximity to the adrenal gland; the remaining 50% are found along neural crest migratory pathways in the thorax and abdomen.[1] Second, although chromogranin A characterizes neuroendocrine cells, it is also present in ganglion cells of the sympathetic nervous system.[50] Taken together, these findings support the hypothesis that neuroblastoma is a cancer of the developing neural crest and that malignant transformation can occur at numerous times and locations during neural crest migration and differentiation.

Cell surface proteins that mediate growth factor and immune responses can also be used to characterize human neuroblastoma cell variants. Of special interest to clinicians has been the finding that neuroblastoma cell lines, and in particular malignant neuroblasts (N-type cells), weakly express HLA class I molecules (ie, HLA-A, -B, and -C) and their associated proteins, β_2-microglobulin and HSP96[20,52] (Table 104-2). Because these molecules mediate the interaction between antigen-bearing cells and cytotoxic T lymphocytes, their absence on the cell surface may be an indication of the embryonic nature of these cells as well as a mechanism whereby neuroblastoma tumors escape immune surveillance. By contrast, S-type cells have normal levels of these immune response marker proteins (see Table 104-2). Although neuroblastoma cells do not require nerve growth factor (NGF) for their survival, similar to early embryonic sympathoblasts, they exhibit the low-affinity receptor on their cell surface. Of recent interest is the finding that more

TABLE 104-2. *Differential Protein Expression in Human Neuroblastoma Cell Variants**

Protein	Cellular phenotype N	I	S
Cytoskeletal proteins			
Neurofilaments	2	2	0
Vimentin	0.5	2	3
β-Tubulin	2	2	0.5
Cell surface & ECM markers			
Nerve growth factor receptor	2	—	0.5
Epidermal growth factor receptor	0.5	2	3
Chondroitin sulfate proteoglycan	0	2	3
Fibronectin	0	0.5	2
Phenotype-specific proteins			
Tyrosine hydroxylase (neuronal)	2	2	0
Tyrosinase (melanocyte)	0	0	0.5
Chromogranin A (neuroendocrine)	3	2	0
Nuclear proteins			
MYCN	3	2	0.5
P53	0.5	1	2
HUD	3	2	0
HASH1	3		0
BCL2	2	2	0.5
Immune response markers			
HLA-A, -B, and -C	0	—	2
β_2-microglobulin	0	0.5	2
HSP96	1	1	3

N, neuroblastic; I, intermediate; S, substrate-adherent; HuD, human neuron-specific RNA-binding protein; HASH1, human aschete-scute homolog.

* Relative amount of protein: 3, abundant; 2, easily detectable; 1, weakly expressed; 0.5, sometimes expressed, 0, not detectable.

Data from Rettig et al, 1987;[20] Ciccarone et al, 1989;[23] Biedler et al, 1988;[46] Hanada et al, 1993;[53] and unpublished findings.

neuronally differentiated neuroblastoma cells can also exhibit other neurotrophin receptors, particularly TRKA, the high-affinity NGF receptor, as well as TRKB, the receptor for brain-derived neurotrophic factor.[54,55]

We have also determined expression of other proteins implicated in neuronal growth or differentiation: MYCN, BCL2, P53, the human aschete-scute homolog (HASH1), and human neuron-specific RNA-binding protein (HUD). A distinguishing feature of about 30% of tumors and more than 90% of human neuroblastoma cell lines is high-level amplification and overexpression of the protooncogene, *MYCN*. Multiple *MYCN* amplicons are either (1) chromosomally integrated and visualizable cytogenetically as one or more long, homogeneously staining region (HSR) or as regions with distinctly abnormal banding patterns (ABRs), or (2) present as small, extrachromosomal chromatin bodies known as double minute chromosomes (DMs). The presence of HSRs and DMs as prevalent features of cell lines[56–58] preceded the discovery of cellular oncogenes and the identification of an amplified *MYC* homolog in neuroblastoma.[59] The exact role of this presumed transcription factor with respect to either malignant transformation or cell differentiation has not been clarified. However, its presence in multiple copies in tumors is indicative of a poor prognosis for the patient.[60] In cell lines that amplify the *MYCN* gene, S cells express at least fourfold less gene product than their N-cell counterparts, even if both cell types contain the same number of *MYCN* genes. This difference may account, in part, for the tumorigenicity of N-type cells and the limited growth and abrogated tumorigenic potential of S cells.

Other proteins that may play a role in either expression of the cellular phenotype or malignant potential of human neuroblastoma cell variants are those encoded by the protooncogene *BCL2* and the tumor suppressor gene *P53*. Both proteins play a role in cell growth and survival; BCL2 has been shown to block programmed cell death in a variety of cultured cells, whereas wild-type P53 blocks progression through the cell cycle in response to DNA damage.[61,62] Elevated BCL2 and low P53 protein levels in N-type cells may be indicative of the neuroblastic phenotype or may provide these cells with a growth advantage in culture as well as in the patient[53] (unpublished results). Conversely, low levels of BCL2 and elevated P53 protein levels in S-type cells could explain their limited lifespan in culture and their low malignant potential. Recently, we have also examined neuroblastoma cell variants for the expression of two genes whose homologs in *Drosophila* have been reported to indicate commitment to the neuroblast cell phenotype.[63] As expected, HASH1 and HUD are expressed in N- and I-type cells and not in S cells. The specific function of these nucleotide-binding proteins in determining the neuronal phenotype is unknown.

The morphologic and biochemical properties of N-type cells substantiate their embryonic neuronal differentiation lineage. Identification of S-cell variants has been more difficult, for these cells generally fail to express proteins specific for a mature cellular phenotype. However, biochemical studies of cell-specific enzymes (tyrosinase and 2′,3′-cyclic nucleotide 3′-phosphohydroxylase), cytoskeletal and extracellular matrix proteins (eg, interstitial collagens, fibronectin, intermediate filaments such as vimentin and glial fibrillary acidic protein), and cell surface antigens (A2B5, epidermal growth factor receptor, and NGF receptor) by ourselves and others have provided convincing evidence that the S cell does not represent a dedifferentiated cell that arises as an artifact of cell culture, but instead represents the nonneuronal neural crest precursor cell that can give rise to Schwann, glial, and melanocytic cells.[19,20,23,39] Whereas Schwann cells and melanocytes have been identified in neuroblastoma tumors, the presence of S cells (ie, Schwann-melanocyte precursor cells of tumor origin) in the tumors of patients has not been shown. Although it has been proposed that S cells may represent the stromal component observed in some neuroblastoma tumors (stages I and II), certain findings do not support this contention. First, Ambros and associates[64] have recently shown in 13 stroma-rich neuroblastoma tumors that the stromal elements arise not from the tumor but from surrounding normal tissue. Second, because S cells express the immune response markers (HLA-A, -B, and -C and β_2-microglobulin), they could be recognized and destroyed by T-cell lymphocytes. Whether S cells, because of their ability to migrate within the extracellular matrix, may escape this surveillance system is not known.

The I-type cell is the third predominant cell type found in neuroblastoma cell lines. This cell type expresses morphologic and biochemical traits of both N and S cells (see Table 104-2). I cells do not show contact inhibition, have short neurites, and contain the cell-surface receptors, cytoskeletal proteins, and enzymes that are characteristic of N-type cells. I cells attach well to the substrate and also have many of the cytoskeletal and cell-surface proteins characteristic of S cells (eg, vimentin, chondroitin sulfate proteoglycan, β_2-microglobulin, epidermal growth factor receptor). Based on these features, we have proposed that I cells represent malignant stem cells from which both N and S cells can arise.[23]

EXPERIMENTALLY INDUCED DIFFERENTIATION

As discussed in the preceding section, human neuroblastoma cell variants can spontaneously differentiate or transdifferentiate in culture. In addition, these cells can also be experimentally manipulated to differentiate along one or more specific, divergent neural crest cell lineages. Studies of experimentally induced differentiation have used two model systems. One exploits the capacity of multipotent I-type neuroblastoma cells to differentiate along either a neuroblastic or nonneuronal lineage. The other system focuses on the differentiation of neuroblastic cells along the same pathway toward a mature neuronal phenotype.

One of the best characterized model systems with which to examine changes accompanying human neuroblastoma cell differentiation consists of the I-type, BE(2)-C clonal cell line. In response to all-*trans* retinoic acid (RA), these cells become more neuronal and exhibit an increased number and length of neurites and formation of pseudoganglia, an increased expression of neuronal proteins, and a coordinate decrease in S-cell marker proteins. Conversely, treatment with 5-bromo-2′-deoxyuridine (BUdR) induces an S-cell phenotype in BE(2)-C cells, seen both morphologically, as increased cell flattening and contact inhibition and loss of neuritic processes, and biochemically, by the loss or decreased expression of neuron-associated proteins and increased expression of nonneuronal proteins.[35] A subsequent study with multiple subclones of BE(2)-C showed that differentiation occurred by induction of an altered cellular phenotype and not by selection of spontaneously arising variants, and that the differentiation phenotype was stable in the absence of inducing agents.[65] These and other studies[23] have strongly suggested that human neuroblastoma I-type cells, exemplified by the BE(2)-C cell line, are malignant neural crest stem cells capable of either neuronal or nonneuronal neural crest differentiation. To date, six parental or clonal cell lines with an I-cell phenotype—BE(2)-C, SH-IN, RT-LN-1, GOTO, CHP-126, and NUB-7—have been shown to possess this multipotent differentiation capacity. We speculate that differentiation of malignant stem cells may explain, at least in part, the cellular diversity seen in human neuroblastoma tumors and cell lines.

More commonly, experimentally induced differentiation studies have dealt with the progression of neuroblastic (N) cells along the same differentiation lineage toward a more neuronal phenotype (see Table 104-1). Such differentiation is manifested morphologically and biochemically as pronounced increases in neurite length, cell aggregation, and amounts of neurotransmitter-associated proteins (receptors and biosynthetic enzymes). Whereas neuroblasts are highly proliferative, neuronal differentiation is accompanied by a decrease in the rate or cessation of cellular proliferation. Such experimentally induced neuronal differentiation has been observed for a variety of neuroblastic cell lines (eg, SH-SY5Y, NB-1, LA-N-5, and SMS-KCNR), in response to a diverse group of differentiation-inducing agents.[29,32–34,40,42]

Studies in our laboratory, however, indicate that human neuroblastoma cell lines differ widely in response to commonly used differentiation-inducing agents.[66] In a survey of clones or parental populations from 12 human neuroblastoma cell lines, four lines (IMR-32, CHP-234, SMS-KANR, and LA-N-2) showed no overt morphologic response after a 6-day exposure to eight agents: RA, BUdR, forskolin (FSK), dibutyryl cyclic adenosine monophosphate (dbcAMP), sodium butyrate, phorbol 12-myristate 13-acetate (TPA), phorbol 12, 13-dibutyrate analog or dimethyl sulfoxide. RA and BUdR were the most effective agents, eliciting responses in almost two thirds of lines tested. Both agents induced neuronal and nonneuronal differentiation, depending on the phenotype of the original population. By contrast, sodium butyrate and the two phorbol ester compounds induced differentiation in only one line each. Extent of cytotoxicity or growth inhibition was variable and did not appear to correlate with differentiation induction. The wide differences in differentiation capacity exhibited by neuroblastoma cell lines raise the possibility of a corresponding variation among neuroblastoma tumors, with clinical implications for differentiation-induction therapy.

SUMMARY AND OVERVIEW

A major characteristic of human neuroblastoma cells established in culture is their capacity to differentiate, either spontaneously or in response to appropriate agents, into more mature cell types representative of neural crest derivatives such as neurons, Schwann cells, and melanocytes. This diverse differentiation capacity in vitro may be reflected in both the cellular heterogeneity and the differentiative proclivity sometimes exhibited by tumors in vivo. In a number of recent reviews,[39,67–71] the usefulness of neuroblastoma cell lines for gaining new insights into the cell biology of this tumor and into the differentiation potential of neuroblastoma cells both in vivo and in vitro has been discussed and evaluated. However, new knowledge of the molecular mechanisms controlling growth, differentiation, and malignancy is required, and cell lines provide a useful model in this regard.

Neuroblastoma cells also represent a versatile model of neural crest development. Many cell lines are karyotypically diploid or near-diploid, often with only two or three structurally rearranged or deleted marker chromosomes.[15,56,58] For example, among 22 independently derived cell lines, 18 exhibited modal chromosome numbers in the diploid range.[58] Further, the karyotypes tend to be stable during long-term serial passage. These features contrast with those of the majority of cell lines derived from other tumor types, especially in adults, which are generally heteroploid, with many chromosomal rearrangements, both specific and apparently nonspecific. The often near-normal chromosome constitution of neuroblastoma cells may be indicative of considerable genetic fidelity, despite the malignant phenotype, in terms of representing normal neural crest cells at various stages of development. In support of this notion is the stability of the cells in culture with respect to their biochemical phenotype if cloned or purified populations are maintained carefully as morphologically homogenous populations of N, S, I (and possibly other) cell types.

REFERENCES

1. Brodeur GM. Neuroblastoma and other peripheral neuroectodermal tumors. In: Feinbach DJ, Vietti TJ, eds. Clinical pediatric oncology, 4th ed. St Louis, Mosby–Year Book, 1991:437.
2. Brodeur GM, Seeger RC, Barret A, et al. International criteria for diagnosis, staging, and response to treatment in patients with neuroblastoma. J Clin Oncol 1988;6:1874.
3. LeDouarin NM, Smith J. Development of the peripheral nervous system. Annu Rev Cell Biol 1988;4:375.
4. Patterson PH. Control of cell fate in a vertebrate neurogenic lineage. Cell 1990;62:105.
5. Stemple DL, Anderson DJ. Isolation of a stem cell for neurons and glia from the mammalian neural crest. Cell 1992;71:973.
6. Murray MR, Stout AP. Distinctive characteristics of the sympathicoblastoma cultivated in vitro. Am J Pathol 1947;23:429.
7. Goldstein MN. Neuroblastoma cells in tissue culture. J Pediatr Surg 1968;3:166.
8. Tumilowicz JJ, Nichols WW, Cholon JJ, Greene AE. Definition of a continuous human cell line derived from neuroblastoma. Cancer Res 1970;30:2110.
9. Biedler JL, Helson L, Spengler BA. Morphology and growth, tumorigenicity, and cytogenetics of human neuroblastoma cells in continuous culture. Cancer Res 1973;33:2643.
10. Seeger RC, Rayner SA, Banerjee A, et al. Morphology, growth, chromosomal pattern, and fibrinolytic activity of two new human neuroblastoma cell lines. Cancer Res 1977;37:1364.
11. Brodeur GM, Sekhon GS, Goldstein MN. Chromosomal aberrations in human neuroblastomas. Cancer 1977;40:2256.
12. Biedler JL, Roffler-Tarlov S, Schachner M, Freedman LS. Multiple neurotransmitter synthesis by human neuroblastoma cell lines and clones. Cancer Res 1978;38:3751.
13. Sekiguchi M, Oota T, Sakakibara K, Inui N, Fujii G. Establishment and characterization of a human neuroblastoma cell line in tissue culture. Jpn J Exp Med 1979;49:67.
14. Schlesinger HR, Rorke L, Jamieson R, Hummeler K. Neuronal properties of neuroectodermal tumors in vitro. Cancer Res 1981;41:2573.
15. Reynolds CP, Biedler JL, Spengler BA, et al. Characterization of human neuroblastoma cell lines established before and after therapy. J Natl Cancer Inst 1986;76:375.
16. West G, Uki J, Herschman HR, Seeger R. Adrenergic, cholinergic, and

inactive human neuroblastoma cell lines with the action-potential Na + ionophore. Cancer Res 1977;37:1372.
17. Biedler JL, Spengler BA, Ross RA. Chromosomal and biochemical properties of human neuroblastoma lines and clones in cell culture. Gaslini 1979;11:128.
18. Ross RA, Joh TH, Reis DJ, Spengler BA, Biedler JL. Neurotransmitter-synthesizing enzymes in human neuroblastoma cells: relationship to morphological diversity. In: Evans AE, D'Angio GJ, Seeger RC, eds. Advances in neuroblastoma research. New York, Raven Press, 1980: 151.
19. Ross RA, Biedler JL. Presence and regulation of tyrosinase activity in human neuroblastoma cell variants in vitro. Cancer Res 1985;45:1628.
20. Rettig WJ, Spengler BA, Garin Chesa P, Old LJ, Biedler JL. Coordinate changes in neuronal phenotype and surface antigen expression in human neuroblastoma cell variants. Cancer Res 1987;47:1383.
21. DeClerck YA, Bomann ET, Spengler BA, Biedler JL. Differential collagen biosynthesis by human neuroblastoma variants. Cancer Res 1987; 47:6505.
22. Sadée W, Yu VC, Richards ML, et al. Expression of neurotransmitter receptors and *myc* protooncogenes in subclones of a human neuroblastoma cell line. Cancer Res 1987;47:5207.
23. Ciccarone V, Spengler BA, Meyers MB, Biedler JL, Ross RA. Phenotypic diversification in human neuroblastoma cells: expression of neural crest lineages. Cancer Res 1989;49:219.
24. Veillette A, O'Shaughnessy J, Horak ID, et al. Coordinate alteration of pp60$^{c\text{-}src}$ abundance and c-*src* RNA expression in human neuroblastoma variants. Oncogene 1989;4:421.
25. Sidell N, Sarafian R, Kelly M, et al. Retinoic acid–induced differentiation of human neuroblastoma: a cell variant system showing two distinct responses. Exp Cell Biol 1986;54:287.
26. Foley J, Cohn SL, Salwen HR, et al. Differential expression of N-*myc* in phenotypically distinct subclones of a human neuroblastoma cell line. Cancer Res 1991;51:6338.
27. Sugimoto T, Ueyama H, Hosoi H, et al. Alpha–smooth-muscle actin and desmin expressions in human neuroblastoma cell lines. Int J Cancer 1991;48:277.
28. Sugimoto T, Kato T, Sawada T, et al. Schwannian cell differentiation of human neuroblastoma cell lines in vitro induced by bromodeoxyuridine. Cancer Res 1988;48:2531.
29. Sano K, Motoike T, Nakamura H, Matsui Y, Teranishi Y, Takai Y. Differential expression of the N-*myc*, c-*fos*, and smg p25A genes in human neuroblastoma cells during neuronal and schwannian differentiation. Molec Brain Res 1991;9:149.
30. Sugimoto T, Horii Y, Hino T, et al. Differential susceptibility of HLA class II antigens induced by γ-interferon in human neuroblastoma cell lines. Cancer Res 1989;49:1824.
31. Feyles V, Dixon WT, Sikora LKJ, McGarry RC, Jerry LM. Human melanoma-associated antigen expression on human neuroblastoma cells: effects of differentiation inducers. Cancer Immunol Immunother 1991;32:261.
32. Påhlman S, Ruusala A-I, Abrahamsson L, Mattsson MEK, Esscher T. Retinoic acid–induced differentiation of cultured human neuroblastoma cells: a comparison with phorbolester-induced differentiation. Cell Differ 1984;14:135.
33. Shea TB, Beermann ML. Staurosporine-induced morphological differentiation of human neuroblastoma cells. Cell Biol Int 1991;15:161.
34. Jensen LM. Phenotypic differentiation of aphidicolin-selected human neuroblastoma cultures after long-term exposure to nerve growth factor. Dev Biol 1987;120:56.
35. Ross RA, Bossart E, Spengler BA, Biedler JL. Multipotent capacity of morphologically intermediate (I-type) human neuroblastoma cells after treatment with differentiation-inducing drugs. In: Evans AE, D'Angio GJ, Knudson AG, Seeger RA, eds. Advances in neuroblastoma research 3. New York, Wiley-Liss, 1991:193.
36. Reynolds CP, Perez-Polo JR. Nerve growth factor induces neurite outgrowth in a clone derived from an NGF-insensitive human neuroblastoma cell line. Int J Dev Neurosci 1989;7:125.
37. Slack R, Lach B, Gregor A, Al-Mazidi H, Proulx P. Retinoic acid- and staurosporine-induced bidirectional differentiation of human neuroblastoma cell lines. Exp Cell Res 1992;202:17.
38. Sidell N, Altman A, Haussler MR, Seeger RC. Effects of retinoic acid on the growth and phenotypic expression of several human neuroblastoma cell lines. Exp Cell Res 1983;148:21.
39. Tsokos M, Scarpa S, Ross RA, Triche TJ. Differentiation of human neuroblastoma recapitulates neural crest development: study of morphology, neurotransmitter enzymes, and extracellular matrix proteins. Am J Pathol 1987;128:484.
40. Thiele CJ, Reynolds CP, Israel MA. Decreased expression of N-*myc* precedes retinoic acid induced phenotypic differentiation of human neuroblastoma. Nature 1985;313:404.
41. Dimitroulakos J, Squire J, Pawlin G, Yeger H. NUB-7: a stable I-type human neuroblastoma cell line inducible along N- and S-type cell lineages. Cell Growth Differ 1994;5:373.
42. Pence JC, Shorter NA. In vitro differentiation of human neuroblastoma cells caused by vasoactive intestinal peptide. Cancer Res 1990;50:5177.
43. Matsushima H, Bogenmann E. Bi-modal differentiation pattern in a new human neuroblastoma cell line in vitro. Int J Cancer 1992;51:250.
44. Biedler JL, Spengler BA, Ross RA. Expression of catecholamine-synthesizing enzymes in human neuroblastoma lines with unique chromosomal abnormalities. In: Usdin E, Kopin IJ, Barchas J, eds. Catecholamines: basic and clinical frontiers, vol 1. New York, Pergamon Press, 1979:192.
45. Ross RA, Spengler BA, Biedler JL. Coordinate morphological and biochemical interconversion of human neuroblastoma cells. J Natl Cancer Inst 1983;71:741.
46. Biedler JL, Spengler BA, Chang T-D, Ross RA. Transdifferentiation of human neuroblastoma cells results in coordinate loss of neuronal and malignant properties. In: Evans AE, D'Angio GJ, Knudson AG, Seeger RC, eds. Advances in neuroblastoma research 2. New York, Alan R Liss, 1988:103.
47. Reynolds CP, Tomayko MM, Donner L, et al. Biological classification of cell lines derived from human extracranial neural tumors. In: Evans AE, D'Angio GJ, Knudson AG, Seeger RC, eds. Advances in neuroblastoma research 2. New York, Wiley–Liss, 1988:291.
48. Eguchi G, Kodama R. Transdifferentiation. Curr Opin Cell Biol 1993; 5:1023.
49. Ross RA, Biedler JL, Spengler BA, Reis DJ. Neurotransmitter-synthesizing enzymes in 14 human neuroblastoma cell lines. Cell Mol Neurobiol 1981;1:301.
50. Hsiao RJ, Seeger RC, Yu AL, O'Connor DT. Chromogranin A in children with neuroblastoma. J Clin Invest 1990;85:1555.
51. Cooper MJ, Hutchins GM, Cohen PS, Helman LJ, Mennie RJ, Israel MA. Human neuroblastoma tumor cell lines correspond to the arrested differentiation of chromaffin adrenal medullary neuroblasts. Cell Growth Differ 1990;2:149.
52. Lampson LA. Biological significance of HLA-A,B,C expression in neuroblastoma and related cell lines. In: Evans AE, D'Angio GJ, Knudson AG, Seeger RC, eds. Advances in neuroblastoma research 2. New York, Alan R Liss, 1985:409.
53. Hanada M, Krajewski S, Tanaka S, et al. Regulation of *Bcl-2* oncoprotein levels with differentiation of human neuroblastoma cells. Cancer Res 1993;53:4978.
54. Azar CG, Scavarda NJ, Nakagawara A, Brodeur GM. Expression and function of the nerve growth factor receptor (TRK-A) in human neuroblastoma cell lines. In: Evans AE, Biedler JL, Brodeur GM, D'Angio GJ, Nakagawara A, eds. Advances in neuroblastoma research 4. New York: Wiley-Liss, 1994:169.
55. Lucarelli E, Kaplan D, Matsumoto K, Sickafuse S, Thiele CJ. Retinoic acid induced differentiation is mediated by trkb receptors. In: Evans AE, Biedler JL, Brodeur GM, D'Angio GJ, Nakagawara A, eds. Advances in neuroblastoma research 4. New York: Wiley-Liss, 1994:185.
56. Biedler JL, Spengler BA. A novel chromosome abnormality in human neuroblastoma and antifolate-resistant Chinese hamster cell lines in culture. J Natl Cancer Inst 1976;57:683.
57. Biedler JL, Ross RA, Shanske S, Spengler BA. Human neuroblastoma cytogenetics: search for significance of homogeneously staining regions and double minute chromosomes. In: Evans AE, D'Angio GJ, Seeger RC, eds. Advances in neuroblastoma research. New York: Raven Press. 1980:151.
58. Biedler JL, Meyers MB, Spengler BA. Homogeneously staining regions and double minute chromosomes: prevalent cytogenetic abnormalities of human neuroblastoma cells. In: Federoff S, Hertz L, eds. Advances in cellular neurobiology, vol 4. New York, Academic Press, 1983:267.
59. Schwab M, Alitalo K, Klampnauer K-H, et al. Amplified DNA with limited homology to *myc* cellular oncogene is shared by human neuroblastoma cell lines and a neuroblastoma tumor. Nature 1983;305:245.
60. Brodeur GM, Seeger RC, Schwab M, Varmus HE, Bishop JM. Amplifi-

cation of N-*myc* in untreated human neuroblastomas correlates with advanced stage disease. Science 1984;223:1121.

61. Vaux D, Cory S, Adams J. *Bcl-2* gene promotes haematopoietic cell survival and cooperates with c-myc to immortalize pre–B-cells. Nature 1988;335:440.
62. Diller L, Kassel J, Nelson CE, et al. *P53* functions as a cell cycle control protein in osteosarcomas. Mol Cell Biol 1990;10:5772.
63. Szabo A, Dalmau J, Manley G, et al. HuD, a paraneoplastic encephalomyelitis antigen, contains RNA-binding domains and is homologous to elav and sex-lethal. Cell 1991;67:325.
64. Ambros IM, Zellner A, Stock C, Amann G, Gadner H, Ambros PF. Proof of the reactive nature of the Schwann cell in neuroblastoma and its clinical implications. In: Evans AE, Biedler JL, Brodeur GM, D'Angio GJ, Nakagawara A. Advances in neuroblastoma research 4. New York: Wiley-Liss, 1994:331.
65. Ross RA, Spengler BA, Rettig WR, Biedler JL. Differentiation-inducing agents stably convert human neuroblastoma I-type cells to neuroblastic (N) or nonneuronal (S) neural crest cells. In: Evans AE, Biedler JL, Brodeur GM, D'Angio GJ, Nakagawara A, eds. Advances in neuroblastoma research 4. New York: Wiley-Liss, 1994:253.
66. Spengler BA, Domènech C, Porubcin M, Biedler JL. Human neuroblastoma lines respond differently to diverse differentiation-inducing agents. In: Evans AE, Biedler JL, Brodeur GM, D'Angio GJ, Nakagawara A, eds. Advances in neuroblastoma research 4. New York: Wiley-Liss, 1994:261.
67. Abemayor E, Sidell N. Human neuroblastoma cell lines as models for the in vitro study of neoplastic and neuronal cell differentiation. Environ Health Perspect 1989;80:3.
68. Påhlman S, Mamaeva S, Meyerson G, et al. Human neuroblastoma cells in culture: a model for neuronal cell differentiation and function. Acta Physiol Scand Suppl 1990;140:25.
69. Biedler JL, Spengler BA, Ross RA. Cellular maturation and oncogene expression during drug-induced differentiation in vitro: a brief review. In: Ragaz J, Simpson-Herrn L, Lippman ME, Fisher B, eds. Effects of therapy on biology and kinetics of the residual tumor. New York, Wiley-Liss, 1990;354A:287.
70. Thiele CJ. Biology of pediatric peripheral neuroectodermal tumors. Cancer Metastasis Rev 1991;10:311.
71. Israel MA, Thiele CJ. Tumor cell lines of the peripheral nervous system. In: Hay RJ, Park J-G, Gazdar A, eds. Atlas of human tumor cell lines. San Diego, Academic Press, 1994:43.

Principles and Practice of Genitourinary Oncology, edited by Derek Raghavan, Howard I. Scher, Steven A. Leibel, and Paul H. Lange. Lippincott-Raven Publishers, Philadelphia, © 1997.

CHAPTER 105

Neuroblastoma

Biomarkers

Judith G. Villablanca and Stuart E. Siegel

A variety of markers have been described for neuroblastoma that are useful in diagnosis, determining prognosis (Table 105-1), and monitoring response to therapy. Many of these markers have been studied retrospectively, and data regarding important molecular genetic markers such as *MYCN*[1] and *TRK*[2,3] have not been included. The results of ongoing, prospective studies that include some of the critical markers described here as well as molecular genetic data will help determine the most significant markers for defining biologic subgroups of patients in regard to determination of prognosis and stratification for therapy. Some of these markers may also be used as therapeutic targets for the treatment of neuroblastoma.

URINARY CATECHOLAMINE METABOLITES

Neuroblastoma, which originates from the embryonal neural crest, is associated with elevated levels of the dopamine metabolite homovanillic acid (HVA) in 90% to 92% of patients, and of the norepinephrine metabolites vanillylmandelic acid (VMA) in 72% to 95% of patients and 3-methoxy-4-hydroxyphenoglycol (MHPG) in 97% of patients.[4,5] HVA and VMA levels normalized to urinary creatinine can be evaluated by a single random sample of urine, with a positive predictive value of 100% and a negative predictive value of 93%,[4] an equivalent reliability to 24-hour urine collections.[6] Epinephrine and norepinephrine levels are normal or only minimally elevated in most patients.[7,8]

A higher ratio of VMA to HVA at diagnosis has been shown to correlate with a better prognosis in Evans[3a] stage IV disease.[9] Higher VMA levels are associated with more differentiated tumors that express dopamine β-hydroxylase, which converts dopamine to norepinephrine.[10] Gitlow and colleagues[11] found that lower HVA excretion at diagnosis correlated with a better prognosis and was more frequently found in younger patients. The incidence of catecholamine excretion is lower in more mature tumors.[12] Serial VMA and HVA levels are also a useful monitor of disease response to therapy.[13–15]

Mass screening for neuroblastoma at 6 to 7 months of age using spot urine values of VMA was first studied by Sawada in Japan in 1973.[16] Those infants diagnosed by screening had a high survival rate, compared with children missed by screening. However, the screening program was associated with an increased incidence in neuroblastoma, suggesting that screening was detecting cases that may not have developed clinical manifestations.[17] Another screening study was performed in 1981 by Takeda and colleagues[18] in Japan using HVA and VMA. This study found a decrease in mortality from neuroblastoma compared with previous rates in Japan, but these lower mortality rates were equivalent to outcomes in North America and Europe, where mass screening was not being performed.[17] Two additional studies, in Northern England and in Quebec,[17] detected 2 and 23 patients, respectively, by screening; most of them had low-stage tumors with favorable biologic markers. Three patients detected clinically after negative screening tests in the English study had unfavorable, higher-stage disease. These data support the hypothesis that there may be two forms of neuroblastoma. The evaluation of mass screening is still ongoing. It will be critical to thoroughly evaluate biologic features of tumors detected, and to obtain accurate normative mortality data to determine the usefulness and future role of screening children for neuroblastoma.

FERRITIN

Ferritin, a tissue iron-binding protein, is correlated with neuroblastoma and returns to normal levels with disease response to therapy. Ferritin is secreted into the serum by the tumor.[19] However, elevations of ferritin are not usually found in ganglioneuroblastomas, or in Evans stage I, II, or IVS tumors.[20] Hann and associates[21] reported that serum ferritin levels lower than 142 ng/mL are correlated with a significant increase in the progression-free survival rate for patients with Evans stage III disease (76% versus 23%; Fig. 105-1) or stage IV disease (27% versus 3%) independent of stage and age; however, *MYCN* (for-

TABLE 105-1. *Prognostic markers in subgroups of neuroblastoma*

Marker	Value associated with poor prognosis
Ferritin	>142 ng/mL
VMA:HVA ratio	HVA > VMA
Neuron-specific enolase	>100 ng/mL
Lactate dehydrogenase	>1500 U/L
G_{D2} ganglioside	>568 pmol/mL
Chromogranin A	>190 mg/mL

HVA, homovanillic acid; VMA, vanillylmandelic acid.

merly N-*myc*) was not evaluated in this study. By combining the factors of age (greater or less than 2 years), stage (I, II, or IVS versus III/IV), serum ferritin (normal versus greater than 150 ng/mL), and histology (favorable versus unfavorable), Evans and colleagues defined two risk groups, one with a 2-year survival rate of better than 80% and one with a rate of less than 20%.[22] Ongoing studies in the Children's Cancer Group are evaluating the prognostic significance of ferritin in neuroblastoma in a prospective manner, with multivariate analysis for *MYCN* as well as the factors previously analyzed by Evans. Isoferritins from neuroblastomas have been reported to suppress immune function through inhibition of mitogen responses,[23,24] rosette formation by T lymphocytes,[25,26] and granulocyte function.[27]

LACTATE DEHYDROGENASE

Serum lactate dehydrogenase is a useful, although nonspecific, marker for monitoring disease activity, and it can easily be determined in clinical practice. Levels greater than 1500 U/L have been reported to be associated with poorer outcome.[28,29]

NEURON-SPECIFIC ENOLASE

Neuron specific enolase (NSE), an isoenzyme of a glycolytic enzyme, is expressed by neuronal and neuroendocrine cells of the central and peripheral nervous system[30–31] and by tumors of the peripheral neuroendocrine system, including neuroblastoma.[32] NSE levels greater than 100 ng/mL have been reported as a significant adverse prognostic factor for Evans stage IV tumors in patients diagnosed before 1 year of age, and for Evans stage III tumors in patients younger than 2 years of age.[33–34] As observed with ferritin, NSE levels are not elevated in stage IVS tumors.[34] NSE levels have also been correlated with response to therapy,[35] although the measurement is not specific for neuroblastoma.[36]

G_{D2} GANGLIOSIDE

G_{D2} ganglioside is a sialic acid–containing glycosphingolipid that is located primarily on the cell membrane and was found in all primary untreated neuroblastomas evaluated by Wu and associates,[37] irrespective of tumor stage. Very low or undetectable levels were noted in ganglioneuroblastomas and ganglioneuromas, suggesting a correlation with tumor differentiation. In contrast to other markers that stratify tumors for prognosis, the expression of G_{D2} in all neuroblastomas has made it useful for bone marrow purging of neuroblastoma tumor cells[38] and as a target antigen for monoclonal antibody–based tumor imaging[39] and immunotherapy.[40,41] G_{D2} is shed into the circulation by

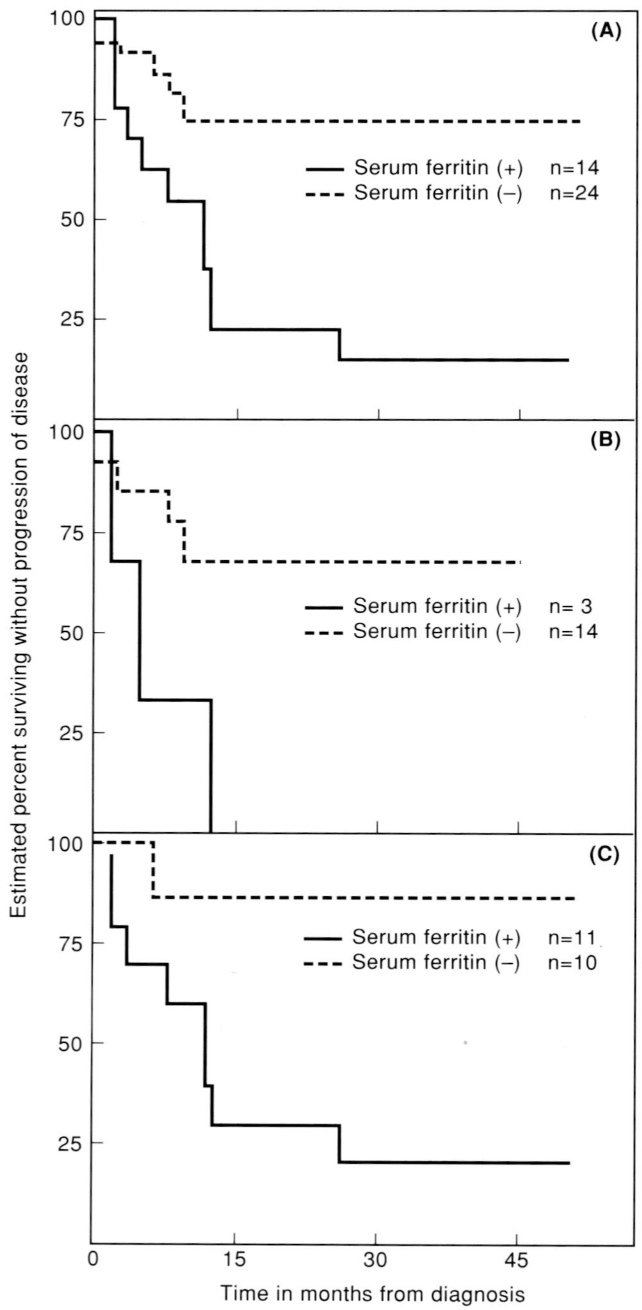

FIG. 105-1. Chart of progression-free survival for patients with stage III neuroblastoma in relation to normal (−) or elevated (+) serum ferritin. Patients were grouped as follows according to age at diagnosis: A, patients of all ages (P = .002); B, patients younger than 2 years of age (P = .03); and C, patients 2 years of age or older (P = .02). The median follow-up period was 30 months, and the range was 3 to 52 months.

neuroblastomas, and levels of this ganglioside have been found to be inversely correlated with progression-free survival in stage III and IV patients.[42] A possible mechanism for the association of G_{D2} levels with outcome is suggested by the observation that gangliosides derived from neuroblastomas can depress cellular immunity in vitro[43] and therefore may enhance tumor progression by host immunosuppression.

TUMOR DETECTION IN MARROW AND PERIPHERAL BLOOD STEM CELLS

A panel of monoclonal antibodies against cell-surface antigens, including G_{D2}, that reacts with neuroblastoma tumor cells but not normal bone marrow cells, has been developed by Seeger and coworkers.[44] This panel can detect as few as 1 tumor cell in 100,000 normal mononuclear cells in bone marrow, and can detect marrow metastases in patients with stage I, II, or III disease by routine marrow histology.[44] A subgroup of patients with stage II or III tumors diagnosed after 1 year of age who had detectable marrow metastases at diagnosis by immunocytologic analysis had a lower progression-free survival rate (Fig. 105-2). Patients with stage IV tumors diagnosed before 1 year of age also had a more unfavorable outcome if more than 0.02% tumor cells were present by immunocytologic evaluation of the marrow. Immunocytologic quantitation of marrow tumor content on serial marrow sampling during therapy may define prognostic subgroups of patients with lower progression-free survival rates among the group with marrow metastases that persist after therapy.[45] Circulating neuroblastoma cells can be detected by immunocytologic analysis in the blood of some patients at diagnosis, and their presence is predictive of relapse if tumor cells are still noted during therapy.[46]

Monoclonal antibodies can be used to purge residual tumor from bone marrow before autologous marrow rescue from myeloablative therapy and to determine the efficacy of tumor removal after completion of purging.[47] Neuroblastoma cells have also been detected by immunocytologic examination of peripheral blood stem cell collections in patients with minimal or no marrow tumor cells.[48] A more sensitive method of neuroblastoma tumor cell detection, which can detect 1 tumor cell in 10^7 peripheral blood mononuclear cells, determines the expression of the neuroendocrine protein PGP 9.5 by reverse transcriptase-polymerase chain reaction.[49] PGP 9.5 is expressed in all neuroblastoma cell lines evaluated, and it is not found on normal mononuclear cells in the peripheral blood or bone marrow.[49] Sensitive detection methods for tumor are critical for analysis of either marrow or peripheral blood collections used for hematopoietic rescue from myeloablative chemotherapy, in order to determine whether tumor cells will be reinfused into the patient.[48]

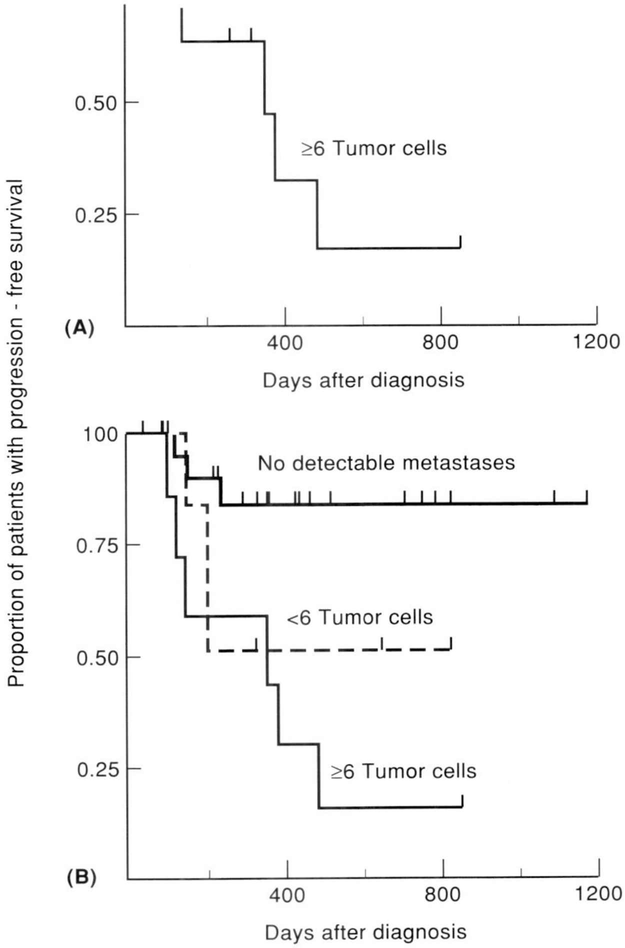

FIG. 105-2. Chart of progression-free survival in patients with localized or regional disease (stage I, II, or III), according to the number of neuroblastoma cells per 100,000 marrow cells on immunocytologic analysis. The top panel shows survival rates for all 65 patients ($P = .001$), and the bottom panel shows survival rates for 37 patients who were older than 1 year of age at diagnosis ($P = .003$). Tick marks represent individual patients.

NEUROPEPTIDES

Several neuropeptides have been reported as markers in neuroblastoma. Circulating levels of vasoactive intestinal peptide (VIP) may be elevated in neuroblastoma, ganglioneuroblastoma, and ganglioneuroma and may be associated with a syndrome of severe intractable diarrhea and hypokalemia.[50–52] Levels of VIP should be measured in patients with neuroblastoma who present with these symptoms. Increased VIP levels in primary tumors at diagnosis are correlated with cellular differentiation and favorable disease stage,[53] whereas somatostatin levels correlate only with differentiation. VIP receptors were expressed in 12 of 15 neuroblastomas studied by O'Dorisio and colleagues, and in vitro studies suggest that VIP may function as an autocrine growth factor in neuroblastoma.[54] Somatostatin receptor expression is found in tumors with less advanced stages at diagnosis and was downregulated in a small sample of tumors studied after disease progression.[55]

Elevated plasma levels of neuropeptide Y, a regulatory peptide present in the human central nervous system and the sympathetic chain, have been found in patients with neuroblastoma at diagnosis and correlated with the clinical response to therapy.[56] In the human adrenal medulla, neuropeptide Y expression occurs from 7.5 weeks to 18 weeks of gestation, and then not again until 8 months after birth.[57] Expression of neuropeptide

Y was found in 0 of 4 stage IV tumors but 15 of 15 stage IVS tumors diagnosed in children younger than 1 year of age, suggesting that it may correlate with prognosis and that these two subgroups of tumors may arise from different populations of cells at distinct maturational time points.[57]

OTHER MARKERS

Chromogranin A,[58] a protein that is stored with catecholamines and released with them from storage vesicles in the adrenal medulla by exocytosis,[59] has a sensitivity of 91% and a specificity of 100% for the diagnosis of neuroblastoma.[60] Higher serum levels (>190 mg/mL) of chromogranin A at diagnosis were correlated with higher tumor stage and lower progression-free survival rate (0% versus 54%; $P < 0.005$) in patients older than 1 year of age.[60]

The alpha subunit of one of the guanosine triphosphate–binding proteins, G_0, is found in significantly higher levels in neuroblastomas than in other pediatric solid tumors. Higher levels are also correlated with lower disease stage and age younger than 1 year at diagnosis for patients with neuroblastoma.[61]

Elevated urinary levels of the amino acids cystathionine and aminoisobutyric acid have been reported in patients with neuroblastoma but have not found to have significant associations with outcome.[12,62,63]

The multiple markers described for neuroblastoma have been a valuable asset for determining prognosis (see Table 105-1) and for designing therapeutic approaches to this tumor, because they define biologically characterized subgroups of patients and their associated clinical behavior. The application of this approach to other solid tumors should advance our understanding of tumor biology and allow the rational design of novel therapies, some of which may target specific tumor markers.

REFERENCES

1. Seeger RC, Brodeur GM, Sather H, et al. Association of multiple copies of the N-*myc* oncogene with rapid progression of neuroblastomas. N Engl J Med 1985;313:1111.
2. Nakagawara A, Arima-Nakagawara M, Scavarda NJ, Azar CG, Cantor AB, Brodeur GM. Association between high levels of expression of the *TRK* gene and favorable outcome in human neuroblastoma. N Engl J Med 1993;328:847.
3. Miyake M, Suzuki T, Shimada H, Stram D, Seeger RC. High affinity nerve growth factor receptor expression (gp140trkA), N-*myc* amplification, histopathology, and survival in neuroblastoma. Prog Clin Biol Res 1994;385:163.
4. Tuchman M, Ramnaraine MLR, Woods WG, Krivit W. Three years of experience with random urinary homovanillic and vanillylmandelic acid levels in the diagnosis of neuroblastoma. Pediatrics 1987;79:203.
5. Gitlow SE, Bertani LM, Rausen A, Gribetz D, Dziedzic SW. Diagnosis of neuroblastoma by qualitative and quantitative determination of catecholamine metabolites in urine. Cancer 1970;25:1377.
6. LaBrosse EH, Com-Nougue C, Zucker JM, et al. Urinary excretion of 3-methoxy-4-hydroxymandelic acid and 3-methoxy-4- hydroxyphenylacetic acid by 288 patients with neuroblastoma and related neural crest tumors. Cancer Res 1980;40:1995.
7. Isaacs H, Medalic M, Politzer WM. Noradrenaline-secreting neuroblastomas. Br Med J 1959;1:401.
8. Mason GA, Hart-Mercer J, Millar EJ, Strang LB, Wynne NA. Adrenaline-secreting neuroblastoma in an infant. Lancet 1957;2:322.
8a. Evans AE, D'Angio GJ, Randolph J. A proposed staging for children with neuroblastoma. Cancer 1971;27:374.
9. Laug WE, Siegel SE, Shaw KNF, Landing B, Baptista J, Gutenstein M. Initial urinary catecholamine metabolite concentrations and prognosis in neuroblastoma. Pediatrics 1978;62:77.
10. Kontras SB. Urinary excretion of 3-methoxy-4-hydroxy-mandelic acid in children with neuroblastoma. Cancer 1962;15:978.
11. Gitlow SE, Dziedzic LB, Strauss L, Greenwood SM, Dziedzic SW. Biochemical and histologic determinants in the prognosis of neuroblastomas. Cancer 1973;32:898.
12. Bore KE, McAdams J. Composite ganglioneuroblastoma. Arch Pathol Lab Med 1981;105:325.
13. Labrosse EH, Comoy E, Bohuon C, Zucker JM, Schweisguth O. Catecholamine metabolism in neuroblastoma. J Natl Cancer Inst 1976;57:633.
14. Liebner EJ, Rosenthal IM. Serial catecholamines in the radiation management of children with neuroblastoma. Cancer 1973;32:623.
15. Moyano MB, Bergada C, Becu L. Significance of catecholamine excretion in the follow-up of sympathoblastomas. Cancer 1971;27:228.
16. Sawada T, Todo S, Fujita K, et al. Mass screening of neuroblastoma in infancy. 1982;136:710.
17. Tuchman M, Woods WG. Introduction: neuroblastoma screening, laboratory, clinical and epidemiological aspects. Am J Pediatr Hematol Oncol 1992;14:95.
18. Takeda T, Shimada M, Iizuka S, Takasugi N. Effects of mass screening for neuroblastoma and the presumptive natural history of this tumor. Prog Clin Biol Res 1994;385:383.
19. Hann HL, Stahlhut MW, Evans AE. Source of increased ferritin in neuroblastoma: studies with concanavalin A-sepharose binding. J Natl Cancer Inst 1986;76:1031.
20. Hann HL, Levy HM, Evans AE. Serum ferritin as a guide to therapy in neuroblastoma. Cancer Res 1980;40:1411.
21. Hann HL, Evans AE, Siegel SE, et al. Prognostic importance of serum ferritin in patients with stages III and IV neuroblastoma: the Childrens Cancer Study Group experience. Cancer Res 1985;45:2845.
22. Evans AE, D'Angio GJ, Propert K, Anderson J, Hann HL. Prognostic factors in neuroblastoma. Cancer 1987;59:1853.
23. Matzner Y, Hershko C, Polliack A, Konijin AM, Izak G. Suppressive effect of ferritin on in vitro lymphocyte function. Br J Haematol 1979;42:345.
24. Niitsu Y, Kohgo Y, Ohtsuka S, et al. Ferritins in serum and tissue and their implications in malignancy. In: Fishman WH, Sell S, eds. Oncodevelopment gene expression. New York, Academic Press, 1976:757.
25. Hann HL, Stahlhut MW, Chung LC. Inhibitory effect of isoferritins from tumor and non-tumor tissues on E-rosette formation. Lancet 1984;1:43. Letter.
26. Moroz C, Giler S, Kupfer B, Urca I. Lymphocytes bearing surface ferritin in patients with Hodgkin's disease and breast cancer. N Engl J Med 1977;296:1172.
27. Hann HWL, Stahlhut BA, Evans AE. Serum ferritin as a prognostic indicator in neuroblastoma: biological effects of isoferritins. Prog Clin Biol Res 1985;175:331.
28. Berthold F, Trechow R, Utsch S, et al. Prognostic factors in metastatic neuroblastomas: a multivariate analysis of 182 cases. Am J Pediatr Hematol Oncol 1992;14:207.
29. DeBernardi B, Pianca C, Boni L, et al. Disseminated neuroblastoma (stage IV and IVS) in the first year of life. Cancer 1986;57:1230.
30. Marangos PJ, Schmechel DE. The neurobiology of the brain enolases. In: Youdim MBH, Lovenberg W, Sharman ER, Lagnado JR, eds. Essays in neurochemistry and neuropharmacology. New York, John Wiley, 1980:211.
31. Marangos PJ, Zis AP, Cleark RL, Goodwin FK. Neuronal, non-neuronal, and hybrid forms of enolase in brain: structural, immunological and functional comparisons. Brain Res 1978;150:117.
32. Tapia FJ, Polak JM, Barbosa AJA, et al. Neuron-specific enolase is produced by neuroendocrine tumours. Lancet 1981;1:808.
33. Zeltzer PM, Parma AM, Dalton A, et al. Raised neuron-specific enolase in serum of children with metastatic neuroblastoma. Lancet 1983;2:361.
34. Zeltzer PM, Marangos PJ, Evans AE, Schneider SL. Serum neuron-specific enolase in children with neuroblastoma: relationship to stage and disease course. Cancer 1986;57:1230.
35. Ishiguro Y, Kato K, Takahiro I, Nagaya M, Yamada N, Sugito T. Nervous system-specific enolase in serum as a marker for neuroblastoma. Pediatrics 1983;72:696.
36. Tsuchida Y, Honna T, Iwanaka T, et al. Serial determination of serum

neuron-specific enolase in patients with neuroblastoma and other pediatric tumors. J Pediatr Surg 1987;22:419.
37. Wu ZL, Schwartz E, Seeger R, Ladisch S. Expression of G_{D2} ganglioside by untreated primary human neuroblastomas. Cancer Res 1986; 46:440.
38. Cheung NKV, Saarinen UM, Neely JE, Landmeir B, Donovan D, Coccia PF. Monoclonal antibodies to a glycolipid antigen on human neuroblastoma cells. Cancer Res 1985;45:2642.
39. Miraldi FD, Nelson AD, Kraly C, et al. Diagnostic imaging of human neuroblastoma with radiolabeled antitumor antibody. Radiology 1986; 161:413.
40. Cheung NKV, Lazarus H, Miraldi FD, et al. Ganglioside G_{D2} specific monoclonal antibody 3F8: a phase I study in patients with neuroblastoma and malignant melanoma. J Clin Oncol 1987;5:1430.
41. Handgretinger R, Baader P, Dopfer R, et al. A phase I study of neuroblastoma with the anti-ganglioside G_{D2} antibody 14.G2a. Cancer Immunol Immunother 1992;35:199.
42. Valentino L, Moss T, Olson E, Wang HJ, Elashoff R, Ladisch S. Shed tumor gangliosides and progression of human neuroblastoma. Blood 1990;75:1564.
43. Floutsis G, Ulsh L, Ladisch S. Immunosuppressive activity of human neuroblastoma tumor gangliosides. Int J Cancer 1989;43:6.
44. Moss TJ, Reynolds CP, Sather HN, Romansky SG, Hammond GD, Seeger RC. Prognostic value of immunologic detection of bone marrow metastases in neuroblastoma. N Engl J Med 1991;324:219.
45. Ozkaynak MF, Gallego R, Hong W, et al. Immunocytologic quantitation of tumor in marrow during induction chemotherapy predicts tumor progression in neuroblastoma. Proc Am Soc Clin Oncol 1994;13:415. Abstract.
46. Moss TJ, Sanders DG. Detection of neuroblastoma cells in blood. J Clin Oncol 1990;8:736.
47. Reynolds CP, Moss TJ, Seeger RC, Black AT, Woody JN. Sensitive detection of neuroblastoma cells in bone marrow for monitoring the efficacy of marrow purging procedures. In: Evans AE, D'Angio GJ, Seeger RC, eds. Advances in neuroblastoma research. New York, Alan R Liss, 1985:425.
48. Moss TJ, Sanders DG, Lasky LC, Bostrom B. Contamination of peripheral blood stem cell harvests by circulating neuroblastoma cells. Blood 1990;76:1879.
49. Mattano LA, Moss TJ, Emerson SG. Sensitive detection of rare circulating neuroblastoma cells by the reverse transcriptase-polymerase chain reaction. Cancer Res 1992;52:4701.
50. Scheibel E, Rechnitzer C, Fahrenkrug J, Hertz H. Vasoactive intestinal peptide (VIP) in children with neural crest tumours. Acta Paediatr Scand 1982;71:721.
51. Cooney DR, Voorhees ML, Fisher JE, Brecher M, Karp MP, Jewett TC. Vasoactive intestinal peptide producing neuroblastoma. J Pediatr Surg 1982;17:821.
52. El-Shafie M, Samuel D, Klippel CH, Robinson MG, Cullen BJ. Intractable diarrhea in children with VIP-secreting ganglioneuroblastomas. J Pediatr Surg 1983;18:34.
53. Qualman SJ, O'Dorisio MS, Fleshman DJ, Shimada H, O'Dorisio TM. Neuroblastoma: correlation of neuropeptide expression in tumor tissue with other prognostic factors. Cancer 1992;70:2005.
54. O'Dorisio MS, Fleshman DJ, Qualman SJ, O'Dorisio TM. Vasoactive intestinal peptide: autocrine growth factor in neuroblastoma. Regul Pept 1992;37:213.
55. O'Dorisio MS, Chen F, O'Dorisio TM, Wray D, Qualman SJ. Characterization of somatostatin receptors on human neuroblastoma tumors. Cell Growth Differ 1994;5:1.
56. Kogner P, Bjork O, Theodorsson E. Neuropeptide Y as a marker in pediatric neuroblastoma. J Pediatr Pathol 1990;10:207.
57. Cohen PS, Cooper MJ, Helman LJ, Thiele CJ, Seeger RC, Israel MA. Neuropeptide Y expression in the developing adrenal gland and in childhood neuroblastoma tumors. Cancer Res 1990;50:6055.
58. Smith WJ, Kishner N. A specific soluble protein from the catecholamine storage vesicles of bovine adrenal medulla I: purification and chemical characterization. Mol Pharmacol 1967;3:52.
59. Sage JH, Smith WJ, Kirshner N. Mechanism of secretion from the adrenal medulla: I. A microquantitative immunologic assay for bovine adrenal catecholamine storage vesicle protein and its application to studies of the secretory process. Mol Pharmacol 1967;3:81.
60. Hsiao RJ, Seeger RC, Yu Al, O'Connor DT. Chromogranin A in children with neuroblastoma: Serum concentration parallels disease stage and predicts survival. J Clin Invest 1990;85:1555.
61. Ishiguro Y, Kato K, Asano T, et al. The alpha subunit of GTP-binding protein G_o in neuroblastoma: correlation with advanced disease stage. Cancer Res 1994;54:2334.
62. Giessing LR. Cystathionuria and vanil-lactic-acid-uria. In: Bohuoun C, ed. Recent results in cancer research; neuroblastoma-biochemical studies. Berlin, Springer-Verlag, 1966:26.
63. Gesser CG, Efron ML. Cystathioninuria in patients with neuroblastoma or ganglioneuroblastoma: its correlation to vanillylmandelic acid excretion and its value in diagnosis and therapy. Cancer 1968;22:856.

Principles and Practice of Genitourinary Oncology, edited by Derek Raghavan, Howard I. Scher, Steven A. Leibel, and Paul H. Lange. Lippincott-Raven Publishers, Philadelphia, © 1997.

CHAPTER 106

Pathology of Neuroblastoma

Hiroyuki Shimada and Vijay V. Joshi

Tumors of the neuroblastoma group include neuroblastoma, ganglioneuroblastoma, and ganglioneuroma. These tumors are usually diagnosed in early life, before 5 years of age; some congenital cases can be diagnosed before birth. Neuroblastomas are reported to be associated with congenital malformations, such as defects of the adrenal gland,[1,2] heterochromia,[3] aganglionosis of the colon,[4] anencephaly, trisomy 13, and partial trisomy 15.[5] They are also found in association with various disease conditions, such as Ondine's curse syndrome,[4] fetal hydantoin-alcoholic syndromes,[6] cystic fibrosis,[7] von Recklinghausen's disease,[8] tuberous sclerosis,[9] and Beckwith-Wiedemann syndrome.[10] Rare cases of familial neuroblastoma have been reported in the literature,[11] suggesting a hereditary predisposition. However, no constitutional abnormalities or specific congenital-anomaly syndromes, such as the aniridia or hemihypertrophy found in patients with Wilms tumor, have been identified in neuroblastoma patients.

Differential diagnoses include the so-called small blue cell tumors of childhood[12]: malignant lymphoma, rhabdomyosarcoma, osseous and extraosseous Ewing's sarcoma or peripheral primitive neuroectodermal tumor (PNET), and esthesioneuroblastoma. Identifying the neural phenotype in tumor tissue is important for the diagnosis of neuroblastoma. However, because proliferating cells in PNET and esthesioneuroblastoma also have a neural phenotype, pathologists may face difficulty in differentiating neuroblastoma from these other entities.

Unique biologic characteristics, including involution, spontaneous regression, and maturation, are well documented in this group of tumors. Involution is frequent. In situ neuroblastoma,[13,14] found incidentally as a microscopic nodule larger than 2000 μm in the adrenal gland during neonatal autopsy, is estimated to occur approximately 40 to 50 times more frequently than clinically detectable neuroblastoma; most in situ neuroblastomas therefore are destined to involute without clinical manifestation. One of the examples of spontaneous regression is well illustrated in stage IVS (special) neuroblastoma.[15] Tumors in this category are typically diagnosed during the first year of life as small primary lesions, usually in the adrenal gland, with widespread metastasis to liver, bone marrow (without bony destruction), and/or subcutaneous tissues. More than 75% of children with this type of neuroblastoma experience spontaneous regression of the disease and enjoy favorable clinical courses without treatment or with minimal therapy.

For the pathologist, the most interesting characteristic of this group of tumors is the potential of histologic maturation. Occasionally, pathologic examination of sequential surgical specimens from the same patient demonstrates histologic maturation during the clinical course, from undifferentiated neuroblastoma toward a less aggressive form or even toward a benign ganglioneuroma.[16] Furthermore, tumors of this group can be defined as a spectrum of neoplastic conditions showing different stages of histologic maturation. In other words, the individual tumor categories (neuroblastoma, ganglioneuroblastoma, and ganglioneuroma) can be illustrated according to the histology of continuous and sequential steps of maturation.[17]

In this chapter, the pathology of the tumors of the neuroblastoma group, including histogenesis and morphologic features, is described. Histopathologic features of prognostic significance and brief descriptions of nonmorphologic prognostic factors are also included in the latter portion.

HISTOGENESIS

Tumors of this group originate from the neural crest. Neural crest cells are located in the crests of the neural folds of the neural groove. The cells migrate and disperse in the body to form the sympathetic ganglia and adrenal medulla. The tumors of the neuroblastoma group are found in the normal anatomic sites for neural crest cells according to the embryonic pattern, such as the adrenal gland (40%), the abdominal sympathetic ganglia including the organ of Zuckerkandl (25%), the sympathetic ganglia of the posterior mediastinum (15%), the cervical sympathetic ganglia (5%), and the pelvis (5%). Unusual primary tumors have been reported in the kidney[18] and ovary, with or without other teratomatous elements.[19] Some paraspinal tumors showing a dumbbell-type of growth pattern with extradural extension into the spinal canal may be made up of cells originating in the dorsal root ganglion.

Cellular types derived from the neural crest and found during the development of the sympathetic nervous system include neuroblastic cells (neuroblasts, maturing neuroblasts, ganglion cells) and stromal cells (Schwann cells, perineurial cells, and satellite cells). The tumors of the neuroblastoma group recapitulate the development of the sympathetic ganglion and therefore

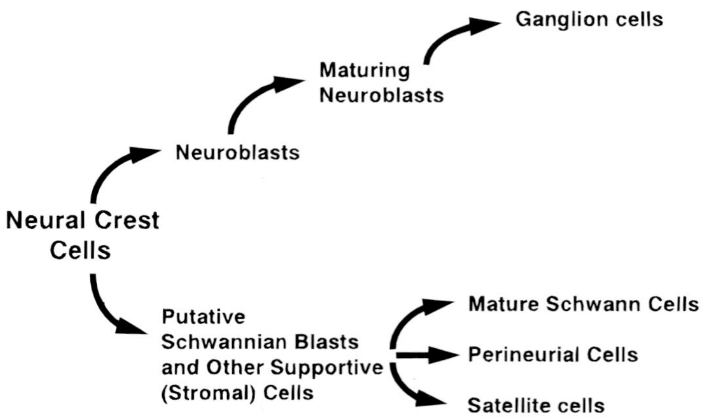

FIG. 106-1. Development of neural crest cells in sympathetic nervous system.

contain both cell types, showing neuroblastic and stromal differentiation (Fig. 106-1).

BASIC MORPHOLOGY

Tumors of the neuroblastoma group show various morphologic appearances according to maturational grade, from the most primitive form of undifferentiated neuroblastoma to the final stage of maturation of a ganglioneuroma. Between these extremes, there is a spectrum of intermediate tumors which can be described as differentiating neuroblastoma from ganglioneuroblastoma.[17]

Gross Appearance

Gross morphology varies depending on the maturational grades of the tumors. Cut surfaces of neuroblastoma tissue appear friable, hemorrhagic, and partially necrotic and may or may not have calcification and cystic formations. Ganglioneuroblastoma and ganglioneuroma specimens usually have smooth or slightly trabeculated cut surfaces that are glistening, homogeneously gray-tan or yellowish-white, and somewhat elastic. Direct local extension to the kidney and liver is considered an indicator of aggressive tumor growth and poor clinical outcome. Retroperitoneal and pelvic tumors occasionally involve the great vessels and other vital organs and may be subjected to incomplete surgical resection. Patients presenting with paraspinal tumors having the dumbbell-type intraspinal extension may require emergent surgical intervention for neurologic symptoms. Metastatic dissemination can occur by lymphatic and vascular routes to bone, lymph nodes, and liver. Neuroblastoma also spreads to the dura mater and leptomeninges, but intracerebral metastasis is very rare, as is intrapulmonary metastasis, though diffuse spreading on the pleural surface can occur. Soft tissue metastasis is virtually nonexistent.

Maturational Sequences

Because the tumors of the neuroblastoma group arise from neural crest cells, which have the potential for a broad spectrum of differentiation, the individual tumors contain a mixture of cell types with differing degrees of maturation. The cells show both neural phenotypes (neuroblasts, maturing neuroblasts, and ganglion cells) and stromal phenotypes (putative Schwannian blasts, mature Schwann cells, perineurial cells, and satellite cells). The three subcategories of neuroblastoma, ganglioneuroblastoma, and ganglioneuroma are more precisely defined morphologically as described in the following sections.

Neuroblastoma

In the subcategory of neuroblastoma (stroma-poor tumor), routine hematoxylin and eosin staining shows no stromal development evident in the tumor tissue. The tumor is composed of proliferating neuroblasts with or without active production of neuritic processes. The neuroblasts are characteristically arranged in lobules surrounded by fibrovascular septa. Some tumors are densely cellular, whereas others are relatively hypocellular within an abundant neurofibrillary background of eosinophilic meshwork. Homer Wright rosettes are seen in about one third of cases. Stromal elements comprised of putative Schwannian blasts may be present in the thin fibrovascular septal area of this stroma-poor tumor, but they can be detected only by immunohistochemical staining with anti–S-100 protein antibody.[20,21]

The stroma-poor tumor can be separated into two subsets, undifferentiated and differentiating, based on the grade of neuroblastic differentiation. The undifferentiated stroma-poor tumor includes prototypic neuroblastoma and is mainly or exclusively composed of primitive neuroblastic cells measuring 7 to 10 μm in diameter with dense hyperchromatic nuclei and scanty cytoplasm (Fig. 106-2*A*). The appearance of maturing neuroblasts is the first morphologic change in the maturational sequence of the tumors. If more than 5% of neuroblasts have a maturing appearance, the tumor is classed as differentiating stroma-poor (see Fig. 106-2*B*). A maturing neuroblast is defined as one that exhibits cellular enlargement with cytoplasmic eosinophilia, distinct cellular borders, easily recognizable neuritic production, and nuclear enlargement with a discrete nucleolus clearly evident in sections routinely stained with hematoxylin and eosin. Some maturing neuroblasts are binucleated or multinucleated.

Neuroblastoma, of even the most primitive form, can usually be diagnosed by transmission electron microscope identifica-

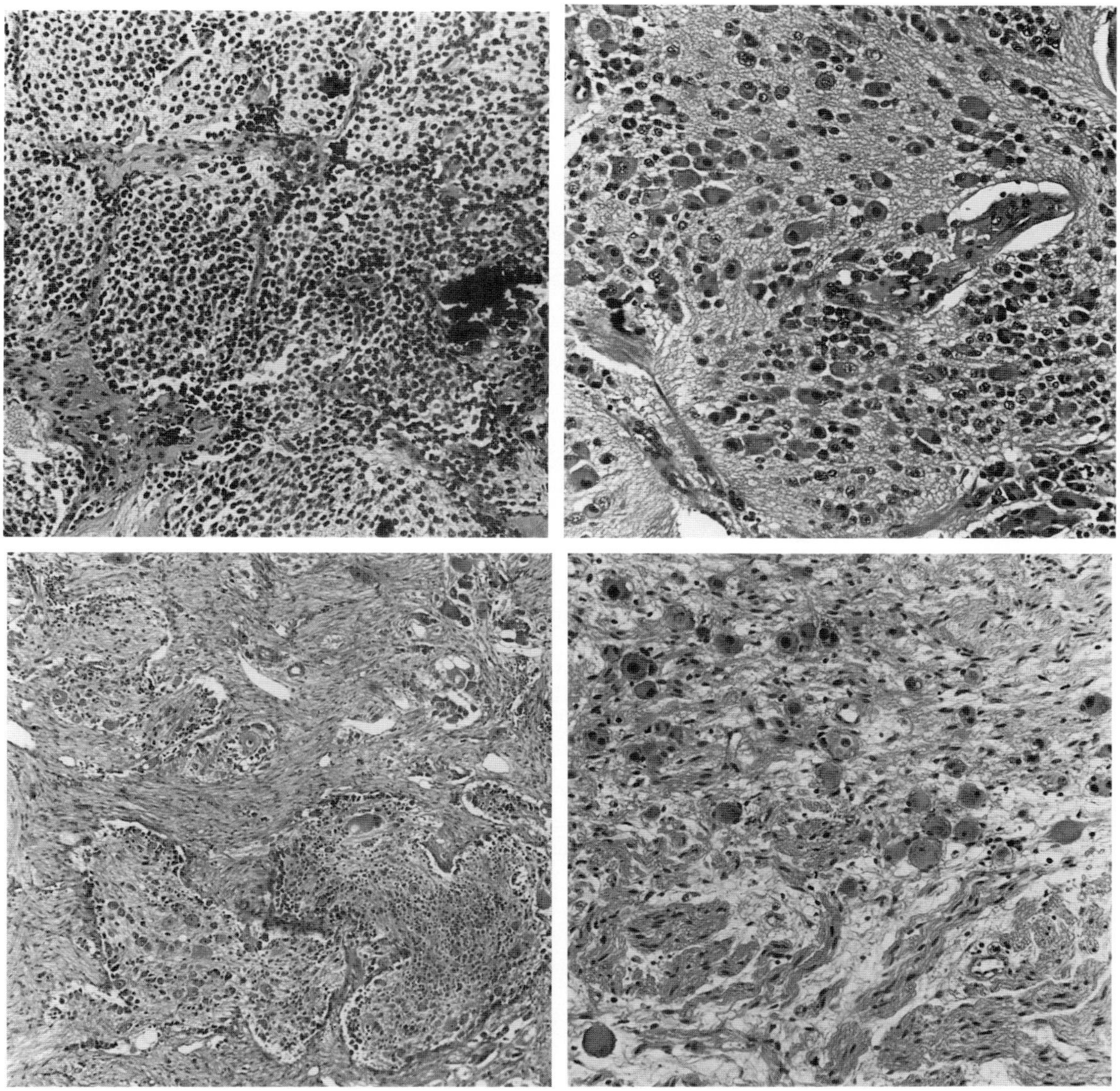

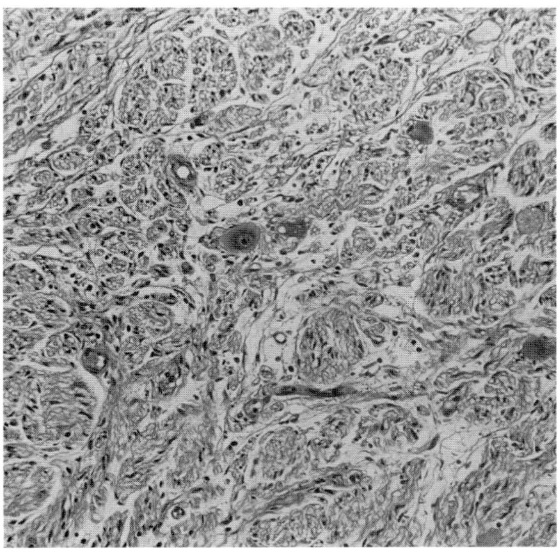

FIG. 106-2. Morphology of the tumors of the neuroblastoma group according to the maturational sequences. (**A**) Neuroblastoma (stroma-poor), undifferentiated with calcification. (**B**) Neuroblastoma (stroma-poor), differentiating. (**C**) Ganglioneuroblastoma (stroma-rich), intermixed. (**D**) Ganglioneuroblastoma (stroma-rich) well-differentiated. (**E**) Ganglioneuroma. (H&E stains; magnification ×200 [**A, B, D**], ×40 [**C**], ×100 [**E**].)

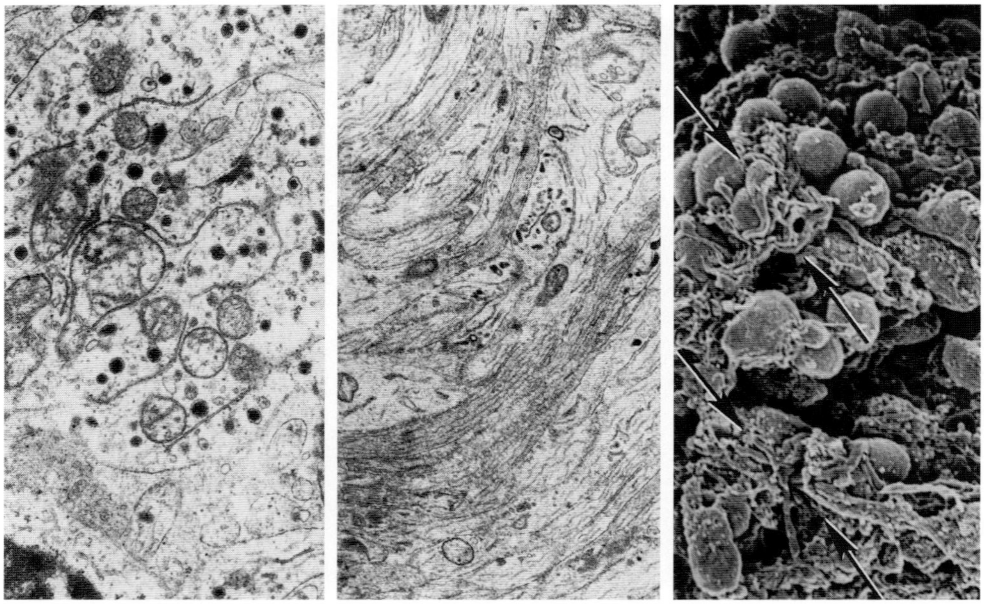

FIG. 106-3. Electron microscopic features of neuroblastoma. (**A**) Numerous neurosecretory granules (transmission electron microscope, magnification × 18,000). (**B**) Area showing longitudinal sections of multiple neuritic processes corresponding to a neurofibrillary background of eosinophilic meshwork by light microscopy (transmission electron microscope, magnification × 12,000). (**C**) Neuroblastic cells and neuritic processes (*arrows*) (scanning electron microscope, magnification × 720).

tion of neurosecretory granules and neuritic processes.[22] The neurosecretory granules are membrane-bound dense-core granules measuring 150 to 200 nm in diameter that are found in the neuritic processes and in the cell bodies as well (Fig. 106-3*A*). The neuritic processes contain microtubules arranged in a parallel fashion (see Fig. 106-3*B*). The neuritic processes in the stroma-poor tumors are naked, without Schwannian protection. By contrast, neurites in the normal human peripheral nervous system are always found in either myelinated or unmyelinated form with protection by Schwann cells.

Viewed with the scanning electron microscope, the undifferentiated neuroblastoma is composed of mixtures of neuroblasts showing different patterns of neurite projection: they are apolar, monopolar, bipolar, or multipolar (see Fig. 106-3*C*)[22] Occasionally, rudimentary attachment structures are seen between individual neuroblastic cells and between neuroblasts and neuritic processes. Varying numbers of glycogen particles are seen in about 10% of undifferentiated neuroblastoma tumors. The maturing neuroblasts seen in differentiating neuroblastomas have an eccentrically located nucleus with one or a few nucleoli and increased numbers of cytoplasmic organelles. They always show a multipolar type of neuritic projection.[22] Putative Schwannian blasts seen in the perivascular areas have an ultrastructural morphology of complicated cellular surfaces or infoldings, pinocytotic vesicles, and external lamina.[20–22]

Ganglioneuroblastoma

The step of maturation known as ganglioneuroblastoma (stroma-rich tumor) is characterized by extensive development and proliferation of Schwannian stromal cells, originating most likely from the putative blasts in perivascular areas. Septal tissue surrounding the lobules of neuroblastic cells gradually thickens, and the proliferating Schwann cells steadily increase in percentage of total cells within the tumor. The neuroblastic cells, advancing their maturation into ganglion cells, are now grouped into small foci or nests separated by and embedded in a bulky stroma of mature Schwann cells. Tumor tissue at this stage of maturation is categorized as intermixed; it is distinguished by Schwannian "neurofibromatous" stroma studded with scattered, variably differentiated neuroblastic cell nests (see Fig. 106-2*C*).

Further maturation of the tumor leads to the stage designated well-differentiated stroma-rich, or borderline, ganglioneuroblastoma. This tumor is only one step from the fully mature form of ganglioneuroma (see Fig. 106-2*D*). In tumor sections at this stage of maturation, no microscopically distinguishable foci of neuroblastic nests are seen. Instead, a few randomly distributed maturing neuroblasts or immature ganglion cells, along with fully mature ganglion cells surrounded by diffusely proliferating Schwannian stromal cells, are observed. Some ganglion cells are surrounded by satellite cells. Both types of ganglioneuroblastoma, intermixed and well-differentiated, demonstrate occasional stromal areas in which multiple fascicular formations are established by close structural association between Schwann cells and perineurial cells.

Ultrastructural examination of the stromal portion of ganglioneuroblastoma clearly demonstrates the presence of mature Schwann cells. They usually show a lack of myelin, but they are covered by continuous external lamina and incorporate multiple neuritic processes originating from cell bodies of neuroblasts, maturing neuroblasts, and ganglion cells. Occasional fascicles in the stromal area represent a well-organized structure of pure unmyelinated nerve fibers.[17,22]

Ganglioneuroma

In the final stage of maturation, ganglioneuroma, scattered, fully mature ganglion cells surrounded by satellite cells are embedded in a bulky stromal tissue (see Fig. 106-2*E*). The ganglion cells contain an eccentrically located large nucleus with a single prominent nucleolus and abundant cytoplasmic organelles, including Nissl bodies of peripherally distributed rough endoplasmic reticulum and free ribosomes. Completely developed synaptic structures can be observed. The stromal portion dominating the histologic appearance of the tumor has a "neurofibromatous" appearance and is completely organized into multiple fascicles, which are bundles of unmyelinated nerve fibers composed of Schwann cells, endoneurial connective tissue, and perineurial cells.[17,22]

Immunohistochemistry

A battery of selected antibodies for neural elements is used for the diagnostic evaluation of neuroblastoma. These antibodies are against, for example, neuron-specific enolase (NSE); neurofilaments (NF) of 68, 150, or 200 kd; synaptophysin; chromogranin A; Lue-7; and S-100 protein.[20,21,23–26] There are also monoclonal antibodies[27–30] such as UJ13, 3F8 (against the ganglioside G_{D2}), SOS 13, FMG 25, BA1, BA2, HNK1, A2B5, and HSAN 1.2, and monoclonal antibodies against the tetanus toxin receptor, microtubule-associated proteins (MAP1 and MAP2), and neural cell adhesion molecules (NCAM), to name a few. Despite its questionable specificity,[31] NSE is still the most popular and useful antibody and should be included in the routine workup for diagnosis.

Although many monoclonal antibodies have been raised against human neuroblastomas, a truly neuroblastoma-specific antigen has not been defined. Some of the monoclonal antibodies listed share their antigenic determinants with normal and neoplastic nervous tissue, and others also share determinants with blood cells.[32] For the purpose of differential diagnosis, it is useful to note that neuroblastic cells in neuroblastoma are usually negative for antibody against glycoprotein p 30/32,^{MIC2}, differentiating them from the cells of most peripheral PNETs, which react positively.[33]

Unusual Histologic Features

Pleomorphic neuroblastoma is a rare tumor that carries a poor prognosis; it is composed of diffuse pleomorphic neuroblastic cells with bizarre giant cells.[34] Occasionally, neuroblastomas show an angiomatoid pattern of pooled erythrocytes.[35] One neuroblastoma has been reported to contain abundant melanin pigment in the tumor tissue.[36]

HISTOPATHOLOGIC CLASSIFICATION OF PROGNOSTIC SIGNIFICANCE

The amounts or percentages of mitotic activity, lymphoid infiltration, neuropil, anaplastic cells, calcification, necrosis, foam cells, and neuroblastic differentiation or maturation have been evaluated by various investigators in attempts to correlate the variables with prognosis. In this section, two histopathologic classification systems, the Shimada classification[37] and the low-risk and high-risk grouping by histologic grade,[38] are outlined. The Shimada classification is applicable to both stroma-poor and stroma-rich tumors. The low-risk and high-risk grouping developed by Joshi and colleagues covers neuroblastomas only. Each of these classification systems requires extensive pathologic review of specimens from material untreated before surgery for informed evaluation.

Shimada Classification for Neuroblastomas and Ganglioneuroblastomas

The Shimada classification scheme is based on the conceptual framework of an age-linked maturational sequence in the tumors of the neuroblastoma group.[37,39,40] The histologic changes in the tumor tissue during the maturational steps have already been described. Neuroblastomas are divided into favorable and unfavorable prognostic groups according to the patient's age, grade of neuroblastic differentiation (undifferentiated or differentiating subset), and nuclear abnormalities. The nuclear abnormalities are determined by counting mitotic cells and karyorrhectic cells (ie, those having a ruptured nucleus with spilling chromatin condensed as formless granules) in tumor tissue and recording these figures as the mitosis-karyorrhexis index (MKI) per 5000 neuroblastic cells.[40] Each tumor is evaluated as having a high (>200), intermediate (100 to 200) or low (<100) MKI.

If the patient is younger than 1.5 years of age, the grade of neuroblastic differentiation has no prognostic significance: only nuclear abnormalities correlate with clinical behavior for such infant tumors. In other words, in very young children, both undifferentiated and differentiating tumors can carry a good prognosis, unless they have a high MKI. Tumors with high MKI scores have a poor prognosis regardless of the grade of neuroblastic differentiation (see Fig. 106-4*A*). If the patient's age is between 1.5 and 5 years, both the grade of neuroblastic differentiation and the MKI are prognostically significant, and only the differentiating tumor with low MKI has a good prognosis. In this age group, neuroblastomas behave aggressively because of an immaturity of neuroblastic cells (undifferentiated stroma-poor), an increased number of nuclear abnormalities (intermediate or high MKI), or a combination of these factors. Patients older than 5 years of age with stroma-poor tumors have a poor prognosis regardless of the maturational grade of neuroblastic cells and the number of nuclear abnormalities. For the child older than 5 years of age, a good prognosis depends on the tumor being at a histologically advanced stage of maturation—that is, a stroma-rich ganglioneuroblastoma.

Stroma-rich tumors usually occur in older children and are rarely seen in infants and children younger than 1 year of age. Ganglioneuroblastomas are divided into two prognostic groups. One group includes intermixed and well-differentiated stroma-rich tumors, transitional forms in the maturational sequence toward ganglioneuroma; this group has an excellent prognosis. The second group is a composite tumor characterized by the presence of one or a few grossly visible, discrete nodules, usually hemorrhagic and composed of the stroma-poor type of neuroblastic proliferation (see Fig. 106-4*B*). This tumor is designated nodular stroma-rich. The nodules are considered a sign of malignant

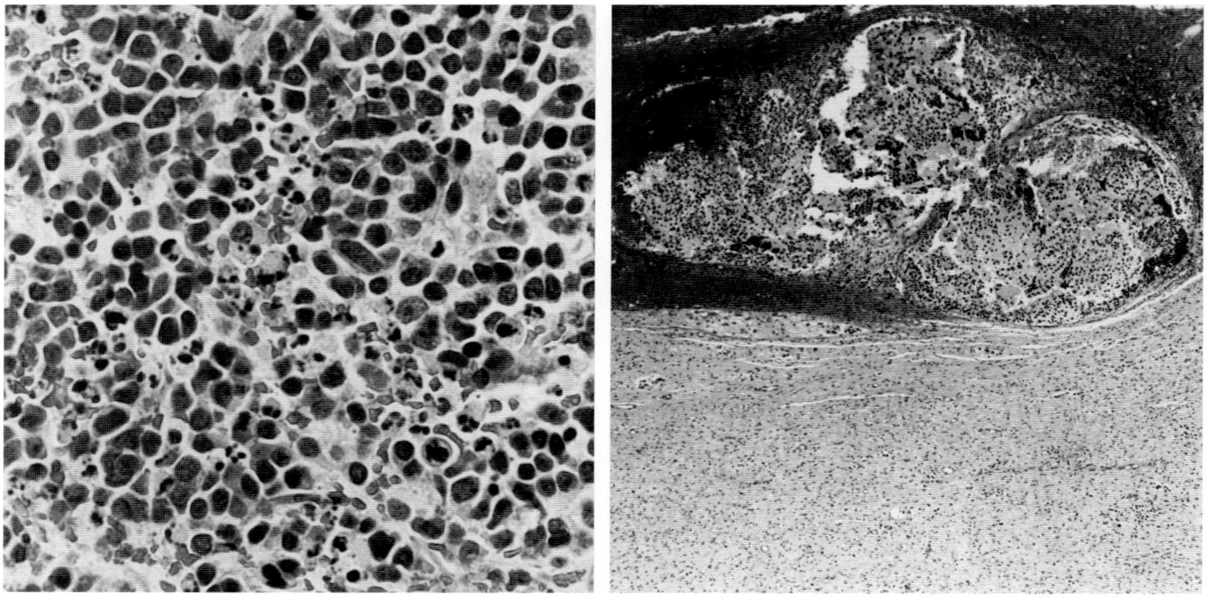

FIG. 106-4. Examples of unfavorable tumors. (**A**) Neuroblastoma (stroma-poor), "undifferentiated" and high MKI. (**B**) "Nodular" ganglioneuroblastoma (stroma-rich, "nodular") composed of stroma-rich tumor (*lower half*) with stroma-poor nodule (*upper half*). H&E stain, original magnification (**A**) ×400, (**B**) ×20.

clonal evolution arising during the maturational processes of intermixed or well-differentiated tumor; they have a high potential for distant metastasis and often cause a fatal outcome.

Table 106-1 summarizes the Shimada classification system. Tumors in the favorable group show histologic changes in a continuous maturational process, advancing from undifferentiated and differentiating neuroblastoma (stroma-poor) to intermixed and well-differentiated ganglioneuroblastoma (stroma-rich) according to the patient's age at diagnosis. Tumors in the favorable group therefore show morphologic changes within an age-matched maturational sequence. On the other hand, tumors with any histologic indicators, such as abnormally increased MKI, maturational arrest (or inappropriate degree of maturation for patient's age), or abnormal evolution of aggressive clones, are classified into the unfavorable group. This classification system is now being used as one of the front-end prognostic indicators for assignment of treatment protocols for patients with newly diagnosed neuroblastoma who are enrolled in the Children's Cancer Group studies.

Low-Risk and High-Risk Grouping for Neuroblastomas

This is also an age-linked prognostic categorization. Two parameters, mitotic rates and calcification, are used for histologic grading. Grade 1 tumors have both low mitotic rate (fewer than 10 mitotic cells per 10 high-power fields) and calcification; grade 2 tumors have either low mitotic rate or calcification; and grade 3 tumors lack both low mitotic rate and calcification. The low-risk or high-risk status is determined by correlating the histologic grade with patient age. The low-risk group is composed of (1) patients with grade 1 tumors and (2) patients younger than 1 year with grade 2 tumors. The high-risk group

TABLE 106-1. *Shimada classification for neuroblastoma and ganglioneuroblastoma*

Favorable histology	Unfavorable histology
Stroma-poor tumors	Stroma-poor tumors
Patients <1.5 years of age:	Patients <1.5 years of age:
All tumors with low or intermediate MKI	All tumors with high MKI
Patients 1.5–5 years of age:	Patients 1.5–5 years of age:
Differentiating tumors with low MKI	Undifferentiated tumors with any MKI
	Differentiating tumors with intermediate or high MKI
	Patients >5 years of age:
	All stroma-poor tumors
Stroma-rich tumors	Stroma-rich tumors
Intermixed	Nodular
Well-differentiated	

MKI, mitosis-karyorhexis index. See text for other definitions.

TABLE 106-2. *Low-risk and high-risk grouping for neuroblastoma based on histologic grades* and patient's age*

Low-risk group:
Patients with grade 1 tumors
Patients younger than 1 year of age with grade 2 tumors
High-risk group:
Patients with grade 3 tumors
Patients older than 1 year of age with grade 2 tumors

* Histologic grading: grade 1, mitotic rate per 10 high-power fields <10, plus calcification; grade 2, mitotic rate <10 or calcification; grade 3, mitotic ratre >10, without calcification.

includes (1) patients with grade 3 tumors and (2) patients older than 1 year with grade 2 tumors. Table 106-2 summarizes the high-risk and low-risk classification scheme.[38]

In this system, only two histologic parameters are used. Degree of neuroblastic differentiation is not used as an indicator for prognostic evaluation. The high-risk and low-risk grouping based on age and histologic grading was developed after a retrospective analysis of 211 neuroblastoma cases from the Pediatric Oncology Group studies. Additional study of this method of evaluation for a new data set is needed, as is a test of its prognostic significance for newly diagnosed neuroblastomas.

NONMORPHOLOGIC PROGNOSTIC FACTORS

Predictions of the clinical behavior of tumors of the neuroblastoma group have been reported using many indicators and prognostic factors other than histopathology. Indicators of good prognosis include: (1) younger patients, especially those younger than 1 year of age at diagnosis; (2) low clinical stage of tumor; (3) primary sites other than adrenal gland or abdomen; and (4) clinical symptoms of opsoclonus-myoclonus.[41] Biochemical markers, such as NSE,[42], lactate dehydrogenase,[43], ferritin,[44], and G_{D2},[45] are also of prognostic value; elevated levels of these markers indicate poor prognosis.

Genetic and molecular markers are important for biologic as well as prognostic analysis of the neuroblastoma tumors. Partial deletion of the short arm of chromosome 1 distal to 1p32,[46] the presence of double minute chromosomes, and the presence of homogeneously staining regions of chromatin[47] are known cytogenetic indicators of poor prognosis. A DNA index of diploid pattern also predicts poor outcome.[48] Tumors with amplification of the *MYCN* gene behave aggressively and progress poorly.[49] In contrast, tumors expressing the gene for the high-affinity nerve growth factor receptor, *TRKA*, are reported to confer a good prognosis.[50] Because the morphology of tumors of the neuroblastoma group probably reflects the summation of their molecular and biologic properties, analyses of the correlations between these indicators and the classic histopathologic indices are of great importance to prediction of outcome.

REFERENCES

1. Blatt J, Lee PA, Taylor SR. Neuroblastoma associated with adrenocortical defects. Pediatrics 1988;82:790.
2. Sy WM, Edomonson JH. The developmental defects associated with neuroblastoma etiologic implications. Cancer 1968;22:234.
3. Jaffe N, Cassady R, Filler RH, Petersen R, Traggis D. Heterochromia and Horner syndrome associated with cervical and mediastinal neuroblastoma. J Pediatr 1975;87:75.
4. Bower RJ, Adkins JC. Ondine's curse and neurocristopathy. Clin Pediatr 1980;19:665.
5. Sanger WG, Howe J, Fordyce R, Purtilo DT. Inherited partial trisomy 15 complicated by neuroblastoma. Cancer Genet Cytogenet 1984;11:153.
6. Seeler RA, Israel JN, Royal JE, Kaye Cl, Rao S, Abulaban M, Ganglioneuroblastoma and fetal hydantoin-alcohol syndromes. Pediatrics 1979;63:524.
7. Moss RB, Blessing-Moore J, Bender SW, Weibel A. Cystic fibrosis and neuroblastoma. Pediatrics 19185;76:814.
8. Bolande RP, Towler WF. A possible relationship of neuroblastoma to von Recklinghausen's disease. Cancer 1970;26:162.
9. Miller DR, Patel K, Allen JC, Horten B. Neuroblastoma, tuberous sclerosis, and subependymal giant cell astrocytoma. Am J Pediatr Hematol Oncol 1983;5:213.
10. Emery LG, Shields M, Shah NR, Garbes A. Neuroblastoma associated with Beckwith-Wiedermann syndrome. Cancer 1983;52:176.
11. Kushner BH, Gilbert F, Helson L. Familial neuroblastoma: case reports, literature review, and etiologic considerations. Cancer 1986;57:1187.
12. Triche TJ, Askin FB. Neuroblastoma and the differential diagnosis of small-, round-, blue-cell tumors: part II. Hum Pathol 1983;14:569.
13. Beckwith JB, Perrin EV. In situ neuroblastomas: a contribution to the natural history of neural crest tumors. Am J Pathol 1963;43:1089.
14. Bolande RP. Developmental pathology. Am J Pathol 1979;94:627.
15. D'Angio GJ, Evans AE, Koop CE. Special pattern of widespread neuroblastoma with a favorable prognosis. Lancet 1971;1:1046.
16. McLaughlin JE, Ulrich H. Maturation of neuroblastoma and ganglioneuroblastoma: a study of four cases with long survival. J Pathol 1977;121:19.
17. Shimada H. In: Williams RA, ed. Pathology: State of the art reviews. Topics in pediatric pathology. Philadelphia, Hanley & Belfus, 1993;2:43.
18. Shende A, Wind ES, Lanzkowsky P. Intrarenal neuroblastoma mimicking Wilms' tumor. N Y State J Med 1979;79:93.
19. Kleinman GM, Young RH, Scully RE. Primary neuroectodermal tumors of the ovary: a report of 35 cases. Am J Surg Pathol 1993;17:764.
20. Shimada H, Aoyama C, Chiba T, Newton WA. Prognostic subtypes for undifferentiated neuroblastoma: an immunohistochemical study with anti-S-100 protein antibody. Hum Pathol 1985;16:471.
21. Hachitanda Y, Tsuneyoshi M. Neuroblastoma with a distinct organoid pattern: a clinicopathologic, immunohistochemical, and ultrastructural study. Hum Pathol 1994;25:67.
22. Shimada H. Transmission and scanning electron microscopic studies on the tumors of neuroblastoma group. Acta Pathol Jpn 1982;32:415.
23. Osborn M, Dirk T, Kaser H, et al. Immunohistochemical localization of neurofilaments and neuron specific enolase in 29 cases of neuroblastoma. Am J Pathol 1986;122:433.
24. Pelc C, Gompel C, Simonet M-L. S-100 protein expression in satellite and Schwann cells in neuroblastoma: an immunohistochemical and ultrastructural study. Virchows Arch B Cell Pathol Incl Mol Pathol 1986;51:487.
25. Hachitanda Y, Tsuneyoshi M, Enjoji M. Expression of pan- neuroendocrine proteins in 53 neuroblastic tumors: an immunohistochemical study with neuron-specific enolase, chromogranin, and synaptophysin. Arch Pathol Lab Med 1989;113:381.
26. Carter RL, Al-Sam SZ, Corbett RP, Clinton S. A comparative study of immunohistochemical staining for neuron-specific enolase, protein gene product 9.5 and S-100 protein in neuroblastoma, Ewing's sarcoma and other round cell tumors in children. Histopathology 1990;16:461.
27. Kemshead JT. Monoclonal antibodies to the small round cell tumors of childhood: an international workshop. Prog Clin Biol Res 1988;271:535.
28. Berliner P, Unisicker K. Tetanus toxin labeling as a novel rapid and highly specific tool in human neuroblastoma differential diagnosis. Cancer 1985;56:419.
29. Artlieb U, Krepler R, Wiche G. Expression of microtubule-associated proteins, Map-1 and Map-2, in human neuroblastomas and differential diagnosis of immature neuroblasts. Lab Invest 1985;53:684.
30. Garin-Chesa P, Fellinger FJ, Huvos AG, et al. Immunohistochemical

analysis of neural cell adhesion molecules: differential expression in small round cell of childhood and adolescence. Am J Pathol 1991;139: 275.

31. Pahlman S, Esscher T, Milsson K. Expression of gamma-subunit of enolase, neuron-specific enolase in human non-neuroendocrine tumors and derived cell lines. Lab Invest 1986;54:554.
32. Sugimoto T, Tatsumi E, Kemshead JT, et al. Determination of cell surface membrane antigens common to both human neuroblastoma and leukemia-lymphoma cell lines by a panel of 38 monoclonal antibodies. J Natl Cancer Inst 1984;73:51.
33. Weidner N, Tjoe J. Immunohistochemical profile of monoclonal antibody O13: antibody that recognizes glycoprotein p30/32[MIC2] and is useful in diagnosing Ewing's sarcoma and peripheral neuroepithelioma. Am J Surg Pathol 1994;18:486.
34. Cozzuto C, Carbone A. Pleomorphic (anaplastic) neuroblastoma. Arch Pathol Lab Med 1988;112:621.
35. Koppersmith DL, Powers JM, Hennigar GR. Angiomatoid neuroblastoma with cytoplasmic glycogen: a case report and histogenetic considerations. Cancer 980;45:553.
36. Mullins JD. A pigmented differentiating neuroblastoma: a light and ultrastructural study. Cancer 1980;46:522.
37. Shimada H, Chatten J, Newton WA, et al. Histopathologic prognostic factors in neuroblastic tumors: definition of subtypes of ganglioneuroblastoma and an age-linked classification of neuroblastomas. J Natl Cancer Inst 1984;73:405.
38. Joshi VV, Canter AB, Altshuler G, et al. Age-linked prognostic categorization based on a new histologic grading system of neuroblastomas: a clinicopathologic study of 211 cases from the Pediatric Oncology Group. Cancer 1992;69:2197.
39. Chatten J, Shimada H, Sather HN, et al. Prognostic value of histopathology in advanced neuroblastoma: a report from the Childrens Cancer Study Group. Hum Pathol 1988;19:1187.
40. Joshi VV, Chatten J, Sather HN, et al. Prognostic value of the Shimada classification in advanced neuroblastoma with a special reference to mitosis karyorrhexis index: a report from Childrens Cancer Group Study. Mod Pathol 1991;4:139.
41. Altman AJ, Baehner RL. Favorable prognosis for survival in children with coincident opso-myoclonus and neuroblastoma. Cancer 1976;37: 846.
42. Zeltzer PM, Marangos PJ, Evans AE, Schneider SL. Serum neuron-specific enolase in children with neuroblastoma: relationship to stage and disease course. Cancer 1986;57:1230.
43. Joshi VV, Canter AB, Brodeur GM, et al. Correlation between morphologic and other prognostic markers of neuroblastoma: a study of histologic grade, DNA index, N-*myc* gene copy number, and lactic dehydrogenase in patients in the Pediatric Oncology Group. Cancer 1993;71: 3173.
44. Silber JH, Evans AE, Fridman M. Models to predict outcome from childhood neuroblastoma: the role of serum ferritin and tumor histology. Cancer Res 1991;51:1426.
45. Valentino L, Moss T, Olson E, et al. Shed tumor gangliosides and progression of human neuroblastoma. Blood 1984;73:406.
46. Weith A, Martinsson T, Cziepluch C, et al. Neuroblastoma consensus deletion maps to chromosome 1p36.1–2. Genes Chromosom Cancer 1989;1:159.
47. Biedler JL, Meyers MB, Spengler BA. Homogeneously staining regions and double minute chromosomes: prevalent cytogenetic abnormalities of human neuroblastoma cells. Adv Cell Neurobiol 1983;4: 267.
48. Brenner DW, Barrance SC, Winslow BH, Shaeffer J. Flow cytometric analysis of DNA content in children with neuroblastoma. J Pediatr Surg 1989;24:204.
49. Seeger RC, Brodeur GM, Sather H, et al. Association of multiple copies of the N-*myc* oncogene with rapid progression of neuroblastomas. N Engl J Med 1985;313:1111.
50. Nakagawara A, Arima M, Scavarda NJ, Azar CG, Cantor AB, Brodeur GM. Association between high levels of expression of the *trk* gene and favorable outcome in human neuroblastoma. N Engl J Med 1993;328: 847.

Principles and Practice of Genitourinary Oncology, edited by Derek Raghavan, Howard I. Scher, Steven A. Leibel, and Paul H. Lange. Lippincott-Raven Publishers, Philadelphia, © 1997.

CHAPTER 107

Clinical Presentation, Patterns of Spread, Diagnosis, Staging, and Prognosis

Robert P. Castleberry, Jr.

CLINICAL PRESENTATION AND PATTERNS OF SPREAD

Neuroblastomas are malignant neoplasms derived from primordial neural crest cells that ultimately populate the sympathetic ganglia and adrenal medulla. The variety of tumor locations and degrees of histopathologic differentiation result in an array of tumors demonstrating diverse clinical and biologic characteristics and behavior. The frequency of primary tumor site is related to age at diagnosis (Table 107-1).[1] Most primary tumors occur within the abdomen (65%). The frequency of adrenal tumors is slightly higher in children (40%) than in infants (25%), and infants also have more thoracic and cervical primary tumors. In about 1% of patients, a primary tumor cannot be found.

Ninety percent of neuroblastoma cases are diagnosed by the age of 5 years, and more than 50% are detected in the first 2 years of life (Fig. 107-1).[1] Typically, the incidence shows a slight male predominance.

Both lymphatic and hematogenous metastatic spread of neuroblastoma occur. Regional lymph node metastases are noted in 35% of patients with apparently localized tumors. Spread of tumor to lymph nodes outside the cavity of origin is considered to be disseminated disease. These children may have a better outlook if there is no other metastatic disease.[2] Bone marrow, bone, liver, orbit, and skin are the most frequent sites of hematogenous spread. Rarely, disease may spread to lung and brain parenchyma, usually as a manifestation of relapsing or end-stage disease.

The proportion of patients presenting with localized, regional, or metastatic disease depends on age (Table 107-2).[1] the incidences of localized tumors, regional lymph node spread, and disseminated disease are 39%, 18%, and 25% (plus 18% stage IVs), respectively, in infants and 19%, 13%, and 68%, respectively, in older children.

The signs and symptoms of neuroblastoma reflect the location of primary, regional, and metastatic tumor deposits. Abdominal disease is associated with complaints of fullness, discomfort and, rarely, gastrointestinal tract dysfunction. A fixed, hard abdominal mass is commonly noted on physical examination. Primary tumors arising from the organ of Zuckerkandl often result in bladder and bowel symptoms related to organ compression. Massive involvement of the liver in metastatic disease (Pepper syndrome) is particularly frequent in infants and may result in respiratory compromise. Occasionally, the size of primary or metastatic abdominal tumor can result in compression of venous and lymphatic drainage from the lower extremities, leading to scrotal and lower extremity edema. Renin-mediated hypertension caused by compromise of renal vasculature is a rare event.[3,4] Because of the type of catecholamine metabolites released from most neuroblastomas, hypertension, tachycardia, flushing, and sweating are uncommon. Primary thoracic tumors are commonly diagnosed coincidentally when chest radiographs are obtained to evaluate patients for other reasons. High thoracic and cervical masses can be associated with Horner's syndrome (unilateral ptosis, myosis, and anhydrosis) or, if large, with mechanical obstruction and resultant superior vena cava syndrome.

Paraspinal tumors in the thoracic, abdominal, and pelvic regions may extend into the neuroforamina of the vertebral bodies (so-called dumbbell tumors) and result in symptoms related to compression of nerve roots and spinal cord. The range of symptomatology includes radicular pain, subacute or acute paraplegia, and bladder or bowel dysfunction. Most of these tumors have a low incidence of recurrent disease.

There are several classic signs and symptoms associated with metastatic disease. Retrobulbar and orbital infiltration with tumor are frequent, resulting in proptosis and periorbital ecchymoses. Widespread bone marrow and bone disease (Hutchinson syndrome) causes bone pain, which leads to limping and to irritability in the younger child. Skin involvement, characterized by variable numbers of nontender, bluish nodules, is seen exclusively in infants with Evans stage IVS tumors.[5] Constitutional symptoms associated with disseminated disease may include failure to thrive and fever, the latter observed most often in the presence of bone metastases.

Several unique paraneoplastic syndromes have been associated with both localized and disseminated neuroblastoma. Up to

TABLE 107-1. *Primary sites of neuroblastoma according to age*

Site	Age at diagnosis ≤1 year		Age at diagnosis >1 year		Total	
	No.	Percentage	No.	Percentage	No.	Percentage
Cervical	7	4	2	0.5	9	1
Thoracic	58	29	59	14	117	19
Abdominal						
Adrenal	50	25	171	40	221	35
Non-adrenal	51	26	136	32	187	30
Pelvic	5	3	11	2.5	16	2
Other	26	13	38	9	64	12
Unknown	0		8	2	8	1
Total	197		425		622	

Courtesy J. J. Shuster, PhD, Pediatric Oncology Group Statistical Office, Gainesville, FL. From Brodeur GM, Castleberry RP. Neuroblastoma. In: Pizzo PA, Poplack DG, eds. Principles and practice of pediatric oncology. Philadelphia, JB Lippincott, 1993:739.

4% of patients demonstrate opsomyoclonus (myoclonic jerking and random eye movement) or cerebellar ataxia, or both.[6–8] These symptoms often disappear with successful therapy and may be associated with a more favorable outcome.[7,8] Intractable secretory diarrhea, associated with hypokalemia and dehydration (Kerner-Morrison syndrome), is a manifestation of tumor secretion of vasoactive intestinal peptides.[9,10] More frequently associated with ganglioneuroblastomas or ganglioneuromas, these symptoms resolve only after eradication of the offending tumor.

DIAGNOSIS

By international agreement, a diagnosis of neuroblastic tumor must at a minimum meet one of the following criteria: (1) unequivocal pathologic diagnosis from tumor tissue by light microscopy with or without immunohistology, electron microscopy, and increased urine or serum catecholamines or metabolites; or (2) bone marrow aspirate or trephine biopsy containing unequivocal tumor cells, and increased urine or serum catecholamines or metabolites.[11,12] Random urine samples for homovanillic acid and vanillylmandelic acid are recommended because age-related normal values standardized per milligram of creatinine are available. Levels that are three standard deviations or more above the mean for age are considered elevated. Strict adherence to these criteria could discourage the sampling of primary or metastatic tumors for biologic characterization, which is becoming increasingly important in treatment planning. Minimally invasive procedures, such a ultrasound-guided needle biopsies, have proven to be safe and reliable ways to obtain tissue for diagnosis and for biologic studies if open biopsy is not required or feasible.[13,14]

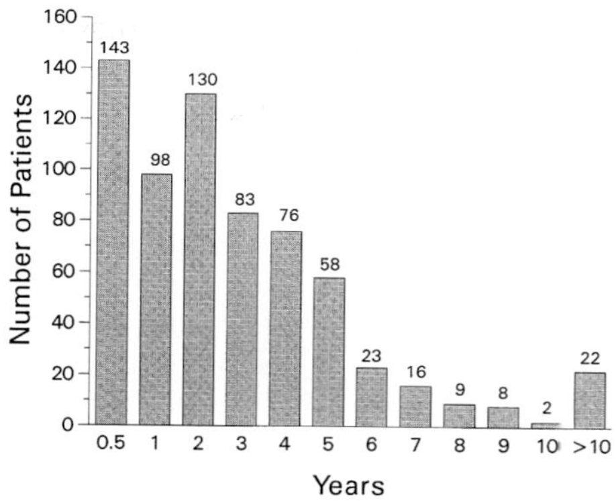

FIG. 107-1. Age at diagnosis for 668 consecutive patients with neuroblastoma treated in the Pediatric Oncology Group between 1981 and 1989. More than 50% of cases are detected by 2 years of age, and 90% by age 5 years. (Courtesy of J.J. Shuster, PhD, Pediatric Oncology Group Statistical Office, Gainesville, FL).

The typical histopathologic features of neuroblastoma include uniformly sized cells with dense, hyperchromatic nuclei and scant cytoplasm and the presence of neuritic processes, or neuropil (see Chap. 106). In 15% to 50% of tumors, Homer Wright rosettes are observed.[15] Immunohistochemistry and electron microscopy are often helpful for differentiating neuroblastoma from other "small blue round cell" neoplasms of childhood, such as Ewing's sarcoma, non-Hodgkin lymphoma, primitive neuroectodermal tumor, and undifferentiated soft tissue sarcoma such a rhabdomyosarcoma.[16–19]

Diagnostic imaging is both supportive of the diagnosis of neuroblastoma and helpful in determining extent of disease. Computed tomography, magnetic resonance imaging, and ultrasound scanning allow three-dimensional assessment of primary and metastatic tumor volumes. Bony involvement should be ascertained with both plain radiographs and ^{99m}Tc-diphosphonate scanning.[20,21] If available, ^{131}I- or ^{123}I-metaiodobenzylguanidine (MIBG) scintigraphy may be informative regarding deposits of tumor. International convention suggests that bone marrow infiltration be assessed with bilateral posterior iliac crest marrow aspirates and trephine bone marrow biopsies.[12] Immunohistologic methods to detect neuroblastoma in bone marrow are currently under investigation to determine the meaning of positive results at diagnosis and after therapy.[22,23]

STAGING

Several systems for the clinical or surgicopathologic staging of neuroblastoma are currently being used. The prevailing methods are the clinical system reported by Evans and colleagues[24] and now employed by the Children's Cancer Group (CCG), the surgicopathologic staging developed at St. Jude Children's

TABLE 107-2. *Extent of disease at diagnosis according to age*

Site at diagnosis	Age at diagnosis ≤1 year		Age at diagnosis >1 year		Total	
	No.	Percentage	No.	Percentage	No.	Percentage
Localized	93	39	83	19	176	26
Regional	43	18	54	13	97	15
Disseminated	61	25	290	68	351	52
Stage IVS	44	18	0	0	44	7
Total	241		427		668	

Courtesy J. J. Shuster, PhD, Pediatric Oncology Group Statistical Office, Gainesville, FL. From Brodeur GM, Castleberry RP. Neuroblastoma. In: Pizzo PA, Poplack DG, eds. Principles and practice of pediatric oncology. Philadelphia, JB Lippincott, 1993:739.

Research Hospital and subsequently modified for use by the Pediatric Oncology Group (POG),[25] and the tumor-nodes-metastasis method adopted by the Union International Contre le Cancer.[26] Although most staging schema agree regarding the definitions of completely resected, localized tumors or widely disseminated disease, there is diversity in criteria for and natural history implications of localized unresected tumors, regional lymph node spread, and large midline tumors. These discrepancies have impeded the comparison of data among therapeutic trials and biologic studies. A comparison of the CCG and POG methods, for example, reveals problematic differences (Table 107-3).[1] A tumor extending in continuity across the midline but completely removed and with no involved lymph nodes would be scored a CCG stage III but a POG stage A. Similarly, interpretation of the prognostic impact of nonadherent, ipsilateral and contralateral lymph node metastases cannot be resolved between the CCG and POG criteria.

In 1987, representatives from eleven countries met[11,12] to develop standard criteria for staging that would have universal appeal and acceptance: the International Staging System, or INSS (see Table 107-3). The INSS combined the effective portions of other clinical and surgicopathologic systems with several definitions that deal specifically with the staging controversies mentioned previously. Stage 1 allowed for both the presence of microscopic residual disease and involvement of adherent lymph nodes, a feature not thought to affect outcome.[27] Localized unresected tumors were divided into two categories (stages 2A and 2B) to clearly distinguish between patients with and without positive ipsilateral or contralateral, nonadherent lymph nodes. The inference of midline tumors was clarified to indicate infiltration across, and not simply hanging over, the midline. Midline tumors without regional lymph node involvement or disseminated disease were classified stage 1, 2A, or 3 depending on degree of surgical resection. Although not addressing all contingencies, the INSS has been validated to identify prognostic subsets of patients.[28] The universal implementation of INSS has made possible the creation and assessment of risk groups based on age, INSS stage, and biologic characteristics. The prognostic strength of selected biologic features in neuroblastoma should reduce reliance on age and stage alone to determine treatment.

PROGNOSTIC CONSIDERATIONS

Clinical Features

After the classic report by Breslow and McCann,[29] stage of disease and patient age have proved to be the most influential factors regarding treatment planning based on risk for recurrent disease. Patients with localized or limited regional disease (INSS stages 1, 2A, and 2B) experience statistically significantly better survival than those with extensive unresected tumors or metastatic disease (INSS stages 3 and 4). Further, patients younger than 1 year of age at diagnosis have, in general, a superior outcome compared with older children having the same stage of disease.

The site of primary tumor may also affect outcome, with tumors arising in the adrenal gland being associated with higher risk for recurrent disease than those in the thorax.[30–33] If other clinical and biologic factors are considered, however, it is unclear whether primary tumor site is an independent prognostic variable.[33]

Histopathologic features, scored according to the Shimada classification[34] and its modification by Joshi,[35] have prognostic importance. The presence of opsomyoclonus may portend a better outlook.[7,8]

Elevated serum levels of lactate dehydrogenase (>1500 U/mL),[36] ferritin (>142 ng/dL),[37,38] and neuron-specific enolase (>100 ng/mL),[39,40] most likely reflecting rapid tumor cell turnover, have been associated with inferior survival rates. Although these markers are not observed exclusively in neuroblastoma, evaluation of them may assist in treatment planning and monitoring of disease activity. The utility and prognostic impact of other peptides released from neuroblastic tumors, chromogranin A,[41] the ganglioside G_{D2},[42–44] and neuropeptide Y[45,46] are still being investigated.

Biologic Features: Clinical Implications

The protooncogene, *MYCN* (formerly N-*myc*), is amplified in approximately 30% of neuroblastomas and is associated with advanced disease at diagnosis and poor survival prognosis, regardless of stage or patient age[47–49] (see also Chaps. 105 and 106). Almost all tumors cells with amplified *MYCN* also have increased *MYCN* expression, but *MYCN* expression in the absence of amplification is not necessarily associated with poor outcome.[50,51] *MYCN* copy number is a stable feature between primary tumor and metastatic deposits and does not appear to change over time.[52]

Tumor DNA content (ploidy), is a powerful independent predictor of response to therapy and outcome in infants (<1 year of age) and to some extent in children between 1 and 2 years of age.[53–56] Tumors exhibiting hyperdiploid or increased DNA content are associated with lower stages of disease at diagnosis

TABLE 107-3. *Comparison of staging systems for neuroblastoma*

Extent of disease	Children's Cancer Group System	Pediatric Oncology Group System	International Staging System
Localized, resected	Stage I. Tumor confined to the organ or structure of origin.	A. Complete gross resection of primary tumor, with or without microscopic residual tumor; intracavitary lymph nodes not adhered to and removed with the primary tumor must be histologically free of tumor; if primary is in abdomen/pelvis, liver must be histologically free of tumor.	1. Localized tumor confiend to the area of origin; complete gross excision with or without microscopic residual disease; identifiable ipsilateral and contralateral lymph nodes negative microscopically.
Localized, unresected	Stage II. Tumor extending in continuity beyond the organ or structure of origin, but not crossing the mid-line; regional lymph nodes on the ipsilateral side may be involved.	B. Grossly unresected primary tumor; lymph nodes/liver as for stage A.	2A. Unilateral tumor with incomplete gross excision; identifiable ipsilateral and contralateral lymph nodes negative microscopically.
Regional lymph node	Stage II. Tumor extending in continuity beyond the organ or structure of origin, but not crossing the mid-line; regional lymph nodes on the ipsilateral side may be involved Stage III. Tumor extending in continuity beyond the mid-line. Regional lymph nodes may be involved bilaterally.	C. Complete or incomplete resection of primary; intracavitary lymph nodes not adhered to and removed with the primary tumor histologically positive for tumor; liver as in stage A.	2B. Unilateral tumor with complete or incomplete gross excision; with positive ipsilateral regional lymph nodes; identifiable contra-lateral lymph nodes negative microscopically. 3. Tumor infiltrating across the midline with or without regional lymph nodes involvement; or, unilateral tumor with contralateral regional lymph node involvement; or midline tumor with bilateral regional lymph node involvement.
Metastatic	Stage IV. Remote disease involving the skeleton, bone marrow, soft tissue and distant lymph node groups.	D. Any dissemination of disease beyond cavitary nodes.	4. Dissemination of tumor to distant lymph nodes, bone, bone marrow, liver and or other organs.
Special metastatic	Stage IVS. As defined in stage I/ II, except remote disease confined to the liver, skin, or bone marrow (without bone metastases).	Ds. Infants with IVS disease as defined by CCG.	4s. Localized primary tumor as defined for stage I or 2A with dissemination limited to liver, skin or bone marrow.

From Brodeur GM, Castleberry RP. Neuroblastoma. In: Pizzo PA, Poplack DG, eds. Principles and Practice of Pediatric Oncology. Philadelphia, JB Lippincott, 1993:739.

and a more favorable outlook. In contrast, those with diploid or normal DNA content have lower response rates to cyclophosphamide and doxorubicin and an inferior disease-free survival rate.[56] Ploidy has limited predictive ability in children older than 2 years of age at diagnosis.[53,56] Because the presence of *MYCN* amplification or diploid DNA content identifies almost all infants who are destined to have recurrent or progressive disease, therapeutic trials in infant neuroblastoma are now being conducted in which treatment is based on these two biologic variables.[57]

There appears to be a strong correlation between deletions of chromosome 1p and poor prognosis.[58–61] Because this feature is often associated with *MYCN* amplification, it remains to be proven conclusively that 1p deletions are independently prognostic.

The *TRK* protooncogene encodes for a family of transmem-

TABLE 107-4. *Genetic subtypes of neuroblastoma*

Feature	Type 1	Type 2	Type 3
Age	Usually <12 mo	Usually ≥12 mo	Usually ≥12 mo
INSS stage	Usually 1, 2, 4s	Usually 3, 4	Usually 3, 4
Ploidy	Hyperdiploid or triploid	Near-diploid or near-tetraploid	Near-diploid or near-tetraploid
MYCN gene	Normal	Normal	Amplified
Chromosome 1p	Normal	Normal	±LOH
TRK expression	High	Intermediate	Low or absent
Survival rate	>95%	25%–50%	About 5%

INSS, International Staging System; LOH, loss of heterozygosity.

From Brodeur GM, ar C, Brother M, et al. Neuroblastom: effect of genetic factors on prognosis and treatment. Cancer 1992;70:1685.

TABLE 107-5. *Proposed prognostic strata for neuroblastoma based on INSS stage,* MYCN *copy number, and DNA ploidy*

Risk category (survival rate)	Age (years)	INSS stage	*MYCN* copy no.	DNA index
Low (>90%)	<1	1, 2A, 2B, 3, 4, 4s	1	>1
	≥1	1, 2A	1	NA
Intermediate (30%–50%)	<1	2A, 2B, 3, 4, 4s	1	>1
	≥1	2B, 3	1	NA
High (>20%)	<1	2A, 2B, 3, 4, 4s	>1	1 or >1
	≥1	2B, 3	>1	NA
	≥1	4	1	NA
Unclear	<1	1	>1*	1*
	≥1	1	>1	NA

INSS, International Staging System; NA = not applicable.
* Either >1 *MYCN* copy number or DNA index of 1, or both of these characteristics.
From Castleberry RP. Clinical and biologic features in the prognosis and treatment of neuroblastoma. Curr Opin Oncol 1992;4:116.

brane tyrosine kinases that serve as receptors for a number of neurotrophic factors. Of particular interest in neuroblastoma is *TRKA,* which encodes for the high-affinity receptor for nerve growth factor (NGF).[62] If expressed in high levels, *TRKA* is associated with lower stage tumors, younger age, and normal *MYCN* copy number and is strongly predictive of favorable outcome.[63–66] A similar relation is suggested from preliminary studies of *NGFR*, the low-affinity NGF receptor.[65]

With the frequency of drug resistance observed in high-risk neuroblastoma, studies of the expression of P-glycoprotein, a transmembrane efflux protein encoded by *PGY1* (formerly *MDR1*), have produced conflicting results regarding correlation with outcome.[67–71] The technical difficulties inherent in determining P-glycoprotein expression and the absence of prospective, longitudinal studies are contributing factors to these observations. Further prospective investigations regarding the prognostic impact of P-glycoprotein expression in neuroblasotma are required before assessing the therapeutic value of *PGY1* reversing agents such as cyclosporine.

Other molecular and cell biologic features currently under investigation include microtubular associated proteins,[72,73] loss of heterozygosity of chromosome 14,[60,74–76] smg-p25A,[77] *SRC*,[78] and *HRAS* (formerly c-Ha-*ras*).[79–81] These studies will probably provide further insight into the biologic heterogeneity of neuroblastoma and may be useful for developing future treatment strategies.

Prognostic Groups

Based on current clinical and laboratory data, three biologic subtypes of neuroblastoma have been suggested (Table 107-4).[82] Type 1 usually occurs in infants, and it is associated with low-stage disease, hyperdiploid, *MYCN*-nonamplified, *TRK*-expressing, biologically favorable tumors and survival rates of more than 95%. Type 2 is seen in older children with biologically favorable tumors but more advanced clinical disease and has a predicted long-term survival rate of 25% to 50%. Type 3 is observed in older children with advanced clinical disease and biologically unfavorable tumors; the survival rate is typically less than 5%.

Although hypothetical and continually evolving, biologic groupings of this nature serve as a foundation for determining treatment according to predicted risk for recurrent disease. One such risk stratification that combines age, INSS stage, *MYCN* copy number, and tumor DNA content is currently being employed in the POG (Table 107-5) to route patients into therapeutic studies in which patients of similar risk receive similar therapy.[83] The INSS committee is currently developing a statistically valid and universally accepted set of prognostic groupings in neuroblastoma, the International Neuroblastoma Risk Groups or INRG,[12] which employs the most powerful clinical and biologic prognostic features available to date. Inherent to the INRG is the flexibility to periodically modify these prognostic subsets to account for new biologic information. The INRG affords the ability for working groups worldwide to collaborate in clinical trials and to compare data as has not been possible before.

REFERENCES

1. Brodeur GM, Castleberry RP. Neuroblastoma. In: Pizzo PA, Poplack DG, eds. Principles and practice of pediatric oncology. Philadelphia, JB Lippincott, 1993:739.
2. Rosen EM, Cassady JR, Frantz CN, et al. Neuroblastoma: The Joint Center for Radiation Therapy/Dana-Farber Cancer Institute/Children's Hospital experience. J Clin Oncol 1984;2:714.
3. Kedar A, Glassman M, Voorhess ML, et al. Severe hypertension in a child with ganglioneuroblastoma. Cancer 1981;47:2077.
4. Weinblatt ME, Heisel MA, Siegel SE. Hypertension in children with neurogenic tumors. Pediatrics 1983;71:947.
5. D'Angio GJ, Evans AE, Koop CE. Special pattern of widespread neuroblastoma with a favorable prognosis. Lancet 1971;1:1046.
6. Roberts KB, Freeman JM. Cerebellar ataxia and "occult neuroblastoma" without opsoclonus. Pediatrics 1975;56:464.
7. Altman AJ, Baehner RL. Favorable prognosis for survival in children with coincident opsomyoclonus and neuroblastoma. Cancer 1976;37:846.
8. Pranzatelli MR. The neurobiology of the opsoclonus-myoclonus syndrome. Clin Neuropharmacol 1992;15:186.
9. Kaplan S, Holbrook C, McDaniel H, Buntain W, Crist W. Vasoactive intestinal peptide secreting tumors of childhood. Am J Dis Child 1980;134:21.
10. El Shafie M, Samuel D, Klippel CH, et al. Intractable diarrhea in children with VIP-secreting ganglioneuroblastoma. J Pediatr Surg 1983;18:34.
11. Brodeur GM, Seeger RC, Barrett A, et al. International criteria for diagnosis, staging, and response to treatment in patients with neuroblastoma. J Clin Oncol 1988;6:1874.
12. Brodeur GM, Pritchard J, Berthold F, et al. Revisions of the interna-

tional criteria for neuroblastoma diagnosis, staging, and response to treatment. J Clin Oncol 1993;11:1466.
13. Parker SH, Hopper KD, Yakes WF, Gibson MD, Ownbey JL, Carter TE. Image directed percutaneous biopsies with a biopsy gun. Radiology 1989;171:663.
14. Hedborg F, Lindgren PG, Johansson I, et al: N-*myc* gene amplification in neuroblastoma: a clinical approach using ultrasound guided cutting needle biopsies collected at diagnosis. Med Pediatr Oncol 1992;20: 292.
15. Russell DS, Rubenstein LJ. Tumors of peripheral neuroblasts and ganglion cells. In: Russell DS, Rubenstein LJ, eds. Pathology of tumors of the central nervous system. Baltimore, Williams & Wilkins, 1989: 900.
16. Shimada H. Transmission and scanning electron microscopic studies on the tumors of neuroblastoma group. Acta Pathol Jpn 1982:32:415.
17. Dehner LP: Pathologic anatomy of classic neuroblastoma: including prognostic features and differential diagnosis. In: Pochedly C, ed. Neuroblastoma: tumor biology and therapy. Boca Raton, FL, CRC Press, 1990:111.
18. Delellis RA. The adrenal glands. In: Sternbert SS, ed. Diagnostic surgical pathology. New York, Raven Press, 1989:445.
19. Triche TJ, Askin FB, Kissane JM. Neuroblastoma, Ewing's sarcoma, and the differential diagnosis of small-, round-, blue-cell tumors. In: Finegold M, ed. Pathology of neoplasia in children and adolescents. Philadelphia, WB Saunders, 1986:145.
20. Heisel MA, Miller JH, Reid BS, Siegel SE. Radionuclide bone scan in neuroblastoma. Pediatrics 1983;71:206.
21. Kaufman RA, Thrall JH, Keyes JW, et al. False negative bone scans in neuroblastoma metastatic to the ends of long bones. Roentgenology 1978;130:131.
22. Donner K, Triche TJ, Israel MA, et al. A panel of monoclonal antibodies which discriminate neuroblastoma from Ewing's sarcoma, rhabdomyosarcoma, neuroepithelioma, and hematopoietic malignancies. Prog Clin Biol Res 1985;175:347.
23. Moss TJ, Seeger RC, Kindler-Rohrborn A, et al. Immunohistologic detection and phenotyping of neuroblastoma cells in bone marrow using cytoplasmic neuron specific enolase and cell surface antigens. Prog Clin Biol Res 1985;175:367.
24. Evans AE, D'Angio GJ, Randolf JA. A proposed staging for children with neuroblastoma: Children's Cancer Study Group A. Cancer 1971; 27:374.
25. Nitschke R, Smith EI, Altshuler G, et al. Postoperative treatment of nonmetastatic visible residual neuroblastoma: a Pediatric Oncology Group study. J Clin Oncol 1991;9:1181.
26. American Joint Committee on Cancer. Neuroblastoma. In: Manual for staging of cancer, 2nd ed. Philadelphia, JB Lippincott, 1983:237.
27. Smith IE, Nitschke R, Shochat S, et al. Lack of significance of involved lymph nodes attached to localized neuroblastoma: a Pediatric Oncology Group study. Proc Amer Soc Clin Oncol 1987;6:219.
28. Castleberry RP, Shuster JJ, Smith EI. The Pediatric Oncology Group experience with the international staging system criteria for neuroblastoma. J Clin Oncol 1994;12:2378.
29. Breslow N, McCann B. Statistical estimation of prognosis of children with neuroblastoma. Cancer Res 1971;31:2101.
30. Coldman AJ, Fryer CJH, Elwood JM, Sonley MJ. Neuroblastoma: influence of age at diagnosis, stage, tumor site, and sex on prognosis. Cancer 1980;46:1896.
31. Carlsen NLT, Christensen IJ, Schroeder H, et al. Prognostic factors in neuroblastomas treated in Denmark from 1943 to 1980: a statistical estimate of prognosis based on 253 cases. Cancer 1986;58:2726.
32. Evans AE, D'Angio GJ, Propert K, Anderson J, Hann H-WL. Prognostic factors in neuroblastoma. Cancer 1987;59:1853.
33. Adams GA, Shochat SJ, Smith EI, et al. Thoracic neuroblastoma: a Pediatric Oncology Group study. J Pediatr Surg 1993;28:372.
34. Shimada H, Chatten J, Newton WA, et al. Histopathologic prognostic factors in neuroblastic tumors: definition of subtypes of ganglioneuroblastoma and an age-linked classification of neuroblastomas. J Natl Cancer Inst 1984;73:405.
35. Joshi VV, Cantor AB, Altshuler G, et al. Age-linked prognostic categorization based on a new histologic grading system of neuroblastomas. Cancer 1992;69:2197.
36. Shuster JJ, McWilliams NB, Castleberry RP, et al. Serum lactate dehydrogenase in childhood neuroblastoma: a Pediatric Oncology Group recursive partitioning study. Am J Clin Oncol 1992;15:295.
37. Hann HWL, Evans AE, Siegel SE, et al. Prognostic importance of serum ferritin in patients with stages III and IV neuroblastoma: The Children's Cancer Study Group experience. Cancer Res 1985;45:2843.
38. Hann HWL, Stahlhut MW, Evans AE. Serum ferritin as a prognostic indicator in neuroblastoma: biological effects of isoferritins. Prog Clin Biol Res 1985;175:331.
39. Marangos P. Clinical studies with neuron specific enolase. Prog Clin Biol Res 1985;175:285.
40. Tsuchida Y, Honna T, Iwanaka T, et al. Serial determination of serum neuron-specific enolase in patients with neuroblastoma and other pediatric tumors. J Pediatr Surg 1987;22:419.
41. Hsiao RJ, Seeger RC, Yu AL, O'Connor DT. Chromogranin A in children with neuroblastoma. J Clin Invest 1990;85:1555.
42. Ladisch S, Wu Z-L. Circulating gangliosides as tumor markers. Prog Clin Biol Res 1985;175:277.
43. Schengrund CL, Repman MA, Shochat SJ. Ganglioside composition of human neuroblastomas: correlation with prognosis. A Pediatric Oncology Group study. Cancer 1985;56:2640.
44. Valentino L, Moss T, Olson E, Wange HJ, Elashoff R, Ladisch S. Shed tumor gangliosides and progression of human neuroblastoma. Blood 1990;75:1564.
45. Kogner P, Theodorsson E, Bjork O. Plasma neuropeptide Y (NPY): a novel marker of neuroblastoma. Prog Clin Biol Res 1991;366:367.
46. Kogner P, Bjork O, Theodorsson E. Neuropeptide Y in neuroblastoma: increased concentration in metastasis, release during surgery, and characterization of plasma and tumor extracts. Med Pediatr Oncol 1993; 21:317.
47. Brodeur GM, Seeger RC, Schwab, Amplification of N-*myc* in untreated human neuroblastomas correlates with advanced disease stage. Science 1984;224:1121.
48. Seeger RC, Brodeur GM, Sather H, et al. Association of multiple copies of the N-*myc* oncogene with rapid progression of neuroblastomas. N Engl J Med 1985;313:1111.
49. Brodeur GM: Molecular biology and genetics of human neuroblastoma. In: Pochedly C, ed. Neuroblastoma: tumor biology and therapy. Boca Raton, FL, CRC Press, 1990:32.
50. Schwab M, Ellison J, Busch M, et al. Enhanced expression of the human gene N-*myc* consequent to amplification of DNA may contribute to malignant progression of neuroblastoma. Proc Natl Acad Sci U S A 1984;81:4940.
51. Seeger RC, Wada R, Brodeur GM, et al. Expression of N-*myc* by neuroblastomas with one or multiple copies of the oncogene. Prog Clin Biol Res 1988;271:41.
52. Brodeur GM, Hayes FA, Green AA, et al. Consistent N-*myc* copy number in simultaneous or consecutive neuroblastoma samples from sixty individual patients. Cancer 1987;47:4248.
53. Look AT, Hayes FA, Nitschke R, et al. Cellular DNA content as a predictor of response to chemotherapy in infants with unresectable neuroblastoma. N Engl J Med 1984;311:231.
54. Oppedal BR, Storm-Mathisen I, Lie SO, Brandtzaeg P. Prognostic factors in neuroblastoma: clinical, histopathologic immunohistochemical features and DNA ploidy in relation to prognosis. Cancer 1988;72:772.
55. Cohn SL, Rademaker AW, Salwen HR, et al. Analysis of DNA ploidy and proliferative activity in relation to histology and N-*myc* amplification in neuroblastoma. Am J Pathol 1990;136:1043.
56. Look AT, Shuster JJ, Douglass EC, Castleberry RP, Brodeur GM. Clinical relevance of tumor cell ploidy and N-*myc* gene amplification in childhood neuroblastoma: a Pediatric Oncology Group study. J Clin Oncol 1991;9:581.
57. Bowman LC, Castleberry RP, Altshuler G, et al. Therapy based on DNA index (DI) for infants with unresectable and disseminated neuroblastoma (NB): preliminary results of the Pediatric Oncology Group "better risk" study. Med Pediatr Oncol 1990;18:364.
58. Fong CT, Dracopoli NC, White PS, et al. Loss of heterozygosity for the short arm of chromosome 1 in human neuroblastomas: correlation with N-*myc* amplification. Proc Natl Acad Sci U S A 1989;86: 3753–3757.
59. Hayashi Y, Kanda N, Inaba T, et al. Cytogenetic findings and prognosis in neuroblastoma with emphasis on marker chromosome 1. Cancer 1989;63:126.
60. Fong CT, White PS, Peterson K, et al. Loss of heterozygosity for chromosomes 1 or 14 defines subsets of advanced neuroblastomas. Cancer Res 1992;52:1780.
61. Christiansen H, Schestag J, Christiansen NM, Grzeschik KH, Lampert

F. Clinical impact of chromosome 1 aberrations in neuroblastoma: a metaphase and interphase cytogenetic study. Genes Chromosom Cancer 1992;5:141.

62. Persson H, Ibanex CF. Role and expression of neurotropins and the *trk* family of tyrosine kinase receptors in neural growth and rescue after injury. Curr Opin Neurol Neurosurg 1993;6:11.
63. Nakagawara A, Arima M, Azar CG, Scavarda NJ, Brodeur GM. Inverse relationship between *trk* expression and N-*myc* amplification in human neuroblastomas. Cancer Res 1992;52:1364.
64. Nakagawara A, Arima-Nakagawara M, Scavarda NJ, Azar CG, Cantor AB, Brodeur GM. Association between high levels of expression of the *trk* gene and favorable outcome in human neuroblastoma. N Engl J Med 1993;328:847.
65. Kogner P, Barbany G, Dominici C, Castello MA, Raschella G, Persson H. Coexpression of mRNA for *trk* protooncogene and low affinity nerve growth factor receptor in neuroblastoma with favorable prognosis. Cancer Res 1993;53:1.
66. Suzuki T, Bogenmann E, Shimada H, Stram D, Seeger RC. Lack of high-affinity nerve growth factor receptors in aggressive neuroblastomas. J Natl Cancer Inst 1993;85:377.
67. Goldstein LJ, Fojo AT, Ueda K, et al. Expression of the multidrug resistance, *MDR1*, gene in neuroblastomas. J Clin Oncol 1990;8:128.
68. Bourhis J, Hartmann O, DeVathaire F, et al. Expression of *MDR1* and *GST* pi genes in 35 advanced neuroblastomas. Prog Clin Biol Res 1991; 366:127.
69. Chan HS, Haddad G, Thorner PS, et al. P-glycoprotein expression as a predictor of the outcome of therapy for neuroblastoma. N Engl J Med 1991;325:1608.
70. Bates SE, Shieh CY, Tsokos M. Expression of *mdr-1*/P-glycoprotein in human neuroblastoma. Am J Pathol 1991;139:305.
71. Favrot M, Combaret V, Goillot E, et al. Expression of P-glycoprotein restricted to normal cells in neuroblastoma biopsies. Br J Cancer 1991; 64:233.
72. Loomis PA, Howard TH, Castleberry RP, Binder LI. Identification of nuclear isoforms in human neuroblastoma cells. Proc Natl Acad Sci U S A 1990;87:8522.
73. Sternberg H, Mesco G, Cole G, Timiras PS. Tau protein: its presence and metabolism in human neuroblastoma cells. Adv Exp Med Biol 1990;265:283.
74. Suzuki T, Mugishima H, Fujisawa T, et al. Loss of heterozygosity on chromosome 14 in neuroblastoma. Prog Clin Biol Res 1991;366:135.
75. Srivatsan ES, Murali V, Seeger RC. Loss of heterozygosity for alleles on chromosomes 11q and 14q in neuroblastoma. Prog Clin Biol Res 1991;366:91.
76. Takayama H, Suzuki T, Mugishima H, et al. Deletion mapping of chromosomes 14q and 1p in human neuroblastoma. Oncogene 1992; 7:1185.
77. Sano K, Nakamura H, Mabuchi S, et al. Expression of the smg p25A (a ras p21-like GTP-binding protein) gene in human neuroblastoma cell lines and tumor tissues. Cancer Res 1990;50:7242.
78. Matsunaga T, Takahashi H, Ohnuma N, et al. Expression of N-*myc* and c-*src* protooncogenes correlating to the undifferentiated phenotype and prognosis of primary neuroblastomas. Cancer Res 1991;51:3148.
79. Bjelfman C, Hedborg F, Johansson I, Nordenskjold M, Pahlman S. Expression of the neuronal form of pp60c-*src* in neuroblastoma in relation to clinical stage and prognosis. Cancer Res 1990;50:6908.
80. Tanaka T, Slamon DJ, Shimada H, et al: A significant association of Ha-*ras* p21 in neuroblastoma cells with patient prognosis: a retrospective study of 103 cases. Cancer 1991;68:1296.
81. Moley JF, Brother MB, Wells SA, Spengler BA, Biedler JL, Brodeur GM. Low frequency of *ras* gene mutations in neuroblastomas, pheochromocytomas, and medullary thyroid cancers. Cancer Res 1991;51: 1596.
82. Brodeur GM, Azar C, Brother M, et al. Neuroblastoma: effect of genetic factors on prognosis and treatment. Cancer 1992;70:1685.
83. Castleberry RP. Clinical and biologic features in the prognosis and treatment of neuroblastoma. Curr Opin Oncol 1992;4:116.

Principles and Practice of Genitourinary Oncology, edited by Derek Raghavan, Howard I. Scher, Steven A. Leibel, and Paul H. Lange. Lippincott-Raven Publishers, Philadelphia, © 1997.

CHAPTER 108

Low-Risk and Intermediate-Risk Neuroblastoma

Brian H. Kushner, Nai-Kong V. Cheung, and Michael P. LaQuaglia

Neuroblastoma stands out among pediatric solid tumors because of its relative frequency, enigmatic natural history, distinctive biologic features, and challenging therapeutic demands. It derives from precursors of the sympathetic nervous system. Neuroblastoma is the most common extracranial solid tumor of childhood[1] and the most common neoplasm of infants.[2] More than 90% of the 500 cases diagnosed annually in the United States involve children 5 years old or younger.[1] Many cases no doubt escape detection because of spontaneous regression or maturation into benign lesions.[3]

At diagnosis, neuroblastoma, unlike most solid cancers, is usually already disseminated beyond the primary site. Cure rates of patients diagnosed when older than 1 to 2 years of age with metastases to bone and bone marrow are lower than 20% despite aggressive multimodality therapy. In sharp contrast, patients with localized disease and infants with widespread disease have high cure rates, often with little or no therapeutic intervention other than surgery. No other well-defined oncologic entity includes subtypes that are cured without further treatment when documented disease is left behind after surgery or the disease process involves multiple sites (stage 4S, discussed later). Biologic markers clearly distinguish good-risk from poor-risk forms of neuroblastoma, allowing identification of patients who, despite a favorable clinical profile (e.g., localized tumor), are likely to develop lethal metastatic disease.

PATHOGENESIS

The young age of most patients with neuroblastoma and the postmitotic state of cells comprising the mature sympathetic nervous system suggest that causative insults occur early in life or affect parental germ cells. Although some epidemiologic studies and case reports implicate environmental teratogenic-oncogenic events,[4] the fairly uniform worldwide incidence of neuroblastoma suggests that most cases result from random genetic mutations. No excessive association with idiopathic developmental defects, other than a possible increased frequency of skull and brain anomalies,[5] has been noted. The synchronous occurrence of neuroblastoma and other neurocristopathies (i.e., entities of neural crest origin), such as neurofibromatosis,[6] are intriguing in terms of implicating a common genetic origin, but its rarity suggests a random association. The same conclusion applies to the occasional development of neuroblastoma in patients with nonneural genetic disorders such as cystic fibrosis[7] or Beckwith-Wiedemann syndrome.[8] Concordance for neuroblastoma in monozygotic siblings during infancy implicates hereditary pathogenetic factors, whereas discordance in older twins favors random mutations as underlying events.[9]

Familial aggregations of neuroblastoma and the phenomenon of multifocal tumors were the basis for Knudsen's "two-hit hypothesis," which states that two genetic abnormalities in a single cell are prerequisites for malignant transformation.[10,11] In this scheme, oncogenic events involve deletion or mutation of a critical allele, followed by the inactivation or loss of the homologous gene on the sister chromosome. In sporadic or random cases, both mutations are postzygotic events. In familial cases, the first hit is an inherited germ-line mutation; this predisposes to early tumor development and the occurrence of multiple primary tumors. Knudsen's model is compatible with the antioncogene or suppressor gene theory of tumorigenesis. Definitive identification of an antioncogene is being sought, with particular attention focused on the short arm of chromosome 1 because of the increased frequency of chromosome 1p deletions in established neuroblastoma cell lines and in tumors from patients who died of disease.[12]

DIAGNOSIS AND CLINICAL PRESENTATION

Neuroblastoma is diagnosed by characteristic histopathologic findings (i.e., neural or ganglionic features) or the presence of tumor cell clumps or syncytia in the bone marrow, plus elevations of one or more urinary catecholamines; vanillylmandelic acid (VMA) and homovanillic acid (HVA) are the two most commonly measured.[13]

Neuroblastomas usually present with symptoms and signs attributable to local effects of primary or metastatic tumor. Although metastatic neuroblastoma arises most often in the retroperitoneum, 50% or more of localized neuroblastomas occur in extraabdominal locations, particularly the posterior mediastinum. Paraspinal neuroblastomas have a tendency to grow through intervertebral foramina (i.e., "dumbbell" tumors); spinal cord compression may result. Pelvic tumors may cause obstructive genitourinary problems. Upper thoracic or cervical involvement may be confused with infectious lymphadenitis, impinge on the upper airway, and cause Horner's syndrome. Multiple primary lesions can occur and may reflect an inherited predisposition.[10,11] Infants with low-risk or moderate-risk forms of widespread neuroblastoma typically come to medical attention because of tumor nodules in skin or, more often, abdominal distention from large liver tumors.

Elevated levels of catecholamines may cause hypertension,[14] but marked paroxysmal effects from catecholamine release, as seen in pheochromocytomas, are uncommon in neuroblastoma. Hypertension in patients with neuroblastoma is more commonly renin associated, the consequence of ureteral obstruction by tumor.

Unsuspected neuroblastomas may be detected during routine physical examination, by screening for urinary catecholamines as in neonatal screening programs, or when imaging studies are performed for other reasons (e.g., antenatal ultrasonography or x-ray for suspected pneumonia).[15] Neuroblastomas occasionally present with paraneoplastic syndromes, which are clinical findings not directly resulting from mass effect. These remote effects include watery diarrhea and opsoclonus-myoclonus (i.e., ''dancing eyes, dancing feet''), which occasionally cause neuroblastoma to be mistaken for intestinal malabsorption disease or primary neurologic disorders. The diarrhea, which results from vasoactive intestinal peptide production by tumor cells,[16] resolves after complete tumor removal, but neurologic deterioration may not; myoclonic encephalopathy may develop after tumor resection.[17] The pathogenesis of the neurologic effects of neuroblastoma is not known. Long-term neurodevelopmental deficits have been documented in as many as 50% of these patients. Paraneoplastic syndromes most commonly occur with prognostically favorable forms of neuroblastoma, but exceptions do occur.[18]

CLINICAL STAGING

Age at diagnosis and pattern of disease involvement are long-established independent prognostic variables for neuroblastoma.[19] Infants have a better prognosis than older patients. This derives partly from the greater percentage of infants who present with localized, prognostically favorable forms of neuroblastoma; however, the pattern holds for widespread disease as well.[20] Patients older than 2 years with metastatic disease to bone and bone marrow constitute the worst prognostic subgroup. The favorable prognosis associated with neuroblastomas arising in the chest or pelvis may be the result of the rarity of primary extraabdominal tumors in classic poor-risk metastatic disease.

As with other cancers, clinical staging in neuroblastoma is useful for prognostication and for comparing results of treatments carried out by different groups. The system devised by Evans and colleagues[21] was the first to gain widespread acceptance. The staging system subsequently developed by Hayes and colleagues[22] and modified by the Pediatric Oncology Group (POG)[23] placed greater emphasis on surgicopathologic findings. An international effort to develop a single, readily applicable system culminated in the International Neuroblastoma Staging System (INSS),[13] which combines features of the Evans and the POG systems (Table 108-1).

The INSS categorizes patients according to clinical patterns of disease as determined by radiographic and scintigraphic studies, surgical findings, and bone marrow status.[13] Localized tumors are divided into stages 1, 2, and 3, depending on regional lymph node findings and features of the primary tumor. Regarding the primary tumor, the INSS borrows from the Evans system, which highlights infiltration across the midline, and from the POG system, in which resectability takes precedence over site and size. All patients older than 12 months of age diagnosed with neuroblastoma in distant sites have stage 4 disease. Widespread disease in infants is classified as either stage 4 or stage 4S, depending on the presence of skeletal metastases, the amount of bone marrow disease, and the stage of the primary tumor.

Clinical findings that suggest an ominous prognosis are skeletal metastases, which must be distinguished from disruption of bone by an adjacent soft tissue mass, and substantial involvement of bone marrow, which contrasts with the minimal involvement seen in stage 4S. Clinical findings that have less certain prognostic import include tumor resectability and regional or distant lymph node involvement. Infiltration across the midline is often considered synonymous with a large, locally invasive tumor that encases or entraps vital structures, thus impeding tumor resectability. This problem most typically occurs with retroperitoneal neuroblastomas engulfing celiac vasculature or with tumors invading the spinal canal. Resectability is also impeded when thoracic paraspinal tumors encase mediastinal vasculature, cervical tumors impinge on the larynx or entrap the brachial plexus, and pelvic tumors adhere to the ureters, bladder, and rectum.

Approximately two thirds of localized neuroblastomas involve regional lymph nodes. Based on data from POG,[24] the INSS distinguishes between involved lymph nodes that are adherent to and surgically removed with the primary tumor (stage 1) versus involved regional lymph nodes that are separate from the primary tumor (stage 2B or 3). INSS stage 2 is subdivided because of the possibility that nodal involvement has prognostic significance. Involvement of distant nodes confers stage 4 status, even when no other metastatic lesions are present.

Classic stage 4 neuroblastoma is one of the most obvious and dramatic clinical pictures in oncology: a previously well child becomes irritable and is found to harbor a large abdominal tumor, sizable metastatic deposits in bones, and numerous syncytial clumps of tumor cells in bone marrow. However, more subtle clinical forms of stage 4 neuroblastoma also occur; therefore, when a child appears to have a localized neuroblastoma, a multitude of studies must be performed to ensure accurate determination of the extent of disease. The essential studies for clinical staging include the following:

- computed tomography of the chest, abdomen, pelvis, head, and orbits
- magnetic resonance imaging of spine if epidural extension is suspected
- bone marrow aspirates and biopsy specimens from the bilateral posterior iliac crests
- bone scan (if normal, a radiographic skeletal survey is necessary)
- metaiodobenzylguanidine (MIBG) scan

TABLE 108-1. *Comparison of staging systems for neuroblastoma*

CCSG system[21]	POG system[23]	INSS[13]
Stage I: tumor is confined to the organ or structure of origin.	Stage A: complete gross resection of the primary tumor, with or without microscopic residual disease. Intracavitary lymph nodes not adhered to the primary tumor must be histologically free of tumor. Nodes adhered to the surface of or within the primary may be positive.	Stage 1: localized tumor confined to the area of origin; complete gross excision with or without microscopic residual disease; identifiable ipsilateral and contralateral lymph nodes negative microscopically.
Stage II: tumor extends in continuity beyond the organ or structure of origin but does not cross the midline. Regional lymph nodes on the ipsilateral side may be involved.	Stage B: grossly unresected primary tumor. Nodes and nodules as in stage A.	Stage 2A: unilateral tumor with incomplete gross excision; identifiable ipsilateral and contralateral lymph nodes negative microscopically. Stage 2B: unilateral tumor with complete or incomplete gross excision; positive ipsilateral regional lymph nodes; identifiable contralateral lymph nodes negative microscopically.
Stage III: tumor extends in continuity beyond the midline. Regional lymph nodes may be involved bilaterally.	Stage C: complete or incomplete resection of primary tumor. Intracavitary nodes not adhered to primary must be histologicaly posiitve for tumor. Liver as in stage A.	Stage 3: tumor infiltrating across the midline with or without regional lymph node involvement, unilateral tumor with contralateral regional lymph node involvement, or midline tumor with bilateral lymph node involvement.
Stage IV: remote disease involves the skeleton, bone marrow, soft tissue, and distant lymph node groups (see stage IVS). Stage IVS: as defined in stage I or II, except for the presence of remote disease confined to the liver, skin, or bone marrow without bone metastases.	Stage D: dissemination of disease beyond intracavity nodes (i.e., extracavitary nodes, liver, skin, bone marrow, bone marrow, bone). Stage DS: infants <1 year of age with stage IVS disease (see CCSG).	Stage 4: dissemination of tumor to distant lymph nodes, bone, bone marrow, liver, or other organs, except as defined in stage 4S. Stage 4S: localized primary tumor as defined for stage 1 or 2 with dissemination limited to liver, skin, or bone marrow.

CCSG, Children's Cancer Study Group; INSS, International Neuroblastoma Staging System; POG, Pediatric Oncology Group.

- surgical sampling of regional lymph nodes for histopathologic examination

In the absence of classic stage 4 disease, the importance of ruling out metastatic involvement of cortical bone and bone marrow is of such paramount prognostic significance that special attention must be focused on these organs. For example, if a standard technetium-99m bone scan shows no lesions, a skeletal survey is necessary. Although extensive bone marrow invasion is frequent, spotty involvement also occurs; sampling of multiple sites is a necessity for adequate evaluation of bone marrow status.[25] Imaging with radiolabeled MIBG, an analog of catecholamine precursors that is taken up by catecholamine-producing cells, may also help identify unsuspected distant metastatic disease.

The available staging systems rely exclusively on clinical parameters; however, in terms of prognostic significance, intrinsic biologic properties may complement the clinical pattern of disease involvement. Future revisions of staging systems will likely exploit this critical insight into the natural history of neuroblastoma.

BIOLOGIC PROGNOSTIC FACTORS

The markedly divergent natural histories of subsets of neuroblastoma are strongly associated with specific biologic markers (Table 108-2). Readily available tests of tumor tissue can identify those patients who have clinically favorable forms of neuroblastoma but are destined to develop lethal metastatic disease. Chromosomal features in particular have already proven their worth in this regard. The presence of multiple copies, or amplification, of the *NMYC* protooncogene is an adverse prognostic factor regardless of age or clinical stage.[26,27] Chromosomal diploidy or pseudodiploidy portends refractory disease in infants.[28,29] Chromosome 1p deletions are common in poor-risk disease, although their independent prognostic significance is obscured by a strong association with *NMYC* amplification.[12,30,31] The basis for the relation between these cytogenetic abnormalities and tumor cell behavior awaits elucidation.

Additional biologic features have been identified that, in preliminary studies, have proved helpful in defining prognostic subsets of neuroblastoma. A good outlook is associated with high expression of *TRKA*, which is a nerve growth factor receptor.[32,33] One hypothesis is that nerve growth factor receptors mediate differentiation, maturation, or senescence of neuroblasts. The study of these molecules may yield critical insights into the underlying biology of neuroblastomas, from which novel therapeutic approaches may ensue.

CD44 is another surface molecule that is highly expressed on low-risk neuroblastomas and is absent on poor-risk forms.[34,35] This finding is at odds with the strong association of CD44 expression with metastasis in other neoplasms. Survival is poor among patients whose neuroblastoma cells can be cultured in vitro.[36]

Histologic variability among neuroblastomas has long spurred efforts at defining clinical correlates. The histopathologic classification developed by Shimada and colleagues[37] provides a valuable prognostic system based on age at diagnosis

TABLE 108-2. *Biologic prognostic factors*

Biological parameter	Adverse finding	References
TUMOR CELL FEATURES		
NMYC protooncogene	>10 copies	26, 27
Chromosomal ploidy	Near diploid or near tetraploid	28, 29
Chromosome 1p36 region	Loss of heterozygosity	12, 30, 31
Nerve growth factor receptor (*TRKA*)	Not expressed	32, 33
CD44	Not expressed	34, 35
In vitro growth	Cell line established	36
Histopathology	Unfavorable by Shimada criteria or by Joshi criteria	37, 38
BIOCHEMICAL MARKERS		
Serum ferritin	>142 ng/mL	39
Serum lactate dehydrogenase	>1500 U/L	40
Serum neuron specific enolase	>100 ng/mL	41
Urine VMA:HVA ratio	Low (<1)	42

HVA, homovanillic acid (HVA); VMA, vanillylmandaelic acid.

and histologic features of the untreated primary tumor: stromal organizational pattern, degree of neuroblast maturation, and nuclear morphology (aggressive tumors have a high mitotic-karyorrhexis index. A modification of the Shimada system developed by Joshi and colleagues[38] is also useful.

Several biochemical findings in serum or urine of patients with neuroblastoma are associated with prognosis (see Table 108-2). The basis for the relation between high levels of serum ferritin and adverse prognosis in neuroblastoma is not known.[39] The ferritin appears to originate in neuroblasts, because neuroblastoma cell lines produce ferritin in vitro and circulating human ferritin is detected in nude mice bearing human neuroblastomas.[40] High serum lactate dehydrogenase levels may reflect tumor burden or rapid growth of tumor.[41] Serum neuron-specific enolase (NSE) level is of prognostic value in patients younger than 2 years who have Evans stage III disease and in infants who have widespread disease.[42] Tumor burden is not obviously a determinant of serum NSE levels, because these can vary widely in patients with apparently similar amounts of tumor. Pretreatment levels of urinary catecholamines are not predictive of outcome, but in one study, low VMA and high HVA excretion was associated with short survival.[43] Because HVA is an early metabolite of the catecholamine pathway, this finding was interpreted as suggesting that biochemically primitive neuroblastomas are more aggressive.

TREATMENT

The INSS has only recently come into use; however, many reports provide enough clinical information to allow its retrospective application. This is useful because, for example, an Evans stage III tumor without nodal involvement is INSS stage 1 if it is totally excised, and an Evans stage II tumor may be INSS stage 1, 2A, or 2B (see Table 108-1).

Localized Tumors With no Regional Spread

Surgery alone has proven to be adequate treatment for the 10% of patients with neuroblastoma whose tumors have no nodal or distant spread and are grossly excised.[22,23,44–51] This is true regardless of whether or not microscopic residual disease is left behind (INSS stage 1).

Retrospective[22,44–46,49,52] and prospective[23,47,50,51,53] studies of patients with well-circumscribed neuroblastoma have shown near 100% survival regardless of postoperative management (Table 108-3). For example, in an early prospective Children's Cancer Study Group (CCSG) study in which surgery alone was used to treat patients with Evans stage I disease, there was only one late death among 26 patients followed for a minimum of 45 months.[47] In a POG study noteworthy for its large size, prospective design, and use of staging criteria identical to those of INSS stage 1 (including the postoperative presence of microscopic residual disease), there were only three deaths in 101 patients who were treated with surgery alone.[23]

Regionally Invasive Localized Tumors

Patients with regionally advanced neuroblastomas (INSS stage 2 or 3) traditionally receive chemotherapy, local radiotherapy, or both. These are patients whose neuroblastoma involves regional lymph nodes apart from the main mass and in whom gross total resection of tumor is not achieved. Several factors confound analysis of results. First, many reports are retrospective reviews covering long periods of time during which staging procedures and treatments evolved considerably. Second, documentation of lymph node involvement is incomplete. Third, quantitative definitions of postoperative residual disease are imprecise; commonly used terms such as "microscopic," "minimal," or "grossly visible" residual tumor may not be uniformly interpreted. Finally, few reports present critical biologic prognostic factors.

Patients in INSS stage 2 or 3 with relatively confined tumors have had long-term survival rates approaching those of patients with INSS stage 1 tumors (Table 108-4). Although most of these patients receive chemotherapy, radiotherapy, or both, in a retrospective CCSG study of Evans stage II disease reported by Matthay and colleagues,[54] 75 of 156 patients received no postoperative therapy, whereas 66 received local radiotherapy and no systemic therapy.

Studies of Evans stage II disease included a number of patients with INSS stage 1 tumors. For example, in the review

TABLE 108-3. *Localized neuroblastoma with no regional spread (INSS stage 1)*

Investigators	Period of study	Clinical stage	Treatment	Survival
Evans et al, 1976[53]	1970–1974, prospective	Evans stage I	S ± RT ± CPM	27/27
Evans et al, 1984[47]	1975–1978, prospective	Evans stage I	S alone	25/26
Adams and Hochholzer, 1981[46]	1944–1978, retrospective	Evans stage I	S alone	18/18
			S ± RT ± CT	18/19
Hayes et al, 1983[22]	1962–1980, retrospective	Stage I and IIA by St. Jude system	S alone	15/15
			S + RT + CPM/VCR	12/12
			S + RT	6/6
Berthold et al, 1986[50]	1979–1985 prospective	Evans stage I	S alone	27/27
De Bernardi et al, 1987[51]	1979–1984, prospective	Stage I, by Italian system	S alone	15/17
			S + pepti ± RT	19/19
Nitschke et al, 1988[23]	1981–1986, prospective	POG stage A	S alone	98/101

CPM, cyclophosphamide; CT, chemotherapy; pepti, peptichemio; POG, Pediatric Oncology Group; RT, radiotherapy; S, surgery; VCR, vincristine.

by Matthay and colleagues,[54] 43 of 156 patients had "complete removal of tumor with clear margins and no positive lymph nodes," which is clearly INSS stage 1, and 62 had "microscopic residual disease" defined as "tumors at the surgical margins or positive lymph nodes," node-negative tumors would be INSS stage 1. Nevertheless, the studies no doubt included a substantial number of patients with INSS stage 2 disease. The excellent prognosis for such patients was also evident in a prospective POG study that showed 87% 3-year survival among 61 patients with localized, visible residual neuroblastoma after surgery, but without regional lymph node involvement (POG stage B).[56] Postoperative treatment initially consisted of low-dose cyclophosphamide-doxorubicin (CPM/DOX).

In 1979, their single-institution experience with localized thoracic neuroblastoma and a literature review of the treatment of localized disease led Castleberry and colleagues[45] to question "the efficacy of adjunctive therapy following partial or complete surgical excision of the primary lesion in [Evans] stage I or II neuroblastoma." There is still no conclusive evidence that cytotoxic therapy has had an impact on the favorable outcome of patients with relatively confined neuroblastomas.

The uniformly excellent survival rates of INSS stage 1 or 2A patients stands in marked contrast to the variable survival rates reported for patients with regional lymph node involvement and for those with extensive but localized neuroblastomas (Evans stage III; POG stage C). These patients are therefore considered to be at intermediate risk for poor outcome. Studies assessing the impact of nodal involvement have yielded contradictory findings (Table 108-5).[22,49,57–62] In two, large, single-insitution retrospective reviews,[22,58] nodal involvement was a statistically significant adverse prognostic factor.[58] In contrast, Rosen and colleagues,[59] in a review of their single-institution experience, found that nodal involvement had no prognostic impact; survival was 84% (21 of 25 patients) for node-positive patients and 95% (18 of 19 patients) for node-negative patients with Evans stage II or III disease. These authors speculated that more aggressive therapy, including repeated surgery, extensive irradiation fields, and greater reliance on adjuvant chemotherapy (many different combinations were used) canceled out the potential adverse prognostic effects of nodal invasion. It should be noted, however, that four of the node-positive patients received no postoperative therapy; their outcomes were not presented.

POG has undertaken prospective studies of patients with localized neuroblastoma involving regional lymph nodes. In a study of 44 infants with POG stage C,[60] postoperative treatment consisted of low-dose CPM/DOX. The 3-year survival was

TABLE 108-4. *Localized neuroblastoma without nodal involvement (INSS stage 2A)*

Investigators	Period of study	Clinical stage	No. of patients	Treatment (no. of patients)	Survival (%)
Evans et al, 1984[47]	1970–1978, prospective	Evans stage II	126	S ± RT alone (29) S + RT + CPM (23) S + RT + COD (74)	89
Rosen et al, 1984[55]	1970–1982, retrospective	Evans stage II	32	S alone (5), S + RT (7), S + RT + CT (20)	94
Berthold et al, 1986[50]	1979–1985, prospective	Evans stage II	41	S + CPM/DOX	97
Matthay et al, 1989[54]	1978–1985, retrospective	Evans stage II	156	S alone (75), S + RT (66), S + CT ± RT (15)	96
Nitschke et al, 1995[56]	1981–1987, prospective	POG stage B	61	S + CPM/DOX alone (48) or + CT ± RT (13)	87

COD, cyclophosphamide, vincristine, and dacarbazine; CPM, cyclophosphamide; CT, chemotherapy; DOX, doxorubicin; POG, Pediatric Oncology Group; RT, radiotherapy; S, surgery.

TABLE 108-5. *Localized neuroblastoma with lymph node involvement*

Investigators	Clinical stage	Period of study	Treatment	Survival: Infants	Survival: >12 mo	Survival: Total
Hayes et al, 1983[22]	Stage IIIA(N) by St. Jude system	1974–1980, retrospective	CPM/DOX ± P/ VM-26	7/12 (58%)	4/14 (29%)	11/26 (42%)
Ninane et al, 1982[58]	Evans stage II	1970–1977, retrospective	Various	Not given	Not given	7/13 (54%)
Rosen et al, 1984[59]	Evans stage II and III	1970–1980, retrospective	Various	9/10 (90%)	12/15 (80%)	21/25 (85%)
De Bernardi et al, 1987[51]	Evans stage II and III	1979–1984, prospective	Pepti ± RT	7/7 (100%)	6/10 (60%)	13/17 (76%)
Castleberry et al, 1992[80]	POG stage C (Evans stage II and III)	1980–1987, prospective	CPM/DOX	41/44 (93%)		
Castleberry et al, 1991[61]	POG stage C	1981–1989, prospective	Initial CPM/DOX Initial CPM/DOX + RT		12/29 (41%) 24/33 (73%)	
Kushner et al, 1996[62]	INSS stage 2B and 3	1987–1993, prospective	Initial S alone	7/7 (100%)	7/7 (100%)	14/14 (100%)*

* One patient received cytotoxic therapy for recurrence.

CPM, cyclophosphamide; DOX, doxorubicin; INSS, International Neuroblastoma Staging System; P, cisplatin; POG, Pediatric Oncology Group; RT, radiotherapy; S, surgery; VM-26, teniposide.

93%, which is comparable to results in infants with stage B disease treated in the same manner.[56] The conclusion was that lymph node involvement may not have prognostic significance in infants with localized disease. For older stage C patients, POG conducted a randomized study of low-dose CPM/DOX and cisplatin/teniposide (VM-26), with or without radiotherapy, to the primary site and draining lymph node groups.[61] Doses were 2400 to 3000 cGy for the primary site, and 1800 to 2400 cGy for nodes. Survival in the radiotherapy arm was 73% (24 of 33 patients) compared to 41% (12 of 29 patients) in the chemotherapy-alone arm; these results were interpreted as supporting a role for local radiotherapy and showing the prognostic significance of lymph node involvement in this subset of patients. This is the only study that demonstrates a benefit from local radiotherapy. No benefit from radiotherapy for node-positive localized tumors was found in a prospective Italian study in which 13 of 17 patients, all of whom received minimal postoperative chemotherapy, were survivors.[51] Several attempts to determine the role of radiotherapy in localized neuroblastoma were retrospective and inconclusive.[63–65] Recommended doses, which are largely based on tissue tolerance for age combined with a reasonable chance of tumor control, have varied from 1200 cGy in infants to more than 5000 cGy in older children. An ongoing follow-up study by POG examines whether high-dose cisplatin can obviate the need for local radiotherapy. In this study, preliminary results show excellent survival for patients without *NMYC*-amplified tumors, regardless of treatment.[66]

At Memorial Sloan-Kettering Cancer Center, New York, we use surgery alone to treat all patients with non–stage 4 disease lacking *NMYC* amplification. Of 14 consecutive patients with non–stage 1 localized disease with documented regional lymph node involvement (INSS stage 2B or 3), only one received chemotherapy (after relapsing with a biologically unfavorable tumor), and all survived with a median follow-up of 43 months (range, 16 to 81 months).[62]

In studies dating from the 1970s, survival rates for patients with Evans stage III neuroblastoma were in the range of 50% to 75%.[47,50,53,67–71] Earlier studies showed lower survival rates.[44,72] Improvements in outcome have been attributed to advances in surgical technique, radiotherapy, and chemotherapy. An equally plausible explanation, however, is the phenomenon of stage migration. Studies of localized neuroblastoma from before the mid-1980s are flawed because disease extent was established by bone marrow or imaging studies deemed inadequate by subsequently defined standards. The impact of this deficiency on results with relatively confined tumors (e.g., Evans stage I or II) would be minimal, because the likelihood of metastases with such tumors is small. With more extensive tumors, the risk of missing metastatic disease is much greater and could have a considerable impact on survival rates. The confounding effect of simultaneous changes in staging procedures and treatment is evident in an Italian multiinstitutional retrospective study of 145 patients with localized but unresectable neuroblastoma (mainly Evans stage III) diagnosed in 1979 and in 1990.[71] Improved outcome was attributed to the use, beginning in 1985, of high-dose chemotherapy. In that year, however, bone marrow assessment as part of the extent-of-disease evaluation was expanded from one aspirate to four aspirates and two biopsies; furthermore, MIBG scintigraphy was used in some patients from 1987 onward. Prior to 1985, a number of patients may have had stage 4 disease that was missed because of suboptimal staging procedures.

The importance of categorizing patients with localized neuroblastoma by biologic parameters is well recognized. As with improvements in clinical staging, the use of biologic findings for prognostication is particularly critical for those with more extensive, intermediate-risk tumors. In the previously cited ongoing POG study of children with stage C disease[66] and in a retrospective study of patients with Evans stage III neuroblastoma,[70] patients with *NMYC*-amplified tumors did poorly. These studies illustrate the need for interpreting treatment results in conjunction with critical biologic factors.

Stage 4S Neuroblastoma

Stage 4S neuroblastoma is a well defined clinical entity (see Table 108-1) that often resolves with minimal or no cytotoxic therapy; however, it can cause death from complications of enlarging liver tumors or by progressing to classic stage 4 disease with osseous metastases and extensive bone marrow involvement.[27,50,73–85] This highly variable natural history has complicated management decisions, as has death from sequelae of cytotoxic therapies in at least 10% of these patients. Clinical features found in some studies to have prognostic implications include age younger than 2 to 3 months, which was unfavorable, and skin nodules, which were favorable. It has become evident that, as discussed previously in regard to extensive localized tumors, biologic features (e.g., *NMYC* amplification, DNA index) identify with a high degree of accuracy those stage 4S patients who are at risk of developing lethal stage 4 disease.[27,29,80,81,86] Biologic markers predictive of uncontrollable hepatic enlargement have not been found.

In published reports, most patients with stage 4S disease received cytotoxic therapy.[27,50,73–85] However, the reliability of *NMYC* copy number and DNA index for discriminating between low-risk and high-risk infantile neuroblastoma has spurred general acceptance of the management recommendations for stage 4S of Evans and colleagues dating from 1971.[73] Standard current practice in infants with widespread disease is to ensure that there are no osseous metastatic lesions, process tumor specimens for biologic studies, and monitor for signs of hepatic complications. If *NMYC* is amplified, cytotoxic therapy is instituted. Those with hepatic complications are initially managed with supportive care, but low-dose radiotherapy using lateral fields in an attempt to spare the kidneys and spine may be necessary. Chemotherapy is added if radiotherapy is ineffective.

Moderate-Risk Stage 4 Neuroblastoma

Survival rates of infants with stage 4 neuroblastoma have increased from 10% to 50%[44,50,72,74,77,79,83] to 75% to 85%.[20,83,85] If the small number of infants with *NMYC*-amplified stage 4 disease are excluded, the survival rates may be even higher, which suggests that these patients comprise the one neuroblastoma subgroup for whom chemotherapy has clearly had a major impact on prognosis. The improved outlook holds even if patients who in retrospect may actually have had stage 4S disease are excluded from the analysis.[75] This improvement has been noted with several different chemotherapy regimens and stands in marked contrast to the failure of intensive and myeloablative therapies to have a significant impact on the survival rates of older patients with stage 4 neuroblastoma involving bone and bone marrow (see Chap. 110).

Among patients older than 1 year of age, those categorized as having stage 4 disease because of distant lymph node involvement may have an intermediate prognosis. Rosen and colleagues[87] called this clinical picture "stage IV-N" and noted that at their institution, 3 of 6 such patients were long-term survivors, compared with 0 of 40 patients with extranodal metastatic disease. Stage IV-N disease merits special attention in future studies correlating biologic prognostic factors and outcome. These patients may have a highly favorable outlook if, for instance, *NMYC* is not amplified.

CONCLUSIONS

Surgery alone is sufficient treatment for INSS stage 1 neuroblastoma. Conservative treatment is widely accepted for stage 4S disease as well. It is possible that surgery alone may suffice for virtually all patients with non–stage 4 disease. Exceptions include the rare non–stage 4 patient whose tumor either has *NMYC* amplification or causes mechanical problems not amenable to surgical correction (e.g., surgically unapproachable cervical tumors causing airway obstruction, life-threatening enlargement of liver tumors).

Among patients with stage 4 disease, infants with hyperdiploidy do well with chemotherapy,[86] and older patients with distant disease limited to lymph nodes may also have a good prognosis.[87] Key issues in stage IV-N patients include investigating biologic prognostic markers and defining adequate therapy.

A number of considerations favor surgical treatment alone in non–stage 4 patients. First, an analysis of the literature suggests that cytotoxic therapies have had little impact on cure rates of unselected patients with neuroblastoma; most patients ultimately die even after myeloablative regimens[88] (see Chap. 110), whereas the remainder do well, often with little or no cytotoxic therapy. Second, a limited potential for malignant progression of non–stage 4 neuroblastoma is indicated by the survival with minimal therapy of many stage 4S patients and of patients left with microscopic residual disease after surgery (INSS stage 1). Third, conflicting assessments of the prognostic value of lymph node involvement by neuroblastoma and the variable prognosis of extensive but localized neuroblastomas can be accounted for by the inclusion of patients who had *NMYC*-amplified tumors or had stage 4 disease that was missed because of suboptimal bone marrow or imaging studies. Fourth, late effects of cytotoxic therapy are especially worrisome in patients with long projected survival. In addition, patients with non–stage 4 neuroblastoma who develop recurrent disease can still be salvaged.[45,46,62,89] These observations and uncertainties undermine the logic of treating stage 2 or 3 patients differently from those with stage 1 or stage 4S disease.

Biologic findings reinforce arguments against the use of cytotoxic therapy in non–stage 4 disease. The striking differences in chromosomal features of lethal versus low-risk forms of neuroblastoma constitute a biologic basis for the radical dichotomy in prognosis.[28–30] Furthermore, progression of non–stage 4 tumors with low-risk biologic features (e.g., triploidy, unamplified *NMYC*) to lethal stage 4 disease with its characteristic chromosomal features (e.g., diploidy, amplified *NMYC*) appears to be a rare event.[31,90]

Results of neuroblastoma screening programs support the hypothesis that non–stage 4 neuroblastoma without *NMYC* amplification rarely, if ever, evolves into lethal disease. Thus, screening has led to the detection of increased numbers of low-risk cases, whereas the incidence of stage 4 or *NMYC*-amplified neuroblastoma has not changed.[91] These findings are consistent with the long-held view that many cases of neuroblastoma escape detection through spontaneous regression or maturation.

This chapter focuses on the subset of patients with neuroblastoma who lack clinical characteristics that connote a poor prognosis (e.g., unresectable primary tumor, cortical bone metastases, extensive bone marrow involvement). Involvement of bone and bone marrow are objective findings, but resectability is partly dependent on subjective, nonquantifiable factors. A treatment plan that includes chemotherapy, regardless of the extent of tumor resection, may make it unjustifiable to undertake a difficult procedure to achieve a gross total excision. An aversion to performing major surgery may be strengthened by imaging studies showing extensive disease. Resectability, however, can be definitively assessed only during surgery. Low-risk tumors are characterized by a firm consistency that makes resection a feasible option, even if large size and bilateral extension necessitate more than one surgical procedure. In contrast, primary tumors in patients with classic stage 4 disease are often impossible to mobilize and resect because of their hemorrhagic friability and adhesiveness to neighboring tissues. Differences in tumor consistency probably reflect biologic differences; therefore, a distinction should be made between tumors that are difficult to resect because they happen to entrap vital structures and tumors that are unresectable because of hemorrhagic friability. Although low-risk neuroblastomas may be potentially resectable in their entirety, complete resections sometimes entail the risk of unwanted sequelae (e.g., brachial plexopathy with a cervical tumor). Under these circumstances, partial resection followed by observation alone is reasonable, given the very small risk that residual, biologically favorable tumor may evolve into lethal metastatic disease.

In contrast to a growing worldwide trend toward minimizing the use of cytotoxic therapy in non–stage 4 patients,[62,89,92] several groups have recently advocated intensive cytotoxic therapy for some subsets of these patients. However, studies interpreted as showing a benefit from this approach[61,70,71] have the same drawbacks as early studies: inadequate extent-of-disease evaluations (e.g., single bone marrow aspirate and biopsy) and no discrimination by *NMYC* status. In addition, two of the studies were 12-year retrospective reviews,[70,71] one of which included patients with INSS stage 1 tumors and patients with *NMYC*-amplified tumors. The potential impact of patient heterogeneity on outcome is evident in POG's ongoing study of extensive but localized neuroblastoma; as might be expected, patients with *NMYC* amplification do poorly, whereas the remainder do well.[66]

The use of comprehensive staging studies and the categorization of patients on the basis of key biologic prognostic markers promise to yield more homogeneous patient subgroups, particularly with regard to large, regionally invasive tumors, than has been the case in most past studies. Studies that base management on *NMYC* amplification, DNA index, Shimada histopathology, serum ferritin level, or some combination of these are in progress. It is predicted that the moderate-risk group of patients will break down into low-risk and poor-risk subgroups. The eventual result promises to be further reduction in the use of cytotoxic therapy in infants and children, an exciting prospect in view of their lengthy projected survival.

REFERENCES

1. Young JL Jr, Miller RW. Incidence of malignant tumors in U.S. children. J Pediatr 1975;86:24.
2. Bader KL, Miller RW. US cancer incidence and mortality in the first year of life. Am J Dis Child 1979;133:157.
3. Evans AE, Gerson J, Schaufer L. Spontaneous regression of neuroblastoma. Natl Cancer Inst Monogr 1976;44:49.
4. Brodeur GM, Castleberry RC. Neuroblastoma. In: Pizzo PA, Poplack DG, eds. Principles and practice of pediatric oncology. Philadelphia: JB Lippincott, 1993:739.
5. Sy WM, Edmonson JH. The developmental defects associated with neuroblastoma: etiologic implications. Cancer 1968;22:234.
6. Kushner BH, Hajdu SI, Helson L. Synchronous neuroblastoma and von Recklinghausen's disease: a review of the literature. J Clin Oncol 1985; 3:117.
7. Moss RB, Blessing-Moore J, Bender SW, Weiberl A. Cystic fibrosis and neuroblastoma. Pediatrics 1985;76:814.
8. Emery LG, Shields M, Shah NR, Garbes A. Neuroblastoma associated with Beckwith-Wiedemann syndrome. Cancer 1983;52:176.
9. Kushner BH, Helson L. Monozygotic siblings discordant for neuroblastoma: etiologic implications. J Pediatr 1985;107:405.
10. Knudson A, Strong LC. Mutation and cancer: neuroblastoma and pheochromocytoma. Am J Hum Genet 1972;24:514.
11. Kushner BH, Gilbert F, Helson L. Familial neuroblastoma: case reports, literature review, and etiologic considerations. Cancer 1986;57:1887.
12. Fong C-T, White PS, Peterson K, et al. Cytogenetic findings and prognosis in neuroblastoma with emphasis on marker chromosome 1. Cancer Res 1992;52:1780.
13. Brodeur GM, Pritchard J, Berthold F, et al. Revisions of the international criteria for neuroblastoma diagnosis, staging, and response to treatment. J Clin Oncol 1993;11:1466.
14. Weinblatt ME, Heisel MA, Siegel SE. Hypertension in children with neurogenic tumors. Pediatrics 1983;71:947.
15. Ho PTC, Estroff JA, Kozakewich H, et al. Prenatal detection of neuroblastoma: a ten-year experience from the Dana-Farber Cancer Institute and Children's Hospital. Pediatrics 1993;92:358.
16. Mendelsohn G, Eggleston JC, Olson JL, et al. Vasoactive intestinal peptide and its relationship to ganglion cell differentiation in neuroblastoma. Cancer 1976;37:846.
17. Mitchell WG, Snnodgrass SR. Opsoclonus-ataxia due to childhood neural crest tumors: a chronic neurologic syndrome. J Child Neurol 1990; 5:153.
18. Hiyama E, Yokoyama T, Ichikawa T, et al. Poor outcome in patients with advanced stage neuroblastoma and coincident opsomyoclonus syndrome. Cancer 1994;74:1821.
19. Evans AE. Staging and treatment of neuroblastoma. Cancer 1980;45: 1799.
20. Paul SR, Tarbell NJ, Korf B, et al. Stage IV neuroblastoma in infants. Long-term survival. Cancer 1991;67:1493.
21. Evans AE, D'Angio GJ, Randolph JA. A proposed staging for children with neuroblastoma: Children's Cancer Study Group A. Cancer 1971; 27:374.
22. Hayes FA, Green A, Hustu HO, Kumar M. Surgicopathologic staging of neuroblastoma: prognostic significance of regional lymph node metastases. J Pediatr 1983;102:59.
23. Nitschke R, Smith EI, Shochat S, et al. Localized neuroblastoma treated by surgery: a Pediatric Oncology Group Study. J Clin Oncol 1988;6: 1271.
24. Smith EI, Haase GM, Seeger RC, et al. A surgical perspective on the current staging in neuroblastoma: the International Neuroblastoma Staging System proposal. J Pediatr Surg 1989;24:386.
25. Franklin IM, Pritchard J. Detection of bone marrow invasion by neuroblastoma is improved by sampling at two sites with both aspirates and trephine biopsies. J Clin Pathol 1983;36:1215.
26. Seeger RC, Brodeur GM, Sather H, et al. Association of multiple copies of the N-myc oncogene with rapid progression of neuroblastomas. N Engl J Med 1985;313:1111.
27. Bourhis J, Dominici C, McDowell H, et al. N-myc genomic content and DNA ploidy in stage IVS neuroblastoma. J Clin Oncol 1991;9: 1371.
28. Kaneko Y, Kanda N, Maseki N et al. Different karyotypic patterns in early and advanced stage neuroblastomas. Cancer Res 1987;47:311.

29. Look AT, Hayes FA, Shuster JJ, et al. Clinical relevance of tumor cell ploidy and N-myc gene amplification in childhood neuroblastoma: a Pediatric Oncology Group study. J Clin Oncol 1991;9:581.
30. Hayashi Y, Inaba T, Hanada R, et al. Similar chromosomal patterns and lack of N-myc gene amplification in localized and IV-S stage neuroblastomas in infants. Med Pediatr Oncol 1989;17:111.
31. Caron H. Allelic loss of chromosome 1 and additional chromosome 17 material are both unfavourable prognostic markers in neuroblastoma. Med Pediatr Oncol (in press).
32. Suzuki T, Bogenmann E, Shimada H, et al. Lack of high-affinity nerve growth factor receptors in aggressive neuroblastomas. J Natl Cancer Inst 1993;85:377.
33. Nakagawara A, Arima-Nakagawara M, Scavarda NJ, et al. Association between high levels of expression of the TRK gene and favorable outcome in human neuroblastoma. N Engl J Med 1993;328:847.
34. Favrot MC, Combaret V, Lasset C. CD44: a new prognostic marker for neuroblastoma. (Letter) N Engl J Med 1993;329:1965.
35. Gross N, Beretta C, Peruisseau G, Jackson D, Simmons D, Beck D. CD44H Expression by human neuroblastoma cells: relation to MYCN amplification and lineage differentiation. Cancer Res 1994;54:4238.
36. Reynolds CP, Frenkel EP, Smith RG. Growth characteristics of neuroblastoma in vitro correlate with patient survival. Trans Assoc Am Phys 1980;93:203.
37. Shimada H, Chatten J, Newton WA Jr, et al. Histopathologic prognostic factors in neuroblastic tumors: definition of subtypes of ganglioneuroblastoma and an age-linked classification of neuroblastomas. J Natl Cancer Inst 1984;73:405.
38. Joshi VV, Cantor AB, Altshuler G, et al. Recommendations for modification of terminology of neuroblastic tumors and prognostic significance of Shimada classification. Cancer 1992;69:2183.
39. Evans AE, D'Angio GJ, Propert K, et al. Prognostic factors in neuroblastoma. Cancer 1987;59:1853.
40. Schuster JJ, McWilliams NB, Castleberry R, et al. Serum lactate dehydrogenase in childhood neuroblastoma. Am J Clin Oncol 1992;15:295.
41. Zeltzer PM, Marangos PJ, Evans AE, et al. Serum neuron-specific enolase in children with neuroblastoma: relationship to stage and disease course. Cancer 1986;57:1230.
42. Laug WE, Siegel SE, Shaw KNF, et al. Initial urinary catecholamine metabolite concentrations and prognosis in neuroblastoma. Pediatrics 1978;62:77.
43. Hann HL, Stahlhut MW, Millman I. Human ferritins present in the sera of nude mice transplanted with human neuroblastoma for hepatocellular carcinoma. Cancer Res 1984;44:3898.
44. Zucker JM. Retrospective study of 462 neuroblastomas treated between 1950 and 1970. Maandschr Kindergeneesk 1974;42:369.
45. Castleberry RP, Crist WM, Cain WS, Holbrook T, Malluh A, Salter MM. Management of localized thoracic neuroblastoma. Med Pediatr Oncol 1979;7:153.
46. Adam A, Hochholzer L. Ganglioneuroblastoma of the posterior mediastinum: a clinicopathologic review of 80 cases. Cancer 1981;47:373.
47. Evans AE, Brand W, de Lorimier A, et al. Results in children with local and regional neuroblastoma managed with and without vincristine, cyclophosphamide, and imidazole-carboxamide: a report from the Children's Cancer Study Group. Am J Clin Oncol 1984;6:3.
48. Evans AE, D'Angio GJ, Koop CE. The role of multimodal therapy in patients with local and regional neuroblastoma. J Pediatr Surg 1984; 19:77.
49. Le Tourneau JN, Bernard JL, Hendren WH, Carcassonne M. Evaluation of the role of surgery in 130 patients with neuroblastoma. J Pediatr Surg 1985;20:244.
50. Berthold F, Brandeis WE, Lampert F. Neuroblastoma: diagnostic advances and therapeutic results in 370 patients. Monogr Paediatr 1986; 18:206.
51. De Bernardi B, Rogers D, Carli M, et al. Localized neuroblastoma: surgical and pathologic staging. Cancer 1987;60:1066.
52. Coldman AJ, Fryer CJH, Elwood JM, Sonley MJ. Neuroblastoma: influence of age at diagnosis, stage, tumor site, and sex on prognosis. Cancer 1980;46:1896.
53. Evans AE, Albo V, D'Angio GJ, et al. Cyclophosphamide treatment of patients with localized and regional neuroblastoma: a randomized study. Cancer 1976;38:655.
54. Matthay KK, Sather HN, Seeger RC, Haase GM, Hammond GD. Excellent outcome of stage II neuroblastoma is independent of residual disease and radiation therapy. J Clin Oncol 1989;7:236.
55. Rosen EM, Cassady JR, Frantz CN, et al. Improved survival in neuroblastoma using multimodality therapy. Radiother Oncol 1984;2:189.
56. Nitschke R, Smith EI, Altshuler G, et al. Postoperative treatment of nonmetastatic visible residual neuroblastoma: a Pediatric Oncology Group study. J Clin Oncol 1991;9:1181.
57. O'Neill JA, Littman P, Blitzer P, Soper K, Chatten J, Shimada H. The role of surgery in localized neuroblastoma. J Pediatr Surg 1985;20: 708.
58. Ninane J, Pritchard J, Jones PMM, Mann JR, Malpas JS. Stage II neuroblastoma: adverse prognostic significance of lymph node involvement. Arch Dis Child 1982;57:438.
59. Rosen EM, Cassady JR, Kretschmar C, Frantz CN, Levey R, Sallan SE. Influence of local-regional lymph node metastases on prognosis in neuroblastoma. Med Pediatr Oncol 1984;12:260.
60. Castleberry R, Shuster JJ, Altshuler G, et al. Infants with neuroblastoma and regional lymph node metastases have a favorable outlook after limited postoperative chemotherapy: a Pediatric Oncology Group study. J Clin Oncol 1992;10:1299.
61. Castleberry RP, Kun LE, Shuster JJ, et al. Radiotherapy improves the outlook for patients older than 1 year with Pediatric Oncology Group stage C neuroblastoma. J Clin Oncol 1991;9:789.
62. Kushner BH, Cheung NV, LaQuaglia MP, et al. Survival from locally invasive or metastatic neuroblastoma without cytotoxic therapy. J Clin Oncol 1996;14:373.
63. Jacobson HM, Marcus Jr RB, Thar TL, et al. Pediatric neuroblastoma: postoperative radiation therapy using less than 2000 rad. Int J Radiat Oncol Biol Phys 1983;9:501.
64. Jacobson GM, Sause WT, O'Brien RT. Dose response analysis of pediatric neuroblastoma megavoltage radiation. Am J Clin Oncol 1984;7: 693.
65. Halperin EC, Cox EB. Radiation therapy in the management of neuroblastoma: the Duke University Medical Center experience 1967-1984. Int J Radiat Oncol Biol Phys 1986;12:1829.
66. Strother D, Cantor A, Halperin E, et al. Treatment of Pediatric Oncology Group (POG) stage C neuroblastoma (NBL): a preliminary POG report. (Abstract) Proc Am Soc Clin Oncol 1993;12:415.
67. Ikeda K, Nakagawara A, Yano H, et al. Improved survival rates in children over 1 year of age with stage III or IV neuroblastoma following intensive chemotherapeutic regimen. J Pediatr Surg 1989;24:189.
68. Hasse GM, Wong KY, deLorimier AA, et al. Improvement in survival after excision of primary tumor stage III neuroblastoma. J Pediatr Surg 1989;24:194.
69. Tsuchida Y, Yokoyama J, Kaneko M, et al. Therapeutic significance of surgery in advanced neuroblastoma: a report from the Study Group of Japan. J Pediatr Surg 1992;27:616.
70. West DC, Shamberger RC, Macklis RM, et al. Stage III neuroblastoma over 1 year of age at diagnosis: improved survival with intensive multimodality therapy including multiple alkylating agents. J Clin Oncol 1993;11:84.
71. Garaventa A, De Bernardi B, Pianca C, et al. Localized but unresectable neuroblastoma: treatment and outcome of 145 cases. J Clin Oncol 1993; 11:1770.
72. Breslow N, McCann B. Statistical estimation of prognosis for children with neuroblastoma. Cancer Res 1971;31:2098.
73. D'Angio GJ, Evans AE, Koop CE. Special pattern of widespread neuroblastoma with a favourable prognosis. Lancet 1971;1:1046.
74. Grosfeld JL, Schatzlein M, Ballantine TVN, Weetman RM, Baehner RL. Metastatic neuroblastoma: factors influencing survival. J Pediatr Surg 1978;13:59.
75. Evans AE, Baum E, Chard R. Do infants with stage IV-S neuroblastoma need treatment? Arch Dis Child 1981;56:271.
76. Stokes SH, Thomas PRM, Perez CA, Vietti TJ. Stage IV-S neuroblastoma: results with definitive therapy. Cancer 1984;53:2083.
77. Jereb B, Bretsky SS, Vogel R, Helson L. Age and prognosis in neuroblastoma: review of 112 patients younger than 2 years. Am J Pediatr Hematol Oncol 1984;6:233.
78. Nickerson HJ, Nesbit ME, Grosfeld JL, Baehner RL, Sather H, Hammond D. Comparison of stage IV and IV-S neuroblastoma in the first year of life. Med Pediatr Oncol 1985;13:261.
79. Stephenson SR, Cook BA, Mease AD, Ruymann FB. The prognostic significance of age and pattern of metastases in stage IV-S neuroblastoma. Cancer 1986;58:372.
80. Nakagawara A, Sasazuki T, Akiyama H, et al. N-myc oncogene and

stage IV-S neuroblastoma: preliminary observations on ten cases. Cancer 1990;65:1960.
81. Wilson PCG, Coppes MJ, Solh H, et al. Neuroblastoma stage IV-S: a heterogeneous disease. Med Pediatr Oncol 1991;19:467.
82. Suarez A, Hartman O, Vassal G, et al. Treatment of stage IV-S neuroblastoma: a study of 34 cases treated between 1982 and 1987. Med Pediatr Oncol 1991;19:473.
83. Bowman LC, Hancock ML, Santana VM, et al. Impact of intensified therapy on clinical outcome in infants and children with neuroblastoma: The St. Jude Children's Research Hospital experience, 1962 to 1988. J Clin Oncol 1991;9:1599.
84. Martinez DA, King DR, Ginn-Pease ME, Haase GM, Wiener ES. Resection of the primary tumor is appropriate for children with stage IV-S neuroblastoma: an analysis of 37 patients. J Pediatr Surg 1992;27:1016.
85. De Bernardi B, Pianca C, Boni L, et al. Disseminated neuroblastoma (stage IV and IV-S) in the first year of life: outcome related to age and stage. Cancer 1992;70:1625.
86. Bowman L, Castleberry R, Altschuler G, et al. Therapy based on DNA index (DI) for infants with unresectable and disseminated neuroblastoma (NB): the Pediatric Oncology Group "better risk" study. (Abstract) Proc Am Soc Clin Oncol 1992;11:365.
87. Rosen EM, Cassady JR, Frantz CN, Kretschmar CS, Levey R, Sallan SE. Stage IV-N: a favorable subset of children with metastatic neuroblastoma. Med Pediatr Oncol 1985;13:194.
88. Philip T, Zucker JM, Bernard JL, et al. Improved survival at 2 and 5 years in the LMCE1 unselected group of 72 children with stage IV neuroblastoma older than 1 year of age at diagnosis: is cure possible in a small subgroup? J Clin Oncol 1991;6:1037.
89. Matthay KK, Stram D, Seeger RC, et al. A prospective Children's Cancer Group study of stage II neuroblastoma treated with surgery alone. Proc Am Soc Clin Oncol 1993;12:414. abstract
90. Brodeur GM, Hayes FA, Green AA, et al. Consistent N-myc copy number in simultaneous or consecutive neuroblastoma samples from sixty individual patients. Cancer Res 1987;47:4248.
91. Murphy SB, Cohn SL, Craft AW, et al. Do children benefit from mass screening for neuroblastoma? Lancet 1991;337:344.
92. Rubie H, Plantaz D, Michon J, et al. Localized neuroblastoma: N-myc gene amplification is the main prognostic factor and post-operative treatment can be deleted in infants. (Abstract) Med Pediatr Oncol 1993;21:582.

Principles and Practice of Genitourinary Oncology, edited by Derek Raghavan, Howard I. Scher, Steven A. Leibel, and Paul H. Lange. Lippincott-Raven Publishers, Philadelphia, © 1997.

CHAPTER 109

High-Dose Chemotherapy in Advanced Neuroblastoma

D. Frappaz and Thierry Philip

The therapy of advanced neuroblastoma in children older than 1 year of age at diagnosis remains a major challenge. In the 1980s, less than 40% of children achieved a response using conventional combined chemotherapy, and this complete or partial remission was usually of short duration: median disease-free survival was less than 2 years, and only 10% to 15% of children became long-term survivors.[1,2] The prolongation of conventional chemotherapy for up to 2 years did not increase the survival rate.[3] The addition of cisplatin, its derivative carboplatin, or epipodophylloxins (i.e., etoposide or teniposide) to the classic conventional drugs cyclophosphamide, doxorubicin, vincristine, and dacarbazine has altered these figures, with more than 70% of patients achieving a complete or partial response. Dose increases and schedule modifications have not provided further major breakthroughs, although the most recent figures show a 35% 7-year overall survival (Fig. 109-1).[4–11] Some increase in survival rates may be the result, in part, of the introduction of high-dose chemotherapy following induction. The rationale for delivering high-dose therapy followed by hematopoietic progenitor cell rescue is based on laboratory data indicating that alkylating agents have a steep dose-response curve[12] and that hematopoietic toxicity may be overcome by progenitor reinfusion. Multiagent high-dose chemotherapy, radiotherapy, or both may also be delivered, provided that the agents are individually active at conventional doses against neuroblastoma, are synergistic or at least not cross-resistant, and have nonadditive extrahematopoietic toxicities.

HOW SHOULD HIGH-DOSE CHEMOTHERAPY BE PERFORMED?

The first convincing clinical evidence for the efficacy of high-dose therapy came from the randomized European Neuroblastoma Study Group trial, which compared high-dose melphalan versus no further therapy after induction. A significantly longer progression-free survival and a survival advantage for the former group was initially published, although further follow-up showed less impressive results.[13] Most conditioning regimens proposed since this study combine melphalan with other drugs, radiotherapy, or both. Proposed combination therapy regimens for the treatment of neuroblastoma include the following:

- VM26, BCNU, and melphalan,[14]
- BCNU, cisplatin, VP16, and melphalan or Thiotepa[15]
- vincristine, melphalan, VP16, carboplatin (OMEC[16] or rapid OMEC[17])
- melphalan and total-body irradiation (TBI)[18,19]
- VM26, doxorubicin, cisplatin, melphalan, and TBI[20,21]
- vincristine, melphalan, and TBI[22–24]

The acute hematologic toxicity is similar for all these regimens. The rate of toxic death as a result of gastrointestinal toxicity[16] or venoocclusive disease[14] seems lower for melphalan alone (3% to 6%) than for other regimens. However, the European Bone Marrow Transplant (EBMT) analysis does not show any significant difference in overall toxic death rate among these protocols.[25] The long-term toxicity of TBI and the lack of obvious survival advantage explains why many centers have abandoned its use. Some have advocated the use of local irradiation instead of TBI,[15] because nearly 70% of relapses are local (20% isolated, 50% associated with other sites), and there is an association between incomplete resection of the primary lesion and relapse at that site.[26]

The type of progenitors to be reinfused also remains an issue. Marrow as well as peripheral blood samples may be contaminated by malignant cells at diagnosis or after induction at the time of progenitor cell collection.[27,28] Attempts to remove tumor cells were proposed using immunomagnetic procedures,[29] cyclophosphamide derivatives,[30] and soybean agglutinin.[31] Positive selection of CD34-positive progenitor cells has been proposed.[32] All of these methods are effective in vitro, but there is no clear demonstration of the usefulness of these purging methods in vivo.

An attempt to purge in vivo in the double-graft program of the Lyon, Marseille, Curie, and East of France Group (LMCE2) included marrow collection with immunomagnetic purging before and after the first high-dose therapy. This study showed that the microenvironment may be altered by the first dose,

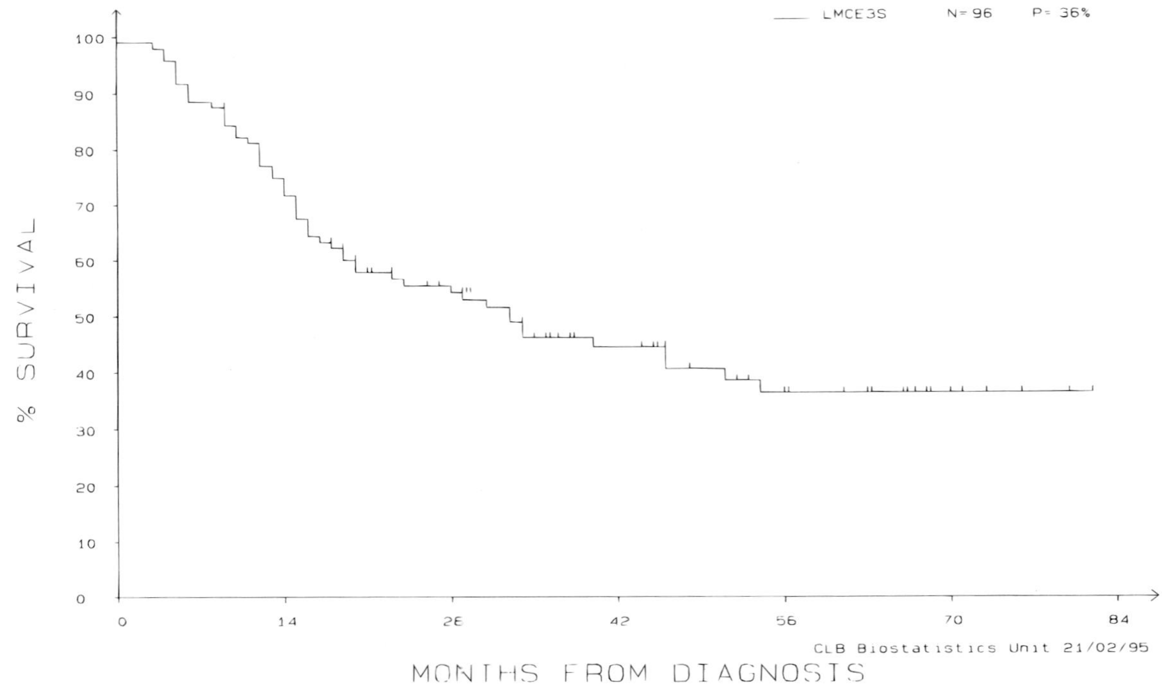

FIG. 109-1. Overall survival of 96 patients in the LMCE3 study.

leading to delayed engraftment after the second procedure.[24] A retrospective comparison between two groups of patients who received similar induction and high-dose therapy regimens with either purged or nonpurged marrow failed to show any significant difference in the outcome.[33] The most convincing evidence that any contaminated marrow may be at least partially responsible for relapse comes from the demonstration of the *NEOR* transfected gene in tumor cells at relapse when the reinjected bone marrow was pretransfected with such genes.[34] However, a clear demonstration by a clinical randomized study is lacking.

The use of alternative progenitor sources such as peripheral blood stem cells, allogenic bone marrow transplantation, or allogenic umbilical cord–derived progenitors has no proven advantage.[18,35] An EBMT registry case-control study comparing allogenic and autologous transplant has shown no significant difference in outcome between the two groups. This may be because the lower risk of graft-versus-host disease in young children limits any graft-versus-tumor effect of allogenic bone marrow transplant.[36] The use of growth factors during the rapid upswing of white blood cells following conventional chemotherapy results in the enriched collection of peripheral blood stem cells. However, the use of growth factors after peripheral blood stem cell transplant is associated with only modest clinical benefit in neutrophil recovery.[37,38]

WHO WILL BENEFIT FROM SUCH TREATMENT?

Overall survival using modern induction therapy and high-dose therapy now reaches 45% at 2 years posttherapy but decreases to 20% at 5 years and to 15% at 7 years as a result of late relapses.[22,23,39] The last LMCE study upgrades these results to 35% at 7 years (T. Philip, unpublished data, August 1995). With improved survival, new prognostic factors can be applied and help to determine which are good-prognosis groups that may benefit from some modifications of the current strategy and which are bad-prognosis groups that require completely new strategies. Some criteria may be obtained at diagnosis, but the most discriminative one is response to therapy, particularly complete response in metaiodobenzylguanidine (MIBG)-defined bone metastases after induction, as shown by our group[22] and confirmed by EBMT studies (40% versus 15% 5-year survival; Fig. 109-2).[25] At diagnosis, age appears to be a prognostic factor; 1- to 2-year-old children have a 41% 5-year overall survival compared with 24% for older children. The size of the tumor (<10 cm) and female gender are also associated with favorable outcome. Single-center data have suggested that the lack of bone involvement at diagnosis based on technetium scintigraphy increased 6-year progression-free survival after autologous bone marrow transplant (50% versus 5%),[22] but this was not confirmed in EBMT data.[25]

Numerous characteristics of the tumor at diagnosis have been assessed, including serum concentration of ferritin, neuron-specific enolase, morphologic features defined by the Shimada classification, DNA ploidy, deletion of chromosome 1p, and *NMYC* oncogene copy number.[40,41] Of these, the rise in lactate dehydrogenase (LDH; 10% event-free survival versus 36% for normal levels; $P < .0001$)[42] and CD44-positive staining (29% versus 83% progression-free survival in stage III-IV patients; $P < .001$) are the most discriminating prognostic factors in multivariate analyses. However, only 15% of patients initially show low levels of LDH, which is insufficient to separate two prognostic groups. Insufficient numbers of patients have been studied to confirm unequivocally or refute the prognostic importance of biologic characteristics[43]; however, a nonran-

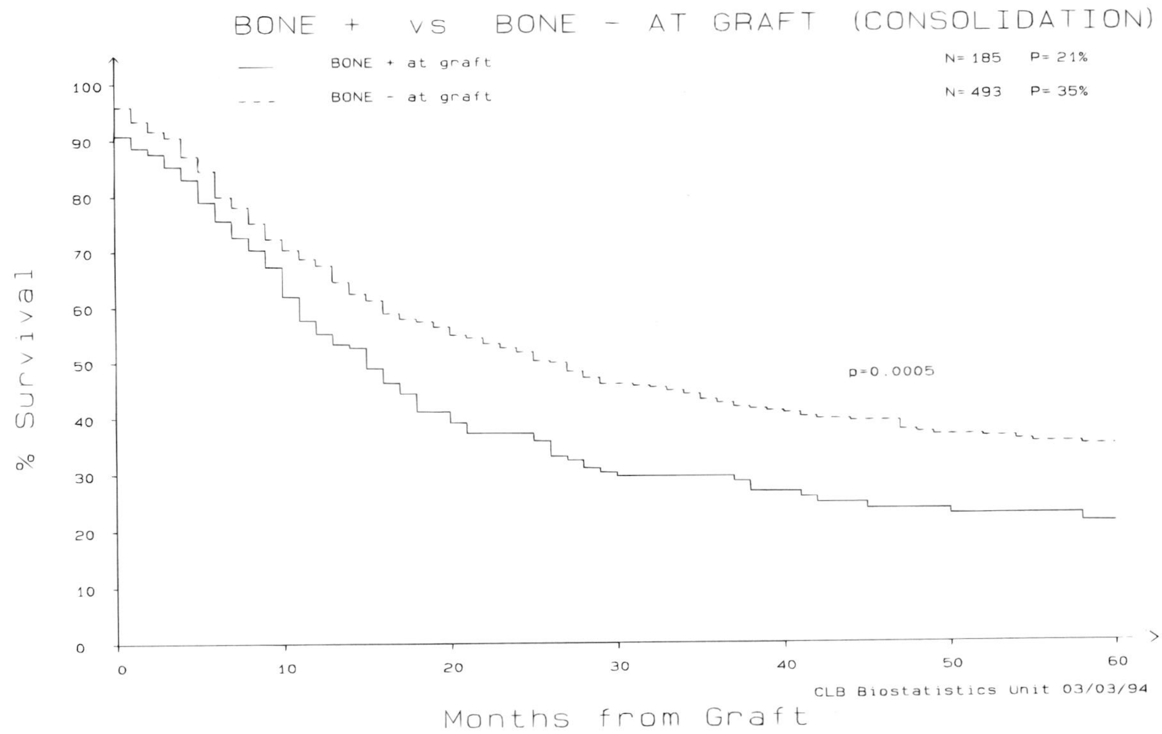

FIG. 109-2. Overall survival of 678 neuroblastoma patients in the European Bone Marrow Transplant Registry according to skeletal involvement at time of high-dose therapy.[46]

domized study by the U.S. Children's Cancer Study Group (CCSG) suggests that autologous bone marrow transplant is more effective for patients with genomic amplification of *NMYC*.[44]

It is not possible to be certain whether such improvement is the result of more aggressive induction, consolidation by high-dose therapy, or both. In the nonrandomized CCSG study, autologous bone marrow transplant seems to benefit children who fail to respond completely after induction therapy, and there is no clear difference between children who still have abnormal bone marrow after induction therapy in this study.[45] However, the overall response to induction chemotherapy and surgery as assessed by the International Neuroblastoma Response Criteria has no significant influence on the outcome of patients who receive high-dose therapy; 29% of patients with an incomplete response versus 30% of those in good partial or complete re-

TABLE 109-1. *Analysis of risk factors in 550 stage 4 neuroblastoma patients older than 1 year of age at diagnosis, consolidated by megatherapy and bone marrow transplant*

Univariate factors		Before or during 1986 n	Before or during 1986 *P*	After 1986 n	After 1986 *P*	Total group n	Total group Five-year overall survival (%)	Total group *P*
Pre-MGT skeleton lesions	+	82	.03	84	.047	166	16	.001
(^{99m}Tc+MIBG)	−	150	M	214	M	364	34	M
Pre-MGT skeleton lesions	+	40	.036	76	.07	116	10	.007
(MIBG)	−	83		189		272	34	
Boys		147	.04	178	NS	325	20	.05
Girls		93	M	132		225	37	M
Pretreatment durations	>12 mo	28	.004	16	NS	44	46	.006
	≤12 mo	212	M	294		506	27	M
Primary tumor size	<10 cm	128	.002	138	NS	266	29	.11
	>10 cm	79	M	120		199	31	M
Patients included in MA (%)		200	(83)	277	(89)	441	(80)	

+, positive; −, negative; M, factors remaining in the multivariate analysis model; MA, multivariate analysis; MIBG, metaiodobenzylguanidine; MGT, megatherapy; NS, not significant.

From Ladenstein R, et al. (Abstract 1440) Annual Meeting of the American Society of Clinical Oncology, May 16–18, 1993.

sponse are 5-year survivors.[25] This may simply reflect the fact that those called complete responders (i.e., those who show no sign of disease with the criteria and methods currently used to assess response) still have minimal residual disease that is not detected. Attempts to treat minimal residual disease with immunotherapy (i.e., interleukin 2) have been disappointing.[45] The efficacy of differentiating agents (i.e., retinoic acid) is currently under investigation.

The complete disappearance of metastases, regardless of primary tumor status at graft, increases the 5-year progression-free survival from 12% to 38%.[22] The clearance of bone marrow deposits have no significant value in the EBMT registry. The most discriminatory response feature is the disappearance of bone metastases on MIBG scintigraphy at the end of induction: nearly 40% of patients are in such a situation, and their 5-year overall survival is 40%, as opposed to 15% for those who retain bone metastases. Thus, these criteria may currently be the only ones available for separating the two prognostic group of patients (Table 109-1).

WHEN SHOULD THERAPY BE PERFORMED?

As stated previously, there is little clear evidence that high-dose programs with autologous bone marrow transplantation are compulsory as a first-line therapy. It could be argued that such treatment be proposed only for patients who relapse after conventional chemotherapy. The LMCE2[24] and EBMT registry[46] data suggest a 27% 2-year survival in relapsed patients who had not received high-dose therapy previously versus 0% for those who had received such a treatment previously. These data support the need for an international randomized study that could accrue a sufficient number of patients to compare the overall survival of patients systematically grafted as first-line therapy following induction versus a group treated conventionally and grafted only in the case of relapse.

In addition to stage IV disease in patients older than 1 year of age at diagnosis, high-dose therapy should probably also be considered for those with nonmetastatic disease with *NMYC* amplification. There are, however, insufficient data to support such a recommendation.

CONCLUSIONS

Obvious improvements in overall survival have been obtained in the past 15 years, and major progress has been achieved in the understanding of tumor resistance mechanisms in neuroblastoma. The real role of high-dose therapy in such improvements cannot yet be defined, and the results of ongoing randomized protocols on high-dose therapy as a first-line treatment are urgently awaited before additional protocols can be designed.

ACKNOWLEDGMENT

We are indebted to C.R. Pinkerton, Royal Marsden Hospital, London, England for editorial assistance.

REFERENCES

1. Leiken S, Evans A, Hein R. The impact of chemotherapy on advanced neuroblastoma: survival of patients diagnosed in 1956–1962 and 1966–1988 in Children's Cancer Study Group. Am J Pediatr 1974;84:131.
2. Hartmann O, Slopinario M, Tournade MF, et al. Neuroblastomes traités à l'Institut Gustave Roussy de 1979 à 1979: cent soixante treize cas. Arch Fr Pediatr 1983;40:15.
3. Rosen EM, Cassady JR, Frantz CN, et al. Neuroblastoma: the Joint Center for Radiation Therapy/Dana Farber Institute/Children's Hospital experience. J Clin Oncol 1984;2:719.
4. Ranck A, Newton W, O'Dorisio MS, et al. Survival of 131 children with stage IV neuroblastoma at Colombus Children's Hospital 1945–1992. Proc Am Soc Clin Oncol 1994;13:427.
5. Hartmann O, Pinkerton CR, Philip T, et al. Very-high dose cisplatin and etoposide in children with untreated advanced neuroblastoma. J Clin Oncol 1988;6:44.
6. Shafford EA, Rogers DW, Pritchard J. Advanced neuroblastoma: improved response rate using multidrug regimen (OPEC) including sequential cisplatinum and VM26. J Clin Oncol 1984;2:742.
7. Kushner BH, Helson L. Coordinated use of sequentially escalated cyclophosphamide and cell-cycle specific chemotherapy (N4SE protocol) for advanced neuroblastoma: experience with 100 patients. J Clin Oncol 1987;5:1746.
8. Bernard JL, Philip T, Zucker JM, et al. Sequential cisplatin/VM26 and vincristine/cyclophosphamide/doxorubicin in metastatic neuroblastoma: an effective non cross resistant regimen? J Clin Oncol 1987;5:1952.
9. Pinkerton CR, Zucker JM, Hartmann O, et al. Short duration, high dose, alternating chemotherapy in metastatic neuroblastoma (ENSG 3C induction regimen). Eur J Cancer 1990;62:319.
10. Philip T, Shalie R, Pinkerton R et al. A phase II study of the high-dose cisplatin and VP16 in neuroblastoma: a report from the Société Française d'Oncologie Pédiatrique. J Clin Oncol 1987;9:941.
11. Frappaz D, Michon J, Hartmann O, et al. VP16-carboplatin in neuroblastoma: a SFOP phase II study. J Clin Oncol 1992;10:1592.
12. Frei E III, Teicher BA, Holden SA, et al. Preclinical studies and clinical correlations of the effect of alkylating dose. Cancer Res 1988;48:6417.
13. Pinkerton CR, Pritchard J, De Krater J, et al. ENSG 1: randomised study of high dose melphalan in neuroblastoma. In: Dicke KA, Spitzer G, Jacannath S, eds. Autologous bone marrow transplantation. Houston: University of Texas Press 1987:401.
14. Hartmann O, Benhamou E, Beaujan F, et al. Repeated high dose chemotherapy followed by purged autologous bone marrow transplantation as consolidation therapy in metastatic neuroblastoma. J Clin Oncol 1987;5:1205
15. Kushner BH, O'Reilly RJ, Mandell LR, et al. Myelo-ablative combination without total body irradiation for neuroblastoma. J Clin Oncol 1991;9:274.
16. Corbett R, Pinkerton CR, Pearson ADJ, et al. High dose vincristine, melphalan, etoposide, and carboplatin (OMEC) with autologous bone marrow transplantation in the treatment of advanced neuroblastoma. Med Pediatr Oncol 1990;18:388
17. Gordon SJ, Pearson ADJ, Reid MM, et al. Toxicity of a single day high dose vincristine, melphalan, etoposide and carboplatin consolidation with autologous bone marrow rescue in advanced neuroblastoma. Eur J Cancer 1992;28A:1319
18. August CA, Gerota FT, Koch PA, et al. Treatment of advanced neuroblastoma with supralethal chemotherapy, radiation and allogenic or autologous marrow transplantation. J Clin Oncol 1984;2:609.
19. Pole JG, Casper J, Elfrenbein L, et al. High dose chemoradiotherapy supported by marrow infusion for advanced neuroblastomas: a pediatric oncology group study. J Clin Oncol 1991;9:152.
20. Seeger RC, Moss TJ, Feig SA, et al. Bone marrow transplantation for poor prognosis neuroblastoma. In: Evans AE, D'Angio GJ, Knudson AG, et al, eds. Advances in neuroblastoma research, 4th ed. New York: Liss, 1988:201.
21. Lam-Po-Tang PRL, Lowage GB, Vowels MR. Teniposide, doxorubicin, melphalan, cisplatin, and total body irradiation with autologous bone marrow transplantation for advanced neuroblastoma. Transplant Proc 1993;25:2881.
22. Philip T, Zucker JM, Bernard JL et al. Improved survival at 2 and 5 years in the LMCE1 unselected groups of 72 children with stage IV

neuroblastoma older than 1 year of age at diagnosis: is cure possible in a small subgroup? J Clin Oncol 1991;9:1037.
23. Dini G, Lanino E, Garaventa A, Rogers D, et al. Myelo-ablative therapy and unpurged bone marrow transplantation for poor prognosis neuroblastoma: report of 34 cases. J Clin Oncol 1991;9:962.
24. Philip T, Ladenstein R, Zucker JM, et al. Double megatherapy and autologous bone marrow transplantation for advanced neuroblastoma: the LMCE2 study. Br J Cancer 1993;67:119.
25. Ladenstein R, Hartmann O, Pinkerton CR. The role of megatherapy with autologous bone marrow rescue in solid tumours of childhood. Ann Oncol 1993;4(Suppl 1):45.
26. Matthay KK, Aktinson JS, Stram DO, et al. Pattern of relapse after autologous purged bone marrow transplantation for neuroblastoma: a Children's Cancer Study Group pilot study. J Clin Oncol 1993;11:2226.
27. Favrot MC, Frappaz D, Maritaz O, et al. Histological, cytological and immunological analyses are complementary for the detection of neuroblastoma cells in the bone marrow. Br J Cancer 1986;54:637.
28. Mi Yajima Y, Numata S, Matsumoto K, et al. Detection of neuroblastoma cells in bone marrow and peripheral cell harvests by reverse transcriptase chain reaction using typosine kinase RNA. Am Soc Clin Oncol Proc 1994;13:419.
29. Favrot MC, Philip T. Bone marrow purging. In: Magrath I, ed. New directions in cancer treatment. New York: Springer Verlag, 1989:343.
30. Beaujean F, Hartmann O, Pico J, et al. Incubation of autologous bone marrow graft with ASTA-Z-7557. Pediatr Hematol Oncol 1987;4:105
31. Kapelushnik J, Nagler A, Or R, et al. Autologous bone marrow transplantation for stage IV neuroblastoma: the role of soybean agglutinin purging. Transplant Proc 1993;25:2375.
32. Fruchauf S, Haas R, Zeller WJ, et al. CD 34 selection for purging in multiple myeloma and analysis of CD 34 + B cell precursors. Stem Cells 1884;12:95.
33. Garaventa A, Ladenstein R, Chauvin F, et al. High-dose chemotherapy with autologous bone marrow rescue in advanced stage IV neuroblastoma. Eur J Cancer 1993;29A:487.
34. Brenner MK, Rill DR, Moen RC, et al. Gene marking to trace origin of relapse after autologous bone marrow transplantation. Lancet 1993; 341:85.
35. Vanlemmens P, Plouvier E, Amsallem D, et al. Transplantation of umbilical cord blood in neuroblastoma. Nouv Rev Fr Hematol 199;34: 243.
36. Ladenstein R, Lasset C, Hartmann O, et al. Comparison of auto versus allografting as consolidation of primary treatments in advanced neuroblastoma over one year of age at diagnosis: report from the European group for bone marrow transplantation. Bone Marrow Transplant 1994; 14:37.
37. Quinones RR. Hematopoietic engraftment and graft failure after bone marrow transplantation. Am J Pediatr Hematol Oncol 1993;15:3.
38. Spitzer G, Adkins DR, Spencer V, et al. Randomized study of growth factors post peripheral blood stem cell transplant: neutrophil recovery is improved with modest clinical benefit. J Clin Oncol 1994;12:661.
39. Zucker JM, Philip T, Bernard JL, et al. Single or double consolidation treatment according to remission status after initial therapy in metastatic neuroblastoma: first results of LMCE study in 40 patients. In: Evans AE, D'Angio GJ, Knudson AG, Seeger RC, eds. Advances in neuroblastoma research, 5th ed. New York: Wiley-Liss, 1991:543.
40. Brodeur GM, Azar C, Brother M, et al. Neuroblastoma: effect of genetic factors on prognosis and treatment. Cancer 1992;70:1685
41. Favrot MC, Combaret V, Lasset C. CD 44: a new prognostic marker for neuroblastoma. Lancet 1994;329:1965
42. Berthold F, Trechow R, Utsch S, et al. Prognostic factors in metastatic neuroblastoma. Am J Pediatr Hematol Oncol 1992;14:207.
43. Combaret V, Wang Q, Favrot MC, et al. Clinical value of N-myc oncogene amplification in 52 patients with neuroblastoma included in recent therapeutic protocols. Eur J Cancer Clin Oncol 1989;25:1607.
44. Stram DO, Matthay KK, O'Leary M, et al. Myeloablative chemoradiotherapy versus continued chemotherapy for high risk neuroblastoma. (Abstract 133) Proceedings of advances in neuroblastoma research N·6, Philadelphia, May 1993.
45. Favrot MC, Michon J, Floret D, et al. Interleukin-2 immunotherapy in children with neuroblastoma after high dose chemotherapy and autologous bone marrow transplantation. Pediatr Hematol Oncol 1990;7:275.
46. Ladenstein R, Lasset C, Hartmann O, et al. Impact of megatherapy on survival after relapse from stage 4 neuroblastoma in patients over 1 year of age at diagnosis: a report from the European Group for Bone Marrow Transplantation. J Clin Oncol 1993;11:2330.

Principles and Practice of Genitourinary Oncology, edited by Derek Raghavan, Howard I. Scher, Steven A. Leibel, and Paul H. Lange. Lippincott-Raven Publishers, Philadelphia, © 1997.

CHAPTER 110

Treatment of Advanced-Stage Neuroblastoma

Nai-Kong V. Cheung, Brian H. Kushner, Michael P. LaQuaglia, and Karen Lindsley

Neuroblastoma arises from neural crest cells that are progenitors of the adrenal medulla and the sympathetic nervous system. It is the most common extracranial solid tumor of childhood[1] and the most common neoplasm diagnosed in the first month and first year of life.[2] The median age at diagnosis is 2.5 years, and 90% of cases are diagnosed in children 5 years old or younger. In Britain, although survival from this disease improved from 1971 through 1985, an unexpected increase in age-standardized mortality from 1986 through 1990 suggests an increase in the incidence of poor-risk neuroblastoma and a halt in the improvement in the treatment.[3]

The diagnosis is established by characteristic histopathologic findings or by elevations in urinary catecholamines such as vanillylmandelic acid; occasionally, more sophisticated techniques are required to rule out other small round cell tumors such as Ewing's sarcoma, primitive neuroectodermal tumor, rhabdomyosarcoma, and, occasionally, lymphoma.[4] In contrast to other solid tumors, 60% of neuroblastomas are already metastatic at the time of diagnosis. Massive primary tumors and metastatic disease give neuroblastoma its dismal reputation because, despite experiencing marked tumor regressions with cytotoxic therapy, most of these patients die of disease.

Neuroblastoma is uncommon among adults, in contrast to esthesioneuroblastoma. Unlike neuroblastoma, this tumor of the olfactory nerve typically has a chromosome 11–22 translocation, pathognomonic for Ewing's sarcoma or primitive neuroectodermal tumor; its biology and treatment approach also differ from those of classic neuroblastoma.

AN OVERVIEW OF STANDARD TREATMENT FOR POOR-RISK NEUROBLASTOMA

Early combination chemotherapy regimens using low doses of cyclophosphamide, doxorubicin, vincristine, and agents with less activity against neuroblastoma (eg, dacarbazine [DTIC]) produced response rates of less than 50% in patients with stage 4 neuroblastoma.[5–7] The median time from diagnosis to disease progression was approximately 8 months, and few patients were cured. Despite this discouraging experience, there was optimism in the early 1980s that significant numbers of patients with stage 4 neuroblastoma could benefit[8] from (1) the addition of cisplatin and epipodophyllotoxins to the antineuroblastoma chemotherapeutic armamentarium[9]; (2) the coordinated use of cell cycle–nonspecific agents (cyclophosphamide and cisplatin) and agents most active against cells in the S phase (doxorubicin and epipodophyllotoxins)[10]; (3) supralethal chemoradiotherapy with exogenous bone marrow support[11]; and (4) newly available ex vivo systems for purging possible contaminating malignant neuroblasts from harvested bone marrow.[12,13]

Most combination chemotherapy regimens for the initial control of stage 4 (INSS) neuroblastoma have included all or most of the principal antineuroblastoma drugs: cyclophosphamide, doxorubicin, etoposide (VP-16), and cisplatin (Table 110-1). Substantially improved progression-free survival (PFS) rates have been observed. However, curative cytoreduction with these regimens are rare, as shown by findings on comprehensive extent-of-disease evaluations and by eventual relapse in most patients. Consequently, the use of myeloablative chemoradiotherapy to consolidate tumor regressions or to achieve complete remissions has gained widespread acceptance.

Alkylating agents, particularly melphalan, have remained the centerpiece of transplant programs for neuroblastoma (Table 110-2). High-dose melphalan rather than cyclophosphamide was chosen for remission consolidation, in conjunction with bone marrow rescue, because of bladder toxicity concerns and because most patients had previously received cyclophosphamide.[11,14] Most experience has been with autologous bone marrow transplantation (ABMT) (see Chap. 109). The drawbacks of allogeneic bone marrow transplantation in neuroblastoma include the lack of donors—a reminder that the median age of patients with neuroblastoma is 2.5 years—and the risks of using nephrotoxic agents such as methotrexate or cyclosporin to prevent graft-versus-host disease in patients who have compromised renal function because of extensive prior use of cisplatin and antibiotics. Furthermore, although the allogeneic graft itself may have therapeutic potential in the treatment of leukemias (by virtue of a T-cell–mediated graft-versus-leukemia reaction), this so-called allogeneic advantage does not apply to neuroblastoma because neuroblasts have low to absent expression of cell-surface HLA and adhesion molecules required for T-cell–mediated cytotoxicity.[15]

TABLE 110-1. *Chemotherapy regimens for Stage 4 neuroblastoma*

Investigators	Regimen	Drugs	Dosage	Schedule
Pearson et al, 1990[126]	Napoleon	(sequential)		
		Cisplatin*	200 mg/m^2	d 0 and d 40
		VP-16	500 mg/m^2	d 0 and d 40
		Vincristine	—	d 10, d 30, d 50, and d 70
		Cisplatin	80 mg/m^2	d 10, d 30, d 50, and d 70
		Vincristine	—	d 20 and d 60
		VP-16	300 mg/m^2	d 20 and d 60
		Cyclophosphamide	1000 mg/m^2	d 20 and d 60
O'Leary et al, 1989[167]	CCG 321P2	Cisplatin	60 mg/m^2	d 1
		VP-16	100 mg/m^2	d 3 and d 6
		Doxorubicin	30 mg/m^2	d 3
		Cyclophosphamide	900 mg/m^2	d 4 and d 5
Bouvier et al, 1989[118]	N6	(alternating)		
		Cyclophosphamide	70 mg per kg	d 1 and d 2
		Doxorubicin*	25 mg/m^2	d 1–3
		Vincristine*	1.0 mg/m^2	d 1–3
		Cisplatin	50 mg/m^2	d 1–4
		VP-16	200 mg/m^2	d 1–3
Campbell et al, 1993[129]	CCG 3891	Cisplatin*	40 mg/m^2	d 1–4
		VP-16*	125 mg/m^2	d 1–4
		Doxorubicin*	10 mg/m^2	d 1–4
		Ifosfamide	2500 mg/m^2	d 1–4
Castleberry et al, 1987[130]	POG 8742	Cisplatin	40 mg/m^2	d 1–5
		VP-16	200 mg/m^2	d 2–4
		Cyclophosphamide	150 mg/m^2	d 21–27
		Doxorubicin	35 mg/m^2	d 28

VP-16, etoposide.
* Administered by continuous infusion.

A major weakness of autografting in patients with neuroblastoma is contamination by occult tumor cells. That contaminated marrow is at least partly responsible for marrow relapse is clearly shown by gene-marking experiments.[16] The high frequency of bone marrow invasion by neuroblastoma has prompted the routine use of ex vivo immunologic[17–19] or pharmacologic[20] purging of harvested bone marrow. Peripheral blood stem cell harvest has been applied widely in ASCT for various

TABLE 110-2. *Bone marrow transplantation regimens for neuroblastoma*

Investigators	Drugs	Dosage	Schedule
Hartmann et al, 1987[26]	BCNU	300 mg/m^2	d −8
	VM-26	250 mg/m^2	d −7, −6, −5, −4
	Melphalan	180 mg/m^2	d −3
Seeger et al, 1991[57]	Cisplatin	30 mg/m^2	d −8, −7, −6, −5
	VP-16	100 mg/m^2	d −8, −7, −6, −5
	Melphalan	140 mg/m^2	d −7
		70 mg/m^2	d −6
	TBI	333 cGy	d −3, −2, −1
Phillip et al, 1991[19]	Vincristine	1.5 mg/m^2	d −6
	Vincristine, CI	0.5 mg/m^2	d −5, −4, −3, −2, −1
	TBI	400 cGy	d −5, −4, −3
	Melphalan	180 mg/m^2	d −1
Graham-Pole et al, 1991[18]	Melphalan	60 mg/m^2	d −7, −6, −5
	TBI	200 cGy	d −4, −3, −2
Kushner et al, 1991[27]	Carboplatin	500 mg/m^2	d −19, −18
	Local RT	150 cGy	2x/d, x7d
	BCNU	200 mg/m^2	d −9
	Melphalan	60 mg/m^2	d −8, −7, −6
	VP-16	250 mg/m^2	d −5, −4, −3

BCNU, carmustine; CI, continuous infusion; RT, radiotherapy; TBI, total body irradiation; VM-26, teniposide; VP-16, etoposide.

malignancies. However, peripheralization of clonogenic neuroblasts is common in neuroblastoma,[21] and ex vivo purging is necessary. The emphasis on purging efficacy in neuroblastoma rests on the assumption that the transplant regimen can eradicate all residual tumor cells in the patient. However, if the regimen in question is not significantly different from the preceding induction treatments, it may not assure total tumor ablation. Under these circumstances, ex vivo purging efficacy may be a moot point, because residual disease in the patient leads to relapse, no matter how tumor-free the autograft has been rendered by the ex vivo treatment.

The standard approach is 6 to 12 months of moderate-dose combination chemotherapy, followed by alkylator-based myeloablative consolidation with bone marrow transplantation. This approach has significantly prolonged the event-free survival times of patients with poor-risk neuroblastoma, compared with results in the pretransplantation era. The precise contribution of myeloablative regimens to the longer event-free survival time is obscured by concurrent improvements in induction chemotherapy. Two retrospective analyses did not show any statistical benefit of ABMT compared with continued chemoradiotherapy.[22,23] The only randomized study reported to date found that high-dose melphalan prolonged the event-free survival time but probably did not increase the overall cure rate.[24] Similar conclusions emerge from reviews of unselected patients who were consecutively entered at diagnosis on treatment protocols consisting of moderate-dose combination chemotherapy plus myeloablative regimens for consolidation of remission.[19,25,26]

Although event-free survival time is prolonged in comparison with historical controls, the survival rate declines steadily with time, reaching only 12% to 18% in the studies with the largest number of patients and the longest follow-up. Length of follow-up is important, because relapses are not uncommon in patients who have been off all therapy and in complete remission for more than 2 years.[19] Myeloablative regimens have not improved the outcome of patients with refractory or gross disease and only rarely have achieved long-term survival of patients in second remission.[14,18,27–29] The impact of myeloablative treatments on the cure rate of patients with poor-risk neuroblastoma therefore remains uncertain. The US Children's Cancer Study Group is conducting a prospective, randomized study with the aim of comparing the efficacy of myeloablative treatment with that of intensified conventional chemotherapy in poor-risk neuroblastoma. The cost-benefit ratio of this modality, especially in comparison with other, less toxic approaches, has yet to be definitively resolved.

NOVEL STRATEGIES FOR TREATING POOR-RISK NEUROBLASTOMA

A number of recent clinical advances and laboratory findings, in conjunction with clinically valid hypotheses, suggest promising strategies for a curative approach to poor-risk pediatric neuroblastoma. These include dose intensification of active agents (especially alkylators), the combined modality approach (chemotherapy, surgery, radiotherapy, immunotherapy, and differentiation therapy), and selective targeting to minimal residual disease. Also under investigation is early detection by neonatal screening for abnormal urinary catecholamine excretion. However, large scale screening has so far not decreased the incidence of stage 4 neuroblastoma in children older than 12 months of age.[30]

Chemotherapy

At diagnosis, children with stage 4 neuroblastoma typically have large primary tumors, sizable metastatic deposits in bones, liver, or lymph nodes, and extensive bone marrow involvement. Chemotherapy is unsurpassed at producing dramatic disease regressions. Nevertheless, the clinical emergence of drug resistance has been a frustrating hallmark of treatment of neuroblastoma. Drug resistance is a complex phenomenon related in part to the enormous tumor burden characteristic of stage 4 neuroblastoma. Goldie and Coldman proposed a model for understanding and approaching the problem of drug resistance in cancer.[31] This model, which appears to be applicable to neuroblastoma, posits that spontaneous mutations confer drug resistance and that the number of drug-resistant clones is a function of the tumor size, the rate of mitosis, and a permissive (ie, subtherapeutic) environment. Patients with a large tumor burden at diagnosis have probably already developed resistant clones. Rapid elimination of sensitive cells, however, reduces the risk of new drug-resistant mutants. The model predicts that the initiation at diagnosis of maximal dosing and dose-rate therapy, using active and noncross-resistant chemotherapeutic agents, will yield improved clinical results.

Support for early dose-intensive use of chemotherapy also comes from a retrospective analysis of 44 published neuroblastoma clinical trials.[32] This study showed that major response rates, median survival rates, and PFS rates correlated strongly with the amount of four drugs (cyclophosphamide, doxorubicin, cisplatin, epipodophyllotoxins) given during the first 21 weeks after diagnosis. Vincristine and DTIC dose intensities did not contribute to improved clinical outcome. Alkylating agents, including cyclophosphamide, constitute a large class of effective agents against neuroblastoma.[33] Features accounting for the clinical efficacy of alkylating agents include their cell-cycle nonspecificity, their activity against hypoxic as well as oxygenated tumor cells, and their small size, all important attributes when treating large tumors with poor vascular perfusion and relatively dormant subpopulations of tumor cells.[34] Properties of cyclophosphamide that set it apart from other alkylators in terms of potential for maximizing dose intensity include its negligible extramedullary toxicity (in contrast to ifosfamide, for example) and its relative sparing of hemopoietic stem cells (in contrast to melphalan, thiotepa, busulfan, and carmustine). Multiple courses of high-dose cyclophosphamide can therefore be administered within a short time frame, which translates into increased dose intensity.[35] In addition, this use of cyclophosphamide does not preclude subsequent harvesting of bone marrow for future transplantation.[20]

Alkylating agents have a log-linear dose-response effect against tumor cells in vitro that is maintained through four to five logs of tumor cell kill,[36] providing an experimental rationale for maximizing dose intensity. Enhanced chemotherapeutic efficacy can be achieved, not only through escalating dosage and increasing dose rate, but also through modulating mechanisms of drug resistance operative at the cellular level. These mechanisms include drug uptake, efflux, and detoxification systems.

Alkylating agents are chemically heterogeneous and have diverse modes of action; the underlying cellular mechanisms of resistance to these agents appear to be varied and complex.

Potential methods to modulate such resistance are being tested. For example, intracellular glutathione and glutathione S-transferase activities have been implicated in alkylator resistance. Depletion of glutathione by carmustine or inhibition of its synthesis by buthionine sulfoximine may be methods that can enhance alkylator cytotoxicity.[37,38]

The other commonly used classes of antineuroblastoma drugs are anthracyclines, epipodophyllotoxins, and vinca alkaloids. Although they are a seemingly disparate group of chemotherapeutic agents, they share the underlying property of being derived from naturally occurring substances. They may be affected by P-glycoprotein, which is a specific membrane constituent that is present in many tissues and is thought to function as a pump to impede the absorption of environmental toxins. Amplification or overexpression of the MDR1 gene, which code for P-glycoprotein, can increase the resistance of tumor cell lines (including neuroblastoma lines) to all agents affected by the pump by several hundred or thousand times.[39] Clones of tumor cells with this pleomorphic resistance probably develop de novo but are expanded under the selection of repeated sublethal drug treatments. The clinical significance of MDR1 and MRP (multidrug resistance-associated protein) overexpression in neuroblastoma is being tested.[40–42]

Surgery

Chemotherapy, which is highly effective against small metastases, may not be as useful against the large primary tumors characteristic of neuroblastoma. These tumor masses contain mixed populations of both rapidly proliferating and relatively dormant cells. Rapid proliferation enhances the likelihood of mutations that result in resistance to therapy; the slow metabolism of relatively dormant subpopulations blunts the lytic effects of cytotoxic treatment. The compromised blood supply to areas within these tumor masses protects neuroblastoma cells from lethal concentrations of chemotherapy drugs. Exposure of tumor cells to sublethal concentrations of cytotoxic agents in vitro is associated with the emergence of drug resistance.[43] Poor perfusion may also impair the penetration of macromolecules (eg, monoclonal antibodies) and cytotoxic leukocytes into tumors and thereby blunt the efficacy of biologic therapies.[44]

A solution to these problems is surgical removal of primary neuroblastoma. The Goldie-Coldman hypothesis favoring rapid cytoreduction suggests that this step be taken as soon as chemotherapy-induced tumor regressions have made resection feasible. Gross total resection has clearly prolonged survival time among stage 3 patients.[45] The impact of gross total resection on patients with stage 4 neuroblastoma remains controversial, possibly because of the usually short duration of remission of their systemic disease. Among infants and those receiving intensive therapies, including ABMT, in which PFS rates are prolonged, gross total resection appears to be important.[46–48] However, surgical complications, particularly renal compromise, can adversely affect the timing or dosage of chemotherapy.[46,49,50] Most studies that tested the role of surgery in stage 4 neuroblastoma involved patients who received chemotherapy that was suboptimal by current standards. As a result, overall survival times were too short to assess the impact of surgery (early or late) on the appearance of late resistant clones. More recently, a retrospective analysis of patients diagnosed with stage 4 neuroblastoma diagnosed after 1 year of age clearly demonstrated a positive impact of gross total resection on survival by univariate analysis.[48] However, the close correlation between dose intensity of induction chemotherapy and the ability to achieve gross total resection weakened any conclusion regarding an independent role of surgery on long-term survival.

Radiotherapy

The third traditional cancer treatment modality, radiotherapy, has a critical role not fully realized in the treatment of stage 4 neuroblastoma. Although curative radiation dosages have not been firmly established, neuroblastoma is radiosensitive, as manifested clinically by rapid tumor shrinkage and relief of pain after radiotherapy. In patients with stage 4 disease, radiotherapy in doses of 2000 to 3500 cGy improves local control of primary tumors.[51] Because tumor masses have poor blood supply and the antitumor effect of irradiation is oxygen dependent, radiotherapy cannot be relied on to ablate bulk disease. It may best be exploited for consolidation of tumor regressions after by chemotherapy and surgery. Administration of radiotherapy after chemotherapy has been completed can also prevent radiation-induced bone marrow suppression and toxicities to organs that may compromise the optimal delivery of the drugs required for eradication of distant metastases. Hyperfractionation of radiation dosage is reasonable, because this method has been shown to reduce toxicity to normal tissues while retaining antineuroblastoma efficacy in laboratory models. Neuroblastoma cell lines and xenografts have a limited repair capability for sublethal damage and have equivalent sensitivity to a given total radiation dosage whether it is administered singly or in multiple fractions.[52,53]

The radiosensitivity of neuroblastoma, plus the unsatisfactory results with chemotherapy alone, has stimulated efforts to develop systemic radiotherapeutic approaches to stage 4 neuroblastoma. These include both external beam total body irradiation (TBI) and targeted radiotherapy using radiolabeled tumor-seeking agents such as metaiodobenzylguanidine (MIBG) or monoclonal antibodies.

Total Body Irradiation

Early studies of TBI or hemibody external beam irradiation, using nonmyeloablative doses, did not improve on results obtained with chemotherapy alone.[54–56] In a pilot study of myeloablative therapy combining melphalan, other drugs, and fractionated TBI 1000 cGy, 4 of 8 patients with relapsed stage 4 neuroblastoma achieved long-term remissions.[14] This highly encouraging clinical experience, along with laboratory studies of neuroblastoma cell lines suggesting that fractionated TBI may be beneficial in a transplant setting,[53] provided the rationale for the inclusion of TBI in many myeloablative regimens for stage 4 neuroblastoma. However, a decade of experience has shown approximately comparable event-free survival rates for patients undergoing myeloablative consolidation of first remission, whether they did[18,19,57] or did not[26,27,58] receive TBI. This result can be explained by inadequate radiation dosage to tumor cells and by increased mortality from radiation-related toxicities such as venoocclusive disease of the liver.

Metaiodobenzylguanidine

Targeting of radiation to neuroblastoma, using MIBG or monoclonal antibodies, has the potential of increasing radiation dosage delivered while minimizing toxic effects on normal tissues. MIBG is concentrated by the neurosecretory granules of both normal and neoplastic tissues of neural crest origin.[59] Iodine-131–MIBG accumulates in the thyroid, salivary glands, lung, myocardium, liver, gastrointestinal tract, contents of the urinary bladder, and, occasionally, the adrenal glands. MIBG uptake can be blocked by common drugs, including sympathomimetics, antipsychotics, tricyclic antidepressants, calcium channel blocking agents, long-acting β-blockers, and other drugs such as cocaine.[59] It is metabolized by the liver, and only a small amount is secreted in bile; most of the injected MIBG is excreted unchanged in the urine. The average total body half-life is 24 hours. MIBG is quite specific for neuroblastoma and other amine precursor uptake tumors.[60] However, its known uptake in ganglioneuroma,[61–64] a benign tumor that often accompanies neuroblastoma, can render non–biopsy-proven tumor responses uninterpretable.

Primary and metastatic tumors are heterogenous in their ability to accumulate MIBG, and there is a quantitative difference among tumors with various degrees of differentiation,[65] a clinical finding reflected in laboratory studies showing that some neuroblastoma cell lines do not take up MIBG.[66] Although MIBG can detect tumors in more than 90% of patients with neuroblastoma, its ability to detect marrow and lymph node soft tissue disease on a site-by-site basis is approximately 63%. Whether MIBG can detect all bone lesions is controversial, because the many sites commonly detected by bone and MIBG scans cannot be biopsied to confirm disease.[67–70] In one study, 2 mCi (approximately 5 mCi/1.73 m^2) of monoclonal antibody specific for ganglioside G_{D2} was able to detect significantly more lesions than what was obtained with the standard imaging dose (0.5 mCi/1.73 m^2) of ^{131}I-MIBG.[71]

Many pilot studies using radiolabeled MIBG in relapsed patients have shown response rates of 10% to 57%; durations of response have usually been brief for disease with unequivocal poor-risk biologic or clinical features (Table 110-3).[72–76] Hematologic, hepatic, renal, and adrenal toxicity have been observed, but marrow suppression is the dose-limiting toxicity.[73,75,76] Eighty percent of patients treated with therapeutic doses of ^{131}I-MIBG developed grade 3/4 myelotoxicity at a total body dose of 2.5 Gy. However, the achievement of even transient clinical improvement in heavily pretreated patients has prompted consideration of this treatment modality in patients whose disease has not progressed. Early results of ^{131}I-MIBG treatment after ABMT did not change the 15% to 20% long-term PFS rate[72]; this result may relate to the uncertainties regarding optimal dosing and scheduling. Furthermore, marrow suppressive effects, which are especially severe if the marrow is invaded by neuroblasts, may preclude subsequent use of dose-intensive chemotherapy. Perhaps the most disturbing predictions derive from microdosimetry studies, which suggest that ^{131}I-MIBG may be ineffective for microscopic disease (as in bone marrow) of micron-size diameters.[77,78] In vitro attempts to upgrade or induce cellular mechanisms of MIBG uptake by using differentiation inducers have largely been unsuccessful.[79] Radionuclides (eg, alpha-emitting astatine-211–MIBG)[80] with dosimetric features more favorable for eradication of microscopic tumor deposits or carrier-free ^{131}I-conjugates[81] may improve the tumor control potential of MIBG.

Radiolabeled Antibody Therapy

Targeted radioimmunotherapy[82,83] exploits the specificity of antibodies to deliver radioisotopes (eg, iodine-131) directly to tumor cells. Neuroblastoma has a limited number of target antigens that are tumor specific; most are glycoproteins, to which only a few antibodies have been tested clinically. UJ13A, an antibody specific for human NCAM,[84] and CE7, which binds to a 190-kd glycoprotein,[85,86] have been tested in patient radioimmunotherapy trials with some success.

The glycolipid antigen ganglioside G_{D2} is abundantly expressed in neuroblastoma, and several antibodies to it have been tested. These include 14.G2a (a mouse IgG_{2a} class switch variant from 14.18), ch14.18 (a human-mouse chimeric form of 14.18) and 3F8 (mouse IgG_3). Disialoganglioside G_{D2} is well suited for targeting therapy because of the following reasons: (1) it is expressed at a high density in human neuroblastomas (5 to 10 $\times$ 10^6 molecules per cell) and is restricted to neuroectodermal tissues; (2) although it circulates in serum, it does not interfere with the biodistribution of specific antibody (eg, 3F8), allowing excellent tumor localization;[87] (3) as is characteristic of carbohydrate antigens, it is not modulated from cell surface on binding to antibodies;[88] and (4) it is expressed homogeneously in human neuroblastoma, with little heterogeneity within tumors and among patients.[89]

The potential for tumor targeting was tested in 42 neuroblastoma patients imaged with ^{131}I-3F8. Radiolocalization was demonstrated in primary tumors of the mediastinum and abdomen and in metastatic disease of the lymph nodes, bone marrow, and bone.[71,87] The specificity was validated by tumor and marrow biopsies, as well as by computed tomography, magnetic

TABLE 110-3. *Results of treatment with ^{131}I-MIBG in patients with chemoresistent neuroblastoma*

Investigators	No. patients	Stage	Dose	CR/VGPR	PR
Hutchinson et al, 1992[76]	36 11	IV III	8.9 mCi/kg	9/47	13/47
Lashford et al, 1992[75]	22 3	IV III	1–2.5 /Gy /TBD	—	8/25
Garaventa et al, 1991[73]	19 12	IV III	2.8–6 GBq/kg	2/31	4/31

MIBG, metaiodobenzylguanidine; CR, complete remission; VGPR, very good partial remission; PR, partial remission; TBD, total body dose.

resonance imaging, and bone scans. A comparison with ^{131}I-MIBG suggested that ^{131}I-3F8 was more sensitive in detecting metastatic sites of disease.[71] The radiologic toxicities of ^{131}I-3F8 were defined in a phase I dose escalation study.[83] Twenty-four patients with refractory neuroblastoma (23 stage 4, 1 stage 3 unresectable) were treated with ^{131}I-3F8 at seven dose levels, ranging from 6 to 28 mCi/kg. Twenty-two patients were rescued with cryopreserved autologous bone marrow; 1 patient received granulocyte-macrophage colony-stimulating factor; 1 died of progressive disease before marrow reinfusion. Acute toxicities of ^{131}I-3F8 treatment included pain during the infusion (20 of 24 patients), fever (20 of 24 patients), and mild diarrhea. All patients developed grade 4 myelosuppression. Thyroid uptake occurred despite oral administration of saturated solution of potassium iodide and led to hypothyroidism in 4 patients. Subsequently, patients were treated with Synthroid or Cytomel to suppress thyroid functions. Six patients survived longer than 20 months from the time of ^{131}I-3F8 treatment, and none encountered late extramedullary toxicities. Responses were seen in both soft tissue masses and bone marrow. Dose estimates based on conjugate planar images and plasma activity over time were favorable. The average doses to body organs and marrow were between 1.9 and 2.5 rad/mCi, and the average dose to tumor was 13.7 rad/mCi. Although extramedullary toxicities in the acute phase were not severe, the late effects of this treatment modality have not yet been defined.

Treatment of Microscopic Residual Disease

Organ toxicity is a major limitation on the curative potential of increases in chemotherapy dose intensity. The use of hemopoietic growth factors may facilitate treatment intensification by reducing the duration of myelosuppression and thereby shortening the interval between courses of chemotherapy.[90] However, the enhanced acute toxicity to vital organs that accompanies intensified use of most drugs remains an obstacle. Furthermore, although an aggressive program of dose-intensive chemotherapy plus early surgical intervention and local radiotherapy to previous sites of bulk disease may achieve complete remissions in a high percentage of patients with stage 4 neuroblastoma, the concept of log kill and the Goldie-Coldman model predict the persistence of microscopic disease resistant to the traditional treatment modalities. Definitive ablation of microscopic residual disease resistant to conventional chemotherapy therefore poses a pressing therapeutic challenge.

Biologic therapies of potential use for this purpose fall into two general categories, differentiation induction and immunologic maneuvers. Immunologic approaches to controlling neuroblastoma have involved the in vivo administration of biologic response modifiers and of monoclonal antibodies directed against neuroblastoma-associated antigens.

Differentiation Induction

Although a variety of agents induce morphologic differentiation of neuroblastoma cell lines in vitro, only *cis*-retinoic acid is currently being used in large clinical trials designed to evaluate antineuroblastoma activity.[91] In vitro, this vitamin A derivative decreases the expression of *MYCN* and modulates the proliferative capacity of neuroblastoma cell lines.[92] However, clinical efficacy against gross disease is not substantial.[93] Whether this relatively nontoxic agent will prove to be clinically helpful for eradication of minimal residual disease awaits the results of randomized trials.[94]

Biologic Response Modifiers

In heavily pretreated patients with resistant disease, interleukin-2, with or without lymphokine-activated killer (LAK) cells produced no significant clinical responses.[95,96] These patients all had profound immunologic defects, including expanded CD8-positive T-cell populations that may have inhibited effector cell function. An alternative strategy under study is to administer interleukin-2 at some point after myeloablative therapy and bone marrow transplantation,[97] when a preferential outgrowth of natural killer cells occurs and when tumor burden is at a minimum. The lack of prolonged remissions when patients were treated with these regimens may relate in part to the complexities of cell trafficking and neuroblastoma recognition by natural killer and LAK cells in vivo. The absence of adhesion molecules on subsets of neuroblastoma cells[15] may render them resistant to these kinds of cell-mediated cytotoxicity mechanisms.

Interferon gamma (IFN-γ) is another biologic response modifier that has produced no antitumor effect in children with chemotherapy-resistant neuroblastoma.[98] Biologic effects of IFN-γ included the activation of natural killer cells and induction of HLA expression on neuroblastoma cells. The latter effect, however, may not alter the resistance of neuroblastoma cells to T-cell–mediated lysis, which requires other intercellular adhesion molecules that are lacking on neuroblastoma cells.[15]

Monoclonal Antibody Targeted Immunotherapy

Monoclonal antibodies can mediate efficient tumor cell kill by human complement[99] and by human lymphocytes,[100,101] neutrophils,[102,103] and activated monocyte/macrophages.[104] Neuroblastoma has poor expression of decay-accelerating factor and is therefore unable to resist complement activation and cytotoxicity.[105] Complement may be critical for the initiation of inflammation that can attract leukocytes and increase vascular permeability to proteins, including passively administered monoclonal antibodies.

A number of phase I studies have been carried out to define the acute toxicities of unconjugated antibodies. At dose levels of 5 mg/m^2 to 500 mg/m^2, there were significant toxicities, including severe pain, hypertension, hypotension, hyponatremia, sensory and autonomic neuropathy, papilledema without increase in intracranial pressure, visual symptoms, and optic atrophy (Table 110-4). The toxicity spectrum appeared to be more severe among adults, and it was not consistently associated with a human antimouse antibody (HAMA) response. Antitumor activity was observed in patients with chemorefractory neuroblastomas and melanomas, although responses were few and not durable. Although the antitumor effect appears to be associated with complement-mediated cytotoxicity and antibody-dependent cell-mediated cytotoxicity (ADCC), additional mechanisms are likely, given the length of time required for

TABLE 110-4. *Anti-G_{D2} antibodies in the treatment of human neuroblastoma*

Antibody	T1/2β	Dose/Cycle	CR	PR	HAMA	Side effects	Investigators
14.G2a	30–53†	100–400	2/6	2/6	9/9	—	Handgretinger et al, 1992[131]
14.G2a	—	25–500	1/15	—	6/7	Papilledema Fixed dilated pupils without increased intracranial pressure	Yu et al, 1991[132]
14,G2a	46	50–200	—	2/5	5/5	Hyponatremia Severe postural hypotension Severe paresthesia	Murray et al, 1994[116]
14G.2a	42	10–120‡	—	—	12/12	Hyponatremia Neuropathy	Saleh et al, 1992[133]; Dropcho et al, 1992[134]
ch14.18	66.6	5–200	3/7	1/7	—		Yu et al, 1991[135]
ch14.18	185§	5–50‡	—	—	8/13	—	Saleh et al, 1992[136]
3F8	43	5–100	—	1/8	2/8	Paresthesia	Cheung et al, 1987[122]; Cheung et al, 1992[123]

CR, complete remission; PR, partial remission.
† T1/2α (initial plasma half-life) = 0.66–2.0
‡ Total mg given to each patient, not per m^2
§ T1/2α (terminal plasma half-life) = 23

response (weeks after the initiation of treatment) and the continued response long after treatment has ended.

Antiidiotype network[106,107] or T-cell response against antibody-modified tumors[108,109] may have contributed to the tumor regression. Antiidiotypic antibodies are clearly effective in inducing antigen-binding antibodies that protect animal systems from various infectious agents and tumors.[110,111] Their role in human cancer is much less definitive.[107,109,112–115] Among patients treated with the murine antiganglioside G_{D2} monoclonal antibodies (Ab1), a substantial portion of the HAMA response was directed against the $F(ab')_2$ portion of the mouse antibody, uninhibitable by IgG-class–matched myelomas, a result most consistent with antiidiotype antibodies (Ab2). Patients who developed antiidiotypic[116] or anti-antiidiotypic antibodies[107] demonstrated more responses or longer PFS times. These observations suggest that monoclonal antibody–mediated antitumor effects can proceed in at least two phases. Although the initial rapid phase uses complement-mediated cytotoxicity and ADCC, the second or delayed phase may involve an antiidiotype network. Although previously postulated,[113,117,118] the importance of the antiidiotype network (Ab3 production), especially in patients receiving antiganglioside monoclonal antibodies, has been difficult to demonstrate. Although much effort is devoted to developing antiidiotype antibodies as vaccines, the fine specificities of idiotypic network in patients receiving clinically active monoclonal antibodies have remained largely unexplored and the immunologically relevant epitopes undefined.[107]

The formation of HAMA and the inefficiency of most murine IgG subclasses in binding to human Fc receptors have stimulated a large effort to genetically engineer chimeric and humanized antibodies. For murine antibodies of the IgG_1 or IgG_{2a} subclasses that are unable to activate human complement or mediate ADCC with human leukocytes, there would seem to be a significant advantage to chimeric and humanized forms.[119,120] However, some murine anti-G_{D2} IgG_3 antibodies, such as 3F8, are unusually efficient in activating human complement, compared with their chimeric constructs, whereas leukocyte-mediated ADCC is quite comparable.

Although most attention has been focused on monoclonal antibody Fc functions, there are other biologic factors that are often overlooked in choosing antibodies for clinical development. Because the in vivo antitumor mechanism of a monoclonal antibody is complex, common parameters such as antibody affinity, nonspecific uptake by reticuloendothelial system, tumor penetration, toxicity, and antiidiotypic network are not usually appraised. In initial clinical development of antibodies, an excellent tumor uptake (both in tumor-to-nontumor ratio and in absolute uptake in percent injected dose per gram) is critical whether the murine antibody or chimeric form is being used. Other factors often overlooked are the spectrum of toxicities encountered and the potentials for late complications.

Clinical experience with monoclonal antibodies in neuroblastoma is still limited. Although no neurologic damage has been detected among the more than 50 children who have been treated with 3F8, after some have been monitored for more than 2 years (maximum, 8 years), the definitive toxicity spectrum can be determined only among long-term survivors. The apparent differences among anti-G_{D2} antibodies (see Table 110-4) may be dose related. Nevertheless, they highlight the caution that is needed, because the spectrum of toxicities in children can differ from those in adults, and because differences in antibody fine specificities can affect toxicity and efficacy.

Use of Monoclonal Antibodies in Combined Modality Therapy for Poor-Risk Neuroblastoma

Although unmodified monoclonal antibodies have not demonstrated significant antitumor activity against bulky tumors, their role in treating microscopic disease appears promising.[121] In phase I through phase II studies,[122–124] acute self-limited toxicities of 3F8 treatment included severe pain requiring analgesics, fever, urticaria, hypertension, hypotension, anaphylactoid reactions of the respiratory tract, and significant but rapidly reversible decreases in blood counts and serum complement levels. The absence of neurologic damage has prompted the use of this agent in patients with minimal residual disease. Among

22 patients with stage 4 neuroblastoma diagnosed at more than 18 months of age who had shown progression while off therapy and were successfully reinduced to achieve complete remission or very good partial remission (CR/VGPR) or minimal residual marrow disease, >30% remained progression-free during a median follow-up period of 56 months after 3F8 treatment. Of 18 newly diagnosed patients with similar poor-prognosis neuroblastomas (stage 4, >18 months of age at diagnosis) who were treated with 3F8 after they achieved their first CR/VGPR, >30% remained alive with no evidence of disease, during a median follow-up period of 32 months after diagnosis, without ABMT.

Although these sample sizes are small, they suggest that a treatment strategy that combines dose-intensive induction (rapid bulk tumor ablation) and antibody targeting (selective removal of minimal residual disease) can significantly extend the survival times of a substantial number of patients. Recent refinements of antibody-based therapies using antibody-toxin conjugates, novel radionuclide conjugates, and antibody-cytokine fusion proteins have shown promising results in preclinical and early clinical trials.[125] Further understanding of the biology of cell differentiation and programmed cell death may provide additional targets for elimination of microscopic residual disease. A multimodality approach is probably necessary for reducing the lethality of this neuroblastoma.

REFERENCES

1. Young JLJ, Miller RW. Incidence of malignant tumors in U.S. children. J Pediatr 1975;86:254.
2. Bader KL, Miller RW. US cancer incidence and mortality in the first year of life. Am J Dis Child 1979;133:157.
3. Stiller CA. Trends in neuroblastoma in Great Britain: incidence and mortality, 1971–1990. Eur J Cancer 1993;29A:1008.
4. Triche TJ, Askin FB. Neuroblastoma and the differential diagnosis of small round blue cell tumors. Hum Pathol 1983;14:569.
5. Finklestein JZ, Klemperer MR, Evans A, et al. Multiagent chemotherapy for children with metastatic neuroblastoma: a report from Childrens Cancer Study Group. Med Pediatr Oncol 1979;6:179.
6. Ninane J, Pritchard J, Malpas JS. Chemotherapy of advanced neuroblastoma: does adriamycin contribute? Arch Dis Child 1981;56:544.
7. Green A, Hayes FA, Hustu HO. Sequential cyclophosphamide and doxorubicin for induction of complete remission in children with disseminated neuroblastoma. Cancer 1981;48:2310.
8. Simone JV. The treatment of neuroblastoma. J Clin Oncol 1984;2: 717. Editorial.
9. Hayes FA, Green AA, Casper J, Cornet J, Evans WE. Clinical evaluation of sequentially scheduled cisplatin and VM26 in neuroblastoma. Cancer 1981;48:1715.
10. Hayes FA, Green AA, Mauer AM. Correlation of cell kinetic and clinical response to chemotherapy in disseminated neuroblastoma. Cancer Res 1977;37:3766.
11. McElwain TJ, Hedley DW, Gordon MY, et al. High dose melphalan and non-cryopreserved autologous bone marrow: treatment of malignant melanoma and neuroblastoma. Exp Hematol 1979;7(Suppl 5): 360.
12. Treleaven JG, Ugelstad J, Philip T, et al. Removal of neuroblastoma cells from bone marrow with monoclonal antibodies conjugated to magnetic microspheres. Lancet 1984;1:70.
13. Reynolds CP, Reynolds DA, Frenkel EP, Smith RG. Selective toxicity of 6-hydroxydopamine and ascorbate for human neuroblastoma in vitro: a model for clearing marrow prior to autologous transplant. Cancer Res 1982;42:1331.
14. August CA, Serota FT, Koch PA, et al. Treatment of advanced neuroblastoma with supralethal chemotherapy, radiation, and allogeneic or autologous marrow reconstitution. J Clin Oncol 1984;2:609.
15. Foreman NK, Rill DR, Coustan-Smith E, Douglass EC, Brenner MK. Mechanisms of selective killing of neuroblastoma cells by natural killer cells and lymphokine activated killer cells: potential for residual disease eradication. Br J Cancer 1993;67:933.
16. Brenner MK, Rill DR, Holladay MS, et al. Gene marking to determine whether autologous marrow infusion restores long-term haemopoiesis in cancer patients. Lancet 1993;342:1134.
17. Seeger RC, Moss TJ, Feig SA, et al. Bone marrow transplantation for poor prognosis neuroblastoma. In: Evans, AE, D'Angio GJ, Knudsen AG, Seeger RC, eds. Prog Clin Biol Res 271: Advances in neuroblastoma research 2. New York, Alan R Liss, 1988;203.
18. Graham-Pole J, Casper J, Elfenbein G, et al. High-dose chemoradiotherapy supported by marrow infusions for advanced neuroblastoma: a Pediatric Oncology Group study. J Clin Oncol 1991;9:152.
19. Phillip T, Zucker JM, Bernard JL, et al. Improved survival at 2 and 5 years in the LMCE1 unselected group of 72 children with stage IV neuroblastoma older than 1 year of age at diagnosis: is cure possible in a small subgroup? J Clin Oncol 1991;9:1037.
20. Kushner BH, Gulati SC, O'Reilly RJ, Heller G, Cheung NKV. Autografting with bone marrow exposed to repeated courses of very high dose cyclophosphamide in vivo and to 4-hydroperoxycyclophosphamide in vitro. Med Pediatr Oncol 1990;18:454.
21. Moss TJ, Cairo M, Santana VM, et al. Clonogenicity of circulating neuroblastoma cells: implications regarding peripheral blood stem cell transplantation. Blood 1994;83:3085.
22. Shuster JJ, Cantor AB, McWilliams N, et al. The prognostic significance of autologous bone marrow transplant in advanced neuroblastoma. J Clin Oncol 1991;9:1045.
23. Stram DO, Matthay KK, O'Leary M, Reynolds CP, Seeger RC. Myeloablative chemoradiotherapy versus continued chemotherapy for high risk neuroblastoma. In: Evans AE, Biedler JL, Brodeur GM, D'Angio GJ, Nakagawara A, eds. Prog Clin Biol Res 385: Advances in neuroblastoma research 4. New York, Wiley-Liss, 1994;287.
24. Pinkerton CR, Hartmann O, Dini G, Philip T. ENSG 1: randomized study of high-dose melphalan in neuroblastoma. In: Dicke KA, Spitzer G, Jagannath S, eds. Autologous bone marrow transplantation: proceedings of the third international symposium, Houston. The University of Texas MD Anderson Hospital and Tumor Institute, 1989;401.
25. Pritchard J, Kiely E, Rogers DW, et al. Long-term survival after advanced neuroblastoma. N Engl J Med 1987;317:1026.
26. Hartmann O, Benhamou E, Beaujean F, et al. Repeated high-dose chemotherapy followed by purged autologous bone marrow transplantations as consolidation therapy in metastatic neuroblastoma. J Clin Oncol 1987;5:1205.
27. Kushner BH, O'Reilly RJ, Mandell LR, et al. Myeloablative combination chemotherapy without total body irradiation for neuroblastoma. J Clin Oncol 1991;9:274.
28. Pinkerton CR, Philip T, Biron P, et al. High-dose melphalan, vincristine, and total-body irradiation with autologous bone marrow transplantation in children with relapsed neuroblastoma: a phase II study. Med Pediatr Oncol 1987;15:236.
29. Ladenstein R, Lasset C, Hartmann O, et al. Impact of megatherapy on survival after relapse from stage 4 neuroblastoma in patients over 1 year of age at diagnosis: a report from the European Group for Bone Marrow Transplantation. J Clin Oncol 1993;11:2330.
30. Woods WG, Lemieux B, Leclerc J-M, et al. Screening for neuroblastoma in North America: The Quebec Project. In: Evans AE, Biedler JL, Brodeur GM, D'Angio GJ, Nakagawara A, eds. Prog Clin Biol Res 385: Advances in neuroblastoma research 4. New York, Wiley-Liss, 1994:377.
31. Goldie JH, Coldman AJ. The somatic mutation theory of drug resistance: The "Goldie-Coldman" hypothesis revisited. In: Devita HR, ed. Cancer: principles and practice of oncology, 3rd ed, vol 3. Philadelphia, JP Lippincott, 1989:1.
32. Cheung NK, Heller G. Chemotherapy dose intensity correlates strongly with response, median survival and median progression-free survival in metastatic neuroblastoma. J Clin Oncol 1991;9:1050.
33. Carli M, Green AA, Hayes FA, Rivera G, Pratt CB. Therapeutic efficacy of single drugs for childhood neuroblastoma: a review. In: Raybaud C, Clement R, Lebreuil G, Bernard JL, eds. Proceedings of the 13th meeting of the International Society of Pediatric Oncology, ICS 570. Amsterdam, Excerpta Medica, 1982:141.
34. Frei E III, Teicher BA, Holden SA, Cathcart KNS, Wang Y. Preclinical studies and clinical correlation of the effect of alkylating dose. Cancer Res 1988;48:6417.
35. Kushner BH, O'Reilly RJ, LaQuaglia M, Cheung NK. Dose intensive

use of cyclophosphamide in ablation of neuroblastoma. Cancer 1990; 66:1095.
36. Teicher BA, Cucchi CA, Lee JB, et al. Alkylating agents: in vitro studies of cross-resistance patterns in human cell lines. Cancer Res 1986;46:4379.
37. Waxman DJ. Glutathione S-transferases: role in alkylating agent resistance and possible target for modulation chemotherapy. A review. Cancer Res 1990;50:6449.
38. Hamilton TC, Ozols RF, Dabrow MB. Multidrug resistance to alkylating agents and platinum compounds: state of our knowledge. Oncology 1990;4:101.
39. Van der Bliek AM, Baas F, Van der Velde-Koerts T, et al. Genes amplified and overexpressed in human multidrug-resistant cell lines. Cancer Res 1988;48:5927.
40. Bourhis J, Benard J, Hartmann O, et al. Correlation of *MDR1* gene expression with chemotherapy in Neuroblastoma. J Natl Cancer Inst 1989;81:1401.
41. Goldstein LJ, Fojo AT, Ueda K, et al. Expression of the multidrug resistance, *MDR1*, gene in neuroblastomas. J Clin Oncol 1990;8:128.
42. Chan HSL, Thorner PS, Haddad G, et al. P-glycoprotein (P170) status predicts outcome of therapy in advanced neuroblastoma and soft tissue sarcoma. Proc Am Soc Clin Oncol 1990;9:290.
43. Teicher BA, Frei E III. Development of alkylating agent-resistant human tumor cell lines. Cancer Chemother Pharmacol 1988;21:292.
44. Jain RK. Delivery of novel therapeutic agents in tumors: physiological barriers and strategies. J Natl Cancer Inst 1989;81:570.
45. Hasse GM, Wong KY, deLorimier AA, Sather HN, Hammon GD. Improvement in survival after excision of primary tumor in stage III neuroblastoma. J Pediatr Surg 1989;24:194.
46. Le Tourneau JN, Bernard JL, Hendren WH, Carcassonne M. Evaluation of the role of surgery in 130 patients with neuroblastoma. J Pediatr Surg 1985;20:244.
47. Matsumura M, Atkinson JB, Hays DM, et al. An evaluation of the role of surgery in metastatic neuroblastoma. J Pediatr Surg 1988;23: 448.
48. LaQualia MP, Kushner BH, Heller G, et al. Stage 4 neuroblastoma diagnosed at more than one year of age: gross total resection and clinical outcome. J Pediatr Surg 1994;29:1162.
49. Sitarz A, Finklestein J, Grosfeld J, et al. An evaluation of the role of surgery in disseminated neuroblastoma: a report from the Children's Cancer Study Group. J Pediatr Surg 1983;18:147.
50. Azizkhan RG, Shaw A, Chandler JG. Surgical complications of neuroblastoma resection. Surgery 1985;97:514.
51. Rosen EM, Cassady RJ, Frantz CN, et al. Neuroblastoma: The Joint Center for Radiation Therapy/Dana-Farber Cancer Institute/Children's Hospital experience. J Clin Oncol 1984;2:719.
52. Deacon JM, Wilson PA, Peckham MJ. The radiobiology of neuroblastoma. Radiother Oncol 1985;3:201.
53. Wheldon TE, O'Donoghue J, Gregor A, Livingstone A, Wilson L. Radiobiological considerations in the treatment of neuroblastoma by total body irradiation. Radiother Oncol 1986;6:317.
54. Green AA, Hustu HO, Palmer R, Pinkel D. Total body sequential segmental irradiation and combination chemotherapy for children with disseminated neuroblastoma. Cancer 1976;38:2250.
55. Kun LE, Casper JT, Kline RW, Piaskowski VD. Fractionated total body irradiation for metastatic neuroblastoma. Int J Radiat Oncol Biol Phys 1981;7:1599.
56. Helson L, Jereb B, Vogel R. Sequential hemi-body irradiation in treatment of advanced neuroblastoma: a pilot study. Int J Radiat Oncol Biol Phys 1981;7:531.
57. Seeger RC, Villablanca JG, Matthay KK, et al. Intensive chemoradiotherapy and autologous bone marrow transplantation for poor prognosis neuroblastoma. In: Evans AE, D'Angio GJ, Knudson AG, Seeger RC, eds. Prog Clin Biol Res, vol 366: Advances in neuroblastoma research 3. New York, Wiley-Liss, 1991;527.
58. Shafford EA, Rogers DW, Pritchard J. Advanced neuroblastoma: improved response rate using a multiagent regimen (OPEC) including sequential cisplatin and VM26. J Clin Oncol 1984;2:742.
59. Gelfand MJ. Meta-iodobenzylguanidine in children. Semin Nucl Med 1993;23:231.
60. Beierwaltes WH. Application of I-131 metaiodobenzylguanidine. Nucl Med Biol 1987;14:183.
61. Caballero O, Ferris J, Verdeguer A, et al. Visualization of a ganglioneuroma by means of scintigraphy with 131-I-MIBG. Eur J Nucl Med 1986;12:351.
62. Pritchard J, Gordon I, Lashford L, Dicks-Mireaux C. Specificity of iodobenzylguanidine scanning in neuroblastoma. Lancet 1988;1:479.
63. Clerico A, Jenkner A, Castello MA, et al. Functionally active ganglioneuronma with increased plasma and urinary catecholamines and positive iodine 131-metaiodobenzylguanidine scintigraphy. Med Pediatr Oncol 1991;19:329.
64. Hoefnagel CA, Voute PA, de Kraker J, Marcuse HR. Radionuclide diagnosis and therapy of neural crest tumors using iodine-131-metaiodobenzylguanidine. J Nucl Med 1987;28:308.
65. Moyes JS, Babich JW, Carter R, et al. Quantitative study of radioiodinated metaiodobenzylguanidine uptake in children with neuroblastoma: correlation with tumor histopathology. J Nucl Med 1989;30: 474.
66. Montaldo PG, Lanciotti M, Casalaro A, Cornaglia-Ferraris P, Ponzoni M. Accumulation of *m*-iodobenzylguanidine by neuroblastoma cells results from independent uptake and storage mechanisms. Cancer Res 1991;51:4342.
67. Bouvier JF, Philip T, Chauvot P, et al. Pitfalls and solutions in neuroblastoma diagnosis using radioiodine-MIBG: our experience about 50 cases. In: Evans AE, D'Angio GJ, Knudsen AG, Seeger RC, eds. Prog Clin Biol Res 271: Advances in neuroblastoma research 2. New York, Alan R Liss, 1988:707.
68. Schmiegelow K, Siimes MA, Agertoft L, et al. Radio-iodobenzylguanidine scintigraphy of neuroblastoma: conflicting results, when compared with standard investigation. Med Pediatr Oncol 1989;17:126.
69. Gordon I, Peters AM, Gutman A, et al. Skeletal assessment in neuroblastoma: the pitfalls of iodine-123–MIBG scans. J Nucl Med 1990; 31:129.
70. Sautter-Bihl ML, Bihl H, Heinze HG, et al. Stellenwert der 99mTc-MDP-skelettszintigraphie beim neuroblastom: 1st eine neubewertung notig? Nuklearmedizin 1991;30:7.
71. Yeh SD, Larson SM, Burch L, et al. Radioimmunodetection of neuroblastoma with iodine-131-3F8: correlation with biopsy, iodine-131-metaiodobenzylguanidine (MIBG) and standard diagnostic modalities. J Nucl Med 1991;32:769.
72. Klingebiel T, Berthold F, Treuner J, et al. Metaiodobenzylguanidine (MIBG) in treatment of 47 patients with neuroblastoma: results of the German Neuroblastoma Trial. Med Pediatr Oncol 1991;19:84.
73. Garaventa A, Guerra P, Arrighini A, et al. Treatment of advanced neuroblastoma with I-131 meta-iodobenzylguanidine. Cancer 1991; 67:922.
74. Voute PA, Hoefnagel CA, de Kraker J, et al. Results of treatment with 131-I-metaiodobenzylguanidine in patients with neuroblastoma: future prospects of zetotherapy. In: Evans AE, D'Angio DJ, Knudson AG, Seeger RC, eds. Prog Clin Biol Res 366: Advances in neuroblastoma research 3. New York, Wiley-Liss, 1991;439.
75. Lashford LS, Lewis IJ, Fielding SL, et al. Phase I/II study of iodine 131 metaiodobenzylguanidine in chemoresistant neuroblastoma: a United Kingdom Children's Cancer Study Group investigation. J Clin Oncol 1992;10:1889.
76. Hutchinson RJ, Sisson JC, Shapiro B, et al. 131-I-metaiodo-benzylguanidine treatment in patients with refractory advanced neuroblastoma. Am J Clin Oncol 1992;15:226.
77. O'Donoghue JA, Wheldon TE, Babich JW, et al. Therapeutic implications of the uptake of radiolabelled mIBG for the treatment of neuroblastoma. In: Evans AE, D'Angio DJ, Knudson AG, Seeger RC, eds. Prog Clin Biol Res 366: Advances in neuroblastoma research 3. New York, Wiley-Liss, 1991:455.
78. Humm JL. Dosimetric aspects of radiolabelled antibodies for tumour therapy. J Nucl Med 1986;27:1490.
79. Matthay KK, Gaudin P, Calzolari P, et al. Effect of differentiation inducers and calcium channel blockers on 125I-metaiodobenzylguanidine uptake by neuroblastoma. Proc Am Assoc Cancer Res 1990; 31:412.
80. Vaidyanathan G, Zalutsky MR. *meta*-[211-At]Astatobenzylguanine: synthesis via astatodemetallation and preliminary in vitro and in vivo evaluation. Bioconjug Chem 1992;3:499.
81. Vaidyanathan G, Zalutsky MR. No-carrier-added synthesis of meta-[131]-iodobenzylguanidine. Int J Radiat Appl Instrum 1993;44:621.
82. Cheung NK. Biological and molecular approaches to treatment: immunotherapy. In: Pizzo, PA, Poplack, DG, eds. Principles and practice of pediatric oncology, 2nd ed. Philadelphia, JB Lippincott, 1992:357.

83. Larson SM, Cheung NK, Leibel S. Antibodies in cancer therapy: basic principles of monoclonal antibodies. Radioisotope conjugates. In: DeVita VT, Hellman S, Rosenberg SA, eds. Biologic therapy of cancer. Philadelphia, JB Lippincott, 1991:496.
84. Kemshead JT, Malpas JS, Pritchard J, Breatnach F. Targeted radiation therapy to neuroblastoma cells using 131-I conjugated to monoclonal antibody UJ13A. In: Evans AE, ed. Prog Clin Biol Res: Advances in neuroblastoma research. New York, Allan R Liss, 1984.
85. Amstutz H, Rytz C, Novak-Hofer I, et al. Production and characterization of a mouse/human chimeric antibody directed against human neuroblastoma. Int J Cancer 1993;53:147.
86. Novak-Hofer I, Amstutz HP, Haldemann A, et al. Radioimmunolocalization of neuroblastoma xenografts with chimeric antibody chCE7. J Nucl Med 1992;33:231.
87. Miraldi FD, Nelson AD, Kraly C, et al. Diagnostic imaging of human neuroblastoma with radiolabeled antibody. Radiology 1986;161:413.
88. Kusano A, Ohta S, Shitara K, Hanai N. Immunocytochemical study of internalization of anti-carbohydrate monoclonal antibodies. Anticancer Res 1993;13:2207.
89. Sariola H, Terava H, Rapola J, Saarinen UM. Cell-surface ganglioside G_{D2} in the immunohistochemical detection and differential diagnosis of neuroblastoma. Am J Clin Pathol 1991;96:248.
90. Furman WL, Fairclough DL, Huhn RD, et al. Therapeutic effects and pharmacokinetics of recombinant human granulocyte-macrophage colony-stimulating factor in childhood cancer patients receiving myelosuppressive chemotherapy. J Clin Oncol 1991;6:1022.
91. Wilbur JR, Shurin SB, Seeger RC. Response of neuroblastoma bone marrow metastases to 13-*cis*-retinoic acid. Proc Am Soc Clin Oncol 1990;9:64.
92. Thiele CJ, Reynolds CP, Israel MA. Decreased expression of N-*myc* precedes retinoic acid–induced morphological differentiation of human neuroblastoma. Nature 1985;313:404.
93. Finkelstein JZ, Krailo MD, Lenarsky C, et al. 13-*cis*-Retinoic acid (NSC 122758) in the treatment of children with metastatic neuroblastoma unresponsive to conventional chemotherapy: report from the Children's Cancer Study Group. Med Pediatr Oncol 1992;20:307.
94. Villablanca JG, Avramis VI, Khan AA, et al. Phase I trial of 13-*cis*-retinoic acid (*cis*-RA) in neuroblastoma patients following bone marrow transplantation. Proc Am Soc Clin Oncol 1992;11:366.
95. Favrot M, Floret D, Michon J, et al. A phase II study of adoptive immunotherapy with continuous infusion of interleukin-2 in children with advanced neuroblastoma: a report on 11 cases. Cancer Treat Rev 1989;16(Suppl A):129.
96. Negrier S, Michon J, Floret D, et al. Interleukin-2 and lymphokine-activated killer cells in 15 children with advanced metastatic neuroblastoma. J Clin Oncol 1991;9:1363.
97. Michon J, Negrier S, Coze C, et al. Administration of high dose recombinant interleukin-2 after autologous bone marrow transplantation in patients with neuroblastoma: toxicity, efficacy, and survival. A Lyons-Marseille-Curie-East of France Group Study. In: Evans AE, Biedler JL, Brodeur GM, D'Angio GJ, Nakagawara A, eds. Prog Clin Biol Res 385: Advances in neuroblastoma research 4. New York, Wiley-Liss, 1994:293.
98. Evans AE, Main E, Zier K, et al. The effects of gamma interferon on natural killer and tumor cells of children with neuroblastoma: a preliminary report. Cancer 1989;64:1383.
99. Saarinen UM, Coccia PF, Gerson S, et al. In vitro eradication of neuroblastoma (NB) cells by monoclonal antibody (Mab) and human complement (C′): a method for purging autologous bone marrow (BM). Proc Am Assoc Cancer Res 1985;26:291.
100. Munn DH, Cheung NK. Interleukin-2 enhancement of monoclonal antibody-mediated cellular cytotoxicity (ADCC) against human melanoma. Cancer Res 1987;47:6600.
101. Gillies SD, Reilly EB, Lo KM, Reisfeld RA. Antibody-targeted interleukin-2 stimulates T-cell killing of autologous tumor cells. Proc Natl Acad Sci U S A 1992;89:1428.
102. Kushner BH, Cheung NK. GM-CSF enhances 3F8 monoclonal antibody–dependent cellular cytotoxicity against human melanoma and neuroblastoma. Blood 1989;73:1936.
103. Barker E, Mueller BM, Handgretinger R, et al. Effect of a chimeric anti–ganglioside G_{D2} antibody on cell-mediated lysis of human neuroblastoma cells. Cancer Res 1991;51:144.
104. Munn DH, Cheung NK. Phagocytosis of tumor cells by human monocytes cultured in recombinant macrophage colony-stimulating factor. J Exp Med 1990;172:231.
105. Cheung NKV, Walter EI, Smith-Mensah WH, et al. Decay-accelerating factor protects human tumor cells from complement-mediated cytotoxicity in vitro. J Clin Invest 1988;81:1122.
106. Koprowski H, Herlyn D, Lubeck M, DeFreitas E, Sears HF. Human anti-idiotype antibodies in cancer patients: is the modulation of the immune response beneficial for the patient? Proc Natl Acad Sci U S A 1984;81:216.
107. Cheung NK, Cheung IY, Canete A, et al. Antibody response to murine anti-G_{D2} monoclonal antibodies: correlation with patient survival. Cancer Res 1994;54:2228.
108. Lanzavecchia A, Abrignani S, Scheidegger D, et al. Antibodies as antigens: the use of mouse monoclonal antibodies to focus human T cells against selected targets. J Exp Med 1988;167:345.
109. Fagerberg J, Frodin JE, Ragnhammar P, et al. Induction of an immune network cascade in cancer patients treated with monoclonal antibodies (ab1): II. Is induction of anti-idiotype reactive T cells (T3) of importance for tumor response to mAb therapy? Cancer Immunol Immunother 1994;38:149.
110. Sikorska HM. Therapeutic applications of antiidiotypic antibodies. J Biol Resp Modif 1988;7:327.
111. Kennedy RC, Zhou EM, Lanford RE, Chanh TC, Bona CA. Possible role of anti-idiotypic antibodies in the induction of tumor immunity. J Clin Invest 1991;80:1217.
112. Yamamoto S, Yamamoto T, Saxton RE, Hoon DSB, Irie RF. Anti-idiotype monoclonal antibody carrying the internal image of ganglioside G_{M3}. J Natl Cancer Inst 1990;82:1757.
113. Lichtin A, Iliopoulos D, Guerry D, et al. Therapy of melanoma with an anti-melanoma ganglioside monoclonal antibody: a possible mechanism of a complete response. Proc Am Soc Clin Oncol 1988;7:958.
114. Mittelman A, Chen ZJ, Kageshita T, et al. Active specific immunotherapy in patients with melanoma. J Clin Invest 1990;86:2136.
115. Robbins RA, Denton GWL, Hardcastle JD, et al. Antitumor immune response and interleukin 2 production produced in colorectal cancer patients by immunization with human monoclonal anti-idiotypic antibody. Cancer Res 1991;51:5425.
116. Murray JL, Cunningham JE, Brewer H, et al. Phase I trial of murine monoclonal antibody 14G2a administered by prolonged intravenous infusion in patients with neuroectodermal tumors. J Clin Oncol 1994;12:184.
117. Irie RF, Matsuki T, Morton DL. Human monoclonal antibody to ganglioside G_{M2} for melanoma treatment. Lancet 1989;1:786.
118. Herlyn D, Wettendorff M, Schmoll E, et al. Anti-idiotype immunization of cancer patients: modulation of the immune response. Proc Natl Acad Sci U S A 1987;84:8055.
119. Morrison SL. Transfectomas provide novel chimeric antibodies. Science 1985;229:1202.
120. Roberts S, Cheetham JC, Rees AR. Generation of an antibody with enhanced affinity and specificity for its antigen by protein engineering. Nature 1987;328:731.
121. Riethmüller G, Schneider-Gädicke E, Schlimok G, et al. Randomised trial of monoclonal antibody for adjuvant therapy of resected Dukes' C colorectal carcinoma. Lancet 1994;343:1177.
122. Cheung NK, Lazarus H, Miraldi FD, et al. Ganglioside G_{D2} specific monoclonal antibody 3F8: a phase I study in patients with neuroblastoma and malignant melanoma. J Clin Oncol 1987;5:1430.
123. Cheung NK, Lazarus H, Miraldi FD, et al. Reassessment of patient response to monoclonal antibody 3F8. J Clin Oncol 1992;10:671.
124. Cheung NKV, Kushner BH, Yeh SJ, Larson SM. 3F8 monoclonal antibody treatment of patients with stage IV neuroblastoma: a phase II study. In: Evans AE, Guillio JD, Biedler JL, Brodeur G, Nakagawara N, eds. Prog Clin Biol Res 385: Advances in neuroblastoma research, vol 4. New York, Wiley-Liss, 1994:319.
125. De Vita VT, Hellman S, Rosenberg SA, eds. Biologic therapy of cancer: principles and practice, 2nd ed. Philadelphia, JB Lippincott, 1995.
126. Pearson ADJ, Pinkerton CR, Gerard M, et al. High dose rapid schedule chemotherapy for disseminated neuroblastoma. Med Pediatr Oncol 1990;18:284.

127. O'Leary M, Sather H, Ramsay NKC, et al. Intensive chemotherapy for stage IV neuroblastoma (NB) over one year of age. Proc Am Soc Clin Oncol 1989;8:307. Abstract.
128. Bouvier JD, Seyfried TN. Ganglioside composition of normal and mutant mouse embryos. J Neurochem 1989;52:460.
129. Campbell LA, Seeger RC, Harris RE, et al. Escalating dose of continuous infusion combination chemotherapy for refractory neuroblastoma. J Clin Oncol 1993;11:623.
130. Castleberry RP, Green AA, Casper J, et al. A pilot study of high dose cisplatinum (HDP) and high dose VP16 (HVP) in children with recurrent neuroblastoma (NB). Proc Am Soc Clin Oncol 1987;6:218. abstr.
131. Handgretinger R, Baader P, Dopfer R, et al. A phase I study of neuroblastoma with the anti-ganglioside G_{D2} antibody 14.G2a. Cancer Immunol Immunother 1992;35:199.
132. Yu AL, Reisfeld RA, Gillies SD. Immune response to monoclonal anti-G_{D2} antibody therapy. Proc Am Assoc Cancer Res 1991;32:263.
133. Saleh MN, Khazaeli MB, Wheeler RH, et al. A phase I trial of the murine monoclonal anti-G_{D2} antibody 14.G2a in metastatic melanoma. Cancer Res 1992;52:4342.
134. Dropcho EJ, Saleh MN, Grizzle WE, Oh SJ. Peripheral neuropathy following treatment of melanoma with a murine anti-G_{D2} monoclonal antibody (MoAb). Neurology 1992;4:457.
135. Yu AL, Gillies SD, Reisfeld RA. Phase I clinical trial of ch14.18 in patients with refractory neuroblastoma. Proc Am Soc Clin Oncol 1991;10:318.
136. Saleh MN, Khazaeli MB, Wheeler RH, et al. Phase I trial of the chimeric anti-GD2 monoclonal antibody ch 14.18 in patients with malignant melanoma. Hum Antibod Hybridomas 1992;3:19.

SECTION XI

Wilms' Tumor/Nephroblastoma

Principles and Practice of Genitourinary Oncology, edited by Derek Raghavan, Howard I. Scher, Steven A. Leibel, and Paul H. Lange. Lippincott-Raven Publishers, Philadelphia, © 1997.

CHAPTER 111

Biology and Management of Wilms' Tumor

Daniel M. Green, Giulio J. D'Angio, J. Bruce Beckwith, Norman E. Breslow, Paul E. Grundy, Michael L. Ritchey, and Patrick R. M. Thomas

Wilms' tumor provides the paradigm for multimodal treatment of a pediatric malignant solid tumor. Developments in surgical techniques and postoperative care, recognition of the sensitivity of Wilms' tumor to irradiation, and the availability of several active chemotherapeutic agents have led to a dramatic improvement in the prognosis for most patients with this once uniformly lethal malignancy.

The clinical research on which these new treatments were based was initially conducted by individual institutions. Subsequently, randomized trials were conducted by multiinstitutional cooperative clinical trials groups. These studies contributed to the accurate categorization and increased understanding of the clinical evolution of Wilms' tumor and several other rare renal tumors of childhood and the development of more effective therapeutic strategies for these malignancies.[1,2] Equally promising are the advances being made in epidemiology, molecular biology, and genetics.[3–5]

The success of the studies conducted by the National Wilms' Tumor Study (NWTS) Group has resulted in the availability of a large population of uniformly treated patients who are available for study of the late effects of therapy,[6] and one or more models of Wilms' tumorigenesis have been confirmed through observation of the occurrence of Wilms' tumor in family members and in some of the patients' offspring.

EPIDEMIOLOGY AND GENETICS

Wilms' tumor is the most common malignant renal tumor in children and adolescents. In the United States, the annual incidence is 8.1 cases per million in white children younger than 15 years of age.[7] In 1991, Wilms' tumor represented 5% to 6% of childhood cancers in the United States, and the total incidence was estimated to be 460 cases per year.[8] The incidence rate is approximately three times higher for American and African blacks than for East Asians, and rates for Caucasian populations in Europe and North America fall between these extremes.[9] The median age at diagnosis is 35 months for boys and 42 months for girls with unilateral tumors, and 23 months for boys and 28.5 months for girls with bilateral tumors.[10]

Wilms' tumor shows a strong association with certain congenital anomalies, notably aniridia, hemihypertrophy, and malformations of the genitalia (e.g., cryptorchidism, hypospadias, pseudohermaphroditism, gonadal dysgenesis), especially in boys.[11,12] The disease occurs in conjunction with the Beckwith-Wiedemann syndrome; Denys-Drash syndrome, consisting of pseudohermaphroditism, glomerulopathy, and Wilms' tumor; and Perlman familial nephroblastomatosis malformation syndrome, consisting of bilateral renal hamartomas, macrosomia, islet cell hypertrophy, and unusual facies.[12–15]

Epidemiology

Several studies have analyzed parental occupations of patients with Wilms' tumor in comparison with those of patients with other childhood cancers and with unaffected children, usually with negative results.[16–18] Other research has indicated an increased risk for children whose fathers are occupationally exposed to hydrocarbons or lead[19] or work as mechanics or machinists.[20–22]

Nonoccupational risk factors, including maternal exposure to hormones, tobacco, and hair dyes during pregnancy; complications of pregnancy; and use of penthrane anesthesia have been investigated in association with Wilms' tumor incidence, but no consistent positive findings have emerged.[23–26]

Genetics

Wilms' tumor is an important model for the study of fundamental mechanisms of carcinogenesis. The inheritance of Wilms' tumor was initially thought to follow the pattern of retinoblastoma, in which approximately 10% of patients with sporadic unilateral tumors and all patients with bilateral tumors were thought to carry a germline mutation. The tumor would arise only if a second event occurs (i.e., the so-called second hit).[27] The first event may be constitutional—either a new germinal mutation transmitted from the father[28,29] or transmitted from a carrier or affected parent,[30] or it may be somatic. In either case, it results in loss of function of one of the alleles of the retinoblastoma (*RB1*) gene. Subsequently, the function of the remaining normal allele may be lost by one of several mechanisms, resulting in absence of normal RB1 gene product within the affected retinal cell.[31]

The genetics of Wilms' tumor, however, are more complex. Analysis of the epidemiologic and clinicopathologic features of patients with Wilms' tumor led the NWTS investigators to suggest that some bilateral and multicentric tumors may arise from somatic mosaicism rather than germline mutation.[3,11] They also suggested that the disease comprises at least two pathogenetic entities that are identifiable on the basis of distinct precursor lesions.[32]

The first evidence that a specific chromosomal locus was associated with Wilms' tumor was the demonstration that patients with aniridia and Wilms' tumor usually had an interstitial deletion at 11p13.[33] This deletion occurs preferentially in the paternal allele,[34] as is the case for new germinal mutations at 13q14.[28] Subsequently, several laboratories reported that about one third of Wilms' tumors have undergone tumor-specific loss of heterozygosity for polymorphic DNA markers on 11p13.[35,36] Isolation of the Wilms' tumor gene located at 11p13 (*WT1*)[37,38] allowed the sequence of the normal gene to be determined. Germinal mutations within the *WT1* gene have been identified in patients with Wilms' tumor who also have the rare Denys-Drash syndrome[39] and in a few patients with bilateral Wilms' tumor.[40] However, constitutional or even tumor-specific mutations of *WT1* have been found in far fewer cases than would be expected.[41,42] Furthermore, in some patients with a tumor-specific *WT1* mutation of one allele, the remaining allele is normal.[41]

A second Wilms' tumor locus was found to map to chromosome 11p15.5 based on tumor-specific loss of heterozygosity restricted to this region.[36] The Beckwith-Wiedemann syndrome, which is associated with a predisposition to embryonal tumors including Wilms' tumor, also maps to this location,[36] but it is not yet known whether a single gene or adjacent genes are involved in both the tumor and the syndrome. The copy of 11p15 lost in Wilms' tumor is invariably that which was derived from the mother.[35,43,44] This evidence suggests that the 11p15 Wilms' tumor locus is subject to genomic imprinting, resulting in a functional difference between the two alleles. *IGF2*, an embryonal growth factor, is a candidate gene for both Wilms' tumor and Beckwith-Wiedemann syndrome because it maps to 11p15.5,[45] is imprinted such that it is expressed only from the paternal allele,[46] and is highly expressed in Wilms' tumors.[47] Tumor-specific loss of imprinting at the *IGF2* locus has been found in many Wilms' tumors that did not show loss of DNA heterozygosity for 11p15,[46,48] and constitutional loss of the imprint is associated with both generalized somatic overgrowth and Wilms' tumor.[49] This epigenetic alteration may result in increased levels of *IGF2* and hence a possible autocrine stimulation pathway. Loss of heterozygosity for 11p15, which usually results from mitotic recombination rather than deletion, may not represent loss of a tumor suppressor allele but rather duplication of the only active *IGF2* allele. It is not yet known whether a separate Wilms' tumor suppressor gene may exist adjacent to *IGF2*. Finally, linkage studies of rare but large Wilms' tumor pedigrees have excluded linkage to 11p13 and 11p15[44,50] as well as linkage to 16q.[51]

The development of Wilms' tumor involves at least two genes on chromosome 11p, an as yet unidentified familial locus, and both genetic and epigenetic mechanisms.

PATHOLOGY

The gross appearance of the kidney, distorted by the presence of the tumor, seldom gives external evidence pointing to the underlying histopathology. Any associated congenital anomalies such as a bifid collecting system point more toward Wilms' tumor, which is associated with genitourinary anomalies.[52–54] Tumor multifocality or nephrogenic rests, which manifest as subcapsular, pale pink areas or nodules in the non–tumor-bearing kidney substance, are strongly suggestive of Wilms' tumor.[32]

An obvious multicystic lesion may be a manifestation of the multicystic–Wilms' tumor complex, whereas a tumor with a firm, rubbery consistency in an infantile kidney is more likely to be mesoblastic nephroma.[55,56]

HISTOPATHOLOGY

Wilms' Tumor

The classic nephroblastoma is made up of three cell types—blastemal, stromal, and epithelial; however, they are not all present in every case (Fig. 111-1). If anaplastic nuclear changes (described later) are not present, the histology is termed favorable (FH) by the NWTS Pathology Center because of the generally good outcome in these patients.[57]

The neoplastic elements often reflect their renal origin, forming primordial tubules and glomeruli with associated supporting tissues. Although there is much diversity from one tumor to the next, and often within a single tumor, the diagnosis is seldom difficult. Special stains and preparations are usually not required. Because of small sample size or extreme lack of differentiation of cellular components, ultrastructural study is sometimes needed. Wilms' tumor usually shows many well developed desmosomes, prominent cilia, and a distinctive flocculent material, possibly an embryonic adhesion molecule, surrounding the tumor cells.[58] Immunohistochemical analyses are useful primarily for exclusion of other small round cell tumors of childhood, notably the intrarenal neuroblastoma.

Anaplasia

Extensive research has been conducted to identify gross and histopathologic patterns that correlate with outcome. These are used both for staging purposes (Table 111-1) and for tumor type categorization. The excellent survival rates currently achieved with modern combined modality therapy make it difficult to detect features intrinsically associated with an especially favorable outlook.[59] Rather, cytohistopathology serves to identify those patients with a more ominous prognosis.

Anaplasia is recognized by the presence of gigantic polyploid nuclei within the tumor sample. Recognition of this change requires nuclei with major diameters at least three times those of adjacent cells, with increased chromatin content and the presence of multipolar or otherwise recognizably polypoid mitotic figures (Fig. 111-2). Both of these features must be identified in the sample. Occasionally, if only a small biopsy specimen is available, the presence of a single multipolar mitotic figure

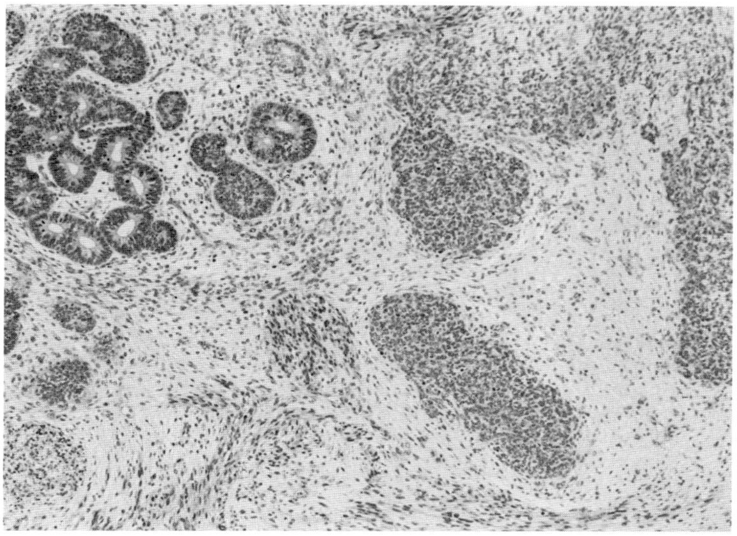

FIG. 111-1. Wilms tumor. Low-magnification photomicrograph showing three distinct cell types. Tubular structures, groups of densely packed blastemal cells, and loosely aggregated spindled stromal cells are seen. Nuclei are regular and without multipolar mitoses, in contrast to those seen in anaplastic Wilms tumor.

TABLE 111-1. *National Wilms Tumor Study clinicopathologic staging system*

Stage I
Tumor limited to kidney and completely excised. The surface of the renal capsule is intact. Tumor was not ruptured before or during removal. There is no residual tumor apparent beyond the margins of resection.
Stage II
Tumor extends beyond the kidney but has been completely removed. There is regional extension of the tumor (ie, penetration through the outer surface of the renal capsule into the perirenal soft tissues). Vessels outside the kidney substance are infiltrated or contain tumor thrombus. The tumor may have been biopsied or there has been local spillage of tumor confined to the flank. There is no residual tumor apparent at or beyond the margins of excision.
Stage III
Residual nonhematogenous tumor confined to the abdomen with one or more of the following: (a) lymph nodes on biopsy are found to be involved in the hilus, the periaortic chains or beyond; (b) there has been diffuse peritoneal contamination by tumor, such as spillage of tumor beyond the flank before or during surgery, or by tumor growth that has penetrated through the peritoneal surface; (c) implants are found on the peritoneal surface; (d) the tumor extends beyond the surgical margins either microscopically or grossly; and (e) the tumor is not completely resectable because of local infiltration into vital structures.
Stage IV
Hematogenous metastases. Deposits beyond stage III (eg, lung, liver, bone or brain).
Stage V
Bilateral renal involvement at diagnosis. An attempt should be made to stage each side according to these criteria on the basis of the extent of disease before biopsy.

or an unequivocally gigantic tumor cell nucleus suffices to diagnose anaplasia.

Anaplastic changes can be either focal or diffuse. The criteria distinguishing focal from diffuse anaplasia were modified in 1993.[60] The original definition of focal anaplasia was based on the amount of anaplasia present. Anaplastic nuclear changes present in fewer than 10% of microscopic fields was originally designated as focal anaplasia. This criterion permitted the inclusion of tumors in which anaplasia was present throughout the tumor, albeit at low density, and cases with anaplasia in extrarenal sites or in metastatic deposits. The new definition of focal anaplasia emphasizes distribution and requires that cells with anaplastic nuclear changes be confined to sharply restricted foci within the primary tumor.

Diffuse anaplasia is diagnosed if one or more of the following criteria are met:

- Anaplasia is present in any extrarenal site, including vessels of the renal sinus, extracapsular infiltrates, and nodal or distant metastases.
- Anaplasia is present in a random biopsy specimen.
- Anaplasia is unequivocally expressed in one region of the tumor, but with extreme nuclear pleomorphism approaching the criterion of anaplasia (extreme nuclear unrest) elsewhere in the lesion.
- Anaplasia is present in more than one tumor slide, unless it is known that every slide showing anaplasia came from the same region of the tumor or anaplastic foci on the various slides are minute and are surrounded on all sides by nonanaplastic tumor.

This topographic definition of focal anaplasia makes it mandatory that pathologists carefully document the exact site from which every section is obtained on a diagram, specimen photocopy, or Polaroid photograph of the gross specimen.

Anaplasia was present in 4.5% of cases entered in the NWTS-3 trial and was related to patient age (unpublished data). It is rare in the first 2 years of life (8 of 362 such patients; 2%); the incidence increases after age 2 years to a relatively stable rate of about 13% in those 5 years of age or older.[61] More recent

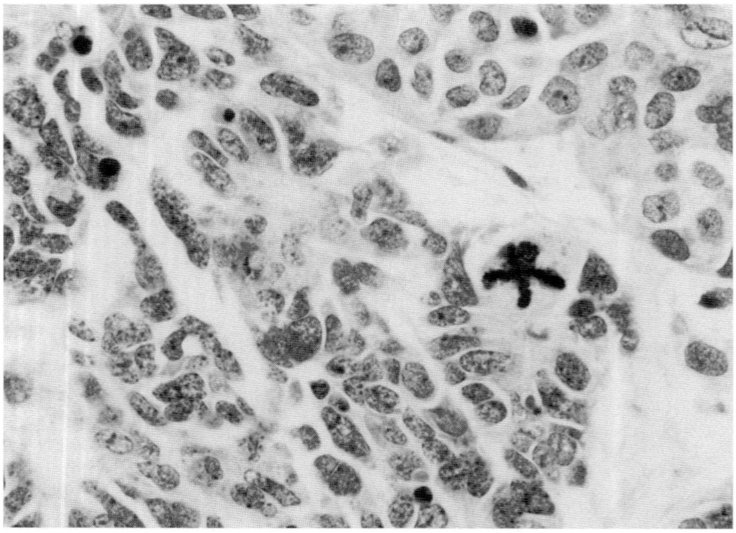

FIG. 111-2. Anaplastic Wilms tumor. Nuclei are variable in size, and a star-shaped multipolar mitotic figure is seen. Multipolar mitotic figures are the most important indicator of anaplasia.

NWTS data show only a slight increase in incidence of anaplasia in black patients than in white patients.[7,61]

Anaplasia in only one or a few small foci of a Wilms' tumor is sufficient to impart a poor prognosis. Stage II, III, and IV Wilms' tumor specimens must therefore be sampled thoroughly. The NWTS Pathology Center recommends that a minimum of one generous section be obtained for each centimeter of tumor diameter and that each individual tumor be sampled in multicentric or bilateral cases. Meticulous attention to details of tissue preservation and slide preparation is necessary. Poor fixation, sectioning, or staining can easily lead to false-positive or false-negative interpretations.

Clear Cell Sarcoma of the Kidney

Although not currently thought to be a Wilms' tumor variant, clear cell sarcoma of the kidney (CCSK) is an important entity to consider. Its site of origin and age distribution are identical to those of Wilms' tumor, yet it is associated with a significantly higher rate of relapse and death than FH Wilms' tumor. CCSK also displays a distinctively high rate of skeletal metastasis. This variant was first recognized in the literature by Kidd in 1970,[62] and in 1978 it was independently identified by pathologists of the NWTS and the United Kingdom Medical Research Council Nephroblastoma trial.[57,63] The descriptive term CCSK was used by the NWTS; British researchers referred to ''bone-metastasizing renal tumour of childhood.'' Several points concerning CCSK deserve emphasis.

In contrast to stage I anaplastic Wilms' tumor, stage I CCSK is associated with a very high rate of tumor relapse, suggesting that micrometastases occur early with this tumor. For example, in NWTS-2, five of seven stage I CCSK children relapsed and died with tumor. The use of doxorubicin (ADR) seems to be associated with a significantly improved outcome for CCSK.[64] This underscores the importance of correct identification of CCSK and places a major responsibility on pathologists. CCSK has been found to be associated with both brain and bone metastases.[64,65]

Most CCSK specimens have a distinct and easily recognized

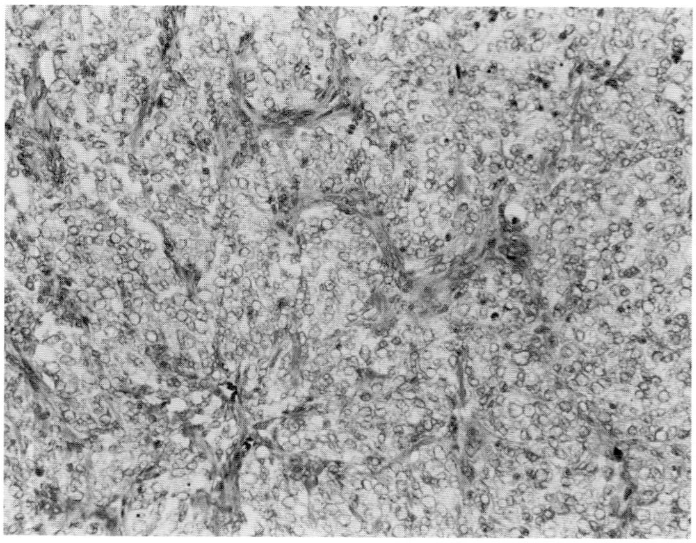

FIG. 111-3. Clear cell sarcoma of kidney. This lesion has a distinctive pattern, with cell cords subdivided by delicate vascular septa. Tumor cells have extremely pale, empty-appearing nuclei, and inconspicuous, pale-staining cytoplasm.

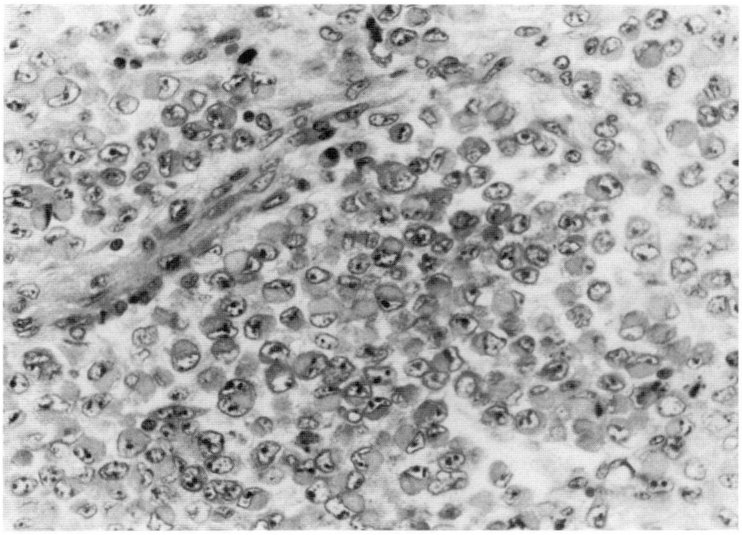

FIG. 111-4. Rhabdoid tumor of kidney. Tumor cells have abundant cytoplasm with vesicular nuclei and prominent nucleoli. Many cells contain pale, rounded cytoplasmic inclusions.

histologic appearance (Fig. 111-3), but a number of variant patterns, such as epithelioid, spindling, myxoid, and cystic patterns, invite confusion with Wilms' tumor or other tumor types.[66–69] Detailed descriptions and illustrations of both the classic and variant patterns are provided elsewhere.[63,70]

Rhabdoid Tumor of Kidney

A distinctive and highly malignant tumor type, rhabdoid tumor of the kidney (RTK), was identified for the first time in 1978 by NWTS pathologists.[57] The neoplasm, previously confused with Wilms' tumor, is a monomorphous tumor, as is CCSK. RTK tumor cells, unlike those of CCSK, characteristically have prominent acidophilic cytoplasm that often resembles that of myoblasts but is negative for ultrastructural or other markers of skeletal muscle (Fig. 111-4). The term rhabdomyosarcomatoid, used in the original description, was shortened to rhabdoid in a subsequent paper.[71] The cell of origin for this distinctive tumor remains unknown. It is not a variant of Wilms' tumor and is not encountered as a focal change in a conventional Wilms' tumor. Several points regarding this important entity deserve emphasis.

RTK is characteristically seen in the infant or very young child. The median age of patients seen in the NWTS Pathology Center is 13 months (range, 2 months to 5 years). It is associated with relapse and death rates higher than 80% and thus is one of the most malignant neoplasms in the pediatric population. The more aggressive therapeutic protocols used in NWTS-3 did not significantly improve the outlook for patients with this tumor. Stage I lesions, like those of CCSK, are associated with a high rate of relapse and death from advancing disease; unlike CCSK this pattern has not been altered by more aggressive therapies.[72]

Several cases have been reported in which apparently separate primary neuroectodermal tumors of the brain have developed in children with rhabdoid tumor.[73] A few clear cases of rhabdoid tumor do occur in extrarenal sites, but the majority of extrarenal rhabdoid tumors and RTK in patients older than 5 years of age represent other neoplasms. They can mimic RTK closely, both at the light microscopic and ultrastructural level. Many of these "pseudorhabdoid" entities can, however, be identified by immunohistochemistry or other techniques as carcinomas, melanomas, histiocytic tumors, or myosarcomas. Immunohistochemical studies of RTK have not clarified the cell of origin.[74]

PATTERNS OF SPREAD

Wilms' Tumor

The lung is the most common site of metastatic involvement (Tables 111-2 and 111-3).[75] Pulmonary deposits are present in most patients with stage IV disease at the time of diagnosis and are the first signs of relapse in those with stage I to III tumors who develop recurrent disease. The liver is the second most commonly affected organ; other regions are affected far less frequently. Intraabdominal relapses are unusual in children with

TABLE 111-2. *Third National Wilms Tumor Study: Metastases present at diagnosis among 1757 children with kidney tumors, by site and histology*

Site	FH (173/1550)* N (%)	Anaplastic (16/85)* N (%)	CCSK (4/76)* N (%)	RTK (10/46)* N (%)
Lung only	142 (82)	13 (81)	2 (50)	5 (50)
Liver only	10 (6)	1 (6)	0	0
Bone only	0	0	2 (50)	0
Lung and other	21 (12)	2 (13)	0	3 (30)
Other	0	0	0	2 (20)

FH, favorable histology; Ana, anaplasia; CCSK, clear cell sarcoma of the kidney; RTK, rhabdoid tumor of the kidney.
* Number of patients with metastases/total number observed.

Adapted from Weeks DA, Beckwith JB, Mierau GW, Luckey DW. Rhabdoid tumor of kidney. Am J Surg Pathol 1989;13:439.

TABLE 111-3. *Third National Wilms Tumor Study: Sites of initial relapse by histology among 1554 children with renal tumors without metastases at diagnosis*

Site†	FH (174/1377)* N (%)	Ana (25/69)* N (%)	CCSK (26/72)* N (%)	RTK (26/36)* N (%)
Lung	114 (66)	10 (40)	5 (19)	14 (54)
Liver	18 (10)	5 (20)	1 (4)	3 (12)
Bone	1 (1)	1 (4)	13 (50)	1 (4)
Brain	0	0	5 (19)	3 (12)
Flank/ Abdomen	31 (18)	12 (48)	2 (8)	13 (50)
Kidney	18 (10)	0	0	0
Other	20 (11)	3 (12)	4 (15)	4 (15)

FH, favorable histology; Ana, anaplasia; CCSK, clear cell carcinoma of the kidney; RTK, rhabdoid tumor of the kidney.
* Number of patients with relapse/total number observed.
† More than one site might have been involved.

Adapted from Weeks DA, Beckwith JB, Mierau GW, Luckey DW. Rhabdoid tumor of kidney. Am J Surg Pathol 1989;13:439.

early stage FH tumors; they are more commonly associated with stage III FH disease and anaplastic tumors. Metastases to bone and brain are rare. Metachronous involvement of the opposite kidney is more likely in children who have nephrogenic rests in one or both kidneys at the time of original surgery.[32]

Clear Cell Sarcoma of the Kidney

As in Wilms' tumor, the lung is a common site of metastatic involvement, either at diagnosis or at the time of relapse. In addition, the bone-metastasizing renal tumor of childhood, lives up to its name[63]: although bone metastases were not commonly present at the time of diagnosis in NWTS-3 children, they were found in 50% of those who had relapses. The brain is another site of potential involvement. This has become evident only in the past few years, as improvements in chemotherapy result in longer life for CCSK patients.[61]

Rhabdoid Tumor of Kidney

Like the other renal malignant neoplasms, RTK metastasizes to the lung most frequently. It is also associated with brain lesions, either as coexisting or metachronous primary neoplasms or as metastases.[73]

CLINICAL PRESENTATION

Most children with Wilms' tumor come to medical attention because of abdominal swelling or because an abdominal mass is felt, often first by a family member. Abdominal pain, gross hematuria, hypertension, and fever are other frequent findings at diagnosis. Microscopic hematuria has been documented more often than gross hematuria (Table 111-4).[76]

Hypertension was reported in 121 (26.4%) of 458 children with Wilms' tumor.[76] Hypertension may be caused by ectopic production of adrenocorticotropic hormone or elevated serum renin levels.[77,78]

Hypercalcemia, sometimes severe, can be present at diagnosis, but only in babies with congenital mesoblastic nephromas and RTK. It appears to be secondary to parathormone or prostaglandin E_2 secretion by the tumor cells,[55,79] and nephrectomy corrects the abnormality.

During the physical examination, it is important to note the location and size of the abdominal mass and its movement with respiration, to help differentiate Wilms' tumor from splenomegaly or from neuroblastoma, which often arises in the celiac axis or extends across the midline because of lymph node involvement. A varicocele secondary to obstruction of the spermatic vein may be associated with the presence of a tumor thrombus in the renal vein or inferior vena cava. Persistence of the varicocele when the child is supine is highly suggestive of venous obstruction. It is also important to note specifically any signs of the Wilms' tumor–associated syndromes marked by the presence of aniridia, partial or complete hemihypertrophy, and genitourinary abnormalities such as hypospadias or cryptorchidism.

Evaluation

Laboratory studies should include a complete blood count and differential analysis, liver and kidney function tests, serum calcium determination, and urinalysis.

Imaging Studies

The main purpose of the imaging studies is to assist the physicians, primarily the surgeon, in planning management. They are performed to establish the presence of a renal tumor and a normally functioning contralateral kidney, document the patency of the inferior vena cava, and demonstrate the presence or absence of pulmonary metastases. The initial study is often an abdominal ultrasonographic examination. Ultrasonography is a quick, noninvasive study that can confirm the presence of a mass and determine whether it is solid or cystic.

TABLE 111-4. *Presenting complaints of children with Wilms tumor*

Complaint	Percentage	Number with complaint/total observed
Abdominal mass	75.4%	(1347/1785)
Abdominal pain	28.2%	(401/1419)
Hypertension	26.4%	(121/458)
Hematuria (gross)	18.2%	(325/1779)
Hematuria (microscopic)	24.4%	(102/417)
Fever	22.1%	(137/618)
Urinary frequency	3.9%	(18/454)

Adapted from Bonnin JM, Rubinstein LJ, Palmer NF, Beckwith JB. The association of embryonal tumors originating in the kidney and in the brain. Cancer 1984;54:2137.

Intravenous urography or contrast-enhanced computed tomography of the abdomen is performed to further evaluate the nature and extent of the mass. Computed tomography may suggest apparent extension of the tumor into adjacent structures such as the liver, spleen, or colon. However, most patients identified as having possible invasion of the liver on computed tomography are found at the time of surgical exploration to have no hepatic invasion.[80] In addition, the examination may demonstrate small lesions, which may be nephrogenic rests or Wilms' tumor, in the opposite kidney.[81] Small, superficial or intrarenal lesions are frequently not identified even if computed tomography is employed.[81] When computed tomography is used, it is important that the radiologist obtain a supine view of the abdomen after contrast injection, because this view is necessary for planning and review of radiotherapy.

The patency of the inferior vena cava may be demonstrated relatively inexpensively with the use of real-time ultrasonography. Management decisions are clearly affected if caval thrombi are identified.[82,83] Very rarely, sudden death has been reported after dislodgment and mobilization of tumor lying within the draining vessels at laparotomy.[84] The inferior vena cava of children with Wilms' tumor was visualized by ultrasonography in 14 (77%) of 18 patients in one report.[85] If tumor is identified within the vessel, the proximal extent of the thrombus must be established before operation, because extension of thrombus even to the right atrium may not be suspected preoperatively because there are few if any clinical signs.[82,83]

The results of the radiographic studies and real-time ultrasonography provide sufficient information to make a decision for laparotomy in most children, although no imaging study unequivocally establishes the histologic diagnosis of Wilms' tumor. A number of other neoplasms, benign and malignant, can mimic the clinical and radiographic findings of Wilms' tumor (Table 111-5).

Plain chest radiographs should be obtained to determine whether pulmonary metastases are present. Computed tomography has been compared with conventional radiographic studies in Wilms' tumor patients in two studies. In the first, only 11 (9.4%) of 117 computed tomography scans demonstrated densities not identified on a plain chest radiograph, and none of these patients underwent open lung biopsy for confirmation of the putative malignant nature of the lesion.[86] In the other study, only 2 (2.4%) of 83 computed tomography scans demonstrated densities not identified by four-view chest radiography. One of the lesions was shown pathologically to be a granuloma, not a metastasis.[87] Others have reported that four of five biopsied solitary lesions from the lungs of children with Wilms' tumor identified only by computed tomography were actually pulmonary metastases.[88]

A radionuclide bone scan and radiographic skeletal survey should be obtained postoperatively on all children with CCSK and all other children with pulmonary or hepatic metastases who have suggestive symptomatology. Plain radiographs of the bones involved with CCSK can demonstrate lytic lesions that may not be seen on bone scan.[89]

A magnetic resonance image of the head should be obtained on all children with CCSK or malignant RTK, because both are associated with intracranial metastases.[1] Second primary malignant brain tumors of varying histologic type, often arising in the posterior fossa, are also found in RTK patients.[73,90]

TABLE 111-5. *Diagnoses in children with suspected Wilms tumor*

Diagnosis	NWTS	SIOP	Total
Neuroblastoma	9	19	28
Mesoblastic nephroma	10	4	14
Renal cyst	—	11	11
Renal cell carcinoma	1	5	6
Polycystic kidney	5	—	5
Multicystic kidney	3	—	3
Hydronephrosis	—	3	3
Hypernephroma	2	—	2
Extrarenal fibrosarcoma	1	1	2
Renal carbuncle	1	—	1
Benign teratoma	1	—	1
Adrenal hemorrhage	1	—	1
Renal thrombosis	1	—	1
Renal rhabdomyosarcoma	1	—	1
Renal leiomyosarcoma	1	—	1
Dysplastic kidney	1	—	1
Extrarenal leiomyosarcoma	1	—	1
Multilocular cyst	1	—	1
Lymphangiosarcoma	—	1	1
Incorrect diagnosis	40/586 (6.8%)	44/442 (9.9%)	84/1028 (8.1%)

NWTS, National Wilms Tumor Study; SIOP, International Society of Pediatric Oncology.

Adapted from Green DM. Diagnosis and management of malignant solid tumors in infants and children. Boston, Martinus Nijhoff, 1985: 129.

Prognostic Factors

Tumor size, the age of the patient, histology, lymph node metastases and local features of the tumor, such as capsular or vascular invasion, have in the past been predictive of outcome. Modern treatments have been so successful that some of these no longer pertain.

The results of the first three NWTS series were each evaluated by logistic regression analysis. Children entered on NWTS-1 who were younger than 24 months of age had a significantly better prognosis than those who were older. The relapse rate was 14.8% for the former group, compared with 34.7% for those between 2 and 4 years old and 27.6% for those older than 4 years of age.[91]

The histology of Wilms' tumor was identified as the most important determinant of prognosis. More recent analyses have confirmed the importance of histopathology and lymph node involvement, whereas the prognostic significance of such other factors as age and tumor size change as treatment efficacy improves.[91–93]

Possible chromosomal prognostic factors have been identified by Grundy and colleagues,[94] who evaluated DNA gain and loss using markers for several chromosomal segments. In a study of 232 children with Wilms' tumor registered on NWTS-3 and NWTS-4, he showed that loss of heterozygosity of 16q, which had occurred in tumor tissue from 17.2% of those with FH or anaplastic Wilms' tumor, was associated with statistically significantly poorer 2-year relapse-free and overall survival percentages (Table 111-6).[94] The difference remained after the analysis was adjusted for stage or histology. Loss of heterozy-

TABLE 111-6. *Loss of heterozygosity 16q in Wilms tumor*

Loss of heterozygosity	Number of patients	Relapses		Deaths		% at 2 Years	
		Obs	Exp	Obs	Exp	RFS	Alive
Absent	169	12	16.1	3	7.6	89.5	97.4
Present	35	7	2.9	6	1.4	77.6	84.4
		(P = 0.01)		(P < 0.0001)			

Obs, observed; Exp, expected.

Adapted from Grundy PE, Telzerow PE, Breslow N, et al. Loss of heterozygosity for chromosomes 16q and 1p in Wilms' tumors predicts an adverse outcome. Cancer Res 1994;54:2331.

gosity of chromosome 1p, present in tumor tissue from 11% of children with Wilms' tumor, was associated with poorer relapse-free and overall survival rates, but these results were of borderline statistical significance (P = .08 and .12, respectively) (Table 111-7). By contrast, loss of heterozygosity for 11p and duplication 1q, present in 33% and 25% of cases, respectively, were not associated with any difference in outcome.[94]

Mutations of the *P53* tumor suppressor gene have been reported in 0% to 9.5% of Wilms' tumors.[95–97] Mutations appear to be more frequent in tumors with anaplastic histology (12 of 14; 8.6%)[95,96] than in those with favorable histology (1 of 125; 0.8%),[95–97] suggesting that mutation of this gene may contribute to the anaplastic phenotype.

Partin and colleagues[98] demonstrated in univariate analyses that the skewness of the nuclear roundness factor and the mean of the lowest five values for elipticity measured by the feret diameter provided the best separation of Wilms' tumor patients into those with favorable prognoses and those with unfavorable prognoses. When these factors were combined with age at diagnosis, a discriminant function was developed that separated the patients into two prognostic groups. Those in the adverse-prognosis group comprised 45% of the total. The 4-year relapse-free survival percentages for the two prognostic groups differed by approximately 40%.[98]

SURGERY

The transabdominal approach to the tumor has become standard procedure because it allows inspection of the regional lymph nodes, a very important criterion for staging.[99,100] It also permits mobilization of the opposite kidney, which should be inspected on all its surfaces for evidence of a synchronous bilateral tumor or evidence of nephrogenic rests. These may not be identified on preoperative imaging studies, especially if they are small or flat. Radical or modified radical nephrectomy is employed to remove the affected kidney. Heroic attempts to excise all or parts of adjoining organs that may be implicated are not warranted. Colectomy or partial pancreatectomy should not be performed, although wedge resection of an infiltrated portion of the liver is advisable if the lesion can be removed in toto. Such a patient is thus rendered stage II rather than stage III, and radiotherapy is not required.[101]

The tumor can grow into the renal vein and extend retrograde down the gonadal vein in the case of left-sided tumors, or anterograde into the inferior vena cava and beyond. There may be preoperative clinical or imaging signs of tumor in the renal vein, propagating to obstruct the inferior vena cava wholly or in part. The tumor thrombus can extend to the right atrium.[82,83] Attempts at primary surgical excision of the tumor and caval extension are associated with increased surgical morbidity.[102] Preoperative chemotherapy should be administered to patients who have intravascular extension of tumor thrombus to the intrahepatic vena cava or more proximally, including the right atrium.[83] Tumor shrinkage usually follows, making the standard transabdominal approach feasible, thereby avoiding thoracoabdominal incisions, cardiac bypass, and the other maneuvers necessary to extract the tumor from the heart.[82] Preoperative chemotherapy may also be advisable in children for whom anesthesia or surgery poses a risk, such as children who are emaciated and anemic and those who have very large tumors. Prevailing North American practice, however, has been to proceed with surgery after appropriate workup. This is because treatments can best be modulated in their intensity according to accurate histopathologic and staging criteria, which are obscured if preoperative treatments are given.

Bilateral Tumors

Blute and colleagues[103] reviewed 145 patients with synchronous bilateral tumors and reported several important features.

TABLE 111-7. *Loss of heterozygosity 1p in Wilms tumor*

Loss of heterozygosity	Number of patients	Relapses		Deaths		% at 2 Years	
		Obs	Exp	Obs	Exp	RFS	Alive
Absent	155	12	14.2	5	6.3	88.4	96.0
Present	21	4	1.8	2	0.7	64.2	81.8
		(P = 0.08)		(P = 0.12)			

Obs, observed; Exp, expected.

Adapted from Grundy PE, Telzerow PE, Breslow N, et al. Loss of heterozygosity for chromosomes 16q and 1p in Wilms' tumors predicts an adverse outcome. Cancer Res 1994;54:2331.

The 76% overall 3-year survival expectancy was good for these patients, 62% of whom did not have total removal of all tumor-bearing tissue. This indicates that bilateral nephrectomy should be reserved for patients who fail to be brought under control after chemoradiotherapy of escalating intensity coupled with subtotal excisions as feasible. It also was found that 15 patients (10%) had anaplastic tumors on one or both sides, of whom 6 (4%) had discordant histology (i.e., FH on one side and anaplastic histology on the other).

These data, together with the wish to preserve as much renal tissue as possible, led Blute and colleagues[103] to propose the following approach.

- Exploratory laparotomy is performed for staging (primarily to evaluate the status of regional lymph nodes) and biopsy of both kidneys. Nephrectomy on either side is not performed initially. The more severely affected kidney may have a greater response to chemotherapy plus radiotherapy and therefore may be the kidney preserved at the time of eventual definitive surgery. Partial nephrectomy may be performed, however, if two thirds or more of the total renal volume can be preserved.
- Chemotherapy with dactinomycin (AMD), vincristine (VCR), and ADR is administered in one or more courses; the regimen depends on the stage of disease. Those with stage II or III anaplastic neoplasms require more aggressive therapy, including early nephrectomy.
- Second-look surgery is performed if the response to therapy has been sufficient that partial nephrectomy on one or both sides can be performed.
- Radiotherapy is reserved for patients who fail to respond to the chemotherapy regimen and for those who have stage III FH or stage II or III anaplastic tumors on one or both sides.

The outlook for children with metachronous bilateral tumors is worse. Jones and colleagues reported that only 7 (39%) of 18 patients survived 2 or more years after detection of the second tumor.[104] Reasons for the poorer prognosis are not known. They record that 7 of the 18 children had inadequate exploration of the contralateral side at the time of initial surgery. This emphasizes the need for careful inspection of the second kidney to identify small tumors and precursor lesions. There is also need for accurate physical examination to detect evidence of predisposing genetic conditions such as hemihypertrophy and aniridia. Careful and frequent follow-up is indicated under these sets of circumstances.

RADIOTHERAPY

The role of radiotherapy has evolved over the years.[1,2,105,106]

Abdominal Irradiation

Tumor bed radiotherapy, once given routinely postoperatively to all children with Wilms' tumor in many treatment centers, was believed by many to have produced the improvement in the survival rate to about 50%. There were doubts, however, regarding the need for radiotherapy in all patients.[107] This question was evaluated in NWTS-1. Children with stage I disease were randomly assigned to receive or not receive radiotherapy along with AMD postoperatively.[108] The results demonstrated that among younger children, there was no survival advantage for the irradiated group. Results from NWTS-2 and NWTS-3 suggest that the addition of multiagent chemotherapy suppresses not only distant micrometastases but also any residual disease that may be present postoperatively in the nonirradiated primary tumor site.[1,109] These findings made it clear that radiotherapy could not be viewed as an independent treatment modality in patients with Wilms' tumor. The radiotherapy recommendations that follow are based on those used in NWTS-3 and an analysis of the outcome of NWTS-3 and NWTS-4 patients with anaplastic histology.[110] They are valid only if the surgical and chemotherapeutic components of that study are also being observed.[1]

No postoperative radiotherapy is given to children with stage I or II FH tumors or stage I anaplastic tumors if AMD and VCR are given. Infradiaphragmatic irradiation is given to children with stage III FH lesions and to all those with CCSK. The radiation fields are based on reviews of relapse patterns and are varied according to the extent of disease (Table 111-8).[103] Only the tumor bed and paraaortic lymph nodes are included in those who have regional lymph nodes that are histologically positive for Wilms' tumor. Larger fields are used for children with more extensive disease (e.g., the whole abdomen if massive tumor spillage has occurred). In any case, 1080 cGy given as 180 cGy/day for 6 days or 1050 cGy as 150 cGy/day for 7 days is given, together with 1080 cGy small-field supplements as required for areas of gross residual disease. All such patients also receive AMD, VCR, and ADR.

Similar tumor bed irradiation is also delivered to patients with diffuse anaplastic tumors in the more advanced stages. Age-adjusted doses are no longer considered appropriate because a review of relapses in this group of patients showed no evidence that operative bed relapse was more frequent among patients who received lower radiotherapy doses. These patients also receive AMD, VCR, ADR, and cyclophosphamide (CPM).[110] It is not certain whether whole abdominal irradiation is necessary in patients with tumor spillage that occurs either before or during surgery. Tumor rupture that is believed to be confined to the local site is assigned to stage II in the NWTS, and such patients are not irradiated. Patients who have gross tumor spillage should receive 1050 cGy (150 cGy/day for 7

TABLE 111-8. *National Wilms Tumor Study: Volume of abdominal radiation fields in stage III and IV disease*

Extent of disease	Volume of radiation field required
Hilar nodes Gross* or microscopic residual disease confined to flank	Flank, crossing midline to include bilateral paraaortic nodes
Paraaortic nodes Peritoneal seeding Gross residual abdominal disease* Diffuse spillage at surgery Preoperative intraperitoneal rupture	Whole abdomen

* Local 1080-cGy supplements to be given to volumes measuring 3 cm or more in maximum diameter.

days) to the entire abdomen. Girls seem to be especially prone to pelvic recurrences in the pouch of Douglas area after tumor spillage. In these patients, it is perhaps better to err on the side of overstaging rather than understaging, despite the known consequences of pelvic irradiation in females, until research analyses are completed.

Metastases

Radiotherapy to all metastatic sites, whatever the histology, also is used in the NWTS. Although some advocate other approaches to pulmonary metastases (discussed later), NWTS children with FH tumors and pulmonary metastases currently are given 1200 cGy (150 cGy/day for 8 days) to both lungs, regardless of the number and location of metastases. Bone lesions receive 3060 cGy (180 cGy/day for 17 days) to the tumor and a 3-cm margin. Brain metastases are given the same dose, but the whole brain is included in the irradiated area. The liver is given 1980 cGy (180 cGy/day for 11 days), with local supplements of 540 to 1080 cGy permitted depending on the amount of tumor and volume of liver to be included. Similar doses are used for CCSK, RTK, and anaplastic tumor patients, except that higher doses are allowed for the liver (3060 cGy) because of the poor prognosis associated with tumors in this area.

Preoperative Irradiation

Preoperative irradiation was given some popularity by Silver decades ago.[112] It was used in the first clinical trial by the International Society of Pediatric Oncology (SIOP), which has conducted a series of studies dealing with preoperative therapies.[2,113] Subsequent SIOP trials substituted preoperative chemotherapy (AMD and VCR) for radiotherapy. Postnephrectomy abdominal irradiation is now given only to children found to have disease compatible with stage III distribution after prenephrectomy chemotherapy. SIOP investigators also have attempted to avoid thoracic irradiation in children with pulmonary metastases.[114] Radiotherapy with or without surgery is restricted to children who did not achieve a complete response with chemotherapy or developed recurrent disease thereafter. The occurrence of severe pulmonary toxicity, some of which is lethal, as reported by the NWTS after combined chemoradiotherapy of the chest, is thereby minimized, if not avoided entirely.[115]

The more restricted indications for radiotherapy and the doses employed are well tolerated by most children except for the pulmonary toxicity described previously. In addition, diffuse interstitial pneumonitis after whole-lung irradiation may result from *Pneumocystis carinii* infection. Patients who receive whole-lung radiotherapy should therefore receive prophylactic trimethoprim-sulfamethoxazole.

Rhabdoid Tumor of Kidney

The value of radiotherapy in children with RTK is not clear. There were 13 infradiaphragmatic relapses (excluding the liver) among 26 NWTS-3 children with stage I, II, or III RTK despite the chemotherapy and radiotherapy given to all (see Table 111-3). More effective chemotherapy clearly is needed. Radiotherapy is delayed until 6 or more weeks after diagnosis for this group of children in NWTS-5 to permit administration of more intensive chemotherapy.

CHEMOTHERAPY

The NWTS Group has conducted several randomized trials to evaluate the effect of chemotherapy modifications on outcome. In NWTS-3, treatment was modulated according to the histology of the tumor and the clinicopathologic stage (see Table 111-1). The results of this study demonstrated that patients with stage I FH Wilms' tumor could be treated successfully by a 10-week regimen composed of VCR and AMD without abdominal irradiation. The 4-year relapse-free survival with this regimen in NWTS-3 was 89%, and the 4-year survival was 95.6%.[1]

NWTS-3 patients with stage II FH tumors were randomly assigned to receive either AMD and VCR or AMD, VCR, and ADR. They were also randomly assigned to receive either 2000 cGy of tumor bed irradiation or no radiotherapy (Fig. 111-5). The 4-year relapse-free survival rate for patients who were treated with AMD and VCR and received no abdominal radiotherapy was 87.4%, and the 4-year survival rate was 91.1%. There was no statistically significant difference between these results and those for each of the remaining three treatment regimens[1]; therefore, neither radiotherapy nor ADR can be recommended for patients with stage II FH Wilms' tumor.

NWTS-3 patients with stage III FH tumors were likewise randomly assigned to treatment with either AMD and VCR or AMD, VCR, and ADR. They were also randomly assigned to receive either 1000 cGy or 2000 cGy of radiotherapy. The portals included the flank or the whole abdomen, according to the extent of disease (see Table 111-8). This study demonstrated that children receiving the lower radiotherapy dose benefitted from the addition of ADR to the two-drug combination in that they had the same low frequency of intraabdominal relapses as patients treated with two drugs and 2000 cGy. The 4-year relapse-free survival rate for those patients given three drugs and 1000 cGy abdominal radiotherapy was 82%, and the 4-year survival rate was 90.9%.[1]

Patients with stage IV FH tumors in NWTS-3 were randomly assigned to receive either AMD, VCR, and ADR or these three drugs plus CPM. All patients underwent immediate nephrectomy, and all received both abdominal and whole-lung radiotherapy. The 4-year relapse-free survival percentage for patients treated with three drugs was 71.9%, and the 4-year survival percentage was 78.4%. There was no statistically significant improvement in the 4-year relapse-free or overall survival rate from the addition of CPM to the three-drug regimen.[1] Considerable toxicity was noted, however.[115]

The results of studies conducted by the SIOP and the United Kingdom Children's Cancer Study Group suggest that some patients with stage IV FH Wilms' tumor can be treated successfully without whole-lung irradiation.[114,116] Before firm conclusions can be drawn, however, more thorough analyses of possible prognostic factors are needed. These include delineation of the number of pulmonary metastases, the presence of renal or paraaortic lymph node involvement by tumor, and the time required for chemotherapy to achieve a radiographically complete

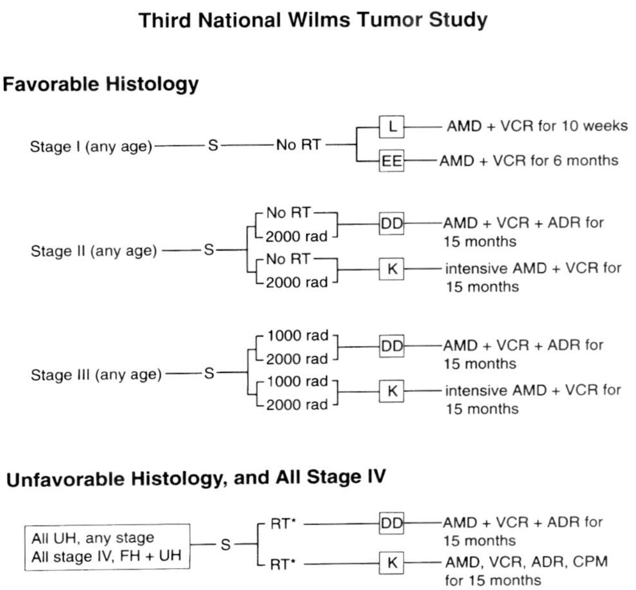

FIG. 111-5. Chemotherapy protocols used in the Third National Wilms Tumor Study. The drug doses employed are as follows: dactinomycin (AMD), 15 μg/kg/d IV; vincristine (VCR), 1.5 mg/m^2/wk IV; doxorubicin (ADR), 20 mg/m^2/d IV; and cyclophosphamide (CPM), 10 mg/kg/d IV. All regimens start with a course of ADM beginning on the first postoperative day and VCR weekly for 10 weeks starting on day 7. Patients treated with regimen L received a second course of AMD at week 5. Patients treated with regimen EE received additional courses of AMD at weeks 5, 13, and 24, and additional doses of VCR on day 1 and day 5 of each 5-day course of AMD at weeks 13 and 24. Patients treated with regimen K received additional courses of AMD at weeks 5, 13, 22, 31, 40, 49, and 58, and additional 6-week courses of VCR at weeks 24, 33, 42, 51, and 60. Patients treated with regimen DD received additional courses of AMD at weeks 13, 26, 39, 52, and 65; courses of ADR at weeks 6, 19, 32, 45, and 58; and additional doses of VCR on day 1 and day 5 of each 5-day course of AMD, at weeks 13, 26, 39, 52, and 65. Patients treated with regimen J received chemotherapy identical to that of regimen DD, with the addition of courses of CPM with each course of AMD or ADR at weeks 6, 13, 19, 26, 32, 39, 45, 52, 58, and 65.

response of the pulmonary metastases. These analyses may allow more accurate identification of those patients who can be treated successfully without whole-lung irradiation.

Children with FH tumors or tumors that contained focal or diffuse anaplasia were randomly assigned in NWTS-2 to the same treatments without stratification.[109] In NWTS-3, patients with anaplastic lesions were randomly assigned to treatment with AMD, VCR, ADR, and CPM, as in Figure 111-5. NWTS-2 results showed that patients with stage I anaplastic tumors had a prognosis not different from that of patients with stage I FH tumors who received the same chemotherapeutic regimen. None of the NWTS-2 stage I Wilms' tumor patients received abdominal radiotherapy, regardless of histology.[109] Early NWTS-3 analyses suggested that patients with stage II through stage IV anaplastic Wilms' tumor, all of whom were irradiated, benefited from the addition of CPM to the combination of AMD, VCR, and ADR.[1] This result for patients with diffuse anaplasia (stages II through IV) has been confirmed with additional patient accrual on NWTS-4.[110] There is no beneficial effect of added CPM in patients with tumors having only focal anaplasia. All NWTS-3 patients with CCSK received abdominal radiotherapy and were randomly assigned to the same three- versus four-drug comparative regimens (see Fig. 111-5). The 4-year relapse-free survival rate for CCSK patients treated with three drugs was 70.6%, and the 4-year survival rate was 74.8%. There was no statistically significant improvement in those given the fourth drug (CPM).[64]

Patients with RTK responded poorly to all the treatments used in the NWTS. The 4-year relapse-free survival rate for all NWTS-3 patients with RTK who were randomly assigned according to Figure 111-5 was about 25%, and the 4-year survival percentage was the same.[1]

Prenephrectomy Chemotherapy

The efficacy of prenephrectomy abdominal radiotherapy, combination chemotherapy, or both for decreasing the frequency of tumor rupture at the time of nephrectomy was investigated by the members of SIOP. Prenephrectomy abdominal radiotherapy decreased the percentage of nephrectomies complicated by tumor rupture from 33% (20 of 60 patients) to 4% (3 of 72 patients).[113] In a subsequent randomized trial, the frequency of tumor rupture was similar among patients treated with prenephrectomy abdominal radiotherapy plus AMD (7 of 76 patients; 8%) and among those treated with prenephrectomy chemotherapy plus VCR and AMD (5 of 88 patients; 6%).[2] The frequency of tumor rupture observed among SIOP patients undergoing nephrectomy without preoperative treatment was higher than that reported by NWTS-1 (92 of 92 patients; 22%) or by NWTS-2 (76 of 626 patients; 12%).[108,109]

The administration of prenephrectomy chemotherapy is associated with several disadvantages, including potential administration of combination chemotherapy to patients with benign or malignant conditions different from Wilms' tumor and loss of staging information. The SIOP and NWTS experience indicates that about one third of patients with an erroneous prenephrectomy diagnosis of Wilms' tumor have a benign disease, although the overall accuracy has improved over the years (see Table 111-5).[2,100,109,113] SIOP investigators designed a clinical trial in which patients treated with prenephrectomy combination chemotherapy who had postchemotherapy Wilms' tumor compatible with stage II disease and without regional lymph node involvement (SIOP definitions) were randomized to receive or not receive postnephrectomy abdominal radiotherapy. This trial was discontinued because there was an excess of intraabdominal recurrences in the nonirradiated patients.[117] The SIOP result suggests that prenephrectomy chemotherapy can obscure perinephric tumor extensions and regional lymph node tumor deposits, leading to false downstaging.[118]

SIOP, like NWTS, is attempting to reduce the need for radiotherapy to a minimum. In a one-arm study, SIOP has elected to substitute epirubicin for radiotherapy in SIOP stage II patients with negative nodal involvement. It is difficult to evaluate the effectiveness of this modification without including a randomized comparison group; however, doing so would expose more SIOP patients to potentially cardiotoxic agents. Those using the SIOP approach must balance the merits of a possible reduction in the number of patients undergoing abdominal radiotherapy against the disadvantages of treating some children unnecessarily and of exposing more children to the cardiac toxicity of an anthracycline.

TREATMENT OF RECURRENT WILMS' TUMOR

Children with relapsed FH Wilms' tumor have a variable prognosis, depending on the initial stage, the site of relapse, the time from initial diagnosis to relapse, and previous therapy. Favorable prognostic factors include no prior treatment with ADR, relapse more than 12 months after diagnosis, and intraabdominal relapse in a patient not previously treated with abdominal irradiation.[119]

Children in this more favorable group should be treated aggressively because they usually have a good response to retrieval therapy. Although surgical excision of pulmonary metastases does not result in an increase in the number of children who do not have a second relapse,[120] surgical biopsy or excision of recurrence should be performed for the purposes of confirming histologically the presence of recurrent disease, accurately documenting the sites of recurrence, and, in the case of intraabdominal recurrence, reducing the tumor burden before the initiation of radiotherapy and combination chemotherapy. The chemotherapy regimen should include agents not previously employed, such as ADR, CPM, etoposide, and carboplatin.

Patients who relapse after prior treatment with a regimen that included ADR or who develop a recurrence in the abdomen (including the liver) after previous irradiation have a poor prognosis. The combination of etoposide and ifosfamide has rarely produced prolonged responses in these children.[121] Several centers have suggested that a more aggressive approach, including the use of autologous bone marrow transplantation, should be employed in the management of patients with adverse prognostic factors at the time of relapse.[122–124] In general, these children should be referred to centers that are conducting research on the role of autologous bone marrow transplantation in the treatment of children with recurrent solid tumors. If this is not possible or is not desired by the family, these patients are usually eligible for phase I or II studies.

Single-agent carboplatin[125–128] and the combination of etoposide and carboplatin[129,130] are active in Wilms' tumor. The response rate for carboplatin has been reported to be 37% in previously treated patients, or 12 of 32 patients, including 4 with complete remission (CR) and 8 with partial remission (PR). Among previously untreated patients with Wilms' tumor, the response rate for carboplatin was 100% (3 CR, 5 PR). The combination of carboplatin and etoposide has been evaluated in two phase II trials in children with Wilms' tumor. In one, which included both children with relapse and those previously untreated, the response rate was 100% (5 CR, 7 PR). The doses employed were etoposide, 100 mg/m^2/day for 3 days, and carboplatin, 560 mg/m^2 for 1 day.[129] The other study included only patients with recurrent Wilms' tumor. The response rate was 69% (8 CR, 8 PR) in patients with FH and 100% (3 PR) in patients with anaplastic histology. All three patients with CCSK responded (1 CR, 2 PR). The dose schedule was etoposide, 100 mg/m^2/day for 5 days, followed by carboplatin, 160 mg/m^2/day for 5 days.[130] There are insufficient phase II studies of this combination in patients with RTK, CCSK, or Wilms' tumor with diffuse anaplasia, although the available data suggest that the regimen has activity in both CCSK and Wilms' tumor with anaplasia.

The combination of etoposide and ifosfamide is highly active in FH Wilms' tumor and CCSK.[121,131] Ifosfamide was administered in combination with etoposide at a higher dose intensity

TABLE 111-9. *Selection of imaging studies for follow-up of children with renal neoplasms of proven histology who are free of metastases at diagnosis*

Tumor type	Study	Schedule after primary therapy
FH Wilms tumor, all patients and stage I anaplastic Wilms tumor	Chest films	6 wk and 3 mo after operation; then every 3 mo for 15 mo, every 6 mo for 18 mo, yearly for 2 y
Irradiated patients only	Bony structure (eg, spine ± pelvis)	Yearly to full growth, then every 5 y indefinitely*
Without NR, stages I and II	Abdominal ultrasound	Yearly for 3 y
Stage III	Abdominal ultrasound	As for chest films
With NR, any stage	Abdominal ultrasound	Every 3 mo for 24 mo, then every 6 mo for 36 mo, then yearly for 5 y
Stage II and III Ana Wilms tumor	Chest films	As for FH
	Abdominal ultrasound	Every 3 mo for 24 mo, then every 6 mo for 36 mo
CCSK	Brain MRI and/or opacified CT	—
	Skeletal survey and bone scan	When CCSK is established; then every 6 mo for 5 y
	Chest films	As for FH
Rhabdoid tumor of the kidney	Brain MRI and/or opacified CT	As for CCSK
	Chest films	As for FH

FH, favorable histology; Ana, anaplastic; NR, nephrogenic rests; CCSK, clear cell sarcoma of the kidney; MRJ, magnetic resonance imaging; CT, computed tomography.

* To detect second neoplasms, benign (osteochondromas) or malignant.

Adapted from Weeks DA, Beckwith JB, Mierau GW, Luckey DW. Rhabdoid tumor of kidney. Am J Surg Pathol 1989; 13:439.

than that used for CPM in combination with VCR, AMD, and ADR in regimen J of NWTS-3 and NWTS-4. The nephrotoxicity of ifosfamide in children with Wilms' tumor discourages its use in previously untreated children.[121,132] CPM is synergistic with etoposide in experimental systems.[133,134] Administration of CPM, using a dose intensity similar to that employed in the phase II trial of ifosfamide and etoposide, may yield evidence of increased therapeutic efficacy, an outcome suggested by the results of two recent phase II trials of etoposide and CPM.[135,136] The mechanism of action of etoposide suggests that a combination that included an alkylating agent and etoposide might exhibit schedule dependence. Administration of etoposide after the alkylating agent would be expected to result in greater activity. The results of a recent trial in small cell lung cancer, in which the sequence of cisplatin followed by etoposide was most effective, supports this concept.[137]

FOLLOW-UP

Children who have been treated for Wilms' tumor should be examined regularly by a physician who is familiar with the natural history of the disease and the complications of therapy. The type, frequency, and total number of imaging examinations depend on the original stage and histology of the tumor (Table 111-9).[75] For example, children with nephroblastomatosis identified in either kidney have a greater risk of developing metachronous contralateral disease and require regular monitoring of the remaining kidney.[32,104] Useful as they are, these studies are not substitutes for frequent careful physical examination, which often first elicits signs of trouble. Enlargement or nodularity of the liver on abdominal palpation should be confirmed with appropriate imaging means; combined chemoradiotherapy can cause liver swelling and produce confusing physical and imaging signs. Bone pain in patients with CCSK should be evaluated first with plain radiographs. Plain radiographs seem to be more sensitive in detecting recurrence than radionuclide bone scans; however, these should be obtained if the plain radiographs are negative. The two studies are complementary.[89]

REFERENCES

1. D'Angio GJ, Breslow N, Beckwith JB, et al. Treatment of Wilms' tumor: results of the Third National Wilms' Tumor Study. Cancer 1989;64:349.
2. Lemerle J, Voute PA, Tournade MF, et al. Effectiveness of preoperative chemotherapy in Wilms' tumor: results of an International Society of Pediatric Oncology (SIOP) clinical trial. J Clin Oncol 1983;1:604.
3. Breslow N, Beckwith JB, Ciol M, Sharples K. Age distribution of Wilms' tumor. Cancer Res 1988;48:1653.
4. Knudson AG Jr, Strong LC. Mutation and cancer: a model for Wilms' tumor of the kidney. J Natl Cancer Inst 1972;48:313.
5. Orkin SH. Wilms' tumour: molecular evidence for the role of chromosome 11. Cancer Surv 1984;3:465.
6. Evans AE, Norkool P, Evans I, Breslow N, D'Angio GJ. Late effects of treatment for Wilms' tumor: a report from the National Wilms' Tumor Study Group. Cancer 1991;67:331.
7. Breslow N, Olshan A, Beckwith JB, Moksness J, Feigl P, Green D. Ethnic variation in the incidence, diagnosis, prognosis and follow-up of children with Wilms tumor. J Natl Cancer Inst 1994;86:49.
8. Crist WM, Kun LE. Common solid tumors of childhood. N Engl J Med 1991;324 (correction 1295).
9. Stiller CA, Parkin DM. International variations in the incidence of childhood renal tumors. Br J Cancer 1990;62:1026.
10. Breslow NE, Olshan A, Beckwith JB, Green DM. Epidemiology of Wilms tumor. Med Pediatr Oncol 1993;21:172.
11. Breslow NE, Beckwith JB. Epidemiological features of Wilms' tumor: results of the National Wilms' Tumor Study. J Natl Cancer Inst 1982; 68:429.
12. Miller RW, Fraumeni JF Jr, Manning MD. Association of Wilms' tumor with aniridia, hemihypertrophy and other congenital malformations. N Engl J Med 1964;270:922.
13. Beckwith JB. Macroglossia, omphalocele, adrenal cytomegaly, gigantism and hyperplastic visceromegaly. In: Bergsma D, McKusick VA, Hall JG, Scott CI, eds. Birth defects: original article series, vol 5. New York, Stratton Intercontinental, 1969:188.
14. Eddy MA, Mauer SM. Pseudohermaphroditism, glomerulopathy and Wilms' tumor (Drash syndrome): frequency in end-stage renal failure. J Pediatr 1985;106:584.
15. Greenberg F, Stein F, Cresick MV, et al. The Perlman familial nephroblastomatosis syndrome. Am J Med Genet 1986;24:101.
16. Fabia J, Thuy TD. Occupation of father at time of birth of children dying of malignant diseases. Br J Prev Soc Med 1974;28:98.
17. Zack M, Cannon S, Lyod D, et al. Cancer in children of parents exposed to hydrocarbon-related industries and occupations. Am J Epidemiol 1980;111:329.
18. Hakulinen T, Salonen T, Teppo L. Cancer in the offspring in hydrocarbon-related occupations. Br J Prev Soc Med 1976;30:138.
19. Kantor AF, McCrea Curren MG, Meigs JW, et al. Occupations of fathers of patients with Wilms' tumor. J Epidemiol Community Health 1979;33:253.
20. Dwa SL, Fine LJ. The association between parental occupation and childhood malignancy. J Occup Med 1980;24:792.
21. Bunin GR, Nass C, Kramer S, Meadows AT. Parental occupation and Wilms' tumor: results of a case-control study. Cancer Res 1989;49: 725.
22. Olshan AF, Breslow NE, Daling JR, et al. Wilms' tumor and paternal occupation. Cancer Res 1990;50:3212.
23. LeMasters GK, Bove KE. Genetic/environmental significance of multifocal nodular renal blastema. Am J Pediatr Hematol Oncol 1980;2: 81.
24. Stjernfeldt M, Berglund K, Lindstern J, Ludvigsson J. Maternal smoking during pregnancy and risk of childhood cancer. Lancet 1986;1: 1350.
25. Lindblad P, Zack M, Adami H-O, Ericson A. Maternal and perinatal risk factors for Wilms tumor: a nationwide nested case-control study in Sweden. Int J Cancer 1992;51:38.
26. Olshan AF, Breslow NE, Falletta JM, et al. Risk factors for Wilms' tumor: report from the National Wilms' Tumor Study. Cancer 1993; 72:938.
27. Knudson AG. Mutation and cancer: statistical study of retinoblastoma. Proc Natl Acad Sci U S A 1971;68:820.
28. Dryja TP, Mukai S, Petersen R, Rapaport JM, Walton D, Yandell DW. Parental origin of mutations of the retinoblastoma gene. Nature 1989;339:556.
29. Ejima Y, Sasaki MS, Kaneko A, Tanooka H. Types, rates, origin and expressivity of chromosome mutations involving 13q14 in retinoblastoma patients. Hum Genet 1988;79:118.
30. Wiggs J, Nordenskjold M, Yandell D, et al. Prediction of the risk of hereditary retinoblastoma, using DNA polymorphisms within the retinoblastoma gene. N Engl J Med 1988;318:151.
31. Cavenee WK, Dryja TP, Phillips RA, et al. Expression of recessive alleles by chromosomal mechanisms in retinoblastoma. Nature 1983; 305:779.
32. Beckwith JB, Kiviat NB, Bonadio J. Nephrogenic rests, nephroblastomatosis and the pathogenesis of Wilms' tumor. Pediatr Pathol 1990; 10:1.
33. Riccardi VM, Sujansky E, Smith AC, Francke U. Chromosomal imbalance in the aniridia-Wilms' tumor association: 11p interstitial deletion. Pediatrics 1978;61:604.
34. Huff V, Meadows A, Riccardi VM, Strong LC, Saunders GF. Parental origin of de novo constitutional deletions of chromosomal band 11p13. Am J Hum Genet 1990;47:155.
35. Mannens M, Slater RM, Heyting C, et al. Molecular nature of genetic changes resulting in loss of heterozygosity of chromosome 11 in Wilms' tumors. Hum Genet 1988;81:41.
36. Koufos A, Grundy P, Morgan K, et al. Familial Wiedemann-Beckwith

syndrome and a second Wilms' tumor locus both map to 11p15.5. Am J Hum Genet 1989;44:711.
37. Call KM, Glaser T, Ito CY, et al. Isolation and characterization of a zinc finger polypeptide gene at the human chromosome 11 Wilms' tumor locus. Cell 1990;60:509.
38. Gessler M, Poustka A, Cavenee W, Neve RL, Orkin SH, Bruns GAP. Homozygous deletion in Wilms' tumours of a zinc-finger gene identified by chromosome jumping. Nature 1990;343:774.
39. Pelletier J, Bruening W, Cashtan CE, et al. Germline mutations in the Wilms' tumor suppressor gene are associated with abnormal urogenital development in Denys-Drash syndrome. Cell 1991;67:437.
40. Huff V, Miwa H, Haber DA, et al. Evidence for *WT1* as a Wilms' tumor gene: intragenic germinal deletion in bilateral WT. Am J Hum Genet 1991;48:997.
41. Haber DA, Buckler AJ, Glaser T, et al. An internal deletion within an 11p13 zinc finger gene contributes to the development of Wilms' tumor. Cell 1990;61:1257.
42. Varanasi R, Bardeesy N, Ghahremani M, et al. Fine structure analysis of the *WT1* gene in sporadic Wilms' tumors. Proc Natl Acad Sci U S A 1994;91:3554.
43. Schroeder WT, Chao L-Y, Dao DD, et al. Nonrandom loss of maternal chromosome 11 alleles in Wilms' tumors. Am J Hum Genet 1987; 40:413.
44. Grundy P, Koufos A, Morgan K, Li FP, Meadows AT, Cavenee WK. Familial predisposition to Wilms' tumour does not map to the short arm of chromosome 11. Nature 1988;336:374.
45. Tricoli JV, Rall LB, Scott J, Bell GI, Shows TB. Localization of insulin-like growth factor genes to human chromosomes 11 and 12. Nature 1984;310:784.
46. Rainer S, Johnson LA, Dobry CJ, Ping AJ, Grundy PE, Feinberg AP. Relaxation of imprinted genes in human cancer. Nature 1993;362: 747.
47. Reeve AE, Eccles MR, Wilkins RJ, Bell GI, Millow LJ. Expression of insulin-like growth factor-II transcripts in Wilms' tumour. Nature 1985;317:258.
48. Ogawa O, Eccles MR, Szeto J, et al. Relaxation of insulin-like growth factor II gene imprinting implicated in Wilms' tumor. Nature 1993; 362:751.
49. Ogawa O, Becroft DM, Morison IM, et al. Constitutional relaxation of insulin-like growth factor II gene imprinting associated with Wilms' tumour and gigantism. Nature Genet 1993;5:408.
50. Huff V, Comptom DA, Chao LY, et al. Lack of linkage of familial Wilms' tumour to chromosomal band 11p13. Nature 1990;336:377.
51. Huff V, Reeve AE, Leppert M, et al. Nonlinkage of 16q markers to familial predisposition to Wilms' tumor. Cancer Res 1992; 52:6117.
52. Franco EL, de Camargo B, Saba L, Marques LA. Epidemiological and clinical correlations with genetic characteristics of Wilms' tumor: results of the Brazilian Wilms' Tumor Study Group. Int J Cancer 1991;48:641.
53. Bonaiti-Pellie C, Chompret A, Tournade MF, et al. Genetics and epidemiology of Wilms' tumor: the French Wilms' Tumor Study. Med Pediatr Oncol 1992;20:284.
54. Pendergrass TW. Congenital anomalies in children with Wilms' tumor. Cancer 1976;37:403.
55. Beckwith JB. Pediatric neoplastic disorders of the kidney. In: Sternberg SS, ed. Diagnostic surgical pathology. New York, Raven Press, 1989:1331.
56. Joshi VV, Beckwith JB. Multilocular cyst of the kidney (cystic nephroma) and cystic, partially differentiated nephroblastoma: terminology and criteria for diagnosis. Cancer 1989;64:466.
57. Beckwith JB, Palmer NF. Histopathology and prognosis of Wilms' tumor. Cancer 1978;41:1937.
58. Mireau GW, Weeks DA, Beckwith JB. Anaplastic Wilms' tumor and other clinically aggressive childhood renal neoplasms: ultrastructural and immunocytochemical features. Ultrastruct Pathol 1989;13:225.
59. Beckwith JB. Grading of pediatric tumors. In: Care of the child with cancer. New York, American Cancer Society, 1979:32.
60. Faria P, Beckwith JB. A new definition of focal anaplasia (FA) in Wilms' tumor (WT) identifies cases with good outcome: a report from the National Wilms' Tumor Study. Mod Pathol 1993;6:3b. Abstract.
61. Bonadio JF, Storer B, Norkool P, Farewell VT, Beckwith JB, D'Angio GJ. Anaplastic Wilms' tumor: clinical and pathological studies. J Clin Oncol 1985;3:513.
62. Kidd JM. Exclusion of certain renal neoplasms from the category of Wilms' tumor. Am J Pathol 1970;59:16a. Abstract.
63. Marsden HB, Lawler W, Kumar PM. Bone metastasizing renal tumor of childhood: morphological and clinical features and differences from Wilms' tumor. Cancer 1978;42:1922.
64. Green DM, Breslow NE, Beckwith JB, Moksness J, Finklestein JZ, D'Angio GJ. The treatment of children with clear cell sarcoma of the kidney: a report from the National Wilms' Tumor Study. J Clin Oncol 1994;12:2132.
65. Beckwith JB, Larson E. Clear cell sarcoma of kidney. Pediatr Pathol 1989;9:211.
66. Haas JE, Bonadio JF, Beckwith JB. Clear cell sarcoma of kidney with emphasis on ultrastructural studies. Cancer 1984;54:2978.
67. Schmidt D, Harms D, Evers KG, et al. Bone metastasizing renal tumor (clear cell sarcoma) of childhood with epithelioid elements. Cancer 1985;56:609.
68. Lamego CMB, Zerbini MCH. Bone-metastasizing primary renal tumors in children. Radiology 1983;147:449.
69. Marsden HB, Lawler W. Bone metastasizing renal tumour of childhood: histopathological and clinical review of 38 cases. Virchows Arch A Pathol Anat Histopathol 1980;387:341.
70. Beckwith JB. Wilms' tumor and other renal tumors of childhood: a selective review from the National Wilms' Tumor Study Pathology Center. Hum Pathol 1983;14:481.
71. Haas JE, Palmer NF, Weinberg AG, Beckwith JB. Ultrastructure of malignant rhabdoid tumor of the kidney: a distinctive renal tumor of children. Hum Pathol 1981;12:646.
72. Weeks DA, Beckwith JB, Mierau GW, Luckey DW. Rhabdoid tumor of kidney. Am J Surg Pathol 1989;13:439.
73. Bonnin JM, Rubinstein LJ, Palmer NF, Beckwith JB. The association of embryonal tumors originating in the kidney and in the brain. Cancer 1984;54:2137.
74. Vogel AM, Gown AM, Caughlan J, et al. Rhabdoid tumors of the kidney contain mesenchymal specific and epithelial specific intermediate filament proteins. Lab Invest 1984;50:232.
75. D'Angio GJ, Rosenberg H, Sharples K, Kelalis P, Breslow N, Green DM. Imaging methods for primary renal tumors of childhood: costs versus benefits. Med Pediatr Oncol 1993;21:205.
76. Green DM. Diagnosis and management of malignant solid tumors in infants and children. Boston, Martinus Nijhoff, 1985:129.
77. Pombo M, Alvez F, Varela-Cives R, Iglesias-Diz JL, Martinon F, Castro-Gago M. Ectopic production of ACTH by Wilms' tumor. Hormone Res 1982;16:160.
78. Voute PA Jr, van der Meer J, Stugaard-Kloosterziel W. Plasma renin activity in Wilms' tumor. Acta Endocrinol (Copenh) 1971;67:197.
79. Jayabose S, Iqbal K, Newman L, et al. Hypercalcemia in childhood renal tumors. Cancer 1988;61:788.7. Ng YY, Hall-Graggs MA, Dicks-Mireaux C, Pritchard J. Wilms' tumour: pre- and post-chemotherapy CT appearances. Clin Radiol 1991;43:255.
80. Ng YY, Hall-Graggs MA, Dicks-Mireaux C, Pritchard J. Wilms tumour: pre- and post-chemotherapy CT appearances. Clin Radiol 1991; 43:255.
81. Ritchey ML, Green DM, Breslow N, Moksness J, Norkool P. Accuracy of current imaging modalities in the diagnosis of synchronous bilateral Wilms' tumor: a report from the National Wilms' Tumor Study Group. J Urol 1994;151:329A. Abstract.
82. Nakayama DK, Norkool P, Delorimier AA, O'Neill JA, D'Angio GJ. Intracardiac extension of Wilms' tumor. Ann Surg 1986;204:693.
83. Ritchey ML, Kelalis PP, Haase GM, Shochat SJ, Green DM, D'Angio GJ. Preoperative therapy for intracaval and atrial extension of Wilms' tumor. Cancer 1993;71:4104.
84. Shurin SB, Gauderer MWL, Dahms BB, Conrad WG. Fatal intraoperative pulmonary embolization of Wilms' tumor. J Pediatr 1982;101: 559.
85. Slovis TL, Philippart AL, Cushing B, et al. Evaluation of the inferior vena cava by sonography and venography in children with renal and hepatic tumors. Radiology 1981;140:767.
86. Wilimas JA, Douglass EC, Magil HL, Fitch S, Hustu HO. Significance of computed tomography at diagnosis in Wilms' tumor. J Clin Oncol 1988;6:1144.
87. Riggs JM, Wooton SL, Ihrke H, Albano EA, Rumack CM, Strain JD. Computed tomography versus chest radiography in the detection of pulmonary metastases in Wilms' tumor. Clin Res 1994;42:30A. Abstract.
88. Green DM, Fernbach DJ, Norkool P, Kollia G, D'Angio GJ. The treatment of Wilms' tumor patients with pulmonary metastases detected only with computed tomography: a report from the National Wilms' Tumor Study. J Clin Oncol 1991;9:1776.

89. Feusner JH, Beckwith JB, D'Angio GJ. Clear cell sarcoma of the kidney: accuracy of imaging methods for detecting bone metastases. Med Pediatr Oncol 1990;18:225.
90. Palmer NF, Sutow WW. Clinical aspects of the rhabdoid tumor of the kidney: a report of the National Wilms' Tumor Study Group. Med Pediatr Oncol 1983;11:242.
91. Breslow NE, Palmer NF, Hill LR, Buring M, D'Angio GJ. Wilms' tumor: prognostic factors for patients without metastases at diagnosis. Cancer 1978;41:1577.
92. Breslow N, Churchill G, Beckwith JB, et al. Prognosis for Wilms' tumor patients with nonmetastatic disease at diagnosis: results of the Second National Wilms' Tumor Study. J Clin Oncol 1985;3:521.
93. Breslow N, Sharples K, Beckwith JB, et al. Prognostic factors in nonmetastatic, favorable histology Wilms' tumor: results of the Third National Wilms' Tumor Study. Cancer 1991;68:2345.
94. Grundy PE, Telzerow PE, Breslow N, Moksness J, Huff V, Paterson MC. Loss of heterozygosity for chromosomes 16q and 1p in Wilms' tumors predicts an adverse outcome. Cancer Res 1994;54:2331.
95. Bardeesy N, Falkoff D, Petruzzi M-J, et al. Anaplastic Wilms' Tumour, a subtype displaying poor prognosis, harbours p53 gene mutations. Nature Genet 1994;7:91.
96. Malkin D, Sexsmith E, Yeger H, Williams BRG, Coppes MJ. Mutations of the p53 tumor suppressor gene occur infrequently in Wilms' tumor. Cancer Res 1994;54:2077.
97. Waber JPG, Chen J, Nisen PD. Infrequency of ras, p53, WT1, or RB gene alterations in Wilms tumors. Cancer 1993;72:3732.
98. Partin AW, Yoo JK, Crooks D, Epstein JI, Beckwith JB, Gearhart JP. Prediction of disease-free survival after therapy in Wilms' tumor using nuclear morphometric techniques. J Pedatr Surg 1994;29:456.
99. Leape L, Breslow N, Bishop HC. The surgical treatment of Wilms' tumor: results of the National Wilms' Tumor Study. Ann Surg 1978; 187:351.
100. Othersen HB Jr, DeLorimier A, Hrabowsky E, Kelalis P, Breslow N, D'Angio GJ. Surgical evaluation of lymph node metastases in Wilms' tumor. J Pediatr Surg 1990;25:330.
101. Thomas PRM, Tefft M, D'Angio GJ, Norkool P for the National Wilms' Tumor Study Committee. Validation of radiation dose reductions used in the Third National Wilms' Tumor Study (NWTS-3). Proc Am Assoc Cancer Res 1988;29:227. Abstract.
102. Ritchey ML, Kelalis PP, Breslow N, Etzioni R, Evans I, Haase GM, D'Angio GJ. Surgical complications after nephrectomy for Wilms' tumor. Surg Gynecol Obstet 1992;175:507.
103. Blute ML, Kelalis PP, Offord KP, Breslow N, Beckwith JB, D'Angio GJ. Bilateral Wilms' tumor. J Urol 1987;138:968.
104. Jones B, Hrabovsky E, Kiviat N, Breslow N. Metachronous bilateral Wilms' tumor. Am J Clin Oncol 1982;5:545.
105. Cassady JR, Tefft M, Filler RM, Jaffe N, Hellman S. Considerations in the radiation therapy of Wilms' tumor. Cancer 1973;32:598.
106. Gross RE, Neuhauser EBD. Treatment of mixed tumors of the kidney in childhood. Pediatrics 1950;6:843.
107. Schneider M. Renal embryoma. In: Buschke F, ed. Radiation therapy. New York, Grune & Stratton, 1958.
108. D'Angio GJ, Evans AE, Breslow N, et al. The treatment of Wilms' tumor: results of the National Wilms' Tumor Study. Cancer 1976;38: 633.
109. D'Angio GJ, Evans A, Breslow N, et al. The treatment of Wilms' tumor: results of the Second National Wilms' Tumor Study. Cancer 1981;47:2302.
110. Green DM, Beckwith JB, Breslow NE, et al. The treatment of children with stages II-IV anaplastic Wilms' tumor: a report from the National Wilms' Tumor Study. J Clin Oncol 1994;12:2126.
111. Thomas PRM, Tefft M, Farewell VT, Norkool P, Storer B, D'Angio GJ. Abdominal relapses in irradiated second National Wilms' Tumor Study patients. J Clin Oncol 1984;2:1098.
112. Silver HK. Wilms' tumor (embryoma of the kidney). J Pediatr 1947; 31:643.
113. Lemerle J, Voute PA, Tournade MF, et al. Preoperative versus postoperative radiotherapy, single versus multiple courses of actinomycin D, in the treatment of Wilms' tumor. Cancer 1976;38:647.
114. DeKraker J, Lemerle J, Voute PA, Zucker JM, Tournade MF, Carli M. Wilms' tumor with pulmonary metastases at diagnosis: the significance of primary chemotherapy. J Clin Oncol 1990;8:1187.
115. Green DM, Finklestein JZ, Tefft M, Norkool P. Diffuse interstitial pneumonitis after pulmonary irradiation for metastatic Wilms' tumor. Cancer 1989;63:450.
116. Pritchard J, Imeson J, Barnes J, et al. Results of the United Kingdom Children's Cancer Study Group (UKCCSG) first Wilms' tumor study (UKW-1). J Clin Oncol 1995;13:124.
117. Tournade MF, Com-Hougue C, Voute PA, et al. Results of the sixth International Society of Pediatric Oncology Wilms' tumor trial and study: a risk-adapted therapeutic approach in Wilms' tumor. J Clin Oncol 1993;11:1014.
118. Green DM, Breslow NE, D'Angio GJ. The treatment of children with unilateral Wilms' tumor. J Clin Oncol 1993;11:1009.
119. Grundy P, Breslow N, Green DM, Sharples K, Evans A, D'Angio GJ. Prognostic factors of children with recurrent Wilms' tumor: results from the second and third National Wilms' Tumor Study. J Clin Oncol 1989;7:638.
120. Green DM, Breslow N, Ii Y, et al. The role of surgical excision in the management of relapsed Wilms' tumor patients with pulmonary metastases. J Pediatr Surg 1991;26:728.
121. Miser J, Krailo M, Hammond GD. The combination of ifosfamide (IFOS), etoposide (VP-16) and MESNA (M): a very active regimen in the treatment of recurrent Wilms' tumor (WT). Proc Am Soc Clin Oncol 1993;12:417. Abstract.
122. Warkentin PI, Brochstein JA, Stranjord SE, et al. High dose therapy followed by autologous stem cell rescue for recurrent Wilms' tumor (WT). Proc Am Soc Clin Oncol 1993;12:414. Abstract.
123. Garaventa A, Hartmann O, Bernard J-L, et al. Autologous bone marrow transplantation for pediatric Wilms' tumor: the experience of the European Bone Marrow Transplantation Solid Tumor Registry. Med Pediatr Oncol 1994;22:11.
124. Kletzel M, Morgan E, Cohn S, Williams L, Camitta B. Autologous bone marrow (BM)/peripheral blood stem cell (PBSC) rescue in children with relapsed Wilms' tumor (WT). Med Pediatr Oncol 1994;23: 201. Abstract.
125. Ettinger LJ, Gaynon PS, Krailo M, et al. A phase II study of carboplatin in children with recurrent or progressive solid tumors. Cancer 1994;73:1297.
126. Zoubek A, Kajtar P, Fink FM, et al. Response to carboplatin (CBDCA) monotherapy in children with stage IV and relapse Wilms' tumors (WT). Proc Am Soc Clin Oncol 1993;12:410. Abstract.
127. Lewis IJ, Stevens MCG, Pearson A, Pinkerton CR, Stevens R. Phase II study of carboplatin in children's tumours. Proc Am Soc Clin Oncol 1993;12:412. Abstract.
128. de Camargo B, Melaragno R, Saba e Silva N, et al. Phase II study of carboplatin as a single drug for relapsed Wilms' tumor: experience of the Brazilian Wilms' Tumor Study Group. Med Pediatr Oncol 1994; 22:258.
129. Malogolowkin M, Feusner J, Steele DA, Lavado MG, Ortega J. Carboplatin (CBDCA)/Etoposide (VP-16) for the treatment of children with high-risk (HR) or recurrent Wilms' tumor (RWT). Proc Am Soc Clin Oncol 1994;13:424. Abstract.
130. Pein F, Tournade MF, Zucker J-M, et al. Etoposide and carboplatin: a highly effective combination in relapsed or refractory Wilms' tumor. A phase II study by the French Society of Paediatric Oncology (SFOP). J Clin Oncol 1994;12:931.
131. Kung FH, Pratt CB, Vega RA, et al. Ifosfamide/etoposide combination in the treatment of recurrent malignant solid tumors of childhood. A Pediatric Oncology Group Phase II study. Cancer 1993;71:1898.
132. Rossi R, Godde A, Kleinebrand A, et al. Unilateral nephrectomy and cisplatin as risk factors of ifosfamide-induced nephrotoxicity: analysis of 120 patients. J Clin Oncol 1994;12:159.
133. Dombernowsky P, Nissen NI. Combination chemotherapy with 4′ Demethylepipodophyllotoxin 9-(4,6-O-ethylidene-beta-D-glucopyranoside), VP-16-213 (NSC 141540) in L1210 leukemia. Eur J Cancer 1976;12:181.
134. Koza I, Balazova E, Ujhazy V. Single versus combination chemotherapy of L1210 leukemia. Neoplasma 1980;27:691.
135. Grana N, Graham-Pole J, Cassano W, et al. Etoposide (VP16) infusion plus cyclophosphamide (CY) pulses: an effective combination for refractory cancer (CA). Proc Am Soc Clin Oncol 1989;8:300. Abstract.
136. White L, McCowage G, Kannourakis G, et al. Dose-intensive cyclophosphamide with etoposide and vincristine for pediatric solid tumors: a phase I/II pilot study by the Australia and New Zealand Childhood Cancer Study Group. J Clin Oncol 1994;12:522.
137. Maksymiuk AW, Jett JR, Earle JD, et al. Sequencing and schedule effects of cisplatin plus etoposide in small-cell lung cancer: Results of a North Central Cancer Treatment Group randomized clinical trial. J Clin Oncol 1994;12:70.

Index

J

K

L

Q

R

U

V